Manual of Dietetic Practice

This book is dedicated to Edith Elliot (BDA member number 001)
for her outstanding and continuing contribution to dietetics.

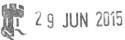

Manual of Dietetic Practice

Fifth Edition

Edited by Joan Gandy

In conjunction with

The British Dietetic Association

WILEY Blackwell

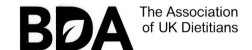

This edition first published 2014 © 2014 by The British Dietetic Association
Other editions © 2007, 2001, 1994 and 1988 by John Wiley & Sons, Ltd.

Registered office: John Wiley & Sons, Ltd, The Atrium, Southern Gate, Chichester, West Sussex, PO19 8SQ, UK

Editorial offices: 9600 Garsington Road, Oxford, OX4 2DQ, UK
The Atrium, Southern Gate, Chichester, West Sussex, PO19 8SQ, UK
1606 Golden Aspen Drive, Suites 103 and 104, Ames, Iowa 50014-8300, USA

For details of our global editorial offices, for customer services and for information about how to apply for permission to reuse the copyright material in this book please see our website at www.wiley.com/wiley-blackwell

Library of Congress Cataloging-in-Publication Data
Manual of dietetic practice / edited by Joan Gandy in conjunction with the British Dietetic Association. – Fifth edition.
    p. ; cm.
   Preceded by: Manual of dietetic practice / edited by Briony Thomas and Jacki Bishop in conjunction with The British Dietetic Association. 4th ed. 2007.
   Includes bibliographical references and index.
   ISBN 978-0-470-65622-8 (cloth : alk. paper)
   I. Webster-Gandy, Joan, editor of compilation.   II. British Dietetic Association, publisher.
   [DNLM: 1. Diet Therapy.   2. Dietetics.   3. Nutritional Physiological Phenomena. WB 400]
   RM216
   615.8'54–dc23
                                            2013024993   1007217636

A catalogue record for this book is available from the British Library.

Wiley also publishes its books in a variety of electronic formats. Some content that appears in print may not be available in electronic books.

Set in 9.5/11.5 pt ITC Garamond by Toppan Best-set Premedia Limited
Printed and bound in Singapore by Markono Print Media Pte Ltd

1 2014

Contents

Contents

Appendices

Contributors

Editor and contributor

Joan Gandy   *Dietetics Department, School of Life and Medical Sciences, University of Hertfordshire, Hatfield, Hertfordshire*
Address for correspondence c/o The British Dietetic Association, 5th Floor Charles House, 148/9 Great Charles Street, Queensway, Birmingham B3 3HT

Contributors

Sarah Adam   *Metabolic Dietitian for Adults with Inherited Metabolic Disorders, Royal Hospital for Sick Children, Glasgow*
Phil Addicott   *Swallow Team Dietitian, Cardiff & Vale University Health Board, Cardiff; Llandough Hospital, Vale of Glamorgan*
Ursula Arens   *Freelance Dietitian, London*
Sarah Armer   *Community Dietitian – Home Enteral Feeding, The Cudworth Centre, Barnsley*
Melanie Baker   *Senior Specialist Dietitian, Nutrition Support Team, Leicester Royal Infirmary, Leicester*
Eleanor Baldwin   *Refsums Dietitian, Chelsea & Westminster NHS Foundation Healthcare Trust, London*
Rachael Barlow   *Clinical Lead: All Wales Enhanced Recovery after Surgery Programme and Lecturer, School of Healthcare Studies, Cardiff University, Cardiff*
Rachel Barton   *Dietetic Manager (Public Health), Leicestershire Nutrition and Dietetic Service, Enderby, Leicestershire*
Julie Beckerson   *Haemato-Oncology Specialist Dietitian, Imperial College Healthcare NHS Trust, London*
Ruth Birt   *Consultant in Regulatory Affairs, Glasgow*
Sarah Boocock   *Specialist Dietitian in Inherited Metabolic Disorders, Queen Elizabeth Hospital, Birmingham*
Lindsey Bottle   *Macmillan Oncology Dietitian, Royal Surrey County Hospital Guildford, Surrey*
Angeline Brookes   *Specialist Dietitian, University College Hospital, London*
Diane Brundrett   *Advanced Specialist Dietitian, St Marks Hospital, Harrow, Middlesex*
Siân Burton   *Head of Nutrition & Dietetics for Learning Disabilities, Directorate of Learning Disability Services, ABMU Local Health Board, Bridgend, Mid Glamorgan*
Gaynor Bussell   *Freelance Dietitian, Llechryd nr Cardigan, Ceredigion*
Helen Campbell   *Dietitian, Diabetes and Nutritional Sciences Division, King's College, London*

Elaine Cawadias   *Clinical Dietitian, ALS Clinic Team, The Ottawa Hospital Rehabilitation Centre, Ottawa, Canada*
Abbie Cawood   *Visiting Research Fellow, Institute of Human Nutrition, University of Southampton, Southampton*
Sarah Cawtherley   *Paediatric Dietitian, Royal Manchester Children's Hospital, Manchester*
Heidi Chan   *Specialist Metabolic Dietitian, University College London Hospital, London*
Saira Chowdhury   *Specialist Upper GI Oncology Dietitian, Guys & St Thomas' NHS Foundation Trust, London*
Alison Coates   *Paediatric Dietitian, Royal Hospital for Sick Children, Edinburgh*
Peter Collins   *Senior Lecturer in Nutrition and Dietetics, Institute of Health and Biomedical Innovation, Faculty of Health, Queensland University of Technology (QUT), Brisbane, Australia*
Claire Conway   *Paediatric Dietitian, Derriford Hospital, Plymouth, Devon*
Lisa Cooke   *Head of Paediatric Dietetics, Bristol Royal Hospital for Children, Bristol*
June Copeman   *Subject Group Lead Nutrition and Dietetics, Faculty of Health and Social Sciences, Leeds Metropolitan University, Leeds*
Kathy Cowborough   *Dietitian and Public Health Nutritionist Retford, Nottinghamshire*
Julie Crocker   *Paediatric Dietitian, Royal Hospital for Sick Children, Glasgow*
Alison Culkin   *Research Dietitian, St Mark's Hospital, Harrow, Middlesex*
Ingrid Darnley   *Policy Officer Clinical Quality, British Dietetic Association, Birmingham*
Janeane Dart   *Senior Lecturer, Department of Nutrition and Dietetics, Monash University, Melbourne, Australia*
Mhairi Donald   *Macmillan Consultant Dietitian in Oncology, Royal Sussex County Hospital, Brighton, Sussex*
Sarah Donald   *Senior Dietitian, Addenbrookes Hospital, Cambridge*
Emma Dresner   *Head of Dietetics, The Royal Hospital for Neuro-disability, Putney, London*
Catherine Dunn   *Clinical Specialist Dietitian for Neurosciences, Royal Free Hampstead NHS Trust, Hampstead, London*
Annette Dunne   *Mental Health Dietetic Lead, Cardiff and Vale University Health Board, Llandough Hospital, Vale of Glamorgan; Whitchurch Hospital, Cardiff*
Jennie Dunwoody   *Senior Dietitian, The Royal Hospital for Neuro-disability, Putney, London*

Pam Dyson *Research Dietitian, Oxford Centre for Diabetes, Endocrinology and Metabolism, Churchill Hospital, Oxford*

Shelley Easter *Specialist Paediatric Dietitian, Bristol Royal Hospital For Children, Bristol*

Lucy Eldridge *Dietetic Team Leader – Nutrition & Dietetics, The Royal Marsden NHS Foundation Trust, Chelsea, London*

Marinos Elia *Professor of Clinical Nutrition and Metabolism, University of Southampton, Southampton*

Clare Ewan *Paediatric Dietitian, NHS North Somerset, Clevedon, Somerset*

Julie Farmer *Former Policy Officer – Education, British Dietetic Association, Birmingham*

Helen Fraser-Mayall *Dietetic Team Lead, West Cumberland Hospital, Whitehaven, Cumbria*

Elaine Gardner *Freelance Dietitian, London; Module Organiser for Nutrition and Infection, Distance Learning Unit, London School of Hygiene and Tropical Medicine, London*

Jenny Gillespie *Dietitian, Children's Weight Clinic, Edinburgh*

Eva Glass *Macmillan Specialist Oncology Dietitian, Velindre Cancer Centre, Cardiff*

Karen Green *Senior Specialist Dietitian (Neurosciences), The National Hospital for Neurology & Neurosurgery, London*

Jane Green *Specialist Community Dietitian, Cambridgeshire Community Services, Doddington Hospital, Doddington*

Poonam Guila *Gastroenterology & Stroke Dietitian, Sandwell General Hospital, West Bromwich, West Midlands*

Catherine Hames *Dietitian, Cambridge University Hospitals NHS Foundation Trust, Cambridge*

Susie Hamlin *Hepatology Specialist/ICU Dietitian, Rehabilitation Department, St James's University Hospital, Leeds*

Catherine Hankey *Senior Lecturer, College of Medical Veterinary & Life Sciences, School of Medicine, University of Glasgow, Glasgow*

Lynn Harbottle *Head of Dietetic Services, Wythenshawe Hospital, Manchester*

Karin Harnden *Research Dietitian, OXLIP, Oxford Centre for Diabetes, Endocrinology and Metabolism, Oxford*

Katie Harriman *Paediatric Dietitian, Bristol Royal Hospital for Children, Bristol*

Kate Harris *Home Enteral Nutrition Dietitian, Lewisham NHS Healthcare Trust, London*

Maryanne Harrison *Team Lead, Senior Specialist Dietitian, Hertfordshire Neurological Service, Abbots Langley, Hertfordshire*

Kathryn Hart *Lecturer in Nutrition & Dietetics, Faculty of Health & Medical Sciences, University of Surrey, Guildford, Surrey*

George Hartley *Renal Dietetic Manager, Freeman Hospital, Newcastle upon Tyne*

Michelle Harvie *Research Dietitian, Nightingale and Genesis Prevention Centre, Wythenshawe Hospital, Manchester*

Sarah Heath *Specialist Paediatric Dietitian, King's College Hospital, London*

Julie Hinchliffe *Cardiac Rehabilitation Dietitian, Salford Royal Hospital Trust, Salford*

Linda Hindle *Consultant Dietitian, Senior Manager Healthy Eating and Activity, Birmingham City Council, Birmingham*

Michelle Holdsworth *Senior Lecturer in Public Health, School of Health & Related Research (ScHARR), University of Sheffield, Sheffield*

Deborah Howland *Head & Neck Dietitian, Torbay Hospital, Torquay, Devon*

Zoe Hull *Specialist Paediatric Dietitian, Bristol Children's Hospital, Bristol*

Karen Hyland *Dietitian, Team Leader, Barnet PCT, Edgware, Middlesex*

Joanna Instone *NHS National Genetics Education and Development Centre, Birmingham*

Camille Jankowski *Specialist Paediatric Dietitian, Bristol Royal Hospital for Children, Bristol*

Yvonne Jeannes *Senior Lecturer, Health Sciences Research Centre, Roehampton University, London*

Fiona Jenkins *Locality Team Manager, Medway Community Healthcare, Kent*

Sue Kellie *Head of Education and Professional Development, British Dietetic Association, Birmingham*

Karen Klassen *HIV Dietitian & PhD Student, University of Melbourne, North West Academic Centre, Melbourne, Australia*

Annemarie Knight *Lecturer in Nutrition and Dietetics, Diabetes and Nutritional Sciences Division, King's College, London*

Edwige Landais *Research Associate/Public Health Nutritionist, UMR NUTRIPASS, Institut de Recherche pour le Développement- IRD, Montpellier, France*

Kelly Larmour *Lead Paediatric Dietitian, Evelina Children's Hospital, Westminster, London*

Anne Laverty *Specialist Dietitian, Learning Disability, Northern Health & Social Care Trust, Coleraine, Northern Ireland*

Katherine Law *Medirest Dietitian, King's College Hospital, London*

Judy Lawrence *Research Officer, British Dietetic Association, Birmingham; Senior Research Fellow, Nutritional Sciences Division, King's College, London*

Julie Leaper *Senior Specialist Dietitian (Liver/ICU), Rehabilitation Department, St James's University Hospital, Leeds*

Miranda Lomer *Consultant Dietitian, Guy's and St Thomas' NHS Foundation Trust and King's College, London; Honorary Senior Lecturer in Nutritional Sciences, Diabetes and Nutritional Sciences Division, King's College, London*

Jacqueline Lowden *Paediatric Dietitian, Therapies and Dietetic Department, Royal Manchester Children's Hospital, Manchester*

Marjory Macleod *Specialist Dietitian – Learning Disabilities Service, NHS Lothian, Scotland*

Linda Main *Dietitian, Heart UK, Drummond Consultants, Slough, Berkshire*

Sara Mancell *Senior Specialist Paediatric Dietitian, Barts and The London NHS Trust, London*

Luise Marino *Paediatric Research Dietitian, Imperial College, London*

Charlé Maritz *Specialist Practitioner, University College London Hospital, London*

Yvonne McKenzie *Specialist Gastroenterology Dietitian, Digestible Nutrition, Chipping Camden, Gloucestershire*

Jennifer McIntosh *Advanced Dietetic Practitioner in CFS/ME, Leeds Partnerships NHS Foundation Trust, Leeds*

Kirsty-Anna Mclaughlin Senior Dietitian, Great Western Hospitals NHS Foundation Trust, Bath

Christina Merryfield *Lead Dietitian, Bupa Cromwell Hospital, Kensington & Chelsea, London*

Rosan Meyer *Principal Paediatric Research Dietitian, Great Ormond Street Hospital For Sick Children, London*

Avril Micciche *Principal Adult Metabolic Dietitian, St Thomas' Hospital, London*

Emma Mills *Freelance Dietitian, Mansfield, Nottinghamshire*

Natalie Mohamdee *Paediatric Dietitian, Northumbria Healthcare Foundation NHS Trust, Northumbria North Shields, Tyne and Wear*

Gemma Moore *Wiltshire Community Health Services, St Martin's Hospital, Bath*

Alison Morton *Clinical Specialist Dietitian, Regional Adult Cystic Fibrosis Unit, St James' Hospital, Leeds*

Linda Murray *Clinical Team Lead – Dietetics, Surgery & Critical Care Team, Greater Glasgow and Clyde*

Alison Nelson *Food and Health Policy Officer, British Dietetic Association, Birmingham*

Kim Novell *Paediatric Dietitian, University Hospital Southampton NHS Foundation Trust, Southampton*

Mary O'Kane *Consultant Dietitian, NHS Foundation Trust, Leeds Teaching Hospitals NHS Trust, Leeds*

Derbhla O'Sullivan *Formerly University College London Hospitals Foundation NHS Trust, London*

Fionna Page *Independent Nutrition Consultant and Registered Dietitian, First Page Nutrition Ltd, Great Somerford, Wiltshire*

Samantha Parry *Senior Dietitian, The Royal Hospital for Neuro-disability, Putney, London*

Dorothy J Pattison *Freelance Dietitian, St Mabyn, Cornwall*

Sue Perry *Deputy Head of Dietetics, Hull Royal Infirmary, Hull*

Dympna Pearson *Consultant Dietitian and Freelance Trainer, Leicester*

Mary Phillips *Advanced Hepato-Pancreatico-Biliary Specialist Dietitian, Regional Hepato-Pancreatico-Biliary Unit (Surrey & Sussex), Royal Surrey County Hospital NHS Foundation Trust, Surrey*

Ursula Philpot *Senior Lecturer, Nutrition & Dietetics, Leeds Metropolitan University, Leeds*

Gail Pinnock *Specialist Bariatric Dietitian, Stone Allerton, Somerset*

Pat Portnoi *Dietitian, Galactosemia Support Group, Sutton Coldfield, West Midlands*

Vicki Pout *Acute Dietetic Team Leader, Kent Community Health NHS Trust, Kent and Canterbury Hospital, Canterbury, Kent*

Jane Power *Macmillan Palliative Care Dietitian, Betsi Cadwaladr University Health Board, Wrexham*

Najia Qureshi *Policy Officer (Professional Development), British Dietetic Association, Birmingham*

Jean Redmond *Dietitian & PhD Student, Medical Research Council Human Nutrition Research, Elsie Widdowson Laboratory, Cambridge*

Gail Rees *Lecturer in Human Nutrition, School of Biomedical and Biological Sciences, Plymouth University, Plymouth*

Katie Richards *Senior Dietitian, The Royal Hospital for Neuro-disability, Putney, London*

Alan Rio *Expert in Nutritional Support, Surrey*

Sarah Ripley *Metabolic Dietitian, Salford Royal Hospital, Salford*

Louise Robertson *Specialist Dietitian in Inherited Metabolic Disorders, Queen Elizabeth Hospital, Birmingham*

Hazel Rogozinski *Specialist Metabolic Dietitian, Bradford Teaching Hospitals, Bradford*

Lisa Ryan *Senior Lecturer & Operations Director of the Functional Food Centre, Faculty of Health & Life Sciences, Oxford Brookes University, Oxford*

Jeremy Sanderson *Consultant Gastroenterologist, St Thomas' Hospital, London*

Inez Schoenmakers *Senior Investigator Scientist, Medical Research Council Human Nutrition Research, Elsie Widdowson Laboratory, Cambridge*

Ella Segaran *Critical Care Dietitian, Imperial College Healthcare NHS Trust, St Mary's Hospital, Paddington, London*

Clare Shaw *Consultant Dietitian, The Royal Marsden NHS Foundation Trust, Chelsea, London*

Isabel Skypala *Director of Rehabilitation and Therapies, Royal Brompton and Harefield NHS Foundation Trust, Chelsea, London*

Julia Smith *Advanced Specialist Paediatric Gastroenterology Dietitian, Cambridge University NHS Foundation Trust, Cambridge*

Laura Stewart *Team Lead, Paediatric Overweight Service Tayside, NHS Tayside, Perth*

Rebecca Stratton *Visiting Research Fellow, Institute of Human Nutrition, University of Southampton, Southampton*

Louise Sutton *Principal Lecturer, Leeds Metropolitan University, Leeds*

Diane Talbot *Dietitian, Uppingham, Leicestershire*

Bella Talwar *Clinical Lead Dietitian, Head & Neck Cancer Service, University College London, London*

Aruna Thaker *Retired Chief Dietitian, Purley, Surrey*

Karen Thomsett *Renal Dietitian, East Kent Hospitals University NHS Trust, Canterbury, Kent*

Alan Torrance *Acting Head Newcastle Nutrition, Newcastle upon Tyne Hospitals NHS Foundation Trust, Newcastle upon Tyne*

Sarah Trace *Specialist Paediatric Dietitian (Nephrology), Bristol Royal Hospital for Children, Bristol*

Kirsten Tremlett *Senior Paediatric Hepatology Dietitian, Leeds Teaching Hospitals NHS Trust, Leeds*

Helen Truby *Professor of Nutrition and Dietetic, Department of Nutrition and Dietetics, Monash University, Melbourne, Australia*

Anthony Twist *Orthopaedic Lead Dietitian, Robert Jones and Agnes Hunt Orthopaedic Hospital NHS Foundation Trust, Oswestry, Shropshire*

Sharon Underwood *Renal Dietitian, East Kent Hospitals University NHS Trust, Canterbury, Kent*

Carina Venter *NIHR Post Doctoral Fellow, University of Portsmouth; Specialist Allergy Dietitian, Isle of Wight, Food Allergy MSc Module Leader, University of Southampton, Southampton*

Diana Webster *Regional Specialist Paediatric Dietitian for Inherited Metabolic Diseases, Bristol Royal Hospital for Children, Bristol*

C Elizabeth Weekes *Consultant Dietitian and Research Lead, Guy's & St Thomas' NHS Foundation Trust, St Thomas' Hospital, London; Honorary Lecturer, Diabetes and Nutritional Sciences Division, King's College, London*

Ailsa Welch *Senior Lecturer, Department of Nutrition, University of East Anglia, Norwich, Norfolk*

Kevin Whelan *Professor of Dietetics, Diabetes & Nutritional Sciences Division, King's College, London*

Rhys White *Principal Oncology Dietitian, Guy's and St Thomas' NHS Foundation Trust, Guy's Hospital, London*

Kate Williams *Head of Nutrition and Dietetics, South London and Maudsley NHS Foundation Trust, The Maudsley Hospital, Denmark Hill, London*

Nicola Williams *Senior Paediatric Dietitian, Royal Manchester Children's Hospital, Manchester*

Sue Williams *Clinical Lead Dietitian, Lewisham NHS Healthcare Trust, London*

Richard Wilson *Director of Nutrition and Dietetics, King's College Hospital NHS Foundation Trust, Denmark Hill, London*

Sarah Wilson *Specialist Dietitian, Princess Grace Hospital, London*

Mark Windle *Nutritional Support Dietitian, Pinderfields General Hospital, Wakefield, Yorkshire*

Samford Wong *Clinical Lead Dietitian – Spinal Injuries, National Spinal Injuries Centre, Stoke Mandeville Hospital, Aylesbury*

Philippa Wright *Paediatric Therapy Lead, Royal Brompton Hospital, Chelsea, London*

Tanya Wright *Allergy Coordinator & Specialist Dietitian, Buckinghamshire Healthcare, Amersham Hospital, Amersham, Buckinghamshire*

Suzy Yates *Senior Specialist Neuroscience Dietitian, The National Hospital for Neurology and Neurosurgery, London*

Additional contributors and acknowledgements

Stavria Achilleos
Jane Alderdice
Mary Ann Among
Arit Ana
Simran Arora
Sue Baic
Arlene Barton
Tahira Bashir
Danielle Bear
Philippa Bearne
Nick Bergin
Catherine Best
Rebecca Brake
Ailsa Brotherton
Helen Brown
Rose Butler
Nina Calder
Elizabeth Campling
Louise Chambers
Echo Chan
Jackie Charlton
Renuka Coghlan
Sue Corbett
Jeanette Crosland
Barbara Davidson
Julie De' Havillande
Emer Delaney
Holly Doyle
Hilary du Cane
Alastair Duncan
Claudia Ehrlicher
Trudie France
Mandy Fraser
Robert Garside
Lynne Garton
Gillian Gatiss
Chris Gedge
Frances Gorman
Azmina Govindji
Clare Gray
Hannah Greatwood
Judith Harding
Lisa Henry
Gemma Hitchen
Anne Holdoway
Lisa Holmes
Sandra Hood
Jenny Hughes
Kalpana Hussain
Bushra Jafri
Sema Jethwa

Jill Johnson
Susanna Johnson
Natasha Jones
Ruth Kander
Nariman Karanjia
Tanya Klopper
Jenny Lee
Seema Lodhia
Christel Lyell
Angela Madden
Amanda Martin
Barbara Martini Arora
Anneka Maxwel
Sarah Mihalik
Thomina Mirza
Kashena Mohadawoo
Melanie Moore
Afsha Mughal
Clio Myers
Kate Nancekivell
Gopi Patel
Katherine Paterson
Christiana Pavlides
Sue Pemberton
Helen Powell
Vivian Pribram
Ellie Ripley
Mark Robinson
Laura Rowe
Nicki Ruddock
Rupindar Sahota
Caroline Sale
Juneeshree S Sangani
Nicola Scott
Reena Shaunak
Bushra Siddiqui
Nathalie Sutherland
Elzbieta (Ela) Szymula
Ravita Taheem
Carolyn Taylor
Stephen Taylor
Angela Tella
Denise Thomas
Nerissa Walker
Sunita Wallia
Eleanor Weetch
Louise Wells
Joanna Weston
Emma Whitehurst
Anthony Wierzbicki
Jo Wildgoose

Kelly Wilson
Sue Wolfe
Joanne Wraight
Priscilla Yan
Nardos Yemane
Ghazala Yousuf

The BDA Specialist Groups:

* Cardiovascular & Respiratory Dietitians.
* Diabetes Management & Education Group.
* Dietitians in Critical Care.
* Dietitians in HIV/AIDS Group.
* DOM UK: Dietitians in Obesity Management.
* Food Allergy and Intolerance Group.
* Food Counts.
* Freelance Dietitians Group.
* Gastroenterology Specialist Group.
* Mental Health Group.
* Multicultural Nutrition Group.

* National Dietetic Management Group.
* Neurosciences Specialist Group.
* Nutrition Advisory Group for Older People.
* Oncology Group and Sub Groups.
* Paediatric Group.
* Parenteral & Enteral Nutrition Group.
* Public Health Nutrition Network.
* Renal Nutrition Group.
* Sport Dietitians UK.

Other groups of dietitians including:

* Department of Nutrition and Dietetics, Royal Surrey County Hospital.
* Dietitians with an Interest in Spinal Cord Injuries.
* Dietitians Working with Adults with Inherited Metabolic Disorders.
* Freelance Fact Sheet Authors.
* South East Neuro Dietitians Group.

Foreword

Good nutritional care has never been so important and, as the British Dietetic Association (BDA) has said, registered dietitians (RDs) are the only *'qualified health professionals that assess, diagnose and treat diet and nutrition problems at an individual and wider public health level'*. Dietitians have, therefore, many crucial roles to play in improving care standards in the new emerging NHS and beyond in improving the health of our nation.

This edition of the *Manual of Dietetic Practice* is an outstanding source of information for both qualified and student dietitians. It takes an exemplary systems approach in its clinical sections, which focus on dietetic practice, beginning with nutritional support and followed by chapters dedicated to specialist areas such as gastroenterology and oncology. It also covers the breadth of dietetic specialties outside healthcare. Dr Joan Gandy should be congratulated for her excellent contribution in managing, collating and editing this leading edge reference work, and clear praise and acknowledgement must also be given to the many authors of the individual chapters without whom the manual could not have been produced.

Providing good nutritional care for all is a matter of quality. During my many years involved with clinical nutrition, including periods chairing the group that developed the National Institute for Health and Care Excellence (NICE) Quality Nutrition Support Standards (2006) as well as the British Association of Parenteral and Enteral Nutrition (BAPEN), I have had the privilege of working with visionary, highly committed and enthusiastic dietitians who make a real difference. This manual should help to guide many more individuals to pursue such dietetic excellence and I hope that for many it will also lead to a commitment to join cross disciplinary efforts to improve the nutritional care delivered to patients, their carers and the public. Only then will we attain unprecedented levels of excellence.

Dr Mike Stroud
Consultant Gastroenterologist, Southampton University Hospitals NHS Trust
Senior Lecturer in Medicine and Nutrition, Southampton University

Preface

This book, the fifth edition of the *Manual of Dietetic Practice*, is intended to be part of a spectrum of resources available to dietitians, dietetic students and others. The spectrum now includes an increasing number of specialist dietetic texts and this edition of the manual is written, as far as possible, to complement these texts; both published works and books currently being prepared, e.g. *Diet and Nutrition for Gastrointestinal Disease*. Inevitably, some specialisms are too small to warrant a separate text and are therefore included in this manual. This edition of the manual is aimed mainly at non-specialist dietitians and dietetic students, and is intended for use as a standard textbook in dietetic departments.

Dietetics is a dynamic profession, which means that knowledge and practice change rapidly and dietitians are working in more diverse areas. Therefore, this edition of the manual includes new topics such as genetics and nutrogenomics, and immunology and health. Areas of interest to dietitians continue to expand and dietitians are specialising in areas such as respiratory medicine that were previously considered as general rather than specialist; another new chapter. Medical advances have resulted in conditions that once resulted in early death being managed differently, with longer survivorship. An example of this is the dietetic management of inherited metabolic disorders. Most people with these conditions now survive well into adulthood and therefore present fresh challenges in management; as a result, this topic has been included in this edition.

Many of the chapters have been totally rewritten, often by pairs or groups of people and with many more involved in reviewing the texts; dietitians of every level of experience have been involved, from students through to professors. The approach of the manual has also changed and is in line with the specialisms of the British Dietetic Association (BDA) specialist groups and other dietetics groups and networks.

However, as this is a text on dietetic practice, general chapters on the nutrients have been removed, although an appendix has been created to provide a ready reference on micronutrients. The *Manual of Dietetic Practice*

is constructed to be cohesive and as such there is considerable cross referencing between chapters. It is divided into two parts encompassing seven sections with appendices:

Part 1. General topics
Section 1 – Dietetic practice
Section 2 – Nutritional status
Section 3 – Nutrition in specific groups
Section 4 – Specific areas of dietetic practice
Section 5 – Other topics relevant to dietetic practice

Part 2. Clinical dietetic practice
Section 6 – Nutrition support
Section 7 – Clinical dietetic practice

The area of paediatric dietetics is always challenging, as well as interesting, and this area has been completely revised in this edition to provide an appropriate level of knowledge for non-paediatric dietitians who work with children in general settings. Working with the BDA's Specialist Paediatric Group and Vanessa Shaw, editor of *Clinical Paediatric Dietetics*, the chapters on developmental stages have been edited and consolidated into one extended chapter, with an introduction to topics in clinical paediatric practice. Hopefully, dietitians will find this useful and student dietitians will be introduced to another exciting and satisfying area of practice.

Another innovation is the inclusion on the Wiley Blackwell Internet site of additional resources, including case study discussion papers and slides of the figures and tables that can be downloaded. In addition, this edition will be available as an electronic book. As the field of dietetic practice has expanded so too has the *Manual of Dietetic Practice* and I suspect that the next edition will be presented in a different, if not multiple, format.

While editing the MDP has been a challenge, the level of support has been overwhelming and inspiring. I am indebted to the many people who have written or revised the chapters, and the many reviewers and other contributors.

Joan Gandy

Check out the

Manual of Dietetic Practice
Companion Website

by visiting
www.manualofdieteticpractice.com

Click now and gain access to:

- Case study vignettes linking theory to practice
- Updates to chapters submitted by authors
- Further reading, references and useful links
- Downloadable versions of the illustrations and tables within the book
- Downloadable versions of the appendices
- The editor's biography

WILEY Blackwell

PART 1
General topics

SECTION 1

Dietetic practice

1.1

Professional practice

Najia Qureshi, Sue Kellie, Ingrid Darnley, Julie Farmer, Judy Lawrence and Joan Gandy

Key points

- In the UK dietitians must be graduates of an approved programme of education and registered with the Health and Care Professions Council.

- The British Dietetic Association is a professional association that aims to inform, protect, represent and support its members.

- Dietitians are autonomous practitioners who work within an ethical framework of conduct.

- The nutrition and dietetic process is central to dietetic practice.

- Dietetics is an evidence based profession with research and outcome evaluation at its core.

- Dietitians engage in continuing professional development throughout their careers to ensure that their practice is robust, efficacious and innovative.

Dietetics is a well respected and established profession, albeit a relatively new profession. The first UK dietitian, Ruth Pybus, a nursing sister, was appointed in 1924 at the Royal Infirmary in Edinburgh. She initially sought to demonstrate that a dietetic outpatient clinic could significantly reduce the number of admissions and therefore benefit the hospital. She was successful; after a 6-month trial, her appointment as a dietitian was confirmed. The development of other dietetic departments quickly followed, especially in London, and in 1928 the first non-nursing dietitians were appointed. From these early days dietetics has been a science based profession and in the 1980s became the first of the allied health professions (AHPs) to become a graduate profession.

In 1936 the British Dietetic Association (BDA) was founded as the professional association for registered dietitians in Great Britain and Northern Ireland. The BDA aims to inform, protect, represent, and support its members.

Dietetics is both an art and a science that requires the application of safe and evidence based practice, reflective practice and systematic clinical reasoning. A dietitian needs to combine these skills with knowledge and experience, together with intuition, insight and understanding of the individual (or specific) circumstance in order to maintain and improve practice. Following several public enquiries at the end of the last century it was recognised that there needed to be greater priority given to non-clinical aspects of care, such as skills in communicating with colleagues and service users, management, develop-

ment of teamwork, shared learning across professional boundaries, audit, reflective practice and leadership. Subsequent legislative changes were implemented with the establishment of the Health and Care Professions Council (HCPC).

Dietetics as a profession

An occupation or trade becomes a profession *'through the development of formal qualifications based upon education, apprenticeship, and examinations, the emergence of regulatory bodies with powers to admit and discipline members, and some degree of monopoly rights on the knowledge base'* (Bullock & Trombley, 1999, p. 689). A degree of responsibility and expectation comes with being a professional. A member of any profession, including dietetics, must, within their practice, agree to be governed by a code of ethics, uphold high standards of performance and competence, behave with integrity and morality, and be altruistic in the promotion of the public good (Cruess *et al.*, 2004). Furthermore, these commitments form the basis of an understanding, or social contract, that results in professions, and their members, being accountable to service users and to society.

Professional regulation

To practise as a dietitian, and to use the title of dietitian, it is mandatory to have completed an approved programme of education and be registered with the HCPC. The HCPC was set up in 2001 to protect the health and wellbeing of people using the services of the health professionals registered with them. It aims to:

- Maintain and publish a public register of properly qualified members of the professions.
- Approve and uphold high standards of education and training and continuing good practice.
- Investigate complaints and take appropriate action.
- Work in partnership with the public and other groups, including professional bodies.

To remain on the HCPC register, dietitians must continue to meet the standards that are set for the profession. The professional standards are:

- Good character of health professionals.
- Health.
- Proficiency (dietetics).
- Conduct performance and ethics.
- Continuing professional development (CPD).
- Education and training.

The HCPC use these standards to determine if a registrant is fit to practise. If the HCPC finds that there are concerns about a dietitian's ability to practise safely and effectively, and therefore fitness to practise is impaired, it has the legal right to take action. This may mean that the registrant is not allowed to practise or that they are limited in what they are allowed to do. The HCPC can legally take appropriate action to enforce this (HCPC, 2010).

The British Dietetic Association as a professional body

The distinction between a regulatory body (HCPC) and a professional body (BDA) is often misunderstood. It is important that dietitians are fully aware of the differences from the beginning of professional training. Much like the HCPC, the BDA is committed to protecting the public and service users. However, the two organisations achieve this is very different ways (Table 1.1.1). The HCPC has the ultimate sanction to prevent a dietitian from practising if, following investigation, they are deemed to be unsafe or untrustworthy. However, the BDA provides guidance, advice, learning and networking opportunities, and professional indemnity insurance cover, all with the aim of supporting the development of safe and effective practitioners. This ultimately helps protect the public and service users. The BDA also provides a trade union function and supports members throughout their working life on issues such as pay and conditions, equal opportunities, maternity rights and health and safety.

Autonomy

Autonomy can be defined as the right of self governance and as independent practitioners, who practice autonomously, dietitians are personally accountable for their

Table 1.1.1 Remit of the Health and Care Professions Council (regulatory body) and the British Dietetic Association (professional body)

Health and Care Professions Council	British Dietetic Association
Protect the public and service users	Protect the public and service users
Set professional standards of practice	Membership support
Approve education programmes that train and educate graduates to meet these standards	Advance the science and practice of dietetics
Register graduates of these programmes	Promote education and training in the science and practice of dietetics
Ensure registrants meet professional standards	Regulate the relationship between dietitians and their employer through the trade union
Sanction registrants who do not meet these standards	Provide professional indemnity insurance

practice (BDA, 2008a). This means they are answerable for their actions and omissions, regardless of advice or directions from another health professional. Dietitians have a duty of care for their service users and clients who are entitled to receive safe and competent care or service.

The HCPC states that as autonomous and accountable professionals, dietitians, '. . . *need to make informed and reasonable decisions about their practice. This might include getting advice and support from education providers, employers, professional bodies, colleagues and other people to make sure that you protect the wellbeing of service users at all times.*' (Health and Care Professions Council, 2008).

It is important that dietitians are aware of the boundaries of their autonomy, which will never be limitless but will always be confined to their scope of practice. As with all health professionals, dietitians must never practise in isolation. Up to date knowledge skills and experience are the cornerstone of safe and effective practice, and as such dietitians should always have access to a support network of leaning, development and peer review. In the National Health Service (NHS) setting, the system for learning and development is usually already established via internal processes, e.g. supervision, appraisal, local training programmes, library services and journal clubs. Outside of the NHS these processes are not automatically in place and it is essential that every healthcare professional actively establishes a network of support and learning to match their scope of practice, e.g. freelance practice (see Chapter 4.1).

Scope of practice

Identifying individual scope of practice is not easy as the boundaries will be different for each practitioner and will

Table 1.1.2 Factors that define dietetic scope of practice

Factor	Example
Occupational role	Clinician, researcher, educator, writer, consultant
Sector	Private practice, industry, higher education, commercial
Environment	Acute, community, GP practice, industry, media
Client group	Children, elderly, people with learning difficulties, public, supermarket
Speciality	Diabetes, public health, obesity, product development
Approaches	Behavioural therapy, group education, anthropometry, cook and eat session
Types of cases for referral elsewhere	Other dietitians or other healthcare professionals, social services

evolve over time (BDA, 2009a). The description of a dietitian's scope of practice is often broad and may describe some or all of the factors shown in Table 1.1.2.

A much more specific scope of practice is described in relation to specific service users. When presented with a service user, the dietitian should undertake a personal risk assessment as part of the overall assessment, asking key questions before proceeding. These questions include:

- Is the service user safe?
- Am I safe?
- Can I justify the decision I have made during the assessment (e.g. has the research, evidence, standards and guidance been considered)?
- Can I identify the most appropriate approach for the service user group?
- Do I have the correct balance of skills, knowledge and experience to be competent in my chosen approach?

Extended scope of practice

The extended roles dietetic practitioner undertake are those outside their core and specialist roles. They are usually (but not exclusively) roles traditionally carried out by other health professionals either as a core duty or role extension. Additional skills and knowledge are acquired through formal training. The extended role practitioner must advance dietetic practice and contribute to improving outcomes. Examples of extended roles include:

- Replacing gastrostomy tubes in the community.
- Inserting peripheral midlines for intravenous feeding.
- Advising on appropriate exercise regimens.

Whatever role a dietitian commits to, extended or otherwise, they must constantly be aware of their individual scope of practice, and practice within this.

Ethics and conduct

Conduct is the manner in which a person behaves, especially in a particular place or situation, while ethics are moral principles that govern a person's or group's behaviour. However, it is essential to put these definitions into context for them to have any meaning. In professional practice, professional ethical conduct is paramount. Outside of their professional role, dietitians have the right to behave how they choose, within the limits of the law, and this will be limited only by personal ethical boundaries. In professional practice, it is the professional codes of conduct that provide the framework for, and the benchmark by which, ethical conduct will be measured.

A major function of a code of conduct is to enable professionals to make informed choices when faced with an ethical dilemma. For the dietetic workforce the key guidance is laid out in the HCPC Standards of Conduct, Performance and Ethics (2008) and Guidance on Conduct and Ethics for Students (2009). These standards are written in broad terms so as to apply to all registrants as far as possible, and are designed not to be overly prescriptive, thereby undermining professional judgement and stifling progress and innovation.

The BDA Code of Professional Conduct (2008a) builds on the generic standards of the HCPC, with more dietetic specific guidance. They apply to the whole dietetic workforce from unregulated students and support workers to qualified dietitians. In practice, however, there will be numerous occasions where, despite guidance, there is no right or wrong answer to everyday dilemmas in practice. The HCPC (2008, p. 5) states that in such situations *'If you make informed, reasonable and professional judgements about your practice, with the best interests of your service users as your prime concern, and you can justify your decisions if you are asked to, it is very unlikely that you will not meet our standards.'*

Through HCPC mandated continuing professional development, a dietitian can ensure they have the technical knowledge, with the right skills and competencies, to be able to function in their role. As an autonomous professional, it is equally important to be an ethically competent practitioner to ensure trust between the professional and user. In addition, this trust is not confined to the individual practitioner but to the profession itself. Interpretation of ethical competence allows the distinction between skill and expertise or technical competence, and professionalism (Friedman, 2007). Friedman describes the acquisition of ethical competence in five stages as shown in Figure 1.1.1.

Model and Process for Nutrition and Dietetic Practice

The primary purpose of the practice of dietetics is to optimise the nutritional health of the service users, be they an individual, group or community, or population. By optimising the nutritional health of the service users the dietitian expects to positively influence health outcomes. In the practice of dietetics it is common for the dietitian to seek to influence or change other aspects of

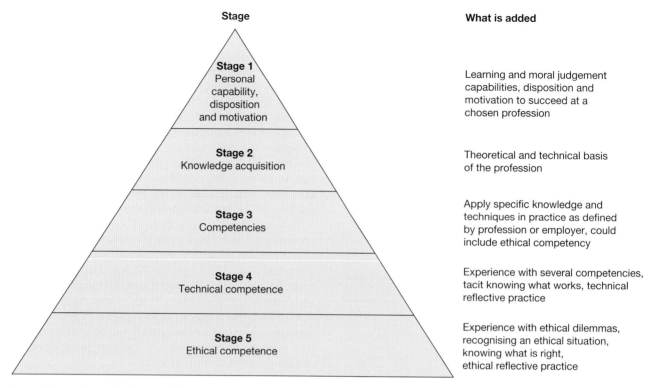

Figure 1.1.1 Stages in the acquisition of ethical competence (adapted from Friedman, 2007)

care or treatment, e.g. medication or the psychological wellbeing of the service user. However, the primary purpose of the dietitian is to identify and take action to improve the nutritional status of the service user and to improve those symptoms that are amenable to dietetic intervention.

Any single consultation or professional activity is incredibly complex and involves a number of different and varied strands of knowledge from biological and social sciences to food and medicine, alongside communication and clinical decision making skills and attributes such as empathy and respect. These are applied within professional and legal frameworks and boundaries and within organisational and social norms and standards. Most of this thought process is invisible to other professionals and often to the user as it takes place rapidly within the dietitian. The model of dietetic practice (MDP) seeks to make this explicit and visible. The BDA's Model and Process for Nutrition and Dietetic Practice (2012) is shown in Figure 1.1.2.

The model for dietetic practice brings together all of these aspects in a single framework that describes dietetic practice whether with individuals, groups or communities. The purpose of the MDP and the nutrition and dietetic process (NDP), which is the key aspect within it, is to help the profession provide safe, effective and consistent services and evidence of this.

Nutrition and dietetic process

At the centre of the NDP is the relationship between the service user and the dietitian. This relationship is key and influences how all the other aspects of the process function. The service user is at the centre of all professional practice and is most often the most important decision maker in any situation. User (person or patient) centred care has been demonstrated to lead to improved outcomes and to improved satisfaction with care (Robinson *et al.*, 2008). There are many and varied definitions, but the Institute of Medicine (2001) definition, '*Providing care that is respectful of, and responsive to individual patient preferences, needs and values and ensuring that patient values guide all clinical decisions*' encompasses all the concepts.

This definition ensures that the dietitian recognises that the service user's values and preferences will influence how the dietetic intervention is received and therefore how the intervention is delivered. This could be as simple as the level of information and choice the service user requests within the consultation or as complex as decisions about which aspects of the possible dietetic intervention plan to participate in or how to receive the service. The NDP developed by the BDA (2012) is shown in Figure 1.1.3.

This core relationship is at the centre of the NDP and is surrounded by other factors that will influence how the dietitian delivers the intervention and how the service user receives it. The inner rings describe what the dietitian, as a professional, brings to the relationship. This includes:

- Ethical frameworks such as the HCPC Code of Conduct, Performance and Ethics and the BDA Code of Professional Practice.

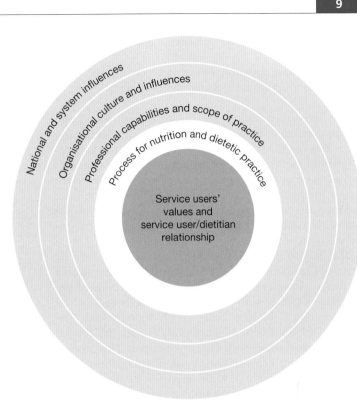

Figure 1.1.2 Model of Nutrition and Dietetic Practice [source: The British Dietetic Association 2013. Reproduced with permission of the British Dietetic Association (www .bda.uk.com)]

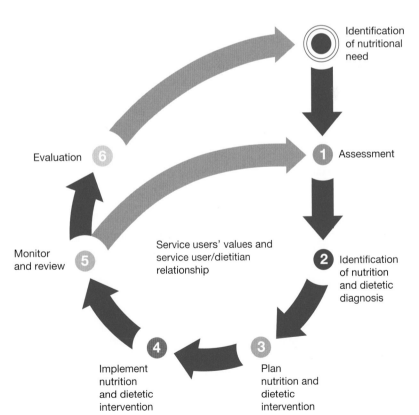

Figure 1.1.3 Nutrition and Dietetic Process [source: The British Dietetic Association 2013. Reproduced with permission of the British Dietetic Association (www.bda.uk.com)]

- Dietitian's scope of practice and professional capabilities.
- Evidence base for professional practice and the dietitian's continuing professional development.

This is surrounded by the organisational, social and environmental influences on practice. An organisation providing health services will require the dietitian to practise within their governance systems that are designed to provide safe and effective practice. There will be health needs and economic analysis, which will determine what services are required to meet the health needs of the local population and where the care is provided, and these can influence how the dietetic service is delivered.

The BDA Model and Process for Nutrition and Dietetic Practice (2012) provides the framework for a nutritional or dietetic intervention and describes the actions of the dietitian, together with the knowledge skills and critical thinking that a dietitian brings to all interventions. The dietitian places decision making skills and the service user's needs at the centre of the intervention. This process supports the implementation of a standard quality of care that is then personalised to the service user. By using the process, the dietitian moves from experience based practice to evidence based practice, explicitly applying the science and social science evidence base to critical decision making; essentially they are influenced by the service users preferences, need and values (Lacey & Pritchett, 2003). The BDA nutrition and dietetic process consists of five steps (Table 1.1.3):

1. Assessment.
2. Nutrition and dietetic diagnosis.
3. Formulation and planning of the intervention.
4. Implementation of the intervention.
5. Monitoring and evaluation.

Dietetic diagnosis

As previously stated, a dietitian is an autonomous professional and therefore responsible for their actions. One of the ways in which a dietitian demonstrates this autonomy is the identification of a nutritional and dietetic diagnosis. The diagnosis step may be considered the most important step in the NDP but it is often the step that is missed. In making a diagnosis the dietitian uses critical reasoning skills to evaluate the assessment information and to make judgements as to the risks to the service user(s) of taking action, or not. The dietitian will prioritise the nutritional issues identified and make a judgement as to whether taking action on these issues will make a difference to the health and outcomes for the service user.

In developing the diagnosis, the dietitian identifies the relevant aspects of the assessment and clearly states the nutritional problems that they and the service user have prioritised and the nutritional issues the dietitian can influence, and by doing so, the impact the nutritional and dietetic intervention will have on the service user's health. The benefits from making a nutritional and dietetic diagnosis include:

- Sharing with others involved with the service user the nutritional issue(s) that the dietitian and service user have prioritised.
- Identifying the specific nutritional issue(s) that the dietitian can influence.
- Identifying the indicators in the assessment process that will form the basis of monitoring and evaluation.
- Demonstrating the thoroughness of the assessment process and clearly communicating this to other professionals.

The diagnostic statement should clearly record for all service providers the problem, its cause (aetiology) and why the dietitian considers that it is a problem (symptoms). This statement also forms the basis of the monitoring and evaluation step as the dietitian will also have identified the most important indicators from their description of the symptoms.

Recording and information management

Another fundamental aspect of professionalism is the accurate recording of the nutrition and dietetic process. The HCPC (2007) Standards of Proficiency require dietitians to be able to maintain records appropriately. The information in records, including dietetic records, is used for many different purposes. Most importantly, it provides a permanent account of the dietetic process, especially the intervention, and a means of communication between all professionals and others involved, including the service user.

Information contained within records is also used for a number of other purposes, including demonstrating the overall effectiveness of the dietetic service and, possibly, organisation, quality monitoring and service improvement, research and public health purposes. While the increasing use of electronic health records will require more systematic record keeping, there is evidence that using a systematic format in any record, paper or electronic, improves the quality of care and service user outcomes (Mann & Williams, 2003). It is therefore important that the information in professional records is recorded accurately, systematically and consistently.

Quality improvement

Quality (Donabedian, 1980) has many dimensions. In the health service, patients, the public and carers expect safe, effective and consistent high quality care and treatment (NHS Scotland, 2003). For the individual dietitian this is a requirement of registration with the HCPC. Quality improvement involves a series of activities undertaken to reduce the gap between current practice and desired practice.

As a result of the need to account for its management and clinical efficiency, effectiveness and value for money, the NHS developed the concept of clinical governance. Clinical governance is defined *as, 'the system through which NHS organisations are accountable for continuously improving the quality of their services and safe-*

Table 1.1.3 Definitions of the steps in the Model and Process for Nutrition and Dietetic Practice

Step	Definition
Assessment	A systematic process of collecting and interpreting information to make decisions about the nature and cause of nutrition-related health issues in an individual, a group or a population
	Its purpose is to obtain adequate and relevant information to identify nutrition related problems and to inform the development and monitoring of the intervention
	It is initiated by the identification of need, e.g. screening, referral by a health professional, self referral, high level public health data, epidemiological data or other similar process
Identification of nutritional and dietetic diagnosis	Identification of nutritional problems that impact on the physical, mental and/or social wellbeing where the dietitian is responsible for action
	Individual
	It requires therapeutic or educational action as determined by the dietitian and service user
	Based on scientific evaluation of physical and psychological signs, symptoms, dietary and medical history, procedures and test results and the priorities of the service user
	Groups
	In a therapeutic group there will be a diagnosis for the individuals in the group (as individuals). In a public health group the diagnosis step will be the same as for the population
	Populations
	Within a public health needs assessment framework the nutritional diagnosis is defined as assessing a nutritional health priority for action. It involves choosing (for action) the nutritional health conditions and determinant factors with the most significant size, impact and severity
	At all levels it includes the identification and categorisation of the occurrence, risk or potential for the development of a nutritional problem that the dietitian will be responsible for treating independently or of leading the strategy to manage
Plan intervention	A set of activities and associated resources that are used to address the identified nutritional and dietetic diagnosis designed with the intent of changing nutrition related behaviours, risk factors, environmental factors or aspect of physical or psychological health or nutritional status of the individual, group or population. All interventions are planned with the communities, service users and carers who are the recipients of the intervention. This client centred approach is a key element in developing a realistic plan that has a high probability of positively influencing the outcome. This will usually involve describing:
	• Overall measurable and specific outcomes
	• Intermediate goals, which will achieve the outcomes, determined by the diagnosis statement and assessment information
	• Plan designed to meet the goals and outcomes – interventions, provision of food, provision of nutritional support, education package, counselling, coordination of care, social marketing campaigns, food availability, food shopping and cooking skills
	• Roles and responsibilities of individuals, professionals and organisations in delivering the plan
Implementation	The action phase of the nutrition and dietetic process. Dietitians may carry out the intervention, delegate or coordinate to another health or social care professional; patient, client or carer; voluntary organisation or member of the nutrition and dietetic team
Monitoring	The review and measurement of the client, group or population's nutritional status at planned intervals with regard to the nutritional diagnosis, intervention plan, goals and outcomes. It includes monitoring the implementation processes of the plan
Evaluation	The systematic comparison of current findings against previous status, intervention goals and outcomes or a reference standard, and usually takes place at the end of the process

guarding high standards of care, by creating an environment in which clinical excellence will flourish' (Scally & Donaldson, 1998, p. 61). The principles of clinical governance are embedded within the organisation and encompass:

- Clinical audit.
- Evidence based practice.
- Information governance (including record keeping).
- Patient and public involvement.
- Patient safety.
- Revalidation and performance.
- Risk management and medicolegal issues.

Latterly, the term clinical effectiveness was developed as a response to demands to provide evidence of effectiveness. Health professionals have developed measures to report on the quality of clinical services and assess the effectiveness of medical interventions. These include:

- Clinical or medical audit.
- Outcome measures.
- Evidence based practice.
- Guidelines.

Clinical audit is carried out locally and nationally, and provides a method for systematically evaluating, reflecting upon and reviewing practice against evidence based standards.

Dietetic outcome measurement

The provision of safe, effective and good quality care, or intervention, is fundamental to dietetic practice and is a HCPC registration requirement. A dietitian needs to know that an intervention is evidence based and effective, i.e. that it achieves the predicted outcome and makes effective use of the available resources. To demonstrate this, the dietitian needs to be able to systematically and consistently identify and predict what the desired outcome of their intervention will be, the timescale involved and to what extent this has been achieved from the viewpoint of both the dietitian and the recipient.

Outcome measurement should use SMART principles (systematic, measurable, achievable, realistic and timely). Much of the information needed will already have been collected and is readily available. Putting the patient at the centre of care is a central feature of health policy across the UK, so measuring the patient experience has to be a key component of outcome measurement. The BDA (2011a) outcomes model is a useful starting point for measuring dietetic outcomes, i.e. capturing the unique contribution of the dietitian.

Measurement of outcomes can take place at the individual, service, multidisciplinary team, organisational or national level. Measuring healthcare outcomes is a developing field and no single methodology is universally applicable to all situations. Patient reported outcome measures (PROMs) are a national, validated and mandated approach to collecting outcome information from the patient's perspective for a small number of elective surgical procedures. This approach is being expanded to cover more situations. The use and development of validated outcome measures is an emerging methodology; however, no single outcome measure will capture every dimension of care. The BDA (2011a) outcomes model provides an introduction and steps for developing dietetic outcome models.

Evidence based practice

Evidence based practice has been defined as, '. . . *the conscientious, explicit and judicious use of current best evidence in making decisions about the care of individual patients'* (Sacket *et al.,* 1996). While evidence based practice was developed in clinical practice, it can be applied to any dietetic discipline or setting and is an essential part of professional practice. The International Confederation of Dietetic Associations (2010) defines evidence based dietetics practice as being, '. . . *about asking questions, systematically finding research evidence, and assessing the validity, applicability and importance of that evidence. This evidence-based information is then combined with the dietitian's expertise and judgement and the client's or community's unique values and circumstances to guide decision-making in dietetics.'*

Evidence based practice is not a 'one off' activity but must be continuous throughout a dietitian's professional career. It is an essential part of being a professional and an essential element in the nutrition and dietetic process. Evidence based practice can be broken down into five key stages which are:

* Formulating the question.
* Finding the evidence.
* Critical appraisal.
* Using and acting on evidence.
* Evaluation and reflection.

At the end of this process it should be possible to identify areas within practice that require evidence; this should be the stimulus to conduct research to fill this gap. Measuring outcomes and audit are essential elements of evidence based practice.

Formulating the question

The first step in evidence based practice is recognising that there is a need for new information. This may be recognised from practice, reading or research. Recognition of need for new information must be converted into an answerable question. This can be broken into four stages that are collectively known as the PICO principle (Glasziou *et al.,* 2003).

The PICO principle

PICO is an acronym that stands for:

* Patients, or population, to which the question applies.
* Intervention being considered in relation to these patients/population.
* Comparison(s) to be made between those receiving the intervention and another group who do not receive the intervention.
* Outcome(s) to be used to establish the size of any effect caused by the intervention.

It is a framework that helps to focus the literature search by clarifying the question, identifying the information needed to be able to answer the question, translating the question into searchable terms and helping to develop and refine the search approach. In research this will be the research question or hypothesis.

Finding the evidence

Choosing the right evidence is of fundamental importance; therefore, it is essential to use PICO to identify search terms, search for evidence systematically and critically appraise the evidence.

Literature searching

A literature search is a systematic approach to retrieving information, i.e. a detailed and organised stepwise search for all the material available on a topic. Choosing the right evidence is of fundamental importance to answering the research question. There are several literature databases available and each has different criteria for the inclusion

Table 1.1.4 Levels of evidence [from Evidence Based Nursing Practice Hierarchy of Evidence (2008)]

Level	Description	Example
1	Strong evidence from at least one systematic review of well designed randomised controlled trials (RCTs)	Meta analyses The Cochrane Collaboration publications
2	Evidence from at least one properly designed RCT of appropriate size	Articles published in peer reviewed journals
3	Evidence from well designed trials without randomisation, e.g. cohort, time series or matched case controlled studies	Articles published in peer reviewed journals
4	Evidence from well designed non-experimental studies from more than one centre or research group	Articles published in peer reviewed journals
5	Opinions from respected authorities, based on clinical evidence, descriptive studies or reports from committees	NICE guidelines Evidence based local procedures and care pathways
6	Views of colleagues/peers	Members of the multidisciplinary team

of articles. The databases include PubMed (MedLine), CINAHL and Web of Science. NHS Evidence, managed by The National Institute for Health and Care Excellence (NICE), provides access to selected quality health and social care evidence and best practice.

Levels of evidence

There are different systems in use to grade evidence, but they all reflect the methodological rigour of studies. A study assigned as level 1 (or A) evidence (a systematic review or meta analysis that has been conducted using Cochrane Library methodology) is considered the most rigorous and least susceptible to bias. A study deemed to be level 4 evidence is considered the least rigorous and more susceptible to bias (Table 1.1.4). Level 1 evidence is limited for dietetic practice due to the ethical constraints of performing the studies.

When searching for evidence it is necessary to identify the best available evidence, which may include evidence from qualitative, observational studies or professional consensus (expert) opinion. Qualitative methods can help to provide answers to the kinds of questions that are not easily answerable by experimental methods (Swift & Tischler, 2010).

Critical appraisal

Each year thousands of articles are published in peer reviewed journals; however, many will not be well written, report robust studies or be relevant to practice. Therefore, it is essential to evaluate the rigour of an article and whether or not it is relevant to practice by critically appraising it. Critical appraisal is the systematic approach to the evaluation and interpretation of a publication in terms of its validity, results and relevance to an individual's practice or further research. It is essential that the approach is systematic so that the entire article is assessed; strengths and weaknesses of the study design, as well as biases within the study design or writing, need to be identified if effective change is to be made to practice. Critical appraisal will also enhance skills in understanding the research and audit process, while being an important CPD activity. The principle of critical appraisal should be used when evaluating any publication.

How to critically appraise an article

There are many examples available of how to do critical analysis; however, with experience, specific study design tools should be used. Recognised tools are available from NHS Solutions for Public Health (www.sph.nhs.uk) or the Scottish Intercollegiate Guidelines Network (SIGN) (www.sign.ac.uk). A generic framework for critical appraisal is shown in Appendix A1.

Using and acting on evidence

Research and evidence is of limited use if it is not translated into effective clinical practice. Dissemination and utilisation of evidence in decision making in healthcare is the key to the provision of quality care. Clinical experience, based on personal observation, reflection and judgement, is also needed to translate scientific results into treatment of an individual service user. After appraising the evidence and deciding that it is sound, it is essential to put it into context. Evidence must be combined with a dietitian's own expertise, experience and knowledge within their own setting before changes are implemented. The benefits and risks of implementing change must be weighed against the benefits and risks of not using alternative approaches. The decision to implement change should be made in collaboration with other members of the team or department, or patient. Involving all stakeholders will ensure that changes are implemented.

Evaluation and reflection

Evidence based practice is a continuing activity, and evaluation and reflection are a fundamental part of practice. This enables dietitians to identify gaps in their knowledge, areas that require further research and continuously to question practise. Any changes must be evaluated by either audit or service evaluation using appropriate outcome measures. To evaluate the effect of change it is essential that baseline information is collected.

Once a sufficient body of evidence is available, practice recommendations, guidelines and their associated standards can be generated. Clinical guidelines are recommendations on the appropriate treatment and care of patients with specific diseases and conditions. Guidelines can be generated at an international level, e.g. The World Health Organization, or nationally by organisations such as NICE or SIGN in the UK, or by other clinical specialist organisations and professional bodies, e.g. BDA, Royal College of Physicians, and associated clinical working groups, e.g. Intercollegiate Stroke Working Group. Some, such as those developed by NICE, also consider cost effectiveness. Guidelines can also be produced at a regional or local level. Evidence can be used to improve the quality and outcomes of care by informing structural changes at national and regional levels, such as Managed Clinical Networks in Scotland and the Regional Cancer Networks.

Practice based evidence in nutrition (PEN) (www .pennutrition.com/bda) is a dynamic knowledge translation subscription service that is based on knowledge pathways providing evidence based answers for food, nutrition and dietetic practice questions. The content is developed by systematically reviewing the evidence base.

Routine activities that aid practitioners include keeping a portfolio and reading and evaluating new evidence. A portfolio is vital evidence of CPD and should be used to reflect and evaluate practice and the effect of any change. Simple electronic tools are available to provide information on new evidence. These include:

- *Application software (Apps)* – these include EBM toolkits from publishers, e.g. BMJ books, journals, searchable databases, e.g. PubMed, and critical appraisal tools.
- *Electronic table of contents (eTOC)* from appropriate journals – current contents pages are sent to subscribers (this is usually a free service).
- *Alerts, updates and newsletters* from professional bodies and organisations, e.g. Bandolier and Centre for Reviews and Dissemination (CRD) York.

Most of these services are available as email alerts or Really Simple Syndication (RSS) Feeds; once set up they are automatic.

Research, audit and service evaluation

The skills required to conduct research can also be applied to conduct audit and service evaluation. However, research is used to generate new evidence whilst audit and service evaluation evaluate care. It is important to remember that a survey conducted in clinical care cannot be called an audit unless the results are compared with a standard; standards are generated by research. An important distinction between research, audit and service evaluation is that research requires ethical approval from the appropriate research ethics committee while audit and service evaluation do not. Within the NHS they all require review and approval by the appropriate department, i.e. research and development or clinical governance. Table 1.1.5 gives a brief summary of the key differences between the categories of studies. If the categorisation of the study is unclear, it is important to consult the appropriate department or committee before commencement.

Research can be defined as the, '*original investigation undertaken in order to gain knowledge and understanding*' (Research Assessment Exercise, 2001). It underpins evidence practice and is a vital component of a dietitian's professional role. The HCPC (2008) requires that dietitians must be able to conduct research and audit and that they continue to use and develop research skills throughout their careers. The essential nature of research and audit as part of professional practice is embedded within both the BDA's Code of Professional Practice (BDA, 2008a) and the Curriculum Framework for the Pre-registration Education and Training for Pre-registration Dietitians (BDA, 2008b). The BDA (2009b) defines four stages of research involvement and details the skills required at each stage. On qualification all dietitians should have the necessary skills to understand, interpret and apply research. If dietitians maintain and build upon these basic skills, some will eventually lead research and supervise others (Whelan, 2007).

The research process

Research consists of three phases: planning, conducting research and disseminating the results (Hickson, 2008), as shown in Table 1.1.6. The phases may overlap, e.g. dissemination may be planned during the planning stage or an application for funding may require a dissemination plan.

Research governance and ethics

Research governance encompasses regulations, standards and principles of good research practice, therefore ensuring that research is conducted to high ethical and scientific standards. It applies to everyone involved in the research process, including researchers at all levels, employers and support staff. In a clinical setting this will include care providers. Every organisation that conducts research or in which research is conducted should have a research governance framework or guide to good research practice, e.g. Department of Health (2005) Research Governance Framework for Health and Social Care; Medical Research Council (2000) Good Research Practice. Such frameworks and guides protect everyone involved in research, including the researcher. The framework or guide should include:

- Principles of good research, including the research culture.
- Responsibilities and accountability of researchers at all levels, institutions and carers if applicable.
- Processes including approval.
- Finance.
- Ethics.
- Gathering, handling and storing data.
- Result reporting.
- Monitoring procedures.

Ethical approval from an appropriate committee is essential for any research involving humans, clinical data, human organs or tissues; it is a legal requirement in the NHS. Informed consent and confidentiality are central to ethical research. The review process will vary depending

Table 1.1.5 The differences between research, audit and service evaluation (source: NHS National Patient Safety Agency 2008. Reproduced with permission)

Research	Clinical audit	Service evaluation
Attempts to derive new knowledge; studies may aim to generate hypotheses or to test them	Designed and conducted to produce information to inform delivery of best care	Designed and conducted solely to define and judge current care
Quantitative research – designed to test a hypothesis	Designed to answer the question: 'Does this service reach a predetermined standard?'	Designed to answer: 'What standard does this service achieve?'
Qualitative research – identifies/explores themes following established methodology		
Addresses clearly defined questions, aims and objectives	Measures against a standard	Measures current service without reference to a standard
Quantitative research – may involve evaluation or comparing interventions, particularly new ones	Involves an intervention in use ONLY (the choice of treatment is that of the clinician and patient according to guidance, professional standards and/or patient preference)	Involves an intervention in use ONLY (the choice of treatment is that of the clinician and patient according to guidance, professional standards and/ or patient preference)
Qualitative research – usually involves studying how interventions and relationships are experienced		
Usually involves collecting data that are additional to those for routine care, but may include data collected routinely. May involve treatments, samples or investigations additional to routine care	Usually involves analysis of existing data, but may include administration of a simple interview or questionnaire	Usually involves analysis of existing data, but may include administration of a simple interview or questionnaire
Quantitative research – study design may involve allocating patients to an intervention group	No allocation to intervention groups; the healthcare professional and patient have chosen intervention before clinical audit	No allocation to intervention groups; the healthcare professional and patient have chosen intervention before service evaluation
Qualitative research uses a clearly defined sampling framework underpinned by conceptual or theoretical justifications		
May involve randomisation	No randomisation	No randomisation

Table 1.1.6 The research process

Phase	Step
Plan research	Develop a research question Use the literature to research the background Choose an appropriate methodology Write a research proposal Formulate aims and objectives If necessary, obtain funding Obtain ethical and institutional approval
Conduct research	Prepare for data collection and management Recruitment and consent participants Collate and analyse data
Dissemination of results	Develop dissemination plan Present findings at a scientific conference Write and submit a manuscript for a peer reviewed journal

on the organisation. Within the NHS the National Research Ethics Service offers a central and consistent service, including the Integrated Research Application System (IRAS) (www.myresearchproject.org.uk). This is a single system of applying for permissions and approvals for health and social care and community research in the UK without unnecessary duplication. Each university will have its own system for ethical approval.

How to do research

This section gives a brief overview of research; more detailed information can be found in Hickson (2008). Further resources are listed at the end of the chapter.

Planning research

The first step in research is developing the question and the PICO principle can be used to generate a concise question. The aims and objectives of the research should relate directly to the research question; the methodology will be determined by the aims and objectives; and when disseminating the results of the research, the discussion and conclusion of a paper or abstract should relate to the question and aims and objectives. The research question may arise from clinical practice or from the literature. A research question will lead to a hypothesis.

Table 1.1.7 Research methodologies

Descriptive	Cross sectional survey Qualitative, e.g. grounded theory, discourse analysis, ethnography, narrative research and phenomenology	
Empirical	Experimental	Randomised parallel groups Randomised cross over
	Observational	Cohort Cross sectional Case control

The research question plays a crucial role in reviewing the literature for the project. The literature review may stem from the aims and objectives or serve to formulate the aims and objectives. The research aim is usually a broad statement outlining the goal and objectives are more detailed statements of how the aim will be achieved. Each objective should be simple, straightforward and achievable. Well thought out objectives suggest a methodology and thus help determine the methodology.

The actual method is how the study will be carried out and includes details such as where the research will take place, who will be involved, how the participants will be recruited, the actual data collection and how the data will be analysed. It is quite acceptable to include both quantitative and qualitative methodologies in a study, but often such a study will be divided into two stages with one stage informing the other. Table 1.1.7 gives an overview of research methodologies.

It is essential to write a research protocol when planning the project and include details of the study rationale, aims and objectives, methods with specific measureable outcomes, statistical analysis, dissemination plans and timeline. The protocol can be used when applying for governance and ethical approval, and funding and will form the basis of the eventual dissemination. When using questionnaires, or other instruments to measure variables, it is important to consider the population for which they are validated and how the results obtained from them will be analysed. If results require statistical analysis, it is sensible to consult a statistician at this stage so that any necessary modifications can be made to the planned data collection.

Conducting research

This stage of the research process is usually constrained by time and money. A Gantt chart detailing delivery dates and deadlines is a useful organisational tool. Difficulties obtaining ethical approval or with recruitment of research staff and participants often delay projects, so sufficient time should be built in at the planning stage to avoid missing deadlines later. Communication is the key to keeping the research process on track, e.g. if recruitment

is slower than anticipated, it is helpful to let funders know before deadlines are missed; funding bodies often have a wealth of research experience and can be a source of help and advice if necessary. Meticulous record keeping will also help the research process to run smoothly. Data collection sheets that are easy to complete will be less likely to contain errors. Data collection methods should be piloted and necessary changes made. Research logs or diaries can act as a cross check to reference dates and times that certain activities took place. Keeping a research diary may be a requirement of an organisation.

Data analysis will probably involve transferring data into a software analysis program and particular care should be taken at this stage to avoid introducing errors. If possible, double data entry should be used where two people enter quantitative data on separate spreadsheets and compare them for differences. Qualitative data often need to be transcribed. This time consuming task can be delegated to professional transcribers, although this step can be a valuable part of the process of becoming familiar with the data.

Dissemination

It is essential that dietitians disseminate all the evidence generated, including research, audit and service evaluation. There are vehicles for every type and size of study; small and negative studies are valuable as they add to the evidence base and may inform others of potential difficulties. Dissemination can occur internally, within the department or institution, or externally at conferences and in peer reviewed journals. Conferences are the best way to disseminate small studies and initial findings. The most important way to disseminate work is as a manuscript published in a peer reviewed journal. Guidance on how to write a conference abstract or a manuscript for publication can be found at www.bda.uk.com/conference/research. Publication guidelines, e.g. CONSORT (Consolidated Standards of Reporting Trials) have been produced in order to improve the quality of research reporting and are available from the Equator Network (www.equator.org.uk).

Continuing professional development

Professional practice develops over time and individual professionals must strive, and expect, to develop and improve their practice so that services and the outcomes for their service users improve. This process is known continuing professional development (CPD). Continuing professional development is an active process by which every day and more formal experiences are critically reflected upon to identify learning points which are then recorded in a useful format. The BDA (2008c) defines CPD as, '. . . *a systematic on-going process which allows individuals to maintain, update and enhance their knowledge and expertise in order to ensure that they are able to carry out work safely and effectively.*'

A dietitian has a responsibility to meet the HCPC Standards for CPD (2011). The HCPC states that, '. . . *CPD is the way health professionals continue to learn and develop throughout their careers so they keep their skills and knowledge up to date and are able to work safely, legally and effectively.*' Dietitians, like other HCPC registrants, are required to reregister every two years and each profession is audited. A random sample of dietitians is required to submit their CPD portfolios for audit. It is not a review of the standard of the CPD activities themselves, but of how the individual meets the HCPC standards for CPD. Registrants must demonstrate a variety of CPD activities and how the activities were used to improve their practice. Further guidance on this process is available both from the BDA and the HCPC.

Continuing professional development activities

An individual's CPD should reflect a wide range of learning activities and be relevant to their current or developing scope of practice. CPD activities may be self directed, work based, professional activities or formal/educational activities. Further examples of CPD are shown in Table 1.1.8. Dietitians working within the NHS may be required to link to the NHS Knowledge and Skills Framework (Department of Health, 2004; NHS Employers, 2010). However, as an individual practitioner, a dietitian should organise and undertake CPD for their own development.

Reflective practice

Reflective practice has been defined as, '*. . . the capacity to reflect on action so as to engage in a process of continuous learning*' (Schon, 1991) and is essential to the development of professional practice in dietetics. The purpose of reflection is to enable a practitioner to use experience to develop practice through a systematic process of analysing experience to learn from it. Reflective practice is the method by which dietitians make sense of practice by analysing a situation or experience, knowledge and skills used, and their reaction to the experience, and by exploring learning, which can be applied in the future. During the process further learning needs are often identified. This reflection on practice is also one method by which a professional may identify new theories of practice and so integrate the technical science basis and the practice and art of dietetics.

Reflection is a skill that requires development and practice. It requires the individual to be open to their feelings and to what they can learn from the experience. There are a number of models that provide a structured process to aid the process of reflection and building a portfolio (Gibbs, 1988; Rolfe *et al.*, 2001).

Practice supervision

A dietitian should also seek practice supervision throughout their professional training and career. Supervision is the process of professional learning and support involving a range of activities. It enables individuals to develop knowledge and competence, assume responsibility for their own practice and enhance service user protection, quality and safety of care (BDA, 2011b). The supervision process can directly influence CPD, providing a structured process of professional support that facilitates life long learning and personal development, and highlights training needs. Practice supervision is integral to delivering a quality service and should be included within working practices where work based scenarios are explored, reflection upon practice takes place and evidence of CPD is gathered. This process of supervision will start as a student in practice education and continue throughout working life. Examining performance, identifying strengths and weaknesses and seeking to improve are key attributes of a professional.

Preceptorship

Professionals in the first year of practice, particularly within the NHS, should work within a structured development programme called preceptorship. The aim of preceptorship is to enhance the competence and confidence

Table 1.1.8 Examples of continuing professional development (CPD) activities

Workbased learning	Professional activity	Formal / educational	Self directed learning
Learning by doing	Involvement in a professional	Courses	Reading journals/articles
Case studies	body	Further education	Reviewing books or articles
Reflective practice	Membership of a specialist	Research	Keeping a file of progress
Clinical audit	interest group	Attending conferences or	
Discussions with colleagues	Lecturing or teaching	seminars	
Gaining, and learning from,	Mentoring	Writing articles or papers	
experience	Being an examiner or tutor	Distance learning	
Work shadowing	Organising journal clubs or	Planning or running a	
Secondments	other specialist groups	course	
Job rotation	Membership of other		
Journal club	professional bodies or groups		
In-service training	Presenting at conferences		
Supervising staff or students	Supervising research		
Analysing significant events	Being promoted		
Project work or project			
management			

of newly registered practitioners as autonomous professionals (Department of Health, 2010). During this time, the new practitioner, supported by a preceptor, will develop their skills, behaviour and attitude to become a more confident practitioner. It is likely to be a structured programme with a mix of theory and guided reflection with a preceptor. Further guidance is available from a number of different sources including the BDA (2011b).

Recording continuing professional development

Dietitians have a responsibility to maintain an accurate, continuous and up to date record or portfolio of CPD activities (HCPC, 2009). The BDA provides tools to support the development of a portfolio and proformas to record CPD, based on the framework for reflective practice of Rolfe *et al.* (2001) which uses the following questions:

- What?
- So what?
- Now what?

These enable the dietitian to describe the CPD activity, explain what is learnt and reflect on the benefits to the service user alongside the use of new skills, as well as investigating any areas for development or improvement.

Conclusion

Dietetics has a proud tradition of upholding safe, effective, evidence based nutritional expertise, and this is fundamentally a result of the professionals who work within the discipline. The profession's commitment to constantly be innovative, whilst striving for the highest standards of technical and ethical competence, have seen it evolve into the internationally respected profession it is today.

Further reading

Greenhalgh T. (2010) *How to Read a Paper: The Basics of Evidence-Based Medicine*. Oxford: Wiley Blackwell.
Hickson M. (2008) *Research Handbook for Health Care Professionals*. Oxford: Wiley Blackwell.

Internet resources

British Dietetic Association   www.bda.uk.com
BDA guidance on writing an abstract   www.bda.uk.com/conference/research
Centre for Evidence Based Medicine   www.cebm.net/
Centre for Reviews and Dissemination (CRD) York   www.york.ac.uk/inst/crd/
EQUATOR Enhancing the Quality Of health Research   www.equator-network.org
Evidence Based Nursing Practice   www.ebnp.co.uk/The%20Hierarchy%20of%20Evidence.htm
Healthcare Improvement Scotland   www.healthcareimprovementscotland.org/welcome_to_healthcare_improvem.aspx
Healthcare Quality Improvement Partnership (HQIP)   www.hqip.org.uk/
Health & Care Professions Council   www.hcpc-uk.org

NHS Evidence   www.evidence.nhs.uk/
Eyes on evidence   www.evidence.nhs.uk/about-us/eyes-on-evidence
NHS Scotland Clinical Governance   www.clinicalgovernance.scot.nhs.uk/
National Institute for Health and Care Excellence (NICE)   www.nice.org.uk
NICE Guidance and Scotland   www.healthcareimprovementscotland.org/programmes/nice_guidance_and_scotland.aspx
National Research Ethics Service   www.myresearchproject.org.uk
Practice-based Evidence in Nutrition (PEN)   www.pennutrition.com/bda
Scottish Intercollegiate Guidelines Network   www.sign.ac.uk
Solutions for Public Health – Critical Appraisal Skills Programme   www.sph.nhs.uk/what-we-do/public-health-workforce/resources/critical-appraisals-skills-programme
Trip Database – Clinical Search Engine   www.tripdatabase.com/

References

NB: BDA documents can be accessed by members via the member's page. Non-members should contact the BDA directly.
British Dietetic Association (BDA). (2008a) *Code of Professional Conduct*. Birmingham: BDA.
British Dietetic Association (BDA). (2008b) *Curriculum Framework for the Pre-registration Education and Training for Pre-registration Dietitians*. Birmingham: BDA.
British Dietetic Association (BDA). (2008c) *Continuing Professional Development Position Statement*. Birmingham: BDA.
British Dietetic Association (BDA). (2009a) *Guidance Document on Extended Scope Practice*. Birmingham: BDA.
British Dietetic Association (BDA). (2009b) *Dietitians and Research: A Knowledge and Skills Framework – Guidance Document*. Birmingham: BDA.
British Dietetic Association (BDA). (2011a) *Model for Dietetic Outcomes*. Birmingham: BDA.
British Dietetic Association (BDA). (2011b) *Practice Supervision*. Birmingham: BDA.
British Dietetic Association (BDA). (2012) *Model and Process for Dietetic Outcomes*. Birmingham: BDA.
Bullock A, Trombley S. (1999) *The New Fontana Dictionary of Modern Thought*. London: Harper-Collins, p. 689.
Cruess SR, Johnston S, Cruess RL. (2004) 'Profession': a working definition for medical educators. *Teaching and Learning in Medicine* 16(1): 74–76.
Department of Health. (2004) The NHS Knowledge and Skills Framework (NHS KSF) and the Development Review Process. Available at http://www.dh.gov.uk/en/Publicationsandstatistics/Publications/PublicationsPolicyAndGuidance/DH_4090843 Accessed 28 July 2011.
Department of Health. (2005) Research Governance Framework for Health and Social Care. Available at www.dh.gov.uk/en/Publicationsandstatistics/Publications/PublicationsPolicyAndGuidance/DH_4108962. Accessed 19 January 2012.
Department of Health. (2010) Preceptorship Framework for Newly Registered Nurses, Midwives and Allied Health Professionals. Available at http://www.dh.gov.uk/dr_consum_dh/groups/dh_digitalassets/@dh/@en/@abous/documents/digitalasset/dh_114116.pdf. Accessed 30 November 2011
Donabedian A. (1980) *The Definition of Quality and Approaches to its Assessment*. Ann Arbor, MI: Health Administration Press.
Friedman A. (2007) *Ethical Competence and Professional Associations*. Bristol: Professional Associations Research Network.
Gibbs G. (1988) *Learning by Doing: A Guide to Teaching and Learning Methods*. Oxford: Further Educational Unit, Oxford Polytechnic.
Glasziou P, Del Mar C, Salisbury J. (2003) *Evidence-based Medicine Workbook*. London: BMJ Books.
Health and Care Professions Council (HCPC). (2007) *Standards of Proficiency – Dietitians*. London: HCPC.

Health and Care Professions Council (HCPC). (2008) *Standards of Conduct, Performance and Ethics*. London: HCPC.

Health and Care Professions Council (HCPC). (2009) *Guidance on Conduct and Ethics for Students*. London: HCPC.

Health and Care Professions Council (HCPC). (2010) *Information for Employers and Managers: The Fitness to Practice Process*. London: HCPC.

Health and Care Professions Council (HCPC). (2011) *Your Guide to our Standards for Continuing Professional Development*. London: HCPC.

Hickson M. (2008) *Research Handbook for Health Care Professionals*. Oxford: Wiley Blackwell.

Institute of Medicine. (2001) *Crossing the Quality Chasm: A New Health System for the 21st Century*. Washington, DC: National Academy Press.

International Confederation of Dietetic Associations (ICDA). (2010). Available at www.internationaldietetics.org/International -Standards/Evidence-based-Dietetics-Practice.aspx. Accessed 18 January 2012.

Lacey K, Pritchett E. (2003) Nutrition Care Process and Model: ADA adopts road map to quality care and outcomes management. *Journal of the American Dietetic Association* 103(8): 1061–1072.

Mann R, Williams J. (2003) Standards in medical record keeping. *Clinical Medicine* 3: 329.

Medical Research Council. (2000) *Good Research Practice*. Available at www.mrc.ac.uk/Utilities/Documentrecord/index.htm?d=MRC 002415. Accessed 19 January 2012.

NHS Employers. (2010) Simplified KSF. Available at http://www .nhsemployers.org/PayAndContracts/AgendaForChange/KSF/ Simplified-KSF/Pages/SimplifiedKSF.aspx. Accessed 28 July 2011.

NHS National Patient Safety Agency. (2008) National Research Ethics Service leaflet: Defining Research Issue 3. London: Health Research Authority.

NHS Scotland. (2003) Partnership For Care. Available at www .scotland.gov.uk/Resource/Doc/47032/0013897.pdf. Accessed 19 January 2012.

Research Assessment Exercise. (2001) Definition of research. Available at www.rae.ac.uk/2001/Pubs/4_01/section2.asp. Accessed 18 January 2012.

Robinson, JH, Callister, LC, Berry, JA, Dearing, KA. (2008) Patient-centered care and adherence: Definitions and applications to improve outcomes. *Journal of the American Academy of Nurse Practitioners* 20: 1745–7599.

Rolfe G, Freshwater D, Jasper M. (2001) *Critical Reflection for Nursing and the Helping Professions – a User's Guide*. Basingstoke: Palgrave.

Sacket DL, Rosenberg WMC, Gray JAM, Richardson WS. (1996) Evidence based medicine: what it is and what it isn't. *BMJ* 312: 71–72.

Scally G, Donaldson IJ. (1998) Clinical governance and the drive for quality improvement in the new NHS in England. *BMJ* 317: 61–65.

Schon D. (1991) *The Reflective Practitioner: How Professionals Think in Action*. Surrey: Ashgate Publishing Limited.

Swift JA, Tischler V. (2010) Qualitative research in nutrition and dietetics: getting started. *Journal of Human Nutrition and Dietetics*. 23(6), 559–566.

Whelan K. (2007) Knowledge and skills to encourage comprehensive research involvement among dietitians. *Journal of Human Nutrition and Dietetics* 20: 291–293.

1.2

Dietary modification

Annemarie Knight and Katherine Law

Key points

■ Dietary modification is defined as the elimination, manipulation or introduction of dietary components to achieve dietary goals.

■ Skillful assessment is required to identify all the factors that may influence the success of dietary intervention.

■ Dietary modification requires the use of a range of dietetic skills, including communication skills and the skills to change health behaviour.

■ A total diet approach should be adopted and dietary advice should be given in terms of food choice not nutrients.

Dietary modification is a cornerstone of dietetic practice and employs a range of dietetic skills. When undertaking dietary modification, dietitians need in depth knowledge of food composition, food availability and factors that determine what people eat. It is well acknowledged that dietary interventions are more likely to be effective when they are based on a sound understanding of the factors influencing the food choice of individuals or communities, not on the principles of changing health behaviour alone. An integrated approach to dietary counselling that considers all the relevant factors can improve compliance, satisfaction and clinical outcomes (Fine, 2006). The emphasis that these factors have on developing the most effective dietary intervention strategies will vary depending on the situation.

In the assessment phase of the nutrition and dietetic care process, the dietitian uses skills in nutritional, dietary and clinical assessment in order to decide the goals of dietary intervention (BDA, 2012) (see Chapter 1.1). Key to deciding how best to achieve these goals is an assessment of the interaction between the individual, or community, and their social situation. This assessment can also aid the identification of potential barriers that may impact the effectiveness of the intervention. Service users can and should be actively involved in their own healthcare, and the dietitian's role is to advise and help facilitate negotiated patient centred goals. When monitoring and evaluating the effectiveness of any dietary intervention, ongoing reassessment of the factors contributing to the achievement of dietary goals will be necessary.

Principles of dietary modification

Dietary modification can be defined as the elimination, manipulation or introduction of dietary components to achieve dietary goals. Dietary interventions are aimed at individuals, groups or communities and vary greatly in complexity. Modifications that are considered simple, e.g. increasing the fruit and vegetable intake of a community, may in fact be very difficult to achieve and require significant dietetic input. Similarly, those considered more complex, e.g. meeting an individual's nutritional requirements via the parenteral route, might be more straightforward to achieve.

Whether total or partial control of an individual's nutritional intake is required, challenges will almost certainly arise. A detailed knowledge of food and its composition is vital, together with an excellent knowledge of the tools and resources to reach achievable results. Once the requirement for dietary modification is highlighted and the level of regulation has been determined, four keys factors should be considered to achieve the required result: knowledge, achievability, motivation and communication.

Knowledge

In order for dietary modification to be effective, both the dietitian and service user (and any other healthcare professionals, or supporting individuals) must be knowledgeable regarding the rationale for the changes

Manual of Dietetic Practice, Fifth Edition. Edited by Joan Gandy.
© 2014 The British Dietetic Association. Published 2014 by John Wiley & Sons, Ltd.
Companion Website: www.manualofdieteticpractice.com

proposed. It is part of the dietitian's role to ensure that all those involved understand why change is necessary and how the proposed dietary modification will contribute to achieving treatment goals. From a service user's perspective, this can encourage compliance and also empower individuals to take some responsibility (Department of Health, 2001) for their own health and lifestyle. This process can be demonstrated through programmes such as Dose Adjustment for Normal Eating (DAFNE) and Diabetes Education and Self-Management for Ongoing and Newly Diagnosed (DESMOND), which focus primarily on the education and empowerment of the patient to allow for ongoing dietary modification that compliments individual lifestyles (see Chapter 7.12).

Thomas (1994) identified a reaction to the development of knowledge, including the development of skills, confidence in one's ability to make dietary changes and response to situational cues; all impacted positively on the service user's ability to take ownership of their diet. It is part of the dietitian's role to be the source of knowledge for the service user, facilitating and promoting dietary change and providing support and encouragement to the empowered individual.

Achievability

It is the dietitian's responsibility to ensure that goals set for diet modification are achievable, both from the clinical and service user's perspectives. The provision of practical, tailored advice and support are useful in this process. Excellent communication and, in some cases, counselling skills are required to assess the service user's lifestyle and level of understanding, to ensure that goals set are appropriate (see Chapter 1.3). Within a clinical or institutional setting, dietary modification is arguably more achievable due to a more controlled environment. Meals are generally provided and nutritionally regulated, so more specific guidance is easily accessible. There may however be barriers to ensuring an individualised approach to dietary modification in an institutional setting. With regard to artificial enteral and parenteral nutrition, a prescribed regimen is normally provided and amended as required, usually resulting in greater compliance.

Working alongside service users in outpatient or community settings can pose different challenges. Dietary interventions may be targeted at individuals or groups and in both cases, the optimum duration and frequency of contact needed to build effective relationships will need to be considered. More frequent or longer consultations may be necessary to ensure that the dietitian can provide adequate support.

Motivation

As is evident within many areas of dietetic practice, the motivation of both the service user and the dietitian is key to success. The Transtheoretical Model (Stages of Change Model) (Prochaska & DiClemente, 1986) demonstrates this process, highlighting those stages where successful dietary modification may be optimised. Identifying that individual service users will differ in terms of their motivation to adopt potential dietary modifications is also key, and in all cases targeting and tailoring of advice will probably increase effectiveness (Thomas, 1994). It may be appropriate to make smaller dietary changes first, allowing additional time and support for the adoption of more substantial dietary changes. The dietitian can use skills such as rapport building, motivational interviewing, reflective listening and problem solving to assess and increase motivation to change (Fine, 2006; Gable, 1997; Hunt & Pearson, 2001).

Communication

Effective, clear communication underpins successful dietetic practice. The way in which dietary advice is communicated can have an important impact on its effectiveness. An individualised approach should be adopted to ensure messages are tailored to the individual or group and that the most effective communication strategies are adopted. Recognising that dietary choices are mostly made on the basis of foods rather than nutrients and communicating actions using food terms enables the individual to take control of their dietary changes. When communicating dietary strategies to individuals, groups or communities, the dietitian may use written, verbal, audiovisual, electronic or interactive forms of communication, although often a combination of these will be used. Knowledge of tools such as dietary exchange systems and resources can also facilitate the communication of dietary modifications. Skills in changing health behaviour and effective communication are central to successful dietary modification (see Chapter 1.3).

Types of dietary modification

Modifying dietary intake can provide a methodical and practical solution to wider health issues, and encourage an individualised and problem solving approach. This can range from the elimination of nutrients through to the reintroduction of dietary components, and can also include the manipulation of foods (Table 1.2.1).

Manipulation of dietary components

Dietary components can be manipulated in the following ways:

Texture

The texture or consistency of the diet may be modified, e.g. in the management of swallowing disorders.

Composition

It may be necessary to alter the chemical composition of the diet in the management of conditions such as food hypersensitivity. Modification may require the use of dietary products whose macronutrient composition has been manipulated, e.g. amino acid or medium chain triglyceride based formulae.

Table 1.2.1 Approaches to dietary intervention

	Dietary intervention	Example of dietary modification to achieve dietary goals
Elimination	Weight management	Eliminate energy dense foods
	Food hypersensitivity	Eliminate foods containing allergen Eliminate foods causing intolerance
Manipulation	Weight management	Manipulation of portion size
	Oral nutritional support	Substitute foods to increase energy density
	Texture modification	As per the Dysphagia Diet Food Texture Descriptors (NPSA Dysphagia Expert Reference Group, April 2011)
	Artificial nutritional support	Manipulation of chemical composition of dietary components, e.g. elemental feed
	Restrict nutrients	Low fat diet, electrolyte restriction in renal disease, metabolic disorders
Introduction or reintroduction	Healthy balanced diet	Ensuring intake is balanced, including all food groups
	Elimination diet	Foods are eliminated and reintroduced slowly, assessing symptoms (e.g. LOFFLEX diet, suspected allergies)
	Weight management	Introduce substitutions for high energy density foods
	Oral nutritional support	Introduce substitutions for low energy density foods

Quantity

When modifying the quantity of a dietary component, it is necessary to consider the frequency of consumption, portion size and any appropriate food substitutions that can be made in the diet to achieve dietary goals.

Elimination of dietary components

Where possible, dietary interventions should always take a total diet approach and focus on the overall pattern of foods eaten rather than on specific foods or nutrients (American Dietetic Association, 2002). In the majority of cases, the elimination of individual foods will not be necessary; instead, modifying the quantity of the food consumed alongside the frequency of consumption will be sufficient to achieve dietary goals. The elimination of dietary components will be necessary in some conditions, e.g. inborn errors of metabolism. Where dietary components are excluded it is important to assess the role they play in the individual's diet and what substitute foods need to be recommended to ensure nutritional requirements are met.

Introduction and reintroduction of dietary components

A starting point for dietary modification is often to base recommendations on an individual's current dietary intake, although achieving dietary goals will involve the introduction of new foods. The introduction of dietary components will range from simple to complex recommendations, all of which should meet individual requirements. Where foods have been eliminated from the diet it will be necessary to plan their reintroduction, e.g. a food challenge with an identified allergen in the management of food hypersensitivity (see Chapter 7.11.2).

Process of dietary modification

Rationale

The first step in dietary modification is to ascertain the purpose of the modification based on a comprehensive assessment and the identification of the nutritional problem. The aim of dietary modification may be to:

- Achieve a nutrient profile that offers greater health benefits.
- Meet dietary needs in a safer way.
- Correct a dietary deficiency or surplus.
- Avoid the consumption of a particular dietary component.
- Achieve symptom relief.
- Achieve specific metabolic or clinical effects.

Key dietetic skills of clinical reasoning and evidence based practice are employed to develop a dietary intervention plan. Dietary modification should provide benefit to the individual or group, but it should be noted that the interactions between foods and nutrients are complex and altering one dietary component may affect another, e.g. increasing the energy density of a diet in oral nutritional support may increase the intake of saturated fat with the associated cardiovascular consequences. A total diet approach allows for an overall view of the likely consequences.

Factors that influence food choice

In deciding the most effective dietary intervention, any factors that will potentially influence adherence to the proposed modification should be identified.

Access to food

This will include factors such as purchasing patterns, budgetary constraints and cooking skills. To achieve dietary change it will be necessary to identify whether the foods that have been recommended are available where the individual shops, if support is needed with shopping or if the individual has the required skills to prepare the foods in the modified diet, e.g. for a texture modified diet, it is important to assess if the necessary equipment is available to modify foods to the correct consistency. At a community level, shopping and leisure facilities available in the local area may influence the effectiveness of interventions.

Taste and food preferences

Individual food preferences and the role food plays in an individual's life need to be considered when making dietary modifications.

Lifestyle influences

The lack of time and the burden of juggling work and home commitments can be a significant constraint in adopting healthy eating practices or dietary advice. It is important that the burden of proposed dietary modification in terms of time and effort is considered.

Cultural background

Developing effective dietary intervention strategies for individuals and groups from minority ethnic backgrounds requires an understanding of their relevant health behaviours (Thomas, 2002). Cultural food practices affect taste preferences and play a role in purchasing patterns. When developing dietary interventions for minority ethnic groups, it is necessary to take account of dietary patterns and acknowledge the variations in health beliefs, attitudes and practices within each cultural group (Bronner, 1994) (see Chapter 3.5).

Religious or ethical beliefs

In order to ensure that dietary modifications are compatible with an individual's or group's beliefs, it is necessary to establish them and the extent to which they are followed. There can be a wide variation in the interpretation of and adherence to the dietary restrictions associated with a particular faith.

Media

The media plays an important role in influencing food choice and shaping beliefs about nutrition and the role of the dietitian. It is important that dietitians keep abreast of media reporting on nutrition and diet in order to ensure that dietary education is effective and targeted, and that incorrect dietary beliefs can be addressed.

Practical aspects of dietary modification

All dietary modifications should be individualised and based on a detailed assessment. How dietary modification can be approached in order to achieve a range of dietary goals is shown in Box 1.2.1.

As well as the food based approaches outlined in Box 1.2.1, a range of other modifications may be used in order to achieve dietary goals and include:

Box 1.2.1   Practical examples of dietary modification strategies

Macronutrient modification
- Aim of dietary modification is to decrease the percentage of dietary fat:
  ○ Identify foods contributing to dietary fat intake
  ○ Limit frequency of consumption of high fat foods
  ○ Limit portion size of high fat foods
  ○ Recommend lower fat alternative foods
  ○ Recommend lower fat cooking methods
- Aim of dietary modification is to increase dietary intake of protein:
  ○ Increase frequency of consumption of high protein foods, including between meal snacks
  ○ Increase portion size of high protein foods
  ○ Fortify commonly consumed foods with additional protein
  ○ Consider need for supplements to achieve dietary aim

Micronutrient modification
- Aim of dietary modification is to increase dietary intake of iron:
  ○ Increase frequency of consumption of high iron foods
  ○ Increase portion size of high iron foods
  ○ Consider foods that increase or decrease the bio-availability of dietary iron
  ○ Consider need for supplements to achieve dietary aim
- Aim of dietary modification is to decrease dietary intake of potassium:
  ○ Eliminate or limit frequency of consumption of high potassium foods
  ○ Recommend cooking methods to reduce potassium content of foods

Single/multiple food exclusion
- Aim of dietary modification is to exclude cow's milk protein and egg:
  ○ Eliminate all foods sources of cow's milk protein and egg, including where these are present as an ingredient
  ○ Advise alternatives to foods eliminated in order to ensure nutritional adequacy
  ○ Consider need for supplements to ensure nutritional adequacy of diet

---

- *Meal patterns* – the timing or frequency of meals may be adjusted, e.g. the provision of small, frequent meals may promote dietary intake. It may also be necessary to modify when foods or fluids are taken together.
- *Meal environment and eating behaviour* – altering the environment in which food is consumed may be an effective modification strategy. Changing feeding behaviour may be an important part of achieving

dietary targets and may involve other healthcare professionals.

Conclusion

Dietary modification underpins many aspects of dietetic practice and it is vital that the dietitian understands the principles detailed in this chapter so that these principles can then be applied to practice.

References

American Dietetic Association. (2002) Position of the American Dietetic Association total diet approach to communicating food and nutrition information. *Journal of the American Dietetic Association* 102: 100–108.

British Dietetic Association (BDA). (2012) Nutrition and dietetic care process. Available at http://members.bda.uk.com/profdev/profpractice/modeldieteticpractice/index.html. Accessed 2 December 2012.

Bronner Y. (1994) Cultural sensitivity and nutrition counselling. *Topics in Clinical Nutrition* 9: 13–19.

Department of Health. (2001) The expert patient: a new approach to chronic disease management for the 21st century. Available at www.dh.gov.uk/prod_consum_dh/groups/dh_digitalassets/@dh/@en/documents/digitalasset/dh_4018578.pdf. Accessed 2 February 2012.

Fine J. (2006) An integrated approach to nutrition counselling. *Topics in Clinical Nutrition* 21: 199–211.

Gable J. (1997) *Counselling Skills for Dietitians*. Oxford: Blackwell Scientific Publications.

Hunt P, Pearson D. (2001) Motivating change. *Nursing Standard* 16: 45–52.

National Patient Safety Agency (NPSA) Dysphagia Expert Reference Group. (April 2011) Dysphagia Diet Food Texture Descriptors. Available at www.bda.uk.com/publications/statements/National DescriptorsTextureModificationAdults.pdf. Accessed 2 February 2012.

Prochaska J, DiClemente C. (1986) Towards a comprehensive model of change. In: Miller W, Heather N (eds) *Treating Addictive Behaviours: Processes of Change*. New York: Plenum.

Thomas J. (1994) New approaches to achieving dietary change. *Current Opinion in Lipidology* 5: 36–41.

Thomas J. (2002) Nutrition intervention in minority ethnic groups. *Proceedings of the Nutrition Society* 61: 559–567.

1.3 Changing health behaviour

Dympna Pearson

Key points

■ The art of dietetic practice is to integrate the science of food and medicine with the psychosocial aspects of people's lives in the context of changing health related behaviours.

■ An integrated approach to changing health related behaviours embraces the underlying theory, principles, skills and processes that are necessary to initiate and maintain changes to lifestyle behaviours.

■ A behavioural approach is directive and client centred. Consultations need to be structured and focused, where both the practitioner's and service user's (client's) agendas are considered through working in a collaborative way.

■ There should be clarity of purpose and it must be ensured that any goals agreed will help the client achieve the desired outcome.

■ Increasing self awareness is an important aspect of becoming an effective change agent, as is working collaboratively with clients.

'I do not understand my own actions. For I do not do what I want, but I do the very thing I hate.'

(Romans 7:15 Revised Standard Version)

Dietetics was originally based on the traditional medical model of expert led, advice giving with the expectation that once people are told what to do, they will follow this advice. However, research has shown that giving advice alone does not automatically change behaviour (Thomas, 1994; Contento *et al*., 1995; Thorogood *et al*., 2002). The challenge for dietitians and other healthcare professionals is to develop an understanding of what influences health behaviour and to acquire the necessary skills that will enable them to facilitate change.

Traditional medical care has moved towards a client centred model that takes into account the psychosocial aspects of care, as well as the clinical picture (Stewart, 1995). Setting the stage psychologically is of prime importance when helping others change their behaviour (Brownell & Cohen 1995a; 1995b). It is necessary to have some understanding of a person's previous experience and how they think and feel about their situation, as this will ultimately influence their health behaviour. Attitudes, beliefs, individual learning styles and the social, cultural, religious and economic situation will also affect their behaviour.

The environment in which somebody lives has a major influence on health. Public health interventions, such as those proposed in *Healthy Lives, Healthy People* (Department of Health, 2011), are designed to make healthy choices easier and are likely to have maximum impact if fully implemented. If people are motivated to change their health behaviour, easy availability of healthy and economic choices will support the process. Dietitians have a key role to play in implementing food health policies, which are of major importance if better health outcomes are to be secured in the future. This chapter focuses on achieving change at an individual level and how interventions can be maximised through enhancing traditional practice to achieve an integrated approach to changing health behaviours.

An integrated approach to changing health behaviour

A range of approaches can be used to facilitate health behaviour change. Different approaches may work for different people at different times. An integrated approach to changing health behaviour in dietetic practice:

• Enables the client to take the next concrete, practical step to change eating or other lifestyle behaviours.
• Combines a directive and non-directive client centred approach by using a guiding style (Rollnick *et al*., 2010).
• Includes a range of tools and approaches adapted from the world of psychology to provide information, strengthen motivation and facilitate behaviour change, taking the client's context into consideration.
• Integrates whichever approach seems most relevant for that individual at any given time, e.g. exploring motivational difficulties or working on modifying behaviour.

- Treats the whole person, taking into account the world in which they live, what matters to them and the factors that are likely to influence their health behaviour. It looks at how diet and activity fit into the client's life.
- Recognises that the skills and mindset of the practitioner will influence how effective they are as a behaviour change agent. It therefore acknowledges that the need for practitioners to engage in ongoing self development and self awareness as part of continuing professional development is just as important as it is for them to facilitate this process in their clients.

Differences between traditional advice giving and an integrated approach to changing health behaviour

The traditional approach often consists of advice giving combined with persuading the client to adopt a preferred course of action. This approach can render the client a passive recipient of expert knowledge, and can reduce client autonomy and create discord in the helping relationship (Heritage & Sefi, 1992). When the client's perspective is not fully taken into account, it is possible that mental and/or emotional harm may be inflicted, which can have long lasting consequences. In an integrated approach to changing health behaviour, *first do no harm* is as applicable as in any other clinical procedure. This means that practitioners need to be mindful of the client's overall situation rather than just following their own agenda (see Chapter 1.1).

A consultation based on an integrated approach to changing health behaviour has the following characteristics:

- The client and practitioner work together as equal partners.
- The client is treated with courtesy and respect at all times.
- Information and ideas are shared.
- The language and approach is collaborative.
- The client is actively involved and there is a two way conversation.
- The practitioner actively listens and interprets what the client says, checking for understanding.
- There is common agreement and a clear plan about the way forward.

Foundations underpinning behaviour change approaches

The foundations of an integrated approach to changing health related behaviours are its theoretical underpinning, guiding principles, good communication skills and ongoing practitioner development.

Theoretical underpinning

Models

A model attempts to understand and describe what factors affect behaviour and from this, specific approaches and

---

Box 1.3.1 Models used to influence health behaviour

The Helping Model (Egan, 1998)
A simple three stage model for use within a consultation which helps guide the dietitian through the interview in a structured way:

- Stage 1 (the assessment) establishes the current scenario and helps both client and practitioner work towards a common agenda as a basis for moving to Stage 2
- Stage 2 involves exploring the options, setting goals and developing a change plan
- Stage 3 is the action stage, which mainly happens outside the consultation, with the sessions used for monitoring, review and follow-up

The Transtheoretical Model (Stages of Change Model) (Prochaska & DiClemente, 1986).
The model can increase understanding of the process people go through to make changes; people who successfully change go through:

- A thought process (weighing up the pros and cons of change) and
- A preparation stage before embarking on
- An action stage of change.

Most people who reach a stage of maintaining change have gone through the process of thinking, preparing, action and relapse several times before eventually changing permanently. This highlights the ongoing nature of change and that many different interventions may be required depending on the stage a person has reached.

The limitation of this model are that, because of the shifting nature of change, it is not possible to identify someone as being in a particular stage. In addition, people may be at different stages for different eating behaviours.

---

applications are developed to effect or influence this behaviour. There are a number of health behaviour models that contribute to the understanding of human behaviour in relation to health. The models that have had most influence on dietetic clinical practice are the Helping Model (Egan, 1998) and the Transtheoretical Model of Change (Prochaska & DiClemente, 1986) (Box 1.3.1). The complexity of human behaviour can never be fully understood; therefore, no model or approach can be complete or definitive. Models can however help understanding of how things function. An integrated approach to changing health related behaviours embraces elements from many different models and approaches.

Psychological approaches

The most commonly used psychological approaches in dietetic practice are motivational interviewing (MI), behaviour therapy (BT) and cognitive behaviour therapy (CBT).

Motivational interviewing

Motivational difficulties are often the greatest challenge for people struggling with change. The task of the dietitian is to tap into the intrinsic motivation that exists within each individual and to help build and strengthen that motivation in order to facilitate change. Clients often express a desire to change but somehow find they cannot. Motivational interviewing (MI) aims to help individuals explore and resolve the discrepancy between where they are and where they want to be in relation to their health behaviour. A collaborative conversation style of consulting is used to strengthen someone's motivation and commitment to change (Miller & Rollnick, 2012). It is part of an integrated approach, rather than a standalone therapy, and consists of a range of therapeutic strategies, which are underpinned by a person centred approach. The use of high level interpersonal skills in this context enables the client to build commitment and reach a decision to change if that is appropriate for them (Miller & Rollnick, 2012; Rollnick *et al.*, 1992).

Behaviour therapy

Behaviour therapy or behaviour modification helps clients to identify unhelpful behavioural patterns and develop ways of modifying these. A wide range of practical behaviour modification strategies are commonly used in dietetics that help clients manage eating and activity behaviours (Pearson & Grace, 2012), as shown in Box 1.3.2.

Cognitive behaviour therapy

Cognitive behaviour therapy includes behaviour modification strategies as well as cognitive restructuring. Cognitive restructuring aims to help clients identify and then change unhelpful thoughts, ideas and beliefs that might maintain undesirable behaviours. The application of these approaches to dietetic practice has been described and explored by Rapoport (1998). It is essential that appropriate clinical supervision is in place for practitioners using this approach.

Box 1.3.2   Examples of behavioural strategies used in dietetic practice

- Do nothing else whilst eating; sit down at a table
- Do not eat when watching TV or reading
- Chew each mouthful thoroughly
- Put your knife and fork down between mouthfuls
- Use a smaller plate or bowl
- Put food away – out of sight
- Plan menus for the week ahead
- Always shop from a list
- Never shop on an empty stomach
- Do not sit for longer than 30 minutes
- Plan activity for the week ahead

Guiding principles

Health professionals ideally base their practice on underlying principles, ethics and beliefs (see Chapter 1.1). Good communication skills play a major role in the outcome of a consultation and underlying these skills are principles that motivate or guide the practitioner and influence the way they apply any skills they may have acquired. These guiding principles provide a foundation for any model, theory or skills that are used. In an integrated approach they include the following:

Person centred approach

A person centred approach forms the basis of the helping relationship. Rogers (1951) described the essential core conditions that need to be present in order to work in a person centred way: empathy, genuineness and acceptance.

Empathy

Empathy involves caring in a truly genuine and accepting way, and developing a sensitive and accurate understanding of the way in which the client perceives their experience. An empathic person shares another person's experience as if it were their own, whilst being aware throughout that it is not. Clients feel they have been heard and understood.

Genuineness (congruence)

Genuineness is important for the formation of a helping relationship, which is built on trust. It means being who we truly are, being honest and matching what we say with how we say it, both verbally and non-verbally.

Acceptance (unconditional positive regard)

Acceptance means having respect for another as a human being, regardless of who they are or what they have done. This means accepting the cleint unconditionally without condoning and being judgemental. Health professionals need to guard against forming judgements about clients who do not adhere to recommended treatment and to seek to understand the client's perspective rather than label them as non-compliant.

The core conditions are often difficult to adhere to but their importance highlights the need for continual reflective practice. When consultations do not go well, a natural response is to blame the client as being difficult, but it may be more productive to reflect and consider if any of the core conditions were absent.

Respecting client autonomy

This is a key element of facilitating health behaviour change; it is accepting the right of the individual to make choices about their own actions. Practitioners need to resist the urge to tell people what to do, in the belief that they know what is best. Experience and expertise need to be shared in a collaborative way in order to achieve the best outcomes, with clients being fully involved in any decisions.

Client responsibility

This principle acknowledges that people are responsible for their own actions. Practitioners need to try to understand the difficulties that people experience with change, whilst at the same time respecting client autonomy.

Social influence

Dietitians have a remit to influence health behaviour and this influence can be very powerful, even when time is limited. Practitioners can sometimes feel that the situation is hopeless when the client has multiple problems, e.g. poor relationships, low income and poor health. It is important to remember that everybody has the ability to change (Miller & Rollnick, 2012); although not everyone will change, they may be able to take some steps towards improving their health.

Collaboration

The principle of collaboration helps to accommodate both the client's and the healthcare professional's agenda. It recognises that two parties with expertise have met; one with expertise about themselves (the client) and one with expertise in the topic area, along with specific helping skills (the healthcare professional). A collaborative helping relationship is built on trust and mutual respect; it considers both parties as equals in exploring the possibilities for change (Pearson, 2010).

Self efficacy

In order to change people need to believe that change is possible. The task of the practitioner is to help people develop self belief in their ability to make changes. This can be achieved by helping to build the client's confidence and competence (Bandura, 1977).

Empowerment

Empowerment for health is a process through which people gain greater control over decisions and actions affecting their health. This principle has especially influenced the development of care offered in diabetes management (Funnell & Anderson, 2003). It recognises that clients are in control of and responsible for the daily self management of their health and that, to succeed, a self management plan has to fit clients' goals, priorities and lifestyle, as well as health problems.

The client centred method

The client centred clinical method (which includes many of the above elements) was developed by Stewart (1995) to address the limitations of the biomedical model. It includes the conventional biomedical approach but extends it to include consideration of the client as a person. The model consists of six interconnecting components:

- Explore both the disease and the illness experience.
- Understand the whole person.
- Find common ground.
- Incorporate prevention and health promotion.
- Enhance the client–practitioner relationship.
- Be realistic.

A client centred approach has been shown to be associated with improved health status and increased efficacy of care (Stewart *et al.*, 2000).

Communication skills

Effective client care relies heavily on good communication skills that can be applied in any setting, e.g. during consultations and when discussing client care with medical staff, relatives, administrators, etc. These skills may be variably described as counselling, consultation, interviewing, active listening, reflective listening and communication or interpersonal skills. Many dietitians are naturally good listeners while others develop their listening skills through years of practice. These skills must be continually developed and refined. Using these skills throughout the consultation can have an enormous impact on facilitating health behaviour change.

There is evidence to support the use of communication skills. Najavits & Weiss (1994) reported that the single most important factor that influences change is the practitioner's possession of strong communication skills. The health practitioner's way of working or therapeutic style can strongly influence the intervention outcome (Miller & Rollnick, 2012). Stewart (1995) showed a positive and significant relationship between communication and client health outcomes, concluding that '*good communication is good evidence-based medicine*'.

Attending behaviour

Actively listening to another person, both verbally and non-verbally, conveys acceptance. Attending also involves being aware of personal verbal and non-verbal behaviour, which reflects personal thoughts, feelings and attitudes.

Non-verbal communication

In addition to words, non-verbal communication gives very powerful messages and may account for as much as 85% of communication (Ivey *et al.*, 1997). The practitioner should also observe clients' non-verbal cues. Important aspects of non-verbal communication include:

- Body language that is appropriate to the context of the conversation. An open, relaxed posture and leaning slightly forward is generally recommended, rather than an unnatural or stiff posture. It is also important to avoid distracting behaviours such as constant nodding, fiddling with pens or looking at a watch. Hand movements are a normal part of non-verbal communication, but they should not be invasive. Sitting at an appropriate distance so as not to invade the other person's space, but equally, not too far away, should be taken into consideration.
- Eye contact that is varied and non-staring.
- Facial expressions that convey empathy and provide encouragement, e.g. an encouraging smile or nod. Facial expressions need to match the mood of the conversation, e.g. not smiling when the person is describing something sad.
- Pace of an interview. Rushed consultations can leave the client feeling confused or unsure about what has

been discussed. It is important to allow time for clients (and practitioners) to think clearly and express their thoughts; a brief silence or a pause can help achieve this.

- Tone of voice and general demeanour make a difference to the meaning of what is said and its interpretation. It is important for dietitians to take note of these factors as clients may be communicating something different from the actual words that are being said. Dietitians also need to be aware that their tone of voice and body language can convey meaning in either a more or less helpful way, e.g. disapproval or encouragement.

Practitioners need to be familiar with and take into account cultural differences, along with the age and gender of the person. Disabilities such as hearing, sight or cognitive impairment will also impact on communication.

Minimal encouragers

These are used to indicate to clients that they are being *actively* listened to and to encourage them to talk. They can include non-verbal language such as nodding, an encouraging smile, or minimal utterances, e.g. 'mm, mm', 'ah hah', 'and', 'so . . .'. Finding the right balance of how and when to use (and not to overuse) minimal encouragers is a skill that needs practise. Some words used in everyday conversations such as 'right' and 'ok' can convey the wrong meaning or become irritating if constantly repeated throughout the conversation.

Verbal following or restating

This consists of a word, a phrase or a sentence (sometimes phrased as a question) that repeats what has just been said (although not verbatim). For example:

> Client: 'I'm really struggling to fit this diet in with the rest of the family.'
> Dietitian: ''Family?' or 'You are struggling to fit the diet in with the family.'
> Client: 'Yes, they all like . . .'

It encourages the person to expand on what they have said; it needs to be used skilfully without overuse, but combined with other skills to convey accurate empathy.

Paraphrasing

Paraphrasing is the skill of rephrasing that conveys the factual essence of what has been said and is used to reflect back the essence of the conversation in 'pieces' of content For example:

> Client: 'This diet is just too hard to follow when I'm eating out.'
> Dietitian: 'You are struggling to manage with eating when you are not at home . . .'

To be effective, a paraphrase requires a level of accuracy that helps provide clarity for both the client and practitioner. A paraphrase should be used tentatively so that the client can agree or correct any inaccuracies. A succinct accurate paraphrase is very powerful in helping clients feel understood.

Reflecting feelings

A reflection of feeling conveys to the client that the practitioner is trying to understand what they are experiencing emotionally. People can show their feelings in different ways: verbally, non-verbally or a combination of both. Asking people how they feel is not always helpful as people can struggle to express their emotions, so avoid *'How do you feel?'* It is more useful to reflect tentatively and at the right intensity what the person appears to be experiencing. For example:

> Client: 'And then he told me that I have got diabetes!'
> Dietitian: 'It sounds as if the news was upsetting for you . . .'

Many dietitians are wary of addressing feelings but to neglect how people are feeling in relation to their health is missing a vital element of what is likely to influence their behaviour. However, dietitians need to recognise their limitations in this area and to know when and how to refer on when appropriate.

Questions

Questions are useful for eliciting important information. Closed questions are an efficient way for gathering specific information, e.g. *'Do you take milk in your tea?'* whereas an open question encourages the client to explain things from their perspective, e.g. *'Can you fill me in on what led up to your doctor suggesting you come to see me?'* Most consultations require a combination of open and closed questions. However, questions need to be used selectively to avoid what can feel like an interrogation. In general, ask open questions (unless specific information is required), avoid asking two questions in a row and for every question, offer at least two responses (Rollnick *et al.*, 2008).

Summarising

Summarising helps to pull things together at different points in the consultation and is especially useful at the beginning and end of the session. Short summaries help to clarify the situation as the consultation proceeds. For example:

> Dietitian: 'Can I check what we have covered so far? You went to see the doctor because you were feeling unwell and the result of all the tests was that he told you that you have diabetes, which was unexpected and the news has left you feeling upset and worried. Is that right? *(Pause)*.
> Is there anything else?'

Longer summaries may be needed to clarify long and complicated stories as they provide a pause, time to think and help give direction on what to focus on next. Summaries are also useful to help dietitians remember what needs to be recorded in the notes.

Potential pitfalls for practitioners

Dietitians and health professionals often feel they have an obligation to make their clients change – we cannot *make* people change. Despite the best of intentions, this can get in the way of facilitating change. In an integrated approach, the dietitian aims to enable the client to choose and implement changes to their health related behaviour. Anything that results in the client feeling disempowered or criticised may inhibit this process and can be a potential pitfall. Examples of common pitfalls are:

- *Trying to persuade or force clients to change*, e.g. 'Your blood pressure is raised; you really must make some lifestyle changes . . .' Using pressure to try and convince or persuade someone to change assumes that the practitioner knows best about what the person should do. If a person feels under pressure, they are less likely to be able to make a free choice.
- *Trying to solve the problem*, e.g. 'What I think you need to do is cut out chocolate and go walking instead'. This is often portrayed as well meaning advice or a solution offered from the practitioner's point of view. In practice, however, clients are their own experts and are best at finding a solution that will work for them. They may need some guidance from the practitioner but this does not mean that the practitioner should lead or dictate rather than facilitate.
- *Underplaying the real health risks*, e.g. 'The situation could be worse . . .' This may take the form of trying to appease clients. It arises from an apparent desire to protect clients and is often due to fear of upsetting them or a fear of not knowing how to cope with a client's distress if they become upset. How information about health risks is presented is of vital importance.
- *Presenting information in a threatening manner*, e.g. 'If you don't lower your cholesterol, you risk getting . . .' Fear can motivate some people, but others may become defensive as a result.
- *Hiding behind or dictating policy*, e.g. 'If you don't lose more than a couple of pounds by your next appointment you will be discharged'. This strategy may be an attempt to control caseload by discharging anyone who is not succeeding according to a predetermined specification, but in practice is likely to reinforce a person's sense of failure and may exert unrealistic pressure. Policies need to incorporate negotiation and flexibility.
- *Interrogating*, e.g. 'Why didn't you follow your eating plan?' This is difficult to answer and may make clients defensive. Asking lots of questions, often in a desire to get to the heart of the problem so that it can be 'fixed', or to try to get the client to 'tell the truth' is counterproductive. It does not encourage clients to talk openly as the agenda is practitioner led and can close down the conversation.
- *Blaming or judging*, e.g. 'You must be eating more than you have said or you would have lost weight'. This assumes that the client is lying and that the practitioner knows better than the client.

Ongoing practitioner development

In psychology and counselling, practitioners routinely receive supervision on developing their own responses and understanding, as well as improving how they work with their clients. This is not generally the case with other health professionals. It is unrealistic to expect anyone to be totally empathic, unconditionally accepting and genuinely collaborative, and also free from judgement, blame and criticism and the desire to want to rescue, protect or fix it for their clients. Although dietitians can aspire to these qualities, they are not necessarily present. Some elements can be acquired through skills training and can be further enhanced through self development (Gable, 1997). Ongoing self evaluation, developing self awareness and life management skills can all help this process. Regular supervision is essential and all health professionals should be involved in ongoing self development as an essential foundation to their practice and as part of continuing professional development (see Chapter 1.2).

The dietetic consultation in practice

Setting

A dietetic consultation has the explicit intention of discussing the person's diet in relation to their health. It is clearly very different from an informal meeting and therefore needs to operate within certain boundaries, but should not be so formal that the client feels uncomfortable. The environment, or setting, in which people are seen needs careful consideration. Is the waiting room arranged in a way that is welcoming, with suitable seating and reading material? Is the consultation room arranged in the best way? Has clutter been removed and telephones or other interruptions been diverted? The dietitian (as the client's advocate) has a professional responsibility to seek optimal consultation settings.

Proposed framework for the consultation

The dietetic consultation is made up of a series of different elements. Suggested frameworks for an initial and follow-up consultation are shown in Figure 1.3.1 and Figure 1.3.2. These should be flexible with different elements being applied interchangeably within each interview, depending on the varying needs of the client. Not all elements are necessarily included in all interviews, e.g. if someone is very ambivalent about making changes, the whole of the first session may involve exploring this. How interpersonal skills link to the elements involved in the consultation and how to manage difficulties that may arise are explored later. It is important to be aware of one's limitations and to refer on appropriately. Difficulties generally outside a dietitian's expertise include psychiatric or psychological problems, relationship problems, bereavement, stress, social and economic problems, and problems that are more properly the remit of other health professionals, e.g. speech and language therapists.

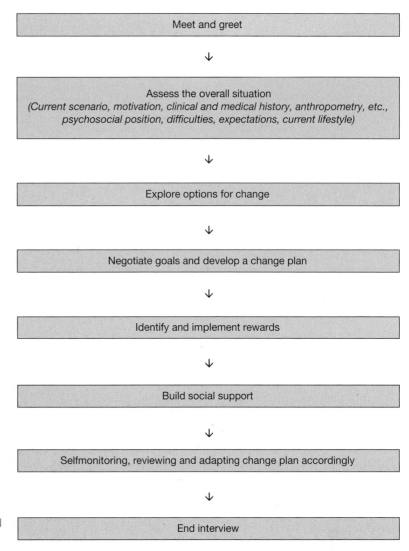

Figure 1.3.1 A suggested framework for an initial dietetic consultation

Elements of the consultation

The following elements within the dietetic consultation form a highly specific focus in an integrated approach to changing health related behaviours. It is essential to skilfully interweave interpersonal skills with specific elements seamlessly. Not all these elements will necessarily be used in each consultation. The skilled practitioner learns to work with different elements flexibly, using the most appropriate one at any given time.

Meeting and greeting the client

It is easy to rush this part of the consultation, but it is important to take time to greet clients in a warm and friendly manner. Introductions are important, including checking how the client wishes to be addressed and stating the amount of time available for the consultation. It is also important to include client relatives or carers, if that is the wish of the client, in the conversation and to treat them in the same respectful manner. The consultation itself should start with an open invitation to talk, allowing clients to state what is on their mind, as well as

giving an indication of their understanding of the reason for the referral. For example:

'Your doctor has written and asked me to see you. Would you like to tell me what has been happening from your point of view that has led up to this?'

Or for a review appointment:

'How have things been going since we last met?'

Assessing the overall picture

Assessment is standard practice and is likely to take up most of the first consultation, but it also needs to continue throughout further consultations as change takes place. It needs to be undertaken in a collaborative manner so that a true picture of the person's situation emerges. Subsequent treatment goals can then be tailored to the individual with the ultimate target of achieving better health outcomes. The initial assessment needs to include the overall clinical and medical situation as well as the client's experiences and circumstances. For example:

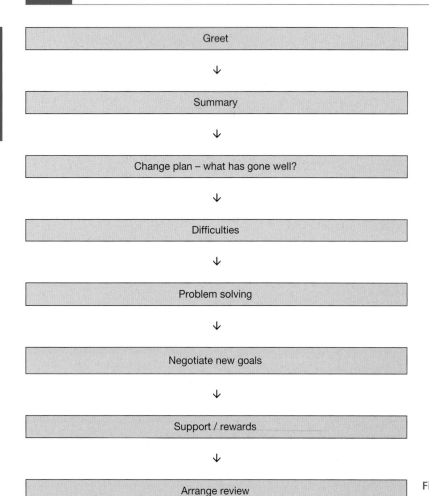

Figure 1.3.2 A suggested framework for a follow-up dietetic consultation

Dietitian: 'Can you tell me a bit about your current situation (family, job, that kind of thing . . .) so that we can see how any dietary or lifestyle changes may fit in . . . ?'
Client: 'I work part-time . . .'
Dietitian: *(paraphrase/reflect this information)*

Try to avoid asking a lot of questions in a row without reflecting back the responses. If a series of closed questions is necessary, it is less intrusive if permission is asked first. For example:

Dietitian (assessing calcium intake): 'Would it be alright with you if we go through a number of questions, so that we both get a clear picture and don't miss anything important?'
Client: 'That's fine.'
Dietitian: 'Can you tell me how much milk you consume? . . . . do you eat cheese? . . . , how often . . . , how much . . . ., what about yogurt?'

Providing information

Exchanging information is a process that needs to be interwoven into all aspect of the consultation. It can either focus on providing information to the client or gathering information about their overall situation. The aim is to assess the client's knowledge about their own condition, biochemistry results, approaches to treatment, etc., and on that basis to give relevant new information that may help in their decision making regarding making changes or managing their condition. Pitfalls in a dietetic consultation include:

* Making assumptions about the client's current levels of knowledge or understanding.
* Interrogating the client.
* Imposing information on the client that they do not want or are unable to assimilate at that particular time. This may make them more resistant to change.

Exchanging information needs to be done in a client centred way, so that the person feels free to disclose relevant information. For example:

* Find out what they know, e.g. about their diabetes:
  Dietitian: 'Has your doctor explained what diabetes is?'
  Client: 'Yes . . .' *(sounding unsure)*
* Ask permission to give them further information:
  Dietitian: 'Would it be helpful if we talked a bit more about that now?' *or* 'Would you like me to go over any of it again?'

Some people do not want or need information because they already know the facts or because the timing is not right. If someone is genuinely not interested or ready to know more, asking permission alerts the dietitian to this and enables the consultation to progress at the client's pace. Information given when someone is not ready can seem like undue pressure and stop people from wanting to know more or from wanting to make a return visit. When clients agree to receive information, they listen more carefully.

- *Provide the information in an objective, neutral manner.* Information should be given in a simple, objective, non-emotional manner and always related to current scientific understanding, e.g. 'There is good evidence that losing weight can help lower blood pressure'.
  Avoid long complicated explanations and the use of jargon or scientific language.
- *Find out what their interpretation is of the information you give them.* 'What do you think about that?' *or* 'Does that make sense?'

Motivation

Motivation is affected by many factors and can fluctuate to a greater or lesser degree. How important the client sees a change in terms of their overall life will affect the likelihood of them implementing it, and therefore needs to be explored. For example:

Dietitian: 'Would you say that making changes to your diet in order to lose weight is a priority for you at the moment?'
Client: 'Oh, yes, I mean if it will help with my blood pressure . . .' or 'I'm not sure it will make any difference . . .'
Dietitian: (reflecting the response and continuing to explore) 'You are keen to get your blood pressure down' or 'You can't see much point in making any changes to your diet . . .'

This is part of establishing a common agenda. It is the responsibility of dietitians to ensure that the client has the correct information at this point. This helps to raise awareness in a non-threatening manner about the unhelpful behaviour and its implications. Increasing concern about the behaviour may increase its importance to the person and therefore make change more likely.

If the health related change is important to the individual, the next step is to explore whether they feel confident in their ability to do so and to offer support. For example:

Dietitian: 'Do you feel able to make some change to your eating at the moment?'
Client: 'I know I should if it will help with my blood pressure, but I have tried lots of times . . .'
Dietitian: (reflecting the response and continuing to explore) 'You have tried lots of times and are feeling a bit disheartened by that experience?'
Client: 'Yes.'
Dietitian: 'Is there anything that we could do together that would help?'

It is possible to use scaling questions to establish levels of motivation, e.g. *'on a scale of 0–10, where 0 is not important/not confident at all and 10 is extremely important/confident, where would you place yourself?'* (Rollnick *et al.*, 1999). This approach however needs to be used with a high level of good interpersonal skills and applied with sensitivity. It can be a helpful way broadly to establish how important change is to the client, but should not be regarded as a precise or rigid assessment tool. The response should be met with reflective statements rather than judgement.

Eliciting information on current health related behaviours

An overview of current eating and activity levels can be undertaken by asking the client to describe a typical day. For example:

Dietitian: 'Can I ask you to describe a fairly typical day, in terms of how food (or activity) fits into that day, starting from when you get up in the morning to last thing at night?'
Client: 'Well, the mornings are always a rush . . .'
Dietitian: *(follow the person's description with reflective responses and summarise to capture what has been said.)*

Taking a diet history is another way of gathering detailed information about current diet. It is traditionally the mainstay of dietetic practice but there are pitfalls:

- As it involves asking lots of questions, it can feel like an interrogation. Intensive questioning, as with any succession of closed questions, risks damaging the helping relationship. People who eat for emotional reasons will be less likely to disclose this with intensive questioning as they often feel vulnerable, and this can expose the vulnerability and increase defensiveness.
- All methods of assessing dietary intake, and especially dietary recall, have inaccuracies (see Chapter 2.3). People are likely to report what they think the professional wants to hear rather than what they actually do.

Initially, general information regarding how the diet fits in with life can be gathered as this is what will ultimately influence change. Further necessary information can then be elicited when options for change are discussed. Self monitoring (see later) is another tool that can be used to gather information about diet and keeping diaries can be informative. Once a supportive relationship is formed, clients are more likely to offer accurate information. By threading the process of exchanging information regarding dietary intake and activity levels into different aspects of the interview, clients are less likely to feel they are being judged.

Exploring options for change and helping decision making

Once someone decides to make changes, it is helpful to explore what options are available. Initially it is helpful to identify the change that is most favoured by the client. This can then be discussed in terms of whether it is realistic to make this change. Focusing on this makes it more likely that the change will be implemented and maintained. In some cases however, it may be necessary to concentrate on the option that will have most impact on the immediate health concern, e.g. reducing saturated fat intake where there is a raised cholesterol level. Generally, the following approach can be helpful:

Dietitian: 'There are a range of possibilities that would help your overall health – changing the types of fat you eat, eating more fruit and vegetables, eating less sugar, etc. Where do you think you would like to start?'

This exploration can be helped in a various ways, e.g. with visual aids. The recommendations can be discussed and further information about a person's dietary practices gathered at the same time. For example:

Dietitian: 'The recommendations are to eat five portions of fruit and vegetables per day – How does that compare with what you are doing at the moment?'

Negotiating goals and developing a change plan

Setting appropriate behavioural goals is the basis of achieving a successful outcome. These need to be negotiated with clients so that they have an active role in deciding what they can realistically achieve. Goals set by health practitioners may not take account of other factors that are affecting people's lives. Unrealistic goals can set clients up for failure and undermine the confidence of both the patient and the practitioner. Clients should be encouraged to use a stepwise approach to achieve a particular goal. Ideally, goals should fulfil SMART (specific, measurable, achievable, relevant and time specific) criteria:

- Specific, e.g. eating less fat might be achieved by spreading fat more thinly on bread.
- Measurable, e.g. eating five portions of fruit and vegetables each day.
- Achievable and realistic, e.g. reducing chocolate intake by consuming one bar each day instead of two.
- Relevant to the goal of treatment, e.g. if the aim of treatment is to decrease fat intake, clients need to concentrate on eating foods that are low in fat.
- Time specific, e.g. setting a goal to be achieved within an agreed time frame.

For a goal to make a difference in the specified time, it needs to be as far reaching as possible. For example, if the main goal is to reduce fat intake, the main dietary source of fat intake needs to be identified and reduced to a level that will make a difference (e.g. if fried foods are eaten daily, an appropriate weekly goal may be to use fat free methods of cooking). This would have a larger effect than a goal of not eating a food that is only consumed once a fortnight.

Only two or three specific, realistic and achievable changes should be chosen. Successful negotiation of each of the smaller steps gives people a sense of achievement and helps keep them motivated in the longer term. Once the precise nature of the goal has been agreed, and ways of implementing it explored, it is helpful to summarise

---

> **Box 1.3.3** Example of a change plan that can be agreed between the dietitian and client
>
> - **What** do I want to achieve overall?
> - **Why** it is important to me?
> - Specific goal (**what** exactly am I going to do?)
> - Steps to achieve this (**how** am I going to do it?)
> - **What** needs to be in place?
> - **What** might get in the way?
> - I will ask for **support** to help me work towards my goal from . . .
> - **What** will help to reinforce new habits (reward or encouragement)?
> - **How** will I keep a record of progress?
> - **When** will I review progress?
> - **When** will I start?

this by completing a change plan (Box 1.3.3). A change plan should be a starting point that is regularly reviewed and updated in the light of what is or is not working. Once goals have been established and a change plan has been agreed, it is important to ensure that the elements that are known to support behaviour change, such as rewards and support, receive due attention.

Identifying and implementing rewards

People can be encouraged to reward themselves on a regular basis for the efforts that they are making. This may make them more likely to repeat the change and is a method of reinforcing new eating habits. Suitable rewards may be enjoyable leisure time activities and hobbies, being with favourite people, buying small things they want, or doing what they find relaxing or fun (Holli & Calabrese, 1998). Rewards need to be something that is truly pleasurable (and non-food based) for the individual and this may need exploring. Practitioners need to avoid making suggestions for rewards that would appeal to them personally. People should also be encouraged to mentally congratulate themselves on every effort and achievement, however small, to help build self esteem and belief in their ability to change. Other methods of reinforcing new habits may not necessarily be pleasurable, e.g. asking the family to remind you to go for a walk each evening, but can still be effective.

Building support

The importance of social support from a range of sources cannot be underestimated. As well as support from the dietitian and other health professionals, family members, friends and colleagues can play key roles. Responsibility for enlisting support from elsewhere lies with the client, but they may need help in how to do it. Family members and carers can be included in consultations and leaflets can be produced for them explaining how to support the person making the changes and, where appropriate, the benefits that changing the diet can have on the health of the client. The client may also need to clarify the type of support that would be most helpful to them. For example:

'I really appreciate your support. What would help me even more would be if you don't nag me, but encourage me, and offer practical support, like helping me with planning and preparation of meals.'

Other sources of support include self help groups, books, telephone help lines, the Internet and social networking. The dietitian may give information on these resources.

Self monitoring and developing self awareness

Self monitoring, e.g. keeping a diary, helps achieve changes in behaviour. This increases self awareness of current behaviour, highlights problem areas and to reinforces success. A willingness to observe behaviour often indicates a willingness to recognise it and to change it if appropriate. Self monitoring can be used in many ways, e.g. to identify:

- Time and place of eating.
- What a person was doing prior to eating.
- Who they are eating with.
- How the person felt and what they were thinking.
- Symptoms.
- Behavioural outcome.

It is unrealistic and inappropriate to ask clients continuously to record all of the above. Diary keeping is a difficult skill that often needs practice in order to focus on the behaviour that is being targeted, e.g. timing of meals. For self monitoring to be effective, care needs to be taken to ensure that the client knows what is expected, and the purpose and benefit of keeping a diary. Diaries need to be used collaboratively; clients must agree to keep the dairy and be able to use their preferred method, e.g. preprinted sheets or their own notebook; they should not be used as a means of checking up on clients. In order to reinforce that self monitoring is for the client's own benefit, it is helpful to ask what they have learnt from the exercise. Monitoring needs to be regularly reviewed by the client in order to use the information to adapt and update their change plan. Difficulty in keeping to the self monitoring process may suggest that unresolved motivational issues exist and need to be addressed (see Managing common difficulties later).

Ending the interview

This is just as important as a good beginning. Sufficient time needs to be allowed to ensure that the main points of the consultation are summarised and that there is clear agreement about goals set, monitoring, review and any follow-up arrangements. The client should be given the opportunity to ask questions to clarify any concerns.

Managing common difficulties

Clients who want advice

Clients usually recognise that the dietitian they are consulting has expertise. It is important to give information when clients are seeking it (this can be an indication of readiness to change), but at the same time it is important to draw on the expertise that clients have about themselves. For example:

Dietitian: 'You would like me to tell you exactly what to eat in order to . . . ?'
Client: 'Yes, what I need is a diet sheet; that is what I have comefor.'
Dietitian: 'It sounds like an eating plan would really help, as well as being clear about which foods are best to avoid and which ones to include. I can certainly give you that information and we can work out together what would be the best eating plan for you. That way, we can make sure that we include some of the foods you really like and make sure that the plan fits in around your life. How does that sound?'

Referred clients who do not want advice

Sometimes clients feel that they have been sent to see the dietitian, rather than choosing to come themselves. A consultation where this is the underlying feeling will only be met with resistance. It can help to find out the client's understanding of what led to the referral being made: it is more helpful to ask *'Can you tell me what led up to your doctor suggesting that you come to see me'* rather than *'Do you know* why *this appointment was made?'* It is useful to find out what their thoughts are about the referral: *'I wonder what your thoughts were when the doctor suggested coming to see me?'*, rather than *'How do you feel about coming here?'*

Clarify that your role is to explore the situation with them and consider any possible options, but do not to tell the client what to do. Ask permission to progress on that basis and explain what service you can offer.

Clients who cannot come up with their own solution

Clients should be given the opportunity to make suggestions, although not all clients have ideas or solutions for their situation. The temptation is to jump in with suggestions; however, there is a risk that the dietitian's ideas might be inappropriate, that clients will feel this as pressure and be inclined to agree without thought, and then find that they cannot do it in practice. In this situation, it can help to present possible solutions in the context of what has worked for others. This still allows the client either to accept or decline a particular suggestion. Always ask permission before making suggestions, e.g. *'Would you like me to tell you about some of the things that have worked for other people?'*

Ambivalence about change and motivational difficulties

Ambivalence about change is normal; clients often feel torn between wanting better health and not wanting to change established eating habits. Exploring ambivalence by looking at all the implications of change, the benefits and disadvantages of change, or no change, can be liberating and help build motivation for change. It should be explored in a non-judgemental way; either verbally or on paper, but writing points down usually clarifies the situation and develops a common understanding between client and practitioner (Miller & Rollnick, 2012). It is important to respect client autonomy if the client decides not to change.

A decision not to make a change at the present time is a viable option. If the client has already tried and failed many times to change, a further half hearted attempt and failure might reinforce low levels of self esteem. Providing unasked for advice in this situation is likely to be met with resistance. Motivation for change can be triggered by helping a person become more aware of the discrepancy between where they are and where they would like to be. Clients need to recognise this (facilitated by a skilled practitioner who highlights the discrepancy between their intentions and their behaviours), rather than having it exposed as a product of their inadequacy. For example, instead of '*You need to keep away from the biscuits, you know the effect it has – you need to work on your will power,*' a reflective response can be more helpful: '*So although you want to lose weight, you are finding it hard to keep away from the biscuits.*'

If a person clearly is unmotivated, many of the strategies already mentioned can help. In addition, increasing their perception of the importance of proposed change can help by raising awareness about the unhelpful behaviour. For example:

Dietitian: 'Are you aware that low calcium intake has certain health risks?'
Client: 'No, tell me more.'
Dietitian: 'It increases your risk of developing osteoporosis. What are your thoughts about that?'

Lack of confidence

A client's level of confidence about their capacity to make and sustain a change is key (Rollnick *et al*., 1999). Self esteem and self efficacy impact on a person's confidence to implement and sustain a change. Supporting self efficacy and self esteem involves encouraging an environment that increases the client's confidence that they will be successful. The dietitian can assist by:

- Exploring what worked in the past and trying to incorporate it into the present change plan.
- Encouraging clients to talk about their past and present successes.
- Drawing attention to success in other areas of their life.
- Helping to devise a change plan (see earlier) with small achievable steps.
- Looking for opportunities to support clients' confidence in their ability to change.
- Conveying optimism in a supportive and realistic manner.

Problems

Problems can arise at all stages of making change and need to be addressed. It is important to address any difficulties related to change and to encourage clients to generate solutions to the perceived difficulties themselves. This helps to increase their sense of confidence and competence. It also emphasises that there is no one right option for change and requires experimentation to find what works best for each person. The following steps have been identified as key elements of the problem solving process. This process can be used at any stage in the intervention:

- Identify the problem.
- Explore all possible options and evaluate the advantages and disadvantages of each option.
- Choose the preferred option(s).
- Develop a plan.
- Implement and monitor the plan.
- Review the plan.

Distractions to the planned change

A number of feelings, thoughts, beliefs, events and situations can initiate a behaviour. The environment can be changed to make new behaviours more likely to happen and undesirable behaviours less likely to happen, e.g. putting away the shopping. Making changes to eating habits usually means changing long established habits related to eating, including shopping and cooking. Planning ahead can aid success by drawing attention to problems or difficulties that the client may be able to resolve in advance. This makes revising the plan easier if the client has clear expectations of themselves. Any changes need to be developed collaboratively with the client, rather than presented as solutions from the practitioner's viewpoint, e.g. '*Why don't you . . .*', '*Do you think you could . . .*', '*How about . . .*'

Examples of strategies for modifying *external* cues to eating used in weight management but that can be adapted for use with other conditions are:

- Plan meals and shopping in advance so that appropriate foods are available to eat regularly.
- Plan daily eating times in advance.
- Carry suitable snacks.
- Ask a friend, partner or workmate to make a change at the same time, or to be encouraging.
- Avoid tasting when cooking, as this may result in overeating.
- Limit the opportunities to see tempting foods other than at meal times, e.g. put things away in cupboards, do not shop when hungry.
- Take a route home that does not involve passing a tempting food shop, e.g. bakery or sweet shop.
- Always make sure there are suitable foods, e.g. fruit and vegetables, available to avoid being tempted to eat less suitable foods if hungry.
- Do not buy, or only occasionally buy, tempting or energy dense foods, such as chocolates, cakes and crisps.

Strategies for modifying *internal* cues include:

- *Ask in response to an urge to eat: 'Am I really hungry?'* Urges to eat or cravings need to be distinguished from hunger. The former are psychological triggers to eating and distinct from physical hunger, which is the real need to eat. Real hunger needs to be responded to, but there are a number of strategies that can be learned to help overcome psychological urges. Some people find it helpful to use a hunger score (*'How hungry am I on a scale of 0–10 where 0 is not at all hungry and 10 is extremely hungry?'*) to check if they are truly hungry. Urges and cravings are sometimes described as being wavelike: they build and build until they peak, but then break and fade away within 15–30 minutes (Brownell, 2004). An urge or craving can be withstood by doing something incompatible with eating until it has faded.

- *Make a list of alternative activities* that make it impossible to give into urges, e.g. walking, reading a novel, running, painting or practising a relaxation exercise.
- *Mood changes can be due to other worries*, e.g. relationship problems, job worries or long term effects of illness. These may need to be addressed and it may be necessary to refer the client for more in-depth counselling or therapy.

Setbacks

Lapsing from a planned change or a made change is normal, but clients frequently see it as a failure (Marlatt & Gordon, 1985). Prevention and management of lapses need to be anticipated and worked with throughout the consultation process. Lapses often lead to feelings of guilt, which makes a person more susceptible to other slips and potentially complete abandonment of changes and a return to previous patterns. How a person thinks about a lapse or setback is likely to determine the outcome. It can be helpful to explain:

- Lapses are a natural and accepted part of change, and can provide a learning experience. Eating an unplanned food is a slip and not a personal failure.
- High risk situations (ones that present an increased and significant risk of returning to old behaviours) are either triggered by internal states, e.g. anxiety, boredom, anger, loneliness, or external events, e.g. social situations, passing a bakery, or a combination of both. An individual can learn to cope by identifying their particular high risk situations and then learning how best to manage them.
- Change is an ongoing process and a goal in itself. The process should be the focus rather than perceived failure or success at any given step. Every small change in behaviour in the desired direction is a step forward and a sign of important progress.
- Even if clients abandon their change plan for now, they can return to it at a later time.

Dietitians can help people to identify what leads to a lapse so the client can plan in advance to prevent them. Coping strategies can be established and accessed when necessary. The way a person copes after a setback can influence the likelihood of further lapses. The six steps shown in Table 1.3.1 can help a client cope with lapses.

Table 1.3.1 Coping strategies for coping with lapses in behaviour change

	Strategy
Stop	Go away from the situation to a safe place to think about what has happened.
Say	It is not a catastrophe – one error does not mean the end of the world.
Learn	What was going on before the lapse? Analyse the situation to see why it happened.
Plan	What can be done in the same situation to avert another lapse? Use the above information to plan in advance to reduce the risk of it happening again. Decide what can be done immediately to stop the slip spiralling out of control. Put these strategies into practice at once.
Be positive	Has anything really changed? Review personal goals and motivation for change.
Ask	Is there anything that can be done to balance out the slip? For example, do some extra exercise. (It is not recommended that clients skip a subsequent meal as a result of a lapse as this in itself can trigger overeating.)

Unhelpful thinking

People can be helped to identify unhelpful thoughts and to replace these with more helpful, coping thoughts. As this process can be complex, further training, accompanied by appropriate supervision is recommended. Referral to specialist practitioners may be necessary. Steps involved in modifying unhelpful thoughts include:

- identifying the unhelpful thoughts through keeping a diary, e.g. *'What were you thinking at that time?'*;
- generating alternative ways of thinking and test out if these alternatives are more helpful in everyday life.

Implications for practice

Integrating a behavioural approach to changing health related behaviours involves using a wide range of skills. Behaviour change intervention has been described as combining art and science (Hunt & Pearson, 2001). In other words, not only the message but also the way in which it is delivered is important. Dietitians need to ensure that they equip themselves with the necessary skills to integrate a behavioural approach into their practice. This includes having appropriate training and clinical supervision, and ensuring that this way of working becomes an integral part of continuing professional development.

Further reading

Bauer K, Sokolik C. (2002) *Basic Nutrition Counselling Skill Development*. Belmont, CA: Wadsworth.
Cooper Z, Fairburn CG, Hawker DM. (2004) *Cognitive-Behavioural Treatment of Obesity. A Clinician's Guide*. New York: Guilford Press.

Egan G. (1998) *The Skilled Helper: A Problem Management Approach to Helping*, 6th edn. USA: Brooks/Cole Publishing Company.

Fairburn C. (1995). *Overcoming Binge Eating*. New York: Guilford Press.

Fairburn CG, Marcus MD, Wilson GT. (1993) Cognitive-behavioural therapy for binge eating and bulimia nervosa: a comprehensive treatment manual. In: *Binge Eating: Nature, Assessment and Treatment*. Fairburn CG, Wilson GT (eds) New York: Guilford Press, pp. 361–404.

Gable J. (1997) *Counselling Skills for Dietitians*. Oxford: Blackwell Science.

Gauntlett-Gilbert J, Grace C. (2005) *Overcoming Weight Problems. Self-help Guide Using Cognitive-Behavioural Techniques*. London: Robinson Publishing Ltd.

Miller WR, Rollnick S. (2012) *Motivational Interviewing: Preparing People to Change Addictive Behaviour*, 2nd edn. New York: The Guilford Press.

Rollnick S, Miller WR, Butler C. (2008) *Motivational Interviewing in Healthcare*. New York: Guilford Press.

Rollnick S, Mason P, Butler C. (1999) *Health Behaviour Change*. Edinburgh: Churchill Livingstone.

Stewart M, Brown JB, Weston WW, McWhinney IR, McWilliam CL, Freeman TR. (2003) *Patient-centered Medicine: Transforming the Clinical Method*, 2nd edn. Abingdon, Oxon: Radcliffe Publishing.

Treasure J, Schmidt U. (1993) *Getting Better Bit(e) by Bit(e)*. Hove: Lawrence Erlbaum Associates.

Wardle J, Liao LM, Rapoport L, Hillsdon M, Croker H, Edwards C. (2001) *Shape-Up – A Lifestyle Programme to Manage your Weight*. London: Weight Concern.

References

Bandura A. (1977) *Social Learning Theory*. Englewood Cliffs, NJ: Prentice Hall.

Brownell KD. (2004) *The Learn Programme for Weight Management*, 10th edn. Dallas, Texas: American Health Publishing Company.

Brownell KD, Cohen LR. (1995a) Adherence to dietary regimens 1: An overview of research. *Behavioural Medicine* 20: 149–154.

Brownell KD, Cohen LR. (1995b) Adherence to dietary regimens 2: Components of effective interventions. *Behavioural Medicine* 20: 155–164.

Contento J, Balch GI, Bronner YL, *et al.* (1995) The effectiveness of nutrition education and implications for nutrition education policy, programs, and research: a review of research. *Journal of Nutrition Education* 27 (6) Nov/Dec Special Issue.

Department of Health. (2011) *Healthy Lives, Healthy People: Update and Way Forward*. London: The Stationery Office. Available at www.official-documents.gov.uk

Egan G. (1998) *The Skilled Helper: A Problem Management Approach to Helping*, 6th edn. USA: Brooks/Cole Publishing Company.

Funnell MM, Anderson RM. (2003) Patient empowerment: a look back, a look ahead. *Diabetes Education* 29: 454–458.

Gable J. (1997) *Counselling Skills for Dietitians*. London: Blackwell Science.

Heritage J, Sefi S. (1992) Dilemmas of advice: Aspects of the delivery and reception of advice in interactions between health visitors and first time mothers. In: Drew P, Heritage J (eds) *Talk at Work*. Cambridge: Cambridge University Press, pp. 359–419.

Holli BB, Calabrese RJ. (1998) *Communication and Education Skills for Dietetics Professionals*. Philadelphia: Williams and Wilkins.

Hunt P, Pearson D. (2001) Motivating change. *Nursing Standard* 16: 45–52.

Ivey AE, Gluckstern N, Ivey MB. (1997) *Basic Attending Skills*, 3rd edn. North Amherst, MA: Microtraining Associates.

Marlatt GA, Gordon JR. (1985) *Relapse Prevention: Maintenance Strategies in Addictive Behaviour Change*. New York: Guilford Press.

Miller WR, Rollnick S. (2012). *Motivational Interviewing*. New York: Guilford Press.

Najavits LM, Weiss RD. (1994) Variations in therapist effectiveness in the treatment of patients with substance use disorders: an empirical review. *Addiction* 89: 679–688.

Pearson D. (2010) *Changing Behaviour in Advancing Dietetics and Clinical Nutrition*. Edinburgh: Churchill Livingstone, Ch 3, pp. 17–22.

Pearson D, Grace C. (2012) *Weight Management: A Practitioners Guide*. Oxford: Wiley Blackwell.

Prochaska JO, DiClemente CC. (1986) Towards a comprehensive model of change. In: Miller WR, Healther N (eds): *Treating Addictive Disorders: Processes of Change*. New York; Plenum, pp. 3–27.

Rapoport L. (1998) Integrating cognitive behavioural therapy into dietetic practice: a challenge for dietitians. *Journal of Human Nutrition and Dietetics* 11: 227–237.

Rogers CR. (1951) *Client-Centered Therapy*. Boston: Houghton Mifflin.

Rollnick S, Healther N, Bell A. (1992) Negotiating behaviour change in medical settings: The development of brief motivational interviewing. *Journal of Mental Health* 1: 25–37.

Rollnick S, Mason P, Butler C. (1999) *Health Behaviour Change*. Edinburgh: Churchill Livingstone.

Rollnick S, Miller WR, Butler C. (2008) *Motivational Interviewing in Healthcare*. New York: Guilford Press.

Rollnick S, Butler C, Kinnersley P, Gregory J, Marsh B. (2010) Motivational interviewing. *BMJ* 340: 1900.

Stewart M. (1995) Effective physician–patient communication and health outcomes: A review. *Canadian Medical Association Journal* 152: 1423–1433.

Stewart M, Brown JB, Donner A, *et al.* (2000) The impact of patient-centered care on outcomes. *Journal of Family Practice* 49: 796–804.

Thomas J. (1994) New approaches to achieving dietary change. *Current Opinion in Lipidology* 5: 36–41.

Thorogood M, Hillsdon M, Summerbell C. (2002) Changing behaviour. *Clinical Evidence* 8: 37–59.

SECTION 2

Nutritional status

2.1

Dietary reference values

Joan Gandy

SECTION 2

Key points

- Dietary reference values (DRVs) are estimates of the nutritional requirements of a particular population and assume that requirements are normally distributed.

- They are based on the best evidence available when they are set and must be regularly reviewed.

- DRVs are applicable to groups and populations and should be used with caution when assessing the nutritional adequacy of individuals.

- DRVs are devised for healthy populations and may not be applicable in some clinical situations.

- Dietitians should understand the guiding principles of establishing DRVs and their limitations.

Dietary reference values (DRVs) are established within a population as a measure of nutritional adequacy. As such they are aimed at preventing deficiencies rather than preventing nutrition related diseases. However, DRVs are used as the basis for dietary based food guidelines, such as the eatwell plate, and dietary recommendations that are aimed at optimising health and preventing disease related to over- and under-nutrition (see Chapter 4.2).

The first DRVs were devised in the late 19th century and international values were established by the League of Nations (the forerunner of the United Nations) in 1936–1938 to prevent deficiencies in a population group (Beaton, 1991). Many countries have their own values and international values have been published by the Food and Agriculture Organization of the United Nations (FAO)/World Health Organization (WHO)/United Nations University (UNU). In Europe the European Food Safety Agency (EFSA) has begun publishing a series of scientific opinions on DRVs, with the most recent being average requirements for energy intake for infants, children, pregnant and breastfeeding women and adults. To date, the EFSA has also published scientific opinions on DRVs for water (see Chapter 6.6), carbohydrates and fats, fibre, and protein.

In a separate initiative, the European Commission funded the EURRECA (EURopean micronutrient RECommendations Aligned) project to harmonise micronutrient recommendations across Europe. This project included scientists from 17 countries and aimed to deliver an aligned set of standards that provided a robust scientific basis for establishing micronutrient requirements and for devising micronutrient recommendations. It focused on

the needs of specific vulnerable groups, e.g. infants, children and adolescents, adults, pregnant and lactating women, the elderly, people with low income and immigrants. In addition, EURRECA evaluated the impact of socioeconomic status, ethnic origin, interindividual variability and vulnerability due to genetics, environmental factors and epigenetic phenomena on dietary requirements. A full list of publications is available at www.eurreca.org.

In the UK, the Department of Health Committee on Medical Aspects of Food Policy (COMA) revised DRVs for nutrients in 1991 (Department of Health, 1991) with the exception of energy, which was revised in 2011 by COMA's successor, the Scientific Advisory Committee on Nutrition (SACN) SACN, 2011a.

Development of dietary reference values

Dietary reference values are developed by an expert group reviewing the evidence; DRVs are then derived by the expert group, e.g. WHO, for a specific population of a country or a group of countries. The values are based on the assumption that individual requirements for a nutrient within a population or group are normally distributed and that 95% of the population will have requirements within two standard deviations of the mean, as shown in Figures 2.1.1 and Figure 2.1.2. They assume that individuals are healthy and also consider gender, age, growth and physiological status, i.e. pregnancy and lactation. Guiding principles for the development of recommendations for micronutrients have been developed by EURRECA (van't Veer *et al.*, 2012).

Manual of Dietetic Practice, Fifth Edition. Edited by Joan Gandy.
© 2014 The British Dietetic Association. Published 2014 by John Wiley & Sons, Ltd.
Companion Website: www.manualofdieteticpractice.com

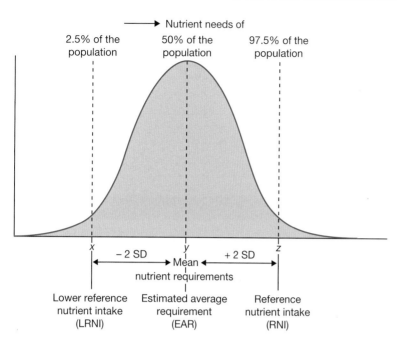

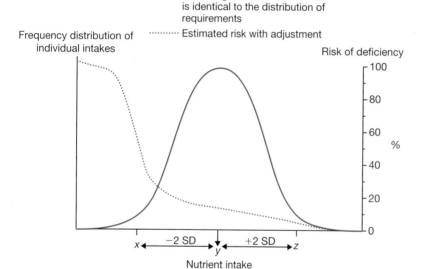

Figure 2.1.1 Derivation and definition of dietary reference values in the UK (source: Public Health England 1991. Reproduced with permission of Public Health England)

Figure 2.1.2 Dietary intakes and risk of deficiency (source: Public Health England 1991. Reproduced with permission of Public Health England)

The first UK dietary reference standards were established in 1950 as a single set of recommended daily amounts (RDA). In 1991, the standards were extensively reviewed and replaced by a range of reference standards for use in different applications (Department of Health, 1991). Several terms were used in this report, with DRVs as the collective term for the standards. The DRVs will vary according to the country or organisation responsible for the recommendation. Table 2.1.1 gives the definitions of the DRVs used in the UK and by other expert groups, such as WHO and the Institute of Medicine (USA).

Limitations

While DRVs are useful, they are open to misuse and the inherent problems associated with developing recommendations for an entire population should be consid-

ered. It is assumed that nutrient requirements are normally distributed for a population; however, the data may be skewed or sufficient data may not be available to establish normality. Robust data are required for the expert group to evaluate requirements; these data may be derived from tissue levels, balance studies, body pool size, etc., amount required to prevent symptoms of deficiency, or a measure of function of the nutrient. However, these data are not always available. When there is insufficient data the expert group will recommend a safe level of intake rather than a recommended intake value. It is important to remember that DRVs are recommended for healthy populations and many factors may affect dietary requirements, as shown in Table 2.1.2.

In particular, it is important to consider bioavailability; while the majority of macronutrient intake is absorbed, the absorption of micronutrients is more variable. This is

Table 2.1.1   Definitions of dietary reference values

Definitions used in the UK (Department of Health, 1991)

Recommended daily amount (RDA)	Average amount of the nutrient that should be provided per head in a group of people if needs of practically all members of the group are to be met (Department of Health, 1979)
Recommended Intakes	Amounts sufficient, or more than sufficient, for the nutritional needs of practically all healthy persons in a population. Intake emphasises that the recommendations relate to food actually eaten (Department of Health, 1969)
Requirement	The amount of a nutrient that needs to be consumed in order to maintain normal nutritional status
Estimated average requirement (EAR)	The mean requirement of a nutrient for a population or group of people. On average, 50% will consume more than the EAR and 50% less (point y in Figure 2.1.2)
Lower reference nutrient intake (LRNI)	The level at which only approximately 2.5% of the population or group will have an adequate intake; it will not be enough for most people. An individual with this intake may be meeting their requirement but it is highly probable that they are not (point x in Figure 2.1.2)
Reference nutrient intake (RNI)	At this level, intake will be adequate for 97.5% of the group or population. It is possible that an individual's intake at this level will not meet their requirement, but it is highly improbable
Safe level	This is given when insufficient information is available to derive requirements. It is an average requirement plus 20% and is believed to be adequate for most people's needs. The panel judged that there is no risk of deficiency at this level and that there is no risk of undesirable effects above this level

Other values used for dietary reference values (DRVs)

Protective nutrient intake (PNI)	Amount >RNI for some micronutrients that may be protective against a specified health or nutritional risk of public health relevance. PNI are expressed as daily value or an amount to be consumed with a meal
Upper tolerable nutrient intake level [upper limit (UI)]	The maximum intake of some micronutrients that is unlikely to pose risk of adverse health effects in almost all (97.5%) apparently healthy individuals in a gender and age specific population
Recommended dietary allowance (RDA)	Average daily dietary intake that meets the requirements of nearly all (97–98%) healthy persons
Adequate intake (AI)	Established for a nutrient when available data are insufficient to estimate an intake that would maintain adequacy. The AI is based on observed intakes by a group of healthy persons
Estimated energy requirement (EER)	The average dietary energy intake that is predicted to maintain energy balance in a healthy adult of a defined age, gender, weight, height and level of physical activity consistent with good health
Dietary reference intake (DRI)	A term used in the USA and Canada to broaden the use of RDAs, particularly in food labelling and fortification
Nutrient reference value (NRV)	A collective term for recommended values; used by some expert groups instead of DRVs (see Chapter 4.5)
Daily value (DV)	These were developed by the US Food and Drug Administration (FDA) to help consumers compare the nutrient contents among products within the context of a total daily diet

Table 2.1.2   Factors affecting dietary requirements

Factor	Example
Metabolic requirements	Age, gender, body size Lifestyle (smoking, obesity, physical activity, etc.) Disease, e.g. fever, catabolism Trauma Growth Pregnancy and lactation
Bioavailability	Malabsorption or altered absorption, e.g. milk calcium is better absorbed than non-milk calcium Reduced utilisation Increased losses, e.g. diarrhoea, burns, renal disease Environment, e.g. heating of nutrients Drugs, e.g. diuretics Dietary concentration Dietary interactions Drug–nutrient interactions

recognised to an extent by DRVs, e.g. DRVs for iron are calculated to reflect the fact that only 15% of dietary iron is absorbed. However, they cannot take into account other factors that affect bioavailability, such as amount consumed, body stores, the presence or absence of other nutrients or dietary constituents, the form of the nutrient, e.g. haem or non-haem iron, and the food source from which it is derived (Hurrell & Egli, 2010). These factors may have considerable impact on the adequacy of dietary intake.

Reference values are devised to cover the requirements of the majority of a population and therefore will overestimate the needs of a significant part of that population. It is important to remember that DRVs reflect the needs of healthy people and may not be appropriate in many clinical circumstances. While they are a useful basis to calculate individual needs, they cannot be used alone and other factors, including those shown in Table 2.1.1, must be considered. This is discussed further in Chapter 6.1.

Uses of dietary reference values

They should be used with caution in the dietary assessment of individuals as it must be remembered that DRVs are based on populations and groups, and the nutritional needs of individuals within that group or population, as well as the factors discussed earlier, will vary. Within a population the nutritional requirements of individuals form a continuum and where a particular individual lies on that continuum will be unknown. It is therefore impossible to determine whether an individual's needs are being met on the basis of a DRV. It is only possible to assess the degree of probability that an individual's needs will or will not have been met. If the estimated average requirement (EAR) for a nutrient is being consumed, there is an approximately 50% chance that needs will be met. If intake is at or above the reference nutrient intake (RNI), it is highly likely that needs are being met (and probably exceeded). If intake is below the lower RNI (LRNI), it is highly unlikely that sufficient is being consumed, unless that person is part of the 2.5% of the population with unusually low requirements.

The diet of groups or populations may be assessed by comparison with DRVs; however, it is important that the group or population is comparable to that for which the recommendations are derived. Dietary reference values are also used for the development of diets for groups of people, e.g. prisoners, and the provision of supplies, e.g. school meals. Nutrient reference values are also used in food labelling, fortification and formulation.

UK dietary reference values for specific nutrients

DRVs have been set for many nutrients but not all have an EAR, RNI and LRNI. It is clearly inappropriate to set a RNI (covering the needs of 97.5% of the population) for energy because such an amount would far exceed the needs of most people and, if consumed, would lead to weight gain and associated health problems. The DRV for energy is therefore only set as an EAR. Similarly, the DRVs for the main energy yielding nutrients, such as fat, carbohydrate, sugars and starch, are also expressed in terms of average needs.

Energy

Estimated average requirements for energy are based on regression analyses of measured basal metabolic rate (BMR) against gender, age and weight. The analyses have been used to generate prediction equations. Numerous equations are available and ideally they should be population specific. In 1991, the Department of Health used the equations of Schofield *et al.* (1985), but in 2010 SACN recommended the use of the Henry (2005) equations for this purpose. Energy prediction equations are discussed further in Chapter 6.1. Appendix A8 shows age and gender specific equations with additional data on men aged 60–70 years (Department of Health, 1991). Increments are also added for the last trimester of pregnancy and for lactation. As energy requirement is given as an average, 50% of a population will need more than the EAR and 50% less.

In healthy populations, the total daily energy expenditure (TEE) is traditionally calculated by the factorial method, where BMR is multiplied by a physical activity level (PAL), e.g. a sedentary 40-year-old man weighing 90 kg with a PAL of 1.4 and BMR, as derived from prediction equations, of 7.973 MJ (1880 kcal) would have a TEE of 11.16 MJ (2665 kcal). In their report on DRVs for energy, SACN (2011b) do not recommend this approach but recognise that there no viable alternative is currently available. In 1991, the Department of Health defined the following PALs:

1.4 – inactive men and women (this applies to most people in the UK)
1.6 – moderately active women
1.7 – moderately active men
1.8 – highly active women
1.9 – highly active men

The methodology for deriving the current UK dietary recommendations for energy is described in more detail by Millward (2012).

Protein

Dietary reference values for protein (EAR and RNI) are based on estimates of the amount needed to maintain nitrogen balance with an allowance for the fact that only about 70% of protein consumed is incorporated into body tissue. Incremental amounts are added to these figures for pregnancy and lactation. It is recommended that protein intakes do not exceed twice the RNI. The DRVs for protein assume that energy requirements are met, as protein will be used preferentially for energy when the body is in negative energy balance. The

DRVs also assume that the protein is of high biological value.

Fat and carbohydrate

These nutrients cannot be given EARs or RNIs as there is no absolute requirement for them (other than for small quantities of essential fatty acids) and they do not cause specific signs or symptoms of deficiency or toxicity. However, it is recognised that the proportion of fat and carbohydrate in the diet has important health implications; therefore, values are given as the percentage of total food energy they should provide. It is assumed that 5% of energy intake is from alcohol and values are expressed as percentage of food only energy. These figures are recommended averages for populations and are not necessarily appropriate for all individuals (see Chapter 4.2).

In 2008 SACN (2008) endorsed the recommendations that total dietary fat should be <35% of food energy, with saturated fat not exceeding 11% of food energy. The Department of Health (1991) recommendations for categories of fatty acids were that monounsaturated fatty acids should provide about 12% of food energy, with 6.5% of food energy from n-3 and n-6 fatty acids (linolenic and alpha-linolenic acid should provide at least 1% and 0.2% of total energy, respectively) and not more than 2% from *trans* fatty acids.

Total carbohydrate should provide 50% of food energy, with non-milk extrinsic sugars providing <11% of food energy. Intrinsic and milk sugars, and starch should provide 39% of food energy.

Non-starch polysaccharides and dietary fibre

By definition, dietary fibre is not a nutrient and therefore no specific requirement exists, although its importance in the diet is unequivocal. However, as there is still much debate regarding the terminology, analysis and physiological significance of what is a heterogeneous group of compounds, recommendations regarding fibre intake are difficulty to formulate.

In the Department of Health (1991) report, the DRV for a specifically defined form of dietary fibre, non-starch polysaccharide (NSP), as analysed by the Englyst and Cummings method, was expressed as a recommended average intake for the adult population (18 g/day). For individuals, recommended minimum (12 g/day) and maximum (24 g/day) intakes of NSP were also given.

However, it should be noted that these recommended intake figures are not comparable with the dietary fibre declared on many food labels (see Chapter 4.5). These are now usually derived from the Association of Official Analytical Chemists (AOAC) method of analysis, which measures a range of components in addition to NSP and results in figures that are about 30% higher than those obtained by the Englyst and Cummings method. As yet, the UK DRVs have not been revised but it is estimated that the recommended average fibre intake for the population based on AOAC analysis would be about 24 g/day, rather than 18 g (see Chapter 2.4).

Minerals and vitamins

For most vitamins and minerals, DRVs are given as the EAR, RNI and LRNI (see Appendix A2). Insufficient information was available for establishing the distribution of requirement for pantothenic acid, biotin, vitamin E, vitamin K, manganese, molybdenum, chromium and fluoride, and guidance only on safe intakes is given. In 2003, in response to concerns for supplemental intakes of some micronutrients, the Food Standards Agency's Expert Group on Vitamins and Minerals (EGVM) has reviewed the available evidence on the safety of 31 vitamins and minerals and has made recommendations on safe upper levels of their consumption (EGVM, 2003).

In 2003 SACN reviewed the evidence on the role of sodium in cardiovascular disease and made recommendations on salt, as opposed to sodium, intake. The recommended intake of salt in adults should be <6 g/day (see Chapter 4.2).

Conclusion

Dietary reference values are based on the best evidence available at the time of publication and should therefore be constantly reviewed. There is a paucity of evidence for some nutrients and the requirements for optimal health are continuously being researched; therefore, it is important to use DRVs as reference rather than definite set values. It is essential that dietitians understand the guiding principles used in the derivation of DRVs and understand their limitations and applications. The DRVs in the UK and other countries are revised periodically and further details can be found on the relevant web sites.

Further reading

Department of Health. (1991) *Dietary Reference Values for Food Energy and Nutrients for the United Kingdom. Report of the Panel on Dietary reference values of the Committee on Medical Aspects of Food Policy.* Report on Health and Social Subjects 41. London: HMSO.

FAO. (1991) Nutrient requirements. Available at www.fao.org/docrep/u5900t/u5900t00.htm.

Institute of Medicine (Food & Nutrition Board). (2000) Dietary reference intakes: applications in dietary assessment. Available at www.nap.edu.

Institute of Medicine (Food & Nutrition Board). (2003) Dietary reference intakes: guiding principles for nutrition labeling and fortification. Available at www.nap.edu.

Institute of Medicine (Food & Nutrition Board). (2003) Dietary reference intakes: applications in dietary planning. Available at www.nap.edu.

Scientific Advisory Committee on Nutrition. (2008) *Dietary Reference Values for Energy.* London: TSO. Available at www.sacn.gov.uk.

Scientific Advisory Committee on Nutrition. (2011) *The Nutritional Wellbeing of the British Population.* London: TSO. Available at www.sacn.gov.uk.

van't Veer P, Hesekerb H, Grammatikakic E, *et al.* (2012) EURRECA/WHO Workshop Report: Deriving Micronutrient Recommendations:

Updating Best Practices. *Annals of Nutrition and Metabolism* 62: 63–67.

Internet resources

UK

Scientific Advisory Committee on Nutrition   www.sacn.gov.uk

Europe

European Food Safety Authority   www.efsa.europa.eu
EURopean micronutrient REcommendations Aligned   www.eurreca .org

USA

Institute of Medicine (USA)   www.iom.edu
US Department of Agriculture (Interactive DRIs for Healthcare Professionals)   http://fnic.nal.usda.gov/dietary-guidance/ dietary-reference-intakes

Australia and New Zealand

National Health and Medical Research Council www.nhmrc.gov.au/guidelines/publications/n35-n36-n37

International

Food & Drink Organization of the United Nations (FAO)   www.fao .org
World Health Organization   www.who.int

References

Beaton GH. (1991) *Derivation, interpretation and application in evolutionary perspective*. Rome: FAO. Available at www.fao.org/ docrep/u5900t/u5900t00.htm. Accessed 15 January 2013.

Department of Health. (1969) *Recommended Intakes of Nutrients for the United Kingdom*. Reports on Health and Social Subjects 120. London: HMSO.

Department of Health. (1979) *Recommended Daily Amounts of Food Energy and Nutrients for Groups of People in the United Kingdom*. Reports on Health and Social Subjects 15. London: HMSO.

Department of Health. (1991) *Dietary Reference Values for Food Energy and Nutrients for the United Kingdom. Report of the Panel on Dietary Reference Values of the Committee on Medical Aspects of Food Policy*. Report on Health and Social Subjects 41. London: HMSO.

Expert Group on Vitamins and Minerals (EGVM). (2003). *Safe Upper Levels for Vitamins and Minerals*. London: Food Standards Agency. Available at http://cot.food.gov.uk/pdfs/vitmin2003.pdf Accessed 15 January 2013.

Henry CJ. (2005) Basal metabolic rate studies in humans: measurement and development of new equations. *Public Health and Nutrition* 8: 1133–1152.

Hurrell R, Egli I. (2010) Iron bioavailability and dietary reference values. *American Journal of Clinical Nutrition* 91: 1461S–1467S.

Millward DJ. (2012) A new approach to establishing dietary energy reference values. *Current Opinion in Clinical Nutrition and Metabolic Care* 15: 413–417.

Scientific Advisory Committee on Nutrition (SACN). (2003) *Salt and Health*. London: The Stationery Office, 2003. Available at www.sacn.gov.uk. Accessed 14 January 2013.

Scientific Advisory Committee on Nutrition (SACN). (2008) *Dietary Reference Values for Energy*. London: TSO. Available at www .sacn.gov.uk. Accessed 14 January 2013.

Scientific Advisory Committee on Nutrition (SACN). (2011a) *Dietary Reference Values for Energy*. London: The Stationery Office.

Scientific Advisory Committee on Nutrition (SACN). (2011b) *The Nutritional Wellbeing of the British Population*. London: TSO. Available at www.sacn.gov.uk Accessed 14 January 2013.

Schofield WN, Schofield C, James WPT. (1985) BMR – review and prediction. *Human Nutrition: Clinical Nutrition* 39 (Suppl): 1–96.

Van't Veer P, Hesekerb H, Grammatikakic E, *et al*. (2012) EURRECA/ WHO Workshop Report: Deriving micronutrient recommendations: Updating best practices. *Annals of Nutrition and Metabolism* 62: 63–67.

2.2 Assessment of nutritional status

Joan Gandy

Key points

- Assessment of nutritional status is fundamental to dietetic practice.

- It is a detailed, specific and in-depth evaluation by a competent health professional of an individual's nutritional status.

- Nutrition assessment encompasses many domains and no single parameter should be used in isolation.

- Nutritional assessment is a continuous process.

- Tools for nutritional assessment can be simple, e.g. visual assessment, or more complex, e.g. anthropometric or biochemical measurements.

- A multidisciplinary approach to nutritional assessment is vital to ensure timely and effective intervention.

Nutritional assessment was first described by the Health Organization of the League of Nation in 1932 and referred to a set of procedures to describe populations at a national level (Gibson, 2005). It now encompasses a number of domains, e.g. physical and dietary assessments, and is used in a variety of settings, e.g. clinical, sport, research. Many countries collect data on the nutritional status of populations and use these data to identify health priorities, and develop public health policies and interventions (see Chapter 4.2). Nutritional assessment of an individual will establish present nutritional status and identify potential concerns that can be dealt with promptly and thereby avoid future problems. It is a continuous process especially in clinical practice. Nutritional status can be defined as *the degree to which the individual's physiologic need for nutrients is being met by the foods he/she is eating. It is the state of balance in the individual between the nutrient intake and the nutrient expenditure or need'* (Krause & Mahan, 1979).

The assessment of nutritional status is a detailed procedure that should be conducted by trained and experienced professionals. As such it should be a fundamental part of dietetic practice. The British Dietetic Association (BDA, 2012) defines assessment as '. . . *a systematic process of collecting and interpreting information in order to make decisions about the nature and cause of nutrition related health issues that affect an individual, a group or a population.'* It is the first step in the nutrition and dietetic process (see Chapter 1.1).

It is important not to confuse nutritional assessment with nutritional screening. Nutritional screening is a simple procedure that uses tools designed and validated for use by all healthcare professionals, specifically to identify individuals at risk of malnutrition (over- and undernutrition) (see Chapter 6.2). Individuals identified as being at risk of malnutrition may then be referred to dietitians, according to local or national guidelines, who are trained and experienced in the full range of nutritional assessment techniques.

Nutritional assessment should be structured and standardised and therefore usually follows the ABCDE format:

- Anthropometry, body composition, functional.
- Biochemical, haematological tests.
- Clinical, physical.
- Dietary.
- Environmental, behavioural and social.

Table 2.2.1 gives examples of what may be assessed in each domain. The tools used and information collected in the assessment will vary depending on the practice setting, i.e. individual, group, community or population. This chapter discusses the assessment of adults; further details of the assessment of children can be found in Chapter 3.8.

An individual's clinical status has the potential to affect nutritional status in many ways; examples are shown in Table 2.2.2. Acute or chronic illness, injury and surgery can have considerable impact on nutritional status, both directly (due to the effects of the disease or injury itself) and indirectly (via possible effects on food intake). These effects may result in increased nutritional requirements, increased nutrient losses and/or impaired

Table 2.2.1 Nutritional assessment domains

Domain	Example procedure
Anthropometry, body composition, functional	Weight, height, body mass index, skinfold thickness, waist circumference Bioelectrical impedance analysis Grip strength dynamometry Physical activity questionnaires
Biochemical and haematological	Vitamin status tests Lipid status Iron status – haemoglobin, ferritin, etc.
Clinical	Physical appearance, blood pressure, medication, indirect calorimetry
Diet	24-hour recall, food frequency questionnaire
Environmental, behavioural and social	Shopping habits, housing, cooking facilities, education

Table 2.2.2 Examples of the effects of illness, injury and surgery on nutritional status

Increased nutrient requirements	Increased nutrient losses	Impaired nutrient ingestion, digestion and/or absorption
The metabolic response to trauma or surgery	Vomiting	Lack of appetite
The metabolic costs of repairing tissue damage, e.g. wounds, pressure ulcers	Diarrhoea	Lack of digestive enzymes, e.g. pancreatitis
Sepsis or infection	Renal excretion	Loss of absorptive surfaces, e.g. resection of any part of the gastrointestinal (GI) tract, coeliac disease
Involuntary activity, e.g. tremors, spasms	Surgical drains	Effects of treatments on GI tract, e.g. radiotherapy
Certain conditions, e.g. cystic fibrosis	Bleeding	Effects and symptoms of other conditions on food intake, e.g. dysphagia, breathlessness
	Wound or fistula exudates	Difficulty self feeding, chewing or maintaining food in the mouth

nutrient ingestion, digestion and/or absorption. Drug therapy may further affect nutrient intake, absorption, metabolism and excretion (see Chapter 5.3). Each chapter in Section 7 details assessment of nutritional status, the effect of the title condition on nutritional status and monitoring as appropriate.

Anthropometry, body composition and function

Anthropometry is one of the most frequently used assessment methods, with weight and height forming the most basic of anthropometric assessment. Historically, body composition and functional assessments were confined to the research setting. However, with increasing availability of the necessary equipment, e.g. dynamometry and bioelectrical impedance, dietitians are increasingly including these techniques in nutritional assessment.

Anthropometry

Anthropometry is the external measurement of the human body and reflects health and nutritional status; it can be used to predict performance (Shetty & James, 1994) and survival. Anthropometry is affected by nutritional and other factors, including age, gender and ethnicity. Anthropometric measurements are frequently compared with standards or used in prediction equations, and it is important to use standards and equations derived from the same or comparable ethnic, gender or age group. The most commonly used anthropometric measures are height, weight, waist circumference and skinfold thickness. All measurements will depend on the expertise of the operator and the quality of the equipment used. It is essential that all equipment be serviced, e.g. weighing scales, or replaced as appropriate, e.g. tape measures as they may stretch with continued use.

Training is essential to ensure that the measurements are performed correctly and are reproducible. The World Health Organization has produced a manual describing techniques (WHO, 1995), although more recent publications are available (Frisancho, 2008). It is essential to establish what, if any, standards are used within the local context, e.g. NHS guidance. It is good practice to periodically check proficiency using methods that assess technical error of measurement (Ulijaszek & Kerr, 1999). In longitudinal studies, using the same operator for specific measurements will improve precision.

Standards and reference ranges are available for many anthropometric measures, e.g. WHO (1995), and classifications such as body mass index (BMI) and waist circumference categories are also available. Increasingly, standards, reference ranges and classifications are available for different ethnic groups; it is important to consider the derivation of the standards, etc. when applying these to an individual, group or population.

Body weight

Weighing scales must be maintained and calibrated (Department of Health, 2008) regularly and should be Class III or above. It is recommended that the maximum weighing interval on adult weighing scales for weight monitoring should be 200 g.

A single measurement of body weight is not particularly useful in assessing nutritional status, other than to determine an individual BMI category. Measurement of body weight at regular intervals is vital to record changes in weight over time and to calculate percentage increase or decrease. Unless weights are recorded daily to measure change in fluid balance, weight over the longer term gives no indication of changes in body composition, since weight does not differentiate between fat, fat free mass (FFM) and fluid. It is important to use the appropriate weight for the clinical status of an individual, e.g. dry weight in renal dialysis patients (see Chapter 7.5.1).

Factors that affect body weight

Fluid retention, oedema or ascites

The causes of fluid retention may include hypoalbuminaemia, certain medications, e.g. steroids, and response to injury, renal, cardiac and hepatic dysfunction. The presence of additional fluid has been estimated by Mendenhall (1992) to contribute between 1 and 14 kg of measured weight (see Table 7.4.22). For barely detectable oedema, a correction of 2–3 kg can be subtracted from the measured weight (Elia, 2003).

Accuracy of scales

As previously stated, scales should be calibrated at regular intervals. Weights can vary between different scales and at different times during the day. For more accurate and useful results, individuals should be weighed on the same set of scales, in similar clothing and at roughly the same time of day.

Amputations

Table 2.2.3 shows the adjustments to weight that should be made if limbs have been amputated (Osterkamp, 1995.).

Plaster casts, splints and replacement joints

These can add significant amounts of weight. Typically, a cast for an upper limb weighs <1 kg, and for a leg can weigh up to 5 kg. Adjustments should be made when using weight to calculate BMI and these noted in the dietetic records. Fibreglass casts will weigh less than plaster of Paris casts. The weight of a replacement joint is not usually significantly different from that of the bone

Table 2.2.3 Weight adjustments for amputations

Body part	Percentage of body weight
Upper limb	5.0
Forearm	1.6
Hand	0.7
Lower limb	16.0
Lower leg	4.4
Foot	1.5

it is replacing. If there are concerns, advice should be sought from a specialist in this area.

When weight cannot be measured

Sometimes it is not possible to obtain a weight for a patient due to their clinical condition or simply due to the lack of accessible, suitable working scales. In these circumstances weight, may be estimated, e.g.:

- Self-reported usual weight from the patient. Studies have shown this results in a certain amount of underestimation in the overweight and obese (Dekkers *et al.*, 2008) and in women (Gunnare *et al.*, 2013), and overestimation in the underweight (Rowland, 1990). The reported figure is unlikely to take into account any change in weight since admission or illness began.
- Estimates are sometimes made by the dietitian, relatives, carers or other health professionals. Reed & Price (1998) showed that first degree relatives can estimate weight to within 3–5% of measured weight.
- Other anthropometric measurements have a linear relationship with weight change, e.g. mid upper arm circumference (MUAC) (see later).

Specialist weighing equipment may be available, such as weighing beds in some clinical settings, e.g. spinal cord injury units (see Chapter 7.17.3).

Percentage weight change

This is calculated as:

$$\% \text{ Weight change} = \left[\frac{\text{Usual or previous weight (kg)} - \text{Actual weight (kg)}}{\text{Usual or previous weight (kg)}} \right] \times 100$$

This equation is used more often for calculating percentage weight loss than weight gain, as this is an important indicator of the risk of malnutrition. Using percentage weight loss as a guide, nutritional support should be considered when someone has experienced unintentional weight loss of more than 10% over a 3–6-month period or the patient has a BMI of <20 kg/m² and unintentional weight loss of more than 5% over a 3–6-month period (NICE, 2006a).

In a clinical situation, weight loss may have a greater detrimental effect in a lean individual than an obese individual, even when the same percentage weight loss has occurred. However, it is important to remember that significant, rapid weight loss in an obese individual also makes them vulnerable to malnutrition associated morbidity. Rapid weight loss over a few days reflects changes in fluid balance rather than body tissue.

Height

Height is usually measured using a stand alone stadiometer or one fixed at the appropriate height to a wall. Subjects must stand straight and stretched, with their heels against the wall or rod. The measurement should ideally be taken with the head in the Frankfort plane (top of external ear canal and top of the lower bone of the eye socket are in a horizontal plane parallel to the floor). The head plate is lowered until it lightly touches the top of the head.

Proxy height measures

When it is not possible to measure a patient's height, this can be estimated using alternative methods.

Self reported height

Studies have shown that people, especially the elderly, are not usually aware of the reduction in height with progressing age and can overestimate their height by approximately 2 cm (Spencer et al., 2002; Rowland, 1990). However, the estimated height is unlikely to affect the BMI category. Self reported height has been shown to be reliable (Wada et al., 2005). For individuals with spine curvature it is advisable to obtain and use reported maximum height as an adult. Measuring recumbent height is accurate but 2% higher than standing height (Gray et al., 1985). This can be estimated if the length of the bed is known. Relatives can usually estimate height to within 1% of actual height (Reed & Price, 1998).

Alternatively, other anthropometric measurements can be taken and from these height can be estimated. These are:

- Ulna length.
- Knee height.
- Demispan.

Ulna length

The use of ulna length as a proxy for height is generally the easiest and quickest measure to use in bed bound patients. It is validated for use on the left side but, as no systematic differences have been found, either side can be used. The arm is bent diagonally across the chest with the palm facing inwards and the fingers pointing towards the shoulder. The measurement is taken between the central and most prominent parts of the styloid process and the centre (tip) of the bony prominence (olecranon) at the elbow (see Appendix A7). Estimates of height from ulna length can also be found in this appendix. However, caution should be used in non-Caucasian populations as predicting height from ulna length has been shown to overestimate height in Asian and Black adults (Madden et al., 2012).

Knee height

Knee height is measured with the leg flexed so that the thigh and calf create a right angle. The fixed blade of a knee height caliper is placed under the heel and the sliding blade moved down to rest on the top of the knee, about 4 cm behind the knee cap. The knee height is then read from a scale to the nearest 0.1 cm. The procedure can be carried out with a tape measure with little loss of accuracy. Height is calculated using the following formulae (Chumlea et al., 1985; 1992; 1994):

Men	18–60 years:	Predicted height (cm) = [knee height (cm) $\times$ 1.88] + 71.85
	60–90 years:	Predicted height (cm) = [knee height (cm) $\times$ 2.08] + 59.01
Women	18–60 years:	Predicted height (cm) = [knee height (cm) $\times$ 1.87] − [age (years) $\times$ 0.06] + 70.25
	60–90 years:	Predicted height (cm) = [knee height (cm) $\times$ 1.91 − [age (years) $\times$ 0.17] + 75.00

Demispan

Demispan can be undertaken on people sitting on a chair or lying in bed. It requires the individual to be able to outstretch their arm perpendicular to their body. It is measured by placing the end of a tape measure between the middle and ring fingers of the person with arm outstretched and running the tape along to the centre of the sternal notch (Kwok & Whitelaw, 1991). It is important to ensure the arm is horizontal and straight, and that the wrist is in natural flexion and rotation. Height is predicted using the following formulae:

Men	16–54 years:	Predicted height (cm) = [demispan (cm) $\times$ 1.3] + 68
	>55 years:	Predicted height (cm) = [demispan (cm) $\times$ 1.2] + 71
Women	16–54 years:	Predicted height (cm) = [demispan (cm) $\times$ 1.3] + 62
	>55 years:	Predicted height (cm) = [demispan (cm) $\times$ 1.2] + 67

There is some evidence suggesting that estimating height from demispan may be less reliable in the elderly.

Body mass index

BMI is a weight for height indicator that may be used to classify overweight and obesity, and is calculated as weight (kg)/height (m^2). However, it does not give any indication of adipose distribution. In addition, it assumes that the relationship of weight to height is constant in adults and therefore may underestimate obesity in individuals with reduced levels of FFM, e.g. the elderly, and overestimate obesity in muscular individuals with high levels of FFM, e.g. athletes. It is a simple measure for use in nutritional assessment of individuals and populations, and forms part of many screening tools. The BMI cut-off ranges are based on the effect body weight has on morbidity and

Table 2.2.4 Classification of body mass index and risk of comorbidities in adults (WHO, 1998; 2004)

Classification	BMI (kg/m²)	BMI (kg/m²) Asian origin	Risk of comorbidities
Underweight	<18.5	<18.5	Low (but risk of other clinical problems increased)
Normal range	18.5–24.9	18.5–22.9	Average
Overweight	25.0–29.9	23–27.4	Increased risk
Obese class I	30.0–34.9	27.5–32.4	Moderate
Obese class II	35.0–39.9	32.5–37.4	Severe
Obese class III	>40.0	>37.5	Morbid obesity

Table 2.2.5 Waist measurements in adults as a predictor of health (WHO, 2008)

	Men	Asian men	Women	Asian women
Waist circumference (cm)				
Increased risk	≥94		≥80	
Substantially increased risk	≥102	≥90	≥88	≥80
Waist to hip ratio				
Increased risk	≥0.9		≥0.85	

mortality (Table 2.2.4). The higher the BMI, the greater the risk of developing certain conditions, including type 2 diabetes, heart disease, osteoarthritis and some cancers (see Chapter 7.13.1). Conversely, the lower the BMI, the greater the risk of osteoporosis and of complications associated with malnutrition. A ready reckoner of BMI can be found in Appendix A7. The BMI classification of WHO (1998; 2004) is shown in Table 2.2.4. BMI is now being superseded as a measure of obesity associated health risks by waist circumference. However, due to its simplicity, BMI is still widely used and is particularly useful in populations.

BMI is affected by many factors including:

- *Ethnicity* – the BMI ranges were primarily developed for use in public health using healthy Caucasian adults. The range for other ethnic groups reflects the differences in body composition between races and the subsequent risk to health (James *et al.*, 2001).
- *Setting* – BMI can be and is used in a clinical setting; however, it must be used as part of the overall assessment and not as a standalone result. Clinical judgement can override BMI category where necessary. It will also be affected by over- or under-estimates of weight or height as discussed earlier.
- *Age* – a BMI value may have different prognostic significance in different age groups, particularly the elderly (Beck & Ovesen, 1998). BMI ranges were derived from people aged between 18 and 65 years, so care should be taken when interpreting calculated values for people above this age range. Adult BMI reference ranges are not appropriate for children as they assume a constant height. BMI age specific centiles should b used in children (see Chapter 3.8).
- *Body composition* – BMI should be used with caution in people who have a distorted fluid balance (oedema, ascites or dehydration) or a high proportion of muscle mass, e.g. athletes, body builders and military personnel (Prentice & Jebb, 2001).

Other indices of obesity are used, e.g. Ponderal index; however, these are not in common practice and have not been researched anywhere near to the extent of BMI.

Demiquet and mindex

Alternative indices to the BMI based on weight and demispan (rather than height) have been derived for use in the elderly (Lehman *et al.*, 1991). In men over 64 years, the demiquet can be used:

$$\text{Demiquet} = \frac{\text{Weight (kg)}}{[\text{Demispan (m)}]^2}$$

In women over 64 years, the mindex is considered more suitable. This is defined as:

$$\text{Mindex} = \frac{\text{Weight (kg)}}{\text{Demispan (m)}}$$

Demiquet and mindex are independent of stature; therefore, they may be useful in studies of the elderly. However, they are not routinely used in clinical dietetic practice. Tables showing the percentile distribution of demiquet and mindex in the elderly are given in Appendix A7, although the limitations of these reference data (which are based on relatively small population samples) should be borne in mind (Bannerman *et al.*, 1997).

Waist circumference and waist to hip ratio

Waist circumference is now considered a more appropriate measure of obesity related morbidity and mortality (Seidell, 2010) as it assesses visceral adiposity. Visceral adipose tissue surrounds organs such as the liver and has a greater effect on health than peripheral adipose tissue. NICE (2006b) recommends the use of BMI and waist circumference in the assessment of obesity related health risks. It is a useful tool for monitoring weight loss programmes and can predict changes in risk, even if weight has remained stable. However, when BMI is >35 kg/m², measuring the waist circumference adds little predictive power. Table 2.2.5 shows the value of waist circumference and waist to hip ratio (WHR) as predictors of health (WHO, 2008).

The waist circumference is measured at the halfway point between the lowest rib and the iliac crest in the midaxillary line. The advantage of this method is that it uses a bony landmark and there is little scope for error provided that the patient can be partially undressed. It is important to ensure that the tape is snug but not tight and is parallel to the ground, and that the patient is not breathing in (Ashwell *et al.*, 1996; Lean, 1998; SIGN, 1996).

Waist to hip ratio (WHR) is used less frequently in individual assessment, mainly due to difficulties in locating the appropriate place to measure hip circumference. However, it is a useful indicator of obesity related health risks.

As with BMI, the risk of morbidity occurs at lower levels of waist circumference and WHR in Asian populations and the WHO cut-offs are therefore lower these populations (see Table 2.2.5). There is a paucity of evidence for different cut-offs in other population groups (Lear *et al.*, 2010), although the International Diabetes Federation (2006) has made recommendations for several ethnic groups for the diagnosis of metabolic syndrome.

Mid–upper arm circumference

When neither weight nor height can be measured, the BMI can be estimated using the mid–upper arm circumference (MUAC). This is a useful tool when oedema is present as the upper arms tend not to be affected. It is also useful during pregnancy as MUAC changes little during gestation when weight obviously increases. This measurement can provide an estimation of BMI but only for the cut-off values for underweight, i.e. BMI $<20\,kg/m^2$, and obesity, i.e. BMI $>30\,kg/m^2$. The measurement is made with the patient sitting or standing. The arm must be bare and the top of the shoulder accessible. With the arm bent at right angles at the elbow and forearm across the body, the midpoint between the top of the shoulder and the tip of the elbow is identified and marked. The arm is then allowed to hang loosely by the side and the circumference is measured at the marked mid point.

If MUAC < 23.5 cm	BMI < 20 kg/m², i.e. underweight
If MUAC > 32 cm	BMI > 30 kg/m², i.e. obese

The reference values for MUAC derived from an American population (Bishop *et al.*, 1981) are given in Appendix A7. More recent data from the USA NHANES survey has been used to produce reference values (McDowell *et al.*, 2008), however their applicability to the UK population is being debated. Data for the UK population are not currently available. Patients with liver disease and alcoholism have greatly reduced arm circumference measurements compared with normal controls (Thuluvath & Triger, 1994).

Skinfold thickness

The relationship between subcutaneous fat and total body fat can be exploited by measuring skinfold thickness at specific sites to estimate adiposity. Durnin & Womersley (1974) produced equations from the relationship between total body fat, as measured by densitometry, and the sum of four skinfold thicknesses (biceps, triceps, subscapular and supra iliac), which can be used to estimate total body fat. To minimise measurement error, three separate readings should be taken and averaged. The same person should make all the measurements for a particular individual.

Triceps skinfold

Measurement should be made on the non-dominant arm, which should be bent at a right angle. The length from the tip of the acromion process on the scapula to the olecranon process of the ulna is measured and the mid point marked. With the arm hanging loosely by the side, the skinfold at the mid point level on the back of the arm over the triceps muscle is picked up between the thumb and forefinger of the left hand. The calipers are placed on the skinfold just below the fingers, the fingers removed, and a reading taken 2–3 seconds later.

Biceps skinfold

Measurement is as for the triceps, but over the biceps muscle on the front of the arm.

Subscapular skinfold

This measurement is made about 2.5 cm in and below the angle of the scapula towards the midline, and at an angle of approximately 45 degrees to the spine along the natural line of skin cleavage. Alternatively, the skinfold is picked up just below the tip of the right scapula. The natural potential crease that is lifted to form this fold runs at an angle of about 45 degrees downwards from the spine.

Supra iliac skinfold

This is measured midway between the anterior superior iliac spine crest and the lowest point of the ribs, horizontal to the floor, or just above the iliac crest in the midaxillary line. Alternatively, the vertical skinfold can be picked up immediately above the anterior superior iliac spine in the midaxillary line.

In clinical practice, and especially in the bed bound patient, triceps skinfold thickness alone is most commonly used as an indicator of endogenous fat stores and, in conjunction with MUAC (see earlier), is a useful way of evaluating body composition in patients with ascites or peripheral oedema, or who cannot be weighed. Selected reference values of triceps skinfold thickness in a normal adult population (Bishop *et al.*, 1981) are given in Appendix A7.

Problems associated with measurement of skinfold thickness include:

- *Measurement error* – subcutaneous fat is compressible and it is difficult to determine at which pressure the reading should be taken. It takes time and practice to acquire a measurement technique that gives reproducible recordings. Measurements differ substantially when made on the same person by different observers (Ulijaszek & Kerr, 1999).
- *Measurement difficulties* – the correct anatomical site is difficult to establish, and in some cases the site may be inaccessible due to burns, bandages, etc. The jaws of the calipers may not be wide enough to encompass the fat fold in people who are obese.
- *Errors due to individual variation in fat distribution* – although the relationship between subcutaneous fat

and total body fat is relatively constant, there are variations between individuals, or within an individual, at different points in time. In addition it is assumed that the arm is a symmetrical cylinder, which is clearly not entirely true. The relationship of skinfold thickness to total body fat changes with age; as people get older, a greater proportion of body fat is deposited internally rather than subcutaneously. It should also be noted that loss of body weight results in non-proportional changes in muscle and fat stores at different sites (Katch & Hortobagyi, 1990).

- *Population differences in body fat distribution* – people of Afro-Caribbean origin tend to have more visceral and upper body fat deposition than Caucasians (Zillikens & Conway, 1990; Conway *et al.*, 1995). Asian adults have also been shown to have more upper body subcutaneous fat and a higher body fat to BMI ratio than Caucasian adults, a finding more pronounced in women (Wang *et al.*, 1994). Ethnic specific equations should be used, e.g. Ortiz *et al.* (1992) and Schutte *et al.* (1984) developed equations for Afro-Caribbean women and men.
- *Insensitivity* – small changes in body fat (<0.5 kg) cannot be measured by anthropometry (Heymsfield & Matthews, 1994). This therefore limits the value of the technique as a short term monitoring tool. However, serial measurements of skinfold thickness can be a useful way of monitoring nutritional status long term.

Mid arm muscle circumference (MAMC)

An estimate of muscle mass, an indicator of protein stores, can be derived from measurement of MUAC and triceps skinfold thickness (TSF) using the formula:

$$MAMC\,(cm) = MUAC\,(cm) - [TSF\,(mm) \times 0.314]$$

Standards for interpreting the MAMC are given in Appendix A7.

Body composition

Dietitians most frequently use skinfold thicknesses to evaluate body composition; however, increasingly other techniques such as bioelectrical impedance (BIA) are being used. In research settings, other techniques such air displacement plethysmography (BodPod; used to estimate body density) or dual energy X ray absorptiometry are used. However, it is important that dietitians understand the underlying principles of these techniques as they are used to derive many standards, reference ranges and equations, e.g. under water weighing was used in the derivation of the Durnin & Womersley (1974) equations. A summary of methods used for the determination of body composition is shown in Table 2.2.6. Further details of the techniques can be found in Heymsfield *et al.* (2005).

Bioelectrical impedance analysis

Bioelectrical impedance analysis is an easy, non-invasive bedside measure used to estimate total body water and body composition. Analysers incorporate sophisticated software to interpret the measurements. It is based on the principle that fat does not contain water and that the water content of FFM is a constant. Body fat can be determined by subtracting the estimate of FFM from total body weight. An electrical current flows predominantly through tissues containing water and ions but not through fat, which is an insulator. Body resistance or impedance was originally used as an index of total body water (TBW). However, because of the complex electrical properties of tissues and the lack of uniformity of body shape and dimensions, an easy approach was adopted.

Table 2.2.6 Summary of methods for the determination of body composition (source: M.J. Gibney 2009. Reproduced with permission of Wiley-Blackwell Publishing)

Method	Accuracy	Cost	Radiation	Time	Convenience for subject
IVNAA	+++	–	–	++	++
Densitometry	++	+		++	±
Dilution	++	±	(–)	+	++
TBK	++	–		++	++
DEXA	+++	±	–	++	++
CT scanning	++	–	–	++	++
MRI scanning	++	–		++	+
Anthropometry	+	+++		++	+
Infrared interactance	+	++		++	++
BIA	+	+		+++	+++
TOBEC	+	–		++	++
Urinary metabolites	+	+		–	–

+++, excellent; ++, very good; +, good; ± reasonable; – bad.
IVNAA, *in vivo* neutron activation analysis; TBK, total body potassium; DEXA, dual energy X ray absorptiometry; CT, computer assisted tomography; MRI, magnetic resonance imaging; BIA, bioelectrical impedance analysis; TOBEC, total body electrical conductivity.

Whole body impedance was regressed against reference measures of TBW, and this then extended to FFM and fat, producing equations to estimate body composition. The equipment can be hand held (arm to arm current), requires electrodes to be placed on specific parts of the body (total body analysis), or foot to foot current can be measured using stand-on scales that incorporate the software.

Impedance is commonly adjusted for height and an equation is derived that is used to estimate body composition. The equations contain anthropometric data, such as weight and height, and different equations are used. It is difficult to establish the equations used by a particular manufacturer and therefore caution should be expressed.

Bioelectrical impedance analysis is useful for large population studies, due to portability and low cost. It can be useful when making serial measurements of an individual, but it is not recommended by some for single measurements in individual patients (Buchholz et al., 2004) as it may be insensitive to underlying variability between individuals due to factors such as gender, age and disease state. However, other studies have shown it to be a useful tool in clinical practice (Desport et al., 2003; Lammersfeld et al., 2004).

Bioelectrical impedance analysis can be a useful tool, providing that the operator is aware of its limitations, which include:

- Inaccuracies in the measurement or inputting of body weight.
- It is important to standardise conditions, e.g. fasting or non-fasting state, and the consumption of drinks high in electrolytes can perturb the system.
- Many machines require data entry about exercise levels or have a different setting for standard or athletic. Variations in levels entered or setting chosen can greatly affect individual results.
- The assumed hydration of FFM is relatively constant in the healthy population, but significant variation can occur in subjects with abnormalities of water balance.
- Variation in body geometry – the contribution of different segments of the body to whole body impedance is assumed to be relatively standard. Significant individual variation in body shape and fat distribution may distort these conversion factors.

Bioelectrical impedance analysis can be useful for assessing nutritional status in seriously ill patients where anthropometric methods are less practical. Sequential BIA measurements may be used to monitor hydration status in the critically ill. However, the measurements are of limited use in patients with grossly abnormal fluid balance, e.g. severe dehydration or ascites, or at extremes of the BMI ranges (Kyle et al., 2004a; 2004b). Bioelectrical impedance analysis has been used to monitor changes in body composition in patients during refeeding (Pencharz & Azcue, 1996).

Increasingly bioelectrical spectral analysis is being used to study fluid status and fluid shifts.

Table 2.2.7 Dynamometry (grip strength) [data derived from Griffith and Clark (1984) and Klidjian et al. (1980)]

	Normal values (kg)	85% of normal (values at or below this level are indicative of protein malnutrition) (kg)
Men		
18–69 years	40.0	34.0
70–79 years	32.5	27.5
80+ years	22.5	19.0
Women		
18–69 years	27.5	23.0
70–79 years	25.0	21.0
80+ years	20.0	17.0

Functional assessment

The functional test most frequently used by dietitians is grip strength dynamometry. An individual is asked to grip the handle of a dynamometer as tightly as possible and the exerted pressure is read off the scale; usually expressed in kilograms. Hand grip strength is a measure of muscle strength. Normal values are available and a reading of 85% or less is indicative of protein malnutrition. Hand grip strength is used in a variety of settings, including sport, and has been used as a measure of recovery following surgery. A recent review by Norman et al. (2011) concluded that impaired grip strength was an indicator of poor postoperative recovery, including increased complication rates and length of hospital stay. In the elderly, loss of grip strength was related to loss of independence. Grip strength is increasingly being used in nutritional research. Normal values and 85% values are shown in Table 2.2.7.

When assessing lifestyle, especially for energy balance issues, dietitians should also consider physical activity levels. Many tools are available to assess physical activity, including logs and pedometers. The tools most widely used by dietitians are physical activity questionnaires. Many validated questionnaires are available in the literature for specific groups.

Biochemical and haematological markers

Clinical chemistry can provide objective results for use during the nutritional assessment process and in the monitoring of nutritional status and nutritional support. Biochemical and haematological measurements have limited value in the assessment of nutritional status as many of these parameters are dynamic and change on a daily basis, and are compensated by homeostatic mechanisms, influenced by underlying disease and vary with age. However, clinical chemistry is essential to determine the status of specific nutrients, e.g. vitamin B_{12} or iron deficiency in anaemia. Laboratory tests are not carried out on every individual but are patient specific as guided by the clinical situation or research protocol. Appendix A9 gives reference ranges for some parameters; however, these ranges will vary depending on local laboratory standards and protocols. It is essential to use reference ranges that refer to the local setting.

The chapters in Section 7 discuss biochemistry and haematological tests for each clinical condition as appropriate.

Visceral protein status

The majority (30–50%) of body protein is found in skeletal muscle (also called somatic protein). Skeletal muscle wastes in ill people due to disease, malnutrition and inactivity. The remaining protein (visceral protein) is found in organs such as the liver, heart, pancreas and kidneys, and in serum proteins, e.g. albumin, blood cells. Other proteins found in the body are the non-structural proteins, e.g. in cartilage. These are not affected by trauma or stress and play no role in nutritional assessment.

Serum proteins, such as albumin, prealbumin, transferrin, thyroxine-binding prealbumin and retinol binding protein, are sometimes measured as an indicator of visceral protein status and hence clinical outcome. Synthesis of these proteins is compromised in malnutrition. However, it should also be borne in mind that non-nutritional factors such as trauma, sepsis, liver disease, and altered fluid state can have a much greater effect than nutritional influences.

Serum albumin

Serum albumin has a long half life of 14–20 days; therefore, it is not very sensitive to short term changes in protein status. Normal albumin levels in short term starvation and severe anorexia nervosa have been reported (Broom et al., 1986). Albumin levels are affected by age, infection, zinc depletion (causing a decrease) and dehydration (causing an increase), and low levels correlate poorly with nutritional status (Anderson & Wochos, 1982; Friedman & Fadem, 2010). However, an albumin level of <35 g/L does indicate the body's impaired ability to cope with major illness, surgical intervention or sepsis, and can be a useful part of a nutritional assessment (Scott et al., 1998).

Prealbumin

This has been used to monitor nutritional status and can be a sensitive index of early response to nutritional support due to its short half life of <2 days. It is affected by changes in hydration status and acute changes in liver and renal function, but the fluctuations are limited and smaller than is the case with albumin. Levels may be depressed in inflammatory states independently of nutritional status. It is wise to consider prealbumin results with C-reactive protein (CRP) values to distinguish between reduction due to illness or malnutrition (Robinson et al., 2003).

Serum transferrin

Serum transferrin has a shorter half life than albumin (8–10 days), so responds more rapidly to changes in protein status. However, it is also affected by other factors such as metabolic stress, so it is not a sensitive marker of nutritional status. Transferrin is an iron transport protein and is markedly affected by changes in iron status, e.g. anaemia, use of iron supplementation, severe blood loss or blood transfusion. Transferrin tends not to be measured routinely in the acute setting.

Thyroxine binding prealbumin (2–3-day half life) and retinol binding protein (12-hour half life) are much more sensitive to protein depletion, but are of little value in assessing nutritional status as they are extremely sensitive to changes in stress or disease (Casati et al., 1998).

Nitrogen balance

Measurement of nitrogen excretion over a period of time will reflect the nitrogen balance and changes in total body protein mass. It is a useful tool to assess and monitor catabolism. In practice, urinary urea nitrogen is measured using a 24-hour urine collection and the nitrogen output calculated, taking into account renal and other losses, e.g. from skin or faeces.

Vitamin, mineral and trace element status

Serum levels of trace elements are of limited value as indicators of nutritional inadequacy because body stores must be severely depleted before circulating levels are affected. Compensatory homeostatic mechanisms may mask nutrient deficiencies until an advanced stage of depletion. Periodic measurements of blood levels are, however, useful as a way of monitoring long term nutritional support, e.g. in home enteral feeding. Webster-Gandy et al. (2011) discuss the measurement of vitamin, mineral and trace element status further.

Calcium status can be monitored by measuring blood levels. However, total plasma calcium is a measure of both ionised and non-ionised calcium (the latter being calcium bound to albumin, citrate or phosphate). When plasma albumin is low, total calcium will also appear low. The biochemistry result for corrected calcium takes into account the reduction in circulating calcium secondary to low circulating protein levels, and is the better value to use. Plasma pH will influence calcium binding. In acidosis, less calcium is albumin bound and more exists in the ionised form. Calcium balance is influenced by hormonal and biochemical factors, including parathyroid hormone (PTH), calcitonin and calcitriol (the active metabolite of vitamin D) (see Chapter 7.9.1).

Hydration status and serum electrolytes

Iatrogenic, dietetic and clinical interventions can all influence these factors (see Chapters 6.6 and 7.17.1). Commonly used markers of hydration status include sodium, potassium and urea. However, results need to be interpreted alongside fluid balance charts and clinical examination for indications of over- or under-hydration. Urinary sodium levels can be measured to check salt depletion. This is useful in conditions with large fluid loss, e.g. Crohn's disease.

Dehydration

This concentrates the extracellular fluid, reflected in the blood results as hypernatraemia, uraemia and raised serum haemoglobin. If sodium and urea rise concurrently, dehydration should be suspected even in the presence of fluid overload, e.g. oedema. Fluid balance can be monitored by daily measurement of body weight. Dehydration with raised urea may occur without raised sodium levels if patients are losing both sodium and fluid, yet are having a low sodium diet, e.g. diarrhoea while being enterally fed.

Refeeding syndrome

Prior to starting feeding an at-risk patient, blood levels of potassium, calcium and phosphate should be checked. If these are low, magnesium should also be measured and all acted upon according to local protocols. Once feeding has commenced, low blood levels of phosphate, potassium and magnesium should alert to refeeding syndrome (see Chapter 6.4).

Other parameters

Other parameters that may be used include:

* Renal function tests, e.g. creatinine, urea.
* Inflammation markers, e.g. CRP.
* Infection markers, e.g. white blood cells.

Clinical assessment

The clinical assessment should include medical history, test results and current medicines, including prescribed and over the counter medicines. It is important to consider drug–nutrient interactions (see Chapter 5.3). These factors can be ascertained from the medical or nursing notes or the patient, family and/or carers.

It is not possible to overestimate the importance of physical observations. Examples of physical signs of nutritional problems are shown in Table 2.2.8 (Shaw & Lawson, 2007). Other examples include:

* Physical appearance – does the person look thin, of acceptable weight or overweight? Emaciation, pale complexion and hair loss suggest long term undernutrition. Loose clothing, rings and ill fitting dentures indicate weight loss. Sunken eyes, dry mouth and fragile skin are indicative of dehydration. Is there evidence of fluid retention, e.g. swollen ankles? Badly damaged nails and surrounding tissue may be an indication of self induced vomiting in bulimia nervosa.
* Breathlessness may be a symptom of anaemia or due to a clinical condition, and can make it more difficult to eat.
* Poor wound healing may reflect impaired immune function as a consequence of undernutrition and/or vitamin deficiencies, and/or lack of mobility.
* Oedema may reflect underlying disease, or heart failure secondary to prolonged protein or thiamine deficiency. The presence of oedema may mask loss of lean tissue.

Table 2.2.8 Examples of physical signs of nutritional problems (source: Shaw and Lawson 2007, table 1.6, p. 9. Reproduced with permission of Wiley-Blackwell Publishing)

Assessment	Clinical sign	Possible nutrient(s)
Hair	Thin, sparse / Colour change – flag sign / Easily plucked	Protein and energy, zinc, copper
Skin	Dry, flaky / Rough 'sandpaper' texture / Petechiae, bruising	Essential fatty acids, B vitamins / Vitamin A / Vitamin C
Eyes	Pale conjunctiva / Xerosis, keratomalacia	Iron / Vitamin A
Lips	Angular stomatitis / Cheilosis	B vitamins
Tongue	Colour changes	B vitamins
Teeth	Mottling of enamel	Fluorosis (excess fluoride)
Gums	Spongy, bleed easily	Vitamin C
Face	Thyroid enlargement	Iodine
Nails	Spoon shape, koilonychias	Iron, zinc, copper
Subcutaneous tissue	Oedema, over hydration / Depleted subcutaneous fat	Protein, sodium / Energy
Muscles	Wasting	Protein, energy, zinc
Bones	Craniotabes / Parietal and frontal bossing / Epiphyseal enlargement / Beading of ribs	Vitamin D

- Adverse effects of illness or drug treatment, such as nausea, vomiting, diarrhoea.
- Physical problems affecting eating, e.g. poor dentition, dry mouth, sore or painful mouth, orofacial surgery.
- Repeated medical investigations, treatments and medications requiring fasting or dietary change.

Some vitamin deficiencies have clear visible signs, such as xerophthalmia (failure to produce tears), which is indicative of vitamin A deficiency, and the distinctive appearance of Casal collar in pellagra (niacin deficiency).

Dietary assessment

Dietary assessment is discussed in detail in Chapter 2.3. Establishing the extent to which nutritional needs are being met is core to the nutritional assessment. Factors that need to be considered include:

- Current food and fluid intake.
- Duration and severity of any changes in appetite and oral intake.
- Presence of factors affecting food and fluid intake.

The findings need to be interpreted in the context of the individual's nutritional requirements (see Chapter 2.1).

In clinical settings it is also important to consider recent changes in intake, including:

- Increase or decrease in appetite.
- Alterations in meal pattern or timings.
- Changes in food choice or food consistency.

The greater the extent and duration of these changes, the more marked the effect on nutritional status will be.

Environmental, behavioural and social assessment

These factors can have a significant impact on nutritional status. Factors that may affect food and fluid intake include:

- *Psychological status:*
  ○ Depression or apathy, bereavement.

Table 2.2.9 Monitoring nutritional status in clinical settings

Assessment parameter	Rationale	Method	Frequency
Weight	Assess change in body mass – intentional or unintentional Calculate percentage change Calculate BMI Determine whether nutritional goals are achieved	Scales Surrogate measures e.g. self reported usual weight from patient, family, carer	At initial assessment then as clinically indicated. Twice a week initially reducing to monthly Daily to assess change in fluid balance
Weight history	To assess recent weight loss or gain and over longer periods Ascertain normal weight for an individual	Medical notes Dietetic records Patient or carer recall	At initial assessment
Height	To calculate BMI	Stadiometer Self reported height Tape measure Surrogate measure, e.g. demi span	Once only unless shrinkage has occurred, e.g. osteoporosis
Other anthropometric measurements	Assessing fat or muscle status Monitor nutrition support	MUAC TSF Hand grip dynamometry Waist circumference	Monthly Monthly Weekly As necessary
Drug and medical history	Assess risk to nutritional intake, metabolism and requirements	Relevant notes Pharmacy chart	Every 2–3 days acutely, weekly long term
Clinical biochemistry	To assess hydration and protein status Monitor nutrition support	Medical notes Pathology systems	Daily initially then twice weekly Longer intervals, e.g. monthly according to individual circumstances
Nutritional intake	To establish usual intake To ensure oral and/or artificial intake are meeting requirements	Interview Food diary Food intake chart Fluid balance chart Discussion with patient, carer, family, ward staff	At assessment, then at considered intervals thereafter Dependent on patient's condition
Social history	Establish factors affecting nutritional intake	Dietetic record cards Consultation with patient, family, carer	Initial assessment and thereafter as required

BMI, body mass index; MUAC, mid upper arm circumference; TSF, triceps skinfold thickness.

○ Confusion and or memory loss, e.g. in people with dementia.

• *Ability to buy, prepare and cook food* should also be considered. Especially when there is a sudden change in social condition, e.g. bereavement, particularly if it was the partner who organised the meals, or moving from a catered institution into the community. Mobility will affect the ability to shop, prepare and cook food. Weakness and impaired movement may result from loss of muscle mass.

• *Social factors:*
  ○ Living conditions and recent changes, e.g. an elderly person moving from their own home to sheltered accommodation or a care home.
  ○ Cultural and religious beliefs.
  ○ Low income and recent changes in income, e.g. redundancy, recent immigration.
  ○ Alcoholism.
  ○ Education, e.g. the inability to read or severe dyslexia will influence the ability to read nutrition labelling and understand health messages.

Nutritional requirements

In order to determine whether an individual's nutritional intake is meeting their needs it is important to consider their requirements. Nutritional requirements are available for population groups (dietary reference values) or can be estimated for an individual, taking into account age, gender, level of physical activity and clinical condition (see Chapters 2.1 and 6.1).

Monitoring nutritional status

In clinical settings nutritional status must be assessed on a regular basis to ensure that treatment, including nutritional support, is appropriate and effective. Monitoring can be carried out by the patient, dietitian or other health professional according to the stability and location of the patient. Suitable methods and suggested frequency of assessment are summarised in Table 2.2.9.

The nutritional status of groups and populations may be monitored for public health surveillance purposes (see Chapter 4.2) or epidemiological studies, e.g. the European Perspective Investigation into Cancer and nutrition project (EPIC). The parameters measured will be determined by set protocols.

Further reading

Frisancho AR. (2008) *Anthropometric Standards: An Interactive Nutritional Reference of Body Size and Body Composition for Children and Adults.* Ann Arbor: The University of Michigan Press.

Gibson RS. (2005) *Principles of Nutritional Assessment,* 2nd edn. Oxford: Oxford University Press.

Heymsfield S, Lohman TG, Wang ZM, Going S. (2005) *Human Body Composition by Human Kinetics.* Illinois: Champaign.

Heyward VH, Wagner D. (2004) *Applied Body Composition Assessment,* 2nd edn. Illinois: Champaign.

Internet resources

National Obesity Observatory   www.noo.org.uk
World Health Organization   www.who.int

References

Anderson CF, Wochos DN. (1982) The utility of serum albumin values in the nutritional assessment of patients. *Mayo Clinic Proceedings* 57(3): 181–184.

Ashwell M, Cole TJ, Dixon AK. (1996) Ratio of waist circumference to height is strong predictor of intra-abdominal fat. *BMJ* 313: 559–560.

Bannerman E, Reilly JJ, MacLennan WJ, Kirk T, Pender F. (1997) Evaluation of validity of British anthropometric reference data for assessing nutritional state of elderly people in Edinburgh: cross sectional study. *BMJ* 315: 338–341.

Beck AM, Ovesen L. (1998) At which body mass index and degree of weight loss should hospitalized elderly patients be considered at nutritional risk? *Clinical Nutrition* 17(5): 195–198.

Bishop CW, Bowen PE, Ritchley SI. (1981) Norms for nutritional assessment of American adults by upper arm anthropometry. *American Journal of Clinical Nutrition* 34: 2530–2539.

Broom J, Fraser MH, McKensie K, Miller JDB, Fleck A. (1986) The protein metabolic response to short-term starvation in man. *Clinical Nutrition* 5: 63–65.

Buchholz AC, Bartok C, Schoeller DA (2004) The validity of bioelectrical impedance models in clinical populations. *Nutrition in Clinical Practice* 19: 433.

Casati A, Muttini S, Leggieri C, Colombo S, Giorgi E, Torri G. (1998) Rapid turnover proteins in critically ill ICU patients. Negative acute phase proteins or nutritional indicators? *Minerva Anesthesiologica* 64: 345–350.

Chumlea WC, Guo S. (1992) Equations for predicting stature in white and black elderly individuals. *Journal of Gerontology* 47(6): M197–M203.

Chumlea W, Roche AF, Steinbaugh ML. (1985) Estimating stature from knee height for persons 60 to 90 years of age. *Journal of the American Geriatric Society* 33: 116–120.

Chumlea WC, Guo SS, Steinbaugh ML. (1994) Prediction of stature from knee height for black and whilte adults and children with application to mobility-impaired or handicapped persons. *Journal of the American Dietetic Association* 94: 1388–1391.

Conway JM, Yanovski SZ, Avila NA, Hubbard VS. (1995) Visceral adipose tissue differences in black and white women. *American Journal of Clinical Nutrition* 61: 765–771.

Dekkers J, van Wier MF, Hendriksen IJM, Twisk JWR, van Mechelen W. (2008) Accuracy of self-reported body weight, height and waist circumference in a Dutch overweight working population. *BMC Medical Research Methodology* 8: 69.

Department of Health. (2008) Weighing scales alerts. Available at www.dh.gov.uk/en/Publicationsandstatistics/Lettersandcirculars/Estatesalerts/DH_085720 Accessed 7 March 2013.

Desport JC, Preux PM, Bouteloup-Demange C, *et al.* (2003) Validation of bioelectrical impedance analysis in patients with amyotrophic lateral sclerosis. *American Journal of Clinical Nutrition* 77: 1179–1185.

Durnin JVGA, Wolmersley J. (1974) Body fat assessed from total body density and its estimation from skinfold thickness: measurements on 481 men and women aged from 16 to 72 years. *British Journal of Nutrition* 32: 77–97.

Elia M. (2003) *The 'MUST' Report: Nutritional screening of Adults: a multidisciplinary responsibility.* Malnutrition Advisory Group, A standing committee of BAPEN. Redditch: BAPEN.

Friedman AN, SZ Fadem SZ. (2010) Reassessment of Albumin as a Nutritional Marker in Kidney Disease. *Journal of the American Society of Nephrology* 21: 223–230.

Frisancho AR. (2008) *Anthropometric Standards: An Interactive Nutritional Reference of Body Size and Body Composition for Children and Adults*. Ann Arbor: The University of Michigan Press.

Gibney MJ, Lanham-New SA, Cassidy A, Vorster HH. (2009) *Introduction to Human Nutrition*, 2nd edn. Oxford: Wiley Blackwell.

Gibson RS. (2005) *Principles of Nutritional Assessment*, 2nd edn. Oxford: Oxford University Press.

Gray DS, Crider DS, Kelley C, Dickinson LC. (1985) Accuracy of recumbent height measurement. *Journal of Parenteral and Enteral Nutrition* 9: 712–715.

Griffith CDM, Clark RG. (1984) A comparison of the 'Sheffield' prognostic index with forearm muscle dynamometry in patients from Sheffield undergoing major abdominal and urological surgery. *Clinical Nutrition* 3: 147–151.

Gunnare NA, Silliman K, Neyman Morris M (2013) Accuracy of self-reported weight and role of gender, body mass index, weight satisfaction, weighing behavior, and physical activity among rural college students. *Body Image* 10: 406–410.

Heymsfield SB, Matthews D. (1994) Body composition: research and clinical advances. *Journal of Parenteral and Enteral Nutrition* 18: 91–103.

Heymsfield S, Lohman TG, Wang ZM, Going S. (2005) *Human Body Composition by Human Kinetics*. Illinois: Champaign.

International Diabetes Federation (2006) The IDF consensus worldwide definition of the metabolic syndrome. Available at www.idf.org. Accessed 7 March 2013.

James PT, Leach R, Kalamara E, Shayeghi M. (2001) The worldwide obesity epidemic. *Obesity Research* 9 (Suppl 4): 228S–233S.

Katch FI, Hortobagyi T. (1990) Validity of surface anthropometry to estimate upper-arm muscularity, including changes with body mass loss. *American Journal of Clinical Nutrition* 52: 591–595.

Klidjian AM, Foster KJ, Kammerling, RM, Cooper A, Karran SJ. (1980). Relation of anthropometric and dynamometric variables to serious post-operative complications. *BMJ* 281: 899–901.

Krause MV, Mahan LK. (1979) Assessment of nutritional status. In: *Nutrition and Diet Therapy*, 6th edn. Philadelphia: WB Saunders, pp. 220–241.

Kwok T, Whitelaw MN. (1991) The use of armspan in nutritional assessment of the elderly. *Journal of the American Geriatric Society* 39: 492–496.

Kyle UG, Bosaeus I, De Lorenzo AD, *et al.*; Composition of the ESPEN Working Group. (2004a) Bioelectrical impedance analysis – part 1: review of principles and methods. *Clinical Nutrition* 23: 1226–1243.

Kyle UG, Bosaeus I, De Lorenzo AD, *et al.*; ESPEN. (2004b) Bioelectrical impedance analysis – part 2: utilization in clinical practice. *Clinical Nutrition* 23: 1430–1453.

Lammersfeld CA, Gupta D, Dahlk S, *et al.* (2004) Bioelectrical impedance analysis (BIA) as a nutritional assessment tool in advanced colorectal cancer. *Journal of Clinical Oncology* 22 (14S): 6121.

Lean MEJ. (1998) *Clinical Handbook of Weight Management*. London: Martin Dunitz.

Lear SA, James PT, Ko GT, Kumanyika S. (2010) Appropriateness of waist circumference and waist-to-hip ratio cutoffs for different ethnic groups. *European Journal of Clinical Nutrition* 64(1): 42–61.

Madden AM, Tsikoura T, Stott DJ. (2012) The estimation of body height from ulna length in healthy adults from different ethnic groups. *Journal of Human Nutrition and Dietetics* 25: 121–128

McDowell MA, Fryar CD, Ogden CL, Flegal KM. (2008) Anthropometric Reference Data_for_Children and Adults: United States, 2003–2006. National Health Statistics Reports 10. Available at www.cdc.gov/nchs/data/nhsr/nhsr010.pdf Accessed 7 March 2013.

Mendenhall CL. (1992) Protein-calorie malnutrition in alcoholic liver disease. In: Watson RR, Watzl B (eds): *Nutrition and Alcohol*. Boca Raton: CRC Press, pp. 363–384.

National Institute for Health and Care Excellence (NICE) (2006a) *Nutrition Support in Adults: Oral Nutritional Support, Enteral Tube Feeding and Parenteral Nutrition*. Clinical Guideline 32. London: NICE.

National Institute for Health and Care Excellence (NICE). (2006b) *Obesity Guidance on the Prevention, Identification, Assessment and Management of Overweight and Obesity in Adults and Children*. Clinical Guideline 43. London: NICE.

Norman K, Stobäus N, Gonzalez MC, Schulzke JD, Pirlich M. (2011) Hand grip strength: outcome predictor and marker of nutritional status. *Clinical Nutrition* 30(2): 135–142.

Ortiz O, Russell M, Daley TL, Baumgartner RN. (1992) Differences in skeletal muscle and bone mineral mass between black and white females and their relevance to estimates of body composition. *American Journal of Clinical Nutrition* 55(1): 8–13.

Osterkamp LK. (1995) Current perspective on assessment of human body proportions of relevance to amputees. *Journal of the American Dietetic Association* 95(2): 215–218.

Pencharz PB, Azcue M. (1996) Use of bioelectrical impedance analysis measurements in the clinical management of malnutrition. *American Journal of Clinical Nutrition* 64: 485S–488S.

Prentice AM, Jebb SA. (2001) Beyond body mass index. *Obesity Reviews* 2(3): 141–147.

Reed DR, Price RA. (1998) Estimates of the heights and weights of family members: accuracy of informant reports. *International Journal of Obesity and Related Disorders* 22: 827–835.

Robinson MK, Trujillo EB, Mogensen KM, Rounds J, McManus K, Jacobs DO. (2003) Improving nutritional screening of hospitalized patients: The role of prealbumin. *Journal of Parenteral and Enteral Nutrition* 27: 389–395.

Rowland ML. (1990) Self-reported weight and height. *American Journal of Clinical Nutrition* 52: 1125–1133.

Schutte JE, Townsend EJ, Hugg J, Shoup RF, Malina RN, Blomquist GC. (1984) Density of lean mass is greater in blacks than in whites. *Journal of Applied Physiology* 56(6): 1647.

Scott A, Skerratt S, Adam S. (1998) *Nutrition for the Critically Ill: A Practical Handbook*. London: Arnold.

Seidell JC. (2010) Waist circumference and waist/hip ratio in relation to all-cause mortality, cancer and sleep apnea. *European Journal of Clinical Nutrition* 64: 35–41.

Shaw V, Lawson M. (2007) Nutritional assessment, dietary requirements and feed supplementation. In: Shaw V, Lawson M (eds) *Clinical Paediatric Dietetics*, 3rd edn. Oxford: Blackwell Science.

Shetty PS, James WPT. (1994) *Body Mass Index – A Measure of Chronic Energy Deficiency in Adults* (FAO Food and Nutrition Paper 56). Rome: Food and Agriculture Organization of the United Nations.

Scottish Intercollegiate Guidelines Network (SIGN). (1996) *Obesity in Scotland*. Edinburgh: SIGN, pp. 52–53.

Spencer EA, Appleby PN, Davey GK, Key TJ. (2002) Validity of self-reported height and weight in 4808 EPIC-Oxford participants. *Public Health Nutrition* 5: 561–565.

Thuluvath PJ, Triger DR. (1994) Evaluation of nutritional status by using anthropometry in adults with alcoholic and nonalcoholic liver disease. *American Journal of Clinical Nutrition* 60: 269–273.

Ulijaszek SJ, Kerr DA. (1999) Anthropometric measurement error and the assessment of nutritional status. *British Journal of Nutrition* 82: 165–177.

Wada K, Tamakoshi K, Tsunekawa T, *et al.* (2005)Validity of self-reported height and weight in a Japanese workplace population. *International Journal of Obesity (London)* 29(9): 1093–1099.

Wang J, Thornton JC, Russell M, Burastero S, Heymsfield S, Pierson RN Jr. (1994) Asians have lower body mass index (BMI) but higher percent body fat than do whites: comparisons of anthropometric measurements. *American Journal of Clinical Nutrition* 60: 23–28.

Webster-Gandy J, Madden A, Holdsworth M. (2011) *Oxford Handbook of Nutrition and Dietetics*, 2nd edn. Oxford: Oxford Univeristy Press.

World Health Organization (WHO). (1995) *Physical Status: The Use and Interpretation of Anthropometry*. Report of a WHO Expert Committee. Technical Report Service 854. Geneva: WHO.

World Health Organization (WHO). (1998) *Obesity: Preventing and Managing the Global Epidemic*. Report of a WHO consultation on obesity. Geneva: WHO.

World Health Organization Expert consultation. (2004) Appropriate body mass index for Asian Populations and its implications for policy and intervention strategies. *Lancet* 363: 157–164.

World Health Organization (WHO). (2008) Waist circumference and waist–hip ratio. Report of a WHO expert consultation. Available at www.who.int. Accessed 16 February 2013.

Zillikens MC, Conway JM. (1990) Anthropometry in blacks: applicability of generalized skinfold equations and differences in fat patterning between blacks and whites. *American Journal of Clinical Nutrition* 52: 45–51.

SECTION 2

2.3

Dietary assessment

Ailsa Welch

Key points

- A wide variety of methods are available for measuring dietary intake.

- Methods for estimating dietary intake in individuals can be retrospective measures, e.g. 24-hour recalls, diet histories or food frequency questionnaires, or current measures, e.g. weighed or estimated food records.

- The differences between methods and the impact of measurement error need to be considered when intending to use dietary methods.

- It is essential to understand the advantages and limitations of dietary assessment methods both for use in clinical practice and when reading and interpreting the scientific literature.

only talk about individual's intake

Dietary assessment methods are used for a variety of purposes from individual assessments in clinical situations, through to use in epidemiology. In epidemiology they are used to estimate intakes of populations and establish associations between nutrition and disease. They are also used as a basis for developing dietary guidelines and health policy, for monitoring change in intervention studies and for monitoring the effectiveness of public health interventions. Dietary assessments are traditionally used to estimate intakes of foods and nutrients, but more recent interest has arisen in estimating intake of bioactive phytochemicals, e.g. flavonoids, additives and contaminants. Ideally, assessment methods should have a low burden on respondents and investigators, and be rapid and cheap, but also result in accurate, precise data with minimal measurement error.

There are a number of dietary assessment methods for measuring food consumption at the national, household and individual level. This chapter focuses on assessment methods suitable for individual intakes. At the national level, food balance sheets can be used to assess dietary intakes. Household level methods include the food account method, inventory method, household record method and list recall methods, and further information on these methods can be found in Gibson (2005).

Table 2.3.1 describes the advantages and limitations of the main types of dietary assessment methods used for individuals. Although many methods are available for estimating dietary intake in individuals, they can mainly be divided into two types; retrospective measures of intake, such as 24-hour recalls (24 HR), diet history or food frequency questionnaires (FFQs), or current measures of

intake, such as weighed or estimated food records. Qualitative information is available from all methods, but quantitative estimates for nutrient consumption are possible only if data for weighed or estimated portion weights are available.

Weighed records, estimated food records, 24 HR and dietary histories are the most intensive methods. The quantity of food consumed may be weighed directly or estimated using household measures such as cups and spoons, photographs, standard units or average portions (Food Standards Agency, 2001; Nelson *et al.*, 1997). Data for portion sizes should be derived from weighed intakes, government surveys and research groups in populations similar to the one to be studied. Food models/replicas (three dimensional models representing foods) can also be used, particularly in clinical practice.

More recently, methods are being developed that utilise photographs of portion size recorded with mobile phone or digital camera technology (Penn *et al.*, 2010). For all methods the amount consumed can be measured or described either including or excluding wastage material usually discarded during food preparation, e.g., outer leaves and peel from vegetables or bones from cuts of meat. A number of newer methods for recording food intake are being developed involving online methods.

Number of days of recording

The number of days of report required for adequate measures of nutrients using 24 HRs, weighed or estimated records varies depending on the day to day variability of nutrient consumption (Nelson *et al.*, 1989;

Table 2.3.1 Characteristics of dietary assessment methods

Method	Advantages	Limitations
Retrospective methods		
24-hour recall (24 HR) (single or multiple days)	Not reliant on long term memory; interview length 20–45 minutes	Single 24 HRs can be used for group assessments but not for estimating intake of individuals
Diet history	Respondent literacy not required	Report of past intake is influenced by current diet; trained interviewers required
Food frequency questionnaire (FFQ) (if portion estimates included, termed semiquantitative FFQ)	Useful for large sample sizes; relatively straightforward to complete	Need to be developed for specific population group to ensure important food items are covered and requires updating to accommodate changes to supply of foods; responses governed by cognitive, numeric, and literacy abilities of respondents, also by length and complexity of the food list. Not easy to develop for clinical practice since specific computer programs need to be developed.
Short frequency questionnaires	Targeted to specific food types, administration simpler and easier than long questionnaires	Need to be developed for specific population group to ensure questions are relevant
Current methods		
Weighed food record (weighed inventory technique)	No requirement for memory retrieval as it records current intake; food intake weighed so estimates of quantity consumed not required	Literate, cooperative respondents required as burden is high; possible that respondents change usual eating patterns to simplify the record; high data entry costs
Food record with estimated weights	No requirement for memory retrieval as it records current intake	Literate, cooperative respondents required as burden is high; possible that respondents change usual eating patterns to simplify the record
Duplicate analysis	Greater accuracy	Very labour intensive; requires laboratory to do food composition analysis
Records using electronic equipment, e.g. mobile phones, digital cameras	Visual records of foods. Avoids need for paper records. Data can be sent to investigators electronically	Currently involves labour intensive programs to convert to usable data, i.e. quantities and types of foods, although systems are in development to deal with this. Limited use in older people who experience difficulties with using newer technology

Mennen *et al.*, 2002; Lanigan *et al.*, 2004). The number of days is partly dependent on the variation in nutrient concentration in foodstuffs. The concentration of macro-nutrients such as protein and carbohydrate in foods varies less than that of micronutrients such as vitamin C or iron. The number of days required to classify adult individuals into the correct third of the percentage distribution for usual intake for 80% of individuals has been calculated (Nelson *et al.*, 1989; Mennen *et al.*, 2002). Up to 7 days of recall are required for energy, protein, sugars and calcium. Nutrients with greater variability, including alcohol, vitamin C, riboflavin, and iron, require between 4 and 14 days of records. Fewer days of data collection are required to capture habitual diet in children (Lanigan *et al.*, 2004). More recent estimates of the number of days to estimate energy intake (using the doubly labelled water technique) suggest that 3 days of record are optimal of which 1 day should be a weekend day (Ma *et al.*, 2009).

Dietary assessment methods

24-hour recalls

Twenty-four-hour recalls determine intake during the preceding 24 hours and can be recorded on paper or using interactive computerised software (Slimani *et al.*, 1999). Day to day variability in nutrient intake is large and a single day will not categorise individuals correctly within a distribution of intake. Particular issues are the capture of episodic (infrequently eaten) foods such as fish and liver; therefore, single 24 HRs are better used for group assessments than estimates for individuals. However, multiple 24 HRs can be used to overcome this problem. Newer methods of online recording of 24 HRs are under development. The 24 HR method is useful for assessment in clinical situations, but the difficulty with assessment and accurately reporting intake due to the variation in nutrient concentration of foodstuffs needs consideration. This will affect the number of days required to obtain adequate measures of nutrient intakes.

Diet history

The diet history consists either of an interview administered 24 HR or establishing usual eating pattern over a 1-week period, followed by a frequency questionnaire to provide additional information. The dietary history provides a representative pattern of usual intake and is interview administered only. Diet histories are traditionally used in clinical practice and may take up to 1.5 hours to complete.

Food frequency questionnaires

Food frequency questionnaires (FFQs) consist of a list of specific foods or food types associated with frequency of consumption to record average consumption over the previous month or year. They are termed semiquantitative if portions are included. Food frequency questionnaires are thought to provide estimates of habitual intake and are widely used in nutritional epidemiology (Welch et al., 2005; Cade et al. 2004). They need to be specific to a population group to ensure coverage of important foods and the population must be literate and numerate, as some mathematical ability is necessary to calculate relative frequencies (Smith, 1993). Factors influencing response to FFQs are the length and complexity of the food list and current diet (Smith, 1993). For clinical use it is necessary to develop specific software and databases to obtain nutrients and therefore record methods are likely to be preferable (Welch et al., 2005).

Short frequency questionnaires

Short frequency questionnaires have been developed to estimate intakes of specific foods or nutrients and can be useful in clinical practice to determine where eating habits require change; examples are the Dietary Instrument for Nutrition Education (DINE) and the 5 A DAY Community Evaluation Tool (FACET) questionnaires (Roe et al., 1994; Ashfield-Watt et al., 2007; Welch et al., 2006).

Weighed food record inventory and estimated food record

For weighed food records (WRs) all food and drink consumed over a period is weighed and recorded on forms or in booklets, with details of food type and method of preparation, to obtain consumption over a period of days. Portable scales need to be supplied. Leftover food should be weighed and deducted. The recommended time period for records is 4–7 days or more, although the number of days depends on the nutrient of interest, study population and objectives of the study. As some populations have different eating habits at weekends, weekend days should be included proportionately. For estimated food records all foods consumed over a period of days are recorded with details of food type, method of preparation and estimated portion sizes. If recorded over 7 days, this is often called a 7-day diary.

Both these methods have a high respondent burden and need cooperative, literate respondents. Respondents require training in the level of detail needed to describe foods. It is also possible that respondents may change usual eating patterns to simplify the process of the record and may also find this method tedious. It is also beneficial to include a review of weighed records during the period of recording either after the first day or at the end.

Duplicate sample technique

Duplicate samples of all foods consumed are made and the nutrient content analysed chemically. This method is used for metabolic studies and, though providing greater accuracy than other methods, its use is only feasible for certain purposes. Studies are conducted in hospital metabolic units or research centres; they are expensive, time consuming and require considerable technical support.

Use of methods in clinical practice versus research

Dietary methodology for clinical practice requires rapid assessments of nutritional intake in order to prescribe dietary change or to improve nutritional status. Traditionally, 24 HRs of usual intake or diet histories have been used for this purpose. Food frequency questionnaires and weighed or estimated food records are not generally used due to the more intensive burden on respondents and on the resources required for coding and processing the data. For research purposes a number of methods may be used from FFQs to multiple 24 HRs. When designing a study, it is advisable to obtain expert advice to decide on the optimum method.

Recall of remote diet – current intake biases recall of past diet

When designing studies or reading the literature, dietitians need to be aware that recall of diet in the remote past is heavily influenced by current dietary habit. Studies have found that the correlations between recalled past diet and current diet are higher than the correlations between actual past diet and recall of past diet (Willett, 1998). The onset of diseases such as cancer may affect appetite and dietary assessment, as recall of remote diet is strongly related to current diet. Therefore, studies where diet was measured prior to the onset of disease are less likely to suffer from bias than, for instance, case–control studies in which the diet of cases with disease is compared with controls.

Use of data and conversion of reported intake to nutrients and food types

Qualitative data

Dietary method data can be used qualitatively, e.g. during the process of reviewing nutritional intake for the purpose of dietary treatment, as in clinical practice. However, the majority of uses of dietary methods are targeted towards quantitative analyses.

Quantitative data

Food composition databases, data entry and nutrient calculation systems

The data collected by dietary methods are converted into food and nutrient consumption by calculating the amount of food eaten and linking this to a database with values for the nutrient composition of foods. The governments of many countries provide the databases of nutrient composition of foods. The UK National Nutrient Database consists of *McCance and Widdowson's The Composition of Foods* (2002) and its supplements. It is essential to read the information distributed with the printed or electronic versions of databases to determine the uses and limitations of the data (see Chapter 2.4).

Nutrient databases vary in the coverage and comprehensiveness of the foods and nutrients, and in the conversion factors used for certain nutrients. Care should be taken when comparing values from different sets of food tables because the definition and expression of nutrients may not always be the same. Different conversion factors may have been used to prepare the values, e.g. to calculate protein from nitrogen or to convert the major nutrients to energy. The same nutrient may be quoted in different ways, e.g. carbohydrate may be expressed as monosaccharide equivalents, actual weights or by difference. In the UK food tables, carbohydrate is expressed as monosaccharide equivalents but for food labelling purposes carbohydrate should be provided as actual weight.

The nutrient values provided in food tables are generally averages of representative samples of foods or selected values from literature surveys. However, like any other biological material, the composition of food can vary considerably and so the values in food tables are only representative of the true biological range of values and should not be considered as having the accuracy of atomic weights. Values in nutrient composition databases are expressed as either per 100g of food or per common household measure. Most up to date information in the UK, European, US and international nutrient databases can be found at the Food Standards Agency (FSA) (www.food.gov.uk), European Food Information Resource Network (EuroFIR) (www.eurofir.org), USA Department of Agriculture http://ndb.nal.usda.gov) and the Food and Agriculture Organization of the United Nations (www.fao.org/infoods).

Several steps are involved in calculating nutrient intake (also known as coding or processing). The first is to choose the item in the database that corresponds most closely with the food consumed. If the food consumed is not in the database, a suitable alternative can be chosen by considering food type, general characteristics and likely nutrient profile. Once the food has been chosen, the nutrient composition of the food quoted in the database is multiplied by the amount of food eaten. To calculate daily intake for an individual, the contribution of each food is calculated and all the foods for a day summated. If more than one day's data have been collected, it is usual to calculate the average for the number of days recorded. Although it is possible to compute intake by hand, using a calculator and a printed copy of a nutrient database, this is very labour intensive and in practice, has been superseded by computerisation for most purposes. A number of computerised data entry systems and nutrient calculation programs exist to calculate nutrient intakes (Welch *et al.*, 2001). Prior to purchasing a new

entry system, it is important to know on which version or food composition database it is based.

Dietitians should be aware that the UK food tables are not adequate for estimating salt intake because the nutrient intakes for recipe or composite dishes do not include salt and therefore calculations are systematic underestimates.

Estimated food quantities

To obtain quantitative information for nutrients or food groups, actual or estimated food weights are used. For methods using estimated food weights, values also need to be found for the foods described, such as standard units, average portions or household measures. Sources of data are national publications, surveys of weighed dietary assessments, and food manufacturers. Data may also be included in nutrient calculation programs.

Additional sources of nutrients

Proprietary medicines may contain sources of nutrients, and vitamin and mineral supplements can contain considerable amounts of nutrients. Therefore, they should be taken into account when assessing total nutrient intakes (Lentjes *et al.*, 2010). Current estimates of prevalence of supplement intakes are around 40% in the UK population aged over 40 years (Lentjes *et al.*, 2010).

Measurement error

Measurement error can be defined as the difference between the measured exposure (or measure of dietary assessment) and the true exposure; it is now known that there is measurement error associated with using dietary methods. Measurement error reduces the likelihood that true values have been measured with accuracy and in nutritional epidemiology, associations between dietary intake and disease outcomes will be affected (Schatzkin & Kipnis, 2004). As the proportion of measurement error increases, the scale of the relationship relating diet to disease status will tend towards no relationship. Overall the effect of measurement error would be to misclassify an individual within a range of intake.

The existence of measurement error also impacts on the interpretation of the scientific literature. For instance, it is known that FFQs tend to produce systematically greater estimates of fruit and vegetable intake and of vitamin C intake than record methods such as 7-day diaries (Dehghan *et al.*, 2007). As a result, fruit and vegetable intake for individuals and populations will be overestimated using an FFQ; more individuals measured with this method will appear to have sufficient intakes than if a record method had been used.

The technique of validation can be used to estimate measurement error. Although full detail of the impact, scale and detection of measurement error is beyond the scope of this chapter, an awareness of the differences between dietary methods and the potential pitfalls when using them is helpful to clinicians in interpreting the scientific literature.

Methods of detecting measurement error

There are four major methods of detecting measurement error:

1. *Comparison with other diet methods*, but this is not advisable since individuals report in the same way with all methods and the errors are correlated (Black & Cole, 2001; Kipnis *et al.*, 2003).
2. *Predictor reference methods*, such as the Goldberg equations, or percentile cut points to detect energy misreporting and potentially statistical model the effects of misreporting (Stubbs, 2002).
3. *Biomarkers* (biological markers) in blood or urine, quantitative recovery biomarkers (quantitative estimates of intake over a specific time period) and concentration biomarkers (measure relative concentrations over a distribution) are thought to be independent of errors when measuring intake (Potischman & Freudenheim, 2003). Examples of quantitative markers are urine nitrogen excretion over 24 hours (to estimate protein intake) and energy expenditure measured using the doubly labelled water technique (DLW). Examples of concentration markers are plasma concentrations of n-3 polyunsaturated fatty acids and fish consumption (Welch *et al.*, 2006).
4. *Comparison with disease risk biomarkers*, e.g. saturated fat and low density lipoprotein (LDL) cholesterol (Bingham *et al.*, 2008).

Examples of validation studies are those performed within EPIC Europe and the Observing Protein and Energy Nutrition Study (OPEN) in the US (Kipnis *et al.*, 2003; Slimani *et al.*, 2003).

Although biomarkers are useful in the detection of measurement error, it should be noted that a number of factors influence their interaction with nutrition, e.g. differences in gender or genetics and homeostatic or behavioural influences. Not all associations are linear, e.g. vitamin C concentrations in the blood plateau since additional concentrations are excreted, and smoking impacts on circulating concentrations of vitamin C.

Sources of measurement error in dietary assessment

Sources of measurement error when using dietary assessment are many. They may occur both during data collection and processing. Systematic bias, interviewer bias, recall bias and social desirability bias have been identified, but there are likely to be other sources of error. Bias can be defined as the modification of a method of measurement by a factor that influences the measurement in one or more directions. Measurement error associated with dietary methods may consist of one or more types of error.

Systematic bias is a systematic mismeasurement of data and can occur, for instance, if an interviewer consistently fails to use questions to probe for consumption of snacks and additional foods. If systematic bias is identified, it can be overcome by interviewer training and monitoring interviewers.

The behaviour of interviewers can influence the response of interviewees or clients and introduce interviewer bias. It is important to develop rapport between interviewers and respondents and for questions to be asked in an open ended, neutral manner without value judgements.

Social desirability bias can influence dietary assessment methods as respondents strive to report what they think is required, not what was actually consumed, e.g. reporting less alcohol consumption or greater consumption of foods with perceived health benefits, such as fish, fruit or vegetables. This is likely to be the cause of misreporting, under reporting or low energy reporting, which occurs in certain respondents and can affect clinical practice.

Conclusion

A wide variety of methods for measuring dietary intake exist and it is essential to understand their advantages and limitations, both for use in clinical practice and when reading and interpreting the scientific literature.

Further reading

Cameron ME, Van Staveren WA (1988) *Manual on Methodology for Food Consumption Studies*. Oxford: Oxford University Press.

Feskanich D, Sielaff BH, Chong K, Buzzard IM. (1989) Computerized collection and analysis of dietary assessment information. *Computer Methods and Programs in Biomedicine* 30: 47–57.

Gibson RS. (2005) *Principles of Nutritional Assessment*, 2nd edn. Oxford: Oxford University Press.

Margetts BM, Nelson M. (1997) *Design Concepts in Nutritional Epidemiology*, 2nd edn. Oxford: Oxford University Press.

Pao EM, Cypel YS. (1996) Estimation of dietary assessment. In: Zeigler EH, Filer LJ, eds. *1996. Present Knowledge in Nutrition*, 7th edn. Washington, DC: ILSI Press, pp. 498–507.

Potischman N, Freudenheim JL. (2003) Biomarkers of nutritional exposure and nutritional status: an overview. *Journal of Nutrition* 133 (Suppl 3): 873S–874S.

Thompson FE, Byers T. (1994) Dietary assessment resource manual. *Journal of Nutrition* 124: 11S.

Willett W. (1998) *Nutritional Epidemiology*, 2nd edn. Oxford: Oxford University Press.

Internet resources

EuroFIR Project website with information on European food composition databases   www.eurofir.net

FAO – INFOODS information for nutrient database compilers and suppliers   www.fao.org

USA Department of Agriculture (USDA) National Nutrient Database for Standard Reference Release 24   www.ars.usda.gov/Services/docs.htm?docid=8964

References

Ashfield-Watt PA, Welch AA, Godward S, Bingham SA. (2007) Effect of a pilot community intervention on fruit and vegetable intakes: use of FACET (Five-a-day Community Evaluation Tool). *Public Health and Nutrition* 10: 671–680.

Bingham S, Luben R, Welch A, *et al.* (2008) Associations between dietary methods and biomarkers, and between fruits and vegetables and risk of ischaemic heart disease, in the EPIC Norfolk Cohort Study. *International Journal of Epidemiology* 37: 978–987.

Black AE, Cole TJ. (2001) Biased over- or under-reporting is characteristic of individuals whether over time or by different assessment methods. *Journal of the American Dietetic Association,* 101: 70–80.

Cade JE, Burley VJ, Warm DL, Thompson RL, Margetts BM. (2004) Food-frequency questionnaires: a review of their design, validation and utilisation. *Nutrition Research and Review* 17: 5–22.

Dehghan M, Akhtar-danesh N, Mcmillan CR, Thabane L. (2007) Is plasma vitamin C an appropriate biomarker of vitamin C intake? A systematic review and meta-analysis. *Nutrition Journal* 6: 41.

Food Standards Agency (2001) *Food Portion Sizes.* London: The Stationery Office.

Gibson RS. (2005) *Principles of Nutritional Assessment.* Oxford: Oxford University Press.

Kipnis V, Subar AF, Midthune D *et al.*(2003) Structure of dietary measurement error: results of the OPEN biomarker study. *American Journal of Epidemiology* 158: 14–21; discussion 22–26.

Lanigan JA, Wells JC, Lawson MS, Cole TJ, Lucas A. (2004) Number of days needed to assess energy and nutrient intake in infants and young children between 6 months and 2 years of age. *European Journal of Clinical Nutrition* 58: 745–750.

Lentjes MA, Bhaniani A, Mulligan AA, Khaw KT, Welch AA. (2010) Developing a database of vitamin and mineral supplements (ViMiS) for the Norfolk arm of the European Prospective Investigation into Cancer (EPIC-Norfolk). *Public Health Nutrition* 13: 1–13.

Ma Y, Olendzki BC, Pagoto SL., *et al.* (2009) Number of 24-hour diet recalls needed to estimate energy intake. *Annals of Epidemiology* 19: 553–559.

McCance RA, Widdowson EM. (2002) *McCance and Widdowson's The Composition of Foods*, 6th ed. Cambridge: Royal Society of Chemistry.

Mennen LI, Bertrais S, Galan P, Arnault N, Potier de Couray G, Hercberg S. (2002) The use of computerised 24 h dietary recalls in the French SU.VI.MAX Study: number of recalls required. *Europea Journal of Clinical Nutrition* 56: 659–665.

Nelson M, Black AE, Morris JA, Cole TJ. (1989) Between- and within-subject variation in nutrient intake from infancy to old age: estimating the number of days required to rank dietary intakes with desired precision. *American Journal of Clinical Nutrition* 50: 155–167.

Nelson M, Atkinson M, Meyer J. (1997) *A Photographic Atlas of Food Portion Sizes.* London:, MAFF Publications.

Penn L, Boeing H, Boushey CJ, *et al.* (2010) Assessment of dietary intake: NuGO symposium report. *Genes and Nutrition* 5: 205–213.

Potischman N, Freudenheim JL. (2003) Biomarkers of nutritional exposure and nutritional status: an overview. *Journal of Nutrition* 133 (Suppl 3): 873S–874S.

Roe L, Strong C, Whiteside C, Neil A, Mant D. (1994) Dietary intervention in primary care: validity of the DINE method for diet assessment. *Family Practice* 11: 375–381.

Schatzkin A, Kipnis V. (2004) Could exposure assessment problems give us wrong answers to nutrition and cancer questions? *Journal of the National Cancer Institute* 96: 1564–1565.

Slimani N, Deharveng G, Charrondiere RU, *et al.* (1999) Structure of the standardized computerized 24-h diet recall interview used as reference method in the 22 centers participating in the EPIC project. European Prospective Investigation into Cancer and Nutrition. *Computer Methods and Programs in Biomedicine* 58: 251–266.

Slimani N, Bingham S, Runswick S, *et al.* (2003) Group level validation of protein intakes estimated by 24-hour diet recall and dietary questionnaires against 24-hour urinary nitrogen in the European Prospective Investigation into Cancer and Nutrition (EPIC) calibration study. *Cancer Epidemiology, Biomarkers and Prevention* 12: 784–795.

Smith AF. (1993) Cognitive psychological issues of relevance to the validity of dietary reports. *European Journal of Clinical Nutrition* 47 (Suppl 2): S6–18.

Stubbs J. (2002) Detecting and modelling MIS-reporting of food intake in adults. Available at www.foodbase.org.uk/results.php?f_category_id=&f_report_id=289.

Welch AA, McTaggart A, Mulligan AA, *et al.* (2001) DINER (Data Into Nutrients for Epidemiological Research) – a new data-entry program for nutritional analysis in the EPIC-Norfolk cohort and the 7-day diary method. *Public Health and Nutrition* 4: 1253–1265.

Welch AA, Luben R, Khaw KT, Bingham SA. (2005) The CAFE computer program for nutritional analysis of the EPIC-Norfolk food frequency questionnaire and identification of extreme nutrient values. *Journal of Human Nutrition and Dietetics* 18: 99–116.

Welch AA, Bingham SA, Ive J, *et al.* (2006) Dietary fish intake and plasma phospholipid n-3 polyunsaturated fatty acid concentrations in men and women in the European Prospective Investigation into Cancer-Norfolk United Kingdom cohort. *American Journal of Clinical Nutrition* 84: 1330–1339.

Willett W. (1998) *Nutritional Epidemiology, 2nd edn.* Oxford: Oxford University Press.

Food composition tables and databases

Edwige Landais and Michelle Holdsworth

Key points

- Food tables are a vital resource, but to avoid errors from their use, it is essential to understand their strengths and limitations.

- The composition of a particular food can vary as a result of differences in plant and animal genetics, strain and breed variety, farming practices, soil quality, climate, storage conditions and the way in which food has been processed, manufactured or cooked.

- Food tables do not take account of bioavailability (the extent to which a nutrient present in a food will be absorbed).

- In the UK, food composition data are recorded in a National Nutrient Databank maintained by the Food Standards Agency and published in book form as *McCance and Widdowson's The Composition of Foods* or electronically.

Food composition data provide information on the nutritional composition of foods and are available in print (referred to as food composition tables) and computerised formats (food composition databases). Food composition tables are generally used to calculate the food intake of individuals and groups from information gathered during dietary assessment (see Chapter 2.3). They are used in different settings, including clinical practice, research, health promotion and the food and agriculture industry, as shown in Table 2.4.1.

Data in food composition databases come from different sources:

- Original analytical values obtained from chemical analysis of food samples.
- Analytical values from scientific literature or food labels for branded foods.
- Imputed values derived from analytical values of a similar food.
- Calculated values derived from recipes using yield and nutrient retention factors.
- Borrowed values taken from other tables or databases.
- Presumed values which are presumed as being null or at a certain level.

National food tables

UK food tables

Tables of food composition have been published in the UK since the 1920s, stimulated by concerns over food shortages in the First World War (Church, 2006). They were continued by the pioneering work of McCance and Widdowson, initially conducted under the auspices of the Medical Research Council and subsequently the Ministry of Agriculture, Fisheries and Food (MAFF). In 1987 MAFF, in conjunction with the Royal Society of Chemistry, began the production of a computerised UK National Nutrient Databank (UKNND) from which the fifth edition of *McCance and Widdowson's The Composition of Foods* (Holland *et al.*, 1991a) and a number of detailed supplements were produced. In 2000, responsibility for the maintenance of the UKNND was transferred to the Food Standards Agency (FSA), which published the most recent sixth summary paper edition in 2002.

The printed form of the summary edition of *McCance and Widdowson's The Composition of Foods* (FSA, 2002) is widely used; however, it should be appreciated that, whilst convenient, the single volume edition does not contain the complete set of data available, but only a subset of foods and nutrients. The most comprehensive information is contained within the separately published supplements, as shown in Table 2.4.2, and a complete collection of these should be regarded as the definitive UK food tables. Most of these are now in electronic form and have been integrated into the UKNND (www .food.gov.uk), and are regularly updated as part of a rolling programme of food analysis and analytical reports.

A range of nutrient analysis software programs using the UKNND is available for dietitians and nutritionists (see Chapter 2.3). Some less sophisticated nutrient analysis software programs, particularly those designed for the general public or schools which comprise summarised data derived from the main food tables, need to be used with caution. Data for groups of foods may either be averaged or confined to a few selected options, e.g. data for

Table 2.4.1 Role of food composition tables

Use	Clinical practice	Health education and promotion	Research	Food and or agriculture industry
Assessing nutritional status at individual, community and national levels	√	√	√	
Preparing educational materials	√	√		√
Designing therapeutic diets, e.g. hospitals, schools	√		√	
Devising food and nutrition labelling				√
Assessing the diet–disease link	√		√	
Developing food products and recipes				√
Monitoring food and nutrient availability		√	√	√
Developing food and nutrient guidelines	√	√	√	
Monitoring food legislation and safety – consumer protection		√		√
Completing missing values in a data set	√	√	√	√

Table 2.4.2 UK food tables and supplements

Single volume summary	
McCance and Widdowson's The Composition of Foods 6th edition	FSA (2002)
Supplements	
Amino acid composition and fatty acid composition	Paul et al. (1980)
Immigrant foods	Tan et al. (1985)
Cereals and cereal products	Holland et al. (1988)
Milk products and eggs	Holland et al. (1989)
Vegetables, herbs and spices	Holland et al. (1991b)
Fruit and nuts	Holland et al. (1992a)
Vegetable dishes	Holland (1992b)
Fish and fish products	Holland et al. (1993)
Miscellaneous foods	Chan et al. (1994)
Meat, poultry and game	Chan et al. (1995)
Meat products and dishes	Chan et al. (1996)
Fatty acids	MAFF (1998)
Others	
Foods commonly consumed by South Asians	Judd et al. (2000)

Details of the analysis of specific food products and nutrients, e.g. salt in bread, are available at www.food.gov.uk.

meat may be confined to a few possible choices from the hundreds cited in the main food tables. Dietary estimates based on such generalised figures can be misleading.

Food tables used in other countries

In order to be useful and accurate, food tables need to reflect the foods consumed in the culture in which they are used. Dietary investigations carried out in other parts of the world should use the appropriate local data. Many other countries worldwide produce national food com-

position tables. Several European Union countries publish food composition tables, and the first European food composition table was published in Germany in the 1800s (Church, 2006). The USA also began producing food composition tables in the 1800s and has continued to produce widely accessible electronic food tables (www.ars.usda .gov). In the late 1970s, the Center for Food Safety and Applied Nutrition (CFSAN) of the United States Food and Drug Administration (FDA) developed a standardised system for describing food. This system, called LanguaL (Langua aLimentaria) (www.langual.org), facilitates links to many different food databases and enables data exchange of over 40 000 food products so far.

In 1984, the United Nations University's Food and Nutrition Programme set up the International Network of Food Data Systems (INFOODS), coordinated by the Food and Agriculture Organization of the United Nations (FAO), to improve the quality of food data and also worldwide access. The website of INFOODS (www.fao.org/infoods) provides information about all existing food composition tables, some of which are directly accessible through the website. More recently, a European initiative, called the European Food Information Resource project (EuroFIR), was established. The main objective of this was to deliver a comprehensive and validated European databank for nutrients and bioactive compounds for 27 European Countries (www.eurofir.net). In the USA, the Department of Agriculture maintains the nutrient database (www .ars.usda.gov).

Food tables are an extremely valuable resource, but it is important to understand their limitations and some of the associated problems.

Derivation of food table data

Before using food table data, it is essential to read the introduction explaining how the values in the tables were derived. This is particularly important if food composition data from more than one source, e.g. food labelling information, or food tables from other countries are used alongside standard food table data, because the definition and expression of the nutrients may not be the same. The following factors should be considered when using food composition tables or databases.

Analytical methodology

Different analytical techniques can be used to obtain estimates of the same nutrient. Historically, food analysis consisted of determining the percentage of water, fat, nitrogen and ash (minerals) in a food. Protein content was derived by multiplying the percentage of nitrogen by 6.25 as protein is on average 16% nitrogen. While the latter is still widely used in food composition tables and databases, it is now recognised that the amount of nitrogen depends on the protein source (FAO, 2003). Carbohydrate content was estimated by difference; the percentage of other nutrients was calculated and carbohydrate was assumed to be the remaining percentage needed to give 100%. This derived figure for carbohydrate included the contribution from dietary fibre or other dietary components.

More recently, chemical analyses methods have become more sophisticated, so different types of sugars (glucose, fructose, galactose, sucrose, maltose, lactose and oligosaccharides) and complex carbohydrates (dextrins, starch and glycogen), amino acids and fatty acids, as well as individual minerals and vitamins can now be determined. Information on manufactured foods not included in the food tables can increasingly be obtained from food labels or food manufacturers, but much commercial food analysis is still carried out using simpler analytical techniques. The use of different methodologies will result in different estimates of nutrient content.

- *Carbohydrate* may be determined as monosaccharide equivalents, actual weights or by difference as described earlier. Monosaccharide equivalents, the usual form of expression in UK food tables, result in slightly higher estimates of carbohydrate content (due to the fact that disaccharides and polysaccharides gain water when hydrolysed) than when expressed as actual weight, as on most food labels. Direct determination of carbohydrates is used in the UKNND.
- *Dietary fibre* can be analysed using different methods that give differing estimates of fibre content. The McCance and Widdowson tables and the UKNND give figures for non-starch polysaccharides (NSP) based on the Englyst method (Englyst and Cummings, 1988). However, the food industry measures fibre by the AOAC enzymatic gravimetric method, which is now recommended for food labelling purposes. The AOAC method usually gives much higher estimates of fibre content, particularly for cereal foods because it includes lignin (or substances measuring as lignin) and resistant starch. The sixth edition of *McCance and Widdowson* (FSA, 2002) includes a comparative table of the fibre content of a limited number of foods measured by both the Englyst and AOAC methods.
- Many *vitamins* are composites of substances with variable degrees of activity and either some or all of these may be cited depending on the type of analysis performed. For example, vitamin A may be expressed as retinol and beta-carotene separately, or as retinol equivalents. Different units may also be used, e.g. micrograms or International Units (IU).

Energy conversion factors used to calculate data

The energy content of food may be measured by bomb calorimetry, but not all food energy is metabolisable; therefore, conversion factors which account for this are used to calculate the energy yield. Atwater and colleagues derived these factors from meticulous human studies over a 100 years ago (Atwater & Benedict, 1902). It is important to remember that slightly different Atwater factor systems may be used and the energy content of foods may vary between McCance and Widdowson tables or the UKNND and those required for food labelling declarations (Table 2.4.3).

The two components of vitamin A are given separately as retinol (RET) and carotene (CAREQU). Retinol is expressed as the weight of all *trans* retinol equivalent, i.e. the sum of all *trans* retinol plus contributions from the other forms after correction to account for their relative activities.

Sampling procedure

Food composition data are derived from a sample of foods and, therefore, their accuracy depends on how

Table 2.4.3 Energy conversion factors (source: Webster-Gandy 2011, table 1.2, p. 11. Reproduced with permission of Oxford University Press)

Nutrient	kcal/g	kJ/g	Comments
Protein	4	17	For food labelling purposes, protein content is derived by multiplying the nitrogen content in all foods by 6.25 UK food tables use specific conversion factors for different types of foods
Fat	9	37	The original Atwater factor was 8.9 kcal, but the lower kJ figure is preferable
Carbohydrate	3.75	16	If carbohydrate is expressed directly or by difference, 4 kcal/g is used, which is the figure used on food labels Values for available carbohydrate are expressed as monosaccharides
Sugar alcohols	2.4	10	Food labeling uses mean value
Ethyl alcohol	7	29	
Glycerol	4.31	18	Complete metabolism assumed

representative the sample is; the UK food tables are designed to be as representative as possible. Significant numbers of food samples are purchased from different retail outlets and pooled before analysis. Market share information is used to assess which brands of a particular type of food are included, and recipes are chosen to be as similar as possible to those used in the normal domestic setting. Other sources of food composition data may not be based on such high standards. Details of the samples used in analysis are given for each food item in the tables and database.

Currency of data

Food composition tables need to be regularly updated for the following reasons:

- *New manufactured foods* are constantly developed and the composition of existing ones may change as a result of product reformulation, altered manufacturing processes, fortification and use of nutrients such as beta-carotene or vitamin C as colourings or antioxidants.
- *Changes in farming practices* can alter the composition of both plant and animal products over a period of time. For example, the fat content and fatty acid profile of meat has changed considerably in the last 20 years as a result of selective breeding programmes to produce leaner animals, changes in feeding techniques and modern butchery techniques which remove a greater proportion of carcass fat. Development of new varieties of agricultural crops or changes in the level of usage of fertilisers can also affect nutritional composition.
- *Domestic preparation and cooking practices* may change, e.g. vegetables may be steamed rather than boiled and bread may be made from a mix in a domestic bread making machine.
- *Previously unfamiliar foods* are now available in shops.
- *More accurate methods of analysis* are developed.

Use of old analytical data will considerably increase the likelihood of errors, which will introduce significant errors in even the most detailed dietary assessment. However, in some circumstances, e.g. the analysis of dietary information obtained many years ago, it may be necessary to use composition data that were contemporary at the time in order to obtain realistic figures of nutrient intake. It is particularly important that those engaged in dietary survey work are aware of the implications of using data from older editions and supplements of *The Composition of Foods* (Black & Paul, 1999). There are also a number of differences in code numbers between different editions of food tables, which can have implications in computerised analysis; a summary of these can be found in the introduction to the sixth summary edition (FSA, 2002). Data for food tables are updated on a rolling basis; it is also important to know which data have been incorporated into any nutrient analysis programmes purchased.

Limitations of food composition data

Food tables and databases will always have limitations for several reasons, including variability between foods consumed and food table values and bioavailability.

Variability between foods consumed and food table values

Despite careful sampling the resultant values will be representative of a particular food, but there will still be some variation from foods actually consumed. A number of factors, such as plant or animal species, seasonal changes in feeding practices or growing conditions, or the effects of storage on water content, affect the composition of natural foods such as meat, milk and eggs or plant crops. Further variability is likely to occur as a result of differences in food manufacture, catering or domestic cooking practices. For example, a lasagne may be a manufactured ready meal, an item prepared by a restaurant or made at home. All will differ in composition and probably none will exactly match the values given in food tables. In western diets, comparisons of the nutrient content of diets calculated from food tables and analysed by direct analysis have been shown to range between 2% and 20% (Bingham, 1987).

This variability is most likely to occur with micronutrients, i.e. vitamin and minerals content due to:

- The soil in which a plant was grown, e.g. this can markedly affect selenium content.
- Agricultural practices, e.g. antagonism between soil fertilisation using nitrogen and vitamin C content.
- Stage of maturity, e.g. in plant foods vitamin C content decreases during ripening, whereas carotenoid content increases.
- Duration and conditions of storage before being eaten, e.g. water soluble vitamin content will diminish with time.
- The way the food is cooked, e.g. the potassium content of boiled vegetables will depend on the amount of water used and length of the cooking time.
- Use of food fortification in some but not all brands of a particular food, e.g. folate or iron added to breakfast cereals.
- Use of food additives that are also nutrients, e.g. beta-carotene (colour) or vitamin C (antioxidant; may be unexpectedly present in foods such as meat products).

It should be noted that vitamin C and folic acid naturally vary widely in foods and that both heat and light affect them. It should also be noted that in food table analyses, vegetables would usually have been cooked in distilled water and without added salt. This means that the measured content of sodium, chloride and calcium (present in tap water) will be much lower than is likely in the typical domestic setting.

For most dietetic purposes, the importance of any differences between theoretical and actual nutrient composition may be relatively insignificant in the average mixed diet. However, for metabolic studies based on the consumption of very few foods, or where extreme precision is required, duplicates of the actual foods concerned must be prepared for direct laboratory analysis.

Bioavailability

Bioavailability is defined as the proportion of a nutrient that can be absorbed and hence available to the human body. The bioavailability of a particular nutrient can vary according to a number of factors:

- Source of origin, e.g. calcium in milk is absorbed more readily than calcium in bread.
- Chemical form, e.g. haem iron absorption is greater than that of non-haem iron.
- Ease with which the nutrient can be released from the food structure, e.g. some carbohydrate in fibrous foods cannot be digested and is lost in faeces.
- Presence of factors that inhibit absorption, e.g. phytates in cereal foods can reduce calcium absorption.
- Presence of factors that enhance absorption, e.g. vitamin C enhances the absorption of non-haem iron.
- Physiological factors – absorption may be increased in states of nutritional depletion or at times of increased need, e.g. during pregnancy.

Bioavailability is most likely to impact on minerals and trace elements such as calcium, magnesium, iron, zinc, copper, manganese and selenium, and vitamins such as folate and B_6. Since these interactions are so variable, UK food tables take no account of bioavailability and the nutrient content given in the food table is the amount present in the food. The only exception is the allowance made for the reduced activities of the different forms of some vitamins, e.g. 13-*cis* retinol and retinaldehyde (vitamin A), carotenes other than beta-carotene, and tocopherols and tocotrienes other than alpha-tocopherol (vitamin E). It is important to check if the food composition data nutrient values have been modified to take account of their bioavailability.

Error associated with the use of food composition data

Coding errors

In addition to inherent error in the food table data, additional errors may be introduced into nutrient analysis programmes in a number of ways:

- Missing nutrient values in food composition tables may be treated as zero values during calculation, resulting in an underestimation of nutrient intake.
- There may not be a suitable code for the food consumed or an inappropriate code may be chosen.
- There may be incorrect entry of food code numbers into the computing system.
- Errors can occur in the measurement, recording and estimation of food weights.
- Misclassification can result from a food having different names in different parts of the country. For example,

in some parts of the UK, roast potatoes may be entered on a dietary record as baked potatoes. This is particularly important when working with other nationalities, e.g. in the USA, chips refer to potato crisps rather than fried potatoes.

Interpretation errors

Food tables are useful to help identify good and poor food sources of nutrients, but are not always used for this purpose in an appropriate way. The values given in the tables will identify foods that are particularly concentrated sources of a specific nutrient, but this does not necessarily mean that a food is an important source of that nutrient in the typical diet. The contribution that a particular food makes to nutrient intake depends on the:

- Concentration of nutrient in the food (content per 100 g) and its bioavailability.
- Amount of the food consumed, i.e. portion size.
- Frequency with which that food is consumed.

For example, parsley is a highly concentrated source of vitamin C, but is unlikely to be a significant dietary source because it is usually only eaten infrequently and in small quantities. In contrast, potatoes are a much less concentrated source of vitamin C, but because they are a regular feature of many UK diets, they may make a major dietary contribution to vitamin C intake in the UK. When giving dietary advice it is important to remember that however valuable a food may be as a source of a particularly nutrient, it will make only a small contribution to dietary intake if it is rarely eaten.

Further reading

Greenfield H, Southgate DAT. (2003) *Food Composition Data: Production, Management and Use*, 2nd edn. Rome: FAO.

Klensin JC, Feskanich D, Lin V, Truswell AS, Southgate DAT. (1989) *Identification of Food Components for INFOODS Data Interchange*. Hong Kong: The United Nations University.

Rand WM, Pennington JAT, Murphy SP, Klensin JC. (1991) *Compiling Data for Food Composition Data Bases*. Hong Kong: The United Nations University,.

Internet resources

EuroFIR Project website with information on European food composition databases   www.eurofir.net

FAO – INFOODS information for nutrient database compilers and suppliers   www.fao.org

USDA nutrient data laboratory   http://www.ars.usda.gov/main/site_main.htm?modecode=12-35-45-00

References

Atwater WO, Benedict FG. (1902) *Experiments on the Metabolism of Matter and Energy in the Human Body, 1898–1900*. US Office of Experiment Stations Bulletin No. 109. Washington, DC: Government Printing Office.

Bingham S. (1987) The dietary assessment of individuals: methods, accuracy, new techniques and recommendations. *Nutrition Abstracts and Reviews* 57: 705–742.

Black AE, Paul AA. (1999) McCance & Widdowson's Tables of Food Composition: origins and clarification of the fifth edition. *Journal of Human Nutrition and Dietetics* 12: 1–5.

Chan W, Brown J, Buss DH. (1994) *Miscellaneous Foods: Fourth Supplement to The Composition of Foods*, 5th edn. Cambridge: Royal Society of Chemistry/MAFF.

Chan W, Brown J, Lee SM, Buss DH. (1995) *Meat, Poultry and Game: Fifth supplement to McCance and Widdowson's The Composition of Foods*, 5th edn. Cambridge: Royal Society of Chemistry/MAFF.

Chan W, Brown J, Church SM, Buss DH. (1996) *Meat Products and Dishes: Sixth Supplement to McCance and Widdowson's The Composition of Foods*, 5th edn. Cambridge: Royal Society of Chemistry/MAFF.

Church SM. (2006) The history of food composition databases. *Nutrition Bulletin* 31, 15–20.

Englyst HN, Cummings JH. (1988) An improved method for the measurement of dietary fibre as the non-starch polysaccharides in plant foods. *Journal of the Association of Official Analytical Chemists* 71: 808–814.

Food and Agriculture Organization of the United Nations (FAO). (2003) Food energy – Methods of Analysis and Conversion Factors (Technical report). Rome: FAOUN.

Food Standards Agency (FSA). (2002) *McCance and Widdowson's The Composition of Foods*, 6th summary edn. Cambridge/London: Royal Society of Chemistry/FSA.

Holland B, Brown J, Buss DH. (1993) *Fish and Fish Products: Third Supplement to the Composition of foods*, 5th edn. Cambridge: Royal Society of Chemistry/MAFF.

Holland B, Unwin ID, Buss DH. (1988) *Cereals and Cereal Products: Third Supplement to McCance and Widdowson's The Composition of Foods*, 4th edn. Cambridge: Royal Society of Chemistry/MAFF.

Holland B, Unwin ID, Buss DH. (1989) *Milk Products and Eggs: Fourth Supplement to McCance and Widdowson's The Composition of Foods*, 4th edn. Cambridge: Royal Society of Chemistry/MAFF, 1989.

Holland B, Welch AA, Unwin ID, Buss DH, Paul AA, Southgate DAT. (1991a) *McCance and Widdowson's The Composition of Foods*, 5th edn. Cambridge: Royal Society of Chemistry/MAFF.

Holland B, Unwin ID, Buss DH. (1991b) *Vegetables, Herbs, and Spices: Fifth Supplement to McCance and Widdowson's The Composition of Foods*, 4th edn. Cambridge: Royal Society of Chemistry/MAFF.

Holland B, Unwin ID, Buss DH. (1992a) *Fruit and Nuts: First Supplement to McCance and Widdowson's The Composition of Foods*, 5th edn. Cambridge: Royal Society of Chemistry/MAFF.

Holland B, Welch A, Buss DH. (1992b) *Vegetable Dishes: Second Supplement to McCance and Widdowson's The Composition of Foods*, 5th edn. Cambridge: Royal Society of Chemistry/MAFF.

Judd PA, Kassam-Khamis T, Thomas JE. (2000) *The Composition and Nutrient Content of Foods Commonly Consumed by South Asians in the UK*. London: The Aga Khan Health Board for the United Kingdom.

Ministry of Agriculture, Fisheries and Food (MAFF). (1998) *Fatty Acids: Seventh Supplement to The Composition of Foods*, 5th edn. Cambridge: Royal Society of Chemistry/MAFF.

Paul AA, Southgate DAT, Russell J. (1980) *Amino Acid Composition (mg per 100 g food) and Fatty Acid Composition (g per 100 g food): First supplement to McCance and Widdowson's The Composition of Foods*, 4th edn. London/Cambridge: HMSO/Royal Society of Chemistry.

Tan SP, Wenlock RW, Buss DH. (1985) *Immigrant Foods: Second supplement to McCance and Widdowson's The Composition of Foods*, 4th edn. London/Cambridge: HMSO/Royal Society of Chemistry, 1985.

Webster-Gandy J, Madden A, Holdsworth M. (2011) *Oxford Handbook of Nutrition and Dietetics*, 2nd edn. Oxford: Oxford University Press.

SECTION 2

SECTION 3

Nutrition in specific groups

3.1.1 Polycystic ovary syndrome
Yvonne Jeannes

Key points

- Polycystic ovary syndrome (PCOS) presents as a range of symptoms that vary in severity.

- Weight management should be the primary therapy in overweight women with PCOS.

- Dietary modification should aim to improve insulin resistance.

- A patient centred approach is needed to improve symptoms as well as reduce the risk of developing diabetes and cardiovascular disease.

- Binge eating behaviour is common in PCOS.

Polycystic ovary syndrome (PCOS) is a heterogeneous condition and women may present with one or several of the following symptoms: menstrual irregularity and fertility problems, excess male pattern hair (hirsutism), male pattern alopecia, acne, central adiposity, insulin resistance and depression (Azziz *et al.*, 2006; Dokras *et al.*, 2011). Symptoms vary in severity and can change over the lifecycle; PCOS often becomes clinically apparent during adolescence (Ojaniemi *et al.*, 2010). The diagnostic criteria for PCOS involve the presence of two of the following features and exclusion of other endocrine disorders (ESHRE and ASRM, 2004):

- Oligo-ovulation leading to oligomenorrhoea (fewer than nine menses per year), or anovulation leading to amenorrhoea.
- Hyperandrogenism – clinically (hirsutism, male pattern alopecia, acne) or biochemically.
- Polycystic ovaries.

It is important to note that women can be diagnosed with PCOS from the presence of oligo-ovulation and clinical signs of hyperandrogenism without polycystic ovaries. A woman with polycystic ovaries without the other symptoms should not be diagnosed with PCOS.

The aetiology of PCOS is complex, with a genetic heritability that is enhanced by environmental factors, especially obesity (Pasquali *et al.*, 2011). Hyperandrogenism is present in 60–80% of women, either clinically (hirsutism, male pattern alopecia, acne) or biochemically (elevated total or free testosterone) (Azziz *et al.*, 2006). Although insulin resistance is not among the diagnostic criteria for PCOS, most women with PCOS, both the lean and overweight, have a form of insulin resistance intrinsic to PCOS (Baptiste *et al.*, 2010). Hyperinsulinaemia promotes ovarian hyperandrogenism and reduces hepatic production of sex hormone binding globulin (SHBG), thus increasing free testosterone levels. Together hyperinsulinaemia and hyperandrogenaemia disrupt follicle growth, which leads to menstrual irregularity, anovulatory subfertility and accumulation of immature follicles (Goodarzi *et al.*, 2011).

Disease consequences

It is the most common endocrine disorder in women of reproductive age, affecting up to 10% (March *et al.*, 2010). South Asian women have the highest prevalence (Rodin *et al.*, 1998) followed by Black women (Azziz *et al.*, 2004). Between 30% and 70% of women with PCOS are obese (Barr *et al.*, 2011) and frequently exhibit central obesity (Amato *et al.*, 2011; Cascella *et al.*, 2008) that is linked to greater insulin resistance (Barber *et al.*, 2006).

Obese women with PCOS are generally more symptomatic and are at greater health risk compared with lean women with PCOS (Majumdar & Singh, 2009). Up to 50% of women with PCOS develop impaired glucose tolerance or type 2 diabetes by the age of 40 years (Ehrmann et al., 1999) and there is a greater incidence of gestational diabetes (Bals-Pratsch et al., 2011) (see Chapter 7.12). South Asian patients tend to exhibit greater insulin resistance and are at an increased risk of type 2 diabetes (Wijeyaratne et al., 2002). Up to 47% of women with PCOS exhibit features of the metabolic syndrome (Ehrmann et al., 2006). Women with PCOS have a greater prevalence of cardiovascular disease (CVD) risk factors, including hypertriglyceridaemia, low high density lipoprotein (HDL) cholesterol, hypertension and endothelial dysfunction (Wild et al., 2010). They are also more likely to develop cancer of the endometrium (Chittenden et al., 2009; Fearnley et al., 2010).

The symptoms associated with PCOS have been shown to lead to a reduction in health related quality of life (Jones et al., 2008). Depression and anxiety are common in PCOS (Dokras et al., 2011). Studies have indicated a higher prevalence of eating disorders in women with PCOS (Morgan et al., 2008; Kerchner et al., 2009). Anecdotal reports suggest women with PCOS may have increased binge eating, food cravings and symptoms of postprandial hypoglycaemia (Herriot et al., 2008). However, there remains a paucity of well designed studies investigating the eating behaviours or food cravings in women with PCOS.

It is important to consider the psychological impact of PCOS when advising sufferers and to involve them in every part of the care process.

Clinical management

Management of PCOS focuses on treating the presenting symptoms. Lifestyle management is advocated as the primary therapy in overweight and obese women with PCOS. A modest weight loss of just 5–10%, without medical intervention, has been shown to improve many of the symptoms associated with PCOS (Moran et al., 2009; 2011), including lower fasting insulin levels, reduced free testosterone and increased SHBG, improved reproductive function, less hirsutism and an improvement in risk factors for diabetes and CVD.

Medical treatments are available for hirsutism, acne and infertility. Metformin is commonly prescribed for women with PCOS as it reduces serum insulin levels in insulin resistant individuals (Diamanti-Kandarakis et al., 2010). Several studies have revealed some reproductive benefits of metformin and a beneficial effect on serum testosterone concentration has also been observed (Tang et al., 2010).

Nutritional consequences

There are no known nutritional consequences specific to PCOS.

Nutritional assessment

Anthropometric measurements include determining body mass index (BMI) and waist circumference to inform risk of comorbidities and dietary management. A dietary assessment to determine habitual dietary habits should also aim to detect any binge eating behaviour (see Chapter 7.10.1). Due to the increased prevalence of impaired glucose tolerance and type 2 diabetes in PCOS, an oral glucose tolerance test may be performed, and due to the increased prevalence of cardiovascular risk factors, measurements of blood pressure, plasma total, low density lipoprotein (LDL) and HDL cholesterol as well as triglycerides are recommended (Wild et al., 2010).

Nutritional management

Weight loss through dietary restriction and increased physical activity are key management strategies for overweight and obese women with PCOS (Moran et al., 2009). The optimal method of achieving sustainable weight loss is under constant debate; the aforementioned studies demonstrating clinical benefit of weight loss in women with PCOS incorporated a variety of methods to reduce energy intake and achieve the weight loss. A range of weight loss strategies are available and a patient centred approach that addresses the needs and preferences of patients is important when managing PCOS. Behaviour change strategies have long been recognised as instrumental in managing chronic conditions, particularly weight management (see Chapter 7.13.2).

Dietary modification to improve insulin resistance may produce benefits greater than those achieved by weight loss alone and would also be suitable for lean women with PCOS (Marsh & Brand-Miller, 2005). Modifying carbohydrate and fatty acid content of the diet have both been proposed as methods to improve insulin sensitivity. The concept of a low glycaemic index (GI) diet aims to reduce the glycaemic load and hence insulin response to ingested foods and drinks. As previously mentioned, hyperinsulinaemia has a detrimental effect on symptoms and thus reducing the body's exposure to insulin may be beneficial. The delivery of a low GI diet should incorporate healthy eating principles to additionally reduce risk factors for CVD (see Chapter 7.14.1).

At present only a couple of studies have investigated the impact of a low GI diet independent of weight loss in women with PCOS. Marsh et al. (2010) reported greater improvement in insulin sensitivity and regular menses after weight loss with a low GI approach compared to weight loss through conventional healthy eating. Both diets were designed to provide reduced energy, low fat, low saturated fatty acids and moderate to high fibre; the low GI diet additionally modified the quality of carbohydrate. Twenty-nine women with PCOS followed the low GI diet and 20 completed the healthy eating regimen, and women were followed for 12 months or until they achieved 7% weight loss. Barr et al. (2010) demonstrated an improvement in insulin sensitivity through an isocaloric diet with a reduction in dietary GI in 21 women with

PCOS over a 12-week intervention period. These studies provide some evidence to support dietary advice to lean women with PCOS, many of whom are also insulin resistant. These studies are in agreement with studies that have indicated enhanced insulin sensitivity in individuals with type 2 diabetes (Rizkalla *et al.*, 2004). Herriot *et al.*, (2008; 2009) reported that an isocaloric low glycaemic load diet in lean women with PCOS resulted in a reduction in waist circumference. In addition, a reduction in carbohydrate craving and general hunger was observed.

Fatty acid intake has been shown to influence glucose metabolism by altering insulin signalling and cell membrane function, with a diet high in saturated fatty acids associated with a decrease in insulin sensitivity when compared to a high monounsaturated fatty acid diet (Galgani *et al.*, 2008). Furthermore, a review by Risérus (2008) concluded that saturated and *trans* fatty acids should be replaced with poly- (PUFAs) and monounsaturated fatty acids to improve insulin sensitivity and prevent type 2 diabetes. Phelan *et al.* (2011) indicated a role for PUFAs in modulating hormones, whereby supplementation with n-3 PUFA improved the androgenic profile. Further studies are required to substantiate the evidence in this area.

Increasing physical activity has been shown to improve glucose metabolism and insulin sensitivity, and to reduce abdominal adiposity independent of weight loss (Ross *et al.*, 2004). Benefits are seen without weight loss, and thus should be encouraged in all women with PCOS, irrespective of weight. Eighty-four per cent of women with PCOS self reported improvements in PCOS symptoms when they increased their level of physical activity (Jeannes *et al.*, 2009). Barriers to participating in physical activity, above and beyond those experienced by overweight women without PCOS, include: excess body and facial hair, acne, unpredictable menses, body shape concerns, low self esteem and feelings of being unfeminine.

A high proportion of women with PCOS report taking nutrient or herbal supplements, which many felt had a beneficial effect on their symptoms (Jeannes *et al.*, 2009). *Agnus castus* has been proposed to help relieve some PCOS symptoms, including restoring menses; however, at present there are no studies to support this in women with PCOS. Saw palmetto has been proposed to reduce circulating testosterone and hirsutism, but again there is inadequate evidence to support this.

A holistic approach to dietary management with consideration of immediate goals (improvement of symptoms and fertility, and weight loss) as well as reducing the long term health risks, e.g. of diabetes and CVD, should be incorporated. Women who are trying to conceive should also be following a nutritionally adequate diet with folic acid supplements.

Drug–nutrient interactions

Oral contraceptives may negatively impact upon insulin sensitivity and dyslipidaemia. Metformin can cause gastrointestinal side effects such as nausea and diarrhoea.

Further reading

Bailey S. (2011) *Nutrition and Polycystic Ovary Syndrome.* available from PCOS UK.

Bailey S. (2011) *Successful Lifestyle Change and Polycystic Ovary Syndrome*. Available from PCOS UK.

Elsheikh M, Murphy C. (2008) *Polycystic Ovary Syndrome. The Facts*. Oxford: Oxford University Press.

Internet resources

Verity (a self-help group for women with PCOS) www.verity-pcos .org.uk

PCOS UK www.pcos-uk.org.uk

References

Amato MC, Verghi M, Galluzzo, A, Giordano C. (2011) The oligomenorrhoic phenotypes of polycystic ovary syndrome are characterized by a high visceral adiposity index: a likely condition of cardiometabolic risk. *Human Reproduction* 26: 1486–1494.

Azziz R, Woods KS, Reyna R, Key TJ, Knochenhauer ES, Yildiz BO. (2004) The prevalence and features of the polycystic ovary syndrome in an unselected population. *Journal of Clinical Endocrinology and Metabolism* 89: 2745–2749.

Azziz R, Carmina E, Dewailly D, Diamanti-Kandrarakis E, *et al.* (2006) Criteria for defining polycystic ovary syndrome as a predominatly hyperandogenic syndrome. *Journal of Clinical Endocrinology and Metabolism* 91: 4237–4245.

Bals-Pratsch M, Großer B, Seifert B, Ortmann O, Seifarth C. (2011) Early onset and high prevalence of gestational diabetes in PCOS and insulin resistant women before and after assisted reproduction. *Experimental and Clinical Endocrinology & Diabetes* 119(6): 338–342.

Baptiste CG, Battista M-C, Trottier A, Baillargeon J-P. (2010) Insulin and hyperadrogenism in women with polycystic ovary syndrome. *Journal of Steroid Biochemistry and Molecular Biolgy* 122:, 42–52.

Barber TM, McCarthy MI, Wass JAH, Franks S. (2006) Obesity and polycystic ovary syndrome. *Clinical Endocrionology* 65: 137–145.

Barr S, Reeves S, Sharp K, Jeanes Y. (2010) Efficacy of a low-glycaemic index diet in women with polycystic ovary syndrome. *Proceedings of the Nutrition Society* 69: E404.

Barr S, Hart K, Reeves S, Sharp K, Jeanes Y. (2011) Habitual dietary intake, eating pattern and physical activity of women with polycystic ovary syndrome. *European Journal of Clinical Nutrition* 65: 1126–1132.

Cascella T, Palomba S, De Sio I, *et al.* (2008) Visceral fat is associated with cardiovascular risk in women with polycystic ovary syndrome. *Human Reproduction* 23: 153–159.

Chittenden BN, Fullerton G, Maheshwari A, Bhattacharya S. (2009) Polycystic ovary syndrome and the risk of gynaecological cancer: a systematic review. *Reproductive BioMedicine Online* 19: 398–405.

Diamanti-Kandarakis E, Christakou CD., Kandaraki E, Economou FN. (2010) Metformin: an old medicine of new fashion: evolving new molecular mechanisms and clinical implications in polycystic ovary syndrome. *European Journal of Clinical Endocrinology* 162: 193–212.

Dokras A, Clifton S, Futterweit W, Wild R. (2011) Increased risk for abnormal depression scores in women with polycystic ovary syndrome: a systematic review and meta-analysis. *Obstetrics & Gynecology* 117: 145–152.

Ehrmann DA, Barnes RB, Rosenfield RL, Cavaghan ML, Imperial J. (1999) Prevalence of impaired glucose tolerance and diabetes in women with polycystic ovary syndrome. *Diabetes Care* 22: 141–146.

SECTION 3

Ehrmann D, Liljenquist DR, Kasza K, Azziz R, Legro RS, Ghazzi MN; PCOS/Troglitazone Study Group (2006) Prevalence and predictors of the metabolic syndrome in women with PCOS. *Journal of Clinical Endocrinology and Metabolism* 91: 48–53.

ESHRE and ASRM Sponsored PCOS Consensus Workshop Group (2004) Revised 2003 consensus on diagnostic criteria and long-term health risks related to polycystic ovary syndrome. *Fertility and Sterility* 81: 19–25.

Fearnley EJ, Marquart L, Spurdle AB, Weinstein P, Webb PM; Australian Ovarian Cancer Study Group & Australian National Endometrial Cancer Study Group. (2010) Polycystic ovary syndrome increases the risk of endometrial cancer in women aged <50 years: an Australian case-control study. *Cancer Causes Control* 21: 2303–2308.

Galgani JE, Uauy RD, Aguirre CA, Díaz EO. (2008) Effect of the dietary fat quality on insulin sensitivity. *British Journal of Nutrition* 100: 471–479.

Goodarzi MO, Dumesic DA, Chazenbalk G, Azziz R. (2011) Polycystic ovary syndrome: etiology, pathogenesis and diagnosis. *Endocrinology* 7: 219–231.

Herriot A, Whitcroft S, Jeanes Y. (2008) A retrospective audit of patients with polycystic ovary syndrome: the effects of a reduced glycaemic load diet. *Journal of Human Nutrition and Dietetics* 21: 337–345.

Herriot AM, Whitcroft S, Jeanes Y. (2009) A low glycaemic load diet reduces risk factors for the metabolic syndrome and type 2 diabetes in lean and overweight menopausal women and women with polycystic ovary syndrome (PCOS). *Journal of Human Nutrition and Dietetics* 22: 595.

Jeannes Y, Barr S, Smith K, Hart KH. (2009). Dietary management of women with polycystic ovary syndrome in the United Kingdom: the role of dietitians. *Journal of Human Nutrition and Dietetics* 22: 551–558.

Jones GL, Hall JM, Balen AH, Ledger WL. (2008) Health-related quality of life measurement in women with polycystic ovary syndrome: a systematic review. *Human Reproduction Update* 14: 15–25.

Kerchner A, Lester W, Stuart SP, Dokras A. (2009) Risk of depression and other mental health disorders in women with polycystic ovary syndrome: a longitudinal study. *Fertility and Sterility* 91: 207–212.

Majumdar A, Singh TA. (2009) Comparison of clinical features and health manisfestations in lean vs. obese Indian women with polycystic ovarian syndrome. *Journal of Human Reproductive Sciences* 2: 12–17.

March WA, Moore VM, Willson KJ, Phillips DIW, Norman RJ, Davies MJ. (2010) The prevalence of polycystic ovary syndrome in a community samples assessed under contrasting diagnositc criteria. *Human Reproduction* 25: 544–51

Marsh K, Brand-Miller J. (2005) The optimal diet for women with polycystic ovary syndrome? *British Journal of Nutrition* 94: 154–165.

Marsh K, Steinbeck KS, Atkinson FS, Petocz P, Brand-Miller JC (2010) Effect of a low glycaemic index compared with a conventional healthy diet on polycystic ovary syndrome. *American Journal of Clinical Nutrition* 92: 83–92.

Moran LJ, Pasquali R, Teede HJ, Hoeger KM, Norman RJ. (2009) Treatment of obesity in polycystic ovary syndrome: a position statement of the androgen Excess and Polycystic Ovary Syndrome Society. *Fertility and Sterility* 92: 1966–82.

Moran LJ, Hutchison SK, Norman RJ, Teede HJ. (2011) Lifestyle changes in women with polycystic ovary syndrome. *Cochrane Database of Systematic Reviews* 2: CD007506.

Morgan J, Schotz S, Lacey H, Conway G. (2008) The prevalence of eating disorders in women with facial hirsutism: An epidemiological cohort study. *International Journal of Eating Disorders* 41: 427–431.

Ojaniemi M, Tapanainen P, Morin-Papunen L. (2010) Management of polycystic ovary syndrome in childhood and adolescence. *Hormone Research in Paediatrics* 74: 372–375.

Pasquali R, Stener-Victorin E, Yildiz BO, *et al.* (2011) Research in polycystic ovary syndrome today and tomorrow. *Clinical Endocrinology* 74: 424–433.

Phelan N, O'Connor A, Tun TK, *et al.* (2011) Hormonal and metabolic effects of polyunsaturated fatty acids in young women with polycystic ovary syndrome: results from a cross-sectional analysis and a randomized, placebo-controlled, crossover trial. *American Journal of Clinical Nutrition* 93: 652–662.

Risérus U. (2008) Fatty acids and insulin sensitivity. *Current Opinion in Clinical Nutrition & Metabolic Care* 11: 100–105.

Rizkalla SW, Taghrid L, Laromiguiere M, *et al.* (2004) Improved plasma glucose control, whole body glucose utilization, and lipid profile on a low glycemic index diet in type 2 diabetic men: a randomized controlled trial. *Diabetes Care* 27: 1866–1872.

Rodin DA, Bano G, Bland JM, Taylor K, Nussey SS. (1998) Polycystic ovaries and associated metabolic abnormalities in Indian subcontinent Asian women. *Clinical Endocrionology* 49: 91–99.

Ross R, Jansen I, Dawson J, *et al.* (2004). Exercise-induced reduction in obesity and insulin resistance in women: a randomized controlled trial. *Obesity Research* 12: 789–798.

Tang T, Lord JM, Norman RJ, Yasmin E, Balen AH. (2010) Insulin-sensitising drugs (metformin, rosiglitazone, pioglitazone, D-chiro-inositol) for women with polycystic ovary syndrome, oligo amenorrhoea and subfertility. *Cochrane Database of Systematic Reviews* 1: CD003053.

Wijeyaratne C, Balen AH, Barth JH, Belchetz PE. (2002). Clinical manifestations and insulin resistance (IR) in polycystic ovary syndrome (PCOS) among South Asians and caucasians: is there a difference? *Clinical Endocrinology* 57: 343–350.

Wild RA, Carmina E, Diamanti-Kandarakis E, *et al.* (2010) Assessment of cardiovascular risk and prevention of cardiovascular disease in women with the polycystic ovary syndrome. *Journal of Clinical Endocrinology & Metabolism* 95: 2038–2049.

3.1.2 Premenstrual syndrome

Gaynor Bussell

Key points

■ Most women experience premenstrual symptoms; for 8–20% it is severe.

■ Premenstrual symptoms is cyclical and does not occur in anovulatory cycles, but it is unrelated to hormonal levels.

■ A healthy diet and lifestyle can help relieve mild symptoms.

■ Adequate dietary sources of calcium and vitamin D are important. For other supplements, the evidence is equivocal.

Premenstrual syndrome (PMS) is cyclical and occurs during the luteal phase of the cycle (1–2 weeks before menstruation); symptoms are relieved by the onset of or during menstruation. Most women experience mild symptoms, but for 8–20% its severity can prompt them to seek medical treatment (Chocano-Bedoya et al., 2011); the most severe form affects 3–5% of women.

Symptoms of PMS vary between and within individuals, and include mood swings, irritability, increased appetite, carbohydrate and alcohol cravings, breast tenderness, headaches and bloating. Women with chronic disease, e.g. diabetes, irritable bowel syndrome (IBS) or allergies, may have a low threshold for developing PMS (Bussell, 1998). Good control of chronic medical conditions may reduce the severity of symptoms.

Aetiology

The cause of PMS is unknown, but it is believed to be due to an increased sensitivity to circulating progesterone and its metabolites (Brown et al., 2009). Progesterone production by the corpus luteum of the ovary may provoke symptoms; cyclicity disappears in anovulatory cycles when a corpus luteum is not formed. It has also been suggested that a lack of prostaglandin E1 (PGE1) production from n-6 fatty acids (O'Brien, 1987) may be a contributing factor.

Management

It is difficult to diagnose PMS; the most definitive method is a symptom diary as symptoms will start in the luteal phase and cease at the start of or during menstruation (Ugarriza et al., 1998).

There is no universally recognised single treatment for PMS and women will often use diet, supplements and alternative approaches to relieve symptoms. For mild to moderate symptoms, lifestyle changes and a healthy diet can substantially reduce, if not alleviate, the symptoms (Stewart, 1993). For those who are treated with drugs, a healthy lifestyle may make the treatment more successful (Bussell, 1998).

Nutritional management

A healthy diet, regular physical activity and stress reduction techniques can help to reduce symptoms (Andrews, 1994; Ugarriza et al., 1998). Sustained dietary change is necessary for symptom relief.

Low glycaemic diet

Anecdotally, PMS sufferers complain of hypoglycaemia and sugar and carbohydrate cravings. An increased sensitivity to the fall in blood glucose after a fast acting carbohydrate and sugar load has been observed premenstrually (Benton, 2002), but low glucose blood levels are rarely observed. A low GI diet is anecdotally reported to be effective, particularly in the luteal phase.

Micronutrients

Sufferers frequently use supplements, although there is little evidence to support their use (Royal College of Obstetrics & Gynaecology, 2007). Only calcium has good quality evidence to support its use (Whelan et al., 2009).

Calcium and vitamin D

A diet rich in calcium and vitamin D is associated with a lower incidence of PMS. Lower fat versions of dairy foods reduce the incidence of PMS (Bertone-Johnson et al.; 2005). Calcium (1000 mg/day) and vitamin D (10 μg) may be useful in treating premenstrual pain and emotional symptoms associated with PMS (Thys-Jacobs et al., 1989; Alvir & Thys-Jacobs, 1991; Thys-Jacobs, 1994). Dietary vitamin D has been shown to reduce the risk of PMS in young women (Bertone-Johnson et al., 2010). Women with PMS who consumed at least 100 IU/day of vitamin D had a significantly reduced prevalence of PMS compared with women who consumed less than this amount.

Magnesium

Low intake and blood levels of magnesium have been found in PMS sufferers (Posaci et al., 1994; Quaranta et al., 2007). An improvement in PMS symptoms with magnesium supplementation has been observed (Quaranta et al., 2007). However, more recent reviews have concluded that there is little evidence for the effectiveness of magnesium in PMS (Labruzzo et al., 2009; Whelan et al., 2009).

B vitamins

Historically, vitamin B_6 supplements were used to treat PMS, but a pharmacological dose of 50–100 mg was required and such doses may induce neuropathy (Labruzzo et al., 2009). As a consequence, in the UK B_6 supplements are only sold in 10 mg ineffective doses. Recently, an observational study showed that higher intakes of thiamine and riboflavin may reduce the incidence of PMS by 35% (Chocano-Beoya et al., 2011).

Vitamin E, evening primrose oil and essential fatty acids

Recent studies have shown the efficacy of vitamin E combined with evening primrose oil for premenstrual breast pain (Pruthi et al., 2010). A supplement containing a mixture of essential fatty acids (gamma linolenic acid, linolenic acid, oleic acid) and vitamins (including vitamin E) significantly reduced the symptoms of PMS, with the 2-g highest level supplement having the greatest effect (Filho et al., 2011). Evening primrose oil was prescribable for PMS due to the presence of gamma linolenic acid. However, many trials were poorly designed and/or showed no reduction in breast pain or other PMS symptoms (Kleijnen, 1994); therefore, it was withdrawn as a prescribable product.

Fibre

Increasing dietary fibre can help to alleviate the constipation that may occur premenstrually (Bussell, 1998). Appropriate treatment for IBS is helpful in the premenstrual period (Kane et al., 1998).

Alcohol

Alcoholics are prone to PMS (Allen, 1996) and alcohol aggravates symptoms (Gold *et al.*, 2007). Some PMS sufferers have alcohol cravings premenstrually (Bryant *et al.*, 2006); alcohol metabolism may also be impaired (Perry *et al.*, 2004).

Soya

A phyto-oestrogen rich diet has been shown to prolong the follicular phase of the menstrual cycle (Patisaul & Jefferson, 2010). However, the evidence is equivocal (Kim *et al.*, 2006).

Weight gain

Obesity is associated with PMS (Masho *et al.*, 2005). Many women report an increase in appetite during the luteal phase (Bryant *et al.*, 2006; Tucci *et al.*, 2009). Women with PMS have been shown to eat significantly more fat, carbohydrates and simple sugars premenstrually (Cross *et al.*, 2001). Conversely, energy expenditure has been shown to increase premenstrually in some women (Henry *et al.*, 2003).

Herbal treatments

Although herbal medicines are used, their effectiveness has not been fully evaluated in randomised controlled trials (Jing *et al.*, 2009). Single trials of Jingqianping, *Vitex agnus castus*, *Ginko biloba* and *Crocus sativus* have shown efficacy; however, more trials are needed (Dante & Facchinetti, 2010).

Internet resources

National Association for Premenstrual Syndrome   www.pms.org.uk

References

Allen D. (1996) Are alcoholic women more likely to drink premenstrually? *Alcohol* 31(2): 145–147.

Alvir JM, Thys-Jacobs S. (1991) Premenstrual and menstrual symptom clusters and response to calcium treatment. *Psychopharmacology Bulletin* 27(2): 145–148.

Andrews G. (1994) Constructive advice for a poorly understood problem: treatment and management of PMS. *Professional Nurse* 9: 364–370.

Benton D. (2002) Carbohydrate ingestion, blood glucose and mood. *Neuroscience & Biobehavioral Reviews* 26(3): 293–308.

Bertone-Johnson ER, Hankinson SE, Bendich A, Johnson SR, Willett WC, Manson JE. (2005) Calcium and vitamin D intake and risk of incident premenstrual syndrome. *Archives of Internal Medicine* 165(11): 1246–1252.

Bertone-Johnson ER, Chocano-Bedoya PO, Zagarins SE, Micka AE, Ronnenberg AG. (2010). Dietary vitamin D intake, 25-hydroxyvitamin D3 levels and premenstrual syndrome in a college-aged population. *Journal of Steroid Biochemistry and Molecular Biology* 121(1–2): 434–437.

Brown J, O'Brien PMS., Marjoribanks J, Wyatt K. (2009) Selective serotonin reuptake inhibitors for premenstrual syndrome. *Cochrane Database of Systematic Reviews* 2: CD001396. Bryant M, Truesdale KP, Dye L. (2006) Modest changes in dietary intake across the menstrual cycle: implications for food intake research. *British Journal of Nutrition* 96(5): 888–894.

Bussell G. (1998) Pre-menstrual Syndrome and Diet. *Journal of Nutritional & Environmental Medicine* 8: 65–75.

Chocano-Bedoya PO, Manson JE, Hankinson SE, *et al.* (2011) Dietary B vitamin intake and incident premenstrual syndrome. *American Journal of Clinical Nutrition* 93: 1080–1086.

Cross GB, Marley J, Miles H, Willson K. (2001) Changes in nutrient intake during the menstrual cycle of overweight women with premenstrual syndrome. *British Journal of Nutrition* 85(4): 475–482.

Dante G, Facchinetti F. (2010). Herbal treatments for alleviating premenstrual syndrome: a systematic review. *J Psychosomatic Obstetrics & Gynecology* 32(1): 42–51.

Filho R, Lima JC, Pinho N, Montarroyos U. (2011) Essential fatty acids for premenstrual syndrome and their effect on prolactin and total cholesterol levels: a randomized, double blind, placebo-controlled study. *Reproductive Health* 8(1): 2.

Gold EB, Bair Y, Block G, *et al.* (2007) Diet and lifestyle factors associated with premenstrual symptoms in a racially diverse community sample: Study of Women's Health Across the Nation (SWAN). *Journal of Women's Health (Larchmt)* 16(5): 641–56.

Henry CJ, Lightowler HJ, Marchini J. (2003) Intra-individual variation in resting metabolic rate during the menstrual cycle. *British Journal of Nutrition* 89(6): 811–817.

Jing Z, Yang X, Ismail KMK, Chen XY, Wu T. (2009) Chinese herbal medicine for premenstrual syndrome. *Cochrane Database of Systematic Reviews* 1: CD006414.DO1.

Kane SV, Sable K, Hanauer SB. (1998) The menstrual cycle and its effect on inflammatory bowel disease and irritable bowel syndrome: a prevalence study. *American Journal of Gastroenterology* 10: 1867–1872.

Kim HW, Kwon MK, Kim NS, Reame NE. (2006) Intake of dietary soy isoflavones in relation to perimenstrual symptoms of Korean women living in the USA. *Nursing & Health Sciences* 2: 108–113.

Kleijnen J. (1994) Evening primrose oil. *BMJ* 309: 824–825.

Labruzzo BA, Chasuk R, Kendall S. (2009) Which complementary therapies can help patients with PMS? *Journal of Family Practice* 58(10): 552–559.

Masho SW, Adera T, South-Paul J. (2005) Obesity as a risk factor for premenstrual syndrome. *J Psychosometric Obstetrics & Gynecolgy* 26(1), 33–39.

Perry BL, Miles D, Burruss K, Svikis DS. Premenstrual symptomatology and alcohol consumption in college women. *Journal of Studies on Alcohol and Drugs* 65(4): 464–468.

O'Brien PMS. (1987) *Pre-menstrual Syndrome*. Oxford: Blackwell Scientific.

Patisaul HB, Jefferson W. (2010) The pros and cons of phytoestrogens. *Frontiers in Neuroendocrinology* 31(4): 400–419.

Posaci C, Erten O, Uren A, Acar B. (1994) Plasma copper, zinc and magnesium levels in patients with premenstrual tension syndrome. *Acta Obstetrica Gynecoligica Scandinavica* 73(6): 452–455.

Pruthi S, Wahner-Roedler DL, Torkelson CJ, *et al.*. (2010) Vitamin E and evening primrose oil for management of cyclical mastalgia: a randomized pilot study. *Alternative Medicine Reviews* 15(1): 59–67.

Quaranta S, Buscaglia MA, Meroni MG, Colombo E, Cella S. (2007) Pilot study of the efficacy and safety of a modified-release magnesium 250 mg tablet (Sincromag) for the treatment of premenstrual syndrome. *Clinical Drug Investigation* 27(1): 51–58.

Royal College of Obstetrics and Gynaecology (RCOG). (2007) *Green Top Guide* (48). London: RCOG.

Stewart AC. (1993) Effect of nutritional programme on premenstrual syndrome and work efficiency. *Complimentary Therapies in Medicine* 1: 68–72.

Thys-Jacobs S. (1994) Alleviation of migraines with therapeutic vitamin D and calcium. *Headache*. 34(10): 590–592.

Thys-Jacobs S, Ceccarelli S, Bierman A, Weisman H, Cohen MA, Alvir J. (1989) Calcium supplementation in premenstrual syndrome: a randomized crossover trial. *Journal of General Internal Medicine* 1989 4(3): 183–189.

Tucci SA, Murphy LE, Boyland EJ, Halford JC. (2009) [Influence of premenstrual syndrome and oral contraceptive effects on food choice during the follicular and luteal phase of the menstrual cycle]. *Endocrinologia y Nutricion* 56(4): 170–175.

Ugarriza DN, Klingner S, O'Brien S. (1998) Premenstrual syndrome: diagnosis and intervention. *Nurse Practitioner* 23(9): 40, 45, 49–52.

Whelan AM, Jurgens TM, Naylor H. (2009) Herbs, vitamins and minerals in the treatment of premenstrual syndrome: a systematic review. *Canadian Journal of Clinical Pharmacology* 16(3): e407–429.

3.1.3 Menopause

Gaynor Bussell

Key points

- The menopause can be accompanied by weight gain, an increased risk of osteoporosis, cardiovascular disease and diabetes.

- Controlling weight and increasing physical activity can help to reduce menopausal symptoms.

- Menopausal women frequently increase their phytoestrogens intake, but evidence for its effectiveness is equivocal.

The menopause occurs when ovulation ceases and the production of oestrogen decreases. This results in the cessation of menstruation and other changes associated with the menopause. It is a gradual change (perimenopause) that usually happens between 40 and 58 years of age (Roberts, 2007); the average age is 51 years. Approximately 75–80% of women suffer menopausal symptoms; 45% find the symptoms distressing while 20–30% find them severe (Royal College of Physicians Edinburgh, 2003). The menopause is self limiting (usually 2–5 years), although for some women it can extend over a longer period.

The most common menopausal symptoms include hot flushes, night sweats, vaginal dryness, sleep disturbance, mood swings, forgetfulness and lack of concentration (Roberts, 2007). Menopausal and postmenopausal women are at increased risk of several conditions, including osteoporosis, hypertension, heart disease and stroke.

Nutritional problems and their management

Weight gain

Lean body mass and metabolic rate decrease in both older men and women. The menopause is associated with an average weight gain of 2–2.5 kg over 3 years (Polotsky & Polotsky, 2010). Weight is more likely to be deposited abdominally, so increasing the risk of insulin resistance, dyslipidaemia and metabolic syndrome (Mastorakos *et al.*, 2010). Weight gain can exacerbate hot flushes and night sweats (Whiteman, 2003), especially if the weight is carried centrally (Raeme, 2008). To prevent weight gain energy intake may need to be reduced and physical activity increased. Physical activity is also associated with fewer menopausal symptoms and may help to reduce central adiposity (Leite *et al.*, 2010; Seo *et al.*, 2010).

Metabolic syndrome and heart disease

Oestrogen is cardioprotective; by the age of 65 years, the risk of heart disease in women is the same as that in men. Falling oestrogen levels lead to central adiposity, a risk factor for heart disease and insulin resistance (Llaneza *et al.*, 2010). The incidence of metabolic syndrome increases substantially during the perimenopause and leads to an increase in cholesterol and triglycerides, hypertension and risk of diabetes (Polotsky & Polotsky, 2010). Reducing the level of saturated fat in the diet is associated with an improved lipid profile and a reduced incidence of heart disease postmenopausally (Davidson *et al.*, 2002). The role of soya foods in improving the lipid profile is controversial (Beavers *et al.*, 2010; Llaneza *et al.*, 2010). Reducing glycaemic load (GL) has been shown to increase HDL cholesterol levels in postmenopausal women (Shikany *et al.*, 2009).

Bone health

Postmenopausal women are at risk of osteoporosis. The rate of bone calcium loss is escalated during the menopause, as osteoclast activity exceeds osteoblast activity due to falling oestrogen levels, and this continues for up to 10 years [North American Menopause Association (NAMA), 2010]. Menopausal women who are at risk of osteoporosis should be assessed and may need to receive specific dietary counselling (NAMA, 2010). The National Osteoporosis Society (2011) recommends a daily intake of 700 mg of calcium in postmenopausal women, which should be increased to 1000–1200 mg in women with osteoporosis. Postmenopausal women considering taking calcium supplements should seek medical advice due the risk of heart disease (Bolland *et al.*, 2011).

Vitamin A is associated with an increased risk of osteoporosis; therefore, vitamin A or retinol supplements should be used with caution (Dennehy & Tsourounis, 2010). The results of studies on the benefits of isoflavones on bone mineral density are conflicting (Liu *et al.*, 2009; NAMA, 2010). Unfortunately, weight loss of as little as 5% of body weight is associated with increased bone turnover in postmenopausal women, even when combined with low impact, weight bearing exercise (Rector *et al.*, 2009). Weight loss programmes should be combined with high impact exercise (Engelke *et al.*, 2006) (see Chapter 7.9.1).

Breast cancer

Although oestrogen production decreases during the menopause, SHBG also deceases, leading to a rise in free circulating oestrogen, which increases the risk of developing hormone sensitive breast cancers and some other cancers (see Chapter 7.15.4). This may be modulated by the increased consumption of brassicas (Fowke *et al.*, 2000) and fibre (Park *et al.*, 2009; Suziki *et al.*, 2008). The evidence for the role of isoflavone is conflicting (Kang *et al.*, 2010; Steinberg *et al.*, 2011).

Hot flushes

Hot flushes are one of the most common symptoms of the menopause and can be treated with hormone replacement therapy (HRT). Reducing the intake of alcohol, spicy food and caffeine, and losing weight if overweight or obese (Roberts, 2007) have been shown to be beneficial. There is no evidence to support the use of herbal supplements, including black cohosh, dong quai, evening primrose oil and ginseng. A recent review has shown that 400 IU of vitamin E for 4 weeks reduced hot flush frequency and severity (Dennehy & Tsourounis, 2010).

Phyto-oestrogens for the relief of menopausal symptoms

Eastern populations that consume a diet high in isoflavones appear to have lower rates of menopausal associated problems (Avis *et al.*, 2001). However, a systematic review concluded that there was no evidence for the effectiveness of phyto-oestrogen treatments in the alleviation of menopausal symptoms (Lethaby *et al.*, 2007).

Many women use complementary and alternative therapies for menopausal symptoms and may seek advice from dietitians (Lunny & Fraser, 2010).

Internet resources

Menopause Exchange   www.menopause-exchange.co.uk
Menopause Matters   www.menopausematters.co.uk
National Osteoporosis Society   www.nos.org.uk

References

Avis NE, Stellato R, Crawford S, *et al.* (2001) Is there a menopausal syndrome? Menopause status and symptoms across racial. ethnic groups. *Social Science & Medicine* 52: 345–356.

Beavers KM, Serra MC, Beavers DP, Hudson GM, Willoughby DS. (2010). The lipid-lowering effects of 4 weeks of daily soymilk or dairy milk ingestion in a postmenopausal female population. *Journal of Medicinal Food* 13(3): 650–656.

Bolland MJ, Grey A, Avenell A, Gamble GD, Reid IR. (2011). Calcium supplements with or without vitamin D and risk of cardiovascular events: reanalysis of the Women's Health Initiative limited access dataset and meta-analysis. *BMJ* 342: 2080.

Davidson, MH, Maki KC, Karp SK, Ingram KA. (2002). Management of hypercholesterolaemia in postmenopausal women. *Drugs & Aging* 19(3): 169–178.

Dennehy C, Tsourounis C. (2010) A review of select vitamins and minerals used by postmenopausal women. *Maturitas* 66(4) 370–380.

Engelke K, Kemmler W, Lauber D, Beeskow C, Pintag R, Kalender WA. (2006) Exercise maintains bone density at spine and hip EFOPS: a 3-year longitudinal study in early postmenopausal women. *Osteoporosis International* 17(1): 133–142.

Fowke JH, Longcope C, Hebert JR. (2000) Brassica vegetable consumption shifts estrogen metabolism in healthy postmenopausal women. *Cancer Epidemiology, Biomarkers & Prevention* 9(8): 773–779.

Kang X, Zhang Q, Wang S, Huang X, Jin S. (2010) Effect of soy isoflavones on breast cancer recurrence and death for patients receiving adjuvant endocrine therapy. *CMAJ* 182(17): 1857–1862.

Llaneza P, Gonzalez C, Fernandez-Iñarrea J,*et al.* (2010). Soy isoflavones, Mediterranean diet, and physical exercise in postmenopausal women with insulin resistance. *Menopause* 17(2): 372–378.

Leite RD, Prestes J, Pereera GB, Shiguemoto GE, Perez SE. (2008) Menopause, highlighting the effects of resistance training. *International Journal of Sports Medicine* 31(11): 761–767.

Lethaby AE, Brown J, Marjoribanks J, Kronenberg F, Roberts H, Eden J. (2007) Phytoestrogens for vasomotor menopausal symptoms. *Cochrane Database of Systematic Reviews* 17(4): CD001395.

Liu J, Ho SC, Su YX, Chen WQ, Zhang CX, Chen YM. (2009) Effect of long-term intervention of soy isoflavones on bone mineral density in women: a meta-analysis of randomized controlled trials. *Bone* 44(5): 948–953.

Lunny CA, Fraser SN. (2010) The use of complementary and alternative medicines among a sample of Canadian menopausal-aged women. *Journal of Midwifery & Women's Health* 55(4): 335–343.

Mastorakos G, Valsamakis G, Paltoglou G, Creatsas G. (2010) Management of obesity in menopause: diet, exercise, pharmacotherapy and bariatric surgery. *Maturitas.* 65(3):, 219–224.

North American Menopause Society (NAMA) (2009). The role of isoflavones in menopausal health. *Menopause* 7(4), 215–229.

North American Menopause Society (NAMA) (2010) Management of osteoporosis in postmenopausal women. *Menopause: The Journal of the North American Menopause Society* 17(1): 25–54.

National Osteoporosis Society (NOS) (2011) All about osteoporosis. Available www.nos.org.uk. Accessed 8 February 2012.

Park Y, Brinton LA, Subar AF, Hollenbeck A, Schatzkin A. (2009) Dietary fiber intake and risk of breast cancer in postmenopausal women: the National Institutes of Health-AARP Diet and Health Study. *American Journal of Clinical Nutrition* 90(3): 664–671.

Polotsky HN, Polotsky AJ. (2010) Metabolic implications of menopause. *Seminars in Reproductive Medicine* 28(5): 426–434.

Rector RS, Loethen J, Ruebel M, Thomas TR, Hinton PS. (2009) Serum markers of bone turnover are increased by modest weight loss with or without weight-bearing exercise in overweight premenopausal women. *Applied Physiology, Nutrition, and Metabolism* 34(5), 933–941.

Raeme NK. (2008) Adiposity and hot flashes: one more tree in the forest. *Menopause* 15(3): 408–409.

Roberts H. (2007) Managing the menopause. *BMJ* 334: 736–741

Royal College of Physicians, (2003) Consensus Conference on Hormone Replacement Therapy. Available at www.rcpe.ac.uk/clinical-standards/standards/hrt_03.php. Accessed 23 July 2013.

Seo DI, Jun TW, Park KS, Chang H, So WY, Song W. (2010) 12 weeks of combined exercise is better than aerobic exercise for increasing growth hormone in middle-aged women. *International Journal of Sport, Nutrition and Exercise Metabolism* 20(1): 21–26.

Shikany JM, Tinker LF, Neuhouser ML, *et al.* (2010) Association of glycemic load with cardiovascular disease risk factors: the Women's Health Initiative Observational Study. *Nutrition* 6: 641–647.

Steinberg FM, Murray MJ, Lewis RD, *et al.* (2010) Clinical outcomes of a 2-y soy isoflavone supplementation in menopausal women. *American Journal of Clinical Nutrition* 93(2): 356–367.

Suzuki R, Rylander-Rudqvist T, Ye W, Saji S, Adlercreutz H, Wol, A. (2008), Dietary fiber intake and risk of postmenopausal breast cancer defined by estrogen and progesterone receptor status–a prospective cohort study among Swedish women. *International Journal of Cancer* 15(122): 403–412.

Whiteman MK. (2003) Smoking and Obesity Increase risks of severe Hot Flashes. *Obstetrics & Gynecology* 101: 264–272.

SECTION 3

3.2 Preconception and pregnancy

Gail Rees

> ## Key points
>
> ■ A healthy diet and limited alcohol consumption should be advised during the preconceptional period.
>
> ■ Supplements of folic acid (usually 400 μg/day) should be taken preconceptually and until the 12th week of pregnancy.
>
> ■ Being under- or over-weight can affect the outcome of pregnancy.
>
> ■ A healthy balanced diet is important for maternal and foetal health.
>
> ■ A 10 μg supplement of vitamin D should be advised for all women throughout pregnancy and lactation.

Preconception

Body weight and fertility

Low body weight can affect reproductive function by causing hormone imbalances and anovulation; the relative risk of infertility increases in women who are underweight (Homan *et al.*, 2007). Compared with a reference body mass index (BMI) of 20–21.9 kg/m², the relative risk of infertility at 18 years of age at a BMI 16–17.9 kg/m² was 1.1 and 1.2 at a BMI of less than 16 kg/m² (Rich-Edwards *et al.*, 1994). Conversely, obesity also adversely affects ovulation and obese women have lower natural and assisted fertility rates. Relative rates of infertility gradually increase in women with a BMI greater than 25 kg/m² (Homan *et al.*, 2007). In women aged 18 years, the relative risk of infertility was 2.4 at a BMI 18–19.9 kg/m² and 2.7 at a BMI of greater than 32 kg/m² (Rich-Edwards *et al.*, 1994).

Polycystic ovary syndrome (PCOS) is the most common cause of anovulation and this is more common in obese women (see Chapter 3.1.1). High levels of body fat, particularly around the abdominal region, are linked to insulin resistance and this increases ovarian androgen secretion and abnormal development of follicles. Raised insulin levels also lower production of sex hormone binding globulin (SHBG) from the liver, resulting in high free androgen activity. High levels of androgens give rise to amenorrhoea, infertility, hirsutism, acne and alopecia (Ramsay *et al.*, 2006).

Weight loss is the first line therapy for obese women with PCOS wishing to become pregnant (The Thessalo-

niki Consensus, 2007). Studies clearly show a benefit from modest weight loss (5%). A systematic review of the literature on lifestyle changes and PCOS found that lifestyle intervention improves body composition, hyperandrogenism and insulin resistance. However, there was no evidence of effect for lifestyle intervention on improving glucose tolerance or lipid profiles, and there was no literature assessing clinical reproductive outcomes, quality of life and treatment satisfaction (Moran *et al.*, 2011).

A restrictive diet prior to conception or during pregnancy is not recommended as this may increase the likelihood of poor micronutrient intakes, which could have an adverse effect on foetal development, maternal nutrient stores and breast milk composition. Therefore, advice should focus on a varied, nutrient rich diet following healthy eating guidelines, with an active lifestyle to encourage a gradual weight loss before conception is attempted.

Male fertility and body weight

Undernutrition and obesity can affect steroid hormone production in men. Obesity in males is associated with reduced insulin sensitivity and decreased testosterone secretion (Pasquali *et al.*, 2007). A systematic review by MacDonald *et al.*, (2010) found no evidence for a relationship between BMI and average sperm concentration or total sperm count. Obesity is, however, associated with erectile dysfunction, which may be treated with weight loss (Pasquali *et al.*, 2007).

Alcohol

Female fertility

The relationship between alcohol and female fertility is equivocal. Some studies have shown that alcohol consumption reduces female fertility and some prospective cohort studies suggest that there is a dose–response relationship between alcohol and infertility. However, other studies find no effect on fertility or only find an effect at high levels of alcohol intake (Homan *et al.*, 2007). However, alcohol is known to be harmful to the foetus, especially during early pregnancy when the foetus is most susceptible to teratogens (compounds that are harmful to the foetus and cause malformations), and so alcohol is best limited or avoided preconceptually.

Male fertility

A meta analysis of social and behavioural factors and semen quality in men reviewed 57 cross sectional studies with 29914 participants from 26 countries and regions, and concluded that alcohol consumption was a risk factor for lower semen volume (Li *et al.*, 2011).

Folic acid and neural tube defects

The link between folic acid supplementation and a reduction in risk of neural tube defects (NTD) is well established (Czeizel & Dudas, 1992; MRC, 1991) Current advice from the Department of Health is to take a dietary supplement of folic acid (400 µg/day) from the time contraception is stopped until the 12th week of pregnancy. To prevent recurrence of NTDs in the offspring of women or men with a NTD, or for those who have previously had a child with a NTD or have a family history of NTDs, women who may become pregnant should take a daily supplement of 5mg of folic acid (available on prescription) until the 12th week of pregnancy. Women with diabetes, obesity or coeliac disease or who are taking medication for epilepsy are also advised to take 5mg of folic acid/day.

Despite campaigns to increase awareness, supplement use preconception (or prior to neural tube closure) continues to be low, especially in the socially disadvantaged and in ethnic minorities (Brough *et al.*, 2009). Therefore, opportunities to encourage preconception folic acid supplementation should be sought and women should also be advised to consume both naturally rich sources of folate and fortified foods. A good dietary intake is needed throughout pregnancy and lactation as requirements are increased. Women who have not taken folic acid supplements preconception should be advised to start immediately and continue until the 12th week of pregnancy. Many countries throughout the world (but not the UK) have introduced mandatory fortification of flour with folic acid. It is estimated that this produces a reduction in NTD incidence of 46% (Blencowe *et al.*, 2010). Table 3.2.1 shows the folic acid content of some foods.

Table 3.2.1 Folic acid content of some foods

Food source (portion size)	Folate per portion (µg)
Broccoli – boiled (85 g)	54
Spinach – boiled (90 g)	73
Baked beans in tomato sauce (135 g)	30
Orange juice (150 g)	27
Wholemeal bread – one slice (36 g)	14
Chicken – roast (100 g)	10
Fortified cereals:	
Cornflakes (Tesco) (30 g)	120
Cheerios (Nestle) (30 g)	51
Weetabix Bitesize (40 g)	68

Pregnancy

Basal metabolic rate and energy requirements

Energy requirements vary greatly between individuals according to body size and level of activity. During pregnancy additional energy is needed to support the increase in body tissues of the mother and foetus. Therefore, energy requirements increase due to increases in metabolically active tissues, and the increased energy cost of moving a heavier body (Butte *et al.*, 2004). Hytten & Leitch (1971) calculated theoretical estimates of the components of average pregnancy weight gain. A mean weight gain of 13 kg was calculated (uterus 0.9 kg; breasts 0.4 g; blood 1.2 kg; extracellular fluid 1.2 kg; fat 3.5 kg; plus the products of conception 5.8 kg). It should be remembered that this is a theoretical value and a wide range of weight gains are associated with a healthy pregnancy.

There are differences in changes in basal metabolic rate (BMR) during pregnancy between women in developed and developing countries. Generally, women in developed countries have been shown to have increased BMR, whilst in developing countries BMR decreases (Prentice *et al.*, 1996). Research also suggests that while the mean BMR for women in the UK changes little during early pregnancy, some women show increases in BMR at this stage and some show reductions in BMR, making it difficult to recommend an ideal energy intake (Prentice *et al.*, 1989). The UK estimated average requirement (EAR) for energy intake during pregnancy is therefore unchanged until the third trimester when there is an increment of 190 kcal (800 kJ)/day, but with the recognition that those who are underweight at the start of pregnancy and those who do not reduce their activity levels may require more (Scientific Advisory Committee for Nutrition, 2011).

Obesity and weight gain

Maternal obesity is increasing in the UK. In a 19-year period between 1989 and 2007, obesity doubled from 7.6% to 15.6% and the percentage of women in early pregnancy with a normal range BMI has decreased from 66% to 54% (Heslehurst *et al.*, 2010). Obesity during pregnancy has been associated with many adverse outcomes

SECTION 3

Table 3.2.2 USA guidelines for weight gain during pregnancy (Institute of Medicine/National Research Council. 2009)

BMI category	Total weight gain (kg)
Underweight (BMI <18.5 kg/m²)	13–18
Normal weight (BMI 18.5–24.9 kg/m²)	11–16
Overweight (BMI 25–29.9 kg/m²)	7–11
Obese (BMI 30 kg/m² or above)	5–9

BMI, body mass index.

Table 3.2.3 Summary of nutritional requirements during pregnancy (females 19–50 years) (Department of Health, 1991)

Nutrient	Reference nutrient intake	Increment for pregnancy
Protein (g/day)	45	6
Thiamine (mg/day)	0.8	0.1
Riboflavin (mg/day)	1.1	0.3
Niacin (mg/day)	13	No increment
Vitamin B$_6$ (mg/day)	1.2	No increment
Vitamin B$_{12}$ (µg/day)	1.5	No increment
Folate (µg/day)	200	100
Vitamin C (mg/day)	40	10
Vitamin A (µg/day)	600	100
Vitamin D (µg/day)	–	10
Minerals	Various	No increment

for the mother, including gestational diabetes, thromboembolism, pre-eclampsia, caesarean sections, haemorrhage and wound infections. It is also associated with miscarriage, congenital abnormality, stillbirth, preterm birth and neonatal death (Sebire *et al.*, 2001a; Yu *et al.*, 2006; McDonald *et al.*, 2010; Vasudevan *et al.*, 2011). A recent enquiry into maternal and child health recognised obesity as a risk factor for maternal death [Centre for Maternal and Child Enquiries (CMACE), 2011].

There are currently no UK recommendations for weight gain during pregnancy as a wide range of weight gain is associated with a healthy pregnancy outcome. However, American guidelines provide guidance for weight gain based on prepregnancy body weight, as shown in Table 3.2.2 (Institute of Medicine/National Research Council, 2009). There is currently a renewed interest in weight gain due to the increasing number of obese women of childbearing age worldwide. Gestational weight gain has also been found to predict postpartum weight retention (Kac *et al.*, 2004). Thus, it is important that excess weight gain is avoided to prevent postpartum obesity and prevent women conceiving again when obese. The Royal College of Obstetricians and Gynaecologists (RCOG/CMACE) (2010) have called for research to determine the optimal weight gain during pregnancy for women in different BMI categories.

Current guidance from the National Institute for Health and Care Excellence (NICE) (2008) in the UK does not recommend routine monitoring of weight gain unless clinical management is likely to be influenced. However, it does recommend that height and weight are measured and recorded for all pregnant women at the first booking clinic (before 12 weeks' pregnant) (NICE, 2010). Body mass index (BMI) should also be calculated. The guidance also states that all obese, pregnant women should be given advice about diet and activity levels, and have the opportunity for referral to a dietitian (or other trained health professional) for further advice.

Several intervention programmes have been developed to prevent excessive weight gain during pregnancy. However, a systematic review of randomised controlled trials found that the trials were of insufficient quality to develop evidence based recommendations for clinical

practice in antenatal care (Ronnberg & Nilsson, 2010). More recently, a randomised controlled trial of a behavioural intervention aiming for adherence to US weight gain guidelines compared with standard care, showed that the intervention increased the percentages of normal weight, overweight and obese women who returned to their prepregnancy weights or less by 6 months postpartum (Phelan *et al.*, 2011).

Dietary management should ensure that the diet follows general healthy eating principles to provide sufficient micronutrients and protein, with supplementation of folic acid up to the 12th week of pregnancy and vitamin D throughout pregnancy. The diet should avoid those foods thought to be hazardous to the foetus (Table 3.2.3) and weight gain should be controlled by avoidance of high energy drinks and snacks, and limiting portion sizes where necessary. In the absence of evidence based UK guidelines for weight gain, US guidelines may be used if appropriate.

Underweight

It has been estimated in England that 5% of pregnant women are underweight (BMI <18.5 kg/m²) in the first trimester (Heslehurst *et al.*, 2010). Underweight women are at less risk of gestational diabetes and pre-eclampsia, but are significantly more at risk of anaemia, preterm birth and a birth weight less than the fifth centile (Sebire *et al.*, 2001b). A dietary assessment should be undertaken to ensure nutrient requirements are covered and advice given to ensure weight gain is appropriate. Discussion with midwifery colleagues to ensure adequate foetal growth may also be helpful.

Nutritional requirements during pregnancy

Protein

The current UK dietary reference values (DRVs) recommend an increment of 6 g/day of protein during pregnancy. For women aged 19–50 years this would mean an increase in the reference nutrient intake (RNI) from 45 g/day to 51 g/day. Most women in the UK exceed this amount and so do not need to alter their protein intake.

Fat

There are no recommendations to change the percentage of energy derived from fat during pregnancy. It is assumed that there will be some increment in fat intake as energy needs increase in the third trimester. There has however been debate about the requirements for long chain n-3 fatty acids. Long chain n-3 fatty acids, particularly docosahexaenoic acid (DHA), are required for brain growth and development of the retina, and so requirements are increased in pregnancy and lactation, but the exact amounts are difficult to quantify. An increase in intake however, needs to be balanced with advice to moderate oily fish consumption. While limited, there is some evidence that seafood intake (>340 g/day) in pregnancy has beneficial effects on child development (Hibbeln *et al.*, 2007). Higher n-3 intake has also been associated with longer gestation, higher birth weight and lower rates of postpartum depression (Genuis, 2008). However, in countries where fish is more common in the diet, mercury (high levels are associated with nerve damage in the foetus) in blood, placenta and cord blood has exceeded recommended levels and the levels were highest in those who ate fish more than three times a week (Hsu *et al.*, 2007). Therefore, women who could become pregnant or who are pregnant should be encouraged to eat oily fish within the guidelines offered by the Department of Health (Table 3.2.4). Fish oil supplements should be avoided during pregnancy due to their high vitamin A content. A pregnancy specific DHA supplement may be taken if it does not contain retinol.

Vitamins

There are modest increments in the dietary requirement for vitamins, as shown in Table 3.2.4 (Department of Health, 1991). Other than vitamin D and folate, vitamins should be provided by a diet following usual healthy eating guidelines – see also Micronutrient supplementation and Healthy Start.

Minerals and trace elements

In the UK there are no recommended increments in mineral or trace element intakes; recommendations for non-pregnant women therefore apply. This is due to physiological changes whereby there is an increased intestinal absorption of minerals. This assumes that there are sufficient minerals in the diet and the woman has a good nutritional status prepregnancy, so stores can be mobilised. Iron is the mineral most likely to be deficient, and although there are some savings of iron during pregnancy from the cessation of menstruation, it is sensible to ensure that adequate dietary sources are consumed throughout pregnancy (see Appendix A2). Haem iron is better absorbed than non-haem iron and so regular consumption of lean red meat is useful. If meat is not eaten, absorption of iron from vegetable and cereal sources can be improved if consumed with a source of vitamin C and if inhibitors of iron absorption (especially tea) are avoided with meals. Retinol is teratogenic and pregnant women will require advice on how to avoid excessive amounts (Table 3.2.4).

Micronutrient supplementation

Supplementation of some micronutrients is recommended in pregnancy. Folic acid supplementation is discussed earlier – Folic acid and neural tube defects.

Vitamin D

The Department of Health recommends that all pregnant and breastfeeding women take a supplement of 10 µg/day of vitamin D. (See Appendix A2 for sources of Vitamin D.) Vitamin D insufficiency has been found in pregnant women of different ethnic groups. Brough *et al.* (2010) showed that 70% of women in the first trimester in a diverse ethnic group in London had 25-hydroxy vitamin

SECTION 3

Table 3.2.4   Food to avoid in pregnancy

Risk	Sources – avoid
Listeriosis	Mould ripened soft cheeses, e.g. brie, camembert Soft blue vein cheeses, such as Danish blue Unpasteurised cow's, goat's or sheep's milk or soft cheese made from them All types of pâté including vegetable pâté
Salmonella and other food-borne infections	Raw, undercooked eggs and products containing, for example, homemade or restaurant-made mayonnaise, mousse, cold soufflés, etc. Raw or under cooked meat, poultry Raw shellfish
Toxoplasmosis	Unwashed fruit, vegetables and salad
Vitamin A toxicity	Liver, liver products such as liver pâté, liver sausage Supplements containing retinol, including fish liver oils
Mercury toxicity	Shark, marlin and swordfish Limit tuna to a max of two tuna steaks a week (140 g cooked) or four cans of tuna a week (140 g drained) Max of two portions of oily fish per week

D below 50 nmol/L, indicating insufficiency. There were significant differences between ethnic groups with 91% of Asian, 85% of African, 71% of Caribbean and 47% of Caucasian women having insufficient vitamin D. Vitamin D is synthesised under the skin from the actions of ultra-violet light, but in the UK (depending on the latitude) sunlight is at the correct wavelength to produce vitamin D only in summer months. At particular risk are women who cover themselves for religious or cultural reasons or who have limited time outside. Sunscreens also reduce the action of sunlight on the skin. Groups of women that are particularly vulnerable to vitamin D insufficiency include:

- South Asian, African, Caribbean and Middle Eastern Origin.
- Limited sunlight exposure.
- Diet containing no meat, oily fish, eggs, margarine or breakfast cereal.
- A prepregnancy BMI over 30 kg/m^2 – obese – have a lower bioavailability of vitamin D as it is sequestered in the body fat.

Iron

Iron demands increase in pregnancy and the mother is put at risk of anaemia by the demands of the foetus. Historically, all pregnant women were offered supplementation, but increasing understanding of changes in metabolism in pregnancy, such as haemodilution in the mother, has lead to changes in routine practice. NICE guidance (2008) recommends that iron supplementation should not be routinely offered to pregnant women and is only advised where there is a clinical need. Haemoglobin levels are measured at the booking appointment and usually in the second and third trimester according to local policy. Women with haemoglobin levels less than 11 g/100 mL at booking or less than 10.5 g/100 mL at 28 weeks' gestation should be investigated and iron supplementation offered if indicated. Iron supplementation may result in constipation; appropriate dietary advice should be given.

Multivitamins

Currently, it is not standard advice to recommend universal multivitamin supplementation in the UK, as it is in other countries, e.g. the USA. The most recent Cochrane review found that there is insufficient evidence to recommend multiple micronutrient supplementation to improve birth outcomes, apart from folic acid and iron supplementation (Haider & Bhutta, 2006). The studies included in this review were based in low and middle income countries and, therefore, their applicability in wealthier countries is open to debate. For example, a placebo controlled trial carried out in London, in a multiethnic population, did not show an effect of supplementation on mean birth weight or numbers of low birth weight babies. However, fewer small for gestational age babies were born in the group receiving multi micronutrient supplementation compared with the placebo group. This analysis was based on a small number of women who

were compliant with taking the supplements and the results need confirmation in larger studies (Brough *et al.*, 2010).

A multi micronutrient supplement specifically manufactured for pregnancy should be considered in all those who are suspected of having an inadequate intake of micronutrients. Appropriate dietary advice should be given, but nutrients are needed quickly in a short time-frame for pregnancy and dietary changes may take time to adopt. Pregnant teenagers are particularly at risk of inadequate diets and may have additional requirements to support the growth of the mother as well as the foetus. A pregnancy specific micronutrient supplement should be advised to ensure that it does not contain retinol, and has the required dose of folic acid and suitable amounts of other nutrients for pregnancy. If insufficient calcium is consumed, a calcium supplement may be needed, as calcium is often not present in multi micronutrient supplements. Retinol containing supplements should be avoided due to the teratogenic effects of large doses of retinol (vitamin A).

Healthy start

In the UK the NHS scheme Healthy Start provides vouchers for mothers on low incomes to purchase milk, fresh and frozen fruit and vegetables or infant formula. Women can apply for vouchers at their booking appointment with their midwife and receive them until their child is 4 years old. Teenagers under the age of 18 years are eligible for the scheme even if they or their parents are not on government benefits. Pregnant women and those with children aged from 1 to 4 years receive one voucher each week (currently worth £3.10); two vouchers are given each week for children under 1 year. To qualify for Healthy Start vouchers, mothers must have an annual family income of below £16 190 (20011/12) or receive one of the following government benefits:

- Income Support.
- Income based Jobseeker's Allowance.
- Income related Employment and Support Allowance.
- Child Tax Credit.

Vitamin tablets containing folic acid (400 μg), vitamin C (70 mg) and vitamin D (10 μg) are available free during pregnancy and until the child is 1 year old under this scheme. Further details can be found at www.healthystart.nhs.uk.

Food safety

During pregnancy the mother is relatively immunocompromised and thus may be more susceptible to infections, including foodborne infections. More care should be taken with food hygiene to avoid infections such as salmonella by ensuring thorough cooking of eggs, meat, poultry and ready meals, and proper storage of chilled foods. Good kitchen hygiene practices should also prevent the cross contamination of cooked food from raw meat and poultry.

Toxoplasmosis

The bacteria *Toxoplasma gondii* can cause severe foetal abnormalities. It can be transmitted by unwashed fruit and vegetables and is avoided by careful washing of produce, cleaning kitchen surfaces and hand washing. Protective gloves should be worn for gardening and handling cat litter trays. It can also be found in raw meat and unpasteurised milk.

Listeria

Listeria monocytogenes is able to grow at low temperatures and may be present in cook–chill foods, mould ripened cheeses and pâté. Certain foods should be avoided as a precaution (Table 3.2.4). Listeria infection in pregnancy, although rare, can cause miscarriage, stillbirth and severe illness in the newborn.

Mercury and polychlorinated biphenyl

The Department of Health advises pregnant and lactating women (and those trying to conceive) to avoid or limit certain oily fish due to mercury and polychlorinated biphenyl (PCB) contamination. These contaminants are present in marine life and subsequently become concentrated up the food chain. Large oily fish, shark, marlin and swordfish should be avoided since a relatively small amount contains sufficient mercury to be potentially neurotoxic to the foetus. Tuna also contains significant amounts of mercury and advice is to limit the amount consumed (Table 3.2.3).

Caffeine

In the UK, the Department of Health recommends that pregnant women should restrict caffeine intakes to below 200 mg/day. High caffeine intakes have been linked to foetal growth restriction. The Committee on Toxicity (COT, 2008a) reviewed the evidence from a number of research studies, including a study by Konje *et al.* (2008), which found a positive association between caffeine intake and increased risk of foetal growth restriction, which was maintained throughout pregnancy. More than 60% of the caffeine consumed during pregnancy in this study was from tea, and only 14% from coffee and 12% from cola. The mean intake of caffeine in this study of 2635 women was 159 mg/day. Exceeding the limit occasionally is not likely to cause problems because the risks are likely to be very small. There is still the possibility that the association is not causal due to the influence of confounding factors, but a cautious approach is advised. The COT committee also states that there may be a positive association between caffeine intake and miscarriage, but the evidence is unclear.

The amount of caffeine in drinks and foods will vary depending on the manufacturer and personal preferences. The following examples of drinks and food contain roughly 200 mg:

- Two mugs of instant coffee (100 mg each).
- One and a half mug of filter coffee (140 mg each).
- Two to three mugs of tea (75 mg each).
- Five cans of cola (up to 40 mg each).
- Two and a half cans of energy drink (up to 80 mg each).
- Four (50 g) bars of plain chocolate (up to 50 mg each) – milk chocolate contains approximately 50% of the caffeine in plain chocolate.

Alcohol

Current advice from the Department of Health is not to drink alcohol during pregnancy, but if a woman chooses to drink, then the maximum intake should be one to two units of alcohol once or twice a week. The National Institute for Health and Care Excellence (NICE, 2008) advises avoidance of alcohol in the first 3 months in particular, because of the increased risk of miscarriage, but alcohol at any stage of pregnancy can cause foetal alcohol syndrome (FAS) (restricted growth, facial abnormalities, learning and behavioural disorders). There are various degrees of FAS, and for some women, drinking >1–2 units once or twice a week may cause learning and behavioural disorders that may only become more obvious later on in childhood. Results of a systematic review and meta analysis show that the risks of low birth weight and small for gestational age gradually increase in mothers who consume an average of one or more alcoholic drinks a day. Risks of preterm birth increase by 23% in those who consume three or more drinks per day (Patra *et al.*, 2011).

Peanuts

There is no clear evidence that eating peanuts during pregnancy affects the chances of the infant developing a peanut allergy. Results from research in humans are limited and it is not clear whether consumption of peanuts during pregnancy increases or decreases the risk of peanut allergy in offspring, or whether there is any effect at all. It is also possible that the effect could differ according to the level of intake. Therefore, current advice is that there is no need to avoid peanuts unless the mother herself is allergic to them (COT, 2008b) (see Chapter 7.11.2).

Nutrition related problems

Nausea and vomiting in pregnancy

Nausea and vomiting are common symptoms of pregnancy that usually begin at 4–8 weeks' gestation and last for the first trimester. Although often termed morning sickness, these symptoms can occur at any time of the day and can last all day. Approximately 50–90% of women experience nausea and vomiting, but only a minority experience this after 20 weeks' gestation. Symptoms range from periodic nausea to severe vomiting (Jarvis & Nelson-Piercy, 2011). Most women manage to keep hydrated and eat an adequate diet by avoiding foods and smells that precipitate the symptoms. Small, frequent, high carbohydrate snacks (such as sandwiches and breakfast cereals) and fluids such as milk or fruit juice can help to keep the patient nourished and hydrated. Reassurance can be given that during the first trimester energy

SECTION 3

requirements are not increased and large hot meals can be avoided if these precipitate vomiting.

A Cochrane review considered several interventions for nausea and vomiting in early pregnancy and found a lack of robust evidence for any interventions. There was limited evidence of the effectiveness of acupressure, but acupuncture showed no significant benefit. The evidence for the effectiveness of ginger, vitamin B_6 and several antiemetics was limited and inconsistent (Matthews *et al.*, 2010). Although not evidence based, the following tips may be beneficial:

- Small frequent snacks – avoid getting very hungry.
- Drink liquids between meals rather than with meals.
- Dry foods may be better tolerated, e.g. dry biscuits, bread, toast, cereal, especially early morning.
- Avoid cooking smells and keep rooms well ventilated.
- Avoid high fat and highly spiced foods.
- Fizzy drinks and ginger flavoured drinks have anecdotally been reported as helpful.

Hyperemesis gravidarum is a severe form of vomiting which affects less than 1% of pregnant women. It is a serious condition often requiring hospital admission. It is characterised by intractable vomiting and weight loss of >5% of prepregnancy weight, dehydration, electrolyte imbalances and ketosis. Patients require intravenous rehydration, antiemetics and vitamin supplementation. Thiamine deficiency can occur if vomiting is prolonged, which can result in Wernicke's encephalopathy, and so thiamine administration may be required. Dextrose containing fluids can increase requirements for thiamine and should be avoided (Bottomley & Bourne, 2009). Although trials of efficacy for antiemetics are lacking, many are safe to use (antihistamines, phenothiazines and metaclopromide). The aetiology of hyperemesis is not fully understood and management aims to relieve symptoms and avoid complications (Bottomley & Bourne, 2009). Foetal complications can include foetal growth restriction (Jarvis & Nelson-Piercy, 2011).

Constipation

Constipation is a common problem during pregnancy and is probably caused by changes to gut transit time mediated by hormonal changes associated with pregnancy. Standard dietary treatment for constipation can be advised; high fibre containing cereals, fruit and vegetables and ensuring plenty of fluid (see Chapter 7.4.11). Faecal bulking agents can be used and changing the type of iron supplementation may be beneficial.

Heartburn

Heartburn and gastrointestinal reflux are also common problems experienced in pregnancy. Symptoms result from increased abdominal pressure and changes in gut transit time. Symptoms are usually more severe in the final trimester but can start from early pregnancy. Milk based foods can alleviate the symptoms and small frequent meals and snacks are sometimes better tolerated that large meals. Some foods may exacerbate the symp-

toms, such as spicy, fatty or acidic foods and drinks. Antacids are commonly prescribed.

Cravings and pica

Pregnant women frequently report cravings for certain foods and food aversions. Common food aversions include tea, coffee and alcohol. There are no reported patterns to the type of foods craved and no reports that cravings for foods adversely affect the nutritional intake of women. Pica is the craving and consumption of substances other than food and has been reported worldwide. Substances consumed include earth (geophagy), stones or pebbles (lithophagia), ice (pagophagia) and raw starches (amylophagy). It has been associated with both negative effects on health, e.g. heavy metal poisoning, micronutrient imbalances ad transmission of parasites, and positive health effects, e.g. providing micronutrients and relieving gastrointestinal discomfort (Young *et al.*, 2010). Pica is more common in developing countries than in developed countries. A study of well nourished Danish women reported an incidence of 0.02% (Mikkelsen *et al.*, 2006).

Internet resources

Committee on Toxicity   http://cot.food.gov.uk/cotstatements/
Department of Health – Nutrition for pregnancy and early life   www.dh.gov.uk/en/Publichealth/Nutrition/Nutritionpregnancyearly years/DH_127622
Go Folic   www.gofolic.co.uk
Health Start   www.healthystart.nhs.uk
NICE Guidelines   www.nice.org.uk
   Antenatal care: Routine care for the healthy pregnant woman CG62 Dietary interventions and physical activity interventions for weight management before, during and after pregnancy PH27 Maternal and child nutrition low income & disadvantaged groups to improve nutrition in pregnancy and breast feeding women PH11

References

Bottomley C, Bourne T. (2009) Management of hyperemesis. *Best Practice and Research Clinical Obstetrics and Gynaecology* 23: 549–564.

Blencowe H, Cousens S, Modell B, Lawn J. (2010) Folic acid to reduce neonatal mortality from neural tube disorders. *International Journal of Epidemiology* 39(Suppl 1): i110–i121.

Brough L, Rees GA, Crawford MA, Dorman, EK. (2009) Social and ethnic differences in folic acid use preconception and during early pregnancy in the UK: effect on maternal folate status and birth outcome. *Journal of Human Nutrition and Dietetics* 22(2): 100–107.

Brough L, Rees GA, Crawford MA, Morton H, Dorman E. (2010) Effect of multiple-micronutrient supplementation on maternal nutrient status, infant birth weight and gestational age at birth in a low income multi-ethnic population. *British Journal of Nutrition* 104: 437–445.

Butte NF, Wong WW, Treuth MS, Ellis KJ, O'Brian Smith E. Energy requirements during pregnancy based on total energy expenditure and energy deposition. *American Journal of Clinical Nutrition* 2004; 79(6): 1078–1087.

Centre for Maternal and Child Enquiries (CMACE). (2011) Saving Mothers' Lives: reviewing maternal deaths to make motherhood safer: 2006–08. The Eighth Report on Confidential Enquiries into Maternal Deaths in the United Kingdom. *British Journal of Obstetrics and Gynaecology* 118 (Suppl 1): 1–203.

Committee on Toxicity (COT). (2008a) Statement on the reproductive effects of caffeine. COT statement. Available at http://cot.food.gov.uk/cotstatements. Accessed 12 April 2012.

Committee on Toxicity (COT). (2008b) Statement on the review of the 1998 COT recommendations on peanut avoidance. COT Statement. Available at http://cot.food.gov.uk/cotstatements. Accessed 12 April 2012.

Czeizel AE, Dudas I. (1992) Prevention of the first occurrence of neural tube defects by peri-conceptional vitamin supplementation. *New England Journal of Medicine* 327: 1832–1835.

Department of Health. (1991) *Dietary Reference Values for Food Energy and Nutrients for the UK. Report of the Panel on Dietary Reference Values of the Committee on Medical Aspects of Food Policy*, 41. London: HMSO.

Genuis S. (2008) A fishy recommendation: omega-3 fatty acid intake in pregnancy. *British Journal of Obstetrics and Gynaecology* 115: 1–4.

Haider BA, Bhutta ZA. (2006) Multiple-micronutrient supplementation for women during pregnancy. *Cochrane Database of Systematic Reviews* 4: CD004905.

Heslehurst N, Rankin J, Wilkinson JR, *et al.* (2010) A nationally representative study of maternal obesity in England, UK: trends in incidence and demographic inequalities in 619 323 births, 1989–2007. *International Journal of Obesity* 34: 420–428.

Hibbeln JR, Davis JM, Steer C, Emmett P, Rogers I, Williams C, Golding J. (2007) Maternal seafood consumption and neurodevelopment outcomes in childhood (ALSPAC study): an observational cohort study. *Lancet* 369: 578–585.

Homan GF, Davies M, Norman R. (2007) The impact of lifestyle factors on reproductive performance in the general population and those undergoing infertility treatment: a review. *Human Reproduction Update* 13: 209–223.

Hsu C-S, Liu P-L, Chien L-C, Chou S-Y, Han B-C. (2007) Mercury concentration and fish consumption in Taiwanese pregnant women. *BJOG* 114: 81–85.

Hytten FE, Leitch I. (1971) *The Physiology of Human Pregnancy.* Oxford: Blackwell Scientific Publications.

Institute of Medicine/National Research Council (Committee to Re-examine IOM Pregnancy Weight Guidelines, Food and Nutrition Board and Board on Children, Youth, and Families). (2009) *Weight Gain During Pregnancy: Reexamining the Guidelines.* Washington, DC: National Academy Press.

Jarvis S, Nelson-Piercy C. (2011) Management of nausea and vomiting in pregnancy. *BMJ* 342: d3606.

Kac G, Benicio MHDA, Velasquez-Melendez, Valente JG, Struchiner CJ. (2004) Gestational weight gain and prepregnancy weight influence postpartum weight retention in a cohort of Brazilian women. *Journal of Nutrition* 134: 661–666.

Konje JC, CARE Study Group. (2008) Maternal caffeine intake during pregnancy and risk of foetal growth restriction: a large prospective observational study. *BMJ* 337: a2332.

Li Y, Lin H, Li Y, Cao J. (2011) Association between socio-psycho-behavioral factors and male semen quality: systematic review and meta-analyses. *Fertility and Sterility* 95(1): 116–123.

MacDonald AA, Herbison GP, Showell M, Farquhar CM. (2010) The impact of body mass index on semen parameters and reproductive hormones in human males: a systematic review with meta-analysis. *Human Reproduction Update* 16: 293–311.

Matthews A, Dowswell T, Haas DM, Doyle M, O'Mathúna DP. (2010) Interventions for nausea and vomiting in early pregnancy. *Cochrane Database of Systematic Reviews* 9: CD007575.

McDonald SD, Han Z, Mulla S, Beyene J. (2010) Overweight and obesity in mothers and risk of preterm birth and low birth weight infants: systematic review and meta-analysis. *BMJ* 341: c3428.

Mikkelsen TB, Andersen AM, Olsen SF. (2006) Pica in pregnancy in a privileged population: myth or reality. *Acta Obstetrica Gynecologica Scandinavica* 85(10): 1265–1266.

Moran LJ, Hutchison SK, Norman RJ, Teede HJ. (2011) Lifestyle changes in women with polycystic ovary syndrome. *Cochrane Database of Systematic Reviews* 7: CD007506.

MRC Vitamin Study Research Group. (1991) Prevention of neural tube defects: results of the MRCs vitamin study. *Lancet* 338: 131–149.

National Institute for Health and Care Excellence (NICE). (2008) *Antenatal Care: Routine Care for the Healthy Pregnant Woman.* Clinical Guideline no. 62. London: NICE.

National Institute for Health and Care Excellence (NICE). (2010) *Dietary Interventions and Physical Activity Interventions for Weight Management Before, During and After Pregnancy*. Public health guidance 27. London: NICE.

Pasquali R, Patton L, Gambineri A. (2007) Obesity and infertility. *Current Opinion in Endocrinology, Diabetes & Obesity* 14(6): 482–487.

Patra J, Bakker R, Irving H, Jaddoe VWV, Malini S, Rehm J. (2011). Dose-response relationship between alcohol consumption before and during pregnancy and the risks of low birth weight, preterm birth and small for gestational age (SGA) – a systematic review and meta-analyses. *BJOG* 118: 1411–1421.

Phelan S, Phipps MG, Abrams B, Darroch F, Schaffner A, Wing RR (2011). Randomized trial of a behavioral intervention to prevent excessive gestational weight gain: the Fit for Delivery Study. *American Journal of Clinical Nutrition* 93: 772–779.

Prentice AM, Goldberg GR, Davies HL, Murgatroyd PR, Scott PR. (1989) Energy sparing adaptations in human pregnancy assessed by whole body calorimetry. *British Journal of Nutrition* 62: 5–22.

Prentice AM, Spaaij CJ, Goldberg GR, *et al.* (1996). Energy requirements of pregnant and lactating women. *European Journal of Clinical Nutrition* 50 (Suppl 1): s82–s118.

Ramsay JE, Greer I, Sattar N. (2006) Obesity and reproduction. *BMJ* 333: 1159–1162.

Rich-Edwards JW, Goldman MB, Willet WC, *et al.* (1994) Adolescent body mass index and infertility caused by ovulatory disorder. *American Journal of Obstetrics & Gynecology* 171: 171–177.

Ronnberg AK, Nilsson K. (2010). Interventions during pregnancy to reduce excessive gestational weight gain: a systematic review assessing current clinical evidence using the Grading of Recommendations, Assessment, Development and Evaluation (GRADE) system. *British Journal of Obstetrics and Gynaecology* 117: 1327–1334.

Royal College of Obstetricians and Gynaecologists (RCOG)/CEMACE. (2010) *The Management of Women with Obesity in Pregnancy.* London: RCOG. Available at www.rcog.org.uk/womens-health/clinicalguidance/management-women-obesity-pregnancy. Accessed 12 April 2012.

SACN. (2011) Dietary reference values for energy. TSO, London.

Sebire NJ, Jolly M, Harris JP, *et al.* (2001a) Maternal obesity and pregnancy outcome: a study of 287,213 pregnancies in London. *International Journal of Obesity & Related Metabolic Disorders* 25(8): 1175–1182.

Sebire NJ, Jolly M, Harris J, Regan L, Robinson S. (2001b). Is maternal underweight really a risk factor for adverse pregnancy outcome? A population-based study in London. *British Journal of Obstetrics and Gynaecology* 108: 61–66.

The Thessaloniki Consensus. (2007) Consensus on infertility treatment related to polycystic ovary syndrome. *Human Reproduction* 23: 462–477.

Vasudevan C, Renfrew M, McGuire W. (2011) Foetal and perinatal consequences of maternal obesity. *Archives of Diseases in Childhood Foetal Neonatal Edition* 96: F378–382.

Young SL, Khalfan SS, Farag TH, *et al.* (2010) Association of pica with anemia and gastrointestinal distress among pregnant women in Zanzibar, Tanzania. *American Journal of Tropica Medicine and Hygiene* 83(1): 144–151.

Yu CKH, Teoh TG, Robinson S. (2006) Obesity in pregnancy. *British Journal of Obstetrics and Gynaecology* 113: 1117–1125.

3.3

Older adults

Vicki Pout

Key points

- The older population is diverse with a wide range of nutritional issues and needs.

- Food has biological, social, psychological and economic roles, and these aspects will affect food patterns of older people.

- Intakes of energy, protein, vitamin C, vitamin D, folate, iron, zinc and fibre are of most concern in older people.

- Good nutrition contributes to health and ability to recover from illness, may lessen health costs by promoting independence for as long as possible and improve overall quality of life.

- The biggest challenge is to maintain adequate nutrition when multiple factors conspire to reduce appetite and food consumption.

- A patient centred approach to care planning should be followed to establish individual dietary problems and formulate effective interventions.

- Team working can improve nutritional status in older adults.

There is no standard definition for when a person becomes elderly or old. Most developed countries take the age when pension benefits can be claimed as the starting point for old age. However, although it is common to use chronological age as a marker for old age, this is not synonymous with biological age. In the UK, the age of 65 years is usually taken as old, with age ranges after this of 65–74, 75–85 and 85+ years. The World Health Organization classifies 45–59 years as middle aged, 60–74 years as elderly, 75–89 years as old and 90+ years as very old.

The UK population was estimated to be 62.3 million in 2010, of which 10.5 million (17%) were 65 years and older and 1.4 million (2.3%) were 85 years and older [Office for National Statistics (ONS), 2010]. The UK population is growing older and is projected to age: those aged 65 years and over increased from 15% in 1985 to 17% in 2010 (an increase of 1.7 million people). In addition, the population aged <16 years decreased from 21% to 19% over the same time period. By 2035 23% of the population is projected to be aged 65 years and over compared with 18% aged <16 years (Older People's Day, ONS (2011)).

Within this ageing population there is also an ageing of the older population itself. The 'oldest old' in the UK have increased in number and proportion from 690 000 people aged over 85 years (1% of total population) in 1985 to 1.4 million in 2010 (2% of total population). It is estimated that in 2033 there will be 3.2 million people in the UK aged 85 years and older (5% of total population) (ONS, 2011). Similarly, the number of centenarians in the UK has grown from 2500 in 1980 to an estimated 12 640 in 2010. This includes an estimated 10 supercentenarians (people aged 110 years or more). It is projected that the number of centenarians in the UK in 2035 will be approximately 100 000 (ONS, 2011).

The World Health Organization (2011) has stated that the ageing of the world's population, in developing and developed countries, is an indicator of improving global health. Currently, the world's population aged 60 years and over is 650 million; by 2050 this population is forecast to reach 2 billion.

The ratio of women to men aged over 65 years is changing. It has fallen from 154 women for every 100 men in 1985 to a current ratio of 127 women for every 100 men. By 2035 it is projected that the sex ratio will have changed to 118 women for every 100 men. This change is also seen among centenarians, with nine women to every one man in 2000 to six women to every one man in 2009 and five women to every one man in 2010. The change in ratio is due largely to recent improvements in male mortality (ONS, 2011).

Currently life expectancy in the UK has reached its highest level on record for both men and women: 78.1

Manual of Dietetic Practice, Fifth Edition. Edited by Joan Gandy.
© 2014 The British Dietetic Association. Published 2014 by John Wiley & Sons, Ltd.
Companion Website: www.manualofdieteticpractice.com

years for newborn boys and 82.1 years for newborn girls (ONS, 2011). Women continue to live longer than men but the gap between the sexes has narrowed from 6 years to 4.1 years. In the UK, life expectancy varies by country. England has the highest life expectancy at birth (78.4 years for males and 82.4 years for females), while Scotland has the lowest (75.8 years and 80.3 years, respectively) (ONS, 2011).

This ageing population poses a challenge for the future. Society needs to prepare to meet the needs of older people, including health promotion, management of age related chronic diseases, long term and palliative care and age friendly services. As the population ages there is also a change in ethnographic make-up. Within minority ethnic groups there is a trend towards a younger age structure; however, this too may change as the population as a whole grows older.

Older people occupy up to two-thirds of NHS beds and as many as 60% of these will have mental health needs, mainly delirium and depression (Royal College of Psychiatrists, 2005).

Over the last 20 years the spectrum of accommodation available for older people has grown enormously and now encompasses extra care housing, very sheltered housing, assisted living as well as residential and nursing homes. Approximately 5% of over 65s live in residential or nursing care and of this population around 20% are aged over 80 years (Office of Fair Trading, 2005). In 2009 the British Association for Parenteral and Enteral Nutrition (BAPEN) reported that 700 000 older people were resident in sheltered housing in England.

The ageing process and nutrition

Ageing is a natural process that has effects on many body systems (see Table 3.3.1). The anorexia of ageing is seen where appetite and intake are reduced due to changes related to the ageing process (Morley, 1997).

Food habits and nutritional status of older people

The National Diet and Nutritional Survey of People Aged 65 Years or Over (Finch *et al.*, 1998; Steele *et al.*, 1998) explored the eating habits and nutritional status of people aged 65 years and older. Eating habits and nutritional status of older people are summarised in Table 3.3.2. Intakes of energy, protein, vitamin C, vitamin D, folate, iron, zinc and fibre are of most concern in older people. There are many factors that influence dietary intake and thus nutritional status. Food has biological, social, psychological and economic roles within life and these aspects will all affect food patterns of older people. If appetite is affected, this will lead to a change in intake. Table 3.3.3 gives examples of factors associated with dietary intake in older people.

Dietary recommendations for older people

Older people are a diverse group and as such have a wide range of nutritional needs. When making recommendations it is important to consider biological as well as chronological age. Good nutrition contributes to health and ability to recover from illness, may lessen burden of health costs by promoting independence for as long as possible and improves overall quality of life (King's Fund Centre, 1992).

Older people should be eating for health, which is not the same as healthy eating. People age at different rates and each individual needs to eat a diet that meets their own health and nutritional needs. For many people this will be traditional healthy eating but others will need increased levels of energy and nutrient dense foods and fluids. Older people should be encouraged to consume a variety of nutrient dense foods and maintain an active lifestyle where possible (Department of Health, 1992).

Appetite often declines with advancing age but other than energy requirements, most other requirements remain at the recommended levels for younger adults (Scientific Advisory Committee for Nutrition (SACN), 2011). Where appetite is decreased, the focus should be on nutrient dense, appealing and palatable meals and snacks. The emotional and social aspects of food and the role that food and drink plays in life's events must not be underestimated. The impact of acute or chronic illness and disability should be considered as this can quickly compromise food intake, nutritional status and body weight. Although older people are at higher risk of nutrient deficiencies, the population is diverse and this may not always be the case with individuals. Low intake may not always lead to deficiency due to individual variations in requirements or adaptation. Conversely, some nutrient intakes may appear adequate when compared with reference nutrient intakes (RNIs), but may be inadequate for individuals with higher requirements (see Appendix A3).

Energy

Older people should be advised to consume enough energy to maintain a healthy body weight. There is only a small age related decline in energy requirements, as shown in Table 3.3.4.

Calcium and vitamin D

Calcium, sunlight exposure and dietary vitamin D are important for bone health. Osteoporosis and associated fractures are a major cause of morbidity and mortality in older people. For those aged 50 years and over, osteoporosis is a contributory factor in at least 85% of fractures at all sites, most of which occur in the wrist, spine or hip (Department of Health, 2001). An intake of 700 mg/day of calcium is recommended for the elderly. Most of this will be consumed from milk and milk based foods, white fortified flour products and vegetables (Department of Health, 1998). An intake of 10 μg/day of vitamin D is recommended (Department of Health, 1998). Older people are particularly vulnerable to deficiency as they tend to have less sunlight exposure than younger people and there is a reduced efficiency of skin synthesis with age. In addition, oily fish consumption may be poor,

SECTION 3

Table 3.3.1 Effects of ageing on body systems (Copeman & Hyland, 1999; Department of Work and Pensions, 2012)

System	Changes produced by ageing
Skin	Wrinkling, thinning, reduced strength and elasticity Increased fragility and susceptibility to damage with elongated wound healing time Touch and pain thresholds increase Loss of hair, slowing of hair and nail growth Loss of pigment cells leading to the appearance of paler skin with age spots Reduced function of sweat and sebaceous glands Reduced synthesis of vitamin D (MacLaughlin & Holick, 1985)
Heart	Loss of heart muscle with increased fibrous tissue Decreased cardiac output
Renal function	20–30% decrease in weight and volume affecting nephrons, decreased filtration rate and increased glucose threshold Impaired renal function and fluid balance Less concentrated urine Benign enlargement of the prostate gland in 25–50% of men over 65 years leads to incomplete emptying of the bladder and a weak stream of urine, or signs of irritation with frequency of urination
Bone	Increased resorption Skeletal changes Osteoporosis
Immune system	Impaired T cell function leading to greater susceptibility to viral infections
Small and large intestine	Decreased motor function and muscle tone, constipation is more common Impaired digestive capacity Diverticula
Muscle	Sarcopaenia (decreased muscle strength and power, and lean body mass and increased fat body mass) resulting in decreased functional capacity
Hearing	Elevated sound threshold Loss of perception of high frequencies Degenerative changes in the inner ear may lead to balance impairment
Taste and smell	Decreased number of taste buds and loss of taste sensitivity Reduced number of nasal sensory cells
Vision	Diminished colour fidelity and peripheral vision Decreased visual acuity Decreased ability to focus on near objects Diminished ability to see in low or dim light and to distinguish objects of low contrast
Nervous system	Changes in central and peripheral nervous system Decreased size and mass of the brain Loss of neurones with fewer connections in the brain and spinal cord Slower thought processes Slower reaction time Decreased vibration and position sense Reduced sensitivity to temperature changes
Homeostatic regulation	Reduced ability to maintain homeostasis
Whole body composition	Sarcopaenia and frailty Physical fitness and strength reduced Loss of muscle and bone strength lead to increased risk of falls and resulting fracture Changes to muscles, bones and joints lead to height loss

especially in those in institutions. A supplement of 10 µg/day is recommended, especially in the winter for older people in residential care settings and those who are housebound or rarely go outside (Department of Health, 1998) (see Chapter 7.9.1).

Vitamin C

An intake of 40 mg/day is recommended for adults (Department of Health, 1998), but in older people consumption of fruit and vegetables may be insufficient to achieve this. This is of particular concern in those individuals who have a poor appetite, are frail or are dependent on institutional catering. Recommendations for vitamin C fortified drinks or supplements may need to be made. Where supplementation is advised, it should not greatly exceed the RNI.

Folate

Intake of folate is of concern in people who are frail or depend on institutional catering. A daily intake of 200 µg/day is recommended (FSA, 2006).

Table 3.3.2 Eating habits and nutritional status of people aged 65 years or over

Free living	Institutions	All
Lower socioeconomic status correlated with significantly lower average intakes of energy, protein, carbohydrate, fibre, some vitamins (especially vitamin C) and minerals	Oral health poor compared with free living individuals Poor oral hygiene and root decay especially prevalent	Better oral health, including the number of natural teeth, linked with better diet and nutritional status
People heavier than people of same age 30 years previously but recorded food energy intake lower	Vitamin D status poor in some people especially those in institutions in winter	Presence of root decay showed strong relationship with frequency of intake of high sugar foods independent of age, gender, social class and region of origin
90% of people had seven of 10 staple items from a list in their home	Residents were more likely to consume sugar, preserves, buns, cakes, pastries and cereal based milk puddings	As a group, people met COMA recommendations for total fat as opposed to national adult average, but had above recommended intakes of saturated fat and non-milk extrinsic sugars and below recommended intakes of fibre
86% visited shops but 55% said food shopping was sometimes done by someone else		For most people, biochemical status of most vitamins and minerals was adequate as measured by blood levels
53% had milk delivered where this was available		Folate status poor in a significant proportion of older people, especially in those aged 85+ years
One in three reported taking non-prescribed dietary supplements; the most common was cod liver oil		A traditional diet was common, especially as age increased and in those in institutions Most commonly consumed foods were tea, boiled/mashed/baked potatoes, white bread and biscuits
		Traditional meal pattern was for three meals a day plus smaller snacks in between. For some, nutritional contribution from snacks and drinks was considerable

Vitamin B$_{12}$

Dietary deficiency is uncommon and pernicious anaemia is usually caused by absorptive problems. However, low intake may be found in those with restricted intakes, e.g. vegetarians or vegans. Particular attention should also be paid to people who have intestinal conditions such as Crohn's disease and achlorhydria or have had a gastrectomy (Finch et al., 1998).

Iron

The RNI for iron is 8.7 mg/day for those aged over 50 years (Department of Health, 1991). A lower iron intake may be sufficient to maintain iron status in older people, especially postmenopausal women, compared with younger individuals. Iron intake can be of particular concern in those individuals who do not have a varied diet or who need texture modification, especially men aged 65 years and over living in institutions and free living men and women aged 85 years and over.

Gastrointestinal blood loss is the most common cause of iron deficiency in older people. This can be caused by a range of factors, including diseases of the genitourinary system, colorectal cancer, anti-inflammatory drugs, e.g. aspirin, or frequent blood tests. In 2010 SACN produced a report on iron and health and recommended that emphasis should be placed on a healthy balanced diet including a variety of iron containing foods. Less empha-

sis should be placed on the inclusion or avoidance of enhancers or inhibitors of iron absorption.

Zinc

Wound healing may be delayed with overt zinc deficiency. Decreased taste acuity in older people has been associated with zinc deficiency (Prasad, 1995; Prasad et al., 1993). Again, zinc intake can be of particular concern in those individuals who do not have a varied diet or who need texture modification.

Fluid and hydration

Older people are at greater risk of dehydration and a fluid loss of 20% can be fatal. Up to 10% of older people admitted to community hospitals suffer from clinical dehydration and up to 25% of immobile older people have chronic mild dehydration (Rolls & Phillips, 1990). Restoring normal hydration increases sense of wellbeing and comfort. Common causes of dehydration in older adults are shown in Table 3.3.5. The effects of dehydration on older people can compound the problem and lead to further reduction in fluid intake (Ritz & Berrut, 2005). The effects of dehydration in older adults include:

- Loss of appetite.
- Increased risk of development of pressure sores.
- Constipation.

Table 3.3.3 Examples of factors associated with dietary intake in older people

Theme	Factors
Availability of food	Loss of control over food when shopped for or in care Out of town supermarkets may restrict food choice if no car or unable to use public transport or carry heavy shopping Lack of help with shopping or food and beverage preparation Carers may not appreciate/ realise importance of nutrition
Finances	Low finances and limited budget. Food may be available but not able to afford nutritionally adequate diet Supermarkets usually offer best value and special offers on larger pack sizes of food, which may cost too much or not be able to be stored or used Concerns about paying bills, e.g. fuel bills in winter
Cooking	Time available to prepare and eat food Cooking for self and/or others Eating alone or with others Cooking and living facilities
Sensory perception	Loss of or altered sense of taste, sight, hearing, smell and thirst
Health issues	Decreased mobility or physical or mental illness affects ability to shop, prepare and consume food and may affect appetite Pain – chronic or acute Constipation Confusion or dementia Drug side effects or interactions may affect appetite, cause taste changes or constipation or affect absorption of nutrients. May be compounded by polypharmacy Impaired communication skills, e.g. dementia, loss of hearing or dysphasia Dysphagia especially if a modified texture diet is required Constipation Altered nutritional requirements due to medical conditions
Food provision	Unfamiliar or culturally inappropriate foods or menu terminology Repeated investigations and periods of fasting Poor nutritional content of food Lack of provision for second helpings Inappropriate mealtimes with long gaps when no food or drinks are offered
Lack of interest in food	Poor appetite Anorexia Nausea Depression, dementia, confusion or cognitive impairment, drowsiness, anxiety, side effects of drugs Secondary to malnutrition Illness and anxiety
Inappropriate food	Cultural/religious restrictions Dietary misconceptions, food myths and incorrect media messages Unfamiliar foods or menu items, Lack of patient/resident choice and poor menu planning
Previous experience	Cooking skills – skills needed to prepare a varied diet, reliance on prepared foods Budgeting skills Education and nutritional knowledge Personal likes and dislikes, cultural and religious needs Habit Fear of complaining about food or asking for food or beverages or assistance in case care is compromised Lack of appreciation of importance of food in treatment of illness and rehabilitation
Mealtime experience	Narrow range of foods eaten and reluctance to try new foods Unprotected mealtimes where staff breaks coincide with resident mealtimes, medical or drug rounds at meal times Poorly served food Inappropriate portion sizes Lack of garnishes and condiments Food served at incorrect temperature or kept warm for long periods Lack of choice as to whether to join others for meals Monotonous menus
Assistance with food	Unable to unwrap food Unable to use cutlery Reduced manual dexterity Poor hand to mouth coordination Inadequate assistance with eating and drinking Afraid to ask for assistance or feel they may be bothering busy staff, poor positioning
Oral problems	Sore or dry mouth Oral thrush Ill fitting dentures Poor oral hygiene, mouth care or dentition Reduced number of or no teeth (chewing ability is related to the number of teeth) Gum disease

- Electrolyte imbalance.
- Falls.
- Altered cardiac function.
- Unpleasant taste in mouth.
- Headaches.
- Drowsiness and confusion.
- Urinary tract infections.
- Irritability.
- Loss of skin elasticity.

Older people should be encouraged to maintain an adequate fluid intake. Although there is no set recommended amount in the UK, for most individuals this will be between 1500 and 2000 mL daily, which equates to six to eight drinks (FSA, 2009). The European Food Safety Agency (2010) recommends adequate daily intakes of water of 2000 mL for adult women and 2500 mL for adult men; the value is the same for adults of all ages. Awareness that all fluids count towards this target should be promoted. Where poor appetite or nutritional intake is of concern, nourishing fluids should be advised. In cases where there is inability or reluctance to consume enough fluid, additional sources of fluid can be promoted, e.g. soup, sauces and gravy, jelly, milk puddings, custard and ice cream. Often an additional drink in the form of fruit juice is accepted at breakfast as well as tea or coffee. Drinks are often not taken towards the end of the day due to a perceived increase in micturition at night. If an individual is concerned, encouragement should be given to maximise fluid intake during the day. Fluid intake is of particular concern in individuals who require thickened fluids (Whelan, 2001) (see Chapter 6.6).

Physical activity

Older people should be encouraged to maintain an active lifestyle where possible. Weight bearing exercise promotes bone health. Being active promotes weight maintenance, appetite, cardiovascular health and mental wellbeing as well as reducing falls (Health Education Authority, 1999).

Nutritional challenges in older people

Older people suffer from the same illnesses and nutritional assaults as younger adults. However, there are some conditions that present more often with advancing age, such as stroke, dementia and cognitive impairment, osteoporosis and falls. Older people may present with more diffuse symptoms such as falls, immobility, incontinence, acute confusion or weight loss, making diagnosis and treatment more difficult. There may also be a reluctance by an older person to visit their GP due to the misconception that disease is a natural part of ageing, not wanting to bother a busy health professional or thinking that there is nothing that can or will be done to help at their age. Often the biggest challenge when working with older people is to maintain adequate nutritional intake in the face of multiple factors conspiring to reduce appetite and food consumption.

Malnutrition

Malnutrition affects physical and mental function and the outcome of disease. These consequences of malnutrition include weight loss, reduced muscle strength, impaired immune response and delayed recovery from illness. The adverse effects of malnutrition in older adults are shown in Table 3.3.6 (NICE, 2006).

Table 3.3.4 Changes in energy requirements with age [based on SACN, (2011)]

Age (years)	Men (MJ/day)	Women (MJ/day)
45–54	10.8	8.8
55–64	10.8	8.7
65–74	9.8	8.0
Over 75	9.6	7.7

Table 3.3.5 Common causes of dehydration [based on Copeman & Hyland (1999)]

Pathological causes	Effects of ageing	Iatrogenic causes
Confusion – unable to ask for a drink, do not recognise thirst, may forget to drink	Altered thirst perception –thirst mechanism less sensitive so may not feel thirsty	Drugs, e.g. diuretics
Depression	Increased skin losses – thinner skin therefore more water lost via skin	Fluid restriction
Drowsiness	Reduced total body water	Institutionalisation – lack of availability of drinks
Decreased mobility or dexterity – unable to procure a drink or drink unaided. Lack of assistance given with drinking	Reduced renal function – kidneys not able to concentrate urine to the same degree as both renal plasma flow and glomerular filtration rate decrease with age	Physical environment, e.g. poor access to drinks, high room temperature
Conditions that affect fluid requirements or fluid losses, e.g. pyrexia or renal failure		Urinary incontinence or perceived increase in micturition after drinking, especially in the evening

Table 3.3.6 Adverse effects of malnutrition (NICE, 2006)

Adverse effect	Related consequences
Impaired immune response	Compounded by age related decrease in immunity Increased risk of infection including pneumonia and other respiratory tract infections Delayed recovery from infections
Muscle wasting	Decreased muscle strength and increased fatigue leads to delayed rehabilitation from illness Decreased mobility and increased risk of thromboembolism Decrease in ability to perform activities of daily living and increased burden on carers Increased risk of falls and consequent fracture more likely Increased risk of heart failure due to wasting of heart muscle compounding age related decline in cardiac function
Reduced respiratory muscle function	Increased breathing problems and less effective coughing mechanism Reduced cough pressure affects recovery from chest infection
Impaired thermoregulation	Increased risk of hypothermia
Impaired wound healing	Increased risk of wound infection and ununited fractures Increased risk of pressure sores
Psychological effects	Apathy, depression, anorexia, anxiety, fatigue and self neglect, impaired psychosocial function, low self esteem
Increased risk of vitamin and other deficiencies	Increased risk of refeeding syndrome Increased risk of specific nutrient deficiencies, e.g. iron deficiency anaemia
Overall	Delayed recovery from illness Greater risk of mortality

Table 3.3.7 Malnutrition prevalence rates in different settings [based on BAPEN (2010)]

Group	Rate of malnutrition
General population	5% (BMI <20 kg/m^2)
Free living older people	14%*
GP and outpatient attendees	18–30%*
Chronic disease	12% (underweight)
Care homes	16–29% (underweight) 20–50%*
Hospital admissions general	15–40%* (underweight)
Hospital admissions medical, surgical, elderly and orthopaedic wards	20–60%*

*using Malnutrition Universal Screening Tool ('MUST').

Groups of people who are more vulnerable to malnutrition include older people, and those with longstanding conditions, recently discharged from hospital, socially isolated or with a low income. Prevalence rates of malnutrition are shown in Table 3.3.7.

It has been shown using the Malnutrition Universal Screening Tool ('MUST') that older people at risk of malnutrition [body mass index (BMI) <20 kg/m^2] have 25% more hospital admissions, 6% more GP visits and 9% more prescriptions than individuals within the normal weight range (BMI 20–25 kg/m^2). For patients in hospital, it has been shown that those at risk of malnutrition have a significantly longer length of stay and are more likely to be discharged to a care destination other than their own

home (Elia, 2005). Risk of malnutrition increases with age. Older people may well have multiple factors that lead to inadequate nutritional intake and individual problems must be ascertained in order to develop a targeted nutritional care plan. Davies (1998) identified four types of malnutrition that are pertinent to older people and help to identify nutritional strategies to improve nutritional status:

- *Specific malnutrition* – a deficiency of a specific nutrient or nutrition related disease, e.g. scurvy or osteomalacia.
- *Long standing malnutrition* – often linked with general neglect. Clinical appearance of energy and nutrient deficiencies following period of inadequate intake.
- *Sudden* – a sudden marked change in food intake. Often after significant life event, e.g. major fall or bereavement.
- *Recurrent* – an older person with barely adequate nutritional status who, following a period of illness, enters a cycle of poor nutrition and repeated episodes of illness.

There are four main causes of malnutrition:

- Impaired intake.
- Altered nutrient requirements.
- Impaired digestion and/or absorption.
- Increased nutrient losses.

Specific factors affecting intake have been shown in Table 3.3.3 and factors affecting requirements, digestion and absorption and nutrient losses are shown in Table 3.3.8.

Table 3.3.8 Factors affecting nutrient requirements, digestion, absorption and nutrient losses in older people

Cause of malnutrition	Factors
Altered nutrient requirement	Increased energy requirements, e.g. due to involuntary movements or wandering, drug–nutrient interactions
Impaired digestion and/or absorption	Drug–nutrient interactions, polypharmacy, bacterial overgrowth, achlorhydria, medical or surgical problems affecting stomach, intestine, pancreas and liver
Increased nutrient losses	Gastrointestinal losses, e.g. vomiting; diarrhoea; fistulae, stomas, exudate from wounds or pressure sores.

Common issues

Osteoporosis is a common condition in older people. When assessing an individual nutritionally, their weight and level of physical activity should be taken into account. Being overweight can impair mobility and hence lead to increased risk of falls. However, being underweight also increases the likelihood of falling and consequent fracture.

Dementia and cognitive impairment are an important factor in nutritional problems. Individuals may have a number of challenging issues that impact on ability to prepare and consume food, and communicate thoughts and feelings related to food to other people. Food is an emotive issue for patients and carers and is seen as a very important part of the care process. Comprehensive and effective communication with patients and relatives is needed when addressing feeding difficulties in this area. Similarly, stroke also poses challenges to maintaining nutritional status.

Polypharmacy can compound the drug–nutrient interactions or side effects of a single medication. Older people often take a range of medications, including prescribed, over the counter, vitamin and mineral supplements, and complementary remedies. It is important to take into account any implications of an individual's medication regimen when performing a dietetic consultation. Common side effects include nausea, dry mouth, altered taste sensation, constipation, diarrhoea and drowsiness.

Nutritional care planning

Older people often have multiple comorbidities. It is important to consider their combined effect on nutritional status and function when devising a nutritional strategy. Box 3.3.1 illustrates a checklist for good nutritional care of older people.

Free living and sheltered accommodation

The majority of older people live in the community. The aim of nutritional intervention is usually to promote independence for as long as possible and maintain nutritional

---

Box 3.3.1   Checklist for good nutritional care of older people

- Ensure that the patient is involved as far as possible with their nutritional care. Follow best practice in decision making if an older person does not have capacity regarding nutritional care
- Older people are a diverse population with a range of factors affecting nutrition. Ensure an individual's circumstances are fully explored when planning nutritional care
- Check that national regulatory standards for food, fluid and nutritional care are being adhered to
- There is a need for a local healthcare wide strategy for good nutritional care of older people
- Follow local policies for malnutrition or risk of malnutrition and appropriate prescribing of oral nutritional supplements
- Regular nutritional screening should occur in all health settings to identify those at risk of malnutrition. A validated screening tool should be used. Results of screening and nutritional care plans should be communicated across care settings. Ensure that there is regular monitoring of weight and food and fluid intake
- A food first approach to improving nutritional intake is advised where possible
- Work towards a positive mealtime experience in all settings. Food should be a highlight of the day
- In institutional care settings ensure protected mealtimes are implemented. Give consideration to timing of meals, appropriate menus and drink and snack provision
- Ensure modified texture meals are used only when appropriate
- Set realistic goals and desired outcomes
- Ensure adequate and effective training on nutritional issues for health and social care staff working with older people. Many health professionals and carers have had very little nutrition training other than education about healthy eating

Table 3.3.9 Risk factors for poor nutrition for older people living in the community [based on Davies (1981)]

Theme	Risk factor
Food habits	Fewer than eight main meals, hot or cold, eaten in a week Minimal consumption of milk, fruit and vegetables Wastage of food, even when supplied ready to eat Long periods during the day without food or drink
Physical or mental factors	Depression or loneliness Unexpected weight changes either up or down Indications in medical records of disabilities including alcohol abuse or dependence
Social	Problems shopping Poverty

status to avoid admission to hospital or another care setting. In the community, care is often provided informally by a relative or carer or by a paid care package. It is important to ensure that carers as well as older people themselves are given sufficient information about specific nutritional issues and strategies to enable them to provide appropriate care. There are some specific risk factors for poor nutrition that are particularly pertinent to older people living in the community [based on Davies, (1981)] and should be considered when assessing nutrition in older people (Table 3.3.9).

Community meals

There are no national standards for nutritional content of community meals. The National Association of Care Catering (2003) and the Caroline Walker Trust (2004) both give guidelines for meal specification, but they are not the same. Community meals should meet the dietary needs of a variety of groups of people, from traditional healthy eating, to energy and nutrient dense in a small serving, to modified texture and therapeutic diets. One meal a day should aim to provide 40–50% of daily nutrient requirements in a realistic volume. There should be sufficient variety to reduce menu fatigue. Some meals are very low in salt, which can reduce its tastiness, but if a meal is not eaten it provides no nutrition. The energy content of meals can also be low. Individuals should be easily able to choose suitable dishes to meet their needs. Provision needs to be made for those with reduced appetites to ensure that suitable meals are nutrient and energy dense.

It must be remembered that community meals only provide one meal a day and not always 7 days a week. Overall meal, snack and beverage provision must be taken into consideration when working with older people as well as the need for encouragement and assistance. The human contact involved in delivered hot meals is very important as for some people this may be the only contact

they ... ay. However, delivery staff need to be train ... t the older people to whom they deliver.

C ... er factor in community meals and care pac ... eral. Some individuals will only order a me ... r day due to the expense. Food is not seen as ... mportant as there is a widely held misconce ... eople will lose weight and become more malnourished as they get older, but this is not a normal part of ageing.

Institutions (care home and hospital)

Regulation and monitoring of food and nutritional care in hospitals and other care settings has changed and strengthened. In England this is monitored by the Care Quality Commission, with Outcome 5 of the Essential Standards for Quality and Safety (2010) relating to meeting nutritional needs. The Health Inspectorate Wales monitor this through dignity and essential care inspections. Healthcare Improvement Scotland monitors nutrition and runs the Improving Nutritional Care Programme. Standards of nutritional care for Scotland are laid out in Food Fluid and Nutritional Care in Hospitals (2003). In Northern Ireland the Regulation and Quality Improvement Authority has produced Minimum Standards for Care in Nursing Homes, Residential Care and Day Care settings, which include standards for nutrition (Department of Health, Social Services and Public Safety, 2008; 2011; 2012).

The recent Care Quality Commission report into Dignity and Nutrition (2011) found that in hospitals, where there were problems, the recurrent themes were:

- Patients were not given the help they needed to eat, which meant they struggled to eat or were physically unable to eat meals.
- Patients were interrupted during meals and had to leave their food unfinished.
- Needs of patients were not always assessed properly, which meant they did not always get the care they needed, e.g. specialist diets.
- Records of food and drink were not kept accurately, so progress was not monitored.
- Many patients were unable to wash their hands before meals.

These themes are not new and have been the subject of high profile campaigns and media coverage e.g. Hungry to be Heard (Age Concern, 2006) and Still Hungry to be Heard (Age UK, 2010).

Care must be taken to promote a positive approach to food and the mealtime experience in all healthcare settings. Table 3.3.10 lists some examples of factors that will contribute to positive nutritional care. There should be a team approach to caring for older people. Working with this group will often entail being part of one or more multidisciplinary teams. The exact make up of each team will vary according to setting, speciality and funding. Good, effective team working can improve patients' nutritional status as each team member understands the role

SECTION 3

Table 3.3.10 Factors promoting nutritional care

Factor	Comment
Snacks	Snacks should be available between meals. Patients may often only be able to manage small portion sizes and rely on snacks to make up their nutritional deficit. Nourishing drinks should be available, e.g. milky drinks
Appropriate meals	Dishes, timings and dining arrangements should be appropriate to the population they are for. Routines should be flexible enough to be able to cope with individual needs. There should be a choice of portion sizes and the provision of seconds for those who are still hungry. A range of drinks should be available during and after the meal. Meals should be culturally appropriate and meet religious requirements where necessary. If required there should be the ability to fortify foods to increase nutritional content
Assistance	Appropriate assistance with eating and drinking should be available when needed from appropriately trained staff. The need for assistance should be assessed on admission and reviewed regularly
Team work	Nutritional care of patients is the responsibility of the entire health and social team. There should be effective communication between the team members and the patient and their relatives to ensure a consistent message
Eating area	Where there is a dining room it should be comfortable, clean and tidy and have appropriate furniture for the older people who will be using the room. Where there is no dining room, bed tables should be cleared and cleaned prior to meal times
Hygiene	People should be given the opportunity to use the toilet and wash their hands prior to meal service. Good oral hygiene should be promoted
Adaptations	Eating and drinking aids should be available for those people who require them. Modified texture diets should only be used where this will benefit the patient

Table 3.3.11 Range of services available in the community setting

Services to prevent hospital admission or provide support post discharge	Social services or private care packages Community meals – may be hot meals on wheels or regular delivery of frozen meals Rapid response teams to reduce admission Early supported discharge teams to provide immediate post discharge support and reduce readmission Intermediate care teams to provide rehabilitation at home Day hospital Respite care
Local community services	Over 60s clubs Retirement clubs Lunch clubs Community centres Day centres Cultural and religious activities
Shopping services	Dial a Ride Free bus laid on by supermarket Internet or telephone shopping and delivery
Voluntary services	Age UK Disease specific groups, e.g. Alzheimer's Society, Stroke Association and stroke clubs, Parkinson's Society Carers UK Citizens Advice CRUSE – bereavement care Ex services groups, e.g. Royal British Legion Admiral Nurses – Dementia UK

that they perform and the contribution to nutritional care that they bring.

Promoting independence and rehabilitation

There is a range of community based services to promote independent living for older people. Providers range from local authorities to private companies and the voluntary sector. The services available in any one area differ, as do access routes and eligibility criteria. Much support for older people is provided by family and friends who may be of a similar age to the person they are helping. Table 3.3.11 shows the range of services available in the community setting.

Further reading

Association of Community Health Councils. (1997) *Hungry in Hospital*. Available at www.achcew.org.uk

British Association of Parenteral and Enteral Nutrition (BAPEN) Improving nutritional care and treatment: Perspectives and recommendations from population groups, patients and carers. Available at www.bapen.org.uk

SECTION 3

British Association of Parenteral and Enteral Nutrition (BAPEN). Nutrition Screening Survey in the UK in 2008. Available at www.bapen.org.uk

British Association of Parenteral and Enteral Nutrition (BAPEN). (2005) The cost of disease-related malnutrition in the UK and economic considerations for the use of oral nutritional supplements (ONS) in adults. Available at www.bapen.org.uk

British Dietetic Association. (1996) Malnutrition in Hospital.1996. Available from www.bda.org

British Medical Association. (2001) *Withholding and Withdrawing Life Prolonging Medical Treatment: Guidance for Decision Making*. London: British Medical Association.

Copeman J. (1999) *Nutritional Care for Older People* London: Age Concern.

Council of Europe Resolution. (2003) *Food and nutritional care in hospitals*. Strasbourg: Council of Europe Publishing. Available at https://wcd.coe.int/ViewDoc.jsp?id=85747.

Crawley H. (2002) Food, drink and dementia. How to help people with dementia to eat well. Available from www.stir.ac.uk/dsdc

Department of Health. (2006) Dignity in care campaign. Available at www.dh.gov.uk.

Department of Health. (1998). *Nutrition and Bone Health. Report of the Working Group of the Committee on Medical Aspects of Food Policy*. Report on Health and Social Subjects 49. London: HMSO.

Department of Health. (2001) The National Service Framework for Older People. Available at www.dh.gov.uk.

European Nutrition for Heath Alliance. (2006) Malnutrition among older people in the community: Policy recommendations for change. Available at www.european-nutrition.org/publications.cfm.

European Society of Parenteral and Enteral Nutrition. (2006) Nutrition in Ageing: A call to action. Available at www.espen.org.

Food Counts Group. (2006) *Delivering Nutritional Care Through Food and Beverage Services – A Tool Kit for Dietitians*. London: British Dietetic Association Available at www.bda.uk.org.

Gurcharan SR (ed). (2004) *Medical Ethics and the Elderly*. Oxford: Radcliffe Medical Press.

Healthcare Commission. (2007) Caring for Dignity: A National Report on Dignity in Care for Older People while in Hospital. Available at www.cqc.org.uk.

Lennard Jones JE. (2012) *Ethical and Legal Aspects of Clinical Hydration and Nutritional Support*. London: BAPEN.

Malnutrition Advisory Group (MAG) of the British Association for Parenteral and Enteral Nutrition (BAPEN). (1999) *Hospital Food as Treatment*. London: BAPEN

National Collaborating Centre for Mental Health Dementia (2006) Supporting people with dementia and their carers in Health and Social Care. NICE Clinical Guideline 42. Available at www.nice.org.uk/Cg042.

National Patient Safety Agency. 10 key characteristics of good nutritional care. Available at www.nrls.npsa.nhs.uk.

National Quality Improvement Scotland (NQIS). (2002) Standards: Nutrition for Physically Frail Older People. Available at www.nhshealthquality.org.

Royal College of Nursing. Nutrition Now campaign Available at www.rcn.org.uk.

Royal College of Physicians. (2004) National Clinical Standards for Stroke. Available at www.rcplondon.ac.uk.

Scottish Executive National Care Standards. (2005) Care Home for Older People. Available at www.scotland.gov.uk.

Scottish Intercollegiate Guideline Network (SIGN) 78 Management of patients with stroke: identification and management of dysphagia. Available at www.sign.ac.uk/guidelines/published/index.html.

Stratton RJ, Green CJ, Elia M. (2006) *Disease Related Malnutrition – An Evidence Based Approach*. Wallingford: Cabi Publishing.

VOICES. (1998) Eating Well For Older People With Dementia. Available at www.cwt.org.uk.

Volkert D, Berner YN, Berry E, *et al*. (2006) ESPEN Guidelines on Enteral Nutrition; Geriatrics. *Clinical Nutrition* 25: 330–360.

World Health Organization. (2002) Keep Fit for Life: Meeting the nutritional needs of older people. Available at www.who.int.

Internet resources

Age UK   www.ageuk.org.uk

Alzheimer's Society   www.alzheimers.org.uk

Alzheimer Scotland – Action on Dementia   www.alzscot.org

Arthritis Care   www.arthritiscare.org.uk

British Geriatrics Society   www.bgs.org.uk

Care for Older People Portal   www.knowledge.scot.nhs.uk/home/portals-and-topics/care-for-older-people-portal.aspx

Carers UK   www.carersuk.org

Caroline Walker Trust   www.cwt.org.uk

Centre for Policy on Ageing   www.cpa.org.uk

Cruse Bereavement Care   www.crusebereavementcare.org.uk

Disabled Living Foundation   www.dlf.org.uk

Dementia UK   www.dementiauk.org

International Longevity Centre – UK   www.ilcuk.org.uk

National Osteoporosis Society   www.nos.org.uk

Nutrition Advisory Group for Older People (NAGE) – a specialist group of the British Dietetic Association (BDA) providing support, education and specialist information for dietitians and other Health Professionals working with older people   www.bda.uk.com NAGE resources can be purchased from Nutrition & Diet Resources UK   www.ndr-uk.org

Parkinson's Disease Society   www.parkinsons.org.uk

Relatives and Residents Association   www.relres.org

Stroke Association   www.stroke.org.uk

References

Age Concern. (2006) Hungry to be heard. The scandal of malnourished older people in hospital. Available from www.ageuk.org. Accessed 5 December 2012.

Age UK. (2010) Still hungry to be heard. The scandal of people in later life becoming malnourished in hospital. Available from www.ageuk.org. Accessed 5 December 2012.

British Association of Enteral and Parenteral Nutrition (BAPEN). (2009) *Screening for Malnutrition in Sheltered Housing*. British Association of Parenteral and Enteral Nutrition. Available at www.bapen.org.uk. Accessed 5 December 2012.

British Association of Enteral and Parenteral Nutrition (BAPEN). (2010) Malnutrition matters meeting quality standards in nutritional care. Available from www.bapen.org.uk. Accessed 5 December 2012.

Care Quality Commission. (2010) Guidance about compliance. Essential standards of quality and safety. Available at www.cqc.org.uk. Accessed 5 December 2012.

Care Quality Commission. (2011) Dignity and Nutrition Inspection Programme. National overview Available at www.cqc.org.uk. Accessed 5 December 2012.

Caroline Walker Trust. (2004) Eating well for older people – Practical nutritional guidelines for food in residential and nursing homes and community meals. Available from www.cwt.org.uk.

Copeman JP, Hyland K. (1999) Nutrition issues in older people. In: Corley G (ed). *Older People and Their Needs*. London: Whurr Publishers, pp. 35–53.

Davies L. (1981) *Three Score Years . . . and Then?* London. Oxford: Heinemann Medical Books.

Davies L. (1998) Practical nutrition for the elderly. *Nutrition Reviews* 46: 83–87.

Department of Health. (1991) *Dietary Reference Values for Food, Energy and Nutrients for the UK. Report of the Working Group of*

the Committee on Medical Aspects of Food Policy. Report on Health and Social Subjects 41. London: HMSO.

Department of Health. (1992) The Nutrition of Elderly People. Report of the Working Group on the Nutrition of Elderly People of the Committee on Medical Aspects of Food Policy. Report on Health and Social Subjects 43. London: HMSO.

Department of Health (1998). Nutrition and Bone Health. Report of the Working Group of the Committee on Medical Aspects of Food Policy. Report on Health and Social Subjects 49. London: HMSO.

Department of Health (2001). The National Service Framework for Older People. London: The Stationery Office.

Department of Health, Social Services and Public Safety. (2008) Nursing home minimum standards. Available at www.rqia.org.uk.

Department of Health, Social Services and Public Safety. (2011) Residential care minimum standards. Available at www.rqia.org.uk.

Department of Health, Social Services and Public Safety. (2012) Day care settings minimum standards. 2012. Available at www.rqia.org.uk.

Department for Work and Pensions. (2012) Ageing. Available at www.dwp.gov.uk. Accessed 5 December 2012.

Elia M. (2005) Economic implication of malnutrition. Available at www.bapen.org.uk. Accessed 5 December 2012.

European Food Safety Authority. (2010) Scientific opinion on reference values for water. EFSA Journal 8(3): 1459–1507.

Finch S, Doyle W, Lowe C, et al. (1998) National Diet and Nutrition Survey: People Aged 65 years and Over. Volume 1: Report of the Diet and Nutrition Survey. London: The Stationery Office.

Food Standards Agency (FSA). (2006) FSA Nutrient and Food Based Guidelines for UK Institutions. Available at www.food.gov.uk. Accessed 5 December 2012.

Food Standards Agency (FSA). (2009) The good life. Available at www.food.gov.uk. Accessed 5 December 2012.

Heath Education Authority. (1999) Guidelines. Promoting physical activity with older people. Available at www.nice.org.uk. Accessed 5 December 2012.

King's Fund Centre. (1992) A Positive Approach to Nutrition as Treatment. London: King's Fund Centre.

MacLaughlin J, Holick MF. (1985) Aging decreases the capacity of human skin to produce vitamin D3. Journal of Clinical Investigation 76: 1536–1538.

Morley JE. (1997) Anorexia of ageing: Physiologic and pathologic. American Journal of Clinical Nutrition 66: 760–763.

National Association of Care Catering. (2003) A recommended standard for community meals. Available at www.thenacc.co.uk/.

National Institute for Health and Care Excellence (NICE). (2006) Guideline 32. Nutritional Support in Adults. Available at www.nice.org.uk.

NHS Quality Improvement Scotland. (2003) Clinical Standard. Food, Fluid and Nutritional Care in Hospitals. Available at www.nhshealthquality.org.

Office for Fair Trading. (2005) Care homes for older people in the UK – a market study. Annexe K, consumer behaviour and care homes – a literature assessment. London: Office of Fair Trading.

Office for National Statistics (ONS). (2010) Annual Mid Year Population Statistics 2010. London: ONS.

Office for National Statistics (ONS). (2011) Older People's Day. Statistical Bulletin. London: Office for National Statistics.

Prasad AS. (1995) Zinc: an overview. Nutrition 11: 93–99.

Prasad AS, Fitzgerald JT, Hess JW, Kaplan J, Penlan F, Dardenne M. (1993) Zinc deficiency in elderly patients. Nutrition 9(3): 218–224.

Ritz P, Berrut G. (2005) The importance of good hydration for day-to-day health. Nutrition Reviews 63(6 Pt 2): S6–S13.

Rolls BJ, Phillips PA. (1990) Aging and disturbances of thirst and fluid balance. Nutrition Reviews 48: 137–144.

Royal College of Psychiatrists. (2005) Who Cares Wins, Improving the outcome for older people admitted to the general hospital: Guidelines for the development of Liaison Mental Health Services for older people. London: Royal College of Psychiatrists.

Scientific Advisory Committee on Nutrition (SACN). (2010) Iron and Health. London: The Stationery Office.

Scientific Advisory Committee on Nutrition (SACN). (2011) Dietary Reference Values for Energy. London: The Stationery Office.

Steele JG, Sheiham A, Marcenes W, Walls AWG. (1998) National Diet and Nutrition Survey: People Aged 65 years and Over. Volume 2: Report of the Oral Health Survey. London: The Stationery Office.

Whelan K. (2001) Inadequate fluid intakes in dysphagic acute stroke. Clinical Nutrition 20(5): 423–428.

World Health Organization. (2011) Global Health and Ageing. Geneva: World Health Organization.

Rachel Barton and Diane Talbot

Key points

- The links between poverty, poor health and diet related inequalities in health are well recognised, and dietitians need to be aware of these.

- Dietitians need to understand the issues for people living in poverty and the impact on food choice when offering any dietary advice.

- Dietitians need to be involved in policy development in relation to food and health strategies. They have a role in helping to ensure that issues of poverty, and their impact on the ability to make healthier food choices, are understood and taken into account by policy makers.

- Working with individuals and communities living on a low income poses challenges for dietitians. These may require the dietitian to use new and varied ways of working, leading to the development of new skills and competencies, particularly in the field of public health.

Whilst the developed world does not experience the same level of poverty related malnutrition as the developing world, there are still clear links between diet and inequalities in health. This chapter considers why those with the lowest income have the poorest diet and examines some of the difficulties people on a low income encounter in relation to food. It discusses the size and nature of the problem; the barriers to eating a healthy diet and some of the ways in which the problems people experience may be overcome.

It is estimated that 60% of premature deaths in Britain are due to non-communicable diseases, including coronary heart disease and cancer. Poor nutrition is estimated to be a contributory factor in one-third of all cancers (Department of Health, 1998), nearly 30% of deaths from coronary heart disease (Peterson & Rayner, 2003) and 30% of years are lost due to disability or early death (WHO, 2002). The Department of Health has estimated that if diets followed nutritional guidelines, around 70 000 deaths in the UK could be prevented each year and that the health benefits [in terms of quality adjusted life years (QALYs)] would be as high as £20 billion each year (Cabinet Office, 2008).

Within the last two decades numerous policy documents, including *Choosing a Better Diet: A Food and Health Action Plan* (Department of Health, 2005a) and more recently Healthy *Lives, Healthy People: Our Strategy for Public Health in England* (Department of Health, 2010a) have highlighted areas for action to improve the diets of individuals, and set out strategies to reduce fat, sugar and salt consumption, and to increase intakes of fruit and vegetables. All of these documents recognise the links between poor diet and deprivation.

The Marmot Review (2010) extensively highlighted a systematic pattern of declining health linked to socioeconomic status: the social gradient. Shorter life expectancy and greater disability are concentrated in some of the poorest areas of England. This means that people living in disadvantaged areas are more likely to bear a higher burden of ill health (Department of Health, 2010b). Inequalities are not limited to life expectancy and are also present for diseases and conditions that impact on a person's quality of life. Marmot (2010) noted a gap in life expectancy of 7 years between the richest and poorest neighbourhoods and a gap in disability free life expectancy of up to 17 years.

Whilst dietitians cannot alleviate poverty directly, they can, by means of sensitive and appropriate advice, help to minimise some of the nutritional consequences. Dietitians also have a responsibility to highlight to policy makers and planners the nutrition related inequalities in health that can result from low income.

Links between low income, diet and health

Evidence shows that there is a wide health divide between the richer and poorer sections of society in the UK (Acheson, 1998; Marmot, 2010). People in lower income

Table 3.4.1 Observed prevalence of disease and risk factors within social class, in men and women of all ages [Reproduced from James *et al.*, (1997), with permission]

	Social class					
	I	II	IIINM	IIIM	IV	V
Men						
Ischaemic heart disease (%)	5.1	5.4	6	7.7	7	6.4
Stroke (%)	1.3	1.6	1.7	2.3	2.7	2.1
Mean blood pressure (mmHg)	136/76	137/77	138/76	139/77	138/77	139/77
Cholesterol >6.5 mmol/L (%)	26	28	27	27	27	26
Smoking >20 cigarettes/day (%)	31	31	33	44	40	40
Obesity (BMI >30 kg/m^2) (%)	9.9	13.5	13.7	15	15	14
Physically inactive (%)	14	14	15	20	21	21
Women						
Ischaemic heart disease (%)	1.8	3.4	5.2	4.4	5.9	7.2
Stroke (%)	0.5	0.9	2.3	1.5	2.0	2.5
Mean blood pressure (mmHg))	130/72	132/72	136/73	134/73	136/73	141/75
Cholesterol >6.5 mmol/L (%)	26	29	35	33	33	36
Smoking >20 cigarettes/day (%)	24	24	23	28	30	30
Obesity (BMI >30 kg/m^2) (%)	11.8	14.3	15	19.7	21.9	22.6
Physically inactive (%)	15	15	17	24	22	22

SECTION 3

groups have a higher prevalence of diet related conditions such as obesity, hypertension, high serum cholesterol and anaemia, and are more likely to suffer a premature death from coronary heart disease or cancer (Table 3.4.1). Children from lower income groups are more likely to have a low birth weight, birth abnormalities, poor growth, poor oral health or die in the perinatal period (see Chapter 3.2). Data from the UK National Child Measurement Program 2009/10 showed an almost linear relationship between the prevalence of obesity in children and deprivation. Among children in the first year (reception) of school, obesity prevalence ranged from 6.6% in the least deprived tenth of the population to 12.2% in the most deprived tenth. In Year 6 (10–11 years), this range was 12.6–22.8% (Health & Social Care Information Centre, 2010).

While many factors contribute to the increased risk of certain diseases, it is now widely accepted that dietary factors play an important role. Many UK dietary surveys (Gregory *et al.*, 1990; 2000) show the same pattern: lower income groups consume a diet containing fewer essential nutrients but more fat and sugars than those in higher income groups. The more recent National Diet and Nutrition Survey (NDNS) (Henderson *et al.*, 2002) confirmed this and highlighted that people in receipt of benefit were less likely to eat oily fish, whole grain and high fibre breakfast cereals, and more likely to consume less healthy alternatives, such as chips, table sugar, burgers, kebabs, meat pies, pastries and whole milk.

Increased concern in relation to dietary intake and low income led to the commission of a nutritional survey specifically focusing on low income groups. The Low Income Diet and Nutrition Survey (Nelson *et al.*, 2007a) included over 3600 adults and children from throughout the UK and living in households that fell into (approximately) the bottom 15% of the population in terms of material deprivation. The results were similar to those found in other surveys and broadly showed that those surveyed failed to meet population dietary targets, had poor micronutrient intakes, high body mass index (BMI) and blood pressure, and low reported levels of physical activity.

Size and nature of the problem

Unlike most other European countries, the UK does not have an official poverty line below which people are defined as poor. However, there are a range of measures that are frequently used to identify those in society with insufficient resources. While each measure of poverty has advantages and disadvantages, it is important to note that each often produces different estimates and identifies different groups as poor. *'Minor changes in available income can be critical in determining how much households can afford for food, which is an essential but flexible budget item'* (Dowler, 2008).

It would be wrong to assume that poverty is a static phenomenon and that the poor are a homogeneous group. There have always been groups in societies who are vulnerable, such as the elderly, disabled, chronically ill and those from ethnic minorities. Often these groups have fewer resources and many have struggled to make ends meet. However, over the last decade, the proportion of children and pensioners in poverty has fallen, while the proportion of working age adults in poverty has remained unchanged. As a result, more than half the people who live in poverty are working aged adults (Palmer *et al.*, 2007) and 53% of children have one or both parents in work (Department of Works and Pensions, 2010). Research suggests that individuals or households may enter poverty either because they are excluded from employment or their wages are insufficient to provide their families with adequate resources. People move in and out of poverty; some experience repeated spells in poverty as, while they may move out of poverty, this escape is short lived and they oscillate between being in and out of poverty. This movement affects the financial and other resources to which individuals have access and in turn limits their opportunities for adopting a healthy diet.

There has been a rise in the number of poor people and a widening of the gap between the rich and the poor (Hills, 1995; Babb, 2005). A common threshold of low income is one <60% of the median income. In 2005–2006, approximately 13 million people (22% of the population) in Great Britain were living in households below this income threshold and until 2004–2005; about 15% of the population (nine million individuals) had been in this category for 2 of 3 years, i.e. living in what might be termed persistent low income poverty (New Policy Institute, 2008). Parents living in poverty are more likely to be experiencing poor mental and/or physical health, to be disabled or to be caring for a disabled relative; this has an impact on children's immediate health and future life chances.

Disabled adults are twice as likely to live in low income households. While the number of children living in poverty has reduced by 6% since 1998–1999, it was estimated that 20% of children (2.6 million) in the UK were living in low income households in 2009–2010 (Department of Work and Pensions, 2011). This may be an underestimate; e.g. the Children's Commissioner cited 3.5 million children in low income families in 2010. Ethnicity also plays a part in childhood poverty with 63% of children from Pakistani or Bangladeshi families living in poverty compared with 25% of white children. The average risk of a child being poor is 28%.

It is also important to note that while half of those people living on low income live in the most deprived areas of the country, the other half live outside these areas and may not benefit from policies that target poverty in areas of known deprivation. Although poverty levels have been falling in recent years, the difference between rich and poor households is still significant.

A number of studies have investigated the effects of living in poverty. A 2003 survey for the National Children's Home (NCH, 2004) found that:

- Almost half of parents (46%) had gone short of food during the previous 12 months to meet the needs of someone else in their family.
- Over one-third (36%) said that they had gone without food so that others in the family could eat.

- One in five (20%) families said that they did not have enough money for food, with a further 40% saying that they had only just enough money for food.
- Of the families on income support, several said that they had been so desperate for money they had considered doing something illegal.

In the UK, social security benefit levels are sometimes used as an indicator of those living on a low income as, in theory, they represent the safety net:, the amount of income required to live on. In 2005, 4.25 million people were in families that were reliant on means tested benefits. However, the amount of income that a family living on benefit receives is not generous. This money has to cover all household and family expenses such as food, utility and other bills, school costs, travel, household consumables as well as larger items such as furniture, birthday and other celebrations, and presents. The Low Income Diet and Nutrition Survey (LIDNS) found the median spend on food was £28 per person per week, which included eating out, but excluded alcoholic drinks (Nelson *et al.*, 2007a). Given the limited income of families in this study, it is not surprising that they were unable to afford to follow healthy eating guidelines. '*Food poverty is worse diet, worse access, worse health, higher percentage of income on food and less choice from a restricted range of foods. Above all food poverty is about less or almost no consumption of fruit and vegetables*' (Lang, 2009).

Food poverty is defined as those households that '*do not have enough food to meet the energy and nutrient needs of all their members*' (DeRose *et al.*, 1998) and this is influenced not only by the cost of healthy food, but also the availability of healthy food in a local area as well. Evidence has shown that a healthy diet is more expensive than a diet that is based mainly on foods that are considerably higher in fats and sugars (Drenowski & Darman, 2005). It has also been found that the cost of a diet that adhered to nutritional standards was 88% more expensive in small local shops compared to the same diet bought in an out of town supermarket (O'Neill, 2005). Many people living on a low income rely heavily on local shops, as they cannot readily access out of town supermarkets. This illustrates an inequality in the affordability of healthy food for people living on a low income and thus a limited amount of money to spend on food, and is one of the reasons healthy eating guidelines are not followed (see Chapter 4.2).

Nutritional consequences of low income

The LIDNS (2007) set out to assess the diets of the low income population to determine the extent to which they vary from expert recommendations, whilst also providing data on height, weight and blood pressure for a representative sample of low income individuals and examining relationships between diet and risk factors in later life. The broad conclusions drawn from the study were that the dietary patterns of many low income households were falling short of those recommended for health and that there were reasons to be concerned about the health consequences of following such a diet (Nelson *et al.*, 2007b). More detailed results are summarised below:

- The average number of fruit and vegetable portions eaten daily was: men 2.4, women 2.5, boys 1.6, girls 2.0.
- Compared with adult National Diet and Nutrition Survey (NDNS) data, adults in the LIDNS were less likely to eat wholemeal bread and vegetables, and more likely to drink more soft drinks (but not more low calorie diet drinks) and eat more processed meats, whole milk and sugar.
- Non-milk extrinsic sugars accounted for 14% and 17% of food energy for adults and children, respectively.
- Percentages of food energy from total fat were 35.9% (men), 35.2% (women), 36.1% (boys) and 35.7% (girls).

Average daily intakes of most vitamins and minerals from food sources were found to be above or close to the reference nutrient intake (RNI). There was a proportion of the population whose intake fell well below the RNI for iron, magnesium, potassium and zinc, and the intake for some was lower than the lower RNI. This was especially noticeable for iron.

The LIDNS was the first to use a food security questionnaire in a national survey. About 30% of households within this low income population lived in food insecure households, which meant they had reported that during the previous year their access to enough food that was both sufficiently varied and culturally appropriate to sustain an active and healthy lifestyle had been limited by lack of money or other resources. Thirty-nine per cent reported having worried that their food would run out before they had money for more and 22% reported that they reduced or skipped meals regularly because of lack of money, with 5% reporting not eating for a whole day because they did not have enough money to buy food.

Low income issues and dietetic practice

When working with low income households, dietitians have to address a very complex situation in which access to food and shops, prices, budgeting strategies, patterns of food choice as well as the need for social and cultural acceptability all interact. The challenge for dietitians is to find ways of maximising the opportunities available to people on a low income to incorporate a healthier diet into their daily lives. Dietitians must understand how these factors interact in order to ensure that the information and the advice that they give is appropriate, and that the particular individual or family has the resources to implement the guidance given. Dietitians working with low income groups should have a knowledge of available benefits and be able to direct clients as appropriate. The Citizen's Advice Bureau is a good starting place (www.adviceguide.org.uk).

The UK Child Poverty Action Group (CPAG) looked at the causes of food poverty (Dowler *et al.*, 2001) and

highlighted its complexity and the multifactorial nature of what determines food security for households and individuals within the UK (Figure 3.4.1). Factors that contribute to food poverty in people living on low income include:

- Food affordability.
- Food access and availability.
- Food access through institutions, e.g. schools.
- Food usage.

An earlier study by Dobson *et al.*, (1994) examined the food choices of families and identified some of the difficulties and barriers faced when eating on a limited budget. All families who participated in this study struggled to make ends meet and their main concern was feeding their families and preventing children from going hungry. They had all changed their food buying habits in an attempt to economise and the cost of food took precedence over issues of taste, cultural acceptability and healthy eating. The responsibility for budgeting and feeding the family rested with the mother. Many found themselves having to ration food to ensure that there would be enough. Families tended to shop little and often at local discount supermarkets as they could not commit income to buying in bulk or in advance from large supermarkets or food cooperatives. In addition, families resisted radical changes and tried to maintain conventional eating patterns, often eating cheaper versions of familiar mainstream meals. They had worked out that it was cheaper to buy prepared foods from discount supermarkets than to buy raw ingredients. A limited income also discouraged experiments with new foods in case children and partners did not like them and so refused to eat them. Parents were concerned that their children should not appear different from their peers; having crisps or chocolate to take to school was not seen as a luxury but as a way of participating in conventional behaviour. Families were aware of the need to eat healthily but the difficulty for many was how to achieve this given the constraints of a limited income. It was often considered infeasible to adopt advice on healthy eating or this advice could only be partially carried through. The advice that many families received would have involved making substantial changes to their diet, which few could risk or afford.

This study did not include travellers, the homeless or those living in temporary accommodation such as hostels or bed and breakfasts. For these individuals and families, the difficulties are even more severe as many will not have access to cooking or storage facilities. Therefore, the advice given to these groups needs to reflect the realities of their everyday life.

In order to work with groups to enable them to change their dietary behaviour, the complexities surrounding food choice and its multifactorial nature, as outlined earlier, must be acknowledged. Health behaviour is deeply embedded in people's social and material circumstances and their cultural context. In 2007, the National Institute for Health and Care Excellence (NICE) published guidelines on promoting health related

SECTION 3

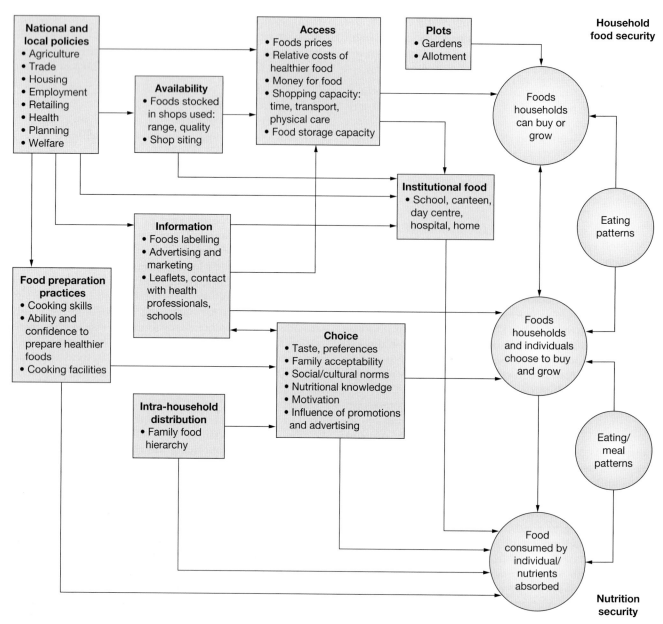

Figure 3.4.1   Framework of the barriers to healthy eating on a low income [source: Dowler *et al.* 2001. Reproduced with permission of the Child Poverty Action Group (CPAG)]

behavioural change. The guidance is for interventions at population, community and individual level. It identifies certain features that should be characteristic of interventions designed to promote health related behaviour change:

- They should be based on a needs assessment or knowledge of the target audience.
- They should take into account the circumstances in which people live, especially the socioeconomic and cultural context.
- They should be tailored to tackle the individual beliefs, attitudes, intentions, skills and knowledge associated with the target behaviour, e.g. healthy eating.
- Work should be developed in collaboration with the target population and take into account lay wisdom about barriers and change.

- Messages should be consistent with other national and local interventions.
- Key life stages or times when people are more open to change (such as pregnancy, starting or leaving school and entering or leaving the workforce) should be used.

Policy response to low income issues

The link between diet, poverty and health has been well documented, together with overwhelming evidence that a poor diet increases the risk of certain diseases. In addition, Marmot (2010) recently recognised the need for ensuring a healthy standard of living for all in order to reduce health inequalities. The NHS Plan (Department of Health, 2000) referred directly to the need to increase the intake of fruit and vegetables by improving availability and affordability; it launched the 5 A DAY programme. The programme included:

- School fruit and vegetable scheme.
- Local 5 A DAY initiatives.
- 5 A DAY programme, including a communications programme.
- Work with industry.

In 2004, the government launched Healthy Start as a replacement for the welfare food scheme, which targeted low income families and provided milk and vitamins to expectant and nursing mothers, babies and children under the age of 5 years. A review of the original scheme carried out by the Committee on Medical Aspects of Food and Nutrition Policy (Department of Health, 1999) concluded that the scheme did not meet the wider nutritional needs of pregnant and nursing mothers and young children. It concluded that the original scheme acted as a disincentive to breast feeding by providing up to twice as much infant formula as a 6–12-month-old baby required, and also provided more milk than children aged 1–5 years required. The current scheme targets pregnant women and families with children under the age of 4 years who are in receipt of some key means tested benefits and all pregnant women under the age of 18 years. Recipients now receive weekly vouchers to exchange in registered shops for modest quantities of milk, fresh fruit or vegetables or infant formula, and for vitamin supplements from health distribution points (Department of Health, 2004) (see Chapter 3.2).

Recognition of the impact of diet related inequalities in health led to the UK government including improving nutrition within low income and socially excluded groups as a key commitment in tackling health inequaliti,es (Department of Health, 2003; 2005b; 2005c). These policies recognised the role that all government departments can play in tackling inequalities in health. Alongside this, the Department of Health Food and Health Action Plan was published (Department of Health, 2005a). Although there was no explicit focus on inequalities, population wide interventions were advocated, including social marketing, public food procurement, food labelling, restrictions on food marketing to children and processed food reformulation, which potentially benefit low income households alongside the majority (Dowler, 2008). In 2004, the National Heart Forum produced a tool kit *Nutrition and food poverty* (Press, 2004) that was aimed at supporting people who were developing or implementing local nutrition and poverty strategies.

Dietitians have increasingly looked for alternative ways of encouraging people to make changes to their diets since empirical research has shown that, for low income groups, nutrition education has a limited role (Kennedy *et al.*, 1999). The reasons for this are summarised in Box 3.4.1. A number of community projects involving dietitians have adopted a community development approach or have used methods such as social marketing to ensure local communities are involved in the development of project methodology more commonly seen within social

---

Box 3.4.1 Reasons the for the limited role of nutrition education for low income groups [Kennedy *et al.* (1999)]

- Traditional approaches to nutrition education have shown limited success in changing food consumption patterns of low income households
- The main barrier to change is not ignorance of nutrition but the sum effect of social, cultural and economic factors
- The unidimensional model of knowledge, attitudes and behaviour is too simplistic
- The combination and interrelationship of factors has a more powerful effect on the individual's ability to exercise informed choice
- Nutrition education is clearly only part of the solution
- Even using more contemporary methods of nutrition education, people with limited resources are less likely to adopt recommended dietary changes unless other barriers to healthy eating are also dealt with
- More comprehensive approaches are needed
- Evaluation of the effectiveness of nutrition education and health promotion work at the community level is urgently required

---

sciences. Community development is an interactive and iterative process that should involve genuine partnership between local people, local workers and professionals. It is a process that has been described as *'working to stimulate and encourage communities to express their needs'* and then to work with all those concerned to address these needs (Ewles & Simnett, 1995).

Dietitians have used community development to ensure initiatives include the needs and food concerns of local people. Community based food projects use familiar foods that are available locally and dietitians work with local people to identify dietary changes that they can achieve, afford and are acceptable to the whole family (Dobson *et al.*, 2000).

An interesting development has been the use of non-dietetic workers in food projects, i.e. members of the communities in which the projects are based. The emergence of these new practitioners has necessitated the development of training programmes to enable these workers to go into communities and work with local people to address their food concerns (Le Cornu *et al.*, 2010; Kennedy *et al.*, 2008). Their involvement has included running a number of different sessions including 'cook and eat' and food tastings, as well as providing healthy eating advice and supporting food related community activities.

In recent years the Department of Health (2011) has introduced social marketing to facilitate change in health behaviours. Health related social marketing is the systematic application of commercial marketing concepts and techniques, such as insight generation and customer segmentation, to promote healthy behaviour in an appropriate way to the appropriate group of people. Essentially, social marketing is about understanding people's starting point in relation to an issue, e.g. healthy eating (Medical Research Council, 2007). The key questions are:

- What in their behaviours places them at risk?
- What drives their current behaviours?
- How might they be motivated to change?
- Who might be able to influence them?
- What might act as barriers to change?

Examples of using social marketing to change behaviours in relation to childhood obesity are the Change4Life project in the UK and the EPODE (Ensemble, Prévenons l'Obésité des Enfants or 'Together, let's prevent obesity in children) programme in France. The Change4Life campaign developed tools and messages aimed at specific groups of families identified as at risk of childhood obesity. Using research into food and physical activity behaviours (insight generation), families were split into six distinct groups, each with different characteristics, including socioeconomic class, age of mother, awareness of risk and intent to change (customer segmentation). Specific campaigns were developed using this insight generation and customer segmentation, which could be used by local health workers, businesses and community groups (Department of Health, 2008) The Change4Life evaluation indicated that 30% of mothers with children aged 2–11 years claimed to have changed at least one thing in their children's diets and activity levels as a direct result of Change4Life (Department of Health, 2010c) Dietitians can incorporate these techniques into targeted interventions with hard to reach groups, including those living on a low income. The EPODE programme in France used a whole town approach to social marketing and, alongside school based activities, different promotions were designed for different locations across the town but all with the same message. Over the course of 5 years, children aged between 5 and 12 years were weighed and measured. Results from the programme showed a reduction in mean BMI in participating towns compared with control towns (Ramon *et al.*, 2009).

Although community development and social marketing offer dietitians innovative ways to work with local people to change eating behaviour, they also present them with a number of challenges that must be addressed if these approaches are to prove effective. Dietitians need to be involved in the development of policy to address food security and food poverty work with communities and within public health departments and settings.

Further reading

Dowler E. (2008) Policy initiatives to address low-income households' nutrition needs in the UK. *Proceedings of the Nutrition Society* 67: 289–300.
Leather S. (1996) *The Making of Modern Malnutrition: An Overview of Food Poverty in the UK*. London: The Caroline Walker Trust.
Pantazis C, Gordon D, Levitas R (eds). *Poverty and Social Exclusion in Britain: The Millennium Survey*. Bristol: *University* of Bristol.

Internet resources

Child Poverty Action Group   www.cpag.org.uk
Citizen's Advice Bureau   www.adviceguide.org.uk
Supports to encourage low-income families   www.selfhelps.org
The Poverty Site   www.poverty.org.uk

References

Acheson D. (1998) *Inequalities in health: An Independent Inquiry*. London: The Stationery Office.
Babb P. (2005) *A Summary of Focus on Social Inequalities*. London: Office of National Statistics.
Cabinet Office – The Strategy Unit. (2008) *Food Matters. Towards a Strategy for the 21st Century*. London: Cabinet Office.
DeRose L, Messer E, Milman S. (1998) *Who's Hungry? And How do we Know? Food Shortage, Poverty and Deprivation*. New York: United Nations University Press.
Department of Health. (1998) *Nutritional Aspects of the Development of Cancer. Report on Health and Social Subjects No. 48*. London: Stationery Office.
Department of Health, Committee on Medical Aspects of Food Policy (COMA). (1999) *Scientific review of the welfare food scheme. Report on Health and Social Subjects 51*. London: HMSO, 1999.
Department of Health. (2000) *The NHS Plan: A Plan for Investment a Plan for Reform*. London: Department of Health.
Department of Health. (2003) *Tacking Health Inequalities: A Programme for Action*. London: Department of Health.
Department of Health. (2004) *Healthy Start: Government Response to Consutation Exercise*. London: Department of Health, 2004b.
Department of Health. (2005a) *Choosing a Better Diet: A Food and Health Action Plan*. London: Department of Health.
Department of Health. (2005b) *Tackling Health Inequalities: Status Report on the Programme for Action*. London: Department of Health.
Department of Health. (2005c) *Delivering Choosing Health: Making Healthier Choices Easier*. London: Department of Health.
Department of Health. (2008) *Healthy Weight, Healthy Lives: Consumer Insight Summary*. London: Department of Health.
Department of Health. (2010a) *Healthy Lives, Healthy People: Our Strategy for Public Health in England*. London: Department of Health.
Department of Health. (2010b) *Our Health and Well-being Today*. London: Department of Health.
Department of Health. (2010c) *Change4Life: One Year On*. London: Department of Health.
Department of Health. (2011) *Changing Behaviour, Improving Outcomes: A NSocial Marketing Strategy for Public Health*. London: Department of Health.
Department for Work and Pensions. (2010) *Households Below Average Income: An Analysis of the Income Distribution 1994/1995–2008/2009*. London, Department for Work and Pensions. Available at http://research.dwp.gov.uk. Accessed 5 December 2012.
Department for Work and Pensions. (2011) *Households Below Average Income (HBAI)*. London, Department for Work and Pensions. Available at http://research.dwp.gov.uk. Accessed 5 December 2012.
Dobson B, Beardsworth A, Keil T, Walker R. (1994) *Diet, Choice and Poverty: Social, Cultural and Nutritional Aspects of Food Consumption Among Low Income Families*. London: Family Policy Studies Unit.
Dobson B, Kellard K, Talbot D. (2000) *The Saffron Food and Health Project: An Evaluation*. Loughborough: Centre for Research in Social Policy.
Dowler E. (2008) Policy initiatives to address low-income households' nutrition needs in the UK. *Proceedings of the Nutrition Society* 67: 289–300.

Dowler E, Turner S, Dobson B. (2001) *Poverty Bites*. London: Child Poverty Action Group.

Drenowski A, Darman N. (2005) Diet choices and food costs: an economic analysis. *Journal of Nutrition* 135: 910–912.

Ewles L, Simnett I. (1995) *Promoting Health: A Practical Guide*. London: Scutari Press.

Gregory J, Foster K, Tyler H, Wiseman M. (1990) *The Dietary and Nutritional Survey of British Adults*. London: The Stationery Office.

Gregory J, Lowe S, Bates CJ, *et al.* (2000) . *National Diet and Nutrition Survey: Young People Aged 4 to 18 Years. Volume 1. Report of the Diet and Nutrition Survey*. London: The Stationery Office.

Health and Social Care Information Centre. (2010) *National Child Measurement Programme England 2009/10 School Year*. Available at www.noo.org.uk

Henderson L, Gregory J, Swan G. (2002) *National Diet and Nutrition Survey: Adults Aged 19 to 64 Years. Volume 1: Types and Quantities of Food Consumed*. London: The Stationery Office.

Hills J. (1995) *Inquiry into Income and Wealth*. York: Joseph Rowntree Foundation.

James W, Nelson M, Ralph A, Leather S. (1997) The contribution of nutrition to inequalities in health. *BMJ* 314: 1545–1549.

Kennedy L, Ubido J, Elhassan S, Price A, Sephton J. (1999) Dietetic helpers in the community: The Bolton Community Nutrition Assistants project. *Journal of Human Nutrition and Dietetics* 12(6): 501–512.

Kennedy LA, Milton B, Bundred P. (2008) Lay food and health worker involvement in community nutrition and dietetics in England: roles, responsibilities and relationship with professionals. *Journal of Human Nutrition and Dietetics* 21: 210–224.

Lang T. (2009) *What is food poverty?* Available at www.sustainweb .org/foodaccess/what_is_food_poverty/. Accessed 25 June 2012.

Le Cornu KA, Halliday DA, Swift L, Ferris LA, Gatiss GA. (2010) The current and future role of the dietetic support worker. *Journal of Human Nutrition and Dietetics* 23: 230–237.

Marmot M. (2010) *Fair Society; Healthy Lives: Strategic Review of Health Inequalities in England post 2010*. Available at www.marmotreview.org.

Medical Research Council (MRC). (2007) *The 'Healthy Living' Social Marketing Initiative: A review of the evidence*. London: Department of Health.

National Children's Home (NCH). (2004) *Going Hungry: The Struggle to Eat Healthily on a Low Income*. London: NCH.

National Institute for Health and Care Excellence (NICE). (2007) *Behaviour Change at Population, Community and Individual Levels. NICE Public Health Guidance 6*. London: NICE.

Nelson M, Ehrens B, Bates B, Church S, Boshier T. (2007a) *Low Income Diet and Nutrition Survey, vol. 1: Summary of Key Findings*. London: The Stationery Office.

Nelson M, Ehrens B, Bates B, Church S, Boshier T. (2007b) *Low Income Diet and Nutrition Survey, vol. 2: Food Consumption Nutrient Intake*. London: The Stationery Office.

New Policy Institute. (2008) Persistent low income. Available at www.poverty.org.uk/08/index.shtml. Accessed 25 June 2012.

O'Neill M. (2005) *Putting Food Access on the Radar*. London: National Consumer Council.

Palmer G, MacInnes T, Kenway P. (2007) *Monitoring poverty and social exclusion*. London: Joseph Rowntree Foundation.

Peterson S, Rayner R. (2003) *Coronary Heart Disease Statistics. British Heart Foundation Statistics Database 2003*. London: British Heart Foundation.

Press V. (2004) *Nutrition and Food poverty: A Tool Kit*. London: National Heart Forum.

Ramon M, Lommez A, Tafflet M, *et al.* (2009). Downward trends in the prevalence of childhood overweight in the setting of 12-year school- and community-based programmes. *Public Health Nutrition* 12(10): 1735–1742.

World Health Organization (WHO). (2002) *Reducing Risk, Promoting Healthy Life*. Geneva: WHO.

SECTION 3

3.5 Dietary patterns of black and minority ethnic groups

Aruna Thaker

Additional contributors: Heidi Chan, Ruth Kander, Christina Merryfield and Elzbieta Szymula

Key points

- The traditional diet of first generation Black and minority ethnic groups was well balanced, high in fibre and low in saturated fats.

- Most migrants adopt western eating habits, whilst maintaining some of their traditional eating habits.

- Over the years, the adoption of unhealthy western eating patterns and changes in lifestyle has resulted in a rise of chronic diseases in ethnic groups.

- There is robust evidence that diet, with other lifestyle changes, plays an important part in maintaining optimum health and in the treatment of chronic disease, but no systematic research has been undertaken for Black and minority ethnic groups in the UK to support this.

- Dietitians need to make a careful individual assessment of where a client is in the process of dietary acculturation before tailoring dietary advice.

The UK is a multicultural, multiracial society. Over many years, migration to the UK, mainly from Europe, was driven by political upheaval or war. However, during the 1950s and 1960s, due to expansion in different manufacturing and infrastructure sectors, young men were systematically recruited from British colonies such as the West Indies, India, Pakistan, Bangladesh, China and Hong Kong to fill an increasing shortage of labour that was created by the Second World War. Due to their status as British subjects, these young men settled with their families in the UK. Migration of Black and minority ethnic (BME) groups peaked during 1970s, as there were changes in the migration law and deportation of South Asians from Uganda, a former British colony. It has been shown that these migrants have contributed to the economic development of the UK over the last 60 years. For example, the British curry industry, which is Bangladeshi dominated, contributes approximately £4.5 billion to the British economy (Federation of Bangladeshi Caterers, 2008). In recent years, many cultural groups have arrived from the European Union as well as war zones of the world as asylum seekers or refugees, e.g. Tamils, Somalis and Iranians.

In the 2001 census, the size of the BME population in the UK was 4.6 million (7.9% of the total population) (ONS, 2004a). The largest category was South Asians, accounting for 2 million people or 3.6% of the UK population. The second largest group was comprised of 1.0%

Black Caribbean and 0.8% Black African people. Their geographical distribution in England was uneven with most living in Greater London, the West Midlands and other metropolitan counties (ONS, 2004a,b). The first generation of migrants mostly stayed within their communities in the large cities, as there were ample job opportunities. However, the second generation, who were born and educated in this country, are much more mobile and are more willing to move to different parts of the UK where there are job prospects.

The profiles for Scotland, Wales and Northern Ireland differ substantially from England. In Scotland, the BME population is just over 2%, with the main concentrations in the four largest cities. The South Asian population totals nearly 1% of the Scottish population, whilst the next largest BME group is Chinese at 0.3% (ONS, 2004a,b).

It is now acknowledged that the BME population is generally disadvantaged in terms of health (Erens *et al.*, 2001; Balarajan & Raleigh, 1995). The prevalence of disorders such as diabetes, heart disease, hypertension, stroke, cancer and mental illness tends to be higher in BME groups; good nutrition is important in the prevention of these diseases. Despite increased health needs, uptake of healthcare services tends to be low. Health problems are often compounded by factors such as poverty, unemployment, poor housing, communication difficulties and social isolation, in particular for women. Figure 3.5.1 shows the deprivation index of some BME

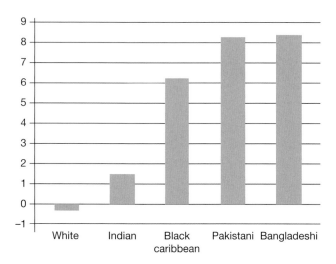

Figure 3.5.1 Relative deprivation of some ethnic groups in the UK (source: Cabinet Office Strategy Unit, *Ethnic Minorities and the Labour Market: Final Report*, 2003, figure 2.1, p. 15. Reproduced with permission under the Open Government Licence v2.0)

groups in the UK. This index combines several indicators, including unemployment rate, children in low income households, households that lack amenities (bath/shower/toilet) or a car, children in unsuitable accommodation and educational participation (Cabinet Office, 2003).

About half of those of BME origin were born in the UK, a proportion that will steadily increase and, as a result, western influences have affected traditional eating patterns to a considerable extent. Some people consume a diet that is no different from that of their indigenous peers, while others, particularly older people or those who have recently migrated, retain their traditional eating practices. This presents a major challenge in the UK, as there is enormous diversity in culture, traditions and food habits, both between and within different ethnic groups, and within a single family.

Dietitians are well placed to advise ethnic minority patients. It is erroneous to make assumptions about an individual's food habits simply based on their ethnic origin. Dietary needs should be tailored to take account of cultural factors, such as food preferences, religious dietary requirements and spoken and written language. It is vital that dietitians understand and are familiar with these factors when offering dietary guidance.

Collecting information

Dietitians can enhance their understanding by collecting information about and familiarising themselves with different ethnic groups and foods. The later section on Arabic diets should be used an example of how to gather this information. It is important to find out about traditional foods, and the availability and affordability of the following:

- Starchy foods.
- Fruit and vegetables.
- Meat, fish, pulses, dals, nuts and seeds.
- Fats and oils.

- Milk and dairy foods.
- Sugary and fatty foods.

It is important to also consider these points:

- Try to be objective about the quality of the diet and recognise the healthy aspect of traditional foods.
- Try to find out the ethnic names of the traditional foods that form a normal part of the diet.
- Try to find out how migration, religion and culture has affected food choices, e.g. fasting and alcohol intake, as well as smoking and physical activities.
- Try to find out who is responsible for making decisions about the diet at home, e.g. shopping, different cooking methods and portion size.
- Suggest healthier acceptable western foods, which can be cheaper as some of traditional foods in the UK may be quite expensive, e.g. tropical fruit and vegetables.
- Find out how much the client is motivated to make changes and what support is received from the family members, especially, if living within an extended family.
- Find out what are the barriers for making dietary and life style changes and how these can be overcome.
- Find out what is the best way to get your message across effectively so that adherence to dietary changes is more effective and easier to achieve.
- Find out which language the client fluent in and what resources are available.
- Do not be reluctant to question the client if you are unsure about any foods or if any clarification is needed.

The aim of this chapter is to provide a short introduction to well established cultural groups, some which have only recently arrived in the UK, and to describe how to find out relevant information about these ethnic groups before consultation. This chapter can only give an introduction to this topic and more detail can be found in Thaker & Barton (2012). The cultural groups' diets that are covered are:

- South Asian sub-continent: Gujarati, Punjabi, Pakistani, Bangladeshi, Sri Lanka.
- Arabic.
- Jewish.
- African–Caribbean.
- West African.
- Chinese.
- Polish.
- Turkish.
- Greek.

South Asian sub-continent

The term South Asian defines many ethnic groups with distinctive regions of origin, languages, religions and customs, and includes people born in India, Bangladesh, Pakistan and Sri Lanka (Fox, 2004). Figure 3.5.2 shows the cultural and religious diversity of South Asians living in the UK.

The Indian sub-continent was considered the jewel in the crown of the British Empire and young Indian men were recruited to different parts of the British Empire as

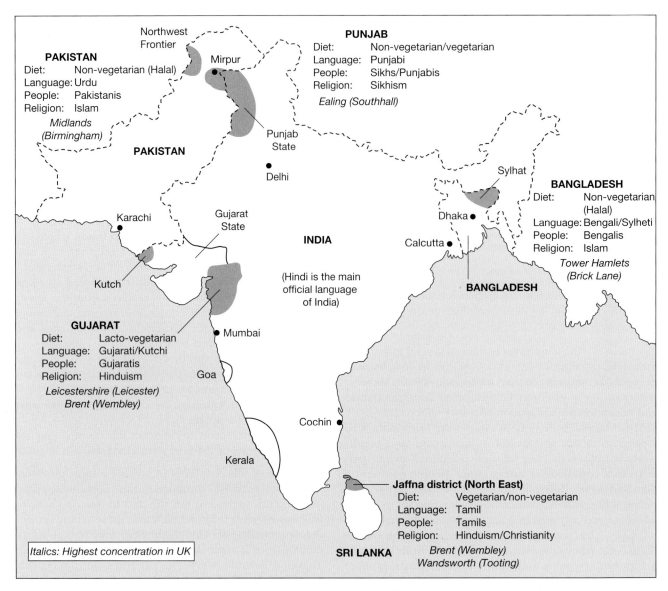

Figure 3.5.2   Cultural and religious diversity of South Asians living in the UK ([source: Thomas B, Bishop J (eds). (2007, Fig. 3.10.1, p. 361) *Manual of Dietetic Practice*, 4th edn. Oxford: Blackwell Scientific. Figure reproduced with permission of A. Thaker])

work force to develop the British colonies. In early 1900, young men from Gujarat and Punjab were recruited to lay a railway line from Mombasa in Kenya to Kampala in Uganda. After the completion of the line, these men settled with their families and helped in the development of these East African countries (Figure 3.5.3). They were able to maintain their culture and traditions in East Africa, as they were a very close knit community. In 1960, East African countries were granted independence, but after the deportation of South Asians from Uganda in 1972, the South Asians in other African countries felt unsafe and as a result many subsequently migrated to the UK. Young men from Pakistan and Bangladesh came directly to the UK after 1950. After 1980, many Tamil families migrated to the UK as refugees because of the civil war in Jaffna, the northern most region of Sri Lanka.

Due to the heterogeneity of diets consumed by South Asians, it is impossible to generalise about the nutritional implications. These will vary from person to person depending on the nature of the diet and the extent to which it meets individual nutritional needs and provides overall dietary balance. In the UK, older South Asian people are more likely to be first generation immigrants and follow traditional customs, although this is now happening to a lesser extent. Some may not read or speak English. In contrast, the younger generation may have adopted many aspects of the westernised way of life, including dietary habits.

Religious influences on diet

Religion is an integral part of the life of South Asians and each religion has its specific dietary restrictions. The four main religions of South Asians living in the UK are Hinduism, Sikhism, Islam and Buddhism. Table 3.5.1 shows the traditional diets of the South Asian ethnic groups.

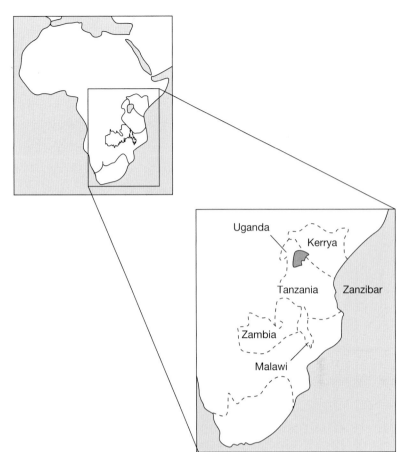

SECTION 3

Figure 3.5.3 African origins of South Asian migrants to the UK [source: Thomas B, Bishop J (eds). (2007, Fig. 3.10.2, p. 353) *Manual of Dietetic Practice*, 4th edn. Oxford: Blackwell Scientific. Figure reproduced with permission of A. Thaker]

What is a curry?

In the UK, many people now enjoy eating South Asian foods including curry, which has become a household name. This is one of the most institutional and best loved foods in the UK but there is no dish in the Indian, Pakistani, Bengali or Sri Lankan home called curry. Curry is an Anglicised version of the Tamil word *kari*, which refers to a dish made with vegetables or meat cooked in spices with or without a sauce in the south of India. The way it is pronounced is the most likely derivation of the word curry. Curry is now generically used to describe a variety of spiced dishes from the Indian sub-continent.

It is also likely that the word was adopted during the British Raj in India when British personnel stationed in India acquired a taste for the spicy foods. These dishes and recipes were brought back and adapted to suit the British palate and personal taste. A typical British curry originally included ingredients such as sultanas, spices and sugar in a sauce and was very mild in comparison with its Indian counterpart.

The first appearance of curry on a menu in the UK was at the Coffee House in Norris Street, Haymarket, London in 1773, but the first establishment dedicated to Indian cuisine was the Hindostanee Coffee House at 34 George Street, Portman Square, London in 1809. In <200 years this industry has grown from one restaurant to approximately 9500 restaurants with a £3.2 billion annual turnover (www.tandoorimagazine.com).

India consists of 28 states, all of which have their own regional cuisine, and people who migrated from the Indian sub-continent to the UK brought their traditional local dishes with them and these are recognised by specific names in South Asian households. As previously stated, the word curry is not used in South Asian homes.

In Hindi, this dish is known as masalaydar, which indicates that fresh herbs and spices (masala) are used in the cooked dish. Masala is a shallow fried mixture, cooked in fat or oil, that consists of cumin seeds, onions, ginger, green chillies, garlic, tomatoes and spices, such as turmeric (haldi), chilli powder, garam masala and salt. This was one of the cooking methods used to preserve food due to the hot climate of the Indian sub-continent. Dishes that are dry are sukhi and those that are liquid are tari. These dishes will include vegetables, pulses, dals, meat, poultry, seafood and paneer (unprocessed cheese). The precise name of the dish is dependent on which of these main food ingredients is used. The following terms are used:

- Gujarati dish made with vegetables – shaak:
  - Dry vegetable dish – koroo shaak.
  - With sauce – rasa varoo shaak.
  - Stuffed – bhareloo shaak.
  - Fried – tareloo shaak.
  - Potatoes – known as batata and according to the way it is cooked, e.g. batata nu karoo shaak, batata nu rasa varoo shaak or batata nu bharelloo shaak.

SECTION 3

Table 3.5.1 Traditional diet of South Asian ethnic groups ([from Thomas B, Bishop J (eds). (2007, Fig. 3.10.1, p. 354) *Manual of Dietetic Practice*, 4th edn. Oxford: Blackwell Scientific]

	Gujarat		Punjab		Pakistan	Bangladesh	Sri Lanka
	Hindus	Muslims	Sikhs	Hindus	Muslims	Muslims	Christians Buddhists Hindus
Main staple cereals	Rotali made from whole wheat flour Millet/Jowar/cornflour White rice	Chapattis/roti made from whole wheat flour White rice	Chapattis/roti made from whole wheat flour or corn flour	Chapattis/roti made from whole wheat flour or corn flour	Chapattis/roti made from whole wheat flour White rice	White rice Rice flour	Red rice Red rice Flour Whole wheat flour White rice
Vegetables and fruit	Vegetables cooked in oil with spices Raita/pickles Fresh fruit	Vegetables cooked in oil with spices Raita/pickles Fresh fruit	Vegetables cooked in oil with spices Raita/pickles Fresh fruit	Vegetables cooked in oil with spices Raita/pickles Fresh fruit	Vegetables cooked in oil with spices Raita/pickles Fresh fruit	Vegetables cooked in oil with spices Salad/pickles Fresh fruit	Vegetables cooked in oil with spices Salad/pickles Fresh fruit
Meat	No beef Might eat meat	No pork Halal meat: chicken, mutton, lamb	No beef Mainly chicken and mutton	No beef. Might eat meat	No pork Halal meat: chicken, mutton, lamb, beef	No pork Halal meat: chicken, mutton, lamb	Pork Chicken Mutton Lamb Or lacto vegetarian diet
Fish	White fish	Little if any fish	—	—	Little fish	White/oily/dried	White/oily
Eggs	Not eaten by strict lacto vegetarians	Usually hard boiled, fried or omelette	Not a major part of the diet	Not eaten by strict lacto vegetarians	Usually hard boiled, shallow fried or omelette	Usually hard boiled, shallow fried or omelette	Hard boiled or omelette
Pulses and dals	Major source of protein	Important	Major source of protein	Major source of protein	Important	Important	Major source of protein
Dairy products	Semi skimmed milk, yoghurt, paneer	Semi skimmed milk, yoghurt	Semi skimmed milk, yoghurt, paneer (used for making savoury dishes)	Semi skimmed milk, yoghurt, paneer	Full fat milk or semi skimmed milk, yoghurt	Full fat milk or semi skimmed milk, yoghurt, paneer(used for making sweet dishes)	Full fat milk or semi skimmed milk, yoghurt
Fats/oils	Ghee Butter Groundnut/sesame oil	Ghee Butter Groundnut/sesame oil	Ghee Butter Mustard oil	Ghee Butter Mustard oil	Ghee Butter Groundnut oil	Ghee Butter Groundnut/mustard oil	Ghee Butter Coconut/sesame oil
Cooking methods	Breads are cooked in a frying pan or on a griddle (tava) Shallow frying Deep frying Steaming Baking	Breads are cooked in a frying pan or on a griddle (tava) Shallow frying Deep frying	Breads are cooked in a frying pan or on a griddle (tava) Shallow frying Deep frying	Breads are cooked in a frying pan or on a griddle (tava) Shallow frying Deep frying	Breads are cooked in a frying pan or on a griddle (tava) Shallow frying Deep frying Tandoor (type of open oven)	Breads are cooked in a frying pan or on a griddle (tava) Shallow frying Deep frying	Breads are cooked in a frying pan or on a griddle (tava) Shallow frying Deep frying Steaming

Fresh herbs and spices are used by all the cultural groups in cooking and as garnish

Note: South Asian communities in East Africa follow the traditional diet that is largely based on the area of the sub-continent from which they emigrated but might include some African starchy foods, e.g. green banana (matoke) and cassava in their diet.

- A Punjabi dish – sarson ka saag – is made with spinach and mustard leaves and served with corn flour chapattis (makke di roti).
- A Pakistani dish made with vegetables is sabji and saalan is made with meat, e.g. mutton or chicken.
- Rasam or saaru is a South Indian soup which is dal based and served with boiled rice.
- Jhol – the Bengali dish usually made with seafood or fish.

Gujarati diet

Gujaratis constitute the largest cultural group of South Asians in the UK. They migrated from Gujarat on the Northwest coast of India, but significant numbers also came via East Africa where Gujaratis became prominent in the business community. Idi Amin expelled a large number of Ugandan Gujaratis in 1972, and the majority came to the UK. Gujarati or Kachi is likely to be their first language. Most Gujaratis follow the Hindu religion and the remainder are Muslims following Islam.

Hindu religion

The Hindu religion (Dharma) is the oldest religion in the world, having existed for over 5000 years. Hinduism is founded on reverence for life, non-violence and a belief in reincarnation. Dietary restrictions were laid down in the Hindu holy book, the *Bhagavat Gita* (chapter 17, verses 2–22).

Dietary restrictions

The Hindu dietary restrictions are:

- Hindus like Buddhists and Jains are lacto vegetarians and believe in Ahimsa, meaning non-violence to all forms of life. They avoid beef, as cows are sacred, and other meat and fish. They do not eat eggs since they are potentially a source of life.
- Animal derived fats such as dripping or lard are not acceptable. Foods that contain animal products are not eaten, e.g. rennet and gelatine.
- Milk, yoghurt, paneer and butter are consumed because they do not involve killing an animal. Paneer and yoghurt are made at home with full fat milk.
- Cooking with ghee (clarified butter) is believed to sanctify food. Fruit and cooked foods, especially sweet dishes (prasad) that are offered to the deities in the temples, are made at home with ghee. Ghee and vegetable oils are used in cooking and frying.
- Alcohol is forbidden, but is consumed by some.
- Strict Hindus will be unwilling to eat food unless they are certain that the utensils used in its preparation and service have not been in contact with meat or fish.
- Less strict Hindus may eat lamb, chicken or white fish.

Festivals

The Hindu festivals and religious days are:

- Mahashivratri – the birthday of Lord Shiva (March).
- Holi (March).
- Ram Navmi – the birthday of Lord Rama (April).
- Janmastami – the birthday of Lord Krishna (August).
- Raksha Bandhan (August).
- Navaratri – nine nights (October).
- Diwali – festival of lights and New Year (October/ November).

NB: all dates in this chapter are approximate as they are based on the lunar calendar.

Special sweet and savoury dishes are prepared during festival days and shared with friends and families.

Fasting

Some devout Hindus will fast regularly during the week and on religious days; it is mostly a matter of individual preference. The fast will be observed usually for a single day (24 hours) from dawn to dusk or for several days. Fasting is willingly abstaining from some or all food, drink or both. Some may have one cooked meal a day or only eat *pure* foods such as yoghurt and fruit, whilst others forego all food and may take fluids only.

Punjabi diet

Most Sikhs in Britain originate from the Punjab in India and like Gujaratis most came to the UK via East Africa. Many Sikhs came to the UK after the partition of India and there are now second and third generations in the UK. The mother tongue is Punjabi, but most Sikhs in the UK speak English and many can also converse in Hindi or Urdu.

Sikh religion

Sikhism is a reform movement, which is an offshoot of Hinduism and Islam and has developed into a religion in its own right. It started nearly 300 years ago. Guru Nanak, the first of 10 Sikh Gurus, founded Sikhism. Sikhs believe in one God. A Sikh Gurdwara (place of worship) traditionally serves meals (langar) to anyone at any time regardless of their caste, religion or class. In the UK, langar is cooked on Saturdays and served after evening prayer.

The three main principles of Sikhism are:

- Nam Japna (reciting God's name, e.g. prayers).
- Kirat Karna (honest earning).
- Vand Chhakna (helping the needy or less fortunate people, i.e. charity).

In 1699 the 10th Guru baptised the Sikhs and ordered the baptised Sikhs to wear five Ks, which are Kesh (uncut hair), Kanga (comb) Kara (steel bangle), Kirpan (small sword) and Kachhera (special shorts). Sikh men are meant to wear turbans and grow a beard; however, the majority are now clean shaven.

Dietary restrictions

Sikh dietary restriction include:

- The main food restriction is that Sikhs are not allowed to eat halal or kosher meat.
- For Sikhs this is a matter for each individual's conscience. As a group, they are less strict than Hindus and

SECTION 3

Muslims, but for each Sikh their own self imposed restrictions are binding.

- They are unlikely to eat pork, and beef is forbidden as the cow is considered a sacred animal.
- On the Indian sub-continent, chicken, lamb and sheep are killed by the jatka method (at one stroke); however, this practice is not common in the UK.
- Meat and eggs are included in the diet; however, after the Amrit (baptism) ceremony, individuals will revert to a lacto vegetarian diet.
- It has retained many features of Hinduism, e.g. women still follow a lacto vegetarian diet, even though they cook meat dishes for family members.
- Fasting is forbidden but many Sikhs still practice this Indian tradition and women may fast in the same way as Hindus.
- Alcohol, smoking and taking recreational drugs are also prohibited, although in practice alcohol consumption by men can sometimes be excessive.

Festivals

There are three main festivals in the Sikh calendar:

- Baisakhi – the Sikh New Year's day (April).
- Diwali – the Festival of Light (October/November).
- Birth of Guru Nanak – the founder of Sikhism (November).

Pakistani and Bangladeshi diet

The South Asian Muslim community in the UK came mainly from Pakistan, Bangladesh and East Africa. However, some Muslims in the UK will have originated from the Middle East, Malaysia, Indonesia, Sri Lanka and Africa. Many Muslims of Asian origin will speak Urdu, Punjabi, Mirpuri or Bengali. Muslims who have come from India or via East Africa may also speak Gujarati; they do not speak Kachi.

Islamic religion

The religion of Muslims is Islam; the word Islam is an Arabic word meaning submission. All Muslims acknowledge the obligation to signify their submission in terms of the five pillars of Islam. These are:

- Belief in one God (Allah) and that Mohammed is his true messenger.
- Prayer – five times a day.
- Zakat – giving 2.5% of wealth to the poor and needy.
- Pilgrimage – once in a lifetime Muslims should make a pilgrimage to Mecca if they can afford it.
- Fasting – complete abstention from food and drink from dawn to sunset in the month of Ramadan.

Dietary restrictions

Muslim dietary restrictions laid down in the Holy Qur'an are:

- Animals to be ritually slaughtered while reciting the name of Allah and then blood being allowed to drain (halal meat). (Kosher meat may be acceptable.)

- All wholesome foods are halal unless it is declared unlawful (haram). Unlawful (haram) foods are:
  - Foods and food products from the pig and foods containing ingredients or additives derived from the pig, any animal that has not been ritually slaughtered or any Haram source. Strict Muslims will eat outside home provided it is halal. Halal food is now available in institutions such as schools and hospitals. Ready made halal frozen foods are produced and sold in shops. Catering organisations, e.g. restaurants or other eateries, serve halal foods.
  - In practice, this means that a wide range of manufactured foods containing gelatine, animal fats or emulsifiers derived from animal sources will be avoided.
  - Alcohol, including that used in cooking or for medicinal purposes.
- A Muslim might refuse a food if they cannot be sure that it does not contain unlawful ingredients. Similarly, a devout Muslim will be concerned that the dishes used for cooking have not been in contact with unlawful foods.
- Fish is acceptable providing it has fins and scales and for Bengali Muslims both white and oily fish forms part of the diet.

The Muslim Food Board (UK) produces a regularly updated halal food directory listing halal manufactured foods available in the UK.

Festivals

There are two major festivals in the Muslim calendar:

- Eid-al Fitr (little Eid) marks the end of the fasting month of Ramadan and celebrations are held both in the community and at home.
- Eid-al Adha (big Eid) commemorates the pilgrimage to Mecca that concludes the Hajj.

Both Eids are marked with prayers in addition to the regular daily prayers, mutual visiting by family and friends and celebratory meals. Muslims are required to sacrifice a lamb, sheep, cow or goat after Eid–al Adha. During the celebration this meat is shared amongst family, friends and the poor. In the UK Muslims may contribute financially so that an animal is slaughtered by a halal butcher in the UK or abroad and then distributed to the needy.

Fasting

Muslims are required to fast from dawn to sunset during the month of Ramadan, which is the ninth month of the Muslim (lunar) calendar. Fasting involves abstinence from all food and drink and some Muslims might also stop smoking. It is considered one of the highest forms of worship as it enables people to practise self discipline, and it helps them to appreciate and share the feelings of the poor and hungry. Muslims should rise just before sunrise (sehri), have a meal similar to breakfast and then break their fast again at sunset (iftari). Feelings of weakness and lethargy can occur because of this abstinence and, to help overcome this, some Muslims rise early and eat a substantial high carbohydrate, high fat meal before dawn. Another heavy meal is then taken after sunset.

Elderly people and children under 12 years are exempt from fasting. Women who are pregnant, breastfeeding or menstruating and people who are ill or travelling during Ramadan are also exempt, but are expected to compensate by fasting at some other time. Chronically ill people, such as those with diabetes or heart disease, for whom fasting would be physically harmful, are exempt. However, many Muslims still choose to fast and should be advised accordingly (see Chapter 7.12). Devout Muslims may also fast once or twice a week in addition to Ramadan.

Arabic diet

Arab is the generic term applied to inhabitants of the Middle East and North Africa whose mother tongue is Arabic and who are Muslims. Arabic foods were originally the food of desert nomads. It was simple and carried during travels from one area to another, such as settled farming areas and oases. Animals such as goats and camels travelled with nomadic people and provided meat and milk, often cooked over camp fires. Foods such as flour, dates, spices and vegetables were collected on the way from farms and incorporated into various dishes including bread. Although there are still nomadic people having traditional diets, food consumption has changed to incorporate foods from different parts of the world, including aspects of a western diet. Urbanisation has also played a dramatic role in changes in food consumption patterns and dietary habits.

Traditional foods groups

Bread, rice, potatoes and other starchy foods
Bread (houbus – traditional flat bread made with white wheat flour), rice (roz), couscous and potatoes are all available from supermarkets. Cassava, millet or yam is often pounded into a porridge consistency. Cassava can be made into flour to be used in sauces with meat and vegetables or fried. These are the more traditional foods from North Africa and are now available in most UK supermarkets and ethnic stores.

Fruit and vegetables
Commonly eaten vegetables include aubergines, carrots, onions, okra, courgettes, spinach, green beans and salads (lettuce, tomatoes and cucumber). These are all available, although aubergines and okra may be expensive. Commonly eaten fruit include melon, pineapple, mangoes, grapes, citrus fruit and pomegranate. Most tropical fruit, while available, tend to be expensive. Dried fruit, particularly dates (tamour) and figs, are abundant in most Arabic countries, but although available, again are more expensive in the UK.

Meat, fish, eggs, beans and other non-dairy sources of protein
Meat (lahm) – lamb, mutton and chicken (dajaaj) –are available as halal. However, other meats that are traditionally eaten are not always available in the UK; these include goat and camel.

Many varieties of fish (samak) are eaten, especially in countries such as the Gulf States that are situated on the coast. Salmon, sardines, mackerel (oily fish), prawns and other shellfish are readily available in the UK. However, others are not so available and are likely to be expensive, these include monkfish, mullet, bream and trevally, which are all white fish.

Eggs (baydh) are frequently consumed at meal times, especially breakfast.

Pulses and beans are consumed frequently in main dishes, particularly split lentils in stew (mujaddarah), chickpeas that may be whole or puréed (hummus), broad beans (fool), white kidney beans (fasulya beyda) and green beans (fasulya). A variety of beans or individual pulses may be used in one dish, such as ground broad beans (fool) and ground chickpeas (hummus). Many of these are available in the UK, although ready made foods such as fool and falafel (made from ground chickpeas, sometimes added potato, onion and flour and usually fried) will be more expensive.

Nuts and seeds are a permanent feature on the table, especially pistachios, walnuts, cashews, sunflower and pumpkin seeds (salted). These are often consumed as snacks between meals. Sesame seeds are often added to bread and pastries, often with thyme.

Milk and dairy foods
Arabs consume either full -fat or semi variety cow's milk in the UK; traditional milk is from the goat, sheep and camel. Goat's milk has become more popular in the UK and is available in supermarkets; however, sheep's milk is harder to obtain and more expensive and camel's milk is virtually impossible to buy in the UK. Powdered milk in many Arabic countries is full fat; condensed and Carnation milk (normal or light) are also used, particularly in tea.

The most commonly eaten cheeses (jebnah) are haloumi and feta, which are both usually made from a mixture of sheep's and goat's milk. Haloumi has a high melting point and can be grilled or fried whilst feta cheese is usually eaten cold with salads; both can be quite salty.

The consistency of natural yoghurt (lebneh) is between yoghurt and soft cheese. Strained yoghurt is prepared by removing the whey. This may be made at home or bought and is mostly spread on bread. Full cream cow's or camel's milk is often used.

Foods and drinks high in fat and/or sugar
Sugar (sukkar) and honey (aasat) form the basis of pastries and are used to sweeten drinks (tea and coffee). These are readily available but are often cheaper in Arabic countries. Honey is seen as a having health benefits and frequently consumed. Mostly olive and sunflower oil are used in cooking but groundnut, sesame oil and ghee may are also used.

Traditional diet of first and second generation Arabs

The diet of first generation Arabs is more traditional and second generation people will include more western foods.

First generation

Breakfast may be eaten quite late (around 10–11 am) and can include many of the following items:

- Fruit juice – various.
- Eggs (fried or boiled) one or two.
- Salad such as onions, tomatoes and olives.
- Flatbread with honey or natural or strained yoghurt.
- Cereal – often cornflakes.
- Ground broad beans (fool made with garlic, olive oil and lemon).

Lunch may be eaten at about 2–3 PM and is often the main meal of the day. This is usually a mezze, which is a selection of several dishes. Bread is usually eaten with the main meal or as a starter with ground chickpeas (hummus), natural yoghurt, cracked wheat and parsley (taboulleh), ground aubergine (baba ghannou) or vine leaves stuffed with onion, garlic, tomato, rice, herbs and often minced meat (usually lamb). The meal is usually based on starchy foods, particularly rice (roz); this may be boiled or have meat juices and fat added. Other starchy foods may be specific to specific dishes, such as potatoes, cassava, yam (boiled or fried) and couscous.

Vegetables and meat, fish and pulses, such as chickpeas (hummus), lentils (aadas), broad beans (fool) and peas (basilla), are often mixed with the rice to form a stew-like dish. A salad of leaves, tomatoes, and cucumber is usually included; dressings may simply be lemon juice, garlic and olive oil.

Desserts are mixed fresh fruit or a milk pudding (rice or semolina based; mahalabia) and may be followed by (usually many) dates, often stuffed, or pastries filled with nuts and coated with honey/sugar syrup (baklava), both usually eaten with coffee.

The evening meal may be consumed late (8–9 PM) and is usually a light meal: bread (flat or sliced, white or brown) and cheese made into a sandwich or flat traditional bread filled with red or white meat eaten with cracked wheat, tomato, parsley (tabouli) and a sauce, such as sesame based one (sharwama). Meat or vegetables (usually potato; kibbeh) may be eaten. Salad (tomatoes, lettuce and olives) will accompany the meal.

Fruit juices (aasir), water, tea (shay) or Arabic coffee (ground coffee beans brewed with boiling water to which saffron, ginger and cardamom may be added) tend to be the main fluids consumed. Coffee is usually consumed in small cups and accompanied by dates or other snacks. Tea usually has moderate amounts of sugar added to it.

Second generation

If meals are not be consumed with the rest of the family, they may be skipped. A consequence of meals being eaten outside the family home (often with friends or work colleagues) has been a significant increase in intake of fast foods.

Breakfast may be a traditional breakfast or a croissant. Lunch is commonly fast foods such as, pizza, fried chicken, chips and burgers. Foods from other cultures such as pasta dishes and Chinese food have become more popular.

Desserts may include ice cream, cakes and chocolate. Chocolate bars and crisp are eaten as snacks and fizzy drinks (many diet or low calorie varieties are not available in Arab countries) may be consumed during the day. There has also been the introduction of accompaniments such as ketchup, mayonnaise, chocolate and vegetables such as mushrooms

The evening meal may be eaten with the family and this is likely to be a traditional light or main meal. However, it is common to see many Arabic people eating out with friends and to incorporate fast foods, similar to those constituting lunch. Alternatively, traditional Arabic foods may be consumed at a restaurant.

Diet quality

Healthy aspects of traditional Arabic food habits include:

- Generally meals are not skipped, i.e. three meals a day, with lunch being the main meal.
- Vegetables and/or salad included as part of main meal.
- Pulses included in dishes – olive oil may be added liberally to dishes such as hummus and fool.
- Fruit usually as a dessert, including dried (dates and figs).
- Variety of fish, including oily fish (salmon, mackerel and sardines) particularly in coastal areas. This is usually shallow fried, but oven baking is becoming more frequent.
- Dressings on salad, with the exception of olive oil, are usually low fat (lemon and garlic).
- Particularly with traditional diets, snacks include high fibre foods, e.g. nuts, dates and fruit.

Religion, culture and migration affect food choices and physical activities, e.g. fasting, alcohol intake, smoking and exercise.

Religion

Most of the populations of Arab League countries are practising Muslims, divided mainly into Sunnis and Shia. There are different branches and denominations of Islam, each with its own traditions and practices. However, the basic practices of Islam are universal. There are some Christians in some countries, such as Jordan, Lebanon, Djibouti and Sudan. Restrictions on what Muslims can eat are laid down in the Qur'an and are regarded as the direct command of Allah, as discussed earlier.

Alcohol consumption has increased due to availability and peer pressure; it is not uncommon for many Arabic people to drink alcohol at home or socially. It is unusual for Arabic women to drink alcohol. In many Arabic countries, the prevalence of men smoking cigarettes appears to be higher than among women; however, the Shisha (pipe) may be smoked by men and women and is often seen as a fashionable thing to do and less stigma is attached to women smoking this.

Many people are put off exercising (men and women) due to the hot weather; generally, physical activity is low or not common. Physical activity may be reduced, particularly for women, who cover themselves with the hajib and who may be conscious about wearing sports clothes.

Decisions about the diet at home

These will include shopping, cooking methods and use of herbs and spices. The main female person in the household, wife or mother, usually makes the decisions. If there is more than one wife, the first wife of the household will decide about diet at home. Cooking may be carried out by the main female of the house or by maids. Often Arabic families will have maids who do the shopping and cooks who prepare the food (especially in the Gulf States). Many of these domestic helpers are from Indian or Sri Lanka and hence they may introduce the influence of Indian foods such as biryani. In the UK, women mostly do the cooking; it may be cooked daily (especially if cooks are available) or in bulk. Shallow frying is used frequently for cooking, e.g. for pastries, vegetables such as aubergines, and falafel. Many main dishes use boiling as a cooking method. However, the fat from meats is not removed in this process and other foods will be added to the dish to make stews. There appears to be healthier, low fat methods of cooking in the younger generation. Frequently used seasonings include salt (mileh), mint (nana), parsley (badoonis), nutmeg (basbasa), tumeric (kurkum), cardamom (hail), cinnamon (qurfal), black pepper (filfil aswad) and coriander (kuzbara).

Traditionally, foods such as fruit and vegetables are bought in bulk from market stalls; in the UK, traditional foods may not always be available. Arabic foods will be bought from Arabic shops and other shopping is done from supermarkets.

Dietary components

Some of the following foods tend to be more significant in the diet in Arabic countries compared with the diet in the UK:

- Portions of starchy staple foods such as rice and bread tend to be large. It is not unusual for a portion of rice to cover a full dinner plate, along with bread as an accompaniment, and meals are based around these. Due to social events and hospitality it is usual to have food available and large 'spreads'.
- Dates – these are often consumed in large amounts, e.g. five to 10 may accompany coffee that is more than once a day, usually between or after meals.
- Eggs are consumed frequently at breakfast (boiled or fried); this may be amount to one to two daily.
- Fluids – fruit juices and sugary carbonated drinks in hot climates; sugar free (low calorie) varieties may not be available.
- Fruit – particularly grapes, pineapple, melon and mangoes; however, in some countries fruit may not be widely available.
- Salads are often preferred to cooked vegetables.

Fewer if the following foods may be consumed due to the lack of availability in Arab countries:

- Fruit and vegetables may not always be available, or are seasonal; this includes frozen or tinned.
- Low fat dairy products, particularly milk, may not be available; an alternative to fresh milk may be condensed or powdered milk.
- Sugar free varieties of drinks.

In some countries multicultural outlets have increased the variety of dishes, including Italian, Chinese and Indian foods, as well as western fast foods. In the first generation low fat and sugar free foods may not be accepted, but there is greater acceptance in the second generation.

Cooking methods

Traditionally fat or juices from meat are used in stews and added to rice. Second generation Arabs appear to use less fat in cooking, although the intake of fast foods containing fats can be greater. Olive and vegetable oil are mainly used, although ghee is used for some specific dishes. With education refrying has reduced but may still be carried out by the first generation.

Dietary advice

Healthier western foods should be suggested as traditional foods in the UK are quite expensive. These include:

- Low fat milk and dairy products.
- Oils higher in monounsaturated fats, e.g. olive oil, and polyunsaturated fats, e.g. corn, sunflower and sesame oil.
- Fruit and vegetables in their frozen or tinned form, such as pineapple, mangoes, peas, various beans and tomatoes.
- Sugar free beverages.

The barriers to healthier dietary changes include:

- Eating late – lunch may be around 2–3 PM and the evening meal also late, with food spread out during the evening.
- Misconception that some foods such as honey are good for health and therefore added liberally to foods and beverages.
- Large consumption of dates in some countries due to their availability and the tradition for eating them with coffee.
- Social obligations, visiting friends and being hospitable and generous when friends visit. Welcoming people with food is a common tradition.

The following may help to improve compliance with and ease of dietary changes:

- Diet sheets to reinforce the message – bilingual diet sheets in Arabic and English are very useful as they allow family members to share the information. It is worth noting that a proportion of patients, particularly Bedouin and nomads, may be unable to read and then

SECTION 3

visual diet sheets portraying foods and portion sizes are very useful.

- Discuss portions visually – use hands to demonstrate appropriate portion sizes.
- Quantities in spoons and cups may be better than in grams.

The following changes to the diet may be agreed with the client:

- Reducing the amount of starchy food at the main meal (rice, bread, potatoes, which can be eaten in large quantities) and replacing these with larger portions of vegetables and salad.
- White bread is predominant in Arabic countries; however, in the UK patients should be encouraged to choose wholemeal varieties.
- Although there are alternative high fibre cereals, cornflakes are widely consumed and it is worth educating patients about the availability of and types of cereals higher in fibre.
- Reducing the amount of oil in cooking (measuring oil before using) and changing to one higher in monounsaturated fats and polyunsaturated fats.
- Avoiding the fat and juice of meat in stews and rice and looking at low or non-fat cooking methods, such as oven baking, grilling and boiling foods containing fat (such as meat) initially and discarding the fluid before other ingredients are added to make stews.
- Replacing meat dishes (often lamb is used) with dal or fish. Removing visible fat from meat and skin from chicken before cooking and smaller portions.
- Changing to low fat milk and dairy products.
- Choosing sugar free carbonated drinks and reducing intake of sugar and honey.

African-Caribbean diet

African-Caribbean collectively refers to people of African descent from the many West Indian islands. The majority of people from the Caribbean, notably Jamaicans, moved to the UK during the 1950s and 1960s.

Religion

Religious beliefs influence food choice, preparation and cooking methods. Although African-Caribbean people are generally Christian, there are many faiths in the Caribbean. The two main religions that affect dietary practice are Seventh Day Adventism and Rastafarianism.

Seventh Day Adventists are often vegetarian. If meat and fish are eaten, pork is avoided, as are fish without fins and scales. Alcohol and other stimulants, e.g. coffee and tea, are avoided.

The degree of dietary restriction observed by Rastafarians depends upon the individual; many are vegetarian or vegan. The majority of followers will only eat *ital* foods, which are foods considered to be in a whole and natural state. Processed or preserved foods are excluded. Specific foods not consumed are pork, fish without fins

and scales, vine fruit and stimulants such as alcohol, coffee and tea.

As with people of South Asian origin, it is important to remember that the dietary customs of people from the Caribbean are not uniform and food habits and their cultural context play an important role in every island, with clear differences between islands. The dietary traditions of each island have been influenced by different historical, political, social and geographical factors; the development of the sugar colonies, for example, brought many different cultures to the Caribbean (HEA, 1993). As a result, dietary practices can vary considerably and dishes with similar or the same name can contain different ingredients. Alternatively, the same dish may have several names, e.g. Journey cakes are also called Jonny cakes (Douglas, 1987). There will also be variation in the degree to which individuals follow traditional eating habits; some people will consume a diet indistinguishable from the typical UK diet.

Meal pattern

The meal pattern varies with the individual or family. Traditional dishes may take a long time to prepare and are more likely to be eaten at weekends and evenings. At weekends there is a tendency towards eating two meals, omitting lunch. Popular cooking methods include stewing, braising, steaming, frying and roasting, and very often involve the use of added fat. Food is highly seasoned. Desserts are traditionally only eaten on special occasions, although this trend appears to be changing. Foods such as fruit, fruit salads and ice cream may be eaten quite commonly and other items such as apple pie and gateaux are being increasingly consumed.

Within the African-Caribbean community, beliefs about diet and health may influence dietary practices, e.g. use of herbal (bush) teas as a cure for disease.

West African diet

The majority of West Africans in the UK originate from Nigeria and Ghana and have settled in the major cities.

Traditional dietary practices

The diet consumed by West Africans is generally similar to that consumed by African-Caribbean people, but there are some differences in both food choice and cooking methods (Bailey *et al.*, 2012).

Bread, cereals and other starchy foods
Cassava, green bananas, yam, cocoyam, plantain and sweet potatoes are usually boiled, roasted or fried. Fufu is made by pounding cooked tubers like cassava, yam and cocoyam, and then dried in the sun. These ready made flours are now available in the UK. Other starchy foods include rice, corn, cornmeal millet and sorghum.

Fruit and vegetables

Commonly eaten fruit and vegetables are oranges, pawpaw, mango, ugu (pumpkin leaves), green leafy vegetables and okazi.

Meat, fish and alternatives

Meat, fish and seafoods are eaten at each meal. Among Nigerians, black eyed beans are cooked as a stew. Melon seeds (egusi), pumpkin seeds and groundnuts (peanuts) are used in cooking or as snacks.

Milk and dairy foods

Evaporated, condensed and powered milk are used in tea and coffee.

Other dietary practices

Other dietary practices are:

- One pot meals (stew) are the most common cooking method and can include meat or fish.
- Stew is served with cassava, yam or plantain (possibly pounded), which are mostly boiled but also can be fried.
- Vegetable stew or soup is also served with starchy foods.
- Palm oil is used in cooking to give flavour and colour to the dishes.
- Nuts and seeds, e.g. Ghanaians use peanut butter to make soups.
- Nigerians eat peanuts (roasted or boiled) and cashew nuts as snacks.
- Desserts are not usually served.

Common health problems

The incidence of type 2 diabetes, hypertension and obesity is high in the West African community (Erens *et al.*, 2001). General weight reducing dietary advice is often necessary and aspects that need to be highlighted are:

- Reducing the amount of oil used in stews. Palm oil and palm nut oil are commonly used but are saturated fats; if possible, a limited amount of sunflower, corn or groundnut oil should be used instead.
- Reducing the amount of peanut butter used in soups.
- Reducing the amount of fried foods such as fried fish or meat.
- Fish, e.g. snapper, may be stewed or baked instead of being fried.
- Portion size of green bananas, yam, ground rice and other starchy foods is often quite substantial and may need to be reduced.
- Frequent use of glucose drinks such as Lucozade and other sugar rich drinks should be discouraged.

Chinese diet

The majority of Chinese people in the UK originate from Hong Kong and arrived in the UK in the 1950s and 1960s. This was partly in response to the collapse of traditional agriculture there and partly because of the boom in the Chinese restaurant trade in Britain. Other Chinese people migrated from mainland China, Taiwan and Vietnam; Chinese people from Vietnam came as refugees (boat people) mostly after 1978.

In 2009, the estimated Chinese population in England and Wales exceeded 451 000, which accounted for 0.8% of the total population (ONS, 2009). They had the highest average growth rate compared with all the other ethnic groups at 8.6% annually. The Chinese and white population was the highest amongst Other Mixed descriptors at 10%, whereas Asian and Chinese and Black and Chinese were both reported to be <1% (ONS, 2006). There has been a 21.1% and 3.6% increase in the number of students from China and Hong Kong, respectively, in higher education in the UK (HESA, 2000).

Traditional dietary practices

Although coming from various countries such as China, Taiwan, Hong Kong, Singapore and Malaysia, Chinese people or their ancestors all originate from China. Food has a prominent position in Chinese culture and is used as a to mark family, religious and social events. The dietary pattern is believed to be an important determinant of the body's balance and state of health, and manipulations of this pattern to restore equilibrium lost as a result of disease or changes in physiological status may have considerable influence on food habits.

Festivals

At the beginning of the year, Chinese celebrate their lunar New Year, which is sometime in late January or early February depending on the lunar calendar. A mid Autumn festival usually takes place in late September or early October to coincide with the end of the harvest year. Feasting demands the preparation and consumption of highly calorific foods that people at other times may not be able to afford.

Food preparation

Most of the staple foods in the Chinese diet, e.g. rice or wheat dumplings, are cooked by boiling. Other prominent dietary components such as soups and stews will also be boiled for several hours before serving. More delicately flavoured items such as seafood and dim sum are more likely to be steamed, usually by placing them on slatted wooden or bamboo trays over boiling water. Roasting is used as a cooking method for items such as pork, chicken and duck.

Baking has become more common in areas exposed to western influence with items such as cakes, tartlets and buns being produced. However, in northern China, where wheat consumption has always been common, buns made from wheat flour and sesame seeds have traditionally been baked by sticking them to the sides of a large pot or pot shaped oven. Fried foods are commonly stir fried, although some dishes will be deep fried. Oil is heated until it smokes; meat and vegetables sliced into small pieces are tossed in it and rapidly stirred around the hot wok so that the food cooks without being burnt. This usually only takes a few seconds. Larger pieces of fish, poultry and egg may be cooked for longer with more oil and less stirring.

It is also a common practice to cook a food item by sequential methods. For example, a food may be smoked, then boiled and finally stir fried. Alternatively, it may be partly boiled, then set aside until needed and the cooking process completed by further additional boiling as part of another dish, or by another cooking method.

Meal pattern

Depending on their degree of acculturation, migrant Chinese adopt certain western eating habits while maintaining other traditional Chinese eating habits. For example, in a Chinese American study (Pan *et al.*, 1999), it was noted that rice continued to be an important staple but other traditional foods were replaced by cereal, bread, sandwiches, milk and soft drinks. The evening meal remained the most traditional meal. Breakfast, lunch and snack items were more likely to be replaced by foods more commonly consumed by Americans.

Most children and young adults will consume a western style breakfast and lunch, and only the evening meal is likely to be typically Chinese. Popular foods are white bread, burgers, pork chops, ham, bacon, peas, butter, crisps, chips and those from fast food outlets. Lamb and frozen vegetables are less commonly eaten. Older adults are more likely to maintain traditional customs. Elderly people still consume the more traditional diet but often incorporate western foods such as white bread and breakfast cereals for convenience at breakfast (Chan, 1991). Men are more likely to change their food habits than women as the latter have more experience of preparing traditional cuisines (Pan *et al.*, 1999).

Jewish diet

Many Jewish people were born in the UK and for the majority English is the native language. Jewish people are very diverse, reflecting differing degrees of assimilation and religious observance of Judaism, an ancient religion.

Dietary restrictions

Jewish people, like all other people, have food customs traditionally associated with their daily lives, holidays and festivals. These are in addition to detailed dietary laws (Kashrut) that date back to the Old Testament and define the selection, preparation and consumption of permitted (kosher) food. Self discipline and preservation of Jewish spirituality and religious identity underlie these laws, which are:

- Meat and poultry must not be cooked with milk or milk derivatives, or be served at the same meal. Utensils,

crockery, pots and pans used for milk and meat must be stored, washed and dried separately.
- All meat and milk products must be bought from a kosher shop bearing a kosher stamp.
- Permitted animals are quadrupeds that chew the cud and have cloven hoofs, such as sheep, goats and cattle. All others, including pigs, are forbidden.
- Poultry such as chicken, duck, goose, turkey and some game birds are permitted. Most others, including birds of prey and ostrich, are forbidden.
- Animals and birds must be slaughtered by shechita. This procedure, considered the painless means of slaughtering the animal, must be carried out by a trained and authorised person and entails a rapid cut with a sharp knife to sever the jugular vein and carotid artery. The meat must then be salted and soaked in water to remove the blood and render it kosher (permitted).
- Only fish with scales and fins, such as cod, plaice, salmon, tuna, etc., are allowed. Eels, shark, monkfish and all shellfish are forbidden.

The modern orthodox Jew will follow similar rules but is more integrated with the general population. It is important to establish the level of observance at the time of consultation.

The variety of kosher low fat, low sugar dairy foods are limited. During Shabbat and festivals, high calorie foods are served. Shabbat and festival foods from the Ashkenazi tradition (that of families from Eastern Europe and Russia) tend to be higher calorie than traditional Sephardic foods (those of families from Southern Europe, the Middle East and Asia) due to the different climates where the recipes were developed. A traditional Ashkenazi diet uses large amounts of chicken fat (schmaltz) and may require different dietary modification from that of the traditional Sephardic diet.

Social restrictions

In the ultra orthodox Jewish community a woman runs the house and looks after the children and the husband goes to work. One of the many laws that exists regarding behaviour is that men and women should not mix together or have any bodily contact apart from with their husband, brother or child. If a male dietitian is seeing an ultra orthodox female, she will not want to shake hands or have any contact with him and may feel uneasy being in the same room with him and vice versa.

Festivals and fasting

The seventh day of the week is the Sabbath (Shabbat), a day of prayer at the synagogue and complete rest from work from sundown on Friday to Saturday evening. Writing, operating any electrical equipment, cooking and travelling are amongst the tasks that are forbidden during the Sabbath and many festivals. All food preparation is done in advance and large family meals are traditionally eaten.

The Jewish year is based on lunar calculations. The New Year (Rosh Hashanah) is celebrated in September/October. Ten days later is the Day of Atonement (Yom Kippur), which is the holiest day of the Jewish calendar. It is also a fast day; no food or drink is permitted for 25 hours (from sunset the evening before to sunset the next day).

Passover, which commemorates the exodus of Jews from Egypt, is celebrated for 8 days in April. No foods made with, or in contact with, wheat, barley, oats or rye may be eaten. Unleavened bread (matzo) is eaten in place of normal bread. Cooking and eating utensils that are reserved only for Passover are used.

Polish diet

Slavic and many other culinary traditions, including German, Austro-Hungarian, Jewish, Turkish, French and Italian, have influenced Polish cuisine over several centuries.

Festivals and feasting

The majority of the population, approximately 90%, are Roman Catholics who observe varying degree of strictness. Christmas and Easter are the most celebrated religious festivals. Some people abstain from alcohol or meat during Lent; others may fast on Great (Good) Friday and until late afternoon supper on Christmas Eve. Many people traditionally eat fish on Friday.

Traditional dietary practices

Polish cuisine is abundant in meat and sausages of all kinds, as well as different kinds of pickles, dumplings and pasta shapes, most notably Polish ravioli (pierogi) and kasha (kasza).

Bread, rice, potatoes, pasta and other starchy foods

Many types of bread (chleb) are eaten but the most popular include mixed rye and wheat bread (chleb pszenno-żytni), wheat (pszenny) bread, rye (żytni) bread and wholegrain (pelnoziarnisty) bread. Traditionally, bread is made with a sour dough starter. Poppy, sunflower and caraway seeds are added to some breads and rolls. Potatoes are the most popular accompaniment to the main course. Kasha (kasza), which is made from buckwheat, cracked pearl barley or millet, is an alternative accompaniment to the main course. It is also used in soups, cakes (semolina) or boiled with milk as a type of porridge (millet or semolina). Oats are eaten with milk or can be added to bread. Breakfast cereals, often sugary varieties, are consumed more often nowadays. Rice is used in soups such as tomato or sour cucumber soup, and in stuffed cabbage parcels.

Pasta is eaten in a variety of ways. Pasta shapes are added to soups, e.g. chicken consommé, tomato or mushroom soups; eaten as pasta salads and most importantly as Polish ravioli or stuffed dumplings (pierogi). Pierogi can be filled with a variety of fillings. Savoury fillings include farmer's cheese and potatoes – Russian style, minced meat, cabbage and mushrooms. Sweet fillings include sweetened farmer's cheese or fruit, e.g. apples, wild blueberries, cherries and plums. Pierogi are usually eaten boiled or boiled and then fried. They are served with a variety of toppings such as melted butter, fried onion, fried chopped bacon, sugar and cream. Other types of pasta include dumplings made with flour and potatoes mixed together e.g. kopytka and pyzy. These can be stuffed with meat or served plain. Ready made pierogi and dumplings sold in Polish shops are a quick and easy meal to prepare and hence are very popular with Polish people.

The following foods should be encouraged:

- Wholegrain bread and cereal, e.g. rye bread (chleb żytni), wheat–rye bread (chleb pszenno-żytni), pumpernickel (pumpernikiel), graham or razowy (wholemeal), wholegrain (pelnoziarnisty) and sunflower seed bread (chleb z ziarnami slonecznika).
- Breakfast cereal such as porridge, branflakes or any other unsweetened wholegrain variety, rather than cornflakes.
- Kasha are a good source of soluble fibre but should not be topped with bacon or other fat.
- Pierogi can be served with kefir or maslanka (low fat soured milk drinks) or a small amount of melted vegetable based spread/olive oil with stir fried onion topping instead. Mushroom (grzyby), cabbage (kapusta), Russian style (ruskie) and fruit (owoce) fillings should be encouraged in preference to a meat filling (farsz miesny).

Meat, fish, eggs, beans and alternatives

Meat (pork, beef and lamb in some regions of Poland), sausages and offal are consumed in great amounts in Poland. Fish, both white and oily, is available. Herrings, mackerel, trout, sprats, sardines, tuna, cod and hake are most commonly eaten. Carp is eaten mostly at Christmas. Herrings are usually preserved in oil or vinegar marinade, often consumed with sour cream with the addition of onion, apple, gherkins, dill and spices. The majority of sausages and hams, and some fish, are smoked. Pulses are not eaten to a great extent but are used to make soups or as a main meal accompaniment. Nuts and seeds are used in baking, bread making or as a sweet or savoury snack. Eggs are eaten at breakfast, added to soups and salads.

The following foods should be encouraged:

- To increase the consumption of pulses, the following could be suggested: bean soup (zupa grochowa, fasolowa), adding beans to other vegetable soups and stews to replace some meat, serving beans as a side dish more often, a butter bean casserole in tomato sauce Bretagne style (fasolka po bretonsku) and trying baked beans in tomato sauce. Bean soup and casserole should be made with a limited amount of lean bacon, good quality lean sausage or without meat altogether, and no roux.
- Instead of ordinary sausage (zwyczajna), country sausage (wiejska), grilling sausage (grilowa), pâté (pasztet),

Frankfurters (parówki), bacon (boczek) and black pudding (kaszanka), choose lean ham or pork loin (chuda szynka lub poledwica), chicken or turkey (szynka z kurczaka lub indyka).

- Choose low fat dairy, e.g. cottage cheese (serek ziarnisty) or Polish low fat (ser bialy chudy) or reduced fat white cheese (ser bialy półtłusty) and low fat milk (mleko chude).
- Avoid using cream, sour cream, butter, roux (zasmażka), bacon, ribs or sausages in food preparation, e.g. in soups, sauces and pierogi. Try to use substitute with the following as appropriate: low fat milk (mleko chude), buttermilk (maslanka) or kefir (a type of sour milk, usually low fat) and vegetable oils, including spreads. For example, beetroot soup (barszcz czerwony) can be served clear with boiled egg or mushroom ravioli and sour rye soup (żurek) with boiled egg and/ or potatoes, and without roux. Chicken soup is healthier if the skin is removed prior to cooking and more vegetables and herbs can be used to improve flavour.

Fruit and vegetables

Commonly consumed vegetables are beetroot, cabbage including sauerkraut, cucumbers, tomatoes, peppers, beans, lettuce, onion, leek and mushrooms. Fruits include apples, pears, plums, cherries, berries, bananas and citrus fruit.

Milk and dairy products

Full fat milk (mleko tłuste) is often chosen over low fat. Cream and sour cream are commonly used in soups, sauces, and vegetable and herring salads. Condensed milk is used in baking and creamer in coffee. Hard cheese, often referred to as yellow cheese (ser żółty), and full fat (tłusty) farmer's cheese, referred to as white cheese (ser biały), have been traditionally eaten. Nowadays, reduced and low fat equivalents, as well as a whole range of foreign cheeses, are widely available. Buttermilk (maślanka) and a medium to low fat soured milk (kefir) are consumed especially in summer months; they go well with pierogi. They can be used as a low fat alternative to cream in soups and salads. Similarly, low fat yoghurt could replace sour cream in vegetable and herring salads.

Food and drinks high in fat, sugar or salt

Poles tend to consume large amounts of sugary snacks, sweetened fruit juice drinks, e.g. Kubuś or Tymbark, honey, fruit compote and soft drinks. Energy drinks, coke or Sprite are also often used as mixers in cocktails. Polish fruit compote is a sweet drink made by boiling fruit in water with added sugar. This is traditionally served with main meals.

The following foods should be encouraged:

- Healthy alternatives, including vegetable juice, no sugar added squashes, herbal teas and water could be recommended.
- Vegetable juices, e.g. carrot (sok z marchwi) or tomato juice (sok pomidorowy) could provide an alternative.
- Tinned fruit in fruit juice rather than in syrup.

Ready meal consumption

Polish ready meals are widely available in Polish shops and some supermarkets in the UK. They often contain a high level of fat and salt. Some popular examples of Polish ready meals are Hunters' stew (bigos – sauerkraut and cabbage stewed with a variety of meats, sausages, bacon and spices), stuffed cabbage parcels (gołąbki – cabbage stuffed with rice and pork filling) and meatballs in tomato sauce (pulpety or klopsy). Ready made soups and dumplings also feature heavily on the shelves in Polish delis and some supermarkets. Home made varieties can be made healthier; however, they often require fairly long preparation time and therefore ready made alternatives make an easy option.

Food production and preservation

A wide variety of herbs and spices are used in meal preparation, e.g. dill, parsley, marjoram, paprika, black, cayenne and herb pepper, bay leaf, all spice, caraway seed, cinnamon, nutmeg and cloves. Bacterial and yeast fermentation are widely used in food production and preservation.

Turkish diet

There is a significant Turkish community in the UK; it is the third largest in Europe. Most Turks are Muslim and as such will follow the religious customs and dietary restrictions as described earlier. The Turkish diet is essentially a Mediterranean diet, which may reduce the risk of some non-communicable diseases. However, with acculturation, some Turks, especially those who are second or third generation, are adopting a more western diet.

The main meal is eaten in the evening and traditionally fingers are used instead of cutlery, although cutlery is widely used in the UK. Food is often prepared over a few days due to this being labour intensive and time consuming. The traditional Turkish diet will include a lot of vegetables and fruit. Many traditional varieties are available in the UK, although they may be more expensive. Despite most Turks being Muslims, there is a tradition of starting a meal with mezze, which is eaten with wine or raki (the anise flavoured national drink of Turkey). Dessert is often fresh fruit; desserts most associated with Turkish cuisine are baklava, a sweet filo pastry dish, and milk desserts (muhallebi), which are made with rice flour.

A glossary of Turkish foods, a list of traditional Turkish foods and example meal plans, with examples of the effect of migration, are given by Mirza & Sarwar (2012).

Greek diet

Many Greek emigrants arrived in the UK after the Second World War, with most coming from Cyprus. Most Greek speaking people live in and around London with communities in other large English cities, e.g. Liverpool. The Greek Orthodox Church, a Christian religion, is the main religion of the Greek community and on 180–200 days of the year there are specific dietary restrictions or fasting. These restrictions include:

- Avoiding fish, eggs, meat, cheese and olive oil on Wednesdays and Fridays (except during the week following Christmas, Easter and Pentecost).
- There are three fasting periods:
  - 40 days before Christmas – eggs, dairy products and meat are not allowed. White fish and olive oil are allowed except on Wednesdays and Fridays.
  - Lent – 48 days preceding Easter, which varies each year depending on the time of the full moon on or after the vernal (spring) equinox. Fish is only allowed on the 25th March and Palm Sunday.
  - The Assumption – 15 days in August. The same rules as at Lent apply, except that fish is only allowed on 6th August.

Festivals

The main festivals are Easter, Christmas and New Year. Traditionally, specific foods are associated with each festival including:

- Easter – Easter bread (tsoureki) eaten with boiled eggs that are dyed, Easter soup (mayeritsa) and Easter savoury pastries (flaounes).
- Christmas – rich, sugary cakes are made (e.g. kourabiethes) but other food choices will vary. These may include meat in aspic (saladina). Christmas food is plentiful and shared with family members.
- New year – a vasiloptia cake is made and shared amongst the family.

Like the Turkish diet, the Greek diet is a Mediterranean diet and is therefore associated with reduced risks of some non-communicable diseases, e.g. type 2 diabetes. A glossary of Greek foods, a list of traditional Greek foods and example meal plans, with examples of the effect of migration, are given by Petrides (2012). In addition, advice on foods to be encouraged and discouraged in the Greek diet are listed.

Conclusion

The ethnic and cultural mix of the UK is constantly changing, partly due to the migration. The population of any specific city or location may also change and it is therefore important that dietitians stay abreast of the diversity in the locality in which they work. One example of this is the influx of Somalian migrants to London and other large communities including Liverpool and Cardiff. Details of the diet eaten by Somalian people and some other groups can be found in the *Multicultural Handbook of Food, Nutrition and Dietetics* (Thaker & Barton, (2012)). The resources at the end of this chapter will assist dietitians in finding information relevant to working with specific cultural groups.

Further reading

South Asian Health Foundation. (2005) *Prevention, treatment and rehabilitation of cardiovascular disease in South Asians*. In: Patel KCR, Shah AM (eds). London: The Stationery Office. Available at www.sahf.org.uk. Accessed 3 October 2012.

Thaker A, Barton A. (2012) *Multicultural Handbook of Food Nutrition and Dietetics*. Oxford: Blackwell Science.

Internet resources

The British Dietetic Association – Multi-Cultural Nutrition Group www.bda.uk.com

Chinese National Healthy Living Centre   www.cnhlc.org.uk

Chinese Health Information Centre   www.eastlancshealthyminds .nhs.uk/directory_info.asp?id=82

Federation of Bengali Caterers   www.fobc2008.com

Ismaili Nutrition Centre   www.theismaili.org/nutrition

London Beth Din (for Kosher food enquiries)   www.kosher.org.uk

Muslim Food Board (UK)   www.halaal.org

South Asian Health Foundation   www.sahf.org.uk

Tandoori Magazine   www.tandoorimagazine.com

Additional resources

A number of UK dietetic departments have produced excellent dietary resource material for use with BME groups, often in a variety of languages. Details of material currently available and contacts are available to BDA members from the Multi-Cultural Nutrition Group (www.bda.uk.com).

The British Heart Foundation has developed free booklets and DVDs in English and five South Asian Languages (www.bhf.org.uk).

Diabetes UK produces a number of resources for people with diabetes from BME groups and have resources available in different languages (www.diabetes.org.uk).

The Food Standards Agency has translated diet sheets (www .food.gov.uk).

Local resources

Local community and religious leaders may be able to help with general information, translation of leaflets and the establishment of contacts with relevant individuals or groups. Local temples and religious establishments or local council offices may be a useful starting point of contact.

Local public health departments may have produced resource material relevant to local ethnic minority groups.

Local voluntary organisations in different areas of the UK run luncheon clubs for local relevant communities.

References

Balarajan R, Raleigh VS. (1995) *Ethnicity and Health in England*. London: HMSO.

Bailey L, Cudjoc A, Fraser M, Jackson S, Thompson D. (2012) African-Caribbean Diet. In: Thaker A, & Barton A (eds) *Multicultural Handbook of Food Nutrition and Dietetics* Oxford: Blackwell Science.

Cabinet Office (2003) *Ethnic Minorities and the Labour Market: Final Report*. London: Cabinet Office Strategy Unit.

Chan W. (1991) Concept of illness, dietary beliefs and food related health practices. PhD Thesis, University of London.

Douglas J. (1987) *Caribbean Food and Diet, Food and Diet in a Multiracial Society*. Cambridge: National Extension College.

Erens B, Promatesta P, Prior G. (2001) *Health Survey for England – The Health of Minority Ethnic Groups 1999*. London: TSO. Available at www.dh.gov.uk. Accessed 6 October 2012.

Fox C. (2004) *Heart Disease and South Asians: Delivering the National Service Framework for Coronary Heart Disease*. London: The Stationery Office.

Federation of Bangladeshi Caterers (2008). About Fobc. Available at www.fobc2008.com. Accessed 23 September 2012.

Health Education Authority (HEA). (1993) *Nutrition in Minority Ethnic Groups. Asians and Afro-Caribbeans in the United Kingdom*. Briefing Paper. London: HEA.

Higher Education Statistics Agency (HESA). (2000) *Students in Higher Education Institutions*. Cheltenham: HESA.

Mirza T, Sarwar T. (2012) Turkish diet. In: Thaker A & Barton A (eds) *Multicultural Handbook of Food, Nutrition and Dietetics*. Oxford: Blackwell Science.

Office for National Statistics (ONS) (2004a) *Census 2001*. London: ONS. Available at www.ons.gov.uk. Accessed 28 September 2012.

Office for National Statistics (ONS). (2004b) *Ethnicity and Identity*. London: ONS. Available at www.statistics.gov.uk.

Office for National Statistics (ONS). (2006) *Who are the 'Mixed' Ethnic Group? Social and Welfare*. London: ONS.

Office for National Statistics (ONS). (2009) Population Estimates by Ethnic Group 2002–2009. Statistical Bulletin. London: ONS.

Pan YL, Dixon Z, Himburg S, Huffman F. (1999) Asian students change their eating patterns after living in the United States. *Journal of the American Dietetic Association* 1: 54–57.

Petrides S. (2012) Greek diet. In: Thaker A & Barton A (eds) *Multicultural Handbook of Food, Nutrition and Dietetics*. Oxford: Blackwell Science.

Thaker A, Barton A. (2012) *Multicultural Handbook of Food. Nutrition and Dietetics*. Oxford: Blackwell Science.

SECTION 3

3.6 Vegetarianism and vegan diets

Elaine Gardner

Key points

- Well balanced vegetarian diets are appropriate for all ages.

- Vegetarians consume widely divergent diets; a well balanced vegetarian diet can offer potential health benefits over non-vegetarian diets.

- A vegetarian eating pattern is associated with a lower risk of death from ischaemic heart disease.

- Vegetarians and vegans tend to have a lower body mass index (BMI) than omnivores.

- There is an increased risk of nutrient deficiencies when consuming a vegan diet compared with a vegetarian diet.

- Vegetarian and vegan diets have the potential to be used as treatment for chronic diseases such as type 2 diabetes and metabolic syndrome.

The Vegetarian Society (UK) defines a vegetarian as *'someone who lives on a diet of grains, pulses, nuts, seeds, vegetables and fruits with, or without, the use of dairy products and eggs. A vegetarian does not eat any meat, poultry, game, fish, shellfish or by-products of slaughter'* (www.vegsoc.org). The Vegan Society (UK) defines veganism as *'excluding all animal flesh and animal products, including milk, honey, and eggs and may also exclude any products tested on animals, or any clothing from animals'* (www.vegansociety.com). A number of other definitions are available but these are not *true* vegetarianism or veganism as they include animal consumption in some format. For completeness they are included in Table 3.6.1.

Individual consumers may have their own definitions and understandings of these terms, which can vary depending on their country of origin, culture, views on animal welfare and other factors. If appropriate and practical, especially when consulting with individuals, it is recommended to clearly define any parameters of reference. The UK National Diet and Nutrition Survey 2008/9 reported that 2% of both adults and children reported being vegetarian (Bates *et al.*, 2010). This is lower than previously reported in the Consumer Attitude to Food Standards Survey (FSA, 2003), which reported that 6% of households contained at least one vegetarian member. In 2001, 0.3–0.4% of the UK population was reported as being vegan (FSA, 2006a).

Alternatives to unacceptable foods for vegetarians and vegans

There are a number of alternatives to unacceptable foods, as shown in Table 3.6.2 and Table 3.6.3. These foods are generally found within supermarkets, with the more unusual items available for purchase from health food shops or online shopping.

The labelling of foods as *suitable for vegetarians* or *suitable for vegans* has increased and is making it easier, in some cases, to identify acceptable products (although there are still some problems, e.g. welfare issues such as whether eggs used are free range). Guidance on these terms is provided by the Food Standards Agency (FSA, 2006b) as the labelling is not mandatory and falls under several pieces of legislation (see Chapter 4.5).

Reasons for following a vegetarian or vegan diet

Religion

Some religions advocate avoiding animal products, either partially or fully (see Chapter 3.5 for more details).

Parental and peer influence

Vegetarianism is becoming more common among teenagers, especially among girls. The National Diet and Nutrition Survey of 4–18-year olds found that one in 10 girls

---

Manual of Dietetic Practice, Fifth Edition. Edited by Joan Gandy.
© 2014 The British Dietetic Association. Published 2014 by John Wiley & Sons, Ltd.
Companion Website: www.manualofdieteticpractice.com

Table 3.6.1   Broad definitions regarding vegetarianism and vegan diets

	Meat and meat products	Fish, seafood and their products	Milk and milk products (including cheese and yoghurt)	Eggs and egg products	Other food items that are unacceptable	Comments
Vegetarian [Vegetarian Society (UK)]	×	×	√ Cheese needs to be animal rennet free	Free range eggs only		Sometimes referred to as lacto-ovo-vegetarian
Vegan [Vegan Society (UK)]	×	×	×	×	Honey, beeswax, some alcohol and all products tested on animals	Many products can have hidden animal ingredients so it is recommended to contact the Vegan Society or to use the Vegan Shopping Guide
Lacto-vegetarian	×	×	√ Cheese needs to be animal rennet free	×		
Ovo-vegetarian	×	×	×	Free range eggs only		
Piscatarian	×	√	√ Cheese needs to be animal rennet free	√		

Table 3.6.2   Alternative foods for vegetarians[1,2,3]

Unacceptable foods	Possible vegetarian alternatives
Meat, fish and poultry, and products containing these like pies, sausages	Nuts, seeds, free range eggs, pulses and beans, sprouted beans and seeds, root vegetables, seaweed Soya,[4] tofu, Quorn, TVP (textured vegetable protein) Cereal based foods such as bread, pasta, noodles, couscous, quinoa, rice, bulgar wheat, barley, buckwheat, spelt, millet
Meat and fish stocks, soups and gravies	Vegetable stock, yeast extracts, vegetarian gravy mix
Animal fats and fish oils Fish oils, foods that are 'n-3 enriched by fish oils'	Trex, Pura, 100% vegetable oils and margarines, vegetariaSuet, Trex, Pure, Vitalite, 100% vegetable oils and margarines, vegetable suet. Plant sources of n-3 oils, e.g. hempseed, rapeseed and flax oils
Gelatine and its products, including aspic, jelly, marshmallows, jelly type sweets, gelatine thickened yoghurts	Agar agar, Gelozone, carrageen, pectin
Animal based flavourings, e.g. some brands of Worcester sauce	Yeast extracts, soya sauce, miso, herbs and spices, vegetarian Worcester sauce
Cheese made with animal rennet, including Parmesan, Grana Padano, Gorgonzola	Vegetarian cheese
Animal sources of E numbers: • E120 – cochineal/carmine (from crushed insects) • E452 – edible bone phosphate (from animal bones) Some E numbers may be derived from either plant or animal sources. The Vegetarian Society (UK) provide an online, up to date factsheet.	Foods without animal sources of E numbers
Eggs from caged hens and products prepared with these, e.g. quiche	Free range eggs and products prepared with these
Alcoholic drinks that have been clarified using animal derived products, e.g. chitin, gelatine, isinglass. This includes the majority of real ales; bottled naturally conditioned beers; some ciders; some fortified wines and some wines	Majority of keg beers and lagers, canned beers Ciders that have been produced without gelatine Majority of organic wines and those produced using non-animal alternatives Majority of spirits and liqueurs. Vegetarian alcoholic drinks

[1]The labels and ingredients of all manufactured products must be read carefully.
[2]Care must be taken in the storage and preparation to ensure that the ingredients used do not come into contact with animal products.
[3]Vegetarian foods should not be cooked in oils that have been used for frying animal products.
[4]The term 'soya' is used throughout the chapter; however, it should be noted that in the US they commonly use the term soy.

Table 3.6.3 Alternative foods for vegans[1,2,3]

Unacceptable foods	Possible vegan alternatives
Meat, fish and poultry, and products containing these like pies, sausages.	Nuts, seeds, pulses and beans, root vegetables, sprouted beans and seeds, pure nut and seed butters, seaweed Soya, TVP (textured vegetable protein), tofu Vegan meat substitutes, e.g. vegan sausages, vegan bacon rashers, mock duck Cereal based foods such as bread, pasta, plain noodles, couscous, quinoa, rice, bulgar wheat, barley, buckwheat, spelt, millet
Eggs and cheese and products made from these, e.g. Quorn, mayonnaise, quiche, cakes, egg noodles, pesto	Vegan mayonnaise, vegan cakes, vegan biscuits, rice noodles, vegan pesto
Meat and fish stocks, soups and gravies	Vegetable stock, yeast extracts, miso
Animal fats and products made from these, e.g. chocolate	Vegan chocolate, carob 100% vegetable oils, e.g. soya, sunflower, rapeseed, olive Vegetable suet
Fish oils, foods that are 'n-3 enriched by fish oils' Margarines that contain milk products and/or vitamin D3 Ghee	Plant sources of omega-3 oils, e.g. hempseed, rapeseed and flax oils Pure dairy free spreads, e.g. Vitalite, Pure
Gelatine and its products, including aspic, jelly, marshmallows, jelly type sweets, gelatine thickened yoghurts	Agar agar, Gelozone, carrageen, pectin
Animal based flavourings, e.g. Worcester sauce	Yeast extracts, soya sauce, herbs and spices, vegan worcester sauce, miso
Animal milks, cheese, yoghurt, cream, ice cream Products made from these or manufactured products containing whey powder, casein or lactose, e.g. some crisps	Soya, nut and cereal based milks (vitamin and mineral fortified products are strongly recommended) Soya cheese and alternatives made from nuts and seeds. Nutritional yeast flakes for 'cheese' sauces and for sprinkling on savoury dishes Soya yoghurt, soya based desserts, soya ice cream. Non-dairy creams e.g. soya, nut and rice
E numbers from unacceptable sources (approx. 35 possible E numbers). The Vegan Society (UK) provides online, up to date information	Foods without unacceptable sources of E numbers
Honey, cereal bars containing honey, some breakfast cereals that contain honey/milk/vitamin D$_3$	Maple and agave syrup, sugar, jams. Vegan cereal and fruit bars, pure breakfast cereals not enriched with vitamin D$_3$ and honey
Alcoholic drinks that have been clarified using animal derived products, e.g. chitin, gelatine, isinglass. This includes the majority of real ales; bottled naturally conditioned beers; some ciders; some fortified wines and some wines	Majority of keg beers and lagers, canned beers Ciders that have been produced without gelatine Majority of organic wines and those produced using non-animal alternatives Majority of spirits and liqueurs Vegan alcoholic drinks

[1]The labels and ingredients of all manufactured products must be read carefully.
[2]Care must be taken in the storage and preparation to ensure that the ingredients used do not come into contact with animal products.
[3]Vegan foods should not be cooked in oils that have been used for frying animal products.

aged 15–18 years reported that they were vegan or vegetarian (Gregory *et al.*, 2000). Support for vegetarian practices from mothers and classmates has been shown to be high, although many adolescents reported finding it difficult to avoid eating meat at home (Trew *et al.*, 2006). There are associations between vegetarianism and anorexia nervosa (Aloufy & Latzer, 2006), but while being vegetarian does not cause disordered eating, it may be used to camouflage an existing eating disorder.

Animal welfare

Issues concerning animal welfare that may lead to the adoption of a vegetarian or vegan diet include:

- Conditions in which animals are kept, e.g. restricted space.
- Use of antibiotics and growth promoters to maintain and increase production.
- Intensive breeding and culling programmes.
- Production and killing of animals and fish solely for food purposes.

Environmental issues

Resources required for animal food production have a higher environmental impact than those for growing food from plant sources. With world food security an issue, this inefficient use of land may be viewed as non-sustainable.

In addition, the increased water needs for the production of food from animal as opposed to plant sources is also causing concern. The impact on the environment also encompasses the following issues:

- Quantity of greenhouse gases produced by animals.
- Damage to ecosystems, the environment and other animals.
- Water contamination.
- Higher carbon footprint.

Health reasons

Vegetarians appear to be more health conscious than non-vegetarians (Bedford & Barr, 2005) and a vegetarian eating pattern is associated with a lower risk of death from ischaemic heart disease (Craig et al., 2009; Key et al., 2006). An evidence based review by the American Dietetic Association (Craig et al., 2009) found that vegetarians compared with non-vegetarians had lower:

- Low density lipoproteins (LDL) cholesterol levels (Ferdowsian & Barnard., 2009).
- Blood pressure levels.
- Rates of hypertension.
- Rates of type 2 diabetes (Tonstad et al., 2009. Zaman et al., 2010).
- Risk of metabolic syndrome (Rizzo et al., 2011).
- Body mass index (BMI) (Sabate & Wien, 2010. Tonstad et al., 2009).
- Overall cancer rates and risk (Lanou & Svenson, 2010a).

These findings are supported by the European Prospective Investigation in Cancer (EPIC) and Nutrition Oxford Study that included approximately 65 000 participants of whom 31 000 were non-meat eaters (Key et al., 2009; Spencer et al., 2003, Appleby et al., 2002; Davey et al., 2002).

Bone fracture risk among vegetarians, meat eaters and fish eaters was similar if they consumed at least 525 mg/day of calcium, as measured over a 5.2-year follow-up period in the EPIC Oxford study (Appleby et al., 2007), and normal bone mass has been reported for vegetarians (New, 2004). However, it is acknowledged that there are large variations in factors that may impact on, this including dietary components and lifestyle factors.

Features of a vegetarian diet that may reduce the risk of chronic diseases include lower intakes of saturated fat and a higher consumption of fruit, vegetables, wholegrains, nuts, soya products (the term soya will be used throughout this chapter, rather than soy), fibre, some vitamins and minerals, and phytochemicals (Craig, 2010; Craig et al., 2009). The overall antioxidant status is similar between vegetarians and omnivores, but vegetarians have a 15% higher level of plasma carotenoids (Halder et al., 2007). However, it should be noted that vegetarians consume widely divergent diets and only a well balanced, vegetarian diet offers potential health benefits.

Other lifestyle practices, including activity levels, smoking and drinking habits, may also have an impact on the positive health benefits. Alewaeterers et al., (2005) reported that vegetarians smoked less, drank less alcohol

at the weekends and were engaged in more intensive physical activity compared with a reference population. In the EPIC Oxford study, however, such differences in lifestyle factors accounted for <5% of the difference in mean age adjusted BMI between meat eaters and vegans, whereas differences in macronutrient intake accounted for approximately half of the difference (Spencer et al., 2003).

There have been suggestions that the term vegetarian, often used in research, is not specific and requires fuller clarification. Studies have found that some people who classify themselves as vegetarian actually occasionally eat meat (Haddad & Tanzman, 2003). Robinson-O'Brien et al. (2009) found that approximately one-quarter of those who classified themselves as current vegetarians ate chicken. Inconsistencies in this description may have led to anomalies in findings between studies, such as the differences in the rates of colorectal cancer between British vegetarians and other populations (Key et al., 2009; Sanjoaquin et al., 2004), and as a result findings might need to be interpreted cautiously (Fraser, 2009).

Compared with other vegetarian diets, vegan diets tend to contain less saturated fat and cholesterol and more dietary fibre, but there is an increased risk of nutritional deficiencies (Craig et al., 2009; Key et al., 2006). Lower BMI levels and rates of type 2 diabetes have been seen in those consuming vegan diets as compared with vegetarians and non-vegetarians (Zaman et al., 2010; Spencer et al., 2003). There is, however, a higher fracture risk for vegans, probably as a consequence of lower calcium intakes (Ambroszkiewicz et al., 2010; Appleby et al., 2007).

Nutritional adequacy of a vegetarian or vegan diet

Protein

Vegetarians and vegans in the UK, Europe and North America consume adequate energy as derived from protein, albeit at lower levels than omnivores (Craig et al., 2009; Cade et al., 2004; Davey et al., 2002). The source of protein is important as this dictates its digestibility. Soya protein can meet needs as effectively as animal protein, whereas wheat protein, for example, eaten alone may result in reduced efficiency of nitrogen utilisation. Requirements may therefore vary depending on food selection. Kniskern & Johnston (2011) have suggested that the dietary reference intake (DRI) should be increased to 1.0 g/kg (from 0.8 g/kg) when consuming <50% of protein from animal sources. While it was once thought that combinations of plant foods had to be eaten at the same meal to ensure a sufficient intake of amino acids, it is now known that if energy intake is adequate and a mixture of plant proteins are eaten over the course of the day, requirements for essential amino acids will be met.

Fatty acids

The consumption of alpha-linolenic acid (ALA), an n-3 fatty acid obtained from plants, is relatively low in vegetarian and vegan diets compared with n-6 polyunsaturated fatty acids intakes, mainly linoleic acid, from seed oils (Sanders, 2009; Kornsteiner *et al.*, 2008). This results in an unbalanced n-6 to n-3 ratio in vegetarians and vegans, which may inhibit endogenous production of eicosapentaenoic acid (EPA) and docosahexaenoic acid (DHA). Little, if any, EPA and DHA are obtained from a vegetarian or vegan diet (as they are mainly obtained from fish sources, although some spreading fats, soups and sauces have been found to be the major sources in vegetarians) (Welch *et al.*, 2010; Sanders, 2009). Studies have shown that tissue levels of long chain n-3 fatty acids are depressed in vegetarians and particularly in vegans, irrespective of the duration of the diet (Kornsteiner *et al.*, 2008; Rosell *et al.*, 2005).

This is compounded by an inefficient conversion of ALA by the body to the more active longer chain metabolites (<5–10% for EPA and 2–5% for DHA) (Davis & Kris-Etherton, 2003). Total n-3 requirements may therefore be higher for vegetarians and vegans than for fish and meat eaters as they must rely on conversion of ALA to EPA and DHA. However, Welch *et al.* (2010) found that, although non-fish eating meat eaters and vegetarians have much lower intakes of EPA and DHA than fish eaters, their n-3 status is higher than would be expected, which suggests a greater conversion of ALA to circulating long chain n-3 fatty acids in non-fish eating groups. As yet, there is no documented evidence of adverse effects on health from the lower DHA intake in vegetarians.

The American Dietetic Association (Craig *et al.*, 2009) recommends that '*vegetarians should include good sources of ALA in their diets like flaxseed, walnuts, canola* [rapeseed] *oil and soya. Those with increased requirements of n-3 fatty acids such as pregnant and lactating women, may benefit from DHA rich microalgae*'.

Iron

Vegetarian diets contain mainly non-haem sources of iron, and the iron from these is less efficiently absorbed than haem iron of animal origin. They have generally higher intakes of inhibitors of iron absorption such as phytate, but evidence suggests that the overall effect of enhancers and inhibitors on iron absorption is considerably less than predicted and do not substantially influence iron status (SACN, 2010). Soya contains iron mostly in the form of ferritin, which is easily absorbed despite the presence of phytate, and so iron absorption may be higher than previously thought (Lonnerdal *et al.*, 2006). The Scientific Advisory Committee on Nutrition (SACN, 2010) reviewed a number of studies and found that dietary iron intakes of vegetarians are on average similar, or sometimes higher, than those of non-vegetarians. This is also consistent with regards to vegans in the EPIC study (Davey *et al.*, 2003), for whom intake was higher (14.1 mg/day) than for meat eaters (12.6 mg/day), fish eaters (12.8 mg/day) and vegetarians (12.6 mg/day).

Haemoglobin concentrations in vegetarians and non-vegetarians are similar, but although serum ferritin concentrations can be consistently statistically significantly lower in vegetarians, they are usually within the reference ranges (Haddad *et al.*, 1999). In western societies, incidence of iron deficiency anaemia among vegetarians is similar to that among non-vegetarians, although iron stores are often lower (Hunt, 2002).

Zinc

In the EPIC Oxford study (Davey *et al.*, 2003), vegetarians had lower intakes of zinc than meat eaters (7.67 mg/day versus 9.16 mg/day for women and 8.44 mg/day versus 9.78 mg/day in men), with vegans consuming even lower intakes (7.22 mg/day and 7.99 mg/day for men and women, respectively). The UK Women's Cohort Study (Cade *et al.*, 2004) confirmed this, with vegetarians consuming 10.2 mg/day versus meat eaters consuming 12.0 mg/day, a finding consistent with studies in other countries (de Bortoli & Cozzolino, 2009; Tupe & Chiplonkar, 2010; Chiplonkar & Agte, 2007; Haddad *et al.*, 1999).

The effect of phytates and folic acid on zinc bioavailability also causes concern with regards to vegetarian and vegan diets (Craig, 2009; Chiplonkar & Agte, 2006; Kristensen *et al.*, 2006; Hunt, 2003; Gibson, 1994). Suitable zinc rich foods for vegetarians and vegans include legumes, nuts and soya products. Soaking and sprouting seeds can increase zinc bioavailability. There no evidence has been found for any impact or adverse health effects of these lower intakes and biochemical stores on functional immunity (Hunt, 2003; Haddad *et al.*, 1999).

Iodine

The iodine content of food of plant origin may be lower than that of animal origin due to lower iodine concentration in the soil in some geographical areas. A number of studies have looked at the iodine content of vegetarian and vegan diets and all have found that there is a high potential for deficiency, especially in vegan diets (Leung *et al.*, 2011; Waldmann *et al.*, 2003; Krajcovicova-Kudlackova *et al.*, 2003; Remer *et al.*, 1999; Lightowler & Davies, 1998). Where iodine containing foods are consumed, however, mean iodine intakes can be greatly in excess of the RNI, e.g. if some types of seaweeds are eaten (Lightowler & Davies, 1998). Iodised table salt is a useful contributor to total iodine intake (Davidsson, 1999) and those who do not eat seaweed should be encouraged to consume this, kelp fortified yeast extracts or iodine supplements.

Selenium

Concerns have been raised about the selenium status of non-meat eaters, as the consumption of red meat is a major determinant of serum selenium (Letsiou *et al.*, 2010). Selenium status in vegetarians in studies by De Bortoli & Cozzolino (2009) and Gibson (1994) found that selenium blood levels were adequate. There is, however, currently insufficient evidence to assess the usefulness of biomarkers of selenium status and results as to whether vegetarians and vegans may be selenium deficient or not may depend on the biomarker chosen (Hoeflich *et al.*, 2010). Cereals, nuts and seeds are all suitable sources of selenium, but the actual content will vary depending on the soil in which they are grown.

Calcium

Calcium intakes for vegetarians are similar to those for meat eaters for men and women (Cade *et al.*, 2004; Davey *et al.*, 2003). Intakes of calcium by vegans are much lower, with a mean intake for men of 610 mg/day for men and 582 mg/day for women (Davey *et al.*, 2003), and may fall below the recommended intakes. Calcium enriched soya products are excellent sources of bioavailable calcium for vegans alongside kale and pak choi, tofu, brown and white bread (legally fortified with calcium), sesame seeds, tahini, nuts and dried fruit such as apricots and figs. Some green vegetables such as spinach and Swiss chard are high in calcium, but the calcium is bound to oxolate which makes it poorly absorbed.

Vitamin D

The richest sources of vitamin D are animal foods (with the exception of fortified products), so there is a potential for vegetarians and vegans to be deficient. There are conflicting results with regard to vitamin D status from different populations. The Adventist Health Study-2 found that there was no significant difference in serum 25-hydroxyvitamin D status (Chan *et al.*, 2009), but the EPIC Oxford study found that serum 25-hydroxyvitamin D was lower in vegetarians and vegans than meat eaters (Crowe *et al.*, 2011). A small study from Finland concluded that dietary intake of vitamin D in vegans was insufficient to maintain levels within normal ranges in the winter months at northern latitudes (Outilia *et al.*, 2000). For those with low sun exposure or consuming low intakes of vitamin D, fortified foods (such as margarine, some breakfast cereals and soya milks) or vitamin D supplements are recommended. Vitamin D_3 (cholecalciferol) is obtained from foods of animal origin but vitamin D_2 (ergocalciferol) is obtained from yeast which is an acceptable to vegans.

Vitamin B_{12} (cobalamin)

Vitamin B_{12} occurs in substantial amounts only in foods from animals. There are issues with diagnosing vitamin B_{12} deficiency, but low circulating concentrations and low intakes have been recorded in numerous studies of vegetarians and vegan diets (Gilsing *et al.*, 2010; Waldmann *et al.*, 2003; Herrmann & Geisel, 2002). Megaloblastic anaemia, a symptom of vitamin B_{12} deficiency, can be masked by high intakes of folic acid, with symptoms only detected at a neurological stage. In the EPIC Oxford cohort study, folate concentrations were highest among vegans, intermediate amongst vegetarians and lowest amongst omnivores (Gilsing *et al.*, 2010). Vegetarians can obtain vitamin B_{12} from dairy foods or eggs, but the only reliable source for vegans is fortified foods such as some breakfast cereals, yeast extracts, some plant milks and some soya products (approximately three portions are required per day). Alternatively, a daily supplement can be taken.

Retinol

Retinol is found only in animal foods and intakes for vegetarians and vegans are low (Davey *et al.*, 2003). Intakes of dietary carotenoids enable vegans to obtain an adequate supply of vitamin A, even though the bioavailability of beta-carotene from foods is variable. The most concentrated sources of carotenoids are carrots, red peppers, dark green leafy vegetables, tomatoes and yellow coloured fruit.

Vegetarian or vegan diets as a treatment for chronic diseases

Weight management

Vegetarians tend to have a lower BMI than non-vegetarians (Sabate & Wien, 2010; Appleby *et al.*, 1998) and weight gain over time is lower on a vegetarian diet (Rosell *et al.*, 2006). As vegetarian diets are nutritionally adequate (Farmer *et al.*, 2011), it has been proposed that a vegetarian diet may be a possible approach to treating obesity and weight management. A randomised clinical trial of 176 overweight or obese adults examined whether a prescribed calorie controlled, vegetarian diet had any significant benefits over a prescribed calorie controlled, omnivorous diet (Burke *et al.*, 2007). The vegetarian diet group showed a significant reduction in monounsaturated fat and a marginally significant reduction in total fat intakes at 18 months. Both groups, however, had significant reduction in total energy and fat intakes with reduced body weight, so as yet the evidence for prescribing vegetarian diets *per se* for weight management is inadequate. However, a low fat vegan diet has been compared with the National Cholesterol Education Program (NCEP) on weight loss maintenance and was found to produce significantly greater weight loss (Turner-McGrievy *et al.*, 2007).

Metabolic syndrome and type 2 diabetes

There have been suggestions that a vegetarian or vegan dietary pattern is an appropriate form of treatment for metabolic syndrome and type 2 diabetes (Marsh & Brand-Miller, 2011; Trapp *et al.*, 2010; Trapp & Barnard, 2010; Barnard *et al.*, 2009a). It is believed that the effects are mainly due to the accompanying weight loss, as well as reduced intakes of saturated fats and high glycaemic index food sources, and increased intakes of dietary fibre and vegetable protein.

In a small 24-week trial, 37 patients with type 2 diabetes received a vegetarian, calorie restricted diet and a matched number were assigned a conventional calorie restricted, diabetic diet (Kahleova *et al.*, 2011). Results showed that

43% of participants in the vegetarian group and 5% of participants in the traditional diabetic diet group reduced their antidiabetic medication. Also, body weight decreased more in the vegetarian group than in the traditional group (-6.2 kg versus -3.3 kg), even though the diets were isocaloric. The inclusion of exercise training further improved the outcomes with the vegetarian diet. A similar study with 99 participants compared a low fat vegan diet with a diet following the American Diabetes Association (ADA) guidelines (Barnard *et al.*, 2006). Both diets improved glycaemic control (as measured by HbA1c measurements), and promoted a reduction in body weight and LDL cholesterol levels, but the those on the low fat vegan diet showed greater improvements than those on the diet based on ADA guidelines. Questionnaire responses rated both diets as satisfactory (Barnard *et al.*, 2009b). To assess the quality of the diets, nutrient intake and Alternate Healthy Eating Index (AHEI) scores were collected at baseline and at 22 weeks; the vegan group improved its AHEI score whereas the ADA recommended diet group's AHEI score remained unchanged (Turner-McGrievy *et al.*, 2008).

Cardiovascular disease

Vegetarian and vegan diets have been suggested to be an effective tool for the management of cardiovascular disease (Lanou & Svenson, 2010b). A review by Ferdowsian & Barnard (2009) of both observational and intervention studies concluded that plant based dietary interventions, often in the form of portfolio diets, are effective in lowering plasma cholesterol concentrations to a greater extent than NCEP diets. In conjunction with increased exercise, stress management and group support, a vegetarian diet consumed for 1 year was shown to meet key heart health characteristics (fibre intakes >25 g/day, LDL cholesterol <10 mg/mL, BMI <25 kg/m^2, blood pressure <140/90 mmHg) and reduce risk markers (Marshall *et al.*, 2009). It has been suggested that, if maintained, such an intervention could result in substantial reductions in cardiovascular disease events.

Dietary considerations for different population groups

Pregnancy and lactation

Well planned vegetarian and vegan diets can be adequate in maintaining the health of both mother and child during pregnancy and, in some cases, may even have advantages over omnivorous diets. Gestational weight gain in pregnancy above the recommended ranges can be related to adverse pregnancy outcomes, but consumption of a vegetarian diet is associated with less gestational weight gain (Streuling *et al.*, 2011).

Additionally, vegetarians consume higher intakes of magnesium due to their plant based diet, which can result in slightly improved magnesium status during pregnancy compared with an average western diet (Koebnick *et al.*, 2005). Magnesium is important as a cofactor for many enzyme systems and has a critical role in cell division.

Plasma and red blood cell (RBC) folate concentrations have also been shown to be higher in pregnant vegetarians (probably due to long term, high vegetable intakes) than in those eating an average western diet. This can reduce the risk of folate deficiency if an adequate vitamin B_{12} supply is ensured (Koebnick *et al.*, 2001).

Pregnant vegetarian (and vegan) women, however, are at greater risk of vitamin B_{12} deficiency (Koebnick *et al.*, 2004) and there have been numerous cases cited of severe vitamin B_{12} deficiency with neurological damage in the infant as a result of maternal strict vegetarian/vegan diets (Erdeve *et al.*, 2009; Roed *et al.*, 2009; Mariani *et al.*, 2009; Mathey *et al.*, 2007; Weiss *et al.*, 2004; Smolka *et al.*, 2001). An adequate maternal dietary supply of vitamin B_{12} or a daily supplement is recommended.

A low consumption of red meat was marginally associated with anaemia in pregnant women in Pakistan (Baig-Ansari *et al.*, 2008), but in India there was no significant difference in the prevalence of iron deficiency anaemia between pregnant vegetarians or meat eaters (Sharma *et al.*, 2003). In both studies, prevalence of anaemia was very high in over 95% of the cases. Reference intakes for iron during pregnancy are the same as those for non-pregnant women in the UK (Department of Health, 1991), whether vegetarian or not. The Scientifics Advisory Committee on Nutrition (SACN, 2010) suggested that the high proportion of females with intakes of iron below the lower reference nutrient intake (LNRI) might mean that the iron dietary reference value (DRV) may be set too high. Iron intake recommendations and/or supplements should be based on the standard recommendations for pregnant women (see Chapter 3.2) and be food appropriate.

Vegan diets are devoid of DHA and vegetarian diets that include dairy foods and eggs only provide about 20 mg of DHA/day (Sanders, 2009). Pregnancy is a developmental period during which the n-3 fatty acid supply to the foetus is critical to ensure the optimal development of the brain and visual systems, with the balance between n-3 and n-6 fatty acids present in the perinatal period affecting the development of systems regulating immune function, fat deposition and metabolism (Gibson *et al.*, 2011). The fatty acid composition of breast milk reflects that of the maternal diet and is a major determinant of the n-3 status of a breastfed infant and subsequent immune function (Lauritzen & Carlson, 2011). It has been recommended that all pregnant and lactating women should aim to achieve an average daily intake of at least 200 mg of DHA (Koletzko *et al.*, 2008). Pregnant and lactating vegetarian/vegan women may benefit from DHA rich supplements due to their low intakes and increased requirements.

The American Dietetic Association (ADA, 2009) (now the Academy of Nutrition & Dietetics) has published an evidence based review with regards to vegetarian nutrition in pregnancy with the following summaries in addition to the above:

- Pregnant vegetarians receive statistically lower levels of protein than pregnant non-vegetarians (although none report a protein deficiency), but consume statistically higher levels of carbohydrates (Grade III – limited evidence (see Chapter 1.1).

- No research was identified with regards to macronutrient intakes among pregnant vegans.
- There are no significant health differences in babies born to non-vegan vegetarian mothers versus non-vegetarians (Grade III – limited evidence).
- No research was identified that focussed on the birth outcomes of vegan versus omnivorous mothers.
- Intakes of vitamin B_{12}, vitamin C, calcium and zinc were lower among vegetarians than non-vegetarians. Vegetarians did not meet the dietary standard for vitamin B_{12} and zinc (in the UK), iron (in the US) and folate (in Germany) (Grade III – limited evidence).
- The micronutrient content of a balanced maternal vegetarian diet does not have detrimental outcomes for the health of the child at birth (Grade III – limited evidence).
- Vegetarian diets can be nutritionally adequate in pregnancy and can lead to positive birth outcomes.

Pregnant and lactating vegetarians need to pay attention to the nutritional adequacy of their diets, particularly with regards to vitamin B_{12} and zinc and be mindful about intakes of iron and folate. Supplements normally advised for pregnant women (400 μg folic acid in the first trimester and 10 μg vitamin D) also apply to vegetarians and vegans. There is currently no evidence as to the adequacy of a vegan diet or birth outcomes in pregnant vegans. It has, however, been noted (Amit, 2010) that:

- The calcium content of breast milk is unaffected by a vegan diet in the mother.
- The breast milk from vegan mothers does not contain an adequate amount of zinc for infants after the age of 7 months.
- Soya formula is the only option for non-breastfed vegan infants.

Childhood and adolescence

A review by Sabate & Wien (2010) of the anthropometry of vegetarian youngsters found conflicting data on the height of vegetarian children, with one study finding that vegetarian children were taller than their omnivorous classmates (Sabate et al., 1991), while another showed that they were shorter (Sabate et al., 1990). One study of predominately vegetarian adolescents showed that they had a significantly lower BMI, waist circumference, total cholesterol to high density lipoprotein (HDL) ratio and LDL concentration than their omnivorous classmates (Grant et al., 2008).

There is evidence, however, of inadequate intakes of vitamin D and calcium in vegetarian children aged 2–10 years compared with omnivores, with subsequent lower levels of biochemical bone turnover markers (Ambroszkiewicz et al., 2007). In a small study (n = 56), vitamin B_{12} intake was found to be lower in vegetarian preschool children and their parents compared with omnivores, but both had similar serum vitamin B_{12} concentrations (Yen

et al., 2010). SACN (2010) reported that in young people aged 4–18 years there was no association between a vegetarian diet and lower than average iron intakes, but that girls aged 15–18 years in general, (whether vegetarian or not) were at risk of iron deficiency anaemia. Research from Sweden also found this to be the case for adolescent vegans (Larsson & Johansson, 2002). They did, however, also find that the adolescents had dietary intakes lower than average requirements for riboflavin, vitamin B_{12}, vitamin D, calcium and selenium.

The Canadian Paediatric Society has issued a position statement on vegetarian diets in children and adolescents (Amit, 2010) and concluded that *'a well-balanced vegetarian diet can provide for the needs of children and adolescents'*. It did, however, raise concerns in the following areas:

- Restrictive vegan diets may cause energy deficits (due to low energy density and bulk), which present challenges in feeding smaller children. The inclusion of soya products, nuts (age appropriate) and nut butters can be useful.
- Due to the lower digestibility of plant proteins, some studies have suggested that protein intake may need to be increased for vegans (an increase varying from 30% to 35% for infants up to 2 years of age, 20–30% for 2–6-year olds, 15–20% for those >6 years). Combinations of protein sources from different food groups (nuts and seeds, cereals, legumes) need to be encouraged, but combining complementary proteins at each meal is not believed to be necessary.
- Due to lower bioavailability of iron and increased needs for iron in children, especially during rapid growth periods, it is prudent to ensure that good sources such as fortified cereals are included and supplementation is considered particularly in times of higher needs.
- Zinc requirements in vegans may be higher than in omnivores, due to differences in bioavailability, but additional supplementation is not recommended. Good sources of zinc such as pulses, nuts (age appropriate), yeast leavened bread, fermented soya products and sprouted seeds should be included in the diet.
- Calcium intakes below recommendations have been noted in vegan children and it is essential to ensure an adequate intake of calcium rich and calcium fortified foods (such as soya products, cereals, low oxolate green vegetables). Supplementation may be required.
- Adequate sources of linolenic acid (the precursor of EPA and DHA) are required and supplements may need to be included in the diets of vegetarian and vegan children.
- Supplementation of vitamin B_{12} or a good intake of fortified foods (at least three servings of vitamin B_{12} rich foods per day) is recommended for vegetarian and vegan children. Infants of vegan mothers are particularly at risk from vitamin B_{12} deficiency.

In line with all children who do not consume sufficient vitamin D enriched foods or have limited exposure to sunlight, supplementation is recommended.

Three servings of dietary carotenoids per day (from fruit and vegetable products) are recommended for vegan children. Fibre intake should be monitored to avoid dilution of energy and interference with essential minerals, particularly in young children with potentially high intakes.

The Position Statement from the American Dietetic Association (Craig *et al.*, 2009) supports these points. Guidelines are available for children being weaned onto a vegetarian diet (Di Genova & Guyda, 2007) that reflect these recommendations. The Vegan Society (UK) (www.vegansociety.com) gives details about the introduction of solid foods for vegan children.

Older adults

In ageing, there is a decreased energy need but increased requirements and/or decreased absorption for some nutrients. This combined with a smaller appetite and the physical limitations that may increase with age means that nutrient dense, vegetarian or vegan acceptable foods should be eaten in line with nutritional requirements (see Chapter 3.3). When dietary selection is limited, nutrient supplementation with a low dose multivitamin and mineral supplement can be useful in meeting recommended intake levels.

A study in community living elderly vegetarians in Taiwan found they had significantly lower daily total energy, lower cholesterol, a higher percentage of fat as polyunsaturated fatty acid (PUFA), higher calcium and higher fibre intakes compared with omnivores. Vegetarian diets in this group contained more potassium, calcium, magnesium and fibre than vegan diets (Huang *et al.*, 2011). In China, community living, elderly women consuming a vegetarian or vegan diet had significantly lower bone mineral density at some sites in the hip (although bone mineral density at the spine was similar between vegetarians and omnivores) (Lau *et al.*, 1998). Due to possibly very different types of food consumption, these results should be viewed cautiously and further research is warranted. There appears to be little difference in the dietary intakes, blood values and physical characteristics between the institutionalised vegetarian and non-vegetarian elderly (Deriemaeker *et al.*, 2011).

Athletes

There is no reason why a vegetarian or vegan athlete will perform differently from omnivore athletes as long as they are consuming a well balanced diet. As yet, there is no evidence that a vegetarian or vegan diet will improve performance either (Fuhrman & Ferreri, 2010). There are a number of concerns that vegetarian and vegan athletes must be aware of to ensure optimum intake as an athlete may require more protein than non-athletes, but this generally should not cause any problems unless the diet becomes too bulky. However, vegetarian athletes may be at risk for low intakes of energy, fat, vitamin B_{12}, riboflavin, vitamin D, calcium, iron (particularly in women and during adolescence and pregnancy) and zinc (Rodriguez *et al.*, 2010). There is no current evidence regarding the adequacy of the nutritional intake of vegan athletes (see Chapter 4.3).

Internet resources

British Dietetic Association
   Factsheet 'Vegetarian Diets – Keeping a Healthy Balance' www.bda.uk.com/foodfacts/vegetarianfoodfacts.pdf
Vegan Society (UK) www.vegansociety.com
Vegetarian Society (UK) www.vegsoc.org
Vegetarian for Life www.vegetarianforlife.org.uk

References

Alewaeterers K, Clarys P, Hebbelinck M, Deriemaeker P, Clarys JP. (2005) Cross-sectional analysis of BMI and some lifestyle variables in Flemish vegetarians compared with non-vegetarians. *Ergonomics* 48(11–14): 1433–1444.

Aloufy A, Latzer Y. (2006) Diet or health – the linkage between vegetarianism and anorexia nervosa. *Harefuah* 145(7): 526–531.

Ambroszkiewicz J, Klemarczyk W, Gajewska J, Chelchowska M, Laskowska-Klita T. (2007) Serum concentration of biochemical bone turnover markers in vegetarian children. *Advances in Medical Sciences* 52: 279–82.

Ambroszkiewicz J, Klemarczyk W, Gajewska J, Chelchowska M, Franek E, Laskowska-Klita T. (2010) The influence of vegan diet on bone mineral density and biochemical bone turnover markers. *Pediatric Endocrinology, Diabetes and Metabolism* 16(3): 201–204.

American Dietetic Association. (2009) Vegetarian nutrition in pregnancy. *Journal of the American Dietetic Association* 109: 1266–1282.

Amit M. (2010) Vegetarian diets in children and adolescents. *Journal of Paediatrics and Child Health* 15(5): 303–308.

Appleby PN, Thorogood M. Mann JI, Key TJ. (1998) Low body mass index in non-meat eaters: the possible roles of animal fat, dietary fibre and alcohol. *International Journal of Obesity Related Metabolic Disorders* 22(5): 454–460.

Appleby PN, Davey GK, Key TJ. (2002) Hypertension and blood pressure among meat eaters, fish-eaters, vegetarians and vegans in EPIC Oxford. *Public Health and Nutrition* 5(5): 645–654.

Appleby P, Roddam A, Allen N, Key T. (2007) Comparative fracture risk in vegetarians and non-vegetarians in EPIC Oxford. *European Journal of Clinical Nutrition* 61(12): 1400–1406.

Baig-Ansari N, Badruddin SH, Karmaliani R, *et al.* (2008) Anaemia prevalence and risk factors in pregnant women in an urban area of Pakistan. *Food Nutrition Bulletin* 29(2): 132–139.

Barnard ND, Cohen J, Jenkins DJ, *et al.* (2006) A low-fat vegan diet improves glycaemic control and cardiovascular risk factors in a randomised control trial in individuals with type 2 diabetes. *Diabetes Care* 29(8): 1777–1783.

Barnard ND, Katcher HI, Jenkins DJ, Cohen J, Turner-McGrievy G. (2009a) Vegetarian and vegan diets in type 2 diabetes management. *Nutrition Reviews* 67(5): 255–263.

Barnard ND, Gloede L, Cohen J, *et al.*. (2009b) A low-fat vegan diet elicits greater macronutrient changes, but is comparable in adherence and acceptability, compared with a more conventional diabetes diet among individuals with type 2 diabetes. *Journal of the American Dietetic Association* 109(2): 263–272.

Bates B, Lennox L, Swann G. (2010) NDNS: Headline results from year 1 of the rolling programme (2008/2009), Available at www.food.gov.uk/multimedia/pdfs/publication/ndnsreport0809.pdf. *Accessed* 7 July 2011.

Bedford JL, Barr SI. (2005) Diets and selected lifestyle practices of self-defined adult vegetarians from a population-based sample suggest they are more 'health conscious'. *International Journal of Behavioural Nutrition and Physical Activity* 2(1): 4.

Burke LE, Hudson AG, Warziski MT, Styn Ma, Music E, Elci OU, Sereika SM. (2007) Effects of a vegetarian diet and treatment preference on biochemical and dietary variables in overweight and obese adults: a randomised clinical trial. *American Journal of Clinical Nutrition* 86(3): 588–596.

Cade JE, Burley VJ, Greenwood DC, UK Women's Cohort Study Steering Group. (2004) The UK Women's Cohort Study: comparison of vegetarians, fish-eaters and meat-eaters. *Public Health and Nutrition* 7(7): 871–878.

Chan J, Jaceldo-Siegl K, Fraser GE. (2009) Serum 25-hydroxyvitamin D status of vegetarians and non vegetarians: The Adventist Health Study-2. *American Journal of Clinical Nutrition* 89(5): 1686S–1692S.

Chiplonkar SA, Agte VV. (2006) Predicting bioavailable zinc from lower phytate forms, folic acid and their interactions with zinc in vegetarian meals. *Journal of the American College of Nutrition* 25(1): 26–33.

Chiplonkar SA, Agte VV. (2007) Association of micronutrient status with subclinical health complaints in lactovegetarian adults. *Scandinavian Journal of Food and Nutrition* 51(4): 159–166.

Craig WJ. (2009) Health effects of vegan diets. *American Journal of Clinical Nutrition* 89(5): 1627S–1633S.

Craig WJ. (2010) Nutrition concerns and health effects of vegetarian diets. *Nutrition and Clinical Practice* 25: 613–620.

Craig WJ, Mangels AR, ADA. (2009) Position of the American Dietetic Association: vegetarian diets. *Journal of the American Dietetic Association* 109(7): 1266–1282.

Crowe FL, Steur M, Allen NE, Appleby PN, Travis RC, Key TJ. (2011) Plasma concentrations of 25-hydroxyvitamin D in meat eaters, fish eaters, vegetarians and vegans: results from the EPIC Oxford Study. *Public Health and Nutrition* 14(2): 340–346.

Davey G, Allen N, Appleby P, et al. (2002). Dietary and lifestyle characteristics of meat-eaters, fish-eaters, vegetarians and vegans. *IARC Scientific Publications* 156:113–114.

Davey GK, Spencer EA, Appleby PN, Allen NE, Knox KH, Key TJ. (2003) EPIC Oxford: lifestyle characteristics and nutrient intakes in a cohort of 33 883 meat-eaters and 31 546 non meat-eaters in the UK. *Public Health and Nutrition* 6(3): 259–268.

Davidsson L. (1999) Are vegetarians an 'at risk group' for iodine deficiency? *British Journal of Nutrition* 81: 3–4.

Davis BC, Kris-Etherton PM. (2003) Achieving optimal essential fatty acid status in vegetarians: current knowledge and practical implications. *American Journal of Clinical Nutrition* 78 (3 Suppl): 640S–646S.

de Bortoli MC, Cozzolino SM. (2009) Zinc and selenium nutritional status in vegetarians. *Biological Trace Element Research* 127(3): 228–233.

Department of Health. (1991) *Dietary Reference Values*. London: The Stationery Office.

Deriemaeker P, Aerenhouts D, De Ridder D, Hebbelinck M, Clarys P. (2011) Health aspects, nutrition and physical characteristics in matched samples of institutionalised vegetarian and non-vegetarian elderly (>65yrs). *Nutrition and Metabolism* 8(1): 37.

Di Genova T, Guyda H. (2007) Infants and children consuming atypical diets: Vegetarianism and macrobiotics. *Journal of Paediatrics and Child Health* 12(3):185–188.

Erdeve O, Arsan S, Atasay B, Ileri T, Uysal Z. (2009) A breast-fed newborn with megaloblastic anaemia-treated with vitamin B12 supplementation of the mother. *Journal of Pediatric Hematolgy and Oncology* 31(10): 763–765.

Farmer B, Larson BT, Fulgoni VL, Rainville AJ, Liepa GU. (2011) A vegetarian dietary pattern as a nutrient-dense approach to weight management: An analysis of the National Health and Nutrition Examination Survey 1999–2004. *Journal of the American Dietetic Association* 111(6): 819–827.

Ferdowsian HR, Barnard ND. (2009) Effects of plant-based diets on plasma lipids. *American Journal of Cardiology* 104: 947–956.

Food Standards Agency (FSA). (2003) *Consumer Attitudes to Food Standards Survey*. London: FSA.

Food Standards Agency. (2006a) *Guidance on use of the terms 'vegetarian' and 'vegan' in food labelling*. London: FSA. Available at www.food.gov.uk/scotland/regsscotland/regsguidscot/vegiguidance notes.

Food Standards Agency. (2006b) *Consumer Attitudes to Food Standards Survey*. London: FSA.

Fraser GE. (2009) Vegetarian diets: what do we know of their effects on common chronic diseases?. *American Journal of Clinical Nutrition* 89(5): 1607S–1612S.

Fuhrman J, Ferreri DM. (2010) Fueling the vegetarian (vegan) athlete. *Current Sports Medicine Report* 9(4): 233–241.

Gibson RS. (1994) Content and bioavailability of trace elements in vegetarian diets. *American Journal of Clinical Nutrition* 59 (5 Suppl): 1223S–1232S.

Gibson RA, Muhlhausler B, Makrides M. (2011) Conversion of linoleic acid and alpha-linoleic acid to long-chain polyunsaturated fatty acids (LCPUFAs), with a focus on pregnancy, lactation and the first 2 years of life. *Maternal and Child Nutrition* 7 (Suppl 2): 17–26.

Gilsing AM, Crowe FL, Lloyd-Wright Z, et al. (2010) Serum concentrations of vitamin B12 and folate in British male omnivores, vegetarians and vegans : results from a cross sectional analysis of the EPIC Oxford cohort study. *European Journal of Clinical Nutrition* 64(9): 933–939.

Grant R, Bilgin A, Zeuschner C et al. (2008) The relative impact of a vegetable-rich diet on key markers of health in a cohort of Australian adolescents. *Asia Pacific Journal of Clinical Nutrition* 17: 107–115.

Gregory J, Lowe S, Bates CJ, et al.. (2000) *National Diet and Nutrition Survey: Young People Aged 4 to 18 Years. Volume 1: Report of the Diet and Nutrition Survey*. London: The Stationery Office.

Haddad EH, Tanzman JS. (2003) What do vegetarians in the United States eat? *American Journal of Clinical Nutrition* 78 (3 Suppl): 626S–632S.

Haddad EH, Berk LS, Kettering JD, Hubbarb RW, Peters WR. (1999) Dietary intake and biochemical, hematologic and immune status of vegans compared with non vegetarians. *American Journal of Clinical Nutrition* 70 (Suppl): 586S–593S.

Halder S, Rowland IR, Barnett YA, et al. (2007) Influence of habitual diet on antioxidant status: a study in a population of vegetarians and omnivores. *European Journal of Clinical Nutrition* 61(8): 1011–1022.

Huang CJ, Fan YC, Liu JF, Tsai PS. (2011) Characteristics and nutrient intake of Taiwanese elderly vegetarians: evidence from a national survey. *British Journal of Nutrition* 9: 1–10.

Herrmann W, Geisel J. (2002) Vegetarian lifestyle and monitoring of vitamin B12 status. *Clinica Chimica Acta* 326(1–2): 47–59.

Hoeflich Hollenbach B, Behrends T, Hoeg A, Stosnach H, Schomburg L. (2010) The choice of biomarkers determines the selenium status in young German vegans and vegetarians. *British Journal of Nutrition* 104(11): 1601–1604.

Hunt JR. (2002) Moving toward a plant-based diet: are iron and zinc at risk? *Nutrition Reviews* 60 (5 Pt 1): 127–134.

Hunt JR. (2003) Bioavailability of iron, zinc and other trace minerals from vegetarian diets. *American Journal of Clinical Nutrition* 78 (3 Suppl): 633S–639S.

Kahleova H, Matoulek M, Malinska H, et al. (2011) Vegetarian diet improves insulin resistance and oxidative stress markers more than conventional diet in subjects with Type 2 diabetes. *Diabetes Medicine* 28(5): 549–559.

Key TJ, Appleby PN, Rosell MS. (2006) Health effects of vegetarian and vegan diets. *Proceedings of the Nutrition Society* 65(1): 35–41.

Key TJ, Appleby PN, Spencer EA, Travis RC, Roddam AW, Allen NE. (2009) Cancer incidence in vegetarians: results from the European Prospective Investigation into Cancer and nutrition (EPIC Oxford). *American Journal of Clinical Nutrition* 89(5): 1620S–1626S.

Kniskern MA, Johnston CS. (2011) Protein dietary reference intakes may be inadequate for vegetarians if low amounts of animal protein are consumed. *Nutrition* 27(6): 727–730.

Koebnick C, Heins UA, Hoffmann I, Dagnelie PC, Leitzmann C. (2001) Folate status during pregnancy in women is improved by long-term high vegetable intake compared with the average western diet. *Journal of Nutrition* 131(3): 733–739.

Koebnick C, Hoffmann I, Dagnelie PC, *et al.* (2004) Long-term ovo-lacto vegetarian diet impairs vitamin B12 status in pregnant women. *Journal of Nutrition* 134(12): 3319–3326.

Koebnick C, Leitzmann R, Garcia AL, *et al.* (2005) Long-term effect of a plant based diet on magnesium status during pregnancy. *European Journal of Clinical Nutrition* 59(2): 219–225.

Koletzko B, Lien E, Agostoni C, *et al.* (2008) The roles of long-chain polyunsaturated fatty acids in pregnancy, lactation and infancy: review of current knowledge and consensus recommendations. *Journal of Perinatal Medicine* 36(1): 5–14.

Kornsteiner M, Singer I, Elmadfa I. (2008) Very low n-3 long-chain polyunsaturated fatty acid status in Austrian vegetarians and vegans. *Annals of Nutrition and Metabolism* 52(1): 37–47.

Kristensen MB, Hels O, Morberg CM, Marving J, Bugel S, Tetens I. (2006) Total zinc absorption in young women, but not fractional zinc absorption, differs between vegetarian and meat-based diets with equal phytic acid content. *British Journal of Nutrition* 95(5): 963–967.

Krajcovicova-Kudlackova M, Buckova K, Klimes I, Sebokova E. (2003) Iodine deficiency in vegetarians and vegans. *Annals of Nutrition and Metablism* 47(5): 183–185.

Lanou AJ, Svenson B. (2010a) Reduced cancer risk in vegetarians: an analysis of recent reports. *Cancer Managment Research* 20(3): 1–8.

Lanou AJ, Svenson B. (2010b) Vegetarian dietary patterns as a means to achieve reduction in cardiovascular disease and diabetes risk factors. *Current Cardiovascular Risk Reports* 4: 48–56.

Larsson CL, Johansson GK. (2002) Dietary intake and nutritional status of young vegans and omnivores in Sweden. *American Journal of Clinical Nutrition* 76(1): 100–106.

Lau EM, Kwok T, Woo J, Ho SC. (1998) Bone mineral density in Chinese elderly female vegetarians, vegans, lacto-vegetarians and omnivores. *European Journal of Clinical Nutrition* 52(1): 60–64.

Lauritzen L, Carlson SE. (2011) Maternal fatty acid status during pregnancy and lactation and relation to newborn and infant status. *Maternal and Child Nutrition* 7 (Suppl 2): 41–58.

Letsiou S, Nomikos T, Panagiotakos D, *et al.* (2010) Dietary habits of Greek adults and serum total selenium concentration: the ATTICA study. *European Journal of Nutrition* 49(8): 465–472.

Leung AM, Lamar A, He X, Braverman LE, Pearce EN. (2011) Iodine status and thyroid function of Boston-area vegetarians and vegans. *Journal of Clinical Endocrinology & Metabolism* 96(8): E1303–1307.

Lightowler HJ, Davies GJ. (1998) Iodine intake and iodine deficiency in vegans as assessed by the duplicate-portion technique and urinary iodine excretion. *British Journal of Nutrition* 80(6): 529–535.

Lonnerdal B, Bryant A, Liu X, Theil EC. (2006) Iron absorption from soybean ferritin in nonanemic women. *American Journal of Clinical Nutrition* 83(1): 103–107.

Mariani A, Chalies S, Jeziorski E, Ludwig C, Lalande M, Rodiere M. (2009) Consequences of exclusive breast feeding in vegan mother newborn-case report. *Archives of Pediatrics* 16(11): 1461–1463.

Marsh K, Brand-Miller J. (2011) Vegetarian diets and diabetes. *American Journal of Lifestyle Medicine* 5: 135–143.

Marshall DA, Walizer EM, Vernalis MN. (2009) Achievement of heart health characteristics through participation in an intensive lifestyle change program (Coronary Artery Reversal Study). *J Cardiopulmonary Rehabilitation and Prevention* 29(2): 84–94.

Mathey C, Di Marco JN, Poujol A, *et al.* (2007) Failure to thrive and psychomotor regression revealing vitamin B 12 deficiency in 3 infants. *Archives of Pediatrics* 14(5): 467–471.

New SA. (2004) Do vegetarians have a normal bone mass? *Osteoporosis International* 15(9): 679–688.

Outilia TA, Karkkainen MU, Seppanen RH, Lamberg-Allardt CJ. (2000) Dietary intake of vitamin D in premenopausal, healthy vegans was insufficient to maintain concentrations of 25-hydroxyvitamin D and intact parathyroid hormone within normal ranges during the winter in Finland. *Journal of the American Dietetic Association* 100(4): 434–441.

Remer T, Neubert A, Manz F. (1999) Increased risk of iodine deficiency with vegetarian nutrition. *British Journal of Nutrition* 81(1): 45–49.

Rizzo NS, Sabate J, Jaceldo-Siegl K, Fraser GE. (2011) Vegetarian dietary patterns are associated with lower risk of metabolic syndrome: The Adventist Health Study 2. *Diabetes Care* 34: 1225–1227.

Robinson-O'Brien R, Perry CL, Wall MM, Story M, Neumark-Sztainer D. (2009) Adolescent and young adult vegetarianism: better dietary intake and weight outcomes but increased risk of disordered eating behaviors. *Journal of American Dietetic Association* 109(4): 648–655.

Rodriguez NR, DiMarco NM, Langley S. (2010) Joint position statement from the American Dietetic Association, Dietitians of Canada and American College of Sports Medicine: Nutrition and athletic performance. *Medicine and Science in Sports Exercise* 41(3): 709–731.

Roed C, Skovby F, Lund AM. (2009) Severe vitamin B12 deficiency in infants breastfed by vegans. *Ugeskr Laeger* 171(43): 3099–3101.

Rosell MS, Lloyd-Wright Z, Appleby PN, Sanders TA, Allen NE, Key TJ. (2005) Long-chain n-3 polyunsaturated fatty acids in plasma in British meat-eating, vegetarian and vegan men. *American Journal of Clinical Nutrition* 82(2): 327–334.

Rosell M, Appleby P, Spencer E, Key T. (2006) Weight gain over 5 years in 21966 meat-eating, fish-eating, vegetarian, and vegan men and women in EPIC Oxford. *International Journal of Obesity (London)* 30(9): 1389–1396.

Sabate J, Wien M. (2010) Vegetarian diets and childhood obesity prevention. *American Journal of Clinical Nutrition* 91(5): 1525S–1529S

Sabate J, Linsted KD, Harris RD, Johnston PK. (1990) Anthropometric parameters of schoolchildren with different life-styles. *American Journal of Diseases of Children* 144: 1159–1163.

Sabate J, Linsted KD, Harris RD, Sanchez A. (1991) Attained height of lacto-ovo-vegetarian children and adolescents. *European Journal of Clinical Nutrition* 45: 51–58.

Scientific Advisory Committee on Nutrition (SACN). (2010) *Iron and Health*. London: The Stationery Office.

Sanders TA. (2009) DHA status of vegetarians. *Prostaglandins, Leukotrienes and Essential Fatty Acids* 81(2–3):137–141.

Sanjoaquin MA, Appleby PN, Thorogood M, Mann JI, Key TJ. (2004) Nutrition, lifestyle and colorectal cancer incidence: a prospective investigation of 10998 vegetarians and non-vegetarians in the United Kingdom. *British Journal of Cancer* 90: 118–121.

Sharma JB, Soni D, Murthy NS, Malhotra M. (2003) Effect of dietary habits on prevalence of anaemia in pegnant women of Delhi. *Journal of Obstetrics and Gynaecology Research* 29(2): 73–78.

Smolka V, Bekarek V, Hlidova E, *et al.* (2001) Metabolic complications and neurologic manifestations of vitamin B12 deficiency in children of vegetarian mothers. *Journal of Czech Physicians* 140(23) 732–735.

Spencer EA, Appleby PN, Davey GK, Key TJ. (2003) Diet and body mass index in 38000 EPIC Oxford meat-eaters, fish-eaters,, vegetarians and vegans. *International Journal of Obestric and Related Metabolic Disorders* 27(6): 728–734.

Streuling I, Beyerlein A, Rosenfeld T, Schukat B, von Kries R. (2011) Weight gain and dietary intake during pregnancy in industrialised countries- a systematic review of observational studies. *Journal of Perinatal Medicine* 39(2): 123–129.

Tonstad S, Butler T, Yan R, Fraser GE. (2009) Type of vegetarian diet, body weight and prevalence of type 2 diabetes. *Diabetes Care* 32(5): 791–796.

Trew K, Clark C, McCartney G, Barnett J, Muldoon O. (2006) Adolescents, food choice and vegetarianism. In: Shepherd R, Raats M (eds) *The Psychology of Food Choice*. Cabi Org in association with The Nutrition Society, pp. 247–262.

Trapp CB, Barnard ND. (2010) Usefulness of vegetarian and vegan diets for treating type 2 diabetes. *Current Diabetes Reports* 10(2): 152–158.

Trapp C, Barnard N, Katcher H. (2010) A plant-based diet for type 2 diabetes. *Diabetes Educator* 36(1): 33–48.

Tupe R, Chiplonkar SA. (2010) Diet patterns of lactovegetarian adolescent girls: need for devising recipes with high zinc bioavailability. *Nutrition* 26(4): 390–398.

Turner-McGrievy GM, Barnard ND, Scialli AR. (2007) A two-year randomised weight loss trial comparing a vegan diet to a more moderate low-fat diet. *Obesity* 15(9): 2276–2281.

Turner-McGrievy GM, Barnard ND, Cohen J, Jenkins DJ, Gloede L, Green AA. (2008) Changes in nutrient intake and dietary quality among participants with type 2 diabetes following a low-fat vegan diet or a conventional diabetes diet for 22 weeks. *Journal of the American Dietetic Association* 108(10): 1636–1645.

Waldmann A, Koschizke JW, Leitzmann C, Hahn A. (2003) Dietary intakes and lifestyle factors of a vegan population in Germany: results from the German Vegan Study. *European Journal of Clinical Nutrition* 57: 947–955.

Weiss R, Fogelman Y, Bennett M. (2004) Severe vitamin B12 deficiency in an infant associated with a maternal deficiency and a strict vegetarian diet. *Journal of Pediatric Hematolgy and Oncology* 26(4): 270–271.

Welch AA, Shakya-Shrestha S, Lentjes MA, Wareham NJ, Khaw KT. (2010) Dietary intake and status of n-3 polyunsaturated fatty acids in a population of fish-eating and non-fish-eating meat-eaters, vegetarians, and vegans and the product-precursor ratio [corrected] of alpha-linolenic acid to long-chain polyunsaturated fatty acids: results from the EPIC-Norfolk cohort. *American Journal of Clinical Nutrition* 92(5): 1040–1051.

Yen CE, Yen CH, Cheng CH, Huang YC. (2010) Vitamin B12 status is not associated with plasma homcysteine in parents and their preschool children: lacto-ovo, lacto, and ovo vegetarians and omnivores. *Journal of the American College of Nutrition* 29(1): 7–13.

Zaman GS, Zaman FA, Arifullah M. (2010) Comparative risk of type 2 diabetes mellitus among vegetarians and non-vegetarians. *Indian Journal of Community Medicine* 35(3): 441–442.

SECTION 3

Siân Burton, Anne Laverty and Marjory Macleod

Key points

■ People with a learning disability are nutritionally vulnerable and their needs should be assessed on an individual basis.

■ Dietary guidance for clients should be clear and concise with no more than three key messages or dietary goals at a time.

■ Issues of client consent and involvement in the decision making process must be considered.

■ Multidisciplinary and multiagency collaborative working is essential to ensure consistent messages and continuity of care.

■ Guidelines for the nutritional management of specific learning disabilities, e.g. Down's syndrome and Prader–Willi syndrome, should be used.

NB: The guidance within this chapter is not applicable for people who have a higher level autistic spectrum disorder (ASD) such as Asperger's or other specific learning difficulties (SpLD), e.g. attention deficit disorder (ADD), attention deficit hyperactive disorder (ADHD) dyslexia, dyscalculia, dyspraxia and speech and language delay.

Government policy is aimed at encouraging people with a learning disability (LD) to access mainstream services (Rutter & Carmichael, 2011). Therefore, healthcare professionals (HCP), including dietitians, are more likely to encounter people with a LD in general clinics within primary and secondary care (Powrie, 2003; Sowney & Barr, 2004; Edwards, 2007). There has also been a major move away from institutionalised care so that people with a LD are enabled to live within the community, supported by a variety of healthcare and/or social care services as dictated by individual need. The unforeseen increase in the level of obesity, however, as a consequence of the change in domicile is impacting on people's health and quality of life (Robertson *et al.*, 2000; Emerson, 2005; Yamaki, 2005; Ito, 2006; Rimmer & Yamaki, 2006; Henderson *et al.*, 2008; Melville *et al.*, 2008).

People with a LD experience a higher burden of ill health than the general population, and are more than twice as likely to suffer health problems and four times as many die from preventable diseases (Disability Rights Commission. 2006). The range of health needs includes mental illness, epilepsy, an array of physical and sensory limitations (including impaired sense of touch, tempera-

ture, pain, taste and smell), dental disease, thyroid disorders, heart disease, alopecia, binge eating disorder (BED), dysphagia, undernutrition and obesity [Kennedy *et al.*, 1997; Bryan *et al.*, 2000; Hove, 2004; National Patient Safety Agency (NPSA), 2004; Bernall, 2005; Melville *et al.*, 2005; Wali *et al.*, 2006; Department of Health, 2007; 2009a; Wallace & Schluter, 2008; Carnaby, 2009].

The health gains associated with good nutritional care include enhanced quality of life and improved disease outcomes (Astor & Jeffreys, 2000; Department of Health, 2004). People with a LD must be enabled, as much as possible, to make informed decisions and steps must be taken to ensure that this client group has access to both mainstream and specialist services as and when required (Burton *et al.*, 2011).

Definition of learning disabilities

A universally accepted definition of LDs is not available; however, there is general agreement that the term includes a group of conditions that, as a result of factors occurring prior to birth, at birth, during childhood or up to the age of brain maturity, affect intellectual development and are life long (WHO, 2010). The following definition includes all the requisite dimensions and is useful for practitioners (WHO, 1992):

• A significant intellectual impairment with an intellectual quotient (IQ) of >2 standard deviations below the general population, i.e. <70 on a recognised IQ test.

Manual of Dietetic Practice, Fifth Edition. Edited by Joan Gandy.
© 2014 The British Dietetic Association. Published 2014 by John Wiley & Sons, Ltd.
Companion Website: www.manualofdieteticpractice.com

- Deficits in social functioning or adaptive behaviour that significantly impact on how well a person's coping skills allow for everyday social demands that present within their environment.
  - Formal psychological assessments may include the Vineland Adaptive Behaviour Scales and the AAMR Adaptive Behaviour Scales.
- Are present before 18 years and are life long.

There will be local variations of this definition and it must be remembered that the use of IQ alone is not sufficient to define this population (Health Inspectorate Wales, 2007).

All children and adults with profound and multiple learning disabilities (PMLDs) need high levels of support with most aspects of daily life. They are among the most marginalised people in society, have some of the highest support needs and are the most reliant on services (Pawlyn & Carnaby, 2009). People with PMLDs:

- Have more than one disability.
- Have a profound learning disability.
- Have great difficulty communicating.
- May have additional sensory or physical disabilities, complex health needs or mental health difficulties.
- May have behaviours that are challenging.

All people with a LD have an expectation and a right to access core services as well as specialist LD teams [Scottish Executive, 2000; Learning Disabilities Advisory Group (LDAG), 2001; Bamford, 2005; Department of Health, 2007; 2009b]. Whether living at home, with parents, in supported or assisted accommodation or residential setting, appropriate support should be available from specialist teams that help clients live an ordinary life

within their local community. The division of what is considered core or specialist is not (or indeed should not be) clear cut, and robust working relationships between teams are essential for the provision of a seamless service for this client group; the dietitian is pivotal to service provision.

People with a LD are more nutritionally vulnerable than the general population for a number of reasons, including:

- Restricted income or poverty.
- Inappropriate or poor living conditions.
- Poor or limited availability in disadvantaged areas.
- Difficulties with travel and transport.
- Social isolation.
- Social exclusion.
- Limited training for healthcare staff about LDs.
- Limited nutritional knowledge of person with a LD and their carers.
- Limited budgeting or cooking skills of person with a LD and their carers.
- Reduced ability to understand and apply health messages, and read or understand food labels.
- Reduced ability or opportunity to make informed choices.
- Dependence on others for eating and drinking.

Physiological anomalies, polypharmacy, diagnostic overshadowing, multiple diagnoses and dysphagia are also common amongst this client group (Department of Health, 2007). Additionally, people with PMLDs are totally dependent on a range of carers, many of whom do not have the knowledge or skills to enable them to provide a well balanced diet for their clients (Melville *et al.*, 2009). Figure 3.7.1 shows the factors to consider when assessing

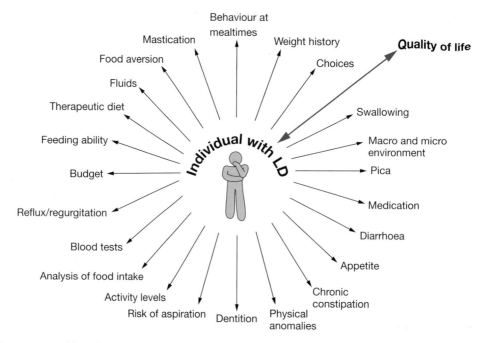

Figure 3.7.1 Factors to consider when assessing nutritional requirements for people with a learning disability (LD) [source: Thomas B, Bishop J (eds). (2007, Fig. 3.12.1, p. 391) *Manual of Dietetic Practice*, 4th edn. Oxford: Blackwell Scientific]

the needs of LD clients; these will also impact on the given intervention.

Capacity to consent

Consent must always be obtained before dietary interventions. When dealing with the general population, consent is customarily obtained verbally; however, for clients with cognitive impairment the issue of capacity to consent needs to be explored fully. In determining capacity to consent, it is essential to involve both clients and carers in the assessment and treatment process, and to communicate openly.

Assessments can be carried out without considering whether the client has the ability to give consent to treatment, but their capacity must be determined if treatment is to be given. Determining capacity to consent must always be time and decision specific. A person should not be viewed as unable to make a decision unless all practicable steps to help them do this have been taken without success. This includes employing alternative forms of communication such as symbolised information or signing. Legislation exists to provide a legal framework for decision making on behalf of adults who lack capacity to make specific decisions. It also provides the means for adults with the capacity to plan ahead in the event of future incapacity. Legislation differs slightly between countries; the relevant legislation for the UK is:

- Scotland – The Adults with Incapacity Act (Scottish Parliament, 2000).
- England and Wales – The Mental Capacity Act (MCA) (Department of Health, 2005).
- Northern Ireland – Seeking Consent [Department of Health, Social Services and Public Safety (DHSSPS), 2003].

Relevant excerpts from the legislation are included here as it is core to the care for a person with a LD. *The Short Reference Guide for Psychologists and Psychiatrists* (British Psychological Society, 2007) is recommended as a brief guide to its implementation for clinicians. This guide is applicable to England and Wales and also reflects the principles underpinning the Scottish Act. The guide includes the following:

- A person must be assumed to have capacity until it is established that they lack capacity.
- A person is not to be treated as unable to make a decision unless all practicable steps to help him or her to do so have been taken without success.
- A person is not to be treated as unable to make a decision merely because they makes an unwise decision.
- When decisions are made on behalf of someone who lacks capacity, they must be made in that person's best interests.
- When decisions are made on behalf of someone who lacks capacity, the less restrictive alternative must be considered to attain the goal specified.

The MCA defines capacity as: an adult can only be considered unable to make a particular decision if:

- They have 'an impairment of, or disturbance in, the functioning of the mind or brain', whether permanent or temporary.

and

- They are unable to undertake any (one or more) of the following steps:
  - Understand the information relevant to the decision.
  - Retain that information (despite use of prompts).
  - Use or weigh that information as part of the process of making the decision.
  - Communicate the decision made (whether by talking, sign language or other means).

A functional approach must be taken so that someone's ability to make a decision is determined by assessing whether they can undertake the steps above; it is not determined by their diagnosis or by the apparent wisdom of their decision. Decision making capacity is decision and time specific.

The functional approach (best interests)

In considering what is in someone's best interests when making a decision, the following should be taken into account:

- Whether and/or when the person is likely to regain capacity and whether the decision or the act to be undertaken can wait.
- How to encourage and optimise the participation of the person in the decision.
- Past and present wishes, feelings, beliefs and values of the person and any other relevant factors.
- Views of other relevant health, family, carer and social representatives. The decision should be perceived to be in the best interest of the client and not that of the family or carers.

When a person lacks the capacity to make decisions and has no family or friends, there is a duty to appoint an Independent Mental Capacity Advocate (IMCA) to help inform the determination of best interests. The dietitian should consult with paid and unpaid carers, and the client's general practitioner (GP) to determine if a dietetic treatment specific or overarching certificate of incapacity has been completed. The latter has generally been put in place for people with PMLDs, as many have permanent cognitive impairment. In some instances the client may have an advocate. It is also recommended that relevant professionals, whose core skills include assessment for capacity, from the specialist community learning disabilities team (CLDT) are approached, e.g. speech and language therapist (SLT), clinical psychologist, psychiatrist, LD community nurse and care manager. In many cases the issue of capacity is generally decided by multidisciplinary working.

If a client does not have capacity to consent, then whether the carer, relative or social worker has legal guardianship or power of attorney, which entitles them to consent on specific issues on behalf of the client, should be considered. In Scotland a welfare guardian may be appointed, who may be granted full or partial powers under the act (Scottish Executive, 2000). If there is no welfare guardian, the GP, in consultation with the team, may complete an Adults with Incapacity form, which enables treatments to take place. In emergency situations the doctor can act without consultation of the team. In Northern Ireland, those close to the incapacitated individual should be involved in the decision making process (DHSSPS, 2003). In instances where there is no legal guardian, the decision should be reached with consultation of all health, family, carer and social representatives. Convening of a multidisciplinary or multiagency meeting is good practice to allow all to participate in decision making; this must be documented as well as any decisions made. The key documents for carers on the issue of consent are:

- *Scotland* – Caring and consent: information for carers (NHS Scotland, 2009).
- *England and Wales*:
  - Making Decisions: A guide for family, friends and other unpaid carers (Department for Constitutional Affairs, 2005a).
  - Making Decisions: A guide for people who work in health and social care (Department for Constitutional Affairs, 2005b).
- *Northern Ireland* – Seeking Consent: Working with people with learning disabilities (DHSSPS, 2003).

Role of advocacy

An advocate enables clients to get their views across and may be a friend, family member or independently appointed representative following a referral to an advocacy group, service or statute. Anyone can advocate on behalf of an individual, but emotional involvement with the client may make impartiality impossible. The advocate should contribute to the decision making process on the client's behalf. Where conflict occurs it should be remembered that their views, whilst listened to, have no legal status in relation to consent. In some cases their views may conflict with others who are involved in the decision making process. As the client's representative, they should be included in client specific multidisciplinary or agency meetings to discuss what is perceived to be in the client's best interests.

In England and Wales statutory Independent Mental Capacity Advocates (IMCAs) undergo formal training as stipulated by legislation (Department of Health, 2005) to enable them to assist with decision making in the best interests of clients who cannot make decisions by themselves or who have no family or friends. In Scotland a Mental Health Officer may be involved in this decision making process. In Northern Ireland family and carers involved with a particular client meet with the relevant health and social care professionals to act in the client's best interests.

Ethical issues

It is essential that any concerns raised about the ethical approach of managing a nutritional intervention in any adult with a LD should be discussed fully at a multidisciplinary/agency meeting. Where appropriate this should include key family members and an advocate to ensure that all are working in a consistent manner to meet the 'best interests' of the client at all times. All discussions and decisions must be fully documented.

Specific health needs of people with learning disabilities

Clinical syndromes associated with LDs include Down's syndrome and Prader–Willi syndrome.

Down's syndrome

Down's syndrome, also known as trisomy 21, is the most widely recognised chromosomal disorder and most common genetic cause of LD. The incidence is approximately 1 in 600–1000 live births with increasing prevalence rates due to increased life expectancy as the result of advancing medical knowledge and improving care. In addition, later pregnancies are increasingly common and the incidence of Down's syndrome rises with increasing maternal age. There are significant differences between various racial and social groups (Shin *et al.*, 2009).

Approximately 12% of neonates with Down's syndrome display congenital gastrointestinal anomalies, which require immediate surgical intervention to facilitate nutrition. Congenital heart disease occurs in approximately 40% of infants and may cause faltering growth. Following surgical repair of heart defects, these children's nutritional status will improve. Hypotonia (poor muscle tone) together with a small oral cavity, enlarged tongue and poor suck reflex can lead to initial feeding difficulties and delayed weaning (see Chapter 3.8.21).

Thyroid dysfunction is more common in people with Down's syndrome, with the incidence increasing with age. Hypothyroidism is most frequently reported but hyperthyroidism can also occur. Thyroid function should be checked every 2 years throughout life (Levy *et al.*, 2006). Obesity is common, but not inevitable, especially among the female population (Melville *et al.*, 2005). Growth retardation, short stature, hypotonia and a low resting metabolic rate (RMR) may all contribute to the problem. Other factors include poor eating behaviour, excessive energy intake and low exercise levels. Individuals should therefore be encouraged to follow healthy eating guidelines and participate in regular physical activity. People with Down's syndrome have an increased incidence of developing type 1 and type 2 diabetes and coeliac disease (Cohen, 2006). Diarrhoea, constipation, abdominal bloating, dyspepsia, mouth ulceration, mood change, arthritis, general fatigue and mild anaemia are common in Down's syndrome.

Nutritional management

Children and adults with Down's syndrome need the same range of nutrients as the general population. Energy intake estimates based on age groups are not appropriate in Down's syndrome and need to be tailored to height, weight and physical activity (Murray & Ryan-Krause, 2010). Growth charts specifically for Down's syndrome have been developed; standard charts are inappropriate due to developmental delay (Down's Syndrome Medical Interest Group, 2000).

Individuals have been found to be at greater risk of reduced bone mineral density as they age, possibly as a consequence of their small stature and sedentary lifestyle (Center *et al*., 1998). For this reason a healthy balanced diet rich in calcium containing foods, regular weight bearing activity and a safe level of sunshine exposure in the summer months is recommended.

Dental anomalies include changes in tooth structure, reduced total number of teeth and delayed or abnormal eruption, as well as the physical abnormalities of the facial appearance and oral cavity, can impact on feeding. Dental disease is common because teeth are more at risk of wear through bruxism (teeth grinding) and decay due to enamel fragility. In addition, gingivitis (gum disease) and oral infections due to mouth breathing can lead to tooth loss and looseness (Hennequin *et al*., 1999). A healthy balanced diet that avoids snacks and fizzy drinks can help preserve teeth.

Problems relating to premature ageing with Alzheimer-like changes in the brain have become more apparent as people with Down's syndrome are living longer. Between the ages of 40 and 50 years some individuals display a rapid deterioration in cognitive function. Possible explanations for this are being linked to the extra genetic material on chromosome 21. Low levels of vitamin E have been found to be associated with dementia in individuals with Down's syndrome, but more research is required into the possible effects of supplementation. In order to increase antioxidant intake, a diet rich in fruit, vegetables and oily fish is recommended. Features of rapid ageing in Down's syndrome include weight loss, reduction in appetite and problems with chewing and swallowing (Lazenby, 2008). If Alzheimer-like symptoms develop, it is important that steps are taken to ensure adequate nutrition and hydration (see Chapter 7.10.2). An individual may lose interest in food, forget to eat or may no longer recognise food or feeding utensils. The following points may help maximise food intake:

- Give assistance with feeding where appropriate but maintain independence for as long as possible.
- Give small frequent meals and snacks.
- Offer food that the individual is familiar with; items should be appetising and of appropriate consistency.
- Offer dessert later rather than present it with the main course, as many will reject savoury foods in preference for sweet items.
- Avoid external distractions and maintain a peaceful quiet environment at meal times.
- Avoid food that is too hot or too cold.

- Do not fill cups, beakers or plates to capacity to avoid spillage.
- Use food fortification for extra nutrition.

Most people with Down's syndrome live in the community, some with parents or carers, but adults often live independently or semi independently and many are able to learn about healthy eating and manage their own diet. A dietitian's role is likely to encompass not only individual assessment but also teaching and educating people with Down's syndrome as well as their parents, carers and other professionals.

Prader–Willi syndrome

Prader–Willi syndrome (PWS) is a relatively rare genetically determined neurodevelopment spectrum disorder with symptoms varying in severity and occurrence. It is believed to be caused by dysfunction of the hypothalamus, which controls bodily functions including hunger and satiety, temperature and pain regulation, fluid balance, puberty, emotions and fertility (van Mil *et al*., 2000a; Whittington *et al*., 2001; Vogels *et al*., 2004; Lindmark *et al*., 2010). It occurs in approximately 1 in 22 000 births, affecting males and females with equal frequency and all races and ethnicities (Prader-Willi Syndrome Association UK, 2010b). This genetic abnormality involves the absence of expression of one or more genes on chromosome 15 and definitive diagnosis is now based on genetic testing. Clients present with mild to severe LD; verbal skills are often better than functional skills. Obsessional characteristics include food related hoarding, ritualistic behaviour and an insatiable appetite, which drives the client to seek food (and sometimes fluids) and means they never feel full even after a large meal. This leads to severe hyperphagia (overeating), which is driven by a physiological abnormality and is highly resistant to motivational change. Prader–Willi syndrome is recognised as the most common genetic cause of life threatening obesity. Physical characteristics in PWS include:

- Short stature.
- Obesity.
- High vomiting threshold, possibly due to poor muscle tone.
- High pain threshold.
- Poor temperature control – erratic behaviour may occur during very cold or very hot weather.
- Decreased motor skills, hypotonia and poor balance.
- Bowel irregularities.
- Dental abnormalities.
- Abnormally thick and sticky saliva, especially in children.

The approach required in PWS is unique and requires close involvement of the multidisciplinary team (MDT). To work effectively with the client, clear boundaries are required, and due to the nature of the syndrome and the inability to self regulate, external management of the eating disorder is mandatory. The ethics of this situation have been fully explored in an application submitted for guardianship within the Adults with Incapacity Act (Scotland), to ensure protection of the client (Healy, 2005). Long term structures and routines in relation to food and behaviours are essential for effective management. This can be seen to be in conflict with the prevailing health and social care ethic, which favours individual choice and decision making, but too much choice in particular situations can be counterproductive and may result in adverse outcomes. People with PWS can usually cope with a choice of two food or drink items at one time; more will lead to uncertainty and heightened anxiety, hampering not only decision making but also general behaviour, and is not recommended. People with PWS do not like sudden change or new experiences; therefore, incremental changes should be made to routines to allow adjustment and acceptance to take place. In order to establish and maintain a successful clinical relationship, the practitioner must give the client:

- Clear expectations and messages: leave no room for misinterpretation.
- Consistent routine and structure that must be followed by everyone.
- Specific feedback.
- Positive reinforcement to help establish new behaviours.
- Avoid confrontation, use eye contact and a gentle manner and wherever possible include the client in decision making.

Medications include growth hormone, which aims to improve growth velocity, and increase lean mass and physical function and ability (van Mil *et al.*, 2001; Haaq *et al.*, 2003; Carrel *et al.*, 2004) and appetite suppressants. However, there is no published evidence that demonstrates their effectiveness.

Nutritional management

The obesity associated with PWS is the result of a chronic imbalance between energy intake (due to hyperphagia) and reduced energy expenditure (due to decreased physical activity as a result of hypotonia and reduced metabolic rate). Individuals have a high ratio of body fat to fat free mass (FFM), where body fat can account for up to 50% of body weight (Butler *et al.*, 2007). Where the appropriate height to weight ratio is satisfactory, body fat can account for up to 40% (Schoeller *et al.*, 1988). As metabolic rate is related to FFM these abnormally high levels of fat result in significantly reduced metabolic rate and therefore energy requirements. Dietitians must structure weight reducing plans reflecting this.

Predictive formulae for estimating basal metabolic rate (BMR) in the general adult population have been shown to overestimate BMR in some populations (Ramirez-Zea, 2005; O'Riordan *et al.*, 2010) and this is further distorted in adults with PWS. Additionally, the standard approach to calculating requirements by subtracting 400–1000 kcal for a decrease in energy stores will not necessarily be effective in PWS. Research suggests that energy requirements in adults with PWS are up to 50% less than those of healthy age matched controls (Schoeller *et al.*, 1988;

Table 3.7.1 Height based energy prescription for Prader–Willi clients aged >16 years [from Hoffman *et al.* (1992)]

Outcome to be achieved	Energy/cm height
Weight loss	7–8 kcal (29–33 kJ)
Weight maintenance	10–14 kcal (42–59 kJ)

van Mil *et al.*, 2000a; Butler *et al.*, 2007). A height based energy prescription for adults with PWS is a practicable guide, as shown in Table 3.7.1. In predicting the energy requirements from BMR equations, the energy expenditure of physical activity should also be considered. The underdevelopment of muscle and any excess weight limits physical activity. One study in children and adolescents reported a mean physical activity level (PAL) of 1.33 (van Mil *et al.*, 2000b). This is significantly lower than that for obese controls and lower than the PAL of 1.4 previously used in calculating estimated average requirements (EAR) for energy in the UK population (Department of Health, 1991).

Predictive energy equations should be used with extreme caution in people with PWS. The recommended energy intake for adults with PWS is around 800–1200 kcal/day, reducing to 800–1000 kcal/day for weight loss (Heinemann, 2010; International Prader-Willi Association, 2010; Prader-Willi Syndrome Association, 2010a,b). At these levels of energy the diet should be planned using low energy, nutrient dense foods to ensure optimal vitamin and mineral intake (Lindmark *et al.*, 2010). As osteoporosis and low bone mineral density are common in PWS, calcium and vitamin D supplementation should be considered (van Mil *et al.*, 2001).

Adherence to dietary regimens may present many challenges. The dietitian should work closely with the MDT, client and carers to overcome obstacles; this may involve the training of all staff in the management strategies that are required to support PWS clients. All involved must adhere strictly to the prescribed diet, agreed structures and routines, which are required for life and cannot be relaxed even when weight is being maintained.

Clear straightforward language is required and the judicious use of terminology, e.g. *free fluids* will be understood literally by the client and may result in fluid intoxication. If food seeking/stealing behaviour is an issue, the team should work together to seek resolutions. Sanctions may be appropriate but at no time should blame be directed towards the client. The need for rules and routines is inherent in this syndrome (Holland *et al.*, 2003) and can be used advantageously in positive reinforcement of healthy eating behaviours and regular exercise plans.

Clients with PWS have particular difficulties with short term memory and processing spoken information, and tend to display rigid thinking. Forward planning for all changes in routine is therefore an essential component to minimise anxiety and associated challenging behaviour. The dietitian plays a pivotal role when working with these clients as they have the knowledge and skills necessary to guide the management of this disorder.

Other syndromes that cause learning disabilities and their nutritional consequences are shown in Table 3.7.2.

Conditions associated with learning disabilities

Autism

Autism is a spectrum of lifelong neurodevelopmental disorders with onset noted in early childhood (see Autism in Chapter 3.8.6). Social and communication skills are affected and there is often, but not always, some degree of LD. The spectrum ranges from those who are high functioning (often referred to as Asperger's) to people who are severely disabled. The term autism spectrum disorder (ASD) is widely accepted though more recently autistic spectrum condition is used. A triad of impairments – social interaction, social communication and imagination – is used to describe the difficulties that people with autism experience to varying degrees (National Autistic Society, 2011). The prevalence is 5 in 1000 births (Baird et al., 2003), with boys four times more likely to be affected than girls. In the majority of cases causation is unknown. Characteristics include obsessive desire for order, rigid thinking, inflexibility, reliance on routines, ritualistic behaviour, poor social skills, and visual and sensory perception difficulties. Common comorbidities include attention deficit hyperactivity disorder (ADHD), food compulsions, food restrictions and gastrointestinal problems. A structured environment, clear boundaries, and rules and routines are essential components to minimise stress. Changes that can be made occur slowly and over a lengthy period.

Nutritional management

Many children with ASD show selective eating and therefore self limiting diets as a direct result of their disorder (Schreck et al., 2004; Williams et al., 2005). This established eating pattern continues into adulthood and may compromise nutritional status, as the individual may be extremely obsessive, selective and restrictive in food choices. Any alterations in the environment or routine may result in behavioural outbursts or food refusal. Gastrointestinal problems may also affect appetite (Williams et al., 2000; Levy et al., 2007a). This is a complex condition that often requires a coordinated multidisciplinary team/agency approach. The following professionals may be involved in the community team:

- Behavioural therapist.
- Clinical psychologist.
- Community nurse.
- Consultant psychiatrist.
- Dietitian.
- Occupational therapist.
- Physiotherapist.
- Social worker/care manager.
- Speech and language therapist – communication.
- Speech and language therapist – dysphagia.

Detailed nutritional assessment by a specialist dietitian should take place for clients who eat fewer than 20 different foods (Isherwood et al., 2011). The dietitian will work closely with the team, advising on any nutritional deficiencies, providing the evidence base for any dietary modifications and offering practical advice as to how any deficiencies can be treated or how dietary modifications can be implemented. Common feeding concerns include:

- Difficulty with transition to textures (especially during infancy).
- Increased sensory sensitivity (including oral).
- Difficulty accepting new foods.
- Restricted intake due to colour, texture, packaging and food temperature.
- Decreased selection of food over time.
- Difficulty with changes in meal time environment, e.g. school versus home.
- Difficulty with meal time presentation, e.g. specific plate and cutlery, positioning of food on a plate.
- Continually eating rather than having set meal times.

A large number of therapeutic approaches have been developed, such as introducing gluten and/or casein free diets (Elder et al., 2006; Wong & Smith, 2006). Anecdotal reports suggest that these may be beneficial in some cases and many parents and carers strongly believe in their effectiveness. There is limited robust evidence to support gluten or casein free diets (Knivsberg et al., 2002). A Cochrane systematic review highlighted the need for robust studies, suitably powered to ascertain the success or otherwise of any dietary modifications (Millward et al., 2008). The British Dietetic Association (BDA) has produced a professional consensus statement on dietary management of ASD (Isherwood et al., 2011).

Cerebral palsy

Cerebral palsy (CP) is the most common physical disability in children and affects 2–2.5 in 1000 births in the UK (Roebroeck & Stam, 2006) and 3.6 in 1000 births in the USA (Yeargin-Allsop et al., 2008). Known possible causes include oxygen starvation, cerebral bleeding and abnormal brain development. Impairment to the immature brain, which can occur before, during or after birth, affects movement, posture and coordination. Depending upon the severity of the underlying condition, CP may not become obvious until early childhood. It is a wide ranging condition and can affect people in many different ways; it is not a LD, though many people with CP also have a LD.

Cerebral palsy is not progressive though some of the effects on the body may become more noticeable and function may deteriorate with age. There are three types of cerebral palsy; spastic, dyskinetic (also known as athetoid or dystonic) and ataxic, and these generally relate to which part of the brain has been affected. The effects vary enormously from one person to another and it is common for an individual to have a combination of two or more types. Some may have this condition so mildly that its effects are barely noticeable, whilst others

Table 3.7.2 Nutritional consequences of other clinical syndromes associated with a learning disability [adapted from Burton et al. (2009)]

Syndrome	Symptoms affecting nutritional status	Nutritional consequences	Issues
Cornelia de Lange syndrome Chromosome 5 abnormality X chromosome and chromosome 10 responsible for milder form	Low birth weight, delayed growth and stature, developmental delay, cleft palate, gaseous distension. May exhibit autistic-like behaviours including self injury	Intermittent poor appetite, vomiting, constipation. GORD. Nutrition intake may be variable as many behaviours are cyclical	MDT approach required. May require a set of nutrition care plans depending on behaviour and ability to eat and drink
Fragile X syndrome Inhibited mental development, moderate to severe learning disability. Autistic-like behaviour with physical and behavioural features and delayed speech	Need very structured environment, obsessive desire for order and familiarity, poor social skills, rigid thinking, inflexible, cannot cope with change, easily distracted from eating, changed visual perceptions	Nutrition intake may be poor and is dependent on degree of food related obsessive behaviour. Need a stable macro- (competent staff, pleasant, calm surroundings – no TV or music to detract from meal times) and micro-environment (correct seating, utensils, adherence to eating and drinking guidelines, time)	MDT approach required. May require a set of nutrition care plans depending on behaviour and ability to eat and drink
Klinefelter's syndrome Affects males with extra X chromosome. Incidence 1 in 1000 males, 1 in 500 have the extra X syndrome without symptoms of the syndrome	Reduced muscle power and stamina. NB: most will have a specific learning difficulty though some may have a degree of learning disability	Prone to depression, thyroid disease, diabetes, osteoporosis, asthma and heart disease	Difficult to feed, get tired easily. Carers need to be patient and persevere with feeding
Rett syndrome Neurodevelopmental disorder characterised by microcephaly, developmental delay, scoliosis, loss of purposeful use of hands, hand flapping, poor muscle tone, gastric abnormalities, seizures and a degree of learning disability. Occurs almost exclusively in girls	Problems with the mechanics of eating. Breathing issues, e.g. hyperventilation and breath holding. Biting, chewing, swallowing and self feeding are all affected by very poor muscle tone	Babies have a poor suck reflex and difficulty meeting their requirements, leading to faltering growth. Breathing irregularities interrupt feeding. Nutritional intake is an issue from birth	Hypotonia with poor food intakes necessitate texture modification of food and thickened drinks. Difficulties in independent eating as a result of poor hand movements – need to be fed. Constipation is very common due to a low intake of fibre and difficulty meeting fluid requirements; may be reduced gut motility
Smith Magenis syndrome Genetic condition characterised by delayed speech, distinctive facial features, sleep disturbances and behavioural problems, especially self injurious behaviour. Individuals tend to be of short stature and may have scoliosis.	Dental agenesis and protruding lower jaw can lead to problems with chewing and ability to manage textures. Feeding difficulties in infancy due to hypotonia causing poor suck reflex and faltering growth. There is also evidence of oral sensory motor dysfunction and GORD. Many become overweight in teens through to adulthood	Poor oral intake, faltering growth, reluctance to progress to more solid textures. Dental problems can necessitate need for a texture modified diet. Obesity can impact on mobility. Behaviour problems can manifest themselves in limited food choices and reluctance to try new foods	Psychological support for challenging behaviours/self injurious behaviour. A healthy balanced diet and good variety of foods should be encouraged but may need texture modification depending on degree of dental abnormality
Tourette's syndrome Neurological disease of unknown origin characterised by chronic muscular tics and vocal tics, and is socially stigmatising. Often combined with obsessive compulsive behaviour and attention deficit disorder	Need very structured environment. Obsessive desire for order and familiarity, rigid thinking, inflexible, inability to cope with change, easily distracted from eating, changed visual perceptions. Poor social skills	Nutritional intakes are likely to be poor. Many clients will have feeding issues	Psychological aspects affecting food intake. Physical problems affecting eating and feeding
Untreated phenylketonuria (PKU) Autosomal recessive genetic condition resulting from a deficiency in the hepatic enzyme phenylalanine hydroxylase. Hyperphenylalaemia is neurotoxic and the damage is irreversible	If not treated early leads to severe intellectual disabilities. Challenging behaviours include self harm and harm to others, food aversions. Weight disturbances	Challenging behaviours affect food intake. Can present as under- or over-weight	A low phenylalanine diet can improve nutritional status and cognitive abilities in some clients. Acceptability may inhibit continuance and QOL issues need to be addressed before considering implementation of diet. Dietetic management depends on symptoms

GORD, gastro-oesophageal reflux disease; MDT, multidisciplinary team; QOL, quality of life.

may be profoundly affected and require help with many or all aspects of daily life. Many children with CP frequently grow poorly due to the underlying disability, malnutrition, endocrinopathy or poor bone growth (Kuperminc & Stevenson, 2008). Other difficulties and medical conditions that can occur more commonly include:

- Chronic constipation.
- Difficulties in chewing and swallowing, especially with advancing age.
- Epilepsy.
- Gastro-oesophageal reflux disease.
- Learning disability – mild, moderate or severe.
- Oral dysfunction.
- Vomiting due to gut dysmotility and activated emetic reflex.

See Chapter 3.8.7 for further details.

Other nutritional considerations in people with learning disabilities

Key nutritional considerations include obesity, underweight, dysphagia, gastro-oesophageal reflux disease (GORD) and *Helicobacter pylori* infection.

Obesity

People with mild LD are more likely to become obese than people with more severe LD (RCN, 2006; Melville *et al.*, 2008). Evidence indicates that people with a LD tend to become overweight at an earlier age and stay overweight, whereas the general population tends to become more overweight with age (Bhaumik *et al.*, 2008; Gale *et al.*, 2009). There are many factors that predispose people with a LD to developing obesity (Jeffreys, 2000; Beart *et al.*, 2001; Draheim *et al.*, 2002; Illingworth *et al.*, 2003; Frey, 2004; Chapman *et al.*, 2005; Frey *et al.*, 2005; Hawkins & Look, 2006; Henderson *et al.*, 2007; Peterson *et al.*, 2008), including:

- Attitudes of carers.
- Boredom.
- Communication difficulties.
- Hypothyroidism.
- Lack of knowledge.
- Lack of skills including literacy.
- Lack of power/control over own life.
- Limited access to exercise.
- Low income.
- Medication (see Table 3.7.3).
- Thyroid disease in Down's syndrome.
- Mental Illness.
- Misuse of food as rewards or motivators to engage in activities.
- Provision of poor diet.
- Poor self esteem.
- Sedentary lifestyle.
- Altered body composition leading to lower BMR.

Table 3.7.3 Weight gain associated with commonly prescribed drugs in learning disabilities (adapted from Leslie *et al.* 2007. Reproduced with permission of Oxford University Press)

Drug	Indicative condition	Weight change (kg)
Sodium valproate	Bipolar/epilepsy	+1.2–5.8
Lithium	Bipolar/depression	+4.0
Clozapine	Schizophrenia	+4.2–9.9
Olanzapine	Schizophrenia	+2.8–7.1
Risperidone	Psychoses	+2.1–2.3
Ziprasidone	Schizophrenia	−2.7–3.2
Prednisolone	Muscle relaxant	+2
Nortriptyline	Depression	+3.7
Doxepin	Depression	+2.7
Amitriptyline	Depression	+1.7

Levels of obesity are less prevalent in adults with PMLDs but can occur. Sometimes weight maintenance may be the best outcome, ensuring that the intake is nutritionally sound, which in itself confers positive benefits such as relief from constipation, better mood and generally feeling better. The impact of medications should not be overlooked as antipsychotic and antidepressant medications may induce undesired and rapid weight gain (Birt, 2003; Khazaal, *et al.*, 2006; Burton *et al.*, 2009), as shown in Table 3.7.3. Weight gains of 14 kg in 1 year have been reported (Leslie *et al.*, 2007).

Abdominal obesity can occur if energy requirements are overestimated during gastrostomy feeding. It is important to note that energy requirements for these individuals are often lower than for the general population of comparable weight and height (Fairclough *et al.*, 2008). People with a LD are often dependent on others for menu planning, shopping and cooking. Frequently, carers have little knowledge about healthy eating themselves, and many myths about nutrition get passed on and become part of custom and practice in the care setting. The role of the carers in the prevention of obesity and other lifestyle conditions as well as in any intervention strategies should not be overlooked. Their own food beliefs, eating experiences and behaviours are imparted to the client, which places an interesting perspective on client choice (Smyth & Bell, 2006).

There is little evidence describing effective weight loss interventions, whether designed for general use and adapted for people with a LD, or targeted specifically for people with a LD. Evidence that people with a LD who are more independent are more likely to be obese (Levy *et al.*, 2006) is contradicted by other studies that suggest those living in supported accommodation are more likely to be overweight or obese (Moore *et al.*, 2004). Also, another study by Levy *et al.* (2007b) found that those living with their family are more likely to be obese. It would seem reasonable therefore that in all settings any weight loss intervention must include support and motivation from carers (Hamilton *et al.*, 2007).

In addition, as a means of preventing obesity, or limiting any further increases in weight, all paid carers should have mandatory induction training regarding implementing healthy lifestyle choices as a routine duty of care (Melville *et al.*, 2009). Training programmes on nutrition under the umbrella of health and social care are becoming more available throughout the UK. Though conventional weight maintenance regimens emphasise a high fibre and high fluid intake, this is of critical importance in this client group as some clients have difficulties consuming sufficient fluid. Therefore encouraging higher intakes of fruit and vegetables, with their naturally high fluid content, may be the preferred option rather than promoting too much insoluble fibre in the form of wholegrain foods.

In a clinic session standard preappointment processes may need to be adapted; it may be more effective and efficient to telephone the client and/or carer to make the appointment. Also, it should be considered if the appointment needs to be at the beginning or end of a clinic session, to help reduce the client's anxiety levels. Partial booking and similar procedures can be confusing, but if contact by telephone is not feasible, a minimum of (straightforward) words should be used in the appointment letter. To aid attendance, the client/carer should be telephoned and reminded on the working day before the appointment. When consulting in a one to one setting it is essential to consider the points shown in Box 3.7.1.

There is some consensus that group sessions for clients and carers are effective (Marshall *et al.*, 2003), as are those that incorporate increased physical activity (Chapman *et al.*, 2008). Mainstream weight loss group interventions can be accessed with support from carers. It is important that the carers reiterate the key messages and make sure the client feels part of the group. The information will also need to be in an accessible format to aid understanding and compliance. Box 3.7.2 gives recommendations when consulting in a group setting.

Monitoring

Regular monitoring is essential for clients with a LD to sustain motivation. Carers should follow the monitoring protocol as advised by the dietitian, which may include weight checks, food and fluid charts, and menu structure. Ongoing dietetic review is not necessary, though some adjustments to the timeline in any local pathways should be considered, as the first appointment may be introductory. Once the key messages have been understood by the client and carer, and actions and targets agreed, further dietetic reviews may be undertaken at the dietitian's discretion but with discharge, not ongoing care, in mind.

Practical monitoring issues

It is more practical to check weight using stand-on scales, but for those with poor mobility or balance problems, seated or hoist scales may be necessary. Wheelchair beam or platform scales are available. Changes to the wheelchair will mean that the chair will have to be reweighed. In cases where it is not feasible to weigh a client, global assessment taking into account fit of clothes and jewellery can be used as indicators of weight change (Burton *et al.*, 2009).

It will be more difficult to measure an accurate height for clients with physical anomalies such as kyphosis or scoliosis. Alternative or surrogate markers of height, e.g. ulna length, knee height and supine length, have been found to be inferior to self or carer reported height if available (BAPEN, 2003).

Body mass index (BMI) must be treated with caution where an individual has altered body composition as it does not assess fat distribution (SIGN, 2010). Clients with PMLDs are more likely to have muscle wasting of their extremities and greater visceral adiposity, and thus a greater risk of coronary heart disease (CHD) and respiratory problems (Draheim, 2006). Mid upper arm circumference (MUAC) and triceps skin fold (TSF) measurements may be inappropriate (Fairclough *et al.*, 2008) for similar reasons. Targets for BMI in clients with PMLDs should be set at the lower end of the normal range. Achieving a weight loss of between 5% and 10% would be a more appropriate, realistic and achievable goal, irrespective of the degree of obesity, and would confer positive health gains for the individual (SIGN, 2010; DOM UK, 2007; NICE, 2006) (see Chapter 7.13.2). The BDA professional consensus statement on weight management for adults with a LD living in the community gives more detailed advice on managing this client group (Burton *et al.*, 2011).

Underweight

Polarisation of weight is common within the LD, with the incidence of underweight ranging from 14% to 75% depending on the severity of the LD (Gravestock, 2000; Emerson, 2005). It is not uncommon for severe undernutrition to go unrecognised by support staff and family members, particularly when it has been longstanding (Crawley, 2007). Underweight is more common in people who are immobile, and unable to feed themselves or tolerate solid foods, or exhibit regurgitation, rumination or chronic vomiting.

For more detailed information, refer to the BDA Professional Consensus Statements on the nutritional care of adults with a LD in care settings (DiMascio *et al.*, 2012) and home enteral tube feeding for adults with a LD (Fairclough *et al.*, 2008) (see Chapter 6.2).

Dysphagia

Despite dysphagia being a significant problem in people with a LD, few robust studies have been published. Reported prevalence rates vary from 36% (Hickman, 1997) to 73% (Rogers *et al.*, 1994) in inpatient populations and 5% (Hickman & Jenner, 1997) to 8% in the community (Chadwick & Jolliffe, 2009). The range of signs and symptoms of dysphagia in people with a LD include:

• Coughing during, and for up to an hour after, eating and drinking;

Box 3.7.1 Recommendations for consultations in a one to one setting

- Expect first appointment to focus on getting to know the client and gaining trust
- Collect information on the client's social and family network so you know the key people with whom to liaise, i.e. care manager, social worker, day service, college, respite, sitters, family, other healthcare workers currently involved
- Allow at least 30 minutes per consultation
- Keep distractions to a minimum
- Discourage accompanying person (if any) from answering for the client and where possible encourage them to sit behind the client
- Use straightforward language
- Pace delivery
- Ask open questions using no more than two information carrying words at a time*
- Count to 10 after each question (if needed) to give the client time to reply
- Rephrase questions to make sure the client is not just repeating your last word
- Use visual aids to reinforce the spoken word, such as food models, photographs and symbols
- Limit any areas for change to a maximum of three
- Use symbols or photographs and font 14, Arial, Comic Sans, Univers, Tahoma or Verdana in written communication
- Obtain the client's consent to send copies of recommendations and any supporting information to the care manager for distribution to day services and respite as appropriate
- Wherever possible review with same accompanying person for consistency

---

Box 3.7.2 Recommendations when consulting in a group setting

- Plan first session solely for getting to know the clients and gaining trust
- Limit membership to no more than 10 clients
- Encourage carers to attend, although it is not necessary to exclude any clients who attend without support
- Two people are needed to facilitate each session
- Allow a maximum of 2 hours per session with a break midway
- Keep to one theme per session
- Plan a maximum of six sessions with no more than three key themes for the whole programme
- Keep distractions to a minimum
- Discourage accompanying people from answering for the clients
- Use straightforward language
- Pace the delivery
- Ask open questions using no more than two information carrying words at a time*
- Count to ten after each question to give clients time to reply
- Rephrase questions to make sure the clients are not just repeating the last word
- Ask clients to repeat tasks given to them
- Use visual aids and activities such as food models, photographs and symbols to reinforce points
- Limit any areas for change in individual action plans to a maximum of three
- Use symbols or photographs and font 14, Arial, Comic Sans, Univers, Tahoma or Verdana in written communication
- Make sure that copies of activities, work completed and any supporting information are available in individual take home files or folders for clients to share with carers
- Review

---

*An information carrying word is any word in a sentence that must be understood in order to follow an instruction, e.g. 'Give me the ball'. The person asking holds out their hand, with only a ball in front of them. The addressee does not have to understand any words, because the person has shown them what they want. This statement has no information carrying words. If there were to be a ball and a book and the same question was repeated, the addressee needs to know the difference between ball and book. This has one information carrying word level. Messages can have varying numbers of information carrying words depending on how they are said and what clues are provided. Close liaison with a SLT is recommended.

- Accumulation of saliva.
- Drooling.
- Choking.
- Food aversion.
- Behaviour changes.
- Rushing food.
- Difficulty taking medications.

These signs are often attributed to the learning disability itself and in many cases are not investigated; such diagnostic overshadowing is unfortunately a common occurrence within this population (Leslie *et al.*, 2009). During a routine nutritional assessment the dietitian is in an ideal situation to observe potential signs and symptoms of dysphagia. Insidious onset of symptoms, such as unexpected weight loss, taking longer to eat and drink, becoming increasingly selective with food choices and hypersalivation, can be missed or not seen as important by carers or the clients themselves (Burton *et al.*, 2012).

Amylase resistant thickeners based on guar gum/guar gum starch combinations have been suggested as beneficial for individuals who hypersalivate, although recent research questions this evidence (Hanson *et al.*, 2012). From a pragmatic point of view, the best thickener to use will be that preferred by the consumer. The addition of thickener to fluids may lead to an increase in energy intake, resulting in weight gain, which may or may not be advantageous. The dietitian should consider the implications of the additional energy component that impacts on weight when choosing the type of thickener to use as the energy content of thickeners varies (see Chapter 7.3).

Oral hygiene is of particular importance in those who eat and drink very little or are nil by mouth. Reduced stimulation of the oral environment leads to dry mouth (reduced saliva production), increased risk of infection, ulceration and increased build-up of plaque or calculus (tartar). The build-up of plaque and calculus can lead to dental decay due to the presence of plaque acids, periodontal disease due to plaque toxins and bacteria, and increased risk of aspiration pneumonia (Wales, 2010). Plaque organisms such as *Pseudomonas aeruginosa* and *Klebsiella pneumoniae* are common causal organisms of chest infections (Langmore *et al.*, 1998). Each client will require specific guidelines for oral care based on the vulnerability of their airway, underlying condition and tolerance of routine interventions such as tooth brushing, dental reviews and required treatments. Following risk assessment, oral care plans may include specific proactive and reactive strategies such as positioning for oral care, suitable equipment (e.g. using a small headed multitufted manual toothbrush or small headed powered toothbrush), low foaming toothpaste, need for suction and use of any oral hygiene adjuncts (e.g. prescribed mouthwash). People with a LD who are dependent on others for oral hygiene are at high risk of having poor oral health.

Gastro-oesophageal reflux disease

Gastroesophageal reflux disease (GORD) is a common problem in people with a LD, with there being a higher incidence in those with PMLDs. More than 50% of institutionalised people with a moderate to severe LD in the Netherlands were shown to have GORD (Böhmer *et al.*, 1999). Higher incidences have been noted in specific syndromes such as fragile X and Rett syndrome and in conditions such as CP. People taking antiepileptic medication and those with a history of rumination also display a high incidence of the disease. It is caused by acid from the stomach entering the oesophagus, resulting in heartburn, painful swallowing, vomiting and haematemesis (Crawley, 2007). The pain can be intense and individuals may not be able to describe what is wrong. This may also contribute to sleep disturbance or challenging behaviour. Many cases are missed with a single oesophagoscopy and diagnosis requires 24-hour oesophageal pHmetry, which is difficult in this client group. There is justification, therefore, to treat with proton pump inhibitors without prior endoscopy. Recommendations for the management of GORD in clients with a LD include:

- Small frequent meals.
- Feed client in an upright position – this may be difficult in those with PMLDs and advice should be sought from the physiotherapist about positioning.
- Feed slowly and encourage chewing if possible.
- Maintain the client in an upright position for at least 30 minutes after meals.

These recommendations can also be used to assist in the treatment of regurgitation and rumination, which are more common in people with PMLDs and those with behavioural problems. Carers and other key professionals require education and training to understand the rationale for careful feeding and the consequences of not adhering to guidelines.

Helicobacter pylori infection

Helicobacter pylori infection is endemic among the LD population due to communal living situations, including group homes or shared tenancies, respite homes and attending adult day centres, where individuals are in close social contact (De Schryver *et al.*, 2007; Clarke *et al.*, 2008). Diagnosis is confirmed by a breath test, which detects the presence of urea; however, people with a LD find this procedure difficult so other methods such as serological testing or stool sampling to check for antigens are recommended (Scheepers *et al.*, 2000). Infection is associated with peptic ulceration and pain, and in people with a LD can present as nausea, vomiting, general malaise and challenging behaviours when the individual cannot describe the nature of the problem. In extreme circumstances the first indication of the severity of the problem can be perforation of a gastric ulcer. It has been postulated that the high prevalence of infection with *H. pylori* in people with a LD leads to a higher prevalence of gastric carcinoma. Treatment includes antibiotics and proton pump inhibitors. Following eradication therapy reinfection can occur and the incidence of this happening is much higher in people with a LD (Wallace *et al.*, 2002).

Other factors to consider when working with clients with learning disabilities

Medication

The impact of medication is often overlooked despite clients with a LD being prescribed a large number of medications to control mood, behaviour and epilepsy on a daily basis as well as required (*pro nata*; also known as rescue medication). Some medications, e.g. anticonvulsants and osmotic laxatives, have a direct impact on nutrient absorption. Neuroleptics (antipsychotics) cause pharyngeal weakness and dystonia, whilst some of the tricyclic antidepressants, e.g. amitriptyline, reduce saliva production resulting in xerostomia (dry mouth). Medication reviews are important to discuss the impact of new drugs as well as the continued combination of current medications. Medication side effects also include chronic constipation, a frequent problem for people with a LD, which increases the risk of seizure activity. Other medications frequently prescribed for clients with a LD that can impact on nutritional status are shown in Table 3.7.4.

Carers

Many carers will have the skills and knowledge to promote good eating habits and should be encouraged to share good practices with their care teams. In some circum-

Table 3.7.4 Medications prescribed for clients with learning disabilities that impact on nutritional status [adapted from Burton *et al.* (2009)]

Medication	Nutrition related side effects
Antipsychotics, e.g. risperidone, aripiprazole	Drowsiness, apathy, confusion, depression Gastrointestinal disturbances, dry mouth, weight gain
Anticonvulsants/antiepileptics, e.g. topiramate, phenytoin	Nausea, vomiting, constipation, diarrhoea, abdominal pain, oedema, appetite changes, confusion, weight gain, dry mouth, weight loss
Antidepressants: Tricyclics, amitriptyline	Loss of appetite, constipation, weight gain, dry mouth
Monoamine oxidase inhibitors (MAOIs)	As above plus strict adherence to special diet as certain foods need to be avoided
Selective serotonin reuptake inhibitors (SSRIs), e.g. fluoxetine	Taste disturbance, increased salivation, rhinitis, changes in blood sugars
Anxiolytics, e.g. diazepam	Salivation changes, constipation, diarrhoea, vomiting
Hypnotics, e.g. temazepam	Drowsiness, confusion, gastric irritation
Antimuscarinics, e.g. hyoscine	Constipation, dry mouth, nausea, vomiting
Mood stabilisers, e.g. lithium	Weight gain, excessive thirst, oedema
Laxatives: Bulk forming, e.g. methyl cellulose	Flatulence, abdominal distension, gastrointestinal obstruction or impaction
Stimulant, e.g. senna	Diarrhoea, hypokalaemia
Osmotic, e.g. Movicol, lactulose	Long term use can interfere with the absorption of fat soluble vitamins, flatulence, abdominal discomfort
Thickeners – starch and gum based	Diarrhoea, constipation, weight gain

SECTION 3

stances there may be a need to address specific issues pertaining to carers including:

- Varying levels of interest in food and exercise.
- Little or no experience in planning healthy menus or adapting menus to accommodate texture modification.
- Understanding that their clients do not require the same amount of food as they do and so providing smaller portions is acceptable.
- Bringing their own theories and idiosyncrasies to the meal provision process.
- Perceiving clients as not having fulfilled lives and seeking to redress this in some way using food.
- Using 'it's the client's choice' as an excuse to provide or allow access to less healthy food from either a nutrient or texture aspect.

Paid carers often struggle to define their role, especially when the issue of choice is so far reaching. Some see their role as protecting the client's long term health, and so work hard to ensure healthier choices are made. Others see their role as promoting choice, and as long as they enable their client to make a choice, or their client can be seen to be making choices (healthy or unhealthy), they have fulfilled their role. The issue of human rights is also cited and interpreted as people with capacity having the right to make unhealthy choices. Staff need to remember that they have a duty of care to ensure their client's health needs are met and should endeavour to facilitate informed choices as much as possible. It is important to have an appreciation and understanding of the skills base, values and belief systems of carers and to use this state of reality for training and support. Empowering carers is as important as empowering their clients.

Information

Information needs to be provided in a format that is easily understood, i.e. in an accessible format incorporating a range of techniques, e.g. symbols, photographs, audio-visual and Talking Mats™ (see useful resources). With regard to verbal communication it is important to remember how information is interpreted. Advice may be taken literally or choice may be limited to a suggestion given, e.g. *'you can have an occasional treat like chocolate'*, could be interpreted as chocolate is only a treat. The term occasional is abstract and subjective, and the same could be said for daily or weekly, or even hourly depending on the client's understanding of time. Clients should be asked to say in their own words what they understand from the information they have been given. There should be no temptation to use the fact that the client can repeat what has just been said to them as a measure of understanding, as many people with a LD are quite adept at recalling the words most recently spoken to them; this is known as the recency effect (Kroese *et al.*, 1998).

Bowel function

A standardised way of describing bowel function using the Bristol stool chart is recommended (Lewis & Heaton, 1997). Constipation in particular is a frequent problem and increases the risk of epileptic seizure activity, but it often goes unrecognised by carers because it is normal for the client (Fairclough *et al.*, 2008). Contributing factors are poor gut motility, chronic inadequate fluid and fibre intake, chronic laxative usage, lack of physical activity and medication side effects. When enteral tube feeding is commenced, there is a risk of faecal impaction and vomiting despite adequate nutrition and fluid. In dysphagia, thickeners have been reported to alter client's bowel function (diarrhoea or constipation or both). Bowel function therefore needs to be monitored to prevent complications and colonisation by *H. pylori* should be considered.

Quality of life

Any intervention should consider the four principles of medical ethics, i.e. respect for autonomy, beneficence, non-malfeasance and justice (Beauchamp & Childress, 2004), as well as the issue of consent, which always needs to be obtained for dietetic interventions. When dealing with the general population, consent is customarily obtained verbally. In clients with cognitive impairment, however, the issue about capacity to consent needs to be investigated thoroughly. In determining capacity to consent, it is essential to involve both the individual and carers in the process and ensure frequent and transparent communication (Burton *et al.*, 2011).

It is important to highlight that people with a LD want to be (and should be) seen as equal citizens in their communities and wherever possible would prefer to access the same health services as everyone else (Mencap, 2010). The label 'learning disability' encompasses a wide range of disabilities from mild to profound and it is important to ensure that choice is available for all. Where it is not possible to meet the specific needs of people with a LD through adapting mainstream services, referral to a local specialist community learning disability team (CLDT) can be considered. Whilst it is important to appreciate the limitations and expectations of this client group, standard outcome measures used in dietetic practice may not be appropriate. Realistic outcome measures based on thorough assessment of need, ability and quality of life are essential in order to work effectively with, and for, this client group. If clinical expectations expressed by the professional are not harmonious with the fundamental processes operating within specific genetic syndromes, failure will ensue. It is incumbent on the practitioner to work within the parameters of a specific syndrome such as PWS or conditions associated with the LD such as autism, working towards outcomes that are practicable, achievable and most importantly, meaningful to the client.

It has been recognised for some time that people with a LD can be informative, critical and reliable service users, provided that effective interview methods are employed (Kroese *et al.*, 1998). Closer working partnerships with primary, secondary, tertiary and specialist teams, together with local advocacy groups could make inclusion a realistic objective for safeguarding health improvements for people with a LD.

Further reading

Dodd K, Turk V, Christmas M. (2010) *Down Syndrome & Dementia – A Resource for Carers and Support Staff*, 2nd edn. Teddington: Down's Syndrome Association.
Gates B. (ed) (2003) *Learning Disabilities- Toward Inclusion*, 4th edn. London: Churchill Livingstone.
Pawlyn J, Carnaby S (eds). (2009) *Profound and Multiple Learning Disabilities*. Oxford: Blackwell Publishing.
Thompson J, Pickering S (eds). (2001) *Meeting the Health Needs of People who have a Learning Disability*. Edinburgh: Baillière Tindall.

Internet resources

Abertawe Bro Morgannwg University Health Board   www.wales.nhs.uk/sitesplus/863/page/41509
British Dietetic Association   www.bda.uk.com
   Centre for Education & Development: Franchised course – Introduction to mental health, learning disabilities and eating disorders. Details available at www.bda.uk.com/ced
   Mental Health Group   www.dietitiansmentalhealthgroup.org.uk
   Professional Consensus Statements
      Burton S, McIntosh P, Jurs A, *et al.* (2011) Weight management for adults with a learning disability living in the community.
      DiMascio F, Hamilton K, Smith L. (2012) The nutritional care of adults with a learning disability in care settings
      Fairclough J, Burton S, Craven J, Ditchburn L, Laverty A, Macleod M. (2008) Home enteral tube feeding for adults with a learning disability
      Isherwood E, Thomas K, Spicer B. (2011) Dietary management of autism spectrum disorder.
British Institute of Learning Disabilities   www.bild.org.uk
British Psychological Association   www.bps.org.uk
   Best interest guidance on adults who lack capacity to make decision for themselves (2011)
   Mental Capacity Act (2005) Short reference guide for psychologists and psychiatrists
Bristol community (LD) dietitians   www.briscomhealth.org.uk/bristollearning-difficulties
Caroline Walker Trust   www.cwt.org.uk
   Eating well: children and adults with learning disabilities
Clear Consultancy. For advice & training regarding making information accessible   www.clearforall.co.uk
Color Library Collection – Food. Visual dictionary   www.winslow-cat.com
Easy Health – Health information in an easy to understand format   www.easyhealth.org.uk
Food, Fitness, Fun! Training pack in weight management for people with learning disabilities, (2000) Pavilion Publishing   www.pavpub.com
Mayer-Johnson Special education source materials – symbols   www.mayer-johnson.com
Mencap   www.mencap.org.uk
   Guidelines for accessible writing
   Death by indifference (2007)
   Getting it right: the charter explained (2010)
Nutrition and Diet Resources UK   www.ndr-uk.org
POMONA Health indicators for people with learning disabilities   www.pomonaproject.org
PMLD LINK.A journal which shares good practice in supporting children and adults with profound and multiple learning disabilities (PMLD)   www.pmldlink.org.uk
Royal College of Nursing   www.rcn.org.uk
   Meeting the health needs of people with learning disabilities.
Scottish Intercollegiate Guideline Network   www.sign.ac.uk
   SIGN 98 (2008) – Assessment, diagnosis and clinical interventions
Talking MatsTM Communication framework   www.talkingmats.com

Education programmes for nutrition and learning disabilities

Agored Cymru   www.ocnwales.org.uk
Highfield Publications   www.highfield.co.uk
Royal Environmental Health Institute Scotland   www.rehis.com
Royal Society for Public Health   www.rsph.org.uk
Qualifications and Credit Framework   www.edexcel.com

References

Astor R, Jeffreys K. (2000) *Positive initiatives with people with learning disabilities; promoting healthy lifestyles*. London: Mac-Millan Press Ltd.

Baird G, Cass H, Soonims V. (2003) Diagnosis of autism. *BMJ* 327: 488–493.

Bamford D. (2005) The Bamford Review of Mental Health and Learning Disability (Northern Ireland). Available at www.dhsspsni.gov.uk/index/bamford/steering.htm. Accessed 18 April 2011.

British Association for Parenteral & Enteral Nutrition (BAPEN) (2003) Malnutrition Universal Screening Tool 'MUST' Report. Malnutrition Advisory Group. Available at www.bapen.org.uk/musttoolkit.html. Accessed 26 March 2012.

Beart S, Hawkins D, Stenfert Kroese B, Smithson P, Tolosa I. (2001) Barriers to accessing leisure opportunities for people with learning disabilities. *British Journal of Learning Disabilities* 29: 133–138.

Beauchamp TL, Childress JF. (2004) *Principles of Biomedical Ethics*, 5th edn. Oxford: Oxford University Press.

Bernall C. (2005) Maintenance of oral health in people with learning disabilities. *Nursing Times* 101: 40–42.

Bhaumik S, Watson LM, Thorpe CF, Tyrer F, McGrother CW. (2008) Body mass index in adults with intellectual disability: distribution, association and service implications: a population based study. *Journal of Intellectual Disability Research* 53: 287–298.

Birt J. (2003) Management of weight gain associated with antipsychotics. *Annals of Clinical Psychiatry* 15: 49–57.

British Psychological Society. (2007) Mental Capacity Act Short Reference Guide. Available at www.bps.org.uk. Accessed 18 April 2011.

Böhmer CJ, Niezen-de Boer MC, Klinkenberg-Knol EC, Deville WL, Nadorp JH, Meuwissen SG. (1999) The prevalence of gastro-esophageal reflux disease in institutionalized intellectually disabled individuals. *American Journal of Gastroenterology* 94: 804–810.

Bryan F, Allan T, Russell L. (2000) The move from a long-stay learning disabilities hospital to community homes: a comparison of clients' nutritional status. *Journal of Human Nutrition and Dietetics* 13: 265–270.

Burton S, Cox S, Sandham SM. (2009) Nutrition and Hydration In: Pawlyn J, Carnaby S (eds) *Profound Intellectual and Multiple Disabilities*. Oxford: Blackwell Publishing.

Burton S, McIntosh P, Jurs A, *et al.* (2011) *Weight management for adults with a learning disability living in the community*. Birmingham: BDA.

Burton S, Laverty A, Macleod M. (2012) The dietitian's role in the diagnosis and treatment of dysphagia. In: Ekberg, O. (ed). *Dysphagia, Diagnosis and Treatment*. New York: Springer Verlag.

Butler MG, Theodoro MF, Bittel DC, Donnelly JE. (2007) Energy expenditure and physical activity in Prader-Willi syndrome: comparison with obese subjects. *American Journal of Medical Genetics* 143A: 449–459.

Carnaby S. (2009) Good healthcare for people with profound and multiple learning disabilities: complex means to meeting complex needs. *PMLD Link* 21: 2–4.

Carrel AL, Moerchen V, Myres SE, Bekx T, Whitman BY, Allen DB. (2004) Growth hormone improves mobility and body composition in infants and toddlers with PWS. *Journal of Paediatrics* 145: 744–749.

Center J, Beange H, McElduff A. (1998) People with mental retardation have an increased prevalence of osteoporosis. *American Journal of Mental Retardation* 103: 19–28.

Chadwick DD, Jolliffe J. (2009) A descriptive investigation of dysphagia in adults with intellectual disabilities. *Journal of Intellectual Disability Research* 53: 29–43.

Chapman MJ, Craven MJ, Chadwick DD. (2005) Fighting fit?: An evaluation of health practitioner input to improve healthy living and reduce obesity for adults with learning disabilities. *Journal of Intellectual Disabilities* 9: 131–144.

Chapman MJ, Craven MJ, Chadwick DD. (2008) Following up Fighting fit: The long-term impact of health practitioner input on obesity and BMI amongst adults with intellectual disabilities. *Journal of Intellectual Disabilities* 12: 309–323.

Clarke D, Vemuri M, Gunatilake D, Tewari S. (2008) *Helicobacter pylori* infection in five inpatient units for people with intellectual disability and psychiatric disorder. *Journal of Applied Research in Intellectual Disabilities* 21: 95–98.

Cohen WI. (2006) Current dilemmas in Down syndrome clinical care: celiac disease, thyroid disorders and atlanto-axial instability. *American Journal of Medical Genetics* 142: 141–148.

Crawley H. (2007) *Eating Well: Children and Adults with Learning Disabilities*. Caroline Walker Trust.

De Schryver A, Cornelius K, Van Winckel M, *et al.* (2007) The occupational risk of helicobacter pylori infection among workers in institutions for people with intellectual disability. *Occupational and Environmental Medicine* 65: 587–591.

Department for Constitutional Affairs (2005a) The Mental Capacity Act – A guide for family, friends and unpaid carers. Available at webarchive.nationalarchives.gov.uk/+/http://www.dca.gov.uk/legal-policy/mental-capacity/mibooklets/booklet02.pdf. Accessed 18 April 2011.

Department for Constitutional Affairs (2005b) The Mental Capacity Act – A guide for people who work in health and social care. Available at http://webarchive.nationalarchives.gov.uk/+/http://www.dca.gov.uk/legal-policy/mental-capacity/mibooklets/booklet03.pdf. Accessed 18 April 2011.

Department of Health. (1991) *Dietary Reference Values for Food Energy and Nutrients for the United Kingdom*. Report 41. London: HMSO.

Department of Health. (2004) *Choosing Health – Making Healthy Choices Easier*. London: The Stationery Office.

Department of Health. (2005) Mental Capacity Act 2005: Code of Practice Department of Constitutional Affairs. Available at www.dca.gov.uk. Accessed 18 April 2011.

Department of Health. (2007) *Guidance on Services for People with Learning Disabilities and Challenging Behaviour or Mental Health Needs*. London: Department of Heatlh.

Department of Health (2009a) *Improving the Health and Well Being of People with Learning Disabilities*. London: Department of Health.

Department of Health. (2009b) *Valuing People Now: A New Three Year Strategy for People with Learning Disabilities*. London: Department of Health.

Department of Health, Social Services & Public Health (DHSSPS). (2003) Seeking Consent: Working with people with learning disabilities. Scotland. Available at www.dhsspsni.gov.uk. Accessed 26 March 2012.

DiMascio F, Hamilton K, Smith L. (2012) The nutritional care of adults with a learning disability in care settings. British Dietetic Association. Available at www.bda.uk.com. Accessed 21 March 2012.

Disability Rights Commission. (2006) *Equal Treatment: Closing the Gap*. London: Disability Rights Commission.

Dietitians in Obesity Management (DOM) UK. (2007) *The Dietetic Weight Management Intervention for Adults in the One to One Setting – Is it Time for a Radical Rethink?* Birmingham: BDA.

Draheim CC. (2006) Cardiovascular disease prevalence and risk factors of person with mental retardation. *Mental Retardation and Developmental Disabilities Research Reviews* 12: 3–12.

SECTION 3

Draheim CC, Williams DP, McCubbin JA. (2002) Physical activity, dietary intake and insulin resistance syndrome in non-diabetic adults with mental retardation. *American Journal of Mental Retardation* 105: 361–375.

Down's Syndrome Medical Interest Group. (2000) The UK (2000) Growth charts. Available at www.dsmig.org.uk/publications/growthchart.html. Accessed18 April 2011

Edwards M. (2007) Caring for patients with a learning disability. *Practice Nurse* 17: 38–41.

Elder JH, Shanker M, Shuster J, Theriaque D, Burns S, Sherrill L. (2006) The gluten-free, casein-free diet in autism: Results of a preliminary double blind clinical trial. *Journal of Autism and Develpomental Disorders* 36: 413–420.

Emerson E. (2005) Underweight, obesity and exercise among adults with intellectual disabilities in supported accommodation in Northern England. *Journal of Intellectual Disability Research* 49: 134–143.

Fairclough J, Burton S, Craven J, Ditchburn L, Laverty A, Macleod M. (2008) *Home Enteral Tube Feeding for Adults with a Learning Disability*. Birmingham: BDA.

Frey GC. (2004) Comparison of physical activity levels between adults with and without mental retardation. *Journal of Physical Activity and Health* 1: 235–245.

Frey GC, Buchanan AM, Rosser Sandt DD. (2005 'I'd rather watch TV': An examination of physical activity in adults with mental retardation. *Mental Retardation* 43: 241–254.

Gale L, Naqvi H, Russ L. (2009) Asthma, smoking and BMI in adults with intellectual disabilities: a community-based survey. *Journal of Intellectual Disability Research* 53: 787–796.

Gravestock S. (2000) Review. Eating disorders in adults with intellectual disability. *Journal of Intellectual Disability Research* 44: 625–663.

Haaq AM, Stadler DD, Jackson RH, Rosenfeld RG, Purnell JQ, LaFranchi SH. (2003) Effects of growth hormone on pulmonary function, sleep quality, behaviour, cognition, growth velocity, body composition and resting energy expenditure in PWS. *Journal of Clinical Endocrinology and Metabolism* 88: 2206–2212.

Hamilton S, Hankey CR, Miller S, Boyle S, Melville CA. (2007) A review of weight loss interventions for adults with intellectual disabilities. The International Association for the Study of Obesity. *Obesity Reviews* 8: 339–345.

Hanson B, O'Leary M, Smith C. (2012) The effect of saliva on the viscosity of thickened drinks. *Dysphagia* 27(1): 10–19.

Hawkins A, Look R. (2006) Levels of engagement and barriers to physical activity in a population of adults with learning disabilities. *British Journal of Learning Disabilities* 34: 220–226.

Health Inspectorate Wales. (2007) *How Well Does the NHS in Wales Commission and Provide Specialist Learning Disability Services for Young People and Adults?* Caerphilly: Health Inspectorate Wales.

Healy M. (2005) awi and the person with a mild learning disability: the ethical and legal dilemmas posed. *Newsletter for mental health officers in Scotland* 9: 3–4.

Heinemann J. (2010) Wound healing with Prader-Willi syndrome – how many calories? Available at www.pwsausa.org/syndrome/foodpyramid.htm. Accessed 16 April 2011.

Henderson A, Lynch SA, Wilkinson S, Hunter M. (2007) Adults with Down's syndrome: the prevalence of complications and health care in the community. *British Journal of General Practice* 57, 50–55.

Henderson CM, Robinson LM, Davidson P, Haveman M, Janicki MP, Albertini G. (2008) Overweight status, obesity and risk factors for coronary heart disease in adults with intellectual disability. *Journal of Policy and Practice in Intellectual Disabilities* 5: 174–177.

Hennequin M, Faulks D, Veyrune J-L, Bourdiol P. (1999) Significance of oral health in persons with Down's syndrome: a literature review. *Developmental Medicine & Child Neurology* 41: 275–283.

Hickman J. (1997) ALD and dysphagia: issues and practice. *Speech & Language Therapy in Practice* Autumn: 8–11.

Hickman J, Jenner L. (1997) AWID and dysphagia: issues and practice. *Speech & Language Therapy in Practice* Winter: 8–11.

Hoffman CJ, Aultman D, Pipes P. (1992) A nutrition survey of and recommendations for individuals with PWS who live in group homes. *Journal of the American Dietetic Association* 92: 823–830.

Holland A, Whittington J, Hinton E. (2003) The paradox of Prader-Willi syndrome: a genetic model of starvation. *Lancet* 362: 989–991.

Hove O. (2004) Prevalence of eating disorders in adults with mental retardation living in the community. *American Journal of Mental Retardation* 109: 501–506.

Illingworth K, Moore K, McGillvray J. (2003) The development of the nutrition and activity knowledge scale for use with people with an intellectual disability. *Journal of Applied Research in Intellectual Disabilities* 16: 159–166.

International Prader-Willi Association. (2010) Dietary management. Available at: www.ipwso.org/dietary-management/. Accessed 3 May 2011.

Isherwood E, Thomas K, Spicer B. (2011) *Dietary Management of Autism Spectrum Disorder*. Birmingham: BDA

Ito Jun-ichi. (2006) Brief research report – Obesity and its related health problems in people with intellectual disabilities. *Journal of Policy and Practice in Intellectual Disabilities* 3: 129–132.

Jeffreys K. (2000) Managing and treating obesity in people with learning disability. *Learning Disability Practice* 2: 30–34.

Kennedy MI, McCombie L, Dawes P, McConnell KN, Dunnigan MG. (1997) Nutritional support for patients with intellectual disability and nutrition / dysphagia disorders in community care. *Journal of Intellectual Disability Research* 41: 430–436.

Khazaal Y, Charpentier C, Rothen S, Frésard E, Zullino D. (2006) Impact of an outpatient intervention on anripsychotic-induced weight gain. Psychiatry on line. Available at www.priory.com/psych/weightgain.pdf. Accessed 4 April 20111.

Knivsberg AM, Reichelt KL, Holen T, Nodland M. (2002) A randomized controlled study of dietary interventions in autistic syndromes. *Nutritional Neuroscience* 5: 251–261.

Kroese BS, Gillott A, Atkinson V. (1998) Consumers with intellectual disabilities as service evaluators. *Journal of Applied Research in Intellectual Disability* 11: 116–128.

Kuperminc MN, Stevenson RD. (2008) Growth and nutrition disorders in children with cerebral palsy. *Developmental Disabilities Research Reviews* 14: 137–146.

Langmore SE, Terpenning MS, Schork A. (1998) Predictors of aspiration pneumonia. How important is dysphagia? *Dysphagia* 13 69–81.

Lazenby T. (2008) The impact of aging on eating, drinking, and swallowing function in people with Down's syndrome. *Dysphagia* 23: 88–97.

Learning Disabilities Advisory Group (LDAG). (2001) *Fulfilling the Promises. Report of the Learning Disabilities Advisory Group*. Cardiff: National Assembly for Wales.

Leslie WS, Hankey CR, Lean MEJ. (2007) Weight gain a san adverse effect of some commonly prescribed drugs: a systematic review. *QJM* 100: 395–404.

Leslie P, Crawford H, Wilkinson H. (2009) People with a learning disability and dysphagia: a Cinderella population? *Dysphagia* 24: 103–104.

Levy JM, Botuck S, Damiani MR, Levy PH, Dern TA, Freeman SE. (2006) Medical conditions and healthcare utilization among adults with intellectual disabilities living in group homes in New York City. *Journal of Policy & Practice in Intellectual Disabilities* 3: 195–202.

Levy JM, Botuck S, Rimmerman A. (2007a) Examining outpatient health care utilization among adults with severe or profound intellectual disabilities living in an urban setting: A brief snap shot. *Journal of Social Work in Disability & Rehabilitation* 6: 33–45.

Levy SE, Souders MC, Ittenbach RF, Giarelli E, Mulberg AE. (2007b) Relationship of dietary intake to gastrointestinal symptoms in children with ASD spectrum disorders. *Psychiatry* 61: 492–497.

Lewis SJ, Heaton KW. (1997) Stool form scale as a useful guide to intestinal transit time. *Scandinavian Journal of Gastroenterology* 32: 920–924.

Lindmark M, Trygg K, Giltvedt K, Kolset SO. (2010) Nutrient intake of young children with Prader-Willi syndrome. *Food and Nutrition Research* 54: 2112.

Marshall D, McConkey R, Moore G. (2003) Obesity in people with intellectual disabilities: the impact of nurse-led health screenings and health promotion activities. *Journal of Advances in Nursing* 41: 147–153.

Melville CA, Cooper SA, McGrother CW, Thorp CF, Collacott R. (2005) Obesity in adults with Down syndrome: a case-control study. *Journal of Intellectual Disability Research* 49: 125–133.

Melville CA, Cooper S, Morrison J. (2008) The prevalence & determinants of obesity in adults with intellectual disability. *Journal of Applied Research in Intellectual Disability* 21: 425–437.

Melville CA, Hamilton S, Millar S, et al. (2009) Carer knowledge and perceptions of healthy lifestyles for adults with intellectual disabilities. *Journal of Applied Research in Intellectual Disability* 22: 298–306.

Mencap. (2010) Getting it right: the charter explained. Available at www.mencap.org.uk/document.asp?id=14971&audGroup=65&subjectLevel2=33&subjectId=&sorter=2&origin=pageType&pageType=112&pageno=&searchPhrase=. Accessed 3 May 2011.

Millward C, Ferriter M, Claver S, Connell-Jones G. (2008) *Gluten- and casein-free diets for autistic spectrum disorder (Cochrane review)*. *Cochrane Library*, Issue 2. Chichester: Wiley.

Moore K, McGillivray J, Illingworth K, Brookhouse P (2004) An investigation into the incidence of obesity and underweight among adults with an intellectual disability in an Australian sample. *Journal of Developmental Disability* 29: 306–318.

Murray J, Ryan-Krause P. (2010) Obesity in children with Down syndrome: Background and recommendations for management. *Pediatric Nursing* 36: 314–319.

National Autistic Society, (2011) Important facts about autism and Asperger syndrome for GPs. Available at www.autism.org.uk/en-gb/working-with/health/information-for-general-practitioners/important-facts-about-autism-and-asperger-syndrome-for-gps.aspx. Accessed 2 May 2011.

National Patient Safety Agency (NPSA). (2004) *Understanding the Patient Safety Issues for People with Learning Disabilities*. London: NPSA.

NHS Scotland. (2009) Caring and consent. Available at www.hris.org.uk/patient-information/information-for-carers/caring-and-consent/. Accessed 18 April 2011.

National Institute for Health and Care Excellence (NICE) (2006) *Clinical Guideline 43: Obesity guidance on the prevention, identification, assessment and management of overweight and obesity in adults and children*. London: NICE.

O'Riordan CF, Metcalf BS, Perkins JM, Wilkin TJ. (2010) Reliability of energy expenditure prediction equations in the weight management clinic. *Journal of Human Nutrition and Dietetics* 23: 169–175.

Pawlyn J, Carnaby S (eds). (2009) *Profound and Multiple Learning Disabilities*. Oxford: Blackwell Publishing.

Peterson JJ, Janz KF, Lowe JB. (2008) Physical activity among adults with intellectual disability living in community settings. *Preventive Medicine* 47: 101–106.

Powrie E. (2003) Primary health care provision for adults with a learning disability. *Journal of Advances in Nursing* 42: 413–423.

Prader-Willi Syndrome Association. (2010a) A Prader-Willi food pyramid. Availabe at www.pwsausa.org/syndrome/foodpyramid.htm. Accessed 16 April 2011.

Prader-Willi Syndrome Association. (2010b) What is prader-willi syndrome? Available at www.pwsa.co.uk. Accessed 16 April 2011.

Ramirez-Zea M. (2005) Validation of three predictive equations for basal metabolic rate in adults. *Public Health Nutrition* 8: 1213–1228.

Royal College of Nursing (RCN). (2006) *Meeting the Needs of People with Learning Disabilities. Guidance for Nursing Staff*. London: RCN.

Rimmer J, Yamaki K. (2006) Obesity and intellectual disability. *Mental Retardation and Developmental Disabilities Research Reviews* 12: 22–27.

Robertson J, Emerson E, Gregory N, et al (2000) Lifestyle related risk factors for poor health in residential settings for people with intellectual disabilities. *Research in Developmental Disabilities* 21 469–486.

Roebroeck ME, Stam HJ (2006). The epidemiology of cerebral palsy: incidence, impairments and risk factors. *Disability and Rehabilitation* 28: 183–191.

Rogers B, Stratton P, Msall M, et al.(1994) Long-term morbidity and management strategies of tracheal aspiration in adults with severe developmental disabilities. *American Journal of Mental Retardation* 98, 490–498.

Rutter H, Carmichael S. (2011) Health care for prople with learning disabilities – how far havr we come? The national picture. *Tizard Learning Disability Review* 16: 14–17.

Schoeller DA, Levitsky LL, Bandini LG, Dietz WW, Walczak A. (1988). Energy expenditure and body composition in Prader-Willi syndrome. *Metabolism* 37: 115–120.

Schreck KA, Williams K, Smith AF. (2004) A comparison of eating behaviours between children with and without autism. *Journal of Autism and Development Disorders* 34: 433–438.

Scottish Executive. (2000) The same as you .A review of services for people with learning disability. Available at www.scotland.gov.uk/ldsr/docs/tsay-00.asp. Accessed 22 April 2011.

Scottish Parliament. (2000) *Adults with Incapacity (Scotland) Act*. Edinburgh: The Stationery Office.

Scheepers M, Duff M, Baddeley P, Cooper M, Houghton M, Harrison J. (2000) *Helicobacter pylori* and the learning disabled. *British Journal of General Practice* 50: 813–814.

Shin M, Besser LM, Kucik JE, Lu C, Siffel C, Correa A. (2009) Prevalence of Down syndrome among children and adolescents in 10 regions of the United States. *Pediatrics* 124: 1565–1571.

Scottish Intercollegiate Guideline Network (SIGN). (2010) SIGN guideline 115 Management of Obesity. Available at www.sign.ac.uk/. Accessed 4 April 2011.

Smyth CM, Bell D. (2006) From biscuits to boyfriends : the ramifications of choice for people with learning disabilities. *British Journal of Learning Disabilities* 34: 227–236.

Sowney M, Barr O. (2004) Equity of access to health care for people with learning disabilities. *Journal of Learning Disabilities* 8: 247–265.

van Mil E, Westerterp KR, Gerver WJ, et al. (2000a) Energy expenditure at rest and during sleep in children with Prader-Willi syndrome is explained by body composition. *American Journal of Clinical Nutrition* 71: 752–756.

van Mil E, Westerterp KR, Kester ADM, et al. (2000b) Acitivity related energy expenditure in children and adolescents with PWS. *International Journal of Obesity* 24: 429–434.

van Mil E, Westerterp KR, Gerver WJ, Van Marken Lictenbelt WD, Kester ADM, Saris WHM. (2001) Body composition in Prader-Willi syndrome compared with non-syndromal obesity: relationship to physical activity and growth hormone function. *Journal of Paediatrics* 139: 708–714.

Vogels A, Van Den Ende J, Keymolen K, et al. (2004) Minimum prevalence, birth incidence and cause of death for Prader-Willi syndrome in Flanders. *European Journal of Human Genetics* 12: 238–240.

Wales L. (2010) Providing oral healthcare for patients with a PRG tube. *Dental Nursing* 6: 565–568.

Wali A, John P, Gul A, *et al.* (2006) A novel locus for alopecia with mental retardation syndrome (APMR2) maps to chromosome3q26.2 -q26.31. *Clinical Genetics* 70: 233–239.

Wallace RA, Schluter P. (2008) Audit of cardiovascular disease risk factors among supported adults with intellectual disability attending an ageing clinic. *Journal of Intelletual Development and Disability* 33: 48–58.

Wallace R, Schluter P, Webb P. (2002) Environmental, medical behavioural and disabilityfactors associated with Helicobacter pylori infection in adults with intellectual disability. *Journal of Intellectual Disability Research* 46: 51–60.

Whittington JE, Holland, AJ, Webb T, Butler J, Clarke D, Boer H. (2001) Population prevalence and estimated birth incidence and mortality rate for people with Prader-Willi syndrome in one UK health region. *Journal of Medical Genetics* 38: 792–798.

Williams PG, Dalrymple N, Neal J. (2000) Eating habits of children with ASD. *Pediatric Nursing* 26: 259–264.

Williams KE, Gibons BG, Schreck KA.(2005) Comparing selective eaters with and without developmental disabilities. *Journal of Developmental and Physical Disability* 17: 299–309.

World Health Organization (1992) *ICD-10 Classification of Mental and Behavioural Disorders: Clinical Depression and Diagnostic Guidelines.* Geneva: World Health Organization.

World Health Organization. (2010) Healthy ageing-adults with intellectual disabilities: summative report. *Journal of Applied Research in Intellectual Disabilities* 14: 256–275.

Wong HHL, Smith RG. (2006) Patterns of complementary and alternative medical therapy use in children diagnosed with autism spectrum disorders. *Journal of Autism and Developmental Disorders* 36: 901–909.

Yamaki K. (2005) Body weight status among adults with intellectual disability in the community. *Mental Retardation* 43: 1–10.

Yeargin-Allsop M, Braun KVN, Doenberg NS, *et al.* (2008) Prevalence of cerebral palsy in 8-year old children in three areas of the United States in 2002; a multisite collaboration. *Pediatrics* 121: 547–554.

3.8

Paediatric clinical dietetics and childhood nutrition

3.8.1 Introduction

Lisa Cooke and Jacqueline Lowden

Key points

- Paediatric dietetics is a medical speciality and dietitians require postgraduate training.

- Children are not small adults; their physical and medical needs are different from those of an adult.

- The nutritional needs for growth must always be considered in addition to any disease related considerations.

Paediatric dietetics is a medical speciality and dietitians require postgraduate training to become a specialist paediatric dietitian. Many medical experts view children as small adults but this a fallacy. Continuous good nutrition during childhood is imperative and lays down the genetic building blocks for a child's future health. Emerging evidence suggests that the child's diet and growth pattern in the first 2 years of life extrapolate to long term health outcomes (Lanigan & Singhal, 2009; Singhal & Lucas, 2004).

There are 22 children's hospitals in the UK with many more paediatric tertiary referral centres (RCPCH, 2011). These specialist centres often manage patient groups on a shared care basis with the local dietitian within the patient's geographical area.

This chapter gives a brief overview of childhood nutrition and paediatric dietetics; the importance of how a child grows and develops, growth monitoring, nutritional assessment, nutritional needs during childhood and the management of clinical diseases and conditions. *Clinical Paediatric Dietetics* (Shaw & Lawson, 2007) should be consulted for more detailed information and dietetic management. Many of the topics also apply to adults and further information can be found in the relevant chapters.

Dietetic care must always be supported by specialist paediatric supervision in clinical practice until dietetic competence has been achieved.

Paediatric dietetics has a clear career pathway and the British Dietetic Association (BDA) (www.bda.uk.com) has an active and supportive paediatric group. This group provides a student manual toolkit so that departments can actively expose student dietitians to the paediatric speciality. As a newly qualified dietitian, or one embarking on a role that involves paediatric medicine, there is a self directed learning pack that needs to be managed by a paediatric dietetic supervisor with relevant experience. The group produces diet sheets through Nutrition and Diet Resources UK (www. ndr-uk.org), position statements and supports guideline production. It is also actively involved with a Masters degree in paediatric dietetics as a distance learning course jointly hosted by Plymouth University and the BDA.

References

Lanigan J, Singhal A. (2009) Early nutrition and long-term health: a practical approach. *Proceedings of the Nutrition Society* 68: 422–429.

Royal College of Peadiatrics and Child Health (RCPCH). (2011) RCPCH Medical Workforce Consensus 2009. Available at www .rcpch.ac. Accessed 24 April 2012.

Shaw V, Lawson M. (2007) *Clinical Paediatric Dietetics*, 3rd edn. Oxford: Blackwell Publishing.

Singhal A, Lucas A. (2004) Early origins of cardiovascular disease: is there a unifying hypothesis? *Lancet* 363: 1642–1645.

3.8.2 Growth, nutritional assessment and nutritional requirements
Sarah Cawtherley and Claire Conway

The growth of an infant or child is very important, as poor growth can be an indicator of underlying disease, poor nutrition, emotional neglect or a combination of these factors. Growth must be regularly and accurately monitored throughout infancy and childhood. In infancy growth is closely related to nutritional adequacy and consequently the measurement of growth relates to nutritional status. Nutritional requirements during infancy, childhood and adolescence are subject to large changes and can be affected by age, weight, activity levels and illness or disease process. Normal human growth can be divided into two distinctive sections; prenatal growth and postnatal growth.

Abnormal growth and development in childhood is associated with morbidity and mortality. Therefore, regular monitoring and plotting of weight, length and head circumference on growth charts can help identify whether a child is growing normally or abnormally when compared with other children of similar age and gender. Anyone who weighs and measures a child or infant and plots these on a growth chart in the infant's *Personal Child Health Record (PCHR)* (colloquially known as the red book) should be suitably trained.

Prenatal growth

The growth of an infant begins at conception, with the fastest growth period being between conception and birth; this accounts for approximately 30% of eventual height (Tasker *et al.*, 2008). Factors that determine growth during this period include maternal size, maternal nutrition and intrauterine environment. Hormonal factors such as insulin, insulin-like growth factor 2 (IGF-2) and human placental lactogen are important regulators of growth during this period (Tasker *et al.*, 2008) (see Chapter 3.2).

Postnatal growth

Postnatal growth can be subdivided into infancy, childhood and puberty.

Infancy

Weight

From birth to 24 months growth is rapid; an infant doubles their birth weight in the first 5–6 months and trebles it in the first year of life. The rate of growth is largely determined by the nutritional adequacy of the diet. The expected weight gain for a healthy term infant is (Shaw & Lawson, 2007):

- 200 g/week for the first 3 months.
- 150 g/week between 4 and 6 months.

- 100 g/week between 6 and 9 months.
- 50–75 g/week between 9 and 12 months.
- 2.5 kg during the second year.

Linear growth

The length of an infant reflects bone growth and therefore is a better indicator of long term growth and nutritional adequacy than weight. Expected linear growth is 25 cm during the first year and 12 cm during the second year of life (Thompson, 1998).

Head circumference

Expected rate of growth in head circumference is 1 cm/month in the first year and 2 cm in total for the second year (Thompson, 1998). This reflects the rapid brain growth and development.

Growth velocity

Growth velocity varies depending on how an infant is being fed. A breastfed infant initially grows at a slower rate than a formula fed infant.

Childhood

From 2 years until the onset of puberty the rate of growth is slower and steadier than during infancy. Children gain approximately 2 kg in weight and 10 cm in height/year, declining to 6 cm/year until puberty when a further growth spurt occurs. During this period growth is primarily dependent upon growth hormone (GH), providing that there is adequate nutrition (Tasker *et al.*, 2008).

Puberty

Puberty is defined as the changes associated with the maturation of the gonads; testes in boys and ovaries in girls. During this period growth is dependent upon the action of GH and the sex hormones testosterone and oestrogen, which induce the characteristic growth spurt of puberty. Puberty starts earlier in females; therefore, they are taller than males between the ages of 10 and 13 years. In males, puberty generally occurs later and at a greater magnitude, resulting in a larger final adult height. On average puberty usually starts at 10.5 years and 12 years in girls and boys, respectively (Tasker *et al.*, 2008). Normal puberty usually occurs gradually over a period of 18 months to 5 years. Once a child's growth spurt has occurred their nutritional requirements become those of an adult (Webster-Gandy *et al.*, 2006).

General development

Children develop at different rates and stages. In the UK the infant's development is recorded in the PCHR. For premature infants developmental age is calculated from the original due date rather than date of delivery (Department of Health, 2009). Physical and verbal developmental milestones are also monitored. Those relating to food are:

- 11–12 months – enjoys finger foods.
- 13–15 months – begins to feed themselves very messily.
- 3–5 years – can use a knife and fork.

Weaning

The European Society for Paediatric Gastroenterology, Hepatology and Nutrition (ESPGHAN) recommends that weaning onto solids should begin by 6 months but not before 4 months (17 weeks) of age. Exclusive breastfeeding for about 6 months is desirable and should be continued throughout weaning, particularly in the early stages (Agostoni et al., 2008). The Department of Health (1994) recommends that weaning should not be delayed beyond 6 months due to the increased risk of nutrient and energy deficiencies. The Scientific Advisory Committee on Nutrition (SACN) is currently reviewing the advice

regarding weaning and UK practices and this should be published by 2014 (www.sacn.gov.uk).

Developmental signs that an infant is ready for solids include:

- Putting objects and toys in the mouth.
- Chewing fists.
- Showing interest when others are eating.
- Being hungry between milk feeds or demanding more feeds and taking larger volumes.
- Able to sit up and support their head.

At around 6 months infants are generally more accepting of new tastes and textures, and learn to accept them quite quickly (Harris, 2000). The process of weaning is a learning process; therefore, infants should be given the opportunity to learn to accept new tastes and textures, which can take up to ten attempts with the same food (Birch & Marlin, 1982). Infants who are given puréed foods for too long and not offered lumps and finger foods by 9 months are more likely to become fussy eaters. Table 3.8.1 shows the developmental stages of weaning and Table 3.8.2 shows the key stages in the

SECTION 3

Table 3.8.1   Developmental stages of weaning [adapted from Shaw & Lawson (2007, Table 27.3, p526)]

Stage	Age guide	Skills to learn	New food textures to introduce
1	6 months, but not before 4 months (17 weeks) if parents choose to begin earlier	Taking food from a spoon Moving food from the front of the mouth to the back for swallowing Managing thicker purées and mashed food	Smooth purées Mashed foods
2	6–9 months	Moving lumps around the mouth Chewing lumps Self feeding using hands and fingers Sipping from a cup	Mashed food with soft lumps Soft finger foods Liquids in a lidded beaker or cup
3	9–12 months	Chewing minced and chopped food Self feeding attempts with a spoon	Hard finger foods Minced and chopped family foods

Table 3.8.2   Key stages in the normal development of eating and drinking skills (Winstock, 2005)

Age	Oral motor skills	Food related play
Birth–3 months	Rhythmical suckle with up and down jaw movements Sensitive gag reflex	Sucks well, calm, watches mother
4–6 months	Touch of spoon elicits suck Spits out food with forward–back tongue movements	Takes things to mouth Blows bubbles with saliva Pats bottle
6–9 months	Jaw begins to stabilise Bites on cup Tongue tip up, munching, gag reduces	Holds food and toys Desire for some control, messy, plays with food
9–12 months	Tongues moves food from side to side Stabilisation of jaw Chewing, closes lips on spoon, spills drink	Enjoys playing with food Can hold a spoon, poor control Squeezes toys and food
12–18 months	Uses a controlled bite on a biscuit Chews efficiently with rotary tongue and jaw movement	Pretends to feed self, large teddy or person Demands food
18–24 months	Chews with lips closed Up and down sucking pattern on cup	Lifts cup to mouth Pretends to feed dolls Self feeds, still messy

normal development of eating and drinking skills (Coulthard *et al.*, 2009; Northstone *et al.*, 2001; Winstock, 2005).

Infants should be offered a variety of foods from the four main food groups on a daily basis to provide the required nutrients. The National Diet and Nutrition Survey (NDNS) (Bates *et al.*, 2011) demonstrates that diet alone now provides close to, or above, the recommended nutrient intake (RNI) for all vitamins except vitamin D. Foods high in fat and sugar should not be included in the early weaning diet.

Food neophobia

By 12 months infants should be eating family foods and be offered a wide range of foods. Food neophobia, when infants become wary of trying new foods, usually peaks at around 18 months. Infants who have a wide variety of family foods by 12 months are usually happy to continue to accept these foods. Between 3 and 5 years children can develop disgust fears and consequently may stop eating foods that they previously enjoyed. They often refuse a food that looks like something they find disgusting. Children can also develop contamination fears; this often occurs at the same time and if a disliked food is put next to a liked food, then the infant may refuse both foods (Shaw & Lawson, 2007).

Nutritional assessment

A nutritional assessment can determine if a child suffers from malnutrition, which has been defined as a state of deficiency, excess or imbalance of nutrition that has an adverse effect on body function (Elia, 2003). In developed countries malnutrition is usually associated with excess weight and inappropriate dietary habits rather than undernutrition. Information required for nutritional assessment should include dietary intake, anthropometric measurements, including height and weight, biochemistry and a clinical assessment that includes a physical examination and medical history (see Chapter 2.2 and Chapter 2.3).

Dietary intake

Methods for assessing dietary intake for children and young people are the same as for adults: 24-hour recall, food frequency questionnaire, dietary history, food diary or weighed food intake. In most cases it is possible to obtain sufficient information from discussing the child's diet with their parent or carer, and the child themselves, if appropriate. Differences between adults and children include meals and snacks at nursery or school, after school clubs, bedtime food and drinks, staying with friends and relatives, and for older children eating out with friends. Assessing dietary intakes for babies and very young children can be difficult, particularly if the infant is breastfed. It is possible to calculate how much milk a breastfed baby consumes by weighing them before and after each feed over 24 hours. In practice, this is rarely

done as it can cause anxiety in the mother and baby. Questions about the length of time the infant feeds for, sleepiness during feeds, frequency of feeds, whether or not the breast is drained and frequency of wet and dirty nappies are more appropriate and, combined with information about weight gain, can provide information about likely milk intake. If mothers express breast milk and bottle feed this to their baby, ingested volumes can be easily determined. This would only be appropriate if the mother is returning to work, the baby is ill and unable to breastfeed or the mother is leaving the baby for any length of time. For infants of weaning age, it can be difficult to assess the contribution from food to their overall intake due to the amount that is spat out or smeared around with their hands. Information on the nutrient content of ready made weaning foods is readily available.

Anthropometry

The most widely used measures are weight, height and head circumference in infants, which are measured up to 2 years. Anthropometric measurements are compared with standards specific for gender and age. An individual measurement is almost meaningless in isolation as it is impossible to determine whether or not a child is following a satisfactory growth pattern [Michaelsen *et al.*, 2000; Royal College of Nursing (RCN), 2010]. Weight and length or height measurements should be taken whenever there are concerns about a child's weight gain, growth or general health, in addition to routine checks (RCPCH, 2009). Sick infants and children who are hospital inpatients should be weighed at least once a week (RCN, 2006). Anthropometric measurements can be expressed as Z scores. A Z score is the standard deviation (SD) score; the deviation of the value for an individual from the median value of the reference population divided by the SD for the reference population:

Z score = (observed value − median reference value)/
            SD reference population

Growth charts

Growth charts are mathematically created reference curves based on population data to represent the normal genetic growth of healthy children living in a specific environment. There are several growth charts available for use in the UK. The World Health Organization (WHO, 2006) has published Child Growth Standards for infants and children up to the age of 5 years, using data from the Multicentre Growth Reference Study (MGRS). Healthy, full term infants exclusively breastfed for the first 4 months and partially for a year and weaned at 6 months (De Onis *et al.*, 2004) were included. These growth charts set breastfeeding as the norm. The WHO growth standards are available in centiles and as Z scores for weight for age, length/height for age, weight/height for age and body mass index (BMI) for age, for children aged 0–5 years in addition to 5–19 years.

In 2007 SACN adopted the WHO growth charts in the UK (Department of Health, 2007) up to 4 years of age, after which the UK1990 charts are used. The Department of Health recommends that the UK–WHO growth charts should be used for all new births after the 11 May 2009 and the UK 1990 charts for all children over the age of 4 years up to 18 years (Cole, 1997; Cole et al., 1998; RCPCH, 2009).

UK–WHO charts

Three versions are available, 0–4-year and 2–18-year growth charts and the Neonatal and Infant Close Monitoring Chart (NICMC), previously known as the Low Birth Weight Chart. The latter is used for births before 32 weeks' gestation, ill neonates born after 32 weeks' gestation and term infants with significant growth and weight faltering (RCPCH, 2009).

UK1990 charts

These growth charts were constructed using data from a large number of different aged children in the UK during the late 1980s and describe typical but not necessarily healthy growing children. They are based on formula fed infants and should be used for children born before 11 May 2009.

Other charts

Charts are available for specific conditions; Down's syndrome, Turner's syndrome, sickle cell disease and Noonan's syndrome. Thrive lines are available for assessing faltering growth; separate charts are also available for plotting BMI and waist circumference. All charts are gender specific and can be obtained from Harlow Printing (Maxwell Street, South Shields NE33 4PU) or downloaded from www.growthcharts.rcpch.ac.uk.

Interpretation of centile lines

The UK–WHO growth charts consist of nine centile lines. The 50th centile represents the median for the population and the 2nd and 98th centiles are two standard deviations (Z scores) above and below the median. The 0.4th centile identifies extremely low measurements and only $1/_{250}$ (0.4%) optimally growing children will fall on this centile (Wright et al., 2004).

Plotting on a growth chart

Growth monitoring requires accurate measurements that are plotted accurately on the growth chart to see patterns of growth over time. This accuracy ensures the pattern of growth can be assessed correctly. The most common error when plotting growth charts is calculating an infant's age incorrectly. Age should be calculated in weeks for at least the first 6 months of life and thereafter in calendar months. If the point marked is within one-quarter of a space of the centile line, the infant is described as being on the centile. However, if they are further away than this, they should be described as being between the two centile lines, e.g. between the 4th and the 9th centile

Plotting and assessing newborn infants

A baby born between 37 and 42 weeks' gestation is considered full term and should be plotted at age 0. All preterm infants (before 37 weeks' gestation) should be plotted in the preterm section of the growth charts. The birth centiles are average values for weight, length and head circumference for full term babies (Cole, 1997). All infants tend to lose weight initially and then begin to regain their birth weight between 3 and 5 days, and 80% will have regained their birth weight by 2 weeks of age (Wright & Parkinson, 2004).

Calculating percentage weight loss

Percentage weight loss is the difference between the actual weight and the birth weight expressed as a percentage of the birth weight. If a baby has a weight loss of 10% or more at or before 2 weeks, they need careful assessment as this may indicate a possible feeding problem or illness (RCPCH, 2009).

Preterm infants

The WHO standard does not include data for preterm infants; therefore, preterm charts have been produced using the UK1990 reference data (Cole, 1997). A preterm infant born after 32 weeks' gestation should be plotted on the preterm section of the 0–1-year growth chart until they have reached their expected date of delivery (EDD) plus 2 weeks, and then be plotted on the 0–1-year chart using gestational correction. Preterm infants born at <32 weeks' gestation should be plotted on the specially designed neonatal and infant close monitoring chart.

Plotting with gestational correction

Gestational correction adjusts the plot for the number of weeks an infant is born premature. Gestational correction should continue for a year for infants born between 32 and 36 weeks' gestation and for 2 years for infants born before 32 weeks' gestation. For example, an infant born at 34 weeks' gestation is 6 weeks' premature and their growth should be corrected by 6 weeks. Once gestational correction has been calculated, it is important to calculate the actual (calendar) age of the infant and plot this on the growth chart with a clear dot. A line is drawn back from this dot by the number of weeks the infant is premature and this point is marked with an arrow. The point of the arrow shows the infant's centile with gestational correction.

Neonatal and infant close monitoring chart

The NICMC has been specifically designed for monitoring the growth of infants born before 32 weeks' gestation and low birth weight infants. It can be used from 23 weeks' gestation to the corrected age of 2 years. It can also be used for term neonates who are small for gestational age and require close monitoring of their growth pattern. A new feature of these charts is the date box system, which helps to calculate gestational age. This avoids errors in calculating the infant's age.

Adult height prediction

The adult height prediction on the UK–WHO growth charts differs from the target height calculation on the UK1990 height chart. Target height compares the child's height with those of their birth parents, and identifies children who are unusually tall or short compared with their parents. The adult height prediction tool provides a good prediction of adult height for most children, including those who are unusually tall or short, but it does not compare them with their parents (RCPCH, 2009). There it is more useful for families where one or both parents are not the biological parent. The adult height prediction is accurate for 80% of children (RCPCH, 2009).

Further information on plotting growth charts and their use can be found at www.growthcharts.rcpch.ac.uk.

Growth assessment recommendations

As part of the Healthy Child Programme children should be routinely assessed to identify the early signs of obesity and offer interventions from an early stage. The Child Growth Foundation (2012) recommends that infants and children should be routinely measured, as shown in Table 3.8.3. If there are concerns, infants and children may be weighed more often, but weighing at intervals too close together is misleading and can cause parental anxiety. Therefore, the recommended frequency of weighing (RCPCH, 2009) is:

- No more than once a month between 2 weeks and 6 months of age.
- Once every 2 months in infants between 6 and 12 months.
- Once every 3 months in children over the age of 1 year.

This frequency of weighing should reflect the progressive slowing of weight gain in the first year (Wright *et al.*, 2010). However, in practice it is common for babies under 6 months to be weighed fortnightly, and those over 6 months monthly if there are concerns about their weight.

Anthropometric measurement techniques

A narrow plastic or disposable paper, non-stretch tape measure should be used where applicable. Three measurements should be made and the average recorded.

Head circumference

A number of genetic and acquired conditions will affect head growth and measurement of head circumference is not a useful indicator of nutritional status in these conditions (RCPCH, 2009). Measurements should be made at

Table 3.8.3 Recommended measurements for infants and children (source: Child Growth Foundation 2012. Reproduced with permission of the Child Growth Foundation (www.childgrowthfoundation.org)

Age	Weight	OFC	Length	BMI	Notes
Birth	X		X or 10 days		**Weight:** assess malnutrition using 5%/95% thrive line acetates or if weight/length centiles differ by over 2 centile bands. To resolve any concern: if infant is <6 months, weigh fortnightly; if >6 months, weigh monthly
24/30 hours		X			
5 days	X				**OFC:** refer ASAP if OFC curve climbs significantly upwards through centile bands. To resolve concern, measure fortnightly
10 days	X		X		
14 days		X			**Length:** use length predominantly to confirm malnutrition and consider referral (for either slow/excess growth) after three measurements. To resolve concern, measure 3-monthly
6–8 weeks	X	X			
12 weeks	X				
16 weeks	X				
6–8 months	X		X		
12–15 months	X		X	X	
2 years	X		X	X	**BMI**: Having monitored weight gain/length during infancy, measure both height and weight from approx 1 year, calculate BMI and refer if indicated. To resolve any concern, calculate BMI 6-monthly and similarly refer
3 years	X		X	X	
4 years	X		X	X	
Primary school Year 1	X		X	X	**BMI** HMG has still not accepted the House of Commons Health Committee's 2004 recommendation that the BMI of every primary school child be assessed annually. Payments for the BMI assessment of all secondary school age children of 16 years or over are available under the quality and outcomes framework (QoF).
Year 2	X		X	X	
Year 3	X		X	X	
Year 4	X		X	X	
Year 5	X		X	X	
Year 6	X		X	X	
Secondary school	X		X	X	

OFC, occipitofrontal circumference; BMI, body mass index; HMG, Her Majesty's Government.

the widest part of the infant's head; hats or bonnets should be removed.

Weight

Only Class III or above clinical electronic scales with a metric setting should be used. These should be maintained and calibrated annually, in line with medical devices standards (Department of Health, 2010; NICE, 2008). Infants and children under 2 years should be weighed naked without a nappy on baby scales, to the nearest 10 g (RCN, 2010). Children over 2 years should be weighed in minimal clothing (ideally vest and pants, without shoes) to the nearest 100 g. Older children and adolescents should be weighed without shoes, wearing indoor clothing and with empty pockets. A child who is unable to sit or stand should be weighed on a hoist scale (RCN, 2010). If it is not possible to weigh a child, tared weighing should be used: an adult is weighed with and without the child and weight calculated by subtraction (RCN, 2010). The method should be recorded.

Length or height

Length is measured in infants and toddlers up to 2 years; height is measured thereafter. Length and height reflect bone growth and are a better indicator of long term growth and nutritional adequacy than weight. Infants under 2 years should be measured without a nappy or footwear while lying on a length board or mat (RCPCH, 2009). A child's height is usually slightly less than their length due to spinal compression; therefore, the centile lines on the UK–WHO chart shift down slightly at age 2 years to allow for this (RCPCH, 2009). Height is measured using a rigid upright measure with a T piece or a stadiometer, without shoes (RCPCH, 2009). The head should be positioned in the Frankfurt plane and the ear hole should be lined up with the bottom of the eye socket (see Chapter 2.2). Alternative methods for estimating height include lower leg length or knee to heel height.

Weight/height indices

Body mass index

Body mass index can be calculated and interpreted by plotting it on a BMI reference chart. Percentage weight for height and percentage height for age are used to identify the degree of malnutrition, although children with anorexia nervosa and chronic diseases, e.g. cystic fibrosis, often have the former calculated.

Body mass index is a useful indicator of fatness and thinness in children from the age of 2 years, when height can be measured with relative accuracy. However, unlike for adults, BMI is age dependent and therefore plotted on centile charts, rather than being read as an absolute number. A child whose weight is average for their height will have a BMI between the 25th and 75th centiles whatever their height centile. The Scottish Intercollegiate Guidelines Network (SIGN, 2010) and NICE (2007) recommend that in the clinical setting a BMI greater than the 91st centile be used to define overweight and a BMI greater than the 98th centile obese (see Chapter 7.13.4).

Waist circumference

Waist circumference is measured at the natural waistline, which is midway between the tenth rib and iliac crest. Waist circumference charts are available for children over 5 years (McCarthy et al., 2001).

Mid upper arm circumference

Mid upper arm circumference (MUAC) indicates body fat distribution and can be used to determine malnutrition in children. It is useful in children younger than 5 years as until then MUAC increases rapidly; standards are available for children aged 1–5 years (Gibson, 2005). It may be used during research or for children with renal or liver disease where the presence of fluid overload or ascites makes weight inaccurate. When combined with the triceps skinfold measurement, upper arm muscle and fat stores can be estimated, and these measures correlate well with total body measures of fat mass and fat free mass (Zemel et al., 1997).

Skinfold thickness

Measurement of skinfold thickness can be used to assess nutrition in young infants and older children, but it can be difficult to do this well. The process is the same as that for adults and prediction equations for skinfold thickness are available for children's triceps skinfold. These measurements are not performed routinely due to the distress it can cause children; however, it is used in research, HIV and renal and liver diseases.

Height age

Height age is the age at which the measured height of the child falls on the 50th centile. Calculation of height age is necessary when determining nutrient requirements for children who are much smaller or taller than their chronological age (Shaw & Lawson, 2007).

Percentage height for age

Height for age is a measure of linear growth and a faltering of linear growth is called stunting. A low height for age results from slowing of skeletal growth. In general, it reflects a chronic process and is used as an index of chronic undernutrition (WHO, 2003).

Percentage weight for height

Weight for height assesses the appropriateness of the child's weight compared with their height. It is sensitive to acute nutritional disturbances, and a low weight for height is described as wasting, resulting from a failure to gain weight or weight loss. It can develop rapidly and be reversed rapidly, and is an index of acute undernutrition reflecting severe weight loss, which is often associated with acute starvation and/or severe illness (Michaelsen et al., 2000). Calculation of percentage weight for height is often used with cystic fibrosis patients, although it has been found to be an unreliable measure of nutritional status (Poustie et al., 2000).

Both percentage weight for height and percentage height for age are used to classify malnutrition, as shown in Table 3.8.4.

SECTION 3

National Child Measurement Programme

Since 2006/07, all children in the UK in the reception school year (4–5 years) and year 6 (10–11 years) have been invited to have their height and weight measured and BMI calculated. Results are sent to parents, which can be of particular benefit as often parents cannot tell if a child is overweight or obese (Carnell *et al.*, 2005; Jeffery *et al.*, 2005). Anonymous results are collated by the Department of Health to establish trends in children's heights and weights.

Clinical assessment

The two major components of clinical assessment are the medical history and the physical examination. The medical history is similar to that of an adult (see Chapter 2.2). In addition, it is usual to obtain information about gestational age and birth weight, infant feeding history (breast or formula fed, age when weaned) and weight trend.

Visible signs and symptoms that suggest nutritional deficiencies are the same as in adults. In addition, bone changes in vitamin D or calcium deficiency (rickets) in children will include craniotabes, parietal and frontal bossing, epiphyseal enlargement and beading of the ribs. A suspected deficiency should be confirmed by biochemical or haematological tests.

Biochemistry and haematology

Laboratory assessment is used primarily to detect subclinical deficiency states, but also to confirm a clinical diagnosis. Age specific normal ranges for biochemical and haematological tests need to be established and used. Table 3.8.5 provides a summary of some biochemical and haematological measurements. Although urine is used for adult investigations, it is not commonly used for infants and children. Many tests require the collection of a 24-hour urine sample, which is difficult in babies and children, and the usefulness of a single urine sample for nutritional tests is limited (Shaw & Lawson, 2007).

Malnutrition screening tools

Malnutrition screening tools specifically for children admitted to hospital have been developed. However, there are currently no validated screening tools for use with infants aged 0–2 years. The British Association for

Table 3.8.4 Classification of malnutrition using weight for height and height for age (Waterlow, 1972)

Grade of malnutrition	Acute malnutrition (wasting)	Chronic malnutrition (stunting + wasting)
	Weight for height	Height for age
Normal	>90%	>95%
Grade 1 (mild)	80–90%	90–95%
Grade 2 (moderate)	70–80%	85–90%
Grade 3 (severe)	<70%	<80%

Table 3.8.5 Biochemical and haematological tests relating to nutritional status in children (source: Shaw 2007, table 1.7, p. 11. Reproduced with permission of Blackwell Publishing)

Nutrient	Test	Normal values in children	Comments
Biochemical tests			
Protein	Total plasma protein Albumin	55–80 g/L 30–45 g/L	Low levels reflect long term, not acute, depletion
Vitamin B_{12}	Plasma B_{12} value	263–1336 pmol/L	Low levels indicate deficiency
Vitamin C	Plasma ascorbate level	8.8–124 µmol/L	Low levels indicate deficiency
Vitamin A	Plasma retinol level	0.54–1.56 µmol/L	Low levels indicate deficiency
Vitamin D	Plasma 25-hydroxy cholecalciferol level	30–110 nmol/L	Low levels indicate deficiency
Vitamin E	Plasma tocopherol level	α-tocopherol 10.9–28.1 µmol/L	Low levels indicate deficiency
Copper	Plasma level	70–140 µmol/L	Low levels indicate deficiency
Selenium	Plasma level Glutathione peroxidise activity	0.76–1.07 µmol/L >1.77 µmol/L	Low levels indicate deficiency
Zinc	Plasma level	10–18 µmol/L	Low levels indicate deficiency
Haematology tests			
Folic acid	Plasma folate Red cell folate	7–48 nmol/L 429–1749 nmol/L	Low levels indicate deficiency Low levels indicate deficiency
Haemoglobin	Whole blood	104–140 g/L	Levels <110 g/L indicate iron deficiency
Ferritin	Plasma level	5–70 µg/L	Low levels indicate depletion of iron stores. Ferritin is an acute phase protein and increases during infection

Parenteral and Enteral Nutrition (BAPEN) (Brotherton *et al.*, 2011) and the Care Quality Commission (CQC, 2010) recommend the use of paediatric malnutrition screening tools, including:

- *STAMP* – the Screening Tool for the Assessment of Malnutrition in Paediatrics, which is a validated nutritional screening tool for use in hospitalised children aged 2–16 years (McCarthy *et al.*, 2012).
- *PYMS* – the Paediatric Yorkhill Malnutrition Score (PYMS) rates BMI, weight loss, changes in nutritional intake and the predicted effect of the current condition on nutritional status to give a score that reflects the degree of the nutritional risk. It can be used in children aged 1–16 years (Gerasimidis *et al.*, 2009).
- *STRONGkids* – this screening tool consists of a subjective clinical assessment of disease risk, nutritional intake and weight loss for children aged 0–18 years (Hulst *et al.*, 2010).
- *SGNA* – the Subjective Global Nutrition Assessment is an adapted version of the Subjective Global Assessment (SGA) tool used in adults, and is for children aged 0–18 years (Secker & Jeejeebhoy, 2007).

Although PYMS, STAMP and SGNA have been compared against each other (Gerasimidis *et al.*, 2010), it is recommended that each tool be compared against dietetic assessment to identify which has better diagnostic validity in a particular setting.

Nutritional requirements in childhood

Infants and children must not be viewed as small adults as they require different nutrients at different levels and a different nutritional balance from adults. The Committee on Medical Aspects of Nutrition (Department of Health, 1991), as shown in Appendix A3, established nutritional recommendations (dietary reference values (DRVs) for infants, children and adolescents in the UK. Values have been set for infants fed on formula milks, whose nutrient intakes are dependent upon the composition of the feed being offered, but not for breastfed infants as breast milk is the best form of nutrition for an infant. As for adults, DRVs are set for normal healthy individuals. Individual requirements will vary due to age, gender, weight, height, stage of development, body stores, activity levels and genetic factors. Disease process is a further consideration in sick infants and children. It is important to remember to calculate energy requirements and nutrient intakes based upon actual weight.

Fluid

Fluid requirements for infants and children are shown in Table 3.8.6. Breastfed babies will regulate fluid intake and demand feeding will ensure that the infant gets the correct volume of milk and therefore nutrients (Shaw & Lawson, 2007). Ideally, formula fed infants should be fed

Table 3.8.6 Recommended intakes of fluid and electrolytes for infants and children

Age			RNI			
	Weight (kg)	Fluid (mL/kg)	Sodium		Potassium	
			(mmol/day)	(mmol/kg/day)	(mmol/day)	(mmol/kg/day)
Males						
0–3 months	5.9	150	9	1.5	20	3.4
4–6 months	7.7	150	12	1.6	22	2.8
7–9 months	8.9	120	14	1.6	18	2.0
10–12 months	9.8	120	15	1.5	18	1.8
1–3 years	12.6	90	22	1.7	20	1.6
4–6 years	17.8	80	30	1.7	28	1.6
7–10 years	28.3	60	50	–	50	–
11–14 years	43.1	50	70	–	80	–
15-18 years	64.5	40	70	–	90	–
Females						
0–3 months	5.9	150	9	1.5	20	3.4
4–6 months	7.7	150	12	1.6	22	2.8
7–9 months	8.9	120	14	1.6	18	2.0
10–12 months	9.8	120	15	1.5	18	1.8
1–3 years	12.6	90	22	1.7	20	1.6
4–6 years	17.8	80	30	1.7	28	1.6
7–10 years	28.3	60	50	–	50	–
11–14 years	43.8	50	70	–	80	–
15–18 years	55.5	40	70	–	90	–

RNI, reference nutrient intake. (Source: Department of Health, 1991)

Table 3.8.7 Estimation of fluid requirements in children over 10 kg

Body weight (kg)	Estimated fluid requirement
11–20	100 mL/kg for the first 10 kg + 50 mL/kg for the next 10 kg
20 and above	100 mL/kg for the first 10 kg + 50 mL/kg for the next 10 kg + 25 mL/kg thereafter

Table 3.8.8 Energy requirements for low physical activity levels in children (FAO/WHO, 1973)

Age	Energy for maintenance and growth as % of total energy expenditure (per kg actual body weight)
<3 months	90
9–12 months	85
2–3 years	77
4–5 years	71
9–10 years	74

on demand, and for those under 6 months a fluid intake of 150 mL/kg is required. After 6 months, once an infant has been weaned, fluid requirement drops to 120 mL/kg as water is also obtained from food. After 1 year, thirst will determine how much fluid is taken (Shaw & Lawson, 2007). In clinical practice, fluid requirements for children over 10 kg are estimated using the equations shown in Table 3.8.7. However, overweight children will require less than the calculated volume per kilogram. For underweight children, fluid requirements should be calculated for the child's actual weight, but they may require increased energy and protein density for catch-up growth (Great Ormond Street Hospital, 2009).

Energy

Feeding infants younger than 6 months old with 150 mL/kg, either with breast milk or formula, will meet their nutritional needs if they do not have raised requirements. Young children continue to have high energy needs, but have a small stomach capacity and often variable appetites (Thompson, 1998). They therefore require a nutrient dense diet to meet needs, although from 2 years the fat content of their diet can be reduced and lower fat dairy products can be used, as long as they are thriving, have a good appetite and consume a well balanced diet. At 5 years, children can use fully skimmed milk if they also meet the above criteria. Energy requirements peak during the adolescent years when the individual is going through their growth spurt. Children with low physical activity levels require less energy. Table 3.8.8 gives an approximate guide to levels of energy intake for maintenance and

growth alone, with no allowance for energy for activity. For older children energy requirements can be estimated by using prediction equations as used in adults (see Chapter 2.1).

In 2011 SACN published a report on DRVs for energy and, following careful consideration of the evidence, recommended a revision to the estimated average requirements (EARs) for food energy for infants, children, adolescents and adults. However, the DRVs are intended only for use in healthy populations, not individuals or groups who require clinical management. Although exclusive breastfeeding is recommended for about the first 6 months of life, it is recognised that infants are fed in a variety of ways. Therefore, separate recommendations have been made for exclusively breastfed infants, breast milk substitute fed infants and those where the method of feeding is mixed or unknown (SACN, 2011; particularly Tables 14 and 15 within this report).

Protein

Protein should provide 7.5–12% of the energy of an infant feed (Koletzko et al., 2005), and 5–15% of the energy intake for older children (Jackson & Wooton, 1990). An adequate energy intake is essential at all ages, otherwise protein is metabolised as energy.

Vitamins and minerals

Vitamin and mineral requirements for normal children are provided by the DRVs. In disease states, requirements for certain vitamins and minerals will be different for each clinical condition. From 6 months infants who are breastfed, or taking <500 mL/day of formula or follow-on formula, should be given Healthy Start vitamins, providing vitamins A, C and D, and these should be continued until the child reaches 5 years of age. Other widely prescribed vitamin and mineral supplements are Abidec, Dalivit and Ketovite liquid and tablets.

Further reading

Great Ormond Street Hospital. (2009) Great Ormond Street nutritional requirements booklet. Available at www.gosh.nhs.uk/parents-and-visitors/clinical-support-services/dietetics/.

Lawson MS. (2005) Children: Nutritional requirements. In: Caballero B, Allen L, Prentice A (eds) Encyclopedia of Human Nutrition, 2nd edn. London: Elsevier.

More J, Jenkins C, King C, Shaw V. (2010) BDA Paediatric Group Position Statement: Weaning infants onto solid foods. Available at www.bda.uk.com.

Platt MPW. (2009) Demand weaning: infants' answers to professional dilemmas. Archives of Disease in Childhood 94: 79–80.

Platt MPW. (2009) Demand weaning: infants' answers to professional dilemmas. Archives of Disease in Childhood 94: 79–80.

Royal College of Nursing (RCN). (2010) Standards for the Weighing of Infants, Children and Young People in the Acute Health Care Setting. London: RCN.

Shaw V, Lawson M. (2007) Clinical Paediatric Dietetics, 3rd edn. Oxford: Blackwell Publishing.

Winstock A. (2005) Eating and Drinking Difficulties in Children. A Guide for Practitioners. Speechmark Publishing Ltd.

Internet resources

Child growth foundation   www.childgrowthfoundation.org

European Society for Paediatric Gastroenterology Hepatology and Nutrition (ESPGHAN)   www.espghan.med.up.pt

Infant and Toddler Forum   www.infantandtoddlerforum.org

Royal College of Paediatrics & Child Health (RCPCH)   www.rcpch.ac.uk

RCPCH Growth Charts   www.growthcharts.rcpch.ac.uk

STAMP screening tool   www.stampscreeningtool.org

World Health Organization (WHO) Child Growth Standards   www.who.int/childgrowth/en

References

Agostoni C, Decsi T, Fewtrell M, *et al.* (2008) Complementary feeding: A commentary by the ESPGHAN Committee on Nutrition. *Journal of Pediatric Gastroenterology and Nutrition* 46: 99–110.

Bates B, Lennox A, Bates C, Swan G. (2011) National Diet and Nutrition Survey. Headline results from year 1 and 2 (combined) of the rolling programme (2008/2009 and 2009/2010. London: Food Standards Agency/DH TSO.

Birch L, Marlin DW. (1982) I don't like it, I never tried it: Effects on exposure to food on two-year-old children's food preferences. *Appetite* 3: 353–360.

Brotherton A, Simmonds N, Stroud M. (2011) *Malnutrition Matters: Meeting Quality Standards in Nutritional Care.* Redditch: BAPEN.

Care Quality Commission and the Royal College of Nursing. (2010) *Observation prompts and guidance for monitoring compliance. Guidance for CQC inspectors. Outcome 5: meeting nutritional needs.* Available at www.cqc.org.uk. Accessed on 26 July 2013.

Carnell S, Edwards C, Croker H, *et al.* (2005) Parental perceptions of overweight in 3-5 year olds. *International Journal of Obesity* 29: 353–355.

Child Growth Foundation (CGF). (2012) *Growth Assessment Recommendations.* London: CGF. Available at www.childgrowthfoundation.org.

Cole TJ. (1997) Growth monitoring with the British 1990 growth reference. *Archives of Disease in Childhood* 76(1): 47–49.

Cole TJ, Freeman JV, Preece MA. (1998) British 1990 growth reference centiles for weight, height, body mass index and head circumference fitted by maximum penalized likelihood. *Statistics in Medicine* 17: 407–429.

Coulthard H, Harris G, Emmett P. (2009) Delayed introduction of lumpy foods to children during the complementary feeding period affects child's food acceptance and feeding at 7 years. *Maternal and Child Nutrition* 5: 75–85.

De Onis M, Garza C, Victora CG, *et al.* (2004) The WHO Multicentre Growth Reference Study: planning, study design and methodology. *Food and Nutrition Bulletin* 25(1): S15–S26.

Department of Health. (1991) Report on Health and Social Subjects No 41 *Dietary Reference Values for Food Energy and Nutrients for the United Kingdom.* London: The Stationery Office.

Department of Health. (1994) Report on Health and Social Subjects No 45 *Weaning and the Weaning Diet.* London: The Stationery Office.

Department of Health. (2007) Application of the WHO Growth Standards in the UK Department of Health. Available at www.sacn.gov.uk/

Department of Health. (2009) Birth to Five. Available at www.nhs.uk/birthtofive

Department of Health. (2010) Estates and facilities alert: Medical patient weighing scales. Ref: EFA/2010/001. Available at www.dh.gov.uk

Elia M. (2003) *Screening for malnutrition: a multidisciplinary responsibility. Development and use of the "Malnutrition Univer-sal Screening Tool" ("MUST") for adults. Malnutrition Advisory Group (MAG).* Redditch: BAPEN.

FAO/WHO. (1973) *Energy and Protein Requirements: Report of a joint FAO/WHO* ad hoc *expert committee.* FAO Nutrition Meetings Report Series No. 52. WHO Technical Report Series No. 522. Rome and Geneva: FAO/WHO.

Gerasimidis K, Keane O, Macleod I, *et al.* (2009) Criterion validity and interrater reliability of the Paediatric Yorkhill Malnutrition Score. *Journal of Paediatric Gastroenterology and Nutrition* 48 (Suppl 3): E47.

Gerasimidis K, Keane O, Macleod I, *et al.* (2010) A four stage evaluation of the Paediatric Yorkhill Malnutrition Score in a tertiary paediatric and district general hospital. *British Journal of Nutrition* 104(5): 751–756.

Gibson RS. (2005) *Principles of Nutritional Assessment,* 2nd edn. Oxford: Oxford University Press.

Great Ormond Street Hospital. (2009) Great Ormond Street nutritional requirements booklet. Available at www.gosh.nhs.uk/parents-and-visitors/clinical-support-services/dietetics/. Accessed 26 July 2013.

Harris G. (2000) Developmental, regulatory and cognitive aspects of feeding disorders. In: Southall A, Schwartz A (eds) *Feeding Problems in Children.* Oxford: Radcliffe Medical Press.

Hulst J, Zwart H, Hop W, *et al.* (2010) Dutch national survey to test the STRONGkids nutritional risk screening tool in hospitalised children. *Clinical Nutrition* 29: 106–111.

Jackson AA, Wooton SA. (1990) The energy requirements of growth and catch-up growth. In: Scrimshaw NS, Scürch B (eds) *Activity, Energy Expenditure and Energy Requirements of Infants and Children.* Lausanne: IDECG, pp. 185–240.

Jeffery AN, Voss LD, Metcalf BS, *et al.* (2005) Parents' awareness of overweight in themselves and their children: cross sectional study within a cohort (EarlyBird 21). *BMJ* 330: 23–24.

Koletzko B, Baker S, Cleghorn G, *et al.* (2005) Global standard for the composition of infant formula: recommendations of an ESPGHAN coordinated international expert group. *Journal of Paediatric Gastroenterology & Nutrition* 41: 584–599.

McCarthy HD, Jarrett KV, Crawley HF. (2001) The development of waist circumference percentiles in British children aged 5.0–16.9 years. *European Journal of Clinical Nutrition* 55: 902–907.

McCarthy H, Dixon M, Crabtree I, Eaton-Evans MJ, McNulty H. (2012) The development and evaluation of the Screening Tool for the Assessment of Malnutrition in Paediatrics (STAMP©) for use by healthcare staff. *Journal of Human Nutrition and Dietetics* 25: 311–318.

Michaelsen KF, Weaver L, Branca F, Roberts A. (2000) *Feeding and Nutrition of Infants and Young Children.* WHO Regional Publications, European Series, No 87. Denmark: WHO.

National Institute for Health and Care Excellence (NICE). (2008) *Improving the Nutrition of Pregnant and Breastfeeding Mothers and Children in Low Income Households.* London: NICE. Available at www.nice.org.uk/PH011.

Northstone K, Emmett P, Nethersole F and the ALSPAC Study Team. (2001) The effect of age of introduction to lumpy solids on foods eaten and reported feeding difficulties at 6 and 15 months. *Journal of Human Nutrition and Dietetics* 14: 43–54.

Poustie VJ, Watling RM, Ashby D, Smyth RL. (2000) Reliability of percentage ideal weight for height. *Archives of Disease in Childhood* 83: 183–184.

Royal College of Nursing (RCN). (2006) *Malnutrition. What Nurses Working with Children and Young People Need to Know and Do. An RCN Position Statement.* London: RCN.

Royal College of Nursing (RCN). (2010) *Standards for the Weighing of Infants, Children and Young People in the Acute Health Care Setting.* London: RCN.

Royal College of Paediatrics and Child Health (RCPCH). (2009) Department of Health Information for health visitors. Available at www.growthcharts.rcpch.ac.uk.

Scientific Advisory Committee on Nutrition (SACN). (2011) *Dietary Reference Values for Energy.* London: The Stationery Office.

Secker DJ, Jeejeebhoy KN. (2007) Subjective Global Nutritional Assessment for children. *American Journal of Clinical Nutrition* 85: 1083–1089.

Shaw V, Lawson M. (2007) *Manual of Paediatric Dietetics,* 3rd edn. Oxford: Blackwell Publishing.

Scottish Intercollegiate Guidelines Network. (2010) *No 115: Management of Obesity. A National Clinical Guideline.* Edinburgh: SIGN.

Tasker R, McClure R, Acerini C. (2008) *Oxford Handbook of Paediatrics.* Oxford: Oxford University Press.

Thompson JM (ed). (1998) *Nutritional Requirements of Infants and Young Children. Practical Guidelines.* Oxford: Blackwell Science.

Waterlow JC. (1972) Classification and definition of protein-calorie malnutrition. *BMJ* 3: 566–569.

Webster-Gandy J, Madden A, Holdsworth M. (eds) (2006) *Oxford Handbook of Nutrition and Dietetics.* Oxford: Oxford University Press.

WHO Multicentre Growth Reference Study Group. (2006) Assessment of differences in linear growth among populations in the WHO Multicentre Growth Reference Study. *Acta Paediatrica* 450 (Suppl): 56–65.

Winstock A. (2005) *Eating and Drinking Difficulties in Children. A Guide for Practitioners.* Speechmark Publishing Ltd.

World Health Organization (WHO). (2003) WHO Child Growth Standards. Available at www.who.int/childgrowth/en.

World Health Organization (WHO). (2006) Child growth standard in the UK: two prospective cohort studies. *Archives of Disease in Childhood* 93(7): 566–559.

Wright CM, Parkinson KN. (2004) Postnatal weight loss in term infants: what is normal and do growth charts allow for it? *Archives of Disease in Childhood Fetal and Neonatal Edition* 89(3): F254–F257.

Wright CM, Williams AF, Elliman D, *et al.* (2010) Using the new UK-WHO growth charts. *BMJ* 340: 1140.

Zemel BS, Riley EM, Stallings VA. (1997) Evaluation of methodology for nutritional assessment in children: Anthropometry, body composition, and energy expenditure. *Annual Review of Nutrition* 17: 211–235.

3.8.3 Growth faltering

Luise Marino and Rosan Meyer

Many terms are used interchangeably for growth failure, including malnutrition, faltering growth and undernutrition, but they do not necessarily describe the same level of undernutrition. Olsen *et al.* (2007) defined protein energy malnutrition (PEM) as nutritional deprivation amongst children in developing countries, whereas faltering growth is a term more commonly used for affluent societies. A variety of different methods with varying cut-offs exist to define these terms (Olsen *et al.*, 2007; Joosten & Hulst, 2011):

- Inadequate growth or weight gain for >1 month in a child under 2 years.
- Weight crossing more than two centiles for >1 month in child under 2 years.
- Weight loss or no weight gain for >3 months in a child older than 2 years.
- Changes in weight/age of >-1 standard deviation (SD) in 3 months for children under 1 year of age on growth charts.
- Change in weight for height of >-1 SD in 3 months for children aged 1 year or older on growth charts.
- Decrease in height velocity of 0.5–1 SD year at under 4 years and 0.25 SD/year at older than 4 years of age.
- Decrease in height velocity of >2 cm from preceding year during early/mid puberty.

The most common definition of growth faltering in the UK is weight crossing more than two centiles downwards over a period of 1 month. This would be equal to –0.68 of a Z score, indicating that a child may have weight faltering, but is not yet malnourished according to the WHO definition, e.g. moderate malnutrition using the WHO definition is $\leq$–2 Z scores.

Prevalence

The prevalence of growth faltering amongst healthy infants in the UK at 6–8 weeks has been reported as 6.1% (McDougall *et al.*, 2009) and it is believed that in the general infant and toddler population between 5% and 9% (McDougall *et al.*, 2009; Grimberg *et al.*, 2009) develop growth faltering. The prevalence of short stature in the general UK population is reported as being 2.3%. Being short in stature as a result of growth faltering has a more detrimental long term effect on health than being acutely undernourished. Acute undernutrition has little impact on cognitive development compared with severe and prolonged malnutrition (Victora *et al.*, 2010; Rudolf & Logan, 2005). Growth faltering in weight is more commonly seen in children under 2 years in developed countries (Panter-Brick *et al.*, 2004).

Chronically ill children have a higher prevalence of growth faltering, with a reported prevalence in hospitalised children in European countries (including the UK) ranging from 14% to 24% (Joosten & Hulst, 2011; Pawellek *et al.*, 2008). In middle income countries such as South Africa and Turkey, it is between 34% and 40% (Joosten & Hulst, 2011; Marino *et al.*, 2006). The prevalence of undernutrition within a hospital setting has remained unchanged for 20 years (Sullivan, 2010). It is therefore important that dietitians recognise growth faltering early and know how to nutritionally manage the condition.

Children considered to be at a greater nutritional risk include:

- Poorer socioeconomic groups (Panter-Brick *et al.*, 2004).
- Ethnic minorities (Panter-Brick *et al.*, 2004).

- An underlying medical condition (Levy *et al.*, 2009; Staiano, 2003).
- Extreme food fussiness (Haas, 2010; Haas & Maune, 2009).

Growth monitoring

Growth monitoring is an essential part of childhood. There are numerous growth charts, as discussed in Chapter 3.8.2, and it is important that the correct ones are used and that a child's measurements are plotted on them.

Normal growth

Optimal growth is one of the most important hallmarks of childhood, as poor growth has consequences impacting on school performance and cognitive development, and in adulthood has been associated with decreased ability to be socioeconomically active (Goulet, 2010). Intrauterine growth is the most rapid of all growth; the average birth weight in the UK is 3.3–3.5 kg. Birth weight loss occurs in the first few days of life (up to 10% is physiologically acceptable) and this is more common in those who are exclusively breastfed (Cole *et al.*, 2011; DeOnis & Onyango, 2003). It can take up to 2 weeks for an infant to regain this weight loss, which is reflected in the UK–WHO growth charts (Cole *et al.*, 2012; Shaw & Lawson, 2007).

Plotting faltering growth on a growth chart

To identify a child at risk of growth faltering it is important to review their growth trend. Figure 3.8.1 shows examples of growth curves (which can be applied to length or height and weight); children with the growth curves b or c would be considered to have malnutrition, with Z scores of <2.

Frequency of monitoring, catch-up growth and follow-up

As would be expected weight gain is one of the dietary goals; all children with growth faltering should be followed up, initially monthly (UNICEF, 2005), and when the child has caught up one to two centiles or has a weight for height of greater than 90% or 1 SD increase has been reached, supplementation should be reviewed.

At this stage the child is considered to be nutritionally rehabilitated (Patel *et al.*, 2005).

Acute and chronic growth faltering

It is important to establish if growth faltering is acute or chronic, as this impacts on the nutritional management. This can be established by the following:

- *Acute growth faltering* – normal length/height but low weight for height or for age. This normally represents an acute event of short duration, e.g. following a short episode of illness.
- *Chronic growth faltering* – short length for age but normal weight for height/length even though underweight for age, e.g. chronic illness such as end stage renal failure.
- *Acute on chronic growth faltering* – short length/height for age but low weight for height/length and underweight for age, e.g. chronic illness such as end stage renal failure with a recent lower respiratory tract infection.

Organic versus non-organic growth faltering

The terms organic and non-organic growth faltering have been used to describe poor growth related to medical disease (i.e. organic) versus non-medical causes (non-organic), including maternal deprivation, maternal depression and a dysfunctional mother–child relationship (Ramsay *et al.*, 2002). There is significant overlap between organic and non-organic faltering growth (Levy *et al.*, 2009). Ramsay *et al.* (2002) found that a significant number of the children who were classified with non-organic growth faltering had subtle neurodevelopmental disorders and pathophysiology (i.e. delayed sucking ability), but were otherwise medically well. It is therefore important to ensure good history taking when establishing the origin of growth faltering and not to exclude subtle organic disease.

Organic growth faltering

The reasons for poor growth in children with chronic disease is multifactorial and linked to increased requirements, reduced intake and disordered feeding. Children with chronic diseases such as chronic lung disease, gastrointestinal disorders and neuromuscular disorders

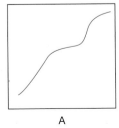
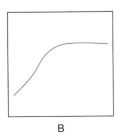
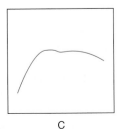

Figure 3.8.1 Examples of growth curves. (A) Growing well; (B) growth faltering; (C) malnutrition (source: WHO 2009. Reproduced with permission of WHO)

A   B   C

often have laboured breathing (Levy *et al.*, 2009; Haas & Maune, 2009), increasing nutrient requirements and/or increased nutrient losses through vomiting.

Non-organic growth faltering

The most common reason for non-organic growth faltering is a disrupted maternal–child relationship, which may occur due to various reasons, including neglect. In addition, toddlers are fussy eaters, as reported by 25–50% of parents (Jacobi *et al.*, 2003). Pickiness narrows the variety of foods consumed by young children (Harding *et al.*, 2010), increasing the risk of being underweight and having nutrient deficiencies, especially in those under 3 years (Ekstein *et al.*, 2010; Bowley *et al.*, 2007; Dovey *et al.*, 2008). A degree of neophobia and pickiness is considered to be developmentally appropriate and usually has no impact on growth (Richman *et al.*, 1975; Wright *et al.*, 2007).

Nutritional assessment

Nutritional assessment should include anthropometry, dietary, biochemical and clinical assessment. In addition, it is important to examine a child for signs of acute weight loss by looking at fat distribution. Some children are thin with no signs of wasting and it is important to distinguish between a well thin child, who is genetically slender, and a child who is growth faltering (UNICEF, 2005). In a child under 5 years, there should be a good layer of subcutaneous fat; therefore it is important to consider the following (Figure 3.8.2):

* What do the arms, shoulder, legs, buttocks look like?
* Is there evidence of temporal or facial wasting?
* Are there bracelets of fat around the wrist?
* Are there rolls of fat on the thighs?
* Looking from the side – are there buttocks or are they flat and sagging?
* Protruding ribs?
* Protruding hips?
* Does the stomach look out of proportion, e.g. is it distended?

Iron deficiency anaemia should be considered. In addition to inadequate iron intake, excessive intake of milk (≥600 mL/day) is also associated with low ferritin and haemoglobin levels (Cowin *et al.*, 2001). Pallor is a sign of anaemia and is easiest to see by looking at a child's palm. Compare the colour of skin on your palm to that of the child, grasping the child's hand gently on either side using one hand, but not bending the child's fingers backwards as this restricts blood flow. If the palm is pale, then there is some evidence of palmar pallor; however, if the child's palm is white, there is severe palmar pallor and iron treatment should be initiated.

Diet history

A complete, detailed dietary history is invaluable, especially questions relating to feeding and dietary intake. Some useful questions to establish dietary and feeding patterns include:

* What type of milk is usually given to the child? How much and how often?
* Are they still breastfed?
* What is the quantity of the main meal eaten? Is it appropriate?
* Did the child eat fish, meat or eggs in the last week and/or any foods excluded for religious or dietary reasons?
* Does the family have good access to food?
* If the child's food intake is poor, it is important to assess whether the child has anticipatory gagging, vomiting, difficulty swallowing or chewing at meal times, has a poor appetite or frequent loose stools (WHO, 2009; Levine *et al.*, 2011).

Dietary management

Nutrition requirements for catch-up growth

Energy and protein requirements

Disease specific recommended energy requirements should be used if available. These generally vary between 120% and 150% energy and protein requirements and the calculations are based on actual body weight (Shaw & Lawson, 2007). The focus should be weight gain and attaining growth with optimal balance between lean and fat mass (73% lean and 27% fat mass) in the new accrued

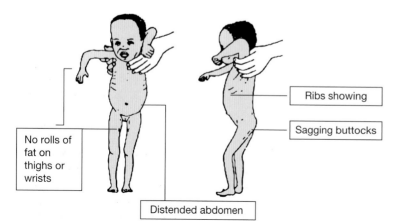

No rolls of fat on thighs or wrists

Ribs showing

Sagging buttocks

Distended abdomen

Figure 3.8.2 Appearance of an infant with severe wasting and growth faltering (source: WHO 2009. Reproduced with permission of WHO)

Table 3.8.9 Theoretical energy and protein intake for 5, 10 and 20 g/kg/day catch-up growth

Catch-up growth (g/kd/day)	Protein (g/kg/day)	Energy (kcal/kg/day)	Protein/energy (%)
5	1.82	105	6.9
10	2.82	126	8.9
20	4.82	167	11.5

tissue. Optimal catch-up growth is not only dependent on sufficient energy delivery, but also adequate protein (see Table 3.8.9). An ideal protein energy (PE) ratio for catch-up growth resulting in lean body mass accretion, rather than deposition of adipose tissue, has been shown to be 8.9–12% (Pencharz, 2010; Golden, 2009). Enriching products with modular additions of fat and carbohydrate alone often results in a PE of 4.5–6%, which does not favour optimal catch-up growth in growth faltering infants (Pencharz, 2010; Clarke *et al.*, 2007).

In younger children (<5 years) with moderate growth faltering, e.g. Z-score >–1, a weight gain of 10 g/kg/day is considered good. In these children for whom weight gain averages 5–10 g/kg/day, it is important to review whether intake targets are being met and/or whether an infection is being overlooked. Poor weight gain is <5 g/kg/day and in these children a review of biochemistry and intake should be considered. In older children (>5 years) weight gain may be slower, but 5–10 g/kg/day should still be achievable (WHO, 1999).

Vitamins and minerals

It is important to ensure that children with growth faltering also receive sufficient vitamins and minerals that aid catch-up growth. Insufficient micronutrients, in particular zinc and vitamin A, can lead to suboptimal catch-up growth. Multiple micronutrient supplementation, including vitamins A and D, zinc and iron, are effective in promoting catch-up growth in children under 5 years and should be considered a routine supplement in growth faltering children (Golden, 2009; Ramakrishnan *et al.*, 2009; Bhaskaram, 2002).

Iron

Even mild iron deficiency anaemia (IDA) can have a long term detrimental influence on mental and psychomotor development (Freeman *et al.*, 1998), although there are many confounders, including poverty, maternal education and prematurity (Aggett *et al.*, 2002). The management of IDA through iron fortified foods or supplementation results in improved growth, although improvements in cognitive outcomes have been harder to define (Domellof, 2009). At risk children should be encouraged to consume iron rich foods as part of their daily diet.

Zinc

Zinc supplementation of 10 mg/day in infants under 6 months and 20 mg/day in infants older than 6 months has been shown to significantly reduce morbidity in those with diarrhoeal disease and pneumonia (Bajait & Tawani, 2011; Baqui *et al.*, 2003, Aggarwal *et al.*, 2007). Zinc supplementation has also been shown to be effective in promoting linear growth (Ramakrishnan *et al.*, 2009; Allen, 1994). Zinc and iron supplementation should be given separately as zinc absorption is affected by iron (Anon, 1982), although this is seen more strongly with non-haem iron foods, e.g. fruit, vegetables, grains and nuts (Solomons & Jacob, 1981).

Nutritional management of infants and children with faltering growth

Nutritional management depends on the severity and type of growth faltering (organic versus non-organic). It is important to have good communication skills and start by exploring the circumstances at home, including the child's early feeding history (UNICEF, 2005). Enriched home foods can initially be tried in those children where growth faltering is not severe; however, if this approach fails, nutritional supplements should be tried. Energy dense ready to feed infant formulae that deliver energy and protein at an appropriate energy to protein ratio have been shown to significantly improve growth and nitrogen status (Clarke *et al.*, 2007). Although it is common practice to increase the nutrient density of standard powdered formulae, attention must be paid to the osmolality and renal solute load (Kin, 2007, Ziegler & Fomon, 1989). The older child may also require nutritionally complete sip feeds if initial nutritional treatment with enriched home foods fails. If this strategy fails, enteral tube feeding should be commenced (King & Davis, 2010). Where weight or length gain is not achieved, the nutrition care plan should include next steps, e.g. moving from home enriched foods to sip feeds and then to enteral tube feeding.

Psychological aspects of growth faltering

A child's intake can be influenced by parental interactions (Harris, 2010). The factors associated with poor intake may relate to poor appetite regulation (Drewett *et al.*, 2003) (early satiety), sensory hypersensitivity, late introduction of complementary foods and/or oral motor dysfunction. They may also have inherited parental traits of food fussiness, making them more likely to be neophobic and picky, which may impact on weight gain (Harris, 2010).

Behavioural management

Fussy eating can have a severe impact on growth, development and behaviour, resulting in significant parental anxiety. For many there may be no apparent medical cause for the child's extreme fussiness; however, parents will often describe early life feeding difficulties relative to reflux (Rommel *et al.*, 2003), food allergies (Haas, 2010), autism (Volkert & Vaz, 2010) and prematurity (especially gestational age <34 weeks' gestation) (Rommel *et al.*, 2003). Feeding skills develop through practise and keen

SECTION 3

observance, along with developmentally appropriate complementary feeding choices within a responsive feeding environment. Any disruption during this period, e.g. through illness, adverse reaction to food, acute or chronic pain, e.g. gastro-oesophageal disease or psychosocial stress, can be disruptive due to reinforcement that avoidance of food means pain or discomfort, etc. is avoided. This can lead to regression of feeding skills, non-acceptance of new foods and/or textures, altered motivation and feeding practices, leading to parental frustration and anxiety, which is mirrored back to the child (Haas, 2010; Rommel et al., 2003).

In children who have been unable to acquire age appropriate feeding skills, meal time avoidance strategies are commonly apparent, e.g. tantrums, volume limiting eating patterns to avoid pain, discomfort or anxiety, habitual gagging or vomiting, mouth sealing and food refusal, or limited variety of foods consumed (Haas, 2010; Kessler et al., 2010). Feeding difficulties, especially those severe enough to result in growth faltering, are usually managed within a multidisciplinary team (MDT) involving a physician, dietitian, speech and language therapist, psychologist, nurse, social worker and others (Rommel et al., 2003; Davis et al., 2010; Harding et al., 2009). The management strategy applied is individualised and dependent on the severity of the type of feeding difficulty and the level of involvement the family is able to make. Treatment may take the form of individual counselling sessions, group feeding programmes and/or a monitored home programme (Haas, 2010).

Behavioural management aspects in this programme aim to address hypersensitivity issues to texture, smell and taste of food through imaginative and messy play, with the aim of promoting sensory integration and building the child's confidence around new food experiences in addition to practising chewing skills. When trying to address issues related to texture and taste, changes should be implemented slowly and independently of each other, e.g. change one aspect of a meal at a time. It is also imperative to provide support to the parents. Video diaries of meal times provide insight into behavioural patterns of the child and caregiver (Harding et al., 2010). Useful techniques for parents at meal times include; limiting the length of meal times to 30 minutes or less, and reduction in reprimands, coercion and/or coaxing; the approach should be less directive or reprimanding in nature (Davis et al, 2010; Harding, 2009).

Severe to moderate malnutrition

Undernutrition in low and middle income countries affects a significant proportion of the paediatric population, resulting in an estimated 2.2 million deaths each year. The WHO has management plans for both severe and moderate malnutrition, describing the use of products such as F75 and F100 in addition to ready to use therapeutic food (RTUF). These are pastes made from peanut butter to which oil, sugar, milk or soya powder, and a micronutrient mix is added. The benefit of RTUF over liquid feeds such as F75 and F100, which are recon-

stituted from powdered milk, is that the high fat content of the paste retards microbial growth (WHO, 1999; WHO/UNICEF, 2009). Bacterial contamination of powdered milk feeds is a significant problem and increases the risk of morbidity and mortality (Andresen et al., 2007; Marino et al., 2007; FAO/WHO, 2007).

Where possible, severely malnourished children are managed within a community environment with the aim of reducing the incidence of hospital acquired infections (Phuka et al., 2009; Manary et al., 2004; Linneman et al., 2007). Many studies during the last decade have considered the benefits of RTUF at preventing growth faltering in high risk communities, in addition to their use in severe acute malnutrition and famine relief settings (Golden, 2010; Isanaka et al., 2009). The benefit of RTUF is high community acceptance, good taste, better catch-up growth, decreased bacterial contamination and no requirement for water (Phuka et al., 2009; Manary et al., 2004; Linneman et al., 2007, Matilsky et al., 2009).

Internet resources

Growth charts
   Cerebral Palsy growth charts www.lifeexpectancy.org/articles/GrowthCharts.shtml
   UKWHO growth charts www.rcpch.ac.uk/child-health/research-projects/uk-who-growth-charts-early-years/uk-who-growth-charts-early-years
   USA Center for Disease Control growth charts www.cdc.gov/growthcharts/cdc_charts.htm
   WHO child growth standards www.who.int/childgrowth/standards/en/
Infant & Toddler forum Little Peoples Plates www.littlepeoplesplates.co.uk/
Nutrition and Diet Resources www.ndr-uk.org

References

Aggarwal R, Sentz J, Miller MA. (2007) Role of zinc administration in prevention of childhood diarrhea and respiratory illnesses: a meta-analysis. *Pediatrics* 119(6): 1120–1130.

Aggett PJ, Agostoni C, Axelsson I, et al. (2002) Iron metabolism and requirements in early childhood: do we know enough?: a commentary by the ESPGHAN Committee on Nutrition. *Journal of Pediatric Gastroenterology and Nutrition* 34(4): 337–345.

Allen LH. (1994) Nutritional influences on linear growth: a general review. *European Journal of Clinical Nutrition* 48 (Suppl 1): S75–89.

Andresen E, Rollins NC, Sturm AW, Conana N, Greiner T. (2007) Bacterial contamination and over-dilution of commercial infant formula prepared by HIV-infected mothers in a Prevention of Mother-to-Child Transmission (PMTCT) Programme, South Africa. *Journal of Tropical Pediatrics* 53(6): 409–414.

Anon. (1992) Inhibition of zinc absorption by inorganic iron. *Nutrition Reviews* 40(3): 76–77.

Bajait C, Thawani V. (2011) Role of zinc in pediatric diarrhea. *Indian Journal of Pharmacology* 43(3): 232–235.

Baqui AH, Zaman K, Persson LA, et al. (2003) Simultaneous weekly supplementation of iron and zinc is associated with lower morbidity due to diarrhea and acute lower respiratory infection in Bangladeshi infants. *Journal of Nutrition* 133(12): 4150–4157.

Bhaskaram P. (2002) *Micronutrient malnutrition, infection, and immunity: an overview. Nutrition Reviews* 60(5 Pt 2): S40–45.

Bowley NA, Pentz-Kluyts MA, Bourne LT, Marino IV. (2007) Feeding the 1 to 7-year-old child. A support paper for the South African paediatric food-based dietary guidelines. *Maternal and Child Nutrition* 3(4): 281–291.

Clarke SE, Evans S, Macdonald A, Davies P, Booth IW. (2007) Randomized comparison of a nutrient-dense formula with an energy-supplemented formula for infants with faltering growth. *Journal of Human Nutrition and Dietetics* 20(4): 329–339.

Cole TJ, Wright CM, Williams AF. (2012) Designing the new UK-WHO growth charts to enhance assessment of growth around birth. *Archive of Disease in Childhood Fetal and Neonatal Edition* 97: F219–F222.

Cowin I, Emond A, Emmett P. (2001) Association between composition of the diet and haemoglobin and ferritin levels in 18-month-old children. *European Journal of Clinical Nutrition* 55(4): 278–286.

Davis AM, Bruce A, Cocjin J, Mousa H, Hyman P. (2010) Empirically supported treatments for feeding difficulties in young children. *Current Gastroenterology Reports* 12(3): 189–194.

de Onis M, Onyango AW. (2003) The Centers for Disease Control and Prevention 2000 growth charts and the growth of breastfed infants. *Acta Paediatrica* 92(4): 413–419.

Domellof M. (2009) Benefits and harms of iron supplementation in iron-deficient and iron-sufficient children. *Nestle Nutrition Workshop Series Pediatric Program* 65: 153–165.

Dovey TM, Staples PA, Gibson EL, Halford JC. (2008) Food neophobia and 'picky/fussy' eating in children: a review. *Appetite* 50(2–3): 181–193.

Drewett RF, Kasese-Hara M, Wright C. (2003) Feeding behaviour in young children who fail to thrive. *Appetite* 40(1): 55–60.

Ekstein S, Laniado D, Glick B. (2010) Does picky eating affect weight-for-length measurements in young children? *Clinical Pediatrics (Philadelphia)* 49(3): 217–220.

FAO/WHO. (2007) *Safe Preparation, Storage and Handling of Powdered Infant Formula: Guidelines.* Geneva: FAO/WHO.

Freeman VE, Mulder J, van't Hof MA, Hoey HM, Gibney MJ. (1998) A longitudinal study of iron status in children at 12, 24 and 36 months. *Public Health and Nutrition* 1(2): 93–100.

Golden MH. (2009) Proposed recommended nutrient densities for moderately malnourished children. *Food and Nutrition Bulletin* 30 (3 Suppl): S267–342.

Golden MH. (2010) Evolution of nutritional management of acute malnutrition. *Indian Pediatrics* 47(8): 667–678.

Goulet O. (2010) Growth faltering: setting the scene. *European Journal of Clinical Nutrition* 64 (Suppl 1): S2–4.

Grimberg A, Ramos M, Grundmeier R, *et al.* (2009) Sex-based prevalence of growth faltering in an urban pediatric population. *Journal of Pediatrics* 154(4): 567–572 e2.

Haas AM. (2010) Feeding disorders in food allergic children. *Current Allergy and Asthma Reports* 10(4): 258–264.

Haas AM, Maune NC. (2009) Clinical presentation of feeding dysfunction in children with eosinophilic gastrointestinal disease. *Immunology and Allergy Clinics of North America* 29(1): 65–75, ix.

Harding C. (2009) An evaluation of the benefits of non-nutritive sucking for premature infants as described in the literature. *Archives of Disease in Childhood* 94(8): 636–640.

Harding C, Faiman A, Wright J. (2010) Evaluation of an intensive desensitisation, oral tolerance therapy and hunger provocation program for children who have had prolonged periods of tube feeds. *International Journal of Evidence Based Healthcare* 8(4): 268–276.

Harris G. (2010) The psychology behind growth faltering. *European Journal of Clinical Nutrition* 64 (Suppl 1): S14–16.

Isanaka S, Nombela N, Djibo A, *et al.* (2009) Effect of preventive supplementation with ready-to-use therapeutic food on the nutritional status, mortality, and morbidity of children aged 6 to 60 months in Niger: a cluster randomized trial. *JAMA* 301(3): 277–285.

Jacobi C, Agras WS, Bryson S, Hammer LD. (2003) Behavioral validation, precursors, and concomitants of picky eating in childhood.

Journal of the American Academy of Child and Adolescent Psychiatry 42(1): 76–84.

Joosten KF, Hulst JM. (2011) Malnutrition in pediatric hospital patients: current issues. *Nutrition* 27(2): 133–137.

Kessler DB, Fortune EL, Werner EG, Stein MT. (2010) 11 month-old twins with food avoidance. *Journal of Developmental and Behavioral Pediatrics* 31(3 Suppl): S112–116.

King C, Davis T. (2010) Nutritional treatment of infants and children with faltering growth. *European Journal of Clinical Nutrition* 64 (Suppl 1): S11–13.

Levine A, Bachar L, Tsangen Z, *et al.* (2011) Screening criteria for diagnosis of infantile feeding disorders as a cause of poor feeding or food refusal. *Journal of Pediatric Gastroenterology and Nutrition* 52(5): 563–568.

Levy Y, Levy A, Zangen T, *et al.* (2009) Diagnostic clues for identification of nonorganic vs organic causes of food refusal and poor feeding. *Journal of Pediatric Gastroenterology and Nutrition* 48(3): 355–362.

Linneman Z, Matilsky D, Ndekha M, Manary MJ, Maleta K, Manary MJ. (2007) A large-scale operational study of home-based therapy with ready-to-use therapeutic food in childhood malnutrition in Malawi. *Maternal and Child Nutrition* 3(3): 206–215.

Manary MJ, Ndkeha MJ, Ashorn P, Maleta K, Briend A. (2004) Home based therapy for severe malnutrition with ready-to-use food. *Archives of Disease in Childhood* 89(6): 557–561.

Marino LV, Goddard E, Workman L. (2006), Determining the prevalence of malnutrition in hospitalized paediatric patients. *South African Medical Journal* 96 (9 Pt 2): 993–995.

Marino LV, Goddard E, Whitelaw A, Workman L. (2007) Prevalence of bacterial contamination of powdered infant feeds in a hospital environment. *South African Medical Journal* 97(7): 534–537.

Matilsky DK, Maleta K, Castleman T, Manary MJ. (2009) Supplementary feeding with fortified spreads results in higher recovery rates than with a corn/soy blend in moderately wasted children. *Journal of Nutrition* 139(4): 773–778.

McDougall P, Drewett RF, Hungin AP, Wright CM. (2009) The detection of early weight faltering at the 6-8-week check and its association with family factors, feeding and behavioural development. *Archives of Disease in Childhood* 94(7): 549–552.

Olsen EM, Petersen J, Skovgaard AM, Weile B, Jørgensen T, Wright CM. (2007) Failure to thrive: the prevalence and concurrence of anthropometric criteria in a general infant population. *Archives of Disease in Childhood* 92(2): 109–114.

Panter-Brick C, Lunn PG, Goto R, Wright CM.. (2004) Immunostimulation and growth faltering in UK infants. *American Journal of Human Biology* 16(5): 581–587.

Patel MP, Sandige HL, Ndekha MJ, Briend A, Ashorn P, Manary MJ. (2005) Supplemental feeding with ready-to-use therapeutic food in Malawian children at risk of malnutrition. *Journal of Health, Population and Nutrition* 23(4): 351–357.

Pawellek I, Dokoupil K, Koletzko B. (2008). Prevalence of malnutrition in paediatric hospital patients. *Clinical Nutrition* 27(1): 72–76.

Pencharz PB. (2010) Protein and energy requirements for 'optimal' catch-up growth. *European Journal of Clinical Nutrition* 64(S1): S5–S7.

Phuka J, Thakwalakwa C, Maleta K, *et al.* (2009) Supplementary feeding with fortified spread among moderately underweight 6-18-month-old rural Malawian children. *Maternal and Child Nutrition* 5(2): 159–170.

Ramakrishnan U, Nguyen P, Martorell R. (2009) Effects of micronutrients on growth of children under 5 y of age: meta-analyses of single and multiple nutrient interventions. *American Journal of Clinical Nutrition* 89(1): 191–203.

Ramsay M, Gisel EG, McCusker J, Bellavance F, Platt R. (2002) Infant sucking ability, non-organic failure to thrive, maternal characteristics, and feeding practices: a prospective cohort study. *Developmental Medicine and Child Neurology* 44(6): 405–414.

Richman N, Stevenson JE, Graham PJ. (1975) Prevalence of behaviour problems in 3-year-old children: an epidemiological study in a London borough. *Journal of Child Psychology and Psychiatry* 16(4): 277–287.

Rommel N, De Meyer AM, Feenstra L, Veereman-Wauters G. (2003) The complexity of feeding problems in 700 infants and young children presenting to a tertiary care institution. *Journal of Pediatric Gastroenterology and Nutrition* 37(1): 75–84.

Rudolf MC, Logan S. (2005) What is the long term outcome for children who fail to thrive? A systematic review. *Archives of Disease in Childhood* 90(9): 925–931.

Shaw V, Lawson LM (eds). (2007) *Clinical Paediatric Dietetics*, 3rd edn. Oxford: Blackwell Publishing.

Solomons NW, Jacob RA. (1981) Studies on the bioavailability of zinc in humans: effects of heme and nonheme iron on the absorption of zinc. *American Journal of Clinical Nutrition* 34(4): 475–482.

Staiano A. (2003) Food refusal in toddlers with chronic diseases. *Journal of Pediatric Gastroenterology and Nutrition* 37(3): 225–227.

Sullivan PB. (2010) Malnutrition in hospitalised children. *Archives of Disease in Childhood* 95(7): 489–490.

UNICEF. (2005) *Handbook : IMCI Integrated Management of Childhood Illness*. Geneva: WHO.

Victora CG, de Onis M, Hallal PC, Blössner M, Shrimpton R. (2010) Worldwide timing of growth faltering: revisiting implications for interventions. *Pediatrics* 125(3): e473–480.

Volkert VM, Vaz PC. Recent studies on feeding problems in children with autism. *Journal of Applied Behavior Analysis* 43(1): 155–159.

World Health Organization. (1999) *Management of Severe Malnutrition: A manual for Physicians and other Senior Health Workers*. Geneva: World Health Organisation.

World Health Organization. (2009) Rollins N (ed). *Guidelines for an Integrated Approach to the Nutritional Care of HIV-infected Children (6 months-14 years). Preliminary Version for Country Introduction. Chart Booklet*. Geneva: WHO.

World Health Organization/UNICEF. (2009) *WHO Child Growth Standards and the Identification of Severe Acute Malnutrition in Infants and Children A Joint Statement by the World Health Organization and the United Nations Children's Fund*. Geneva: WHO.

Wright CM, Parkinson KN, Shipton D, Drewett RF. (2007) How do toddler eating problems relate to their eating behavior, food preferences, and growth? *Pediatrics* 120(4): e1069–1075.

Ziegler EE, Fomon SJ. (1989) Potential renal solute load of infant formulas. *Journal of Nutrition* 119 (12 Suppl): 1785–1788.

3.8.4 Nutritional care of the preterm infant

Kelly Larmour

In 2009 the Department of Health published a toolkit detailing how neonatal services should be delivered in England (Department of Health, 2009). It supported the existing principle that neonatal services should be organised into managed clinical networks with hospitals working as teams to ensure that babies are cared for in appropriate settings. The 23 networks in England are comprised of three types of unit:

- Special care units (SCU).
- Local neonatal units (LNU).
- Neonatal intensive care units (NICU).

Currently not all units have access to a dietitian. It is hoped that recent recommendations may drive change in staffing levels [British Association of Perinatal Medicine Standards (BAPM), 2010].

The UNICEF/WHO definition of prematurity is given in Table 3.8.10. In England and Wales 9% of live births are preterm (Office for National Statistics, 2007). Preterm infants have missed some, or all, of the third trimester of pregnancy, which is a period of rapid growth when nutrient stores are laid down. Consequently, these infants have higher nutritional requirements compared with term infants. Preterm infants are born with immature organ systems and so establishing enteral feed tolerance can take some time.

Aims of dietetic intervention

The aims of the dietetic intervention are:

- To meet preterm nutritional requirements.
- To promote a postnatal growth rate equivalent to utero-foetal nutrient accretion (~15 g/kg/day).
- To establish enteral feeds as early and as safely as possible.
- To ensure that human milk is used wherever possible.

Methods of feeding preterm infants

Preterm infants are usually fed enterally or parenterally initially and transferred to oral feeding when appropriate.

Parenteral nutrition

Most babies weighing <1500 g will require parenteral nutrition (PN). The purpose of PN is to support growth while enteral feeds are being established. The Tsang *et al.* (2005) and ESPGHAN (Koletzko *et al.*, 2005) guidelines give details of the nutritional requirements for preterm PN.

Table 3.8.10 Definition of prematurity (UNICEF/WHO, 2004)

Preterm infant	Born before 37 weeks' gestation
Low birth weight	<2500 g
Very low birth weight	<1500 g
Extremely low birth weight	<1000 g

Enteral nutrition

One of the biggest challenges in neonatal dietetics is establishing enteral nutrition while minimising feed associated risks for developing necrotising enterocolitis (NEC).

Necrotising enterocolitis

This is a potentially life threatening gastrointestinal disease in which the bowel becomes inflamed and damaged to varying extents. Treatment varies from conservative management to extensive bowel resection. No single aetiological factor has been identified, but up to 95% of cases of NEC occur after enteral feeding has been introduced; osmolality, rate of feed advancement and choice of milk have been implicated. Neonatal units with enteral feeding guidelines have a lower incidence of NEC compared with units without them (Patole *et al.*, 2005).

Starting and advancing enteral feeds

Feeding guidelines will often categorise babies according to the risk of NEC. It is increasingly accepted that enteral feeds should be started on day 1 of life in stable preterm infants, but a more cautious approach is taken with babies considered to be high risk. The latter group are more likely to receive a period of minimal enteral feeding before feeds are advanced, while bigger, healthier babies start at larger volumes and progress to full feed volumes more quickly. Enteral feeds are given via orogastric or nasogastric (NG) tubes, with most units preferring bolus to continuous administration as this is more physiological and does not appear to affect the length of time it takes to achieve full enteral feeds (Premji & Chessell 2011).

Oral feeding

Babies must be able to coordinate their suck, swallow, breathe pattern before oral feeds are considered (usually ~33–36 weeks' gestational age). Early involvement of a neonatal speech and language therapist is essential in promoting appropriate oral feeding behaviour. Maternal expressed breast milk (MEBM) is the feed of choice for preterm infants; it confers advantages in terms of neurodevelopmental outcome and immune protection. In addition, preterm infants given MEBM are up to ten times less likely to develop NEC than those fed exclusively with formula milk (Guy *et al.*, 1997). The high nutritional requirements of preterm infants are not met by MEBM unless fed with large volumes and even then, it may not be adequate depending on the composition. In this case, breast milk fortifier can be added to breast milk. Some units routinely add fortifier when babies reach a certain intake, while others prefer to consider each baby individually.

If MEBM is not available, or contraindicated, donor milk is the second choice, as it has been shown to reduce the risk of NEC and is better tolerated compared with feeding formula milk. Due to heat treatment donor milk has slightly reduced immunological components and heat labile nutrients. In addition, fat is not so well absorbed; therefore, it is used in the short term as a tool for establishing enteral feed tolerance and babies are then weaned onto preterm formula in order to meet their requirements.

Preterm formula milks are designed to meet the needs of preterm infants if fed at 150 mL/kg/day. Term formula milks are not suitable to meet the needs of preterm infants and should be avoided. However in practice, some specialist term formula milks are used, as there is no preterm equivalent, e.g. hydrolysed formula and amino acid formula. Care should be taken to check nutritional composition against preterm requirements and manipulations such as supplementation or increasing feed concentration should be undertaken where necessary. NB: The composition of formula milk and breast milk fortifier may change; therefore, it is important to use up to date company information.

Preterm enteral nutritional requirements

Full details of enteral nutritional requirements are given by ESPGHAN (Agostoni *et al.*, 2010) and Tsang (2005). A summary of selected preterm enteral feeding requirements is shown in Table 3.8.11.

Growth

The most common reason for referral to a dietitian is poor growth. The causes are multifactorial and do not always relate solely to nutrition. Points to consider include:

- Check fluid allowance and consider increasing volume before making feed additions or changing feeds.
- Avoid use of energy supplements such as fat emulsions and glucose polymers as these add extra energy without increasing protein.
- Only make single changes at a time, e.g. increase feed volume before making feed additions such as breast milk fortifier.

Table 3.8.11 Preterm enteral nutritional requirements (Agostoni *et al.*, 2010)

Nutrient	Recommended intake	
	Infant <1 kg	Infant 1–1.8 kg
Fluid (mL/kg/day)	135–200	
Energy (kcal/kg/day)	110–135	
Protein (g/kg/day)	4–4.5	3.5–4
Sodium (mmol/kg/day)	3–5	
Calcium (mmol/kg/day)	3–3.5	
Phosphate (mmol/kg/day)	1.9–2.9	
Vitamin A (µg retinol equivalents/kg/day)	400–1000	
Vitamin D (µg/day)	20–25	
Folic acid (µg/kg/day)	35–100	
Iron (mg/kg/day)	2–3	

Vitamin and mineral supplementation

There are no national guidelines on vitamin and mineral supplementation for preterm infants and local policy should be adhered to. The nutrients that are most commonly given in this patient group are sodium, phosphate, fat soluble vitamins, folic acid and iron; zinc and selenium are also required by some infants.

Monitoring

Preterm infants should have their weight and head circumference measured weekly and their length fortnightly. The measurements should be plotted on the UK–WHO low birth weight growth charts as described in Chapter 3.8.2.

Post discharge formula

The Advisory Committee on Borderline Substances (ACBS) approves prescription of post discharge formula milks for catch-up growth in preterm infants (<35 weeks' gestation at birth) and small for gestational age infants up to 6 months corrected age. However, there is debate about indications for their use (Greer, 2007).

Weaning

The first evidence based weaning guideline for preterm infants was published in 2009 (King, 2009). Weaning should be considered in preterm infants between 5 and 8 months uncorrected age to ensure that sensitive periods for the acceptance of solids are not missed and to allow development of appropriate feeding skills. A practical guide for parents can be downloaded from the Bliss website (www.bliss.org.uk).

Neonatal dietitians' interest group

This is a sub group of the Paediatric Group of the British Dietetic Association providing an informal network for neonatal dietitians from the UK and Ireland. Further details can be found on the British Dietetic Association (BDA) web site.

Further reading

Jones E, King C. (2005) *Feeding and Nutrition in the Preterm Infant.* Edinburgh: Elsevier, Churchill Livingstone.

Internet resources

Bliss – for babies born too soon, too small, too sick   www.bliss.org.uk
British Association for Perinatal Medicine   www.bapm.org
  Neonatal Dietitians Interest Group   www.bapm.org/nutrition

British Dietetic Association   www.bda.uk.com
European Society for Paediatric Gastroenterology, Hepatology, and Nutrition   www.espghan.org
Royal College of Paediatrics & Child Health   www.rcpch.ac.uk
  Presentations, training materials and fact sheets on plotting preterm growth

References

Agostoni C, Buonocore G, Carnielli VP, *et al.* (2010) Enteral nutrient supply for preterm infants: Commentary room the European Society for Paediatric Gastroenterology, Hepatology, and Nutrition Committee on Nutrition. *Journal of Paediatric Gastroenterology and Nutrition* 50: 1–9.

British Association of Perinatal Medicine. (2010) Service Standards for hospitals providing neonatal care, 3rd edn. Available at www.bapm.org/publications/documents/guidelines/hosp_standards.pdf. Accessed 26 April 2012.

Department of Health. (2009) Toolkit for high quality neonatal services. Available at http://webarchive.nationalarchives.gov.uk. Accessed 26 April 2012.

Greer FR. (2007) Post-discharge nutrition: what does the evidence support? *Seminars in Perinatology* 31(2): 89–95.

Guy M, Nicoll A, Lynn R (eds). *British Paediatric Surveillance Unit – 11th Annual Report, 1996–97.* London: Research Division, Royal College of Paediatrics and Child Health, 1997. Summary available at www.inopsu.com/bpsu/publications/reports/nnec.html. Accessed 26 April 2012.

King C. (2009) An evidence based guide to weaning preterm infants. *Paediatrics and Child Health* 19(9): 405–414.

Koletzko B, Goulet O, Hunt J, *et al.* (2005) Guidelines on paediatric parenteral nutrition of the European Society of Paediatric Gastroenterology, Hepatology and Nutrition (ESPGHAN) and the European Society for Clinical Nutrition & Metabolism (ESPEN), supported by the European Society of Paediatric Research (ESPR). *Journal of Paediatric Gastroenterology and Nutrition* 41 (Suppl 2): S1–87.

Office for National Statistics. (2007) Preterm births Available at www.ons.gov.uk/ons/rel/child-health/preterm-births/preterm-births-data/index.html. Accessed 1 August 2013

Patole SK, de Klerk N. (2005) Impact of standardised feeding regimens on incidence of neonatal necrotising enterocolitis: a systematic review and meta-analysis of observational studies. *Archives of Disease in Childhood Fetal and Neonatal Edition* 90: F147–F151.

Premji S, Chessell L. (2011) Continuous nasogastric milk feeding versus intermittent bolus milk feeding for premature infants less than 1500 grams. *Cochrane Database of Systematic Reviews* CD001819

Tsang R, Uauy R, Koletzko B, *et al.* (2005) *Nutrition of the Preterm Infant: Scientific Basis and Practical Guidelines*, 2nd edn. Cincinnati: Digital Educational Publishing.

United Nations Children's Fund and World Health Organization (UNICEF/WHO). *Low Birthweight: Country, Regional and Global Estimates.* UNICEF, New York, 2004. Available at www.unicef.org/publications/files/low_birthweight_from_EY.pdf. Accessed 26 April 2012.

3.8.5 Community paediatrics
Clare Ewan

Paediatric community dietetics can be entirely based in the community or can cover both acute and community

work. For example, in a district general hospital the paediatric dietitian may cover both acute and community work for general paediatrics. Some posts may cover a particular speciality and be responsible for its caseload both in and out of hospital. Community paediatrics covers a wide range of work, and paediatric dietitians can be involved in many different activities. These can broadly be divided into clinical and health promotion work.

Clinical community dietetics

Clinical community work in paediatrics includes:

- *General dietetic outpatient clinics* – including one to one assessments, treatment and education around diet and nutrition specific to the particular child. They can be held in hospital outpatient departments, GP surgeries or health centres.
- *Multidisciplinary clinics* – these are held in a number of places, and can cover a variety of disciplines and conditions, e.g. diabetes clinics (jointly with diabetes specialist nurse and consultant), coeliac clinics (jointly with consultant) and feeding clinics held in hospital or special schools (jointly with speech and language therapist, community consultant, and other healthcare professionals).
- *Working with staff in child development services*, e.g. involvement in child centred assessments for children with special needs, in association with consultants and other healthcare professionals; ongoing involvement in multidisciplinary review meetings for children with special needs.
- *Home visiting* – this provides a service for children at home and school.
- *Training for mainstream and special schools* around particular nutritional issues for a child.
- *Home enteral tube feeding services* – services vary; some have a dedicated paediatric dietitian and some have access to a paediatric dietitian.

A smooth transition between acute and community dietetic care of the child is important; therefore, any dietetic plans must be practical and appropriate for the home and school environments. It requires good communication between all members of what can be a very large team of involved carers and healthcare professionals.

Health promotion community dietetics

Health promotion community work includes:

- Involvement in the development of local nutrition guidelines, e.g. development of weaning guidelines.
- Involvement in wellness programmes, e.g. community food initiatives such as food cafés and cooking skills classes.
- Working with community staff in children's centres and Sure Start facilities to provide information and support around promoting healthy eating for families (see Chapter 3.2).
- Working with schools in their delivery of the National Healthy Schools programme, e.g. school meals and packed lunch advice.
- Working with public health nursing teams (health visitors and school nurses) to provide education and training.
- Involvement in the development of local care pathways, e.g. for care of allergy patients and management of medical issues such as constipation.
- Working with public health agencies on the development and delivery of weight management programmes (see Chapter 7.13.4).
- Working at a strategic level to develop national programmes.

These areas rely on good communication and working between the different teams and agencies, to deliver services to benefit their communities (see Chapter 4.2).

Internet resources

British Dietetic Association   www.bda.uk.org
Dietitians: working to improve public health through nutrition (2008)

3.8.6 Autism

Emma Mills

Autism, or autistic spectrum disorder (ASD), is a neurodevelopmental disorder affecting social skills and communication, and is often characterised by stereotypic behaviours, including strict routines and desire for sameness. The spectrum ranges from individuals who are high functioning (Asperger's) to children with very severe disability. The prevalence is estimated at 5 per 1000 with four times more boys affected than girls. The incidence is increasing partly due to better diagnosis but mostly due to unknown environmental factors that trigger autism in those with a particular genetic susceptibility. It can occur in infancy, or later in life (>18 months), which is termed regressive autism. There is growing evidence that there are significant metabolic and nutritional differences between autistic and neurotypical (NT) children and this knowledge should improve management (Adams *et al.*, 2011). The key features of autism in children are shown in Table 3.8.12.

Dietetic evaluation and treatment

Children who have difficult feeding behaviours, significant GI symptoms and are under- or over-weight are likely to be referred to a hospital or community clinic. It is useful to request parents to complete a 7-day food diary of their child's current intake.

Gastrointestinal disturbance

Assuming tests for gastrointestinal disorders, e.g. coeliac disease, are negative, the full extent of gastrointestinal disturbance should be evaluated by taking a full and detailed history, including questions about constipation, diarrhoea, abdominal bloating and abdominal pain. Children with significant gastrointestinal disturbance may respond positively to a gluten and casein free diet (Knivsberg, 2001; Knivsberg et al., 2002; Millward et al., 2004). It is very important to explain to parents the commitment involved in following such a restrictive diet and that an improvement in symptoms may not occur. A trial period (minimum 3 months) should be started with a full evaluation of symptoms pre and post trial to assess effectiveness. A symptom score chart can be used to assess each symptom, i.e. 0 = symptom free and 5 = most severe. Telephone consultations can be done every 2–4 weeks, depending on how much support the family require, until the diet is established.

Selective eating

This will often be the biggest concern for parents and their attitude will influence future progress. Parents should be encouraged to keep meal times relaxed and enjoyable, and explain the need for different strategies with autistic children than those for regular fussy eaters. It is important to assess the diet for possible deficiencies and to supplement appropriately. Long term restrictive eating patterns in autistic children can have serious consequences, including permanent blindness (McAbee et al., 2009), optic neuropathy (Pineles et al., 2010) and reduced bone thickness (Hediger et al., 2008), especially for those following a restricted dairy diet.

Food exchanges

Food exchanges, which match new foods to accepted foods in terms of their sensory characteristics, may increase variety into the diet. Table 3.8.13 illustrates the food exchange system.

Growth and weight

Faltering growth is frequently a problem in young autistic children, often due to selective eating and or gastrointestinal disturbance. Many older children become overweight due to a chronically unbalanced diet rich in processed carbohydrates, salty and sweet foods, with a significant lack of fruit, vegetables, fish and wholegrain foods. The challenge is to stabilise gastrointestinal symptoms and increase the range of acceptable, healthier food choices (see Chapter 7.13.4).

Nutritional supplements

Autistic children with inadequate nutrient intakes on a restricted diet, either because of self selection or a casein and gluten free therapeutic diet, will require nutritional supplementation. Many supplements may be rejected because of their taste or smell so unflavoured supplements, e.g. paediatric Seravit (SHS) is often used, although this does not contain essential or long chain fatty acids. This should be combined with a liquid fish oil supplement, e.g. Ideal Omega Swirl (Barlean's) or Lem-0-3 (Cytoplan), or capsules, e.g. MorEPA and MorDHA (Nutritional Intelligence) according to individual tolerance.

Internet resources

British Dietetic Association   www.bda.uk
   Dietitians in Autism
   A Step-by-Step Guide to Food Acceptance
   Managing Eating & Mealtimes for Children with ASD

Table 3.8.12 Key features in autistic spectrum disorder

Key feature	Example
Major impairment in social skills/relationships	No cuddles or signs of affection with parents Difficulty making friends
Major impairment in communication	Avoidance of eye contact Limited verbalisation
Stereotypic behaviours	Insistence on certain daily rituals Repetitive behaviours
Gastrointestinal disturbance	Diarrhoea Constipation Abdominal bloating* Abdominal pain*
Selective eating	Limited range of acceptable foods Hypersensitivity to bitter and sour tastes Hyposensitivity to sweet and salty Pica
Growth and weight issues	Failure to thrive Overweight/obesity

*Non-verbal clues to look for are walking on tip toes, lying on stomach, leaning stomach against a hard surface, e.g. arm of a chair.

Table 3.8.13 Sensory characteristics of food exchange system

Acceptable food	Colour	Shape	Texture	Taste	Temperature	Exchange food
Bacon	Pink–brown	Rounded flat	Firm crispy	Salty	Hot	Pastrami Gammon Prawns
Cheese balls	Orange	Round	Crunchy	Salty	Ambient	Homemade salted popcorn

Brain and Body Nutrition

Food and Behaviour Research   www.fabresearch.org

National Autistic Society   www.autism.org.uk

References

Adams JB, Audhya T, McDonough-Means S, *et al.* (2011) Nutritional and metabolic status of children with autism vs neurotypical children and the association with autism severity. *Nutrition and Metabolism* 8: 34.

Hediger ML, England LJ, Molloy CA, Yu KF, Manning-Courtney P, Mills JL. (2008) Reduced bone cortical thickness in boys with autism or ASD. *Journal of Autism and Developmental Disorders* 38: 848–856.

Knivsberg AM. (2001) Reports on dietary intervention in autistic disorders'. *Nutritional Neuroscience* 4(1): 25–37.

Knivsberg AM, Reichelt KL, Høien T, Nødland M. (2002) A randomised controlled study of dietary intervention in autistic spectrum. *Nutritional Neuroscience* 5(4): 251–261.

McAbee GN, Prieto DM, Kirby J, Santilli AM, Setty R. (2009) Permanent visual loss due to dietary vitamin A deficiency in an autistic adolescent. *Journal of Child Neurology* 24(10): 1288–1289.

Millward C, Ferriter M, Calver SJ, Connell-Jones GG. (2004) .Gluten and casein free diets for ASD. *Cochrane Database and Systematic Reviews* 2: CD003498.

Pineles SL, Avery RA, Liu GT. (2010) Vitamin B12 optic neuropathy in autism. *Pediatrics* 126(4): 967–970.

3.8.7 Special needs

Clare Ewan

The term special needs covers a wide range of conditions, which can be related to a congenital problem or to an acquired injury. A paediatric dietitian has a role to play in many areas of the care of these children in both hospital and in the community. The impact on nutrition will vary depending on the condition:

- Lack of, or problems with, the physical aspects of feeding.
- Neurodevelopmental delay with a consequent delay in feeding abilities.
- Nutritional requirements that differ from the general paediatric population.
- Diet that needs to be manipulated for treatment and control of the condition.

These children have different nutritional requirements and there is a wide variation between children with the same condition, e.g. a child with Down's syndrome may be able to eat normally, whilst another may have significant difficulties managing foods within their mouth because of tongue thrust (involuntary pushing forward of the tongue). Dietetic needs can change over time, e.g. children with Prader–Willi syndrome frequently have faltering growth and may need tube feeding in their first year of life, whilst in later life their unrestricted eating means they are at greater risk of becoming obese.

Cerebral palsy

Cerebral palsy (CP) is a relatively common disorder that often requires paediatric dietetic input. It is a condition in which impairment to the immature brain affects movement, posture and coordination. (see Chapter 3.7). Problems in children with CP that affect their feeding and require dietetic support include:

- *Sucking and swallowing problems* leading to poor intake, with consequent faltering growth:

  ○ Energy supplementation may be needed.
  ○ Aspiration, with a risk of chest infections, can occur and therefore food textures may need to be modified or the child may need to be tube fed.
- *Gastro-oesophageal reflux*:
  ○ Feeds may need to be thickened.
  ○ Antireflux medication may be prescribed.
  ○ In severe cases fundoplication may be performed (see Chapter 3.8.27).
- *Faltering growth* – this may be due to a combination of poor intake, and increased requirements because of the involuntary movements.
- *Constipation* is common; advice around fluid and food intake may be needed in addition to medication.

Dietetic management

The paediatric dietitian will provide support to families and other carers, nursery and school staff, and respite carers. They work with other healthcare professionals in relation to the child's feeding, sometimes in multidisciplinary feeding clinics. These include:

- *Speech and language therapists* – advise on which types of fluids and foods should be offered to the child, e.g. thickening fluids and/or solids; using special teats (Habermann) or cups (Doidy); and on specific textures of foods to offer.
- *Physiotherapists* – advise on seating and posture that benefit feeding and improve muscle tone.
- *Occupational therapists* – advise on adaptations to the child's environment, e.g. seating and cutlery.

Children with special needs are usually measured and plotted on standard or condition specific growth charts. For many children with special needs, there are challenges around weighing and measuring height. Sitting scales or hoist scales may be used. For children who cannot stand, a supine stadiometer suitable for older children can be used (Stewart *et al.*, 2006). Lengths can be difficult to obtain in children with scoliosis or contractures, so alternative estimates of linear growth are sometimes used (Spender *et al.*, 1989). Down's syndrome specific growth charts are available in the UK (see Chapter 3.8.2). Clinical growth charts for children with CP have recently been developed in the US (Brooks *et al.*, 2011).

Other conditions that are classified as special needs and in which paediatric dietitians can be involved include autism, epilepsy, neurological problems, e.g. Parkinson's disease and multiple sclerosis, and inherited metabolic diseases. If a child presents with a rare condition, the charity Contact a Family (www.cafamily.org.uk) may be helpful for parents and healthcare professionals.

Internet resources

Cerebra   www.cerebra.org.uk
   A charity that aims to help improve the lives of children with brain related conditions.
Contact a Family   www.cafamily.org.uk
   Information on rare conditions and general advice on long term conditions.

Dietitians interested in special children
   A network for paediatric dietitians working with children with complex physical needs and learning disabilities. Joanna .Mankelow@sash.nhs.uk
Down's Syndrome Association   www.downs-syndrome.org.uk
Down's Syndrome Medical Interest Group   www.dsmig.org.uk
Harlow printing   www.healthforallchildren.co.uk
   Growth charts for children with Down's syndrome, Turner's syndrome, Williams' syndrome, Noonan syndrome and homozygous sickle cell disease.
SCOPE   www.scope.org.uk
   Charity supporting disabled people.

References

Brooks J, Day S, Shavelle R, Strauss D. (2011) Low weight, morbidity, and mortality in children with cerebral palsy: new clinical growth charts. *Pediatrics* 128: e299.
Spender QW, Cronk CE, Charney EB, Stallings VA. (1989) Assessment of linear growth of children with cerebral palsy: use of alternative measures to height or length. *Developmental Medicine and Child Neurology* 31: 206–214
Stewart L, McKaig N, Dunlop C, *et al.* (2006) *Guidelines on Dietetic Assessment and Monitoring of Children with Special Needs with Faltering Growth.* Birmingham: BDA. Available at www.bda.uk.com. Accessed 26 April 2012.

3.8.8 Paediatric general medicine
Katie Harriman

Paediatric general medicine is the initial point of contact for a child's medical care after consultation with a GP. Children are assessed in outpatients or if an emergency, on a paediatric emergency assessment unit or general ward within a hospital setting. Children can be admitted for a number of reasons but the main ones are bronchiolitis, faltering growth and general assessment. Most district general hospitals (DGHs) have a paediatric ward and this is where most dietitians will have their first experience of working with children. Referrals to the dietitian are made by the consultant, a member of the acute medical team or by the ward nursing staff after nutritional screening to assess the nutritional risk of the patient.

Care Quality Commission (2010) standards ensure that patients are nutritionally screened within 24 hours of admission and that all patients are provided with adequate hydration and nutritious foods to meet their needs. It is imperative to support those who may require extra help with eating and drinking by providing adapted cutlery and closed lidded cups at ward level. This enables children's hospitals to reduce the risk of poor nutrition and dehydration by encouraging and supporting children to receive adequate nutrition and hydration.

The range of patients seen will differ depending on whether the paediatric dietitian is working in a DGH or a tertiary children's hospital (TCH). The paediatric dietitian working within a DGH will encounter a wide range of medical conditions, including food behavioural problems, constipation, breastfeeding advice, weaning advice, toddler diarrhoea, food allergy and intolerances, feeding problems in newborn babies and infants, gastro-oesophageal reflux, growth faltering, type 1 diabetes, obesity, neurological conditions, respiratory diseases and enteral tube feeding. The paediatric dietitian will see other specialities often with shared care with a TCH. Conditions including metabolic diseases and cystic fibrosis may be managed at these centres. These children may still be admitted to their local medical ward and therefore a good working relationship with the tertiary specialist dietetic team is essential in supporting the care of these children and families. The paediatric dietitian working within a TCH will assess acute general patients, including those with all the above conditions, through to patients with complex syndromes with feeding difficulties.

A nutritional assessment will be carried out following a trigger from the nutritional screening process or medical referral. This involves translating individual nutritional requirements into practical dietary and feeding practices or regimens, to optimise health, growth and development within the parameters of the child's particular condition. It is essential to design a practical plan tailored to the individual, so that families and carers can achieve the desired dietary changes.

Paediatric dietitians will be required to work closely with the MDT to provide advice regarding nutritional assessment and an appropriate working plan for the patient to be implemented with the help of nursing staff. Other professionals that may be involved in an acute setting include speech and language therapists, play specialists, food provision staff and specialist nurses. Upon discharge, it is vital to liaise with health visitors, pharmacists, community children's nurses, social workers, GPs, school and home enteral tube feeding (HETF) services to provide a safe discharge and continuity of care in the community.

Complex discharges are common on a general medical or paediatric ward. Some patients have multiagency care and it is therefore critical to attend multidisciplinary meetings to work effectively with these professionals to provide a safe discharge. The general medical dietitian will also promote education and training at ward level to promote awareness on topics such as effectiveness of nutritional screening, policies around bringing food from home into hospital, accurate use of growth charts, accurate measuring and recording of anthropometric measurements, discharging a patient home on HETF, the range of nutritional supplements and enteral feeds available and their uses, and improving awareness of standard operating procedures.

General medical paediatric dietetics also means seeing patients in regular outpatient clinics both in hospital and the community. Patients should be seen within 18 weeks of the initial referral date (Department of Health, 2012).

Internet resources

Care Quality Commission. (2010) Provider compliance assessment outcome 5 (Regulation 14): Meeting nutritional needs. Available at www.cqc.org.uk/search/apachesolr_search/PCA%205. Accessed 16 May 2012.

References

Department of Health. (2012) Referral to treatment waiting times. Available at www.dh.gov.uk. Accessed 11 December 2012.

3.8.9 Paediatric oral nutritional support
Sara Mancell

A focus on oral nutrition is particularly important in young children as this is when oral motor skills and appropriate feeding behaviours are developed (Chailey Heritage, 1998). When planning oral nutritional support, it is important to be aware of the different settings where children eat. It is often useful to involve extended family members, schools or nurseries in planning.

Methods for supporting oral nutrition

These include:

- Regular meals and snacks.
- Food fortification.
- Energy dense foods.
- Supplements.
- Concentrating formula or feed (used primarily for infants on formula milk or older children on specialist powder based feeds).

Regular meals and snacks

Children should be offered regular meals and snacks to avoid grazing on snacks throughout the day. It may help to have set meal and snack times with at least 2 hours between each. It is important to persist with offering snacks at set times even if they are often refused as children may agree to eat these on some of the days if the opportunity is presented to them. The timing of drinks offered should be considered as many young children find it easier to drink than to eat; it may be better to have drinks after eating.

Food fortification

The nutrient density of a child's usual dietary intake can be increased by adding in foods such as butter, margarine, oil, double cream, jam, syrup, honey, sugar, skimmed milk powder or cheese (see Chapter 6.3).

Energy dense foods

High energy snacks may improve the nutritional status of children with faltering growth (Kasese-Hara et al., 2002). It is, however, important that children continue to have a nutritious, balanced diet, especially those who require long term nutritional support. Examples of high energy snacks are shown in Table 3.8.14. High energy snacks can be an inexpensive method of boosting energy intake.

Supplementation

Children's diets can be supplemented with ready made sip feeds or modules based on fat, carbohydrate or protein. Sip feeds are easy to use, time saving and avoid the risk of reconstitution errors. In contrast, recipes using feed modules must be followed very carefully to maintain the correct balance of nutrients. However, they can be used to achieve precise, tailor made macronutrient profiles.

High energy formulae and sip feeds

High energy formulae and sip feeds are shown in Appendix A10.

Supplement modules based on protein, energy and carbohydrate

Appendix A10 lists protein and energy modules that can be added to foods and drinks. The protein to energy ratio (PER) must be preserved when using these products, particularly in preweaned infants relying solely on formula. The PER should be approximately 7–12% in infants (Koletzko et al., 2005) and 5–15% in older children (Jackson & Wooton, 1990).

Table 3.8.14 Examples of energy dense snacks for children

Name	Individual portion size (g)	Energy (kcal/portion)	Protein (g/portion)	Average cost [per 100 kcal (418 kJ)]
Sesame Snack Bar	30	158	5.0	0.09
Shortbread biscuit	12	65	0.9	0.04
Flapjacks	33	150	1.9	0.11
Oatcakes	8	35	0.8	0.06
Mars bar	58	259	2.4	0.11
Alpen strawberry with yoghurt cereal bar	29	121	1.7	0.30
Dairylea Strip cheese	21	73	4.4	0.39
Babybel cheese	20	63	4.5	0.47
Houmous	50	160	3.7	0.15
Sunmaid Raisin pack	42.5	129	1.3	0.31
Nestle Rolo Dessert	70	172	2.2	0.29
Cadbury Flake Twinpot	90	216	4.0	0.36
Avocado wedges	80	155	1.5	0.22
Yeo Valley Greek Yoghurt with honey	100	152	4	0.22

Concentrating feeds or formulae

Another method of increasing the nutrient density is to concentrate infant formulae or specialist powder based feeds. Adjusting the concentration by adding more powder per 100 mL and maintaining the total fluid volume, increases the nutrient density of the feed. It is important that care is taken when adjusting the concentration of a feed and must only be done by an experienced paediatric dietitian.

Cost of oral nutritional support

Oral nutritional support products are expensive and compliance can be poor; therefore, energy dense snacks may be more suitable. The aim should always be to tailor nutritional support individually to maximise compliance and, therefore, effectiveness of treatment.

Internet resources

British Dietetic Association www.bda.uk.com
    Paediatric group publication

Help my child gain weight: Advice for children who need extra calories
British National Formulary for Children (BNFC) www.bnfc.org
London Procurement Program www.lpp.nhs.uk
    Paediatric nutritional products – cost per 100 kcal (2011)

References

Chailey Heritage. (1998) *Eating and Drinking Skills for Children with Motor Disorders.* Lewes: Chailey Heritage.
Jackson AA, Wooton SA. (1990) The energy requirements of growth and catch-up growth. In: Scrimshaw NS, Scurch B. (eds) *Activity, Energy Expenditure and Energy Requirements of Infants and Children.* Lausanne: IDECG, pp. 185–214.
Kasese-Hara M, Wright C, Drewett R. (2002) Energy compensation in young children who fail to thrive. *Journal of Child Psychology and Psychiatry* 43: 449–456.
Koletzko B, Baker S, Cleghorn G *et al.* (2005) Global standard for the composition of infant formula: recommendations of an ESPGHAN coordinated international expert group. *Journal of Paediatric Gastroenterology & Nutrition* 41: 584–599.

3.8.10 Paediatric enteral tube nutrition

Kate Harris and Sue Williams

The main principles of enteral nutrition are similar for children and adults (see Chapter 6.4). Enteral nutrition is suitable for infants and children who have a partially functional gastrointestinal tract but who are unable to meet their nutritional requirements orally. Table 3.8.15 outlines indications for enteral tube nutrition. Enteral support can be short or long term and it can provide complete or partial nutrition, or used for fluid or medica-tion provision only. Enteral nutrition must always be tailored to meet the child's individual needs.

Enteral formulae

The type of enteral formulation or feed chosen will depend on age, weight, gut function, (e.g. absorption capacity) and dietary restrictions (e.g. allergy or metabolic

Table 3.8.15 Indications for enteral feeding in children (adapted from Braegger *et al.* 2010, table 2, p. 112. Reproduced with permission of the *Journal of Pediatric Gastroenterology and Nutrition*)

Indication	Examples
Inadequate oral intake due to unsafe swallow or poor suck	Prematurity, neurological disorders, e.g. cerebral palsy, congenital disorders such as tracheo-oesophageal fistula, oncology tumours, trauma and burns
Malabsorption and digestive disorders	Cystic fibrosis, short bowel syndrome, food allergy
Gastrointestinal motility disorders	Gastro-oesophageal reflux, chronic pseudo-obstruction
Increased nutritional requirements and losses	Extensive burns, liver disease, heart disease
Growth failure or chronic malnutrition	Anorexia nervosa, non-organic growth faltering
Disease treatment	Crohn's disease
Metabolic diseases	Type 1 glycogen storage disease

conditions). Assessing the requirements for each individual child is important when choosing which feed to use. A generic guide to feeds is summarised in Table 3.8.16 and further details are available in Appendix A10. NB: Age and weight parameters will vary between feed suppliers. Due to a European Union Commission Directive (1999/2006) most feeds for children over 1 year are nutritionally complete.

Routes of enteral feeding

As in adults tubes can be placed in the stomach (gastric) or the jejunum for feeding. The choice of access is determined by gastrointestinal function, feeding duration and aspiration risk. The advantages, disadvantages and contraindications for nasogastric (NG), gastrostomy and jejunostomy feeding routes are summarised in Table 3.8.17.

Gastric feeding

Orogastric feeding

This route is primarily used in neonatal units.

Nasogastric feeding

This type of tube is often used when feeding is likely to be short term (<6–8 weeks). These tubes are considered non-invasive and relatively quick to place. However, they can be traumatic to place and are associated with impaired body image in older children. Younger children may experience oral food aversion secondary to NG tube use (Mason *et al.*, 2005, Byron, 2007). Aspiration due to misplacement or tube dislodgement is a safety risk. See Chapter 6.4 for details on placement checking.

Gastrostomy

This tube is used for longer term feeding, but is indicated in the short term when NG tube placement is not feasible. The most common is percutaneous endoscopic gastrostomy (PEG), but radiologically inserted gastrostomy (RIG) or surgical placements are also available. They may be replaced for a low profile skin level device once the stoma tract is formed, normally after 3 months. They are associated with exacerbating gastro-oesophageal reflux disease (GORD) and so a fundoplication may be created at the

same time as placement (Vernon-Roberts & Sullivan, 2007) (see Chapter 3.8.27).

Jejunal feeding

Jejunal feeding is indicated when gastric feeding is not viable, e.g. in gastroparesis, severe GORD, gastric outlet obstruction.

Nasojejunal feeding

These tubes are difficult to place and can migrate into the stomach or higher in the gastrointestinal tract. They are very vulnerable to blocking and are not replaceable at home.

Jejunostomy

Surgical percutaneous endoscopic jejunostomy (PEJ) or jejunal extensions through a PEG (PEG-J) may be indicated longer term. Traditionally, feeding has used continuous provision of a hydrolysed feed. However, polymeric formulae are increasingly being used due to good tolerance (ESPHGAN, 2010). The main complications for this type of feeding are dumping syndrome, abdominal pain and diarrhoea, especially if a hyperosmolar feed is used (see Table 3.8.17).

Regardless of feeding routine, time needs to be taken with the child and family to explain the planned procedure and aftercare. Communication aids can be used, e.g. cartoons, toys, videos, play therapist and specialist literature, as available (GOSH, 2009).

Feed initiation

Feed initiation will depend on the child's clinical status. Infants may start feeding with 1 mL/hour whilst adolescents may tolerate 100 mL/hour or higher. Refeeding risk must be assessed prior to initiation (ESPHGAN, 2010). Careful monitoring of anthropometry, biochemistry and tolerance is vital.

Feeding methods

There are two main methods of feed delivery; continuous and intermittent (bolus). Intermittent feeding has been

Table 3.8.16 Generic guide to paediatric enteral feeds**

Age	Weight (kg)	Comments	Type of feed				
			Standard	High energy	Low energy	Fibre	Impaired gut function or allergy
<12 months	Up to 8		Expressed breast milk Pasteurised donor breast milk Standard infant formula*	Specialist formula, e.g. Infatrini (Nutricia), Similac (Abbott), SMA High Energy			Hydrolysed or amino acid feeds
1–12 years	8–45	Milk based Premixed, sterile, ready to use packs Lactose free Gluten free Nutritionally complete	1 kcal/mL Suitable for most children, promoting adequate fluid intake+	1.5 kcal/mL Useful when fluid is restricted	0.75 kcal/mL May be used for children with low energy requirements, e.g. neurological conditions++ 8–10 years: alternatively low volumes of adult feeds can be used but use with caution due to increased protein and micronutrient content+++	Available ± fibre Fibre may promote improved bowel function@	Hydrolysed or amino acid feeds
>12 years	>45	Use feeds designed for 7–12 years if small stature Normal stature – adult feeds NB: Caution needed to avoid excessive amounts of protein and micronutrients					Adult elemental feeds introduced gradually due to high osmolality NB: Adult partially hydrolysed feeds are not suitable for allergies

*See BDA Paediatric Group (2010)
**See Appendix A1 for details of available paediatric feeds
+Diamante (2010)
++Sullivan et al. (2006)
+++ESPHGAN (2010)
@NICE, (2010)
NB: Weight and age parameters will vary depending on the feed company.

Table 3.8.17 Advantages, disadvantages and contraindications of different feeding routes

	Nasogastric feeds	Gastrostomy feeds	Jejunostomy
Advantages	Non-invasive Relatively cheap Placement taught to carer/older child	No need to reinsert Devices can be discrete Less associated oral aversion	Reduced aspiration risk No frequent tube reinsertion
Disadvantages	Nasal and throat irritation/ulceration Irritation to cheek Misplacement on passing tube Easy displacement, need to replace frequently Need to check position frequently Gastric pH affected by milk, medications, etc. Can be difficult to aspirate Aspiration risk Visible Traumatic to place Difficult to unblock Oral aversion and difficulty reinstating oral intake Nausea and vomiting Change in bowel habits – short term only	Can exacerbate GORD May pull at tube Local infection risk Leakage can damage surrounding skin Over granulation Buried bumper Aspiration risk Can block Nausea and vomiting Change in bowel habits – constipation/diarrhoea Difficulty reinstating oral intake and tube dependency	Tube blockage Easily dislodged Placed with general anaesthetic Nausea and vomiting Bloating Dumping syndrome Continuous feeds only Change in bowel habits – constipation or diarrhoea Difficulty reinstating oral intake
Contraindications	Severe vomiting Intestinal/ gastric obstruction Uncontrolled GORD	Gross ascites Severe obesity Clotting abnormalities Ventriculo-peritoneal shunt GI obstruction Severe GORD	Complete intestinal obstruction Clotting abnormalities Gross ascites Severe obesity

SECTION 3

shown to be more physiologically normal and allows greater mobility. However, continuous feeding is often better tolerated in those with GORD and can be less labour intensive. Flexibility is key to ensure that the feed plan suits the patient's lifestyle. A combinations of both methods is also possible.

Overnight feeding

Caution must be used to reduce risks of aspiration, especially in children with neurological impairment (Health Improvement Scotland, 2007). Many community teams no longer use NG night feeds, unless clinically indicated and risk assessed.

Complications

Common complications are the same as those seen in adults and include gastrointestinal disturbances, refeeding risk and potential drug–feed interactions (BAPEN, 2004) (see Chapter 6.4).

Equipment

Pumps, giving sets, pH strips, reservoirs and syringes may be needed. All equipment should be National Patient Safety Agency (NPSA) compliant to avoid confusion between intravenous and enteral equipment.

Home enteral nutrition

Moving from hospital to home is a very chaotic time for families and a smooth discharge to the community team for ongoing support is vital. Delivery services from feed manufacturers provide feed, plastics and service pumps, and are used by most home fed children (BAPEN, 2010). These services should be set up before the patient leaves hospital. Liaison with and training of family members as well as nursery and school staff is vital to ensure the feeding plan is safe and achievable. Training should cover reasons for enteral nutrition, goals and outcomes, safety issues, infection control, feeding equipment, social and practical issues, emergency procedures and contact details, oral guidelines and information on equipment deliveries (Vernon-Roberts, 2009). Contact with charities such as PINNT (Patients on Intravenous and Nasogastric Nutrition Therapy; www.pinnt.com/Half-PINNT.aspx) may provide support for families.

Further reading

Baker SS, Baker RD, Davis AM. (2007) *Pediatric Nutritional Support*. Burlington: Jones and Bartlett Learning.
BDA Paediatric Group. (2010) Infant milk formulas in the UK. Available at http://members.bda.uk.com/groups/paediatric/Formulas Table.pdf. Accessed 1 July 2011.
Braegger C, Decsi T, Dias JA, *et al*. (2010) Practical approach to paediatric enteral nutrition: A comment by the ESPGHAN Committee on Nutrition. *Journal of Paediatric Gastroenterology and Nutrition* 51(1): 110–122.

Sullivan PB. (2009) *Feeding and Nutrition in Children with Neu-rodevelopmental Disability*. London: Mac Keith Press.

Internet resources

British Dietetic Association   www.bda.uk.com
  National Patient Safety Alert   www.nhs.npsa.uk
    Reducing the harm caused by misplaced nasogastric feeding tubes in adults, children and infants (2011)   www.nrls.npsa.nhs.uk/alerts/?entryid45=129640
Patients on Intravenous & Nasogastric Nutrition Therapy (PINNT) www.pinnt.com
  Half PINNT For our younger feeders   www.pinnt.com/Half-PINNT.aspx
UK Association for Milk Banking   www.ukamb.org

References

BAPEN. (2004) Advancing clinical nutrition, drug administration via enteral feeding tubes: A guide for general practitioners and community pharmacists. Available at www.bapen.org.uk/pdfs/d_and_e/de_gp_guide.pdf. Accessed 10 July 2011.
BAPEN (2010) Annual BANS report. Available at www.bapen.org.uk/pdfs/bans_reports/bans_report_10.pdf. Accessed 1 July 2011.
Braegger C, Decsi T, Dias JA, *et al.* (2010) Practical approach to paediatric enteral nutrition: a comment by the ESPGHAN committee on nutrition. *Journal of Pediatric Gastroenterology and Nutrition* 51(1): 110–122.
Byron M. (2007) Interventions with children who are tube-fed. In: Southall A, Schwartz A. (2007) *Feeding Problems in Children*. Oxford: Radcliffe Medical Press.
Diamante A. (2010) Enteral formulas in children: which is the best choice? *Nutritional Therapy & Metabolism* 28(1): 40–45.
ESPGHAN. (2010) Practical approach to paediatric enteral nutrition. *Journal of Pediatric Gastroenterology and Nutrition* 51: 110–122.

European Union Commission Directive (1999/2006) Commission directive on dietary foods for special medical purposes (1999/21/EC & 2006/141/EC). Available at http://ec.europa.eu/food/food/labellingnutrition/medical/index_en.print.htm Accessed 18 July 2011.
Great Ormond Street Hospital for Children (GOSH). (2009) Naso-gastric and oro-gastric tube management guidelines. Available at www.gosh.nhs.uk/health-professionals/clinical-guidelines. Accessed 14 July 2011.
Health Improvement Scotland. (2007) Caring for children and young people in the community receiving enteral tube feeding. Available at www.healthcareimprovementscotland.org/previous_resources/best_practice_statement/enteral_tube_feeding.aspx. Accessed 2 July 2011.
Mason SJ, Harris G, Blissett J. (2005) Tube feeding in infancy: implications for the development of normal eating and drinking skills. *Dysphagia* 20(1): 46–61.
NICE. (2010) Constipation in children and young people; Diagnosis and management of idiopathic childhood constipation in primary and secondary care. Available at www.nice.org.uk/nicemedia/live/12993/48741/48741.pdf . Accessed 15 July 2011.
Sullivan PB, Alder N, Bachlet AM, *et al.* (2006) Gastrostomy feeding in cerebral palsy: too much of a good thing? *Developmental Medicine and Child Neurology* 48: 877–882.
Vernon-Roberts A. (2009) The multidisciplinary team and the practicalities of nursing care. In: Sullivan PB (ed) *Feeding and Nutrition in Children with Neurodevelopmental Disability*. London: Mac Keith Press, Chapter 5.
Vernon-Roberts A, Sullivan PB. (2007) Fundoplication versus post-operative medication for gastro-oesophageal reflux in children with neurological impairment undergoing gastrostomy. *Cochrane Database of Systematic Reviews* 1: CD006151.

3.8.11 Paediatric parenteral nutrition
Kim Novell

Parenteral nutrition (PN) is an expensive form of nutrition and incurs a number of risks; therefore, it is only indicated when adequate nutrition cannot be provided by enteral nutrition alone. Demand for paediatric PN varies between institutions and is likely to be highest in the tertiary setting, particularly in clinical areas of neonatology, gastrointestinal surgery, oncology and intensive care. To expedite hospital discharge, home PN is on the rise; however, this is dependent on the availability of community services (see Chapter 6.5).

The decision to commence PN should be made as part of an experienced multidisciplinary nutrition support team (NST), and depends on the child's age, weight and clinical diagnosis. Members of the NST should include, as a minimum, a senior paediatrician, pharmacist, nutrition nurse and a dietitian (Agostoni *et al.*, 2005). The dietitian's role is to ensure the child is receiving adequate nutrition to achieve appropriate growth, and to recommend changes to feeding regimens to optimise feed tolerance. Some paediatric indications for PN are listed in Table 3.8.18.

Early initiation of PN should therefore be considered if the enteral route has been exhausted, to minimise the risk of malnutrition and prevent permanent adverse effects on growth and development.

Nutritional requirements

Parenteral nutritional requirements vary widely within the paediatric population. Guidelines based on the most

Table 3.8.18 Indications for parenteral nutrition in children

Absolute indications	Potential indications
Premature infants	High stoma output
Congenital defects, e.g. gastroschisis, a condition in which a baby has a small hole in the front of the abdomen, through which part of the intestine protrudes	Active inflammatory bowel disease
	Pseudo-obstruction
	Intractable vomiting
	Protracted diarrhoea
Short bowel syndrome	Hypercatabolism
Necrotising enterocolitis	Postoperative gastrointestinal
Malabsorption syndromes	surgery
Intestinal failure secondary to radiation/cytotoxic therapy	Long periods of nil by mouth

current evidence available have been developed however; nutritional requirements need to be adapted according to the clinical situation, enteral intake and whether catch-up growth, which relates to rapid growth following a period of growth failure, is required.

Energy

Energy supply should meet the total needs of the child, whilst avoiding excessive energy intake. Average daily parenteral energy intakes per kilogram body weight considered adequate for the majority of children are shown in Table 3.8.19.

Amino acids

The amino acid preparations available for children are Primene, based on the amino acid profile of cord blood, and Vaminolact, based on the profile of breast milk (Grogan, 2007). A minimum of 1.0–1.5 g/kg/day is necessary to prevent a negative nitrogen balance; however higher intakes are required to achieve protein deposition (Koletzko et al., 2005). Average amino acid requirements are detailed in Table 3.8.20.

Lipids

A range of 10%, 20% and 30% lipid emulsions are used in paediatric PN and contain soyabean oil (Intralipid), soyabean oil and coconut oil (Lipofundin), soyabean oil and olive oil (ClinOleic), and soyabean oil, medium chain triglycerides, olive oil and fish oil (SMOFlipid). Lipid intake should provide 25–40% of non-protein calories in fully parenterally fed patients (Grogan, 2007). A minimum of 0.25 g/kg/day for preterm infants and 0.1 g/kg/day for term infants and older children is required to prevent essential fatty acid deficiency. Parenteral lipid intake

should be limited to a maximum of 3–4 g/kg/day in infants and 2–3 g/kg/day in older children (Koletzko et al., 2005).

Carbohydrates

Dextrose provides 60–75% of total non-protein energy intake (Koletzko et al., 2005). The type of intravenous (IV) access limits maximum dextrose concentrations of solution. Central lines, inserted into large veins in the neck, chest or groin, can accommodate a dextrose concentration of up to 20%, compared with a maximum of 12% with peripheral lines, which are inserted into smaller veins (Koletzko et al., 2005). Maximum carbohydrate requirements are detailed in Table 3.8.21.

Micronutrients and electrolytes

The optimal parenteral micronutrient requirements for infants and children have yet to be determined. Requirements for vitamins and trace elements are based upon standard recommendations, whereas electrolytes are typically based on individual patient requirements adjusted according to serum levels. A detailed review of parenteral vitamin, trace element and electrolyte requirements can be found in Koletzko et al. (2005).

Standard and individually compounded bags

Standardisation of PN formulas reduces prescribing and compounding time, and can limit the risk of errors. However, due to the wide variability of paediatric nutritional requirements, individualised PN is still widely used (Kochevar et al., 2007). Individually compounded bags are based on weight, and combine amino acid and glucose; separate lipid components are produced. Individual bags are beneficial as concentrating the PN, within the maximum carbohydrate concentration, can vary volumes without compromising nutrition. Standardised all in one bags, usually based on adult requirements, are otherwise available. A portion of the bag should be prescribed to meet the child's nutritional and fluid requirements as closely as possible. To prevent the risk of over infusion it is recommend that the child's nutritional requirements be met in no less than three-quarters of the total bag.

Table 3.8.19 Energy requirements for parenteral nutrition in children (Koletzko et al., 2005)

Age (years)	kcal/kg/day	kJ/kg/day
Preterm	110–120	460–500
0–1	90–100	380–420
1–7	75–90	315–380
7–12	60–75	275–315
12–18	30–60	125–275

Table 3.8.20 Amino acid requirements for parenteral nutrition in children (Koletzko et al., 2005)

Age	g/kg/day
Preterm infants	1.5–4.0
Term infants	1.5–3.0
Second month to third year	1.0–2.5
Third to 18th year	1.0–2.5

Table 3.8.21 Maximal parenteral glucose supply for children (Koletzko et al., 2005)

Weight (kg)	g/kg/day
Up to 3	18
3–10	16–18
10–15	12–14
15–20	10–12
20–30	<12
>30	<10

Complications

Two major potential complications of PN are catheter related sepsis and PN associated liver disease. The pathogenesis of PN associated liver disease is multifactorial and is thought to arise from an interaction of many factors, including prematurity, recurrent sepsis, PN duration, lack of enteral nutrition, excessive calories, lipid source or overload, and continuous or excessive glucose supply (Koletzko *et al.*, 2005; Drongowski & Corain, 1989; Bresson *et al.*, 1989; Colomb *et al.*, 2000). Administration of PN by trained staff using a sterile technique can minimise the risk of catheter related sepsis (NICE, 2007). To reduce the risk of liver dysfunction, the introduction of maximally tolerated enteral nutrition should be a priority. The lipid source should be considered, as there is emerging evidence that a change of lipid preparation to one containing fish oils can reverse liver disease over a 4–6 week period (Cheung *et al.*, 2009; Diamond *et al.*, 2008; Ekemaa *et al.*, 2008; Gura *et al.*, 2006; 2008). Cyclical PN, where the PN is administered over intermittent periods, may also be beneficial; however, it should only be used in children who are able to maintain their blood sugar levels during an infusion break (Koletzko *et al.*, 2005). To prevent rebound hypoglycaemia the glucose containing component of the PN should be weaned to half rate for 2 hours prior to stopping. A more detailed account of PN complications can be found in Koletzko *et al.* (2005).

Monitoring

To ensure the PN regimen is suitable for the child's clinical needs and to minimise the risk of complications, it is recommended that an experienced member of the NST carries out regular clinical assessment of patients. A suggested monitoring protocol can be seen in Table 3.8.22. Further information on the rationale and interpretation of results can be found in the NICE guidelines on nutritional support (NICE, 2007).

Weaning off parenteral nutrition

It is useful to assess feed tolerance before weaning off PN, especially in infants and toddlers, in order to prevent nutritional and growth deficits. Children who have had an acute episode of intestinal failure may tolerate a rapid reintroduction of enteral and/or oral feeds. In contrast,

Table 3.8.22 Suggested protocol for monitoring paediatric patients on parenteral nutrition (adapted from National Institute for Health and Care Excellence 2007. Guidelines current as of 2013. Reproduced with permission of NICE)

Parameter	Frequency
Sodium, potassium, urea, creatinine	Baseline Daily until stable then 1–2 times/week
Blood glucose	Baseline 1–2 times/day until stable, then weekly
Magnesium, phosphate	Baseline Daily if risk of refeeding syndrome Or three times a week until stable, then weekly
Liver function tests	Baseline Twice weekly until stable, then weekly
Cholesterol/triglyceride	Baseline Daily whilst grading in lipid, then weekly
Calcium, albumin, C-reactive protein	Baseline, then weekly
Zinc, copper	Baseline, then every 2–4 weeks
Selenium	Baseline if risk of depletion, then further testing depending in result
Manganese	3–6 monthly
Vitamin D	6 monthly
Iron, ferritin	Baseline, then 3–6 monthly
Folate, vitamin B_{12}	Baseline, then 2–4 weekly
Full blood count	Baseline 1–2 times/week until stable, then weekly
Urinary glucose, sodium, potassium	Weekly
Fluid balance charts	Daily until stable, then twice weekly
Weight	Daily if concerns regarding fluid balance, then 1–2 times per week
Length/height, head circumference, BMI	Baseline, then monthly
Signs of infection, drug interactions	Daily
Gastrointestinal function, enteral intake	Daily initially, then twice weekly

BMI, body mass index

children with a primary gut diagnosis may require a more gradual reintroduction.

Internet resources

European Society of Paediatric Gastroenterology, Hepatology and Nutrition (ESPGHAN) www.espghan.org

European Society for Clinical Nutrition and Metabolism (ESPEN) www.espen.org

Patients on Intravenous & Nasogastric Nutrition Therapy (PINNT) www.pinnt.com

Half PINNT *For our younger feeders* www.pinnt.com/Half-PINNT.aspx

References

Agostoni C, Axelson I., Colomb V, *et al.* (2005) The need for nutrition support teams in pediatric units: A commentary by the ESPGHAN Committee on Nutrition. *Journal of Pediatric Gastroenterology and Nutrition* 41: 8–11.

Bresson J, Narcy P, Putet G, Ricour C, Sachs C, Rey J. (1989) Energy substrate utilisation in infants receiving total Parenteral nutrition with different, glucose fat ratios. *Pediatric Research* 25(6): 645–648.

Cheung H, Lam H, Tam Y, Lee K, Ng P. (2009) Rescue treatment on infants with intestinal failure and parenteral nutrition associated cholestasis using a parenteral fish-oil based lipid. *Clinical Nutrition* 28(2): 209–212.

Colomb V, Jobert-Giraud A, Lacaille F, Goulet O, Fournet J, Ricour C. (2000) Role of lipid emulsions in cholestatsis associated with long term parenteral nutrition in children. *Journal of Parenteral and Enteral Nutrition* 24(6): 345–350.

Diamond I, Sterescu A, Pencharz P, Wales P. (2008) The rationale for the use of parenteral omega-3 lipids in children with short bowel syndrome and liver disease. *Pediatric Surgery International* 24: 773–778.

Drongowski R, Corain A. (1989) An analysis of factors contributing to the development of parenteral nutrition induced cholestasis. *Journal of Parenteral and Enteral Nutrition* 13: 604–606.

Ekemaa G, Falchetti D, Boroni G, *et al.* (2008) Reversal of severe parenteral nutrition-associated liver disease in an infant with short bowel syndrome using parenteral fish oil (omega-3 fatty acids). *Journal of Pediatric Surgery* 43(6): 1191–1195.

Grogan J. (2007) Parenteral nutrition. In: Shaw V, Lawson M (eds) *Clinical Paediatric Dietetics*, 3rd edn. Oxford: Blackwell Publishing.

Gura K, Duggan C, Collier S, *et al.* (2006) Reversal of parenteral nutrition-associated liver disease in two infants with short bowel syndrome using parenteral fish oil: implications for future management. *Pediatrics* 118(1): 197–201.

Gura K, Lee S, Valim C, *et al.* (2008) Safety and efficacy of a fish-oil based fat emulsion in the treatment of parenteral nutrition-associated liver disease. *Pediatrics* 121: e678–e686.

Kochevar M, Guenter P, Holcombe B. ASPEN Board of Directors and Task Force on Parenteral Nutrition. (2007) ASPEN statement on parenteral nutrition standardization. *Journal of Parenteral and Enteral Nutrition* 31(5): 441–488.

Koletzko B, Goulet O, Hunt J, Krohn K, Shamir R. (2005) Guidelines on paediatric parenteral nutrition of the European Society of Paediatric Gastroenterology, Hepatology and Nutrition (ESPGHAN) and the European Society for Clinical Nutrition and Metabolism (ESPEN), Supported by the European Society of Paediatric Research (ESPR). *Journal of Pediatric Gastroenterology and Nutrition* 41: S1–S4.

National Institute for Health and Care Excellence (NICE). (2007) Nutrition support in adults: Oral nutrition support, enteral tube feeding and parenteral nutrition. Available at http://guidance .nice.org.uk/CG32/Guidance/pdf/English. Accessed 27 April 2012.

3.8.12 Paediatric gastroenterology

Julia Smith

Infants and children with common gastroenterology disorders often present to the GP initially and are then referred to their local hospital. Those with more complex conditions can warrant a referral to a tertiary unit or children's hospital (see Chapter 7.4).

Infants

Reflux

Simple reflux, where gastric contents reflux back into the oesophagus, is common in infants. Severe and persistent, gastro-oesophageal reflux disease (GORD) can cause vomiting, pain, discomfort and an aversion to feeding. First line advice is to position upright during and after feeding to allow gravity to minimise the reflux. Feed volumes and frequency should be reviewed to ensure that the infant is not receiving too much feed at any one time. A prethickened formula can also be used, e.g. SMA Staydown or Enfamil AR, or a thickener can be added to the regular formula, e.g. Instant Carobel (Cow and Gate) or Thick and Easy. These can be used alongside antireflux medications, which reduce acid production and promote gastric motility. Thickened feeds may be more difficult for the infant to suck than standard formula and they may require a faster flowing teat. If there is faltering growth, an atopic family history, worsening of symptoms on the introduction of formula or cow's milk protein, associated diarrhoea or constipation, non-IgE mediated cow's milk protein allergy should be considered.

Transient lactose intolerance

Transient lactose intolerance can present following an episode of gastroenteritis and should not be confused with congenital lactose intolerance, which is rare. Typically, diarrhoea continues after vomiting has stopped post gastroenteritis. Stools are fermentative and often described as sweet smelling. The infant's buttocks can be excoriated and sore, but they are otherwise well and are unlikely to have faltering growth. Treatment is with a lactose free formula and diet for 6 weeks (MacDonald, 2007) to allow for the return of the lactase enzyme activity. After this time, the infant should resume a normal lactose containing diet. If the symptoms do not settle, non-IgE mediated cow's milk protein allergy should be considered (see Chapter 7.4.6).

Toddlers

Altered stool patterns

Toddlers have stool patterns that vary according to their dietary intake, but symptoms of persistent diarrhoea or constipation can initiate a referral. Toddler diarrhoea is associated with the fast transit of food that can often be seen undigested in the stool. This diagnosis is made if the child is otherwise well and thriving. Diet histories often reveal a high fibre intake, including wholegrains, excess fruit and/or vegetables, and fruit juice. Manipulation of fruit and vegetable intake to appropriate amounts and portion sizes, and limiting fruit juice and squash intake can often help limit symptoms. Constipation is also common in toddlers. Ensuring adequate fibre and fluid intake is essential and there can often be a behavioural component with stool holding and toilet avoidance. Constipation can also be associated with non-IgE mediated cow's milk protein allergy (MacDonald, 2007).

Non-IgE mediated food allergy

Many infants and children with a non-IgE mediated food allergy present with gastrointestinal symptoms, including vomiting, GORD, constipation, enterocolitis enteropathy, eosinophilic oesophagitis, proctitis (inflammation of the rectum and anus) and proctocolitis. The presentation of non-IgE mediated allergy (T cell mediated) is often delayed (24–48 hours), and symptoms and signs typically affect the skin or gastrointestinal tract (Grimshaw, 2007). Cow's milk protein allergy is one of the most common food allergies reported in infants and children, with an estimated prevalence of 2–7.5% in the UK and Europe (Vandenplas et al., 2007). Typically, it presents in early infancy soon after initial exposure to cow's milk protein formula or weaning solids. It can also present in exclusively breastfed infants, although the incidence is much lower (0.5%) (Grimshaw, 2007). The prognosis is good with a remission rate of approximately 85% by 3 years (Vandenplas et al., 2007) (see Chapter 3.8.18).

Coeliac disease (see chapter 7.4.7)

Coeliac disease can present at any age following the introduction of gluten (NICE, 2009). Symptoms can be gastrointestinal: vomiting, diarrhoea and constipation, with faltering growth, abdominal distension, poor appetite and a miserable or clingy child. Dietary treatment is the same as in adult practice but in addition, some children may present with secondary lactose intolerance. It is recommended that gluten free oats are also avoided at diagnosis, although local policy may suggest introduction at a later stage and monitoring of symptoms (British Society of Paediatric Gastroenterology, Hepatology and Nutrition, 2006).

Annual review is essential for these children (Ciclitira, 2002) and should include:

- A dietary review, including micronutrient intakes – especially iron and calcium.
- Age appropriate education to allow independence, e.g. parties, eating out, school meals, cooking for themselves.
- Advice on gluten free products available on prescription (Codex Alimentarius Commission, 1983).
- Monitoring of growth and pubertal assessment.
- Assessment of compliance.

Inflammatory bowel disease

Inflammatory bowel disease (IBD) commonly presents during adolescence. Children with ulcerative colitis have fewer nutritional complications, but may require nutritional support for disease related malnutrition. However, nutrition is key in the treatment and management of Crohn's disease. Features can include raised inflammatory markers, hypoalbuminaemia, loose stools, abdominal pain, nausea, vomiting, weight loss, poor appetite, mouth ulcers, erythema nodosum, iron deficiency anaemia and delayed puberty. These have often been present for some time and children can present with significant growth failure (Wiskin et al., 2007). It is also common for dietary restriction to have been tried before diagnosis and this may also impact on nutritional status (Rigaud et al., 1994).

At diagnosis children with Crohn's disease should be offered exclusive enteral nutrition to induce remission (Beattie et al., 1994; BSPGHAN, 2008; Wiskin et al., 2007). Traditionally these were elemental feeds (E028 Extra SHS Nutricia), but there is no evidence to support that these are more effective than polymeric (whole protein feeds) (Zachos et al., 2001), e.g. Modulen IBD (Nestle Nutrition) or Alicalm (SHS Nutricia). Feed is given exclusively for a period of 4–8 weeks depending on local policy (BSPGHAN, 2008; Johnson et al., 2006). Most children will require 120% of estimated average requirement (EAR) for energy (BSPGHAN, 2008). The daily feed volume should be calculated according to requirements, split into around six drinks/day and introduced over 2–5 days depending on tolerance and risk of refeeding syndrome (Rigaud et al., 1994). Drinks should be taken slowly over 20–30 minutes to prevent osmotic diarrhoea and abdominal cramps. Nasogastric feeding can be used if the child is unable to take sufficient volumes by mouth. Flavourings, chewing gum, mints and flavoured water may aid compliance, but use varies according to local policy. Regular contact and support during this period can also help with compliance. Adolescents can be encouraged to access appropriate support websites.

Further reading

Vandenplas Y, Brueton M, Dupont C, et al. (2007) Guidelines for the diagnosis and management of cow's milk protein allergy in infants. *Archives of Disease in Childhood* 92: 902–908.

Internet resources

Adolescent Crohn's Treatment (ACT) Support Programme www .actzone.co.uk

British Gastroenterology Society www.bsg.org.uk
Guidelines for the management of patients with coeliac disease www.bsg.org.uk/clinical_prac/guidelines/coeliac.htm
British Society Paediatric Gastroenterology, Hepatology and Nutrition www.bspghan.org.uk
Guidelines for the diagnosis and management of coeliac disease in children (2006). www.bspghan.org.uk/document/coeliac/BSPGHANcoeliacguidelinesFINAL.pdf
Guidelines for the management of Inflammatory Bowel Disease (IBD) in children in the United Kingdom (2008). www.bspghan.org.uk/working_groups/documents/IBDGuidelines.pdf
Children with Crohn's and colitis www.cicra.org
Coeliac UK www.coeliacuk.co.uk
Crohn's and Colitis UK www.nacc.org.uk
Living with Reflux Disease www.livingwithreflux.org
Primary Care Society for Gastroenterology www.pcsg.org.uk

References

Beattie M, Schiffrin EJ, Donnet-Hughes A, *et al*. (1994) Polymeric nutrition as the primary therapy in children with small bowel Crohn's disease. *Alimentary Pharmacology and Therapy* 8: 609–615.

British Society of Paediatric Gastroenterology Hepatology and Nutrition. Guidelines for the diagnosis and management of coeliac disease in children. (2006). Available at www.bspghan.org.uk/document/coeliac/BSPGHANcoeliacguidelinesFINAL.pdf. Accessed July 2011.

BSPGHAN. (2008) Guidelines for the management of inflammatory bowel disease (IBD) in children in the United Kingdom. Available at www.bspghan.org.uk/working_groups/documents/IBDGuidelines_000.pdf.

Ciclitira P. (2002) Guidelines for the management of patients with coeliac disease. Available at www.bsg.org.uk/clinical_prac/guidelines/coeliac.htm

Codex Alimentarius Commission, (1983) *Codex Standard for 'Gluten-Free Foods*. Codex standard 118–1981 (amended 1983). Codex Alimentarius Commission.

Grimshaw K. (2007) Food hypersensitivity. In: Shaw V, Lawson M (eds) *Clinical Paediatric Dietetics*, 3rd edn. Oxford: Blackwell Publishing.

Johnson T, Macdonald S, Hill SM, Thomas A, Murphy MS. (2006) Treatment of active Crohn's disease in children using partial enteral nutrition with liquid formula: a randomised controlled trial. *Gut* 55: 356–361.

MacDonald S. (2007) Gastroenterology. In: Shaw V, Lawson M (eds) *Clinical Paediatric Dietetics*, 3rd edn. Oxford: Blackwell Publishing.

National Institute for Health and Care Excellence (NICE). (2009) Coeliac disease: recognition and assessment of coeliac disease. Available at www.nice.org.uk/nicemedia/pdf/CG86FullGuideline.pdf. Accessed 1 August 2013.

Rigaud D, Angel LA, Cerf M, *et al*. (1994). Mechanisms of decreased food intake during weight loss in adult Crohn's patients without obvious malabsorption. *American Journal Clinical Nutrition* 60: 775–781.

Vandenplas Y, Brueton M, Dupont C, *et al*. (2007) Guidelines for the diagnosis and management of cow's milk protein allergy in infants. *Archives of Disease in Childhood* 92: 902–908.

Wiskin AE, Wooton SA, Beattie RM. (2007) Nutrition Issues in pediatric Crohn's disease. *Nutrition in Clinical Practice* 22(2): 214–222.

Zachos M, Tondeur M, Griffiths AM. (2001) Enteral nutritional therapy for induction of remission in Crohn's disease. *Cochrane Database of Systematic Reviews* 3: CD000542.

3.8.13 Cystic fibrosis

Alison Coates and Julie Crocker

The majority of infants with cystic fibrosis (CF) are identified through the national screening programme. Diagnosis is confirmed by a sweat test and/or genetic mutation analysis. Most families will be advised of the diagnosis within 3 weeks of their baby's birth; early diagnosis allows treatment to be commenced promptly. One in 10 babies with CF is born with the bowel obstruction meconium ileus (MI). Meconium is a thick, black material present in the bowels of newborns and in CF it is so thick that it can block the bowel instead of passing through. The obstruction may be managed conservatively, but some babies may require urgent surgery to relieve and bypass the blockage, which may require a gut resection (Patchell, 2007) (see Chapter 7.4.13).

Newly diagnosed infants should be seen for dietetic review every 1–2 weeks until treatment is established, malabsorption symptoms are controlled and the infant is thriving. Subsequent follow-up is usually monthly for babies up to 1 year, then every 8 weeks, although more frequent review may be required. Children will either receive full care from a specialist CF centre or shared care within an agreed designated network (Cystic Fibrosis Trust, 2011). A paediatric dietitian is most likely to see children with CF at a MDT clinic or as an inpatient, particularly during admission for respiratory exacerbations. All children with CF should have an annual assessment, which includes specialist investigations, including a full dietary report that should include a care plan for the coming year.

Pancreatic insufficiency

Up to 90% of CF patients will be pancreatic insufficient and will require pancreatic enzyme therapy. Following diagnosis, measuring faecal pancreatic elastase assesses pancreatic function. Enteric coated microspheres are most commonly used in infants. Many factors affect the efficacy of pancreatic enzymes; therefore, doses should be advised individually and reassessed regularly depending on weight gain and symptoms of fat malabsorption.

Nutritional requirements

Energy requirements

The energy requirements of children with CF are variable and generally increase with age and disease severity. Fat malabsorption and increased energy expenditure both

SECTION 3

increase energy requirements. Therefore, an infant with good absorption control may have normal energy requirements. A teenager with poor respiratory function may have significantly higher energy requirements than expected for age. Many factors may inhibit a child with CF from meeting their increased requirements, including chronic poor appetite, infection related anorexia, gastro-oesophageal reflux, vomiting, low mood and feeding behaviour problems. Regular review by a dietitian experienced in the management of children with CF is essential. A normal to high fat diet should be encouraged (Cystic Fibrosis Trust, 2002).

Vitamins

In CF, there is usually loss of vitamins in the stools, particularly fat soluble vitamins; therefore, regular vitamin supplements are required. The daily supplement should include 4000–8000 IU of vitamin A, 400–800 IU of vitamin D and 50–200 mg of vitamin E. From 8 years a calcium intake of 1300–1500 mg/day is recommended to optimise intake during the child's growth spurt (Cystic Fibrosis Trust, 2007).

Fibre and fluid

Adequate fibre and fluid is important as part of a balanced diet to help maintain normal bowel function and prevent constipation. Salt depletion can occur in children with CF with increased sweating and in infancy when dietary intake is normally low. Salt supplementation should be considered and some centres routinely recommend salt supplementation. However, generous additions of salt to the child's food is not recommended unless advised by the CF team.

Evaluation of growth

Weight and height, and body mass index (BMI) at a later age, should be recorded at each clinic visit and plotted on the appropriate growth chart. Children with CF often show delayed puberty, which may lead to an overestimation of malnutrition. Assessment of pubertal stages is therefore important when interpreting growth data.

Feeding

Infants and toddlers

Most infants with CF will thrive on either breast milk or a standard infant formula if malabsorption is controlled; breastfeeding should be encouraged. High energy formulae can be useful in infants with poor weight gain. Infants who have had a surgical resection for MI usually require a protein hydrolysate feed. Normal weaning practices are advised with support on modifying pancreatic enzyme doses. If weight gain is poor, advice on the use of higher energy or high fat foods should be given (Cystic Fibrosis Trust, 2002). Feeding behaviour problems such as food refusal and inappropriate parental responses are more common in young children with CF. These issues should be addressed at an early stage to prevent unhelpful behaviour patterns becoming entrenched. Joint dietetic and psychology input can be very effective.

School age children

As children get older, there is an increased likelihood of worsening chest symptoms, leading to greater energy requirements. Close monitoring of growth and nutritional status continues to be essential. The need for enzymes can highlight to a child with CF that they are different from their peers. This can result in problems of acceptance of their condition and adherence to treatment. Advice should be given to parents on how best to deal with this.

Adolescence

Adolescence is a challenging time in the dietary management of CF. The main growth spurt occurs during this period and weight gain and growth can decline dramatically. In addition, poor adherence to enzyme, vitamin and nutritional supplementation is common. It is essential to acknowledge what is important to the teenager. Motivational interviewing for goal setting, together with compromise can be helpful.

Nutrition support

Intervention for poor weight gain should start with improving food and energy intake. The use of dietary supplements, e.g. high energy sip feeds, may be required. Care needs to be taken that these are used in addition to current intake and not as a meal replacement as children's appetites can be small. They may be more useful short term during periods of acute illness rather than as a long term intervention. Tube feeding may be required if growth is failing (Cystic Fibrosis Trust, 2002). Families should be involved early in the decisionmaking process and their views and individual circumstances taken into account regarding choice of intervention and timing of feeds. An overnight continuous feed via a gastrostomy is usually the preferred option. Energy dense feeds are often used to reduce the volume required and usually provide 30–50% of energy requirements.

Complications

The progressive nature of CF means that complications increase in prevalence as children age and move into adulthood. Complications include diabetes, liver disease, bone disease and distal intestinal obstruction syndrome. Investigations to screen for these complications are carried out during the child's annual review, including a dual energy X ray absorptiometry (DEXA) scan from 10 years old to monitor bone density. From 12 years of age, children with CF are screened for CF related diabetes.

Internet resources

Cystic Fibrosis Trust   www.cftrust.org.uk

References

Cystic Fibrosis Trust. (2002) Nutritional management of cystic fibrosis. Available at www.cftrust.org.uk. Accessed 17 May 2012.

Cystic Fibrosis Trust. (2007) Bone mineralisation in cystic fibrosis. Available at www.cftrust.org.uk. Accessed 17 May 2012.

Cystic Fibrosis Trust. (2011) Standards for the clinical care of children and adults with CF in the UK. 2nd edn. Available at www.cftrust.org.uk. Accessed 17 May 2012.

Patchell C. (2007) Cystic fibrosis. In: Shaw V, Lawson M (eds) *Clinical Paediatric Dietetics*, 3rd edn. Oxford: Blackwell Publishing.

3.8.14 Paediatric liver disease
Kirsten Tremlett

Liver disease in children differs significantly from in adults. The major differences (Klein *et al.*, 1997):

- Less frequent occurrence per capita in paediatric patients.
- A much wider range of causes.
- Diseases or defects that are present at birth may prove fatal before adulthood if not diagnosed early in life.
- A greater prevalence of inborn errors of metabolism, biliary tract disease, primary infections and autoimmune disorders.
- A higher likelihood of more nutritional deficiencies; these will generally be caused by the higher anabolic needs for growth, compounded by the catabolic effects of the liver disease.

The nutritional management of infants and children with liver disease will be governed largely by whether the presenting condition is acute, chronic or has been caused by an inherited metabolic disease.

Acute presentations may be due to hepatitis, the onset of autoimmune liver disease or the ingestion of a toxic substance, e.g. paracetamol. Infants tend to present with symptoms of biliary tract disorders that can progress to a chronic condition, e.g. biliary atresia.

Specific inherited metabolic disorders within the liver may present undiagnosed as an acute liver failure, including tyrosinaemia, fatty acid oxidation disorders, urea cycle defects, glycogen storage disease, galactosaemia and fructosaemia. These disorders require specific dietary treatment as outlined in Chapter 3.8.16 and Chapter 7.8.

Chronic presentations with significant nutritional implications include Alagille's syndrome and progressive familial intrahepatic cholestasis (PFIC).

Nutritional assessment

A thorough nutritional assessment is essential, including anthropometry, biochemistry, clinical, social and dietary assessment (Smart *et al.*, 2011). The presence of organomegaly and/or ascites will often mask actual body weight and make the screening for malnutrition meaningless. Regular weights can give an indication of ascites progression. Similarly, length or height is not a sensitive short term marker, but can be useful as a long term measure of chronic malnutrition. More reliable indicators include serial measurements of mid upper arm circumference (MUAC) and triceps skinfold thickness (TSF), and therefore arm muscle mass, which is thought to be more sensitive to the patient's nutritional state (Taylor & Dhawan, 2005; Paul *et al.*, 1998; Battler & Roberts, 2000). Percentiles published by the World Health Organization (WHO, 2006) provide a reference for plotting MUAC and TSF (Taylor & Dhawan, 2005; Frisancho, 2008). There is a strong correlation between liver disease severity, when evaluated by liver function tests, and poor nutrition status, as evaluated by anthropometry (Hurtado-Lopez *et al.*, 2007). Although this is a useful general rule, careful interpretation is needed when complications such as peripheral oedema are present, as these may mask the child's true nutritional state. The situation may be further complicated when nutrition related problems are present, e.g. nausea, vomiting, diarrhoea or anorexia (France, 2007). Anthropometry and biochemistry should be considered together with clinical features when deciding upon nutritional management of paediatric liver disease.

Acute liver failure

Acute liver failure describes a severe impairment of liver function in association with hepatocellular necrosis, where there is no underlying chronic liver disease. The term fulminant is usually used when the failure is associated with encephalopathy. Infants and children are often well nourished if they present immediately after onset. In these cases, nutritional management is aimed at maintaining the patient's nutritional status until the liver function improves. However, if the onset is dramatic, there is a possibility of the critical life threatening complication of cerebral oedema; such patients are often treated in intensive care. It is possible for an undiagnosed chronic liver disease to present acutely and all possible causes must be investigated thoroughly, in order to exclude this possibility (France, 2007).

Dietary management

Current practice is to provide maximum nutritional support. However, dietary management lacks consensus and some aspects of treatment are regarded as controversial. Nevertheless, as the cause of acute liver failure in infants could be an undiagnosed inherited metabolic disorder, the introduction of feed should be delayed until these have been excluded. This is less likely in an older child or adolescent, so they may be given a standard enteral formula.

Chronic liver disease

There are many causes of chronic liver disease in paediatrics and it can present at any age. It is particularly important to diagnose treatable causes of liver disease that present in early infancy. These include sepsis, galactosaemia, tyrosinaemia, endocrine disorders, biliary atresia and choledochal cyst. Dietary management depends on the presenting symptoms, which can include the following:

• Cholestatic jaundice and fat malabsorption – the presence of cholestasis in infants usually indicates that a medium chain triglyceride formula should be used, with fat soluble vitamins and essential fatty acid supplements.
• Hypoglycaemia.
• Failure to thrive.
• Ascites.
• Hepatomegaly.
• Portal hypertension and malabsorption.
• Chronic encephalopathy.
• Oesophageal varices.

A detailed description of the management of these symptoms has been reviewed by Smart et al. (2011).

Paediatric liver transplantation

Advancements in the selection of donor organs, together with the wider availability of immunosuppressive therapy and the increased expertise of specialised paediatric transplant teams, have all contributed to the success of paediatric solid organ transplantation. Survival rates at 5 years post cadaveric transplantation are 78–88% and for living related donor grafts are slightly higher at 83–87%. Children aged 6–10 years have the best 5-year post transplant survival rate (88%) (Tolan, 2011). Patients often have to wait for extended periods before receiving a transplant, owing to the shortage of suitable donor organs. During this period, aggressive nutritional management is essential in order to achieve an optimum outcome (Tolan, 2011).

Ensuring an optimum outcome has been shown to improve the post transplantation survival rate, resulting in fewer infections and a reduction in the frequency and severity of surgical complications (McDiarmid, 2001). Post transplant feeding usually commences in the first 72

hours if the patient is stable. If enteral feeds are indicated, a normal standard age appropriate feed may be introduced. The length of time enteral feeding is required will usually depend on the patient's nutritional status prior to transplant, the underlying diagnosis and presence of postoperative complications. However, most patients should expect to require feeds for up to 2 months after transplant, with normal diet for age being achieved within 6 months.

All paediatric liver transplants and hepatobiliary surgery is carried out at one of three paediatric supraregional liver centres in the UK (King's College Hospital, London; Birmingham Children's Hospital; Leeds General Infirmary). All have specialist paediatric dietitians working as part of the MDT.

References

Battler J, Roberts K. (2000) Nutrition assessment of the critically ill child. *AACN Clinical Issues* 11: 498–506.

France S. (2007) The liver and pancreas. In: Shaw V, Lawson M (eds) *Clinical Paediatric Dietetics*, 3rd edn. Oxford: Blackwell Publishing.

Frisancho A. (2008) *Anthropometric Standards: An Interactive Nutritional Reference of Body Size and Body Composition for Children and Adults.* Ann Arbor, MI: The University of Michigan Press.

Hurtado-Lopez EF, Larrosa-Haro A, Vasquez-Garibay EM, Macias-Rosales R, Troyo-Sanroman R, Bojorquez-Ramos MC. (2007) Liver function test results predict nutritional status evaluated by arm anthropometric indicators. *Journal of Pediatric Gastroenterology and Nutrition* 45: 451–457.

Klein S, Kinney J, Jeejeebhoy K, *et al.* (1997) Nutritional support in clinical practice. Review of published data and recommendations for future research directions. *J Parenteral and Enteral Nutrition* 21: 133–154.

McDiarmid SV. (2001) Management of the paediatric liver transplant patient. *Liver Transplantation* 7 (11 Suppl1): S77–86.

Paul AA, Cole TJ, Ahmed EA, Whitehead RG. (1998) The need for revised standards for skinfold thickness in infancy. *Archives of Disease in Childhood* 78: 354–358.

Smart KM, Alex A, Hardikar W. (2011) Feeding the child with liver disease: A review and practical guide. *Journal of Gastroenterology and Hepatology* 26: 810–815.

Taylor R, Dhawan A. (2005) Assessing nutritional status in children with chronic liver disease. *Journal of Gastroenterology and Hepatology* 20: 1817–1824.

Tolan RW Jr. (2011) Nutritional requirements of children prior to transplantation. *Medscape*. Available at http://emedicine.medscape.com/article/1014361-overview. Accessed 2 August 2013.

World Health Organization. (2006) The WHO child growth standards. Available at www.who.int/childgrowth/standards/en/. Accessed 2 August 2013.

3.8.15 Paediatric nephrology
Sarah Trace

Established renal failure requiring renal replacement therapy (RRT) is a rare but significant cause of long term morbidity and mortality in children (Singa *et al.*, 2010). In the UK there are 13 specialist centres for paediatric

nephrology with 10 providing transplantation services. Many children live a significant distance from their renal centre, so may access some of their care at their local hospital. Dietetic care at a local hospital will be on a shared care basis, led by the specialist dietitians at a specialist centre. The specialist dietitian will have an important role within the MDT; the renal team therefore will not only meet the clinical needs of the child, but will also support their social, psychological and educational needs (see Chapter 7.5.1).

Common presentations

The most common primary presentation of acute kidney injury (AKI) in children is haemolytic uraemic syndrome (HUS) associated with *Escherichia coli* infection, which has an annual incidence of 1–2 in 100 000. Acute kidney injury may also present secondary to a multifactorial illness in a severely unwell child. The annual incidence of established chronic kidney disease (CKD) requiring renal replacement therapy (RRT) is 5–10 children per million (Singa *et al*., 2010). Congenital disorders, including congenital anomalies of the kidney and urinary tract and hereditary nephropathies, are responsible for about two-thirds of CKD in developed countries (Harambat *et al*., 2012).

Nutritional assessment

In addition to the usual considerations made during a paediatric nutritional assessment, nutritional care planning for children with kidney disease will depend on the nature and severity of the disease, the resulting biochemical changes and medical management, including RRT methods and fluid status. In CKD a detailed assessment is complex to perform and needs to be carried out by an experienced renal paediatric dietitian (Royle, 2007). The USA National Kidney Foundation Kidney Disease Outcomes Quality Framework Initiative (KDOQI), Clinical Practice Guideline for Nutrition in Children with CKD is a useful resource (The National Kidney Foundation, 2008).

Dietary management

Acute kidney injury

These children are very unwell, usually unable to eat anything significant, are highly catabolic and usually require dialysis. Nutritional support will aim to prevent catabolism and control biochemical disturbances. The choice of support is dependent on intake and children many require tube feeding. Feed choice and regimen is dependent on the previously described factors and general clinical condition, including the presence of vomiting and or diarrhoea (Royle, 2007).

Chronic kidney disease

Most children with CKD will require specialist renal paediatric dietetic monitoring and advice when the kidney function declines to a glomerular filtration rate (GFR) of 30–60 mL/min/1.73 m² (CKD stage 3) and below.

Poor growth and weight gain is a major problem. Malnutrition and resulting hypoalbuminaemia is associated with increased mortality (Wong *et al*., 2002). Dietary restrictions must only be instigated when absolutely necessary. Many will require tube feeding, but this itself can be problematic due to the increased incidence of gastro-oesophageal reflux (Ruley *et al*., 1989). Feeding problems are common in children; those who have a feeding tube placed before 1 year of age are much more likely to develop feeding difficulties (Dello Strologo *et al*., 1997). As with any chronic disease, an infant can miss key developmental stages during repeated periods of illness. There is frequently a decline in food intake. As renal function falls, food intake decreases further, with one study demonstrating a fall of to 85% of the estimated average requirement (EAR) when the GFR was <25 mL/min/1.73 m² (Norman *et al*., 2000). Uraemia, caused by the accumulation of waste products, leads to loss of appetite and taste changes (Bellisle *et al*., 1995). Frequent nausea and vomiting may lead to food refusal, even when a child is well.

Dietary aims

Optimal nutritional status to promote growth and wellbeing, whilst aiding control of biochemical disturbances, is the aim of dietary management. There is no evidence that children consume more energy than their EAR, although energy dense diets and feeds may be needed due to vomiting, or poor or restricted intake. In order to achieve adequate growth, the child's reference nutrient intake (RNI) for protein is the minimum amount that needs to be achieved. In non-dialysed children with good appetites, there may be a need to reduce usual protein intake if there are symptoms of uraemia. In dialysed children, requirements are additionally determined by dialysis method and biochemical assessment (Royle, 2007).

Control of phosphate, calcium and parathyroid hormone levels will help to prevent calcification of the vessels and renal bone disease. Dietary phosphate intakes usually need to be limited to less than the RNI, which is usually achieved by phosphate binding therapy. Fluid and electrolyte requirements depend on disease, biochemical control and RRT. Fluid requirements and restriction or supplementation of sodium and potassium need to be individually tailored. Dietary restriction of electrolytes, combined with phosphate, severely limits food choice. More research is needed to determine other micronutrient requirements. Folic acid, iron and water soluble vitamins are commonly recommended (Royle, 2007; The National Kidney Foundation, 2008; Warady *et al*., 1994). A paediatric renal specific micronutrient supplement, Paediatric Dialyvit (Vitaline Pharmaceuticals), has been developed which also provides some trace elements (Dixon *et al*., 2004).

Transplantation

Many children will receive a kidney from a live related donor, usually a parent. Immediately following transplant the child and their family will need advice on basic food safety for a short period whilst on high doses of immunosuppressant drugs, due to an increased risk of food poisoning. There can be an increase in appetite due to steroids, so weight gain should be monitored.

SECTION 3

Long term aims are for the child to have a healthy balanced diet; however, 13% of transplanted children become obese (Hanevold *et al.*, 2005). The importance of healthy eating is stressed as the impact of CKD on cardiovascular health is high. A child with CKD has a 1000 times higher risk of cardiovascular death than the healthy age adjusted population (Foley *et al.*, 1998), so the importance of lifelong healthy living is paramount.

References

Bellisle F, Dartois AM, Kleinknecht C, Broyer M. (1995) Alteration of the taste for sugar in renal insufficiency: study in the child. *Nephrologie* 16: 203–868.

Dello Strologo L, Principato F, Sinibaldi D, *et al.* (1997)n Feeding dysfunction in infants with severe chronic renal failure after long-term nasogastric tube feeding . *Paediatric Nephrology* 11(1): 84–86.

Dixon P, Iurilli J, Watson A, Neill E, Foy J, Martin M. (2004) Acceptability of a reformulated renal specific micronutrient supplement. *Paediatric Nephrology* 19: 1433–1434.

Foley RN, Parfre PS, Sarnack MJ. (1998) Clinical epidemiology of CVD in chronic renal disease. *American Journal of Kidney Disease* 32 (Suppl): S112–Ss119.

Hanevold CD, Ho PL, Talley L, Mitsnefes MM. (2005) Obesity and renal transplant outcome: a report of the North American pediatric renal transplant cooperative study. *Pediatrics* 115(2): 352–356.

Harambat J, Van Stralen KJ, Kim JJ, Tizard EJ. (2012) Epidemiology of chronic kidney disease in childhood. *Paediatric Nephrology* 27(3): 363–373.

Norman LJ, Coleman JE, Macdonald IA, Tomsett AM, Watson AR. (2000) Nutrition and growth in relation to severity of renal disease in children. *Pediatric Nephrology* 15: 259–265.

Royle J. (2007) The kidney. In: Shaw V, Lawson M. *Clinical Paediatric Dietetics*, 3rd edn. Oxford: Blackwell Science, Chapter 12.

Ruley EJ, Bock GH, Kerzner B, Abbott AW. Majd M, Chatoor I. (1989) Feeding disorders and gastroesophageal reflux in infants with chronic renal failure. *Pediatric Nephrology* 3(4): 424–429.

Singa MD, Castledine D, Van Schalkwyk D, Hussain F, Lewis M, Inward C. (2010) *Demography of UK Paediatric Renal Replacement Therapy Population in 2009*. Bristol: UK Renal Registry UK Renal Registry Bristol. Available at www.renalreg.com/Report-Area/Report%202011/Chap05_Renal11_web.pdf. Accessed 2 August 2013.

The National Kidney Foundation. (2008) Kidney Disease Outcomes Quality Initiative (NKF KDOQI ™). *American Journal of Kidney Diseases* 53 (Suppl 2): S1–S124.

Warady BA, Kriley M, Uri SA, Hellerstein S. (1994) Vitamin status of infants receiving long term peritoneal dialysis. *Paediatric Nephrology* 8: 354–356.

Wong CS, Hingorani S, Gillen DL, *et al.* (2002) Hypoalbuminemia and risk of death in pediatric patients with end-stage renal disease. *Kidney International* 61: 630–637.

3.8.16 Neurology and the ketogenic diet
Camille Jankowski

One of the more common neurological disorders in childhood is epilepsy. Epilepsy is defined as a brain disorder in which normal brain function is disrupted by epileptic seizures (Fisher *et al.*, 2005). An epileptic seizure is the result of excessive and disorderly neurone activity in the brain (Fisher *et al.*, 2005). There are different types of epileptic seizures and an individual child may present with a variety of different seizures. Epilepsy is estimated to affect between 260 000 and 416 000 people in England and Wales (NICE, 2012).

Children with epilepsy will be under the care of a specialist paediatric neurology consultant and they may also have the support of a clinical epilepsy nurse. The majority of children will have their epilepsy successfully controlled through the use of antiepileptic drugs (NICE, 2012). Children whose seizures do not respond to antiepileptic drugs should be referred to a tertiary care centre for consideration of the use of the ketogenic diet under the care of a paediatric dietitian who specialises in it (NICE, 2012).

In 1921 it was reported that fasting patients with uncontrolled epilepsy could lead to an improvement in their seizure control (Freeman *et al.*, 2007). During starvation the body mobilises fat to produce ketone bodies and these can pass through the blood–brain barrier for the brain to use as an alternative energy source. As starvation is not a long term solution for patients with epilepsy, the ketogenic diet was developed to mimic the metabolic effects of starvation (Freeman *et al.*, 2007). The aim of the high fat content and limited carbohydrate intake with this diet is to drive the process of ketogenesis so that ketone bodies will be the body's main source of energy.

The ketogenic diet can be used to treat a range of different types of epilepsy in patients of all ages. It has been noted to be more effective in certain epilepsies, such as severe myoclonic epilepsy of infancy, myoclonic astatic epilepsy and tuberous sclerosis complex (Kossoff *et al.*, 2009). The ketogenic diet is a high fat diet, with controlled amounts of protein that meet requirements for growth and a limited amount of carbohydrate. Fat provides between 80% and 90% of the total energy (Zupec-Kania & Zupanc, 2008). Fat is mainly provided from foods, e.g. butter, cream and oil, enough protein for growth by, for example, poultry, fish and meat. The remaining energy is provided by carbohydrate from fruit and vegetables. Foods high in carbohydrate, e.g. bread, pasta and rice, are often not allowed in the diet (Zupec-Kania & Zupanc, 2008). The diet plan is usually based on –three to four meals with snacks if required. There are currently four different types of the ketogenic diet.

Classical ketogenic diet

The classical ketogenic diet is based on long chain fats and a ratio system of fat to protein and carbohydrate combined. The main ratios used are 4:1 and 3:1; for every

4 or 3 g of fat, there is 1 g of protein and carbohydrate. The amount of protein is kept to a safe minimum for growth and development, and carbohydrate is limited to achieve the appropriate level of ketosis (Cross *et al.*, 2010). The classical ketogenic diet can be provided to patients who are enterally fed with the use of the enteral feed Ketocal (SHS Nutricia).

Medium chain triglyceride ketogenic diet

An alternative to the classical ketogenic diet is the medium chain triglyceride (MCT) ketogenic diet, where MCT is used as a fat source. MCTs are more effective at producing ketone bodies than long chain triglycerides, allowing more protein and carbohydrate to be consumed, thus improving palatability (Cross *et al.*, 2010).

Modified Atkins diet

The classical and MCT ketogenic diets are very restrictive and adherence is difficult in older children. A modified Atkins diet (MAD), which is similar to the classical ketogenic diet with a ratio of 1:1, can be successful (Hartman & Vining, 2007). The MAD enables the patient to consume more protein and carbohydrate, making it more appealing and easier to plan meals (Kossoff *et al.*, 2009).

Low glycaemic index diet

Low glycaemic index (GI) treatment was developed following the observation children on the ketogenic diet tended to have stable blood glucose levels, which may be a reason for its effectiveness (Kossoff *et al.*, 2009). It allows carbohydrate intake of up to 40–60 g/day as long as the carbohydrate integrated into the diet has a GI of <50 (Kossoff *et al.*, 2009).

Monitoring

The ketogenic diet is not balanced and requires close monitoring by the specialist dietitian to ensure sufficient growth and nutritional adequacy. It is important that patients and parents are informed of the adverse effects of the diet, including constipation, vomiting, kidney stones, poor bone mineralisation and poor growth. The diet does not work for everyone and parents are asked to commit to a trial for 3 months while keeping a seizure diary. This information is used to determine diet effectiveness and the child's quality of life. Typically, a child stays on a ketogenic for 2 years. If after 2 years the family want to remain on the diet and the child is not experiencing any adverse effects, this should be supported with con-tinued dietetic follow-up; such diets have been used for up to 12 years (Kossoff *et al.*, 2009).

Discontinuation

The child must be weaned slowly over a 2–3-month period as stopping suddenly can induce a life threatening seizure. The fat to protein and carbohydrate ratio is reduced from 4:1 to 3:1 to 2:1, and once ketosis stops, high carbohydrate foods can be reintroduced (Kossoff *et al.*, 2009).

Illness

If a child becomes unwell while on the ketogenic diet, the illness must be treated and this may mean the diet has to stop for a short period of time. If appetite is decreased and meals are not completely eaten, an emergency ketogenic milkshake can be given as a replacement.

Internet resources

International League Against Epilepsy   www.ilae-epilepsy.org
Matthew's Friends (dietary Treatments for Epilepsy) www .matthewsfriends.org
The Charlie Foundation   www.charliefoundation.org
The Daisy Garland   www.thedaisygarland.org.uk

References

Cross JH, Mclellan A, Neal EG, Philip S, Williams E, Williams RE. (2010) The ketogenic diet in childhood epilepsy: where are we now?. *Archives of Disease in Childhood* 95: 550–553.

Fisher RS, van Emde Boas W, Blume W, *et al.* (2005) Epileptic Seizures and Epilepsy: Definitions proposed by the international league against epilepsy (ILAE) and the international bureau for epilepsy (IBE). *Epilepsia* 46: 470–472.

Freeman JM, Kossoff EH, Freeman JB, Kelly MT. (2007) *The Ketogenic Diet: A Treatment for Children and Others with Epilepsy*, 4th edn. New York: DemosHelth.

Hartman AL, Vining PG. (2007) Clinical aspects of the ketogenic diet. *Epilepsia* 48: 31–42.

Kossoff EH, Zupec-Kania BA, The International Ketogenic Diet Study Group. (2009) Optimal clinical management of children receiving the ketogenic diet: Recommendations of the international ketogenic diet study group. *Epilepsia* 50: 304–317.

National Institute for Health and Care Excellence (NICE). (2012) The epilepsies: the diagnosis and management of the epilepsies in adults and children in primary and secondary care (CG137). Available at www.nice.org.uk/. Accessed 23 June 2011.

Zupec-Kania B, Zupanc ML. (2008) Long-term management of the ketogenic diet: Seizure monitoring, nutrition, and supplementation. *Epilepsia* 49(Suppl.8): 23–26.

3.8.17   Inherited metabolic disorders

Diana Webster

There are over 500 known inherited metabolic disorders (IMD) (Burton, 2005) and many are diagnosed in infancy or early childhood. A significant proportion of those that affect carbohydrate, lipid or protein metabolism require

Table 3.8.23 Inherited metabolic disorders affecting carbohydrate, lipid and protein metabolism that require significant dietary treatment

Carbohydrate metabolism disorders	Lipid metabolism disorders	Protein metabolism disorders
Galactosaemia	Medium chain acyl-CoA dehydrogenase deficiency (MCADD)	Amino acid disorders: Phenylketonuria (PKU) Maple syrup urine disease (MSUD) Homocystinuria (HCU) Tyrosinaemia
Glycogen storage diseases (GSD)	Long chain acyl-CoA dehydrogenase deficiency (LCADD)	Urea cycle disorders: Ornithine transcarbamylase deficiency(OTC) Carbamyl phosphate synthase deficiency (CPS) Citrullinaemia Arginosuccinic aciduria (ASA) Arginase deficiency
Fructose-1,6-biphosphatase deficiency	Very long chain acyl-CoA dehydrogenase deficiency (VLCADD)	Organic acidaemias: Glutaric aciduria type 1 (GA1) Methylmalonic acidaemia (MMA) Propionic acidaemia (PA) Isovaleric acidaemia (IVA)
Hereditary fructose intolerance	Multiple acyl-CoA dehydrogenase deficiency (MADD) Carnitine transporter disorders Peroxisomal disorders Familial hypercholesterolaemia (FH)	

specialist dietetic support as a major part of their ongoing management (Table 3.8.23).

The majority of children with IMD will be seen in a tertiary level specialist children's hospital. However, some children may be seen in a district general hospital (DGH) with local shared care, based on a hub and spoke model. In tertiary care the patients will be under the care of a metabolic paediatrician as part of a specialist MDT. The IMDs that are most likely to be seen in a DGH are phenylketonuria (PKU) and medium chain acyl CoA dehydrogenase deficiency (MCADD). Both of these conditions can be identified by newborn (heel prick) blood spot screening, which is carried out on all newborn babies between days 5 and 8 of age. The aim of this screening is to diagnose these conditions early, so they can be treated quickly to prevent severe disability or, in the case of MCADD, even death. This test is performed irrespective of feeding times, gestational age and medical state. Expanded newborn screening is currently under discussion in the UK to include maple syrup urine disorder, homocystinuria, glutaric aciduria type 1, isovaleric acidaemia and long chain 3-hydroxyacyl CoA dehydrogenase deficiency.

The incidence of each inherited metabolic disorder is very low. For example, one of the commonest, PKU, has an incidence in the UK of 1 in 10 000 live births. As a result, families with a child affected by an IMD can feel very isolated and often experience great difficulty in explaining the needs of their child's management to a wide range of people, including healthcare professionals, social services and educational establishments. Families are encouraged to become members of charities such as Children Living with Inherited Metabolic Disorders

(CLIMB) and the National Society for Phenylketonuria (NSPKU), which provide a wide range of resources.

The diagnosis of an IMD means some level of care will probably be needed for life, with the paediatric dietitian being a significant member of the care team for many years. The degree of disability for a particular child is extremely variable, depending on the particular condition and the severity of the individual genetic mutation. Some children will be able to lead a normal life, whereas others will be severely disabled or die at a young age.

Dietary management

At the time of diagnosis the paediatric dietitian will discuss information on the dietary management of the particular disorder, prescribe any essential dietary products, e.g. alternative infant formulae, and provide written information for the family. This will be followed by regular contact, on a daily basis at certain crisis times, to ensure the child is adhering to the diet and growing well. Contact with other members of the MDT, other health professionals and agencies, e.g. health visitor, home enteral tube feeding team, and education and social services will also be necessary. The child will be seen at all clinic visits and for an annual nutritional assessment. Biochemistry will be regularly monitored and abnormal results may indicate a need for dietary adjustments. For example, carers of a child with PKU will need to send a blood spot on the newborn blood spot card at regular intervals to the clinical biochemistry laboratory; twice weekly to monthly, dependent on the child's age and current level of control. If blood phenylalanine levels are out of the normal range for age, it may be necessary for the dietitian to increase or decrease the phenylalanine content of the diet by adjusting the daily protein intake.

There are manufacturing companies that produce specialist dietary supplements and low protein foods used in the management of many of the IMDs. They are continually developing new products to make adherence to the diet more manageable. Protein substitutes are an essential component of the diet in the management of protein disorders for provision of adequate protein and other essential nutrients without the amino acid(s) affected by the particular disorder. Low protein prescribable foods, e.g. flour, pasta, egg replacer, milk, chocolate, biscuits, bread, dessert mixes, burger mixes, savoury snacks and cakes are an essential component of the management of a disorder of protein metabolism for the provision of energy and variety.

Emergency regimens

Children with some of the IMDs can become acutely unwell if they have an intercurrent infection. If not treated promptly, this can lead to metabolic decompensation, encephalopathy or possibly death. The treatment for any suspected intercurrent infection is usually to stop the usual diet and commence an emergency regimen for a period of 24–48 hours. The emergency regimen is based on a glucose polymer solution, which provides an exogenous supply of energy and prevents a catabolic response that could potentially become toxic. Each child requiring an emergency regimen should have written information from the dietitian and the parents are encouraged to carry this at all times. The concentration of the glucose polymer is age dependent and will be checked when the child comes to their outpatient visits to ensure it is still age appropriate and that the family still understands its importance. Preparation of emergency regimens when a child is unwell at home can be extremely inaccurate and inappropriate volumes can be given (Gokmen-Ozel et al., 2010). It is important that carers are taught how to prepare the drinks, and have relevant written information and in-date product available, which should be carried with them at all times. The children should be offered the drink when they are well so they remain familiar with the flavour. Palatability can be improved by the addition of commercial drinks to a specified recipe.

Professionals working with IMDs can gain support by becoming members of the British Inherited Metabolic Diseases Group (BIMDG) and Scientific Society for Inherited Errors of Metabolism (SSIEM). With improved screening and treatment, children with these disorders now have extended life expectancies and require dietetic management in adulthood (see Chapter 7.8).

Internet resources

British Inherited Metabolic Diseases Group (BIMDG)   www.bimdg .org.uk
Children Living with Inherited Metabolic Disorders (CLIMB)   www .climb.org.uk
National Society for Phenylketonuria (NSPKU)   www.nspku.org
NHS New born blood spot screening   www.newbornbloodspot .screening.nhs.uk
Scientific Society for Inherited Errors of Metabolism (SSIEM)   www .ssiem.org

References

Burton H. (2005) *Metabolic Pathways: Networks of Care*. Cambridge: Public Health Genetics Unit. Available at www.phgfoundation.org/ file/2222/. Accessed 2 August 2013.
Gokmen-Ozel H, Daly A, Davies P, Chahal S, MacDonald A. (2010) Errors in emergency feeds in inherited metabolic disorders: a randomised controlled trial of three preparation methods. *Archives of Diseases in Childhood* 95: 776–780.

3.8.18   Paediatric food hypersensitivity
Sarah Heath

It is estimated that 6–8% of children up to the age of 3 years are affected by food hypersensitivity, with one study showing the prevalence to be between 2.2% and 5.5% in the first year of life (Venter et al., 2006). The most common hypersensitivities are to milk and egg. Children are much more likely to outgrow a food allergy than adults, with reported levels of tolerance development being 85–90% for milk by 3 years (Høst, 1994), and 66% to egg by 5 years (Boyano-Martínez et al., 2002). Allergies to fish, shellfish and nut are more likely to persist into adult life, although some will still be outgrown.

Most simple paediatric food hypersensitivity will present and be managed in primary care; therefore, dietitians running general paediatric clinics are likely to be involved in the management of some food hypersensitivity. Children with multiple food hypersensitivity or complex disease may be managed in secondary care or tertiary clinics.

Diagnosis in children is similar to that in adults and involves an allergy focused history in conjunction with tests such as skin prick or specific IgE testing, diagnostic exclusion diets or food challenges (NICE, 2011). Due to the likelihood of changes in food hypersensitivity status, children will need regular reviews. There are no specific guidelines, although in practice children under 5 years are likely to be reviewed every 6–12 months. Chapter 7.11.2 provides more information on both testing and food reintroduction.

Treatment

Currently the treatment of food hypersensitivity is avoidance of the offending food and treatment of reactions should they occur. A promising new area is oral immunotherapy. It involves giving very small doses of a food to which a child is hypersensitive and increasing this over a prolonged period of time. It should be noted that this is still in a fairly experimental stage and due to the possibility of severe reactions should only be used as part of an appropriate hospital led protocol.

Nutritional aspects

Children with food hypersensitivities do not have special nutritional requirements, but the impact of food exclusions can increase the risk of malnutrition. Diets that necessitate the avoidance of a whole food group (e.g. dairy foods), staple food items (e.g. wheat) or multiple foods will have the most impact. In addition, any child with other coexisting dietary restrictions, e.g. vegetarianism, cultural or religious restrictions, and fussy eating will be at a higher risk of deficiencies.

Where possible, replacement of nutrients lost through food exclusions should be managed by dietary manipulation initially. This is likely to include a combination of alternate normal foods as well as some specialist free from foods. Vitamin supplements should continue to be recommended as per Department of Health guidelines, see Appendix 3. This may be particularly important in cases where acceptance of hypoallergenic formula is poor. Other nutritional supplements may be necessary following dietetic assessment, e.g. calcium supplements for children with milk hypersensitivity. For cow's milk hypersensitivity, a suitable replacement will be essential where breastfeeding is not available. The following is a summary of the main points [see Chapter 7.11.2 and the World Allergy Organization DRACMA (Fiocchi *et al.*, 2010) guidelines for further details]:

- Non-breastfed infants and children under 2 years should be given a suitable infant formula as a main milk replacement:
  - An extensively hydrolysed or amino acid based formula is suitable for most infants.
  - Soya infant formula is not recommended for infants under 6 months except in a few circumstances (BDA, 2011). Care should also be taken to check for coexisting soya allergy.
  - When intake of infant formula is adequate, a ready made milk substitute could be used in cereals or cooking from 6 months.
- In children over 2 years of age a ready made milk may be suitable as a main milk replacement if the child has a good diet, this can include:
  - Alpro soya©, a product aimed at children over 1 year of age.
  - Calcium fortified versions of these milks should be encouraged (NB: organic brands are not fortified).
  - Rice milk is not recommended for any child under 4.5 years due to the possible increased arsenic content (FSA, 2009).
- Most children with cow's milk allergy will also react to goat's and sheep's milk; therefore. these milks should not be recommended.

Dietary management

The main aspects of managing food exclusion are similar to those in adults. Chapter 7.11.2 provides an outline of allergen avoidance, food labelling and eating out. There are additional considerations when managing paediatric food exclusion and these include the following:

- *Other carers* – extended families, nurseries, child minders and schools may all be involved in food provision. They will require education and support to safely manage the child's diet whilst in their care, especially whilst the child is young and unable to understand their dietary restrictions.
- *Parties or playgroups* – in these situations food is often readily accessible to children who may not understand the need for restrictions. Advising parents on practical ways of managing these situations can help maintain a good quality of life for both the parent and child.
- *Specialist free from foods* can play an important role in maintaining a varied diet whilst allowing children to eat a similar diet to their peers. Advice on suitable products should be made available to parents, taking into account factors such as cost and nutritional adequacy of the foods, e.g. salt content, as well as considering other less specialist alternatives.

Weaning

The weaning period is a time of nutritional risk as infants move from formula or breast milk onto solids. Parental anxiety around managing food hypersensitivities can, in some situations, lead to delayed or restricted weaning. Dietetic advice, including written supporting information, can help to ensure that the infant meets their nutritional needs as well as developing age appropriate eating skills. Parents will need to be advised on which foods they can safely introduce to their child's diet; in some situations, testing may support this. It should be noted that whilst it is important to avoid foods a child is known or suspected to be sensitive to, there is no evidence that delaying weaning or the introduction of specific foods will prevent food hypersensitivities developing (Agostoni *et al.*, 2008).

Adolescence

Older children should be encouraged to become gradually more involved in their dietary management and use of emergency medications. As with many chronic conditions, the teenage years may be particularly challenging with regards to compliance and more input may be required from the team at this stage.

Internet resources

BDA   www.bda.uk.com

The BDA Food Allergy & Intolerance Group has a number of resources on their group page and members will also benefit from regular email updates.

British Society of Clinical Allergy & Immunology (BSACI)   www.bsaci.org

European Academy of Allergy & Clinical Immunology (EAACI)   www.infoallergy.com

World Allergy Organisation (WAO)   www.worldallergy.org

References

Agostoni C, Decsi T, Fewtrell M, *et al.*; ESPGHAN Committee on Nutrition. (2008) Complementary feeding: a commentary by the ESPGHAN Committee on Nutrition. *Journal of Pediatric Gastroenterology and Nutrition* 46(1): 99–110.

Boyano-Martínez T, García-Ara C, Díaz-Pena JM, Martín-Esteban M. (2002) Prediction of tolerance on the basis of quantification of egg white-specific IgE antibodies in children with egg allergy. *Journal of Allergy and Clinical Immunology* 110(2): 304–309.

British Dietetic Association (BDA). (2011) Paediatric Group Position Statement, Use of infant formulas based on soy protein for infants. Available at www.bda.uk.com. Accessed 2 August 2013.

Fiocchi A, Brozek J, Schünemann H, *et al.* World Allergy Organization (WAO). (2010) Diagnosis and rationale for action against cow's milk allergy (DRACMA) guidelines. *WAO Journal* 3(4): 57–161.

Food Standards Agency. (2009) Arsenic in rice drinks. Available at www.foodbase.org.uk/results.php?f_category_id=&f_report_id=322. Accessed 12 July 2012.

Høst A. (1994) Cow's milk protein allergy and intolerance in infancy, Some clinical, epidemiological and immunological aspects. *Pediatric Allergy and Immunology* 5: 5–36.

NICE. (2011) *Food Allergy in Children and Young People*. Guideline 116. London: NICE.

Venter C, Pereira B, Grundy J, *et al.* (2006) Incidence of parentally reported and clinically diagnosed food hypersensitivity in the first year of life, *Journal of Allergy & Clinical Immunology* 117(5): 1118–1124.

3.8.19   Paediatric human immunodeficiency virus

Lisa Cooke

There are approximately 1500 children with human immunodeficiency virus (HIV) in the UK [Collaborative HIV Paediatric Study (CHIPS), 2011]. Most children are of sub-Saharan descent and have acquired the virus from mother to child transmission. The majority of children living with HIV in the UK live in and around central London and are cared for in three major centres: Great Ormond Street Hospital for Sick Children, St Mary's, and St George's. These three hospitals form the hub centres for the hub and spoke network of care for children around the rest of the UK [the Children's HIV National Network (CHINN)]. Smaller numbers of patients are seen within the spoke areas of the network within a defined radius surrounding their locality. Each team caring for these children should consist of a paediatrician, (usually an immunology specialist), specialist nurse, dietitian, psychologist, social worker and pharmacist.

There is still much stigma attached to this condition and this brings challenges to its management. In the majority of cases family members also have HIV and the mothers of these children often carry much guilt from the fact they have infected their child. Due to an excellent antenatal screening pathway now in place, there is <1% transmission of the virus from mother to child within the UK.

Dietetic management

Since the introduction of highly active antiretroviral therapy (HAART) treatment in the late 1990s, all children, if well managed, should live a full and physically active life. Some of the medications can have gastrointestinal side effects, e.g. nausea. For long term health and wellbeing it is essential that they do not miss a dose of medication as the HIV virus can become resistant to the drugs. The main dietetic interventions centre on supporting a healthy lifestyle and diet, avoidance of being over- or under-weight and careful management of lipidaemia.

HIV affects blood cholesterol levels, which are often naturally higher in individuals with the condition. Certain antiretroviral drugs can also raise blood lipid levels. The mini DHIVA (Paediatric Dietitians working in HIV) arm of DHIVA have developed a lipid algorithm to support lipid management. This has been accepted by the Children's HIV Association (CHIVA, www.chiva.org.uk) and is available on their website. Mini DHIVA has also produced on annual assessment form that all paediatric dietitians working in HIV are encouraged to use with their patients. This can also be found at CHIVA.

Many children are from black and ethnic minority groups and due to the high latitude of the UK, vitamin D status is often poor. Levels of this vitamin should be measured and supplementation prescribed. CHIVA have developed prescribing guidelines that are available on its website(ww.chiva.org.uk).

The aims of the dietetic intervention are to:

- Monitor growth and development, optimising it where necessary. Awareness of clinical condition, past medical history, parental heights and current treatment status is necessary to inform the child's predicted growth.
- Measure mid upper arm circumference (MUAC) and waist measurement.
- Assess serum lipid levels, $CD_4\%$ (cell count), renal function, vitamin D levels, blood pressure and insulin levels.
- Assess diet using dietary recall and be guided by the annual assessment form.

- Focus on a cardioprotective style diet.
- As this is a chronic condition aim for behavioural change management throughout the child's life.

It is vitally important that the dietitian is an integrated member of the MDT and is aware of the child's knowledge of their condition through close working with this team. Due to the stigma surrounding the condition, it is important that disclosure of the diagnosis is done slowly, age appropriately and fully supported by the parents, within the MDT and supported by all members.

Many children will eat a traditional diet at home. Therefore, a good knowledge of the sub-Saharan African diets is essential (see Chapter 3.5 and Chapter 7.11.3).

Further reading

Collaborative HIV Paediatric Study (CHIPS). (2011) Annual report 2010/2011 Available at www.chipscohort.ac.uk/documents/CHIPS _Annual_Report_2010_11.pdf. Accessed 12 July 2012.

Internet resources

Children's HIV Association   www.chiva.org.uk
Mother to child transmission   www.chiva.org.uk/professionals/ health/guidelines/mtct/index.html
Clinical audit forms   www.chiva.org.uk/professionals/health/ guidelines/forms/index.html
Management of dyslipidaemia   www.chiva.org.uk/professionals/ health/guidelines/followup/management-dyslipidaemia.html
Children's HIV National Network   www.chiva.org.uk/professionals/ health/networks/index.html
Collaborative HIV Paediatrics Study (CHIPS)   www.chipscohort .ac.uk/default.asp
Dietitians working in HIV/AIDS (DHIVA) A group of the BDA   http:// dhiva.org.uk/

3.8.20   Paediatric diabetes

Shelley Easter and Natalie Mohamdee

The incidence of childhood type 1 and type 2 diabetes is increasing (Ma & Chan, 2009). The current estimate of prevalence of type 1 diabetes in children in the UK is 1 per 700–1000. Prevalence figures for children with type 2 diabetes are limited, but as many as 1400 children may have this diagnosis in the UK (Diabetes UK, 2010).

A recent Department of Health (2011/12) guidance document has outlined best practice in caring for children with diabetes. A child should be offered four multidisciplinary clinics per year, one of which should be an annual review clinic. There should be eight additional support sessions (which can be by phone) of 15 minutes each by any team member. The annual review clinic should include a dietary assessment and other clinical investigations, including thyroid function, retinopathy screening, microalbuminaemia and blood pressure from the age of 12 years (NICE, 2004).

To ensure that the special needs of children and young people with diabetes are met, the MDT based in secondary care should include a paediatrician, diabetes specialist nurse and paediatric dietitian. Access to a psychologist and social worker should be available. Parents of young children should be actively involved, as well as other carers: school, nursery, child minders, etc. (Department of Health, 2001; Smart *et al.*, 2009; SIGN, 2001; NICE, 2004). For each clinic visit the child or young person's weight and height should be measured and plotted on the appropriate growth chart, along with calculating and plotting BMI. This will help identify normal growth and/ or any significant changes in weight as these may reflect changes in glycaemic control (NICE, 2004).

The dietitian's role is to balance the necessity of strict glycaemic control with the family diet and to convert scientific theory about food into practical and sensible advice (Couper & Donaghue, 2009). The aims of dietetic management are to:

- Provide an appropriate energy intake for optimal growth, BMI and health.
- Encourage lifelong healthy eating habits, which preserve social, cultural and psychological wellbeing.
- Achieve a balance between food intake, requirements and insulin profiles to obtain optimal control.
- Achieve lipid levels in a desirable range.
- Prevent and treat acute complications of diabetes: hypoglycaemia, illness and exercise.
- Reduce the risk of micro- and macro-vascular complications.

Type 1 diabetes mellitus

There is a preference for intensive insulin regimens, such as multiple daily injections or pump therapy, where education on matching insulin to desired carbohydrate intake is required. Such regimens allow maximum flexibility of food choices. An individual insulin to carbohydrate ratio allows the adjustment of the premeal insulin according to the estimated carbohydrate content of the meal or snack. Visual resources can be very useful when educating the family on carbohydrate counting, especially if mathematical skills are not strong or a bolus advisor or expert meter is not used. *Carbs and Cals* (Cheyette & Balolia, 2013) is a visual guide to carbohydrate and calorie counting and a useful teaching aid.

Conventional therapy may still be used, if this is the best treatment option for the family. Twice daily insulin injections are given, which contain a mix of short and long acting insulin. This therapy requires a day to day consistency in carbohydrate intake to prevent hypoglycaemia during periods of hyperinsulinaemia. Snacks are required and particular attention should be paid to the energy profile of meals and snacks to prevent excessive weight gain.

Type 2 diabetes mellitus

Type 2 diabetes is increasingly recognised in children. It is more prevalent in the developed world where there is an increased prevalence of childhood obesity.

Features associated with the diagnosis are (Couper & Donaghue, 2009):

- Obesity.
- Age >10 years.
- Strong family history of type 2 diabetes.
- Acanthosis nigricans – a brown/black velvety hyperpigmentation of the skin.
- High risk racial or ethnic group.
- Undetectable pancreatic autoantibodies.
- Normal to high C-peptide levels.

Aims of nutritional management are to prevent acute and chronic complications by achieving normoglycaemia, and addressing the child's weight in those with a BMI greater than the 95th percentile and any comorbidities, such as dyslipidaemia. The family should be involved in lifestyle changes and encourage the parents should be encouraged to act as positive role models. Oral antidiabetic agents to reduce glucose absorption, increase insulin secretion and action, and reduce gluconeogenesis and/or insulin may be used. Regular follow-up with monitoring of weight, glycaemic control and treatment is essential.

Other nutritional considerations

Type 1 diabetes is an autoimmune condition; therefore, there is an increased risk of other autoimmune conditions. Coeliac disease occurs in 1–10% of children with diabetes (Smart et al., 2009). All newly diagnosed children should be screened for coeliac disease. Further screening is no longer included in guidance documents (NICE, 2004), but many centres will screen for coeliac disease in the annual review clinic. The gluten free diet is the only accepted treatment. It is common for those with diabetes who develop coeliac disease not to adhere to the gluten free diet, as they may be asymptomatic and dietary manipulation for both disease states is difficult. These children and their families will require additional dietetic support, with realistic, family centred advice.

Health professionals should be aware that children and young people with type 1 diabetes, in particular young women, have an increased risk of eating disorders. Those in whom eating disorders are identified should be offered joint management involving their diabetes care team and child mental health professionals (NICE, 2004).

Age group specific advice

Infant and toddlers

Breastfeeding to 12 months should be encouraged alongside a healthy weaning diet, which encourages a variety of tastes, colours and textures of foods. Frequent, small meals may promote better glycaemic control, depending on the insulin regimen, and may also avoid food refusal. Insulin pump therapy has been shown to be effective when difficulties arise with food refusal. Parental anxiety is common; consideration of this is a priority when deciding upon the insulin regimen.

School children

The diabetes regimen should fit into the school day. Advice should be given on food portion size, healthy food choices, low fat snacks, reduced fat dairy products and physical activity to reduce the risk of inappropriate weight gain and cardiovascular disease. Sleepovers, parties and trips away from home should be discussed. Continuing diabetes nutritional education with the child and family, including problem solving techniques, may be useful.

Adolescents

Lifestyle advice, support and education targeted towards the teenager are required as the teenager starts to take over their diabetes management. Focused surveillance of weight monitoring is also required, as excessive weight gain may be associated with attempts to obtain excellent glycaemic control; weight loss or poor weight gain may be a sign of insufficient intake, inappropriate insulin administration, disordered eating and/or poor glycaemic control. Careful review of insulin dose, food intake and activity is advisable and the association between weight loss or failure to gain weight and disordered eating needs to be recognised. Rebellion, binges and erratic eating behaviour may require psychological support and counselling. Going out with peers, parties or holidays and a healthy lifestyle need to be discussed. Advice on the safe consumption of alcohol and its prolonged glycaemic effect should be discussed, along with advice on increased appetite with alcohol, and information given on the nutritional content of takeaways and shop bought foods. Careful planning of exercise and sport should be encouraged. Young people may wish to be seen alone or in small intervention groups that provide a forum for support and guidance, which can lead to improvement in knowledge, self care and blood glucose control. The planned transfer of care of young people from paediatric to adult services promotes diabetes self care and improves outcomes (Department of Health, 2001) (see Chapter 7.12).

Further reading

Cheyette C, Balolia Y. (2013) *Carbs and Cals, A Visual Guide to Carbohydrate and Calorie Counting for Those with Diabetes*, 4th edn. Chello publishing.

Hanas R. (2009) *Type 1 Diabetes in Children, Adolescents and Young Adults: How to Become an Expert on Your Own Diabetes*, 4th edn. London: Class Publishing.

Internet resources

Diabetes and Sport   www.runsweet.com
Diabetes Net   www.diabetesnet.com
Diabetes UK   www.diabetes.org.uk
International Diabetes Federation   www.idf.org
Nutrition and Diet Resources   www.ndr-uk.org
Quality Institute for Self Management and Education & Training   www.qismet.org.uk
SWEET project (Better control in Pediatric and Adolescent diabetes: working to create Centres of Reference)   www.sweet-project.eu

Insulin pump companies

Accu–chek   www.accu-chek.co.uk
Advanced Therapeutics   www.advancedtherapeuticsuk.com
Animas   www.animascorp.co.uk
Medtronic   www.medtronic-diabetes.co.uk

References

Cheyette C, Balolia Y. (2013) *Carbs and Cals, A Visual Guide to Carbohydrate and Calorie Counting for Those with Diabetes*, 4th edn. Chello Publishing.

Couper J, Donaghue K. (2009) ISPAD Clinical practice consensus guidelines 2009 compendium: Phases of diabetes in children and adolescents. *Pediatric Diabetes* 10 (Suppl 10): 13–16.

Department of Health. (2001) National service framework for diabetes: standards. Available at www.dh.gov.uk/en/Publicationsand statistics/Publications/PublicationsPolicyAndGuidance/DH _4002951. Accessed on 7 August 2011.

Department of Health. (2011/12) Payment by results guidance for 2011-12. Available at www.dh.gov.uk/prod_consum_dh/groups/ dh_digitalassets/documents/digitalasset/dh_126157.pdf. Accessed on 10 August 2011.

Diabetes UK. (2010) Diabetes in the UK 2010, key statistics on diabetes. Available at www.diabetes.org.uk/Documents/Reports/ Diabetes_in_the_UK_2010.pdf. Accessed on 10 August 2011.

Ma R, Chan J. (2009) Incidence of childhood type 1 diabetes: a worrying trend. *Nature Reviews in Endocrinology* 5(10): 529–530.

National Institute for Health and Care Excellence (NICE). (2004) *Type 1 Diabetes Diagnosis and Management of Type 1 Diabetes in Children and young People*. London: NICE. Updated April 2010. Available at www.nice.org.uk/guidance/CG15.

Scottish Intercollegiate Guidelines Network (SIGN). (2001) *Management of Diabetes,* Publication No55. Edinburgh: SIGN.

Smart C, Aslander-van Vilet E, Waldron S. (2009) ISPAD Clinical practice consensus guidelines (2009) ISPAD Clinical practice consensus guidelines 2009 compendium: Nutritional management in children and adolescents with diabetes. *Pediatric Diabetes* 10 (Suppl 12): 100–117.

3.8.21   Cardiology

Philippa Wright

Congenital heart disease (CHD) describes defects in the structure of the heart that are present at birth. It affects 1 in every 145 births (www.BHF.org.uk) and there are a number of associated genetic syndromes, e.g. Down's syndrome. Children with CHD are usually of normal weight for gestational age at birth but are particularly vulnerable to malnutrition due to a combination of severe fluid restriction, inefficient absorption of nutrients and high metabolic demands (Avitzur *et al.*, 2003) (Table 3.8.24).

Children are looked after in designated children's cardiac centres, with shared care arrangements with their local district general hospitals and community, both pre- and post-operatively.

Physiology

Congenital heart disease is defined according to its haemodynamic effects, which fall into two groups; cyanotic and acyanotic. These types of cardiac malformations can have an effect upon outcomes regarding growth and nutritional intake. Cyanosis refers to a reduced level of oxygen in the blood and cyanotic lesions have been found to cause the greatest degree of stunting (Jacobs *et al.*, 2000). The acyanotic group of lesions can be further divided into obstructive malformations and left to right shunt malformations. These lesions have been observed to affect weight rather than height, especially in the presence of pulmonary hypertension (Mehziri & Drash, 1962;

Umansky & Hauck, 1962). In this situation blood is pumped to the lungs under greater pressure, preventing effective oxygenation. As a result the heart pumps faster and the child's breathing increases in an attempt to improve oxygenation. This ultimately increases the child's energy requirements and results in weight loss.

For detailed descriptions of all cardiac lesions, see the British Heart Foundation website (www.BHF.org.uk).

Congestive heart failure

Congestive heart failure (CHF) is the main concern in children with CHD. It occurs when the heart can no longer meet the metabolic demands of the body. Signs include tachycardia, fatigue on feeding and early satiety, all resulting in growth faltering. Diuretic therapy relieves CHF but commonly used diuretics can cause sodium, potassium, chloride and calcium losses. While losses can be replaced, it is important to note that persistent hyponatraemia can result in poor growth and must be corrected.

Anaemia can also mimic the signs of CHF; cyanotic children can have higher iron requirements as they have an increased red cell mass. These infants should be screened for iron deficiency using ferritin, red cell indices and total iron binding saturation, as haemoglobin may be within normal range even though the patient is iron deficient (Premer& Georgieff, 1999).

Table 3.8.24   Factors that may influence the development of malnutrition and growth failure in infants with congenital heart disease (Nydegger & Bines, 2006)

Causative factors	Physiological impact
Type and clinical impact of cardiac disease	Cyanotic versus acyanotic defects Shunts Congestive heart failure Operative status: age at surgery, type of surgery, complications
Disturbances in energy metabolism	Increased energy expenditure: Cardiac hypertrophy Abnormalities in body composition Increased sympathetic nervous system activity Increased haematopoietic tissue Increased basal temperature Recurrent infections Pharmacological agents
Decreased nutritional intake	Anorexia, early satiety Pharmacological agents Decreased gastric volume caused by hepatomegaly
Disturbances in gastrointestinal function	Malabsorption: Oedema and chronic hypoxia of the gut Interference with drugs Compressive hepatomegaly Decreased gastric volume Increased gastro-oesophageal reflux
Prenatal factors	Chromosomal disorders Intrauterine factors Birth weight

SECTION 3

Mechanisms of malnutrition in congenital heart disease

Malnutrition can be caused by fluid restriction, poor absorption and fatigue on feeding, causing a reduced total intake, gastro-oesophageal reflux disease, increased metabolic expenditure, early satiety, anorexia and frequent infections. Energy for growth is diverted to meet the child's increased metabolic demands. Studies give a range of energy requirements from 120 to 170 kcal/kg/day (Yahav et al., 1985; Unger et al., 1992; Barton et al., 1994; Ackerman et al., 1998; Waterlow, 1992). To facilitate weight gain it is therefore advisable to first aim for 120 kcal/kg and to increase this if weight gain is not achieved (Lawson & Shaw, 2001).

Surgery

After surgery children will be admitted to the paediatric intensive care unit (PICU). Postoperative requirements have been shown to be much lower than previously thought, especially in the immediate postoperative ventilated patient. No difference has been observed between cyanotic and acyanotic lesions; the only statistical difference was for those children requiring cardiopulmonary bypass. The non-bypass group appears to need less energy than the bypass group. This could be related to inflammatory response to bypass, but further studies are needed (De Wit et al., 2010).

When calculating requirements in the immediately postoperative ventilated cardiac child, it is important to understand the amount of sedation, paralysis and ventila-

tory support they are receiving. The Schofield equation is currently used to calculate postsurgical requirements; however, the addition of a stress factor of 20% relates to calorimetry findings (Jackson, 2000).

Postoperative weight gain

After discharge from the PICU the growth faltering child may need to return to preoperative requirements until catch-up growth has been facilitated. Enhanced energy content feeds and, in some cases, nasogastric or gastrostomy feeds may be necessary to maintain the patient's growth pre- and post-operatively. If fluid is restricted, then high energy formula or fortified expressed breast milk will be required. Breast milk can be fortified using commercially available fortifiers or by adding 3–5% of standard infant powdered formula. If breast milk is not available, then the following high energy formulae are available:

- SMA High Energy: 91 kcal/100 mL (2 g/100 mL).
- Infatrini: 100 kcal/100 mL (2.6 g protein/100 mL).
- Similac High Energy: 101 kcal/100 mL (2.6 g protein/100 mL).

If weight gain is still not achieved once 150 kcal/kg is provided, then additional energy can be given through the addition of a glucose and fat polymer. The protein to energy ratio of 9–14% must be preserved (Jackson, 2000; Wharton, 1994). However, the 24-hour urinary sodium balance should be measured if weight continues to falter. As these infants are often fluid restricted, which ultimately impacts on energy intake, it is important to ask the medical team if an increase of fluids is possible in order to increase nutritional intake.

Feed administration

The method of feed administration is important and the following steps should be employed, if required, in order to meet the child's dietary requirements for growth or catch-up:

- Offer smaller volumes and more frequent feeds orally.
- Give unfinished feeds via a NG tube if required.
- Give small frequent bolus feeds via a NG tube.
- Give overnight continuous feeds via an enteral feeding pump in addition to small frequent daytime feeds (always refer to local policies and guidelines when advising overnight tube feeding).
- Give feeds continuously over 20 hours via a feeding pump, allowing the gut time to rest and pH to return to normal.

Anthropometry

Anthropometric data is essential and accurate weights must be recorded on growth charts (syndrome specific charts should be used where appropriate) from the point of referral. Be aware that fluctuating fluid balances can mislead weight records so patients at risk may have daily weights recorded.

Expected weight gain

Expected weight gain values are difficult to achieve in children with CHD; therefore, an average gain of 10–20 g/ day would be more appropriate in children under 6 months and 120–210 g/week in children aged 6–12 months (17–30 g/day) (Forchielli *et al.*, 1994).

Complications

Complications that can occur after surgery include:

- *Chylothorax* – the accumulation of chyle in the pleural space. Conservative management involves the reduction of long chain fats (Chan *et al.*, 2005) to <1 g per year of life to a maximum of 5 g/day.
- *Protein losing enteropathy* – there is limited evidence regarding specific diet therapy; however, it is suggested that the diet should consist of 5–10 g/day of fat and be high in protein, with additional fat replaced with a medium chain fat source to improve overall energy intake (Shaw & Lawson, 2007).
- *Necrotising enterocolitis (NEC)* – specific lesions and surgeries may increase the risk of NEC in the child with

CHD. Reduced gut perfusion can occur and the patient will require extremely slow reintroduction of feeds in conjunction with parenteral nutrition if considered at risk.

References

Ackerman IL, Karn CA, Denne SC, *et al.* (1998) Total but not resting energy expenditure is increased in infants with ventricular septal defects. *Pediatrics* 102: 1172–1177.

Avitzur Y, Singer P, Dagan O, *et al.* (2003) Resting energy expenditure in children with cyanotic and noncyanotic congenital heart disease before and after open heart surgery 1. *Journal of Parenteral and Enteral Nutrition* 27: 47–51.

Barton J, Hindmarsh P, Scrimgeour C, *et al.* (1994) Increased energy expenditure in congenital heart disease. *Archives of Disease in Childhood* 70: 5–9.

Chan E, Russell J, William G, Van Arsdell G. (2005) Postoperative chylothorax after cardiothoracic surgery in children. *Annals of Thoracic Surgery* 80: 1864–1871.

De Wit B, Meyer R, Desai A, Macrae D, Pathan N. (2010) Challenge of predicting resting energy expenditure in children undergoing surgery for congenital heart disease. *Paediatric Critical Care Medicine* 11: 496–501.

Forchielli MC, McColl R, Walker WA, Lo C. (1994) Children with congenital heart disease: a nutritional challenge. *Nutrition Reviews* 52(10): 348–353.

Jackson J. (2000) Protein requirements for catch up growth. *Proceedings of the Nutrition Society* 49: 507–516.

Jacobs ECJ, Leung MP, Karlberg JP. (2000) Postnatal growth in southern Chinese children with symptomatic congenital heart disease. *Journal of Paediatric Endocrinology and Metabolism* 11: 195–202.

Lawson M, Shaw V. (2001) *Clinical Paediatric Dietetics*, 2nd edn. Oxford: Blackwell Publishing.

Mehziri A, Drash A. (1962) Growth disturbances in congenital heart disease. *Journal of Paediatrics* 61: 418–429.

Nydegger A, Bines A. (2006) Energy metabolism in infants with congenital heart disease. *Nutrition* 22: 697–704.

Premer D, Georgieff M. (1999) Nutrition for ill neonates. *NeoReviews* 20(9): e56–62.

Shaw V, Lawson M. (2007) *Clinical Paediatric Dietetics*, 3rd edn. Oxford: Blackwell.

Umansky R, Hauck AJ. (1962) Factors in the growth of children with patent ductus arteriosus. *Pediatrics* 30: 540–550.

Unger R, de Kleermaeker M, Giddings S, Kaufer-Christoffel K. (1992) Calories count: improved weight gain with dietary intervention in congenital heart disease. *American Journal of Diseases of Children* 146: 1078–1084.

Waterlow JC. (1992) *Protein Energy Malnutrition*. London: Edward Arnold, pp. 231–232.

Wharton B. (1994) International recommendations on protein intake in infancy: some points for discussion. *Nestle Workshop Series* 33: 67–83.

Yahav J, Avigad S, Frand M, *et al.* (1985) Assessment of intestinal and cardiorespiratory function in children with congenital heart disease on high calorie formulas. *Journal of Pediatric Gastroenterology and Nutrition* 4: 778–785.

3.8.22 Paediatric cancers
Nicola Williams

Approximately 1500 children are diagnosed with cancer in the UK every year. Survival of childhood cancer has

more than doubled since the 1960s with survival now in about 70% of those affected (Children with Cancer UK,

Table 3.8.25 Relative contributions of main diagnostic groups of childhood cancer to overall incidence among children aged 0–14 years (*National Registry of Childhood Tumours*, http://www.ccrg.ox.ac.uk/datasets/registrations.shtml)

Type of cancer	%
Leukaemia	31
Central nervous system	25
Lymphoma	10
Soft tissue sarcoma	7
Neuroblastoma	6
Renal	6
Bone	4
Retinoblastoma	3
Germ cell	3
Liver	1
Other carcinomas and melanomas	
Other	

Table 3.8.26 Types of childhood cancers associated with high or low nutritional risk (source: Shaw & Lawson 2007, table 22.3, p. 466. Reproduced with permission of Blackwell Publishing)

High nutritional risk diagnoses	Low nutritional risk diagnoses
Advanced diseases during initial intense treatment Stages III and IV Wilms' tumour and unfavourable histology Wilms' tumour Stages III and IV neuroblastoma Ewing's sarcoma Pelvic rhabdomyosarcoma Some non-Hodgkin's lymphoma Multiple relapse leukaemia Acute lymphoblastic leukaemia (graded high risk) Medulloblastoma	Acute lymphoblastic leukaemia (graded low risk) Non-metastatic solid tumours Advanced diseases in remission during maintenance treatment

www.childrenwithcancer.org.uk; The Children's Cancer and Leukaemia Group, www.cclg.org.uk). Cancer in children differs from that in adults in terms of the body areas affected and how it responds to treatment. Table 3.8.25 shows the types of cancer seen in children (National Registry of Childhood Tumours, http://www.ccrg.ox.ac.uk/datasets/registrations.shtml). Depending on the type of cancer diagnosed, treatment will usually comprise of chemotherapy with or without surgery and/or radiotherapy.

Nutritional implications

Nutrition support is a key part of supportive care for children with cancer to ensure normal growth and development. Children may present malnourished or cachexic at diagnosis; in addition treatment side effects impact on nutritional status. It is recognised that good nutrition may reduce treatment complications and infection rates, and improve response to intensive anticancer treatments (NICE, 2005; RCN, 2010). Table 3.8.26 shows the types of childhood cancers associated with high or low nutritional risk (Shaw & Lawson, 2007).

Dietetic management

Nutritional assessment

There is no specific nutrition screening tool for children with cancer, although a diagnostic tool for malnutrition in these children has been designed to use alongside the Screening Tool for the Assessment of Malnutrition in Paediatrics (STAMP) (McCarthy *et al.*, 2012). For further information see the Royal College of Nursing (2010).

Nutrition support

Management is determined by nutritional risk of diagnosis, nutritional status, symptoms and anticipated gut func-

tion. Symptoms relating to treatment that may impact upon nutritional status include infection, diarrhoea, nausea and vomiting, mucositis, anorexia, xerostomia and constipation.

Oral nutritional support may be adequate when nutritional status is stable, but intake is reduced. If nutritional status deteriorates, enteral tube feeding should be started early to prevent a further decline in weight and health. Parenteral nutrition is reserved for when gut function is compromised for >5 days. Whole protein feeds are usually the first choice; however, during treatment causing severe gastrointestinal toxicity, a hydrolysate or elemental feed is recommended.

Monitoring and follow-up

The child's tolerance to nutritional support may change significantly depending on the type of anticancer therapy they receive. Frequent monitoring of the feeding regimen and anthropometry will ensure nutritional requirements for normal growth continue to be achieved. As treatment reduces in intensity (called maintenance chemotherapy) or is completed, nutritional support can be weaned, with the aim to progress towards a balanced diet (see Chapter 7.15).

Internet resources

British Dietetic Association   www.bda.uk.com
   Paediatric Oncology Dietitians Interest Group (PODIG)
British Society of Blood and Bone Marrow Transplantation
   http://bsbmt.org
Cancer Research UK   www.cancerresearchuk.org
Children with Cancer UK   www.childrenwithcancer.org.uk
Children's Cancer and Leukaemia Group   www.cclg.org.uk
CLIC Sargent   www.clicsargent.org.uk
Macmillan Cancer Support   http://www.macmillan.org.uk
STAMP   www.stampscreeningtool.org/stamp.html

References

McCarthy H, Dixon M, Crabtree I, Eaton-Evans MJ, McNulty H. (2012) The development and evaluation of the Screening Tool for the Assessment of Malnutrition in Paediatrics (STAMP©) for use by healthcare staff. *Journal of Human Nutrition and Dietetics* 25: 311–318.

National Institute for Health and Clinical Excellence (NICE). (2005) *Improving Outcomes in Children and Young People with Cancer.* London: NICE.

Royal College of Nursing (RCN). (2010) *Nutrition in Children and Young People with Cancer. RCN Guidance.* London: RCN.

Shaw V, Lawson M. (2007) *Clinical Paediatric Dietetics,* 3rd edn. Oxford: Blackwell Publishing.

3.8.23 Paediatric haematopoietic stem cell and bone marrow transplantation
Zoe Hull

Bone marrow transplantation (BMT) [more accurately known as haematopoietic stem cell transplantation (HSCT)] is a highly intensive, life saving therapy available to treat malignant and non-malignant diseases of the bone marrow. High doses of chemotherapy and radiotherapy are given to improve the chances of curing the malignant disease, particularly for cancers with a high risk of relapse. For non-malignant disease, the poorly functioning bone marrow is removed and replaced with stem cells of normal function (Kline, 2006). However, the resulting toxicities and complications, including severe immune suppression, predispose a child to malnutrition (see Chapter 7.15.8). Mortality rates are much improved and more children are surviving transplantation as a consequence of improved donor or recipient matching and supportive care. The role of the dietitian is to help maintain nutritional status before, during and after the transplant, and to maximise quality of life and growth (Ward, 2007).

Transplant procedure

In the UK there are 16 specialist paediatric units where transplantation is carried out (British Society of Blood and Bone Marrow Transplantation, http://bsbmt.org/). The main types of transplant are:

- *Autologous* – the child's own marrow or stem cells are frozen (cryopreserved) and returned after treatment with high dose chemotherapy (stem cell rescue).
- *Allogenic* – the child receives donor marrow or stem cells, ideally from a sibling or close relative to enable a close tissue type match. This is a more complicated, high toxicity procedure with a longer recovery period.
- *Syngeneic* – marrow or stem cells are donated from an identical twin, enabling a perfect genetic match and reduced toxicities.

Prior to admission, stem cells are collected from the bone marrow or peripheral blood, or umbilical cord blood donation is used (Lipkin *et al.*, 2005). After admission high dose chemotherapy with or without total body irradiation (TBI) destroys the remaining cancer cells and the marrow and immune system. The child becomes sick and profoundly immune suppressed. The stem cells are returned to the child intravenously and they are isolated for 5–6 weeks to monitor side effects and recovery until they produce new blood cells (engraftment).

Dietetic management

The transplant process can cause severe oral and gastrointestinal toxicity. The majority of children require nutritional support (Muscaritoli *et al.*, 2002). Side effects leading to compromised nutritional status include:

- Prolonged anorexia.
- Mucositis.
- Nausea and vomiting.
- Diarrhoea and abdominal cramping.
- Malabsorption.
- Bacterial and viral infections
- Prolonged taste changes.
- Xerostomia.
- Gastroparesis.
- Acute and chronic graft versus host disease (GvHD).
- Hyperglycaemia as a result of steroid treatment.
- Fatigue.
- Depression.
- Neutropenia (low level or absent neutrophil count).
- Food aversions.

Children may have increased metabolic requirements resulting from infection, protein losing enteropathy, GvHD or veno-occlusive disease of the liver (Kline, 2006). Enteral nutrition via nasogastric, nasojejunal and gastrostomy feeding is preferred using a semi elemental or elemental feed to protect the gut and aid tolerance during periods of gastrointestinal mucositis (Ward, 2007). Temporary gastrointestinal failure is common and if enteral feeding is not successful, parenteral nutrition is (Murray & Pinderia, 2009). Advice should be given to minimise the risk of food borne illness and gastrointestinal infection while the child is immunosuppressed. A low microbial diet is recommended and all food must be prepared and cooked safely Yokoe *et al.*, 2009). The degree of dietary restriction and duration that must be followed differs between specialist centres.

Internet resources

British Dietetic Association www.bda.uk.com
Paediatric Oncology Dietitians Interest Group (PODIG)

British Society of Blood and Bone Marrow Transplantation   http://bsbmt.org
Cancer Research UK   www.cancerresearchuk.org
Children with Cancer UK   www.childrenwithcancer.org.uk
Children's Cancer and Leukaemia Group   www.cclg.org.uk
CLIC Sargent   www.clicsargent.org.uk
Macmillan Cancer Support   www.macmillan.org.uk

References

Kline RM. (2006) *Pediatric Hematopoietic Stem Cell Transplantation*. New York: Informa Healthcare USA, Inc.

Lipkin AC, Lenssen P, Dickson BJ. (2005) Nutrition issues in hematopoietic stem cell transplantation: State of the art. *Nutrition in Clinical Practice* 20(4): 423–439.

Murray SM, Pindoria S. (2009) Nutrition support for bone marrow transplant patients. *The Cochrane Library*, Issue 1. Chichester: John Wiley and Sons Ltd.

Muscaritoli M, Grieco G, Capria S, Iori AP, Fanelli FR. (2002) Nutritional and metabolic support in patients undergoing bone marrow transplantation. *American Journal of Clinical Nutrition* 75(2): 183–190.

Ward E. (2007) Childhood cancers. In: Shaw V, Lawson M (eds) *Clinical Paediatric Dietetics*, 3rd edn. Oxford: Blackwell Publishing.

Yokoe D, Casper C, Dubberke E, *et al.* (2009) Safe living after hematopoietic cell transplantation. *Bone Marrow Transplantation* 44: 509–519.

3.8.24   Nutrition support in the critically ill child

Luise Marino and Rosan Meyer

During the last few decades, advances in anaesthetic and intensive care have improved outcomes in critical illness (Rittirsch *et al.*, 2008). On average 0.1% of the childhood population in England and Wales is admitted to a paediatric intensive care unit (PICU) per annum, of whom 50% are under 1 year of age. The mean stay is between 1 and 2 days (range 1–35 days) (Parslow *et al.*, 2009). Sixty per cent of admissions are a result of unplanned emergencies, including neurological injuries, cardiac disorders and respiratory distress (O'Donnell *et al.*, 2010). Although this represents only a small number of children admitted for a short period of time for a variety of diagnoses, undernutrition is common (Hulst *et al.*, 2004a,b), which impacts on morbidity, mortality and therefore length of stay in hospital (Goiburu *et al.*, 2006; Kyle *et al.*, 2005; Coss-Bu *et al.*, 2001). It is important to ensure optimal nutritional support from admission to discharge based on anthropometrical and biochemical parameters, clinical assessment and previous dietary intake.

Determining a nutrition care plan

Anthropometry

The rate of acute or chronic malnutrition within the PICU is between 24% and 55% (Delgado *et al.*, 2008). The causes of malnutrition are multifactorial and include pre-morbid disease, e.g. cystic fibrosis, congenital heart disease, acute or chronic suboptimal nutritional support in addition to increased protein breakdown and reduced protein synthesis, especially in the acute phase of an illness (Hulst *et al.*, 2006a). Every child should be weighed on admission to calculate their energy and protein requirements. The clinical condition must be considered as some children are too unstable to be weighed and weight may also be inaccurate due to oedema, ascites or tumour masses. It is usually impossible to perform an accurate length measurement (Feferbaum *et al.*, 2009). It is useful to consult the child's growth chart in their Personal Child Health Record to give an insight into how well they have been growing and whether they are at risk of malnutrition on admission (Shaw & Lawson, 2007).

Biochemistry

Biochemical abnormalities are common in critically ill children and may impact on nutritional support. The most important indices to consider include serum urea, glucose, albumin, C-reactive protein, magnesium, calcium, phosphorus, selenium, zinc, manganese and lactate acidosis. It is essential to refer to Clinical Paediatric Dietetics (Shaw & Lawson, 2007) as biochemistry, and abnormalities in children will differ from those in adults (Table 3.8.27).

Clinical factors

Critical illness can have a profound impact, resulting in increased glucose synthesis, protein breakdown, fat oxidation and the risk of metabolic derangement (Hulst *et al.*, 2006b). A nutritional assessment should take into account these factors and others, including the impact ascites or oedema may have on actual weight and/or enteral feeding tolerance, in addition to protein and energy requirements relative to wound healing.

Dietary intake

Children and infants have significantly less fat and protein stores compared with adults and are unable to tolerate prolonged periods of starvation, e.g. 3–5 days or longer. In addition, the need to support continued growth and development is important, and nutritional support should be started as soon as possible (Skillman & Wischmeyer, 2008). There are many challenges within a PICU setting that impact on the actual delivery of nutrients (Feferbaum *et al.*, 2009; Hulst *et al.*, 2006b):

Table 3.8.27   Relevance of biochemical indices in critical illness

Biochemical index	Comment
Serum urea	Indicative of catabolism and protein breakdown associated with trauma, impaired renal function, dehydration, polyuria or severe sweating impacting on fluid management (Hulst et al., 2006b) Although linked with muscle mass, it is not a reliable marker to assess nutritional support
Glucose	Debatable as to whether it has a positive impact on outcome, decreasing morbidity and mortality Important to monitor, especially in children receiving IV preparations and PN (Skillman & Wischmeyer, 2008)
Albumin	Likely to be low especially if receiving intravenous saline (McClave et al., 1999) Not a good nutritional index, due to long half life. A marker of inflammation, intravascular or extravascular fluid shifts and catabolism (Evans et al., 2006)
C-reactive protein (CRP)	An index of the acute phase response, usually measured serially Serum prealbumin and CRP are inversely related, i.e. serum prealbumin levels decrease and CRP levels increase in proportion to the severity of illness, returning to normal once the illness has resolved, e.g. <0.5 mg/mL In infants, <0.2 mg/mL associated with a return of anabolism, with a concomitant rise in prealbumin (van Waardenburg et al., 2009)
Magnesium	Hypomagnesaemia is commonly found in critically ill children (Braegger et al., 2010)
Calcium	Strongly associated with hypokalaemia and hypocalcaemia (Hulst et al., 2006b)
Phosphorus, selenium, zinc, manganese	Hypophosphataemia (up to 61% of critically ill children) (Santana e Meneses et al., 2009) Low serum levels of selenium, zinc and manganese are also commonly found in critical illnesses (Hulst et al., 2006b)
Lactate acidosis	Common in critically ill children, reflecting hypoperfusion, including diabetic ketoacidosis, septic shock and cardiogenic shock (Zamberlan et al., 2011) Lactic acidosis, base excess and a strong anion gap are associated with increased risk of death (Zamberlan et al., 2011) A level >2 mmol/L may be used as a crude proxy for cell function. Resolution correlates with survival (Zamberlan et al., 2011)

PN, parenteral nutrition.

- *Fluid volume restriction* is the main barrier to adequate nutrition delivery (Feferbaum *et al.*, 2011).
- *Procedural interruptions* can account for 11–57% of total interruptions and affect up to 62% of patients (McClave *et al.*, 1999). Often, feeding rates are not increased to compensate for time lost during the interruption, making it challenging to achieve nutrition goals (Feferbaum *et al.*, 2011) and resulting in large energy and protein deficits which negatively impact on weight (Hulst *et al.*, 2004a).
- *Interruption due to gastrointestinal intolerance*, especially where there is vomiting, diarrhoea, large gastric residuals and abdominal distension, may occur in up to 57% of patients.
- *Mechanical problems* such as nasojejunal tube dislodgement, nasogastric tube blockage and/or enteral feeding pump dysfunction can impact on the amount of feed delivered (Feferbaum *et al.*, 2009).

There is little published data on energy or protein requirements in critically ill children. Table 3.8.28 summarises some recommendations.

Type of feed

Ready to use paediatric specific enteral or infant feeds should be used to decrease the risk of bacterial contamination. The use of energy and nutrient dense infant formulae have been especially useful in critically ill infants (<1 year) (Evans *et al.*, 2006) where there are fluid restrictions, thus improving energy and nitrogen balance (van Waardenberg *et al.*, 2009).

Polymeric fibre containing feeds are appropriate for the majority of critically ill children and are associated with fewer episodes of diarrhoea. A 1 kcal/mL feed will meet the requirements of most children, but where there is fluid restriction, a 1.5 kcal/mL feed may be more appropriate. A small minority of patients with malabsorption syndromes will require hydrolysed, elemental feeds and/or specialist feeds when indicated (Braegger *et al.*, 2010).

Initiation of enteral feeds

Most centres aim to start feeds within 12–24 hours of admission (Briassoulis *et al.*, 2001; Meyer *et al.*, 2009) with the aim of achieving the goal rate as soon as possible (Zamberlen *et al.*, 2011). Early enteral feeds, using a stepwise approach, i.e. feeding algorithms or protocols, is well tolerated in critically ill children and is associated with improved nutritional outcome (Skilman & Wischmayer, 2008; Briassoulis *et al.*, 2001; Meyer *et al.*, 2009). Most children should tolerate nasogastric tube

Table 3.8.28 Recommendations for energy and protein requirements of critically ill children

	Recommendations
Energy requirements	70% EAR – no evidence (Meyer et al., 2009) Schofield equation – without stress addition or activity factor, shown to deliver the closest value to measured REE (Hulst et al., 2006, Briassoulis et al., 2001; Mehta & Compher, 2009; Oosterveld et al., 2006) In long term PICU patients (>7 days), especially where not using muscle relaxants and where there is active physiotherapy, a higher calorie intake may be required (van der Kuip et al., 2007) Ventilated children can be overfed, especially if liberalising fluid volumes. Overfeeding can result in fatty liver, hyperglycaemia, increased CO_2 production and increased length of hospital stay (Skillman & Wischmeyer, 2008)
Protein requirements	0–2 years, 2–3 g/kg/day 2–13 years, 1.5–2 g/kg/day 13–18 years, 1.5 g/kg/day (Mehta et al., 2009) 4 g/kg should not be exceeded (excluding for extremely low birth weight preterm infants) as increases the risk of hypertonic dehydration and exceeds maximal protein oxidation rates (Klein et al., 1998)
Glucose oxidation rate	5 mg/min/kg/day (7.2 g/kg/day) – maximal oxidation rate Excessive glucose intake will increase risk of hepatic steatosis (fatty liver) and CO_2 production Amounts will vary for critically ill neonates and infants (Koletzko et al., 2005)
Feed composition	10–15% energy from protein (Clarke et al., 2007) 50–55% energy from carbohydrate 35% energy from fat (Flaring & Finkel, 2009)

REE, resting energy expenditure.

SECTION 3

feeding, but there will be cohort of patients for whom a nasojejunal feeding tube is indicated, i.e. feed intolerances with nasogastric tube feeding, or at higher risk of aspiration (Mehta et al., 2009; Braegger et al., 2010). Although bolus feeding is more physiological, continuous feeds delivered via a volumetric pump may be better tolerated as they have less impact on clinical indices such as hyperglycaemia, although the research in this area is limited and not equivocal, with some reports showing no difference between tolerance, e.g. diarrhoea and vomiting (Horn & Chaboyer, 2003).

Refeeding syndrome

As the prevalence of malnutrition within the PICU population is high, the risk for refeeding syndrome should be considered. When enteral or parenteral nutrition is commenced in children who have not received optimal nutritional support for some time, e.g. 3 days or more, it is important to ensure there is a multidisciplinary approach to determine the risk of refeeding syndrome, in addition to an appropriate management strategy regarding electrolyte replacement, vitamin supplementation, and energy and protein restriction (Braegger et al., 2010; Byrnes & Stangeness, 2011; Afzal et al., 2002; Solomon & Kirby, 1990; Crook et al., 2001).

Critically ill children represent a nutritionally vulnerable population who may already be malnourished on admission. Nutritional support in this population group requires attention to detail to ensure the challenge of meeting nutritional requirements occurs early in their PICU stay with a focus on achieving equilibrium and not over- or under-feeding.

Internet resources

Paediatric Intensive Care Audit Network (PICANET)   www.picanet.org.uk/index.html

References

Afzal NA, Addai S, Fagbemi A, Murch S, Thomson M, Heuschkel R. (2002) Refeeding syndrome with enteral nutrition in children: a case report, literature review and clinical guidelines. *Clinical Nutrition* 21(6): 515–520.

Braegger C, Decsi T, Dias JA, et al. (2010) Practical approach to paediatric enteral nutrition: a comment by the ESPGHAN committee on nutrition. *Journal of Pediatric Gastroenterology and Nutrition* 51(1): 110–122.

Briassoulis GC, Zavras NJ, Hatzis MT. (2001) Effectiveness and safety of a protocol for promotion of early intragastric feeding in critically ill children. *Pediatric Critical Care Medicine* 2(2): 113–121.

Byrnes MC, Stangenes J. (2011) Refeeding in the ICU: an adult and pediatric problem. *Current Opinion in Clinical Nutrition and Metabolic Care* 14(2): 186–192.

Clarke SE, Evans S, Macdonald A, Davies P, Booth IW. (2007) Randomized comparison of a nutrient-dense formula with an energy-supplemented formula for infants with faltering growth. *Journal of Human Nutrition and Dietetics* 20(4): 329–339.

Coss-Bu JA, Klish WJ, Walding D, Stein F, Smith EO, Jefferson LS. (2001) Energy metabolism, nitrogen balance, and substrate utilization in critically ill children. *American Journal of Clinical Nutrition* 74(5): 664–669.

Crook MA, Hally V, Panteli JV. (2001) The importance of the refeeding syndrome. *Nutrition* 17(7–8): 632–637.

Delgado AF, Okay TS, Leone C, Nichols B, Del Negro GM, Vaz FA. (2008) Hospital malnutrition and inflammatory response in critically ill children and adolescents admitted to a tertiary intensive care unit. *Clinics (Sao Paulo)* 63(3): 357–62.

Evans S, Twaissi H, Daly A, Davies P, Macdonald A. (2006) Should high-energy infant formula be given at full strength from its first day of usage? *Journal of Human Nutrition and Dietetics* 19(3):

191–197; quiz 199–201.Feferbaum R, Delgado AF, Zamberlan P, Leone C. (2009) Challenges of nutritional assessment in pediatric ICU. *Current Opinion in Clinical Nutrition and Metabolic Care* 12(3): 245–250.

Flaring U, Finkel Y. (2009) Nutritional support to patients within the pediatric intensive setting. *Paediatric Anaesthesia* 19(4): 300–312.

Goiburu ME, Goiburu MM, Bianco H, *et al.* (2006) The impact of malnutrition on morbidity, mortality and length of hospital stay in trauma patients. *Nutrition in Hospital* 21(5): 604–610.

Horn D, Chaboyer W. (2003) Gastric feeding in critically ill children: a randomized controlled trial. *American Journal of Critical Care* 12(5): 461–468.

Hulst JM, van Goudoever JB, Zimmermann IJ, *et al.* (2004a) The effect of cumulative energy and protein deficiency on anthropometric parameters in a pediatric ICU population. *Clinical Nutrition* 23(6): 1381–1389.

Hulst J, Joosten K, Zimmermann L, *et al.* (2004b) Malnutrition in critically ill children: from admission to 6 months after discharge. *Clinical Nutrition* 23(2): 223–232.

Hulst JM, Joosten KF, Tibboel D, van Goudoever JB. (2006a) Causes and consequences of inadequate substrate supply to pediatric ICU patients. *Current Opinion in Clinical Nutrition and Metabolic Care* 9(3): 297–303.

Hulst JM, van Goudoever JB, Zimmermann IJ, Tibboel D, Joosten KF. (2006b) The role of initial monitoring of routine biochemical nutritional markers in critically ill children. *Journal of Nutrition and Biochemistry* 17(1): 57–62.

Klein CJ, Stanek GS, Wiles CE 3rd. (1998) *Overfeeding macronutrients to critically ill adults: metabolic complications. Journal of the American Dietetic Association* 98(7): 795–806.

Koletzko B, Goulet O, Hunt J, Krohn K, Shamir R; for the Parenteral Nutrition Guidelines Working Group. (2005) Carbohydrates. *Journal of Pediatric Gastroenterology and Nutrition* 41: S28–S32.

Kyle UG, Schneider SM, Pirlich M, Lochs H, Hebuterne X, Pichard C. (2005) Does nutritional risk, as assessed by Nutritional Risk Index, increase during hospital stay? A multinational population-based study. *Clinical Nutrition* 24(4): 516–524.

McClave SA, Sexton LK, Spain DA, *et al.* (1999) Enteral tube feeding in the intensive care unit: factors impeding adequate delivery. *Critical Care Medicine* 27(7): 1252–1256.

Mehta NM, Compher C, A.S.P.E.N.B.o. Directors. (2009) A.S.P.E.N. Clinical Guidelines: nutrition support of the critically ill child. *Journal of Parenteral and Enteral Nutrition* 33(3): 260–276.

Meyer R, Harrison S, Sargent S, Ramnarayan P, Habibi P, Labadarios D. (2009) The impact of enteral feeding protocols on nutritional support in critically ill children. *Journal of Human Nutrition and Dietetics* 22(5): 428–436.

O'Donnell DR, Parslow RC, Draper ES. (2010) Deprivation, ethnicity and prematurity in infant respiratory failure in PICU in the UK. *Acta Paediatrica* 99(8): 1186–1191.

Oosterveld MJ, Van Der Kuip M, De Meer K, De Greef HJ, Gemke RJ. (2006) Energy expenditure and balance following pediatric intensive care unit admission: a longitudinal study of critically ill children. *Pediatric Critical Care Medicine* 7(2): 147–153.

Parslow RC, Tasker RC, Draper ES, *et al.* (2009) Epidemiology of critically ill children in England and Wales: incidence, mortality, deprivation and ethnicity. *Archives of Disease in Childhood* 94(3): 210–215.

Rittirsch D, Flierl MA, Ward PA. (2008) Harmful molecular mechanisms in sepsis. *Nature Reviews in Immunology* 8(10): 776–787.

Santana e Meneses JF, Leite HP, de Carvalho WB, Lopes E Jr. (2009) *Hypophosphatemia in critically ill children: prevalence and associated risk factors. Pediatric Critical Care Medicine* 10(2): 234–238.

Shaw V, Lawson M (eds) (2007) *Clinical Paediatric Dietetics*, 3rd edn. Oxford: Blackwell Publishing.

Skillman HE, Wischmeyer PE. (2008) Nutrition therapy in critically ill infants and children. *J Parenteral and Enteral Nutrition* 32(5): 520–34.

Solomon SM, Kirby DF. (1990) The refeeding syndrome: a review. *Journal of Parenteral and Enteral Nutrition* 14(1): 90–97.

van der Kuip M, de Meer K, Westerterp KR, Gemke RJ. (2007) Physical activity as a determinant of total energy expenditure in critically ill children. *Clinical Nutrition* 26(6): 744–751.

van Waardenburg DA, de Betue CT, Goudoever JB, Zimmermann IJ, Joosten KF. (2009) Critically ill infants benefit from early administration of protein and energy-enriched formula: a randomized controlled trial. *Clinical Nutrition* 28(3): 249–255.

Zamberlan P, *et al.* (2011) Nutrition therapy in a pediatric intensive care unit: Indications, monitoring, and complications. *Journal of Parenteral and Enteral Nutrition* 35 (4): 523–529.

3.8.25 Neurosurgery

Luise Marino

Only five centres in England are able to provide access to a full time consultant paediatric neurosurgeon; the remaining centres rely on adult neurosurgeons to make a specialist assessment of the individual child's needs, including surgical intervention (Chumas *et al.*, 2008). Paediatric neurosurgical services in the UK accommodate children with hydrocephalus undergoing shunt insertion and other related procedures, central nervous system (CNS) tumours, spinal surgery (excluding scoliosis), neurovascular conditions (excluding those related to head injury) and other specialist surgical work, e.g. cerebral abscesses, craniofacial surgery, epilepsy surgery and interventions for CNS malformations, e.g. Budd–Chiari syndrome (Parslow *et al.*, 2005). The emergency management of children with intracranial problems is initiated in the local hospital before transfer to a regional centre for intensive care and management of intracranial problems, including surgical intervention where appropriate (Tasker *et al.*, 2011)(see Chapter 7.17.2).

Severe head injury in children is the highest cause of morbidity and mortality over the age of 1 year (Malakouti *et al.*, 2012). Infants have proportionally more head injuries (Shi *et al.*, 2009; Bayreuther *et al.*, 2009) and increased risk of mortality from isolated head injuries (Bayreuther *et al.*, 2009). Early nutritional support is fundamental to recovery (Malakouti *et al.*, 2012). Neurological injury in children has significant morbid sequelae impacting on short and long term memory, in addition to difficulties with executive functioning, resulting in attention deficit disorders with long term implications for social, behaviour and cognitive development (Prins, 2008; Kosoff et al., 2009).

Scoring systems and nutritional support

The most common coma scoring system used in children is the modified child's Glasgow Coma Scale (CGCS) (Kirkham et al., 2008). Children with a CGCS score of 12 or less are likely to require nutritional support via a nasogastric feeding tube, due to either increased risk of aspiration and/or dysphagia.

Secondary brain injury

Whilst the primary insult accounts for some of the early mortality, it is the secondary brain injury, occurring as a result of hypotension, hyperglycaemia and raised intracranial pressure (ICP) that leads to poor outcome. Treatment modalities including nutrition management, have been shown to significantly improve outcome (Sharma et al., 2009).

Nutritional assessment

In order to determine a nutrition care plan for children with neurological injury anthropometry, biochemistry, clinical parameters and diet should be considered.

Anthropometry (see chapter 3.8.23)

It is important to consider how well the child has been growing up to the point of admission.

Biochemistry

- *Glucose* – in a recent study considering the relationship between hyperglycaemia and outcome in children with severe traumatic brain injury (TBI), any hyperglycaemia (persistent or episodic) beyond the first 48 hours was associated with poor outcome (Smith et al., 2012). It is therefore important to ensure that any nutritional support being given does not exceed glucose (g/kg) recommendations.
- *Sodium* – low sodium enteral feeds should not be used in children with TBI. Medical management of TBI is aimed at maintaining sodium levels at the higher end of normal usually (145–150 mEq/L) with the aim of reducing ICP as hyponatraemia is detrimental to the brain as it results in cerebral oedema (Carpenter et al., 2007). However, injudicious use of hypertonic solutions can also result in brain shrinkage, increasing the risk of intra cerebral haemorrhage (Patanwala et al., 2010).

Clinical factors

To understand whether the medical management will impact on the type of nutritional support being provided, it is important to have a basic understanding of the treatment modalities and rationale for their use (Huh & Raghupathi, 2009).

Dietary management

Energy and protein

Energy and protein requirements in neurological injury are not well researched. There are some published recommendations, e.g.:

- The Brain Trauma Foundation proposes providing 130–160% of resting energy expenditure for children with neurological injury (Malakouti et al., 2012).
- The American Society of Parenteral and Enteral Nutrition (ASPEN) guidelines suggest protein requirements as: 2–3 g/kg for 0–2 years; 1.5–2 g/kg for 2–13 years; and 1.5 g/kg for 13–18 years (Mehta & Compher, 2009).

However, other research suggests that energy expenditure in children with TBI is no higher compared with other critically ill children (Briassoulis et al., 2006), so a similar approach to that used in critically ill children may be more appropriate. Muscle relaxants, sedation, mechanical ventilation and malnutrition lead to a reduction in energy requirements as a result of decreased muscle mass activity (Briassoulis et al., 2000; Vizzini & Arando-Michel, 2011). Both over- and under-feeding in neurological injury have negative sequelae, with underfeeding resulting in muscle wasting and weight loss of up to 15%/week (Vizzini & Arando-Michel, 2011; Phillips et al., 1987) and overfeeding resulting in hyperglycaemia and hepatic steatosis (Vizzini & Arando-Michel, 2011).

Initiation of enteral feeds

Children not fed within 5–7 days have a two- to four-fold increased likelihood of dying (Hartl et al., 2008) in contrast to those who are fed within 72 hours (Vizzini & Arando-Michel, 2011). Enteral feeds should be commenced as soon as the child is medically stable (Mehta et al., 2010). For most this is within 4–6 hours post surgery or admission with the aim of achieving the goal rate within 72 hours post admission (Mehta et al., 2010). However, enteral feeding in neurological injury is not effective in preserving muscle protein content, resulting in a negative nitrogen balance and hypoglutaminaemia (Vizzini & Arando-Michel, 2011; Charrueau et al., 2009). The implementation of feeding protocols may help to achieve nutrition goals (Vizzini & Arando-Michel, 2011; Mehta, 2009; Meyer et al., 2009). Children with TBI do not require specialised enteral feeds, but as bowel motility is often affected by TBI, a fibre containing feed can be important, with the aim of producing a daily soft stool. Constipation and straining to defecate should be avoided as this increases the risk of raised ICP.

Complications of nasogastric feeding

Complications that are of particular relevance to children with neurological injury are increased risk of enteral feeding intolerance, which correlates with raised ICP and/or low CGCS (≤8), resulting in delayed gastric emptying (Marino et al., 2003), higher gastric residuals and increased risk of aspiration pneumonitis. Nasojejunal feeds should be considered (Vizzini & Arando-Michel, 2011); nasogastric and nasojejunal tubes ideally should only be placed for a maximum of 4 weeks, after which a gastrostomy or jejunostomy should be considered, especially in children who remain dysphagic or who have a CGCS of 12 or less (Vizzini & Arando-Michel, 2011).

Nutrition support of children with TBI in the future may include the use of acetyl-L-carnitine (Scafidi *et al.*, 2010), n-3 fatty acids (Mills *et al.*, 2011), vitamin E (Aiguo *et al.*, 2010) and a ketogenic diet (Prins, 2008; Prins *et al.*, 2005).

Internet resources

American Society of Parenteral and Enteral Nutrition (ASPEN) Nutrition Support in Paediatric Critical Care   www.nutritioncare.org
The Brain Trauma Foundation   www.braintrauma.org

References

Aiguo W, Zhe Y, Gomez-Pinilla F. (2010) Vitamin E protects against oxidative damage and learning disability after mild traumatic brain injury in rats. *Neurorehabilitation and Neural Repair* 24(3): 290–298.

Bayreuther J, Wagener S, Woodford M, *et al.* (2009) Paediatric trauma: injury pattern and mortality in the UK. *Archives of Disease in Childhood Education in Practice Edition* 94(2): 37–41.

Briassoulis G, Venkataraman S, Thompson AE. (2000) Energy expenditure in critically ill children. *Critical Care Medicine* 28(4): 1166–1172.

Briassoulis G, Filippou O, Kanariou M, Papassotiriou I, Hatzis T. (2006) Temporal nutritional and inflammatory changes in children with severe head injury fed a regular or an immune-enhancing diet: A randomized, controlled trial. *Pediatric Critical Care Medicine* 7(1): 56–62.

Carpenter J, Weinstein S, Myseros J, Vezina G, Bell MJ. (2007) Inadvertent hyponatremia leading to acute cerebral edema and early evidence of herniation. *Neurocritical Care* 6(3): 195–199.

Charrueau C, Belabed L, Besson V, Chaumeil JC, Cynober L, Moinard C. (2009) Metabolic response and nutritional support in traumatic brain injury: evidence for resistance to renutrition. *Journal of Neurotrauma* 26(11): 1911–1920.

Chumas P, Pople I, Mallucci C, Steers J, Crimmins D. (2008) British paediatric neurosurgery–a time for change? *British Journal of Neurosurgery* 22(6): 719–728.

Hartl R, Gerber LM, Ni Q, Ghajar J. (2008) Effect of early nutrition on deaths due to severe traumatic brain injury. *Journal of Neurosurgery* 109(1): 50–56.

Huh JW, Raghupathi R. (2009) New concepts in treatment of pediatric traumatic brain injury. *Anesthesiology Clinics* 27(2): p. 213–240.

Kirkham FJ, Newton CR, Whitehouse W. (2008) Paediatric coma scales. *Developmental Medicine and Child Neurology* 50(4): 267–274.

Kossoff EH, Zupec-Kania BA, Rho JM. Ketogenic diets: an update for child neurologists. *Journal of Child Neurology* 24(8): 979–988.

Malakouti A, Sookplung P, Siriussawakul A, *et al.* (2012) Nutrition support and deficiencies in children with severe traumatic brain injury. *Pediatric Critical Care Medicine* 13(1): e18–24.

Marino LV, Kiratu EM, French S, Nathoo N. (2003) To determine the effect of metoclopramide on gastric emptying in severe head injuries: a prospective, randomized, controlled clinical trial. *British Journal of Neurosurgery* 17(1): 24–28.

Mehta NM, Compher C, A.S.P.E.N. (2009) Clinical guidelines: nutrition support of the critically ill child. *Journal of Parenteral and Enteral Nutrition* 33(3): 260–276.

Mehta NM. (2009) Approach to enteral feeding in the PICU. *Nutrition in Clinical Practice* 24(3): 377–387.

Mehta NM, McAleer D, Hamilton S, *et al.* (2010) Challenges to optimal enteral nutrition in a multidisciplinary pediatric intensive care unit. *Journal of Parenteral and Enteral Nutrition* 34(1): 38–45.

Meyer R, Harrison S, Sargent S, Ramnarayan P, Habibi P, Labadarios D. (2009) The impact of enteral feeding protocols on nutritional support in critically ill children. *Journal of Human Nutrition and Dietetics* 22(5): 428–436.

Mills JD, Bailes JE, Sedney CL, Hutchins H, Sears B. (2011) Omega-3 fatty acid supplementation and reduction of traumatic axonal injury in a rodent head injury model. *Journal of Neurosurgery* 114(1): 77–84.

Parslow RC, Morris KP, Tasker RC, *et al.* (2005) Epidemiology of traumatic brain injury in children receiving intensive care in the UK. *Archives of Disease in Childhood* 90(11): 1182–1187.

Patanwala AE, Amini A, Erstad BL. (2010) Use of hypertonic saline injection in trauma. *American Journal of Health System Pharmacy* 67(22): 1920–1928.

Phillips R, Ott L, Young B, Walsh J. (1987) Nutritional support and measured energy expenditure of the child and adolescent with head injury. *Journal of Neurosurgery* 67(6): 846–851.

Prins M. (2008) Diet, ketones, and neurotrauma. *Epilepsia* 49 (Suppl 8): 111–113.

Prins ML, Fujima LS, Hovda DA. (2005) Age-dependent reduction of cortical contusion volume by ketones after traumatic brain injury. *J Neuroscience Research* 82(3): 413–420.

Scafidi S, Racz J, Hazelton J, McKenna MC, Fiskum G. (2010) Neuroprotection by acetyl-L-carnitine after traumatic injury to the immature rat brain. *Developments in Neuroscience* 32(5–6): 480–487.

Sharma D, Jelacic J, Chennuri R, Chaiwat O, Chandler W, Vavilala MS. (2009) Incidence and risk factors for perioperative hyperglycemia in children with traumatic brain injury. *Anesthesia and Analgesia* 108(1): 81–89.

Shi J, Xiang H, Wheeler K, *et al.* (2009) Costs, mortality likelihood and outcomes of hospitalized US children with traumatic brain injuries. *Brain Injury* 23(7): 602–611.

Smith RL, Lin JC, Adelson PD, *et al.* (2012) Relationship between hyperglycemia and outcome in children with severe traumatic brain injury. *Pediatric Critical Care Medicine* 13(1): 85–91.

Tasker RC, Fleming TJ, Young AE, Morris KP, Parslow RC. (2011) Severe head injury in children: intensive care unit activity and mortality in England and Wales. *British Journal of Neurosurgery* 25(1): 68–77.

Vizzini A, Aranda-Michel J. (2011) Nutritional support in head injury. *Nutrition* 27(2): 129–132.

3.8.26 Burns
Jacqueline Lowdon

Every year in the UK, over 6000 children are admitted to hospital for acute burn care (National Burn Care Committee, 2001). The causes and types of burn injury in children include:

- Thermal – scalds, contact, flame, flash.
- Chemical.
- Electrical.
- Radiation.
- Cold injury.
- Diseases, e.g. vesiculobullous skin disorders, staphylococcal scalded skin syndrome (SSSS).

In the UK, children with a burn injury will be treated either at a burn unit or burn facility, with the burns centres taking the more complex cases and where PICU may be required. A network of care also exists between the units, facilities and centres, to allow for communication and sharing of expertise.

Nutritional support

All children admitted with a burn injury are at nutritional risk. A burn injury causes a hypermetabolic state, increasing nutritional requirements. Nutritional support is therefore one of the most significant aspects of burn injury care. The aims of nutritional support are to promote optimal wound healing and skin graft take, maintain normal growth and development, and maintain immunological competence.

Calculation of requirements

There is no agreed classification for the severity of burn injury. The extent of skin injury is quantified in terms of the extent of the total body surface area (TBSA) involved in the injury, expressed as a percentage. This, together with the depth of the injury, is the most commonly used method of classification. However, other factors also have to be considered when initially assessing nutritional requirements:

- Age.
- Sex.
- Weight.
- Height or length.
- Preadmission nutritional state.
- Pre-existing medical condition.
- Special dietary requirements.
- Site of injury.
- Gastrointestinal function.
- Pyrexia.
- Grafted area.
- extent of healing.

Other factors that will influence whether nutritional requirements are met include pain management, periods of nil by mouth for grafting or change of dressings, and psychological distress.

Minor burns (<10%)

Burn injury in children does not raise the resting energy expenditure (REE) proportionally as much as it does in adults. When normally active, children become inactive due to the burn injury; this partly offsets the increase in REE (Goran et al., 1990; Childs 1994; 1995). Optimal nutritional state and weight maintenance can normally be achieved by aiming for the estimated average requirement (EAR) for a non-burned child. Children with minor burns are usually encouraged to meet their nutritional requirements orally. However, it is important to remember that in some children with an injury of <10% that enteral tube feeding may be required depending on site of the burn (e.g. the face), preadmission nutritional status and surgical management (e.g. grafting).

Major burns (>10%)

In a major burn injury, nasogastric or nasojejunal feeding should be commenced within the first few hours post injury. Early enteral feeding of burns patients, within the first 6 hours, reduces the incidence of paralytic ileus. Paralytic ileus can occur in severe sepsis, where septic diarrhoea causes paralysis of the ileus muscles. Other benefits include (Herndon & Tompkins, 2004; Chiarelli et al., 1990; McDonald et al., 1991; Hansbrough, 1998):

- Moderation of the hypermetabolic response.
- Maintenance of gut integrity; reduction in bacterial translocation.
- Improvements in immune status and wound healing.

Continuous feeding should be commenced initially and the rate increased slowly, to reach full maintenance within the first 24 hours post injury (McDonald et al., 1991). Due to the broad spectrum antibiotics used in paediatric burns patients, diarrhoea occurs frequently. This is not usually related to feed osmolality or volume (Thakkar et al., 2005). Feed volume will need to be titrated when oral intake commences, as long as nutritional requirements are still being met. Bolus feeds can be considered once the child starts to eat.

Energy requirements

Energy requirements are thought to increase in burn injury by >10% and are calculated using the Hildreth formula (Hildreth & Carvajal , 1982; Hildreth et al., 1989; 1990; 1993), as shown in Table 3.8.29.

Table 3.8.29 Hildreth formula for energy requirements in paediatric burn patients (Haycock et al., 1978)

Age (years)	Energy requirements
<1	$2100\,kcal/m^2$ (body surface area) + $1000\,kcal/m^2$ (burn surface area)
<12	$1800\,kcal/m^2$ (body surface area) + $1300\,kcal/m^2$ (burn surface area)
>12	$1500\,kcal/m^2$ (body surface area) + $1500\,kcal/m^2$ (burn surface area)

Surface area = square root of [Height (cm) × weight (kg)]/3600
or
Surface area[14] = weight $(kg)^{0.5378}$ × height $(cm)^{0.3964}$ × 0.024265
Burn = surface area × % burn

Normographs are available for estimating burn surface area (British National Formulary for Children, 2006; McCarthy & Hunt (2001).

Protein requirements

Burn injured children have a higher protein requirement than the recommended nutrient intake (RNI). The BDA Burns Interest Group currently recommends the following as a guide:

- Infants under 1 year, use RNI.
- For children aged 1–3 years, use 2–3 g/kg/day (Cunningham *et al.*, 1990).
- For children aged over 3 years and adolescents, use 1.5–2.5 g/kg/day (Bell *et al.*, 1986).

Fluid requirements

All burns units have fluid resuscitation guidelines and the dietitian will need to work out a feed regimen within this allowance. If the child is pyrexic, an extra 10% will need to be added for every degree rise in temperature.

Micronutrients

There are very few studies that have looked at vitamin and mineral requirements for children with a burn injury. Before considering a supplement, check the nutritional composition and bioavailability of the nutritional intervention in conjunction with the biochemical markers.

Parenteral nutrition

This should only be considered where there is a prolonged paralytic ileus or poor tolerance of enteral feeds. However, trophic feeds should continue to maintain brush border integrity of the gastrointestinal tract.

Monitoring

Daily food and fluid charts need to be maintained accurately in order to monitor and evaluate intake (Vijfhuize *et al.*, 2010). Bowel habits also need to be monitored closely as this may affect feed tolerance, e.g. analgesia and being bed bound can result in constipation. Weight should be reviewed when possible in theatre or when there is a change of dressings. It is important to remember that oedema due to the initial injury may mask a true weight. Nutritional biochemical markers should be requested and monitored as necessary.

Burn injuries are dynamic, as the percentage burn surface area changes due to wound healing or degradation due to infection; therefore, so will a child's nutritional requirements, and these require reassessment as necessary.

Post discharge

During hospitalisation the child and family will have been advised about a high energy, high protein diet. On discharge, this needs to be reassessed on an individual basis.

Internet resources

British Burn Association   www.britishburnsassociation.org

References

Bell SJ, Wyatt MS. (1986) Nutritional guidelines for burned patients. *Journal of American Dietetic Association* 86: 648–653.

British National Formulary for Children (2006) London: Pharmaceutical Press.

Childs C. (1994) Studies in children provide a model to re-examine the metabolic response to burn injuries in patients treated by contemporary burn protocol. *Burns* 20: 291–300.

Childs C. (1995) Feeding the burned patient. Energy requirements, timing and effects of dietary intake. *British Journal of Intensive Care* 5: 157–164.

Chiarelli A, Enzi G, Casadei A, Baggio B, Valerio A, Mazzoleni F. (1990) Very early nutritional supplementation in burned patients. *American Journal of Clinical Nutrition* 51: 1035–1039.

Cunningham JJ, Lydon MK, Russell WE. (1990) Calorie and protein provision for recovery from severe burns in infants and young children. *American Journal of Clinical Nutrition* 51: 553–557.

Goran MI, Peters EJ, Herndon DN, Wolfe RR. (1990) Total energy expenditure in burned children using the doubly labelled water technique. *American Journal of Physiology* 259: E576–585.

Hansbrough JF. (1998) Enteral nutritional support in burn patients. *Gastrointestinal Endoscocpy Clinics of North America* 42: 645–667.

Haycock GB, Schwartz GJ, Wisotsky DH. (1978) Geometric method for measuring body surface area: a height – weight formula validated in infants, children and adults. *Journal of Paediatrics* 93: 62–66.

Herndon DN, Tompkins RG. (2004) Support of the metabolic response to burn injury. *Lancet* 363: 1895–1902.

Hildreth MA, Carvajal H. (1982) Caloric requirements in burned children: A simple formula to estimate daily caloric requirements. *Journal of Burn Care and Rehabilitation* 3(2): 78–80.

Hildreth MA, Herndon DN, Desai MH, Duke MA. (1989) Caloric needs of adolescent patients with burns. *Journal of Burn Care and Rehabilitation* 10(6): 523–526.

Hildreth MA, Herndon DH, Desai MH, *et al.* (1990) Current treatment reduces calories required to maintain weight in paediatric patients with burns. *Journal of Burn Care and Rehabilitation* 11: 405–409.

Hildreth MA, Herndon DH, Desai MH, *et al.* (1993) Calorific requirements of patients with burns under one year of age. *Journal of Burn Care and Rehabilitation* 14: 108–112

McCarthy H, Hunt D. (2001) Burns. In: Shaw V, Lawson M (eds) *Clinical Paediatric Dietetics*, 2nd edn. Oxford: Blackwell Publishing.

McDonald WS, Sharp CW Jr, Deitch EA. (1991) Immediate enteral feeding in burn patients is safe and effective. *Journal of Parenteral and Enteral Nutrition* 15: 578–579.

National Burn Care Committee. (2001) *National Burn Care Review: Standards and Strategy for Burn Care*. A Review of Burn Care in the British Isles. UK: Committee Report.

Thakkar K, Kien CL, Rosenblatt JI, Herndon DN. (2005) Diarrhea in severely burned children. *Journal of Parenteral and Enteral Nutrition* 29: 8–11.

Vijfhuize S, Verburg M, Marino L, van Dijk M, Rode H. (2010) An evaluation of nutritional practice in a paediatric burns unit. *South African Medical Journal* 100(6): 383–386.

3.8.27 General surgery
Shelley Easter

There are many conditions and procedures that affect a child's feeding ability. It is important for dietitians in non-specialised hospitals who receive surgical patients from larger centres to understand surgical practices and, for more complex patients, liaise with the centre's dietitian. For example, district general hospitals may receive infants who have had corrective surgery for gastroschisis or duodenal atresia.

As with any admission, a child's intake can be altered just by being away from home and not receiving their usual food choices. This can be compounded by surgery, even if there is not a specific linked nutritional condition. For example, a child who is nil by mouth prior to surgery and for the remainder of the day following their surgery is unlikely to need dietetic input. However, if a teenage boy, who will have a high energy requirement, does not eat well prior to surgery and takes several days to regain his appetite fully, he may lose weight and need brief but quickly implemented nutritional support. Therefore, nutritional screening with a prompt response to any issues raised is essential.

Common surgical procedures that require dietetic input

Fundoplication

This surgery is a treatment option in severe cases of gastro-oesophageal reflux when medication fails to control symptoms and growth is compromised. The most common type performed is a Nissen's fundoplication when the fundus is wrapped around the lower part of the oesophagus to form a valve between the oesophagus and stomach. This reduces stomach capacity, which has nutritional implications immediately postoperatively. If a child is tube fed, the feed plan will need reviewing, either during admission or after discharge, with their local home enteral feeding team as bolus feeding will now be possible and feeding times could also alter. A reduction in feed may now be indicated if the child is no longer vomiting and absorbing all their feed (Vandenplas *et al.*, 2009).

Gastroschisis and exomphalos

These are abdominal wall defects that require corrective surgery soon after birth; in some cases the bowel is returned to the abdomen in a staged return. Parenteral nutrition is commenced until enteral feeding can be fully established. If breast milk is not available and the gut has had a lot of handling or suspected trauma, a partially hydrolysed feed may be used to establish enteral feeding. On reaching full feeds, the infant should be graded over to a standard formula to check if this is tolerated and thereby avoid inappropriate use of a specialist feed.

Oesophageal atresia and tracheo-oesophageal fistula

Both are congenital defects; in oesophageal atresia the oesophagus ends in a blind pouch rather than connecting continuously to the stomach, and in a tracheo-oesophageal fistula there is a connection between the oesophagus and the trachea. Corrective surgery is done soon after birth and, following the repair, the infant will have a transanastomotic tube *in situ* to keep the area patent. Feeds (expressed breast milk or a standard infant formula) can be given via this tube until oral feeding can start. Other points to consider include:

- Corrective surgery may not be possible soon after birth.
- Feeding difficulties can occur, or become more severe, prior to an oesophageal dilation, where the oesophagus is stretched. As the oesophagus starts to narrow, feeding can be difficult and the infant may fail to meet their needs orally. In some cases, temporary nasogastric feeding is needed.
- At weaning, some foods may be more difficult to tolerate and extra advice and support for parents will be needed at this point.
- Both conditions are frequently associated with other medical conditions and syndromes, such as vertebral, anorectal, cardiac, tracheo-oesophageal, renal and limb defects (VACTERL) and coloboma, heart defects, choanal atresia, retarded development, genital hypoplasia and ear abnormalities (CHARGE).

Duodenal atresia

This congenital condition results in a bowel obstruction as there is a blind pouch or a web preventing any further passage through the intestine; therefore corrective surgery is required. Parenteral nutrition should be started after surgery and enteral nutrition is not commenced until gastric aspirates reduce to minimal levels, indicating that the bowel is functioning appropriately; the surgeons will direct this.

Short bowel syndrome

In short bowel syndrome there is a significant loss in bowel length, resulting in malabsorption. It requires intensive and careful nutritional management and is greatly affected by which part of the bowel is lost. Parenteral nutrition is often needed for a considerable time and effort should be made to ensure appropriate growth with action taken to minimise complications associated with parenteral nutrition. Once enteral nutrition is permitted, feed choice and delivery needs careful consideration, along with the use of agents to slow transit time.

Further reading

Olieman JF, Penning C, Ijsselstijn H, *et al.* (2010) Enteral nutrition in children with short-bowel syndrome: Current evidence and recommendations for the clinician. *Journal of the American Dietetic Association* 110: 420–426.

Tsang R. (2005) *Nutrition of the Preterm Infant, Scientific Basis and Practical Guidelines*, 2nd edn. MacMillan Digital Educational Publishing.

Vandenplas Y, Rudolph CD, Di Lorenzo C, *et al.* (2009) Pediatric Gastroesophageal Reflux Clinical Practice Guidelines: Joint Recommendations of the North American Society of Pediatric Gastroenterology, Hepatology, and Nutrition and the European Society of Pediatric Gastroenterology, Hepatology, and Nutrition. *Journal of Pediatric Gastroenterology and Nutrition* 49: 498–547.

Internet resources

TOFS – support for families born unable to swallow   www.tofs.org.uk

References

Vandenplas Y, Rudolph CD, Di Lorenzo C, *et al.* (2009) Pediatric Gastroesophageal Reflux Clinical Practice Guidelines: Joint Recommendations of the North American Society of Pediatric Gastroenterology, Hepatology, and Nutrition and the European Society of Pediatric Gastroenterology, Hepatology, and Nutrition. *Journal of Pediatric Gastroenterology and Nutrition* 49: 498–547.

SECTION 3

SECTION 4

Specific areas of dietetic practice

4.1

Freelance dietetics

Elaine Gardner

Key points

- Freelance practice can be a rewarding career, has benefits and risks, and requires careful thought and planning.
- Self employment has legal and financial implications, and professional advice is needed.
- Constructing a business plan is essential when establishing a new business to assess its viability and monitor its success.
- Professional standards and codes of conduct must be complied with.
- Help and support will lessen feelings of isolation.

Traditional working patterns are changing and an increasing number of people now work in a freelance capacity. Freelance businesses are credited with contributing 8% of business turnover in the UK (Kitching & Smallbone, 2008). The number of freelance dietitians is increasing. The Freelance Dietitians Group (FDG), a specialist group of the British Dietetic Association (BDA), was formed in 1999 to support dietitians who are (or are planning to) work in a freelance capacity. More information can be found in the members' section at www.bda.uk.com and www.freelancedietitians.org.

The following information is intended as guidance only. Professional codes of conduct and legal requirements change and it is the responsibility of each individual to ensure that these are met. It is recommended that professional expertise be sought for individual circumstances.

Becoming a freelance dietitian

For many practitioners, the idea of becoming a self employed, freelance dietitian is an attractive option. Working freelance usually means becoming self employed and setting up a small business. However, there are financial, emotional and professional risks. Unfortunately, many new small businesses fail in their start-up period. In the UK the small business failure rate is about three in 10 in the first 4 years (Maloney, 2010). In order to become successful there are a number of important issues to address and strategies to develop, which may well fall outside the experience of a previously employed dietitian.

There can be a number of reasons for considering becoming a freelance dietitian. Dietitians need to look honestly at their reasons for considering the freelance option and to take an objective look at themselves. What sort of person are they? What are their strengths and weaknesses? Have they got what it takes, including the motivation and self discipline?

Implications of changing from employed to self employed status

When first considering a career as a freelance dietitian it is worth taking note of what may be lost, e.g. from leaving a full time post. Losses may include:

- *Financial benefits:*
  - A regular salary (which is paid irrespective of whether clients attend for appointments).
  - Annual salary increments, holiday pay, sick pay, maternity/paternity leave.
  - Automatic deductions for National Insurance (NI), tax and pension.
  - Professional indemnity insurance cover.
  - Subsidised canteen, accommodation, car loans, etc.
- *Career benefits:*
  - Recognised career path.
  - Supported continuing professional development (CPD).
  - Paid leave to attend conferences and meetings.
  - Free and ready access to journals and libraries.
  - Immediate support of colleagues.
  - Opportunities to work in a range of areas.

Manual of Dietetic Practice, Fifth Edition. Edited by Joan Gandy.
© 2014 The British Dietetic Association. Published 2014 by John Wiley & Sons, Ltd.
Companion Website: www.manualofdieteticpractice.com

- *Environment:*
  - Equipment, e.g. desk, chair, computer, printer, telephone, pager, etc.
  - Administrative and secretarial support.
  - Consulting rooms and booking in and appointment service.
  - diet sheets, resources and equipment, e.g. scales.

Many of these benefits will not be automatically available to the self employed person. The freelance dietitian therefore has to be prepared to take on the uncertainties and expenses associated with working for themselves. A compromise is part time freelance and part time employment. However, this may have tax implication (see section on taxation).

A freelance dietitian seldom knows when work will be commissioned and this demands good time management, both in the quiet and the busy periods. Working freelance may result in working long hours and at weekends in order to meet deadlines and, conversely, having unwanted, unpaid free time when contracts and projects have not been won or are scarce. Making effective use of quiet periods and keeping motivated, as well as productive time management and organisation are key skills required by a freelance dietitian. The nature of freelance work means that a great deal of energy and time needs to be devoted to building and maintaining the business to provide sufficient commissions to equate to a full time job and salary. Although the number of full time, freelance dietitians is increasing, the majority is working in freelance areas part time.

Required qualifications and experience

Registration with the Health and Care Professions Council (HCPC) is essential. A minimum of 5 years' supervised, clinical experience is needed for private, clinical practice as many private medical insurance companies (PMIs) stipulate this as a requirement for registration. A varied dietetic experience after qualification and a broad background is recommended for other areas of freelance work. In addition to dietetic qualifications, it is beneficial to possess other qualifications, e.g. a teaching certificate in adult education or recognised expertise in sports nutrition. A catering qualification, membership of the Hotel and Catering International Management Association (HCIMA) or work experience in catering or food manufacture can also be useful. If the business includes writing, becoming a member of the Guild of Food Writers or the Guild of Health Writers may be valuable. If the business is to offer advice in a particular speciality, the dietitian must have the necessary additional qualifications and experience to justify this.

New skills such as marketing your business, tendering procedures, contracts and remuneration proposals will probably need to be developed for the business to succeed. The most common reason for small business failure is poor cash flow management (Experian, 2010), and advice and training in financial business skills are highly recommended.

Work opportunities

A freelance dietitian can work in the areas of dietetics and nutrition. The opportunities are wide ranging and extremely varied, covering a broad spectrum of dietetic practice. Figure 4.1.1 provides a sample range of work opportunity areas that were identified by the members of the FDG in 2009.

Specialist skills such as lecturing, giving talks and presentations, counselling and research expertise are all marketable and can be valuable skills in a number of areas including:

- Writing diet related articles and books for both the consumer and professional press.
- Media work such as journalism, broadcasting, press releases, scientific or medical briefings and seminars. resource development.
- Consulting in the field of marketing and project management.
- Specialist dietetics, e.g. allergies, child health, obesity and weight management, diabetes, renal disease, coeliac disease, women or men's health. Expertise in achieving behaviour change will be invaluable.
- Menu planning, calculations and evaluation.
- Recipe development and analysis.
- Catering, food policies and writing or advising on catering tenders.
- Health claims research for food companies.
- Sports nutrition/fitness and health consultation and advice.
- Health promotion session development.
- Workplace nutrition programmes.

Clients

Business can come from a wide variety of sources. The fees commanded are likely to vary between the different areas (see Table 4.1.1). It is appropriate to register with a number of PMIs. Each company has its own requirements and specified payment terms. This may mean that the number of consultations or payment rate may be capped and the balance of payment may need to be obtained from the clients themselves (see www .freelancedietitians.org for further details).

Planning the business

If the reason for becoming freelance is to earn easy money, then disappointment and hard work will soon become the reality. Setting up a freelance business is a venture that must be taken seriously. While the professional work may be similar to that of working as an employee, the freelance environment is quite different and demands a different set of skills and aptitudes. To be successful a business-like approach must be adopted, no matter how little or how much work is done. In the early stages it may be worthwhile asking an experienced freelance dietitian to act as a mentor. In addition to excellent dietetic skills and professionalism, the freelancer

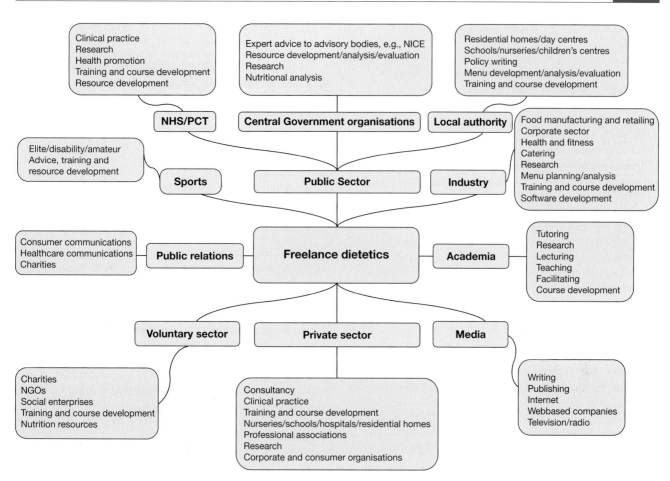

Figure 4.1.1 Work opportunity areas for freelance dietitians (from BDA Freelance Dietitians Group – Where do freelance dietitians work? http://members.bda.uk.com/groups/fdg/files/FDGwheredietitianswork.pdf) [source: The British Dietetic Association 2013. Reproduced with permission of the British Dietetic Association (www.bda.uk.com)]
GP, general practitioner; NHS, National Health Service; NGO, non-government organisation; NICE, National Institute for Health and Care Excellence; PCT, primary care trust

Table 4.1.1 Examples of clients in the public and private sectors

Public sector	Private sector
GP sessions	Private medical insurance companies, private patients
Hospital clinics	Public relations companies – product promotion and support, brochures, customer leaflets, press releases
Research, e.g. for government bodies	
Project management for service providers and area teams within the health services	Food retailers and manufacturers – fact sheets, product development and specifications, customer support, recipe cards, magazine articles
Expert witness	Television, radio and other media – research and consultancy
Education providers, e.g. lecturing, development of programmes and materials	Publishing companies – newspapers, magazines and books
	Medical and health charities – advice and creation of support material
	Catering companies
	Conference and event organisation or management
	Pharmaceutical companies

SECTION 4

needs to set up a business and therefore needs to be able to:

- Work independently and unsupported.
- Be fully committed to the project.
- Demonstrate exceptional organisational and multitasking skills.
- Be proactive:
  - Cope under stress and pressure.
  - Have sufficient funds to set up and survive until work comes in and invoices are settled (these can take 2–4 months to be paid).
  - Live without the security of a regular salary.
  - Take responsibility for tasks previously done by an employer, such as taxation and NI payments, and pension arrangements.
  - Have sufficient experience, confidence and contacts.
  - Write a business plan.

Business plan

The first step in starting any business is to prepare a business plan that outlines the concept of the business and evaluates its strengths and weaknesses, and therefore its viability. It is essential to write a business plan before resigning from employment. A business plan should answer the following questions:

- What is it that is being sold?
  - Dietetic skills and knowledge are now the 'products'. This requires a different mindset.
  - What particular skills and expertise does the business have to sell?
- Who will buy this product?
  - Who will the clients be?
- Where can these clients be found?
  - How will they get to know about the new business?
- How big is this client 'market'?
  - Does it even exist?
  - Can it grow?
- How much will they pay for the services?
  - Will they pay and if so, when?
- What is the competition doing?
  - Who are the competitors?

The business plan should include a month by month plan of the coming year with a realistic estimate of income and expenditure; this can be used as an objective measure of business progress. The plan should be reviewed on a regular basis so that the business can build on its successes and remain profitable. It should set ambitious but realistic goals for the business within a reasonable time frame. A business plan can be viewed as a starting point and can (and should) be reviewed as the business develops. Help in developing a business plan and start up information can be obtained from the business departments of high street banks and the government organisation Business Link (www.gov.uk/business-support-helpline). A number of aspects need to be considered when constructing the business plan.

Type of business

Working practices vary but the majority of freelance dietitians are self employed sole traders. There are alternatives to working alone, such as setting up a formal partnership or group practice. Consideration should also be given to forming a limited company. It is recommended that professional advice be sought as to which option best suits the individual situation and needs of each business; all have different financial implications. Talk to people about the business idea, listen to criticism and negative feedback, as well as doing all the necessary research.

Income and cash flow

Establish the income target that needs to be earned to cover ongoing financial commitments (both business and personal). Factor in standing orders for NI, telephone rental, pension payments, etc. that have to be paid whether there is an income or not. Tax requirements vary (depending on the type of business) and there may be a requirement to pay tax in advance of income receipt. As a safeguard, it is a good idea to set aside contingency monies (consider 4–6 months of requirements) at the outset. Consider that you may need to tender for work, complete the work (or a reasonable proportion of it), invoice the client and then wait for it to be paid before any income is received.

Equipment, resources and paperwork

Take time to consider what hardware is needed to run the business. It is recommended that a computer is dedicated to the business, as is a phone line and broadband access. Consider whether items such as a laptop, scanner or high speed printer are essentials or luxuries at this stage. Software programmes may be needed to write lectures and presentations, to run spreadsheets, or for dietary analysis. Other resources may need to be purchased such as weighing scales, height measures (stadiometers), diet sheets, posters, leaflets, replica foods and audiovisual equipment, depending upon the business focus. Professional documentation such as business cards may need to be obtained and other paperwork such as invoice templates and contracts need to be developed for the business. While there are many examples to be found on the Internet, professional advice regarding specific content may need to be purchased. Membership of professional organisations, both dietetic and business, is an essential expense that also needs to be included.

Office accommodation

Carefully consider whether the business is going to be run from home or an office. Take advice from experts and consider the advantages and disadvantages of each option.

Working from home

It may be that the reason for becoming freelance is to be able to work from home. If this is the case, then ensure that the family are in agreement and will provide full support. The business may need to take precedence over social activities or family events and this must be allowed for. Being at home may bring conflict between family and business, and a proper workspace needs to be allocated and office hours respected by all. Switching off from other activities in the house can be difficult and it is also easy to be consumed by work and difficult to take breaks, especially if there is an urgent deadline. Schedule adequate rest and relaxation as tiredness will slow work, lead to mistakes and reduce creativity.

If private patients are to be seen from home, it will be necessary to consider aspects such as parking facilities, disabled access, waiting areas, toilet facilities, public liability insurance, personal security and disruption to the family. Use of a domestic residence for business purposes may also have implications in terms of house insurance and council tax. If working from home, then the business (and home address) may appear on advertising materials and letterheads. Consider privacy and safety, and perhaps opt for a box number address or similar. If working from home, it is imperative that the business is still run with a professional manner and mindset.

Renting office space

Having a separate work place can be advantageous in keeping work and private life compartmentalised. It may be more professional to use rented accommodation for consultations rather than a room at home. There may also be an opportunity to share a receptionist who can take calls or make appointments. Alternatively, there are call centres that can handle your calls and pass on messages by text or email.

Suitable premises can include private hospitals, clinics and gyms. Alternatively, it may be worth considering linking up with other professionals, e.g. other dietitians, physiotherapy practices, pharmacies, or health and fitness clubs. It is important to find out what will be included in the rental. Does the room contain a telephone, computer, scales and chairs or do these need to be provided? Is there safe storage space for equipment allocated within the rental or does that need to be considered separately? Is the rental per session, week or month? These costs need to be incorporated into the business plan.

Arranging holiday cover

Events such as holidays should be anticipated and strategies developed to minimise their effects on the business, e.g. by informing regular clients that you will be unavailable between certain dates or arranging with colleagues to provide cover. In this way the goodwill of the client will be maintained, which is essential for continued business success.

Professional obligations

Registered dietitians must comply with the professional standards laid down by the HCPC and must make sure that the nature of the business, and the way it is con-ducted and promoted, conforms with these standards (HCPC, 2007) (see Chapter 1.1). Freelance dietitians working in private practice may have self referrals from clients. In such cases, dietitians must adhere to a strict code of professional conduct designed to protect the interests of both client and professional (BDA, 2008). It is important that freelance dietitians understand the circumstances when medical confirmation, or even formal medical referral, should be obtained for a self referred patient. Further guidance is available from the FDG.

Setting up a business

A new set of rules and regulations will apply and a dietitian must think and act as the owner of a business, not as an employee. For example, a dietitian who sees private patients and keeps patient details on a database will need to register in accordance with the Data Protection Act 1988. It is recommended that independent legal and financial advice is sought to help develop and action the business plan. Some of the issues that may need to be discussed are outlined below.

Banking

At least two business accounts should be opened; a cheque or current account for day to day banking and expenses incurred in running the business, and an interest earning reserve or savings account. Money should be put into this account to pay for tax and NI when it becomes due and, given the irregular nature of freelance work, it may be wise to allocate a proportion of earned income to this account to cover quiet periods when there is little work, or during holiday periods or in the event of illness. It is essential that business and personal accounts are kept clearly separate.

Insurance

It is important to know which types of insurance policies are necessary. This will depend on the professional activities of the business, the type of clients and from where the business is being conducted, but may need to include:

- *Additional professional liability insurance* – membership of the BDA includes a certain level of cover with regards to professional liability insurance. Check the extent of the cover and consider whether circumstances dictate a higher level or whether this is adequate. NB: Some areas of freelance work, although covered by this policy, require notification to the insurance providers to ensure adequacy of coverage for the profession. Additionally, it is advised that a provision for dietetic advice that is not face to face, e.g. given via the Internet or text, is discussed with the insurance providers.
- *Public liability insurance* – this is an essential requirement of some contracts but it may also be wise depending on the nature of the business.
- *Additional household insurance* – to protect business hardware.

- *Additional car insurance* – if a car is being used for business purposes, the insurance company must be informed and the premium may need to be adjusted.
- *Income protection* – this may be needed in case of minor illness or injury that means you are unable to work for a period of time.
- *Critical illness cover* – this may be recommended in case of serious health problems. This is useful, even if working part time, as it could provide money to help with childcare or a partner's expenses during a difficult time.
- *Private medical insurance* – this may be advantageous as medical treatment can usually be carried out quickly and can be dove tailed with work commitments, thus minimising disruption to earning capacity.

Pension provision

Retirement may seem a long way away but planning for it is strongly recommended and there are tax advantages in doing so. Retirement planning is a complicated area and it is important to take proper advice from qualified professionals, such as independent financial advisors who specialise in this area.

Taxation and national insurance

An accountant should advise on these and HM Revenue and Customs (HMRC) should be informed as soon as possible after the period of self employment begins. The HMRC provides fact and advice sheets about all areas relating to taxation and NI.

Taxation

Most self employed people will complete an annual self assessment form for the assessment of their tax liabilities. The rules governing the taxation of employed and self employed people differ in some respects and HMRC may not regard regular hospital clinic and lecturing commitments as self employed work. Such details will need to be clarified on an individual basis.

National insurance

Special arrangements apply for self employed people and it is essential to get advice on exactly what is required. Currently, Schedule D Class 2 will need to be paid from the outset and is best done by a standing order from the current business account. Class 4 is liable over a certain profit level and is assessed at the annual tax return.

Corporation tax

This is paid by a limited company on overall taxable profits; it is recommended that an accountant is consulted on this type of taxation.

Setting fees for services

The rate of fees charged for freelance dietetic services is important to the profit and hence sustainability of the business. Charges need to be clearly stated at the outset and clients need to be clear about what they will be getting for their money. Recommending a fee structure is difficult because of differences in the area of expertise, the client (public or private sector), dietetic experience, the amount of work and time involved, and the degree of difficulty. Fees can be set hourly for individual patients or per therapeutic session (perhaps one of three visits); per half day or day, per recipe, for one-off lecture or a series of lectures, for private patients or a regular clinic; or for charities or large companies, a long term project, a retainer, or according to the degree of urgency. Different fees may be necessary according to the region, e.g. fees may be higher in London and the South East of England.

Fees must take full account of the business set up and running costs. These include:

- The time required to prospect for new business and clients, follow up leads, put together bids and proposals, and attend interviews.
- Taxation, NI, pension, accountant's fees, insurance policies, professional memberships, subscriptions, etc.
- Hardware such as computer and printer, laptop and office furniture.
- Rental of office space, telephone (mobile and landline) and Internet access.
- Website development and hosting.
- Administrative and secretarial help to send out invoices and follow up those that remain unpaid.
- Cost of stationery, stamps, printer paper and ink.
- Loss of earnings during holidays or illness, or the costs of providing holiday or sick leave cover.
- Tcosts and travelling time.
- Continuing professional development – costs of subscribing to journals, buying textbooks and attending meetings, including travelling expenses.
- Sundry other expenses.

Approximately, 40% of a fee should be paid into a business reserve or savings account to cover tax, NI, and other expenses so that money will be available when these are due. Fees should be competitive and updated annually. It is important that a proper rate is always charged because undercutting fees devalues professional skills. It is essential that freelancers do not breach competition law by agreeing amongst themselves what they are going to charge for services and they must not discuss their fee structure with competitors.

Book keeping

It is essential that records are kept of all income and receipted expenditure. If the business is not too busy or complicated, it might be possible to run accounts on a spreadsheet or simple accounting software. Employing a bookkeeper and/or an accountant with experience of small businesses may be advantageous, particularly when dealing with HMRC. Invoices need to be sent out regularly to maintain a steady cash flow and any unpaid invoices followed up promptly. Although rare, bad (unpaid) debts can arise, so proper invoicing systems need to be in place to help prevent this. If this does happen, there are a number of options available for dealing with non-payment: invoking the Late Payments Act, the Small Claims Court, or hiring debt collectors.

Contracts

A contract defines the relationship between the business and the client. It needs to reflect and record accurately the joint commercial intentions and visions so that when an invoice is presented there are no surprises for the client. It can be used as a point of reference to help avoid any disputes and also as a tool for discussions with regards to further work or time allowance. It should contain case specific details such as who everybody is, dates, payment basis, services to be provided, the boundaries of these services, e.g. does it include travelling expenses and time? It may also be important to detail what is not included to help define the boundaries. It should also contain legal background details, e.g. terms, responsibilities for defective work, confidentiality and termination of contract. This section may be similar for all work undertaken. A written agreement or contract needs to be signed before work is started.

Advertising and marketing

Potential clients need to know that the business is operating and what services are being provided. Advertising the products and marketing the services are an essential part of the business, but as a registered dietitian there are limitations on what can be said, where it can be said and how it is expressed. Generally, it is recommended that advertisements be accurate and restrained; they must not be false, fraudulent, misleading, deceptive, self laudatory, unfair or sensational. Increasingly new technologies are being utilised by dietitians to market their services and promote their business. Consider establishing a website and registering the business in professional directories or with healthcare providers. It is essential that the right image is communicated via the company name, website and on headed paper and compliment slips, business cards and leaflets. Ensure that these all reflect what the business is about and what is being marketed.

Many jobs are obtained by word of mouth from contacts and by reputation. Some may be advertised in professional magazines or on websites. A specialist healthcare employment agency may also be a source of potential work. Ensure that a *curriculum vitae* (CV) is up to date and relevant for each potential client.

Help and support

There is a lot of help available, much of it free. Until November 2011, the UK government had a one stop website Business Link, which provided free and easy access to information, advice, funding and training for the small business, but this was suspended in November 2011. Details of replacement services are available at www.gov.uk/business-support-helpline. Local newspapers can be a useful source of information on courses and business networks that can provide help and support.

The FDG produces, and continually updates, a series of fact sheets for freelance dietitians on a wide range of topics, including Business Planning, Taxation and Accounting for your Business, Setting up in Private Practice, and Self Referrals. These are an invaluable resource for anyone involved in or contemplating freelance work.

Maintaining and expanding the business

Getting the business up and running may seem a challenge but keeping up the momentum is just as important and can be challenging to a dietitian working alone. It is not easy to look to the future when busy on a daily basis. It is important to maintain a professional approach:

- Keep to deadlines, deliver promptly and always deal with clients in a professional manner.
- Keep up to date.
- Pass on work to other freelance dietitians that is not within the area of expertise of the business, or where there is insufficient time to do the job properly.
- Be proactive – follow up leads and keep in touch with people. Be seen at relevant meetings or perhaps present a paper.
- Consider writing a newsletter for circulation to past and current clients.
- If working from home, dress the part. The freelancer who looks professional will feel more competent when talking to a client on the telephone in the office.

Staying motivated

Working single handed may bring feelings of isolation or even boredom, especially after working in a busy department. It is all too easy to put things off until later, e.g. go shopping rather than follow up client leads. If work does not come in as planned, then there is increased pressure, particularly financial, to succeed. Staying motivated can be one of the most difficult things to do.

Lack of work

It is inevitable as a freelancer that there will be times when there is no work. Be prepared for this, make good use of the time and consider the following:

- Enrolling on a course such as media, cookery, food hygiene, advanced computing, web design, etc. and make use of the newly acquired skills by, for example, writing an article or producing a website.
- Volunteering to be a member of a committee that might be useful and relevant to the business.
- Attending conferences and contacting former colleagues.
- Reviewing the business plan and tidying up paperwork, e.g. expense receipts.
- Updating the CV or the continuing professional development (CPD) portfolio.

SECTION 4

Continuing professional development

Any or all of the range of activities undertaken as a freelance dietitian can be used to provide evidence of how the HCPC's CPD standards are being met. The focus of the freelance business often evolves and changes and this can be excellent material for the portfolio. The CPD activity could show professional development alongside business development and evidence could be details from specific examples. It is important to document and evaluate every piece of freelance work that is done and every meeting that is attended. This document should be regularly updated and reviewed to see what has been learned and how this can be extended. This is an intrinsic and necessary part of being a professional.

Internet resources

British Dietetic Association   www.bda.uk.com
Freelance Dietitians Group (FDG) a specialist group of the BDA
www.freelancedietitians.org

HM Revenue and Customs   www.hmrc.gov.uk
Professional Contractors Group   www.pcg.org.uk
An independent professional association that covers all professions and represents, supports and promotes the freelance community
UK Government Business Support (successor of Business Link)
www.gov.uk/business-support-helpline

References

British Dietetic Association (BDA). (2008) *Code of Professional Conduct*. Birmingham: BDA.

Experian. (2010) Insight Report – Tomorrow's Champions: Finding the Small Business Engines for Economic Growth. Available at www.experian.co.uk/insight-reports/index.html. Accessed 18 May 2011.

Health & Care Professions Council (HCPC). (2007) *Standards of Proficiency: Dietitians*. London: HCPC. Available at www.hcpc-uk.org.

Kitching J, Smallbone D. (2008) *Defining and Estimating the Size of the UK Freelance Market*. London: The Professional Contractors Group. Avaialble at www.pcg.org.uk. Accessed 6 August 2013.

Maloney D. (2010) Small Business Failure Rate- 9 out of 10. Available at www.ezinearticles.com. Accessed 18 May 2011.

4.2

Public health nutrition

Alison Nelson

Key points

■ Public health nutrition is concerned with improving the health of the population and preventing diet related illnesses across that population.

■ There has been increasing recognition that nutrition is a major and modifiable determinant of many chronic diseases; diet can have positive and negative impacts on health throughout life.

■ Obesity and other diet related diseases are an immense health and economic burden in the UK.

■ A consistent evidence based message about good nutrition is important to give consumers confidence to change their food choices and eating behaviours.

Public health is defined as the '*the science and art of preventing disease, prolonging life and promoting health through the organised efforts and informed choices of society, organisations, public and private, communities and individuals*' (Wanless, 2004). Public health aims to improve the health of the population and reduce health inequalities by helping people live longer, healthier and more fulfilling lives, while improving the health of the poorest fastest. It considers the wellbeing of the population, including mental and physical health, while engendering a sense of control over the way people want to live. Public health focuses on the wider environment by influencing those factors that enable people to make healthier choices.

Today there are significant challenges to public health, e.g. two in three adults in the UK are overweight or obese. In addition, inequalities in health remain widespread with people in the poorest areas living on average 7 years fewer than those in the richest areas and spending up to 17 more years living with poor health (Department of Health, 2011c. The most effective way to address public health is considered to be one that addresses the wider social determinants of health (poverty, housing, education, etc.) and health inequalities so that '*no one should be disadvantaged from achieving their full health potential*' (Whitehead, 2000), whilst adopting a life course framework by addressing influences from infancy to old age.

A range of factors within and outside of the individual's control influence the health and wellbeing of individuals and populations across all age groups. The Dahlgren & Whitehead (1991) *Policy Rainbow* is a commonly cited model, which represents the range and interrelationship of factors that influence health (Figure 4.2.1). It describes factors that are fixed (core, non-modifiable factors), e.g. age, sex and genetics, and those that can be modified and expressed as a series of layers of influence. The relative contribution of each layer to improving health, and the actions required to change each of the influencing factors, has become a framework for the development of public health policy. It recognises that behaviour change can only take place in a supportive environment. For example, families wanting to maintain a healthy weight will be able to do so more easily in a supportive environment; an environment in which food production and retail facilitate access to healthy food at an affordable price, education provides the skills and knowledge to buy and prepare healthy food, employment or benefits provide adequate money, the workplace and schools have food policies in place, and housing is adequate to maintain family life.

Public health workforce

The public health workforce is diverse in what it does and the places it works. It is categorised into three distinct groups (Department of Health, 2001):

● *Specialists* – those qualified in public health and operating at senior strategic levels. This will include dietitians who are registered on the voluntary register for

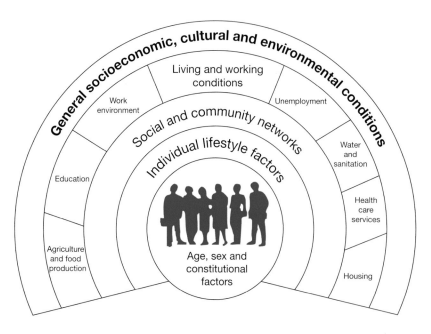

Figure 4.2.1 A social model of health (source: Dahlgren & Whitehead 1991. Reproduced with permission of the Institute for Future Studies, Sweden)

public health consultants or working at a senior strategic level.

- *Practitioners* – those working at an operational level to deliver public health programmes and services, such as public health dietitians, public health nurses, environmental health officers and public health analysts.
- *The wider workforce* – those who are able to influence the health of the population through their roles, including such disparate groups as teachers, spatial planners and directors of finance of health organisations. All dietitians working within a clinical specialty could be included in this group because of their influence on the wider family or community of patients they are working with.

Public health nutrition

Public health nutrition (PHN) is concerned with improving the health of the population by focusing on the wider environment to understand and influence the issues that help or hinder people to make healthy food and lifestyle choices. Public health nutrition aims to improve the population's health and prevent diet related illnesses across that population, rather than treating the diseases of individual patients. It recognises that the way people choose to live their lives is influenced both by individual factors and other factors that may be outside of individual choice. Hence, the work of a public health dietitian could include:

- Identifying need, e.g. using local data to illustrate pockets of increased childhood obesity.
- Planning strategy by engaging partnership groups, e.g. coordinating a group of stakeholders to develop a healthy weight strategy.
- Providing the evidence to support dietary change, e.g. literature review or research.

- Developing programmes, e.g. to increase fruit and vegetable uptake through school cookery clubs.
- Evaluating outcomes.

This chapter outlines the context for PHN and the principles behind the dietary recommendations that support public health policy work. It does not aim to outline the competences required by a public health dietitian or the theoretical models used to underpin ways of working. The history of our food supply and the social and economic influences on the way we eat are fascinating and important for a public health dietitian to understand, but are outside of the scope of this chapter.

Importance of public health nutrition

There has been increasing recognition that nutrition is a major and modifiable determinant of many chronic diseases, and that diet can have positive and negative impacts on health throughout life. The rising rates of obesity in the UK (and around the world) may have been responsible for this resurgence of interest and emphasise the importance of not just addressing micronutrient deficiencies in small groups, but also the need for policies to address whole systems to support people to make changes to the way they choose their food. The implication for health costs, as a result of this obesity and chronic diseases linked to obesity, are now recognised. Improving the population's diet becomes a necessity both for health and the economy. Modelled projections suggest that indirect costs of obesity (including direct NHS costs and loss of earnings) could be as high as £27 billion by 2015 [National Obesity Observatory (NOO), 2010a] (see Chapter 7.13.1).

It was estimated that 70 000 premature deaths in the UK could be prevented each year if diet matched nutritional guidelines (Strategy Unit, 2008). However, this has recently been revised to 33 000 deaths (Scarborough *et al.*, 2011). A third of heart disease and a quarter of cancers are thought to be diet related. The largest number of these deaths could be avoided if fruit and vegetable intakes increased to meet the 5 A DAY target (400 g/day). Reducing average salt intake from 9 g to 6 g could prevent a further 20 000 deaths. A fall in saturated fat intake by 2.5% of total energy intake and added sugar by 1.75% would each make a further reduction of 3500 premature deaths (Strategy Unit, 2008).

There are consistent reports of differences in health in different geographical areas of the UK and diet has a significant impact on these geographical differences (Scarborough *et al.*, 2011). Populations in Scotland and Northern Ireland consume a diet of poorer quality than populations in England. For example, the people of Northern Ireland on average eat a diet that is 4% higher in saturated fat, 7% higher in salt and 20% lower in fruit and vegetables. In Wales, whilst the health risks from diet are similar to those in England, the average diet is higher in fruit and vegetables but also higher in saturated fat and salt.

Although obesity has been the focus for much food and health policy work, it is only one consequence of poor diet. Low levels of breastfeeding, dental caries and constipation in childhood have implications for quality of life. In addition, poor nutrition is common in adults, particularly in older age, with 25% of patients screened on admission to hospital, 41% of residents recently admitted to care homes and 19% of adults admitted to mental health units identified as being malnourished (BAPEN, 2012). The need for consistent and integrated strategies to detect, prevent and treat malnutrition in the community to prevent older people from being admitted to hospital with malnutrition is necessary and has been identified as a major healthcare cost with direct NHS costs higher than those for obesity (BAPEN, 2005) (see Chapter 6.2).

National public health policy and strategy

This section outlines the main policy and strategy documents that have set the direction for public health and PHN, and the key agencies responsible for their implementation in the UK. In the UK, following devolution, the responsibility for formulating and implementing public health policies are under the auspices of the each of the four countries of the UK. The structures, policies and agencies described here may be limited to one country of the UK. More detail of structures in the devolved administrations can be found at:

- NHS Health Scotland   www.show.scot.nhs.uk.
- Health in Wales   www.wales.nhs.uk.
- Department of Health, Social Services and Public Safety in Northern Ireland   www.dhsspsni.gov.uk.

Healthy Lives; Healthy People

This White paper is the UK government's long term vision for the future of public health in England and is part of the reform to the NHS in England introduced in 2010. [For full details of the NHS changes, see Equity and Excellence: Liberating the NHS (Department of Health, 2010a).] It marks a radical change by aiming to deliver a wellness service and to strengthen both national and local leadership. To achieve this vision, the responsibility for public health has moved from the NHS to local authorities that will take the lead in protecting and improving people's health and tackling health inequalities. Local government has the responsibility for commissioning public health services, largely determining local priorities supported by a specific grant. Embedding public health in local authorities enables joint approaches to be taken with other areas of local government work, including housing, transport, planning and children's services, and with other partners, including schools, the police, the NHS, early years services and voluntary organisations, recognised as being influential in determining how and whether people make the best choices for their health. The delivery of the public health system in England creates an unprecedented change to the way many dietitians have worked in the past.

National food and health strategy

A range of expert committees, including the Scientific Advisory Committee on Nutrition (SACN), determines national strategy.

Scientific Advisory Committee on Nutrition

The SACN is an advisory committee of independent experts that provides advice to the Department of Health as well as other government agencies and government departments. Its remit includes the nutrient content of individual foods, advice on diet and the nutritional status of people. This replaced the Committee on Medical Aspects of Food and Health Policy (COMA) in 2000.

National Institute for Health and Care Excellence

The National Institute for Health and Care Excellence (NICE) (England) provides guidance, sets quality standards and manages a national database to improve people's health and prevent and treat ill health.

Food Standards Agency

The Food Standards Agency (FSA) (England) was set up in 2000 as an independent government department to protect the public's health and consumer interests in relation to food. Following the last change of UK government, the FSA (England) is now responsible for food safety and food hygiene. Responsibility for nutrition and food policy issues, other than food safety and food hygiene, moved from the FSA to the Department of Health and Department for Food, Environment and Rural Affairs (Defra) in 2010.

Department of Health – nutrition policy

Since 2010 the Department of Health in England has been responsible for obesity and nutrition policy through the health and wellbeing directorate (Department of Health 2010b). Nutrition schemes managed by this directorate include:

- Healthy Start.
- Nursery milk.
- School fruit and vegetable schemes.
- Breastfeeding, nutritional science and delivery, and obesity programmes (including nutritional labelling, food promotion, and strategy).

Department for Environment, Food and Rural Affairs

The Defra (England) is the government department covering:

- The natural environment, biodiversity, plants and animals.
- Sustainable development and the green economy.
- Food, farming and fisheries – including food labelling.
- Animal health and welfare.
- Environmental protection and pollution control.
- Rural communities and issues.

It is developing the government's commitment to ensuring food procured by government departments, and eventually the whole public sector, meets British standards of production or their equivalent and nutritional quality, wherever this can be achieved without increasing overall costs. The government buying standards for food and catering aim to enhance the competitiveness and resilience of the whole food chain, including farms and the fishing industry, to ensure a secure, environmentally sustainable and healthy supply of food with improved standards of animal welfare (Defra, 2011a).

Health inequalities

The link between inequalities and poor diet is identified in the following strategies; Tackling Health Inequalities: A Programme for Action (Department of Health, 2003) and Fair Society Healthy Lives, A Strategic Review of Health Inequalities in England (Marmot, 2010).

Public health policy structures in devolved governments

All three devolved governments have a specialist public health agency to support the delivery of public health in the country.

Scotland

Food Standards Agency Scotland

Following the transfer of responsibility for nutrition and food labelling in England from the FSA to the Department of Health and Defra, the Scottish government established a review of services. The recommendations of that review have been accepted by the Scottish government which has created a new independent FSA for Scotland responsible for food safety, food standards, nutrition, food labelling and meat inspection.

NHS Health Scotland (National Health Board)

In Scotland, NHS Health Scotland is the national agency for health improvement. The role and direction of NHS Scotland in prioritising health inequalities are described in A Fairer Healthier Scotland – Corporate Strategy 2012–2017(NHS Scotland, 2012).

Wales

Public Health Wales

Public Health Wales is a specialist NHS Trust and it provides an expert public health resource as part of the NHS in Wales. In Wales, the FSA continues to lead on general food labelling policy and food labelling law enforcement, although responsibility for nutrition labelling policy is now with the Welsh government.

Northern Ireland

In Northern Ireland, the FSA has retained responsibility for all aspects of general food labelling and nutrition labelling policy, including liaison with food authorities.

A healthy diet

A healthy diet is one that provides adequate energy and nutrients to promote good health over a life time, delaying or reducing the risk of diet related disease. The goal for healthy living for the population is to promote healthy eating patterns combined with adequate physical activity, and to ensure these health enhancing behaviours become the norm among all individuals. Diets high in salt, saturated fat and sugar, and low in fruit and vegetables and fibre increase the risk of ill health. A poor diet is associated with increased risk of high blood pressure, cardiovascular disease (NICE, 2010) and some cancers (WCRF, 2007). Consuming foods and drinks that are high in fat and/or sugars too frequently can contribute to weight gain, which has many negative effects on health.

Recommendations and key messages for a healthy diet have been remarkably consistent over the last three decades. Quantitative dietary targets for the prevention of a range of diseases associated with affluence were first published in the UK in 1983 (NACNE). The targets outlined a reduced consumption of fat, saturated fat, sugar and salt, and an increase in fibre consumption by the general population. Until this time nutritional policy had focused on reducing the incidence of nutritional deficiencies.

New evidence has added to the understanding of the complexity of the interaction between nutrients and health, and provided answers as to why certain foods seem to be protective. Additional knowledge about the interaction of various nutrients and biologically active compounds in food build on the understanding that a healthy diet should be met by eating a variety of foods in the right amounts. Only in a small number of instances may fortified foods and supplements be required to ensure an optimum nutrient intake.

What is eaten and attitudes to food have however changed markedly in recent years. In the UK, consumers are better informed and are more interested in the provenance, quality and other characteristics of foods and the impact these have on health and on the environment (Strategy Unit, 2008; FSA, 2012). This interest is reflected in the variety of produce in supermarkets, the growth of places to buy or eat food out of the home, the popularity of TV cookery programmes and the media's enthusiastic coverage of food issues (Strategy Unit, 2008). For consumers, many factors compete for a position in the decision of what foods to buy, including price, ingredients, quality, nutrition, provenance, and production and transportation methods.

Role of food price and choice

Changes in consumption and attitude to food have occurred in a period of relative affluence. Food costs, until recently, have been proportionately falling as consumers' disposable income has increased. Food prices have risen more slowly than the retail price index since 1975 and foods are significantly cheaper in real terms than in 1975 (Defra, 2009). Commodity prices are now rising and real food cost increases are starting to add to a family's cost of living. The price of wheat, maize and oilseed crops doubled between 2005 and 2007 and, whilst these prices have seen some falls, there are some permanent factors underpinning prices that will maintain these higher average levels (OECD-FAO, 2008). Recently, food prices have been rising more rapidly than prices generally; they rose by 5.5% on average during 2010 compared with 3.3% for overall inflation (Defra, 2011b). This price increase will hit those with the least income hardest. Households in the lowest income groups spend 16% of their disposable income on food (includes all foods and non-alcoholic drinks), whilst those with the highest income spend only 8% of their income on food (ONS, 2010). This is because low income consumers spend proportionately more on food staples such as milk, eggs and bread, which are hit hard by food price rises. Consumers see some food categories as an essential part of food shopping and will continue to buy them regardless of price; other food categories are more sensitive to price change and have shown a decline in sales; potato and fruit sales have fallen as prices have risen (Defra, 2009). Providing a healthy diet for families will be an additional challenge to those living in low income households who are already suffering a disproportionate amount of diet related ill health.

Environmental impact of food choice

Food not only has an impact on health; the way food is grown, processed, stored, distributed, retailed and disposed of has significant economic and environmental impacts. Concerns about current food consumption in the UK and its impact on health and economic, social and environmental sustainability were raised by the UK government in 2008, which came to the conclusion that the way people currently eat is not sustainable for either health or the environment (Strategy Unit, 2008).

There is an increasing recognition that a healthy diet must also be one that is produced in a sustainable way. Definitions of sustainability differ but generally encompass the three domains of equitable economic development, participatory democratic structures and greater environmental integrity. A much quoted definition of sustainable development is development that '*meets the needs of the present without compromising the ability of the future generations to meet their own needs*' (WCED, 1987).

The Climate Change Act (2008) sets out targets for greenhouse gas emissions (GHGEs). At present it is estimated that 18–20% of GHGEs in the UK come from the food chain (Macdiarmid *et al.*, 2011). Changes in food production and food consumption will be needed to contribute to the necessary reductions in GHGEs.

There is considerable debate about the recommendations for healthy, safe, sustainable, low environmental impact food. A sustainable food system has been defined as '*food associated with high levels of well-being, social justice, stewardship and system resilience*' (NEF, 2011); a vision that fits well with the holistic approach of public health. It is recognised that '*in terms of the environmental impact of household food consumption, the composition of our diet is more important than how and where food items are produced*' (NEF, 2011). Research has shown that diets would not need to change greatly from current recommendations for health to achieve this reduction in GHGEs (Macdiarmid *et al.*, 2011). A single consistent message is needed to prevent confusing consumers. There is general agreement on a set of principles that meets the needs for health and the environment (Table 4.2.1).

The priorities for food and farming are to support and develop British farming and encourage sustainable production by increasing the resilience of the whole food chain, including farming and the fishing industry, to produce a healthy sustainable supply of healthy food with increased standards of animal husbandry (Department of Health, 2011a). The government has a role in encouraging all public sector catering to meet more sustainable standards for the food bought and prepared. More than 50% of the total energy consumption of the UK catering industry is in non-commercial catering such as schools, hospitals and defence organisations (Department of Health, 2011a). Government buying standards are starting to develop criteria to support a more sustainable food system.

Reducing food waste and excessive packaging, and ensuring efficient disposal where waste does occur, are also crucial to reducing the greenhouse gas effect of waste management and meeting the European Union landfill directive to divert biodegradable waste from landfill sites. In the UK 8.3 million tonnes of food and drink are thrown

Table 4.2.1 Principles that meet the needs for health and the environment

Principle	Health benefits	Climate change benefits
Eat more plants	More fruit and vegetables – known risk reduction for coronary heart disease and stroke	Replaces resource intensive animal production
Waste less food	Economic advantages. A healthy diet is perceived as expensive – buying less of better nutritional quality could be achieved	Reduce the 40% of food planted worldwide that is currently wasted
Eat less meat	May reduce saturated fat intake, especially if processed meats. High intakes increase risk of certain cancers. Potential for detrimental reduction in iron intakes must be considered	Reduces resource intensive animal production
Eat less processed foods	Often high in fats, salt and sugars	Resource intensive production, storage and distribution
Choose certified foods	No recognised health benefit	Improved animal welfare, maintenance of stocks

away each year. Most of this is avoidable and could be eaten if planning, storage and management improved [Waste and Resources Action Programme (WRAP), 2009]. Of the avoidable food and drink waste, 2.2 million tonnes is thrown away due to cooking, preparing or serving too much and a further 2.9 million tonnes is thrown away because it was not used in time. This equates to the average UK family spending around £480 per year, increasing to £680 for families with children, on food and drink that could have been used but is thrown away. The GHGEs that this waste food produces is 20 million tonnes; removing this waste is equivalent to the reduction in emissions from taking one in four cars off the roads (WRAP, 2009).

Population dietary guidance that takes nutrition, food safety and sustainability of the food supply into account is urgently needed to ensure that consumers are not confused by competing messages. The public is generally in support of making change to mitigate climate change, but when given a list of possible behaviours to achieve this, adopting a lower impact diet was one they were least likely to try (Defra, 2008). This will be a challenge for public health dietitians in the near future.

Scientific basis for a healthy diet

Clear consistent messages for the general public are important to maintain consumer confidence and support behaviour changes towards a healthier diet. Healthy eating advice for the general public is based on nutrient based guidelines for the population and a set of dietary goals.

Dietary reference values

These are quantified nutrient based guidelines for different population subgroups of the UK for the energy and essential macro- and micro-nutrients to prevent nutritional deficiencies. The COMA (Department of Health, 1991) published dietary recommended values (DRVs) and SACN (2011) revised the reference values for energy in 2011. The European Food Safety Authority (EFSA) sets

European DRVs for nutrients as a basis for consistency across Europe and as reference values in food labelling (EFSA 2010a,b). Recommended daily allowances (RDAs) are used across all European countries to provide a set of standard figures for food labelling. They are based on DRVs, with small differences, and are used only for food labelling.

Dietary reference values are benchmark intakes of energy and nutrients. They indicate the amount of energy or individual nutrients needed by a group of people of a certain age range (and sometimes gender) for good health. They are appropriate for assessing population intakes and should not be used for designing a diet for an individual (see Chapter 2.1).

The DRVs for energy are described as the estimated average requirement (EAR). Most other nutrients have an EAR and also a reference nutrient intake (RNI) and a lower reference nutrient intake (LRNI). These terms are described as:

- *Estimated average requirement (EAR)* – an estimate of the average requirement of energy or a nutrient needed by a group of people. Half the population will have needs greater than this, and half will have needs below this amount.
- *Reference nutrient intake (RNI)* – the amount of a nutrient that is enough to meet the dietary requirements of nearly all of a group of people (about 97%). If people get more than this amount, they will almost certainly be getting enough.
- *Lower reference nutrient intake (LRNI)* – the amount that is sufficient for the 3% of a group of people with the smallest needs. Most people will have needs greater than this.
- *Safe intake* is used where there is insufficient evidence to set an EAR, RNI or LRNI. The safe level is judged to be enough for almost everyone but is below a level that could have undesirable effects.

Nutritional requirements at different life stages are shown in Table 4.2.2 [Public Health Action Support Team (PHAST), 2008].

Table 4.2.2 Nutritional requirements at different life stages [source: Public Health Action Support Team (PHAST) (2008, Table 1). Reproduced with permission of Hannah Pheasant]

Age	Requirements
Infants	First 4–6 months of life (period of rapid growth and development) – breast milk (or infant formula) contains all the nutrients required Between 6–12 months – requirements for iron, protein, thiamine, niacin, vitamin B_6, vitamin B_{12}, magnesium, zinc, sodium and chloride increase Department of Health advice recommends exclusive breastfeeding until 6 months of age, with weaning introduced at 6 months
1–3 years	Energy requirements increase (children are active and growing rapidly) Protein requirements increase slightly Vitamins requirements increase (except vitamin D) Mineral requirements decrease for calcium, phosphorus and iron, and increase for the remaining minerals (except for zinc)
4–6 years	Requirements for energy, protein, all the vitamins and minerals increase, except vitamins C and D and iron
7–10 years	Requirements for energy, protein, all vitamins and minerals increase, except thiamine and vitamins C and A
11–14 years	Requirements for energy continue to increase and protein requirements increase by approximately 50% By the age of 11, the vitamin and mineral requirements for boys and girls start to differ: Boys: increased requirement for all the vitamins and minerals Girls: no change in the requirement for thiamine, niacin and vitamin B_6, but there is an increased requirement for all the minerals. Girls have a much higher iron requirement than boys (once menstruation starts)
15–18 years	Boys: requirements for energy and protein continue to increase, as do the requirements for a number of vitamins and minerals (thiamine, riboflavin, niacin, vitamins B_6, B_{12}, C and A, magnesium, potassium, zinc, copper, selenium and iodine). Calcium requirements remain high as skeletal development is rapid Girls: requirements for energy, protein, thiamine, niacin, vitamins B_6, B_{12} and C, phosphorus, magnesium, potassium, copper, selenium and iodine all increase Boys and girls have the same requirement for vitamin B_{12}, folate, vitamin C, magnesium, sodium, potassium, chloride and copper. Girls have a higher requirement than boys for iron (due to menstrual losses) but a lower requirement for zinc and calcium
19–50 years	Requirements for energy, calcium and phosphorus are lower for both men and women than in adolescents, and there is a reduced requirement in women for magnesium and in men for iron The requirements for protein and most of the vitamins and minerals remain virtually unchanged in comparison to adolescents (except for selenium in men which increases slightly)
Pregnancy	Increased requirements for some nutrients Women intending to become pregnant and for the first 12 weeks of pregnancy are advised to take supplements of folic acid Additional energy and thiamine are required only during the last 3 months of pregnancy Mineral requirements do not increase
Lactation	Increased requirement for energy, protein, all the vitamins (except B_6), calcium, phosphorus, magnesium, zinc, copper and selenium
50+ years	Energy requirements decrease gradually after the age of 50 in women and after age 60 in men as typically become less active and with a reduced basal metabolic rate Protein requirements decrease for men but continue to increase slightly in women The requirements for vitamins and minerals remain virtually unchanged for both men and women After the menopause, women's requirement for iron is reduced to the same level as that for men After the age of 65, there is a reduction in energy needs but vitamins and minerals requirements remain unchanged. This means that the nutrient density of the diet is even more important

Dietary reference values are translated into dietary recommendations as shown in Table 4.2.3 (SACN, 2008). Values for total fat, saturated fat and non-extrinsic milk sugars are set as a percentage of food energy. Additional recommendations are included for maximum daily salt intakes for infants and children (SACN, 2003), as shown in Table 4.2.4.

Dietary guidelines

Dietary guidelines are food based advice for healthy eating. Food based guidelines for the general public translate the recommendations for nutrient intakes based on the DRVs and population goals described earlier into foods. The NHS provides advice on nutrition and healthy eating at www.nhs.uk/homepage.aspx. This advice centres on the eatwell plate and eight tips for eating well, including advice on eating at least five portions of fruit and vegetables a day, the recommended maximum daily intake of salt for children and adults, and hydration.

The recommendations are that everyone should eat a diet that contains:

- Plenty of starchy foods, such as rice, bread, pasta and potatoes (choosing wholegrain varieties when possible).
- Plenty of fruit and vegetables; at least five portions of a variety of fruit and vegetables a day.

Table 4.2.3 Summary of the dietary recommendations for the UK (adapted from Webster-Gandy 2011, table 2.1, p. 26. Reproduced with permission of Oxford University Press)

Recommendation		Population group	Reason for recommendation
Fruit and vegetables	>5 × 80 g/day (400 g)	Adults	↓ Risk of some cancers, CVD and other chronic conditions
Oily fish	>1 portion/week (140 g)	Adults	↓ CVD risk
Red and processed meat	Consider ↓ intake	All red meat consumers	↓ Cancer risk
NMES	<11% food energy*	All	NMES contribute to development of dental caries
Fat	<35% food energy	All	↓ CVD risk, ↓ energy density of diet
Saturated fat	<11% food energy	All	↓ CVD risk, ↓ energy density of diet
Non-starch polysaccharide	>18 g/day	Adults	Improves gastrointestinal health
Alcohol	<3–4 units/day men <2–3 units/day women	Adults (>18 years)	↓ Risk liver disease, CVD, cancer, injury from violence or accidents
Salt	<6 g/day	Adults	↓ Risk hypertension and CVD
Vitamins and minerals	DRVs	All	To prevent deficiencies and promote growth
Dietary vitamin D	DRV for young children, adults >65 years, pregnant and breastfeeding women Others with limited sun exposure also require dietary vitamin D	All	To prevent deficiency
Supplements**	Vitamin D	Older adults, housebound or living in institutions or who eat no meat or oily fish	To achieve adequate vitamin D status and ↓ risk of poor bone health

*Energy consumed as food and drink excluding alcohol.
**Vitamin D supplements are also recommended for pregnant and lactating women.
CVD, cardiovascular disease; DRVs, dietary reference values; NMES, non-milk extrinsic sugars.

Table 4.2.4 Recommended maximum daily salt intakes

Age	Target for average salt intake (g/day)
0–6 months	<1
7–12 months	1
1–3 years	2
4–6 years	3
7–10 years	5
11+ years	6

- Some protein rich foods, such as meat, fish, eggs, beans and non-dairy sources of protein, e.g. nuts and pulses.
- Some milk and dairy products, choosing reduced fat versions or eating smaller amounts of full fat versions or eating them less often.
- A small amount of foods and drinks high in fat and/or sugar.

Avoiding dehydration is also considered with a recommendation that adults drink between six and eight glasses (about 1.2 L) of water, or other fluids. Since this advice was published, the EFSA (2010) has published recommendations on water intake (see Chapter 6.6).

The eatwell plate

The eatwell plate (Department of Health, 2007) is a pictorial representation of the recommendations for a healthy diet for the population and is relevant for all adults and children over the age of 5 years. This food based guidance aims to help consumers understand how to achieve a healthy diet and reflects recommendations for nutrient intake based on advice from COMA and the SACN. The eatwell plate (Figure 4.2.2) gives a visual illustration of the types and proportions of foods needed for a healthy and well balanced diet. The sections of the plate show how much of each food group should contribute to a healthy diet. The sections include:

- Bread, rice, potatoes, pasta and other starchy foods.
- Fruit and vegetables.
- Milk and dairy foods.
- Meat, fish, eggs, beans and other non-dairy sources of protein, and foods and drinks high in fat and/or sugar.

Whether people are eating out, eating at work or cooking food at home, the eatwell plate is designed as a useful reminder of what types of foods to eat more of and which to eat less of.

The eatwell plate does not include references to frequency of serving or recommended portion sizes, other than in relation to:

Use the eatwell plate to help you get the balance right. It shows how
much of what you eat should come from each food group.

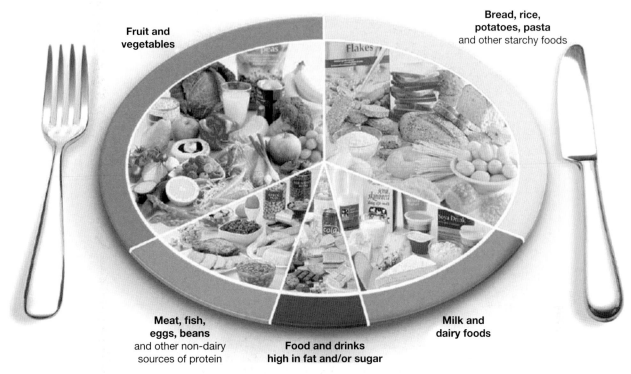

Fruit and vegetables

Bread, rice, potatoes, pasta and other starchy foods

Meat, fish, eggs, beans and other non-dairy sources of protein

Food and drinks high in fat and/or sugar

Milk and dairy foods

Figure 4.2.2 The eatwell plate (source: Department of Health 2012. Reproduced with permission of the Department of Health)

- Fruit and vegetables – at least five portions of a variety a day.
- Fish – eat two portions a week, one of which should be oily.

It is intended as a general educational model for use with most adult population groups (and children over 5 years). The calculation of each segment size was based upon quantitative guidelines for the consumption of foods within each of the five food groups to ensure a national average diet, that is consistent with DRVs. Portion size data were obtained from the Dietary and Nutritional Survey of British Adults (Gregory *et al.*, 1990) and was converted to amounts to be consumed on a weekly basis as a percentage of the total. The five food groups were as follows:

- Bread, other cereals and potatoes (34%).
- Fruit and vegetables (33%).
- Meat, fish and alternatives (15%).
- Milk and dairy products (12%).
- Fatty and sugary foods (7%).

NB: the total is 101% due to rounding of percentages.

The segments represent the proportion that the food group should make towards the whole diet. Individuals differ in the amount of energy they require and energy requirements will affect the total amount of food that an individual needs. However much energy people need, the proportion of food from the different groups should remain the same, as shown in the eatwell plate (Hunt *et al.*, 1994a,b;, 1995a,b; Gatenby *et al.*, 1995).

As the eatwell plate is a general model for the population based on the proportions of food needed, it is not appropriate to include specific frequency or portion advice. However, dietitians working with individuals can tailor advice in consultations, based upon the individual's current diet and food preferences, to include guidance on frequency of servings and appropriate portion size in line with the eatwell plate model, as shown in Table 4.2.5. A suggested number of servings is included but this should be used with caution; a serving is an imprecise measure and will be interpreted very differently by individuals. A good understanding of an individual's eating pattern and cooking habits is needed before offering advice in this way. Different population groups will need different serving sizes. It is the proportion of food on the plate that is important; the total amount will vary with each different population group. The eatwell plate model illustrates the following important key points:

- The need for a change in the proportions of food that should be eaten. Starchy foods and fruit and vegetables are an important part of the meal, and meals should be based on the starchy food supplemented with large amounts of fruit and vegetables and smaller amounts

Table 4.2.5 Suggested proportions of the food groups on which the eatwell plate is based

Food group	Food included	Key messages	Proportion to be eaten	Amount to be eaten	Main source of nutrients
Bread, rice, potatoes, pasta and other starchy foods	Bread, rolls, chapattis, pitta bread, naan bread, crispbread, muffins, scones, crumpets Breakfast cereals Pasta, rice, potatoes	Eat plenty, choose wholegrain varieties when you can	About 33%	For most people this is between six and nine portions/day This is probably more than people commonly consume	Carbohydrate Fibre (particularly insoluble fibre) B vitamins Some calcium (added to bread products) and iron
Fruit and vegetables	All fresh, frozen, tinned, juiced, pulped and dried fruit and vegetables (except potatoes – which are included as a starchy food because of the function they serve in the diet) Includes concentrates and smoothies	Eat plenty, at least five portions of a variety of fruit and vegetables a day	About 33%	At least 400 g of a variety of fruit and vegetables Currently not achieved by many	Vitamin C, carotenes, antioxidants Folate, soluble and insoluble fibre Potassium
Milk and dairy foods	Milk, cheese, yogurt, fromage frais, crème fraiche	Eat some, choose lower fat alternatives whenever possible or eat higher fat versions infrequently or in smaller amounts	About 15%	Two to three servings per day (a serving = 200 mL of milk, a small piece of cheese (40 g) or a small pot of yogurt	Calcium, protein, riboflavin, vitamins A and D (in full fat products only)
Meat, fish, eggs, beans and other non-dairy sources of protein	Meat, poultry, fish, offal, processed meat and fish products Soya, tofu and mycoproteins (Quorn™) Pulses Nuts	Eat some, choose lower fat alternatives whenever possible or eat higher fat versions infrequently or in smaller amounts Aim for at least two portions of fish a week, including a portion of oily fish	About 12%	Two servings per day Maximum of 70 g of red meat At least one portion of oily fish/week Commonly misunderstood as needing to be eaten in larger amounts	Protein, iron, B vitamins, zinc, magnesium
Foods and drinks high in fat and/or sugar	High in fat – butters, margarines, vegetable fat spreads, oils. mayonnaise and dressings, cream/cheese/curry sauces and fatty gravy, pastry, savoury snacks High in sugar – cakes, biscuits, puddings, ice cream, chocolate and other sweets, fizzy drinks	Eat a small amount	8%	Not a nutritional requirement but add variety and interest Most people eat too much	Some vitamins and essential fatty acids but usually combined with excess fat, sugar and/or salt

of protein rich meat or alternatives and dairy produce. The concept of meal planning should not revolve around meat and two vegetables (one of which, in this traditional model, was potato), but rather larger amounts of starchy carbohydrate with a small amount of meat and a large salad.

- All foods can be included as it is the proportion of foods over time. Some foods are eaten in larger amounts or more frequently and others in smaller amounts or less frequently.
- A healthy diet can be flexible and encourages a variety of foods.
- No one food is better than another – it is the balance of all foods that is needed to get the complement of all macro- and micro-nutrients. The concept of good and bad foods is not helpful as all foods can be included if the proportions are right.

An additional key message is to try to choose options that are lower in salt when possible.

The eatwell plate model is now increasingly well recognised. A recent survey exploring food attitudes and behaviours (FSA, 2011) showed that 21% of respondents, when shown a blank plate with the eatwell sections marked but not labelled, could place all the food groups in the correct proportions on the plate. Most respondents (64%) placed three food groups correctly. Younger people were more likely to place all foods correctly, as were people in professional/managerial households. Most people (84%) understood the messages about foods and drinks high in fat and/or sugar and could identify them as fitting in the smallest portion of the eatwell plate.

The most commonly misplaced sections were meat, fish and other sources of protein, which were judged to be eaten in too large amounts (placed in a large section rather than in a medium sized section), and starchy foods, which were judged to be eaten in too small amounts (placed in a medium section rather than in a large section). Fruit and vegetables were placed correctly in one of the largest sections by 82% of respondents. Similarly, 80% correctly placed the milk and dairy foods in a medium section.

Eight tips for eating well

In addition to the eatwell plate, the dietary guidelines include eight tips for healthy eating. The tips are:

1. Base meals on starchy foods.
2. Eat lots of fruit and vegetables.
3. Eat more fish.
4. Cut down on saturated fat and sugar.
5. Try to eat less salt.
6. Get active and try to be a healthy weight.
7. Drink plenty of water.
8. Do not skip breakfast.

Table 4.2.6 summarises the advice for each tip. Full details can be found at www.nhs.uk/Livewell/Goodfood/Pages/eight-tips-healthy-eating.aspx.

Additional guidance

There is additional guidance to support the eatwell plate and the tips for eating well.

Bread, rice, potatoes, pasta and other starchy foods

The advice is to eat plenty of bread, rice, potatoes, pasta and other starchy foods, and to choose wholegrain varieties when possible. Media attention to celebrity diets has resulted in many consumers believing these foods are high in energy or to be avoided to promote weight loss. Consumers' attitude surveys show that the required proportion of carbohydrate foods is often underestimated (FSA, 2011). People may need to be reassured that that they need to increase the amount of these foods in their diet to reach the recommended amount. However, there is no scientific consensus on the optimal macronutrient composition for weight management diets (Abete *et al.*, 2010; SIGN, 2010; Grace, 2011). It has been shown that a reduced energy intake results in weight loss regardless of which macronutrients are emphasised (Sacks *et al.*, 2009). This group provides foods that have a low energy density and a high volume. Choosing foods that are less energy dense results in larger portion size, which helps to control hunger. The intake of total carbohydrate (primarily by this food group) should provide 50% of the total energy intake for both adults and children over the age of 5 years.

Traditionally, these foods are served with added fat, e.g. fried potatoes and butter on bread, and it is this added fat that increases the energy density and leads to a high energy content food item. Advice needs to focus on changing cooking styles and eating behaviours to increase these foods whilst using minimum amounts of fat (e.g. substituting butter for a lower fat spread, oven baking potatoes rather than frying, having larger amounts of rice or pasta and less fatty sauce). Wholegrain cereals and breads, brown rice and whole wheat pasta should be encouraged to increase fibre content, increase satiety and prevent constipation. Most breakfast cereals are fortified with additional micronutrients and can be a valuable dietary source of folic acid, other B vitamins and iron.

Fruit and vegetables

The advice is to eat plenty; at least five portions of a variety of fruit and vegetables a day. Fruit and vegetables are an important component of a healthy diet and if eaten regularly in sufficient amounts, can prevent major diseases such as heart disease, stroke and certain cancers. Low fruit and vegetable intake is estimated to cause 31% of ischaemic heart disease and 11% of strokes worldwide (WHO, 2002). In the UK, the message for 5 A DAY was developed from the joint FAO/WHO global strategy on diet, physical activity and Health (FAO/WHO, 2003). The recommendation was for a minimum of 400 g of fruit and vegetables per day (excluding potatoes and other starchy tubers) for the prevention of chronic diseases such as heart disease, cancer, diabetes and obesity, as well as for the prevention and alleviation of several micronutrient deficiencies, especially in developing countries. The FAO/WHO recommendation added to the already strong

Table 4.2.6 The eight tips for eating well (adapted from NHS Choices. www.nhs.uk/Livewell/Goodfood/Pages/eight-tips-healthy-eating.aspx)

Tip	Details
1. Base meals on starchy foods	Starchy foods include potatoes, cereals, pasta, rice and bread Choose wholegrain varieties when possible; they contain more fibre and can make you feel full for longer. Starchy foods should make up around one-third of the foods you eat Most of us should eat more starchy foods: try to include at least one starchy food with each main meal. Some people think starchy foods are fattening, but gram for gram they contain fewer than half the calories of fat
2. Eat lots of fruit and vegetables	It is recommended that we eat at least five portions of different types of fruit and vegetables a day. This is easier than it sounds. A glass of 100% unsweetened fruit juice can count as one portion, and vegetables cooked into dishes also count. Why not chop a banana over your breakfast cereal or swap your usual mid-morning snack for some dried fruit?
3. Eat more fish	Fish is a good source of protein and contains many vitamins and minerals. Aim for at least two portions a week, including at least one portion of oily fish. Oily fish is high in n-3 fats, which may help to prevent heart disease. You can choose from fresh, frozen and canned; but remember that canned and smoked fish can be high in salt Oily fish include salmon, mackerel, trout, herring, fresh tuna, sardines and pilchards Non-oily fish include haddock, plaice, coley, cod, tinned tuna, skate and hake Anyone who regularly eats a lot of fish should try to choose as wide a variety as possible
4. Cut down on saturated fat and sugar	We all need some fat in our diet. But it is important to pay attention to the type of fat we are eating. There are two main types of fat: saturated and unsaturated. Too much saturated fat can increase the amount of cholesterol in the blood, which increases your risk of developing heart disease. Saturated fat is found in many foods, such as cakes, pies, biscuits, sausages, cream, butter, lard and hard cheese. Try to cut down on these, and choose foods that contain unsaturated rather than saturated fats, such as vegetable oils, oily fish and avocados Most people in the UK eat too much sugar. Sugary foods and drinks are often high in calories and can contribute to weight gain. They can also cause tooth decay, especially if eaten between meals. Cut down on sugary fizzy drinks, cakes, biscuits and pastries, which contain added sugars: this is the kind of sugar we should be cutting down on rather than sugars that are found naturally in foods such as fruit and milk. Food labels can help: use them to check how much sugar foods contain. More than 15 g of sugar/100 g means that the food is high in sugar
5. Try to eat less salt	Even if you do not add salt to your food, you may still be eating too much. About three-quarters of the salt we eat is already in the food we buy, such as breakfast cereals, soups, breads and sauces. Eating too much salt can raise your blood pressure. People with high blood pressure are more likely to develop heart disease or have a stroke. Use food labels to help you cut down. More than 1.5 g of salt/100 g means the food is high in salt. Adults and children over 11 should eat no more than 6 g of salt/day. Younger children should have even less
6. Get active and try to be a healthy weight	Eating well plays an important part in maintaining a healthy weight, which is an important part of overall good health. Being overweight can lead to health conditions such as high blood pressure, heart disease or diabetes. Being underweight could also affect your health. If you are trying to lose weight, healthy food choices will help: aim to cut down on foods that are high in fat and sugar, and eat plenty of fruits and vegetables. If you are worried about your weight, ask your GP or a dietitian for advice Physical activity can help you to maintain a healthy weight. Being active does not have to mean hours at the gym: you can find ways to fit more activity into your daily life. For example, try getting off the bus one stop early on the way home from work and walking
7. Drink plenty of water	Try to drink about six to eight glasses (1.2 L) of water (or other fluids) a day to prevent dehydration. When the weather is warm or when you are active, you may need more. But avoid soft and fizzy drinks that are high in added sugars. Remember: When thinking about alcohol, there is nothing wrong with the occasional drink, but drinking too much can cause serious health problems. Alcohol is also high in calories, so cutting down could help you to control your weight
8. Do not skip breakfast	Some people skip breakfast because they think it will help them lose weight. In fact, research shows that eating breakfast can help people control their weight. A healthy breakfast is an important part of a balanced diet, and provides some of the vitamins and minerals we need for good health. Wholemeal cereal with fruit sliced over the top is a tasty and nutritious breakfast

evidence that fruit and vegetables had important health benefits and gave a quantified target for action. Up until this point, while the health benefits of fruit and vegetables were recognised, advice was to eat more fruit and vegetables with no guidance on the quantities required (Williams, 1995).

As further evidence emerges from large cohort studies, it is becoming clear that specific cancers (head, neck, mouth, larynx, oesophagus, bowel and lung), although not all cancers, may be prevented by higher intakes of fruit and vegetables (Boffeta *et al.*, 2010). There may be additional benefits in eating larger amounts as there is an association between higher intakes of fruit and vegetables and the prevention of heart disease. Results from the large observational European Prospective Investigation into Cancer and Nutrition (EPIC) – Heart study (Crowe et al., 2011) suggested that a higher intake of fruit and vegetables is associated with a reduced risk of ischaemic heart disease (IHD) mortality. Participants consuming at least eight 80-g portions of fruit and vegetables a day had a 22% lower risk of fatal IHD compared with those only consuming three portions a day. As with all observational studies, it remains unclear if this association is the cause of the reduced risk and what the biological mechanism might be.

The message of the 5 A DAY programme has received year on year recognition since it was launched in the UK in 2004. Eating at least five portions of a variety of fruit and vegetables is an important part of healthy eating and is the target for the UK population who, whilst improving their intakes, are still not achieving this recommendation. Current intakes are estimated to be 4.2 portions/day (Bates et al., 2011) for adults (aged 19–64 years) and older adults (aged 65 years and over) consumed 4.4 portions. Thirty per cent of adults and 37% of older adults met the recommendation. There remain wide variations between different socioeconomic groups. Promoting fruit and vegetables as snacks is an important way to achieve the 5 A DAY target. Dried fruit is less suitable for between meal snacks because of its cariogenic potential.

Milk and dairy foods

Lower fat varieties of foods from this group (semi skimmed, 1% and skimmed milk and reduced fat cheeses and yogurts) should be chosen when possible. Lower fat varieties contain the same amounts of calcium, protein and riboflavin as the full fat equivalents, but less fat and energy. Due to their lower energy density and lower content of fat soluble vitamins, which are removed when removing the fat, they are unsuitable for children under 2 years, some older people and those who are nutritionally depleted.

Pregnant women should not drink unpasteurised milk, and should avoid soft blue cheese other soft cheeses such as brie and camembert and others with similar rind, whether they are pasteurised or not. These foods can contain high levels of *Listeria*, bacteria that can cause miscarriage, stillbirth or severe illness in a newborn baby.

Meat, fish, eggs, beans and other non-dairy sources of protein

These foods are all good sources of protein and a range of vitamins and minerals. Around 15% of dietary energy should come from protein.

Meat

Meat is a good source of protein, vitamins and minerals, such as haem iron, zinc and B vitamins; it is one of the main sources of vitamin B_{12}. Farming and butchering practices have changed over the last 20 years to ensure that leaner cuts of meat are available. Lean meat is relatively low in fat and approximately 50% of that fat is monounsaturated in composition. Processed meat products can contain high levels of fat.

In 1998 COMA (Department of Health, 1998) reported possible links between red and processed meat consumption and risk of colorectal cancer. Since that time the accumulating evidence has generally supported that association. The SACN (2010) advised that it is not possible to quantify the amount of red and processed meat that may be associated with increased colorectal cancer risk because of limitations and inconsistencies in the data. However, it advises that adults with relatively high intakes of red and processed meat [defined as those consuming over 90 g (cooked weight) of red and processed meat/day] should consider reducing their intakes. Reducing this intake to the average intake of 70 g/day is thought likely to have little impact on numbers of the population with low iron intakes.

Fish

The majority of the UK population does not consume enough fish, particularly oily fish, and should be encouraged to increase consumption to at least two portions of fish a week, of which one should be oily for the benefit of the n-3 fatty acids that they contain (SACN, 2004). Concerns about the risk of heavy metal contamination in large oily fish (shark, marlin, swordfish) has led to a recommendation that women of reproductive age and girls should not eat more than one to two portions/week of these.

Offal

Liver and kidney are good sources of haem iron. However, pregnant women should avoid liver or liver products due to their high levels of vitamin A; excess vitamin A is harmful to the foetus.

Eggs

Eggs are a good source of protein as well as vitamins and minerals, and can form part of an easily prepared meal. It is important to store, handle and prepare them properly to avoid any risk of food poisoning, particularly for vulnerable groups such as children, anyone who is immune suppressed and older people. There is no limit on the numbers of eggs a healthy person can consume as part of a healthy diet. Although eggs contain dietary cholesterol, this is not a significant concern and eggs consumed within the normal range of intake will have little effect on blood cholesterol. Eggs are relatively low in total and saturated fat.

Pulses

Pulses (beans and lentils) have a high protein content and a low glycaemic index, provide soluble fibre and are a good source of minerals and trace elements. They are useful either to supplement meat products to reduce fat and red meat content or to replace meat. Canned pulses (baked beans, red kidney beans and chickpeas) are a convenient and cheap source of protein. Pulses, despite being a vegetable, are included in the protein food group because of their role as a meat alternative. However, they can also count as one of the 5 A DAY. However, their inclusion is limited to being counted as only one of the five portions, regardless of how many portions are consumed, in recognition that they are less rich in vitamins and other phytochemicals than other vegetables.

Other non-meat alternatives

This includes soya, tofu and mycroproteins (Quorn™), which in their unprocessed forms are relatively low in fat, especially saturated fat, and are suitable alternatives for people wanting to eat less meat or for vegetarians. An increasing number of products are being developed for this expanding market. Although this range of products was developed and aimed at the healthier eater, they may still contain significant amounts of added fat and/or salt.

Foods and drinks high in fat and/or sugar

This group of foods are generally high in energy and add little nutritional value, but can be included in small amounts as they add palatability and variety to a healthy balanced diet. For products high in sugar, the frequency of intake should be low and limited to meal times to reduce dental caries (see Chapter 7.2). Foods high in fat are often highly processed and are also high in salt and sodium based preservatives, e.g. savoury snacks, crisps and pies. The range of lower fat versions of these products may help to reduce the amount of fat eaten, but these products may still have a high salt level. Other low or reduced fat and sugar products are useful alternative choices for some people.

Choosing healthier products – food labelling

Information on the nutritional content of foods is available on the back of most packaged foods in the UK. Full details can be found in Chapter 4.5. The back of pack nutritional information can be difficult for the consumer to interpret; therefore, front of pack (at a glance) information labelling has been developed and has proven to be valued by consumers. Two front of pack labelling scheme are commonly used in the UK to identify the nutritional content of food as a guide for consumers on four key nutrients, namely fat, saturated fat (saturates), salt and sugar, as well as energy. These are guideline daily amounts (GDAs) and the colour coded (traffic light) integrated label. Both systems are detailed in Chapter 4.5.

Current evidence shows that consumers value front of pack labelling (Malam *et al.*, 2009). Although levels of comprehension are generally high for all front of pack labels, standardising to one label format would enhance understanding. The integrated label, using a combination of text and colour codes, is better understood by consumers (Malam *et al.*, 2009) and this model has been advocated by many consumer and health promotion groups and recommended in NICE guidance (NICE, 2010a,b). Recommendations on one consistent scheme were published by the UK governments following a national consultation (Department of Health, 2013).

Nutritional supplements

Nutritional supplements have become increasingly popular and are now widely available in supermarkets. Although most individuals should be able to get all the nutrients they need from following a healthy balanced diet, certain groups within the population may need to take supplements (NHS & Bazian, 2011). These include:

- Pregnant women and those trying to conceive should take 400 μg of folic acid daily until the 12th week of pregnancy. In addition to this, they should also eat folate rich foods such as green vegetables, brown rice and fortified breakfast cereals. Folic acid supplementation reduces the risk of neural tube defects, including spina bifida, in the foetus.
- Pregnant and breastfeeding women should take a daily supplement of 10 μg of vitamin D to ensure the mother's requirements for vitamin D are met and to build adequate foetal stores for early infancy.
- Children aged 6 months to 5 years should be given a supplement containing vitamins A, D and C.
- All infants and children aged 6 months to 5 years should take a daily supplement containing vitamin D in the form of vitamin drops.
- People aged 65 years and over and people who are not exposed to much sun should take a daily supplement containing 10 μg of vitamin D.

Healthy eating for very young children

The eatwell plate is an appropriate model for adults and children over the age of 5 years. It is not appropriate for younger children, as they require foods that are more nutrient dense; very young children have relatively high energy requirements and a small stomach capacity. However, introducing a variety of foods to provide different flavours and textures is an important part of weaning, and the range of foods offered should move gradually towards the model of the eatwell plate so that children are eating foods consistent with the recommendations for adults by 5 years (Department of Health, 2007).

Public health strategies

This section outlines the key issues, guidance and initiatives aimed at improving the health of specific groups through the life course.

Maternal health and the early years (0–5 years)

The nutritional status of a pregnant woman influences the growth and development of the foetus and provides the foundations for the child's later health. The mother's own health, both in the short and long term, is also dependent on how well nourished she is before, during and after pregnancy (NICE, 2008) (see Chapter 3.2).

Public health policy is targeted at women from disadvantaged groups who may find it challenging to meet recommendations for maternal and child health. These mothers are more likely to give birth to low birth weight babies. Breastfeeding is a strong indicator of social inequalities; women who are most disadvantaged are least likely to breastfeed. Less privileged mothers are also more likely to introduce solid foods earlier than recommended and their children are at a greater risk of both faltering growth in infancy and obesity in later childhood. Women from disadvantaged groups have a poorer diet and are more likely to be obese or to show low weight gain during pregnancy.

Initiatives and guidance targeted at maternal health and the early years

Breastfeeding

Current UK policy is to promote exclusive breastfeeding (for the first 6 months) (Department of Health, 2003). Thereafter, it recommends that breastfeeding should continue for as long as the mother and baby wish, while gradually introducing a more varied diet. The continuation of breastfeeding whilst introducing gluten containing complementary foods at 6 months may reduce the risk of coeliac disease, type 1 diabetes and wheat allergies (ESPGHAN, 2008) (see chapter 7.11.2).

Diet during a child's early years also impacts on their growth and development. Poor diet is linked to the incidence of many common childhood conditions such as diarrhoeal disease, dental caries, and iron and vitamin D deficiencies. It may also influence the risk in adult life of conditions such as coronary heart disease, diabetes and obesity (Department of Health, 2003).

Recommendations for health professionals (NICE, 2008) include:

- Providing women with information and advice on the benefits of taking a vitamin D supplement ($10\,\mu g$/day) during pregnancy and while breastfeeding.
- Providing Healthy Start vitamin supplements (folic acid, vitamins C and D) for eligible pregnant women.
- NHS commissioners and managers are advised to implement a structured programme to encourage breastfeeding within their organisations, which should include training for health professionals.
- Encouraging breastfeeding by providing information, practical advice and ongoing support, including the help of breastfeeding peer supporters and advice on how to store expressed breast milk safely.
- Once infants are aged 6 months, encouraging and helping parents and carers to progressively introduce them to a variety of nutritious foods in addition to milk.

Healthy Start

Healthy Start is a UK wide government scheme to improve the health of low income pregnant women and families on benefits and tax credits. It provides free vouchers to eligible families every week to spend on milk, fresh and frozen fruit and vegetables, and infant formula milk. In addition, free vitamins are provided to mothers (Healthy Start vitamin tablets for pregnant and breastfeeding mothers – folic acid and vitamins C and D) and children (Healthy Start children's vitamin drops – vitamins A, C and D) (see Chapter 3.2).

Children's centres

Children's centres provide a variety of advice and support for parents and carers. Their services are available to pregnant women and families with preschool children. They should be developed in line with the needs of the local community; therefore, each children's centre is unique. However, there is a core set of services that must be provided:

- Child and family health services, ranging from health visitors to breastfeeding support.
- Most centres offer high quality childcare and early learning; those that do not can advise on local childcare options.
- Advice on parenting, local childcare options and access to specialist services for families, such as speech therapy, healthy eating advice or help with managing money.
- Help on finding work or training opportunities, using links to local Jobcentre Plus offices and training providers.

Recommendations for nursery food

In England all 3 and 4 year olds are entitled to 15 hours of free nursery education for 38 weeks of the year and so the majority of children will spend some time in early education. The Early Years Foundation Stage framework is a comprehensive statutory framework that sets the standards for the learning, development and care of children from birth to 5 years. It includes a recommendation for guidance on nursery food. The School Food Trust (SFT) has developed voluntary food and drink guidelines for early years settings in England (SFT, 2010). Implementation of this guidance means that children are given the right types of foods in the right portion sizes to meet their nutritional needs, and parents have a national benchmark to help when choosing a childcare place for their child.

Nursery milk scheme

In England (and on behalf of the devolved administrations in Scotland and Wales) the Department of Health administers the nursery milk scheme. The scheme is part of the Welfare Food Scheme and enables children under 5 years to receive, free of charge; 189 mL (1/3 pint) of milk for each day they attend approved day care facilities for 2 hours or more. Babies aged under 1 year may receive infant formula milk (dried baby milk) made up to 189 mL instead. Day care providers who have been approved to supply milk under the scheme are reimbursed the cost of the milk they supply.

Tackling obesity through the healthy child programme

The Healthy Child Programme is the early intervention and prevention programme that begins in pregnancy and continues through childhood. It offers every family a programme of screening tests, immunisations, development reviews, information and guidance to support parenting and healthy choices. Due to its universal reach to all families, it provides an opportunity to identify those families that need to receive additional help and services if they are to achieve optimum health. Tackling obesity through the Healthy Child Programme (Rudolf, 2009) provides supporting evidence, a framework for action and resources for practitioners who are working with families with preschool children.

Start4life

Start4life is a campaign for pregnant women and parents with babies. It is part of the Change4life social marketing campaign to support families in achieving behaviour change for a healthier life.

School aged children

In England 33% of 10–11-year old and 23% of 4–5-year old children are overweight or obese (NCMP, 2010). The importance of preventing obesity in childhood and the consequences of obesity in later adult life has resulted in a significant policy response from the government with the implementation of school based initiatives that have focused much PHN policy on this age group. Policies addressing obesity should also address other diet related problems such as dental disease, constipation and faddy eating.

Initiatives and guidance targeted at school aged children
National Child Measurement Programme (England)

The National Child Measurement Programme (NCMP), established in 2007, is part of the UK government's work programme on childhood obesity, and is operated jointly by the Department of Health and the Department for . Each year children aged 4–5 years (reception year) and 10–11 years (year 6) are weighed and measured during the school year to inform local planning and delivery of services for children; and gather population level surveillance data to allow analysis of trends in growth patterns and obesity. Although designed as a surveillance programme, local areas are encouraged to feed back a child's weight status to parents.

School fruit and vegetable scheme

Since 2004, every child aged 4–6-years old in state schools in England has received a free piece of fruit or vegetable each school day through the Department of Health's school fruit and vegetable scheme. This scheme was introduced as part of wider efforts to increase people's fruit and vegetable intake to the healthy 5 A DAY target.

Food and nutrition standards for schools

Each of the countries of the UK has introduced compulsory changes that prohibit or restrict food served at school that is high in fat, sugar and salt or made with poor quality meat. The UK standards are some of the most detailed and comprehensive in the world (Evans & Harper, 2009). The standards were developed following research showing that children were not making healthy food choices at lunchtime and that school meals did not meet their nutritional needs. The School Food Trust is a national charity and independent advisor to the government in England on school food, children's food and related skills. The Food for Life partnership brings together the expertise of four food focused charities, the Soil Association, Focus on Food Campaign, Health Education Trust and Garden Organic, to help English schools transform their food culture.

European school milk scheme

The aim of the European Union funded school milk subsidy scheme is to encourage children to drink milk and to develop a lasting habit of consuming milk. Milk must be distributed to children as a mid morning or afternoon drink and not used in the preparation of meals. Schools in England may provide subsidised milk to pupils and can claim reimbursement through the local authority, a milk supplier or an organisation specifically set up on behalf of schools. Free milk should be available for children entitled to free school meals. The Welsh government also funds the provision of free school milk for 5–7-year olds (key stage 1) in Wales.

Controlling food and drink TV advertising aimed at children

Television has a relatively modest impact on children's food preferences, and is only one among a number of factors affecting those preferences. Since 2008 the independent regulator and competition authority for the UK communications industries (Ofcom) and its coregulatory partner, the Advertising Standards Association, have had rules in place governing both the scheduling of adverts and their content for foods containing high fat, sugar and salt levels (HFSS); these are amongst the strictest in the world. Advertisements for foods deemed less healthy according to the FSA's Nutrient Profiling Model have not been permitted in or around programmes deemed of particular appeal to under 16-year olds. A programme is defined as being of particular appeal to children if the proportion of children under 16 years of age watching a programme is 20% higher than the general viewing population. These rules apply to all commercial and public service broadcast channels, including all cable and satellite channels.

A review of the advertising restrictions has shown them to reduce significantly the amount of HFSS advertising seen by children, and to reduce the influence of techniques in HFSS advertising that are considered likely to be particularly attractive to children (Ofcom, 2010). However, advertisements, promotions, product placements and sponsorship shown between programmes for older audiences also have a powerful influence on children and young people. Marketing bans have been successfully introduced in several other countries; evidence shows that a 9 pm watershed for such TV advertisements would reduce children and young people's exposure to this type of advertising by 82% (NICE, 2010a,b). Children are exposed to other media such as print and digital media and at present advertising in these media is not restricted.

Change4life

Change4life is a social marketing campaign in England that began in 2009 and is designed to help families make behaviour change and adopt a healthier lifestyle. It is the marketing component of the government's response to the rise in obesity and is supported by partnerships of major food and drink companies; these partnerships have been seen as controversial because of the nature of the behaviour change required.

The adult population

Management of obesity dominates the PHN issues for the adult population because of its impact not only on the health and wellbeing of this group of the population but also because of the economic impact. Care of older people and the importance of preventing malnutrition is an increasingly important public health issue emerging from the dignity in care agenda.

Being overweight has become normal and Britain is an obese society as a response to exposure to a modern lifestyle. The complexities of the obesity epidemic, the challenges in addressing it and the public health policy responses thought to have the greatest impact are addressed in the Foresight Report Tackling Obesities: Future Choices (Foresight, 2007). Public health responses need to be multifaceted and aligned with other major policy issues to ensure the maximum number of potential stakeholders can be involved. Policies linked to climate change and health inequalities have been identified as particularly crucial in developing a strategy to tackle obesity (see Chapter 7.13).

Initiatives and guidance targeted at the adult population

Public Health Responsibility Deal (England)

The English government is aiming for a collaborative approach with businesses and other influential organisations to support lifestyle change. The responsibility deal is a voluntary agreement between businesses and the government to improve public health. There are five networks (alcohol, behaviour change, food, health at work and physical activity), each made up of a high level steering group and task specific working groups as required. The networks have developed a set of core principles and a series of pledges for businesses to demonstrate their commitment to public health. Businesses can sign up to one or more pledges (Department of Health, 2011b). The food network has pledged to encourage the food industry and caterers to remove *trans* fatty acids, reduce salt, label energy at point of purchase, reduce energy and increase fruit and vegetable content. However, health and consumer organisations have criticised the pledges for alcohol as not being robust enough to challenge binge drinking. Evaluation of this voluntary partnership with the food industry has yet to be reported and consumer groups are watching with interest.

Healthy Lives, Healthy People: A Call for Action on Obesity in England

This document sets out how action on obesity will be delivered in England with the ambition of achieving a downward trend in excess weight in both children and adults by 2020 (Department of Health, 2011c).

Front of pack food labelling

Front of pack labelling is seen as a useful way of allowing informed comparisons between convenience foods, par-

ticularly when these have a wide range of nutrient values (Chapter 4.5).

Change4life

As stated earlier this social marketing campaign started with an emphasis on children, but now includes adults and families.

Public health guidance for adults

The NICE has published the following guidelines for some aspects of public health.

Prevention of cardiovascular disease (PH 25)

This guidance includes recommendations for a broad range of policies that require a range of legislative, regulatory and voluntary changes, including the further development of existing policies (NICE, 2010a,b). The guidance addresses reduction of salt, saturated fat and *trans* fatty acids, as well as food marketing, commercial interests, European policies (front of pack labelling and the Common Agricultural Policy) and public sector catering and food from take aways.

Behaviour change (PH6)

This guidance is aimed at those responsible for helping people to change their behaviour to improve their health (NICE, 2007). This includes policy makers and those working in local authorities and the community and voluntary sectors. The guidance gives advice on how to plan and run relevant initiatives.

Maternal and child nutrition (PH 11)

This guidance relates to pregnant women (and those who are planning to become pregnant), mothers and other carers of children aged under 5 years and their children. It is particularly aimed at those on a low income or from a disadvantaged group. It includes recommendations for vitamin D supplementation, Healthy Start, breastfeeding programmes and introduction of a variety of nutritious weaning foods (NICE, 2008).

NICE quality standards

NICE quality standards are a set of standards designed to drive and measure priority improvements in a particular area. They are developed independently by NICE in collaboration with health and social care professionals, their partners and service users. The standards are designed to help professionals, service providers, commissioners and people receiving health and social care to identify the service that delivers the best outcomes. The quality standard for nutrition support in adults has been developed (NICE, 2006).

Common agricultural policy

The Common Agricultural Policy (CAP) is the framework used by countries of the European Union to form their own agricultural policies. The burden of diet related disease has grown considerably since CAP was first implemented. The Common Agricultural Policy reform offers a significant opportunity to address diet related illness. A number of significant distortions in relation to certain food prices and production processes still remain in CAP policies, which potentially increase the burden of disease. Change in these distortions to promote health and wellbeing is recommended for UK policy to address obesity and other diet related illness. Plans for the reform of CAP to strengthen the competiveness and the sustainability of agriculture and guarantee healthy quality food production, to preserve the environment and to help develop rural areas were announced in 2013 (European Commission, 2013).

Measuring change

There is a growing interest in healthy eating with an increasing proportion of the UK population claiming that eating a healthy diet is important to them (FSA, 2011). However, knowing what is good for us does not necessarily lead to a shift in dietary patterns; this requires a long term process of cultural and behavioural change. Consumption patterns still fall far short of aspirations. It is important to measure changes in knowledge and attitudes. Several national surveys are conducted on a regular basis to measure such changes. These are shown in Table 4.2.7. It is also important to measure change when imple-

Table 4.2.7 Key sources of knowledge and attitudes data related to healthy eating (adapted from NOO 2010. Reproduced with permission of Public Health England, Obesity Knowledge and Intelligence)

Survey	Details
Adults	
Health Survey for England	Attitudes to one's own weight; attitudes to healthy eating; knowledge about healthy eating; knowledge about healthy physical activity levels; attitudes to physical activity; self efficacy in relation to physical activity
National Diet and Nutrition Survey	Eating habits and patterns; attitudes to one's eating habits; attitudes to one's own physical activity levels; attitudes to one's own weight; attitudes to dieting
Low Income Diet and Nutrition Survey	Attitudes to organic foods, knowledge of, and competency in, cooking; attitudes to appetite; attitudes to variety of foods consumed; attitudes to physical activity levels at work; weight status over time; attitudes to one's own weight status; influences on food choice; attitudes to one's current diet; attitudes to children's diet; knowledge of healthy eating; self efficacy in relation eating healthily
British Social Attitudes Survey	Attitudes to eating and physical activity as a reliever of stress; attitudes to taking part in games or sports; attitudes to national culture relating to sport; attitudes to individual responsibility and health; attitudes to active transport
Food and You survey (FSA) Consumer Attitudes Survey	Attitudes to importance of healthy eating; self efficacy with regards to cooking; attitudes to convenience foods; attitudes to eating healthily; attitudes to importance of healthy eating for children; knowledge of healthy eating; patterns of eating, including reduction and increase of consumption of certain foods; understanding of food labels; attitudes to food safety and hygiene; sources of information on healthy eating
Sodexo School Food Survey	Parents' attitudes to food provided by school; parental concerns about children's diets; parental attitudes to physical activity; parents' motivation to exercise; parental opinion of own weight status; parental opinion of child's weight status. The latest available survey data are from the 2005 survey
Change4life Tracking Survey	Attitudes to adopting a healthy lifestyle; attitudes to getting children to lead a healthy lifestyle, including healthy eating and being active; attitudes to overweight; knowledge of consequences of overweight; attitudes to changing physical activity and dietary habits; attitudes to changing physical activity and dietary habits of one's child; attitudes to breastfeeding; knowledge about healthy weaning. (Not in the public domain)
Children	
Health Survey for England	Attitudes to one's own weight; attitudes to healthy eating; knowledge about healthy eating; knowledge about healthy physical activity; attitudes to physical activity; self efficacy in relation to physical activity
TellUs	Attitudes to advice on healthy foods; attitudes to how leisure time is spent; attitudes to provision of sports and leisure activities in the local area
Sodexo School Food Survey	Attitudes to one's own diet; knowledge about healthy eating; motivation to eat healthily at school; healthy eating messages at school; attitudes to food provided in school; motivation to exercise outside school
National Diet and Nutrition Survey	Eating habits and patterns; attitudes to one's own eating habits; attitudes to one's own physical activity levels; attitudes to one's own weight; attitudes to dieting
Low Income Diet and Nutrition Survey	School meal entitlement, school provision of food and cooking lessons; competency
Take up of School Meals in England	Annual survey of number of children eating a school meal, catering provision in schools and compliance with school food standards

menting local changes; it is essential that a baseline measurement is made before implementing any intervention aimed at changing knowledge, practice or attitudes.

The key findings of these surveys are:

- People are eating less saturated fat, *trans* fat and added sugar than 10 years ago [National Diet and Nutrition Survey (NDNS)].
- Saturated fat intake in adults has dropped slightly to 12.8% of food energy, but is still above the recommended level of 11%. *Trans* fat intakes, having also fallen slightly, were within recommended levels; mean intake of *trans* fat was 0.7–0.9% of food energy (NDNS).
- People were eating too much non-milk extrinsic sugar (added sugar and sugar released from food during processing); currently 12.5% of food energy intake compared with the recommended 11% (NDNS).
- Adults (aged 19–64 years) consumed on average 4.2 portions per day of fruit and vegetables, older adults (over 65 years) consumed 4.3 portions, and 30% of adults and 37% of older adults met the 5 A DAY recommendation (NDNS).
- People were not eating enough fibre; mean intakes were 14 g/day for adults, below the recommended 18 g (NDNS).
- Families living on low income were less likely to consume wholemeal bread and vegetables, and more likely to consume fat spreads and oils, non-diet soft drinks, beef, veal, lamb and pork dishes, pizza (except males aged 19–64 years), processed meats (children and adults aged 19–64 years), whole milk (children and adults aged 19–64 years) and table sugar [Low Income Diet and Nutrition Survey (LINDNS)].
- Consumption of oily fish, which is the main source of n-3 fatty acids, remained substantially below the recommended one portion per week (LINDNS).
- Adults who consumed alcohol (61% of adults and 53% of older adults) obtained 9% of energy intake from alcohol (NDNS).
- Only 3% of children and 15% of adults reported eating oily fish and dishes containing oily fish (excluding canned tuna) (LINDNS).
- Iron intakes among teenage girls and women were low. However, overall vitamin and mineral intakes among the population are slightly improved (NDNS).
- The majority of respondents rated a variety of factors as important for a healthy lifestyle: 99% reported eating fruit and vegetables was very or fairly important, 94% that eating less salt was important and 92% that limiting foods high in saturated fat was important (Food and You survey).
- About a fifth of respondents were able to identify the types and proportions of foods needed for a healthy balanced diet (based on the eatwell plate) (Food and You).
- Almost one in 10 (9%) correctly stated that the maximum daily intake of salt for an adult was 6 g (Food and You).

Further reading

Donaldson LJ, Scally G. (2009) *Donaldson's Essential Public Health*, 3rd edn. Oxford: Radcliffe Publishing.

Gibney MJ, Lenore A, Margetts B. (2004). *Public Health Nutrition*. Oxford: Blackwell Publishing.

National Audit Office. (2006) *Smarter Food Procurement in the Public Sector*. London: The Stationery Office.

National Institute for Health and Care Excellence (NICE). (2012) Quality standards www.nice.org.uk/guidance/qualitystandards/qualitystandards.jsp.

Pencheon D, Guest C, Melzer D, Muir Gray JA. (2006). *Oxford Handbook of Public Health Practice*, 2nd edn. Oxford: Oxford University Press.

Internet resources

Advertising Standards Association   www.asa.org.uk/

Change4life   www.nhs.uk/Change4Life

Department for Environment, Food and Rural Affairs (Defra)   www.defra.gov.uk

The eatwell plate, eight tips for healthy eating and consumer information on a healthy diet   www.nhs.uk/Livewell/Goodfood

5 A DAY School Scheme   www.nhs.uk/Livewell/5ADAY/Pages/Schoolscheme.aspx

Food for Life   www.foodforlife.org.uk Healthy Start   www.healthystart.nhs.uk

NICE Public health guidance   http://guidance.nice.org.uk/PHG/Published

National Obesity Observatory   www.noo.org.uk

Ofcom   www.ofcom.org.uk

Public Health Action Support Team (PHAST)   www.healthknowledge.org.uk

Scientific Advisory Committee on Nutrition (SACN)   www.sacn.org.uk

School food standards

   School Food Trust England   www.schoolfoodtrust.org.uk

   Scotland – Hungry for success   www.scotland.gov.uk/Publications/2003/02/16273/17566

   Wales – Appetite for Life   www.wlga.gov.uk/english/food-in-schools/

   Northern Ireland   www.deni.gov.uk/index/support-and-development-2/5-schools_meals/nutritional-standards.htm

Start4life   www.nhs.uk/start4life

Surveys of attitudes and knowledge related to healthy eating

British Social Attitudes Survey   www.britsocat.com/Home

Food and You survey (FSA) Consumer Attitudes Survey   www.food.gov.uk/science/socsci/surveys/foodandyou/foodyou10

Health Survey for England   www.dh.gov.uk/en/Publicationsandstatistics/PublishedSurvey/HealthSurveyForEngland/index.htm

Low Income Diet and Nutrition Survey   www.dh.gov.uk/en/Publicationsandstatistics/PublishedSurvey/HealthSurveyForEngland/index.htm

National Diet and Nutrition Survey   www.mrc-hnr.cam.ac.uk/working-with-us/national-diet-and-nutrition-survey

References

Abete I, Astrup A, Martinez J, *et al*. (2010) Obesity and the metabolic syndrome: role of different dietary macronutrient distribution patterns and specific nutritional components on weight loss and maintenance. *Nutrition Reviews* 68: 214–231.

BAPEN. (2005) The cost of disease related malnutrition in the UK and economic considerations for the use of oral nutrition supplements in adults Available at www.bapen.org.uk/pdfs/health_econ_exec_sum.pdf Accessed 10 August 2012.

BAPEN. (2012) Nutrition screening survey in the UK and Republic of Ireland 2011 Hospitals, care homes and mental health units. Data collected April 2011. Available at www.bapen.org.uk/professionals/publications-and-resources/bapen-reports. Accessed 10 August 2012.

SECTION 4

Bates B, Lennox A, Bates C, Swan G. (2011). *The National Diet and Nutrition Survey: Headline results from Year 1 and 2 (combined) of the Rolling Programme (2008/2009 – 2009/10)*. London: Food Standards Agency.

Boffeta P, Couto E, Wichmann J, *et al.* (2010) Fruit and vegetable intake and overall cancer risk in the European Prospective Investigation into Cancer and Nutrition (EPIC) *Journal of the National Cancer Institute* 102: 529–537.

Crowe FL, Roddam AW, Key TJ, *et al.* (2011) Fruit and vegetable intake and mortality from ischaemic heart disease: results from the European Prospective Investigation into Cancer and Nutrition (EPIC) – Heart study. *European Heart Journal* 32(10): 1235–1243.

Dahlgren G, Whitehead M. (1991) *Policies and Strategies to Promote Social Equity in Health*. Stockholm: Institute for Futures Studies.

Defra. (2008) A framework for pro environmental behaviours. Available at www.defra.gov.uk/publications/files/pb13574-behaviours-report-080110.pdf.

Defra. (2009) Family food. Available at www.defra.gov.uk/statistics/files/defra-stats-foodfarm-food-familyfood-2009-110525.pdf. Accessed 16 August 2011.

Defra. (2011a) Government buying standards for food and catering. Available at http://sd.defra.gov.uk/advice/public/buying/products/food/.

Defra. (2011b) Briefing indications for domestic retail food prices following the rise in the FAO food price index. Available at www.defra.gov.uk/statistics/files/defra-stats-foodfarm-monthly-brief-1101-b.pdf.

Department of Health. (1991) *Report on Health and Social Subjects 41 Dietary Reference Values (DRVs) for Food Energy and Nutrients for the UK, Report of the Panel on DRVs of the Committee on Medical Aspects of Food Policy*. London: The Stationery Office.

Department of Health. (2001) *Report of the CMO's Project to Strengthen the Public Health Function in England*. London: Department of Health.

Department of Health. (2003) Infant feeding recommendation. Available at www.dh.gov.uk/en/Publicationsandstatistics/Publications/PublicationsPolicyAndGuidance/DH_4097197.

Department of Health. (1998) *Nutritional Aspects of the Development of Cancer*. Report on Health and Social Subjects, No. 48. London: HMSO.

Department of Health. (2007) The eatwell plate. Available at www.nhs.uk/Livewell/Goodfood/Pages/eatwell-plate.aspx. Accessed 1st December 2013.

Department of Health. (2010a) Equity and excellence: Liberating the NHS. Available at http://www.dh.gov.uk/prod_consum_dh/groups/dh_digitalassets/@dh/@en/@ps/documents/digitalasset/dh_117794.pdf. Accessed 15 June 2011.

Department of Health. (2010b) Healthy Lives, Healthy People: our strategy for public health in England Available at http://www.dh.gov.uk/prod_consum_dh/groups/dh_digitalassets/documents/digitalasset/dh_127424.pdf.

Department of Health. (2011a) Healthier and more sustainable catering: A toolkit for serving foods to adults. Available at http://www.dh.gov.uk/prod_consum_dh/groups/dh_digitalassets/documents/digitalasset/dh_127593.pdf. Accessed 16 June 2011.

Department of Health (2011b) Public Health Responsibility Deal. Available at http://responsibilitydeal.dh.gov.uk/about/. Accessed 12 August 2012.

Department of Health (2011c) Healthy Lives, Healthy People: A call for action on obesity in England. Available at www.gov.uk/government/publications/healthy-lives-healthy-people-a-call-to-action-on-obesity-in-england. Accessed 1st December 2013.

Department of Health. (2013) Guide to creating a front of pack (FoP) nutrition label for pre-packed products sold through retail outlets. Available at www.gov.uk/government/publications/front-of-pack-nutrition-labelling-guidance. Accessed 7 August.

European Commission. (2013) Political agreement on new direction for common agricultural policy. Available at http://ec.europa.eu/agriculture/cap-post-2013/agreement/index_en.htm. Accessed 7 August 2013.

European Food Safety Authority (EFSA). (2010a) Dietary reference values and dietary guidelines. Available at www.efsa.europa.eu/en/topics/topic/drv.htm?wtrl=01. Accessed 13 August 2012.

European Food Safety Authority (EFSA). (2010b) Scientific opinion on reference values for water. *EFSA Journal* 8(3):1459.

ESPGHAN. (2008) Complementary feeding; A commentary by the ESPGHAN committee on nutrition. *Journal of Paediatric Gastroenterology and Nutrition* 46(1): 99–110.

Evans CE, Harper CE. (2009) School meals standards in the UK. *Journal of Human Nutrition and Dietetics* 22: 89–99.

FAO/WHO. (2003) *Diet, Nutrition and the Prevention of Chronic Diseases*. Report of a Joint FAO/WHO Expert Consultation. WHO Technical Report Series, No. 916. Geneva: World Health Organization.

Foresight. (2007) *Tackling Obesities: Future Choices*. London: Government Office for Science.

Food Standards Agency (FSA) Social Science Research Unit.(2011) Exploring food attitudes and behaviours in the UK: Findings from the Food and You Survey 2010. London: FSA. Available at www.foodbase.org.uk/admintools/reportdocuments/641-1-1079_Food_and_You_Report_Main_Report_FINAL.pdf. Accessed 18 April 2011.

Food Standards Agency. (2012) Biannual public attitudes tracker Wave 4 Social Science unit. Available at www.food.gov.uk/multimedia/pdfs/biannualpublicattitudestrack.pdf. Accessed 13 August 2012.

Gatenby S, Hunt P, Rayner M. (1995) The National Food Guide: development of dietetic criteria and nutritional characteristics. *Journal of Human Nutrition and Dietetics* 8: 323–334.

Grace C. (2011) A review of one-to-one dietetic obesity management in adults. *Journal of Human Nutrition and Dietetics* 24: 13–22.

Gregory J, Foster K., Tyler H, Wiseman M. (1990) *The Dietary and Nutrition Survey of British Adults*. Office of Population and Census Surveys, Social Survey Division. London: HMSO.

Hunt P, Rayner M, Gatenby S. (1994a) Pyramid or plate? The development of a National Food Guide for the UK: A preliminary article. *Nutrition and Food Science* 4: 7–12.

Hunt P, Gatenby S, Rayner M. (1994b) The National Food Guide: The tilted plate performs best but what do the health educators think? *Nutrition and Food Science* 5: 5–8.

Hunt P, Rayner M, Gatenby S. (1995a) A national Food Guide for the UK? Background and development. *Journal of Human Nutrition and Dietetics* 8(5): 315–322.

Hunt P, Gatenby S, Rayner M. (1995b) The format for the National Food Guide: performance and preference studies. *Journal of Human Nutrition and Dietetics* 8(5): 335–352.

Macdiarmid J, Kyle J, *et al.* (2011) Livewell; a balance of healthy and sustainable food choices. WWF. Available at http://assets.wwf.org.uk/downloads/livewell_report_corrected.pdf.

Malam S, Clegg S, *et al.* (2009) Comprehension and use of UK nutrition signpost labelling schemes. Prepared for the Food Standards Agency. Available at www.foodwatch.de/foodwatch/content/e10/e13946/e29941/e29948/pmpreport_ger.pdf. Accessed 20 August 2011.

Marmot M. (2010) Fair Society, Healthy Lives. Available at www.marmotreview.org/.

National Advisory Committee on Nutrition Education (NACNE). (1983) A Discussion Paper on Proposals for Nutritional Guidelines for Health Education in Britain. Available at www.dur.ac.uk/publichealth.library/HDA_archive/R%207609%20-%2054007000097782%20-%20NACNE%20REPORT.pdf. Accessed 7 August 2013.

National Child Measurement Programme (NCMP). (2010) National Child Measurement Programme: England 2009/10 school year. Available at www.ic.nhs.uk/ncmp

National Institute for Health and Care Excellence (NICE). (2006) *Nutrition Support in Adults*. Clinical Guideline 32. London: NICE.

National Institute for Health and Care Excellence (NICE). (2007) Behaviour Change PH Guidance 6. Available at http://guidance.nice.org.uk/PH6. Accessed 9 August 2011.

National Institute for Health and Care Excellence (NICE). (2008) Maternal and child nutrition guidance – Guidance for midwives, health visitors, pharmacists and other primary care services to improve the nutrition of pregnant and breastfeeding mothers and children in low income households PH11. Available at http://guidance.nice.org.uk/PH11. Accessed 9 August 2011.

National Institute for Health and Care Excellence (NICE). (2010a) PH 25 Prevention of cardiovascular disease: guidance. Available at http://guidance.nice.org.uk/PH25/Guidance/doc/English.

National Institute for Health and Care Excellence (NICE). (2010b) PH 25 Prevention of cardiovascular disease; guidance. Available at http://guidance.nice.org.uk/PH25/Guidance/doc/English. Accessed 9 August 2011.

National Obesity Observatory (NOO). (2010a) The economic burden of obesity. Available at http://www.noo.org.uk/uploads/doc/vid_8575_Burdenofobesity151110MG.pdf. Accessed 8 August 2011.

National Obesity Observatory (NOO). (2010b) Data source: knowledge of and attitudes to healthy eating and physical activity. p. 3–4. Available at www.noo.org.uk/uploads/doc/vid_10418_Environmental%20%20data%20sources%20FINAL_editedformatted_%20100311.pdf. New Economic Foundation (NEF). (2011) Re-framing the great food debate: the case for sustainable food. Available at www.neweconomics.org. Accessed 10 April 2011.

NHS & Bazian. (2011) Supplements. Who needs them? Available at http://www.nhs.uk/News/2011/05May/Documents/BtH_supplements.pdf. Accessed 20 August 2011.

NHS Scotland. (2012) A fairer healthier Scotland our strategy 2012–2017. Available at http://www.healthscotland.com/uploads/documents/18922-CorporateStrategy.pdf. Accessed 13 August 2012.

Public Health Action Support Team (PHAST). (2008) Dietary reference values (DRVs), current dietary goals, recommendations, guidelines and the evidence for them. Available at www.healthknowledge.org.uk/public-health-textbook/disease-causation-diagnostic/2e-health-social-behaviour/drvs. Accessed 7 August 2013.

OECD-FAO. (2008) Agricultural Outlook 2008–2017. Available at http://www.fao.org/es/esc/common/ecg/550/en/AgOut2017E.pdf.

Ofcom. (2010) HFSS advertising restrictions – Final review (online). Available at http://stakeholders.ofcom.org.uk/market-data-research/tv-research/hfss-final-review/. Accessed 19 August 2011.

Office for National Statistics (ONS). (2010) Living costs and food survey 2009. Available at http://www.statistics.gov.uk/downloads/theme_social/familyspending2010.pdf. Published on website 2011 by BAPEN. www.bapen.org.uk. Accessed 6 June 2011.

Rudolf M. (2009) Tackling obesity through the Healthy Child programme Available at www.nooo.org.uk.

Scientific Advisory Committee on Nutrition (SACN). (2003) *Salt and Health*. London: The Stationery Office. Available at http://www.dietandcancerreport.org/.

Sacks FM, Bray GA, Carey VJ, *et al.* (2009) Comparison of weight-loss diets with different compositions of fat, protein, and carbohydrates. *New England Journal of Medicine* 360(9): 859–873.

Scientific Advisory Committee on Nutrition (SACN). (2004) Advice on fish consumption ; benefits and risks. Available at http://www.sacn.gov.uk/pdfs/fics_sacn_advice_fish.pdf. Accessed 5 May 2011.

Scientific Advisory Committee on Nutrition (SACN). (2010) *Iron and Health*. London: The Stationery Office. Available at http://www.sacn.gov.uk/pdfs/sacn_iron_and_health_report_web.pdf. Accessed 20 May 2011.

Scientific Advisory Committee on Nutrition (SACN). (2008) The nutritional wellbeing of the British population (2008) Avaialble at www.sacn.gov.uk/pdfs/nutritional_health_of_the_population_final_oct_08.pdf. Accessed 6August 2013.

Scientific Advisory Committee on Nutrition (SACN). (2011) *Dietary Reference Values for Energy*. London: The Stationery Office.

Scarborough P, Nnoaham K, Clarke D, Rayner M. (2011) Differences in coronary heart disease, stroke and cancer mortality rates between England, Wales, Scotland and Northern Ireland: the role of diet and nutrition. *BMJ Open*. http://bmjopen.bmj.com/content/1/1/e000263. Accessed 10 August 2012.

School Food Trust (SFT). (2010) Laying the Table. Recommendations for National Food and Nutrition Guidance for Early Years Settings in England. Available at http://www.schoolfoodtrust.org.uk/research/advisory-panel-on-food-and-nutrition-in-early-years.

Scottish Intercollegiate Guidelines Network (SIGN) (2010) Management of obesity. A national clinical guideline 115. Edinburgh: SIGN.

Strategy Unit. (2008) *Food Matters Towards a Strategy for the 21st Century*. London: Cabinet Office.

Wanless D. (2004) *Securing Good Health for the Whole Population: Final Report*. London: Department of Health.

Waste and Resources Action Programme. (2009) Household food and drink waste in the UK. Available at http://www.wrap.org.uk/retail_supply_chain/research_tools/research/report_household.html

Webster-Gandy J. (2011) *Oxford Handbook of Nutrition and Dietetics*, 2nd revised edn. Oxford: Oxford University Press.

Whitehead M. (2000) The concepts and principles of equity and Health, WHO. Available at http://salud.ciee.flacso.org.ar/flacso/optativas/equity_and_health.pdf

Williams C. (1995) Healthy eating: clarifying advice about fruit and vegetables. *BMJ* 310: 1453–1455.

World Commission on Environment and Development (WCED). (1987). Our Common Future [online]. (The Brundtland Report). Available at http://www.un-documents.net/wced-ocf.htm. Accessed 20 July 2011.

World Cancer Research Fund (WCRF). (2007) Food, nutrition, physical activity and the prevention of cancer: a global perspective. Available at http://www.dietandcancerreport.org/. Accessed 20 August 2011.

World Health Organization (WHO). (2002) *The World Health Report, Reducing Risks, Promoting Health*. Geneva: World Health Organization.

Sports nutrition

Louise Sutton

Key points

- An optimal diet for sport is one that assists the athlete to maximise training and competition performance whilst maintaining good health.

- Energy and macronutrient needs, particularly carbohydrate and protein, must be met during training and competition to maintain body mass, recover energy stores and provide adequate protein for tissue growth and repair.

- Fat intake should contribute appropriately to energy demands within the context of weight management.

- Good hydration practices are important to health and performance in sport.

- Vitamins and minerals should be included in the diet to at least the recommended levels for the population as a whole.

- Individualised nutritional plans subsequent to comprehensive nutritional assessment will benefit all athletes, but particularly elite performers.

Sports nutrition remains an emerging discipline within the fields of sports science and dietetic practice. It is now well recognised that physical activity, athletic performance and recovery from exercise are enhanced by optimal nutrition. Individuals participate in sport at different levels and for different reasons, but all athletes, whatever their level, can benefit from making good food choices that support consistent training, maximise performance and maintain good health.

Athletes, especially elite athletes, have widely accepted the need for well designed systematic training programmes, but have seemingly been slower to adopt well planned dietary strategies, with some tempted by the use of supplements or ergogenic aids to boost performance. This is changing with coaches and athletes now clearly recognising that unbalanced and inadequate nutritional intakes can lead to poor training and competition performance, lethargy, increased risk of injury and illness, and unfavourable gains or losses in body mass.

Appropriate selection of foods and fluids, timing of intake and supplement choice, where appropriate, will benefit both health and performance. The foundations of sports nutrition lie in sensible healthy eating approaches. There should be no conflict between eating for health and eating for performance. Nutrition is likely to have its biggest impact on performance by supporting athletes to train consistently and effectively to produce the desired adaptations in response to training. The recreational to elite athlete will benefit from sound nutritional practices,

whilst individualised nutrition direction and advice subsequent to a comprehensive nutritional assessment will particularly benefit elite performers. The recommendations summarised in this chapter relate to performance sport. Due to the diversity of sporting activities and levels of performance, it is beyond the scope of this chapter to provide detailed guidelines for every sport. However, there are some generic sports nutrition principles applicable to all athletes:

- Energy and macronutrient needs, particularly carbohydrate and protein, must be met during training and competition to maintain body mass, recover energy stores and provide adequate protein for tissue growth and repair.
- Fat intake should contribute appropriately to energy demands within the context of weight management and be adequate to supply essential fatty acids and fat soluble vitamins.
- Micronutrient intakes should at least match the requirements for the population as a whole.
- Commence exercise euhydrated and drink enough fluid during and after exercise to balance fluid losses through a customised approach.

The International Olympic Committee (IOC, 2010) advises athletes to adopt specific nutritional strategies before, during and after training and competition to maximise performance. Evidence based guidelines exist on the amount, composition and timing of food intake, and

Manual of Dietetic Practice, Fifth Edition. Edited by Joan Gandy.
© 2014 The British Dietetic Association. Published 2014 by John Wiley & Sons, Ltd.
Companion Website: www.manualofdieteticpractice.com

athletes are advised of the benefits of seeking qualified guidance to formulate sport specific nutritional strategies. Adequate amounts of food and fluid consumed before, during and after exercise will help maintain blood glucose during exercise, maximise performance and speed recovery post exercise.

Energy metabolism during exercise

In order to appreciate the relationship between diet and performance, it is helpful to summarise the effects of exercise on energy metabolism. Energy is largely stored in the body as glycogen and fat. The body stores an average of 375–475 g of glycogen, up to a maximum of approximately 600 g in muscle and a further 100 g in the liver. This is sufficient to run about 20 miles. The body's reserves of fat for all practical purposes are unlimited, even in the leanest of athletes. A third fuel is phospho-creatine. Very small amounts of this are stored in the muscle, sufficient to run for 5 or 6 seconds.

During exercise the working muscles convert stored energy into kinetic energy to fuel movement. The energy needs of the muscles are covered by accelerating the rate of adenosine triphosphate (ATP) resynthesis to match the rate at which ATP is utilised. ATP is produced when muscle cells metabolise carbohydrate and fatty acids in the presence of oxygen; this is aerobic metabolism. It can also be produced without the presence of oxygen, but during this anaerobic metabolism only carbohydrate can be utilised. Therefore, the two main fuels for muscle metabolism are carbohydrate and fat. Fatigue often coincides with depletion of the carbohydrate reserves.

In simple terms, as exercise intensity increases, there is increased reliance on carbohydrate but, as exercise duration increases, there is a declining contribution from carbohydrates. This is partly due to progressively depleted muscle glycogen and glucose as exercise continues, but also to the increased availability of free fatty acids. Training enables the working muscles to take up more oxygen from the blood supply and produce more energy aerobically, i.e. utilising more free fatty acids and therefore sparing the limited glycogen stores.

Energy requirements and availability

Energy expenditure due to physical activity generally accounts for 25–35% of daily energy turnover, but can account for as much as 75% during intense training of long duration. Energy intakes can therefore vary from 1500 kcal/day for young female gymnasts to 6000–7000 kcal/day for competitive cyclists, e.g. Tour de France. In sports where a specific body image is required, e.g. gymnastics, bodybuilding and ballet, or where a sport requires athletes to compete in a weight category, such as judo, boxing or lightweight rowing, athletes may restrict energy intake to lose weight or maintain a particular body composition.

Athletes repeatedly restricting energy intake for competition, then regaining weight afterwards (weight cycling) may find it increasingly hard to lose weight but weight regain is easier. Female athletes who follow intensive training programmes while restricting energy intake may experience other related problems, such as menstrual dysfunction, decreased bone density and iron deficiency anaemia. Lower energy intakes may also be associated with micronutrient intakes below recommended values. The American College of Sports Medicine (ACSM, 2007) has made recommendations for screening, diagnosis, prevention and treatment of the condition known as the female athlete triad.

Beyond the usual factors that affect energy expenditure, energy expenditure for different sports is largely dependent on the duration, frequency and intensity of activity and prior nutritional status of the athlete. Meeting energy requirements should be the main nutritional concern for athletes. During periods of high intensity and/or high duration training, athletes need to consume adequate energy to maintain health, body weight and composition, and to maximise training effects. Low energy intake or availability can result in losses of lean mass, loss or failure to gain bone density, disturbance in menstrual function, increased risk of injury, illness and fatigue, and delayed recovery from training and competition. Inadequate energy intake relative to energy expenditure has the potential to compromise performance and counteract the benefits of training. Losses in lean tissue as a result of inadequate energy intake can result in losses in strength and endurance, as well as compromised musculoskeletal, endocrine and immune function in addition to poor overall nutrient intakes. Most athletes will have a weight management concern whether this is gains in lean mass, losses in fat mass or weight maintenance. As such, energy requirements may need to be considered alongside sensible body weight and composition targets.

The concept of energy availability, the amount of energy available to perform all other functions after exercise training expenditure is subtracted, is defined as dietary intake minus energy expenditure normalised to fat free mass (FFM). It has been proposed that 30 kcal/kg of FFM/day might be the lower threshold of energy availability for women. The IOC (2010) advises that low energy availability be avoided and dieting discouraged, whilst athletes at risk of disordered eating patterns and reproductive disorders should be referred promptly to relevant health professionals for evaluation and treatment.

Macronutrient requirements for sport

Essentially, athletes do not need to eat substantially differently from the recommended diet for the general population; however, for athletes there has been a shift away from using percentage recommendations for carbohydrate and protein intake goals in favour of prescriptions relative to body weight.

Role of carbohydrate in training and recovery

It is important to appreciate that whatever exercise is performed, some carbohydrate will always be used. The longer or harder the exercise, the greater the demands placed on carbohydrate stores to maintain the desired rate of ATP resynthesis. Consequently, without adequate muscle glycogen reserves, the ability to perform high levels of work is markedly impaired.

Muscle glycogen becomes totally depleted after 2–3 hours of continuous exercise at intensities of 60–80% maximal oxygen uptake (VO_2 max). Severe depletion can also be achieved after only 15–30 minutes of exercise at intensities of 90–130% VO_2 max when intervals of 1–5 minutes of exercise followed by rest are repeated. This type of short intermittent, high intensity exercise is a pattern found typically in many individual and team sports, such as football, hockey and tennis, and demonstrates the importance of carbohydrate as a fuel for all types of sport, not just the endurance sports. Athletes who train and compete regularly need to ensure adequate carbohydrate consumption if they are to avoid residual fatigue and poor performance.

Definition of VO_2 max

As an individual moves from rest to running their oxygen uptake increases in an almost linear fashion until they reach a point where there is no further increase in O_2 consumption. This is the maximum O_2 uptake or VO_2 max for the individual. When the exercise intensity is expressed as a percentage, VO_2 max, it is called the relative exercise intensity and it reflects the physiological and psychological demands on the individual.

Glycogen stores are depleted with training. These limited stores must be restocked adequately before the next training bout. Glycogen is restored at a rate of about 5%/hour. After exhaustive exercise, up to and beyond 20 hours may be needed to fully replenish stores. During the first 2 hours after exercise, muscle glycogen resynthesis proceeds at the rate of 7%/hour, making it important that athletes consume sufficient carbohydrate during this time. If glycogen reserves are low, the point at which glycogen becomes limiting may be attained more rapidly. If the process of incomplete refuelling continues, there is a progressive depletion of glycogen stores within the working muscles, resulting in a feeling of continual lethargy. Quality and quantity of training will be impaired, leading to a decrease in overall performance. There is also the potential for blood sugar levels to fall during training, affecting brain function, concentration and coordination, and resulting in an increased injury risk.

Dietary carbohydrate recommendations

Guidelines suggested in The International Olympic Committee Consensus Statement on Sports Nutrition (IOC, 2004) are summarised in Table 4.3.1. These guidelines need to be personalised to take account of total energy needs, phase of training and feedback on performance.

Sufficient foods containing carbohydrate should be consumed on a regular basis to maintain glycogen levels. In most cases, starchy foods are the best choice; however, athletes may also need to include sugary sources of carbohydrate, such as sweets, jam or sugar, or sports food such as drinks, bars and gels, to meet high overall energy

Table 4.3.1 Carbohydrate requirements to aid recovery (IOC, 2004)

Type of training	Carbohydrate requirements for daily recovery (g/kg body weight/day)
Moderate duration/low intensity	5–7
Moderate to heavy endurance training	7–12
Extreme exercise programmes (4–6+ hours/day)	10–12

requirements within the context of achieving an overall balanced intake. As this is where sports nutrition advice can wander from the usual healthy eating message, athletes and parents of younger athletes may require an explanation for the appropriateness of this.

Training versus competition

Different sports operate within different time frames for training and competition, and therefore require distinctive energy and carbohydrate intakes. Generally, endurance athletes such as long distance runners or cyclists and triathletes will train and compete for long periods. Sprinters will compete over very short periods but train for longer periods, and multisprint sports such as rugby, football or netball require training and competition over 1–2 hours, but have periods of relative inactivity within that time period. Each sport will have complex training programmes, including strength and conditioning, endurance, speed and skills specific elements. When assessing requirements before, during and after training, it is important to remember that each training session will affect nutritional requirements differently.

Prior to exercise

Athletes should aim to begin every bout of training and competition fully recovered, with glycogen stores that are adequate to cope with the workload to be undertaken. This may be more difficult to achieve for athletes with multiple bouts of training and/or competition in one day. Eating a meal rich in carbohydrate 3–4 hours prior to exercise increases glycogen stores in the muscles and liver. The quantities of carbohydrate that are appropriate at this time will vary according to the sport, the athlete, their prior nutritional status and overall daily needs.

Endurance events require optimal glycogen stores to maximise performance. The traditional *carbohydrate loading* method popular during the late 1960s and 1970s is no longer used, having been replaced with a tapering of training and an increase in carbohydrate intake over the 3–5 days prior to competition. Subsequent increases in glycogen stores not only benefit the endurance athlete but also may help in sport situations where competition may last for several days. Commencing competition with high glycogen stores may assist in offsetting progressive depletion with each bout of competition. A possible disadvantage of increasing glycogen stores is the commensurate increase in body weight through the associated storage of water with glycogen. This may be an important consideration where an athlete competes in a weight category sport such as judo or in events covering significant distance, e.g. marathon running.

During exercise

The consumption of carbohydrate during competitions of long duration or between bouts of intermittent competition will enhance performance. Muscle glycogen stores and the availability of carbohydrate during exercise are major determinants of endurance performance. The delivery of carbohydrate during exercise becomes more significant when muscle glycogen stores are low at the onset of exercise.

During exercise, the ingestion of carbohydrate is often limited to that which can be taken in fluid form. If exercise duration continues beyond 1 hour, it is recommended that carbohydrates be ingested at a rate of 30–60 g/hour to maintain oxidation of carbohydrates and delay fatigue. Mixing different forms of carbohydrate has been shown to increase carbohydrate oxidation up to 90 g/hour, which may be required to optimise performance in events lasting >3 hours.

Athletes are advised to practise consuming carbohydrate during training and to develop individual strategies, making use of sports foods and drinks containing carbohydrate combinations that will allow for maximal absorption from the gut with minimal gastrointestinal disturbance.

Post exercise

Immediately after exercise, the body resynthesises glycogen at a faster rate. Athletes should aim to consume carbohydrate at the rate of 1.0–1.5 g/kg body weight within 30 minutes and again every 2 hours for 4–6 hours for adequate replacement of glycogen stores. Adequate refuelling is particularly important when there are 8 hours or less before the next training or competition bout. The addition of protein may have additional benefits in enhancing both muscle protein and glycogen synthesis.

Many athletes find solid food immediately after exercise unpalatable, and therefore drinks containing carbohydrate may be useful. Foods with a high glycaemic index (GI) are generally thought to be beneficial during this initial post exercise period. When longer periods of recovery time are available, the athlete may move on to meals containing lower GI foods.

Regular exercise

Regular exercise has been shown to increase protein needs. Athletes should consume daily amounts greater that those recommended for the general population, but a varied diet that meets energy requirements will usually provide a protein intake in excess of requirements. The current consensus evidence suggests that endurance athletes require 1.2–1.4 g of protein/kg body weight/day, whilst strength or speed athletes may require as much as 1.7 g of protein/kg body weight/day. The high energy intakes typical of most athletes make these recommendations easy to attain without dietary manipulation. Athletes with restricted energy intake may require dietary manipulation to achieve their protein requirements. Those who are vegetarian, and particularly vegans, may also need some guidance to ensure adequate protein intake, particularly if also consuming low energy diets.

To maximise protein synthesis foods that contain high quality proteins are recommended to be consumed regularly throughout the day as part of the athlete's total daily consumption. In particular, consumption is recommended soon after exercise in quantities of 15–25 g to aid the repair of damaged tissue and long term maintenance or gain of muscle mass. The consumption of adequate energy, particularly from carbohydrate, is important to protein metabolism to ensure amino acids are spared for protein synthesis.

Fat

Fat (as a source of energy, fat soluble vitamins and essential fatty acids) is an important nutrient in the diet of athletes. However, there is no need to supplement the normal diet with additional fat; intakes of >30% of total energy are likely to indicate an inadequate intake of carbohydrate. In addition intakes of <20% of total energy do not appear to benefit performance.

Athletes should aim to avoid excessive amounts of fat in the diet, and would normally be encouraged to look to lower fat versions of foods where appropriate unless they have exceptionally high overall energy requirements. Athletes, like the general population, should be encouraged to include mono- and poly-unsaturated fats in their diets. Whilst many athletes are familiar with the concepts around the need for carbohydrate in the diet, the issue of including adequate and appropriately healthy fats may not always be fully understood.

Fluid balance

Considerable care should be taken by all athletes to ensure adequate hydration before, during and after exercise to avoid thermal distress. Dehydration, a loss of >2% of body mass, can compromise aerobic performance, particularly in hot and high altitude conditions, and may also impair cognitive performance.

Sweat rates for any given activity, and therefore fluid losses, will vary according to ambient temperature, humidity, body mass, genetics, state of heat acclimatisation, metabolic efficiency and even clothing. Sweat rates can range from as little as 0.3 L/hour to typically maximum rates of 2–3 L/hour. It is important to recognise that large interindividual variation in sweat losses can occur even when the same or similar exercise is carried out in the same conditions.

Where sweat losses greatly exceed replacement, the circulatory system is unable to cope and skin blood flow slows. With this comes a reduction in sweating and the ability to lose heat; thus, body temperature will rise with

SECTION 4

potentially fatal consequences. Although sweating is a very effective way of losing heat, care must be taken to ensure that this process is not impaired through dehydration.

The addition of sodium to sports drinks aids the absorption of water and thus the process of rehydration. Further, this sodium prevents a drop in plasma sodium concentration and plasma osmolality that would occur during exercise with the ingestion of large volumes of plain water. A drop in plasma sodium concentration and plasma osmolality would result in diuresis with an accompanying decline in desire to drink, resulting in a lower fluid consumption. Athletes participating in long endurance events, particularly ultra endurance events, can be at risk of hyponatraemia if they drink copious amounts of plain water. This is most often reported in the non-elite.

The ACSM (2007) position statement on exercise and fluid replacement provides a comprehensive review of research and recommendations for maintaining hydration before, during and after exercise.

Fluid intake

Hydration strategies should be individualised, the ideal strategy covering the athlete's daily fluid requirements plus additional requirements of each bout of training or competition. Drinks used for exercise lasting more than an hour or sports that stimulate heavy sodium losses through sweating should include sodium. There is a range of commercial sports drinks available that athletes can use around training and competition. These contain carbohydrate and electrolytes at levels that will be acceptable for use before, during and after most sports; these will typically be labelled as isotonic. Hypertonic drinks contain more carbohydrate and may be useful where the focus is on refuelling. Where rehydration is a priority, hypotonic drinks may be beneficial where the carbohydrate content is low and sodium content higher. Emphasis should be placed on good oral hygiene when using sports drinks.

Prior to exercise

Euhydration should be strived for prior to training or competition. This can be achieved by:

* Constantly being aware of fluid status and maintaining good fluid intake at all times.
* drinking 5–7 mL/kg body mass of water or sports drink at least 4 hours before exercise.

Markers of urine osmolality, specific gravity and colour can be used as a guide to euhydration.

During exercise

The achievement of fluid balance during exercise is not always possible as a result of maximal sweat rates exceeding maximal gastric emptying. The aim of drinking during exercise is to limit dehydration to <2% of body mass. The amount and rate of fluid replacement achieved will be dependent on individual sweat rate, exercise duration and intensity, and opportunities to consume fluids. The

Table 4.3.2 Weighing before and after sport to ascertain sweat rate

Stage	Procedure
1	Pass urine prior to weighing
2	Wear minimal clothing and remove socks and trainers (preferably nude body mass)
3	Weigh on solid floor with accurate scales prior to exercise
4	Record the amount of fluid consumed during exercise
5	After exercise dry the body of any sweat by rubbing down with a towel
6	Weigh immediately after exercise and drying before passing urine
7	If: Initial weight = a (kg) Final weight = b (kg) Weight difference = c (kg) Fluid drunk during session = d (L) Fluid loss (F) during session is: c = a − b F = c + d This is fluid loss per unit of time measured, e.g. if training session lasts 1 hour, it is loss per hour 1 kg of weight loss equals 1 L of fluid; therefore kg and L can be added or subtracted together

use of beverages containing carbohydrate and electrolytes can help to maintain fluid and electrolyte balance, especially during the performance of endurance exercise. Regular assessment of pre–post exercise body weight can assist dietitians and athletes in determining sweat rates and customising individual hydration programmes (Table 4.3.2).

When exercise lasts less than an hour and temperatures are not high, fluid may not be needed during the exercise period. However, when exercise of long duration or results in excessive sweating, it is advisable to drink during the exercise period. In such cases, hydration strategies during exercise should:

* Aim to match fluid losses through sweat with fluid intake.
* Aim to minimise body weight losses to 1–2% – especially in hot and humid conditions.
* Ensure individualised hydration plans based on the knowledge of sweat rates.
* Encourage consumption of 150–250 mL of fluid every 15–20 minutes during prolonged exercise where practical and within tolerance.
* Use palatable drinks.
* Use training sessions to practice drinking during exercise.

Post exercise

Athletes will complete most exercise bouts with some degree of dehydration. The volume of fluid consumed following exercise needs to replace that lost as sweat, but should also take account of the ongoing sweat losses during the immediate recovery period. Therefore, fluid intake during this period should exceed losses by as much as 50%, i.e. for every litre lost, 1.5 L should be drunk. Strategies implemented following exercise should ensure that:

- Rehydration starts immediately, particularly when repeated bouts of exercise have to be performed.
- Sweat rates calculated from before and after weighing are taken into account.
- Athletes carry their own supply of fluid in their kit bag.
- Drinks contain some sodium to assist rehydration by stimulating thirst.
- Drinks contain some carbohydrate to help replace energy needs where appropriate.

Other considerations

Weight control

In most cases the aim of a weight loss diet for an athlete is to decrease body fat stores without affecting glycogen, water or lean body mass content. The diet must contain sufficient carbohydrate to restock glycogen stores between each bout of training. It will need to be low in fat and may require a proportionately high protein content, as well as providing all essential nutrients in a total energy intake that will achieve the desired weight loss over a sensible period.

If loss of performance due to dehydration and glycogen depletion is to be avoided, rapid weight loss by dietary or non-dietary methods should be discouraged. Despite the importance of maintaining hydration and glycogen stores in preparation for competition, strategies for *making weight* are still practised in some sports by increasing rather than tapering training, fasting, restricting fluids and use of saunas, sweat suits, laxatives and diuretics. Where weight loss is a long term goal, well planned weight reduction programmes are essential if athletes are to maintain training and not impair performance.

Where weight gain is required, the athlete will want to increase lean body mass rather than body fat content. Muscle mass is determined by training effect and adaptation. Advice for the athlete desiring weight gain is to ensure an adequate overall diet with a high proportion of carbohydrate and adequate protein that achieves a 500 kcal/day positive energy balance. A conscious effort may be required to increase food intake. Meals should not be missed and high carbohydrate snacks should be consumed between meals as appropriate.

Micronutrients

Careful selection of nutrient dense foods should reduce the risk of micronutrient deficiencies; however, the vitamins and minerals commonly found to be of concern in the diets of athletes are vitamins D and B group, calcium, iron and zinc. The IOC (2010) warns that athletes should be particularly aware of their needs for calcium, iron and

vitamin D, but that the use of large amounts through supplementation may be harmful.

Micronutrient supplementation will not enhance performance in athletes who are already consuming an adequate diet; however, there may be situations where intakes should be increased by dietary manipulation or recommending the use of supplementation. Supplementation should not compensate for poor food choices, but may provide a short term option when food intake or choice is restricted due to constant travel, giving rise to limited food choice, or restriction of food intake to maintain low body weight.

Single nutrient supplementation may be necessary for specific medical or nutritional purpose, e.g. iron supplementation to correct anaemia. Female athletes with amenorrhoea or dysmenorrhoea have an increased risk of developing osteoporosis due to reduced levels of oestrogen. Improved calcium intakes are particularly important in athletes with low bone density, menstrual irregularities and low calcium intakes, since stress fractures are particularly common in this group of athletes.

Athletes who run the greatest risk of poor micronutrient status are those who restrict energy intake or undertake severe weight loss practices, or through choice or need eliminate one or more food groups, or who repeatedly consume unbalanced low nutrient density diets. These athletes may benefit from a daily low dose multivitamin and mineral supplement. Theories are emerging that supplemental dietary antioxidants may reduce oxidative stress and skeletal muscle damage associated with strenuous exercise, but athletes are advised to maintain an adequate intake through good nutrition.

Supplementation

Sports dietitians need to constantly update their knowledge in this area. The supplement market is worth millions, but the manufacture, processing, labelling and marketing of these products is poorly regulated with variable quality control. The vast array of available products make convincing claims – better recovery, increased strength and size, loss of body fat and enhanced immune function. As such it is easy to appreciate the attraction of such products for the athlete.

The list of supplements is exhaustive, but they can essentially be broken down into two main categories. Nutrient supplements can be used to assist the athlete in meeting their overall nutritional needs. This might be by way of providing a practical alternative to food or to help to meet higher than average requirements for nutrients, in particular carbohydrate and protein. Ergogenic aids are assumed to enhance performance above and beyond that which would normally be expected. Nutritional ergogenic aids generally aim to enhance performance through effects on energy, body composition and alertness.

Nutrient supplements

Nutrient supplements can assist athletes to achieve optimal nutritional requirements. These products include sports drinks, gels and bars, liquid meal and protein supplements, carbohydrate loaders and powders, and multivitamin and mineral supplements. Athletes may find these products useful in helping them to meet their nutritional goals during particularly demanding periods of training and competition. For instance, products such as sports drinks have a genuine role to play, presenting a convenient way to meet the high energy demands of training or competition.

The key question with nutrient supplements is knowing how and when to use them to maximum benefit to support the attainment of nutrition goals. If used appropriately, nutrient supplements can play a role in assisting athletes to train and compete at their best, but the support of a sports dietitian may be required to develop optimum nutritional strategies where these products feature. They are generally more expensive than similar everyday food items, but in some circumstances the extra expense may be worth it.

Nutritional ergogenic aids

There is scientific support for performance enhancement with creatine and caffeine. Other products such as colostrum and HMB (beta-hydroxy-beta-methylbutyrate) are still under scientific scrutiny to assess their benefits or practical uses. Creatine phosphate is used as a fuel source in the first few seconds of a sprint. Creatine supplementation can increase muscle creatine phosphate levels and as such may assist athletes to recover more quickly between repeated bouts of high intensity effort. It may also lead to increases in muscle bulk. Caffeine is a central nervous system stimulant commonly available in a wide range of foods and beverages. Several studies have shown a performance enhancing effect for caffeine during exercise of varying intensities and duration. Sensitivity to caffeine varies between individuals and over consumption can produce a range of side effects, such as insomnia, headache, abdominal discomfort, impaired coordination and muscle tremors, all of which can have a negative impact on training and competition performance. The mild diuretic effect of caffeine needs to be considered when exercising for prolonged duration or in hot and humid conditions.

Points to consider

Supplement use in sport is widespread but the majority of supplements are deemed ineffective or unnecessary. The decision to take supplements is not always a rational one. Not only is supplement usage a common feature, but recommended doses often are exceeded, sometimes simply to outdo whatever the opposition or even team mates are taking. Excessive intakes and cocktails of consumption have the potential to do more harm than good and indiscriminate use carries the risk of contamination and positive doping offences.

Athletes considering the use of a supplement should ensure that it is legal, is backed by sound scientific reason and has sound guidelines for its use, and can be obtained through a reliable source. Indiscriminate use of supplements is unwise. Before deciding to use any supplement,

athletes should be cautioned to undertake a cost–benefit analysis in terms of the potential performance benefits weighed against the costs, not only in terms of finance but also the adverse effects on health and performance and the likelihood of contamination with banned or other undesirable substances.

Contaminated supplements have often been blamed for an athlete testing positive for a banned substance, with subsequent claims that the prohibited substance was not declared in the product list of ingredients. With the inception of the World Anti-Doping Code (World Anti-Doping Agency, 2009) and the implications of strict liability, the athlete is strictly held responsible for any prohibited substance found in their system. As such, athletes are strongly advised to be cautious and vigilant about the use of any supplement and to consider that diet, lifestyle and training should all be optimised before turning to supplements to rectify any shortfall in performance potential. Generally, products manufactured within the food and pharmaceutical industries are safer as standards are more rigorous. If in doubt, athletes should consider asking the manufacturer for a written declaration that the product only contains what is stated on the label and to check carefully where ingredients are sourced from and how and where the product is packaged.

UK Anti-Doping has responsibility for ensuring sports bodies in the UK are compliant with the World Anti-Doping Code through the implementation and management of the UK National Anti-Doping Policy. Athletes are advised to be vigilant in choosing to use any supplement. No guarantee can be given that any particular supplement is free from prohibited substances. A number of initiatives to support athletes have been created globally to identify whether a prohibited substance can be identified in a supplement. In the UK, HFL Sports Science has taken the lead to create a scheme to support athletes in assessing the risk of supplement use. The Informed Sport programme is designed to evaluate the integrity of supplement manufacturer process and screening of supplements and ingredients for the presence of prohibited substances that are cited on the World Anti-Doping Code prohibited list. Further information can be found at www.informed-sport.com.

Practical issues

The general recommendations summarised in this chapter can be adjusted to accommodate the unique concerns of individual athletes regarding health, sports nutrition needs, food preferences, and body weight and composition goals. Athletes will benefit from the guidance of qualified professionals who can advise on individual energy, nutrient and fluid needs to develop sports specific nutritional strategies for training, competition and recovery. To achieve this they may need very practical advice concerning shopping, food preparation and cooking to meet their requirements. On a practical level, one of the greatest difficulties facing the athlete is simply finding time for food, whilst coping with training, travel, competition and employment or education.

Nutritional needs for special populations, including children and young athletes, and those with special needs (e.g. athletes with diabetes, gastrointestinal disorders and disabilities) are beyond the scope of this chapter but are discussed in detail in Burke & Deakin (2010).

Further reading

American College of Sports Medicine. (2007) Exercise and fluid replacement. *Medicine & Science in Sport & Exercise* 39(2): 377–390.

American College of Sports Medicine. (2007) Exertional heat illness during training and competition. *Medicine & Science in Sport & Exercise* 39(3): 556–572.

Burke LM, Deakin V (eds). (2010) *Clinical Sports Nutrition,* 4th edn. North Ryde: McGraw Hill.

International Olympic Committee (IOC). (2010) *IOC Consensus Statement on Sports Nutrition.* Available at www.olympic.org.

Jeukendrup A. (2010) *From Lab to Kitchen.* Meyer & Meyer UK.

Jeukendrup A, Gleeson M. (2010) *Sports Nutrition. An Introduction to Energy Production and Performance,* 2nd edn. Human Kinetics.

Joint Position Statement of the American Dietetic Association, Dietitians of Canada, and the American College of Sports Medicine. (2009) Nutrition and athletic performance. *Journal of the American Dietetic Association* 109(3): 509–527.

Maughan RJ, Burke LM. (2002) *Sports Nutrition: Handbook of Sports Medicine and Science.* Oxford: Blackwell Publishing.

Maughan RJ, Burke LM, Coyle EF. (eds) (2004) *Food, Nutrition and Sports Performance II: The International Olympic Committee Consensus on Sports Nutrition.* Routledge Taylor & Francis Group.

Journals

International Journal of Sport Nutrition & Exercise Metabolism
Journal of the International Society of Sports Nutrition
Medicine & Science in Sport & Exercise

Internet resources

American College of Sports Medicine   www.acsm.org
Australian Institute of Sport   www.ausport.gov.au
Informed Sport Programme   www.informed-sport.com
Sports Dietitians UK   www.sportsdietitians.org.uk
Sport and Exercise Nutrition Register   www.senr.org.uk
UK Anti-Doping   www.ukad.org.uk
UK Sport   www.uksport.gov.uk
World Anti-Doping Agency   www.wada-ama.org

Position papers and references

American College of Sports Medicine. (2007) The female athlete triad. *Medicine & Science in Sport & Exercise* 39(10): 1186–1882.

Burke LM, Deakin V (eds). (2010) *Clinical Sports Nutrition,* 4th edn. North Ryde: McGraw Hill.

International Olympic Committee (IOC). (2010) *IOC Consensus Statement on Sports Nutrition.* Available at www.olympic.org.

International Olympic Committee (IOC). (2004) *IOC Consensus Statement on Sports Nutrition.* Available at www.olympic.org.

World Anti-Doping Agency. (2009) World Anti-Doping Code. Available at www.wada-ama.org. Accessed 6 August 2013.

4.4 Food service

4.4.1 Hospitals and institutions
Richard Wilson

Key points

- Food service is 50% food and 50% service. The service and eating environment elements play an important role in getting food eaten.

- The nutritional value of food not eaten is nil. Above all, food must be attractive, appealing and appetising for the patient if it is to be consumed.

- The menu is the blueprint for success; good menu planning is the key to meeting nutritional goals in institutions.

- The social and rehabilitative value of meal times complements their nutritional importance in the day – make meal times special.

- Modern food production and distribution techniques can be used to improve the patient experience and care or they can be abused to the detriment of the patient experience.

- Getting the right food to the right person at the right time and in perfect condition is an information intensive activity. New technology lends itself to handling that information and enabling its constructive use.

It is important to not lose sight of the fact that 80–100% of patients in hospitals and institutions depend solely on the food provided for their nutritional support (Hiesmayr *et al.*, 2009; Stephen *et al.*, 1997). Ensuring that the food is of good nutritional quality, is appealing to patients and is eaten is a complex and difficult challenge for the dietitian and the caring team. If dietitians do nothing else but maximise the amount of food patients eat while in hospital, they will have achieved a great deal.

General issues

Malnutrition in hospitals

The provision of artificial nutrition has been the focus of much attention in recent decades and has developed considerably. Nutritional support is now possible in all clinical situations but despite these advances, malnutrition in hospitals remains common (Elia, 2009; McWhirter & Pennington, 1994; Stratton *et al.*, 2003) and is often unrecognised (Lennard-Jones *et al.*, 1995).

In the hospital setting, malnutrition is malpractice and it is costly and indefensible (Tucker, 1996; Löser, 2010); managing this risk is an important part of corporate and clinical governance and is widely recognised to be a human rights issue (Kondrup, 2004). In England it is also unlawful, with the Health and Social Care Act: Regulation 14 stating that '. . . *the registered person must ensure that service users are protected from the risks of inadequate nutrition and dehydration . . .*'. The clinical and management team need to recognise this and act when poor food consumption compromises patient nutrition.

Public concern about food in hospitals and institutions

The public and the media are very interested in hospital food. Almost everyone has an anecdote about how a friend or relative *starved* in hospital (Birkett, 2005). Innumerable newspaper articles have highlighted this public concern over the years. The ability of the NHS to deliver this basic human need continues to be a hot topic (Care Quality Commission, 2011; Health Service Ombudsman, 2011). It is clear that food and beverage services in institutions are a *shop window* activity; the funders expect an excellent level of service for the three Cs; catering, cleaning and car parking!

SECTION 4

Why good quality food service is important

Providing food in hospitals and other institutions is fundamental to the success of that organisation. There are no other services delivered to every patient, every day that affect their wellbeing so profoundly. Failures in food service can kill and can close hospitals within hours. If food service fails to nourish, the process of identifying and addressing that failure is complex and difficult (Wheatley, 1999). Patients often cannot tell the difference between good treatment and bad treatment but they can always identify poor food.

Guidance and opinion in the UK

A number of reports regarding food service in hospitals and institutions have been published since 1990 and a summary of their recommendations is given in Table 4.4.1.

Gap between guidance and implementation

Operating and maintaining the performance of high quality food service is a dynamic and iterative process. More research on the cost efficiency of improving food intake in hospitals and institutions is needed (Council of Europe, 2002; NICE, 2006). Although the work that has been published is very convincing (Ödlund-Olin et al., 1996; Gall et al., 1998; Kondrup et al., 1998; Teal et al., 2012), it is difficult and costly to do and the evidence base remains sparse. Public and payer pressure for improvement is an important influencing factor for hospital management teams.

Table 4.4.1 Guidance and opinion on food service in the UK: a review of documents produced since 1990

Year	Organisation and report title	Main recommendations
1992	Department of Health Committee on Medical Aspects of Food Policy *The Nutrition of Elderly People*	Health professionals should be made aware of the often inadequate food intake of elderly people in institutions Effective methods of ensuring adequate nutrition need to be developed and evaluated for elderly people in hospital or institutions
1992	King's Fund (Lennard-Jones, 1992) *A Positive Approach to Nutrition as Treatment*	Every hospital should organise its nutrition services to link management, catering and all the clinical disciplines involved Managers should take account of the potential cost of complications and increased hospital stay due to malnutrition when assessing the cost of nutritional support
1993	British Dietetic Association/Nutrition Advisory Group for Elderly People (NAGE) *Dietetic Standards of Care for the Older Adult in Hospital*	The dietitian advises on nutritionally adequate food which is acceptable to patients and appropriate to patient needs The dietitian advises on hospital policies that affect nutritional care of the older adult
1993	Royal College of Nursing *Nutrition Standards and the Older Adult*	The client has an initial assessment made of their food and fluid intake and eating and drinking patterns The ward/unit team works towards ensuring that the organisation of the ward and staff is responsive to and meets the requirements of the client in order to satisfy their eating and drinking needs The nutritional goals set for the client and the care received are continually evaluated and revised
1993	South East Thames Regional Health Authority *Service Standards: Nutritional Guidelines: The Food Chain*	Best practice guidelines on hospital food service Recommendations aiming to get as much food eaten by patients in hospital as possible
1993	South East Thames Regional Health Authority *Service Standards: Nutritional Guidelines: Menu Planning*	Help and advice on menu planning in the institutional setting Recommendations aiming to ensure that an appealing and attractive menu is constructed which can be delivered and will be eaten
1993	The Patients Association (1993) *Catering for Patients in Hospital*	Meals should be served at times that reflect the normal eating patterns of the majority of patients Patients should be able to order as close to the time of serving the meal itself as possible The children's menu should reflect the foods they are used to at home Snacks should be available There should be adequate staffing so that patients who cannot feed themselves, or who need encouragement, have the full attention of a member of staff Staff should have responsibility to monitor and report on patients' intake of food and liquid Nurses should collect trays from patients for monitoring of intake There should be a regular evaluation of food and catering services, looking at quality, content and presentation

(Continued)

Table 4.4.1 (*Continued*)

Year	Organisation and report title	Main recommendations
1994	British Association for Parenteral and Enteral Nutrition (BAPEN) *Organisation of Nutrition Support in Hospitals*	All UK hospitals should have a nutrition support team (NST) All major UK hospitals or hospital groups should appoint a Nutrition Steering Committee Nutrition Steering Committees should be responsible for setting standards for catering services, dietary supplements and nutritional support All Nutrition Steering Committees should appoint at least one NST to implement standards of nutritional support they recommend
1994	Health of the Nation Nutrition Task Force *Nutrition and Health: A Management Handbook for the NHS*	Makes suggestions for managers about how they can develop and improve nutrition services in their institution
1995	English National Board for Nurse Education (ENB) *Nutrition for Life: Issues for Debate in the Department of Education Programmes*	Nutrition themes should be integrated through both preregistration and continuing postregistration programmes Every student should be able to conduct a detailed nutritional assessment of a healthy person
1995	Health of the Nation Nutrition Task Force *Nutrition Guidelines for Hospital Catering*	Makes recommendations on the nutritional content of hospital food based on the Committee on Medical Aspects of Food Policy recommendations for healthy individuals Provides guidance on best practice in food service and delivery, aimed at getting as much food eaten as possible
1996	BAPEN *Standards and Guidelines for Nutritional Support of Patients in Hospitals*	Purchasers of healthcare should insist on standards for the organisation and provision of nutrition support There should be an interdepartmental and multidisciplinary Nutrition Steering Committee There should be a catering liaison group with representative caterers, doctors, nurses and dietitians
1996	BDA/Parenteral and Enteral Nutrition Group (PENG) *Dietetic Standards for Nutritional Support*	Dietitians should actively promote the identification and treatment of protein energy malnutrition and increase awareness of this issue among other healthcare professionals Managers of nutrition and dietetic services ensure that resources are available for the provision of nutritional support within both the hospital and community
1996	National Health Service Executive *Hospital Catering: Delivering a Quality Service*	Contractors should provide meals which meet patients' dietetic and nutritional requirements Catering procedures should comply with the Nutrition Task Force's guidelines for hospital caterers Chefs should be trained in nutrition to meet dietary needs Contractors should keep prescribed records to demonstrate that nutrition and dietetic requirements are monitored and met The Trust's dietetic manager should ensure that nutrition standards are satisfactory An annual independent audit should be conducted to show meal quality to be satisfactory and to meet patients' needs A guide should be provided for each patient explaining the hospital's catering policies and catering services Patients' meals should not be ordered more than two meals in advance The catering managers name should be made available to patients Help should be readily available for patients where required to allow them to make use of the catering service
1996	British Dietetic Association (BDA) *Malnutrition in Hospitals*	Dietitians should be actively involved in menu planning to ensure that a nutritionally adequate diet is provided in hospital and that patients requiring special or therapeutic diets are catered for Patients who require artificial nutritional support or a supplemented diet should have access to a dietitian Adequate resources should be available to ensure that high quality nutritional care, whether via the oral, enteral or parenteral route, can be delivered and monitored Dietitians should foster close links with other healthcare professionals involved in the detection and management of malnutrition
1997	Association of Community Health Councils for England and Wales *Hungry in Hospital?*	Accusations that patients are starving to death must be investigated Roles and responsibilities at meal times must be defined Existing guidance with regard to hospital catering must be enforced

Table 4.4.1 (Continued)

Year	Organisation and report title	Main recommendations
1997	Centre for Health Services Research, University of Newcastle upon Tyne (Bond, 1997) *Eating Matters*	Meal provision should be responsive to the patients' needs Patients should be asked for their opinions about the meals provided Multidisciplinary and cross departmental dietary care groups should be created All other ward activities should stop when meals are being eaten Audits of dietary care should be carried out regularly
1997	United Kingdom Central Council for Nursing and Midwifery (UKCC) *Responsibility for Feeding of Patients*	Nurses have an implicit responsibility for ensuring that patients are appropriately fed
1997	British Dietetic Association *National Professional Standards for Dietitians Practising in Health Care*	Dietitians will liaise with catering concerning the production of food to specified nutritional standards, the development of menus (including choice), food delivery systems (inhouse or outside caterers), and that the food service encourages and enables the client to eat the food provided Dietitians will be involved in documentation relating to the provision of food and its service to clients Dietitians will advise on the provision of nutritionally adequate food specific to clients' needs and in accordance with national standards Dietitians will ensure catering and other staff have accurate information and receive appropriate training Dietitians will liaise with other members of the multiprofessional team to ensure that all aspects of the individuals care are considered in the nutrition care plan
1999	The Nuffield Trust *Managing Nutrition in Hospital: A Recipe for Quality*	Makes recommendations on the management of nutrition services to the Department of Health, NHS Executive, National Institute for Health and Care Excellence (NICE), The Audit Commission, health professional bodies, research funding agencies, health authorities and primary care groups and hospital trusts Food provision should be managed as an integral component of clinical care rather than a 'hotel' function
1999	BAPEN *Hospital Food as Treatment*	Doctors should acknowledge a responsibility for patient nutrition as an important part of overall management The chief dietitian should have an executive, not just an advisory, input into the catering services Consideration should be given to a new Nutrition Directorate with overall responsibility for all aspects of nutritional care Consideration should be give to transferring the catering and nutritional care service from the hotel/facilities directorate to the clinical support and treatment service budget
2001	*Department of Health* *Better Hospital Food*	This 4-year campaign produced a wide range of resources which are now archived and available for download on the Hospital Caterers Association website (www.hospitalcaterers.org)
2002	Council of Europe *Food Service and Nutritional Care in Hospitals: How to Prevent Undernutrition*	Undernutrition is common in hospitals across Europe Action to improve the identification and treatment of undernutrition Action to improve the training of staff providing nutritional care Action to improve the provision of hospital food Action to understand the health economics of food and nutritional care in hospitals
2002	Royal College of Physicians (Kopelman and Lennard-Jones, 2002) *Patient Nutrition: A Doctor's Responsibility*	Recognition of the important role doctors have to play in ensuring that their patients are adequately nourished Recognition that more emphasis on nutrition is needed in undergraduate and postgraduate training of doctors in the UK
2002	British Dietetic Association *Food Service a Consensus Statement*	Standard methodologies for the nutritional analysis of recipes and menus using food tables
2003	Quality Improvement Scotland (Scottish Executive, 2003) *Food, Fluid and Nutritional Care*	Set of standards covering assessment, screening and nutritional care planning; and the provision of food and fluid to patients
2003	Council of Europe Resolution ResOP (2003)3	The 19 Council of Europe member states that participated in the 2002 report *Food Service and Nutritional Care in Hospitals: How to Prevent Undernutrition* formally endorsed the recommendations of the report This commits governments to implementing the recommendations
2003	*Catering Services for Children and Young Adults*	This report was produced as part of the Department of Health 'Better Hospital Food' campaign Resources are produced by the BDA Paediatric Dietitians specialist group

(Continued)

SECTION 4

Table 4.4.1 *(Continued)*

Year	Organisation and report title	Main recommendations
2004	British Dietetic Association, Hospital Caterers Association and Royal College of Nursing *10 Key Characteristics of Good Nutritional Care*	This short report distils the 100+ recommendations made in the Council of Europe report and resolution into 10 simple actions that can be understood clearly at operational and managerial levels
2004	Hospital Caterers Association and Royal College of Nursing *Protected Meal times Policy*	Ensuring that meal times are a priority in the hospital day and are recognised as an important part of care and treatment delivery
2006	*Hospital Caterers Association* *Good Practice Guide Healthcare Food and Beverage Services*	This is a useful guide to the team working required at ward level if food and beverage services are to be successful
2006	British Dietetic Association *Delivering Nutritional Care Through Food And Beverage Services, A Toolkit for Dietitians*	This report was produced by the Food Counts Interest group of the British Dietetic Association It includes a whole set of useful tools for those charged with delivering food and beverage services in hospitals and other institutions
2007	*Improving Nutritional Care, A Joint Action Plan from the Department of Health and Nutrition Summit stakeholders*	This report was produced following two1-day conferences of stakeholder groups facilitated by the Department of Health in England The report makes many recommendations for joint action to improve nutritional care
2010	Nutrition Action Plan Delivery Board *End Of Year Progress Report*	The Delivery Board was convened to ask stakeholders how the recommendations made in the *Joint Action Plan* could be implemented There are recommendations on screening, training and the provision of information resources Many of the resources produced can be found on the website of the Social Care Institute for Excellence (www.scie.org.uk)
2010	Department of Health *Government Response to the Nutrition Action Plan Delivery Board End of Year Progress Report*	The government broadly endorsed the recommendations of the Delivery Board
2010	Essence of Care *Benchmarks for the Fundamental Aspects of Care*	This guidance on the delivery of nursing care includes a section on standards for the delivery of nutrition and hydration
2011	*All Wales Nutrition and Catering Standards for Food and Fluid Provision for Hospital Inpatients*	Sets out quality standards for food and beverage provision in hospitals in Wales
2011	*Care and compassion? Report of the Health Service Ombudsman on Ten Investigations into NHS Care of Older People*	Report raises concerns about the basic level of care delivered to older people and calls for improvements, particularly in the provision of nutritional care (help and assistance with eating and drinking).
2011	*Promoting Good Nutrition. A Strategy for good nutritional care for adults in all care settings in Northern Ireland 2011–2016*	A strategy document for the improvement of nutritional care in hospitals in Northern Ireland
2011	*Dysphagia Diet Food Texture Descriptors*	This report produced by the National Patient Safety Agency and endorsed by the BDA, RCN and RCSLT defines textures of food for the management of dysphagia
2011	Care Quality Commission *Dignity and Nutrition Inspection Programme National Overview*	This report presents the results of the inspection of nutritional care at 100 hospitals in England; 55 of 100 were found to be below the standard expected
2012	BDA *The Nutrition and Hydration Digest: Improving Outcomes through Food and Beverage Services*	• A comprehensive source for standards, coding, guidance and good practice • An evidence document for tenders and specifications • A tool providing a common language for clinicians, caterers, industry, etc. • The definitive approach in food service in care settings for professional (and other) bodies • A quick reference document on a multitude of food related topics

How to get more food eaten

Getting the food that is served eaten by the intended consumer is the principal goal of any food service system as the nutritional value of food not eaten is nil. The dietitian must understand the principles of food service in order to help achieve this goal. The process begins with menu planning.

Menu planning

The menu is the blueprint of food service and time spent planning the menu is never wasted. A dietitian's expertise is their knowledge of the nutritional requirements of the client group to be served and understanding how these might be met by the food supplied.

Knowing the client group

The first step in menu planning is gathering information about the client group:

- What do they like to eat?
- What are their cultural and religious preferences?
- What are their physical needs and personal preferences?
- When do they like to eat?
- How do they like to eat?
- What assistance will they need with eating?

Knowing what resources are available

It must be possible to deliver the menu you are planning:

- Can it be afforded?
- Is the kitchen equipment needed to produce the recipes available, i.e. enough oven space, crockery, cutlery, serving utensils?
- Is the necessary staffing and expertise available?
- Are the food storage facilities sufficient?
- Are food supplies secure?
- Can the items required be delivered in time and on a regular basis?
- Can the food be distributed to the patients accurately and safely?

Nutrition support team and policy

Menu planning is best practised as a team. Input from the dietitian, caterer, nurse, doctor, pharmacist, speech and language therapist and patients' representative is required to bring the necessary knowledge and expertise to the planning process. This core team will be recognisable to most dietitians as the core membership of the nutrition support team (NST). The reports of the Nuffield Trust (Maryon-Davis & Bristow, 1999), the British Association for Parenteral and Enteral Nutrition (BAPEN, 2007) and the Council of Europe (2002) all recommend that such a group be formed to oversee the nutritional health of the inpatient population in all hospitals or groups of hospitals.

It is recommended that such a cross department and interdisciplinary team develops nutritional policy for the hospital and oversees the implementation and monitoring of the effectiveness of that policy. It is further recommended that nutritional support policy extends to policy related to the provision of food. The NST's involvement in menu planning ensures that this responsibility is executed.

Menu structure

Once the team has gathered the information on policy, patient requirements and resources, the next step is to plan the structure of the menu:

- Over how many days will the menu run?
- Will the menu change daily over a cycle or will it be 'à la carte'?
- How many meals are to be provided each day?
- Will the meals be hot or cold?
- What is the structure of each individual meal?
- Will a starter be offered?
- How many choices will be offered?
- What types of dish are to be offered, i.e. meat, fish, vegetarian, egg, cheese, salad, sandwiches, soft choices, etc.?
- Can each item of the meal be chosen separately or is a meal to be offered as a single choice?

Developing the structure of the menu is the most difficult part of the planning process and it is important to spend time getting it right. Regardless of the dishes offered, a menu with a poor structure will not meet the patient's needs and desires (Table 4.4.2).

Selection of suitable dishes

Once the structure of the menu is determined, decisions can be made about individual dishes that will make up

Table 4.4.2 Outline structure of a menu for a large hospital

Breakfast	Lunch	Supper
Fruit juice	Fruit juice	Fruit juice
Fresh fruit	Soup	Soup
Wholemeal cereal	Main meat or fish dish	Main meat or fish dish
Low residue cereal	Soft dish (suitable for those with no teeth)	Snack dish
Porridge		Soft dish
	Vegan dish	Vegan dish
Wholemeal bread	Salad	Sandwich
White bread	Suitable staple	Suitable staple
Butter	Mashed potato	Mashed potato
Low fat spread		
	Vegetable 1	Vegetable 1
Boiled egg	Vegetable 2	Vegetable 2
Jam	Baked pudding	Baked pudding
Marmalade	Milk pudding	Milk pudding
	Custard	Ice cream
Milk	Fresh fruit	Cheese and biscuits

the menu. It is useful to put the menu structure on a large sheet of paper on the wall at this stage, write the names of the dishes available on sticker notes and assemble the menu. This visual technique allows a degree of interactivity within the planning team and highlights the way in which individual dishes complement one another. A visual prompt such as this will also bring to light any repetitions in the menu, particularly at the beginning and end of the menu cycle.

Information required for each dish

Detailed information about nutritional composition, cost and availability of preprepared dishes and standard recipes for dishes that are to be prepared on site will be needed. The British Dietetic Association (BDA, 2006) provides consensus guidance on the calculation of nutritional composition of recipes from food tables. This process requires professional judgement and interpretation at several stages, and variation and error can be introduced. The guidance aims to standardise methodology and reduce variation and error.

Nutrition information

Nutrition information required by the menu planner will depend on the requirements of the client group. A renal dietitian will be more interested in the electrolyte composition of foods than a dietitian responsible for the care of elderly people, whose focus of interest is more likely to be food consistency and energy density. Information about other aspects of food composition, such as whether it contains gelatine, gluten, milk, nuts or peanuts, etc., is also likely to be required. The menu planning team should agree on information requirements at an early stage in the planning process.

An increasing amount of nutrition information is demanded by a food and health conscious public. The planning team have a duty to meet these needs, e.g. this means knowing if any food item on the menu contains ingredients derived from genetically modified organisms. The NHS Supply Chain (www.supplychain.nhs.uk) provides comprehensive information on food purchased on NHS contracts.

Ratification of the menu

Once the first draft of the menu has been agreed, it will need to be ratified by analysis of its nutritional composition and cost. It is recommended that nutritional analysis is carried out and interpreted by a registered dietitian. The BDA provides consensus guidance on the methodologies involved in this process (BDA, 2006). The dietitian needs to be sure that the menu will meet the nutritional requirements of the client group, including the needs of those requiring modified diets. The ratification process will lead to a fine tuning of the menu, ensuring that the final menu represents the best available in terms of nutritional content, cost and practical deliverability.

Publishing the menu

Once completed, the menu needs to be published. At this point the team needs to consider how patients are going to make their choice from the menu. It is important to make sure that patients understand what is being offered to ensure their active participation in food choice. Patients are much more likely to eat food they have chosen themselves.

Systems and food service

The chain of events from provisions arriving at the hospital gate to completed dishes being presented to the patient is often referred to as the food chain. The best planned menu can fail at any point if the food delivery system is not robust. No one wants to eat cold food that should be hot or hot food that should be cold, or food which is poorly presented.

There are many new systems and technologies available to assist in the delivery of food service in hospitals. Different types of food service systems together with a summary of their benefits and drawbacks are summarised in relation to the following areas:

* Ways in which food can be prepared and stored (Table 4.4.3).
* Ways in which food can be distributed to the ward (Table 4.4.4).
* Methods of food service at ward level (Table 4.4.5).

Ward hostesses

Well trained and dedicated staff at ward level can dramatically improve food service (Stephen *et al.*, 1997). Staff whose main function is to ensure that patients are fed appropriately can make a great deal of difference to the amount of food eaten. By ensuring that all the administration related to securing patient meal choices is carried out, liaising with the kitchen in a timely manner, having time to discuss meal choices with patients and reporting food intake to nursing staff, a significant input to patients' nutritional support can be made. In addition, trained staff can implement food hygiene regulations on the ward and assure food safety.

Eating environment

The environment and ambience on the ward can make a dramatic difference to the acceptability of food and the amount eaten. Meal times should be regarded as special and important times in a patient's day and every effort should be made by ward staff to ensure that patients are uninterrupted and have time to enjoy their meals. Protected meal times give staff on the ward explicit permission to focus all their efforts on nutritional care, allowing other responsibilities to take a lower priority.

Decisions made at the time when new buildings or new food service systems are being planned can have considerable influence on the subsequent quality of food provision. Particular thought should be given to the amount of space required on wards for food preparation, service and consumption; inadequacies in these respects can ultimately affect the amount of food eaten (Bond, 1997).

Table 4.4.3   Food service systems ways in which food can be prepared and stored

System of food preparation and storage	Benefits	Concerns
Cook/serve 75% of hospitals in the UK prepare most food on site from fresh, raw ingredients. Increasingly items such as pies, puddings, preprepared vegetables and cooked meats are used	Flexibility, capable of adaptation to most situations Food preparation skills maintained on site Recipes can be adapted quickly to meet unusual requirements Traditional and regional variability	Depends on a well trained, skilled and motivated workforce Production facilities are expensive to maintain and take up a lot of space
Cook/chill Food is cooked and blast chilled to between 0 and 4°C. Food can be stored and distributed at this temperature for up to 5 days after production. It is then reheated (regenerated) ready for food service	Requirement for skilled cooks is reduced Requirement for expensive cooking equipment is reduced Can reduce 'hot holding' of food and improve nutritional value when served Fewer peaks and troughs in the kitchen working day Can increase variety of food available on the menu	Food costs increase to pay for preprepared food Regeneration must be done skilfully to optimise food quality 5-day shelf life Greater distribution leads to increased food safety risks Increased dependence on outside supplier Some dishes are not suitable for this type of service, e.g. pastry Less flexible service if no production facilities are maintained on site
Steamplicity© This is a variation on cook/chill in that the food is plated and packed in an outer container that includes a patented valve. The whole package is regenerated in a microwave oven and the valve enables steam pressure cooking to take place	Requirement for skilled cooks is reduced Requirement for expensive cooking equipment is reduced Reduces 'hot holding' of food and improves nutritional value when served Can increase variety of food available on the menu Food waste is reduced as a result of the 'plated system'	Food costs increase to pay for preprepared food Regeneration must be done skilfully to optimise food quality 5-day shelf life Increased dependence on outside supplier Some dishes are not suitable for this type of service, e.g. pastry Less flexible service if no production facilities are maintained on site
Cook/freeze. Food is cooked and quickly chilled to –18°C. Food can be stored and distributed at this temperature for periods of up to 3 months. It is then reheated (regenerated) ready for food service	As per cook/chill Increased shelf life makes distribution logistics easier	As per cook/chill Energy costs associated with freezing, storage and regeneration
Cook/conserve/*sous vide* Cook/chill and cook/freeze are often described as cook/conserve systems. This term is also used to describe *sous vide* systems. Food is cooked, sealed in an air free, oxygen impermeable, multilayered plastic bag. It is then chilled or frozen prior to storage and distribution. The food is then reheated (regenerated) ready for service	As per cook/chill Sealed package makes handling easier and safer Increased shelf life makes distribution logistics easier	As per cook/chill Increased cost of packaging

Table 4.4.4   Food service systems: ways in which food can be distributed to the ward

Method	Benefits	Concerns
Plated service Food is served onto the plate centrally and distributed	Good portion control Food safety risks contained in one area Fewer staff required on the ward Tight control of waste	Difficult to maintain food temperature and quality during distribution Logistics of collecting data on patient choice Difficult to cater for out of hours requirements Serving staff do not know who they are serving
Bulk food service Food is distributed in large containers and is served onto the plate at ward level	Food choice takes place at bedside Food temperature and quality easier to maintain during distribution 'You can have your gravy where you want it' Greater flexibility in terms of portion size Serving staff get to know the patients Patients can participate in the food service process	More space required at ward level More food handling risks at ward level Portion control more complex More ward based time required More staff required at ward level

Table 4.4.5 Food service systems: methods of food service at ward level

Method	Benefits	Concerns
Trayed service Food is assembled on a tray and the patient eats at the bedside or in bed	No communal ward areas needed Tight control of modified diets more practicable May be preferred by patients with eating difficulties Privacy Suitable for bedbound patients	Second helpings more difficult to provide Lack of social interaction Monitoring of food intake more difficult Problems unpacking some food items If whole meal is served, parts of it may go cold
Cafeteria style service	More normal Flexibility of service and portion size available at point of service Possibility of social interactions Food choice at point of service	Communal eating area needed Patients need to be mobile
Family meal service	As above Meal times more of an occasion, breaking up the ward day Mealtime can be used as a rehabilitative activity	More food service equipment needed at ward level Requires a degree of patient independence or increased staffing Communal eating area needed

Food waste

Up to 40% of food provided to patients is wasted (Stephen et al., 1997; Edwards & Nash, 1997; Fenton et al., 1995; Kelly, 1999). Full dustbins and empty patients are not successful nutritional support and care! Systems for the monitoring of food waste are a valuable performance indicator and act as a proxy measure for the amount of food that is being eaten. It is important to distinguish between plate waste, i.e. where a patient has attempted to eat a meal and not eaten all of it, and trolley or tray waste, i.e. food that was surplus to requirements and was never offered to patients.

High levels of plate waste may indicate either that the patient has a poor appetite, in which case a different approach to nutritional support needs to be considered, or that the taste, presentation or temperature of the food was at fault.

High levels of tray or trolley waste indicate that there is a food delivery problem. Information on needs may be poor, meal times may be inappropriate or portion control may need to be studied more carefully. *Managing Food Waste in the NHS* is a useful guide (Department of Health, 2005).

Audit of food service

Food service is a large scale, hospital wide operation, and the monitoring and auditing procedures are complex. It is important at the policy setting stage or the contract specification stage that patient centred output measures are agreed that will truly reflect the quality of the service. The NST should play a pivotal role in receiving, reviewing and recommending Hospital Board action on these output measures. Closing the audit loop in food service is difficult and resource intensive, but it is an important part of ensuring that the food service plays its full role in the nutritional support of patients. Developments in information technology are improving the ability to capture data on a large scale and interpret them appro-

priately. These developments need to be applied to food service monitoring to make it operationally practicable (Teal et al., 2012).

Future of food service in the NHS

Each of the UK home countries recognises the important role of food in the nutritional support of patients in hospital and all are signatories to the Council of Europe Resolution ResAP 2003(3), which makes recommendations for the improvement of food and nutritional care in hospitals in 19 Council of Europe member states. The recommendations are being implemented through the setting of quality standards in each of the home countries. The Care Quality Commission is the regulatory body responsible for standards of healthcare provision in England and Northern Ireland. In Wales, inspection is carried out by Healthcare Inspectorate Wales and Healthcare Improvement Scotland sets and assures the standard in Scotland.

Internet resources

British Association for Parenteral and Enteral Nutrition www.bapen.org.uk
Hospital Caterers Association   www.hospitalcaterers.org
King's Fund   www.kingsfund.org.uk
NHS Supply Chain   www.supplychain.nhs.uk
Nuffield Trust   www.nuffieldtrust.org.uk
Patients Association   www.patients-association.com

References

Bond S. (1997) *Eating Matters*. Newcastle upon Tyne: Centre for Health Services Research, University of Newcastle upon Tyne.
British Association for Parenteral and Enteral Nutrition (BAPEN). (2007) *Organisation of Food and Nutrition Support in Hospitals*. Available at www.bapen.org.uk.
British Dietetic Association (BDA). (2006) *Delivering Nutritional Care Through Food and Beverage Services, A Toolkit for Dietitians*. Birmingham: BDA.

Birkett D. (2005) On why nurses won't help. *Health Service Journal* 115: 17.

Care Quality Commission. (2011) Dignity and Nutrition Inspection Programme, national overview. October 2011. Available at www.cqc.org.uk. Accessed 28 August 2012.

Council of Europe. (2002) *Food and Nutritional Care in Hospitals: How to Prevent Undernutrition.* Report and recommendations of the committee of experts on nutrition, food safety and consumer health. Council of Europe Publishing.

Department of Health (2000). *The NHS Plan.* London: The Stationery Office.

Department of Health (2005). *Managing Food Waste in the NHS.* London: Department of Health.

Edwards J, Nash A. (1997) Measuring the wasteline. *Health Service Journal* 107(Nov): 26–27.

Elia M. (2009) Nutrition, hospital food and in-hospital mortality. *Clinical Nutrition* 28(5): 481–483

Fenton J, Eves A, Kipps M, O'Donnell CC. (1995) The nutritional implications of food wastage in continuing care wards for elderly patients with mental health problems. *Journal of Human Nutrition and Dietetics* 8: 239–248.

Gall MJ, Grimble GK, Reeve NJ, Thomas SJ. (1998) Effect of providing fortified meals and between-meal snacks on energy and protein intake of hospital patients. *Clinical Nutrition* 17(6): 259–264.

Health of the Nation, Nutrition Task Force. (1994) *Nutrition and Health: a management handbook for the NHS.* London: Department of Health.

Health of the Nation, Nutrition Task Force. (1995) *Nutrition Guidelines for Hospital Catering.* London: Department of Health.

Health Service Ombudsman. (2011) Care and Compassion, a report of the Health Service Ombudsman on ten investigations into NHS care of older people. February 2011. Available at www.ombudsman.org.uk. Accessed 28 August 2012.

Hiesmayr M, Schindler K, Pernicka E, *et al.* (2009) Decreased food intake is a risk factor for mortality in hospitalised patients: The Nutrition Day survey 2006. *Clinical Nutrition* 28(5): 484–491.

Kelly L. (1999) Audit of food wastage: differences between a plated and bulk system of meal provision. *Journal of Human Nutrition and Dietetics* 12: 415–424.

Kondrup J. (2004) Proper hospital nutrition as a human right. *Clinical Nutrition* 23: 135–137.

Kondrup J, Bak L, Stenbaek Hansen B, Ipsen B, Ronnenby H. (1998) Outcomes from nutrition support using hospital food. *Nutrition* 14: 319–321.

Kopelman P, Lennard-Jones J. (2002) Nutrition and patients: a doctor's responsibility. *Clinical Medicine* 2(5): 391–394.

Lennard-Jones JE. (1992) *A Positive Approach to Nutrition as a Treatment.* London: King's Fund Centre.

Lennard-Jones JE, Arrowsmith H, Davison C, Denham AF, Micklewright A. (1995) Screening by nurses and junior doctors to detect malnutrition when patients are first assessed in hospital. *Clinical Nutrition* 14: 336–340.

Löser C. (2010) Malnutrition in hospital—the clinical and economic implications. *Deutsches Ärzteblatt International* 107: 51–52.

Maryon-Davis A, Bristow A (eds). (1999) *Managing Nutrition in Hospital: A Recipe for Quality.* London: Nuffield Trust.

McWhirter JP, Pennington CR. (1994) Incidence and recognition of malnutrition in hospital. *BMJ* 308: 945–948.

National Institute for Health and Care Excellence (NICE). (2006). *Nutrition Support in Adults: Oral Supplements, Enteral Tube Feeding and Parenteral Nutrition.* London: NICE.

Ödlund-Olin A, Osterberg P, Hadell K, Armyr I, Jerstrom S, Ljungqvist O. (1996) Energy-enriched hospital food to improve energy intake in elderly patients. *Journal of Parenteral and Enteral Nutrition* 20: 93–97.

Patients Association. (1993) *Catering for Patients in Hospital.* Harrow, Middlesex: The Patients Association.

Scottish Executive. (2003) *Food, Fluid and Nutritional Care.* NHS Quality Improvement Scotland.

Stephen AD, Beigg CL, Elliot ET, MacDonald IA, Allison SP. (1997) Food provision, wastage and intake in medical, surgical and elderly hospitalised patients. *Clinical Nutrition* 16 (Suppl 2): 4.

Stratton RJ, Green CJ, Elia M. (2003) *Disease Related Malnutrition: An Evidence Based Approach to Treatment.* CABI Publishing.

Teal G, Macdonald AS, Bamford C. (2012). Redesigning hospital food services for vulnerable older patients. *Touchpoint, The Journal of Service Design* 3(3).

Tucker H. (1996) Cost containment through nutrition intervention. *Nutrition Reviews* 54: 111–121.

Wheatley P. (1999) Report of a nutritional screening audit. *Journal of Human Nutrition and Dietetics* 12: 433–436.

United Kingdom Central Council for Nursing and Midwifery (UKCC). (1997) *Responsibility for Feeding of Patients.* London: UKCC.

4.4.2 Prisons

Joan Gandy

Key points

- Depending on the category of prison, all food and drink, apart from some snacks and soft drinks, consumed by prisoners is provided by the institution.

- The prison governor has responsibility for catering and enforcing Ministry of Justice instructions.

- Food has a significant role in prisoners' lives; it can be the source of complaints, contribute to dissension and become a catalyst for aggression.

- Prison populations are at particular risk of obesity and associated health risks.

Unlike other institutions, prisons provide all the food and drink, apart from some snacks and soft drinks, consumed by prisoners. This depends on the category of the prison, with prisoners in lower security category prisons, e.g. open prisons, having more opportunity to supplement their intake. The primary objective of prison catering is '. . . *to provide a varied and healthy menu which takes account of prisoners' preferences whilst maintaining compliance with all relevant food safety legislation*' (Department of Justice Northern Ireland, 1995). In

December 2011 there were record numbers of prisoners, including those held in Immigration Removal Centres, of over 88000 in England and Wales. In March 2012 the Scottish prison population was nearly 8500 (Berman, 2012).

Meal provision and dietary quality

The provision of meals and food is seen as a key issue in helping to maintain order in prisons and in improving prisoners' health. In the UK Instruction PS44/2210 (Ministry of Justice, 2010) details prison catering services. All prisons use a preselected, multichoice, cyclical menu for lunch and dinner, which covers a minimum 4-week cycle. Portion sizes are tightly controlled to meet budgetary demands and for consistency. In 2004–2005 the UK Prison Service spent £94 million on catering; £43 million of which was spent on food. The average daily allowance for food is £1.87, although this varies between prisons and the type of prison. In Scotland the prison service spends £1.57 per head on food, compared with £2.50 per head in hospitals [National Audit Office (NAO), 2006].

The Ministry of Justice (2010) instruction on catering states that '*The food provided shall be wholesome, nutritious, well prepared and served, reasonably varied and sufficient in quality*'. The NAO report found that food served to prisoners was in line with national recommendations as given in the Balance of Good Health [this has been superseded by the eatwell plate (see Chapter 4.2)]. The food is varied, different dietary requirements are catered for and at least one meal at each serving is labelled as healthy. Religious and cultural requirements are also considered. Some groups have been set up by prisoners to educate and assist prisoners in obtaining specialist diets, e.g. the Vegan Prisoners Support Group. However, the report highlighted that food is often not served within 45 minutes of preparation, leading to decreased palatability and nutritional content. Meal times vary and some meals are served early, such as 11.15 AM for lunch and 4 PM for the evening meal, resulting in some prisoners exceeding the 14-hour interval standard between meals overnight. The NAO commissioned a survey into the diet of prisoners in England that found that prisoners were able to access and choose a nutritionally balanced diet and that most do so (Edwards *et al.*, 2007). However, there were minor dietary deficiencies in some micronutrients in some prisoners, including of vitamin D and zinc. Some dishes were not as healthy as they could be, with significant amounts of fried food being on offer; annotation was not always accurate.

Food has a significant role in prisoners' lives and sometimes symbolises their experience of prison (Smith, 2002). It can be the source of complaints and contribute to dissension and become a catalyst for aggression (Blades, 2001). It is therefore important that where queuing is inevitable, operational measures are taken to ensure that prisoners at the end of the queue are able to obtain their chosen meals; this reduces conflict and confrontation at the serving point.

The prison governor has overall responsibility for catering standards and the kitchens are inspected daily by the prison governor or an assistant. The catering manager at each prison is responsible for implementing standards. Her Majesty's Inspectorate of Prisons and the Independent Monitoring Board are responsible for monitoring all aspects of prison life including catering.

Non-communicable diseases

The prevalence of non-communicable diseases (NCDs) such as obesity, cardiovascular disease (CVD), diabetes and cancer is increasing and vulnerable groups are especially affected. Prisoners are one such vulnerable group. A recent systematic review by Herbert *et al.* (2012) of studies in 15 countries, including >60000 prisoners, showed an increase in some risk factors for NCDs. They found that women prisoners were more likely to be overweight or obese, although men were less likely to be. However, the heterogeneity of the studies meant that no summary calculations could be reported. Women prisoners consumed more energy than the recommended intake and all prisoners had sodium intake two to three times that recommended. UK prisoners were less physically active than the general population. One of the studies reviewed was that of Plugge *et al.* (2009) which surveyed CVD risk factors in women prisoners in the UK. They found that 30% were obese, 86% did not eat five or more pieces of fruit and vegetables per day, 85% smoked and 87% were insufficiently active. The authors repeated the survey a month into the women's sentences and found few improvements in risk factors.

Plugge *et al.* (2009) highlighted that there are currently no systematic approaches to educate prisoners on healthy lifestyles and address health problems within UK prisons. This is despite the NAO (2006) report recommending that the Prison Service should raise awareness of healthy eating by educating prisoners, using posters and actively promoting healthy eating on a regular basis. Following its report, the NAO produced guidance on promoting healthier lifestyles in prisons. Programmes exist in other countries, e.g. the WISEWOMAN programme in the USA. This programme provides heart disease screening and interventions for low income women and now works in women's prisons (Khavjou *et al.*, 2007). It has helped identify undiagnosed hypertension and dyslipidaemia, and offers interventions to improve health and discharge planning.

Dietetic practice in prisons and with prisoners

Given the rising levels of nutrition related diseases and number of prisoners, it is likely that dietitians will increasingly be asked to advise prisons or to advise prisoners in prisons or hospitals. Currently there is no guidance for dietitians working in prisons on how to deal with situations such as patients in restraints, lack of privacy and the prison regimen. In addition, dietitians may be asked to counsel prisoners as hospital patients; both as in- and out-patients. The British Medical Association (2009) provides guidance on the medical care for prisoners that dietitians may find useful. The guidance states:

- Detained prisoners must have the same standards of care as the rest of society, including respect for patient dignity and privacy.
- Risk assessment must be carried out prior to a prisoner going into hospital to determine the degree of supervision. Risk assessment includes: the prisoner's condition, any medical objection to the use of restraints, nature of the prisoner's offence, security of the consulting room and risk of violence to self or others.
- Where escape is unlikely, escort and bed watch by one prison officer, without restraints, is sufficient.
- Hospitals should be informed in advance about the levels of escort and restraint envisaged, and hospital staff should have the opportunity to discuss when level of restraint is clinically unacceptable.

More recently, prisons are increasingly using telemedicine for consultations between prisoners and healthcare professionals, including dietitians.

Nutrition and behaviour

The relationship between nutrition and criminal or delinquent behaviour is receiving increasing attention; however, evidence is still sparse. In addition, some studies are poorly constructed and there are few intervention trials. Benton (2007) reviewed the evidence and performed a meta analysis looking at the impact of diet on antisocial, violent and criminal behaviour. An analysis of five well designed randomised controlled studies showed that elimination diets reduced hyperactivity related symptoms and polyunsaturated fatty acid supplementation decreased violence in children. Three well designed studies showed that vitamin and mineral supplements reduced antisocial behaviour and aggression was linked to low blood glucose levels in adults. Benton (2007) concluded that the reactions to foods were inconsistent and not observed in all participants. Clearly there is a need for more well designed research in this area.

Diet and nutrition in prisons is an area that will undoubtedly become an increasingly important area of dietetic practice, as there is a need for health screening, promotion and education on healthy lifestyles. Further well constructed research studies are needed to look at the relationship between diet and criminal and delinquent behaviour.

Further reading

Cross M, MacDonald B. (2009) *Nutrition in Institutions*. Oxford: Wiley Blackwell.

Internet resources

Department of Justice Northern Ireland   www.dojni.gov.uk/catering
Inside Time (national newspaper for prisoners)   www.insidetime.org
Ministry of Justice   www.justice.gov.uk
National Audit Office   www.nao.org.uk
Vegan Prisoners Support Group   www.vpsg.info

References

Benton D. (2007) The impact of diet on anti-social, violent and criminal behaviour. *Neuroscience and Biobehavioral Reviews* 31: 752–774.

Berman G. (2012) Prison populations statistics (Standard note SN/SG/4334). Available at www.parliament.uk/briefing-papers/sn04334.pdf. Accessed 8 March 2013.

Blades M. (2001) Food and nutrition in the prison service. *Prison Service Journal* 134: 46–48.

British Medical Association. (2009) Health care of detainees in police stations. Available at www.bma.org.uk/images/healthdetainees0209_tcm41-183353.pdf. Accessed 8 March 2013.

Department of Justice Northern Ireland. (1995) Catering. Available at www.dojni.gov.uk/catering. Accessed 8 March 2013.

Edwards JSA, Hartwell HJ, Reeve WG, Schafields J. (2007) The diet of prisoners in England. *British Food Journal* 109: 216–232.

Herbert K, Plugge E, Foster C, Doll H. (2012) Prevalence of risk factors for non-communicable diseases in prison populations worldwide: a systematic review. *Lancet* 379: 1975–1982.

Khavjou OA, Clarke J, Hofeldt RM, *et al.* (2007) A captive audience. Bringing the WISEWOMAN Program to South Dakota Prisoners. *Women's Health Issues* 17: 193–201.

Ministry of Justice. (2010) Instruction PS44/2210: Catering – meals for prisoners. Available at www.justice.gov.uk/offenders/psis. Accessed 8 March 2013.

National Audit Office (NAO). (2006) HM Prison Service – Serving time: Prisoner diet and exercise. Available at www.nao.gov. Accessed 8 March 2013.

Plugge EH, Foster CE, Yudkin PL, Douglas N. (2009) Cardiovascular disease risk factors and women prisoners in the UK: the impact of imprisonment. *Health Promotion International* 24: 334–343.

Smith C. (2002) Punishment and pleasure: women, food and the imprisoned body. *The Sociological Review* 50: 197–214.

4.4.3 Armed forces

Joan Gandy

Key points

- Food is provided to non-operational, operational and civilian personnel.

- Contractors are expected to conform to a standard to provide choice and follow the healthy eating policy.

- Personnel are provided with nutrition guidance when enlisting and commanders are provided with information in order to support personnel.

- Dietitians in the UK are more likely to work in liaison with forces medical services than be employed by them.

Food is provided in three areas; non-operational (UK bases), operational (overseas bases, active theatres and ration packs) and civilian. The Defence Food Services Team (DFS) is responsible for food provision, meal type and quality for the armed forces in all areas including ships and submarines. The DFS also helps develop operational ration packs (ORPs). The Defence Catering Manual (Joint Services Publication 456) covers every aspect of food provision. Contractors must conform to a quality standard (Ministry of Defence, 2011), and supply products that provide choice and meet the healthy eating policy.

The Pay as You Dine (PAYD) system provides catering for non-operational food service. This system replaced the daily food charge, which was deducted from service personnel's salary regardless of whether or not it was taken. The PAYD system provides three core meals and personnel pay only for food that is taken; they also have access to other foods. The core meals must provide at least six items at breakfast and lunch and a three course dinner. Many members of the armed forces live off base or self cater.

The Ministry of Defence has developed military dietary reference values for macro- and micro-nutrients, but these are not readily available to the general public. All advice is based on the eatwell plate (see Chapter 4.2). The Expert Panel on Armed Forces Feeding (EPAFF) UK produces nutrition and hydration guidance for personnel, which emphasises increasing and maintaining performance, reducing the chance of injury, staying fit and healthy, and quick recovery from activity. All new recruits are provided with nutrition education materials. The emphasis is on the importance of nutrition and the gruelling and physical nature of military training, rather than weight and fat reduction. Recruits are treated as athletes and are given the necessary support and advice to achieve fitness. This is accompanied by the Commander's Guide to Nutrition; a more complex guide aimed at senior personnel. It gives more detail and offers nutritional guidance for operation packs (Wilcox, 2005).

The Armed Forces Nutrition Advisory Service offers expert advice and information on nutrition, diet and military feeding; this is only available to UK military personnel and Ministry of Defence civil servants. Dietitians are rarely employed in the UK Armed Forces, although they may be employed in institutes such as the Institute of Naval Medicine. Other dietitians work in liaison with military medical services in settings such as the Royal Centre for Defence Medicine in Birmingham (formerly Selly Oak Hospital).

In other countries, e.g. the USA, dietitians are members of the armed forces. The US military also conducts research into nutrition and has established research institutions for this, e.g. the U.S. Army Research Institute of Environmental Medicine.

Operational ration packs

All personnel are issued with these packs when operational, although field catering facilities are provided as soon as possible after deployment. The packs provide between 3788 and 4996 kcal with approximately 57% carbohydrate, 33% fat and 10% protein. Vegetarian meals and other specific diets, e.g. kosher and halal, are available. Packs always contain instant coffee, tea, fruit biscuits, brown biscuits, tabasco sauce, chewing gum and water purification tablets. Matches are also included for lighting the hexiburner cooker that every soldier carries.

The NATO Nutrition Science and Food Standards for Military Operations also covers UK military personnel working as part of a North Atlantic Treaty Organization (NATO) force.

Further reading

Bray RM. (2006) *Department of Defence Survey of Health Related Behaviors Among Active Duty Military Personnel: A Component of the Defense Lifestyle Assessment Program*. Barby, Philadelphia: Diane Publishing Co.

Internet resources

Ministry of Defence   www.gov.uk/government/organisations/ministry -of-defence
Food quality standard   www.gov.uk/government/publications/ food-quality-standard
NATO Nutrition Science and Food Standards for Military Operations (RTO-TR-HFM-154)   www.cso.nato.int
U.S. Army Research Institute of Environmental Medicine   www .usariem.army.mil/pages/mnd.htm

References

Ministry of Defence. (2011) Food quality standard. Available at www.gov.uk/government/publications/food-quality-standard. Accessed 12 March 2013.
Wilcox K. (2005) You are what you eat. *Defence Management Journal – Procurement and Material Management* 27. Available at www.defencemanagement.com. Accessed 12 March 2013.

4.5

Food law and labelling

Fionna Page and Ruth Birt

Key points

- Many laws relating to food in the UK, e.g. labelling, additives and claims, are now of European Union (EU) origin.

- The Food Standards Agency (FSA) is responsible for food safety and food hygiene across the UK.

- Responsibilities for food labelling are split between the FSA, the Department of Health and the Department for Environment, Food and Rural Affairs (Defra).

- The European Food Safety Authority (EFSA) is responsible for food safety risk assessment and advises the European Commission (EC) on the scientific aspects of food legislation.

- Legislation and guidelines regarding food and nutrition labelling, and claims are changing, and can be complex. Readers can keep up to date by referring to the Department of Health, Defra, EC, EFSA and FSA websites.

History of food legislation in the UK

After years of attempts at food regulation since 1266, the Food and Drugs Act 1938 was the first to combine specific food legislation with public health measures; at this time, food poisoning became notifiable across the UK. The act introduced controls for new areas such as misleading labelling and advertising, and powers were introduced to regulate the composition and labelling of foods as well as on the sanitary conditions of food on sale for human consumption. The act was suspended for the duration of World War 2, but with concerns about food substitutes being passed off as originals and insufficient nutrition being provided to ensure a staple diet to keep people fit and healthy, emergency powers were introduced. In 1955, a consolidating Food and Drug Act came into being, which was to remain the basis for food legislation until general legislation covering the composition, labelling, hygiene and safety of food in the UK was introduced in 1984 with the Food Act. (The Medicines Act superseded the drug aspect in 1968). However, during the 1980s there was a general increase in the number of reported cases of food poisoning and a number of well publicised food scares linked to *Salmonella* infection in raw eggs, *Listeria* contamination in foods such as soft cheeses and pâtés (believed to increase the number of miscarriages and stillbirths), and an outbreak of botulism caused by hazelnut yoghurt. In July 1989, the government announced far reaching proposals to change the law in its White Paper

Food Safety – Protecting the Consumer. As a result, food legislation underwent its first major review since the 1940s, culminating in the Food Safety Act 1990.

In the UK there is now an extensive array of legislation, codes of practice and guidance covering the whole area of food from production to distribution, packing, labelling and sale, and it may be of UK origin or be influenced or driven by European or international standards.

International food legislation

Since food is both imported into and exported from the UK, legislation on standards of composition and on labelling has to be compatible with, and in some instances comply with, international standards.

The European Union

Membership of the European Union (EU) means that the UK is required to implement European Commission (EC) regulations and directives, and this is now a major influence on UK food legislation.

Codex Alimentarius Commission

Codex, as it is usually known, has a fundamental mandate to develop international standards and norms for consumer health protection and fair practices in the food trade. It is comprised of the two United Nation bodies,

Manual of Dietetic Practice, Fifth Edition. Edited by Joan Gandy.
© 2014 The British Dietetic Association. Published 2014 by John Wiley & Sons, Ltd.
Companion Website: www.manualofdieteticpractice.com

the Food and Agriculture Organization (FAO) and the World Health Organization (WHO), and has a wide membership of the majority of developing and developed countries. Codex recommendations have no statutory force but members are encouraged to apply its norms to the widest extent possible as a basis for domestic regulation and international trade. In general, Codex standards are incorporated into European, and hence UK, legislation and, in recent years, have been important in the resolution of trade disputes across the continents.

Current UK food legislation

An understanding of the different types of legislation gives an insight into how and when food legislation becomes effective in the UK. Since the UK is a member of the EU, all EU regulations and directives have to be implemented into the UK regulatory system. This is possible under the Food Safety Act 1990 (classed as primary legislation), which not only provides the framework for all domestic food legislation, but also the powers to make secondary legislation to implement EU laws.

Regulations and directives

EC regulations are effective in all member states as soon as the EC Council adopts them. EC directives, on the other hand, do not become effective until they are written into a country's own legislation, and in the UK are actually also called regulations. For example, to allow for enforcement and execution of the EU Novel Foods Regulation, EC 258/97, the UK had to introduce its own regulations, called The Novel Foods and Novel Food Ingredients Regulations 1997 (SI 1997/1335). European legislation is denoted by EC followed by the number (in this case 258) and the year of publication. The UK regulation is denoted by SI (Statutory Instrument), the year of publication and the number (in this case 1335). These unique identifying numbers are important for citing the correct piece of legislation.

Most of the key provisions in food law are contained in legislation which sets out the specific details governing matters such as:

- Food labelling.
- Food hygiene.
- Animal, meat and meat products, e.g. those concerned with the examination for residues and maximum residue limits.
- Registration of food premises.
- Regulations on milk and dairies.
- Food composition.
- Use of food additives.
- Use of food packaging materials.

Regulations are kept under review and are subject to change (in the form of amendments), either as a result of that review or in order to harmonise food law within the EC.

Some important regulations are those concerning labelling, sweeteners, colours, flavouring, miscellaneous food additives and organic foods. As well as these general (horizontal) regulations that apply across food categories, there are specific (vertical) regulations applying to the composition of specific foods, such as bread and flour, chocolate and chocolate products, milk and soft drinks. There are also specific hygiene regulations relating to the production of milk, meat and other animal products.

Some categories of foods for particular nutritional uses (dietetic foods) have specific compositional and labelling rules as laid down in the European Foods for Particular Nutritional Uses (PARNUTs) directive. These include foods intended for energy restricted diets for weight reduction such as slimming foods; foods for special medical purposes (FSMPs) such as sip and tube feeds amongst others; foodstuffs suitable for people intolerant to gluten; and infant formulae, follow on formulae and weaning foods. Individual European directives that have been implemented into UK law as regulations currently govern each of these food categories.

Emerging issues

In June 2011 the EC published a proposal to revise the current PARNUTS Framework Directive, which may abolish the concept of dietetic foods and put in place a single regulation covering only food intended for infants and young children, and food for special medical purposes, although this approach is still under debate. General food law could in future cover the remaining food categories.

The Food Safety Act

The Food Safety Act 1990 is the main piece of UK legislation on food safety and consumer protection in Great Britain (GB); a separate but similar law applies in Northern Ireland. The act provides the framework for UK food law but does not, in itself, contain the specific rules governing matters such as the safety, quality, description or labelling of food. These details are set out in regulations and orders (classed as secondary legislation) made under the act. Codes of practice can also be issued under Section 40 of the Food Safety Act 1990. These are documents issued by ministers for the guidance of food authorities, the provisions for which can be enforced by direction and court order.

The aims of the Food Safety Act are to:

- Ensure that all food produced for sale is safe to eat, meets quality expectations and is not misleadingly presented.
- Provide legal powers and penalties.
- Enable the UK to fulfil its responsibilities in the EC.
- Keep pace with technological change.

The Food Safety Act 1990 has four main parts; preliminary, main provisions, administration and enforcement, and miscellaneous and supplemental.

Part I: Preliminary

This sets out the full scope of the act and the responsibilities for those involved in enforcing it. It covers the whole of GB and provides for regulations covering all aspects of food production, processing and selling, from the farm to the retailer. Its definitions of food have been widened to include slimming aids, dietary supplements and tap water, and premises now include most Crown properties, ships and aircraft. The act also sets out the principle that local authorities are responsible for enforcing most aspects of food law.

Part II: Main provisions

The main provisions of the act, namely food safety, consumer protection, regulation making powers and defences, are covered in this part of the act.

Offences

The main offences under the Food Safety Act are:

- Selling, or possessing for sale, food that does not comply with food safety requirements.
- Rendering food injurious to health.
- Selling, to the purchaser's prejudice, food that is not of the nature or substance or quality demanded.
- Falsely or misleadingly describing or presenting food.

Food safety requirements apply to food throughout the food chain, not just that for retail sale. Food is injurious to health if it could harm part of the population either in the short term, e.g. cause food poisoning, or long term, e.g. contaminated with lead. 'Not of the nature or substance demanded' means that it is illegal to sell cod described as haddock, or cola instead of diet cola. A purchaser can range from a customer at a shop to one supplier buying from another. 'Falsely or misleadingly described or presented' applies to written statements or pictorial representations which are untrue. Additional constraints are also laid down in food labelling regulations.

Defences

One significant aspect of food legislation introduced under the 1990 act was that due diligence became grounds for defence. Thus, for example, a retailer who unwittingly sold a contaminated food would not be guilty if it could be shown that the contamination occurred at an earlier stage in the supply chain and that the retailer could not have known that the product was unfit for sale. In practice, this means that the onus is on the food industry and food importers to supply safe food, and is considered to be a far reaching and important aspect of the act.

Novel foods

The act also contains powers to make regulations covering the sale of novel foods, i.e. those that are new or have only been rarely eaten in this country. Another significant piece of legislation then introduced was the EU Regulation (EC) 258/97 concerning novel foods and novel food ingredients, which applies to the placing of novel foods or ingredients onto the EU market that have not previously been used for human consumption to a significant degree. Detailed rules for the authorisation of novel foods, ingredients and processes were laid down, including the introduction of a means of mandatory notification for foods or ingredients containing, consisting or produced from genetically modified organisms (GMOs), subsequently updated over the years.

Part III: Administration and enforcement

This lays down procedures for the sampling and analysis of products, powers of entry, obstruction and enforcement. It also deals with the legal aspects of prosecution and appeal procedures.

Part IV: Miscellaneous and supplemental

This covers the issuing of codes of practice to food authorities on the execution and enforcement of legislation, and directions on specific steps to be taken to comply with a code. Other details pertain to areas of coverage of the act and other aspects of its implementation.

Other food related UK legislation

A number of other Acts of Parliament, and their subsidiary regulations, also impact in various ways on the provision, sale or safety of food. It was the Food Standards Act 1999 that set up the FSA and transferred functions and powers relating to food standards and safety to it. The FSA is an independent department working at arm's length from the government, which provides advice and information to the public and government on food safety from farm to fork. It also protects consumers through effective food enforcement and monitoring. The FSA is accountable to parliament through health ministers, and to the devolved administrations in Scotland, Wales and Northern Ireland for its activities within their areas. The FSA obtains independent expert advice from its scientific advisory committees and commissions research to support its functions.

European legislation on general food safety is contained in the General Food Law Regulation (EC) 178/2002), which introduced many key procedures for food safety matters, including the establishment of the European Food Safety Authority (EFSA). In the UK, the General Food Regulations 2004 No 3279 (and amendments) provides for the enforcement of certain provisions of Regulation (EC) 178/2002 (including imposing penalties) and amends the Food Safety Act 1990 to bring it in line with Regulation (EC) 178/2002. Similar legislation applies in Northern Ireland.

An excellent guide to food law is supplied by the FSA as *The Food Law Guide* (www.food.gov.uk). It covers legislation in effect in the UK and lists Statutory Instruments that apply in only one UK country, but gives the details of any equivalent legislation in the other UK countries. It is updated every 3 months. It also provides a link to relevant guidance documents.

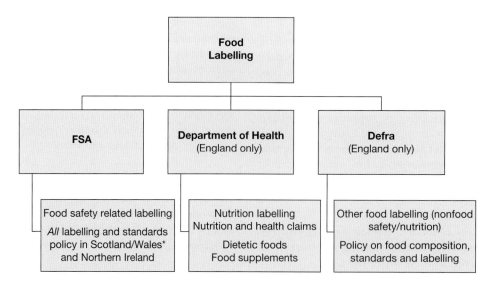

Figure 4.5.1 Food labelling responsibility in the UK

Law enforcement

The FSA works with enforcement officers to ensure that food (and feed) law is applied across the entire food chain as a result of the its statutory powers to strengthen enforcement of food standards, and to ensure national objectives are delivered. The responsibilities of all the enforcement authorities in the UK are set out and agreements are in place that provide a structure to the FSA's supervision of local authority enforcement work.

The Food Law Code of Practice sets out the way local authorities should apply food law, and how they should work with food businesses. The FSA provides guidance on specific regulations that are relevant to enforcement officers and food businesses to ensure that the law is clear. A new body, Local Government Regulation (formerly LACORS, the Local Authorities Coordinators of Regulatory Services), provides one link between local food enforcement and central government, giving advice and guidance to local authorities as well as advising the FSA on food enforcement issues.

Local enforcement officers have wide powers to inspect any stage of the production, manufacturing, distribution and retail chain, and have a responsibility to investigate any food complaints passed on to them by consumers. Food premises are inspected at a frequency dependent upon risk. Frequency of physical inspections can vary from once every 6 months to once every 2 years. Enforcement officers also have the power to take samples of food for testing to ensure compliance with food legislation, as well as powers to take action against a food premise that does not comply with food law. This enforcement action can range from issuing warnings and improvement or prohibition notices, to instigating prosecutions. The courts can inflict heavy penalties for non-compliance, including the closure of a business where conditions are particularly bad.

Food labelling

Food labels are the principle method by which a consumer gets information about their food. Labels must be accurate and must not mislead, so consumers can make informed choices about the food they buy. From October 2010, responsibility for food labelling was divided between three government departments in the UK as illustrated in Figure 4.5.1. The FSA leads on food safety related labelling. Nutrition labelling sits with the Department of Health to help towards a consistent approach to nutrition policy. Other areas of non-safety related food labelling are the responsibility of the Defra whose role also includes coordination of labelling policy across government. NB: Responsibilities for food labelling differ across the UK home countries.

Labelling regulations

Food information regulation

Food labelling in the UK is principally controlled by the Food Labelling Regulations 1996 (and later amendments, incorporating EC directives and regulations) made under the Food Safety Act 1990. However, in November 2011, following a European wide review of general food labelling and nutrition labelling rules, a new Food Information for Consumers Regulation No 1169/2011 (FIR) was published. The FIR consolidates and simplifies existing food labelling legislation and will replace current UK food labelling law after a 3-year transitional period. The general principle of the new FIR remains primarily to provide a basis for consumers to be able to make informed choices about the food they consume and to prevent misleading practices. It also continues to prohibit claims that foods prevent, treat or cure human disease, so-called medicinal claims.

Table 4.5.1   Mandatory information on food labels as required by the Food Information Regulation

Mandatory food information	Notes*
Food name	A legal name, customary name or descriptive name must be used See Product name section for examples
List of ingredients	Must include all the ingredients in the food in descending order of weight (an ingredient list or certain ingredients can be omitted in some circumstances) Annexes to the regulation give detailed rules for listing ingredients by weight, names of ingredients, food additives, enzymes and flavourings, and compound ingredients
Ingredients or processing aids causing allergies or intolerances	Annex II of the regulation lists the substances or products causing allergies or intolerances that must be indicated in the list of ingredients and given special emphasis, e.g. by the use of bold font The rules will extend to foods sold loose and foods sold by caterers
Quantity of ingredients	See Ingredients section for more detail
Net quantity of the food	Continues to allow some foods to be sold by number, e.g. bread rolls or eggs
Date of minimum durability or the use by date	Best before and use by will continue to be used A date of first freezing will be included for foods such as meat or fish See Durability section for more detail
Special storage instructions and/or conditions of use	See Durability section for more detail
Name and address of the food operator marketing or importing the food into the European Union	
Country of origin or place of provenance	The rules have been tightened and will also extend to fresh and frozen meat Scotland and other areas may be referred to without the use of UK on the label
Instructions for use	Particularly where without instructions it would be difficult to make appropriate use of the food
For alcoholic drinks with >1.2% by volume of alcohol	Actual alcoholic strength labelled as X% vol, preceded by the word alcohol or alc
Nutrition declaration	See Nutrition labelling section for more detail

*Refer to Regulation (EU) No1168/2011 and relevant annexes for full details.

The main changes to the legislation include new rules on nutrition labelling, provision of allergen information, labelling clarity, added caffeine in foods and high caffeine drinks, country of origin labelling, the labelling of water content of some meat and fish products, and voluntary calorie labelling on alcoholic drinks. The FIR requires that all foods intended for the final consumer, including foods supplied to or delivered by mass caterers (subject to certain exceptions), be marked or labelled with the mandatory food information shown in Table 4.5.1. A notable change is that by 2016 nutrition labelling will be mandatory on most prepacked foods.

Additional mandatory information is required on some foods, e.g. foods packaged in certain gases, foods containing sweeteners, certain frozen meat and fish products, and foods containing liquorice. Drinks high in caffeine (>150 mg/L) (other than those based on tea or coffee or their extracts will need to show the caffeine content in milligram per 100 mL and carry the warning '*High caffeine content – Not recommended for children or pregnant or breastfeeding women*'. Foods with added caffeine will need to carry the warning '*Contains caffeine – Not recommended for children or pregnant women*' and also show the caffeine content.

The FIR specifies that food information should be available, easily accessible and visible, and where appropriate indelible, but now also places special emphasis on the legibility of the mandatory information on food labels and specifies a minimum font size of 1.2 mm (0.9 mm for small packages).

Product name

This is required to be a clear description of the product, e.g. pilchards in tomato sauce. If the product has a non-descriptive brand name, e.g. Marmite, some indication of its nature must be given, e.g. yeast extract. The name must also indicate if the product has undergone any form of processing, e.g. UHT milk or smoked mackerel. Descriptions must also not be misleading; if a product is described as raspberry yogurt, then it must contain raspberries, not just raspberry flavouring. Some foods have customary names, e.g. cream crackers, which do not contain cream but the name is considered to be sufficiently familiar not to be misleading. Other foods have prescribed names with strict rules governing their use, e.g. margarine has to contain 80% fat; if the product contains less than this, it must be called something else such as a spread.

Ingredients

These are given in descending order of content so, for example, if water is the first item listed, then water is the most abundant ingredient. In the past, food ingredients lists only provided a limited guide to food quality, e.g. whether a hamburger contains cereal filler as well as meat. In 2000, this ability was strengthened by the EC requirement for Quantitative Ingredients Declaration (QUID). Most food products now have to state the quantity of any ingredients that:

- Appear in the name of a food or which are usually associated with that name by consumers.
- Are emphasised on the label in words, pictures or graphics.
- Are essential to characterise the food and to distinguish it from products with which it might be confused because of its name or appearance.

Declarations must appear in, or next to, the name of the food, or in the ingredients list, and must be shown as a percentage (based on the amount of the ingredient used at the manufacturing stage). The aim is to help the consumer compare the quality of similar foods by being able to see how much ham and mushroom is in a ham and mushroom pizza or pork in pork sausages.

Allergens

In the past, substances that were part of a compound ingredient comprising <25% of the finished product did not have to be itemised separately. This meant that potentially allergenic substances, such as small amounts of milk, wheat or gluten, did not appear in the ingredient list, making it difficult for individuals to avoid potentially allergenic substance. New food labelling regulations, implementing a 2003 EU directive, came into force in the UK at the end of 2005. One of the main purposes of the changes was to remove the 25% rule and ensure that all allergenic ingredients, as defined in the directive, are included in ingredient lists (see Chapter 7.11.2). The 14 allergenic food ingredients, and derivatives, that must be declared are:

- Cereals containing gluten.
- Crustaceans.
- Eggs.
- Fish.
- Peanuts.
- Soyabeans.
- Milk (including lactose).
- Nuts (from trees).
- Celery.
- Mustard.
- Sesame seeds.
- Sulphur dioxide >10 ppm.
- Lupin.

Highly processed ingredients derived from these allergens are exempt if they no longer contain allergenic proteins.

The composition and labelling of foodstuffs for people intolerant to gluten is also covered by specific European legislation that came into force in January 2012. It stipulates set levels of gluten that are permitted in foods, making gluten free claims as follows:

- *Gluten free* – the gluten content of foods bearing this claim must not exceed 20 ppm.
- *Very low gluten* – the gluten content of foods bearing this claim must not exceed 100 ppm (only foods with cereal ingredients that have been specially processed to remove the gluten may make this claim).

These rules apply to all foods, including prepacked foods, food sold loose and foods sold in health food shops or catering establishments.

Durability

This must be indicated either by a *use by* or *best before* date, and there is an important difference between the two. Highly perishable fresh foods, e.g. dairy products, must have a use by date, and after this time it should be assumed that the food is no longer safe to eat. To minimise the risk of food poisoning, use by dates should be strictly observed.

The best before date applies to foods with a shelf life of weeks, months or even years, e.g. breakfast cereals or canned foods. After this date there may be some deterioration in the quality of the texture and flavour of the product, but the food will not necessarily be unsafe to eat.

If any special storage conditions such as refrigeration are necessary, these must be shown close to the use by or best before date.

Food additives and E numbers

A food additive is defined as any substance not normally consumed as a food by itself and not normally used as a typical ingredient in a food, which is intentionally added to a food for functional purposes. Types of food additives are preservatives, antioxidants, emulsifiers and stabilisers, colours, sweeteners, flavour enhancers and flavourings. The safety of food additives is rigorously tested and periodically reassessed. The FSA is the responsible authority in the UK for giving advice on the safety of additives. At EU level, all additives currently allowed have been evaluated by the EFSA, or its predecessor, the Scientific Committee for Foods (SCF), and given an E number.

It is perhaps ironic that the E number classification system, originally intended as a way of providing assurance that an additive's safety had been evaluated, came to be regarded by the general public as a symbol of undesirable food. As a result of the bad image associated with E numbers, food manufacturers are increasingly declaring additives in ingredients lists by their chemical name rather than their E serial number (a permitted option under food labelling legislation). From a dietetic viewpoint, this can make it more difficult for any client who may need to avoid particular additives, as they now have to memorise complex chemical names rather than simple numbers. The E number classification system for food additives is summarised in Appendix 5.

The Food Labelling Regulations 1996 determine the way in which additives present in foods are declared on food labels. Those used as ingredients in prepackaged foods must be listed in an ingredients list by:

- The appropriate category name of the function, e.g. preservative.
- This must be followed by their specific name, e.g. sulphur dioxide, or E number, e.g. E220.

If an additive has more than one function, e.g. emulsifier and thickener, the category name that describes its principal function should be used.

Flavourings are slightly different because there are so many of them and they are harder to categorise. They may therefore be declared by the term flavourings, while natural flavourings may be declared if in line with the provisions of the new EU definitions introduced in 2008.

Foods containing artificial sweeteners require a declaration that the food contains sweeteners or, if sugars (any added mono- or di-saccharide) are also present, a declaration of sweeteners and sugars. There are additional labelling requirements for foods containing aspartame (stating that it is a source of phenylalanine) and polyols (excessive consumption of which may have a laxative effect).

Consumer attitude to additives

Many consumers view the presence of additives in foods with great suspicion, believing them to be undesirable in principle, synthetic in nature and a common cause of allergies. However, many of these anxieties are misplaced. Food additives fulfil a useful purpose in retarding microbial spoilage, prolonging shelf life and improving taste, colour and texture. Many food additives are natural or nature identical substances, or even nutrients such as beta-carotene (used as a food colour) or vitamin C (used as an antioxidant). While some people can react to certain additives, this type of food intolerance is relatively rare (see 7.11.2).

The food industry has responded to consumer concerns by carefully assessing the necessity for additives and reducing the level of usage as much as possible, particularly the use of azo food dyes in soft drinks and sweets, and substituting synthetic compounds with more natural alternatives. An interesting development came from the FSA recommendations to government ministers for a ban on the use of certain colours after a study that looked into the effects of six colours and their effect on children's behaviour. The colours are tartrazine (E102), quinoline yellow (E104), sunset yellow (E110), carmoisine (E122), ponceau 4R (E124) and allura red (E129) ((McCann *et al.*, 2007). Over the past few years, the FSA has worked with the UK food industry to voluntarily remove these six colours from food and drink, and to make this information available to consumers. A mandatory warning laid down in EU legislation will make it easier for people to choose products that are free from these colours. Legislation was introduced in 2010 that all food placed on the market containing any of these six colours should carry additional label information that *'consumption may have an adverse effect on activity and attention in children'*.

Nutrition labelling

The Food Labelling Regulations 1996 lay down a prescribed format for the nutrition labelling of foods. Nutrition labelling is currently voluntary under these rules, except where a nutrition or health claim is made. Group 1 or the *Big 4* represents the minimum level of nutrition information that can be given; alternatively, more information can be given using the Group 2 or the *Big 8* format. By 2016 nutrition labelling will be mandatory on the majority of foods under the rules introduced by the new FIR, which also includes new requirements for the content, calculation, expression and presentation of the nutrition declaration.

Table 4.5.2 shows a comparison of the current FLR 1996 and the new FIR nutrition declaration. Due to the

Table 4.5.2 Comparison of the current Food Labelling Regulations (FLR) 1996 and new Food Information Regulation (FIR) nutrition declarations*

FLR 1996 Group 1 (*Big 4*)	FLR 1996 Group 2 (*Big 8*)	FIR 2011 nutrition declaration**
Energy (kJ and kcal)	Energy (kJ and kcal)	Energy (kJ/kcal)
Protein (g)	Protein (g)	Fat (g)
Carbohydrate (g)	Carbohydrate (g)	Of which
Fat (g)	– of which sugars (g)	– saturates (g)
	Fat (g)	– monounsaturates (g)
	– of which saturates (g)	– polyunsaturates (g)
	Fibre (g)	Carbohydrate (g)
	Sodium (g)	Of which (g)
		– sugars (g)
The following nutrients can be included in a nutrition declaration on a voluntary basis, but must be declared if a claim about them is made: sugars, polyols, starch, saturates, monounsaturates, polyunsaturates, cholesterol, fibre, sodium, vitamins, minerals		– polyols (g)
		– starch (g)
		Fibre (g)
		Protein (g)
		Salt (g)
		Vitamins and minerals[†]

*These rules do not apply to food supplements or natural mineral waters.
**Mandatory energy and nutrients shown in bold.
[†]Units are specified in the Annex of the Regulation.

transitional periods in the FIR, a manufacturer who chooses to present nutrition information *voluntarily* on pack could, between 13 December 2011 and 13 December 2014, opt to present nutrition information according to either the rules in the FLR 1996 or the new FIR. However, after 13 December 2014, the FLR 1996 will be repealed, so manufacturers will have to comply with the rules stipulated by the FIR from this date. A nutrition declaration for most foods only becomes *mandatory* in 2016.

The new FIR stipulates seven key nutrients, listed in a different order to the FLR 1996 options. Inclusion of monounsaturates, polyunsaturates, polyols, starch, fibre (previously a requirement in Group 2) and vitamins and minerals are voluntary. Salt is now included in place of sodium to aid consumer understanding. Values per quantified serving may be given as well as, but not instead of, values per 100 g or 100 mL under the FLR 1996. In the FIR there are options for presenting the nutrition declaration on a per portion basis or per consumption unit in certain circumstances.

The new FIR gives the option to express the energy value, fat, saturates, carbohydrate, sugars, protein and salt as a percentage of the reference intakes (Table 4.5.3), which are similar to the guideline daily amounts (GDAs). Under FLR 1996 if a vitamin or mineral is declared in the nutrition labelling panel, or a claim is made, Group 1 nutrition information must be given. If a claim is made relating to a Group 2 nutrient, e.g. high in fibre, information on all Group 2 nutrients should be given.

The rules governing the labelling of vitamins and minerals are more complex. The content of these nutrients can only be declared if a food will provide a significant amount (7.5% for beverages and 15% for products other than beverages) of the nutrient reference values (NRVs) for each vitamin and mineral, as listed in the annex of the regulation (Table 4.5.4). These were previously known as

the recommended daily amounts (RDAs). The EC has committed to look at the issue of *trans* fats and may in due course introduce legislative proposals for the labelling of *trans* fats on foods.

Issues relevant to nutrition labelling in the UK

Aspects of nutrition labelling information that should be noted are:

• *Energy* – for nutrition labelling purposes, energy content is derived using a conversion factor of 4 kcal/g for carbohydrate and sugars, rather than 3.75 kcal/g used by standard UK food tables. The energy content declared on food labels will therefore be slightly higher than food table values. The new FIR also introduces additional new conversion factors for the calculation of energy values for labelling purposes (Table 4.5.5). NB: Fibre now has a conversion factor of 8 kJ/g or 2 kcal/g.

• *Fibre* – a new definition of fibre was introduced in 2008 which expanded the definition to include carbohydrate polymers with three or more monomeric units, which are neither digested nor absorbed in the human small intestine. The Association of Official Analytical Chem-

Table 4.5.4 Nutrient reference values (NRVs)

Nutrient	NRV
Vitamin A (µg)	800
Vitamin D (µg)	5
Vitamin E (mg)	12
Vitamin K (µg)	75
Vitamin C (mg)	80
Thiamine (mg)	1.1
Riboflavin (mg)	1.4
Niacin (mg)	16
Vitamin B_6 (mg)	1.4
Folic acid (µg)	200
Vitamin B_{12} (µg)	2.5
Biotin (µg)	50
Pantothenic acid (mg)	6
Potassium (mg)	2000
Chloride (mg)	800
Calcium (mg)	800
Phosphorous (mg)	700
Magnesium (mg)	375
Iron (mg)	14
Zinc (mg)	10
Copper (mg)	1
Manganese (mg)	2
Fluoride (mg)	3.5
Selenium (µg)	55
Chromium (µg)	40
Molybdenum (µg)	50
Iodine (µg)	150

Table 4.5.3 Comparison of guideline daily amounts (GDAs) (IGD, 2006) with new reference intakes for energy and selected nutrients other than vitamins and minerals (adults). Differences are highlighted in bold

Energy or nutrient	Reference intake	Guideline daily amount*
Energy (kcal)	2000 (8400 kJ)	2000 kcal
Total fat (g)	70	70
Saturates (g)	20	20
Carbohydrate (g)	**260**	**230**
Sugars (g)	90	90
Protein (g)	**50**	**45**
Salt (g)	6	6
Sodium (g)	–	**2.5**
Dietary fibre (AOAC) (g)	–	**25**

*GDA for an adult woman. GDAs for men and children aged 5–10 years are also available (see www.gdalabel.org.uk)

Table 4.5.5 Conversion factors for the calculation of energy for food labelling purposes

Nutrient	Energy value	
	kJ/g	kcal/g
Carbohydrate (except polyols)	17	4
Polyols	10	2.4
Protein	17	4
Fat	37	9
Salatrims	25	6
Alcohol (ethanol)	29	7
Organic acid	13	3
Fibre	8	2
Erythritol	0	0

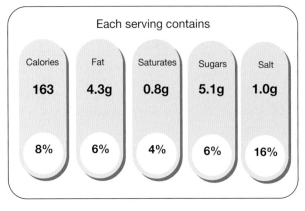

Figure 4.5.2 Example of a front of pack label based on guideline daily amounts (GDAs)

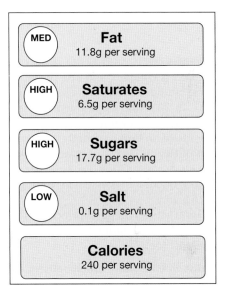

Figure 4.5.3 Example of a front of pack label based on the Food Standards Agency traffic lights system

ists (AOAC) method for analysis of fibre should be used. However, UK food tables mainly give dietary fibre (non-starch polysaccharide) values using the Englyst method and the AOAC method only for a very limited number of foods.

- *Salt* – the FLR 1996 labelling requirement is to list the content of sodium in grams, this will change under FIR to salt in grams to aid consumer understanding. UK food tables provide sodium content in milligrams.
- *Accuracy* – nutrition information on food labels is mainly estimated using published data on food composition as the alternative laboratory analysis is expensive for food manufacturers and is prone to sampling errors, especially for non-homogeneous foodstuffs. There will therefore be some variability between the declared values and those determined by analysis of a sample of the foodstuff. An acceptable margin for error is not specified by law and should reflect the type of foodstuff. For example, a foodstuff consisting of chunks of meat and vegetables in a sauce will be inherently more variable than a homogenous foodstuff such as chocolate and this has to be reflected in the acceptable margin for error.
- *NRVs* – the NRVs for vitamins and minerals, against which the amounts in food are compared in the nutrition panel, are a set of adult data produced specifically for labelling purposes. These were updated in 2008 and were previously known as RDAs.
- *GDAs* – Table 4.5.2 shows what is known as the back of pack nutrition declaration. In the UK manufacturers have been using front of pack labelling for a number of years and several different presentations have emerged, spearheaded by the Institute of Grocery Distribution (Figure 4.5.2) and the FSA traffic light colour coding system (Figure 4.5.3). The new FIR allows the option to continue to voluntarily repeat front of pack information on nutrients of importance to public health (energy value or energy value plus fat, saturates, sugars and salts). It is not yet clear if the term GDAs will be permitted once the FIR is fully in force.

Nutrition and health claims

Nutrition and health claims can be a useful way of conveying information to consumers and help them choose foods with particular nutritional features and health benefits. However, people need to be able to do so without being misled. In December 2006, Regulation No 1924/2006 on nutrition and health claims made on foods was published with the aim of protecting consumers from false or misleading claims, in addition to harmonising the legislation on claims across the EC to facilitate trade. It applies to nutrition and health claims made in commercial communications to the final consumer, including claims made in the labelling, presentation and advertising of food. It also applies to foods supplied to restaurants, hospitals, schools and other mass caterers. The legislation defines what is meant by a claim, and defines the different type of claims (Table 4.5.6).

Table 4.5.6   Key definitions included in Regulation 1924/2006 on Nutrition and Health Claims Made on Foods

Term	Definition
Claim	A claim is defined as *"any message or representation, which is not mandatory under Community legislation or national legislation, including pictorial, graphic or symbolic representation, in any form, which states, suggests or implies that a food has particular characteristics"*
Nutrition claim	Any claim that states suggests or implies that a food has particular beneficial nutritional properties due to the energy it: 1. provides 2. provides at a reduced or increased rate 3. or does not provide and/or the nutrients or other substances it: 1. contains 2. contains in reduced or increased proportions 3. or does not contain
Health claim	Any claim that states, suggests or implies that a relationship exists between a food category, a food or one of its constituents and health
Reduction of disease risk claim	Any claim that states, suggests or implies that the consumption of a food category, a food or one of its constituents significantly reduces a risk factor in the development of a human disease

The regulation is complex and sets out many requirements for the authorisation and use of nutrition and health claims. In 2011 the Department of Health issued an extensive guidance document giving regulatory and best practice advice on how to comply with the regulation (Department of Health, 2011). It covers the whole of the UK. Along with the regulation itself the Department of Health guidance document is essential reading for anyone involved in this area.

The regulation sets out general principles for all claims and further specific conditions for nutrition and health claims, which include:

- Claims must *not* be false, ambiguous or misleading; suggest a balanced and varied diet cannot provide appropriate quantities of nutrients; encourage or condone excess consumption of a food; or refer to changes in bodily functions that could exploit fear in the consumer.
- Claims must be based on generally accepted scientific data and be well understood by the average consumer.
- In most cases if a claim is made, nutrition labelling is mandatory.
- Only nutrition claims listed in the annex to the regulation are permitted and only if they meet the conditions of use stipulated for that claim (Table 4.5.7).
- Only authorised health claims included in the EU Register can be used on food and claims must meet the conditions of use (see Table 4.5.8 for examples of authorised claims).
- Claims must not be made on alcoholic beverages containing >1.2% by volume of alcohol (see regulation for limited exceptions).
- Health claims not permitted include those that suggest that health could be affected by not consuming the food or make reference to the amount or rate of weight loss.

- Health claims that make reference to recommendations of individual doctors or health professionals are not allowed on food labelling. This is covered by Article 12(c) within the regulation and is explained in more detail within the Department of Health guidance document. However, there is still debate about what is permitted. The British Dietetic Association (BDA) has been active on this topic and can provide an update for anyone concerned about the issue.
- Nutrient profiles (restrictions on the use of claims on certain foods or categories of foods based on their nutritional composition) have still not been adopted and are the subject of much debate.

Health claims require authorisation under the regulation. The Panel on Dietetic Products, Nutrition and Allergies (NDA) of the EFSA is responsible for scrutinising the scientific substantiation for health claims submitted by food business operators. Specific rules apply for claims for disease risk reduction and those that refer to children's health and development. ESFA's opinions inform EC decisions about whether a claim will be included in the EU Register. Claims that a food can treat, prevent or cure (medicinal claims) continue to be prohibited.

Addition of nutrients

In December 2006 Regulation (EC) 1925/2006 on the addition of vitamins and minerals and certain other substances to foods was published to provide the same rules throughout the EC. *Other substances* are those, other than vitamins and minerals, that have a physiological effect. The regulation prohibits the addition to unprocessed foods such as fruit, vegetables, meat, poultry and fish, and to beverages containing >1.2% by volume of alcohol. It includes lists of the vitamins and minerals that may be added to foods and the form in which they may be added.

Table 4.5.7 Nutrition claims and conditions applying to them as listed in the Annex of Regulation 1924/2006 on Nutrition and Health Claims Made on Foods

Claim	Condition
Low energy	No >40 kcal (170 kJ)/100 g or 20 kcal (80 kJ)/100 mL
Energy reduced	At least 30% reduction
Energy free	No >4 kcal (17 kJ)/100 mL
Low fat	No >3 g of fat/100 g or 1.5 g/100 mL (1.8 g for semi skimmed milk)
Fat free	No >0.5 g fat/100 g or 100 m:. 'X% fat free' prohibited
Low saturated fat	No >1.5 g/100 g or 0.75 g/10 mL. No >10% of energy
Saturated fat free	No >0.1 g/100 g or 100 mL
Low sugars	No >5 g/100 g or 2.5 g/100 mL
Sugars free	No >0.5 g/100 g or 100 mL
With no added sugars	No added mono- or di-saccharides or any other food used for its sweetening properties. If sugars naturally present, the label should include CONTAINS NATURALLY OCCURRING SUGARS
Low sodium/salt	No >0.12 g of sodium (or the equivalent value for salt)/100 g or 100 mL. Note the rules for waters differ
Very low sodium/salt	No >0.04 g of sodium (or the equivalent value for salt)/100 g or 100 mL. Note not permitted for waters
Sodium or salt free	No >0.005 g of sodium (or the equivalent value for salt)/100 g or 100 mL
Source of fibre	At least 3 g/100 g or 1.5 g/100 kcal
High fibre	At least 6 g/100 g or 3 g/100 kcal
Source of protein	At least 12% of energy
High protein	At least 20% of energy
Source of [named vitamin/s and/or mineral/s]	Significant amount (15% RDA/100 g)
High [named vitamin/s and/or mineral/s]	At least twice the value of source (30% RDA/100 g)
Contains [name of nutrient or other substance]	For vitamins and minerals same level as 'source of'. Article 5 of particular importance for claims relating to other substances and nutrients
Increased [name of nutrient]	Meets requirements for 'source of' and at least 30% more than a similar product
Reduced [name of nutrient]	At least 30% less than a similar product. For micronutrients: 10% difference in reference values. For sodium (or the equivalent value for salt) 25% difference
Light/Lite	As 'reduced'
Natural/naturally	Prefix 'natural/naturally' may be used where food naturally meets the conditions for nutrition claims
Source of n-3 fatty acids	At least 0.3 g of alpha-linolenic acid/100 g and 100 kcal or at least 40 mg of EPA and DHA/100 g and 100 kcal
High n-3 fatty acids	At least 0.6 g of alpha-linolenic acid/100 g and 100 kcal or at least 80 mg of EPA and DHA/100 g and 100 kcal
High monounsaturated fat	>20% energy. At least 45% fatty acids present derived from monounsaturated fat
High polyunsaturated	>20% energy. At least 45% fatty acids present derived from polyunsaturated fat
High unsaturated fat	>20% energy. At least 70% of fatty acids derived from unsaturated fat

See http://ec.europa.eu/nuhclaims/ for a full up to date list of nutrition claims.

SECTION 4

Table 4.5.8 Examples of authorised health claims listed in the EU Register on Nutrition and Health Claims

Claim type	Nutrient, substance, food or food category	Claim	Conditions of use of the claim
Function health claim [Article 13(1)]	Calcium	Calcium is needed for the maintenance of normal bones	The claim may be used only for food which is at least a source of calcium as referred to in the claim SOURCE OF [NAME OF VITAMIN/S] AND/OR [NAME OF MINERAL/S] as listed in the Annex to Regulation (EC) No 1924/2006
Disease risk reduction claim [Article 14(1)(a)]	Oat beta-glucan	Oat beta-glucan has been shown to lower/reduce blood cholesterol. High cholesterol is a risk factor in the development of coronary heart disease	Information shall be given to the consumer that the beneficial effect is obtained with a daily intake of 3 g of oat beta-glucan. The claim can be used for foods that provide at least 1 g of oat beta-glucan per quantified portion
Children's development and health claim [Article 14(1)(b)]	Vitamin D	Vitamin D is needed for normal growth and development of bone in children	The claim can be used only for food that is at least a source of vitamin D as referred to in the claim SOURCE OF [NAME OF VITAMIN/S] AND/OR [NAME OF MINERAL/S] as listed in the Annex to Regulation 1924/2006

See http://ec.europa.eu/nuhclaims/ for a full up to date list of authorised and non-authorised health claims.

Further reading

Thompson K. (1996) *The Law of Food and Drink*. Kent: Shaw & Sons.

Internet resources

Department of Health (DH) www.dh.gov.uk
Department for Environment Food and Rural Affairs (DEFRA) www.defra.gov.uk
European Commission (EC) Register of nutrition and health claims made on foods http://ec.europa.eu/nuhclaims/
European Food Safety Authority (EFSA) www.efsa.europa.eu
Food Standards Agency (FSA) www.food.gov.uk
Food Standards Agency Scotland www.food.gov.uk/scotland
Food Standards Agency Wales www.food.gov.uk/wales
Food Standards Agency Northern Ireland www.food.gov.uk/wales
Institute of Grocery Distribution (IGD) www.igd.com
The Stationery Office (TSO) www.tsonline.co.uk

References

Department of Health. (2011) Nutrition and health claims. Guidance to compliance with Regulation (EC) 1924/2006 on nutrition and health claims made on foods. Available at www.gov.uk. Accessed 6 August 2013.

EU Regulation (EC) 1169/2011 of the European Parliament and of the Council of 25 October 2011 on the provision of food information to consumers. O.J. L304, 22.11.11, 18-61. Available at http://ec.europa.eu/nuhclaims/. Accessed 25 October 2012.

EU Regulation (EC) 1924/2006 of the European Parliament and of the Council of 20 December 2006 on nutrition and health claims made on foods. O.J. L12, 18.1.2007, 3-18. Available at http://ec.europa.eu/nuhclaims/. Accessed 25 October 2012.

Institute of Grocery Distribution (IGD). (2006) *Best Practice Guidance on the Presentation of Guideline Daily Amounts*. Watford: IGD.

McCann D, Barrett A, Cooper A *et al*. (2007) Food additives and hyperactive behaviour in 3-year-old and 8/9-year-old children in the community: a randomised, double-blinded, placebo-controlled trial. *Lancet* 370: 1560–1567.

The Food Safety Act 1990 Chapter 16. Available at www.legislation.gov.uk. Accessed 25 October 2012.

The Food Labelling Regulations 1996 (SI 1996/1499). Available at www.legislation.gov.uk. Accessed 25 October 2012.

SECTION 5

Other topics relevant to practice

5.1 Genetics and nutritional genomics

Joanna Instone and Kevin Whelan

Key points

- Dietitians should be able to recognise modes of inheritance, gather and use multigenerational family history and communicate genetic information relevant to their area of work.

- Modes of inheritance vary for single gene conditions and chromosomal conditions, but patterns can be detected that enable traits to be detected and risk to be estimated.

- Nutritional genomics is the investigation or application of the interaction between genetics, diet and nutrition specifically in relation to the maintenance of health and prevention or treatment of disease.

- Nutrigenomics relates to how diet and nutrients affect gene expression, whereas nutrigenetics relates to how genetic variation modifies an individual's response to diet and nutrients.

- There is increasing evidence for the role for nutritional genomics in dietetic practice, especially in cardiovascular disease, including the use of low fat or low saturated fat diets in people carrying the apolipoprotein ε4 allele.

Genetic activities in clinical dietetic practice

Diet plays a role in the treatment of many conditions that have a genetic component, e.g. phenylketonuria (PKU), cystic fibrosis and familial hypercholesterolaemia. Technological advances enable better understanding of these conditions as well as the discovery of the genetic basis for an increasing number of conditions. Such advances allow the development of new therapies, including in many instances dietary manipulation. To ensure patients have access to genetic advances now and in the future, dietitians must be able to conduct a number of genetic based activities. Examples of such activities include recognising modes of inheritance in families, gathering multigenerational family history information to draw a family tree (pedigree) and communicating genetic information to individuals, families and healthcare staff (Skills for Health/NGEDC, 2007).

Recognising a mode of inheritance

Genes are short sections of deoxyribonucleic acid (DNA) that code for the production of a specific protein. DNA consists of a series of nucleotide molecules bound in a long double helical structure. Nucleotides consist of a five carbon sugar unit bound to one of four potential bases; adenine, guanine, thymine or cytosine. The order of these four nucleotide bases on the DNA is the code responsible for defining the order of amino acids during protein synthesis.

Proteins have a wide range of functions, including transport (e.g. haemoglobin), structure (e.g. actin and myosin) and metabolism (e.g. enzymes such as lipase). Genes come in pairs, which are called an allele (one from each parent), and are located on chromosomes. In a gene, both alleles can be the same (homozygous) or they can be different (heterozygous). A mutation in a gene, or pair of genes, can result in the absence or insufficient amounts of that particular protein, or synthesis of a malformed protein that does not function properly. This can cause disorders such as sickle cell disease, muscular dystrophy or cystic fibrosis, and these can be passed on to future generations via meiosis and fertilisation.

Being able to recognise the mode of inheritance of a particular mutation, and hence a condition, enables the dietitian to give dietary advice to the individual and their family appropriately, e.g. cholesterol lowering advice in familial hypercholesterolaemia, and also to explain the process should a patient ask about the genetic basis of their condition. There are several modes of inheritance and these are explained below. Table 5.1.1 summarises the different conditions that result from the different modes of inheritance, along with an example pedigree for each.

SECTION 5

Table 5.1.1 Examples of inheritable conditions with different modes of inheritance (source: reproduced with permission of the NHS National Genetics Education and Development Centre)

Type of inheritance	Example conditions	Clinical clues and features of inheritance	Probability of having a child with the condition	Example pedigree
Single gene: autosomal dominant	Familial hypercholesterolaemia (FH) Adult polycystic kidney disease Huntington's disease	Males and females are affected in equal proportions The condition is seen in multiple generations All forms of inheritance are observed, e.g. male to male, female to male, etc.	One in two where one parent is affected Autosomal Dominant Inheritance	
Single gene: autosomal recessive	Cystic fibrosis MCADD Haemochromatosis Phenylketonuria	Males and females are affected in equal proportions Affected individuals are usually in a single sibship in one generation Parents of an affected individual will both be carriers for the condition	One in four where both parents are carriers Autosomal Recessive Inheritance	
Single gene: X linked recessive	Adrenoleukodystrophy Duchenne muscular dystrophy Haemophilia	Males are affected almost exclusively The mutation is transmitted through female carriers to their sons Affected males cannot transmit the condition to their sons	One in two in males where the mother is a carrier X-linked inheritance where the mother is a carrier	

SECTION 5

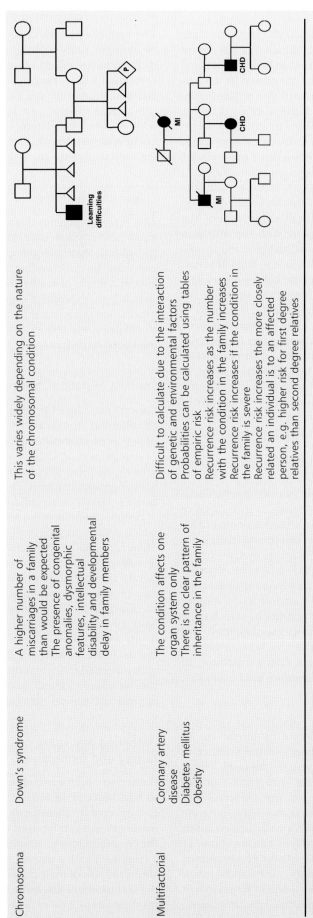

Chromosomal	Down's syndrome	A higher number of miscarriages in a family than would be expected	This varies widely depending on the nature of the chromosomal condition
		The presence of congenital anomalies, dysmorphic features, intellectual disability and developmental delay in family members	
Multifactorial	Coronary artery disease	The condition affects one organ system only	Difficult to calculate due to the interaction of genetic and environmental factors
	Diabetes mellitus	There is no clear pattern of inheritance in the family	Probabilities can be calculated using tables of empiric risk
	Obesity		Recurrence risk increases as the number with the condition in the family increases
			Recurrence risk increases if the condition in the family is severe
			Recurrence risk increases the more closely related an individual is to an affected person, e.g. higher risk for first degree relatives than second degree relatives

MCADD, medium chain acyl CoA dehydrogenase deficiency.

Single gene conditions

Single gene conditions are individually rare, but their high recurrence in affected families means that it is important for people with these conditions to be identified and supported. Single gene conditions are caused by a mutation in one particular gene or pair of genes that significantly affects the production or function of its resulting protein. The probability of children inheriting a single gene condition depends upon the mode of inheritance exhibited by the condition. There are three main modes of inheritance associated with single gene conditions.

In autosomal dominant conditions, if one gene of the pair has a mutation it is sufficient for the condition to be present. At conception, a child will either inherit the usual copy of the gene or the gene with the mutation from the affected parent, therefore having a one in two probability of inheriting the condition, e.g. familial hypercholesterolaemia and adult polycystic kidney disease.

In autosomal recessive conditions, both genes of the gene pairs need to have a mutation for the condition to occur, and therefore a mutated gene is inherited from both parents. When both parents are carriers for the condition (i.e. they each have only one gene with a mutation, so are not affected by the condition), they have a one in four probability of having a child who does not inherit a mutation from either parent, a one in two probability of having a child who is a carrier (but is not affected by the condition) and a one in four probability of having a child who has the condition, e.g. cystic fibrosis, PKU, medium chain acyl CoA dehydrogenase deficiency (MCADD) and hereditary haemochromotosis.

X linked recessive conditions are caused by gene mutations on the X chromosome. Males have one X chromosome (XY) and females have two X chromosomes (XX). Therefore, in X linked recessive conditions, males are affected almost exclusively as the gene mutation only needs to be present on their one X chromosome, whereas females are usually unaffected as they have the usual copy of the gene on their other X chromosome. For a mother who is a carrier for an X linked condition, sons have a one in two probability of inheriting the condition and daughters have a one in two chance of being a carrier. For a father who is affected by an X linked condition, all sons will be unaffected and all daughters will be carriers, e.g. adrenoleukodystrophy.

Chromosomal conditions

Chromosomal conditions are caused by alterations in gene dosage, usually due to changes in the number of copies of genes. They are caused by unusual events during meiosis that results in cells with extra chromosomes (more than two copies), too few chromosomes (fewer than two copies) or chromosomes containing the incorrect amount of DNA, e.g. Down's syndrome is caused by the presence of an extra copy of chromosome 21 [three copies in total (trisomy)]. Whilst chromosomal conditions are usually one-off events, some can be inherited and may be indicated within a family by recurrent miscarriages and clustering of individuals with learning difficulties.

Multifactorial or common complex conditions

The majority of conditions develop due to the interplay of multiple factors. Multifactorial conditions are caused by the additive effects of minor alterations in many genes combined with a range of environmental factors. Multifactorial conditions, e.g. type 2 diabetes, obesity and cardiovascular disease, are seen to cluster in families but with no obvious pattern of inheritance, partly because environmental factors (diet, exercise, smoking behaviour, etc.) also influence the risk of developing the condition.

Epigenetic conditions

The term epigenetic describes heritable influences on gene function that are not accompanied by alteration in the underlying nucleotide sequence on the DNA. Instead, exposure to environmental factors (including diet) can alter the levels of methylation of the DNA and therefore switch gene expression on or off, thus modifying protein production. Epigenetic conditions can still be passed on to offspring and influence their susceptibility to developing those disorders.

Somatic mutations (cancer)

Cancers are caused by gene mutations, but these are not all inherited. Some cancers result from the accumulation of new gene mutations in somatic cells during the lifetime of that person, leading to uncontrolled cell division and growth. As these alterations are not present in the germ cells (reproductive cells, i.e. egg and sperm), they are not usually passed on to children.

People can inherit a cancer risk gene from a parent, which is then present in all cells, including the germ cells. Therefore, this gene mutation can be inherited, resulting in a family with an inherited cancer syndrome. The gene *BRCA1* is expressed in breast tissue and produces breast cancer type 1 susceptibility protein that is involved in repairing faulty DNA. People with this mutation therefore have an impaired ability to repair faulty DNA and as a result are at greater risk of breast cancer. It is important that individuals with the *BRCA1* mutation from families with inherited cancer syndrome are identified so that they can be offered genetic testing, increased screening and appropriate clinical management.

Gathering and using multigenerational family history and family tree

Gathering a multigenerational family history can be useful to healthcare professionals, including dietitians, because it can enable identification of other affected family members and can be used to predict the probability that the condition may be passed on to offspring. Patients with a condition with a genetic component may ask dietitians about the risk of their children also developing the condition. Thus, dietitians must identify the patients in whom taking a family history is an important part of the assessment process.

It is recommended that a genetic family history is gathered and drawn in a particular way to make interpretation easier, as well as to facilitate the sharing of the resultant pedigree with other healthcare professionals. Figure 5.1.1 shows the symbols that are used to draw a pedigree. It also shows the specific order that is recommended for collecting a family history to enable drawing a pedigree, e.g. it is best to ask about and draw the history of the relatives in box 1 before those in box 2, etc. The completed three generation pedigree should be dated and signed by the healthcare professional who recorded it.

Genetic family history information is confidential; recording relevant information (conditions, cause of death, etc.) in a family is permissible without the explicit consent of all those shown on the pedigree, as long as it is necessary to do so for health purposes. Many individuals expressly state that they wish pedigree information to be available to other family members and professionals to assist diagnosis and care, and this consent should be obtained and recorded.

Communicating genetic information

Dietitians may be asked by patients and their families to explain genetic concepts and diagnoses, and must therefore have a thorough understanding of the issues surrounding the communication of information of this nature. The amount of information given at any one time needs to be tailored to the preferences and needs of the individual (Burke *et al.*, 2007). If a patient is dealing with complex emotions that can accompany a diagnosis, e.g. guilt and blame, they may not be able to actively hear, understand and process a great deal of information. The information should be non-directive and non-judgemental. It is important to be sensitive to the emotional impact of the genetic information on the person and their wider family. Simple non-emotive language is preferable, e.g. *altered gene* is preferable to *gene mutation* and *risk* should be replaced by *chance*. Patients may ask to be referred to reliable sources of genetic information, including the internet, support groups and written materials (Burke *et al.*, 2007).

Nutritional genomics

Understanding of human genetics is rapidly increasing, assisted by the use of a range of cutting edge laboratory technologies that enable rapid and accurate determination of gene sequences. This has brought greater understanding of the interaction between genetics and nutrition, and has heralded the advent of nutritional genomics as a scientific discipline.

Nutritional genomics is the investigation or application of the interaction between genetics, genomics, diet, nutrition and other environmental factors specifically in relation to the maintenance of health and prevention or treatment of disease. Some definitions of nutritional genomics are even broader and include the application of genomic technologies to the study of nutritional sciences and food technology (Brown & van der Ouderaa,

2007). In light of this, the importance of nutritional genomics to all aspects of dietetic practice, both now and in the future, is undeniable.

Broadly speaking, nutritional genomics consists of two distinct areas, nutrigenomics and nutrigenetics. Nutrigenomics relates to how diet and nutrients affect gene expression and subsequent protein translation, and therefore metabolism, physiological function and health. In contrast, nutrigenetics relates to how genetic variation within an individual modifies their response to diet and nutrients, and therefore ultimately health or disease. Taken together they can be viewed as two parallel themes that run in opposite directions, one relating to how diet influences gene expression (nutrigenomics) and the other to how genes influence the response to different diets (nutrigenetics) (Brown & van der Ouderaa, 2007).

Five tenets of nutritional genomics have been described (Kaput & Rodriguez, 2004):

1. Common dietary chemicals alter gene expression or structure (nutrigenomics).
2. In some people and in some circumstances, diet can be a serious risk factor for disease.
3. Some diet regulated genes are susceptibility genes, and are likely to play a role in chronic diseases.
4. The influence of diet on the balance between health and disease may depend upon genetic make-up (nutrigenetics).
5. Dietary intervention based on personalised nutrition can be used to prevent, mitigate or cure chronic disease.

It is in the last of these areas where the greatest potential for direct application of nutritional genomics to individual dietetic counselling will eventually be realised. In many areas, dietitians already do this by providing evidence based dietary counselling to people with genetic disorders such as PKU and MCADD. However, this advice is largely based upon a cluster of symptoms and a clinical diagnosis rather than on the patient's genetic profile *per se*. In the future it is likely that dietitians will provide targeted dietary advice for individuals with multifactorial chronic diseases, e.g. cardiovascular disease, based upon their genetic profile (Lovegrove & Gitau, 2008). This may eventually allow the transition from generic nutritional recommendations based upon population health, e.g. reducing saturated fat intake, to personalised nutrition based upon an individual's genetic profile, e.g. reducing saturated fat intake only in those with a specific genotype.

Current evidence

There is mounting evidence for the role of nutrigenetics (the influence of genetic variation on response to diet and nutrients) in cardiovascular disease. The effect of dietary fat on cardiovascular risk factors has been extensively studied in large populations. However, there is wide variation in the effectiveness of low fat/low saturated fat dietary interventions, which is often accounted for by variations in dietary compliance between individuals.

SECTION 5

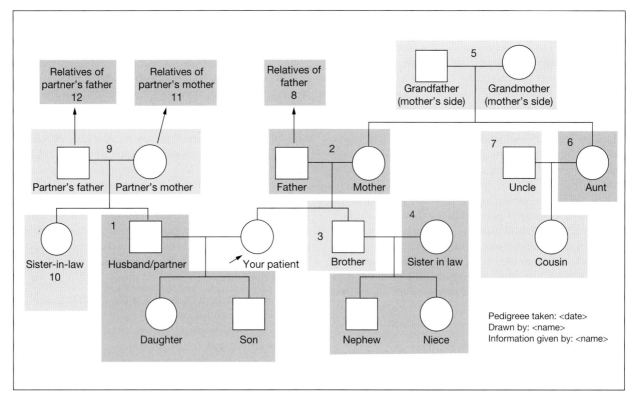

	Male	Female	Sex Unknown
Individual	□	○	◇
Affected individual (symbol coloured in)	■	●	◆
Multiple individuals	5	5	5
Deceased	▨	⊘	◈
Pregnancy	P	P	P
Miscarriage	△ male	△ female	△
Person providing pedigree information	□	○	

Marriage/partnership	□—○
Divorce/separation	□—//—○
Where the partners are blood relatives (consanguineous relationship)	□=○
Children/siblings	Sibship line → Line of descent, Individual line
Identical twins (monozygotic)	
Non-identical twins (dizygotic)	

Key Information

For each key person, record under the pedigree symbol the following information as appropriate:

- Name
- Date of birth (DOBs are preferable to current ages or estimates)
- Relevant symbols and/or diagnoses and age at diagnoses (if known)
- Cause of death and age at death (if known)

Figure 5.1.1 Stepwise approach to drawing a family pedigree (source: reproduced with permission of the NHS National Genetics Education and Development Centre)

However, genotype is a major predictor of response to a low fat/low saturated fat diet. For example, in a study of middle aged healthy people, there was a significant but weak association between total serum cholesterol and dietary intake of total fat and saturated fat. However, when comparing only those people who carried the apolipoprotein E (*apoE*) ε4 allele, there was a significant and stronger correlation between low density lipoprotein (LDL) cholesterol and saturated fat intake (Loktionov *et al.*, 2000).

ApoE is a protein that facilitates the clearance of chylomicrons and very low density lipoproteins from the bloodstream. The gene encoding apoE can have natural variations (polymorphisms) comprising three common versions (ε2, ε3, ε4). As humans carry two alleles (one from each parent), there are a number of different permutations. Therefore, humans can have one of three possible homozygous genotypes (ε2/2, ε3/3, ε4/4) or three heterozygous genotypes (ε2/3, ε2/4, ε3/4). The most common allele is ε3, followed by ε4 and ε2. A meta analysis has indicated that people with an ε2 allele, e.g. ε2/2, ε2/3, have a reduced risk of coronary heart disease, whereas people with an ε4 allele, e.g. ε4/4, ε3/4, have an increased risk of coronary heart disease (Bennet *et al.*, 2007) (Table 5.1.2).

In a controlled feeding study, a low fat/low saturated fat diet resulted in a larger fall in LDL cholesterol concentrations in males with an ε4 allele (13% decrease in ε3/4; 16% decrease in ε4/4) compared with those who were homozygous for ε3 (5% decrease in ε3/3) (Sarkkinen *et al.*, 1998). Large randomised controlled trials are required before widespread application of this evidence in dietetic practice. However, these data highlight the possibility that patients with hyperlipidaemia might one day be screened for carriage of the ε4 allele on their *apoE* gene, in order that they might be targeted with intensive dietary counselling as they may well show the best response in terms of lowering LDL cholesterol.

Another area for the application of nutrigenetics in cardiovascular disease is in relation to the gene coding for the enzyme methylene tetrahydrofolate reductase (MTHFR). The enzyme is involved in folate metabolism, and therefore regulates plasma concentrations of homocysteine, which at high levels are a risk factor for cardiovascular disease. A common polymorphism can occur to one specific nucleotide base of the *MTHFR* gene [hence it is called a single nucleotide polymorphism (SNP)]. This SNP occurs at nucleotide position 677 and involves a cytosine (C) base being replaced by a thymine (T) base; hence it is described as MTHFR 677C>T. Most people have both usual alleles (CC), some have one affected allele (CT) and some have both affected alleles (TT).

This small change in nucleotide sequence still allows the MTHFR enzyme to be produced, but the SNP results in an amino acid change and thus the enzyme activity is lower. People with this SNP have less efficient folate metabolism and an approximately 20% higher plasma homocysteine concentration than those who do not (Jacques *et al.*, 1996). This may explain why people who are homozygous for this SNP (TT) have a 16% higher chance of developing coronary heart disease compared with people who are homozygous wild type (CC) (Klerk *et al.*, 2002).

Dietary intervention with folate supplementation reduces homocysteine concentrations, particularly in those with the *MTHFR* TT genotype. For example, a randomised controlled trial showed that folate supplements (1 mg/day) decreased homocysteine in healthy males, but the greatest decrease was seen in those with the homozygous TT genotype (−6.6 µmol/L) compared to those with the CT or CC genotype (both −2.6 µmol/L) (Miyaki *et al.*, 2005). Nutrigenetic testing for the MTHFR C677T (TT) polymorphism might enable targeted folate supplementation in those most likely to respond. However, a recent meta analysis indicated that although folate supplementation resulted in a 25% reduction in homocysteine concentrations, this did not have an effect on cardiovascular events, cancer or 5-year mortality (Clarke *et al.*, 2010), raising the possibility that elevated plasma homocysteine is a marker of risk rather than a risk itself.

Barriers to nutritional genomics in practice

In the future nutritional genomics is likely to have a major impact on dietetic practice, offering the potential for targeted dietary interventions based upon an understanding of an individual's genotype (personalised nutrition). However, research to support its application is currently in its infancy, and larger scale trials to demonstrate nutritional, metabolic and clinical benefits are required.

A further concern is the focus of research on the evaluation of dietary interventions on single genes. Using cardiovascular disease as an example, many different genes result in elevated susceptibility (it is a polygenic disease) and there are many environmental risk factors as well, such as diet, smoking and physical activity. Therefore, any single nutrigenetic effect, e.g. reducing saturated fat in *apoE* ε4 carriers, in isolation is likely to be small in comparison with those of the many complex gene environment interactions that subsequently result in cardiovascular disease.

Table 5.1.2 Association between *apoE* polymorphisms, coronary risk and diet

Allele	Allele frequency (Masson *et al.*, 2003)	Coronary risk* odds ratio (95% CI)	Impact of low fat diet on LDL cholesterol (Sarkkinen *et al.*, 1998)
ε2	0.08	0.80 (0.70–0.90)	Not measured
ε3	0.77	1.00	5% reduction
ε4	0.15	1.06 (0.99–1.13)	13–16% reduction

*Compared with ε3/ε3 (Bennet *et al.*, 2007).
LDL, low density lipoprotein.

SECTION 5

The potential for ethical, legal and social issues associated with research and practice in genetics and nutritional genomics is emerging. These include how genetic information is analysed, stored and used, particularly in relation to confidentiality, and the avoidance of *genetic discrimination* by those interested in an individual's risk of disease, e.g. health insurers and employers (Reilly & Debusk, 2008).

Finally, studies have shown that dietitians have positive attitudes towards genetics and nutritional genomics, but many have limited knowledge and confidence to enable them to be involved (Whelan *et al*., 2008). Although there is currently limited evidence to support nutritional genomic interventions, clearly dietitians must be competent and skilled to be able to act upon new research evidence as and when it is published.

Further reading

DeBusk RM, Fogarty CP, Ordovas JM, Kornman KS. (2005) Nutritional genomics in practice: where do we begin? *Journal of the American Dietetic Association* 105: 589–598.

Stover PJ, Caudill MA. (2008) Genetic and epigenetic contributions to human nutrition and health: managing genome–diet interactions. *Journal of the American Dietetic Association* 108: 1480–1487.

Internet resources

National Coalition for Heath Professional Education in Genetics – Genetics and nutrition   www.nchpeg.org/nutrition

   National Genetics Education and Development Centre www .geneticseducation.nhs.uk/index.aspx

      Resources for dietitians www.geneticseducation.nhs.uk/ teaching-genetics/dietitians.aspx

Nutrigenomics Organisation (NuGO)   www.nugo.org/everyone

References

Bennet AM, Di Angelantonio E, Ye Z, *et al*. (2007) Association of apolipoprotein E genotypes with lipid levels and coronary risk. *JAMA* 298: 1300–1311.

Brown L, van der Ouderaa F. (2007) Nutritional genomics: food industry applications from farm to fork. *British Journal of Nutrition* 97: 1027–1035.

Burke S, Bennett C, Bedward J, Farndon F. (2007) *The Experiences and Preferences of People Receiving Genetic Information from Healthcare Professionals*. Birmingham: National Genetics Education and Development Centre.

Clarke R, Halsey J, Lewington S, *et al*., B-Vitamin Treatment Trialists' Collaboration. (2010) Effects of lowering homocysteine levels with B vitamins on cardiovascular disease, cancer, and cause-specific mortality: Meta-analysis of 8 randomized trials involving 37485 individuals. *Archives of Internal Medicine* 170: 1622–1631.

Jacques PF, Bostom AG, Williams RR, *et al*. (1996) Relation between folate status, a common mutation in methylene tetrahydrofolate reductase, and plasma homocysteine concentrations. *Circulation* 93: 7–9.

Kaput J, Rodriguez RL. (2004) Nutritional genomics: the next frontier in the postgenomic era. *Physiological Genomics* 16: 166–177.

Klerk M, Verhoef P, Clarke R, Blom HJ, Kok FJ, Schouten EG; MTHFR Studies Collaboration Group. (2002) MTHFR 677C-->T polymorphism and risk of coronary heart disease: a meta-analysis. *JAMA* 288: 2023–31.

Loktionov A, Scollen S, McKeown N, Bingham SA. (2000) Gene-nutrient interactions: dietary behaviour associated with high coronary heart disease risk particularly affects serum LDL cholesterol in apolipoprotein E epsilon4-carrying free-living individuals. *British Journal of Nutrition* 84: 885–890.

Lovegrove JA, Gitau R. (2008) Personalized nutrition for the prevention of cardiovascular disease: a future perspective. *Journal of Human Nutrition and Dietetics* 21: 306–316.

Masson LF, McNeill G, Avenell A. (2003) Genetic variation and the lipid response to dietary intervention: a systematic review. *American Journal of Clinical Nutrition* 77: 1098–1111.

Miyaki K, Murata M, Kikuchi H, *et al*. (2005) Assessment of tailor-made prevention of atherosclerosis with folic acid supplementation: randomized, double-blind, placebo-controlled trials in each MTHFR C677T genotype. *Journal of Human Genetics* 50: 241–248.

Reilly PR, Debusk RM (2008) Ethical and legal issues in nutritional genomics. *Journal of the American Dietetic Association* 108: 36–40.

Sarkkinen E, Korhonen M, Erkkilä A, Ebeling T, Uusitupa M. (1998) Effect of apolipoprotein E polymorphism on serum lipid response to the separate modification of dietary fat and dietary cholesterol. *American Journal of Clinical Nutrition* 68: 1215–1222.

Skills for Health/NGEDC. (2007) Enhancing patient care by integrating genetics in clinical practice UK workforce competences for genetics in clinical practice for non-genetics healthcare staff. Birmingham: National Genetics Education and Development Centre.

Whelan K, McCarthy S, Pufulete M. (2008) Genetics and diet–gene interactions: involvement, confidence and knowledge of dietitians. *British Journal of Nutrition* 99: 23–28.

5.2

Functional foods

Lisa Ryan

Key points

- Functional foods, when consumed regularly as part of the usual diet, have a specific health beneficial effect beyond their basic nutritional value.

- The beneficial health effects are due to the presence of a variety of bioactive components that elicit their effects via a number of different mechanisms.

- Functional foods encompass a very broad range of products, including infant formulas, medical foods, performance foods, probiotics and foods designed to deliver specialised nutrients and non-nutrients.

- The proposed health effects of functional foods must be substantiated.

- In Europe, the assessment of the scientific evidence to support health claims is the responsibility of the European Food Safety Authority (EFSA).

Food has an important role in major chronic diseases such as cardiovascular disease, diabetes, hypertension, some cancers and obesity. Previously, attention has focused on the harmful effects of major food components, e.g. excess saturated fat, or under consumption, e.g. of fibre, vegetables and fruit. Today, certain foods and food ingredients are being studied for their role in preventing and treating various chronic diseases, and for their far reaching benefits in slowing the ageing process and affecting mood and performance. These foods, known as functional foods, have the potential to promote better health and wellbeing, therefore helping to reduce the risk of chronic disease and to improve specific health functions.

History and development

The concept of functional foods first emerged in Japan as a results of escalating healthcare costs. In 1986, the Ministry of Education, Science, and Culture reported that food has three main functions in the body; nutritive value (primary function); sensory appeal (organoleptic properties) and physiological aspects (including regulation of body functions and physical conditions, preventing disease, promoting recovery and general good health). The concept of functional foods grew out of the third function and the Japanese government promoted the idea of functional foods as a possible way of improving the health of their ageing population. In 1991, the Japanese renamed functional foods as foods for specified health use (FOSHU) and defined them as *'processed foods containing ingredients that aid specific bodily functions in addition to being nutritious'*. A regulatory system was established to approve such foods and to evaluate the scientific justification of claims. In Japan, FOSHU foods bear a seal of approval from the Ministry of Health and Welfare, making them easily recognisable to the consumer (Arai, 1996). The area of functional foods is expanding and now represents one of the most dynamic growth categories to have emerged from food science and nutrition.

Definition

In contrast to Japan, no legal definitions are available in either the USA or Europe for functional foods; however, they may be broadly defined as *'foods similar in appearance to conventional foods that are consumed as part of a normal diet and have demonstrated physiological benefits and/or reduce the risk of chronic disease beyond basic nutritional functions'* (Clydesdale, 1997). A functional food may be:

- A natural food.
- A food to which a component has been added.
- A food from which a component has been removed.

Manual of Dietetic Practice, Fifth Edition. Edited by Joan Gandy.
© 2014 The British Dietetic Association. Published 2014 by John Wiley & Sons, Ltd.
Companion Website: www.manualofdieteticpractice.com

- A food where one or more components have been modified.
- A food in which the bioavailability has been modified.
- Any combination of the above.

Functional foods may be classified according to the type of food (Table 5.2.1) or according to the type of bioactive ingredient used (Table 5.2.2).

Ingredients

A food is said to be functional if it contains a food component (whether a nutrient or non-nutrient) that affects one or more targeted functions in the body in a positive way. They are similar in appearance, smell and taste to a conventional food and are consumed as part of the usual diet. Functional foods represent an increasingly diverse collection of foods, e.g. infant formulas, medical foods, performance foods, probiotics and foods designed to deliver specialised nutrients and components (such as fibre, vitamins, minerals, antioxidants, prebiotics, dairy proteins, soya proteins, fats and oils). The beneficial health effects are due to the presence of a variety of bioactive components that elicit their effects via a number of different mechanisms. These substances (bioactives) often originate from plant sources, but some are derived from animals and microorganisms (Table 5.2.2).

Examples

Dairy spreads enriched with plant sterols and stanols

Plant sterols are naturally occurring components of plant wall membranes. Over 40 plant sterols have been identified; the three most abundant plant sterols are beta-sitosterol, campesterol and stigmasterol. Stanols are saturated derivatives of sterols and are less abundant in nature than sterols. The term phytosterols is sometimes used as a generic term to encompass both plant sterols and stanols. In the 1950s, it was recognised that phytosterols lower serum concentrations of cholesterol (Best *et al.*, 1954). Phytosterols reduce the absorption of

Table 5.2.1 Categories of functional foods (source: Arvanitoyannis & Van Houwelingen-Koukaliaroglou 2005. Reproduced with permission of Taylor & Francis)

Category	Example
Basic foods	Tomatoes (rich in natural antioxidant lycopene)
Processed foods	Oat bran cereal
Processed food with added ingredients	Calcium enriched fruit juice
Foods enhanced to have functional component	Oat bran with higher levels of beta-glucan
Isolated, purified preparations of active food ingredients	Soya isoflavones

Table 5.2.2 Examples of bioactive functional food ingredients

Functional ingredient	Food source	Potential effect on health
Beta-glucan	Oats	Lowers blood cholesterol Reduces the postprandial glycaemic response Aids weight control
Conjugated linoleic acid (CLA)	Cheese, meat products	Improves body fat composition Enhances immune system Reduces risk of cancer
Flavonoids, e.g. catechins	Tea, fruit, vegetables	Neutralise free radicals Reduce risk of cancer
Lycopene (carotenoid)	Tomatoes	Reduces risk of prostate cancer
n-3 Fatty acids (ALA/EPA/DHA)	Salmon and fish oils	Reduce risk of cardiovascular disease May improve mental and visual functions
Phytoestrogens, e.g. isoflavones	Soyabeans and soya based foods	Alleviate symptoms associated with the menopause Protect against heart disease and some cancers Lower LDL and total cholesterol Improve bone mineral density
Plant sterols/stanols/stanol esters	Corn, soya, wheat, wood oils	Reduce the absorption of cholesterol in the body Lower blood cholesterol levels (total and LDL cholesterol by ~10%) NB: May interfere with absorption of other fat soluble components from the diet; data on effects of long term consumption at levels >3 g/day are limited
Prebiotics, e.g. inulin, fructo-oligosaccharides	Jerusalem artichokes, shallots, onion powder	Stimulate the growth of certain bacteria in the colon Improve quality of intestinal microflora; gastrointestinal health
Probiotics, e.g. *Lactobacillus acidophilus*	Yoghurt and other dairy products	Improve quality of intestinal microflora; gastrointestinal health

LDL, low density lipoprotein.

cholesterol by competing for incorporation into mixed micelles (and thus inhibiting cholesterol absorption). Therefore, when phytosterols are part of the regular diet, they have an overall lowering effect on serum cholesterol concentrations. The average daily diet contains approximately 0.25 g of plant sterols, though this may be twice as high in a vegetarian diet. Phytosterols at doses of approximately 2 g/day are required to lower low density lipoprotein (LDL) cholesterol. Dairy spreads fortified with phytosterols (~2 g/daily portion) have been developed as functional foods. The added phytosterols in fortified dairy spreads have been shown to reduce the absorption of cholesterol in the gut (both dietary and endogenous) and to lower blood LDL cholesterol by ~7–10.5% (EFSA, 2009).

Omega-3 enriched eggs and bread

Omega (n)-3 fatty acids are polyunsaturated fatty acids, and longer chain derivatives such as eicosapentaenoic acid (EPA) and docosahexaenoic acid (DHA) seem to be consistently associated with health benefits. Plants typically contain the parent n-3 fatty acid, alpha-linolenic acid (ALA), which is essential in humans. Although the longer chain n-3 derivatives can be formed from ALA, research suggests that this is an inefficient process. Furthermore, n-6 fatty acids compete with n-3 fatty acids for metabolising enzymes. Therefore, an excess of n-6 fatty acids in the diet, as is typical of many western diets, will favour the production of longer chain n-6 family derivatives. The main dietary source of eicosapentaenoic acid (EPA) and docosahexaenoic acid (DHA) is oily rich fish. Functional foods containing EPA and DHA, such as enriched eggs and bread, have now been developed as a means of delivering longer chain n-3 fatty acids into the diet.

Oat breakfast cereal rich in beta-glucan

The health importance of dietary fibre has been recognised for decades. However, recently soluble fibres such as beta-glucans have been shown to exert a beneficial effect on health. Beta-glucans are the predominant components of cell walls of cereal grains such as barley and oats. Oat breakfast cereals enriched with oat beta-glucan at doses of at least 3 g/day have shown a statistically significant decrease in LDL cholesterol concentrations (EFSA, 2010). The effect of beta-glucans on other factors and conditions such as the glycaemic response, weight control and certain cancers is also currently under investigation.

Regulation

The effects of functional foods on health must be scientifically proven before claims can be made for a food (see Chapter 4.5). In Europe, the assessment of the scientific evidence to support health claims is the responsibility of the European Food Safety Authority (EFSA). When assessing the evidence, the EFSA considers the extent to which:

- The food/constituent is defined and characterised.
- The claimed effect is defined and is a beneficial physiological effect.
- A cause–effect relationship is established between the consumption of the food/constituent and the claimed effect (for the target group under the proposed conditions of use).

Scientific substantiation requires a favourable outcome to all three statements. If a cause–effect relationship is to be established, the EFSA considers whether:

- The quantity of food and pattern of consumption required to obtain the claimed effect can be consumed within a balanced diet.
- The proposed wording reflects the scientific evidence.
- The proposed wording complies with the criteria for the use of claims specified in the regulation.
- The proposed conditions of use are appropriate.
- Substantiation was dependent on data claimed as proprietary by the applicant.

The process of assessment of claims is continuous and to date positive EFSA opinions on claims have included plant sterols and stanols and cholesterol reduction; xylitol and caries reduction; ALA and brain and nerve tissue development in children; oat beta-glucans and cholesterol reduction, and long chain polyunsaturated fatty acids and visual development in children (Table 5.2.3).

The future

Functional foods constitute a rapidly growing area of product development and research, as well as requiring considerable regulatory efforts. To date, relatively few bioactive ingredients have been substantiated and demonstrated to have a proven beneficial effect on health. Central to the substantiation of functional foods are data from human dietary studies.

An important aspect will also be for functional food manufacturers to communicate health effects reliably to the final consumer. In Europe, the term functional foods is not recognised by the consumer; therefore, approved products may benefit from a specific logo on the label

SECTION 5

Table 5.2.3 Examples of positive health claim evaluations from the European Food Safety Authority

Functional food/ingredient	Health effect
Vitamins, minerals	Cardiovascular, brain, gut, immune, bone, dental, antioxidant, metabolism
Protein, carbohydrate	Muscle, bone, energy
Fatty acids	Brain, cardiovascular, vision
Fibre	Gut, cardiovascular
Other substances – phytosterols/stanols, tomato extract, chewing gum	Cardiovascular, dental

LDL, low density lipoprotein.

identifying them as functional foods. If these products are to be consumed as part of the normal diet, they need to be much more visible and recognisable.

The National Diet and Nutrition Survey (NDNS) (Bates *et al.*, 2011) suggested that while there have been some improvements in the UK diet, there are still certain areas where recommendations are not being met, e.g. dietary fibre and n-3 fatty acids. Functional foods have the potential to improve the health of the population and to address some of the issues identified by the NDNS.

Internet resources

European Food Safety Authority   www.efsa.europa.eu

References

Arai S. (1996) Studies of functional foods in Japan – state-of-the-art. *Bioscience, Biotechnology and Biochemistry* 60: 9–15.

Arvanitoyannis IS, Van Houwelingen-Koukaliaroglou M. (2005) Functional foods: A survey of health claims, pros and cons, and current legislation. *Critical Reviews in Food Science and Nutrition* 45: 385–404.

Bates B, Lennox A, Bates C, Swan G. (2011) *The National Diet and Nutrition Survey: Headline Results from Year 1 and 2 (Combined) of the Rolling Programme (2008/2009 – 2009/10)*. London: Food Standards Agency.

Best MM, Duncan CH, Van Loon EJ, Wathen JD. (1954) Lowering of serum cholesterol by the administration of a plant sterol. *Circulation* 10: 201–206.

Clydesdale FM. (1997). A proposal for the establishment of scientific criteria for health claims for functional foods. *Nutrition Reviews* 55: 413–422.

European Food Safety Authority. (2009) Scientific opinion on plant sterols and plant stanols on blood LDL-cholesterol. *EFSA Journal* 7: 1175 1–9.

European Food Safety Authority. (2010) Scientific opinion on the substantiation of a health claim related to oat beta-glucan and lowering blood cholesterol and reduced risk of (coronary) heart disease pursuant to Article 14 of Regulation (EC) No 1924/2006. *EFSA Journal* 8(12): 1885, 1–15.

5.3 Drug–nutrient interactions

Joan Gandy

Key points

- Nutrition can affect the therapeutic action of many drugs by influences on drug absorption, metabolism and excretion.

- The action and/or side effects of drugs may result in marked changes in food intake. Drugs can also impair nutrient absorption or metabolism, or increase nutrient excretion.

- Prolonged therapeutic drug use may have adverse effects on nutritional status, especially in older people.

- Information about therapeutic drug use, including over the counter medicines, herbs, alcohol consumption and tobacco use, should be obtained during a nutritional assessment.

There are many interactions between drugs and both macro- and micro-nutrients. Drugs and nutrients are absorbed from similar sites and metabolised and excreted in similar ways. Therefore, just as a drug can interfere with the action of another, some drugs may interfere with the action of a nutrient or *vice versa*. It is essential that dietitians have knowledge of these interactions and alert medical personnel to possible problems they may not be aware of. Boullata & Hudson (2012) recently reviewed the implications for dietetic practice of drug–nutrient interactions.

Prescribed drugs are likely to have the greatest nutritional implications since they are the most powerful or high dose forms of medication. However, it is important to consider that people often self administer other types of preparations with pharmacological effects and nutritional implications. These include:

- Over the counter drugs, e.g. analgesics, indigestion remedies, laxatives.
- Herbal remedies, including Chinese herbal remedies (see Chapter 5.4).
- Nutritional supplements, e.g. fish oil capsules, large doses of vitamins.
- Alcohol.
- Tobacco.
- Illegal substances.

Drug abuse can cause many nutritional problems, both directly from the effects of the drug itself and indirectly from the poor dietary habits and living conditions often associated with it.

Drug–nutrient interactions can be broadly categorised into:

- *Effect of nutrition on drugs* – the influence of nutritional factors on drug absorption, action and effectiveness.
- *Effect of drugs on nutrition* – the influence of drugs on nutritional intake, metabolism, excretion and requirements.

Classes of drugs that are most likely to have nutritional implications are shown in Table 5.3.1. Many drugs used in the treatment of mental illness have drug–nutrient interactions and these are summarised in detail in Table 7.10.6. Cytotoxic chemotherapy drugs are also known to have effects on nutritional status and these are discussed further in Chapter 7.15. This chapter gives an overview of the subject with examples; it is not definitive and the titles listed in the resources section of this chapter should be consulted for further detail.

Effects of nutrition on drugs

The metabolism of a drug may involve the following stages, any of which can be influenced by nutrition:

- Transport from the gut lumen to intestinal enterocytes (if the drug is taken orally), sometimes followed by presystemic metabolism prior to absorption into the blood.
- Transport in the blood, usually bound to plasma proteins.

SECTION 5

Table 5.3.1 Classes of drugs that are most likely to have nutritional implications

Class of drug	Possible nutritional implications
Amphetamines	Increased appetite
Antacids	Can bind with minerals such as phosphorus, magnesium, iron and zinc, and reduce their absorption Antacids raise gastric pH and this may also impair the absorption of some trace elements, especially vitamin B_{12}, which requires acid conditions for its release from dietary protein
Antibiotics	Anorexia Altered gut flora and diarrhoea Tetracycline forms complexes with calcium (in foods or mineral supplements), reducing the absorption of both
Anticoagulants	Warfarin action is impaired by vitamin K
Anticonvulsants	Interfere with folate metabolism Interfere with vitamin D metabolism
Antidepressants	Anorexia MAOI type A usage necessitates avoidance of tyramine*
Antihyperlipidaemics	Clofibrate and cholestyramine can result in malabsorption, especially of minerals and fat soluble vitamins
Antipsychotics	Some types markedly increase appetite*
Antirheumatics	Methotrexate inhibits folate metabolism Penicillamine reduces absorption of iron and zinc
Corticosteroids	Anabolic effects and weight gain Glucose intolerance
Cytotoxic (anticancer) drugs	Anorexia Taste changes Sore and painful mouth and tongue Nausea, vomiting and diarrhoea Damage to intestinal villi Interfere with folate metabolism (especially methotrexate) Reduce thiamine status
Dopaminergic drugs (used in parkinsonism)	Levodopa causes nausea and vomiting if taken on an empty stomach Levodopa absorption is inhibited by iron supplements Levodopa can be inhibited by B_6 supplements
Diuretics	Thiazide and loop diuretics can cause excessive urinary loss of potassium, calcium, zinc and water soluble vitamins Dehydration
Hypoglycaemics	Action has to be balanced against carbohydrate intake Alcohol can potentiate their action Chlorpropamide can react with alcohol and cause facial flushing
Laxatives	Reduced absorption of nutrients (liquid paraffin)
Mood stabilisers	Lithium action is affected by dietary sodium*
Non-steroidal anti-inflammatory drugs (NSAIDs)	Gastric irritation and risk of bleeding if taken on an empty stomach Aspirin increases vitamin C excretion
Oral contraceptives	Affect glucose and lipid metabolism Can cause weight gain

*See Chapter 7.10.3.
MAOI,– monoamine oxidase inhibitors.

- Deactivation by a two stage metabolic process:
  - Oxidation by microsomal enzyme systems involving reduced nicotinamide adenine dinucleotide (NADPH) and cytochrome P450, predominantly in the liver but also in other organs including the lungs and small intestine.
  - Conjugation with glucuronic acid, sulphate or glycine.
- Excretion of the conjugate in urine or bile.

Table 5.3.2 gives examples of drug–nutrient interactions that affect drug absorption, metabolism or excre-

tion. NB: This list is not exhaustive; *Stockley's Drug Interactions* or the *British National Formulary* should be consulted for further information.

Drug absorption

The pharmacological effect of an orally administered drug depends on the rate and extent to which it is absorbed from the gastrointestinal tract. This can be either delayed or enhanced by the presence or absence of food. The pres-

Table 5.3.2 Examples of drug–nutrient interactions affecting absorption, metabolism and excretion of drugs (adapted from Webster-Gandy *et al.*, 2011, tables 38.1–38.3, pp. 738–40. Reproduced with permission of Oxford University Press)

Drug or class of drug*	Food and/or nutrient	Effect of interaction and advice
Absorption		
Bismuth Flucloxacillin Phenoxymethylpenicillin Rifampicin	Presence of food in the stomach	Absorption delayed and reduced Advise to take on an empty stomach or 1 hour before food
Ciprofloxacin Norfloxacin Tetracyclines	Milk and dairy products	Absorption reduced Advise to leave 2-hour gap between drug and dairy consumption
Theophylline	High protein diet High carbohydrate diet	Bioavailability reduced by high protein diets Bioavailability increased by high carbohydrate diets
Ciprofloxacin Digoxin Phenytoin Rifampicin Tetracycline Theophylline	Enteral feeds	Absorption reduced Leave time gap between giving medication and enteral feed
Metabolism		
Amiodarone Buspirone Calcium channel blockers Carbamazepine Ciclosporin Colchicine Corticosteroids Coumarins Digoxin Fexofenadine Simvastatin	Grapefruit juice	Metabolism of drug altered due to liver enzyme, cytochrome P450, stimulation Advise to follow manufacturer's instructions
Warfarin	Large amounts of Brussel sprouts, green vegetables, cabbage, lettuce, green tea, excess quantities of ice cream, avocado, mango	Drug metabolism increased and anticoagulant effect of warfarin decreased
	Cranberry juice	Anticoagulant effect of warfarin increased NB: A fatal incident reported
	High doses of vitamin E	Anticoagulant effect of warfarin increased
Levodopa Phenobarbital, phenytoin	Vitamin B_6 (pyridoxine)	Effects of levodopa reduced by concurrent supplementation of pyridoxine Advise to avoid vitamin B_6
Excretion		
Lithium	Salt (sodium)	Excretion affected by increased and decreased salt intake Advise to keep sodium intake constant once stabilised on lithium

*This list is not exhaustive. *Stockley's Drug Interactions* or *British National Formulary* should be consulted for further details.

ence of food in the stomach and proximal intestine may reduce drug absorption as a result of the following:

- Delayed gastric emptying.
- Altered gastrointestinal pH.
- Competition for binding sites with nutrients.
- Chelation of drugs by food cations, e.g. tetracyclines chelate with calcium ions present in milk and dairy products, resulting in reduced absorption of both calcium and antibiotic.

- Dietary fats impeding the absorption of hydrophilic drugs.

Some drugs must therefore be taken on an empty stomach in order to maximise their rate of absorption and therapeutic effect. Conversely, others must be taken with food to achieve a slower, more sustained rate of absorption or to minimise side effects such as gastric irritation, e.g. aspirin and other non-steroidal anti-inflammatory drugs (NSAIDs). Medicines should be taken with water as drinks such as fruit juice, tea and coffee can alter the drug's pH balance and therefore its properties.

Drug transport

Many drugs are transported in blood bound to plasma proteins. Severe malnutrition, or diseases such as liver disease affecting the synthesis of plasma proteins, may reduce the body's ability to transport drugs and hence impair their effectiveness.

Drug metabolism

Factors that affect the deactivation or conjugation of a drug can alter its pharmacological or toxic effects. Periods of short term starvation or prolonged periods of nutritional inadequacy can influence the effectiveness or safety of drugs. The amount of a drug required to produce a certain pharmacological effect is determined by body weight. Sudden reduction in weight or dehydration may therefore result in over dosage. Undernutrition also reduces the activity of microsomal drug metabolising enzymes and this can either diminish a drug's effectiveness (by reducing the rate of synthesis of an active metabolite) or enhance its toxicity (by reducing the rate of its excretion) (Dickerson, 1988). In addition, the metabolism of drugs is affected by the amount of water in the body and this can be perturbed by dehydration or oedema, including that associated with kwashiorkor (protein energy malnutrition) (Oshikoya & Senbanjo, 2009). Some drugs are fat soluble, e.g. barbituates; therefore, their metabolism will be affected by both decreased and increased levels of adipose tissue associated fat. The effects of obesity on drug metabolism vary depending on the pathway by which they are metabolised (Brill *et al.*, 2012). Obviously, decreased or increased clearance rates may lead to potentially impaired drug action or increased possibility of side effects. Doses may need to be adjusted as some are based on ideal body weight rather than actual body weight, e.g. anaesthesia.

It is important to consider that drug–nutrient interactions may be variable, with some individuals being more susceptible than others. An example of this is the interaction between grapefruit juice and simvastatin that results in increased levels of the circulating drug, which has the potential to increase side effects. However, there is debate as to whether or not this potential effect outweighs the potential beneficial effect of simvastatin on cholesterol levels (Pirmohamed, 2013; Backman & Bakhai, 2013).

Drug excretion

Urinary acidity affects drug reabsorption from the renal tubules. Supplemental intakes of nutrients that increase urinary acidity, e.g. large amounts of vitamin C, can decrease the excretion of salicylate drugs such as aspirin.

Potentially serious interactions

The following interactions have the potential to lead to serious events:

- Warfarin and vitamin K containing foods.
- Warfarin and cranberry juice.
- Grapefruit juice and fexofenadine or ciclosporin.
- Angiotensin converting enzyme (ACE) inhibitors or angiotensin II receptor antagonists and potassium supplements or salt substitutes – these drugs may cause potassium retention, which may be exacerbated by potassium supplements and potassium containing salt substitutes, resulting in hyperkalaemia.
- Monoamine oxidase inhibitors (MAOIs) and tyramine – patients taking a MAOI, e.g. phenelzine and moclobemide, should avoid tyramine containing foods, e.g. mature cheese, yeast extracts, soyabean products, pickled herring, red wine, as these may cause a dramatic increase in blood pressure and palpitations.
- Isotretinoin and vitamin A – isotretinoin is a retinoid used for the treatment of acne. Due to the risk of vitamin A toxicity it should not be used with vitamin A supplements.

Effects of drugs on nutrition

Drugs may affect food intake or the absorption, metabolism or excretion of nutrients. This may have implications in terms of food choice and/or nutritional requirements.

Food intake

Food intake may be reduced as a result of drugs that have the following effects:

- Anorexia – either as a direct effect of the drug on appetite, e.g. cytotoxic chemotherapy drugs, or as a result of side effects such as drowsiness or lethargy, e.g. tranquillisers.
- Cause nausea and vomiting – this is a common side effect of many drugs.
- Gastrointestinal tract effects – e.g. NSAIDs often cause gastric irritation and should be taken with, or after, food. Other drugs may cause bloating or early satiety. Chronic abdominal pain or diarrhoea may reduce the desire to eat.
- Taste changes – many drugs, e.g. cytotoxic chemotherapy, make food taste bland (ageusia) or change taste perception (dysgeusia). Many patients receiving some cytotoxic drugs report a metallic taste, often associated with protein consumption.
- Dry mouth (xerostomia) – lack of saliva makes it difficult to masticate and swallow food, especially those of a dry or fibrous consistency.
- Sore or painful mouth (mucositis) or tongue (glossitis) – a common side effect of chemotherapy that can significantly impair food intake.
- Impaired memory or confusion – people may forget to eat.

Drugs may also increase food intake and weight gain if they stimulate appetite or induce cravings. Corticosteroids, insulin and some psychotropic drugs are known to have either or both these effects (see Chapter 7.10.3).

Nutrient absorption

Absorption can be impaired as a result of:

- *Formation of insoluble complexes* – many drugs can chelate with minerals and trace elements, e.g. penicillamine (sometimes used in the treatment of rheumatoid arthritis) chelates zinc; cholestyramine binds with iron; and antacids may bind with phosphorus.
- *Competition for binding sites*, e.g. salicylates (aspirin) compete with vitamin C; and sulphasalazine, used in the treatment of arthritis, impairs folate absorption.
- *Damage to the absorptive surface of the intestinal mucosa* – cytotoxic chemotherapy can cause villous atrophy, resulting in malabsorption.
- *Binding of bile acids* – fat soluble vitamin absorption will be impaired by bile salt binding drugs such as cholestyramine.
- *Lipase inhibitors* that reduce fat absorption and are used to aid weight loss, e.g. orlistat, may impair absorption of fat soluble vitamins.
- *Increased intestinal motility* – drugs that cause diarrhoea or stimulate peristaltic activity, e.g. senna or phenolphthalein laxatives, may result in nutrient losses.

Nutrient metabolism

Some drugs may affect lipid or glucose metabolism. The following drugs may result in dyslipidaemia:

- Beta blockers.
- Corticosteroids.
- Thiazide diuretics.
- Anabolic steroids.
- Some anti-HIV drugs.
- Retinoids.
- Combined oral contraceptives.

Drugs that may affect glucose tolerance, apart from those used to manage diabetes, include thiazide diuretics and corticosteroids.

Micronutrient metabolism

Micronutrients are cofactors and coenzymes in many metabolic pathways, including those that metabolise drugs. Increased activity of these pathways as a result of drug metabolism may increase micronutrient requirements. Drugs can also compete with, or inhibit, the metabolic conversion of some micronutrients to their active metabolites, particularly folate. Some medicines may require nutritional supplements to prevent detrimental effects. These include:

- *Corticosteroids* – long term oral use or high inhaled doses is a risk factor for osteoporosis; therefore, calcium supplements are needed.
- *Methotrexate* – a folate antagonist, so a folate supplement (5 mg/day) is needed to prevent deficiency. It is used in rheumatoid arthritis and in cancer chemotherapy.
- *Isoniazid* – an antibiotic used in the treatment of tuberculosis and may have an antipyridoxine effect; a 10 mg/day supplement of pyridoxine is recommended.

- *Antiepileptic drugs in pregnancy* – many are associated with birth defects; 5 mg/day of folate should be prescribed as women with epilepsy are more likely to have low folate levels.
- *Some cytotoxic antibiotics, imidazole, antifungal agents and anticonvulsants*, e.g. phenytoin, phenobarbitone and primidone, impair vitamin D metabolism by inhibiting the conversion of 25-hydroxyvitamin D to the active form 1,25-dihydroxyvitamin D, with consequent disturbances in calcium metabolism and adverse effects on bone (Expert Group on Vitamins and Minerals, 2003).

Drugs may also affect the metabolism of dietary components. Type A monoamine oxidase inhibitors (MAOI A) exert their antidepressant effect by inhibiting the breakdown of endogenously produced amine neurotransmitters. However, they also inhibit the breakdown of dietary amines such as tyramine, which, if allowed to accumulate, can produce a dangerous rise in blood pressure. Patients on these drugs therefore have to avoid dietary sources of tyramine and other vasoactive amines (see Chapter 7.10.3).

Nutrient excretion

As well as their intended increase in sodium excretion, diuretic drugs can also result in enhanced losses of other elements such as potassium, calcium, magnesium and zinc. Tetracycline increases the urinary excretion of vitamin C.

Clinical significance of drug–nutrient interactions

It is important to remember that poor nutritional status can impair drug metabolism and that drug treatment can have a detrimental effect on nutritional status. However, not all drug–nutrient interactions are clinically significant. In many instances, any losses in nutrient availability or drug action will be small and may be of short duration. Drugs that are most likely to have dietetic implications are those that:

- Have a narrow range between therapeutic effect and toxicity, e.g. lithium and anticoagulants.
- Need to be taken for a prolonged period of time.
- Have implications in terms of the timing of food intake (habitual meal pattern may need to be adjusted).
- Necessitate dietary restrictions or regulation (food choice may need to be altered).
- Have side effects that impact on appetite or gastrointestinal function.
- Directly compete with a nutrient, e.g. vitamin K and warfarin.

Factors that increase the risk from drug–nutrient interactions include:

- Presence of gastrointestinal, liver and/or renal function.
- A nutritionally compromised state due to poor diet, alcoholism or disease.

- Recent weight loss.
- Dehydration.
- Multiple drug therapy.
- Prolonged drug therapy.

Many of these factors are likely to coexist in elderly people. In addition, the physiological changes that occur with age such as a decrease in fat free mass and body water, decreased plasma protein concentration and general decline in renal and liver function mean that the risk of adverse drug reactions is much higher (Klotz, 2009). For this reason, it is a requirement that drug data sheets provide details of suitable dosages for elderly people.

Elderly people are also more likely to be given the types of drugs that have powerful effects and are most likely to impact on nutrition, e.g. anti Parkinson's drugs. Diminished salivation in the elderly may make it more difficult to swallow tablets, and oesophageal motility disorders lead to bulky drugs sticking in the oesophageal mucosa. Other problems such as failing memory, poor hearing and vision, and difficulty with opening containers may mean that drug regimens are not followed correctly, particularly if they are complex. Drug usage is therefore an important consideration in the dietary assessment of elderly people.

Due to the nature of nutrients in enteral tube feeds, drug–nutrient interaction potential is increased. Drugs in liquid form may interact with constituents of the feed preparation, so altering their bioavailability and requiring dose adjustment, e.g. digoxin. There are clinically significant interactions between enteral feeds and phenytoin, theophylline, digoxin, ciprofloxacin, tetracyclines and rifampicin.

Alcohol and drugs

It is important to always assess alcohol intake as part of a nutritional assessment, in part because it can affect drug-nutrient interactions. It may enhance the action of many drugs acting on the brain, e.g. antidepressants, benzodiazepines and antiepileptic drugs, leading to impaired mental ability and increased sedation. It is a misconception that all antibiotics interact with alcohol; however, there are significant interactions with metronidazole and tinidazole, leading to nausea, vomiting and flushing. Even small amounts of alcohol consumed with disulfiram (used to treat alcohol dependence), causing facial flushing, tachycardia, giddiness, hypotension and potentially collapse. Large changes in alcohol consumption will affect the anticoagulant effect of warfarin. NB: Some mouthwashes bought over the counter contain sufficient alcohol to cause this reaction.

Specific drug–nutrient interactions are discussed in chapters in Section 7 as appropriate.

Further reading

Expert Group on Vitamins and Minerals. (2003) *Safe Upper Levels for Vitamins and Minerals*. London: Food Standards Agency. Available at http://cot.food.gov.uk/cotreports/cotjointreps/evmreport/. Accessed 10 March 2013.

Baxter K, Preston CL. (2013) *Stockley's Drug Interactions*, 10th edn. London: Pharmaceutical Press.

Boullata JI, Armenti VT (eds) (2010) *Handbook of Drug Nutrient Interactions*. New York: Humana Press.

Boullata JI, Hudson LM. (2012) Drug–nutrient interactions: A broad view with implications for practice. *Journal of the Academy of Nutrition and Dietetics* 112: 506–517.

Internet resources

British National Formulary   www.bnf.org

Medicines and Healthcare Products Regulatory Agency (MHRA)   www.mhra.gov.uk

Monthly Index of Medical Specialities (MIMS)   www.mims.co.uk

UKMi National Medicines Information for Healthcare Professionals www.ukmi.nhs.uk

References

Backman, WD, Bakhai A. (2013) Drug–grapefruit juice interactions. *BMJ Rapid Response*. Available at www.bmj.com/content/346/bmj.f1/rr/627070. Accessed 9 March 2013.

Boullata JI, Hudson LM. (2012) Drug–nutrient interactions: A broad view with implications for practice. *Journal of the Academy of Nutrition and Dietetics* 112: 506–517.

Brill ME, Jeroen D, van Rongen A, van Kralingen S, van den Anker JN, Knibbe CAJ. (2012) Impact of obesity on drug metabolism and elimination in adults and children. *Clinical Pharmacokinetics* 51: 277–304.

Dickerson JWT. (1988) The interrelationships of nutrition and drugs. In: Dickerson JWT, Lee HA (eds) *Nutrition and the Clinical Management of Disease*, 2nd edn. London: Edward Arnold, pp. 392–421.

Expert Group on Vitamins and Minerals (EVM). (2003) *Safe Upper Levels for Vitamins and Minerals*. London: Food Safety Agency. Available at http://cot.food.gov.uk/cotreports/cotjointreps/evmreport/. Accessed 10 March 2013.

Klotz U. (2009) Pharmacokinetics and drug metabolism in the elderly. *Drug Metabolism Reviews* 41(2): 67–76.

Oshikoya KA, Senbanjo IO. (2009) Pathophysiological changes that affect drug disposition in protein energy malnourished children. *Nutrition & Metabolism (London)* 6: 50.

Pirmohamed M. (2013) Drug–grapefruit juice interactions. *BMJ* 346: f1.

Webster-Gandy J, Madden A, Holdsworth M. (2011) *Oxford Handbook of Nutrition & Dietetics*, 2nd edn. Oxford: Oxford University Press.

SECTION 5

5.4

Alternative and complementary therapies

Joan Gandy

Key points

- Use of complementary and alternative medicine (CAM) therapies is increasing.

- Complementary therapies are used alongside conventional treatment. Alternative therapies are used instead of conventional treatment or advice.

- Dietary supplements are also commonly complementary therapies. Their use should be based on clinical need and underpinned by evidence of efficacy and safety.

- Herbal remedies have potent effects and many interact with conventional drugs.

- Dietitians should ask about the use of CAM, especially dietary supplements, during a nutritional assessment to assess the likely impact on nutrient intake and conventional treatments.

The use of complementary medicine therapies (which includes the use of supplements) and alternative therapies (CAM) is increasing. Therefore, it is essential that dietitians are aware of CAM's efficacy, potential and risks benefits. Dietitians should enquire about their use in every nutritional assessment and are able to advise on their efficacy and safety to enable clients to make informed choices. The Cochrane collaboration (Mannheimer & Berman, 2008) describe CAM as *'a broad domain of healing resources that encompasses all health systems, modalities, and practices and their accompanying theories and beliefs, other than those intrinsic to the politically dominant health system of a particular society or culture in a given historical period. . . . Boundaries within CAM and between the CAM domain and that of the dominant system are not always sharp or fixed'*.

There is a fundamental difference between complementary and alternative therapies, which are defined by the USA National Center for Complementary and Alternative Medicine (NCCAM) (2012) as:

- *Complementary therapies* are used together with conventional treatment, e.g. acupuncture in addition to analgesics to treat pain.
- *Alternative therapies* are used instead of conventional treatment.

In addition, NCCAM defines integrative (integrated) medicine as the combination of conventional medicine and CAM whose safety and effectiveness are supported by some high quality evidence.

There are many forms of CAM and it is not possible to provide a definitive list. However, the Cochrane Collaboration has reviewed this field and considers the following categories:

- Treatments that someone usually self medicates with, e.g. botanicals, nutritional supplements, health food, meditation and magnetic therapy.
- Treatments that are provided by others, e.g. acupuncture, massage therapy, reflexology, laser therapy, balneotherapy, chiropractic and osteopathic manipulations, certain types of psychological counselling, naprapathy and acupressure herbalism.
- Treatments that are self administered under periodic supervision of a therapist, e.g. yoga, biofeedback, Tai Chi, homeopathy, hydrotherapy, Alexander therapy, nutritional therapy and Ayurveda.
- Other interventions including Qi Gong, Doman Delcato patterning, anthroposophical medicine, Unani medicine, traditional African medicine, Bach flower remedies, clinical ecology, colon cleansing or irrigation, and music or sound therapy.
- Diagnostic techniques, e.g. iridology, kinesiology, Vega testing, biofunctional diagnostic testing, electroacupuncture by Voll and hair analysis.

In the UK most CAM practitioners work in private practice; however, some CAM therapies are offered in the NHS (NHS Choices www.nhs.uk/Livewell/complementary-alternative-medicine/Pages/complementary-alternative-medicines.aspx; Wye *et al*., 2009). This is a controversial area and is often hotly debated in the medical press.

SECTION 5

When enquiring about the use of CAM, it is important that the dietitian is respectful of the reasons for their use as these may be cultural or religious, e.g. Ayurveda is commonly used in India. The reasons people use CAM therapies are complex and include the following (Hollander & Mechanick, 2008):

- People feel that symptoms, especially fatigue and chronic pain, are not adequately addressed by conventional practitioners.
- Some prefer to use natural products, as they believe these are safer than man made products such as medicines.
- Some are misled by claims of dramatic improvements in health and cures.
- Many consumers are confused by the often spurious scientific claims of some treatments.
- Terminally ill people and carers who have exhausted conventional treatment may seek further treatments outside conventional medicine.

Dietitians must be aware of the significance of the use of CAM, as while some are innocuous, there are potential problems with some treatments. These therapies are particularly popular in some clinical areas, e.g. multiple sclerosis and cancer, and dietitians specialising in these areas must be conversant with them and any potential problems (see Chapter 7.6.4 and Chapter 7.15.1). These problems include:

- *Lack of nutritional expertise of the practitioner*, including ignorance of biochemistry and physiology (see Professional regulation later in this chapter).
- *Diagnosis of a non-existent nutritional problem*, especially deficiencies. Such deficiencies may be misdiagnosed by the use of tests that have little validity, e.g. hair analysis (Ernst, 2001). Other methods are used that have no credibility or scientific basis, e.g. kinesiology and Vega (electrodermal) testing. Laboratory tests for micronutrients are reviewed by Bender (2003).
- *Lack of informed guidance* – people may obtain information from less reliable resources such as some Internet sites. Schmidt & Ernst (2004) found that many websites endorsed unproven therapies and that a significant proportion of them were giving advice that could be detrimental. They consider that some raised serious concern as they overtly discouraged patients from using conventional therapy.
- *Some therapies may do harm* – elimination diets may be recommended without an in depth understanding of nutrition, resulting in deficiencies (see Chapter 7.11.2). Some alternative therapists advocate stopping conventional treatments, which can have potentially harmful consequences, e.g. advising a type 1 diabetic to stop insulin treatment. Other therapies such as Chinese herbs may cause serious drug interactions.

Some patients, their family or carers may have particularly strong beliefs about the use of CAM therapies and these require careful consideration. This is exemplified by a recent high profile court cases in the UK. Dietitians should explore with clients the reasons for CAM use offering appropriate advice and presenting the evidence base as appropriate.

Professional regulation

Unlike medicine, nursing and the allied health professions, CAM practitioners are poorly, if at all, regulated and there is usually no minimum level of knowledge of expertise. While there are professional bodies for some CAM therapies, e.g. the British Acupuncture Council, these are often self regulatory and the titles are unprotected. In addition, unregulated practitioners will not necessarily be covered by professional indemnity insurance and therefore practice without this protection for themselves and their patients (consumers).

Within the field of nutrition, only the title dietitian (dietician) is protected by law; anyone using the title of dietitian must be registered with the Health and Care Professions Council (HPCP) (Chapter 1.1). Someone using this title without registration is liable to persecution. The titles nutritionist and nutrition therapist are not protected; therefore, these can be used without formal qualifications [British Dietetic Association (BDA), 2012]. However, many nutritionists are registered with the Association for Nutrition (AfN), which has proficiency and competency criteria, and promotes continuing professional development (CPD) and safe conduct. Like the HCPC, the AfN requires registrants to maintain their knowledge and expertise through CPD. Only nutritionists registered with the AfN can use the title Registered Nutritionist. The AfN is working towards making the title nutritionist protected, possibly with the HCPC. Nutrition therapists are not required to be registered, although they do have a professional body (the British Association for Applied Nutrition and Nutritional Therapy). Appropriately trained or qualified nutritional therapists can apply to join the voluntary register held by the Complementary and Natural Healthcare Council (CNHC).

Differences between dietitians, nutritionists and nutrition therapist are discussed further by the BDA (2012).

Nutritional supplements

Nutritional supplements are taken orally as capsules, pills, liquids or powders and in addition to food (Webb, 2006). Supplements may include essential nutrients, e.g. minerals, vitamins and fatty acids, may usually be in the diet and/or have well established functions in the body, e.g. creatine. Alternatively, they may be plant extracts, e.g. garlic. In 2008 a third of adults in the UK reported taking supplement on most days [Food Standards Agency (FSA), 2008]. The three most popular supplements were multivitamins (36%), cod liver oil (35%) and vitamin C (35%). The use of dietary supplements is increasing in many developed countries, including the UK (NHS & BAZIAN, 2011) and the USA (Gahche *et al.*, 2011); over 50% of people surveyed in the USA reported using dietary supplements.

Supplement usage is not necessarily undesirable; fish oils are beneficial for cardiovascular health and people who do not eat oily fish may benefit from taking them as supplements. Folic acid supplementation is recommended for women for the first 12 weeks of pregnancy. There are many circumstances in which vitamin and mineral supplementation may be either necessary or a sensible precaution including:

- People with an identified vitamin or mineral deficiency, e.g. iron.
- People with increased physiological needs, e.g. pregnant women, infants and children.
- People with increased nutrient losses as a result of gastrointestinal disease or resection, other disorders or side effects of drug treatment.
- People with poor appetite, eating or swallowing difficulties due to illness.
- Elderly people, especially those in residential care or with poor wound healing.
- People on either prescribed or self imposed restrictive diets.
- People at high risk of disorders such as osteoporosis or rickets.

There is evidence to suggest that many of those who take vitamin and or mineral supplements are the least likely to need them (Cade *et al.*, 2004). The National Diet and Nutrition survey showed that supplement users often had a higher micronutrient intake from food sources alone than non-supplement users (Henderson *et al.*, 2003). Conversely, people who might benefit from certain supplements may not be taking them. The majority of women of child bearing age do not consume sufficient folate to provide protection against neural tube defects in the event of planned or unplanned pregnancy (Henderson *et al.*, 2003).

The reasons given for supplement usage vary. In general, people choose to take multivitamin and mineral products in the belief that they will boost energy, reduce the effects of ageing, cut the risk of disease such as cancer, extend life or treat specific conditions, e.g. arthritis (FSA, 2008). The marketing of dietary supplements will undoubtedly affect the decision to take dietary supplements, especially for those aimed at particular groups of people, e.g. the elderly. Supplements of single nutrients tend to be chosen for more specific reasons and to prevent or treat a particular condition or symptom (Neuhouser *et al.*, 1999).

Problems associated with their use

While use of some supplements is based on sound evidence of efficacy, e.g. folate in pregnancy to prevent neural tube defects, use of others is based on more dubious claims or misinformation (Satia-Abouta *et al.*, 2003). For example, enzymes present in some supplements cannot be of any benefit as they will be denatured as soon as they come into contact with stomach acid and are rendered ineffective. Some trace elements available in supplements are not essential for human nutrition [Expert Group on Vitamins and Minerals (EVM), 2003].

Safety

The report by the EVM (2003) highlighted the fact that remarkably little is known about the requirements, mode of action, bioavailability and toxicity of many micronutrients. It attempted to determine safe upper levels, but in many cases there was insufficient data to assess the nutritional and toxicological implications. There was a lack of well designed, large comparative human studies of significant duration at different levels of intake and with adequate assessment of possible adverse effects. There was even less information on potentially vulnerable groups, e.g. children or the elderly. The toxicity of some nutrients has only been evaluated in animals and the relevance to humans is uncertain. The EVM set safe upper levels for eight vitamins and minerals; for another 22 the data were limited and only possible guidance levels were set. Neither safe nor guidance levels could be set for three others.

The EVM report concluded that, while current intakes of most vitamins and minerals are not harmful, several may have temporary side effects if taken in high doses. Others may have irreversible adverse effects if taken in large amounts over long periods of time (Table 5.4.1). Concerns over possible risks from prolonged high intakes of vitamin A were also highlighted and, following further review, the Scientific Advisory Committee Nutrition (2005) recommended that people who consume liver (the main dietary source of vitamin A) more than once a week, or older adults who are at risk of osteoporosis, should be cautious about taking retinol containing supplements. Women who are, or may become, pregnant are advised to avoid vitamin A supplements.

Overdosage

Overdosage with vitamins and minerals can occur as a result of taking a preparation that provides many times the reference nutrient intake (RNI) for a nutrient in the belief that it will have more therapeutic benefits. However, inadvertent overdosing may occur as a result of:

- Taking inappropriate combinations of supplements. For example, people may take a multivitamin preparation for bone and joint along with a healthy heart supplement, unaware that each contains more than the RNI for vitamins A and D.
- The vitamin content of some supplements may be significantly higher than the amount stated to be present to allow for natural deterioration during the shelf life of the product (EVM, 2003). This is particularly likely to be the case with supplements containing vitamins A, D and E, which are prone to oxidation.

Fat soluble vitamins are stored in the body and the risks associated with prolonged high intakes, particularly from vitamins A and D, are well documented. The risk of overdosage from water soluble vitamins is much less as excessive intakes are usually excreted in the urine. However,

Table 5.4.1   Possible adverse effects of vitamin and mineral supplements (EVM, 2003; FSA, 2008)

Nutrient	Possible adverse effects
Beta-carotene	Long term intake of >7 mg/day may increase the risk of lung cancer Supplements should not be taken by people who smoke
Nicotinic acid	50-mg doses can cause skin flushing and other reversible side effects such as gastrointestinal disturbances Prolonged intake of higher doses may cause liver dysfunction It is recommended that supplemental intakes do not exceed 17 mg/day
Vitamin A	An excessive intake is teratogenic and may also cause irreversible bone and liver damage Retinol containing supplements should be avoided by people who consume liver more than once a week, or older adults at risk of osteoporosis Pregnant women should avoid taking supplements
Vitamin C	>1000 mg/day may cause abdominal pain and/or diarrhoea
Vitamin B_6	>200 mg/day may cause irreversible neurological damage It is recommended that supplementary intakes do not exceed 10 mg/day
Calcium	>1500 mg/day may cause abdominal pain and/or diarrhoea
Iron	>17 mg/day may cause constipation, nausea and abdominal pain
Magnesium	>400 mg/day may cause osmotic diarrhoea
Manganese	Neurotoxic at high levels of intake It is recommended that supplemental intakes do not exceed 4 mg/day, and in older adults should not exceed 0.5 mg/day
Nickel	Nickel containing products may cause a skin rash in sensitive individuals
Phosphorus	>250 mg/day may cause mild stomach upset in sensitive individuals Long term excessive intake may be detrimental to bone health
Zinc	High intakes impair absorption of iron and copper and may also have gastrointestinal side effects It is recommended that supplemental intakes do not exceed 25 mg/day

the risks are not negligible; irreversible neurological damage can occur following excessive intakes of vitamin B_6. Excessive intakes of some minerals and trace elements (especially iron, copper, fluorine and sodium) can be directly toxic. The threshold between safe upper limits and toxicity may be small in some cases.

Interactions

Although overt toxicity is rare, the long term consequences of excessive high intakes of some vitamins and minerals may be significant. High intake of one, e.g. iron, can impair absorption of another, e.g. zinc, and cause a deficiency. Interactions are particularly likely between elements that are close to each other in the periodic table, e.g. iron, copper, manganese, zinc and chromium (EVM, 2003). Antioxidants also function as part of a coordinated biochemical chain of defence against free radicals; high doses of a single antioxidant supplement such as vitamin E could disturb the antioxidant–pro-oxidant balance and lead to potential risks (Opara, 2002).

Supplemental intakes of some micronutrients can also interact with medicinal drugs, e.g. vitamin B_6 can reduce the therapeutic effect of levodopa used to treat Parkinson's disease and interact with other drugs such as isoniazid, theophylline and phenobarbitone (see Chapter 5.3). It is easy to cause nutritional imbalances by the use of supplements, whereas it is very difficult to do so by consuming food. In order to avoid the potential risks, the use of isolated supplements, particularly in high doses, should therefore be avoided other than in cases of clear clinical need.

Of more concern are the findings that some of these supplements may be associated with long term risks. A meta analysis of seven large randomised trials showed a small but significant increase in all cause mortality and cardiovascular death with beta-carotene therapy (Vivekananthan et al., 2003). Supplemental intakes of beta-carotene may increase the risk of lung cancer in people with a history of smoking (EVM, 2003; Omenn et al., 1996; Albanes et al., 1996). Supplemental intakes of vitamin E in excess of 400 IU/day (268 mg/day) be associated with premature mortality (Miller et al., 2005). Many consumers of megadoses of micronutrients are aware of the potential of overdose but continue to take large doses of supplements (FSA, 2008).

Regulation of supplements

The EU Food Supplements Directive (EC 46/2002) outlines a framework for certain classes of food supplements. It regulates and guarantees legal status of these classes of supplements within the UK and throughout Europe. Vitamin and mineral supplements must be safe and appropriately labelled to enable consumers to make informed choices (see Chapter 4.5). More information on the classification of supplements as food or medicine can be found at the Government Chemist website (www.governmentchemist.org.uk).

Table 5.4.2 Most common herb–drug interactions (source: Webster-Gandy 2001, table 385, p. 744. Reproduced with permission of Oxford University Press)*

Herb	Interacts with	Comment
St John's wort	Antidepressants	Drug plasma concentration reduced, leading to reduced therapeutic effect
	Antivirals: HIV protease inhibitors (atazanavir, indinavir, nelfinavir, ritonavir, saquinavir)	Reduced therapeutic effect
	HIV non-nucleoside reverse transcriptase inhibitors (efavirenz, nevirapine)	Reduced therapeutic effect
	Anticonvulsants (carbamazepine, phenobarbital, phenytoin)	Reduced control of seizures
	Ciclosporin, tacrolimus	Increased risk of transplant rejection
	Digoxin	Reduced therapeutic effect
	Oral combined contraceptives, oestrogen containing patches and vaginal rings	Reduced therapeutic effect
	Voriconazole	Reduced therapeutic effect
	Theophylline	Reduced asthma control
	Warfarin	Reduced anticoagulant effect
	SSRIs (fluoxetine, paroxetine, sertraline)	Increased serotonergic effects
	Triptans (sumatriptan, naratriptan, rizatriptan, zolmitriptan)	Reduced therapeutic effect
Ginkgo biloba	Anticoagulant (warfarin) Antiplatelet (aspirin)	Increased risk of bleeding
Ginseng	Anticoagulant (warfarin)	Increased risk of bleeding
Dong quai	Anticoagulant (warfarin)	Increased risk of bleeding
Echinacea	Immunosuppressant	Possible immune stimulation
Saw palmetto	Anticoagulant (warfarin)	Altered anticoagulation

*This list is not exhaustive. *Stockley's Drug Interactions* or *British National Formulary* should be consulted for further details. SSRI, selective serotonin reuptake inhibitor.

Herbal medicine

Herbal medicine is based on the use of plants or plant extracts to treat disease. Herbal remedies are one of the most powerful forms of complementary therapies and there are considerable risks from their inappropriate use. In the UK, the main systems of herbal medicine practised are western and Chinese. Western herbal medicine is largely, although not exclusively, based on the use of plants native to Britain, Europe and North America. Chinese herbal medicine is part of traditional Chinese medicine (TCM), which may include other CAM therapies, e.g. acupuncture. Other forms of herbal medicine include Ayurveda and Tibetan. Practitioners prescribe herb mixtures based on an individual's symptoms and condition. People can also purchase over the counter herbal remedies from retail outlets or via the Internet.

Problems associated with their use

Herbal medicines are often assumed to be safe as they are natural products. However, herbal remedies can be associated with problems including:

* *Potency* – herbal remedies contain potent pharmacological ingredients that can have similar effects to many conventional drugs. Many conventional drugs were developed following observations of the effects of certain plants, e.g. salicylic acid is found in willow bark and its salts (salicylates) are manufactured as analgesics, e.g. aspirin.
* *Interactions* – herbal ingredients can interact with other herbs, conventional drugs and nutrients in foods (Table 5.4.2).
* *Purity* – herbal medicines made to poor standards may be a health risk. Poor manufacturing practices in some countries have resulted in contamination with heavy metals or toxic herbs, posing a significant risk to health (Goudie & Kaye, 2001). Inadequate labelling or batch to batch variation in ingredient types, levels of active substance and proportions can lead to herbal medicines being used incorrectly (Dunning, 2004).

Some herbal products sold in the UK have to be licensed like other medicines, but many over the counter products are exempt. The Medicines and Healthcare Products Regulatory Agency (MHRA) has a traditional herbal medicines registration scheme to ensure that unlicensed over the counter traditional herbal medicines meet assured standards of safety, quality and patient information. In the UK, suspected adverse reactions to both licensed and unlicensed herbal preparations can be reported using the yellow card system. The MHRA also issues alerts about cases of poisoning and adverse reactions, e.g. as it did for Herbal Flos Lonicerae (Herbal Xenicol) Natural Weight Loss Formula (MHRA, 2013).

Herbal remedies such as feverfew, golden seal, juniper, mistletoe, nutmeg, rosemary and sage are contraindicated in pregnancy due to the increased risk of miscarriage. No herbal preparation should be taken during the first 3 months of pregnancy.

Common herb–drug interactions

The number and availability of herbs as supplements and as complementary therapy are increasing, leading to increased potential for herb–drug interactions. It is important to assess herb intake during a nutritional assessment as, like conventional drugs, they have the potential to enhance or reduce drug action. Examples of common herb–drug interactions are shown in Table 5.4.2. St John's wort (*Hypericum perforatum*) is commonly used as an antidepressant. However, it induces liver enzymes and reduces the effect of several drugs; a physician or pharmacist should be consulted before concomitant use.

Evidence base for CAM therapies

Dietetics is an evidence based practice and dietitians, like other regulated healthcare professionals, have a responsibility to use the best possible practice (see Chapter 1.1). It is therefore reasonable to expect the same level of rigour for all therapies, including CAM (Lewith *et al.*, 2000). There are innate difficulties in conducting this research as funding and support may not be available, and there is resistance from some CAM therapists who question the salience of conventional methods of assessment (Jackson & Scambler, 2007). Perhaps for these reasons, the available evidence is often from studies conducted in small groups of subjects. In addition, studies may not be well constructed. This limits the ability to produce high level evidence such as systematic reviews and meta analyses. However, some high level evidence for the efficacy and safety of CAM is available. For example, Posadzki *et al.* (2012) recently published a systematic review of published case reports and case series on the adverse effects of homeopathy.

As the result of increasing use of CAM in the USA, the National Institute of Health has established the National Center for Complementary and Alternative Medicine (NCCAM) with the mission '. . . *to define, through rigorous scientific investigation, the usefulness and safety of complementary and alternative medicine interventions and their roles in improving health and health care*'. It funds research and produces publications and guidelines on CAM for healthcare professionals and the public.

Dietitians should look for and critically appraise the evidence for CAM as they would conventional medicine (see Evidence based practice in Chapter 1.1 and Appendix A1). The Cochrane Collaboration has a section on CAM and reviews are available on many topics, e.g. aromatherapy for dementia.

While it is understandable that people with incurable or chronic conditions may use CAM, its use should be underpinned by evidence of efficacy and safety. However, when there is no risk to the client, the potential placebo effect should be considered, although vulnerable patients must not be given false hope or have necessary treatments delayed. Ultimately, the patient is responsible for making the decision to follow a complementary or alternative dietary regimen. However, it is the responsibility of the dietitian to ensure that the patient has been given sufficient scientifically based information on which to base that decision.

Further reading

Ernst E. (2008) *Oxford Handbook of Complementary Medicine.* Oxford: Oxford University Press.

Expert Group on Vitamins and Minerals (EVM). (2003) *Safe Upper Levels for Vitamins and Minerals.* London: FSA. Available at http://cot.food.gov.uk/cotreports/cotjointreps/evmreport/

Webb G. (2006) *Dietary Supplements and Functional Foods.* Oxford: Blackwell Publishing.

Internet resources

Cochrane Collaboration   www.cochrane.org

Government Chemist (UK)   www.governmentchemist.org.uk

Information is beautiful www.informationisbeautiful.net/play/snake-oil-supplements

Medicines and Healthcare Products Regulatory Agency www.mhra.gov.uk

National Center for Complementary and Alternative Medicine http://nccam.nih.gov

NHS Choices www.nhs.uk/Livewell/complementary-alternative-medicine/Pages/complementary-alternative-medicines.aspx

NHS Evidence   www.evidence.nhs.uk

Natural medicines comprehensive database   http://naturaldatabase.therapeuticresearch.com

Office of Dietary Supplements (National Institute for Health USA) http://ods.od.nih.gov

References

Albanes D, Heinonen OP, Taylor PR, *et al.* (1996) Alpha-tocopherol and beta-carotene supplements and lung cancer incidence in the Alpha-Tocopherol, Beta-Carotene (ATBC) cancer prevention study: effects of base-line characteristics and study compliance. *Journal of the National Cancer Institute* 88(21): 1560–1570.

Bender DA. (2003) *Nutritional Biochemistry of the Vitamins.* Cambridge: Cambridge University Press.

British Dietetic Association (BDA). (2012) Dietitian, nutritionist, nutritional therapist or diet expert? A comprehensive guide to roles and functions. Available at www.bda.org.uk. Accessed 11 March 2013.

Cade JE, Burley VJ, Greenwood DC. (2004) The UK Women's Cohort Study: comparison of vegetarians, fish-eaters and meat-eaters. *Public Health Nutrition* 7(7): 871–878.

Dunning T. (2004) Complementary therapies: considerations for diabetes care. *Practical Diabetes International* 21(3): 118–125.

Ernst E (ed). (2001) *The Desktop Guide to Complementary and Alternative Medicine – An Evidence-Based Approach.* Edinburgh: Mosby.

Expert Group on Vitamins and Minerals (EVM). (2003) *Safe Upper Levels for Vitamins and Minerals.* London: Food Standards Agency. Available at http://cot.food.gov.uk/cotreports/cotjointreps/evmreport/. Accessed 11 March 2013.

Food Standards Agency (FSA) (2008) Consumer consumption of vitamin and mineral food supplements. Available at http://www.foodbase.org.uk//admintools/reportdocuments/472-1-841_viminsupconsumer.pdf. Accessed 11 March 2013.

Gahche J, Bailey R, Burt V, *et al.* (2011) Dietary supplement use among U.S. adults has increased since NHANES III (1988–1994). *NCHS Data Brief* Apr(61): 1–8.

Goudie A, Kaye JM. (2001) Contaminated medication precipitating hypoglycaemia. *Medical Journal of Australia* 175(5): 256–257.

Henderson L, Irving K, Gregory J, *et al.* (2003). *National Diet and Nutrition Survey: Adults Aged 19 to 64 Years. Volume 3: Vitamin and Mineral Intake and Urinary Analytes.* London: The Stationery Office.

Hollander JM, Mechanick JI. (2008) Complementary and alternative medicine and the management of the metabolic syndrome. *Journal of the American Dietetic Association* 108(3):495–509.

Jackson S, Scambler G. (2007) Perceptions of evidence based medicine: traditional acupuncturists in the UK and resistance to biomedical modes of evaluation. *Sociology of Health & Illness* 29: 412–429.

Lewith GT, Ernst E, Mills S, *et al.* (2000) Complementary medicine must be research led and evidence based. *BMJ* 320: 188.2.

Mannheimer B, Berman B. (2008) Cochrane complementary medicine field. About The Cochrane Collaboration (Fields), Issue 2. Available at: http://www.mrw.interscience.wiley.com/cochrane/clabout/articles/CE000052/frame.html. Accessed 11 March 2013.

Medicines and Healthcare Products Regulatory Agency (MHRA). (2013) Toxic poisoning alert for online Chinese medicines. Available at www.mhra.gov.uk/NewsCentre/Pressreleases/CON239403. Accessed 11 March 2013.

Miller ER 3rd, Pastor-Barriuso R, Dalal D, Riemersma RA, Appel LJ, Guallar E. (2005) Meta-analysis: high-dosage vitamin E supplementation may increase all-cause mortality. *Annals of Internal Medicine* 142(1): 37–46.

National Center for Complementary and Alternative Medicine (NCCAM). (2012) CAM basics. What is complementary and alternative medicine? Available at http://nccam.nih.gov/health/whatiscam. Accessed 11 March 2013.

Neuhouser ML, Patterson RE, Levy L. (1999) Motivations for using vitamin and mineral supplements. *Journal of the American Dietetic Association* 7: 851–854.

NHS & BAZIAN. (2011) Supplements – who needs them? Available at www.nhs.uk/news/2011/05May/Documents/BtH_supplements.pdf. Accessed 11 March 2013.

Opara EC. (2002) Oxidative stress, micronutrients, diabetes mellitus and its complications. *Journal of the Royal Society of Health* 122: 28–34.

Posadzki P, Alotaibi A, Ernst E. (2012) Adverse effects of homeopathy: A systematic review of published case reports and case series. *International Journal of Clinical Practice* 66(12): 1178–1188.

Omenn GS, Goodman G, Thornquist M, *et al.* (1996) Chemoprevention of lung cancer: the beta-Carotene and Retinol Efficacy Trial (CARET) in high-risk smokers and asbestos-exposed workers. *IARC Scientific Publications* 136: 67–85.

Satia-Abouta J, Kristal AR, Patterson RE, Littman AJ, Stratton KL, White E. (2003) Dietary supplement use and medical conditions: the VITAL study. *American Journal of Preventive Medicine* 24(1): 43–51.

Scientific Advisory Committee on Nutrition (SACN). (2005) *Review of Dietary Advice on Vitamin A.* London: The Stationery Office. Available at: www.sacn.gov.uk. Accessed 11 March 2013.

Vivekananthan DP, Penn MS, Sapp SK, Hsu A, Topol EJ. (2003) Use of antioxidant vitamins for the prevention of cardiovascular disease: meta-analysis of randomised trials. *Lancet* 361: 2017–2023.

Webb GP. (2006) *Dietary Supplements and Functional Foods.* Oxford: Blackwell Publishing, pp. 1–37.

Webster-Gandy J, Madden A, Holdsworth M. (2011) *Oxford Handbook of Nutrition & Dietetics*, 2nd edn. Oxford: Oxford University Press.

Wye L, Sharp D, Shaw A. (2009) The impact of NHS based primary care complementary therapy services on health outcomes and NHS costs: a review of service audits and evaluations. *BMC Complementary and Alternative Medicine* 9: 5.

PART 2
Clinical dietetic practice

SECTION 6

Nutrition support

6.1

Nutritional requirements in clinical practice

C Elizabeth Weekes

Key points

- The lack of robust evidence for all prediction methods means that the determination of nutritional requirements requires a significant element of clinical judgement.

- Irrespective of the method used, requirement calculations should be interpreted with care and only used as a starting point.

- Practitioners should regularly review the patient and reassess requirements to take account of any significant changes in clinical condition, nutritional status, physical activity level and goals of treatment.

- The nutritional requirements for a number of clinical conditions have yet to be established.

- The requirements for a number of nutrients in illness and injury have yet to be established.

The aim of devising a nutritional prescription is to provide a patient with their complete requirements either via a single route or any combination of oral, enteral or parenteral nutrition, while avoiding the known complications associated with both under- and over-feeding (ASPEN, 2002; NICE, 2006). The estimation of nutritional requirements is an important part of the patient assessment, yet no single, validated method for estimating requirements exists, and the evidence base for all prediction methods currently in use is poor (Reeves & Capra, 2003). Therefore, practitioners need to exercise a considerable degree of clinical judgement when determining the nutritional requirements of an individual.

All prescriptions for nutritional support should take account of the patient's needs for energy, protein, fluid, electrolytes, micronutrients and fibre (NICE, 2006). However, a number of factors complicate the determination of nutritional requirements in clinical practice (Table 6.1.1) and should be considered prior to estimating the requirements of an individual. Even within a single disease, individual variation, e.g. age, comorbidities, nutritional status, response to surgery or treatment, may make prognosis unpredictable. Furthermore, illness or injury does not have a consistent effect on energy expenditure and this is also likely to be the case for other nutrients. Different treatment modalities, e.g. surgery, chemotherapy or pharmacological agents, may influence requirements in different ways and the same treatment may have very different effects in individuals with the same disease. These differences in response to treatment

may be due, at least in part, to genetic predispositions and environmental influences. The measurement and assay techniques used to assess nutrient status and determine nutritional requirements are not always fully described in the literature and may differ between studies (equipment, timing, protocols, etc.), thus making comparisons difficult. Furthermore, older studies may not be relevant to current practice due to advances in diagnostic procedures and management strategies. Irrespective of the route and likely duration, the aims and objectives of nutritional support should be clearly defined and documented at baseline, reviewed at each stage of the patient's illness and amended accordingly, e.g. minimising losses in acute illness and nutritional repletion in the recovery phase (NICE, 2006).

Energy

Basal metabolic rate and total energy expenditure

In healthy individuals total energy expenditure (TEE) comprises basal metabolic rate (BMR), dietary induced thermogenesis (DIT), i.e. energy expended in the digestion, absorption and transport of nutrients, and physical activity (Figure 6.1.1). Basal metabolic rate, i.e. the metabolic activity required to maintain life, comprises approximately 60% of TEE in any individual; measured BMR is highly reproducible.

The conditions essential for the measurement of BMR are:

Manual of Dietetic Practice, Fifth Edition. Edited by Joan Gandy.
© 2014 The British Dietetic Association. Published 2014 by John Wiley & Sons, Ltd.
Companion Website: www.manualofdieteticpractice.com

SECTION 6

Table 6.1.1 Factors affecting nutritional requirements in illness and injury

Basal requirements	Age
	Sex
	Body weight
	Body composition (proportions of fat and muscle mass)
	Previous and current nutritional intake
	Ambient temperature
Goals of treatment	Diagnosis
	Prognosis
	Likely duration of nutritional support
Disease effects	Metabolic state, e.g. catabolic, normobolic or anabolic
	Severity of illness
	Inflammatory response
	Gastrointestinal function
	Medical interventions, e.g. mechanical ventilation, radiotherapy, chemotherapy, hormone treatment or transplantation
	Surgery
	Pharmacological interventions, e.g. sedation, oral steroid therapy
	Pain
	Psychological state
Activity	Mobility status, e.g. bed bound, mobile on ward
	Level of consciousness
	Neuromuscular function

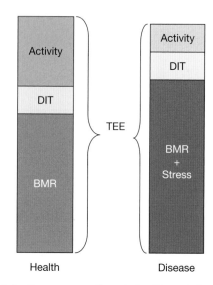

Figure 6.1.1 Energy expenditure in health and disease [source: The British Dietetic Association 2013. Reproduced with permission of The British Dietetic Association (www.bda.uk.com)]

- Postabsorptive (12-hour fast).
- Lying still at physical and mental rest (but not asleep).
- Thermoneutral environment (27–29 °C).
- No stimulants such as tea, coffee or nicotine in the previous 12 hours.
- No heavy physical activity during the previous day.
- Validation gases must be calibrated to ensure measurements are accurate and reliable.
- Steady state must be established, i.e. <10% difference in minute to minute oxygen (VO_2) and carbon dioxide (VCO_2) volume measurements over 5 minutes.

If any of these criteria are not met, then the measurement is defined as resting energy expenditure (REE) or resting metabolic rate (RMR). In the clinical situation it is rarely possible to measure BMR due to the exacting requirements listed above. In sick or injured subjects, REE will comprise BMR plus the effect of any metabolic response to injury or disease. If the patient is not fasted, the REE measurement may also include some proportion of DIT. In some patients, such as those with involuntary movements due to neuromuscular dysfunction, an element of physical activity may also be included during measurements of REE. Conversely, if measurement conditions are strictly controlled, REE may not equate to total energy requirements since neither activity nor DIT will be accounted for.

There are a large number of BMR prediction equations, although the most commonly cited are Harris Benedict (Harris & Benedict, 1919) and Schofield (1985). More

recently, the Henry equations (Henry, 2005) have been evaluated (Ramirez-Zea, 2005; SACN, 2011) and recommended as the most rigorously tested and applicable to modern healthy populations. The Henry equations were derived from a database of 10 552 BMR values in studies conducted from 1914 to 2005, including a larger cohort of elderly subjects than in previous databases. Only studies where conditions met strict criteria for BMR measurements were included.

Inflammatory state

In sick or injured individuals, TEE is influenced by many factors and in any individual patient may be lower, similar to or, in rare cases, higher than requirements in healthy populations (Figure 6.1.1). In the majority of chronic conditions, BMR is usually normal or may be slightly increased. Since any metabolic stress induced increase in BMR is often accompanied by a decrease in physical activity, TEE in chronically ill individuals is usually normal or decreased (Kulstad & Schoeller, 2007; SACN, 2011).

Acute illness increases in BMR above that predicted for healthy individuals of the same age and weight are usually 0–40%, and very rarely, up to 100%. Both the magnitude and duration of the increase are dependent on the presence of an inflammatory response; therefore, an assessment of the patient's inflammatory state is important in the determination of their energy requirements. To avoid the risk of overfeeding in acutely ill individuals, it might be prudent to include a stress factor in any estimate of energy requirements only while there is biochemical and clinical evidence of an inflammatory response, e.g. elevated C-reactive protein or white cell count, low serum albumin, poor appetite or oedema.

In the presence of an inflammatory response, weight gain and other clinical benefits are unlikely to be achieved with nutritional support alone (Streat *et al.*, 1987) and the goal of nutritional support is usually to minimise losses while the patient is in this state. Aggressive nutritional support should only be considered when the patient is more able to utilise the nutrients provided, i.e. during recovery (anabolic phase). A patient is likely to be moving into the recovery phase as oedema resolves and the parameters listed earlier return to the normal range.

Physical activity

Individuals requiring nutritional support range from paralysed and sedated, critically ill patients to fully mobile patients on the ward or in the community. To date however, there is a relative lack of research on the effects of illness and injury on physical activity levels (Elia, 2005), although a recent report concluded that acute illness is usually accompanied by a decrease in physical activity that compensates for any increase in BMR (SACN, 2011). The energy expended in physical activity is lowest in the sickest patients, with sedated, ventilated patients usually expending <10% above BMR on physical activity. This can be highly variable however, especially in agitated patients (Frankenfield, 2006). In hospitalised individuals it is reasonable to assume that physical activity will be lower than habitual levels. For example, in preoperative patients activity accounts for 20% above BMR, while postoperatively physical activity may decrease to 5% BMR in the first few days, increasing to 15% BMR by days 9–12 (Kinney et al., 1968).

While it might be expected that physical activity will be increased in patients receiving active physiotherapy, moving painful or damaged limbs, or in those with abnormal neuromuscular function, this may not result in increased TEE as the patient compensates by resting or sleeping. For example, in patients with involuntary movement due to Parkinson's disease, TEE was not increased due to a reduction in the energy expended in voluntary physical activity (Toth et al., 1997).

As an individual recovers from illness, or once they are discharged from hospital, the component of TEE that is most likely to change is physical activity, assuming there have been no effects on neurological or muscular function. In the community some patients receiving nutritional support, irrespective of feeding route, may have similar activity levels to healthy individuals, whereas house bound or nursing home patients are likely to have physical activity levels similar to those of hospital patients. In the determination of energy requirements, regular assessment of habitual activity is important. However, the best method for assessing physical activity level objectively in clinical practice has yet to be determined (Frankenfield & Ashcraft, 2011). Multiplication factors for physical activity do exist (Taylor, 2007) but are as variable and open to misinterpretation as are stress factors, and thus a considerable degree of clinical judgement is required in their use.

Dietary induced thermogenesis

Dietary induced thermogenesis (DIT) usually accounts for 8–10% of TEE. In healthy individuals the main determinant of DIT is the energy content of the food, followed by the protein fraction (Benedict & Carpenter, 1918). The effects of injury and sepsis on DIT are unclear, although evidence suggests the effects are similar to those in healthy individuals (Westerterp 2004). While differences in DIT might be expected when comparing the parenteral with the enteral route, studies have so far failed to show a significant difference (Stokes & Hill, 1993). When enteral feed is given as a bolus, the effect on DIT is similar to that observed with food, i.e. an increase in total energy expenditure of 8–10%. In contrast, the continuous infusion of nutrients does not significantly increase resting energy expenditure over fasting level (Heymsfield et al., 1987). In the determination of energy requirements, there is rarely a need to make a separate adjustment for DIT as most prediction equations were derived from data collected from subjects who were receiving nutritional support during metabolic measurements. The effects of DIT are therefore already included in the equation.

Prediction methods

The most accurate methods for determining energy requirements are calorimetry and the doubly labelled water technique; however, these methods are generally too expensive and impractical for routine clinical use (Branson & Johannigman, 2004). In clinical practice therefore, energy requirements are usually estimated using published prediction methods. Three main methods for estimating energy requirements exist, all of which use some combination of body weight, age or sex. First, the factorial method involves estimating BMR from prediction equations and then adding factors for metabolic stress, physical activity and DIT (e.g. Taylor, 2007; Todorovic & Micklewright, 2011). Second, a method has been proposed by other organisations (ASPEN, 2002; NICE, 2006) where requirements are based on energy values per kilogram of body weight, adjusted for particular purposes, e.g. 25–30 kcal/kg body weight for bedridden patients (Table 6.1.2). Third, a number of disease specific regression equations have been derived, in particular for intensive care unit (ICU) patients (Frankenfield et al., 2005) and burns (Ireton-Jones et al., 1992).

All three methods are open to criticism, e.g. the Parenteral and Enteral Nutrition Group of the British Dietetic Association (PENG) (Todorovic & Micklewright, 2011) guidelines involve calculating BMR using the Henry equations (Henry, 2005) and adding one factor (0–60%) to take account of metabolic stress and another (10–25%) for activity and DIT. All these steps have the potential to introduce error. All BMR prediction equations were derived for use in healthy populations and therefore, their use in sick individuals is open to criticism. Furthermore, the data used to derive the stress factors are unclear and there is considerable scope for misinterpretation by inexperienced practitioners. While there is a lack of evidence to support this method, the approach is easy and takes account of the main factors that impact on an individual's energy requirements, i.e. weight, age, gender, physical activity level and DIT.

SECTION 6

Table 6.1.2 Guidelines for estimating nutritional requirements in stable patients

Energy (/kg/day)	Protein (/kg/day)	Micronutrients
25–35 kcal (105–147 kJ) (NICE, 2006)*	0.8–1.5 g (NICE, 2006)*	Provision of adequate electrolytes, minerals, micronutrients (allowing for any pre-existing deficits, excessive losses or increased demands) and fibre if appropriate (NICE, 2006)*
20–35 kcal (84–147 kJ) (ASPEN, 2002)†	0.8–2.0 g (ASPEN, 2002)†	Recommendations are made for specific nutrients based on route of administration For enteral nutrition, recommendations are based on the RDA/AI levels and for parenteral nutrition, recommendations were made on the assumption that patients had increased requirements (ASPEN, 2002)†

*For patients who are not severely ill or injured, nor at risk of refeeding syndrome.
†For unstressed adult patients with adequate organ function.
RDA, recommended daily allowance; AI, adequate intake.

While easy to use and based on the parameter with the greatest influence on BMR, the second method (kcal/kg body weight) does not account for changes in energy expenditure with age, gender or metabolic state, and it is unclear for people who are obese whether requirements should be calculated using actual or ideal body weight. Its applicability for depleted individuals has also been questioned. Similarly, there are no defined criteria for when to use 20, 25, 30 or 35 kcal/kg/day.

Disease specific equations are based on physiological variables that may change considerably over a short period of time, e.g. body temperature, heart rate and minute ventilation. While they may be more accurate in the specific population for which they were derived, these equations are also open to similar criticisms regarding validity, and currently there are no indications on how frequently requirements should be reviewed and amended in the light of any changes in these variables. Furthermore, it is yet to be determined if amending feeding regimens in response to changes in physiological variables results in beneficial outcomes.

The data used to derive all prediction methods are difficult to locate and none of the methods described above has been fully validated (Reeves & Capra, 2003). Furthermore, while prediction methods may provide adequate estimates of requirements for groups of patients, they all have a poor predictive value for individuals. Regardless of the method used, all estimates of energy requirements should be interpreted with care and used as a starting point only. Since any one of a number of factors might vary during a patient's illness and recovery, requirements should be reviewed and recalculated regularly to avoid either under- or over-feeding (NICE, 2006).

Protein (nitrogen)

In clinical practice the determination of protein (nitrogen) requirements is complicated by the fact that protein homeostasis is in a state of constant flux. In the healthy individual, protein requirements are dependent to a varying degree on a number of factors, including recent and long term protein and energy intakes, physical activity and the quality of the protein consumed (Calloway & Spector, 1955). A chronic lack of protein (and energy)

results in the body adapting to starvation in order to preserve body protein stores. In illness or injury, determination of protein requirements is further complicated by the metabolic state of the patient and the presence or absence of an inflammatory response. The maintenance of nitrogen balance depends on long term and recent nitrogen and energy intakes and clinical state in injury or illness. As a result, it is very difficult to predict requirements in any one individual at any particular time.

In severe chronic illness, such as cancer, chronic respiratory or cardiac failure, the presence of cachexia may further complicate the picture (see Chapter 7.15.9). Cachexia results in severe and specific loss of skeletal muscle mass, with relative preservation of visceral protein, as the body reprioritises protein metabolism away from the peripheral tissues and towards the liver. This preferential loss of skeletal muscle mass occurs even in the presence of poor dietary intake. In the short term this response may be beneficial as protein stores are liberated to mount the immune response and promote healing. However, in the longer term, or if the loss of muscle mass is excessive, this is detrimental to the patient (WHO/FAO/UNU, 2007).

In clinical practice a prescription consisting of 0.8–1.0 g of protein/kg/day is likely to provide sufficient protein for the majority of patients. In those who are metabolically stressed however, requirements may be higher, although current recommendations suggest that provision of more than 1.5–2.0 g of protein/kg/day is unlikely to be beneficial in terms of clinical outcome and may indeed be detrimental, particularly in patients who have had a prolonged period of poor intake and are therefore at risk of refeeding syndrome (NICE, 2006).

The largest nitrogen losses have been documented in sepsis, major trauma and burns. In these conditions nitrogen balance is almost impossible to achieve in the early catabolic phase post injury and currently there appears to be little to gain from providing nitrogen in excess of 1.5 g of protein/kg body weight in the critically ill (NICE, 2006), although this is open to debate (Frankenfield, 2006). The repletion of protein stores is most likely to be effective once a patient is in the recovery (anabolic) phase, is able to mobilise and when adequate amounts of energy are also provided (WHO/FAO/UNU, 2007).

Fluid

In health, fluid requirements are 25–35 mL/kg body weight. This is approximately 2–3 L for individuals within the normal range for body mass index (BMI). The metabolic response to acute illness and injury results in changes in fluid and electrolyte balance such that water and sodium are retained avidly. This often results in oedema in the early days of illness that may take up to 10 days to return to normal, or longer in the presence of sepsis or other complications. Recovery is accompanied by a return of the capacity to excrete any excess salt and water acquired during the acute phase.

In postsurgical patients there is evidence that poor fluid management (usually administration of excess fluid sodium and chloride) is a common cause of oedema, prolonged ileus and other complications, and has an adverse effect on patient outcome (Lobo et al., 2006). Patients are, therefore, extremely susceptible to errors in fluid prescription early after injury or surgery. The British Consensus Guidelines on Intravenous Fluid Therapy for Adult Surgical Patients (GIFTASUP) (Powell-Tuck et al., 2011) provide evidence based guidelines on the clinical management of fluid balance in surgical patients, those requiring nutritional support and patients with acute kidney injury (see Chapter 7.17.5). The guidelines recommend that food and fluids should be provided orally or enterally and intravenous infusions should be discontinued as soon as possible. In disease or following surgery, estimates of fluid requirements should take into account any losses resulting from pyrexia, drains, diarrhoea, burns, stomas and fistulae, and all sources of fluid should be considered (including fluids given with some intravenous drugs) to minimise the risks of overhydration, especially in patients receiving enteral or parenteral nutrition (see Chapter 6.6).

Currently there is insufficient evidence to provide guidelines on sodium and fluid requirements in very thin or obese individuals; therefore, patients at the extremes of BMI should be monitored closely for signs of over- or under-hydration, and fluid prescriptions adjusted accordingly.

Micronutrients

In the presence of illness or injury, micronutrient deficiencies may occur for a variety of reasons, although blood measurements may not be reliable markers of micronutrient status (Shenkin, 2000):

- Inadequate (or imbalanced) intake.
- Increased metabolic rate and increased number of biochemical reactions.
- Adverse effects of treatment.
- Increased oxidative stress.
- Losses from fistulae, burns, diarrhoea, dialysis.

The effects of micronutrient deficiency are non-specific and insidious, e.g. muscle weakness, anorexia and depression, and are commonly associated with acute and chronic illness. Suboptimal levels may impair function before signs of deficiency become evident and micronutrient deficiencies may therefore go undiagnosed in the presence of illness or injury (see Appendix A2).

In the absence of an adequate evidence base, guidelines for the provision of micronutrients to patients with acute or chronic illness (Arends et al., 2006) are non-specific in that they state that provision should be based on recommended daily amounts (RDAs) or adequate intakes (AIs) (Table 6.1.2). While recognising that these intakes are recommended for healthy populations rather than sick individuals, in the absence of evidence this pragmatic approach appears to be justified. In some patients with long term chronic conditions, e.g. cancer, multiple sclerosis and rheumatoid arthritis, excess micronutrient intake may be of concern, particularly in those taking a number of non-prescription supplements. During assessment the potential adverse effects of self dosing of alternative medicines and/or micronutrient supplements should always be considered.

With regard to nutritional support, most standard oral nutritional supplements and enteral feeds contain sufficient minerals and electrolytes to meet daily requirements for sodium, potassium, magnesium and phosphate (NICE, 2006), but only if the patient is receiving enough of the feed to meet all their energy needs. Since many patients are either receiving less than full nutrition from these products or have pre-existing deficits, high losses or increased demands, additional provision may be required. However, care is needed to avoid excessive provision in some patients, e.g. those with renal or liver impairment. Some specialised feeds are designed specifically to provide adequate electrolytes, vitamins and minerals in lower energy provision for patients with low total energy needs

Premixed parenteral nutrition (PN) bags contain very variable amounts of electrolytes and minerals, and care is needed to avoid giving PN with either inadequate or excessive electrolyte and/or mineral content (NICE, 2006). As with electrolytes and minerals, most standard oral and enteral feeds contain enough vitamins and trace elements to ensure that needs are met if the patient is taking enough feed to meet their daily energy needs. However, when this is not the case, further balanced micronutrient supplementation may be required, especially in those with pre-existing deficits, poor absorption, increased demands or high losses (NICE, 2006). Premixed PN bags invariably contain inadequate levels of some micronutrients and therefore additions need to be made prior to administration. The provision of PN without adequate micronutrient content must be avoided.

Special considerations

Estimating energy and protein requirements in obese patients

Energy

The factor that has the greatest influence on BMR is actual body weight (Horgan & Stubbs, 2003); however, some clinicians have recommended the use of adjusted weights

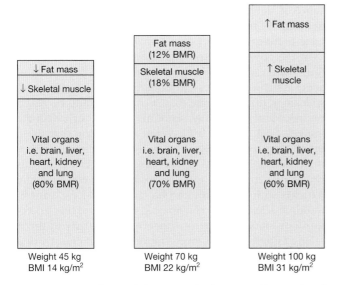

Figure 6.1.2 Effects of changes in body composition on basal metabolic rate

to calculate BMR from prediction equations in subjects at the extremes for BMI. Regardless of BMI, rapid weight loss is associated with increased complications and poor outcome in hospitalised patients (NICE, 2006); therefore, weight loss should not be a nutritional goal during acute illness or following injury, even in the obese. Figure 6.1.2 shows how changes in weight and body composition affect BMR. The excess body weight in obese individuals largely comprises tissue with a low metabolic rate and some clinicians have therefore recommended adjusting weight downwards to calculate BMR, e.g. 25% adjusted weight = (actual body weight × 0.25) + ideal body weight (Ireton-Jones, 2005). Other authors however, recommend the use of actual body weight (Krenitsky, 2005) since BMR prediction equations were derived from data on individuals across the range for BMI and actual rather than adjusted body weight was used to develop the equations. As there is no good evidence to support the use of adjusted body weight or specific cut-offs, clinical judgement is required to minimise the risks of over- or under-estimating energy requirements in obese individuals (BMI >30 kg/m²). In clinical practice, actual body weight should be used to estimate BMR in obese individuals (Frankenfield & Ashcraft, 2011), but the assignment of stress factors should be undertaken with caution (Todorovic & Micklewright, 2011). Alternatively, energy requirements can be calculated using 19–21 kcal/kg actual body weight (Glynn *et al*., 1999). However, it may be beneficial in some conditions, e.g. cancer of the breast and prostate, to aim for weight loss once a full recovery has been made in order to aid mobility and reduce the risk of recurrence (World Cancer Research Fund, 2007).

Protein

Since protein requirements are to a large extent determined by lean body mass, in obese patients there is an argument for using an adjustment to actual body weight

to calculate protein requirements, or to use ideal rather than actual body weight, although original work relating to this suggestion is difficult to locate.

Refeeding syndrome

There are several published regimens for managing patients at risk of refeeding syndrome. The lack of randomised controlled trials in this area however, means that management is based on consensus and expert opinion rather than evidence (Khan *et al*., 2011). Irrespective of which regimen is employed, the common principles are to prevent refeeding syndrome by cautious reintroduction of energy and correction of biochemical abnormalities. While some authors recommend correction of biochemical abnormalities prior to introduction of energy and other macronutrients (Crook *et al*., 2001), others recommend that both can occur in tandem without deleterious effects to the patient (NICE, 2006). There are currently no published randomised trial data to support either view. It is likely that the problems associated with refeeding are less likely to arise with oral nutritional support since starvation is usually accompanied by a loss of appetite; however, care should be taken in the prescription of oral nutritional supplements, particularly in the area of eating disorders (NICE, 2006). Underweight individuals tend to lose muscle and fat stores while preserving tissues with a high metabolic rate, i.e. brain, liver, heart and kidney. On a body weight basis, their metabolic rate is about 25% higher than that of normal weight individuals and some clinicians have used this as a rationale to use ideal or usual body weight instead of actual body weight when calculating BMR. For a full discussion of the management of severely depleted individuals, see the report (MARSIPAN) by the Royal College of Psychiatrists and the Royal college of Physicians (2010) (see Chapter 6.4).

Estimating requirements for patients with abnormal fluid status

Oedema and ascites increase body weight without increasing metabolically active tissue. In the presence of overhydration therefore, dry weight should be measured after paracentesis, drainage of ascites or post dialysis, and used to calculate BMR. In those patients where excess fluid cannot be removed, consider using the last recorded weight prior to developing ascites or oedema or estimating dry weight using the equation:

Estimated dry weight = Actual body weight
    − (Weight of ascites + Weight of oedema)

Estimating energy requirements for critically ill patients

In comparison with other clinical populations, there are considerably more studies measuring the energy expenditure of critically ill patients. The evidence base for protein provision in critically ill patients is more limited however, and for micronutrient provision there is even less evidence. Reported energy requirements for ICU patients vary considerably, in part due to the heterogeneity of the different ICU populations studied and in part due to differences in definitions of critical illness and/or the presence of sepsis. In addition to the factors that affect energy expenditure in general, e.g. age, gender and weight, the determination of energy requirements in ICU patients is complicated by a number of additional metabolic and management factors, such as hyperglycaemia, the presence or absence of sedation, ventilation mode or the fraction of inspired oxygen. In the ICU setting, the estimation of an individual patient's energy requirements can be particularly challenging.

In bed bound artificially ventilated patients, BMR is frequently increased; however, TEE is not usually elevated, mainly because of minimal physical activity and/or sedation (SACN, 2011). In the most acutely ill patients however, e.g. severe burns, TEE may be transiently elevated above normal (Bessey & Wilmore, 1988). For a full discussion of nutritional requirements in critically ill patients, see Chapter 7.17.1.

Further reading

Boullata J, Williams J, Cottrell F, Hudson L, Compher C. (2007) Accurate determination of energy needs in hospitalized patients. *Journal of the American Dietetic Association* 107: 393–401.

British Artificial Nutrition Survey. (2010) *Artificial Nutrition Support in the UK 2000–2009*. Redditch: British Association for Parenteral and Enteral Nutrition.

European Society for Parenteral and Enteral Nutrition (ESPEN). (2007) Guidelines on adult enteral nutrition. *British Journal of Nutrition* 98: 253–259.

Stanga Z, Brunner A, Leuenberger M, *et al.* (2008) Nutrition in clinical practice—the refeeding syndrome: illustrative cases and guidelines for prevention and treatment *European Journal of Clinical Nutrition* 62(6): 687–694.

Weekes CE. (2007) Controversies in the determination of energy requirements. *Proceedings of the Nutrition Society* 66: 367–377.

References

ASPEN Board of Directors and the Clinical Guidelines Task Force. (2002) Guidelines for the use of parenteral and enteral nutrition in adult and paediatric patients. *Journal of Parenteral and Enteral Nutrition* 26 (Suppl 1).

Arends J, Bodoky G, Bozzetti F, *et al.* (2006) ESPEN guidelines on enteral nutrition: non-surgical oncology. *Clinical Nutrition* 25:, 245–259.

Benedict FG, Carpenter TM. (1918) *Food Ingestion and Energy Transformation With Special Reference to the Stimulating Effects of Nutrients*. Pub. No. 261. Carnegie Institution of Washington.

Bessey PQ, Wilmore DW. (1988) The burned patient. In: *Nutrition and Metabolism in Patient Care*. London: WB Saunders, pp. 672–700.

Calloway DH, Spector H. (1995) Nitrogen utilization during caloric restriction. II. The effect of variation in nitrogen intake. *Journal of Nutrition* 56(4): 545–554.

Crook MA, Hally V, Panteli JV. (2001) The importance of the refeeding syndrome. *Nutrition* 17(7–8): 632–637.

Elia M. (2005) Insights into energy requirements in disease. *Public Health Nutrition* 8(7A): 1037–1052.

Frankenfield D. (2006) Energy expenditure and protein requirements after traumatic injury. *Nutrition in Clinical Practice* 21(5): 430–437.

Frankenfield DC, Ashcraft CM. (2011) Estimating energy needs in nutrition support patients> *Journal of Parenteral and Enteral Nutrition* 35(5): 563–570.

Frankenfield DC, Roth-Yousy L, Compher C. (2005) Comparison of predictive equations for resting metabolic rate in healthy non-obese and obese adults: a systematic review. *Journal of the American Dietetic Association* 105(5): 775–789.

Glynn CC, Greene GW, Winkler MF, *et al.* (1999) Predictive versus measured energy expenditure using limits of agreement analysis in hospitalised, obese patients. *Journal of Parenteral and Enteral Nutrition* 23: 147–154.

Harris JA, Benedict FG. (1919) *Biometric Studies of Basal Metabolism in Man*. Publication number 297. Washington, DC: Carnegie Institute of Washington

Henry CJK. (2005) Basal metabolic rate studies in humans: measurement and development of new equations. *Public Health Nutrition* 8(7A): 1133–1152.

Heymsfield SB, Casper K, Funfar J. (1987) Physiologic response and clinical implications of nutrition support. *American Journal of Cardiology* 60(12): 75G–81G.

Horgan GW, Stubbs J. (2003) Predicting basal metabolic rate in the obese is difficult. *European Journal of Clinical Nutrition* 57(2): 335–340.

Ireton-Jones CS. (2005) Adjusted body weight, Con: Why adjust body weight in energy-expenditure calculations? *Nutrition in Clinical Practice* 20: 474–479.

Ireton-Jones CS, Turner WW, Liepa GU, *et al.* (1992) Equations for the estimation of energy expenditure in patients with burns with special reference to ventilatory status. *Journal of Burn Care and Rehabilitation* 13: 330–333.

Khan LUR, Ahmed J, Khan S, MacFie J. (2011) Refeeding syndrome: A literature review. *Gastroenterology Research and Practice* ID 410971.

Kinney JM, Long CL, Gump FE, Duke JH Jr. (1968) Tissue composition of weight loss in surgical patients. I. Elective operation. *Annals of Surgery* 168(3): 459–474.

Krenitsky J. (2005) Adjusted body weight, Pro: Evidence to support the use of adjusted body weight in calculating calorie requirements. *Nutrition in Clinical Practice* 20: 468–473.

Kulstad R, Schoeller DA. (2007). The energetic of wasting diseases. *Current Opinions in Clinical Nutrition and Metabolic Care* 10(4): 488–493.

Lobo DN, Macafee DAL, Allison SP. (2006) How perioperative fluid balance influences postoperative outcomes. *Best Practice and Research Clinical Anaesthesiology* 20(3): 439–455.

National Institute for Health and Care Excellence (NICE). (2006) Nutrition support in adults Oral nutrition support, enteral tube feeding and parenteral nutrition. Clinical Guideline 32. Available at www.nice.org last accessed 21 June 2012.

Powell-Tuck J, Gosling P, Lobo D, *et al.* (2011) British Consensus Guidelines on Intravenous Fluid Therapy for Adult Surgical Patients. Available at www.bapen.org.uk/pdfs/bapen_pubs/giftasup .pdf. Accessed 21 June 2012.

Ramirez-Zea M. (2005). Validation of three predictive equations for basal metabolic rate in adults. *Public Health Nutrition* 8(7A): 1213–1228.

Reeves MM, Capra S. (2003) Predicting energy requirements in the clinical setting: are current methods evidence based? *Nutrition Reviews* 61(4): 143–151.

Royal College of Psychiatrists and the Royal College of Physicians. (2010) Report from the MARSIPAN group. *MARSIPAN: Management of Really Sick Patients with Anorexia Nervosa*. College Report, CR162. London: Royal College of Psychiatrists and Royal College of Physicians.

Schofield WN. (1985) Predicting basal metabolic rate, new standards and review of previous work. *Human Nutrition: Clinical Nutrition* 39: 5–41.

Scientific Advisory Committee on Nutrition (SACN). (2011) Dietary recommendations for energy. Working Group Report. Available at

SECTION 6

www.sacn.gov.uk/pdfs/sacn_energy_report_author_date_10th _oct_fin.pdf. Accessed 22 March 2012.

Shenkin A. (2000) Micronutrients in the severely-injured patient. *Proceedings of the Nutrition Society* 59: 451–456.

Stokes MA, Hill GL. (1993) Total energy expenditure in patients with Crohn's disease: measurement by the combined body scan technique. *Journal of Parenteral and Enteral Nutrition* 17(1): 3–7.

Streat SJ, Beddoe AH, Hill GL. (1987) Aggressive nutritional support does not prevent protein loss despite fat gain in septic intensive care patients. *Journal of Trauma* 27: 262–266.

Taylor SJ. (2007) *Energy and Nitrogen Requirements in Disease States*. London: Smith-Gordon.

Todorovic V, Micklewright A, On behalf of the Parenteral and Enteral Nutrition Group of the British Dietetic Association (PENG). (2011). A pocket guide to clinical nutrition. Available at www .peng.org.uk/publications/pocket-guide.html. Accessed 20 June 2012.

Toth MJ, Fishman PS, Poehlman ET. (1997) Free-living daily energy expenditure in patients with Parkinson's disease. *Neurology* 48(1): 88–91.

Westerterp KR. (2004) Diet induced thermogenesis. *Nutrition and Metabolism* 1(1): 5.

WHO/FAO/UNU Expert Consultation. (2007) *Protein and amino acid requirements in human nutrition, Joint WHO/FAO/UNU Expert Consultation*. World Health Organization Technical Report Series 935 Geneva: World Health Organization.

World Cancer Research Fund. (2007) *Food, Nutrition, Physical Activity, and the Prevention of Cancer: A Global Perspective*. Washington DC: AICR. Available at www.wcrf.org. Accessed 21 December 2012.

6.2

Malnutrition

Rebecca Stratton and Marinos Elia

Key points

■ Malnutrition adversely affects physical and psychological health, and impairs recovery from disease, increasing mortality, complications, hospital stay and use of other healthcare resources.

■ Malnutrition is common and costly but is often unrecognised and untreated.

■ Routine and regular screening is recommended to improve the detection and treatment of malnutrition.

■ Screening should be undertaken using a quick and simple to use, valid, evidence based tool with a care plan attached.

■ Treatment of malnutrition should be undertaken promptly with appropriate nutritional support; energy, protein and other nutrients, including micronutrients, should be considered.

Malnutrition can be defined as '*a state of nutrition in which a deficiency or excess (or imbalance) of energy, protein and other nutrients causes measurable adverse effects on tissue/body form (body shape, size, composition), body function and clinical outcome*' (Elia, 2000, p. 2).

Malnutrition is a broad term that includes not only protein energy malnutrition (both over- and undernutrition), but malnutrition of other nutrients, such as micronutrients. The adverse effects of malnutrition will mostly respond to nutritional treatment. This chapter concentrates on protein energy undernutrition (described here as malnutrition).

Prevalence of malnutrition and at risk groups

Malnutrition is common and is a major clinical and public health problem in the UK (Elia, 2000; Elia & Russell, 2009). At any given point in time, >3 million people in the UK are malnourished with most (~93%) living in the community (Elia & Russell, 2009). Although malnutrition among people in hospitals was identified over three decades ago (Bistrian *et al.*, 1974; Hill *et al.*, 1977), it remains a common and often unrecognised problem (Elia, 2003; Stratton *et al.*, 2003). The British Association for Parenteral and Enteral Nutrition (BAPEN) national screening weeks have shown that approximately one-third of hospital admissions are at risk of malnutrition (Russell & Elia, 2010). Similar estimates of the prevalence

of malnutrition in hospitalised infants and children exist (Stratton *et al.*, 2003; Gerasimidis *et al.*, 2011; Joosten *et al.*, 2011).

The prevalence of malnutrition depends on the criteria used to define it and varies with age, the associated clinical condition and the type of treatments (including surgery) being undertaken. The frequency of malnutrition, and the risk of developing malnutrition, is typically highest in:

• Infants, young children and the elderly.
• Patients with malignancy, gastrointestinal, respiratory or renal disease.
• Those with multiple comorbidities, including the critically ill.
• Individuals undergoing complex surgery, transplantation or treatment for burns.

Once in hospital, deterioration in nutritional status often occurs unless action is taken to prevent it. Studies show that between 30% and 90% of adults and children lose weight whilst in hospital (Stratton *et al.*, 2003). This is partly because malnutrition is often unrecognised and untreated, frequently going undetected. Measurement and documentation of important nutritional information, including body mass index (BMI), unintentional weight loss and recent food intake, in hospital inpatients, outpatients and in many other care settings is often lacking (Elia, 2000; Cawood *et al.*, 2008; Volkert *et al.*, 2010). This is partly due to the absence of formal screening

Manual of Dietetic Practice, Fifth Edition. Edited by Joan Gandy.
© 2014 The British Dietetic Association. Published 2014 by John Wiley & Sons, Ltd.
Companion Website: www.manualofdieteticpractice.com

programmes that link the recognition of malnutrition with treatment plans.

At any point in time, only about 2% of over 3 million adults at risk of malnutrition are in hospital, with 5% in care homes and the remainder in the community (2–3% in sheltered housing) (Elia *et al.*, 2010). National and local surveys suggest 15–30% of outpatients, 5–23% of patients visiting a general practitioner (GP), 25% patients receiving district nursing care, 30–40% of care home residents and 10–14% of individuals in sheltered housing are at risk of malnutrition (Russell & Elia, 2010; Stratton & Elia, 2010). The elderly are a group at particular risk, as suggested by a secondary analysis of a national survey which found that 12% of free living and 21% of institutionalised elderly are at risk of malnutrition and that geographical inequalities exist (higher rates of malnutrition in the North than the South of England) (Elia & Stratton, 2005). In addition, malnutrition is more common in those from more deprived areas (Stratton & Elia, 2006). In community settings, as in hospitals, malnutrition is often undetected and untreated (Cawood *et al.*, 2008; Volkert *et al.*, 2010). An increasingly ageing population, the pressure on healthcare resources (NHS QIPP challenge) (Department of Health, 2010c) and the new community led NHS structure (Department of Health, 2010a) mean a greater proportion of sick and debilitated individuals will be cared for outside hospital, and services for managing malnutrition will be commissioned by community based Clinical Commissioning Groups.

Causes of malnutrition

In the UK, the primary cause of malnutrition is disease, hence the term disease related malnutrition. Other causes for malnutrition include poverty and deprivation, and behavioural problems in children. Disease related malnutrition arises when nutritional intake does not meet nutritional needs because of decreased dietary intake, increased nutritional requirements or an impaired ability to absorb or utilise nutrients.

Insufficient dietary intake is the main reason for malnutrition developing and progressing, and there are many factors that limit nutritional intake (Figure 6.2.1). Broadly these factors can be divided into two types:

- Disease related factors that reduce intake despite availability of food.
- Other factors such as inadequate availability, quality or presentation of foods that reduce intake.

Numerous studies across many different diagnostic groups have documented energy, protein and micronutrient intakes to be insufficient to meet nutritional requirements, particularly in institutionalised patients. Also, studies have shown that food in institutions (hospitals, care homes) is often not consumed and therefore wasted, sometimes because catering practices do not meet the needs of the sick (see Chapter 4.4.1). Nutritional support (oral nutritional supplements, enteral tube feeding, parenteral nutrition) is often not used early enough or

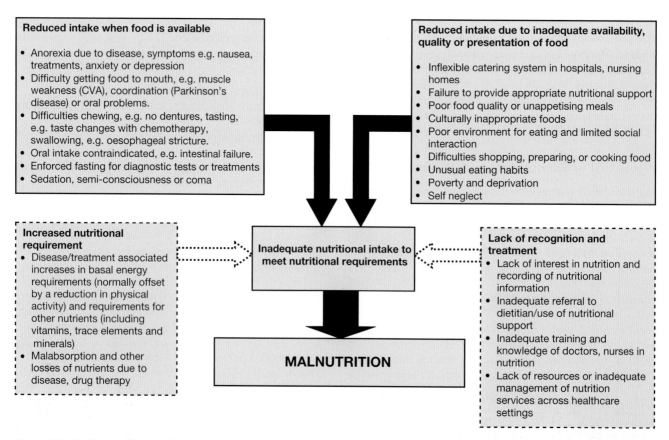

Figure 6.2.1 Causes of malnutrition

frequently enough to prevent or treat malnutrition, despite a large and growing evidence base that suggests benefits when nutritional support is used appropriately. This is increasingly an issue as current economic constraints mean budget holders may choose to withhold prescribed nutritional care, failing to recognise that greater costs result when leaving malnutrition untreated (increased costly hospital admissions and complications such as infections and pressure ulcers).

Malnutrition may also arise if total requirements for energy and nutrients (protein, vitamins, minerals and trace elements) are increased with disease, after trauma and surgery, and with some treatments, e.g. drug therapy and chemotherapy. Increments in basal energy metabolism occur in a number of disease states, postoperatively and in sepsis and burns patients. However, in many cases this is offset by reductions in physical activity (Gibney et al., 1997; Jebb, 1997) so that total energy expenditure is not substantially increased (See Chapter 6.1). Increased nutrient losses and inability to absorb nutrients also elevate requirements, increasing the risk of malnutrition developing.

Consequences of malnutrition

Malnutrition has a diversity of effects, influencing every system of the body. It has many adverse consequences on body structure and function, physical and psychological health, and on recovery and outcome after disease and injury, including surgery (Stratton et al., 2003). Malnutrition results in loss of body structure with weight loss due to loss of fat and lean tissue, including organ mass. In children, malnutrition will also impair growth and development, leading to stunting and/or wasting. However, malnutrition is more than a reduction in nutritional status as there are impairments in physical and psychological health and function that include the following:

- Impaired immune function increasing susceptibility to infection and sepsis.
- Delayed wound healing and increased risk of pressure ulcers.
- Muscle wasting and weakness that may affect:
  - Respiratory function – weakened respiratory muscles may make it difficult for a patient to cough and expectorate effectively, increasing the risk of chest infection. This may also make it harder to wean a patient from artificial ventilation.
  - Cardiac function – this may be impaired, resulting in reduced cardiac output and liability to heart failure.
  - Mobility – weakness of skeletal muscles delays a return to full mobility. Reduced mobility increases the risk of thromboembolism and pressure ulcers.
- Altered gastrointestinal structure and function, impairing digestion, absorption and the gut barrier.
- Apathy and depression, leading to loss of morale and reduced will to recover.
- General sense of weakness and illness, which impairs appetite and physical ability to eat, and hence tends to perpetuate and worsen the state of malnutrition.
- Adverse effects on learning and behaviour in children, with potential long term deficits in cognition.
- Poor libido, fertility, pregnancy outcome and mother–child interactions.

These physical and psychological consequences of malnutrition increase susceptibility to disease, impair clinical outcome and increase healthcare use and costs. Individuals identified as being at risk of malnutrition have:

- Increased risk of mortality and complications during and after hospitalisation.
- Longer hospital stays and greater hospital costs.
- Greater requirement for healthcare post discharge.
- Increased risk of admission to hospital and more visits to the GP.

Consequently, increased use of healthcare resources means malnutrition is very expensive. It is estimated that in 2007 the annual expenditure on disease related malnutrition in the UK exceeded £13 billion, which when extrapolated to the European Union, approximates to €120 billion (Elia & Stratton, 2009; Ljungqvist et al., 2010).

Detection of malnutrition

The rationale for establishing a policy to routinely detect malnutrition is that it:

- Is a common and costly problem.
- Has many adverse short and long term effects on health, function and recovery.
- Is treatable in most cases.

For many years, malnutrition has been under detected and under treated, and for this reason, many national organisations recommend that malnutrition be routinely identified using screening. These include the British Dietetic Association (BDA, 2009), Royal College of Physicians (2002), BAPEN (Elia, 2003), NHS Quality Improvement Scotland (2003), National Institute for Health and Care Excellence (NICE, 2006) and the Department of Health (2008; 2010a; 2010b) Legislation in England [Regulation 14 of the Health and Social Care Act 2008 (Department of Health, 2008)] states that registered organisations have a duty to safeguard service users from malnutrition and dehydration, to identify poor nutrition and dehydration with nutritional screening and to take action to treat it. The Care Quality Commission (CQC) is the regulator in England that continuously monitors registered care providing organisations and their compliance with this aspect of the law.

It has also been suggested that obesity should be routinely identified, ideally using the same screening procedure (Elia, 2003). Obesity has many health risks (see Chapter 7.13.1), but treatment of obesity should not generally be undertaken in those who are acutely unwell. Such patients may still be at risk of malnutrition due to weight loss or limited dietary intake, e.g. nil by mouth post stroke, and should be treated accordingly.

SECTION 6

Table 6.2.1 Important characteristics of a screening tool for malnutrition

Practical	Quick and easy to complete and to understand
	Has a range of alternative measures for when weight or height cannot be measured
Universal	Can be used in all adults of all ages (including the elderly), including the sick and healthy
	Is applicable across different care settings (hospital, GP practice, nursing home, free living)
	Allows continuity of care
	Can be used for public health purposes
Reliable	Good reproducibility between users
	Good internal reliability
Valid	Content, face, internal, concurrent and predictive validity
Evidence based and independently peer reviewed	
Linked to a care plan for treatment	Facilitates nursing and other staff initiating appropriate monitoring or treatment and referral to the dietitian or nutrition support team
Developed by a multidisciplinary group for use by all healthcare professionals	
Acceptable to patients and healthcare professionals	

Screening

Screening is a rapid, simple and general procedure, often carried out at first contact with an individual, to detect those with significant risk of malnutrition, so that action plans for monitoring and/or treatment can be implemented. Some individuals may need help or advice with eating and drinking; others may need special diets and a referral to a dietitian for expert advice. Screening should be routinely and regularly undertaken in hospitals, nursing and residential care and in other primary care settings, e.g. patients seen by district nurses, at risk groups or newly registered patients in GP practices. The frequency of screening and any associated monitoring and treatment will depend on the patient group, the healthcare setting and the resources available.

Screening is a multidisciplinary responsibility and can be undertaken by nurses, doctors, dietitians or other healthcare professionals. Screening, using a test or tool, should be part of a screening programme that includes a full range of activities from identification of risk with the tool, to diagnosis and treatments. Screening can precede nutritional assessment, which is a more in depth and specific evaluation of those individuals at risk and typically undertaken by a dietitian (see Chapter 2.2). Nutritional assessment may be required in the case of serious nutritional problems, to identify micronutrient status or to undertake other detailed dietary investigations. Although dietitians have the expertise, it is neither practical nor cost effective for them to assess the nutritional status of every patient admitted to hospital and they are unlikely to come into direct contact with many of those at risk in the community (often only after problems have arisen). Therefore, identification of people with, or at risk of, malnutrition requires a locally agreed policy and the assistance of other health professionals.

There are many screening tools in use in clinical practice, but it is important to use a tool that meets the important characteristics listed in Table 6.2.1. A screening tool for malnutrition should attempt to establish the following in the most objective way possible:

- Chronic protein energy status, e.g. body mass index (BMI), weight for height, weight and height for age.
- Any recent changes in protein energy status, e.g. weight loss, inadequate dietary intake.
- Any likely future changes in protein energy status, e.g. likelihood of inadequate dietary intake and weight loss.

When objective measures are not feasible, e.g. in an acutely unwell, bed bound individual, or there is concern about their interpretation, e.g. oedema, alternative measures should be considered. As part of the screening programme, the underlying cause of changes in nutritional status, e.g. disease or condition, psychosocial issues and behavioural problems, should also be established and treated if appropriate, e.g. for those who are terminally ill, active treatment may not be undertaken. Although there are many factors that increase an individual's risk of malnutrition, e.g. gastrointestinal symptoms, metabolic stress and pressure ulcers, they do so by affecting the adequacy of nutritional intake relative to an individual's nutritional needs. In most cases, nutritional intake is reduced, nutritional needs are not met and the result is that weight is lost. Therefore, a screening tool is able to assess risk of malnutrition simply by identifying chronic protein energy status, e.g. BMI in adults, and previous and predicted recent changes in status, e.g. weight loss and reduced dietary intake. Thus, screening can reflect aspects of an individual's nutritional status encompassing:

- Past, e.g. unintentional weight loss and lack of nutritional intake.
- Present, e.g. BMI.
- Future, e.g. potential for lack of nutritional intake and weight loss.

The past can be most easily assessed using unintended weight loss over a defined time scale, e.g. 3 months. This is assessed in terms of the extent of unintentional body weight loss, ideally as a percentage of usual body weight, e.g. >10% of weight lost in 3 months. Three to 6 months is the most common time period over which to assess weight loss, although it can be a shorter, e.g. 1 week, or longer, e.g. 1 year, time interval. Weight loss is also a marker for inadequacy of nutritional intake. No nutritional intake for >5 days (without disease) equates to a weight loss of 5–10% (Elia, 2003). Detailed dietary history is not taken as part of screening as it is time consuming and requires a nutritional expert, e.g. dietitian, to undertake (screening is not usually undertaken by dietitians). Detailed dietary information may be obtained as part of nutritional assessment.

The present or current status of an individual can be objectively identified using BMI. This is a simple and reproducible index that reflects body composition and function. A BMI of $<20 \, kg/m^2$ is considered to be underweight and a BMI of $<18.5 \, kg/m^2$ as severely underweight. Individuals with a BMI of $>30 \, kg/m^2$ are considered obese. These are nationally recognised and accepted cut-offs for BMI and are based on the loss of physiological function and wellbeing, and increased clinical risk as BMI decreases. These cut-offs are consistently recommended for all adults, including elderly people. However, these cut-offs denote only risk of malnutrition, as some individuals may be constitutionally thin, fit and well despite having a low BMI.

When screening for risk of malnutrition, particularly in the acute setting, consideration of the future likelihood of deterioration in nutritional status (poor, inadequate nutritional intake leading to weight loss) is needed. For example, a free living individual suffers a stroke and is admitted to hospital, unable to swallow and eat. Despite having a desirable BMI and no history of weight loss, they are at risk of malnutrition as they will be unable to eat for >5 days. During this timeframe, even an individual without disease or injury would lose 5–10% of body weight, feel unwell and lose muscle mass (Elia, 2003). Similarly, those who suffer severe injury are unconscious and have intestinal failure, and many others with severe, acute illness are at risk of malnutrition due to a prolonged inability to eat or drink. These individuals will usually require nutritional assessment by a dietitian or nutrition support team and the provision of artificial nutritional support.

Similar principles apply to screening for malnutrition in paediatrics, although there is more complexity as consideration of growth and development is required. Anthropometric measurements have been widely used to screen for malnutrition in children. These include weight for age, height for age, BMI for age, weight for height and mid upper arm circumference (see Chapter 3.8.2). The new WHO charts for children (aged 0–4 years) are purported to reflect optimal growth in children of all ethnic groups because of the striking similarities in results obtained from the countries that contributed data (the USA, Norway, Oman, Brazil, India and Ghana) (Wright et al., 2010). The charts are based on anthropometric measurements obtained from children who were breast-fed for about 6 months by relatively affluent, non-smoking mothers who experienced a healthy pregnancy. The charts, which have separate sections for preterm babies, infants aged 0–1 years and older children, have been widely adopted in the UK and other countries. Establishing the most appropriate cut-off points for unintentional weight change in children of different ages can be difficult because growth rates vary considerably with age. In contrast to adults, where weight maintenance is considered to be normal, failure to increase weight over even a short period of time, e.g. 1 month, in a rapidly growing child may represent substantial growth failure, and a 5% weight loss over the same period can be of serious concern. In clinical practice, rapid changes in weight, dietary intake and disease related factors might all need to be taken into account. A variety of screening tools have been developed for use in children (mostly in hospital settings), (e.g. Sermet-Gaudelus et al., 2000; Gerasimidis et al., 2010; Hulst et al., 2010), although a universally accepted tool is lacking. Discrepancies between the currently available tools are expected because they incorporate different criteria to detect malnutrition (see Chapter 3.8.2).

Individuals with other nutritional concerns or problems may need to be referred to a dietitian for more detailed evaluation of the extent or risk of nutritional depletion (Chapter 2.2). Particular attention should be paid to the aspects shown in Table 6.2.2. The nature and extent of these problems will determine the way malnutrition is managed or averted. All individuals requiring detailed nutritional assessment and artificial nutritional support need to be referred to a dietitian or nutrition support team (see Chapter 6.3 and Chapter 6.4).

Setting up a screening programme

To facilitate a screening programme, which includes routine screening, monitoring, assessment and treatment plans, and may include referral to the dietitian, the following are suggested:

- Establish a policy locally that ensures that screening is undertaken and repeated as appropriate (and specifies areas, if any, that are exempt from routine screening).
- Agree on the screening tool to be used locally and the resources available for a screening programme across healthcare settings.
- Devise locally agreed care plans for monitoring and treating those identified by screening.
- Ensure equipment required for screening, e.g. weighing scales, stadiometers, tape measure and callipers, is available and regularly calibrated where appropriate.

Table 6.2.2   Aspects relating to malnutrition to be considered in nutrition assessment

Dietary aspects	Adequacy of current intake Recent changes in food intake Appetite Existence of factors likely to impair food intake
Clinical aspects	Presence of factors likely to increase nutrient requirements Presence of factors likely to increase nutrient losses Acute or chronic disease affecting the gastrointestinal tract Use of drugs and other treatments affecting food intake or nutrient utilisation
Physical aspects	Signs of muscle wasting, emaciation or oedema Presence of pressure ulcers (stages I–IV) or other wounds (see Chapter 7.17.5)
Anthropometric aspects	Degree and rapidity of any unintended weight loss BMI, growth (in infants and children) Evidence of muscle wasting, e.g. reduced mid arm muscle circumference or grip strength
Psychosocial aspects	Depression, anxiety or apathy Social isolation Poverty

BMI, body mass index.

- Establish the criteria for those requiring more detailed nutritional assessment and dietetic referral (this will vary locally depending on the resources available).
- Set up systems for the documentation of the results of screening, monitoring and treatment.
- Regularly audit the efficacy of the screening programme.

Malnutrition universal screening tool ('MUST')

Although there are several screening tools available for adults, the Malnutrition Universal Screening Tool ('MUST') is mentioned here as an example because it meets all the key characteristics for a screening tool outlined in Table 6.2.1. 'MUST' was developed by the Malnutrition Advisory Group, a multidisciplinary group of the BAPEN and is supported by the BDA, the Royal College of Nursing, the Registered Nursing Homes Association and the Royal College of Physicians (England). In Scotland, screening of hospital patients is a standard and 'MUST' is the tool suggested for use (NHS Quality Improvement Scotland, 2003). NICE (2006) also recommends the use of 'MUST'. The tool has been extensively peer reviewed by many national organisations and independent healthcare practitioners for use in clinical settings and for public health.

'MUST' (Figure 6.2.2) is an evidence based tool (Elia, 2003) that has been designed to help identify adults who are at risk of malnutrition, as well as those who are obese. It has not been designed to detect poor vitamin and mineral status. 'MUST' involves identification of chronic protein energy status (BMI), change in status (unintentional weight loss) and the presence of an acute disease resulting, or likely to result, in no dietary intake for >5 days. It has been developed for use in all adults, including the elderly, the sick and healthy, free living individuals and those in healthcare, i.e.:

- Hospital wards.
- Outpatient clinics.
- General practice.
- Community settings, e.g. patients receiving care at home and in nursing or other care homes.
- Public health.

'MUST' can be applied to all types of patient groups, is easy and rapid to use and can be used by the multidisciplinary team; it is reproducible, internally consistent and valid. It can be used in situations where weight or height cannot be measured, providing a range of alternatives, including reported or documented measurements, other surrogate measures, subjective criteria and clinical judgement. The tool categorises individuals into low, medium and high risk of malnutrition, and identifies the obese. 'MUST' provides guidelines for care plans, which should be modified to suit local policy and resources.

Practicalities

'MUST' is a five step screening tool to identify adults who are malnourished or at risk of malnutrition, and it includes simple management guidelines that can be used to develop a care plan. The five steps are shown in Figure 6.2.2 and are as follows:

Step 1

Measure height and weight to calculate BMI and a BMI score. If unable to measure weight and/or height, use alternative procedures:

- Recently documented or self reported height and weight (if reliable and realistic).
- If the individual is unable to report their height, a surrogate measure to estimate height, e.g. ulna length (see Appendix A7) or knee height.

if weight and height cannot be obtained, use mid upper arm circumference (MUAC) to estimate BMI. If MUAC is <23.5 cm, BMI is likely to be <20 kg/m². If MUAC is >32.0 cm, BMI is likely to be >30 kg/m².

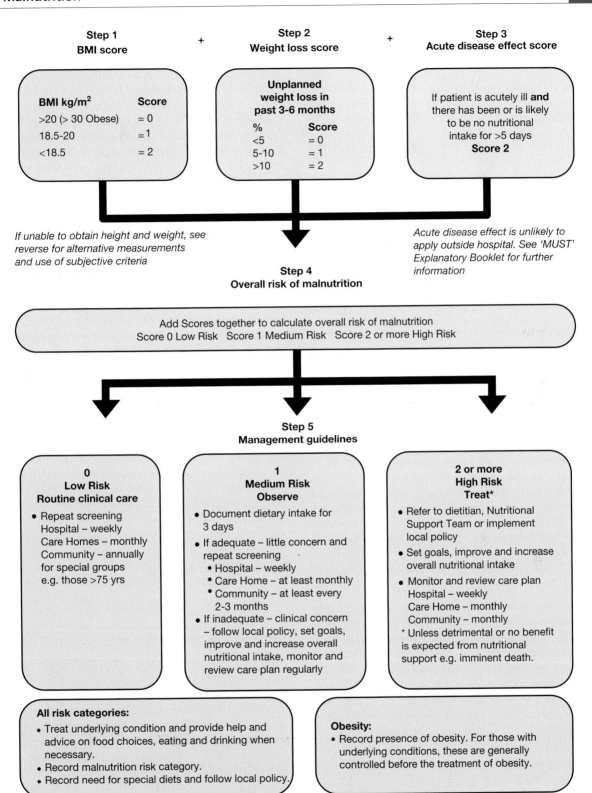

Figure 6.2.2 The Malnutrition Universal Screening Tool ('MUST') [source: BAPEN (British Association for Parenteral and Enteral Nutrition) 2013. Reproduced with permission of the British Association for Parenteral and Enteral Nutrition (www.bapen.org.uk)]

Step 2

Note percentage unplanned weight loss and give a weight loss score. If recent weight loss cannot be calculated:

- Use self reported weight loss (if reliable and realistic).
- Changes in MUAC can also be used as an approximate indication of weight loss, e.g. a 10% reduction in MUAC suggests a weight loss of 10%.

Step 3

Establish if there is an acute disease effect and score (for patients who are acutely ill and for whom there has been or is likely to be no nutritional intake for >5 days – unlikely to apply outside of hospital).

Step 4

Add scores from Steps 1–3 to obtain the overall risk of malnutrition.

Step 5

Use management guidelines and local policy to develop appropriate care plans.

If BMI or weight loss (Steps 1 and 2) cannot be obtained, the following criteria can assist professional judgement of whether an individual is at risk of malnutrition (medium and high risk) or not (low risk):

- *BMI* – obtain a clinical impression of whether the individual is very thin (obvious wasting)/thin, or is of acceptable weight, overweight or obese.
- *Unplanned weight loss* – obtain a clinical impression of whether the individual has lost weight. Have clothes and/or jewellery become loose fitting? Is there a history of decreased food intake, reduced appetite or swallowing problems over the past 3–6 months? Is there evidence of underlying disease, psychosocial problems or physical disabilities that are likely to cause weight loss?

Care should be taken when interpreting BMI or percentage weight loss in individuals with fluid disturbances, plaster casts, amputations and critical illness, and in pregnant or lactating women (Elia, 2003). For more information on undertaking 'MUST', charts to calculate BMI and weight loss scores, electronic applications, use of alternative measures and screening individuals in whom extra care in interpretation is needed, see www.bapen.org.uk and Elia (2003).

Self screening with 'MUST'

A patient friendly version of 'MUST' has been developed for adults to screen themselves for malnutrition. Self screening in outpatients has been shown to be reproducible, have good concurrent validity with healthcare professional screening and to be easy for a wide variety of individuals to complete (Stratton *et al.*, 2011). Self screening with 'MUST' has also been shown to predict patient outcome (Cawood *et al.*, 2011). Further work is ongoing to understand how best to implement self screening within different care settings as part of the overall management of malnutrition.

Benefits of implementing a screening programme

Considering the enormous costs of disease related malnutrition, a condition that is largely treatable, prompt identification with screening, followed by the most appropriate, effective, evidence based treatment is recommended (Elia, 2003; Elia *et al.*, 2005; NICE, 2006). NICE recently released cost saving guidance, within the top four of which was nutritional support (in the form of oral nutritional support, tube feeding and parenteral nutrition). Specifically, NICE suggested that improving systematic screening, assessment and treatment of malnourished patients (NICE CG32 guideline) could lead to an estimated cost saving of £28 472 per 100 000. NICE suggests that If this guidance [CG32] were fully implemented and resulted in better nourished patients, then this would lead to reduced complications such as secondary chest infections, pressure ulcers, wound abscesses and cardiac failure. Conservative estimates of reduced admissions and reduced length of stay for admitted patients, as well as reduced demand for GP and outpatient appointments, indicate that significant savings are possible (NICE, 2009).

A pragmatic programme of screening implementation (using 'MUST') in care homes in Peterborough Primary Care Trust highlighted some such benefits (Cawood *et al.*, 2009). A programme involving education and training on malnutrition, screening and treatment using the framework of 'MUST', locally agreed care plans and monitoring, improved the documentation of nutritional status, the proportion of residents screened and the use of appropriate care plans. After the implementation of the screening programme, reduction in the number and duration of hospital admissions was observed, associated with a significant cost saving. Similar improvements of nutritional care and outcome have been observed in other settings, e.g. hospital wards, where screening has been implemented (Rypkema *et al.*, 2003; Kruizenga *et al.*, 2005).

Treatment of malnutrition

Following the identification of patients at risk of malnutrition with screening, there is a need to implement evidence based treatments. Nutritional treatment of malnutrition (often termed nutritional support) can encompass modification of the diet (dietary fortification), dietetic counselling, use of oral nutritional supplements (single and multinutrient supplements), enteral tube feeding, parenteral nutrition and combinations of these therapies (Figure 6.2.3). The nutritional treatment of malnutrition should be undertaken alongside management of the underlying causes of malnutrition, e.g. disease, symptoms associated with disease and its treatment, and psychosocial problems.

The best strategy for treating malnutrition should be devised for the individual patient, whilst considering a number of factors. First, the type of nutritional treatment chosen will depend on whether the individual is safely and physically able to eat and drink. If they are, consideration is needed of the likely adequacy of intake, which may

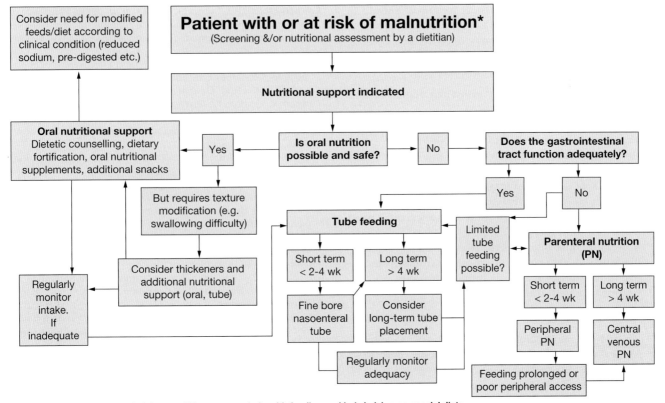

Figure 6.2.3 Algorithm for the treatment of malnutrition

be severely compromised by anorexia, other side effects of disease and any modifications required, e.g. texture, composition (see later). In addition to the diet, oral nutritional supplements and feeding via tube may be required. If the individual is not safely able to eat and drink and oral intake is contraindicated, non-oral means of feeding are required (enteral tube feeding). If feeding into the gastrointestinal tract is contraindicated, then intravenous feeding (parenteral nutrition) is considered (see Chapter 6.3, Chapter 6.4 and Chapter 6.5). For some patients, combinations of treatments will be required.

Second, the method of nutritional support chosen may vary depending on whether an individual will require short or long term support, if they are acutely or chronically ill, in hospital or in the community. In the community, the ability of individuals and their carers/parents to manage nutritional support, e.g. for the very young and old, and their preferences regarding feeding methods need to be considered.

Nutritional treatments may need to be modified (in texture, composition, consistency and quantity) if there are symptoms, e.g. nausea, swallowing problems, severe anorexia, electrolyte disturbances, etc., associated with the disease or its treatment (see Chapter 7.3).

Deficiencies of micronutrients, e.g. vitamins, minerals and trace elements, frequently coexist (Finch *et al.*, 1998; Elia & Stratton, 2005). Nutritional treatment of malnutrition should consider the provision of micronutrients in

addition to energy and protein. All micronutrient deficiencies should be corrected.

Active nutritional treatment may not be considered appropriate in the terminally ill or dying patient. For more information on the ethics of withholding or withdrawing feeding, refer to Lennard-Jones (1998) and Chapter 7.16.

Once the extent of the shortfall between an individual's nutritional requirements and their current or anticipated dietary intake (which could be from food and drink, or may be nothing if intake is contraindicated) has been estimated, the types and quantities of nutritional support can be chosen. Most individuals with malnutrition, both in hospital and in the community, can be managed orally with diet and supplementation. The choice about which form of treatment to use will largely depend on the needs of the individual patient, although local policy and resources need also to be considered. These needs may change during the course of treatment, and so regular monitoring and changes to the types of nutritional support used are required.

Monitoring progress

With any nutritionally compromised individual, it is essential that their condition and the effectiveness of the nutritional support strategy are reviewed at regular intervals. Nutritional support should not be prescribed or provided indefinitely, and goals for treatment should be set and monitored. As a result of monitoring, the type or level of nutritional support may need to be adjusted, dietary guidance amended or reinforced, and new goals set. Monitoring may include assessments of:

- Weight loss, stabilisation or gain (may repeat screening) and growth.
- Body composition, e.g. muscle mass, and function, e.g. strength, ability to walk and quality of life.
- Changes in nutritional (and fluid) intake – quantity, type, variety. Weight change can be a marker of the adequacy of nutritional intake.
- Effectiveness of remedial suggestions, e.g. change in drug therapy or texture of foods, for alleviating problems with food intake.
- Bowel function, fluid and electrolyte balance, swallowing function, skin condition or other symptoms indicative of malnutrition and micronutrient status.
- Compliance with nutritional support.

The frequency of monitoring will depend on the:

- Severity of malnutrition.
- Clinical condition of the individual (stable, deteriorating, improving) and their age.
- Type of nutritional support being used, e.g. patients receiving artificial nutrition may need daily monitoring.
- Setting of an individual (hospital, nursing home, home).
- Resources available for follow-up and monitoring.

Further reading

Elia M (Chairman and Editor). (2003) *Screening for Malnutrition: A Multidisciplinary Responsibility. Development and use of the Malnutrition Universal Screening Tool ('MUST') for Adults*. Redditch: BAPEN.

Elia M, Russell CA. (2009) *Combating Malnutrition: Recommendations for Action*. Redditch: BAPEN.

National Institute for Health and Care Excellence (NICE). (2006) *Nutrition Support in Adults. Oral Nutrition Support, Enteral Tube Feeding and Parenteral Nutrition*. Clinical Guideline 32. London: NICE.

Stratton RJ, Green CJ, Elia M. (2003) Disease-Related Malnutrition: An Evidence Based Approach to Treatment. Oxford: CABI Publishing.

Internet resources

BAPEN
    Further supporting information about 'MUST' and the tool itself can be downloaded from www.bapen.org.uk
Care Quality Commission www.cqc.org.uk
NHS QUIPP programme www.improvement.nhs.uk/qipp

References

Bistrian BR, Blackburn GL, Hallowell E, Heddle R. (1974) Protein status of general surgical patients. *JAMA* 230: 858–860.

British Dietetic Association (BDA). (2009) *A Framework for Screening for Malnutrition*. Birmingham: BDA. Available at www.bda.uk.com.

Cawood AL, Smith A, Dalrymple-Smith J, *et al*. (2008) Prevalence of malnutrition and use of nutritional support in Peterborough Primary Care Trust. *Journal of Human Nutrition and Dietetics* 21: 384.

Cawood AL, Smith A, Pickles S, *et al*. (2009) Effectiveness of implementing MUST into care homes within Peteroborough Primary Care Trust England. *Clinical Nutrition* 4: 81.

Cawood AL, Stratton RJ, Rust S, Walters E, Elia M. (2011) Malnutrition 'self screening' with 'MUST' in hospital outpatients predicts health care outcomes. *Proceedings of the Nutrition Society* 69 (OCE7): E566.

Department of Health. (2008) *Heath and Social Care Act*. London: Department of Health.

Department of Health. (2010a) *Equity and Excellence: Liberating the NHS*. London: Department of Health.

Department of Health. (2010b) *Essence of Care*. London: Department of Health.

Department of Health. (2010c) *The NHS Quality, Innovation, Productivity and Prevention Challenge: An Introduction to Clinicians*. London: Department of Health.

Elia M. (2000) *Guidelines for Detection and Management of Malnutrition*. Maidenhead: Malnutrition Advisory Group (MAG), Standing Committee of BAPEN.

Elia M. (2003) *Screening for Malnutrition: A Multidisciplinary Responsibility. Development and Use of the Malnutrition Universal Screening Tool ('MUST') for Adults*. Birmingham: BAPEN.

Elia M, Russell CA. (2009) *Combating Malnutrition: Recommendations for Action*. Redditch: BAPEN.

Elia M, Stratton RJ. (2005) Geographical inequalities in nutrient status and risk of malnutrition among English people aged 65 years and over. *Nutrition* 21: 1100–1106.

Elia M, Stratton RJ. (2009) Calculating the cost of disease-related malnutrition in the UK. In: Elia M, Russell CA (eds) *Combating Malnutrition: Recommendations for Action*. Redditch: BAPEN.

Elia M, Zellipour L, Stratton RJ. (2005) To screen or not to screen for adult malnutrition. *Clinical Nutrition* 24: 867–884.

Elia M, Russell CA, Stratton RJ. (2010) Malnutrition in the UK: Policies to address the problem. *Proceedings of the Nutrition Society* 69: 470–476.

Finch S, Doyle W, Lowe C, *et al*. (1998) National Diet and Nutrition Survey: People aged 65 years and Over, 1: Report of the Diet and Nutrition Survey. London: The Stationery Office.

Gerasimidis K, Keane O, Macleod I, Flynn DM, Wright CM. (2010) A four-stage evaluation of the Paediatric Yorkhill Malnutrition Score in a tertiary paediatric hospital and a district general hospital. *British Journal of Nutrition* 104: 751–756.

Gerasimidis K, Macleod I, Maclean A, *et al*. (2011) Performance of the novel Paediatric Yorkhill Malnutrition Score (PYMS) in hospital practice. *Clinical Nutrition* 30: 430–435.

Gibney E, Elia M, Jebb SA, Murgatroyd PR, Jennings G. (1997) Total energy expenditure in patients with small-cell lung cancer: results of a validated study using the bicarbonate-urea method. *Metabolism* 46: 1412–1417.

Hill GL, Blackett RL, Pickford I, *et al*. (1977) Malnutrition in surgical patients: An unrecognised problem. *Lancet* i: 689–692.

Hulst JM, Zwart H, Hop WC, Joosten KF. (2010) Dutch national survey to test the STRONGkids nutritional risk screening tool in hospitalized children. *Clinical Nutrition* 29: 106–111.

Jebb SA. (1997) Energy metabolism in cancer and human immunodeficiency virus infection. *Proceedings of the Nutrition Society* 56: 763–775.

Joosten KF, Zwart H, Hop WC, Hulst JM. (2011) National malnutrition screening days in hospitalised children in The Netherlands. *Archives of Disease in Childhood* 95: 141–145.

Kruizenga HM, Van Tulder MW, Seidell JC, Thijs A, Ader HJ, Van Bokhorst-de van der Schueren MA. (2005) Effectiveness and cost-effectiveness of early screening and treatment of malnourished patients. *American Journal of Clinical Nutrition* 82: 1082–1089.

Lennard-Jones JEB. (1998) *Ethical and Legal Aspects of Clinical Hydration and Nutritional Support*. Maidenhead: BAPEN.

Ljungqvist O, van Gossum A, Sanz ML, de Man F. (2010) The European fight against malnutrition. *Clinical Nutrition* 29: 149–150.

National Institute for Health and Care Excellence (NICE). (2006) *Nutrition Support in Adults: Oral Nutrition Support, Enteral Tube Feeding and Parenteral Nutrition*. Clinical Guideline 32. London: NICENICE.

National Institute for Health and Care Excellence (NICE). (2009) *Cost Saving Guidance*. London: NICE. Available at www.nice.org.uk/usingguidance/benefitsofimplementation/costsavingguidance.jsp.

NHS Quality Improvement Scotland. (2003) *Clinical Standards: Food, Fluid and Nutritional Care in Hospitals*. Edinburgh: NHS Quality Improvement Scotland.

Royal College of Physicians (RCP). (2002) *Nutrition and Patients. A Doctor's Responsibility*. Report of a working party of the Royal College of Physicians. London: RCP.

Russell CA, Elia M. (2010) *Nutrition Screening Survey in the UK and Republic of Ireland in 2010*. A Report by the British Association for Parenteral and Enteral Nutrition (BAPEN). Redditch: BAPEN.

Rypkema G, Adang E, Dicke H, *et al.* (2003) Cost-effectiveness of an interdisciplinary intervention in geriatric inpatients to prevent malnutrition. *Journal of Nutrition, Health and Aging* 8: 122–127.

Sermet-Gaudelus I, Poisson-Salomon A-S, Colomb V, *et al.* (2000). Simple pediatric nutritional risk score to identify children at risk of malnutrition. *American Journal of Clinical Nutrition* 72: 64–70.

Stratton RJ, Elia M. (2006) Deprivation linked to malnutrition risk and mortality in hospital. *British Journal of Nutrition* 96: 870–876.

Stratton RJ, Elia M. (2010) Encouraging appropriate, evidence-based use of oral nutritional supplements. *Proceedings of the Nutrition Society* 69: 477–487.

Stratton RJ, Green CJ, Elia M. (2003) *Disease-Related Malnutrition: An Evidence Based Approach to Treatment*. Oxford: CABI Publishing.

Stratton RJ, Cawood AL, Rust S, Walters E, Elia M. (2011) Malnutrition 'self-screening' with MUST in hospital outpatients: concurrent validity and ease of use. *Proceedings of the Nutrition Society* 69 (OCE7): E567.

Volkert D, Saeglitz C, Gueldenzoph H, Sieber CC, Stehle P. (2010) Undiagnosed malnutrition and nutrition-related problems in geriatric patients. *Journal of Nutrition, Health and Aging* 14: 387–392.

Wright CM, Williams AF, Elliman D, *et al.* (2010) Using the new UK-WHO growth charts. *BMJ* 340: c1140.

6.3

Oral nutritional support

Abbie Cawood
Additional contributor: Rebecca Stratton

Key points

- The role of the dietitian is to provide evidence based advice on the most appropriate oral nutritional support for the patient, and tailor dietary advice to the patient's needs.

- Oral nutritional support aims to improve nutritional intake of macro- and micro-nutrients; approaches include fortified food, snacks, nourishing drinks and oral nutritional supplements.

- Dietary strategies improve intake, weight and body composition, but the effect on clinical outcomes and healthcare use has not been fully addressed.

- Oral nutritional supplements have consistently been shown to improve intake, weight, and body composition, with other clinical and economic benefits, e.g. improved function, reduced complications and readmissions to hospital.

- All patients receiving ONS should be monitored regularly against the goals of the intervention.

Oral nutritional support is a collective term used to describe the nutritional options available via the oral route, to manage people who have been identified as malnourished or at risk of malnutrition (see Chapter 6.2). Oral nutritional support should consider macronutrients (energy, carbohydrate protein, fat) and micronutrients (NICE, 2006a). Oral nutritional support options include any of the following methods to improve nutritional intake, as defined by NICE (2006a):

- Fortified food with protein, carbohydrate and/or fat plus vitamins and minerals.
- Snacks.
- Altered meal patterns, practical help with eating.
- Oral nutritional supplements (ONS).
- Provision of dietary advice – including on all of the above and tailoring counselling to the patient's clinical, nutritional, social and psychological needs.

Who should receive oral nutritional support?

Oral nutritional support should be considered for any patient with inadequate food and fluid intakes to meet requirements, unless they cannot swallow safely, have inadequate gastrointestinal function or if no benefit is anticipated, e.g. end of life care (NICE, 2006a) (see Chapter 7.16). For other nutritional support options, see Chapter 6.4 and Chapter 6.5. Healthcare professionals should consider oral nutritional support to improve nutritional intake for people who can swallow safely and are malnourished or at risk of malnutrition (NICE, 2006a) (see Chapter 6.2). This is an A grade recommendation in the National Institute of Health and Care Excellence (NICE) CG32 Nutritional Support in Adults (NICE, 2006a), which is the highest classification of recommendation based on the highest level of evidence. More recently, the Care Quality Commission (2010), as part of the Health and Social Care Act, has highlighted that action should be taken where any risk of poor nutrition or dehydration is identified, and the Department of Health (2010) Essence of Care Framework similarly highlighted that nutritional support be considered for those people who are identified at risk of malnutrition or who are malnourished.

Role of the dietitian in oral nutritional support

The role of the dietitian is to provide evidence based advice on the most appropriate oral nutritional support option for the patient. The dietitian provides tailored dietary advice according to the patient's disease, symptoms and treatment regimen, whilst considering the patient's social, physical, psychological, clinical and nutritional needs. Advice may be given on dietary fortification (in addition to encouragement to eat), food choice and preparation, and how to overcome anorexia or specific difficulties with eating, perhaps due to side effects or symptoms associated with a disease or its treatment.

SECTION 6

Dietary strategies encompass food fortification, extra snacks and nourishing drinks that can be used on their own or in combination with other nutritional support strategies such as ONS and artificial nutrition. Individual patient needs should always be taken into consideration; dietary strategies alone may be adequate for some patients, whereas for others ONS may be the most clinically effective option and should not be delayed.

The effectiveness of dietary advice will depend on many factors, including the method of counselling used, the content and form of the advice given and the patient themselves. The efficacy of dietary advice may be limited in the very sick those with poor consciousness or limited comprehension, and when there are possible time constraints in acute settings. In all settings, dietitians can provide invaluable encouragement and advice (both verbal and written) in the treatment of malnutrition and in the nutritional management of many complex disease states. However, dietetic services can sometimes be thinly spread, which means dietitians are unable to oversee the management of every individual in need of oral nutri-

tional support. Therefore, dietitians have an important role as educators of medical, social care and nursing staff, particularly in the primary and social care sectors, regarding measures that can be taken to improve oral intake. Dietitians can put in place evidence based pathways for oral nutritional support for other healthcare professionals to follow. These pathways should clearly indicate those patients who need more expert dietetic advice or input from a dietitian (BDA, 2009).

Oral nutritional support strategies to improve nutritional intake

There are several oral nutritional support strategies available (Figure 6.3.1).

Fortified food

The aim of food fortification should be to increase the nutrient density of the diet, not the actual amount of food consumed. In practice, food fortification, primarily with

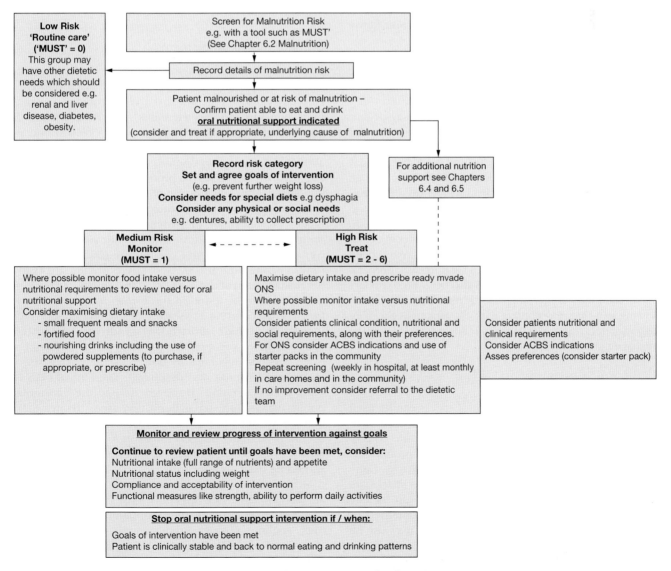

Figure 6.3.1 Algorithm for oral nutritional support in the management of malnutrition

SECTION 6

the addition of energy rich foods, mostly results in increasing energy intakes. Food fortification practices include:

- Fortifying milk by adding four tablespoons of skimmed milk powder to 1 pint of milk. This fortified milk can then be used throughout the day in drinks, on cereals or to make custard, milk puddings, etc.
- Adding grated cheese to soup, savoury dishes and mashed potato.
- Adding double cream to soup, mashed potato, sauces or desserts.
- Adding butter to vegetables, pasta and scrambled egg, and during cooking.
- Adding jam, syrup or honey to breakfast cereals, milk puddings or other desserts.
- Adding sugar to foods or drinks.
- Avoidance of low fat, low sugar and diet foods and drinks.

However, NICE (2006) stated that care should be taken when using dietary fortification in isolation as this approach tends to supplement energy but not other nutrients. Ideally, patients should be encouraged to fortify their diet with foods that are energy and nutrient dense (and not just energy dense).

The use of food fortification may be an attractive option for the patient with anorexia, as the quantity and volume of food consumed does not increase and familiar food ingredients are used. However, dietary fortification may alter the sensory properties of foods, which may or may not be desirable for individual patients. Fortification using high fat foods (especially those with a high saturated fat content like butter, cream and hard cheese) may not be desirable for some patients, e.g. those with high cholesterol levels. There may also be practical difficulties on busy hospital wards or if patients are physically, e.g. disability or fatigue, or mentally unable or unwilling to modify their diet at home without help, so reducing compliance. For all patients the costs of this approach need to be considered, along with issues for purchase, preparation and storage. Thought should also be given to dietary recommendations that other family members may be following and that may conflict with the strategies for managing malnutrition, e.g. weight reducing advice for the management of obesity.

Snacks

Additional food items in the form of snacks can be used in the treatment of malnutrition with the aim of increasing nutritional intake. As with food fortification, consideration should be given to improving energy, protein and micronutrient intakes with the right type of snacks. Compliance with such a strategy may be good, as snacks are familiar and generally well liked. Examples can include cake or malt loaf, yoghurt, custard, toasted crumpets or teacakes with butter, cheese and crackers. It may also be helpful to recommend eating small amounts of food as snacks throughout the day. Snacks may not be effective in patients with anorexia who may be unable to eat more

food, or in patients with physical difficulties with eating (chewing, swallowing). For free living patients, there are also cost considerations and issues of purchase, preparation and storage.

Nourishing drinks

As far as possible, patients should be encouraged to consume drinks that are better sources of nourishment than just tea, coffee or water. Liquids tend to be less satiating than solid foods so can be a good option in patients with very poor appetites. Depending on individual patients and their clinical conditions, suitable suggestions include:

- Milky drinks, e.g. cocoa, drinking chocolate, malted milk drinks, milkshakes, coffee made with full fat milk or fortified milk.
- Soup (especially condensed or *cream of* varieties).
- Fruit juices (or drinks enriched with micronutrients).
- Powdered supplements that can be made up with water or milk, e.g. Complan and Build Up; these can be purchased in pharmacies or supermarkets, although some are available on prescription.

Oral nutritional supplements

Oral nutritional supplements, sometimes referred to as sip feeds, typically contain a mix of macronutrients (protein, carbohydrate and fat) and micronutrients (vitamins, minerals and trace elements). Like tube feeds, ONS are foods for special medical purposes (FSMPs) and as such are regulated under the Commission Directive 1999/21/EC (European Commission, 1999). This directive defines and categorises the products, gives compositional guidelines and sets out labelling requirements. These products are specially formulated, intended for the dietary management of patients and should be used under medical supervision. Oral nutritional supplements can be prescribed in the community (BMJ Group and Royal Pharmaceutical Society of Great Britain, 2011) for the management of disease related malnutrition. Prescribing details can be found in the *British National Formulary (BNF)* section 9.4.2 (www.bnf.org). Other prescribable indications include short bowel syndrome, intractable malabsorption, preoperative preparation of undernourished patients, inflammatory bowel disease, total gastrectomy, bowel fistulae and dysphagia. The cost of ONS is often a consideration. However, despite the enormous public expenditure on malnutrition (see Chapter 6.2), that on treatments including ONS is low (~1% of the overall prescribing budget) (Stratton & Elia, 2010). Nevertheless, ONS, like all forms of oral nutritional support, should be used appropriately.

Most ONS are liquid feeds, but puddings and powders are also available (see Appendix A10). There are a range of types (high protein, fibre containing), styles (juice, milk, yoghurt, savoury, prethickened), energy densities [1–2.4 kcal/mL (4.18–10.0 kJ/mL)] and flavours available to suit a wide range of patient needs. Most provide around 300 kcal (1.25 MJ), 12 g of protein and a full range of vitamins and minerals per serving. Oral nutritional supplement type, dose and duration are used according to clinical judgement. However, most prescriptions range from one to three supplements/day, with clinical benefits typically seen with >300 kcal/day (1.25 MJ/day). Supplementation periods range from weeks in elderly patients who are acutely ill or post surgical, to months for chronically ill patients in the community. Many ONS are nutritionally complete when consumed in a certain volume (range from two to seven servings/day depending on the type of supplement); this means the supplement contains sufficient micronutrients to meet the daily requirements.

Liquid ONS tend not to suppress intake from normal food and in some groups, may help to stimulate appetite (NICE, 2006a; Stratton & Elia, 2007). Oral nutritional supplements should not replace the provision of good food or nutritional care (help with feeding and meal provision) in institutions (hospital and care homes) or in a person's own home. Patients likely to benefit from ONS across both hospital and community settings include acutely ill hospitalised patients (especially the elderly, and hip fracture and gastrointestinal surgical patients), malnourished patients recently discharged from hospital, and those with chronic conditions such as cancer, chronic obstructive pulmonary disease (COPD), neurological conditions, renal and liver disease (NICE, 2006a, Stratton & Elia, 2007). Oral nutritional supplements are also used before and after surgery; perioperatively as part of the nationally recognised ERAS (Enhanced Recovery After Surgery) programme, to improve outcomes after surgery, reduce complications and promote early discharge of patients (Yuill et al., 2005) (see Chapter 7.17.5). Suitability of ONS for specific ethnic groups, people with allergies, vegans and those with other special requirements should always be checked.

Patients find ONS an acceptable form of nutritional support (NICE, 2006a), and compliance with ready made ONS has been shown to be good (78% of prescribed volume consumed), although is variable across settings (Hubbard et al., 2012). It should however be remembered that the efficacy of ONS may be limited if compliance is poor. Optimising compliance with ONS will prevent waste and maximise clinical benefits. Practical tips to aid compliance could include:

- Testing the patient's preferences by offering a variety to try. In the community you may want to try a prescribable starter pack of a range of types and flavours.
- Consider using varied flavours and a choice of different types and consistencies. NB: Some patients are also happy to use only one type and flavour.
- Encouraging ONS to be taken in small doses at intervals throughout the day or as a medication as opposed to a food.
- Using a more energy and nutrient dense ONS (Nieuwenhuizen et al., 2010).
- Consider offering practical advice to patients, e.g. serving ONS chilled or warmed, or using ONS within everyday recipes.

- In some patient groups, e.g. the elderly or those with COPD, the combination of ONS with physical activity programmes (resistance training) may facilitate improvements in intake (Anker et al., 2006; Volkert et al., 2006).

Other strategies

Other strategies that may help to increase dietary intake in the treatment of malnutrition include dining room ambience, sensory enhancement of foods (flavour and odour enhancement), use of music and resistance training or exercise, particularly in the elderly living in long term care settings. In children, behavioural therapy may be useful.

Tailoring dietary advice for oral nutritional support (including practical considerations)

Many factors can impair nutritional intake, with the main factors being disease and its treatment (Stratton et al., 2003). Whenever possible, the underlying cause impairing intake should be identified and addressed. In addition to disease, other factors are social, functional, physical, mechanical and environmental, and may differ depending on where the patient resides (own home, care home, hospital, living alone). Considerations when tailoring dietary advice for oral nutritional support may include:

- Effect of the disease or its management (treatment, surgery), e.g. side effects such as nausea and vomiting, taste changes, dry or painful mouth and the need for modified texture.
- Ability to shop (physical, financial) or collect prescriptions.
- Ability to prepare food or the need for assistance with eating.
- Dentition, loss of appetite, fatigue, early satiety, e.g. stomach resection, abdominal tumours or ascites often result in people feeling full when consuming a small quantity of food.

In addition to advising on the most suitable form of oral nutritional support, dietary advice can also be tailored and personalised for each individual patient. Some of the following practical suggestions may be of help.

Social and functional considerations

These will include factors such as the ability to shop, collect prescriptions or prepare food. Useful strategies include:

- Encourage patients to ask for and accept help from neighbours and friends.
- Encourage patients to make full use of local support services, e.g. social services, home help, meals on wheels and day care facilities, which can provide practical help in terms of shopping, cooking or meal provision and perhaps lessen the social isolation of those who live alone.

- If the patient has limited functional ability and/or no carer or home support, consider ready made meals, snacks, drinks and ONS as appropriate.
- Encourage the use of a pharmacy delivery service if ONS are prescribed.

Physical considerations

Physical considerations include poor appetite, tiredness and early satiety, which may be addressed by considering the following:

- Increase energy and nutrient density and/or decrease amount or volume of food or supplement.
- Offer a smaller portion size and avoid overwhelming platefuls of food (little and often).
- Advise light physical exercise which may improve appetite, e.g. a short walk.
- A small amount of alcohol before or with a meal (if allowed) can stimulate appetite.
- Try spreading meals and snacks throughout the day or try nourishing drinks.
- Consider eating when appetite is best.
- Make use of convenient, simple to prepare foods or meals.
- Choose foods that are particularly fancied, regardless of the time of day.
- Avoid strong cooking smells that could be off putting.
- Take time to eat and relax after meals or between courses.
- Avoid filling up with large volumes of liquid before, during or after meals.
- Some patients (particularly those with early satiety) may find fatty, greasy or rich foods exacerbate their feelings of fullness and would benefit from avoiding these.
- If appetite is poor, e.g. in acute illness or the postoperative period, patients may find nourishing drinks and ONS less satiating than additional food stuffs.

Specific symptoms related to illness or treatment side effects

Nausea and vomiting

Nausea and vomiting can occur for a number of reasons; they are a consequence of many disease states and a common side effect of treatments, e.g. chemotherapy. If nausea and vomiting are severe and food cannot be taken at all, hydration is the first priority. Antiemetics and additional nutritional support can be considered.

Useful strategies include:

- Make use of times when the feeling of nausea is less to eat or prepare foods. Eat anything that is fancied when it is wanted.
- Avoid cooking smells or letting smells linger in the house. Ask someone else to cook or make use of convenience foods, e.g. ready made foods, drinks, snacks and supplements, that create little smell.
- Avoid fatty and fried foods.

- Avoid drinks with meals and serve food relatively dry (unless on a modified consistency diet).
- Sipping drinks and ONS through a straw may be helpful (less likely to detect odour of fluid, resulting in lower taste sensitivity).
- Cold foods, e.g. cold meat, cheese and sandwiches, may be better tolerated than hot foods as they have less smell.
- Savoury foods and drinks may be more acceptable than sweet tasting items.
- Ginger flavoured drinks and foods may be helpful, e.g. ginger ale, ginger beer, ginger biscuits and ginger tea.
- Early morning nausea may be alleviated by dry carbohydrate based foods such as unbuttered toast, cream crackers and plain biscuits.
- Eating or drinking something as soon after vomiting as possible. Ice lollies/ice cubes can clear the mouth.
- Avoid lying down after eating.

Taste problems

Some people are born with taste disorders, but most develop after an illness or injury. People may experience a reduced ability to taste (hypogeusia), an inability to taste (ageusia) or a distorted or altered ability to taste (dysgeusia); many taste disorders are linked to smell disorders. Causes of taste problems include:

- Upper respiratory and middle ear infections.
- Radiation therapy for cancers of the head and neck.
- Medications, including some antibiotics and antihistamines.
- Head injury.
- Some ear, nose and throat surgeries.
- Poor oral hygiene and dental problems.

Useful strategies include:

- Prepare foods with a variety of colours and textures.
- Use aromatic herbs and spices to add more flavour.
- Avoid combination dishes such as casseroles that can hide individual flavours and dilute taste.
- Allow hot food to cool a little before being eaten; high temperatures can accentuate an unpleasant taste sensation.
- If meat tastes unpleasant, try alternatives such as fish, eggs, cheese and dairy products. Cold meats may taste better than hot meats. Marinades can also be helpful.
- Use sharp tasting foods and drinks that are refreshing, e.g. fresh fruit, boiled sweets, mints, lemonade, fruit juice and tonic water.
- If using ONS, consider more tart flavours or a different style, e.g. juice and yoghurt.
- Specific taste problems:
  - Bitterness – avoid foods sweetened with saccharine which can exacerbate this sensation.
  - Metallic – gargle with lemon juice in water before eating.
  - Sweetness – can be offset by adding lemon juice or diluting drinks with soda or mineral water. Adding spices such as ginger, nutmeg or cinnamon to des-

serts and puddings may reduce the sensation of sweetness.
- Saltiness – avoid salt and salty foods or accompaniments, e.g. salted nuts or crisps, packet soups, gravy, sauces, bacon, ham and other types of preserved or canned meat. Adding a pinch of sugar to some foods before serving may be useful.

Dry mouth (xerostomia)

This is a common consequence of damage to the salivary glands, usually as a result of surgery or radiotherapy to the head and neck region. The resulting lack, or even absence, of saliva makes mastication (moving food around the mouth) and swallowing difficult. Lack of saliva can predispose to tooth decay and hence good oral hygiene should be encouraged in all patients. Artificial saliva sprays, gels or salivary stimulant pastilles are prescribable for dry mouth associated with radiotherapy or other conditions.

Useful strategies include:

- Moisten meals with the use of gravy, sauces, butter, cream or evaporated milk.
- Avoid very dry hard foods, e.g. biscuits, crackers or toast.
- Sip drinks frequently, particularly with meals.
- Suck items that help stimulate saliva flow, e.g. boiled sweets, fruit pastilles, pineapple chunks, grapefruit segments and ice cubes (perhaps flavoured with lemon juice or made from fruit juice) – avoid in patients who have a sore mouth (see next section).
- Choose sharp tasting foods, e.g. lemon flavoured food, grapefruit, gooseberry or rhubarb – avoid for patients with sore mouths (see next section).

Sore or painful mouth

This may result from infection, inflammation or ulceration of the oral areas, making eating painful and difficult. Stomatitis (inflammation of the mucous lining of the mouth, e.g. cheeks, gums, tongue, roof or floor of mouth) and mucositis (painful inflammation and ulceration of the gastrointestinal tract, including the mouth) may follow radiotherapy in the head and neck area or as a side effect of some cytotoxic (chemotherapy) drugs. It is important to ensure that these patients are receiving effective pain control at appropriate times to avoid compromising food intake more than is necessary. Appropriate mouth care should be undertaken.

Useful strategies include:

- Eat soft, moist foods by adding sauces, gravy, custard, etc. Some foods may be easier to eat if they are mashed or liquidised.
- Avoid very dry or rough textured foods, e.g. toast, raw vegetables, cereal bars or crisps.
- Avoid foods and drinks at extremes of temperature that can exacerbate pain.
- Avoid salty or highly spiced foods, e.g. salted crackers, salted nuts, crisps, pepper, chilli, curry powder and soya sauce.

- Avoid tart beverages, e.g. pure orange juice and grapefruit juice.
- Use ice lollies, ice cubes or frozen ONS for a soothing effect.

Swallowing difficulties (dysphagia)

Swallowing difficulties may seriously compromise nutritional intake and it is important that dysphagia is properly assessed and managed. Improving nutritional intake in patients with dysphagia can be achieved with oral nutritional support. Dysphagia is a prescribable indication for ONS; a variety of thickeners and prethickened ONS are available. Tube feeds may be necessary if the swallowing difficulty severely limits oral intake (see Chapter 7.3).

Summary of the evidence for oral nutritional support strategies

Dietary fortification

Trials in institutions (including hospitals) have indicated the ability of dietary fortification, using food items, e.g. cream, and glucose polymers, to significantly increase energy intakes (e.g. Gall *et al.*, 1998; Odlund-Olin *et al.*, 2003; Barton *et al.*, 2000). These trials do not assess patient outcomes or the cost effectiveness of this approach. The addition of food snacks can increase energy (Turic *et al.*, 1999, Simmons *et al.*, 2010) and protein intakes (Smoliner *et al.*, 2008) in nursing home residents and children with cystic fibrosis (Hanning *et al.*, 1993). There is a scarcity of data on outcomes (functional or clinical) or the cost effectiveness of these strategies. One trial that assessed functional outcomes found no improvement (Smoliner *et al.*, 2008). For some patient groups, food snacks may be less effective at improving nutritional intakes than liquid ONS, (e.g. Turic *et al.*, 1999; Stratton *et al.*, 2006). Dietary advice (tailored advice from a dietitian) may lead to improvements in weight, body composition and quality of life in some patient groups (COPD, cancer) (Weekes *et al.*, 2009; Ravasco *et al.*, 2005, Baldwin & Weekes, 2011); however, the impact of dietary strategies on clinical outcome and healthcare costs in most patient groups and settings has not been fully addressed in well designed randomised controlled trials and is a research priority.

Oral nutritional supplements

There is a large evidence base for ONS in different patient groups, in both hospital and community settings. Current evidence from systematic reviews and meta analyses (Avenell & Handol, 2010; Baldwin & Weekes, 2011; Cawood *et al.*, 2012; Collins *et al.*, 2012; Elia *et al.*, 2005; 2006; Koretz *et al.*, 2007; Milne *et al.*, 2006; 2009; NICE, 2006a, Potter *et al.*, 1998; Stratton *et al.*, 2003; 2005; Stratton & Elia, 2007) suggest that total nutritional intake is significantly improved by ONS in most patient groups in hospital and community settings. In the community, improvements in intake are more likely in those who are

SECTION 6

underweight [body mass index (BMI) <20 kg/m²]. Food intake tends not to be reduced.

Improvements in body weight and composition (and growth in children) occur with supplementation. Oral nutritional supplements tend to attenuate weight loss in the acutely ill hospitalised patient, and significantly increase weight gain in chronically ill community patients, with weight gain being more likely in those who are underweight (BMI <20 kg/m²) (and most likely to have recently lost weight). Improvements in weight in the acutely ill are related to improvements in physical function observed with consuming ONS.

Functional improvements, which vary according to the patient group, can occur with supplementation. These include increased muscle strength, quality of life, walking distances, activities of daily living, immunological benefits, reduced fatigue and improved wound healing. In those with chronic disease, improvements in function are more likely in those who are underweight (BMI <20 kg/m²) and gain weight with supplementation.

Systematic reviews and meta analyses indicate fewer complications such as infections and pressure ulcers with ONS. These can also prevent pressure ulcers in at risk groups. Reductions in mortality have been consistently shown with ONS versus routine care in acutely ill, hospitalised and elderly patients with a range of conditions.

Oral nutrient supplementation can reduce hospital length of stay and the number of admissions and readmissions to hospital, with potential cost savings. Cost analysis shows intervention with ONS can reduce healthcare costs and be cost effective in those at risk of malnutrition (NICE, 2006b; Cawood et al., 2010). Cost effectiveness analyses take into account the benefits of the intervention balanced against the costs of the intervention, including the use of healthcare professional resources, e.g. for review and monitoring.

Monitoring of all oral nutritional support strategies

Specific targets or goals of oral nutritional support that are appropriate for the individual patient should be recorded. These could include:

- Measures of energy and nutritional intake.
- Appetite.
- Nutritional status.
- Anthropometric measurements (weight, BMI, mid arm muscle circumference, triceps skinfold thickness).
- Functional measures, e.g. strength using hand grip dynamometry.
- Clinically relevant outcomes (pressure ulcer size, infection, quality of life, daily activities).

Regular monitoring of patients receiving oral nutritional support should be undertaken to:

- Assess compliance and acceptability.
- Monitor effectiveness against goals.
- Encourage compliance where appropriate.

- Assess whether current strategy is still required or if other forms of nutritional support, e.g. tube feeding, are warranted.
- Monitor changes in clinical and nutritional status.

Patients receiving oral nutritional support in the community should be monitored every 3–6 months or more frequently if there is any change in clinical condition (NICE, 2006a). Patients receiving oral nutritional support in the hospital setting should be monitored daily initially, reducing to twice weekly when stable (NICE, 2006a).

Discontinuation strategy

Oral nutritional support should be stopped when the patient is established on adequate oral intake from normal food or fed via another route, e.g. enteral or parenteral nutrition.

Further reading

Elia M (ed). (2003) *Screening for Malnutrition: A Multidisciplinary Responsibility. Development and Use of the 'Malnutrition Universal Screening Tool' ('MUST') for Adults.* Redditch: BAPEN.

Elia M, Russell C. (2009) *Combating Malnutrition: Recommendations for Action.* Report from the advisory group on malnutrition, led by BAPEN. Redditch: BAPEN.

Gibney M, Elia O, Ljunggvist J, Dowsett MJ. (2005) *Clinical Nutrition (The Nutrition Society Textbook).* Oxford: Wiley Blackwell.

Sobotka L. (2011) *Basics in Clinical Nutrition,* 4th edn. Prague: Galen.

Internet resources

British National Formulary (BNF) section 9.4.2   www.bnf.org

Malnutrition Pathway   www.malnutritionpathway.co.uk

NICE (2006) Guideline CG32 Nutrition support in adults   http://guidance.nice.org.uk/CG32/NiceGuidance/pdf/English

References

Anker SD, John M, Pedersen PU, et al. (2006) ESPEN guidelines on enteral nutrition: Cardiology and pulmonology. *Clinical Nutrition* 25: 311–318.

Avenell A, Handol HH. (2010) Nutritional supplementations for hip fracture aftercare in older people (review). *Cochrane Database of Systematic Reviews* 1: CD001880.

Baldwin C, Weekes CE. (2011) Dietary advice with or without oral nutritional supplements for disease related malnutrition in adults. *Cochrane Database of Systematic Reviews* 9: CD002008.

Barton AD, Beigg CL, Macdonald IA, Allison SP. (2000) A recipe for improving food intakes in elderly hospitalized patients. *Clinical Nutrition* 19: 451–454.

BMJ Group and the Royal Pharmaceutical Society of Great Britain. (2011) *British National Formulary.* Available at http://bnf.org/bnf/bnf/current/.

British Dietetic Association (BDA). (2009). *A Framework for Screening for Malnutrition.* Available at www.bda.uk.com.

Care Quality Commission (CQC). (2010) *Guidance about Compliance: Summary of Regulations, Outcomes and Judgement Framework.* Available at www.cqc.org.uk.

Cawood AL, Green C, Stratton RJ. (2010) The budget impact of using oral nutritional supplements in older community patients at high risk of malnutrition in England. *Proceedings of the Nutrition Society* 69(OCE7): E544.

Cawood AL, Elia M, Stratton RJ. (2012) Systematic review and meta-analysis of the effects of high protein oral nutritional supplements. *Aging Research Reviews* 11(2): 278–296.

Collins PF, Stratton RJ, Elia M. (2012) Nutritional support in chronic obstructive pulmonary disease (COPD): a systematic review and meta-analysis. *American Journal of Clinical Nutrition* 95(6): 1385–1395.

Department of Health. (2010) *Essence of Care 2010. Benchmarks for Food and Drink.* London: The Stationery Office.

Elia M, Ceriello A, Laube H, Sinclair AJ, Engfer M, Stratton RJ. (2005) Enteral nutritional support and use of diabetes-specific formulas for patients with diabetes: A systematic review and meta-analysis. *Diabetes Care* 28: 2267–2279.

Elia M, Van Bokhorst-de Van der Schueren M, Garvey J, *et al.* (2006) Enteral (oral or tube administration) nutritional support and eicosapentaenoic acid in patients with cancer: A systematic review. *International Journal of Oncology* 28: 5–23.

European Commission. (1999) *Commission Directive 1999/21/EC of 25 March 1999 on Dietary Foods for Special Medical Purposes.* European Commission.

Gall MJ, Grimble GK, Reeve NJ, Thomas SJ. (1998) Effect of providing fortified meals and between-meal snacks on energy and protein intake of hospital patients. *Clinical Nutrition* 17: 259–264.

Hanning RM, Blinkie CJR, Bar-Or O, Lands LC, Moss LA, Wilson WM. (1993) Relationships among nutritional status and skeletal and respiratory muscle function in cystic fibrosis: does early dietary supplementation make a difference? *American Journal of Clinical Nutrition* 57: 580–587.

Hubbard GP, Elia M, Holdoway A, Stratton RJ. (2012) A systematic review of compliance to oral nutritional supplements. *Clinical Nutrition* 31: 293–312.

Koretz R, Avenell A, Lipman T, Braunschweig C, Milne A. (2007) Does enteral nutrition affect clinical outcomes? A systematic review of the randomized trials. *American Journal of Gastroenterology* 102(2): 412–429.

Milne AC, Avenell A, Potter J. (2006) Meta-analysis: protein and energy supplementation in older people. *Annals of Internal Medicine* 144: 37–48.

Milne AC, Potter J, Vivanti A, Avenell A. (2009) Protein and energy supplementation in elderly people at risk from malnutrition. *Cochrane Database of Systematic Reviews* 2: CD003288.

National Institute for Health and Care Excellence (NICE). (2006a) *Nutrition Support in Adults. Oral Nutrition Support, Enteral Tube Feeding and Parenteral Nutrition.* Clinical Guideline 32. London: NICE.

National Institute for Health and Care Excellence (NICE). (2006b) *Nutrition Support in Adults. Oral Nutrition Support, Enteral Tube Feeding and Parenteral Nutrition. Costing Report.* London: NICE.

Nieuwenhuizen WF, Weenen H, Rigby P, Hetherington MM. (2010) Older adults and patients in need of nutritional support: Review of current treatment options and factors influencing nutritional intake. *Clinical Nutrition* 29(2): 160–169.

Odlund-Olin A, Armyr I, Soop M, Ljungqvist E, *et al.* (2003) Energy enriched meals improve energy intake in elderly residents in a nursing home. *Clinical Nutrition* 22(2): 125–131.

Potter J, Langhorne P, Roberts M. (1998) Routine protein energy supplementation in adults: systematic review. *BMJ* 317: 495–501.

Ravasco P, Monteiro-Grillo I, Marques Vidal P, Camilo ME. (2005) Impact of nutrition on outcome: a prospective randomized controlled trial in patients with head and neck cancer undergoing radiotherapy. *Head and Neck* 27(8): 659–668.

Simmons SF, Zhuo X, Keeler E. (2010) Cost-effectiveness of nutrition interventions in nursing home residents: a pilot intervention. *Journal of Nutrition and Healthy Aging* 14: 367–372.

Smoliner C, Norman K, Scheufele R, Hartig W, Pirlich M, Lochs H. (2008) Effects of food fortification on nutritional and functional status in frail elderly nursing home residents at risk of malnutrition. *Nutrition* 24: 1139–1144.

Stratton RJ, Elia M. (2007) A review of reviews: A new look at the evidence for oral nutritional supplements in clinical practice. *Clinical Nutrition Supplements* 2: 5–23.

Stratton RJ, Elia M. (2010) Encouraging appropriate, evidence-based use of oral nutritional supplements. *Proceedings of the Nutrition Society* 69(4): 477–487.

Stratton RJ, Green CJ, Elia M. (2003) *Disease-Related Malnutrition: An Evidence Based Approach to Treatment.* Oxford: CABI Publishing.

Stratton RJ, Ek A-C, Engfer M, *et al.* (2005) Enteral nutritional support in prevention and treatment of pressure ulcers: a systematic review and meta-analysis. *Ageing Research Reviews* 4: 422–450.

Stratton RJ, Bowyer G, Elia M. (2006) Food snacks or liquid oral nutritional supplements as a first line treatment for malnutrition in post-operative patients. *Proceedings of the Nutrition Society* 65: 4a.

Turic A, Gordon KL, Craig LD, Ataya DG, Voss AC. (1999) Nutrition supplementation enables elderly residents of long-term-care facilities to meet or exceed RDAs without displacing energy or nutrient intakes from meals. *Journal of the American Dietetic Association* 98: 1457–1459.

Volkert D, Berner YN, Berry E, *et al.* (2006) ESPEN Guidelines on Enteral Nutrition: Geriatrics. *Clinical Nutrition* 25(2): 330–360.

Weekes CE, Emery PW, Elia M. (2009) Dietary counselling and food fortification in stable COPD: a randomised trial. *Thorax* 64(4): 326–331.

Yuill KA, Richardson RA, Davidson HI, Garden OJ, Parks RW. (2005) The administration of an oral carbohydrate containing fluid prior to major elective upper-gastrointestinal surgery preserves skeletal muscle mass postoperatively – a randomised clinical trial. *Clinical Nutrition* 24: 32–37.

6.4

Enteral nutrition

Sarah Armer and Rhys White

Key points

- The decision to start feeding should consider the ethics of individual patient circumstances, the requirement to do no harm and the potential improvement in quality of life.

- The route of feeding, feeding regimen, including timing and type of feed, should be decided on an individual basis, taking into account clinical indications, treatment plan and nutritional status.

- A specific monitoring plan should be put in place for each patient.

- Effective monitoring will help to ensure that nutritional support is provided safely, complications are detected early and treated effectively, and nutritional objectives are met and/or reviewed to ensure the effectiveness of the nutritional intervention.

- All patients going home on enteral feeding should have an individual discharge plan.

Enteral tube feeding has become a widely used method of ensuring adequate nutrition in patients who have a functioning gastrointestinal tract but are unable to maintain an adequate or safe oral intake. Enteral feeding in both the hospital and community setting is becoming increasingly common, as a range of access and delivery methods have been successfully established. Prior to initiating enteral tube feeding, broader matters such as ethics and consent should be considered (British Gastroenterology Association, 1999), in addition to practical issues such as discharge planning, training and support in the community. Dietitians are uniquely placed to provide guidance and recommendations regarding nutritional support and play a key role within the multidisciplinary team in the treatment of patients requiring enteral nutrition (American Dietetic Association, 1997).

Indications for enteral nutrition

Enteral feeding is indicated when oral intake is insufficient or unsafe (NICE, 2006) and is most commonly used in patients with the following features or disorders (NICE, 2006):

- Unconscious patients.
- Neuromuscular swallowing disorders, e.g. stroke.
- Physiological anorexia.
- Upper gastrointestinal obstruction, e.g. head and neck tumours.
- Gastrointestinal dysfunction or malabsorption, e.g. ~~creatitis, gastrointestinal dysmotility.

- Increased nutritional requirements.
- Psychological problems.
- Specific treatment, e.g. Crohn's disease.

Several factors need to be considered when deciding to initiate enteral tube feeding. These include the risks and benefits of enteral tube placement, the most appropriate method of tube placement and selection of the most suitable feeding tube. The decision should be made following a multidisciplinary discussion and the views and wishes of the patient and/or their family or carers should be considered. A decision to enterally feed a patient may also be influenced by the future treatments required, e.g. surgery or radiotherapy. Nutritional support should be tailored to the clinical state and the perceived best outcome for the patient (see Chapter 2.2 and Chapter 6.1).

Ethics of withholding or withdrawing nutrition

Ethical issues should always be considered before initiating enteral tube feeding and consent must be obtained if a patient has the mental capacity. Often consent and ethics are considered before gastrostomy tube placement, but invariably nasogastric tubes are placed without similar discussions and considerations. Even when only short term nutritional support is thought to be necessary, informed consent should be obtained (if possible) and ethical issues should be considered (RCP, 2010). A multidisciplinary nutrition support team should be available to assess patients and is ideally placed to communicate with patients, carers and the referring team regarding appropriate feeding options. A well functioning nutrition support team can reduce the number of inappropriate gastrostomy placements (Abuksis *et al.*, 2004; Sanders, 2002).

When making a decision regarding enteral feeding, it is essential to first establish what the healthcare professionals are trying to be achieved (RCP, 2010). Whilst offering adequate food and water to patients is a basic duty of care, artificial nutritional support (both enteral and parenteral) is regarded as a medical treatment. In cases where the benefits of nutritional support are uncertain, a time limited trial can be undertaken with clearly agreed objectives. Good open communication with family members and carers and the multidisciplinary team is essential at all times.

The issue of whether to continue feeding severely ill patients who have a poor but not hopeless prognosis is less clear. Where the patient themselves is unable to consent, the consultant (senior medical practitioner) responsible for care has a duty to act in their best interests. Any previous relevant opinions of the patient in the form of an advanced directive must be taken into account. Under the Mental Capacity Act (2005) the medical team is required to obtain the view of family and carers. The patient may have conferred a Lasting Power of Attorney (LPA), giving someone else the authority to make decisions about health and personal welfare. The Royal College of Physicians and the General Medical Council (RCP, 2010) have provided a comprehensive overview of the legal position in the UK regarding the withholding and withdrawing of life prolonging medical treatment, including nutritional support (see Chapter 1.1 and Chapter 7.16).

Routes of enteral feeding

Enteral feeding is preferable to parenteral feeding when the gut is accessible and has adequate, absorptive capacity, as it is more physiological and cheaper (Stroud *et al.*, 2003). Few patients cannot receive some form of enteral nutrition (EN) through the various routes available. The route of enteral feeding is decided on an individual basis according to the clinical indications, treatment plan and nutritional state of the individual patient. Enteral feed may be delivered:

* Directly into the stomach (gastric feeding) via orogastric, nasogastric, gastrostomy or oesophagostomy tube.
* After the stomach (post pyloric feeding) via nasoduodenal or nasojejunal tube, gastrojejunostomy or jejunostomy.

Gastric feeding routes

Nasogastric feeding

This is usually used for short term nutritional support (<4 weeks) or in the longer term when other options such as gastrostomy feeding are contraindicated or inappropriate (McAtear, 1999). All patients should have an individual nutritional risk assessment carried out prior to passing a nasogastric tube [National Patients Safety Agency (NPSA), 2005)].

A fine bore nasogastric tube, usually made from polyvinyl chloride (PVC) or polyurethane, is inserted through the nose and into the stomach. Polyvinyl chloride tubes are suitable for short term feeding (<10 days) and are usually a rigid wide bore (10–18 FG; French gauge – the external circumference of the tube in millimetres; Ryles or Levin's tube). Complications associated with wide bore tubes are well known (nasal erosion, oesophageal ulceration) but, despite this, they should be considered an initial feeding route in patients at high risk of pulmonary aspiration (most commonly critically ill patients), with conversion to a fine bore tube once successful gastric emptying is established. More expensive and durable polyurethane tubes are more suitable for longer term use. In practice, both tubes become dislodged with similar frequency. Some polyurethane tubes can be repassed (marked single patient use); however, most can only be used once only (marked single use). Fine bore feeding tubes are usually of 6–9 FG. Tubes must be radio-opaque throughout their length and have visible markings to ensure accurate identification and documentation of position (NPSA, 2011).

Other methods of gastric placement are:

* Orogastric – used in head injury patients or those with facial trauma.
* Cervical pharyngostomy, oesphagostomy and stoma-gastric tubes – can be placed in head and neck cancer patients.

Confirmation of gastric tube placement

It is vital to establish that the tube tip is positioned in the stomach and not the lungs before each feeding episode, before flushing with water or medication and if there is any doubt about the position of the tube. Deaths resulting from the misplacement of nasogastric tubes have been reported NPSA (2005; 2011). The following methods for confirming nasogastric tube placement are recommended (NPSA, 2005):

* *Stomach aspirate pH* – aspirate stomach contents and check that the contents are acidic, pH ≤5.5 (≤5 on paper that does not have ½ markings) using CE marked pH indicator strips or paper. If the patient is on continuous feeding or receiving drugs such as antacids (including proton pump inhibitors), the pH may be >5.5. If the problem is due to the presence of feed, the pH should be rechecked 1 hour after feeding. If due to antacids, the timing of this medication may need to be reviewed.
* *X ray confirmation* – this should only be carried out if there is any doubt about the position of the tube or difficulty in obtaining aspirate. An X ray only confirms the position of the nasogastric tube tip at the time of the X ray, and as the tip may become dislodged following the X ray, further confirmation of gastric pH will be required.

Alternative methods for placing and confirming position of nasogastric tubes

Electromagnetic sensing devices permit real time tracking of feeding tube position during placement, e.g. Cortrak Enteral Access System™ (Corpak Medsystems). This has been demonstrated to show good reliability in ascertaining gastric and post pyloric tube placement (Rao *et al.*, 2009; Taylor *et al.*, 2010). The guide wire containing the electromagnetic transmitter (stylet) can be reintroduced to confirm tube tip position even after initial placement.

Gastrostomy feeding

A gastrostomy is the creation of an artificial tract between the stomach and the abdominal surface, and is commonly used for long term enteral support. A gastrostomy can be placed endoscopically [percutaneous endoscopic gastrostomy (PEG], surgically or radiologically [radiologically inserted gastrostomy (RIG)]. The terms PEG and RIG describe the actual procedure; however, they are also commonly used to describe the type of tube placed and are most often used to describe a gastrostomy tube with a fixed internal retention device (a disc like bumper). There is often confusion over the definition and terminology used to describe gastrostomy tubes. It is important that dietitians understand the differences between the types of tubes and the correct terminology to describe them.

In order to provide appropriate and safe management of a gastrostomy tube, information regarding when the tube was inserted and how it is retained can be important and help to reduce the risk of complications. Often, how the tube was inserted, e.g. endoscopically or radiologically, is of least importance to the dietitian. Prior to the placement of a gastrostomy tube, a full assessment of the patient, including clinical presentation/medical history, social circumstances and ability to manage the tube, should be carried out. Placement of a gastrostomy is a consented procedure; patients should have the full risks and benefits of placing the tube explained prior to consent being obtained (Westaby *et al.*, 2010). Tubes specifically designed for gastrostomy use should be used; Foley catheters are not designed, or licensed, as enteral feeding devices and may cause duodenal obstruction (Tibbitts & Sorrell, 1999).

Percutaneous endoscopic placement

A PEG is placed under direct visualisation using an endoscope (a camera which is passed down through the mouth and into the gastrointestinal tract). Transillumination of the abdominal wall with the endoscope identifies the appropriate site for insertion. An incision is made into the stomach and a loop of thread introduced. The thread is grasped internally and pulled up to the mouth using the endoscope. A gastrostomy tube is attached to the thread, pulled down through the oesophagus, into the stomach and out through the abdominal wall to lie with its internal bumper against the gastric mucosa. A flange and clamp are then fitted externally. Endoscopic tubes can also be placed using gastropexy and a direct puncture tube inser-

tion. The tube is inserted directly into the stomach through an external puncture and the stomach is sutured to the abdominal wall until the stoma tract matures. This negates the need for a tube to be pulled through the mouth and oesophagus if there is an obstruction. The advantages of using a PEG include:

* Performed as a day care procedure, reducing costs compared with other placement methods.
* High success rate (Wollman *et al.*, 1995).
* Quick – taking <20 minutes.
* General anaesthetic not required.
* Low incidence of complications.

The contraindications and other considerations with PEG placement include:

* Severe obesity.
* Portal hypertension or gastric varices.
* Coagulation abnormalities.
* Active gastric ulceration or malignancy.
* Total or partial gastrectomy.
* Ascites.
* Peritoneal dialysis.
* Oesophageal or gastric tumours that prevent passage of an endoscope.
* Oropharyngeal or oesophageal carcinoma – placement of a PEG tube using the standard pull through technique is associated with a small risk of tumour implantation at the skin site (Cappell, 2007). To reduce this risk, particularly in patients for whom cancer therapy is of curative intent, gastrostomy placement should be achieved by a direct gastric puncture technique (Foster *et al.*, 2007).
* Chronic progressive neurological and neuromuscular disorders, e.g. motor neurone disease. There may be an increased risk associated due to the use of sedation as patients generally have a degree of respiratory compromise. There is some limited evidence to suggest that radiologically placed tubes may confer a survival benefit in these patients because this method avoids the risk of sedation (Shaw *et al.*, 2006).

Removal and replacement of a percutaneous endoscopic gastrostomy tube

Tubes with compressible or deflatable internal bumpers are traction removable and therefore avoid the need for a further endoscopy. Non-traction removable tubes will require endoscopic removal or the tube can be cut and the internal bumper allowed to pass through the gastrointestinal tract naturally. This approach has been widely used and is considered a safe option (Merrick *et al.*, 2008). However, there is an associated, small but recognised risk of bowel obstruction (Coventry *et al.*, 1994) so a risk assessment should be carried out and the patient consented for the procedure.

There are two types of bedside replacement gastrostomy tubes:

* *A balloon retained gastrostomy device* – a balloon is inflated internally with sterile water or saline to hold the tip of the feeding tube against the gastric wall fol-

lowing percutaneous insertion. These gastrostomy tubes usually have a length of tube externally but low profile tubes, or 'buttons', are also available which are flush to the skin and therefore more discreet.
- *A flexible bumper retained gastrostomy device* – held in place by either a flexible internal cage like bumper or an internal bolster that is deployed by cutting an external suture.

Radiological placement

Radiologically inserted gastrotomies are becoming increasingly common. A naso- or oro-gastric tube is required to dilate the stomach with air and, under X ray guidance, gastropexy sutures are inserted to anchor the stomach to the anterior abdominal wall. A gastrostomy is inserted and its position confirmed in the stomach using X ray. Balloon gastrostomies or 'pig tail' tubes are most commonly used. Disc or bumper retained gastrostomies can also be placed radiologically using the pull through technique, where the tube is inserted via a guide wire into the mouth and pulled down through the oesophagus into the stomach and out through the abdominal wall. Tubes inserted using this technique are sometimes referred to as a PIG (per oral image guided gastrostomy) and have the advantage of not requiring gastropexy and allowing insertion of a lower maintenance tube, i.e. bumper/disc retained; however, they are technically more difficult to insert radiologically than endoscopically.

The advantages of RIG placement include:

- Very low risk of tumour seeding from head and neck tumours with direct puncture method as no endoscope required.
- Sedation not required.
- Clear picture of anatomy allowing tube placement in difficult patients where endoscopic placement may have been unsuccessful.

Surgical placement

Surgically inserted gastrostomies are becoming less common with the increasing use of PEGs and RIGs. Surgically placed gastrostomies require a mini laparotomy and general anaesthetic. When a gastrostomy is inserted surgically, it requires a purse string suture around the gastrostomy tube in the stomach wall to keep it in place.

Post insertion instructions

It is safe to commence feeding 4 hours after PEG insertion (NICE, 2006) although local policy may vary. There is no clear consensus on when it is safe to first use a newly inserted RIG for feeding, with some centres feeding after 4 hours and others waiting 24 hours. Like for any interventional procedure, there is potential for complications (including peritonitis, infection, bowel perforation, haemorrhage and aspiration pneumonia), but prompt recognition of these complications with early action reduces the risk of serious harm or death. The NPSA (2010) recommends that all NHS organisations with departments that insert gastrostomy tubes should ensure that:

- Local protocols specify the observations to be taken in the immediate recovery period.
- Medical notes are marked with a high visibility sticker warning of the possible complications that could occur and necessary action.
- Where patients are discharged within 72 hours, equivalent warnings should be communicated to the GP, community nurses, care home nurses, as well as to the patient and/or carers.

Post pyloric feeding routes

Nasoduodenal or nasojejunal feeding

A feeding route bypassing the stomach overcomes the problem of gastroparesis and subsequent aspiration risk. In patients with high gastric aspirates, the small bowel may be working normally. Tubes are most commonly placed endoscopically but can also be placed under X ray guidance or at the bedside. The risk of aspiration is reduced most significantly when the feeding tube is inserted beyond the ligament of Treitz, i.e. intrajejunal placement (Heyland *et al.*, 2001). These tubes often incorporate a lumen for gastric aspiration in these patients (Silk, 2011).

The techniques for bedside placement of nasojejunal tube using different patient positions and prokinetic agents have varying rates of success. Self advancing polyurethane tubes, e.g. Tiger 2™ Tube (Cook Medical, USA), have unique alternating cilia like flaps that allow peristalsis to pull the tube into the small bowel more effectively than standard bedside placements. Endoscopic placement is time consuming and costly, and may not be easily accessible to intensive care patients. A newer bedside technique using a transnasal endoscope for placing nasojejunal tubes has shown promising results, but requires further evaluation (O'Keefe *et al.*, 2003; Zick *et al.*, 2011). Several researchers suggest that at present the X ray guided technique of tube placement is the most successful (Thurley *et al.*, 2008). As with gastric placement, Cortrak® has also been demonstrated to be reliable in ascertaining postpyloric tube placement (Rao *et al.*, 2009). However, it is unknown whether tubes inserted by this method can be positioned beyond the ligament of Treitz.

Gastrojejunostomy

Post pyloric feeding access can be obtained in patients with established gastrostomy access by the insertion of an extension device that threads through the existing gastrostomy lumen into the jejunum. A dedicated gastrojejunostomy combination must be used, as most basic gastrostomies cannot house jejunal extensions. Direct puncture techniques can also be used to place gastrojejunal tubes under X ray guidance. These tubes have a gastric internal retention device that can be either a balloon or disc like bumper.

Jejunostomy

Jejunostomies create a stoma tract between the jejunum and the abdominal surface, and can be placed surgically

SECTION 6

or radiologically. Jejunostomy insertion is indicated when major gastrointestinal or hepatobiliary surgery necessitates post pyloric feeding, e.g. oesophagogastrectomy, or if the clinical condition increases the likelihood of gastric stasis secondary to ileus or pseudo ileus, e.g acute pancreatitis. A feeding jejunostomy should be considered if gastric feeding has failed, and may provide a useful route that avoids parenteral nutrition. There is no internal retention device to avoid bowel obstruction so these tubes must be secured externally. The tubes usually directly puncture the jejunum though some are designed to be tunnelled under the skin and are held in place using a felt like cuff under the skin surface.

A whole protein feed should be well tolerated in jejunostomy feeding. However, if there is pancreatic or biliary insufficiency, or if the jejunostomy has been sited in the lower small bowel, a peptide based or elemental feed may be indicated. Feed usually commences at a low volume (20–30 mL/hour) and is increased slowly until the optimum feeding rate is achieved. Continuous feeding over 24 hours may prevent tube blockage. Jejunostomy tubes often have a thin diameter, e.g. 9 FR, and therefore regular flushing of the tube with water may be necessary to prevent blockage.

Enteral feed delivery

A feeding regimen should be written for nursing staff, or for patients/carers to refer to if enteral feeding takes place in their own homes. The regimen should include the feed to be used, feeding times, drip rate and additional fluid requirements. Timings should include feed breaks to encompass the psychosocial aspects of feeding, together with the influence on other clinical interventions, e.g. physiotherapy and drug–nutrient interactions. Patients wishing to pump feed at home when they are alone or unsupervised should have the risks explained to them, and this should be documented in their care plan, as some local policies may advise against this.

It is usual to start feeding at no more than 50% feed requirements to ensure metabolic and gastrointestinal tolerance to the feed (NICE, 2006). Drip rates can then be increased at regular intervals until the maximum desired drip rate is achieved. Guidance for feeding patients at risk of refeeding syndrome is covered later.

Infusion rate

Bolus feeding

A bolus feed is the delivery of 100–300 mL of feed over a 10–30-minute period. Administration is usually by syringe, using the syringe barrel as a funnel to allow the feed to infuse using gravity or using the plunger. Bolus feeding can also be provided via a feeding pump, although it is important to check the maximum drip rate the feed pump can achieve before considering this option. The tube should be flushed before and after delivery of the feed bolus. Bolus feeding regimens are advantageous in that they can allow greater flexibility for the patient as they fit

with normal eating patterns and may be preferable for patients who do not wish to be restricted by feeding equipment for several hours a day. This type of feeding is also more physiologically normal and may improve blood glucose control in diabetic patients. Bolus feeding may also be the regimen of choice for patients who interfere with tubing and feeding equipment during continuous feeding. Patient positioning should also be considered; it is advisable for patients to remain in a semi upright position during and 1 hour post feeding (Metheny *et al.*, 2006).

Continuous feeding

Continuous feeding usually requires a pump and feeding set for administration and, if ready to hang formulae are not used, a feed reservoir. Continuous feeding usually refers to feeding at rates of 50–150 mL/hour over 16–20 hours, although 24-hour feeding is becoming more common in critical care for patients on sliding scale insulin. A rest period of at least 90 minutes is needed as it allows gastric pH to fall sufficiently to promote antibacterial conditions in the stomach (Bonten *et al.*, 1994). A longer planned rest period allows more flexibility, e.g. to catch up if feeding has been interrupted during the day, or to allow sufficient time for therapy. A rest period can provide an overnight break for those without urinary catheterisation and who may otherwise experience nocturia and interrupted sleep, or a rest period can be given during the day so the patient is unencumbered by enteral feeding equipment.

Continuous feeding is usually the feeding method of choice for patients who are fed via a post pyloric route; however, bolus feeding is not contraindicated for these patients and can be used if tolerated. In deciding whether continuous and/or bolus feeding would be most appropriate, patient preference, risk of tube dislodgement and mobility of the patient should be considered (NICE, 2006).

In patients at risk of pulmonary aspiration (particularly critically ill patients), regular aspiration of the nasogastric tube is routinely undertaken to assess adequacy of gastric emptying. However, recent studies do not support the conventional use of measuring gastric residual volumes (GRVs);, instead, it is suggested to monitor trends to identify any gradual increase in residual volumes, and levels up to 500 mL in the absence of other signs of intolerance (McClave *et al.*, 2005) are acceptable. Poulard *et al.* (2010) found little benefit in stopping enteral feeding in patients who reached a subjectively selected GRV (see Chapter 7.17.1).

Enteral feed formulae

Enteral feeding formulae can be categorised into whole protein (polymeric) feeds, including disease specific feeds, and elemental or peptide feeds (see Table 6.4.1). A summary of enteral feeding products currently available in the UK can be found in Appendix A10.

Whole protein (polymeric) feeds

These require an intact gut for their digestion and absorption. The constituents of whole protein feeds are:

- *Protein* – the source is usually derived from milk or hydrolysed casein, although a soya protein formula is available for those with milk protein intolerance.
- *Carbohydrate* – is usually in the form of maltodextrin, glucose, sucrose or corn syrup solids.
- *Dietary fibre* – various feeds are available containing added soluble and insoluble fibre. Insoluble fibre has most effect on gut barrier function, while soluble fibre can increase short chain fatty acid production (Silk, 1993). Therefore, a mixed fibre source (as is found in most commercially available feeds) is advised. Elia *et al.* (2008) suggest that fibre supplemented enteral formulae have important physiological effects and clinical benefits, and may help to reduce the incidence of diarrhoea in hospital patients.
- *Fat* – the source is usually a vegetable oil derivative, although many feed companies are now reblending fats to alter the ratio of n-3 to n-6 polyunsaturated fatty acids (PUFAs) and increase the monounsaturated fat content. n-3 PUFAs may be provided by the use of canola or rapeseed oil, or by fish oils to provide direct sources of eicosapentaenoic acid (EPA) and docosahexaenoic acid (DHA). Provision of n-3 PUFAs can down regulate the inflammatory response by reducing arachidonic acid (n-6 PUFA) metabolites, but the mechanism to convert n-3 PUFAs to the active EPA and DHA is impaired in the severely ill.
- *Vitamins, minerals and electrolytes* – in the UK, all enteral feeds provide 100% of the recommended nutrient intake (RNIO for micronutrients (excluding electrolytes) in a specified volume of feed (usually within 1–1.8 L of standard enteral feed). Current levels of micronutrients must comply with the European Community (1999) Directive on Dietary Foods for Special Medical Purposes (1999/21/EC).

Types of whole protein feeds can be categorised as:

- *Standard adult formulae* – provide 1 kcal/mL (4.18 kJ/mL) and are suitable for the majority of patients; available with and without fibre.
- *High energy adult formulae* – provide 1.2–2.4 kcal/mL (5.02–10.03 kJ/mL) and are useful for patients on fluid restriction or with increased nutritional requirements, e.g. burns patients. Electrolyte and protein content of these feeds are variable. Fibre containing energy dense feeds are also available, but only up to energy densities of 2 kcal/mL.
- *Low energy formulae* – provide 1–1.2 kcal/mL (4.18–5.02 kJ/mL) and 1000 mL of these usually meets the nutritional needs of patients with low energy and/or fluid requirements, e.g. elderly bed bound patients.
- *Disease specific enteral formulae* – a variety of enteral feeds are provided for a variety of conditions. However, dietitians should consider the use of specific products within the context of the patient's clinical status, and not take the manufacturer's recommended client group as the sole indication for use. A brief overview of some disease specific feeds is given in the Table 6.4.1.

Table 6.4.1 Condition specific feeds

Type of feed	Comment
Renal feeds	Suitable for patients on electrolyte and fluid restrictions Similar or lower protein to energy ratio compared with standard feeds Energy dense versions for fluid restriction are available, with subtle modification of other nutrients, e.g. higher water soluble vitamin content to allow for intradialytic losses
Low sodium feeds	Standard feeds with a sodium content reduced to 10–15 mmol/L. Clinical hypernatraemia is often secondary to dehydration, so the use of a standard feed (providing 35–40 mmol of Na/L) provides less sodium than plasma levels Low sodium feeds may be beneficial for patients with ascitic liver disease
Respiratory feeds	Contain a higher percentage energy content from fat, which reduces the amount of carbon dioxide produced from feed metabolism – may be useful in patients with respiratory failure. However, evidence of the benefit of these feeds is limited and avoidance of overfeeding is as clinically significant as the choice of feed in respiratory failure (Malone, 1997)
Immune feeds	Contain variable amounts of specific amino acids or fats, together with altered levels of specific micronutrients that have an attributed immune benefit, e.g. glutamine, arginine, dietary nucleotides, fish oils, beta-carotene and fructo-oligosaccharides More expensive than standard feeds Evidence that they may benefit some postsurgical or septic patients (Galban *et al.*, 2000)
Elemental/peptide feeds	Provide nitrogen in the form of free amino acids or peptides Indicated in the presence of severe maldigestion or malabsorption The majority of patients can tolerate whole protein feeds even in the presence of some degree of gut malfunction With severe gut impairment, a predigested formula may be indicated. Appropriate use of these feeds may reduce the requirement for parenteral nutrition (Hamaoui *et al.*, 1990) No clinical benefit in using peptide feed rather than whole protein feed in patients with Crohn's disease (Zachos *et al.*, 2006)

Drug–nutrient interactions

Enteral feeding may interfere with the dosage, presentation and action of many drugs. Crushing oral preparations to pass down a tube may compromise their activity, cause tube occlusion and has the potential to cause fatality, particularly if slow release preparations are used. Some medications are not available in liquid form; therefore, alternative formulations or preparations should be sought to deliver the medication safely. Drugs should not be added to the feed infusion, as this may alter the stability of the medication and introduce a potential route of contamination into the enteral feed. Liaison with a pharmacist will ensure optimal enteral feed and drug administration. A practical guide to administration of drugs during enteral feeding can be found on the BAPEN website (www.BAPEN.org.uk).

Common drugs such as phenytoin, ciprofloxacin, tetracyclines, penicillin, sucralfate and theophylline all bind to the feed and/or have altered absorption kinetics, so should be administered during a rest period. Other drugs that can be affected by/affect enteral feeds are digoxin, carbamazepine and antacids. For further reading, see Bradnam & White (2011) and Chapter 5.3.

Enteral feeding monitoring

The main objectives of monitoring nutritional support are to ensure that it is provided safely, complications are detected early and treated effectively, and nutritional objectives are met and/or reviewed, thus ensuring the effectiveness of the nutritional intervention. Close liaison with colleagues, patients and carers is vital when initiating and monitoring enteral nutrition (NICE, 2006) and all have a role to play in the monitoring process. For example, in the community, the patient and/or carer may be responsible for most of the monitoring. In hospital, the dietitian will not be directly responsible for performing all of the monitoring required but it is their responsibility, in conjunction with the wider multidisciplinary team and the patient, to agree an appropriate monitoring plan and to review the results. Table 6.4.2 details the range of parameters that should be considered for monitoring of nutritional support (NICE, 2006).

The frequency and choice of monitoring is dependent on many variables, including the nature and severity of the underlying disease state, whether previous results were abnormal, the type of nutritional support used, the tolerance of nutritional support, the nutritional care setting and the expected duration of the nutritional support (NICE, 2006). Monitoring frequency may need to be more intense at the start of treatment than at a later stage, but should continue throughout the episode of care. Monitoring should be interpreted with caution, as a full understanding of the meaning of a result is needed before any changes are made. There is no one test that will measure nutritional status and therefore a combination of clinical and laboratory results should be used. Additional guidance on monitoring patients on EN can be found in Micklewright & Todorovic (2011) and NICE (2006).

Complications of enteral feeding

Refeeding syndrome

Refeeding syndrome is defined as *'the metabolic and physiological consequences of the depletion, repletion, compartmental shifts and interrelationships of the following: phosphate, potassium, magnesium, glucose metabolism, vitamin deficiency and fluid restriction'* (Solomon & Kirby, 1990). Refeeding syndrome can occur when a patient is fed after a period of starvation. Refeeding triggers include:

- A switch from fat to carbohydrate metabolism.
- Increased insulin release.
- Increased uptake of glucose, phosphate, potassium, magnesium and water into the cells.
- Synthesis of lean tissue.

This can lead to fluid retention and low serum levels of potassium, magnesium and phosphate (Solomon & Kirby, 1990; Brooks & Melnik, 1995). NICE (2006) defines at risk patients as those who have had very little or no food intake for >5 days, especially if already undernourished [body mass index (BMI) <20 kg/m^2; unintentional weight loss of >5% within the last 3–6 months]. High risk patients are those with any one of the following:

- BMI <16 kg/m^2.
- Unintentional weight loss of >15% within the last 3–6 months.
- Very little or no nutrition for >10 days.
- Low levels of potassium, magnesium or phosphate prior to feeding.

or those with two or more of the following:

- BMI <18.5 kg/m^2.
- Unintentional weight loss of >10% within the last 3–6 months.
- Very little or no nutrition for >5 days.
- A history of alcohol abuse or some drugs, including insulin, chemotherapy, antacids or diuretics.

It is important to note that patients with normal levels of potassium, magnesium and phosphate prior to the commencement of feed can still be at risk of refeeding syndrome (Marinella, 2004; NICE, 2006).

Refeeding syndrome can occur in patients fed orally, enterally or parenterally. Although possible, it is less likely to occur in those fed orally (Fung & Rimmer, 2005) since starvation is usually accompanied by a reduction in appetite. However, care should be taken when prescribing oral nutritional supplements. If a patient is considered at risk of refeeding syndrome, they should be fed using the following guidelines (NICE 2006):

- *At risk patients:*
  - Introduce feeding at a maximum 50% of total energy requirements for the first 2 days before increasing to full requirements if no biochemical abnormalities.

Table 6.4.2 Monitoring of patients receiving enteral nutrition

Monitoring parameter	Examples of monitoring	Rationale
Nutritional intake	Food charts, fluid charts, patient reporting	To compare prescribed with actual volume of feed delivered To facilitate transition between different forms of nutritional support To prevent over or under hydration To take account of energy and electrolyte content of IV/enteral fluid infusions
Anthropometry	Weight, body mass index, mid upper arm circumference, triceps skin fold thickness, hand grip dynamometry	To monitor changes in nutritional status To ensure nutritional objectives are met
Clinical chemistry	Biochemistry, haematology	Aids interpretation of hydration status, metabolic stress, specific nutrient deficiencies and metabolic abnormalities.
Clinical condition	Consciousness, swallow status, temperature	To observe changes which may affect nutritional requirements and most appropriate route of access To ensure that the type of nutritional support being provided remains appropriate To monitor for presence of infection
Medications prescribed	Drug charts	To be aware of side effects that may affect tolerance of enteral tube feeding, e.g. nausea/altered bowel habit To be aware of possible drug–nutrient interactions To be aware of drugs that may affect timing of enteral tube feeding To ensure that drugs are in appropriate form for administration via feeding tube To reduce incidence of tube blockage To be aware of the importance of adequate flushing of tubes before and after administration of medication To be aware of medication that may contribute to energy intake, e.g. propofol
Gastrointestinal tolerance	Stool charts, gastric residual volumes	To monitor bowel function and tolerance of feed To assess gastric emptying and therefore determine appropriateness of gastric feeding
Feeding device	Observe position and condition of feeding tube and site of tube insertion	To ensure appropriate position of feeding tube To monitor for signs or infection and or irritation To observe for leaks and cracks in tube
Nutritional goals and outcomes	Dependent on specific goals set but likely to include a measure of nutritional intake and nutritional status	To ensure progress towards agreed objectives of nutritional support To ensure clinical effectiveness of dietetic intervention To ensure objectives remain realistic and achievable To ensure that nutritional interventions remain appropriate to overall care of patients

- ○ Meet full requirements for fluid, electrolytes, vitamins and minerals from day 1 of feeding.
- • *High risk patients:*
  - ○ Consider starting nutrition at a maximum 10 kcal/kg (41.8 kJ/mL) and increase slowly to meet full requirements by 4–7 days. Any increase in feed should be dependent on trends in biochemistry.
  - ○ Potassium, magnesium and phosphate supplementation should be given from the outset (unless blood levels are already high).
  - ○ Give thiamine and a multivitamin.
  - ○ Restore circulatory volume and monitor fluid balance closely.
  - ○ Monitor appropriate biochemistry, including, potassium, phosphate and magnesium.
  - ○ In extreme cases (e.g. BMI <14 kg/m², very little or no nutrition for >15 days or prefeeding hypokalaemia, hypophosphataemia or hypomagnesaemia), consider starting feed at 5 kcal/kg (21 kJ/mL).

Close communication with the medical team is crucial to prevent and recognise refeeding syndrome. A clear plan should be formulated to ensure all team members are aware of their roles and responsibilities in close monitoring and treatment.

Aspiration

Aspiration risk for gastrostomy feeding is the same as for nasogastric feeding. Gastroparesis may be a result of disease management, starvation, or nerve damage, e.g. diabetic neuropathy (see Chapter 7.4.4). Regurgitation of stomach contents and aspiration into the lungs can cause asphyxia; even small amounts increase the risk of pneumonia. The aspiration risk has traditionally been assumed to increase with residual volumes of 200 mL or above (McClave *et al.*, 1992), but more recent evidence suggests this may be an over simplification, particularly in critically ill patients. This subject is discussed in more depth in

Chapter 7.17.1. Failure to establish gastric emptying is not a reason for immediate intravenous nutritional support. Reviewing current medications, e.g. opiates, and the commencement of prokinetic agents should establish adequate emptying (NICE, 2006). Post pyloric feeding should be considered before intravenous nutritional support.

If aspiration is a risk, the following actions may be taken:

- Elevate the head and upper body to at least 30 degrees and maintain this position during and 1 hour after feeding.
- Use prokinetic agents to stimulate gastric emptying, e.g. metaclopromide or erythromycin.
- Consider a post pyloric feeding route – jejunostomy feeding with aspiration of gastric contents by a nasogastric tube is the only safe way to prevent feed aspiration (Elpern, 1997).

Diarrhoea

Diarrhoea is common in enterally fed patients, but is rarely attributable to the enteral feed itself (Bowling & Silk, 1998), although may be attributed to the feeding mechanism. Prolonged use of antibiotics permits *Clostridium difficile* overgrowth and subsequent diarrhoea (Bliss *et al.*, 1998). Enteral administration of magnesium or electrolytes can cause osmotic diarrhoea. Osmolality of the feed is rarely a concern, and feed dilution exacerbates the problem. It is important to consider the following points for enterally fed patients who experience diarrhoea:

- Obtain a stool sample to exclude pathogenic bacteria overgrowth.
- Review the need for, and choice of, antibiotic.
- Ensure adequate hydration – additional fluid may be required as a result of increased losses.
- Reduction in infusion rate of post pyloric feed.
- Use of a peptide feed if malabsorption is suspected.
- Bile acid sequestrants, e.g. cholestyramine, if bile salt diarrhoea is suspected.
- Review medications (drugs in a sorbitol syrup containing ≥15 g of sorbitol can have a laxative effect).
- Consider a fibre feed – a significant reduction in diarrhoea has been shown when using a fibre supplemented enteral feed formula with hospital patients (Elia *et al.*, 2008).

Current evidence to support probiotic use in the management of diarrhoea in critically ill enterally fed patients remains unclear (Jack *et al.*, 2010).

Tube blockage

The small internal diameter (1–2 mm) of fine bore tubes increases the risk of occlusion. The most common cause is coagulation of feed by drug syrups and suspensions, combined with inadequate tube flushing, or obstruction by particles of crushed oral medications. Tube occlusion risk can be minimised by:

- Flushing the tube regularly with water.
- Flushing the tube with water following drug administration (and between drugs).
- Giving medicines individually rather than together, to avoid precipitate formation from drug interactions.
- Using drugs in syrup or dispersible form, rather than crushed tablets.

Consideration should be given to the type of water used to flush enteral feeding tubes. For gastric tubes the choice is tap, cooled boiled or sterile water, but a risk assessment should be undertaken as the choice may be different in the hospital and the patient's home. For post pyloric feeding, sterile water should always be used. Flushing with warm water should be tried initially to unblock a tube, along with manipulation of the tube. Soda water and sodium bicarbonate can also be effective in clearing a blockage. Cola, pineapple juice and lemonade should not be used as the acidity may contribute to occlusion by denaturing the proteins in the enteral feed (Beckwith *et al.*, 2004). Pancreatic enzymes are effective and can unblock a feeding tube blocked with feed within 10–20 minutes (Marcaud & Stegall, 1990); other agents are commercially available. Although gastrostomy tubes are larger in size (usually 12–20 FR), blockages can still occur and therefore measures to minimise risk should still be taken.

Microbiological contamination of feed

Enteral feeds provide an ideal growth medium for microbial contamination, but low counts of non-pathogenic bacteria are clinically unimportant. Bacterial growth within the feed can be minimised by practices such as:

- Using commercially prepackaged, sterile, ready to hang feeds (Beattie & Anderton 1999; 2001). Modular feeds carry a greater risk of microbiological contamination.
- Limiting the hanging time of the feed to a maximum of 24 hours or 4 hours for non-sterile feeds (Payne-James *et al.*, 1992).
- Replacement of reservoir and giving set daily.
- Filling the feeding reservoir with feed for up to 24 hours use rather than for only 4 hours (Patchell *et al.*, 1998).
- Hygienic handling of systems and adequate hand hygiene (Lee & Hodgkiss, 1999).
- Ensuring that systems marked as single use are used only once.
- Ensuring that reuseable equipment for single patient use, e.g. syringes, nasogastric tubes and guide wires, are cleaned, labelled and stored appropriately in accordance with local policy.

Additional care should be taken with jejunal feeds in patients with achlorhydria and immunosuppressed patients as their lack of gastric acidity and impaired immune function, respectively, may increase infection risk.

Accidental tube removal

Feeding tubes can become dislodged or removed accidentally. In the case of nasogastric tubes, the tube should be removed completely and repassed (with the same tube and original guide wire if single patient use) and position reconfirmed. If a gastrostomy tube is accidentally removed, to prevent another procedure, it is important to replace the tube quickly to preserve the stoma tract that can start to heal immediately. Balloon replacement tubes can be used and a spare tube should be routinely supplied to the patient in case of such circumstances. Where there is no spare tube available, a Foley catheter can be used to maintain the tract until an appropriate feeding tube is reinserted, but Foley catheters must not be used for feeding. It is essential that patients and carers are aware of what to do should the feeding tube become dislodged or removed. Adequate training and education for patients, carers and professionals can ensure this is the case.

Stoma site problems

Stoma site complications include leakage, exit site infections, pneumo peritoneum, intra-abdominal abscesses, necrotising fasciitis, problems with self care secondary to poor placement and infection, which can be potentially fatal (Hanlon, 1998). Overgranulation is also a common stoma site problem, but can generally be reduced by correct positioning of the external fixation device (Best, 2004). Minor complications can usually be managed without admission to hospital; a swab of the site may be useful to rule out infection. Thorough hand hygiene and avoiding unnecessary dressings around the stoma site can help minimise the risk of such problems, as can good training for patients and carers regarding tube care. Regular assessment of the stoma site should be integrated into monitoring protocols. A specialist enteral nutrition nurse can also advise regarding treatment for minor gastrostomy related complications and often this service is supplied as part of the enteral nutrition contract for hospitals and community settings.

Buried bumper syndrome

Buried bumper syndrome (BBS) occurs when the gastric mucosa grows over the internal bumper of the gastrostomy tube, resulting in migration through, or into, the abdominal wall. This can result in mechanical feed delivery failure, pain, peritonitis and even death. BBS can be prevented by ensuring the tube is measured and fitted correctly, and regularly introduced into the stomach and rotated. Should BBS occur, the tube must be removed either endoscopically or surgically.

Enteral feeding equipment

The equipment required for enteral tube feeding depends on the method used. Bolus feeding requires only syringes for fluid and feed delivery. Continuous feeding requires a feeding pump, giving sets, syringes and possibly feeding reservoirs if a modular feed or extra water is being administered via the pump. Ambulatory feeding pumps are available for mobile patients. Syringes for enteral feeding are either female luer lock or catheter tipped and must be NPSA compliant (NPSA, 2007). Syringes are available in several sizes from 5 to 60 mL. The largest size is used for water flushes and administration of feed; the smaller sizes can be used for more accurate measurement and administration of medicines.

Weaning from enteral nutrition

Although many patients will rely on enteral feeding as their sole source of nutrition for life, some may be able to resume oral feeding. Once oral feeding has been deemed safe to recommence, enteral feeding can be continued in conjunction with an oral diet during the transitional period. The feeding rate or bolus size can be increased to allow a longer rest period, a higher energy feed can be used or the feed can be reduced to provide <100% of estimated requirements. Bolus feeding or overnight feeding can be useful in ensuring nutritional requirements are met whilst encouraging daytime oral intake during the transitional period. Care should be taken to ensure that patients do not become dehydrated during the weaning process; additional fluid boluses can help to minimise this risk.

Home enteral feeding

Home enteral feeding (HEF) is an expanding area of nutritional support (BAPEN, 2010). The majority of home enterally fed patients have had a stroke, head and neck cancer or a degenerative disorder, e.g. Parkinson's disease or motor neurone disease (BAPEN, 2010). The dietitian's role in the discharge into the community of patients on nutritional support is integral to the process. Local policies and procedures should be in place for training, discharge planning and monitoring of the patient (Elia, 1994). Pressure on hospital beds often leads to early discharge of enterally fed patients, so it is important that patients are reviewed regularly during the initial period to ensure optimal nutritional support is achieved and that plans for discharge are made in an appropriate and timely manner.

Enteral feeds prescribed in the community are available on prescription, but the feeding equipment is financed by the primary care budget. Determination of who pays for the equipment must be confirmed before the patient is discharged. Most UK feed companies provide training, delivery of feeds and equipment, and servicing of pumps to community patients.

The discharge planning process should take into account the knowledge, skills and support network of those who will be responsible for caring for the tube and setting up the feed once the patient is home. The patient and family are usually encouraged to manage these themselves, with adequate training and support provided pre and post discharge. However, if this is not possible, the responsibility often falls to the district nursing teams. Many patients are discharged to nursing homes; therefore, adequate training for care staff should be arranged. The feeding regimen may be altered for discharge home

Table 6.4.3 Discharge planning for patients receiving enteral nutrition at home

Stage of discharge planning	Dietitian's role and responsibility
Decision made to insert feeding tube	Part of the multidisciplinary team; can offer advice regarding what enteral feeding will entail to ensure patients/carers make an informed decision
Decision made to discharge home	Inform home enteral feeding (HEF) dietitian Ensure patient and carers are appropriately trained to use feeding pump and care for the tube Provide written information and contact details Involve other services if required, e.g. district nurse Ensure feeding regimen is suitable for home
On discharge	Ensure patient is discharged with sufficient supply of feed and equipment until repeat prescription and delivery have been confirmed Order supplies, request feed prescription from GP and arrange ongoing delivery of feed and equipment Handover to HEF dietitian
Post discharge	Ensure patient and carers are familiar with management of tube and administration of feed Ensure patient has all necessary equipment Monitor nutritional support intervention and provide a follow-up plan

to best fit with usual home routines and patient/carer preferences. Table 6.4.3 outlines the steps in discharge planning and the dietitian's roles and responsibilities.

The role of the HEF dietitian not only involves the physical, biochemical and anthropometrical monitoring of patients, but also addressing the impact of this potentially life changing intervention. Quality of life issues should be examined, to ensure the feeding regimen is acceptable and suitable for the individual. Patient support groups, such as Patients on Intravenous and Nasogastric Therapy (PINNT), may be useful. Some HEF dietitians also take on the extended role of replacing balloon replacement gastrostomies and nasogastric tubes, and this can help prevent unnecessary hospital admissions, reduce the burden on the acute setting and enable feeding to continue with minimum disruption.

Further reading

Bradnam V, White R, on behalf of the British Pharmaceutical Nutrition Group. (2011) *Handbook of Drug Administration via Enteral Feeding Tubes*, 2nd edn. London: Pharmaceutical Press.

Micklewright A, Todorovic V (eds) and the Parenteral and Enteral Nutrition Group of the British Dietetic Association (PENG). *A Pocket Guide to Clinical Nutrition*, 4th edn. PEN Group Publications.

National Institute for Health and Care Excellence (NICE). (2006) *Nutrition Support in Adults*. Clinical Guideline 32. London: NICE.

Stroud M, Duncan H, Nightingale J, British Society of Gastroenterology. (2003) Guidelines for enteral feeding in adult hospital patients. *Gut* 52 (Suppl 7): vii1–vii12.

Westaby D, Young A, O'Toole P, Smith G, Sanders D. (2010) The provision of a percutaneoulsy placed enteral tube feeding service. *Gut* 59: 1592–1605.

Internet resources

American Society for Parenteral and Enteral Nutrition (ASPEN) www.nutritioncare.org

British Association for Parenteral and Enteral Nutrition (BAPEN) www.bapen.org.uk

European Society for Clinical Nutrition and Metabolism (ESPEN) www.espen.org

Parenteral and Enteral Nutrition Group of the British Dietetic Association (PENG) www.peng.org.uk

Patients on Intravenous and Nasogastric Nutrition Therapy (PINNT) www.pinnt.com

References

Abuksis G, Mor M, Plaut S, Fraser G, Niv Y. (2004) Outcome of percutaneous endoscopic gastrostomy (PEG): comparison of two policies in a 4-year experience. *Clinical Nutrition* 23(3): 341–346.

American Dietetic Association (ADA). (1997) Position Paper. The role of registered dietitians in enteral and parenteral nutrition support. *Journal of the American Dietetic Association* 97: 302–304.

Beattie TK, Anderton DA. (1999) Microbial evaluation of four enteral feeding systems which have deliberately been subjected to faulty handling procedures. *Journal of Hospital Infection* 42: 11–20.

Beattie TK, Anderton DA. (2001) Decanting versus sterile pre-filled nutrient containers – the microbial risks in enteral feeding. *International Journal of Environmental Health Research* 11(1): 81–93.

Beckwith MC, Feddema SS, Barton RG. (2004) A guide to drug therapy in patients with enteral feeding tubes: dosage form selection and administration methods. *Hospital Pharmacy* 39: 225–237.

Best C. (2004) The correct positioning and role of an external fixation device on a PEG. *Nursing Times* 100: 18–50.

Bliss DZ, Johnson S, Savik K, Clabots CR, Willard K, Gerding DN. (1998) Acquisition of *C. difficile* and *Clostridium difficile*-associated diarrhoea in hospitalised patients receiving tube feeding. *Annals of Internal Medicine* 129: 1012–1019.

Bonten MJM, Gaillard CA, van Tiel FH, van der Geest S, Stobberingh EE. (1994) Continuous enteral feeding counteracts preventive measures for gastric colonisation in intensive care unit patient. *Critical Care Medicine* 22: 939–944.

Bowling TE, Silk DBA. (1998) Colonic responses to enteral tube feeding. *Gut* 42: 147–151.

Bradnam V, White R, on behalf of the British Pharmaceutical Nutrition Group. (2011) *Handbook of Drug Administration via Enteral Feeding Tubes*, 2nd edn. London: Pharmaceutical Press.

British Association for Parenteral and Enteral Nutrition (BAPEN). (2010) Artificial Nutrition Support in the UK 2000–2009 A Report by the British Artificial Nutrition Survey (BANS), a committee of

BAPEN (The British Association for Parenteral and Enteral Nutrition). Available at www.bapen.org.uk. Accessed 24 February 2012.

British Society of Gastroenterology (BSG). (1999) *Guidelines for Informed Consent for Endoscopic Procedures*. London: BSG.

Brooks MJ, Melnik G. (1995) The refeeding syndrome: an approach to understanding its complications and preventing its occurrence. *Pharmacotherapy* 15(6): 713–726.

Cappell MS. (2007) Risk factors and risk reduction of malignant seeding of the percutaneous endoscopic gastrostomy track from pharyngoesophageal malignancy: a review of all 44 known reported cases. *American Journal of Gastroenterology* 102: 1307–1311.

Coventry BJ, Karatassas A, Gower L, Wilson P. (1994) Intestinal passage of the PEG end-piece: is it safe? *Journal of Gastroenterology and Hepatology* 9: 311–313.

Elpern EH. (1997) Pulmonary aspiration in hospitalized adults. *Nutrition in Clinical Practice* 12: 5–13.

European Community (EC). (1999) Commission Directive on Dietary Foods for Special Medical Purposes. 1999/21/EC of 25 March 1999. *Official Journal of the European Communities* L91/29–L91/35.

Elia M (ed.) (1994) *Enteral and Parenteral Nutrition in the Community*. BAPEN Working Party Report. Maidenhead: BAPEN.

Elia M, Engfer MB, Green CJ, Silk DBA. (2008) Systematic review and meta-analysis: the clinical and physiological effects of fibre-containing enteral formulae. *Alimentary Pharmacology & Therapeutics* 27: 120–145.

Foster JM, Filocamo P, Nava H, *et al.* (2007) The introducer technique is the optimal method for placing percutaneous endoscopic gastrostomy tubes in head and neck cancer patients. *Surgical Endoscopy* 21: 897–901.

Fung AT, Rimmer J. (2005) Hypophosphataemia secondary to Oral Refeeding Syndrome in a patient with long-term alcohol misuse. *Medical Journal of Australia* 183(6): 324–326.

Galban C, Montejo JC, Mesejo A, *et al.* (2000) An immune-enhancing enteral diet reduces mortality rate and episodes of bacteremia in septic intensive care unit patients. *Critical Care Medicine* 28(3): 643–648.

Hamaoui E, Lefkowitz R, Olender L, Krasnopolsky-Levine E, Favale M, Hoover EL. (1990) Enteral nutrition in the early postoperative period: a new semi-elemental formula versus total parenteral nutrition. *Journal of Parenteral and Enteral Nutrition* 14: 501–507.

Hanlon MD. (1998) Preplacement marking for optimal gastrostomy and jejunostomy tube site locations to decrease complications and promote self-care. *Nutrition in Clinical Practice* 13: 167–171.

Heyland DK, Drover JW, MacDonald S, Novak F, Lam M. (2001) Effect of post-pyloric feeding on gastroesophageal regurgitation and pulmonary microaspiration: results of a randomized control trial. *Critical Care Medicine* 29: 1495–1501.

Jack L, Coyer F, Courtney M, Venkatesh B. (2010) Probiotics and diarrhoea management in enterally tube fed critically ill patients – what is the current evidence? *Intensive and Critical Care Nursing* 26(6): 314–326.

Lee CH, Hodgkiss IJ. (1999) The effect of handling procedures on enteral feeding systems in Hong Kong. *Journal of Hospital Infection* 42: 119–123.

Malone AM. (1997) Is a pulmonary enteral formula warranted for patients with pulmonary dysfunction? *Nutrition in Clinical Practice* 12: 168–171.

Marcaud SP, Stegall KS. (1990) Unclogging feeding tubes with pancreatic enzyme. *Journal of Parenteral and Enteral Nutrition* 14: 198–200.

Marinella MA. (2004) Refeeding syndrome: implications for the inpatient rehabilitation unit. *American Journal of Physical and Medical Rehabilitation* 83: 65–68.

McAtear CA (ed.) (1999) *Current Perspectives on Enteral Nutrition in Adults*. BAPEN Working Party Report. Maidenhead: BAPEN.

McClave SA, Snider HL, Lowen CC, *et al.* (1992) Use of residual volume as a marker for enteral feeding intolerance: prospective blinded comparison with physical examination and radiographic findings. *Journal of Parenteral and Enteral Nutrition* 16: 99–105.

McClave SA, Lukan JK, Stefater JA, *et al.* (2005) Poor validity of residual volumes as a marker for risk of aspiration in critically ill patients. *Critical Care Medicine* 33(2): 324–330.

Merrick S, Harnden S, Shetty S, Chopra P, Clamp P, Kapadia S. (2008) An Evaluation of the 'Cut and Push' method of percutaneous endoscopic gastrostomy (PEG) removal. *Journal of Parenteral and Enteral Nutrition* 32: 78–80.

Metheny NA, Clouse RE, Chang YH, Stewart BJ, Oliver DA, Koller MH. (2006) Tracheobronchial aspiration of gastric contents in critically ill tube fed patients: frequency, outcomes, and risk factors. *Critical Care Medicine* 34(4): 1007–1015.

Micklewright A, Todorovic V (eds). and the Parenteral and Enteral Nutrition Group of the British Dietetic Association (PENG). (2011) *A Pocket Guide to Clinical Nutrition*. PEN Group Publications.

National Institute for Health and Care Excellence (NICE) (2006) *Nutrition Support in Adults*. Clinical Guideline 32. London: NICE.

National Patient Safety Agency (NPSA). (2005) *Reducing the Harm caused by Misplaced Nasogastric Feeding Tubes*. Patient Safety Alert 05. London: NPSA.

National Patient Safety Agency (NPSA). (2007) *Promoting Safer Measurement and Administration of Liquid Medicines via Oral and Other Enteral Routes. Patient Safety Alert* 19. London: NPSA.

National Patient Safety Agency (NPSA). (2010) *Early Detection of Complications after Gastrostomy*. Rapid Response Report NPSA/2010/RRR010. London: NPSA.

National Patient Safety Agency (NPSA). (2011) *Reducing the Harm Caused by Misplaced Nasogastric Feeding Tubes in Adults, Children and Infants*. Patient Safety Alert 002. London: NPSA.

O'Keefe SJ, Foody W, Gill S. (2003) Transnasal endoscopic placement of feeding tubes in the intensive care unit. *Journal of Parenteral and Enteral Nutrition* 27: 349–354.

Patchell CJ, Anderton DA, Holden C, MacDonald A, George RH, Bouth IW. (1998) Reducing bacterial contamination of enteral feeds. *Archives of Diseases in Childhood* 78: 166–168.

Payne-James JJ, Bray J, Rana S, McSwiggan D, Silk DBA. (1992) Retrograde contamination of enteral feeding delivery systems. *Journal of Parenteral and Enteral Nutrition* 16: 369–373.

Poulard F, Dimet J, Martin-Lefevre L, *et al.* (2010) Impact of not measuring residual gastric volume in mechanically ventilated patients receiving early enteral feeding: a prospective before-after study. *Journal of Parenteral and Enteral Nutrition* 34: 125–130.

Rao MM, Kallam R, Arsalanizadeh R, Gatt M, MacFie J. (2009) Placing of enteral feeding tubes by the bedside using an electromagnetic sensing device. *British Journal of Intensive Care* 19: 54–59.

Royal College of Physicians (RCP) and British Society of Gastroenterology. (2010) *Oral Feeding Difficulties and Dilemmas: A Guide to Practical Care Particularly Towards the End of Life*. London: Royal College of Physicians.

Sanders DS, Carter MJ, D'Silva J, *et al.* (2002) Percutaneous endoscopic gastrostomy: a prospective audit of the impact of guidelines in 2 district general hospitals in the United Kingdom. *American Journal of Gastroenterology* 97: 2239–2245.

Shaw AS, Ampong MA, Rio A, *et al.* (2006) Survival of patients with ALS following institution of enteral feeding is related to pre-procedure oximetry: a retrospective review of 98 patients in a single centre. *Amyotrophic Lateral Sclerosis* 7: 16–21.

Silk DBA. (1993) Fibre and enteral nutrition. *Clinical Nutrition* 12 (Suppl 1): 106–113.

Silk DB. (2011) The evolving role of post-ligament of Treitz nasojejunal feeding in enteral nutrition and the need for improved feeding tube design and placement methods. *Journal of Parenteral and Enteral Nutrition* 35(3): 303–307.

Solomon SL, Kirby DF. (1990) The refeeding syndrome: A review. *Journal of Parenteral and Enteral Nutrition* 14(1): 90–97.

Stroud M, Duncan H, Nightingale J. (2003) Guidelines for enteral feeding in adult hospital patients. *Gut* 52 (Suppl 7): 1–12.

Taylor SJ, Manara AR, Brown J. (2010) Treating delayed gastric emptying in critical illness: Metoclopramide, erythromycin, and bedside (Cortrak) nasointestinal tube placement. *Journal of Parenteral and Enteral Nutrition* 34: 289–294.

Thurley PD, Hooper MA, Jobling JC, Teahon K. (2008) Fluroscopic insertion of postpyloric feeding tubes: success rates and complication rates. *Clinical Radiology* 63: 543–548.

Tibbitts GM, Sorrell RJ. (1999) Duodenal obstruction from a gastric feeding tube. *New England Journal of Medicine* 340: 970–971.

Westaby D, Young A, O'Toole P, Smith G, Sanders D. (2010) The provision of a percutaneoulsy placed enteral tube feeding service. *Gut* 59: 1592–1605.

Wollman B, D'Agostino HB, Walus-Wigle JR, Easter DW, Beale B. (1995) Radiological, endoscopic and surgical gastrostomy: an institutional evaluation and meta-analysis of the literature. *Radiology* 197: 699–704.

Zachos M, Tondeur M, Griffiths AM. (2006) Enteral nutritional therapy for induction of remission in Crohn's disease (Review). *Cochrane Database of Systematic Reviews* 1: CD000542.

Zick G, Frerichs A, Ahrens M, *et al.* (2011) A new technique for bedside placement of enteral feeding tubes: a prospective cohort study. *Critical Care* 15: R8.

6.5

Parenteral nutrition

Melanie Baker and Lynn Harbottle

Key points

■ Parenteral nutrition (PN) should only be used when the enteral route is inaccessible or inadequate.

■ Parenteral nutrition can be given peripherally or centrally depending on the predicted length of duration, availability of venous access and nutritional requirements.

■ Electrolytes and micronutrients must be added to all in one and individually compounded bags to meet individual nutritional requirements.

■ Detailed prefeed assessment and close monitoring for metabolic, infectious or mechanical complications is vital.

■ Nutrition teams have an important role in ensuring quality control around the initiation, supply, monitoring and auditing of PN practice and outcomes.

Parenteral nutrition (PN) refers to the delivery of all nutrients, electrolytes and fluid directly into a central or peripheral vein. It is a well established technique for providing nutritional support when the gastrointestinal tract is deemed unsafe or inaccessible, or if absorption via enteral or oral feeding is inadequate to meet full nutritional requirements (NICE, 2006). Previously, PN was considered to have greater complication rates than enteral tube feeding (ETF); however, many of these problems were due to inappropriate use, inadequate line care, unbalanced formulations and significant overfeeding (Koretz *et al.*, 2001). It has subsequently been shown to have similar complication rates to ETF (Woodcock *et al.*, 2001).

Until recently, recommendations regarding the use of PN restricted use to situations where it was to be the sole source of nutrition [and it was therefore referred to as total parenteral nutrition (TPN)]. It was considered that there was no clinical benefit in TPN unless it was to be required for >5 days. However, evidence now supports its wider use where oral feeding or ETF cannot be used and as a supplement to EN when the patient cannot tolerate sufficient EN to meet nutritional requirements (NICE, 2006). Even 1–2 days of PN can improve gastrointestinal tract function and clinical condition and should be considered for short term use in appropriate patients (Austin & Stroud, 2007).

Although PN is an essential and potentially life saving therapy, it is expensive and may be associated with a high risk of serious and, occasionally, life threatening complications, including line infections, micronutrient deficits, electrolyte disturbances, liver dysfunction, hyperglycaemia, hyperlipidaemia and cardiac failure (Austin & Stroud, 2007). It is therefore vital that it is administered appropriately and monitored closely. Where possible, patients should be informed of the potential risks and benefits before treatment, so they can make an informed decision about their treatment.

National and international organisations [British Association for Parenteral and Enteral Nutrition (BAPEN), National Institute for Health and Care Excellence, European Society for Parenteral and Enteral Nutrition, American Society for Parenteral and Enteral Nutrition] have repeatedly recommended the development of multidisciplinary nutrition support teams (NSTs), which include dietitians, to optimise management of patients on PN. Such teams have been shown to improve patient outcomes (Naylor *et al.*, 2004) and save costs (Kennedy & Nightingale, 2005). Despite this, only 60% of hospitals currently have nutrition teams (NCEPOD, 2010) and only 19% of adult PN cases received a good standard of practice, with a significant percentage of cases not receiving any dietetic input. The key recommendations of the NCEPOD study are:

• Multidisciplinary nutrition team management of all PN.
• Only use PN if enteral nutrition has been considered and ruled out.
• Avoid unnecessary delays in recognising the need for and instituting PN.

Manual of Dietetic Practice, Fifth Edition. Edited by Joan Gandy.
© 2014 The British Dietetic Association. Published 2014 by John Wiley & Sons, Ltd.
Companion Website: www.manualofdieteticpractice.com

- Ensure robust assessment is in place and document the purpose and goal of PN.
- Ensure close clinical, biochemical and line monitoring, and clear documentation.
- Active assessment and regular review of intravenous fluid requirements and type.
- Increased education on PN.
- Local proformas and guidelines on use of PN.
- Central record of use and regular audit (a self assessment checklist and audit tool is available from NCEPOD, which can be used as a gap analysis tool in local risk assessments).
- Dedicated central venous catheter (CVC)/peripherally inserted central venous catheter (PICC) service.

Indications

Clinical indications

Parenteral nutrition should only be used when it is not possible to meet nutritional needs via the enteral route. An assessment of gastrointestinal tract function is required, ideally undertaken by a NST; however, some techniques historically used to assess gastrointestinal tract function, e.g. bowel sounds and gastric secretions, have been questioned (Schulman & Sawyer, 2005; Parrish & McClave, 2008). Recent advances have facilitated enteral nutrition use in clinical conditions for which PN was previously favoured, e.g. acute pancreatitis (McClave et al., 2006) and post gastrointestinal surgery (Bozzetti et al., 2001). Advances in ETF delivery techniques, particularly the use of postpyloric feeding tubes, have also reduced the need to give PN, e.g. after upper gastrointestinal tract surgery (Ryan et al., 2006).

Intestinal failure is often short term and self limiting. Indications for short to medium term PN (<14–28 days), whether providing complete or supplementary nutrition, include:

- Major gastrointestinal surgery – where there is no suitable enteral feeding access or it is contraindicated, e.g. intra-abdominal sepsis or perforation.
- Enterocutaneous fistulae – where position, volume or sepsis prevent enteral feeding.
- Gastrointestinal obstruction – where enteral feeding access is not possible.
- Prolonged postoperative ileus.
- Severe malabsorption.
- Severe mucositis following chemotherapy.
- Multiorgan failure.

More prolonged intestinal failure may result in patients remaining PN dependent for months or even permanently [Home Parenteral Nutrition and Intestinal Failure Clinical Network (HIFNET), 2008; Smith et al., 2011]. This may occur in:

- Short bowel syndrome – resulting from Crohn's disease, intestinal ischaemia, surgical complications.
- Motility disorders, e.g. scleroderma.
- Chronic malabsorption.
- Radiation enteritis.

Nutritional indications

Parenteral nutrition should be considered in those who are malnourished [body mass index (BMI) <18.5 kg/m^2, or >10% unintentional recent weight loss, or BMI <20 kg/m^2 and >5% unintentional recent weight loss) or are at risk of becoming so and who fit the clinical indications (NICE, 2006). It is *not* generally indicated in previously well nourished patients (BMI >20 kg/m^2 and <5% recent weight loss) exposed to short periods (up to 5 days) of inadequate nutrition.

Ethical considerations

Parenteral nutrition may not be appropriate if it prolongs an impaired quality of life unnecessarily, e.g. palliative treatment of advanced malignant disease, and the ethical aspects of feeding should be considered before treatment is commenced. If PN is initiated, its appropriateness and the patient's quality of life should be reviewed on a regular basis (Shang et al., 2006).

Treatment goals

A thorough assessment should consider goals of therapy from the outset. The overall aim should be that gastrointestinal tract function will recover to facilitate adequate oral or ETF feeding, although a prolonged period of PN may be required for gastrointestinal tract adaptation or if further surgery is required to restore gut integrity and function. If gut function cannot be restored long term, home PN (HPN) may need to be considered.

Nutrition assessment

A detailed nutrition assessment should be undertaken before initiating PN (see Chapter 2.2). Clinical assessment should consider baseline biochemistry and hydration status, as well as noting concurrent fluids and electrolytes therapy. Table 6.5.1 shows the parameters to be considered.

Access routes

Parenteral nutrition may be administered via a central or peripheral vein, the choice being dictated by availability of venous access (Figure 6.5.1), nutritional requirements and anticipated PN duration. Catheter insertion should be performed according to strict aseptic criteria (Department of Health, 2001); many hospitals now have dedicated vascular access insertion services.

Peripheral catheters

Peripheral catheters are suitable for short term (<14 days) peripheral feeding (PPN) and avoid the clinical risks and costs of CVCs (Kohlhardt et al., 1994). Patients must have good peripheral venous access. Thrombophlebitis is a common problem (Grant, 2001), which may be minimised by avoiding high osmolarity PN regimens. Only regimens clearly designated to be suitable for peripheral

Table 6.5.1 Baseline assessment of a patient requiring parenteral nutrition (PN)

Parameter	Rationale
Indication for PN	Degree of intestinal failure or reasons why enteral nutrition is not appropriate
Goal and expected duration of treatment	Goal of therapy should be determined from considering the overall clinical picture and patient prognosis
Access route for administration	To ensure PN is given via an appropriate route to reduce the risk of complications Central/peripheral route needs to be considered.
Previous nutritional intake	To predict the risk of refeeding syndrome when PN begins
Weight, anthropometry	Assessment of nutritional status and fluid balance
Body mass index (BMI)	Assess nutritional status
Percentage weight loss	Predict degree of malnutrition and refeeding risk
Clinical status – appearance, blood pressure, temperature	General condition, fluid balance, presence of infection, which will help inform on requirements
Drug therapy	Fluid/electrolyte content of concurrent treatment, e.g. IV fluids/medications Whether the patient is on appropriate medication to help promote gut function
Hydration status (fluid balance charts)	Fluid balance, additional gastrointestinal losses that need to be replaced, e.g. vomit, fistula, drain output
Urea and creatinine	Fluid balance, renal function
Electrolytes – sodium, potassium, calcium, phosphate, magnesium	Fluid balance, electrolyte status, refeeding risk
Full blood count and C-reactive protein	Presence of infection and anaemia
Albumin	Used in combination with inflammatory markers to assess catabolic state
Coagulation parameters	Before insertion of line

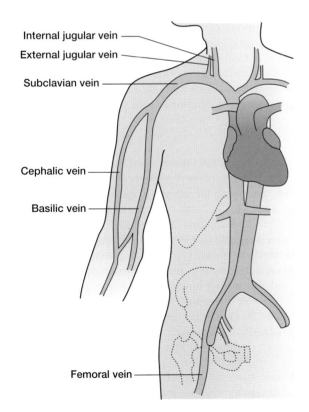

Internal jugular vein
External jugular vein
Subclavian vein
Cephalic vein
Basilic vein
Femoral vein

Figure 6.5.1 Access routes for parenteral nutrition [source: Dougherty L, Lamb J. (eds) 2008, figure 10.1, p. 263. Reproduced with permission of Blackwell Publishing]

use should be infused by this route. Therefore, PPN may not be suitable for patients with high requirements or who on a fluid restriction; there are limits to the additives possible (particularly potassium).

Central venous catheters

Indications for use of CVCs are (NICE, 2006):

- Patient expected to require PN for >14 days.
- Existing central access with a dedicated feeding lumen.
- No suitable veins for peripheral feeding.
- Specialised PN regimen requiring central access.

Central venous catheters should be inserted under ultrasound guidance (NICE, 2002) by experienced personnel and accessed via the subclavian (preferred), jugular or femoral veins. X ray confirmation of correct placement (catheter tip should lie at the junction of the superior vena cava and right atrium) and absence of insertion related complications should be ascertained before feeding is commenced. A variety of CVCs are available for feeding:

- Single or multi lumen.
- Tunnelled or non-tunnelled.
- Antibiotic impregnated.
- Implantable devices (ports).

Ideally, a dedicated single lumen line should be used. If a multi lumen line is used, all other lumens must be handled with the same meticulous attention to aseptic technique (Pittiruti *et al.*, 2009). Tunnelled lines can

SECTION 6

reduce the risk of infection (Randolph *et al.*, 1998), allow easier dressing and reduce the risk of dislodgement (Garden & Sim, 1983). Tunnelled lines with a cuff when used long term tunnelling will allow fibrosis around the line, thus securing it.

Peripherally inserted central catheters

A PICC line is inserted into the antecubital fossa and the proximal end advanced into a central vein; therefore, it can be used to deliver hypertonic solutions. Where short to medium term PN is needed and a CVC is not otherwise required, a PICC can be used (Thompson, 1999). However, PICCs are associated with a higher incidence of placement complications, limit arm movements and can be prone to occlusion or kinking (Cowl *et al.*, 2000).

Administration

Parenteral nutrition bags should be removed from the refrigerator before administration and allowed to adjust to room temperature. Strict aseptic techniques should be applied when setting up and changing PN bags. Local policies for administration, line care and management of complications should be in place and strictly adhered to. All PN must be administered through volumetric pumps with occlusion and air in line alarms to prevent metabolic complications. Most PN is administered continuously over 24 hours, but cyclical infusion may have physiological and psychological advantages and can reduce thrombophlebitis in PPN patients (Kerin *et al.*, 1991). A continuous infusion reduces the number of times the line is accessed and is more appropriate for severely stressed patients, such as those in intensive care where fluid balance is more problematic.

Formulations

Various PN regimens are available and local decision making will depend on compounding facilities, contractual arrangements and the need for specialist feeds to suit specific patient populations, e.g. renal, neonatal. There are three main forms of PN regimen:

* *Ready made three chamber all in one (AIO) bags* where carbohydrate, amino acids and fat sources are in three separate chambers, with or without electrolytes, and are mixed just before use. These bags should never be used alone but should always be administered with a full complement of micronutrients (NICE, 2006).
* *Ready made non-chamber AIO bags* where macronutrients are ready mixed with electrolytes and micronutrients. These tend to have a shorter shelf life and need to be kept refrigerated.
* *Tailored bags* that are made specifically to an individual's requirements. This requires adequately resourced aseptic unit facilities and the number of hospitals equipped to supply such bags is limited.

The stability of PN bags is affected by volume, proportion of different constituents (particularly amino acids and fat), amino acid formulation, glucose and electrolytes. Therefore, the final volume or amount of electrolytes provided may not exactly meet estimated requirements; all formulation requests should be discussed with the pharmacy. Bags should be made under full pharmacy aseptic conditions; it is not appropriate to make additions to bags at ward level.

Constituents

Macronutrients

Requirements for energy and protein should be estimated using standard methods (see Chapter 6.1). The relative contributions of fat, carbohydrate and protein (amino acids) energy provided in relation to requirements should be considered. In AIO regimens, the amount and percentage of macronutrients is fixed, but tailored regimens allow greater flexibility and may be indicated in specific circumstances, e.g. fat content may need to be reduced due to hepatobiliary complications in long term PN.

Protein

Protein is supplied as a balanced mixture of crystalline amino acids, or dipeptides for the less soluble heat labile amino acids, e.g. glutamine. The optimal PN amino acid profile remains unclear. Traditionally, amino acids were classified as indispensable (essential) or dispensable (non-essential); however, the latter are now considered essential under certain conditions (conditionally indispensable), e.g. glutamine (Laidlaw & Kopple, 1987; Grimble, 1993). Glutamine is not present in most commercially available amino acid solutions due to its instability. However, it can be added to a PN bag with other additions prior to administration.

Fat

Fat emulsions in PN commonly contain long chain triglycerides (LCTs) from soyabean or safflower oils and provide an energy dense yet isotonic alternative to dextrose. They also contain essential fatty acids to maintain cell membrane integrity and immune function. Fat emulsions are available in a range of concentrations (10–30%). Fat normally provides <50% of non-nitrogen energy needs in PN, and may help to minimise the risk of hyperglycaemia and abnormally high level of carbon dioxide in blood (hypercarbia). In some cases, e.g. PPN, fat may provide up to 60% of energy requirements. A minimum of 0.5 mg of LCT/kg/day is required to prevent essential fatty acid deficiency (Pullicino & Elia, 2001).

The high content of n-6 polyunsaturated fatty acids in lipid may have adverse effects on immunosuppression and pulmonary complications (Furukawa *et al.*, 1999; Askanazi *et al.*, 1981). Excessive amounts have been implicated in hypertriglyceridaemia and hepatobiliary disease. Increasingly, more diverse lipid preparations containing olive oil, medium chain triglyceride (MCT) and n-3 source appear to offer clinical benefits over soyabean oil based solutions. However, studies are based on small numbers in diverse clinical situations and the optimal lipid profile for different conditions remains unclear.

Carbohydrate

Glucose is available in concentrations of 5–70%. In PPN formulations the concentration and percentage of glucose used is reduced as excess glucose can cause the following problems:

- Contribute to high blood glucose levels. This has been shown to adversely affect outcome in the critically ill (Van den Berghe et al., 2001).
- Increase CO_2 production (Askanazi et al., 1980), aggravating impaired respiratory function, which delays weaning of patients from artificial ventilation (Askanazi et al., 1981).
- Cause hyperinsulinaemia, which prevents the mobilisation of endogenous lipid (Schloerb & Henning, 1998).
- Cause hepatic steatosis (Nightingale, 2003).

A maximum glucose oxidation rate of 4–7 mg/kg/min has been suggested (Burke et al., 1979); by using both glucose and fat energy sources this should not be exceeded.

Electrolytes

The electrolyte content of PN should be based on individual patient requirements, including additional amounts to cover losses (fistula, vomit, refeeding risk) or reductions (renal impairment, fluid overload). Amounts provided should be modified according to serum levels and consideration of other sources, including intravenous fluids and medications. Trends in electrolytes should always be considered rather than one off levels (which may result from taking blood from the catheter during PN administration or haemolysed samples). Table 6.5.2 shows recommendations for making adjustments to standard PN regimens, where increases or reductions in electrolytes are required in response to monitoring (Austin & Stroud, 2007).

Micronutrients

The American Medical Association (1979) recommendations for the provision of micronutrients in PN are used.

However, requirements in the critically ill and metabolically stressed patients remain poorly elucidated. The acute phase response to stress will alter serum levels, thus making monitoring of micronutrient status difficult. Vitamin losses from PN solutions may occur due to oxidation, formation of insoluble precipitates and photodegradation; therefore PN bags should be covered to shield them from sunlight.

The needs of most patients can be met by water and fat soluble vitamins and trace element solutions devised for PN. However, these make little provision for the restoration of body stores. Severely depleted or metabolically stressed patients may therefore need additional amounts, e.g. iron resistant anaemia secondary to copper deficiency has been reported in a patient fed PN secondary to active Crohn's disease (Spiegel & Willenbucher, 1999). Other nutrient deficiencies may include selenium (resulting in cardiomyopathy) and chromium (impairs glucose tolerance factor, exacerbating hyperglycaemia).

Intravenous administration bypasses the normal process of selective absorption and liver processing, so markedly increasing the risk of over dosage of some micronutrients in PN feeding. The risk of toxicity from trace elements such as copper and manganese is high as both are excreted via the biliary tract and their excretion is compromised in the presence of cholestatic syndromes. Excess manganese has been shown to cause neurotoxicity in PN fed patients (Ejima et al., 1992).

Monitoring

Monitoring of clinical state, nutritional requirements, anthropometry, biochemistry and line integrity is essential. The range and frequency of monitoring will depend on the nature and severity of illness, degree of malnutrition and length of time on PN (Austin & Stroud 2007; Micklewright & Todorovic 2005; NICE, 2006; Bowling, 2004).

Complications

Metabolic complications

These include deficiencies and excesses of fluid and nutrients, and occur if insufficient or excess nutrients are given

Table 6.5.2 Adjustments of parenteral nutrition formulations in response to monitoring

Electrolyte	Standard requirement* (not considering replacement of additional losses)	Usual level of adjustment**	Changes unlikely to be clinically significant**
Sodium	1.0–1.5 mmol/kg	Multiples of 40 mmol/day	±10–20 mmol
Potassium	1.0–1.5 mmol/kg	Multiples of 20 mmol/day	±5–10 mmol
Magnesium	0.1–0.2 mmol/kg	5–10 mmol/day	0–5 mmol
Calcium	0.1–0.15 mmol/kg	2.5–5 mmol/day	0–2.5 mmol
Phosphate	0.3–0.5 mmol/kg	10 mmol/day	0–5 mmol

*Elia (1990).
**Austin & Stroud (2007).

Table 6.5.3 Potential metabolic complications of parenteral nutrition

Complication	Possible causes	Prevention
Overhydration, oedema	Provision of excessive fluid, sodium	Detailed assessment of patient needs, including losses Consider other concurrent sources of fluid prior to deciding on PN volume
Hyperglycaemia	Excessive provision of glucose Severe metabolic stress Inappropriate insulin treatment	Max. GOR should not be exceeded Blood glucose should be regularly monitored Insulin should be provided if required
Electrolyte abnormalities, including refeeding syndrome	Inadequate or excessive provision in PN Overfeeding, especially initially	Detailed assessment and monitoring Proactive supplementation according to local guidelines, pharmacy, medical advice
Deranged liver function tests	Common in patients given PN but feed is rarely the main cause (Gabe & Culkin, 2010; Lee, 2006)	Rule out sepsis, medication, underlying liver disease Review total energy to avoid overfeeding from glucose and fat Consider type of fat given Consider cyclical feeding
Hypertriglyceridaemia	If metabolic capacity of the liver to clear fat is exceeded	Avoid excessive lipid provision Monitor and if found, reduce or occasionally remove lipid from PN for 2–3 days (Llop et al., 2003)

GOR, glucose oxidation rate.

or an inappropriate combination of nutrients for that patient is infused, as shown in Table 6.5.3.

Mechanical complications

Insertion related complications include failure to insert, pneumothorax or haemothorax, thrombosis, cardiac arrhythmias and nerve injury (Bowling, 2004). Longer term complications include:

- Thrombus – the risk of thrombus local to the catheter tip increases the longer the catheter is *in situ*.
- Catheter occlusion due to kinking, luminal deposition of fibrin, lipid sludge or debris (after prolonged feeding). Treatment should be as per local protocols.
- Catheter fracture, which can be minimised by the use of connection devices or extension sets that reduce the need to clamp the catheter, and so prolong its life.
- Thrombophlebitis – if there is evidence of phlebitis in peripheral feeding, the feed should be stopped.
- Extravasation can occur when the line displaces from the vessel and nutrition solution infiltrates local subcutaneous tissue.

Infectious complications

Central venous catheter related infections can originate from endogenous skin flora (the most common source of infection), contamination of the catheter hub or contamination of the CVC from a distant site (Krzywda *et al.*, 1999); the exit site tunnel and/or catheter can be infected. Catheter related sepsis is a serious condition and should be treated immediately according to local policies. It can be prevented by:

- Strict adherence to aseptic techniques.
- Only experienced staff being permitted to handle PN lines.
- Using closed systems.
- Using dedicated lines where possible.

Weaning from parenteral nutrition

As intestinal failure resolves, oral or ETF nutrition should be reintroduced, accompanied by a reduction in PN infusion rate to avoid both fluid overload and overfeeding. If electrolyte balance is not an issue, this can be achieved by slowing the infusion rate (some hospitals allow each bag to be hung for >24 hours), which is simpler and cheaper than compounding a series of individually modified bags. Most patients can be transferred entirely onto ETF or oral feeding when intestinal tolerance of more than half of their total nutrient needs is established. Parenteral nutrition should not continue just to supplement a poor oral intake, without consideration of other enteral feeding routes. It should never be stopped abruptly as rebound hypoglycaemia can occur. Supplementary PN may not necessarily impair appetite (Reifen *et al.*, 1999), although many PN patients express early satiety. Weaning from PN is a key dietetic role, and many patients may be anxious about increasing oral intake, particularly after a prolonged period of gut rest.

Home parenteral nutrition

Home parenteral nutrition (HPN) is indicated for ongoing intestinal failure, either permanently or in situations where a prolonged period of PN is required before further surgery to restore gastrointestinal function. In the UK in 2009, Crohn's disease accounted for 22% of new HPN registrations, followed closely by surgical complications (20%) and vascular disease (19%). The use of HPN in cancer patients has been steadily increasing (Smith *et al.*, 2011). A specialist centre with the experience and the required back up facilities should manage HPN patients; this is currently under review in England and Wales (HIFNET, 2008).

The role of a dietitian working with HPN patients encompasses the assessment and monitoring of nutritional status, the contribution of enteral intake to overall nutritional and fluid requirements (considering factors such as malabsorption), the design and monitoring of appropriate regimens, the development of evidence based nutrition education material for patients and carers and participation in audit and research, and should be a point of contact for patients, providing some psychological support (Baker & Farrer, 2006).

Protocols for the training of patients requiring HPN and their carers, and the recognition and management of problems are now readily available. The ability to counsel patients and relatives, and the availability of a 24-hour telephone contact number are important. There is a reported reduction in quality of life (social, psychological and physical parameters) in patients on HPN compared with those with an anatomical or functional short bowel not receiving HPN (Jeppesen et al., 1999).

Regimens should be tailored to suit the patient's requirements and lifestyle, and can differ significantly from inpatient regimens in terms of their composition and frequency, as nutritional needs and activity levels may be vary significantly. Infusions are commonly given over 10–12 hours nightly to allow for increased mobility during the day and to minimise hepatic abnormalities. In addition, to avoid hepatobiliary complications, total energy or lipid content may be reduced and some fat free bags may be indicated. Providing fluid balance is maintained, some patients may not require feeds every day.

Further reading

Bowling T. (2004) *Nutritional Support for Adults and Children: A Handbook for Hospital Practice*. Oxford: Radcliffe Medical Press.

Micklewright A, Todorovic V. (2005) *A Pocket Guide to Clinical Nutrition*. PEN Group Publications.

Nightingale J. (2001) *Intestinal Failure*. London: Greenwich Medical Media Ltd.

Payne-James J, Grimble G, Silk D. (2001) *Artificial Nutrition Support in Clinical Practice*. London: Greenwich Medical Media Ltd.

Powell-Tuck J, Gosling P, Lobo D, et al. (2011) *British Consensus Guidelines on Intravenous Fluid Therapy for Adult Surgical Patients*. Basingstoke: BAPEN.

Internet resources

British Association for Parenteral & Enteral Nutrition (BAPEN) www.bapen.org.uk

National Confidential Enquiry into Patient Outcome and Death www.ncepod.org.uk

Parenteral and Enteral Nutrition Group (PENG) of the British Dietetic Association   www.peng.org.uk

Patients on Intravenous & Nasogastric Nutrition Therapy (PINNT) www.pinnt.com

References

American Medical Association, Department of Foods and Nutrition. (1979) Guidelines for essential trace element preparations for parenteral use – A statement by an Expert Panel. *Journal of the American Medical Association* 241(19): 2051–2054.

Askanazi J, Stanley H, Rosenbaum SW, et al. (1980) Respiratory changes induced by the large glucose loads of total parenteral nutrition. *Journal of the American Medical Association* 243(14): 1444–1447.

Askanazi J, Nordenstrom J, Rosenbaum SH, et al. (1981) Nutrition for the patient with respiratory failure: glucose vs. fat. *Anesthesiology* 54: 373–377.

Austin P, Stroud M. (2007) *Prescribing Adult Intravenous Nutrition*. Pharmaceutical Press

Baker M, Farrer, K. (2006) Dietetics. In: Bozzetti F, Staun M, Van Gossum A (eds) *Home Parenteral Nutrition*. CABI International.

Bowling T. (2004) *Nutritional Support for Adults and Children: A Handbook for Hospital Practice*. Oxford: Radcliffe Medical Press.

Bozzetti F, Braga M, Gianotti L, Cavzzi C, Mariani L. (2001) Postoperative enteral versus parenteral nutrition in malnourished patients with gastrointestinal cancer: A randomised multicentred trial. *Lancet* 358: 1487–1493.

Burke JF, Wolfe RR, Mullany CJ, Mathews DE, Bier DM. (1979) Glucose requirements following burn injury. Parameters of optimal glucose infusion and possible hepatic and respiratory abnormalities following excessive glucose intake. *Annals of Surgery* 190(3): 274–285.

Cowl CT, Weinstock JV, Al Jurf A, Ephgrave K, Murray JA, Dillon K. (2000) Complications and cost associated with parenteral nutrition delivered to hospitalised patients through either subclavian of peripherally-inserted central catheters. *Clinical Nutrition* 19(4): 237–243.

Culkin A, Gabe SM. (2010) Abnormal liver function tests in the parenteral nutrition fed patient. *Frontline Gastroenterology* 1: 98–104.

Department of Health. (2001) Guidelines for preventing infections associated with the insertion and maintenance of central venous catheters. *Journal of Hospital Infection* 47 (Suppl 1): S47–S67.

Ejima A, Imamura T, Nakamura S, Saito M, Matsumoto K, Momomo S. (1992) Manganese Intoxication during total parenteral nutrition. *Lancet* 339: 426

Elia M. (1990) Artificial nutrition support. *Medicine International* 82: 3392–3396.

Furukawa K, Tashiro T, Yamamori H, et al. (1999) Effects of soybean oil emulsion and eicosapentaenoic acid on stress response and immune function after a severely stressful operation. *Annals of Surgery* 229: 255–261.

Garden OJ, Sim AJW. (1983) A comparison of tunnelled and non tunnelled subclavian vein catheters: A prospective study of complications during parenteral feeding. *Clinical Nutrition* 2(1): 51–54.

Grant JP. (2001) Parenteral access. In: Rombeau JL, Rolandelli RH (eds) *Clinical Nutrition: Parenteral Nutrition*. Philadelphia: W.B Saunders Company, pp. 109–117.

Grimble GK. (1993) Essential and conditionally essential nutrients in clinical nutrition. *Nutrition Research Reviews* 6: 97–119.

Home Parenteral Nutrition and Intestinal Failure clinical network (HIFNET). (2008) A strategic framework for intestinal failure and home parenteral nutrition services for adults in England. Available at www.specialisedservices.nhs.uk. Accessed 22 May 2012.

Jeppesen, PB, Langholz E, Mortensen PB. (1999) Quality of life in patients receiving home parenteral nutrition. *Gut* 44: 844–852.

Kennedy JF, Nightingale JMD. (2005) Cost savings of an adult hospital nutrition support team. *Nutrition* 21(11): 1127–1133.

Kerin MJ, Pickford IR, Jaeger H, Couse NF, Mitchell CT, Macfie J. (1991) A prospective and randomised study comparing the incidence of infusion phlebitis during continuous and cyclic peripheral parenteral nutrition. *Clinical Nutrition* 10(6): 315–319.

Kohlhardt SR, Smith RC, Wright CR. (1994) Peripheral versus central intravenous nutrition: comparison of two delivery systems. *British Journal of Surgery* 81(1): 66–70.

SECTION 6

Koretz RL, Lipman TO, Klein S. (2001) AGA Technical Review on parenteral nutrition. *Gastroenterology* 121(4): 970–1001.

Krzywda EA, Andris DA, Edmiston CE. (1999) Catheter infections: Diagnosis, etiology, treatment, and prevention. *Nutrition in Clinical Practice* 14: 178–190.

Laidlaw SA, Kopple JD. (1987) Newer concepts of the indispensable amino acids. *American Journal of Clinical Nutrition* 47: 593–605.

Lee V. (2006) Liver dysfunction associated with parenteral nutrition: What are the options? *Practical Gastroenterology* 45: 49–68.

Llop J, Sabin P, Garaw M, *et al*. (2003) The importance of clinical factors in parenteral nutrition associated hypertriglyceridemia. *Clinical Nutrition* 22(6): 577–583.

Micklewright A, Todorovic V. (2005) *A Pocket Guide to Clinical Nutrition*, 3rd edn. Parenteral and Enteral Nutrition Group (PENG) of the British Dietetic Association. PEN Group Publications.

McClave SA, Chang W, Dhallwai K, Heyland DK. (2006) Nutrition support in acute pancreatitis: A systematic review of the literature. *Journal of Parenteral and Enteral Nutrition* 30(2): 143–156.

National Confidential Enquiry into Patient Outcome and Death (NCEPOD). (2010) A mixed bag. An enquiry into the care of hospital patients receiving parenteral nutrition. Available at www.ncepod.org.uk/2010pn.htm. Accessed 9 August 2013.

National Institute for Health and Care Excellence (NICE). (2002) *Guidance on the Use of Ultrasound Locating Devices for Placing Central Venous Catheters*. No. 49. London: NICE.

National Institute for Health and Care Excellence (NICE). (2006) *Nutrition Support in Adults*. Clinical Guideline 32. London: NICE.

Naylor CJ, Griffiths RD, Fernandez RS. (2004) Does a multidisciplinary total parenteral nutrition team improve patient outcomes? A systematic review. *Journal of Parenteral and Enteral Nutrition* 28 (4): 251–258.

Nightingale JM. (2003) Hepatobiliary, renal and bone complications of intestinal failure. *Best Practice in Research and Clinical Gastroenterology* 17(6): 907–929.

Parrish CR, McClave SA. (2008) Checking residual volumes: A practice in search of science? *Practical Gastroenterology* October: 33–47.

Pittiruti M. Hamilton H, Biffi R, MacFie J, Pertkiewicz M. (2009) ESPEN Guidelines on Parenteral Nutrition: Central Venous Catheters (access, care, diagnosis and therapy of complications). *Clinical Nutrition* 28: 365–377.

Pullicino E, Elia M. (2001) Designing parenteral and enteral regimens. In: Nightingale J (ed) *Intestinal Failure*. London: Greenwich Medical Media Ltd, pp. 325–338.

Randolph AG, Cook DJ, Gonzales CA, Brun-Buisson C. (1998) Tunnelling short-term central venous catheters to prevent catheter-related infection: a meta-analysis of randomised, controlled trials. *Critical Care Medicine* 26(8): 1452–1457.

Reifen R, Khoshoo V, Dinari G. (1999) Effect of parenteral nutrition on oral intake. *Journal of Pediatric Endocrinology and Metabolism* 12: 203–205.

Ryan AM, Rowley SP, Healy LA. (2006) Post-oesophagectomy early enteral nutrition via a needle catheter jejunostomy: 8-year experience at a specialist unit. *Clinical Nutrition* 25(3): 386–393.

Schloerb PR, Henning JF. (1998) Patterns and problems of adult total parenteral nutrition use in US academic medical centers. *Archives of Surgery* 133: 7–12.

Schulman AS, Sawyer RG. (2005) Have you passed gas yet? Time for a new approach to feeding patients post-operatively. *Practical Gastroenterology* October: 82–88.

Shang E, Weiss C, Post S, Kaehler G. (2006) The influence of early supplementation of parenteral nutrition on quality of life and body composition in patients with advanced cancer, *Journal of Parenteral and Enteral Nutrition* 30: 222–230.

Smith T, Micklewright A, Hirst A, Stratton R. and Janet Baxter (2011) Articial nutritiom support in the UK. BAPEN. Available at www .bapen.org.uk/pdfs/bans_reports/bans_report_11.pdf. Accessed 9 August 2013.

Spiegel JE, Willenbucher RF. (1999) Rapid development of severe copper deficiency in a patient with Crohn's disease receiving parenteral nutrition. *Journal of Parenteral and Enteral Nutrition* 23: 169–172.

Thompson SE. (1999) Insertion of peripherally inserted central catheters for the administration of total parenteral nutrition. *Nutrition in Clinical Practice* 14: 191–193.

Van den Berghe G, Wouters P, Weekers F, *et al*. (2001) Intensive insulin therapy in critically ill patients. *New England Journal of Medicine* 345(19): 1359–1367.

Woodcock NP, Zeigler D, Palmer MD, Buckley P, Mitchell CJ, MacFie J. (2001) Enteral versus parenteral nutrition: a pragmatic study. *Nutrition* 17(1): 1–12.

Fluids and electrolytes

Alan Torrance

Key points

- Water has many functions in the body and is essential for survival.

- Regulation of body fluid is under tight homeostatic control; maintenance of fluid balance is an important aspect of dietetic management.

- Disorders of electrolyte and water balance are common in clinical practice, particularly as a result of surgery, trauma, disease and drug therapy.

- Appropriate treatment to correct any disorder needs to be based on a careful physical examination and interpretation of both serum and urine biochemistry.

Water is essential to life and, while humans can survive for several weeks without food, they cannot withstand water deprivation for more than a few days. Water has many vital functions in the body including:

- Solvent for ions and molecules.
- Transport medium, especially for the excretion of osmotically active solutes such as urea and salts.
- Lubricant.
- Temperature regulation.

In the UK there are no nationally agreed, evidence based recommendations for adequate intakes of water for the general public. However, in 2010 the European Food Safety Authority (EFSA, 2010) published dietary reference values for water (Table 6.6.1). The values given are for total water from fluid and water; EFSA estimated that in Europe 20% of water comes from food. It is important to note that this value is variable and can be as high as 40% in some countries, e.g. China where a lot of watery foods, e.g. soup, is consumed.

This chapter concentrates on clinical aspects of fluids and electrolytes. Resources on healthy hydration in the general public are given at the end of the chapter.

Body fluids

Water accounts for approximately 60% of the total body weight of a healthy adult, which is the equivalent of about 42 L in a 70-kg man. Females generally have higher adipose tissue levels than men and the total body water

(TBW) content may be nearer 50% of total body weight. Lean body tissue has a high water content (75%) in contrast to 10–15% in adipose tissue. A newly born infant may have up to 80% of its body weight as water because of minimal fat stores. In contrast, the TBW in the elderly tends to be <50% of total body mass as muscle tissue (with its high water content) decreases with age.

Body fluid compartments

Total body water is generally considered to be divided into two main compartments; intracellular (inside the cells) and extracellular (outside the cells) fluid that are separated by the cell membrane. The extracellular compartment is further subdivided into the interstitial and intravascular (plasma) compartments. Of the 42 L of fluid in a 70 kg adult, 25 L will be intracellular fluid (ICF) and 17 L extracellular fluid (ECF), of which approximately 14 L comprises interstitial fluid and 3 L plasma fluid (Figure 6.6.1).

A number of factors influence and control the movement of fluid and other (substances) between the various compartments. The fluid volume contained in each compartment depends on the quantity of water present and its chemical composition. This is important for two reasons:

- Each fluid compartment contains one principal solute: potassium (intracellular), sodium (extracellular) and plasma proteins (intravascular). The volume of each compartment is controlled by osmotic pressure.

SECTION 6

- Osmotic pressure depends on the total number of particles present in the fluid within a compartment.

Intravascular (plasma) compartment

The intravascular compartment contains proteins in plasma in a concentration of 70–80 g/L. Albumin is the largest single protein component with a concentration of 40–50 g/L, with the globulins (which are more diverse and larger) accounting for the remainder. Due to its higher concentration and low molecular weight, albumin produces almost 80% of plasma oncotic pressure. At the arterial end of the capillaries where hydrostatic pressure is greater than the plasma oncotic pressure, fluid moves from the plasma into the interstitial compartment. At the venous end of the capillaries where the plasma oncotic pressure exceeds the hydrostatic pressure, tissue fluid is drawn back into the intravascular space. The plasma protein concentration allows the heart to pump one-third of the extracellular fluid as the circulating plasma volume and also provides a continuous circulation of the total interstitial fluid, which bathes the cells of the body. Any small quantities of plasma protein and extra fluid that leak from the capillaries are taken up by the lymphatic system and returned to the systemic circulation.

Extracellular compartment

The size of the extracellular compartment (fluid) is determined by homeostatic control of both its tonicity and volume. Changes in tonicity, detected by anterior hypothalamic osmoreceptors in the brain, affect both thirst and levels of arginine vasopressin [AVP; antidiuretic hormone (ADH)], which is produced in the hypothalamus and conveyed to the posterior pituitary where it is stored and subsequently released in response to a number of stimuli that alter both the intake and output of water.

Altered ECF volume can be detected by volume receptors in the circulation. These are present in the large veins and right atrium. The kidney also plays a significant role in controlling the ECF volume. Any reduction in systemic arterial pressure reduces renal blood flow and perfusion pressure. In this situation, renin secretion from the juxtaglomerular apparatus in the kidney is increased, resulting in angiotensin II production, which in turn stimulates aldosterone and AVP release. This causes sodium and water retention.

The sodium content (not concentration) in the ECF determines its volume. Homeostatic mechanisms are directed at controlling the retention or excretion of sodium. If a sodium load is added to the ECF, tonicity will increase, thirst will be stimulated and water retention via the kidneys will occur. This in turn will result in an increase in the ECF volume that will stimulate sodium and water loss, and the ECF volume will return to normal.

Intercellular compartment

The ICF has a volume of 25 L; it contains twice the number of osmotic particles as the ECF and therefore is twice the volume. The cell membrane is freely permeable to water and large macromolecules, but essentially impermeable to electrolytes, although there is movement to a limited degree of sodium and potassium against a concentration and electrical gradient to allow the export of water out of the cell in order to maintain cell stability. The ICF volume is sensitive to changes in the sodium concentration of the ECF. A high ECF (or serum) sodium concentration will result in water moving out of cells by osmosis. The reverse occurs with a low ECF sodium concentration.

Water homeostasis (balance) depends on the control of water intake and output. Water intake is usually dependent on the thirst mechanism that is stimulated by an increased serum osmolality (usually due to hypernatraemia or more rarely hyperglycaemia) or suppressed by a reduction in serum osmolality (normally due to hyponatraemia). Water output depends on water excretion by the kidneys and is influenced by three main factors: urinary dilution and concentration, sodium status and the concentration of circulating AVP.

Table 6.6.1 Reference values for adequate intake of water (EFSA, 2010)

	Age	Water adequate intake (mL/day)
Infants	0–6 months	680
	6–12 months	800–1000
Children	1–2 years	1100–1200
	2–3 years	1100–1200
	4–8 years	1600
	9–13 years	
	Boys	2100
	Girls	1900
	>14 years	As adults
Adults (including elderly)	Men	2500
	Women	2000
Pregnant women		+300
Lactating women		+600–700

28 kg	25 L	14 L	3 L
Proteins, Lipids, Carbohydrate & Minerals	Intracellular Fluid	Interstitial Fluid	Plasma

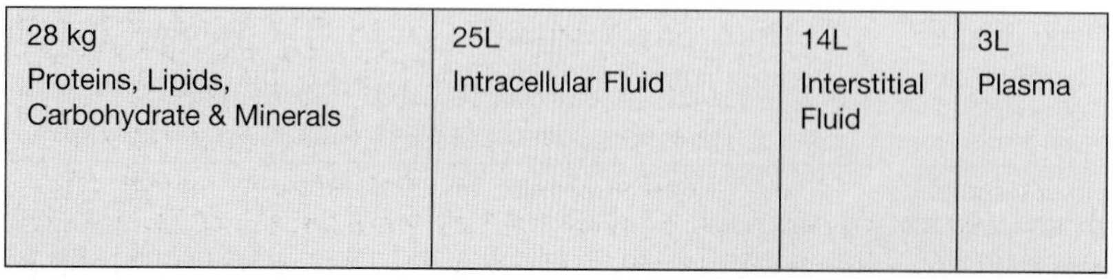

Figure 6.6.1 Body composition and fluid compartments

Sodium homeostasis depends on renal excretion. The average dietary sodium content is in the region of 155 mmol/day. Of this around 2.5 mmol are excreted in sweat and faeces, and 150 mmol via the kidneys. Providing there are no significant extra renal losses, e.g. diarrhoea and vomiting, urinary sodium levels usually reflect dietary sodium intake.

Disorders of sodium and water balance

Disorders of sodium (and other electrolytes) and water balance are common in clinical practice, particularly as a result of surgery, trauma, disease and drug therapy. Appropriate treatment to correct any disorder needs to be based on a careful physical examination and interpretation of both serum and urine biochemistry. Any disorders of sodium and water balance will be reflected in the serum sodium concentration.

Sodium deficit

Sodium cannot be lost from the body without water. A sodium deficit may occur with diarrhoea, diuretic therapy, Addison's disease, diabetic ketoacidosis, ascites and chronic kidney disease. The result is a decrease in the ECF volume with associated hypertension and tachycardia. If the sodium deficit is severe, there is a risk of circulatory failure and renal failure, although ICF levels are unaffected. In the case of a sodium deficit, it is the total amount of ECF sodium that is important. There may be little change in the serum sodium concentration as water loss may increase as a compensatory effect. Sodium deficiency is normally treated with 0.9% sodium chloride.

Sodium excess

This can be caused as a result of a reduced sodium excretion, e.g. kidney usage, primary or secondary aldosteronism; or commonly in the clinical setting, by the administration of 8.4% sodium bicarbonate to correct a metabolic acidosis; or large volumes of 0.9% saline where there are hypotonic losses such as in diabetes mellitus. Where there is sodium retention there is expansion of the ECF volume; there may also be oedema and possibly hypertension. Increased serum sodium may stimulate thirst.

Water deficit

Water deficit usually results from an inadequate intake, often due to the inability to drink or inadequate intravenous fluid or excessive loss. Thirst and oliguria with highly concentrated urine will normally be present. There is less effect on the ECF volume than from the loss of a similar volume of isotonic fluid. Hypernatraemia is usually present.

Water excess

This is usually caused by either impaired water excretion, e.g. inappropriate (increased AVP secretion or renal failure) or excessive water intake usually in association with impaired excretion. If severe, cerebral overhydration and oedema can occur. Hyponatraemia is usually present.

Hyponatraemia

Normal serum sodium is <135 mmol/L; as mentioned, hyponatraemia is usually a result of excess water. It can also occur due to a reduction in the ECF volume with a corresponding loss of total body sodium, although this is uncommon. The main causes of hyponatraemia are shown in Table 6.6.2.

Diagnosis

Diagnosis is based on the following signs:

- *Low serum osmolality* – if a measurement is not available, serum osmolality can be estimated as $2 \times [Na + K] +$ urea + glucose (mmol/L)
- *ECF volume depletion* – weight loss, no oedema and loss of skin elasticity will be present. This is likely to be associated with a loss of total body sodium that will require replacing.
- *Symptoms* – nausea, headache, confusion. Treatment needs to be rapid, usually by administration of small volumes of hypertonic saline, e.g. 100 mL of 1.8% saline with repeated estimations of serum sodium (Piper *et al.*, 2012).

Hyponatraemia can occur with an increased, normal or decreased ECF volume. In cases of an increased ECF, oedema will invariably be present. Cardiac failure, liver cirrhosis or nephritic syndrome renal failure are frequently causative factors.

Where the ECF volume is normal, hypothyroidism, glucocorticoid deficiency (secondary adrenal insufficiency impairs water excretion by increasing AVP release) and stress, pain or drugs (via stimulation of AVP release) are the usual causes. Very occasionally, syndrome of inappropriate ADH secretion (SIADH) may be the cause. The usual cause of both an increased and normal ECF volume is water excess. Treatment will depend on the primary cause, the degree of hyponatraemia present and the severity of symptoms. Specific causes should be treated where possible, e.g. replacement of thyroid or adrenocortical hormones, diuretics for oedema, removal of pain, stress and drugs affecting AVP, etc.

Management

Water restriction is the normal treatment in normal or increased ECF volume causes of hyponatraemia. Water restriction alone, however, will not on its own result in a satisfactory increase in serum sodium and the use of hypertonic saline (as outlined earlier) may be necessary. To be effective, water must be restricted to less than the sum of urine output plus an estimate of insensible losses.

Hyponatraemia and a decreased ECF volume is usually a result of gastrointestinal and third space (non-renal, non gastrointestinal) losses or renal losses of sodium. This is caused byodium depletion and the standard treatment is to administer 0.9% saline at rates that will depend

Table 6.6.2   Main causes of hyponatraemia and hypernatraemia

	Hyponatraemia	Hypernatraemia
Diseases	Severe congestive cardiac failure Liver failure Nephrotic syndrome Acute or chronic kidney disease	
Extrarenal losses	Water losses – vomiting, diarrhoea, pancreatitis, burns	Water losses – respiratory, fever, exercise, insensible losses Sodium losses– diarrhoea, heavy sweating
Renal losses	Water losses – diuretics, salt losing nephritis (e.g. renal tubular acidosis), metabolic alkalosis, ketonuria (e.g. diabetes), alcohol, starvation or osmotic diuresis (e.g. glucose, urea)	Water losses – central or nephrogenic diabetes insipidus Sodium losses – salt losing nephritis, osmotic diuretics
Endocrine	Addison's disease, hypothyroidism, syndrome of inappropriate AVP (ADH) secretion (SIADH)	Primary hyperaldosteronism (Conn's syndrome), Cushing's disease
Others	Pseudohyponatraemia – hyperlipidaemia, myeloma Osmolal shift of sodium, e.g. due to hyperglycaemia	Administration of excess sodium – 8.4% $NaHCO_3$ infusion, salt tablets

AVP, arginine vasopressin; ADH, antidiuretic hormone; SIADH, syndrome of inappropriate ADH secretion.

on whether a patient is asymptomatic or symptomatic. If it is considered necessary to infuse fluids rapidly to replenish a low ECF volume, isotonic fluids must be used to avoid sudden dangerous changes in serum sodium concentrations, which increase the risk of cerebral oedema (Neville *et al.*, 2010; White, 2006).

Hypernatraemia

In hypernatraemia the serum sodium is >135 mmol/L; the usual cause of hypernatraemia is water loss. The main causes are shown in Table 6.6.2.

Diagnosis

Diagnosis of hypernatraemia is based on the following criteria:

* *Increased heart rate and reduced blood pressure* – ICF volume is contracted and the patient is likely to be sodium and water depleted.
* *Urine osmolality* – urine will be concentrated, with a high osmolality of >1200 mOsmol/kg and a low volume. If the osmolality is low or very low, the patient may be receiving diuretics or suffering from diabetes insipidus, respectively.
* *Evidence of ECF expansion*, e.g. oedema and weight gain – an excess of sodium is likely, although this is rare. Hypernatraemia can occur with an increased, normal or low total body sodium. Due to the close relationship between sodium and water balance, the management of hypernatraemia depends on the status of the ECF volume (Piper *et al.*, 2012).

Management

In cases of ECF volume depletion, water should be replaced gradually, ideally by the oral route. If this is not possible (or if the plasma volume needs more rapid repletion, e.g. after blood loss), 0.9% saline is normally infused

intravenously initially and thereafter 5% glucose is the intravenous fluid of choice. Serum sodium levels should not be corrected by >12 mmol/24 hours. Any ongoing losses of water should be addressed, e.g. stopping diuretics, reducing gastrointestinal losses with antidiarrhoeal agents if appropriate or giving ADH if central diabetes insipidus is present.

Expansion of ECF volume is treated with diuretics to remove excess sodium and water. This is also the case when hypernatraemia is a result of excessive sodium administration (Sam *et al.*, 2012).

Potassium

Potassium (K^+) is the principal intracellular cation, with intracellular concentrations of 150 mmol/L. It is important in enzyme and neuromuscular function. Most of the dietary intake (>90%) of potassium is excreted by the kidneys with any excess being excreted in the faeces.

Hypokalaemia

A range of clinical conditions can result in hypokalaemia, which may occur with or without a potassium loss (or deficit). The main causes of hypokalaemia are:

* Hypokalaemia without potassium loss:
  o Alkalosis (results in movement of K^+ into cells in exchange for an equimolar number of H^+).
  o Insulin excess (drives K^+ into cells).
  o Dehydration (often mild hypokalaemia without evidence of K^+ loss) (Armon *et al.*, 2008).
* Hypokalaemia with potassium loss:
  o Decreased dietary intake – alcoholism, anorexia nervosa.
  o Increased cellular uptake (common in hyperalimentation or treatment of megaloblastic anaemia).

Table 6.6.3 Protocol for the correction of hypokalaemia using an infusion of potassium chloride

Serum K (mmol/L)	Max infusion rate (mmol/h)	Max concentration (mmol/L)	Max dose/24 hours (mmol)
>2.5	10	40	200
<2.0	40	80	400

○ Gastrointestinal loss – vomiting, diarrhoea, laxative abuse.
○ Urinary loss – diuretics, leukaemia.

Management

In hypokalaemia where there is no potassium deficit, potassium replacement is usually unnecessary and treatment of the underlying cause will correct plasma levels. In cases of potassium deficit, replacement depends on the severity of the hypokalaemia and the magnitude of potassium loss:

• *Serum K+ >3 mmol/L* – 100–200 mmol of K+ are required for each 1 mmol/L rise in serum K+.
• *Serum K+ <3 mmol/L* – 200–400 mmol of K+ are required for each 1 mmol/L rise in serum K+. Potassium can be given orally but may result in gastrointestinal side effects, e.g. nausea, vomiting and diarrhoea; it is often administered intravenously as potassium chloride (KCl) in a controlled manner to reduce the risk of dangerous hyperkalaemia (Table 6.6.3).

Hyperkalaemia

Hyperkalaemia can occur in a variety of clinical settings, but is usually a result of renal failure. The main causes of hyperkalaemia are:

• Redistribution of K^+ from the ICF – acidosis, glucose loading in diabetes, beta-blockers.
• Potassium excess.
• Diminished excretion – acute or chronic kidney disease, K^+ sparing diuretics, Addison's disease, renal transplant, myeloma, ciclosporin.
• Excess K^+ input – diet, haemolysis, rhabdomyolysis, burns.

Management

In acute hyperkalaemia the aim is to protect the myocardium and move K^+ back into cells. The treatment of choice is normally 10% calcium gluconate (10–30 mL) and 50–150 mmol of sodium bicarbonate, followed by intravenous infusion of 100 mL of 50% glucose and 10 units of soluble insulin over 15–30 minutes. Chronic hyperkalaemia is usually managed using cation binding resins, diuretics (where appropriate) and dietary potassium restriction, e.g. chronic kidney disease, or renal replacement therapy, e.g. dialysis.

Calcium

Calcium is the body's most abundant divalent cation and has important roles in regulating neuromuscular function, myocardial contractility, hormone release and enzyme activity. Normally, about a third of dietary calcium is absorbed, mainly in the jejunum under the control of vitamin D. Disorders of calcium metabolism occur as either hyper- or hypo-calcaemia.

Hypercalcaemia

The main causes of hypercalcaemia are:

• Increased bone resorption:
  ○ Cancer.
  ○ Primary hyperparathyroidism – adenoma, hyperplasia.
  ○ Immobilisation.
  ○ Endocrine – thyrotoxicosis, glucocorticoid deficiency.
• Increased gastrointestinal absorption.
• Vitamin D excess.
• Granulomatous disorders – sarcoidosis, tuberculosis.

Management

Acute hypercalcaemia often occurs in conjunction with ECF depletion, and expansion of the ECF compartment with intravenous normal saline may be sufficient on its own to control the hypercalcaemia and stimulate calcium excretion. Calcitonin and diuretic therapy may also be commenced, providing renal function is adequate. Treatment of chronic hypercalcaemia depends on the primary cause. Sarcoidosis, adenoma and other malignancies, vitamin D excess and immobilisation may all respond to corticosteroids or oral phosphate.

Hypocalcaemia

The main causes of hypocalcaemia are:

• Hypoalbuminaemia.
• Low parathyroid hormone (PTH):
  ○ Hypoparathyroidism.
  ○ Hypomagnesaemia.
• Acute pancreatitis.
• Low vitamin D levels:
  ○ Vitamin D deficiency.
  ○ Malabsorption.
  ○ Alcoholism.
  ○ Hyperphosphataemia.

Management

Acute hypocalcaemia is normally treated with intravenous calcium gluconate. If hypomagnesaemia (which reduces parathyroid hormone secretion) is also present, intravenous magnesium sulphate will be necessary. In chronic hypocalcaemia, treatment is designed to increase intestinal calcium absorption through calcium and vitamin D supplementation.

Phosphate

Phosphate is the body's most abundant divalent anion with an ICF concentration of about 80 mmol/L. Organic phosphates, phospholipids and phosphate containing nucleotides are vital to normal cell function. Inorganic phosphate is a major component of ATP and oxidative metabolism. About 60–65% of dietary phosphate is absorbed throughout the small bowel. Disorders of phosphate metabolism occur as either hyper- or hypo-phosphataemia.

Hyperphospataemia

The main causes of hyperphosphataemia are:

- Renal:
  - Reduced glomerular filtration rate.
  - Acute and chronic kidney disease.
- Increased phosphate intake:
  - Enteral or parenteral nutrition.
  - Phosphate enemas and laxatives.
- Reduced renal excretion:
  - Hypoparathyroidism.
  - Increased growth or thyroid hormone levels.
  - Hypovolaemia.
- Redistribution – cell breakdown:
  - Trauma, haemolysis and burns, rhabdomyolysis.
  - Chemoradiotherapy.

Management

In acute hyperphosphataemia, if renal function is adequate, removal of the cause will resolve the raised serum phosphate level. Chronic hyperphosphataemia is usually due to chronic kidney disease and is treated with a combination of dietary phosphate restriction and oral phosphate binders.

Hypophosphataemia

The main causes of hypophosphataemia are:

- Redistribution:
  - Glucose and insulin administration.
  - Respiratory alkalosis.
  - Catecholamines.
  - Parenteral nutrition and anabolism.
- Gastrointestinal:
  - Reduced phosphate intake, vomiting.
  - Malabsorption, diarrhoea.
- Renal phosphate reabsorption or phosphate loss:
  - Vitamin D deficiency.
  - Hyperparathyroidism.
  - Diabetic ketoacidosis.
  - Renal replacement therapy.
  - Hypervolaemia.

Management

Mild to moderate hypophosphataemia can usually be resolved by treatment of the underlying disease. Severe hypophosphataemia requires phosphate supplementation. This can be given either orally or intravenously, but preferably orally to reduce the risks of hyperphosphataemia and metastatic calcification associated with intrave-

nous administration. Phosphate supplementation should not exceed 200 mmol/24 hours.

Magnesium

Magnesium is the second most abundant intracellular cation after potassium. It plays an important role in neuromuscular and enzyme function. About 50% of dietary magnesium is passively absorbed, mainly in the duodenum and jejunum. Disorders of magnesium metabolism present as either hyper- or hypo-magnesaemia.

Hypermagnesaemia

The main causes of hypermagnesaemia are:

- Kidney disease – acute or chronic.
- Reduced excretion:
  - Sodium depletion (magnesium reabsorption is increased).
  - Mineralocorticoid deficiency and hypothyroidism (both promote magnesium reabsorption).
- Administration of magnesium:
- Tissue breakdown – rhabdomyolysis, burns, diabetic ketoacidosis.

Management

Treatment is initially by removing the underlying cause of the hypermagnesaemia and then by removing excess magnesium. If this is associated with renal disease, dialysis may be necessary. In severe hypermagnesaemia, intravenous calcium may be given to counteract the cardiac effects of magnesium.

Hypomagnesaemia

The main causes of hypomagnesaemia are:

- Reduced intake – decreased oral intake, malnutrition, prolonged intravenous therapy.
- Increased gastrointestinal excretion:
  - Vomiting and diarrhoea/malabsorption.
  - Extrarenal losses, e.g. intestinal or biliary fistulae.
  - Prolonged nasogastric suction.
  - Short bowel.
- Redistribution – glucose, insulin.
- Increased renal excretion:
  - Drugs – diuretics, ciclosporin, cytotoxics, e.g. cisplatin.
  - ECF expansion.
  - Renal tubular acidosis.
- Endocrine:
  - Diabetes, hyperthyroidism, potassium or phosphate deficiency.
  - Hypercalcaemia.
  - Hyperaldosteronism.

Management

Magnesium replacement can be given orally or intravenously (as magnesium sulphate). As a general rule, 1–2 mmol/kg can be used to correct any deficit. Intravenous administration should not exceed 50 mmol in 12 hours.

Further reading

Biesalski HK, Bischoff SC, Boeles HJ, Muehlhoefer A. (2009) Water, electrolytes, vitamins and trace elements – Guidelines on Parenteral Nutrition, Chapter 7. *German Medical Science* 7(Doc 21): 1612–3174.

Elgart H. (2004) Assessment of fluid and electrolytes. *AACN Clinical Issues: Advanced Practice in Acute & Critical Care* 15(4): 607–621.

Powell-Tuck J, Gosling P, Lobo DN, *et al.* (2008) . British Consensus Guidelines on Intravenous Fluid Therapy for Adult Surgical Patients (GIFTASUP). Available at www.bapen.org.uk.

Internet resources

British Association for Parenteral & Enteral Nutrition (BAPEN) www.bapen.org.uk

General hydration websites

European Hydration Institute www.europeanhydrationinstitute .org

Hydration for Health Initiative www.h4hinitiative.com

References

Armon K, Riordan A, Playfor S, Millman G, Khader A. (2008) Hyponatraemia and hypokalaemia during intravenous fluid administration. *Archives of Disease in Childhood* 93(4): 285–287.

European Food Safety Authority. (2010) Scientific opinion on reference values for water. *EFSA Journal* 8(3): 1459–1497.

Neville KA, Sandeman DJ, Rubinstein A, Henry GM, McGlynn M, Walker JL. (2010) Prevention of hyponatraemia during maintenance intravenous fluid administration: a prospective randomised study of fluid type versus fluid rate. *Journal of Paediatrics* 156(2): 313–319.

Piper GL, Kaplan LJ. (2012) Fluid and electrolyte management for the surgical patient. *Surgical Clinics of North America* 92(2): 189–205.

Sam R, Hart P, Haghighat R, Ing TS. (2012) Hypervolemic hypernatremia in patients recovering from acute kidney injury in the intensive care unit. *Clinical & Experimental Nephrology* 16(1): 136–146.

White C. (2006) Managing fluids and electrolytes – a case study. *Canadian Journal of Respiratory Therapy* 42(5): 20–24.

SECTION 6

SECTION 7

Clinical dietetic practice

7.1

Respiratory disease

Peter Collins and C Elizabeth Weekes

Key points

- Malnutrition is common in patients with chronic obstructive pulmonary disease (COPD) and tuberculosis (TB).

- Routine nutritional screening using a validated screening tool should be carried out in all patients to identify those at risk and to initiate treatment.

- Nutritional requirements in COPD and TB have yet to be fully established.

- Nutritional support is an effective treatment in the management of malnutrition in COPD but its role in the management of TB has yet to be determined.

More than 40 different conditions affect the lungs (Table 7.1.1), which impact on breathing ability and cause mortality and morbidity (British Thoracic Society, 2006). In the UK, one person in seven is affected by chronic respiratory disease, most commonly chronic obstructive pulmonary disease (COPD) or asthma. Globally, respiratory disease is the second biggest killer after cardiovascular disease (World Health Organization, 2004).

A number of local symptoms that result from respiratory disease can affect nutritional intake and nutritional status, e.g. dyspnoea, cough and excess sputum production. At any stage in the illness, these symptoms may be compounded by acute exacerbations and increased infection, and influenced by age, the social and psychological effects of chronic illness and the presence of comorbidities. Any patient with respiratory disease may present with malnutrition; however, two respiratory conditions strongly associated with a high prevalence of malnutrition are COPD (Vermeeren *et al.*, 2006) and tuberculosis (TB) (Schwenk & Macallan, 2000). While adequate pharmacological treatment of TB often results in a cure and subsequent improvement in nutritional status (Schwenk *et al.*, 2004), the lack of a cure for COPD means that it is often progressively debilitating with an increasing impact on nutritional status. All respiratory diseases affect lung function to varying degrees but some, particularly COPD and TB, are also associated with chronic systemic inflammation that can have profound effects on skeletal muscle (sarcopenia and cachexia) and bone (osteoporosis).

Chronic obstructive pulmonary disease

The term COPD applies to emphysema, bronchitis or a combination of both. It was recently defined as '. . . *a preventable and treatable disease with some significant extra pulmonary effects that may contribute to the severity in individual patients. Its pulmonary component is characterised by airflow limitation that is not fully reversible. The airflow limitation is usually progressive and associated with an abnormal inflammatory response of the lung to noxious particles or gases*' [Global Initiative for Chronic Obstructive Lung Disease (GOLD), 2010].

Patients usually present with a history of increasing dyspnoea over several years, chronic cough, muscle weakness and poor exercise tolerance secondary to muscle wasting; recurrent bronchial infections or weight loss may also be reported. Although COPD is incurable, early diagnosis and treatment can alleviate symptoms; unfortunately no treatment has modified the rate of decline in lung function (Celli *et al.*, 2004).

Diagnostic criteria and classification

Diagnosis relies on medical history and symptoms at presentation, as well as post bronchodilator spirometry to establish lung function [forced expiratory volume in one second (FEV_1) and forced vital capacity (FVC)]. Lung function results are compared with age and gender specific

Manual of Dietetic Practice, Fifth Edition. Edited by Joan Gandy.
© 2014 The British Dietetic Association. Published 2014 by John Wiley & Sons, Ltd.
Companion Website: www.manualofdieteticpractice.com

SECTION 7

Table 7.1.1 Characteristics of respiratory disease

	Examples
Chronic respiratory diseases	
Obstructive	Chronic obstructive pulmonary disease (COPD) Asthma
Restrictive	Pulmonary fibrosis Sarcoidosis
Vascular	Pulmonary embolism Pulmonary hypertension Cor pulmonale
Infective	Tuberculosis (TB)
Environmental	Pneumoconiosis Asbestosis
Genetic	Cystic fibrosis Alpha-1-antitrypsin deficiency
Acute respiratory disease	
Multiple causes	Adult respiratory distress syndrome (ARDS)
Infective	Pneumonia

Table 7.1.2 Grading of chronic obstructive disease (COPD) obstruction severity

COPD severity classification	Lung function
Stage I: mild	FEV_1/FVC <70%; FEV_1 ≥80% predicted
Stage II: moderate	FEV_1/FVC <70%; FEV_1 50–79% predicted
Sage III: severe	FEV_1/FVC <70%; FEV_1 30–49% predicted
Stage IV: very severe	FEV_1/FVC <70%; FEV_1 <30% predicted*

*Or FEV_1 <50% predicted in the presence of chronic respiratory failure (NICE, 2010); GOLD, 2010).
FEV_1, forced expiratory volume in 1 second; FVC, forced vital capacity.

standards to determine disease severity using the GOLD criteria (Table 7.1.2). A differential diagnosis of bronchitis is made when there is a history of chronic cough productive of sputum present on most days of the month for at least 3 months in 2 consecutive years.

Disease processes

While cigarette smoking and air pollution are the most important factors in the development of COPD, genetic predispositions also play a role (Pauwels, 2003). In addition to airflow limitation, pathological changes and inflammation induced damage in the lungs can lead to excess mucus secretion, ciliary dysfunction, pulmonary hyperinflation and gas exchange abnormalities, and may result in pulmonary hypertension and cor pulmonale.

Patients with COPD have an increased susceptibility to infection and often suffer acute recurrent infective exacerbations of the disease (IECOPD).

Burden of disease

In the UK there are currently 1 million individuals diagnosed with COPD; however, it is estimated 3 million have the disease (NICE, 2010). Around 30000 people die as a result of COPD each year (British Thoracic Society, 2006). With an ageing population, increasing awareness of the disease and improved diagnostic methods, the number of individuals diagnosed with COPD is likely to rise.

Chronic obstructive pulmonary disease is the second largest cause of emergency admissions to UK hospitals, accounting for 130000 admissions/year (British Lung Foundation, 2007), placing a huge operational burden on hospitals by taking up 1 million bed days annually (British Thoracic Society, 2006). Patients with COPD are primarily managed in the community and account for 1.4 million GP consultations/year (Healthcare Commission, 2006).

Social deprivation has been shown to be a significant independent risk factor for malnutrition in COPD (Collins et al., 2010a) and is associated with increased frequency and duration of emergency hospital admissions (Collins et al., 2010b).

Chronic obstructive pulmonary disease is associated with a poor quality of life that significantly declines as disease severity increases (Rutten-van Mölken et al., 2006). In COPD the compounding effect of malnutrition has yet to be fully investigated, but is likely to be significant considering the negative effect of malnutrition on quality of life in other chronic conditions such as cancer (Andreyev et al., 1998).

Nutritional impact

In epidemiological studies, a poor quality diet, especially low in fruit and vegetables and high in meat and potatoes, has been associated with an increased likelihood of developing COPD (McKeever et al., 2010). There is a lack of studies investigating the potential benefits of dietary interventions to prevent the development of COPD in at risk populations and no studies demonstrating that increasing the intake of specific food groups, such as fruit and vegetables, has beneficial effects on outcome in patients with COPD.

Weight loss and being underweight are associated with poor prognosis and increased mortality, independent of disease severity (Landbo et al., 1999). Until recently, weight loss in COPD was seen as inevitable and unresponsive to nutritional intervention. However, studies have shown that weight loss is reversible and a weight gain of kg is associated with a number of functional improvements (Stratton et al., 2003; Collins et al., 2012), as well as reduced mortality (Schols et al., 1998). In malnourished COPD patients, an increase in weight of at least 2 kg should be a therapeutic target.

The exact prevalence of malnutrition in COPD is unknown since an accepted definition of malnutrition does not exist. Reported prevalence rates vary considerably from 9–63% depending on the criteria used to define malnutrition, e.g. <90% ideal body weight (Metropolitan Life Insurance Company, 1959) or >5% recent weight loss, and the population studied, e.g. in- or out-patients (Weekes, 2005). Compared with chronic bronchitis, patients with emphysema are more likely to have a low body mass index (BMI) and to report unintentional weight loss (Guerra *et al.*, 2002). Little has been reported on the pattern of weight loss in patients with COPD; however, Weekes & Bateman (2002) reported significant unintentional weight loss (>5%) in 22% of COPD outpatients. In those who unintentionally lost weight, 41% reported a recent chest infection. Although many patients describe gradual weight loss over a number of years, in a subgroup of patients weight loss and muscle wasting follows a step-wise pattern related to acute illness (Schols & Brug, 2003).

In contrast to observations in the healthy population, survival in COPD appears to be improved in those who are overweight or obese (Landbo *et al.*, 1999; Vestbo *et al.*, 2006). This paradox extends beyond reduced mortality in COPD, with one study finding that overweight patients had lower early readmission rates (Steer *et al.*, 2010) and another that overweight and obese patients had fewer emergency hospital admissions and shorter lengths of stay (Collins *et al.*, 2011a).

Assessment of body weight alone is unlikely to be sensitive enough to detect all of those at nutritional risk, since a subgroup of COPD patients demonstrate loss of fat free mass (FFM) despite maintaining normal weight (Schols *et al.*, 1993; De Benedetto *et al.*, 2000). Depletion of FFM may have more profound effects on functional measures than depletion of body weight *per se* (Schols *et al.*, 1993). The proportion of patients with FFM depletion increases with disease severity (Schols *et al.*, 1993; Vermeeren *et al.*, 2006).

Altered body composition can be attributed to a number of factors, including the disease process itself (systemic inflammation), energy imbalance (positive or negative), medication treatment (oral corticosteroids) and lifestyle (inactivity). Loss of FFM, which often occurs with ageing, can be accelerated in the presence of chronic inflammatory disease.

Nutritional screening and nutritional assessment

As COPD patients readily pass between primary and secondary care, routine nutritional screening should be performed in all patients across both settings. Outpatients with COPD identified as at risk of malnutrition using a validated tool are at increased risk of hospitalisation, longer hospital stays and increased mortality (Weekes *et al.*, 2007; Steer *et al.*, 2010). Studies are needed to establish whether prompt identification and nutritional intervention in these patients reduces their poor clinical outcomes.

Anthropometry

Recent national guidelines for the management of COPD recommend the anthropometric assessment of patients to determine BMI. Unfortunately, the guidelines make no recommendation for formal nutritional screening and the assessment of unintentional weight change (NICE, 2010). Anthropometric assessment in COPD is not straightforward due to changes in body composition and the presence of oedema, which is challenging since there are no agreed adjustment factors for oedema. In the presence of severe oedema, assessment of upper arm anthropometry is useful. A mid upper arm circumference (MUAC) of <23 cm often indicates a BMI of <20 kg/m^2 (Powell-Tuck & Hennessy, 2003). Mid arm muscle area (MAMA) of the non-dominant arm has been reported to be a better predictor of mortality in COPD than BMI (Soler-Cataluña *et al.*, 2005).

Bioelectrical impedance analysis (BIA) is increasingly being used in COPD to assess changes in FFM and as an illness indicator to help predict prognosis. Currently, there is no universal reference population for COPD using this technique and research is ongoing in this area.

Biochemistry

Hospitalised patients should be assessed for hydration status, clinical condition e.g. raised C-reactive protein, white cell count and low serum albumin levels, and nutritional markers. Patients could be at risk of refeeding syndrome if dietary intake has been poor for a prolonged period, and phosphate, potassium, calcium and magnesium levels should be reviewed prior to implementation of nutritional support in all patients with known risk factors (NICE, 2006a).

Clinical condition

Patients with COPD often present with a number of nutritionally relevant comorbidities, e.g. diabetes, gastro-oesophageal reflux, osteoporosis or depression, the management of which may require the patient to take a large number of different drugs (polypharmacy). Assessment of clinical condition should take account of any relevant changes in either comorbidities or pharmacological interventions. Altered swallowing physiology in COPD, particularly around the time of IECOPD, may increase aspiration risk (Teramoto *et al.*, 2002).

Dietary intake

Stable patients with COPD consume close to recommended daily amounts for both energy and protein (Vermeeren *et al.*, 1997; Weekes *et al.*, 2009), however, intake is compromised during IECOPD (Vermeeren *et al.*, 1997; Slinde *et al.*, 2003). Low intakes of calcium and vitamin D have been found in outpatients (Weekes, 2005; Andersson *et al.*, 2007), with a reported non-starch polysaccharide intake of <15 g/day (Weekes, 2005). This together with a sedentary lifestyle and limited fluid intake might predispose to constipation.

Economic and social status

Strong links exist between social deprivation and both the development of COPD and clinical outcome (Prescott *et al.*, 1999). Many patients with COPD are unable to

SECTION 7

continue in employment as their disease progresses or have to decrease their working hours (Eisner et al., 2002). Financial resources therefore may be limited and compromise ability to purchase food. A significant proportion of patients with COPD are housebound (Bestall et al., 1999), which may be accompanied by social isolation and limited access to affordable food. Strategies for improving nutritional intake may need to include the use of meals on wheels type services and socialised eating opportunities such as lunch clubs.

Clinical management

In the absence of a cure, treatments available for the management of COPD rely almost exclusively on symptom management. Infective exacerbations of the disease are usually treated with inhaled and/or oral corticosteroid medication and antibiotics. The increased appetite and food intake that often accompanies courses of oral steroids is usually short term since patients are put on reducing doses as soon as possible to avoid complications of long term therapy. Many patients take medications to counteract osteoporosis. Gastrointestinal disturbances are known complications of antibiotic therapy and may impact on nutritional intake during and immediately after IECOPD.

Recent interest has focused on the levels of vitamin D in COPD patients as the vitamin is not only involved with bone physiology but also plays an important role in muscle function and adaptive immunity (Janssens et al., 2009). Vitamin D deficiency is common in COPD and correlates with disease severity (Janssens et al., 2010). In COPD patients waiting for lung transplantation, 50% were found to be vitamin D deficient (Forli et al., 2004). Immobility, reduced sunlight exposure, reduced capacity of ageing skin to synthesise vitamin D and medications used to manage COPD all influence the osteoporosis risk in COPD. Vitamin D and calcium intakes should be considered in all COPD patients due to the high prevalence of both osteoporosis and vitamin D deficiency.

In patients receiving home oxygen therapy, consideration should be given to the possible effects on mobility, access to food and social life, all of which might impact adversely on nutritional intake. Prolonged periods on oxygen can cause dry mouth and this may affect the ability to taste, chew and swallow foods.

Smoking cessation is a major aim of COPD management. Current smoking status has been shown to be a significant predictor of malnutrition risk (Collins et al., 2011b). An average weight gain of 3.8 kg in females and 2.8 kg in males has been observed in individuals who successfully stopped smoking for >1 year (Williamson et al., 1991). Baseline weight in males did not affect the level of weight gained, but in underweight females the likelihood of gaining 13 kg or more was increased four fold in those who stopped smoking.

An increasing number of patients have lung volume reduction surgery and this has been shown to result in spontaneous weight gain (Christensen et al., 1999), possibly due to a combination of reduced work of breathing, improved gas exchange and reduced post prandial dyspnoea.

Nutritional requirements

The nutritional requirements of an individual with COPD will depend on their nutritional status, clinical condition, physical activity level, nutritional goals and likely duration of nutritional support (NICE, 2006a).

Energy

The energy requirements have yet to be fully characterised and studies of COPD have reported considerable variation in total energy expenditure (TEE) (Slinde et al., 2006). While published prediction methods may provide adequate estimates of requirements for groups of patients, they have a poor predictive value for individuals (see Chapter 6.1). Weight stable outpatients with COPD may have requirements similar to others of their age and gender, but if their physical activity levels are compromised, energy requirements may be lower than for healthy individuals of the same age and gender (Slinde et al., 2011). In stable outpatients, a modest increase in energy intake of 200–300 kcal/day has been shown to result in weight gain (Weekes et al., 2009; Collins et al., 2012) and therefore energy requirements are unlikely to be much above normal.

In IECOPD, resting energy expenditure (REE) may be up to 15–20% above predicted basal metabolic rate (BMR) (Schols et al., 1991; Vermeeren et al., 1997; Nguyen et al., 1999), but since acute illness is usually accompanied by a decrease in physical activity, TEE may be similar to, or even slightly lower than, normal. During IECOPD, some patients may be identified as at high risk of refeeding syndrome; however, this is less likely with oral nutritional support than enteral or parenteral nutrition since acute illness is usually accompanied by a loss of appetite that limits spontaneous dietary intake. Practitioners should however take care not to over prescribe nutritional support (NICE, 2006a) and to follow national or evidence based local protocols for the management of refeeding in those patients identified as high risk.

There is little evidence that disease specific oral nutritional supplements (ONS) are more effective than standard ONS in this group of patients. There is a growing body of evidence demonstrating the effectiveness of immune modulatory enteral feeds in patients with acute respiratory distress syndrome (Gadek et al., 1999) and acute lung injury (Singer et al., 2006) who are ventilated. However, the efficacy of such feeds during the acute phase in COPD patients remains to be established.

Protein

While elevated protein turnover rates have been reported in COPD (Engelen et al., 2000), there is currently no evidence to support prescribing protein intakes above general recommendations for chronic or acute illness (Table 7.1.3). It has been suggested that protein intakes at the upper end of those recommended by NICE (2006a), i.e. 1.5 g/kg/day, might be optimal during IECOPD (Vermeeren et al., 1997).

Table 7.1.3 Nutritional management of chronic obstructive pulmonary disease (COPD)

	Treatment goals	Requirements	Interventions
Stable COPD (outpatients)	Maintain nutritional status *or* Improve nutritional status, e.g. post IECOPD	NICE guidelines (NICE, 2006a)* 25–35 kcal/kg/day 0.8–1.5 g protein/kg/day 30–35 mL of fluid/kg/day *For patients who are not severely ill or injured, nor at risk of refeeding syndrome* Alternatively use PENG guidelines (Todorovic & Micklewright, 2011)	Patients identified as at risk of malnutrition or as malnourished should either be managed by referral to a dietitian or by staff using protocols drawn up by dietitians, with referral as necessary (NICE, 2006a); provision of ONS should be considered in those with a BMI <20 kg/m² (NICE, 2010; Collins et al., 2012).
Acute exacerbation (inpatients)	Minimise effects on nutritional status	No specific recommendations can be made for energy due to the heterogeneity of the patient group and the changing clinical course during the acute phase. Intakes up to 1.5 g of protein/kg/day may be justified in exacerbating COPD patients (Vermeeren et al., 1997)	Maximise oral intake within limits of patient's clinical condition using low volume ONS between meals (Anker et al., 2006) Consider supplementary tube feeding if unlikely to meet requirements for more than 5 days (NICE, 2006a)
Mechanical ventilation (ICU/HDU)	Minimise effects on nutritional status while avoiding complications of overfeeding	No specific recommendations can be made in this setting as conditions leading to the requirement for ventilation are often highly changeable Monitoring in this setting is vital in order to meet the nutritional needs of the patient In patients requiring prolonged ventilation, avoid overfeeding [see PENG guidelines (Todorovic & Micklewright, 2011) for maximal energy and macronutrient profiles for ventilated patients]	Commence enteral tube feeding as soon as possible; if high risk of delayed gastric emptying and aspiration use post-pyloric feeding (Heyland et al., 2001). In acute respiratory distress disorder (ARDS) and acute lung injury (ALI), consider formulas containing n-3 fatty acids and antioxidants (Kreymann et al., 2006)

IECOPD, infective exacerbations of chronic obstructive lung disease; ONS, oral nutritional supplements; ICU, intensive care unit; HDU, high dependency unit; PENG, Parenteral and Enteral Nutrition Group.

Micronutrients

Micronutrient intake is likely to be compromised in individuals who have diets deficient in energy and protein. Prescriptions for nutritional support should provide adequate electrolytes, minerals and other micronutrients, accounting for pre-existing deficits, excessive losses or increased demands (NICE, 2006a). It may therefore be necessary to advise the use of a multivitamin and mineral supplement if intake from diet and/or ONS is unlikely to be adequate.

Nutritional support

The reversibility of weight loss in COPD is dependent on the ability to address the underlying cause. An imbalance between energy intake and expenditure, which commonly occurs during IECOPD, should be amenable to targeted nutritional support. However, during the acute phase, in the face of significant inflammation, improvements with nutritional support are hard to achieve. Studies have shown that ONS are able to overcome energy and protein deficits at this time, whilst not affecting oral intake (Vermeeren et al., 2004), and lead to significant improvements in respiratory function and a tendency for improved general wellbeing (Saundy-Unterberger et al., 1997).

At different periods during the course of their disease, patients may experience one or any number of symptoms that could adversely affect intake. The most frequently reported symptoms likely to affect nutritional intake in COPD are anorexia, early satiety and dyspnoea (Cochrane & Afolabi, 2004). Patients with anorexia and post prandial dyspnoea may benefit more from low volume, high energy/protein ONS and/or advice on food fortification. In the presence of early satiety, small, frequent meals and snacks and/or energy dense ONS are recommended (Anker et al., 2006).

While some symptoms experienced by patients with COPD may be amenable to nutritional intervention alone, others may require a combination of nutritional intervention and other therapeutic and/or pharmacological strategies. For example, in the management of eating related dyspnoea, liaison with the medical team or respiratory nurse could optimise oxygen therapy if appropriate, while nutritional interventions should be tailored to minimise the effects on dyspnoea of preparing and eating food.

Since most patients report experiencing several symptoms that affect dietary intake at any time, a range of dietetic strategies may be required to achieve an increase in intake. In a progressive, debilitating disease such as COPD, strategies may have to change over time to avoid

SECTION 7

Table 7.1.4 Factors influencing progression from latent to active tuberculosis (TB) (Adapted from Bates *et al.*, 2004)

Individual	Household/community	Environmental
Age	Socioeconomic status	Availability of health services
Gender	Migrant status	Quality of healthcare
Nutritional status	Place of residence	Availability of appropriate treatment
Immune status	Access to health services	Drug resistance
Genetic predisposition	Access to treatment	Public policy
Behaviour	Informal care arrangements	Public awareness
Poverty	Access to formal care services	
Education		
Knowledge and attitudes		
Diet		
Employment status		

taste fatigue and/or take into account changes in clinical, psychological or social status (Table 7.1.4).

Evidence base for nutritional support

The efficacy of nutritional support in COPD is controversial as a previous Cochrane Collaboration review concluded that nutritional support has no effect on anthropometry, lung function and exercise capacity (Ferreira *et al.*, 2005). However, other reviewers have suggested otherwise (Stratton *et al.*, 2003) and the most recent systematic review and meta-analysis found that nutritional support in stable COPD (non-exacerbating) is effective (Collins *et al.*, 2012). Further trials are required to examine the cost-effectiveness of nutritional support in improving clinical outcomes. There is a need for robust trials around food fortification and dietary counselling as these are often recommended as a first line treatment for malnutrition in COPD despite a paucity of evidence.

One randomised trial showed individualised dietary counselling by a dietitian together with a 6-month supply of whole milk powder (WMP) to be effective in improving intake and body weight in COPD (Weekes *et al.*, 2009). An important finding from this trial was that simply providing patients with dietary advice literature, without dietetic input tailoring advice, failed to result in any improvements. The efficacy of tailored dietary advice delivered by a dietitian and the provision of supportive literature in the absence of WMP remains unknown and urgently needs addressing. A *post hoc* cost analysis suggests it might be cost-effective for a dietitian to provide dietary counselling to individuals with COPD (Weekes *et al.*, 2006), but this needs to be supported by larger, adequately powered studies.

The current evidence for nutritional support is almost entirely based on ONS and is lacking for other forms of nutritional intervention. There is a need for trials comparing different nutritional intervention strategies, and their effects on mortality, clinical outcomes and cost-effectiveness (Collins *et al.*, 2012). Since ONS presumably produce clinical benefits through increased nutrient intake, a similar increase in nutrient intake achieved by dietary counselling should result in similar benefits

(NICE, 2006a). Confirmation of this should be a priority in dietetic research as it underpins many of the principles of the profession (Baldwin & Weekes, 2011).

The most effective setting for nutritional intervention in COPD is likely to be in outpatients, as these patients tend to be metabolically stable, less acutely unwell and more mobile. The nutritional enhancement of pulmonary rehabilitation (PR) is an area that is receiving increasing interest as multimodal therapy has been found to result in significant improvements not only in malnourished patients but also adequately nourished patients with COPD, suggesting a role for nutrition beyond simply treating malnutrition (Schols *et al.*, 1995; Steiner *et al.*, 2003).

Tuberculosis

Tuberculosis (TB) is an infectious bacterial disease caused by *Mycobacterium tuberculosis* and is transmitted via droplets from the throat and lungs of people with active TB. It most commonly affects the lungs but can affect almost any part of the body, infections of the central nervous system and abdomen being the most severe.

The global prevalence of TB was 14 million in 2004, with >60% of cases in sub-Saharan Africa and Asia (WHO, 2008). Although in Europe active TB cases have declined over the past 50 years, since the 1990s there has been an increase in some countries, including the UK (Health Protection Agency, 2010). Globally, 9.2 million new cases and 1.7 million deaths from TB occurred in 2006, and while the number of new cases per capita is falling in some regions of the world, this is not the case in Africa and Europe (WHO, 2008).

Diagnostic criteria

Tuberculosis is diagnosed by sputum smear microscopy followed by culture testing (NICE, 2006b). Patients with active TB usually present with symptoms of persistent cough, fever, night sweats, dyspnoea, haemoptysis (coughing up blood), weight loss and chest pain.

Disease processes

Following TB exposure, healthy individuals mount a cell mediated immune response involving T cells, macrophages and cytokines, which usually controls the infection. The majority of individuals remain in this asymptomatic (latent) phase and only about 10% go on to develop active TB, usually when their immunity is compromised. Worldwide more than 13 million individuals are coinfected with HIV and TB and in many individuals infected with HIV, development of active TB is the first sign of AIDS.

A number of individual factors such as genetic predisposition (Malik & Godfrey-Faussett, 2005) interact with community and environmental factors, e.g. poverty and poor housing, to influence susceptibility to infection and progression to active TB (Table 7.1.4).

Disease consequences

Tuberculosis is amongst the top 10 causes of illness, disability and death, and is the leading cause of death from a curable infectious disease (WHO, 2008). It is currently estimated that about one-third of the world's population is infected. The main burden of disease in the UK is concentrated in certain urban areas, with 38% of cases in London (Health Protection Agency, 2010). The majority of cases occur in young adults and among non-UK born black African and South Asian ethnic groups. Since most cases occur during the economically productive years of life (19–49 years), the earning capacity of patients can be severely compromised (Frieden et al., 2003). With the advent of effective anti-TB therapy in recent decades, mortality rates have decreased dramatically in industrialised countries.

Nutritional impact

The nutritional consequences of active TB are well recognised; yet little is understood of the complex interactions between TB treatment and nutritional status. Many patients experience severe weight loss and vitamin and mineral deficiencies. People with TB/HIV coinfection have a worse nutritional status as TB worsens malnutrition and malnutrition weakens immunity, thereby increasing the likelihood of progressing from latent to active disease.

Similar to other chronic diseases, a consistent relationship exists between TB incidence and BMI, with one review reporting that TB incidence increases exponentially as BMI decreases (Lönnroth et al., 2010). Patients presenting with active TB are more likely to be wasted or have a low BMI than healthy controls (Paton & Ng, 2006). Nutritional status usually improves with anti-TB therapy, although recent evidence suggests that those who fail to put on weight during the early phase of treatment are more likely to suffer poorer outcomes, including death (Khan et al., 2006; Bernabe-Ortiz et al., 2011).

Nutritional management

The evidence surrounding best practice for nutritional management of TB is very limited, particularly in developed countries. Pragmatically, the underlying principles of nutritional screening and assessment would be the same as for any patient with the potential to benefit from nutritional support (NICE, 2006a). Patients with HIV/TB coinfection face particular challenges and poorer outcomes than those with either infection alone. For more information on the nutritional management of HIV/TB coinfection, see Houtzager et al., (2010) and Chapter 7.11.3.

In patients with active TB, dietary intake is likely to have been poor for some time prior to diagnosis, and in those with disordered lifestyles, e.g. substance abusers, or limited access to food and drink, e.g. the shelter living homeless, nutritional intervention will need to include strategies for ensuring adequate intake throughout the treatment period. Similarly, exploration of the diet of recent immigrants and their potential access to traditional versus native foods may be necessary in order to provide appropriate advice to which patients are likely to adhere.

Clinical investigations and management

In confirmed smear positive cases, the standard treatment is short course chemotherapy for 6–8 months. A combination of drugs and high adherence is necessary to achieve a cure, and treatment usually takes place in two phases; the initial phase lasts 2–3 months and aims to kill active and dormant bacilli, and is followed by the continuation phase, which usually lasts 4–6 months. Patients with HIV coinfection will also be prescribed a variety of antiretroviral drugs that will significantly increase the pill burden, potentially impacting negatively on adherence.

Nutritional requirements

Energy

No studies designed to determine the energy requirements of patients with TB have been published. In the early acute phase of illness, any increase in BMR secondary to the inflammatory response is likely to be accompanied by a decrease in physical activity; thus, TEE may be similar to, or even slightly lower than, normal.

Protein

Protein loss occurs due to the catabolism induced by infection and this loss should be made good through the provision of additional protein. The capacity to retain protein is enhanced during the recovery phase of infection and it is essential that needs are met during this time (NICE, 2006a).

Micronutrients

At the time of diagnosis, patients with active TB may have low levels of several micronutrients, including vitamins C and E, retinol, zinc, iron and selenium (Papathakis, 2008). Daily micronutrient supplementation may be beneficial in those who have deficiencies, especially during the early months of therapy (Abba et al., 2008), but, in the case of vitamin D, possibly only those with specific genotypes will benefit (Martineau et al., 2011).

SECTION 7

Nutritional support

Benefits in terms of weight gain and increased energy intake have been reported (Kennedy *et al.*, 1996; Paton *et al.*, 2004; Schwenk *et al.*, 2004; Sudarsanam *et al.*, 2011); however, it is difficult to distinguish whether improvement in nutritional status was due to control of the disease or to nutritional support, since nutritional status is related to both effective TB treatment and increased dietary intake. Currently, there is a lack of evidence regarding the effects of nutritional support in patients with active TB on outcomes such as hospitalisation, quality of life or functional measures (Sinclair *et al.*, 2011).

References

Abba K, Sudarsanam TD, Grobler L, Volmink J. (2008) Nutritional supplements for people being treated for active tuberculosis. (2008) *Cochrane Database of Systematic Reviews* 4: CD006086.

Andersson I, Grönberg A, Slinde F, Bosaeus I, Larsson S. (2007) Vitamin and mineral status in elderly patients with chronic obstructive pulmonary disease. *Clinical Respiratory Journal* 1(1): 23–29.

Andreyev HJN, Norman AR, Oates J, Cunningham D. (1998) Why do patients with weight loss have a worse outcome when undergoing chemotherapy for gastrointestinal malignancies? *European Journal of Cancer* 34(4): 503–509.

Anker SD, John M, Pederson PU, *et al.* (2006) ESPEN Guidelines on Enteral Nutrition: Cardiology and Pulmonology. *Clinical Nutrition* 25: 311–318.

Baldwin C, Weekes CE. (2011) Dietary advice with or without oral nutritional supplements for disease-related malnutrition in adults. *Cochrane Database of Systematic Reviews* 2: CD002008.

Bates I, Fenton C, Gruber J, *et al.* (2004) Vulnerability to malaria, tuberculosis and HIV/AIDS infection and disease. Part 1: determinants operating at individual and household level. *Lancet Infectious Diseases* 4(5): 267–277.

Bernabe-Ortiz A, Carcamo CP, Sanchez JF, Rios J. (2011) Weight variation over time and its association with tuberculosis treatment outcome: A longitudinal analysis. *PLoS ONE* 6(4): e18474.

Bestall JC, Paul EA, Garrod R, Garnham R, Jones PW, Wedzicha JA. (1999) Usefulness of the Medical Research Council (MRC) dyspnoea scale as a measure of disability in patients with chronic obstructive pulmonary disease. *Thorax* 54: 581–586.

British Lung Foundation. (2007) *Invisible lives: Chronic Obstructive Pulmonary Disease (COPD): Finding the Missing Millions.* London: British Lung Foundation.

British Thoracic Society. (2006) *The Burden of Lung Disease*, 2nd edn. London: British Thoracic Society.

Celli BR, MacNee W, Agusti A, *et al.* (2004) Standards for the diagnosis and treatment of patients with COPD: a summary of the ATS/ERS position paper. *European Respiratory Journal* 23: 932–946.

Christensen PJ, Paine R, Curtis JL, Kazerooni EA, Iannettoni MD, Martinez FJ. (1999) Weight gain after lung volume reduction surgery is not correlated with improvement in pulmonary mechanics. *Chest* 116: 1601–1607.

Cochrane WJ, Afolabi OA. (2004) Investigation into the nutritional status, dietary intake and smoking habits of patients with chronic obstructive pulmonary disease. *Journal of Human Nutrition and Dietetics*, 17: 3–11.

Collins PF, Elia M, Kurukulaaratchy R, Smith TR, Cawood AL, Stratton RJ. (2010a) The influence of deprivation on malnutrition risk in outpatients with chronic obstructive pulmonary disease. *Clinical Nutrition* 5; (Suppl 2): 165–166.

Collins PF, Stratton RJ, Kurukulaaratchy R, Elia M. (2010b) Deprivation is associated with increased healthcare utilisation in patients

with chronic obstructive pulmonary disease. *Thorax* 65 (Suppl IV): A140.

Collins PF, Stratton RJ, Kurukulaaratchy R, Elia M. (2011a) The 'Obesity Paradox' in chronic obstructive pulmonary disease. *Thorax* 65: A74.

Collins PF, Stratton RJ, Elia M. (2011b) The influence of smoking status on malnutrition risk and 1-year mortality in outpatients with chronic obstructive pulmonary disease. *Journal of Human Nutrition and Dietetics* 24(4): 382–383.

Collins PF, Stratton RJ, Elia M. (2012) Nutritional support in chronic obstructive pulmonary disease: a systematic review and meta-analysis. *American Journal of Clinical Nutrition* 95(6): 1385–1395.

De Benedetto F, Del Ponte A, Marinari S, Spacone A. (2000) In COPD patients, body weight excess can mask lean tissue depletion: a simple method of estimation, Monaldi. *Archives of Chest Diseases* 55(4): 273–278.

Eisner MD, Yelin EH, Trupin L, Blanc PD. (2002) The influence of chronic respiratory conditions on health status and work disability. *American Journal of Public Health* 92: 1506–1513.

Engelen MPKJ, Deutz NEP, Wouters EFM, Schols AMWJ. (2000) Enhanced levels of whole-body protein turnover in patients with chronic obstructive pulmonary disease. *American Journal of Respiratory and Critical Care Medicine* 162: 1488–1492.

Ferreira IM, Brooks D, Lacasse Y, Goldstein RS, White J. (2005) Nutritional supplementation for stable chronic obstructive pulmonary disease. *Cochrane Database of Systematic Reviews* 18(2): CD000998.

Forli L, Halse J, Haug E, *et al.* (2004) Vitamin D deficiency, bone mineral density and weight in patients with advanced pulmonary disease. *Journal of Internal Medicine* 256: 56–62.

Frieden TR, Sterling TR, Munsiff SS, Watt CJ, Dye C. (2003) Tuberculosis. *Lancet* 362: 887–899.

Gadek J, DeMichele S, Karlstad M, *et al.* (1999) Effect of enteral feeding with eicosapentaenoic acid, gamma-linolenic acid, and antioxidants in patients with acute respiratory distress syndrome. *Critical Care Medicine* 27(8): 1409–1420.

Global Initiative for Chronic Obstructive Lung Disease (GOLD). (2010) *Pocket Guide to COPD Diagnosis, Management and Prevention.* Available at www.goldcopd.org. Accessed October 2011.

Guerra S, Sherrill DL, Bobadilla A, Martinez F, Barbee RA. (2002), The relation of body mass index to asthma, chronic bronchitis and emphysema, *Chest* 122(4): 1256–1263.

Healthcare Commission. (2006) *Clearing the Air: A National Study of Chronic Obstructive Pulmonary Disease.* London: Healthcare Commission.

Health Protection Agency. (2010) *Tuberculosis in the UK: Annual Report on Tuberculosis Surveillance in the UK.* London: Health Protection Agency.

Heyland DK, Drover JW, MacDonald S, Novak F, Lam M. (2001) Effect of postpyloric feeding on gastroesophageal regurgitation and pulmonary microaspiration: results of a randomized controlled trial. *Critical Care Medicine* 29(8): 1495–1501.

Houtzager L, Barnes M, Matters K. (2010) The nutritional management of patients living with tuberculosis and HIV co-infection. In: Pibram V (ed) *Nutrition and HIV.* Oxford: WileyBlackwell.

Janssens W, Lehouck A, Carremans C, Bouillon R, Mathieu C, Decramer M. (2009) Vitamin D beyond bones in chronic obstructive pulmonary disease. *American Journal of Respiratory and Critical Care Medicine* 179: 630–636.

Janssens W, Bouillon R, Claes B, *et al.* (2010) Vitamin D deficiency is highly prevalent in COPD and correlates with variants in the vitamin D-binding gene. *Thorax* 65: 215–220.

Kennedy N, Ramsay A, Uiso L, Gutmann J, Ngowi FI, Gillespie SH. (1996) Nutritional status and weight gain in patients with pulmonary tuberculosis in Tanzania. *Transactions of the Royal Society of Tropical Medicine and Hygiene* 90(2): 162–166.

Khan A, Sterling TR, Reves R, Vernon A, Horsburgh CR. (2006) Lack of weight gain and relapse risk in a large tuberculosis treatment trial. *American Journal of Respiratory and Critical Care Medicine* 174: 344–348.

Kreymann KG, Berger MM, Deutz NEP, *et al.* (2006) ESPEN Guidelines on Enteral Nutrition: Intensive Care. *Clinical Nutrition* 25: 210–223.

Landbo C, Prescott E, Lange P, Vestbo J, Almdal TP. (1999) Prognostic value of nutritional status in chronic obstructive pulmonary disease. *American Journal of Respiratory and Critical Care Medicine* 160: 1856–1861.

Lönnroth K, Williams BG, Cegielski P, Dye C. (2010) A consistent log-linear relationship between tuberculosis incidence and body mass index. *Lancet* 375: 1814–1829.

Malik ANJ, Godfrey-Faussett P. (2005) Effects of genetic variability of Mycobacterium tuberculosis strains on the presentation of disease. *Lancet Infectious Diseases* 5: 174–83.

Martineau AR, Timms PM, Bothamley GH, *et al.* (2011) High-dose vitamin D3 during intensive-phase antimicrobial treatment of pulmonary tuberculosis: a double-blind randomised controlled trial. *Lancet* 377: 242–250.

McKeever TM, Lewis SA, Cassano PA, *et al.* (2010) Patterns of dietary intake and relation to respiratory disease, forced expiratory volume in 1 s, and decline in 5-y forced expiratory volume. *American Journal of Clinical Nutrition* 92: 408–415.

Metropolitan Life Insurance Company. (1959) New weight standards for men and women. *Statistical Bulletin – Metropolitan Life Insurance Company* 40: 1–10.4.

National Institute for Health and Care Excellence (NICE). (2006a) *Nutrition Support in Adults: Oral Nutrition Support, Enteral Tube Feeding and Parenteral Nutrition.* Avaiable at www.nice.org.uk/cg32. Accessed 12 August 2013.

National Institute for Health and Care Excellence (NICE). National Clinical Guideline Centre for Acute Care. (2006b) *Tuberculosis: Clinical Diagnosis and Management of Tuberculosis, and Measures for its Prevention and Control.* Available at www.nice.org.uk/nicemedia/pdf/cg033niceguideline.pdf. Accessed 12 August 2013.

National Institute for Health and Care Excellence (NICE). (2010) *Chronic Obstructive Pulmonary Disease: Management of Chronic Obstructive Pulmonary Disease in Adults in Primary and Secondary Care.* Clinical Guideline 101. Available at www.nice.org.uk/cg101. Accessed 12 August 2013.

Nguyen LT, Bedu M, Caillaud D, *et al.* (1999) Increased resting energy expenditure is related to plasma TNF-alpha concentration in stable COPD patients. *Clinical Nutrition* 18: 269–274.

Papathakis P; for the United States Agency for International Development (USAID) (2008) *Nutrition and Tuberculosis: A review of the Literature and Considerations for TB Control Programs.* USAID.

Paton NI, Ng YM. (2006) Body composition studies in patients with wasting associated with tuberculosis. *Nutrition* 22(3): 321–331.

Paton NI, Chua YK, Earnest A, Chee CB. (2004) Randomized controlled trial of nutritional supplementation in patients with newly diagnosed tuberculosis and wasting. *American Journal of Clinical Nutrition* 80(2): 460–465.

Pauwels R. (2003) *Global Strategy for the Diagnosis, Management and Prevention of Chronic Obstructive Pulmonary Disease (GOLD).* Bethesda, MD: National Institutes for Health; National Heart, Lung and Blood Institute.

Powell-Tuck J, Hennessy EM. (2003) A comparison of mid upper arm circumference, body mass index and weight loss as indices of undernutrition in acutely hospitalised patients. *Clinical Nutrition* 22: 307–312.

Prescott E, Lange P, Vestbo J, and the Copenhagen City Heart Study Group. (1999) Socioeconomic status, lung function and admission to hospital for COPD: results from the Copenhagen City Heart Study. *European Respiratory Journal* 13(5): 1109–1114.

Rutten-van Mölken MP, Oostenbrink JB, Tashkin DP, Burkhart D, Monz BU. (2006) Does quality of life of COPD patients as measured by the Generic EuroQol Five-Dimension Questionnaire differentiate between COPD severity stages? *Chest* 130: 1117–1128.

Saundy-Unterberger H, Martin JG, Gray-Donald K. (1997) Impact of nutritional support on functional status during an acute exacerbation of chronic obstructive pulmonary disease. *American Journal of Respiratory and Critical Care Medicine* 156: 794–799.

Schols AMWJ, Brug J. (2003) Efficacy of nutritional intervention in chronic obstructive pulmonary disease. *European Respiratory Monograph* 8(24): 142–152.

Schols AMWJ, Soeters PB, Mostert R, Saris WHM, Wouters EFM. (1991), Energy balance in chronic obstructive pulmonary disease. *American Review of Respiratory Diseases* 143: 1248–1252.

Schols AM, Soeters PB, Dingemans AM, Mostert R, Frantzen PJ, Wouters EF. (1993). Prevalence and characteristics of nutritional depletion in patients with stable COPD eligible for pulmonary rehabilitation. *American Review of Respiratory Disease* 147: 1151–1156.

Schols AMWJ, Soeters PB, Mostert R, Pluymers RJ, Wouters EFM. (1995), Physiologic effects of nutritional support and anabolic steroids in patients with chronic obstructive pulmonary disease. *American Journal of Respiratory and Critical Care Medicine* 152: 1268–1274.

Schols AMWJ, Slangen S, Volovics L, Wouters EFM. (1998) Weight loss is a reversible factor in the prognosis of chronic obstructive pulmonary disease. *American Journal of Respiratory and Critical Care Medicine* 157: 1791–1797.

Schwenk A, Macallan DC. (2000) Tuberculosis, malnutrition and wasting. *Current Opinions in Clinical Nutrition and Metabolic Care* 3: 285–291.

Schwenk A, Hodgson L, Wright A, *et al.* (2004) Nutrient partitioning during treatment of tuberculosis: gain in body fat mass but not in protein mass. *American Journal of Clinical Nutrition* 79: 1006–1012.

Sinclair D, Abba K, Grobler L, Sudarsanam TD. (2011) Nutritional supplements for people being treated for active tuberculosis. *Cochrane Database of Systematic Reviews* Issue 11: CD006086.

Singer P, Thiella M, Fisher H, *et al.* (2006) Benefit of an enteral diet enriched with eicosapentaenoic acid and gamma-linolenic acid in patients with acute lung injury. *Critical Care Medicine* 34(4): 1033–1038.

Slinde F, Ellegard L, Gronberg AM, Larsson S, Rossander-Hulthen L. (2003) Total energy expenditure in underweight patients with severe chronic obstructive pulmonary disease living at home. *Clinical Nutrition* 22(2): 159–165.

Slinde F, Kvarnhult K, Grönberg AM, Nordenson A, Larsson S, Hulthen L. (2006). Energy expenditure in underweight chronic obstructive pulmonary disease patients before and during a physiotherapy programme. *European Journal of Clinical Nutrition* 60: 870–876.

Slinde F, Grönberg AM, Svantesson U, Hulthe'n L, Larsson S. (2011) Energy expenditure in chronic obstructive pulmonary disease – evaluation of simple measures. *European Journal of Clinical Nutrition* 65(12): 1–5.

Soler-Cataluña JJ, Sánchez-Sánchez L, Martínez-García MÁ, Sánchez PR, Salcedo E, Navarro M. (2005) Mid-arm muscle area is a better predictor of mortality than body mass index in COPD. *Chest* 128: 2108–2115.

Steer J, Norman E, Gibson GJ, Bourke SC. (2010) Comparison of indices of nutritional status in prediction of in-hospital mortality and early readmission of patients with acute exacerbations of COPD. *Thorax* 65: A127.

Stratton RJ, Green CJ, Elia M. (2003) Disease-related malnutrition: an evidence-based approach to treatment. Oxford: CABI Publishing.

Steiner MC, Barton RL, Singh SJ, Morgan MD. (2003) Nutritional enhancement of exercise performance in chronic obstructive pulmonary disease: a randomised controlled trial. *Thorax* 58(9): 745–751.

Sudarsanam TD, John J, Kang G, *et al.* (2011) Pilot randomized trial of nutritional supplementation in patients with tuberculosis and HIV-tuberculosis coinfection receiving observed short-course

SECTION 7

chemotherapy for tuberculosis. *Tropical Medicine and International Health* 16(6): 699–670.

Teramoto S, Kume H, Ouchi Y. (2002) Altered swallowing physiology and aspiration in COPD. *Chest* 122(2): 1104–1105.

Todorovic V, Micklewright A. On behalf of the Parenteral and Enteral Nutrition Group of the British Dietetic Association. (2011). *A Pocket Guide to Clinical Nutrition*. Available at www.peng.org.uk/publications/pocket-guide.html.

Vermeeren MAP, Schols AMWJ, Wouters EFM. (1997) Effects of an acute exacerbation on nutritional and metabolic profile of patients with COPD. *European Respiratory Journal* 10: 2264–2269.

Vermeeren MA, Wouters EF, Geraerts-Keeris AJ, Schols AM. (2004) Nutritional support in patients with chronic obstructive pulmonary disease during hospitalization for an acute exacerbation: a randomized controlled feasibility trial. *Clinical Nutrition* 23(5): 1184–1192.

Vermeeren MA, Creutzberg EC, Schols AM, *et al.*; on behalf of the COSMIC Study Group. (2006) Prevalence of nutritional depletion in a large out-patient population of patients with COPD. *Respiratory Medicine* 100(8): 1349–1355.

Vestbo J, Prescott E, Almdal T, *et al.* (2006) Body mass, fat-free body mass, and prognosis in patients with chronic obstructive pulmonary disease from a random population sample: findings from the Copenhagen City Heart Study. *American Journal of Respiratory and Critical Care Medicine* 173: 79–83.

Weekes CE. (2005) *Nutritional Strategies in the Management of Chronic Obstructive Pulmonary Disease; Nutrition Screening, Dietary Counselling and Food Fortification*. PhD Thesis. London: King's College.

Weekes CE, Bateman NT. (2002) Weight change in chronic obstructive pulmonary disease; not just a problem of undernutrition. *Thorax* 57 (Suppl III): 60.

Weekes CE, Emery PW, Elia M. (2006) Dietary counselling and food fortification in malnourished outpatients with chronic obstructive pulmonary disease: a post hoc cost analysis. ESPEN Conference, Istanbul 19–22 Oct. 2006, p237 (abstract).

Weekes CE, Emery PW, Elia M. (2007) A nutrition screening tool based on the BAPEN four questions reliably predicts hospitalisation and mortality in respiratory outpatients. *Proceedings of the Nutrition Society* 66: 9A.

Weekes CE, Emery PW, Elia M. (2009) Dietary counselling and food fortification in stable COPD: a randomised trial. *Thorax* 64(4); 326–331.

Williamson DF, Madans J, Anda RF, Kleinman JC, Giovino GA, Byers T. (1991) Smoking cessation and severity of weight gain in a national cohort. *New England Journal of Medicine* 324: 739–745.

World Health Organization. (2004) The Global Burden of Disease 2004 Update. Available at www.who.int/healthinfo/global_burden_disease/GBD_report_2004update_full.pdf.

World Health Organization. (2008) Global Tuberculosis Control: surveillance, planning, financing. www.who.int/tb/publications/global_report/2008/en/.

7.2

Dental disorders

Kathy Cowborough and Ursula Arens

Key points

■ Dental disease has a significant impact on food intake, nutritional status and general health, particularly in older people.

■ Damage to, or loss of, teeth may result from dental caries, acid erosion or periodontal disease.

■ Prevalence is highest in children from socioeconomically disadvantaged groups. In older adults, root caries is a significant contributor to tooth loss.

■ Dietary acid (mainly from soft drinks) causes dental erosion, resulting in irreversible tooth enamel loss and tooth destruction. The tooth enamel of young children is more susceptible and easily damaged.

■ Fluoride, reducing frequency of consumption of sugar containing products and acidic drinks, and good oral hygiene are the most important preventative measures for dental health.

Dental disease is a major public health problem in the UK. Dental diseases can result in acute pain, disfigurement and tooth loss. It can affect food intake, nutritional status and general health, particularly in older people (Steele *et al.*, 1998) and therefore an important aspect of dietary assessment. Dental disease is mainly preventable and should not be viewed in isolation from other aspects of health (Moynihan, 2005). Damage to or loss of teeth may result from dental caries, acid erosion and periodontal disease.

Dental caries

Between 1993 and 2003 There was a decrease in dentine decay prevalence in 15-year-old children from 42% to 13%. Approximately half were found to be caries free, compared with just over one-third in 1993 and fewer than 10% in 1983 (Lader *et al.*, 2005). There were significant improvements in 5–8-year-old children with obvious decay in the primary milk teeth between 1993 and 2003. However, early childhood caries (ECC) affected one in 10 of 3–4-year olds in the UK. Improvements were also seen in the Adult Dental Health Survey 1998 compared with previous surveys (Kelly *et al.*, 2000), but mainly in younger adults (16–44 years). Decreases in the prevalence of caries have occurred largely as a result of the effects of fluoride and better oral hygiene. Over half of young people aged 4–18 years had evidence of dental caries in primary or secondary teeth (Walker, 2000), with caries being more common in children from some minority ethnic groups (Holt *et al.*, 1996). There were regional variations in the prevalence of dental caries and an association with social and economic deprivation (Jones *et al.*, 1997; Walker, 2000). Dental health is particularly poor amongst immigrants and refugees (Davies, 1998; Gussy *et al.*, 2006; Sheiham, 2001).

Causation

Dental caries occur when carbohydrate from food and drinks reacts with dental plaque, a sticky film of bacteria that forms on all surfaces of the teeth, to produce acid. Within minutes of exposure of the bacteria to a carbohydrate, fermentation occurs, which results in acid production. At a pH of <5.5, tooth enamel begins to be demineralised and become porous. At this stage, surface damage to tooth enamel can be repaired as enamel is constantly dissolved (demineralisation) and reformed (remineralisation). Acid produced by bacterial action dissipates after about 30 minutes and, once the pH rises above 5.5, enamel is remineralised with calcium and phosphate released from saliva. However, remineralisation requires acidity to remain above pH 5.5 for a period of time. If carbohydrate is eaten frequently, there will insufficient time for remineralisation to take place. This results in continually repeated, gradual loss of enamel and damage to the dentine. Eventually, the enamel collapses to form a cavity and the tooth is progressively

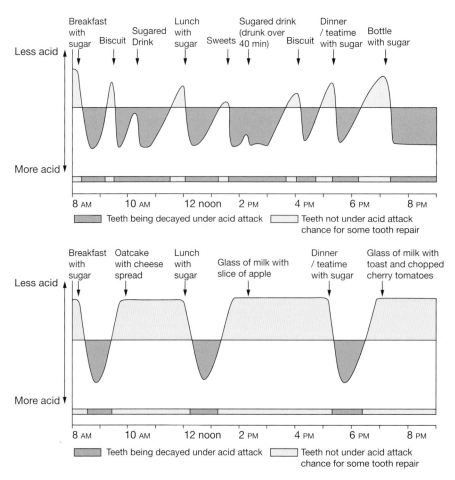

Figure 7.2.1 Stephan curve demonstrating the effect of eating frequency on mouth acidity (source: NHS Scottish Executive 2011 www .child-smile.org.uk/professionals/childsmile-manual.aspx Appendix 5 – Stephan Curve – Example 1. Reproduced with permission of NHS Scottish Executive. Information licensed under the Open Scottish Parliament Licence v. 1.0)

destroyed. This is illustrated in a Stephan curve as shown in Figure 7.2.1.

Children's teeth are particularly vulnerable to this process during the first 6 years of life when tooth enamel is being developed and is relatively soft. Caries can also attack the roots of teeth if they become exposed due to gum recession, which is a common problem in older adults. The National Diet and Nutrition Survey (NDNS) of older adults found a strong relationship between the presence of root decay and the frequency of intake of sugar rich foods (Steele *et al*., 1998).

Factors affecting caries development

Several factors influence the formation of dental caries.

Type of carbohydrate

All carbohydrates are cariogenic, although there is considerable variation. Sucrose, glucose, maltose and fructose are most cariogenic as they are a readily available substrate for oral bacteria. Sugars such as lactose or galactose are less cariogenic; in addition, they are found in foods high in protein, calcium and phosphates, which help neutralise acids. The sugars that are potentially damaging to dental health are classified as non-milk extrinsic sugars (NMES); these include all added sugars, and sugars

in fresh fruit juice, honey and syrups. Starch can contribute to caries as saliva contains amylase, which breaks it down to glucose and maltose in the mouth. However, this varies with the type of starch and the way it has been processed (Grenby, 1997; WHO/FAO, 2003). Fructo-oligosaccharides may be as acidogenic as sucrose (Moynihan *et al*., 2001). Sugar alcohols, e.g. xylitol, mannitol and sorbitol, are not fermentable and hence are non-cariogenic.

Frequency of exposure

Both total sugar intake and the consumption frequency are associated with caries development. However frequency of consumption may be the more significant factor (Holt, 1991; Touger-Decker & van Loveren, 2003). Small, frequent amounts of sugars cause more damage than the same quantity consumed on a single occasion. Acid conditions in the mouth are perpetuated, preventing remineralisation and permitting longer periods of demineralisation to occur. In young children, the combination of poor oral hygiene, limited exposure to fluoride and frequent exposure to sugary snacks and drinks results in ECC, particularly in infants who continually suck a bottle containing sugar containing drinks (Ismail, 1998; Levine & Stillman-Lowe, 2009). Frequency of sugar consumption is an important aspect of dental health, but its contribution to caries development is less if there is good dental hygiene.

Food texture

Small particles of sticky foods may be left wedged between the teeth, so allowing continual acid production. Therefore, foods such as dried fruit, e.g. dates and raisins, have a much greater cariogenic potential than fresh fruit (Edgar, 1993).

Oral hygiene

Failure to clean teeth regularly results in the build up of tooth plaque and the accumulation of food debris in teeth crevices, providing substrate for continuous bacterial acid production. Poor oral hygiene in children has a greater impact on the levels of caries associated microorganisms than the frequency or amount of sugar consumed (Beighton *et al.*, 1996). In the 1998 NDNS, an association between caries and consumption of sugar confectionery was only seen in children whose teeth were brushed less than twice a day (Gibson & Williams, 1999). Lack of oral hygiene measures is likely to account for a significant proportion of the excessive caries prevalence in deprived groups.

Salivary flow

Saliva helps protect against dental caries by removing food particles from teeth, neutralising acids and delivering minerals to the tooth to enhance rates of remineralisation. Salivary flow can be stimulated by eating foods that require chewing or which stimulate saliva production, e.g. hard cheeses (Rugg-Gunn & Nunn, 1999) or chewing sugar free gum (Murray *et al.*, 2003). Reduced saliva production may be associated with the development of root caries in older adults. Saliva flow may be reduced in poorly controlled diabetes.

Tooth decay resistance

There is considerable individual variability in the resistance of tooth enamel to decay due to the influence of genetic factors on tooth production. Children and the elderly (with worn enamel) are at greater risk. Fluoride markedly increases enamel resistance as it results in the formation of fluorhydroxyapatite crystals in the tooth matrix, which are more resistant to acid erosion than unfluoridated hydroxyapatite.

Dental erosion

There is a gradual loss of tooth outer substance, particularly of the very hard outer enamel layer, with ageing. This can be due to a triad of factors:

- *Attrition* – wearing away of teeth by tooth to tooth contact during normal chewing.
- *Abrasion* – wearing away of teeth as a result of external objects applied to the tooth surface, e.g. brushing teeth too strongly or using a toothbrush with hard bristles.

- *Erosion* – wearing away of teeth due to acids in the mouth from foods consumed. This is in contrast to acids of bacterial origin.

The signs of dental erosion are changes to the appearance of the tooth and at a later stage, increased sensitivity of the tooth, leading to pain when eating foods that are very hot or very cold, sweet or acidic. In the last two decades there has been an increased awareness of dental erosion, particularly in children and teenagers. An increase in the observation of dental erosion in young people may be associated with recent changes to diet. The survey Children's Dental Health in the UK (O'Brien, 1994) showed that half of all 6 year olds were found to have erosion, and in one-quarter of children, erosion had resulted in some exposure of dentine. One-third of 14-year-old children had some erosion of their permanent teeth. Wear of permanent teeth is a lifelong process; therefore, the extent and severity of damage can be highest in older people. However, because the most damaged teeth may have been lost or removed, there may be lower occurrence figures in remaining teeth. In the 1998 report NDNS of people aged 65 years and over, severe wear of teeth was recorded in 15% of the dentate (having natural teeth) free living participants (Steele *et al.*, 1998). This figure for tooth wear included, but was not exclusively due to, damage from acid erosion.

Some sources of acid affecting teeth can be intrinsic. Gastric reflux (the regurgitation of stomach acids) increases the acidity of the mouth, and may occur occasionally during illness, or more regularly in people who are obese or alcoholic, or during pregnancy. The observation of tooth damage from acid may be a sign of bulimia. Regurgitated acids from the stomach are very erosive to teeth, and some treatments are available to inhibit reflux or neutralise the acidity of gastric juice, if this occurs regularly (O'Sullivan & Milosevic, 2008).

Extrinsic sources of acid are mainly from foods and drinks consumed in the diet. Acidic foods include many fruits, particularly citrus fruits and their juices; vinegars, salad dressings and pickles; alcoholic drinks, including wines, ciders and alcopops; fruit teas; carbonated drinks, especially those with flavourings such as citric and phosphoric acid; and sour flavoured sweets. Although there is some decrease in pH in carbonated water compared with still water, in practice fizzy waters seem not to affect oral acidity.

Other factors affecting erosion

In addition to the acidity of the food, other factors may influence the risk of dental erosion to teeth.

Titratable acidity

There may be differences in pH values of foods and values obtained when adding buffering solutions to different foods (titratable acidity); the latter is thought to be a better measure of the erosive risk of the food. Buffering capacities have been shown to be high for fruit juices and fruit based carbonated drinks, and lower for non-fruit flavoured and sparkling waters (although still water and milk have the lowest capacities) (Edwards *et al.*, 1999; Dugmore & Rock, 2004).

Frequency and timing of consumption

The frequency of exposure has a greater effect than the quantities of the risk factor. Because the production of saliva is lowest during sleep, the consumption of acidic foods just before rest may result in greater erosive damage.

Consumption in relation to tooth brushing

If teeth are brushed after consuming acidic foods, components of the dissolved enamel will be removed, reducing subsequent remineralisation. Tooth brushing should not be before half an hour after consuming acidic foods; rinsing with water may be an alternative way to support mouth freshness after meals.

Method of consumption

Frequent sipping and swishing of acidic drinks may increase acid erosion of tooth enamel; consuming drinks through a straw may reduce tooth contact with acid liquids.

Other foods

The consumption of dairy foods may prevent the demineralisation that occurs after consuming acid foods. Eating very small amounts of cheese after consuming acid drinks supports remineralisation of the enamel; possibly due to the alkaline properties of dairy foods or their promotion of salivary flow.

Periodontal disease

Gingivitis is the initial stage of periodontal disease when the gums become inflamed by plaque that accumulates next to the gum margin. In its early stages, gingivitis can be slowed by regular dental treatment to remove plaque and tartar (calcified plaque) from the gum margins. If gingivitis persists, periodontal disease develops beneath the gum surface, leading to destruction of bone and loosening of the tooth, which may eventually fall out. There is little evidence for an association between diet and periodontal disease (WHO/FAO, 2003), Periodontal disease and resultant tooth loss impairs the ability to chew and can restrict food choice (Sheiham *et al.*, 1999), and for older adults this can have a significant impact on their nutritional status. People with natural teeth are more likely to consume foods that require chewing, such as fresh fruit and vegetables, and as a result have higher intakes of some vitamins (Steele *et al.*, 1998). The 2003 Children's Dental Health Survey (Lader *et al.*, 2005) showed that the prevalence of periodontal disease was increasing; 68% of teenage boys and 56% of teenage girls had signs of dental plaque and gingivitis.

Dental and oral health promotion

Dental disease is not inevitable and can be prevented by changes in behaviour. Effective and evidence based messages to prevent dental disease should incorporate good oral hygiene practices, dietary practices and fluoride protection, as shown in Table 7.2.1.

Table 7.2.1 Practical measures to provide dental protection

Protective factors	Practical measures
Reducing the frequency of consumption of sugars	Consume sugar containing foods and drinks with meals Limit between meal snacks containing sugars, particularly sticky foods like dried fruit Use sugar free medicines wherever possible
Reducing exposure to acid erosion	Limit consumption of acidic drinks between meals – water, tea/coffee without sugar, or plain milk are suitable Avoid acidic food or drink immediately before brushing teeth or after brushing teeth at night
Ending a meal with foods that buffer acids	Cheese and milk assist remineralisation
Good oral hygiene	Children's teeth should be brushed with a small pea sized amount of low dose fluoride toothpaste when teeth erupt Correct brushing and flossing teeth and gums to remove plaque and debris at base of teeth Avoid brushing teeth immediately after consumption of acidic food or drink as this may hinder remineralisation; it should not be overlooked in those unwell or require care Essential for patients undergoing radiotherapy for head or neck cancer or chemotherapy, who may be more susceptible to dental caries (Bothwell, 1987; Dreizen *et al.*, 1977)
Exposure to fluoride	Topical application, e.g. toothpastes, mouth rinses or tooth coating Flouridated drinking water Fluorides supplements should only be prescribed by a dental practitioner on an individual basis (SIGN, 2005)
Increasing salivary flow	Consuming foods that require mastication, e.g. wholegrain foods Eating foods that increase salivation, e.g. cheese, peanuts Chewing sugar free gum
Regular dental checks	To correct early problems To remove build up of plaque and tartar

Specific guidance for particular population subgroups

Dental health promotion is relevant to the whole population, but is particularly important for those in high risk groups, such as infants, especially at the time of weaning, children and adults living in deprived circumstances, and elderly people.

Infants

Dental health in infants can be improved by adhering to the following recommendations:

- Prolonged bottle feeding should be discouraged and discontinued after 1 year.
- From the age of 6 months, infants should be introduced to drinking from a non-valve, free flowing cup as well as use of a bottle.
- Infants and young children should never be given a bottle or beaker containing sugary drinks as a comforter.
- Dummies or comforters should not be dipped into honey or sugary drinks (Armstrong *et al.*, 2008).
- Soya based formulae can cause tooth decay as they contain sugars (SIGN, 2005).
- Weaning practices can have a major influence of both immediate and future dental health (Holt & Moynihan, 1996) and should be low in sugars and acids.
- Milk or water are the preferred drinks; other drinks, e.g. fruit juices and concentrates, should be limited and given only at main meals. They should not be given in bottles or at bedtime.

Children

Parents and carers can improve a child's dental health by:

- Limiting sugar containing and acidic drinks, especially between meals.
- Making the majority of drinks milk or water.
- Restricting sugary or acidic drinks at bedtime or during the night.
- Supervising teeth cleaning (ideally up to the age of 6 years) with a fluoride containing toothpaste (SIGN, 2005).
- Ensuring children have regular dental check ups.

Elderly people

Elderly people experience changes that may affect good dental health, including:

- Decreased salivary flow.
- Decreased manual dexterity.
- Impaired cognitive function.
- Polypharmacy.
- Swallowing difficulties.
- Reduced thirst and fluid intake.

Factors that should be considered in this age group include:

- Daily tooth or denture cleaning, especially in those unable to do this themselves.
- Avoiding frequent consumption of sugary foods, while still maintaining enjoyment of food.
- Encouraging the consumption of foods that promote salivary flow.
- Monitoring use of over the counter medicines such as cough sweets, laxatives, antacids and various tonics – these should be taken at meals only, if possible.
- Having regular dental checks to identify problems and ensure that dentures fit properly.

Further reading

British Nutrition Foundation (BNF). (1999) *Oral Health. A Task Force Report*. London BNF.

Levine RS, Stillman-Lowe CR. (2009) *The Scientific Basis of Oral Education*, 6th edn. London: British Dental Journal (BDJ) Books.

Internet resources

The British Dental Health Foundation   www.dentalhealth.org

Scottish Intercollegiate Guidelines Network (SIGN)   www.sign.ac.uk
  Prevention and management of dental decay in the preschool child (2005) SIGN guidance 83
  Preventing dental caries in children at high caries risk targeted. Targeted prevention of dental caries in the permanent teeth of 6–16 year olds presenting for dental care (2000) SIGN guidance 47

References

Armstrong A, Freeman R, McComb A, Speedy P. (2008) Nutrition and Dental Health. Health Promotion Agency for Northern Ireland. Available at: www.healthpromotionagency.org.uk/Resources/nutrition/pdfs/Nutrition_and_Dental_Health.pdf. Accessed 22 June 2012.

Beighton D, Adamson A, Rugg-Gunn A. (1996) Associations between dietary intake, dental caries experience and salivary bacterial levels in 12 year old English schoolchildren. *Archives of Oral Biology* 41(3): 271–280.

Bothwell RB. (1987) Prevention and treatment of the orofacial complications of radiotherapy. *Journal of the American Dental Association* 114(3): 316–322.

Davies GN. (1998) Early Childhood caries- a synopsis. *Community Dentistry and Oral Epidemiology* 26 (Suppl 1): 106–116.

Dreizen S, Daly TE, Drane JB, Brown LR. (1977) Oral complications of cancer radiotherapy. *Postgraduate Medicine* 62(2): 85–92.

Dugmore CR, Rock W.P. (2004) A multifactorial analysis of factors associated with dental erosion. *British Dental Journal* 196: 283–286.

Edgar WM. (1993) Extrinsic and intrinsic sugars: a review of recent UK recommendations on diet and dental caries. *Caries Research* 27(1): 64–67.

Edwards SL, Creanor RH, Hoyle W. (1999) Buffering capacities of soft drinks: the potential influence on dental erosion. *Journal of Oral Rehabilitation* 26(12): 923–927.

Gibson S, Williams S. (1999) Dental caries in pre-school children: associations with social class, toothbrushing habit and consumption of sugars and sugar-containing foods. Further analysis of data from the National Diet and Nutrition Survey of children aged 1.5–4.5 years. *Caries Research* 33(2): 101–113.

Grenby TH. (1997) Summary of the dental effects of starch. *International Journal of Food Sciences and Nutrition* 48: 411–416.

SECTION 7

Gussy MG, Waters EG, Walsh O, Kilpatrick NM. (2006) Early child-hood caries: Current evidence for aetiology and prevention. *Journal of Paediatrics and Child Health* 42(1,2): 37–43.

Holt RD. (1991) Foods and drinks at 4 daily intervals in a group of young children. *British Dental Journal* 170(4): 137–143.

Holt RD Moynihan PJ. (1996) The weaning diet and dental health. *British Dental Journal* 181(7): 254–259.

Holt RD, Winter GB, Downer MC, Bellis WJ, Hay IS. (1996) Caries in pre-school children in Camden in 1993/4. *British Dental Journal* 181: 405–410.

Ismail AI. (1998) Prevention of early childhood caries. *Community Dentistry and Oral Epidemiology* 26(1): 49–61.

Jones CM, Taylor GO, Whittle JG, Evans D, Trotter DP. (1997) Water fluoridation, tooth decay in 5 year olds, and social deprivation measured by the Jarman score: analysis of data from British dental surveys. *BMJ* 315: 514–517.

Kelly M, Steele J, Nuttall N, *et al.* (2000) *Adult Dental Health Survey: Oral Health in the United Kingdom 1998*. London: The Stationery Office.

Lader D, Chadwick B, Chestnutt I, *et al.* (2005) *Children's Dental Health Survey in the United Kingdom, 2003. Summary Report*. London: Office for National Statistics.

Levine RS, Stillman-Lowe CR. (2009) *The Scientific Basis of Oral Education*, 6th edn. London: British Dental Journal (BDJ) Books.

Moynihan PJ. (2005) The interrelationship between diet and oral health. *Proceedings of the Nutrition Society* 64: 571–580.

Moynihan PJ, McIlmoyle S, Rowshanaei R, Moxon R, Russell RRB. (2001) Acidogenic potential of fructo-oligosaccharides: incubation studies and plaque pH studies. *Caries Research* 35: 265–316.

Murray JJ, Nunn JH, Steele JG. (2003) *Prevention of Oral Disease*, 4th edn. Oxford: Oxford University Press.

O'Brien M. (1994) *Child Dental Health in the United Kingdom 1993*. Office of Population Census and Surveys, Social Survey Division. London: HMSO.

O'Sullivan E, Milosevic A. (2008) UK National Clinical Guidelines in Paediatric Dentistry: diagnosis, prevention and management of dental erosion International *Journal of Paediatric Dentistry* 18: 29–38.

Rugg-Gunn AJ, Nunn JH. (1999) *Nutrition Diet and Oral Health*. Oxford: Oxford University Press.

Sheiham A. (2001) Dietary effects of dental disease. *Public Health Nutrition* 4(2B): 569–591.

Sheiham A, Steele JG, Marcenes W, Finch S, Walls AW. (1999) The impact of oral health on stated ability to eat certain foods: findings from the National Diet and Nutrition Survey of older people in Great Britain. *Gerodontology* 16(1): 11–20.

Scottish Intercollegiate Guidance Network (SIGN). (2005) Preventing dental caries in children at high caries risk: targeted prevention of dental caries in the permanent teeth of 6–16 year olds. A national clinical guideline 83 Avaialble at www.sign.ac.uk/pdf/qrg83.pdf. Accessed 22 May 2012.

Steele JG, Sheiham A, Marcenes W, Walls AWG. (1998) *National Diet and Nutrition Survey: People Aged 65 Years and Over*, Volume 2: Report of the oral health survey. London: The Stationery Office.

Touger-Decker R, van Loveren C. (2003) Sugars and dental caries. *American Journal of Clinical Nutrition* 78(4): 881S–892S.

Walker A. (2000) *National Diet and Nutrition Survey: Young People Aged 4 to 18 Years*, Volume 2. Report of the oral health survey. Office for National Statistics. London: The Stationery Office.

WHO/FAO. (2003) Recommendations for preventing dental diseases. In: *Joint Expert Consultation on Diet, Nutrition and Prevention of Chronic Diseases*. Geneva: World Health Organization, pp. 105–108.

7.3

Dysphagia

June Copeman and Karen Hyland

Key points

■ People with dysphagia cannot swallow food or fluid effectively.

■ Potential consequences of dysphagia include choking, aspiration, dehydration, malnutrition and death.

■ Food suitable for inclusion in an individual's diet depends on the assessed grade of consistency required. Single texture foods are easier to eat than foods with multiple textures. It is important that adequate nutrients and energy are consumed at all times.

■ Frequent monitoring is required because the individual's condition may change.

■ People with dysphagia may become dehydrated if they cannot swallow normal fluids; thickened drinks may be needed.

Swallowing is a highly complex process requiring appropriate posture of the head and neck, good lip and tongue movement, and the presence of the swallow reflex. Many factors can impair the ability to swallow and the physical and nutritional consequences of this can be profound, even life threatening.

Dysphagia is defined as difficulty in swallowing caused by neurological or structural damage, which interferes with the efficient movement of food and fluid from the mouth to the stomach. It is a common consequence of many different types of illness or injury resulting in mechanical or neurological impairment of the swallowing process (Table 7.3.1). Dysphagia is most likely to be encountered in patients with stroke, progressive neurological disorders, e.g. Parkinson's disease, motor neurone disease and multiple sclerosis, anoxic brain injury, other conditions such as learning disabilities, some cancers or injury affecting the head and neck. The specific feeding difficulties that arise depend on the precise motor function, behaviour or cognitive deficit that has occurred. This chapter refers to dysphagic people over the age of 5 years. The normal swallow does not mature fully until this age, and details of the management of dysphagia in infants and young children should therefore be sought in paediatric textbooks.

The normal swallow

The normal swallow can be divided into four main stages and impairment in any one of these can result in dysphagia:

1. *Preparatory stage* – this stage is mainly under voluntary control, comprising the transfer of food (or liquid) into the mouth. As food or liquid approaches the mouth, the head moves forward, the tongue protrudes and the lips and jaws open in preparation. Food and drink is placed in the mouth and the lips and jaw close to seal the mouth. The sight, smell and taste of the food will have stimulated saliva production.

2. *Oral stage* – this stage, where food is prepared for passage from the mouth into the pharynx, is also mainly under voluntary control. The tongue moves the food and positions it between the teeth. Chewing (mastication) is achieved by up and down, and rotary movements of the jaw in order to grind the food and mix it with saliva. The tongue forms a central groove to collect the food, with its tip sealed against the hard palate. The resulting bolus is propelled backwards by the posterior movement of the tongue.

3. *Pharyngeal stage* – this is an involuntary stage where the food bolus passes from the mouth through the pharynx and into the oesophagus. At the same time, the airway is temporarily sealed off to prevent the entry of food or fluid into the lungs. The process is initiated when sensation of the bolus at the anterior faucal arch (towards the back of the mouth) stimulates the swallowing centre in the brain stem. The swallow reflex is then triggered:
   ○ The soft palate elevates to seal off the nasopharynx.
   ○ The larynx elevates and so forces the epiglottis down to cover the larynx.
   ○ The vocal cords (within the larynx) close.

Table 7.3.1   Common causes of dysphagia

Mechanical	Oesophageal stricture Oesophageal spasm Cancers in the head, neck and oesophageal areas Cancer treatment including radiotherapy/ surgery to head and neck area Pharyngeal pouch Injury or surgery to the tongue, lips, mouth or jaw Severe infections of the mouth or throat, e.g. oral thrush or ulcers Postural problems, e.g. severe kyphosis (curvature of the spine)
Neurological	Stroke Parkinson's disease Motor neurone disease Head injury Multiple sclerosis Cerebral palsy Dementia Huntington's disease Drug induced (psychotropic drugs)
Psychological	Globus hystericus Severe anxiety Severe depression

○ Respiration stops momentarily.

Foods pass through the pharynx mainly by peristalsis, i.e. the muscles of the pharynx contract and move the bolus through, although gravity has some effect. The crico-pharyngeal sphincter relaxes and is opened by the upward pull of the larynx; the food bolus then passes into the oesophagus.

4. *Oesophageal stage* – this stage is also involuntary. The food bolus passes down the oesophagus into the stomach by peristalsis (wave like muscle contractions) and gravity, the cardiac sphincter relaxes and food enters the stomach.

Consequences of dysphagia

Dysphagia is potentially fatal. For example, the presence of dysphagia following a stroke increases the likelihood of subsequent malnutrition (Foley *et al.*, 2009), mortality and disability at 90 days (Paciaroni *et al.*, 2004), with increased institutionalisation (Smithard *et al.*, 2007).

Attempting to swallow foods or liquids without the ability to do so carries a high risk of aspiration (foods or liquids entering the lungs). This, if extensive, can cause acute asphyxiation and in lesser degrees is a major contributor to chest infections, lung abscesses and aspiration pneumonia (Gordon *et al.*, 1987; Ramsey *et al.*, 2003; Ney *et al.*, 2009). Aspiration may also be silent, causing no outward signs of distress but still capable of causing pulmonary complications (Teasell *et al.*,1996; Marik & Kaplan, 2003).

An impaired ability to swallow has many nutritional implications. The physical effects of dysphagia make the process of feeding slow, difficult and tiring, and as a result food intake is often inadequate in terms of both quantity (sometimes further compromised by food leakages from the mouth) and variety of food consumed. Fear of choking (especially if there has been an unpleasant experience of aspiration) may cause food aversions or panic attacks at meal times. Other psychological factors such as depression or anxiety (stemming from the patient's reaction to the illness and its effects) may further depress appetite. Embarrassment, vulnerability and loss of enjoyment of eating as a social function should not be underestimated (Ekburg *et al.*, 2001; Martino *et al.*, 2009).

Physiologically, inadequate intake of food and fluid will lead to undernutrition, weight loss, compromised immune function and a high risk of dehydration. These may in turn lead to deterioration of the patient's physical or mental condition and delay recovery or hasten death. The consequences of dysphagia can be compounded by concurrent:

- General illness and frailty.
- Other comorbidities, e.g. diabetes.
- Difficulties with positioning.
- Ill fitting or absent dentures.

The dysphagia care team

Effective treatment of dysphagia, whether in primary or secondary care (own home, community centre, care home, hospital), requires multidisciplinary care with good communication mechanisms in place. Coordinated multidisciplinary pathways for the assessment of dysphagia and feeding problems, with subsequent agreed intervention, will facilitate cost efficient, appropriate care. Different professionals will have specific roles within the joint treatment plans, as shown in Figure 7.3.1.

Active participation of the client and carers, whenever possible, in any decision making is essential. Short and long term prognosis, ethical issues and quality of life should be considered as an integral part of this discussion. Agreed joint treatment plans should enable the client to be transferred between hospital, intermediate and community locations without appropriate interventions being compromised. In the community, liaison with social workers and support personnel, such as home carers, meals on wheels providers or commercial ready meal home delivery services, may be essential.

Management

Dysphagia requires prompt and skilled remedial action in order to reduce the risk of aspiration and minimise nutritional deterioration, particularly if the onset has been acute (Odderson *et al.*, 1995; Finestone *et al.*, 1995). Nearly half of all stroke patients admitted to hospital will have swallowing difficulties (NICE, 2008; SIGN, 2010) and considerably more among people with other neurological conditions. The primary aims of management by the team are to:

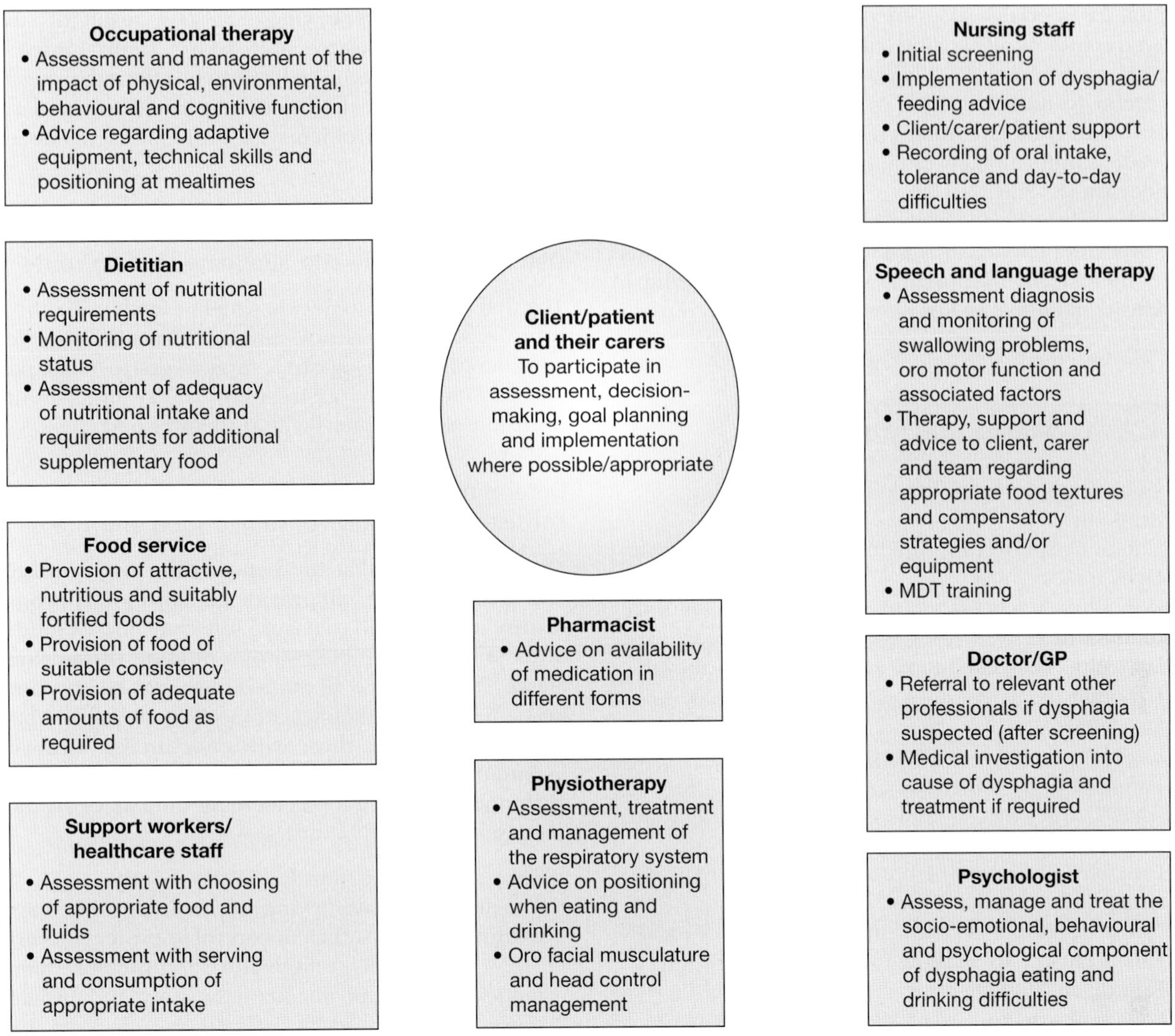

Occupational therapy
- Assessment and management of the impact of physical, environmental, behavioural and cognitive function
- Advice regarding adaptive equipment, technical skills and positioning at mealtimes

Nursing staff
- Initial screening
- Implementation of dysphagia/feeding advice
- Client/carer/patient support
- Recording of oral intake, tolerance and day-to-day difficulties

Dietitian
- Assessment of nutritional requirements
- Monitoring of nutritional status
- Assessment of adequacy of nutritional intake and requirements for additional supplementary food

Client/patient and their carers
To participate in assessment, decision-making, goal planning and implementation where possible/appropriate

Speech and language therapy
- Assessment diagnosis and monitoring of swallowing problems, oro motor function and associated factors
- Therapy, support and advice to client, carer and team regarding appropriate food textures and compensatory strategies and/or equipment
- MDT training

Food service
- Provision of attractive, nutritious and suitably fortified foods
- Provision of food of suitable consistency
- Provision of adequate amounts of food as required

Pharmacist
- Advice on availability of medication in different forms

Doctor/GP
- Referral to relevant other professionals if dysphagia suspected (after screening)
- Medical investigation into cause of dysphagia and treatment if required

Support workers/ healthcare staff
- Assessment with choosing of appropriate food and fluids
- Assessment with serving and consumption of appropriate intake

Physiotherapy
- Assessment, treatment and management of the respiratory system
- Advice on positioning when eating and drinking
- Oro facial musculature and head control management

Psychologist
- Assess, manage and treat the socio-emotional, behavioural and psychological component of dysphagia eating and drinking difficulties

Figure 7.3.1 The role of the multidisciplinary team in the management of swallowing and feeding disorders [modified from King's College Hospital, Multi-disciplinary Working Party (2000)]
MDT, multidisciplinary team

- Assess the nature of the swallowing problem.
- Determine a safe and adequate feeding route.
- Determine the appropriate texture and consistency of orally consumed food and fluids.
- Ensure nutritional needs are met.
- Ensure fluid needs are met.
- Educate the patient, carers and other member of the care team.
- Monitor progress.
- Ensure continuity of care.

Warning signs of dysphagia

Early recognition of dysphagia is important to prevent unnecessary patient distress and for effective intervention. Typically, when several of the signs listed in Box 7.3.1 occur, the individual is likely to be experiencing swallowing difficulties and an assessment is required. This is particularly important in chronic long term condi-

tions such as Parkinson's disease where dysphagia gradually develops as the disease progresses.

Assessment of the swallowing problem

Suspected dysphagia should always be expertly assessed so that it can be managed most effectively (Finestone & Greene-Finestone, 2003). Following a stroke, it is recommended that all patients be given an assessment of swallowing ability using a validated tool and local guidelines administered by designated personnel (RCP, 2008). Patients with suspected difficulties should be referred to a speech and language therapist (SLT). If the initial assessment is inconclusive (difficulties at the pharyngeal stage can be particularly difficult to ascertain), videofluoroscopy (radiological examination of the swallowing process) may be carried out.

In primary care, a dysphagic patient identified by a GP, or district or community nurse should be referred to a hospital for specialist assessment if this cannot be done within the community setting (care home, day centre, day hospital, own home). Dysphagia is a significant contributory factor to undernutrition in elderly people living in the community or care homes (Finch *et al.*, 1998), but its presence is unfortunately often regarded as being of little significance (BAPEN, 2011).

The first three stages of the normal swallow (preparatory, oral and pharyngeal) are most likely to be disrupted when there is neuromuscular dysfunction resulting in weakness, paralysis and/or sensory loss in the muscles associated with swallowing, e.g. as a result of stroke, motor neurone disease and anoxic brain injury. The oesophageal stage is more likely to be affected by mechanical problems such as stricture, e.g. oesophageal carcinoma. The type of problems that can result are summarised in Table 7.3.2.

Determining a safe and adequate feeding route

The first priority is to decide whether feeding via the oral route is safe. If it is not, alternative routes have to be considered, e.g. nasogastric, surgical gastrostomy, percutaneous endoscopic gastrostomy (PEG) and parenteral nutrition (see Chapter 6.4 and Chapter 6.5).

Determining the appropriate texture and consistency of orally consumed food and fluids

After establishing that the patient can safely manage an oral intake, the SLT will provide guidance on appropriate texture modification to ensure safe transport of food and drink and minimise the risk of aspiration (Rosenvinge & Starke, 2005). Liquid or puréed diets may be appropriate for patients with dysphagia of mechanical origin who are unable to chew, e.g. those with a fractured jaw. However, in patients with oropharyngeal disorders, diets comprised of thinned and fluid foods increase the risk of aspiration because:

- They cannot be controlled in the mouth.
- The disordered swallowing mechanism cannot respond in time and with sufficient control to protect the airway.
- They lack the taste, temperature and pressure requirements to elicit an adequate swallow and protective reflex.

Foods and liquids therefore need to be modified to a consistency that provides the patient with best control over the rate at which they pass through the pharynx (Curran & Groher, 1990).

A comprehensive review by Penman & Thomson (1998) highlighted wide variation among dietitians, SLTs and other health professionals in their description of different food textures. They suggested that collaboration between

---

Box 7.3.1 Warning signs of dysphagia

- Coughing/spluttering/choking during or after drinking
- Coughing/spluttering/choking during or after eating
- Dehydration
- Difficulty chewing/manipulating food and drink in the mouth
- Difficulty controlling food and drink in the mouth
- Drooling
- Dry mouth
- Easily distracted – forgetting to swallow
- Frequent chest infections
- Gurgly voice or altered voice after eating and drinking
- Increased shortness of breath/change in breathing after swallowing
- Not being able to swallow mixed consistency meals
- Not been able to swallow/food sticking in mouth
- Pain on swallowing
- Poor oral hygiene
- Pouching of food in the mouth
- Sensory loss and weakness in muscles of mouth and face
- Spilling of food/drink from the mouth
- Unable to clear own saliva/secretions
- Very poor physical posture with neck touching chest
- Vomiting after meals
- Weight loss

Table 7.3.2 Disruption of the normal swallowing process

Stage of the normal swallow	Affected by	Consequences
Preparatory stage	Reduced range of movement of facial muscles, lips, tongue and jaw Loss of sight, smell and/or taste	Difficulty in getting food/liquid into the mouth Difficulty in sealing the mouth Reduced saliva production
Oral stage	Reduced range of movement of facial muscles, lips, tongue and jaw, and lack of saliva Postural problems	Difficulty in mastication Difficulty in forming a food bolus Difficulty in controlling a food bolus Difficulty in swallowing a food bolus
Pharyngeal stage	Absence of swallow reflex	Inability to swallow safely
Oesophageal phase	Impaired peristalsis or obstruction	Food fails to move into the stomach Aspiration after the swallow

the SLT and dietetic professions was needed to produce national guidelines on the use of textured diets in the management of dysphagia. In 2002, a Joint Working Party of the British Dietetic Association (BDA) and Royal College of Speech and Language Therapists (RCSLT) (2002, reviewed in 2009) published the National Descriptors for Texture Modification in Adults. This was in response to the desire to standardise understanding of particular food and fluid consistencies between health professionals to aid effective communication and enhance patient care.

Poor use nationally and concerns relating to patient safety involving recorded incidents and deaths from aspiration pneumonia resulted in a collaborative venture led by the National Patient Safety Agency (NPSA, 2011). The expert reference group with representatives from the BDA, RCSLT, National Nurses Nutrition Group (NNNG) and Hospital Caterers Association (HCA) developed Dysphagia Diet Food Texture Descriptors, endorsed by all organisations to be used by health professionals and food providers (NPSA, 2011). The texture consistencies are described as:

B = thin purée dysphagia diet;
C = thick purée dysphagia diet;
D = premashed dysphagia diet;
E = fork mashable dysphagia diet.

The food texture descriptor tables are comprehensive and include the full range of textures required to manage different types of dysphagia in adults. The tables are intended as a resource and do not in any way distract from an individual professional's own clinical judgement with regard to a particular client, and patient informed choice. The audit checklists produced enable food items to be measured against the standards for each texture. The NPSA group recommendations for future action include:

- A review of descriptors should be undertaken including health professionals and industry.

- All professional organisations should encourage their members to comply with the terminology and language used.
- Pictorial training aids should be developed to support texture descriptors for patients, carers and professionals.
- Industry should be encouraged to review their packaging to reflect colour codes proposed for each texture descriptor.

Commercial thickening agents derived from food starch are Advisory Committee on Borderline Substances (ACBS) prescribable for dysphagia and can be added to foods or liquids to provide the desired consistency and thickness (Box 7.3.2) or prethickened ready to use versions can be utilised (Table 7.3.3).

Foods suitable or unsuitable for inclusion in an individual's diet depend on the grade of consistency required. As a general guideline, single texture foods such as well mashed potato, semolina, custard, Greek yogurt, instant desserts and sieved soup are more appropriate than combination foods such as stews or risotto. Certain foods are considered high risk (Table 7.3.4) either because of their physical structure, e.g. beans with a skin, or difficulty of manipulation within the mouth, e.g. toffees or pie crust. Foods that change consistency from solid to liquid in the mouth, e.g. ice cream and sorbet, may also be unsuitable for patients dysphagic to liquids.

In addition to appropriate texture modification, the SLT may suggest other measures that may assist those with oropharyngeal disorders; for example, the use of cold or stimulating foods in those with delayed triggering of the pharyngeal swallow, or alternate mouthfuls of hot and cold foods for those with reduced oral awareness (Penman & Thomson, 1998). Other members of the care team, e.g. physiotherapist or occupational therapist, may provide guidance on the best posture or sitting position for eating, or the most appropriate eating utensils and drinking vessels. Use of drinking vessels that encourage the head

---

Box 7.3.2 Commercial proprietary thickeners

The following products, available in the form of powders comprised of modified food starch (generally maize), are ACBS prescribable to thicken foods and liquids in the management of dysphagia:

- Multi-thick (Abbott Nutrition)
- Nutilis (Nutricia Advanced Medical Nutrition)
- Resource Thicken Up Clear (Nestles Healthcare Nutrition)
- SLO Drinks (SLO Drinks)
- Thick and Easy Instant Food Thickener (Fresenius Kabi Ltd)
- Thixo-D (Sutherland Health Ltd)
- Vitaquick (Vitaflo International Ltd)

NB: The above products are *not* normally suitable for infants and young children.
Thickeners based on carob seed flour such as Carobel instant powder (Cow & Gate) are used to thicken infant feeds for the treatment of recurrent vomiting. They are *not* suitable for the management of dysphagia.
Full composition details of these products and prescribing indications can be found in the *British National Formulary* or the *Monthly Index of Medical Specialties (MIMS)* or obtained directly from the manufacturers.

Table 7.3.3 Prethickened commercial proprietary prescribable products

	Product (manufacturer)
Thickened desserts	Ensure Plus Crème (Abbott Nutrition) Forticreme Complete (Nutricia Advanced Medical Nutrition) Fortisip Fruit Dessert (Nutricia Advanced Medical Nutrition) Fresubin Creme (Fresenius Kabi Ltd)
Thickened drinks	Fresubin Thickened Stage 1 (Fresenius Kabi Ltd) Fresubin Thickened Stage 2 (Fresenius Kabi Ltd) Nutilis Complete Stage 1 (Nutricia Advanced Medical Nutrition) Resource Thickened Drink (Nestles Healthcare Nutrition) Resource Dessert Energy (Nestles Healthcare Nutrition) Resource Dessert Fruit (Nestles Healthcare Nutrition) Thick and Easy Thickened Juice Drink (Fresenius Kabi Ltd) SLO Cold Juice Drinks, Hot Chocolate, White Coffee (SLO Drinks Ltd)

NB: The above products are *not* normally suitable for infants and young children.
Thickeners based on carob seed flour such as Carobel instant powder (Cow & Gate) are used to thicken infant feeds for the treatment of recurrent vomiting. They are *not* suitable for the management of dysphagia.
Full composition details of these products and prescribing indications can be found in the *British National Formulary* or the *Monthly Index of Medical Specialties (MIMS)* or obtained directly from the manufacturers.

Table 7.3.4 High risk foods in dysphagia [modified from Joint Working Party of the British Dietetic Association and Royal College of Speech and Language Therapists (2002, reviewed 2009) and Dietitians Association of Australia and The Speech Pathology Association of Australia Ltd (2007)]

Food types	Examples
Chewy foods	Chewy sweets and toffees Marshmallows Chew bars, breakfast bars Chewing gum Chewy or crispy meat, e.g. crispy duck, bacon Cooked hard cheese, e.g. cheddar
Crumbly items	Bread crusts, pie crusts Crumble Dry biscuits/cakes
Crunchy foods	Toast Flaky pastry Dry biscuits Crisps, popcorn
Floppy texture	Lettuce, cucumber, uncooked spinach leaves
Hard foods	Boiled and hard sweets and toffees Nuts and seeds Raw vegetables
Husk	Sweetcorn Granary bread, bread with grains and seeds
Mixed consistency foods	Cereals which do not blend with milk, such as muesli Mince with thin gravy Soup with lumps, e.g. minestrone
Stringy, fibrous texture	Pineapple, runner beans, celery, rhubarb Steak
Vegetable and fruit skins (including bean skins)	Broad, baked, soya and black eyed beans, peas, grapes, sweetcorn, apple with peel

to tip back, e.g. feeder beakers, should be avoided. It is also important that patients and their carers are provided with specific guidance on texture modification measures and compensatory swallowing techniques to help minimise problems such as aspiration (DePippo *et al.*, 1994; Elmståhl *et al.*, 1999).

Meeting nutritional needs

As well as being of the appropriate consistency, the diet also has to be capable of meeting the individual's nutritional needs, with consideration of any other medical conditions, e.g. diabetes, coeliac disease, renal failure and dyslipidaemia, as well as cultural requirements. (Brody *et al.*, 2000). Where dysphagia is managed without dietetic input, these aspects are sometimes overlooked.

Key factors to consider in improving nutritional and fluid intake for modified texture diets are:

- Presentation and temperature of food.
- Flavour, taste and palatability.
- Texture of food.
- Nutrient dilution.
- Food fortification and or enrichment.
- Between meal snacks.
- Adequate fluid.
- Appropriate use of thickener.
- Posture and physical access to eating and drinking.

People with dysphagia often consume a very limited variety of foods, either because of the constraints imposed by the need for texture modification or because patients themselves limit their intake to the few foods they know they can tolerate. Retextured food can also look unappetising. Foods such as bread, fresh fruit, meat, pulses and nuts are often absent from the diet (Table 7.3.4) and as a result, intake of dietary fibre and micronutrients, e.g. some vitamins and minerals such as B_{12}, zinc and iron, may be inadequate. In addition, because dysphagia inevitably makes the process of eating difficult and a physical effort, the total quantity of food consumed may be insufficient to meet total energy and nutrient needs.

If intake remains inadequate, additional energy and nutrient supplementation may need to be considered (see Chapter 6.3). Sip feed supplements may, if necessary, be thickened to an appropriate texture with commercial thickeners (Box 7.3.2), or one of the more semi solid fortified dessert supplements may be used (Table 7.3.3) The adequacy of these measures should be continuously reviewed along with the progress of the dysphagia itself (see Monitoring progress later).

Ensuring fluid needs are met

Dehydration is a high risk in the dysphagic patient, so steps need to be taken to ensure that fluid intake is adequate. Speech and language therapist guidance on the appropriate degree of thickening should be followed. It should be borne in mind that the consistency of unthickened drinks may change with time and temperature. Some liquids become thicker as they cool, e.g. gravy,

home made custard and sauces, while others become more watery, e.g. manufactured custard from cartons or cans.

Most liquids, both hot and cold, can if necessary be thickened with one of the commercial thickeners available (Box 7.3.2) or alternatively a ready prepared thickened drink can be offered (Table 7.3.3). It is important that appropriate guidance with supporting written treatment plans, in line with a fluid texture modification table, are given to patients, carers and health and social care professionals. Potential issues include:

- Thickening fluids to the correct consistency can be difficult to achieve.
- Different commercial thickeners work differently.
- Mixing techniques and timing need to be taught to achieve the best results.
- Prethickened drinks and prethickened nutritional support drinks can be a useful choice to increase fluid and nutritional intake.

Rather than focus on thickening fluids with low palatability, it may be better to ensure sufficient fluid intake from foods of modified consistency (Vivanti *et al.*, 2009).

Educating the patient, carers and other member of the care team

People with dysphagia often need to be encouraged to eat. Factors such as anxiety or depression (often as a consequence of the underlying illness), confusion (perhaps as a result of stroke or dementia), fear (of choking) plus the sheer physical effort of consuming food all tend to act as barriers to eating. There are a number of difficulties inherent in producing/providing both texture modified food and fluids to a good standard, as well as meeting the aesthetic, cultural and nutritional requirements of the patient. The finished puréed product is not always acceptable due to the following:

- Some foods cannot be successfully puréed to a consistent smooth texture.
- Food served is not aesthetically acceptable due to poor appearance, presentation, colour and flavour.
- Inconsistent preparation of puréed foods so that the finished product is the wrong texture; this can still increase the risk of aspiration.
- Food items being diluted with non-nutritional fluid, e.g. water and gravy, that also increases the volume needed to meet energy and nutrient requirements.

To improve nutritional intake, consider the following:

- Use high energy liquids when puréeing to avoid diluting flavour and nutrient value e.g. oil, glucose and honey.
- Provide puréed between meal snacks, e.g. strained yoghurt, suitable dessert, fruit purées or cake, biscuits and sandwiches prepared using a thickener soaking solution.
- Enhance flavour of puréed main meals with condiments, sauces, spices, etc.

SECTION 7

- Employ food fortification/enhancement, e.g. fats, sugar and protein – oils, honey, glucose, skimmed milk powder.
- Present food attractively – purée all components, i.e. protein, carbohydrate and vegetables separately, preferably using food moulds.
- Keep food at an appetising temperature (use plate warmers and heated dishes).
- Provide food and fluids that are hot or very cold, with or without being highly flavoured, as they can stimulate a stronger swallow.

Monitoring progress

In some patients, dysphagia may be regarded as stable, i.e. the level of dysphagia remains unchanged for a considerable period of time, but in most instances this is not the case. Following stroke or acute brain injury, there is nearly always some improvement or even complete resolution of dysphagia. Conversely, in progressive neurological disorders or terminal illness, dysphagia may gradually (or suddenly) worsen. Management of dysphagia should therefore be regarded as a dynamic process, which is likely to change with time, rather than as a static solution to a clinical problem (Finestone & Greene-Finestone, 2003). For this reason, frequent monitoring is essential to assess whether current measures are appropriate for the level of dysphagia and to identify when they need to be modified. This monitoring process requires close collaboration between all members of the care team, from carers or nursing staff who may be the first to notice feeding problems or improvements, to SLTs, dietitians and medical staff who can assess the situation and modify the care plan.

If dysphagia is resolving, patients may gradually progress towards a more normal diet in a stepwise process utilising the audit checklist (NPSA, 2011) and local guidelines. If dysphagia is worsening, or there are signs of aspiration such as choking or recurrent chest infection, a different grade of texture modification may be required. In some cases, it may be necessary to change to an alternative feeding route such as enteral feeding, sometimes as a temporary measure until a certain amount of recovery or remission has occurred.

Ensuring continuity of care

Measures need to be in place to ensure that the dysphagic patient in hospital receives continuing assessment and support following discharge back into the community. Many areas now have a liaison nurse who acts as a link between the primary and secondary care sectors, liaising with ward staff to ascertain a patient's needs and ensuring that district nursing services are aware of and able to meet these needs.

Community dietetic provision is variable. In some areas, community dietetic services are an integral part of primary care support teams; in others, liaison with hospital based dietetic departments will be required. When responsibility for dietetic care is transferred from second-ary to primary care, it is vital that this is accompanied by the provision of relevant information. The community dietitian will require details of the following:

- Patient, including relevant medical and contact details.
- Discharge date.
- Discharge location.
- Details of the patient's GP.
- Details of the patient's carer and home circumstances.
- Details of the initial and most recent nutritional assessment, weight, and texture requirement and prescription.
- Details of dietary measures implemented (together with their acceptability and effectiveness).
- Type of follow-up required.

The patient's GP will require:

- A summary of the dietetic management of the patient to date.
- Details of any proprietary thickeners or supplements prescribed and predicted usage.
- An indication of likely future dietetic needs.

The patient (or carer) will require:

- Name and contact details of the dietitian responsible for their care.
- Written details of any dietary guidance they have been given.

Internet resources

British Association for Parenteral and Enteral Nutrition (BAPEN) www.bapen.org.uk
British Dietetic Association (BDA) www.bda.uk.com
Dysphagia.org.uk www.dysphagia.org.uk
Hospital Caterers Association www.hospitalcaterers.org
National Patient Safety Agency (NPSA) www.npsa.nhs.uk
Royal College of Speech and Language Therapists www.rcslt.org

Companies

Companies that provide products that may assist someone with dysphagia

Abbott Nutrition www.abbottnutrition.com
Fresenius Kabi Ltd www.fresenius-kabi.co.uk
Nestle Healthcare Nutrition www.nestlenutrition.co.uk/healthcare
Nutricia Advanced Medical Nutrition www.nutricia.co.uk

Companies that provide texture modified meals

Anglia Crown www.anglia-crown.co.uk
Brakes Bros www.brake.co.uk/your-business/sector-expertise/healthcare
Oakhouse Foods www.oakhousefoods.co.uk
Tillery Valley www.tilleryvalley.com/uktv/our-prime-markets/healthcare/healthcare.asp
Wiltshire Farm Foods www.wiltshirefarmfoods.com

References

British Association of Parenteral and Enteral Nutrition (BAPEN). (2011) *Nutrition Screening Survey in the UK and Republic of Ireland. Hospitals, Care Homes and Mental Health Units*. Basingstoke: BAPEN.

Brody RA, Touger-Decker R, VonHagen S, Maillet JO. (2000) Role of Registered Dietitians in Dysphagia Screening. *Journal of the American Dietetic Association* 100(9): 1029–1037.

Curran J, Groher ME. (1990) Development and dissemination of an aspiration risk reduction diet. *Dysphagia* 5: 6–12.

DePippo KL, Holas MA, Reding MJ, Mandel FS, Lesser ML. (1994) Dysphagia therapy following stroke: a controlled trial. *Neurology* 44(9): 1655–1660.

Dietitians Association of Australia and The Speech Pathology Association of Australia Ltd. (2007) Texture-modified foods and thickened fluids as used for individuals with dysphagia: Australian standardised labels and definition. *Nutrition and Dietetics* 64 (Suppl 2): S53–76.

Ekburg O, Hamdy S, Woisard V, Wuttge-Hanng A, Ortega P. (2001) Social and psychological burden of dysphagia: Its impact on diagnosis and treatment. *Dysphagia* 17(2): 139–146.

Elmståhl S, Bülow M, Ekberg O, Petersson M, Tegner H. (1999) Treatment of dysphagia improves nutritional conditions in stroke patients. *Dysphagia* 14(2): 61–66.

Foley NC, Martin RE, Salter KL, Teasell RW. (2009) A review of the relationship between dysphagia and malnutrition following stroke *Journal of Rehabilitation Medicine* 41(9): 707–713.

Finestone HM, Greene-Finestone LS. (2003) Rehabilitation medicine: 2. Diagnosis of dysphagia and its nutritional management for stroke patients. *Canadian Medical Association Journal* 169(10): 1041–1044.

Finestone HM, Greene-Finestone LS, Wilson ES, Teasell RW. (1995) Malnutrition in stroke patients on the rehabilitation service and at follow-up: prevalence and predictors. *Archives of Physical Medicine and Rehabilitation* 76(4): 310–316.

Finch S, Doyle W, Lowe C, Bates CJ, Prentice A, Smithers G, Clarke PC. (1998) *National Diet and Nutrition Survey: people aged 65 years and over. Volume 1: Report of the Diet and Nutrition Survey*. London: The Stationery Office.

Gordon C, Langton Hewer R, Wade DT. (1987) Dysphagia in acute stroke. *BMJ* 295: 411–414.

Joint Working Party British Dietetic Association and Royal College of Speech and Language Therapists Working Group. (2002, reviewed 2009) *National Descriptors for Texture Modification in Adults*. Birmingham: British Dietetic Association.

King's College Hospital, Multi-disciplinary Working Party. (2000) *A Multi-disciplinary Approach to the Management of Swallowing Disorders*. London: Kings College Hospital.

Marik PE, Kaplan D. (2003) Aspiration pneumonia and dysphagia in the elderly *Chest* 124(1): 328–336.

Martino R, Beaton D, Diamant NE. (2009) Perceptions of psychological issues related to dysphagia differ in acute and chronic patients. *Dysphagia* 25: 26–34.

Ney D, Weiss J, Kind A, Robbins JA. (2009) Senescent Swallowing: Impact, Strategies, and Interventions. *Nutrition in Clinical Practice* 24: 395–413.

National Institute for Health and Care Excellence (NICE). (2008) Clinical Guideline 68 *Stroke: Diagnosis and Initial Management of Acute Stroke and Transient Ischaemic Attack*. London: NICE.

National Patient Safety Agency Dysphagia Expert Reference Group. (NPSA) (2011) *Dysphagia Diet Food Texture Descriptors*. NSPA.

Odderson IR, Keaton JC, McKenna BS. (1995) Swallow management in patients on an acute stroke pathway: quality is cost effective. *Archives of Physical Medicine and Rehabilitation* 76(12): 1130–1133.

Paciaroni M, Mazzotta G, Corea F, *et al.* (2004) Dysphagia following stroke. *European Neurology* 51(3): 162–167.

Penman JP, Thomson M. (1998) A review of the textured diets developed for the management of dysphagia. *Journal of Human Nutrition and Dietetics* 11: 51–60.

Ramsey DJ, Smithard DG, Kalra L. (2003) Early assessments of dysphagia and aspiration risk in acute stroke patients. *Stroke* 34(5): 1252–1257.

Rosenvinge S, Starke ID. (2005) Improving care for patients with dysphagia. *Age and Ageing* 34(6): 587–593.

Royal College of Physicians. (RCP) Intercollegiate Working Party for Stroke (2008) *National Clinical Guidelines for Stroke*, 3rd edn. London: RCP.

Scottish Intercollegiate Guidelines Network (SIGN). (2010) *Management of Patients with Stroke: Identification and Management of Patients with Dysphagia. SIGN Guideline 119*. SIGN.

Smithard DG, Smeeton NC, Wolfe CD. (2007) Long-term outcome after stroke: does dysphagia matter? *Age and Ageing* 36(1): 90–94.

Teasell RW, McRae M, Marchuk Y, Finestone HM. (1996) Pneumonia associated with aspiration following stroke. *Archives of Physical Medicine and Rehabilitation* 77(7): 707–709.

Vivanti AP, Campbell KL, Suter MS, Hannan-Jones MT, Hulcombe JA. (2009) Contribution of thickened drinks, food and enteral and parenteral fluids on fluid intake in hospitalised patients with dysphagia. *Journal of Human Nutrition and Dietetics* 22: 148–155.

7.4.1 Disorders of the upper aerodigestive tract
Poonam Gulia

Key points

- Patients with disorders of the upper aerodigestive tract are nutritionally vulnerable and pose exceptional nutritional management problems.

- Patients with oesophageal disorders may have an increased risk of developing malnutrition, and dietary advice may be required for altered food texture and to ensure nutritional adequacy.

Damage to or disease of the oral cavity, pharynx, hypopharynx and oesophagus can impair the normal swallowing mechanism. This has the potential to compromise nutritional intake because it can affect the amount and types of food consumed, and impact on the time and effort experienced by the patient at each stage of the normal swallow. Even minor disorders can have a major impact on nutritional status, particularly if they are persistent and occur in people whose nutritional status is already poor. As a result, food choice and consumption can be profoundly affected in both the short and long term. The upper aerodigestive tract can be affected by cancer (see Chapter 7.15.3) and several benign disorders that are described here.

Benign disorders of the aerodigestive tract

Micronutrient deficiencies

The rate of epithelial cell turnover of the oral mucous membrane is much more rapid than that of skin (3–7 days compared with up to 28 days). As a result, the oral cavity often demonstrates early signs and symptoms of systemic diseases and nutritional deficiencies (Thomas & Giant, 2010). The presence of minor oral disorders may suggest underlying micronutrient deficiency and poor nutritional status. Both iron deficiency anaemia and pernicious anaemia (B_{12} deficiency) can result in the tongue becoming very red, sore and smooth. Deficiencies of most of the B group vitamins affect the soft tissues of the mouth, e.g. angular stomatitis (riboflavin deficiency) and cheilosis (angular stomatitis). Although cheilosis is a classic symptom of pellagra (niacin deficiency), in the UK it is more likely to be a sign of generalised vitamin B deficiency and undernutrition. Vitamin A deficiency can cause xerostomia (dry mouth) and in children, can result in hypoplasia in tooth enamel and dentine, increasing the susceptibility to caries.

Fractured jaw

Most fractured jaws are treated by open reduction and internal fixation using titanium miniplates and microplates without the need to keep the jaws wired together (Perry *et al.*, 1999). Patients are encouraged to mobilise the jaw gently to avoid stiffness or trismus (contraction of the jaw muscles), but are advised to have a soft diet with adequate fluid replacement. The use of nutritionally complete liquid feeds is advisable to ensure that energy and nutrient needs are met, and that scrupulous oral hygiene can be maintained for the weeks following fixation. On the rare occasions of intermaxillary fixation, when the jaws remain wired for approximately 4–6 weeks, a liquid diet will be necessary. As the wires are relaxed and ultimately removed, the diet should be regraded from a liquid to a soft or semi solid diet, with protein and energy supplements if indicated, until a normal diet can be taken.

Oesophagitis

Oesophagitis is inflammation of the mucosal lining of the oesophagus and is usually a consequence of gastro-oesophageal reflux (GORD) (see Chapter 7.4.3). Symptoms develop if reflux becomes frequent and the mucosa of the oesophagus becomes sensitive to the acidic reflux material. Dietary management is as for GORD, with the patient being advised to consume soft, bland and non-irritant foods and liquids whilst the symptoms are acute.

Achalasia

Achalasia is characterised by weak peristalsis of the oesophagus and the inability of the lower oesophageal sphincter to relax after a swallow; it is relatively uncommon. Food collects in the oesophagus, causing discomfort, and eventually may pass through the sphincter by the action of gravity and the weight of food consumed. Regurgitation of food is common but lacks the bitter taste of acid or bile that is characteristic of reflux. Aspiration of food from the oesophagus may lead to pneumonia. Repeated collection of food in the oesophagus can irritate the mucosa, resulting in secondary oesophagitis and pain. Loss of weight is uncommon unless the patient becomes fearful of eating. Relief may be obtained by advising the patient to:

- Consume small, frequent meals.
- Avoid fried foods or any other foods that aggravate dyspepsia.
- Avoid very hot or cold foods (these tend to increase the intake of air into the stomach).
- Avoid strong tea, coffee, large amounts of alcohol.

The patient may also find that standing up during a meal, drinking a glass of water and exhaling hard may help to force food into the stomach. If dietary measures are ineffective, surgical myotomy or mechanical dilatation may be necessary.

Oesophageal perforation

If the oesophagus perforates spontaneously or is perforated as a result of dilatation, oesophagoscopy or caustic burns, any food or liquid consumed would enter the thoracic cavity with potentially fatal consequences. The perforation may be allowed to heal naturally or may need surgical repair. Patients should not be fed orally; enteral tube feeding or parenteral feeding may be necessary.

Benign oesophageal stricture

Benign stricture usually results from mucosal injury, either as a consequence of chronic GORD or damage following intubation with wide bore gastric tubes. Stricture may initially be due to muscular spasm, or it may result from physical scarring and thickening of the oesophageal wall. The first symptom is usually difficulty in swallowing solid foods or foods sticking, particularly items such as doughy bread or tough meats, which tend to remain as a bolus as they pass down the oesophagus. Dysphagia with solid foods may soon progress to dysphagia with semi solids or liquids. Appetite is usually reduced and severe weight loss may be reported. Patients may suffer these difficulties for some time before seeking help, and may be dehydrated and malnourished on presentation. Some patients who are depleted may need intravenous rehydration and nutritional support prior to treatment, which is usually by oesophageal dilatation. If GORD has been a contributory factor, it is important that this is corrected to prevent recurrence of the stricture.

Internet resources

British Gastroenterology Society   www.bsg.org.uk
Society of Thoracic Surgeons (USA)   www.sts.org

References

Perry M, Evans C, Peel K. (1999) *Maxillofacial Care*. London: Arnold.
Thomas DM, Giant WM. (2010) Nutrition and oral mucosal diseases. *Clinics in Dermatology* 28: 426–431.

7.4.2   Orofacial granulomatosis

Helen Campbell, Jeremy Sanderson and Miranda Lomer

Key points

- Orofacial granulomatosis (OFG) is a rare condition defined by chronic granulomatous inflammation of the lips, oral cavity and sometimes the face.

- It is predominantly an idiopathic disease, although approximately one-quarter of patients present with concurrent Crohn's disease.

- The management of OFG requires a multidisciplinary approach.

- A cinnamon and benzoate free diet is the primary treatment of choice and assumes an increased sensitivity to these compounds.

- It is important that patients are closely monitored and regularly reviewed.

Orofacial granulomatosis (OFG) is a rare condition defined by chronic granulomatous inflammation of the lips, oral cavity and sometimes the face (Wiesenfeld *et al.*, 1985). The typical presentation involves lip swelling and erythema (Campbell *et al.*, 2011; Wiesenfeld *et al.*, 1985). Inside the mouth, the buccal mucosa (inside of the cheeks), gingivae (gums), buccal sulcus (adjoining areas between the gingivae and buccal mucosa) and floor of the mouth can all be affected with swelling, erythema, nodular swelling, tags and ulcers. Lip fissures (cracking) are common and can be prone to bacterial or candida infections that often exacerbate symptoms. Intraoral fissuring can also be present. The tongue, palate and throat are less commonly involved and overall the disease is generally painless except when ulcers are present. Patients are most upset by the physically disfiguring and chronic nature of the disease, which is often difficult to treat and can last for months or even years.

Orofacial granulomatosis predominantly exists as an idiopathic disease, although approximately one-quarter of patients can also present with concurrent Crohn's disease (Campbell *et al.*, 2011). Consequently, OFG is often called oral Crohn's disease. Other more historical nomenclature can include chelitis granulomatosa and Mischer's chelitis. A small proportion also present as Melkersson Rosenthal syndrome, diagnosed when the additional features of a fissured tongue and facial palsy are present (Rogers, 1996).

Diagnosis

Expertise in this condition is rare and often patients undergo a variety of ineffectual treatments, allergy testing and other investigations for prolonged periods prior to an accurate diagnosis. The diagnosis is made through expert examination and exclusion of other granulomatous conditions (such as sarcoidosis and tuberculosis) (Grave *et al.*, 2009). Confirmation of the diagnosis is normally made from histopatholological findings that identify non-caseating granulomas from biopsies taken from the affected sites. Patients with OFG are normally diagnosed as young adults, although it can present at any age (Campbell *et al.*, 2011).

Aetiology and epidemiology

The cause of OFG is unknown, but is thought to involve an allergic component. The heterogeneous nature of the condition indicates a number of different causes and early studies identified an array of foods believed to be dietary triggers, exclusion of which often improved symptoms (Ferguson & MacFadyen, 1986; Wray *et al.*, 2000). Due to the rarity of OFG, there are no epidemiological studies. Most reports are UK based with higher patient numbers being reported in Scotland (Gibson *et al.*, 2000) and Ireland (Fitzpatrick *et al.*, 2011), suggesting a Celtic predominance.

Management

Ideally, the management of OFG requires a multidisciplinary approach. Patients are referred mainly from specialists in oral medicine, gastroenterology, dermatology, allergy clinics and dentists (Campbell *et al.*, 2011). Close collaboration with medical colleagues in oral medicine can be helpful, particularly for expertise in objective examination and documentation of progression or regression of clinical features. In the event of gastrointestinal symptoms, patients should receive an opinion from a gastroenterologist.

The treatment of OFG is challenging and patients often suffer from episodes of relapse and recurrence that can be upsetting and frustrating. The cinnamon and benzoate free diet is the primary treatment of choice and assumes an increased sensitivity to these compounds (Campbell *et al.*, 2011). The mechanism remains unclear, but the diet originates from a retrospective study investigating patch test data from a series of patients with oral mucosal disorders (Wray *et al.*, 2000). Patients with OFG had increased sensitivity to cinnamon, benzoates and chocolate. A subsequent study demonstrated significant benefit from dietary elimination of cinnamon and benzoate in up to 72% of patients (White *et al.*, 2006). Other dietary measures include use of liquid enteral feeds (taken orally) and, in particular, elemental diet has proven beneficial, particularly in children (Kiparissi *et al.*, 2006).

In the event of dietary failure, topical immunosuppression (e.g. beclamethosone mouthwash), topical hydrocortisone or topical tacrolimus can be used (Casson *et al.*, 2000; Leao *et al.*, 2004). Intralesional steroids can also be used, but recurrence is common, although reportedly less so with successive injections (Al *et al.*, 2009). Occasionally, systemic corticosteroids may be given, although again often only resulting in short term improvement. For refractory OFG, patients may require long term systemic immunosuppression, most commonly with a thiopurine (azathioprine or mecarptopurine). Antitumour necrosis alpha antibody infusions (infliximab and abdulimab) have been used if other treatment is unsuccessful (Elliott *et al.*, 2011; Leao *et al.*, 2004). In severe fibrotic disease, it may be necessary for patients to undergo a cheiloplasty to surgically debulk the lips (Kruse-Losler *et al.*, 2005).

Dietary management

The cinnamon and benzoate free diet can be used to treat OFG and offers a non-invasive therapy which provides benefit in up to 72% of patients and can avoid the need for systemic immunosuppression in approximately 25% of patients (Campbell *et al.*, 2010; White *et al.*, 2006). For this reason, dietary treatment is commonly used first, with other therapies being employed either in refractory OFG or when diet fails to provide sufficient benefit. Compliance can be difficult, although motivation is often sufficiently high to overcome this, particularly in those troubled by the disfiguring nature of the disease. However, data on sources and levels of cinnamon and benzoates are scarce and so patients are likely to be inadvertently exposed to sources for which the existence of these compounds may be elusive. This could explain why patients often complain of recurrence despite strict adherence to the diet.

It is important to provide a structure for patients undertaking a cinnamon and benzoate restricted diet. Improvement in symptoms can take some time and can be frustrating, although some patients may see improvement within a few weeks. For this reason, it is important that patients are closely monitored and regularly reviewed. A diet history will identify the patient's current exposure to cinnamon and benzoates. Those regularly drinking soft drinks are most likely to be receiving the highest levels of benzoates as added preservatives. It is not uncommon for patients to be already avoiding foods they feel contribute to their symptoms. Consequently, nutritional adequacy could be challenged with further restrictions and this needs to be considered.

The cinnamon and benzoate free diet

Sources of cinnamon

Cinnamon (*Cinnamomum zeylanium N.*) is a spice originating primarily from Sri Lanka, and is commonly added to both sweet and savoury foods (Singletary, 2008). The main compound that provides the flavour and aroma is cinnemaldehyde and this is often cited as being the component to which patients demonstrate sensitivity on patch testing (Gruenwald *et al.*, 2010; Wray *et al.*, 2000). It is often used in Asian cuisine and curries, but can also be added to chewing gums, sweets, chocolates, alcoholic beverages, fizzy drinks, cereals and bakery products such as cakes and breads. Other products that may include cinnamon include toothpastes, mouthwashes, perfumes, perfumed creams or make up, soaps and medicines. A food product that contains <2% of a spice is not required to be specifically labelled and can instead use the term spices or mixed spices (Food Standards Agency, 2008a; 2008b; HMSO, 1996) (see Chapter 4.5). Consequently, it is necessary to avoid products labelled with these terms. In addition, products labelled as allspice, mixed spices, curry powder and garam masala (a mix of spices used in Indian curries, which could include cinnamon or cassia) need to be avoided.

Cassia (*Cinnamomum cassia Presi*) is a close relative of cinnamon and is often used as a cheaper alternative. Sourced mainly from China, Indonesia and Vietnam, it has recently received some interest as it contains substantial quantities of coumarin, which is thought to be hepatotoxic and carcinogenic (Abraham *et al.*, 2010). It also contains cinnamaldehyde but in lesser quantities than cinnamon. Cassia therefore needs to be avoided on the cinnamon and benzoate free diet.

Sources of benzoates

Rich sources of naturally occurring benzoates requiring avoidance include a number of fruits, predominantly berries, vegetables and spices (Table 7.4.1) (Cressey & Jones, 2009; Heimhuber & Herrmann, 1990; Sieber *et al.*; 1989; Toyoda *et al.*, 1983a; 1983b). Cinnamon is also a naturally occurring source of benzoates. In addition to avoidance of these foods, it is necessary to exclude products that might contain them, e.g. soups, juices, sauces,

Table 7.4.1 Natural benzoates to exclude and some suitable alternatives

Benzoate rich foods to exclude	Alternatives
Fruit	
Dried fruit, fruit sauce Berries, e.g. blackberries, cranberries, blueberries, strawberries, raspberries Prunes, peaches, papaya, nectarines	All other fresh and frozen fruit, e.g. apple, orange, pear, banana, satsuma, tangerine, melon, pineapple, grapefruit, lemon, lime, grape, mango, rhubarb
Vegetables	
Avocado, pumpkin, kidney beans, soya beans, spinach Any juices, sauces, jams, pickles or other food products containing the above fruit and vegetables	Other vegetables, e.g. broccoli, cauliflower, cabbage, carrots, green beans, runner beans, broad beans, spring greens, lettuce, cucumber, onion, peppers, bean sprouts
Spices	
Cinnamon sticks, cinnamon powder, cassia sticks, cassia powder, cloves, nutmeg, 'spices', 'mixed spices'	Salt, pepper, all other fresh herbs, e.g. basil, parsley, mint, coriander, etc., clearly labelled single spices
Teas	
Any tea leaves, tea bags, chai tea, green tea, rooibos tea, fruit or herbal teas with tea leaves	Herbal infusions, coffee
Dairy	
Blue cheeses, gorgonzola, cheese with added fruit or spices listed above	All other cheeses, e.g. cheddar, feta, mozzarella, parmesan, brie, camembert, cottage cheese, etc.

Table 7.4.2 Preservatives to be avoided

E number	Benzoate
E210	Benzoic acid
E211	Sodium benzoate
E212	Potassium benzoate
E213	Calcium benzoate
E214	Ethyl 4-hydroxybenzoate or ethyl para-hydroxybenzoate
E215	Ethyl 4-hydroxybenzoate, sodium salt or sodium ethyl para-hydroxybenzoate
E216*	Propyl 4-hydroxybenzoate or propyl para-hydroxybenzoate
E217*	Propyl 4-hydroxybenzoate, sodium salt or sodium para-hydroxybenzoate
E218	Methyl 4-hydroxybenzoate or methyl para-hydroxybenzoate
E219	Methyl 4-hydroxybenzoate, sodium salt or sodium methyl-hydroxybenzoate

*Banned in foods produced within the European Union, but may be found in products in other countries.

pickles, breads and other baked goods. Vigilance with reading labels is therefore very important.

The highest contributors are benzoates used as preservatives added to foods, drinks, medicines and cosmetics. Table 7.4.2 lists the E numbers of the preservatives that should be avoided. The main foods to which these may have been added include soft drinks, pickles, jams, biscuits, cakes, preprepared ready meals, pickled fish, sauces, dips, yoghurts and confectionary (European Parliament and Council Directive, 1995). Therefore, all food labels need to be checked for the addition of benzoates.

A further source of benzoates and derivatives of cinnamon can include cosmetic and hygiene products. There is no evidence that currently suggests that these contribute to symptoms in OFG, but absorption of benzoates through the skin has been proven (Nair, 2001). Anecdotally, patients often complain of sensitivity to cosmetic products. Consequently, the recommendation is currently to limit exposure to cosmetics that contain cinnamates and benzoates, particularly products that come into direct contact with the lips or face, such as lip balms, make up, face cleansers, soaps, creams and sunscreens. Most high street products contain cinnamates and/or benzoates. However, it is possible to find cinnamon and benzoate free products in specialist health food shops or on the Internet.

Other considerations

Soya

Soya is a natural source of benzoates and should be avoided in the cinnamon and benzoate free diet. In recent years, soya has been increasingly used in many products;

soya flour is added to bread or other baked goods and soya lecithin is added as an emulsifier to many foods. The benzoate content in these foods has not been measured but, previously, the recommendation was to avoid all products with added soya flour and lecithin (E322) that could have been sourced from soya. More recently, this recommendation has been increasingly challenged and a recent enquiry of manufacturers suggests that the contribution of benzoates from these sources is comparatively low and perhaps negligible (Nagarajah et al., 2008). Consequently, this recommendation has been changed and baked goods with added soya flour and products with soya lecithin no longer requires avoidance.

Tomato

Patients with OFG often complain of sensitivity to tomato, in particular cooked tomato sauces. The reason for this is unclear, but tomato does contain small amounts of benzoic acid (Sieber et al., 1989). It is likely that concentrated sources of tomato, such as tomato purée, could have a higher concentration of benzoic acid. Consequently, the recommendation is to avoid concentrated sources of tomato and to use fresh tomato only in salads and cooking. Tomato ketchup also often has benzoates added to it as a preservative.

Chocolate

Patients often complain of sensitivity to chocolate and patch test studies have identified chocolate hypersensitivity in OFG (Wray et al., 2000). Chocolate or cocoa has not been identified as a rich source of benzoic acid or other benzoates, although certain additions such as dried fruit and cinnamon could be contributing factors. Patients should be advised to avoid chocolate for the duration of the elimination diet.

Flavourings

Flavourings do not need to be specifically named on foods labels (Food Standards Agency, 2008b), but they may be derivatives of both cinnamon and benzoates (European Council and Commission Directives, 1992). Consequently, the recommendation is to exclude foods labelled as containing flavourings or natural flavourings.

Monitoring

Objective measures are helpful as change can be subtle. Photographs (both external and intraorally) can prove helpful and can be encouraging for many patients so that progression can be demonstrated. A structured oral examination and documentation of disease activity and severity can also be useful and should be a routine part of the multidisciplinary approach to this condition. The cinnamon and benzoate free diet should be tried for 12 weeks. In the event that significant benefit is demonstrated, this can be extended to maximise improvement. Prolonged or open ended time frames on this restrictive diet are not recommended and will contribute to apathy and non-compliance. If no (or limited) improvement is demonstrated, then it may be necessary to consider other approaches, such as those described previously.

Dietary reintroduction

Following a 12-week dietary restriction, foods are reintroduced. Only one food should be reintroduced at a time. As symptom recurrence is often reported as delayed, it is useful to undertake the challenge over 2–3 consecutive days before commencing with another food. A structured symptom diary can be useful to help identify likely triggers. The highest sources of benzoates are from soft drinks and these are therefore often left until last (if they are reintroduced at all). Similarly, chocolate is often left until later. It is not uncommon to find that patients need to remain on a partially restricted diet long term, limiting exposure to overt sources of cinnamon, fizzy drinks and chocolate.

Further reading

Campbell HE, Escudier MP, Patel P, Challacombe SJ, Sanderson JD, Lomer MCE. (2011) Review article: cinnamon and benzoate free diet as a primary treatment for orofacial granulomatosis. *Alimentary Pharmacology & Therapeutics* 34(7): 687–701.

White A, Nunes C, Escudier M, *et al.* (2006) Improvement in orofacial granulomatosis on a cinnamon- and benzoate-free diet. *Inflammatory Bowel Disease* 12(6): 508–514.

References

Abraham K, Wohrlin F, Lindtner O, Heinemeyer G, Lampen A. (2010) Toxicology and risk assessment of coumarin: focus on human data. *Molecular Nutrition & Food Research* 54(2): 228–239.

Al JK, Moles DR, Hodgson T, Porter SR, Fedele S. (2009) Onset and progression of clinical manifestations of orofacial granulomatosis. *Oral Diseases* 15(3): 214–219.

Campbell HE, Patel P, Escudier M, Challacombe SJ, Sanderson JD, Lomer MCE. (2010) The relevance of patch testing and a clinical review of the cinamon and benzoate free diet in orofacial granulomatosis. Food Feeding and Malnutrition. *Journal of Human Nutrition and Dietetics* 23(4): 443.

Campbell H, Escudier M, Patel P, *et al.* (2011) Distinguishing orofacial granulomatosis from crohn's disease: Two separate disease entities? *Inflammatory Bowel Disease* 17(10): 2109–2115.

Casson DH, Eltumi M, Tomlin S, Walker-Smith JA, Murch SH. (2000). Topical tacrolimus may be effective in the treatment of oral and perineal Crohn's disease. *Gut* 47(3): 436–440.

Cressey P, Jones S. (2009) Levels of preservatives (sulfite, sorbate and benzoate) in New Zealand foods and estimated dietary exposure. *Food Additities & Contaminants Part A Chemistry, Analysis, Control, Exposure & Risk Assessment* 26(5): 604–613.

Elliott E, Campbell H, Escudier M, *et al.* (2011) Experience with anti-TNF-alpha therapy for orofacial granulomatosis. *Journal of Oral and Pathology & Medicine* 40(1): 14–19.

European Council and Commission Directives. (1992) *Statutory Instrument 1992 No. 1971, The Flavourings in Food Regulations.* European Council and Commission.

European Parliament and Council Directive. (1995) *European Parliament and Council Directive No 95/2/ EC on Food Additives Other than Colours and Sweeteners.* European Parliament and Council Directive.

Ferguson MM, MacFadyen EE. (1986). Orofacial granulomatosis – a 10 year review. *Annals of Academic Medicine Singapore* 15(3): 370.

Fitzpatrick L, Healy CM, McCartan BE, Flint SR, McCreary CE, Rogers S. (2011) Patch testing for food-associated allergies in orofacial granulomatosis. *Journal of Oral Pathology & Medicine* 40(1): 10–13.

Food Standards Agency (FSA). (2008a) *Food Labelling: Clear Food Labelling Guidance.* London: FSA.

Food Standards Agency (FSA). (2008b) *The Food Labelling Regulations 1996: Guidance Notes on Quantitative Ingredients Declerations ('QUID').* London: FSA.

Gibson J, Wray D, Bagg J. (2000) Oral staphylococcal mucositis: A new clinical entity in orofacial granulomatosis and Crohn's disease. *Oral Surgery, Oral Medicine, Oral Pathology, Oral Radiology, and Endodontology* 89(2): 171–176.

Grave B, McCullough M, Wiesenfeld D. (2009) Orofacial granulomatosis–a 20-year review 161. *Oral Diseases* 15(1): 46–51.

Gruenwald J, Freder J, Armbruester N. (2010) Cinnamon and health. *Critical Reviews in Food Science and Nutrition* 50(9): 822V834.

Heimhuber B, Herrmann K. (1990). Benzoe-, Phylessig-, 3-Phenylpropan- und Zimtsaure sowie benzoglucosen in einigen Obst-und Fruchtgemusearten. *Deutsche Lebensmittel-Rundschau* 86 jahrg. Heft 7.

HMSO. (1996). *Statutory Instrument No.1599. The Food Labelling Regulations.* London: HMSO.

Kiparissi F, Lindley K, Hill S, Milla P, Shah N, Elawad M. (2006) Orofacial granulomatosis is a separate entity of Crohn's disease comprising and allergic component. *Journal of Pediatric Gastroenterology and Nutriton* 42(5): E3.

Kruse-Losler B, Presser D, Metze D, Joos U. (2005). Surgical treatment of persistent macrocheilia in patients with Melkersson-Rosenthal syndrome and cheilitis granulomatosa. *Archives of Dermatology* 141(9): 1085–11091.

Leao JC, Hodgson T, Scully C, Porter S. (2004) Review article: orofacial granulomatosis. *Alimentimentary Pharmacology & Therapeutics* 20(10): 1019–1027.

Nagarajah R, Campbell H, Sanderson JD, Lomer MC. (2008) Dietary management of orofacial granulomatosis: quantification of benzoates in foods and cosmetics. *Journal of Human Nutrition and Dietetics* 21(4): 397–398.

Nair B. (2001) Final Report on the Safety Assessment of Benzyl alcohol, Benzoic Acid, and Sodium Benzoate. *International Journal of Toxicology* 20(Suppl 3): 23–50.

Rogers RS, III. (1996) Melkersson-Rosenthal syndrome and orofacial granulomatosis. *Dermatology Clinics* 14(2); 371–379.

Sieber R, Butikofer U, Bosset JO, Ruegg M. (1989) Benzoic acid as a natural component of foods – a review. *Mitteilungen aus dem Gebiete der Lebensmitteluntersuchung und Hygiene* 80(3): 345–362.

Singletary K. (2008) Cinnamon: overview of Health Benefits 160. *Nutrition Today* 43(6): 263–266.

Toyoda M, Ito Y, Isshiki K, Onishi K, *et al.* (1983a) Estimation of daily intake of many kinds of food additives according to the market basket studies in Japan. *Journal of the Japanese Society of Nutrition and Food Science* 36(6): 489–497.

Toyoda M, Ito Y, Isshiki K, *et al.* (1983b) Daily intake of preservatives, benzoic acid, dhydroacetic acid, propionic acid and their salts, and esters of *p*-hydroxybenzoic acid in Japan. *Journal of Japanese Society of Nutrition and Food Science* 36(6): 467–480.

White A, Nunes C, Escudier M, *et al.* (2006) Improvement in orofacial granulomatosis on a cinnamon- and benzoate-free diet. *Inflammatory Bowel Disease* 12(6): 508–514.

Wiesenfeld D, Ferguson MM, Mitchell DN, *et al.* (1985) Oro-facial granulomatosis-a clinical and pathological analysis. *Quarterly Journal of Medicine* 54(213): 101–113.

Wray D, Rees SR, Gibson J, Forsyth A. (2000) The role of allergy in oral mucosal diseases. *Quarterly Journal of Medicine* 93(8): 507–511.

SECTION 7

7.4.3   Disorders of the stomach and duodenum
Poonam Guila

Key points

■ Disorders of the stomach and duodenum can have a significant effect on dietary intake and nutritional status.

■ Management of disorders is often a combination of medical or surgical intervention alongside dietary changes.

■ Dietary advice is based on control of symptoms and ensuring nutritional adequacy.

Cancers of the stomach and duodenum (see Chapter 7.15.3) and gastroparesis (see Chapter 7.4.4) are described in separately. Nausea and vomiting are symptoms, rather than conditions, and are included here for completeness.

Nausea and vomiting

Nausea and vomiting can be the pathological consequences of disease or its treatment (e.g. chemotherapy), physiological (e.g. morning sickness in pregnancy), drug induced (e.g. antibiotics) or psychological (e.g. bulimia nervosa) in origin. In healthy individuals, nausea and vomiting caused by infection or food poisoning usually resolve spontaneously. Eating should be ceased until acute symptoms have eased and replaced with frequent consumption of small volumes of water, sugar containing soft drinks or oral rehydration solutions.

Profuse or persistent nausea and vomiting may compromise intake of both food and fluids, and exacerbate an already poor nutritional status resulting from underlying disease. Dietetic management depends on the nature of the underlying problem. Measures that may help alleviate symptoms and other strategies to improve oral nutritional intake are described in Chapter 6.3.

Gastro-oesophageal reflux disease

Gastro-oesophageal reflux disease (GORD) is a term used to describe a range of symptoms, including acid reflux (with or without pain), heartburn and oesophagitis. Heartburn is a common accompaniment to indigestion and is characterised by a sharp, burning pain either just below the sternum or between the shoulder blades. This chest pain may be so severe that it may be mistaken for angina. It is caused by the reflux of the stomach contents (containing acid and enzymes) into the oesophagus, some of which may reach the mouth or be sensed in the back of the throat (Figure 7.4.1). This irritates the oesophageal mucosa, causing pain, and repeated attacks may cause mucosal damage and inflammation (oesophagitis). This in turn increases the risk of developing Barrett's oesophagus and possibly adenocarcinoma of the oesophagus (NICE, 2004). Reflux may occur as a result of the following conditions (Figure 7.4.2):

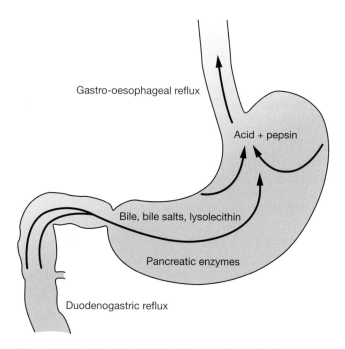

Figure 7.4.1   Constituents of gastro-oesophageal reflux

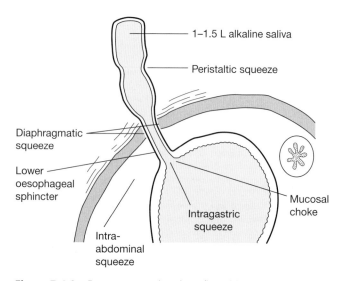

Figure 7.4.2   Factors preventing the reflux of food and regurgitation of food from the stomach

- Weakness of the sphincter at the junction of the oesophagus and stomach.
- High pressure within the stomach, e.g. consumption of a large quantity of food or liquid.
- High pressure from the abdominal area, e.g. obesity, pregnancy.
- Hiatus hernia resulting in impairment of the pinchcock mechanism of the diaphragm (see later).

Although not well supported by clinical data, diet and lifestyle factors remain important instruments for the overall management of GORD (Tytgat *et al.*, 2008). The effectiveness of commonly advised measures, such as reduction of intake of heavily spiced or fatty foods, alcohol intake and smoking cessation, in relieving gastro-oesophageal reflux *per se* have not been conclusively established in well controlled trials. There is sufficient evidence that supports the fact that obesity, in particular abdominal obesity, plays a key role in determining GORD. Controlled weight loss (by diet or surgery) is effective in improving GORD symptoms and risk of oesophageal adenocarcinoma (Festi *et al.*, 2009). Measures that are generally accepted as being helpful are:

- Eating smaller volumes at regular intervals.
- Avoiding rich or fatty foods.
- Avoiding highly spiced or irritant foods known to exacerbate symptoms.
- Avoiding excessive consumption of tea, coffee or alcohol.
- Chewing foods well.
- Avoiding eating late at night.
- Avoiding bending, lifting or lying down after meals.
- Reducing weight if obese.
- Avoiding excessive consumption of tea, coffee or alcohol.
- Avoiding smoking.
- Sleeping in a semi upright position or with the head of the bed raised a few inches to help prevent nocturnal symptoms of reflux.

Additional symptom relief is obtained by use of H_2 receptor antagonists (e.g. cimetidine, ranitidine), proton pump inhibitors (e.g. lansoprazole, omeprazole), prokinetics (e.g. metoclopramide, domperidone) and alginates. Patients with more severe symptoms refractory to lifestyle and drug therapy may be offered surgery, e.g. Nissen fundoplication where the fundus of the stomach is wrapped around the distal end of the oesophagus to create a one way valve.

Dyspepsia

Dyspepsia (indigestion) is a condition characterised by abdominal discomfort, bloating or early satiety on eating. It is important to establish the cause as it may be due to GORD, poor eating habits or a symptom of underlying, possibly serious, disease. Simple indigestion can nearly always be alleviated by the diet and lifestyle measures described earlier for GORD.

Hiatus hernia

The diaphragm has several openings through which the abdominal viscera can enter the thorax. The opening for the oesophagus, the hiatus, is loosely attached to the oesophagus. In middle age this attachment weakens and abdominal pressure may cause the hiatus to herniate (tear). This is likely to happen as a result of becoming overweight, but may also occur as a consequence of pregnancy, chronic coughing or chronic constipation due to straining. The major symptoms are pain and discomfort as a result of reflux and oesophagitis. Patients may also complain of the sensation of foods such as doughy bread or fibrous foods, e.g. salad, nuts or seeds, sticking in the gullet.

In some patients, the priority is weight loss, which will reduce abdominal pressure and may also be advisable if surgical repair is necessary. Symptom relief from GORD may be obtained by following the preventive measures listed earlier. If particular foods cause dysphagic symptoms, they should be avoided. Patients with chronic constipation should be encouraged to increase their fibre and fluid intake.

Gastritis

Gastritis, inflammation of the gastric mucosa, may be acute erosive or chronic atrophic gastritis. Alcohol, non-steroidal anti-inflammatory drugs (NSAIDs), chemical irritants and exposure to certain pathogens may trigger acute gastritis that results in pain, nausea and vomiting; usually of short duration. No particular dietary changes are usually required, although adequate hydration is important during any period of vomiting, and small meals should be taken at regular intervals.

Chronic gastritis may follow repeated attacks of acute gastritis and is closely associated with *Helicobacter pylori* infection, which is treated by eradication therapy, usually along with a proton pump inhibitor. Dietary advice should be based on the following:

- Identifying and attempting to correct dietary and lifestyle factors that are contributing to the condition, e.g. alcohol, smoking, drugs and poor eating habits.
- Encouraging a balanced diet based on healthy eating principles together with a sensible meal pattern.
- Correcting deficiencies, e.g. iron, vitamin B_{12}, that have resulted from repeated bleeding and reduced production of intrinsic factor.

Peptic ulcer

A peptic ulcer is erosion in the mucosal lining of the stomach or duodenum. Duodenal ulcers are more common and often occur in the duodenal cap; duodenitis (inflammation) is invariably present. Ulceration may also occur in the pyloric antrum and the resultant scar tissue may cause pyloric stenosis, resulting in delayed gastric emptying and the accumulation of fermenting food debris in the stomach, causing discomfort, nausea, vomiting and halitosis (bad breath). If untreated, ulcers can eventually result in perforation of the gastric or duodenal wall, a potentially fatal complication.

The principle cause of peptic ulcer is the bacterium *H. Pylori* and NSAID use (Yeomans, 2011). Factors such as a stressful lifestyle, irregular meals, eating too quickly, inadequate mastication and smoking exacerbate ulcer formation and may adversely affect the healing process. Treatment of peptic ulcer has been transformed by the use of antibiotic treatment to eradicate *H. pylori*. To promote healing, this is usually accompanied by a 4–8-week course with an H_2 receptor antagonist or proton pump inhibitor to reduce gastric acid production. Most patients will benefit from healthy diet and lifestyle advice to minimise the risk of recurrence.

Gastric resection and reconstruction

Gastric surgery can have a considerable impact on subsequent food intake, weight recovery and quality of life. Pouch and Roux-en-Y reconstruction following gastrectomy is associated with improved quality of life and reduced complications of gastrointestinal function postoperatively, i.e. reduced reflux symptoms and dumping effects (Zong *et al.*, 2011). Increasingly, laparoscopic techniques are being used for the removal of early gastric cancers.

As a result of the combination of cachexia and chronic symptoms, such as nausea, vomiting or discomfort on eating, gastric carcinoma patients often present in a significantly malnourished state and nutritional support measures should be instituted early, preferably perioperatively, via the enteral rather than parenteral route (see Chapter 7.15.3). Early postoperative enteral nutritional support can be established via a jejunostomy or nasojejunal tube placed intraoperatively. Jejunal feeding may also be required for certain patients receiving palliative treatment for gastric outlet obstruction (see Chapter 6.4).

Disturbances in gastrointestinal function often occur following gastric resection and reconstruction that may affect nutritional intake and nutritional status (see Chapter 7.17.5). Some of these problems occur soon after eating; others result from the long term consequences of disturbed gastric function and include:

- Rapid emptying of the stomach remnant or increased intestinal motility.
- Reduced secretion of intrinsic factor (check vitamin B_{12} status).
- Reduced secretion of pancreatic enzymes.
- Inadequate mixing of food with enzymes and bile.
- Reduced absorption of certain foods, especially protein and fat.
- Rapid absorption of glucose (dumping syndrome).
- Abolition of the normal pH gradient in the small intestine.

Early symptoms

Small stomach syndrome

The majority of patients experience early satiety and may feel distended and uncomfortable during or after eating.

This is particularly likely after total and partial gastrectomy, but may also occur after vagotomy and pyloroplasty. Small, frequent meals should be eaten and fluids consumed separately from solid foods (see Chapter 6.3).

Dumping syndrome

Early dumping occurs soon after eating and involves sweating, dizziness, faintness, a rapid, weak pulse and hypotension as a response to the rapid and early delivery of a hyperosomolar load into the jejunum. The symptoms, which usually recede 2–3 months after surgery, may be relieved by consuming small meals, limiting the consumption of rapidly absorbed carbohydrate (low glycaemic index) and avoiding liquids with meals.

Late dumping may make patients feel weak, faint, cold and sweaty about 2 hours after a meal as a result of over production of insulin in response to the rapid absorption of glucose. The symptoms can be managed by following the advice for early dumping along with regular consumption of starchy carbohydrates.

Diarrhoea

Diarrhoea frequently occurs following vagotomy or total gastrectomy, but may reduce with increasing time after surgery. Antidiarrhoeal agents such as codeine phosphate or loperamide may alleviate the problem.

Bile vomiting

Pancreatic and biliary secretions may accumulate in the afferent loop and, after a meal has left the stomach, can enter the gastric remnant, causing nausea and vomiting. It may be treated by prokinetics and, if refractory, may need surgical correction.

Long term consequences of gastrectomy

Several long term consequences of gastrectomy impact on nutrition.

Weight loss and undernutrition

Weight loss and nutritional inadequacy are common and nearly always reflect poor dietary intake. This may be precipitated by early satiety, dumping syndrome and side effects of treatments such as radiotherapy or chemotherapy. Dietary guidance should aim to improve meal frequency and nutrient density via appropriate food choice and enrichment measures; supplementation may also be indicated.

Malabsorption

Malabsorption of fat may cause steatorrhoea. Energy intake should be increased to compensate for faecal energy losses and to ensure that intake of iron, calcium and fat soluble vitamins are not compromised. Steatorrhoea should not be treated by dietary fat restriction alone. If symptoms are particularly troublesome, a proportion of dietary fat can be isocalorically substituted by either glucose polymers or medium chain triglycerides (MCTs). Medical management involves the use of antidiarrhoea medication, bile acid binders and possibly pancreatic enzyme replacements.

Anaemias

Iron deficiency anaemia can occur as a result of poor iron intake and reduced absorption; therefore, haematological status should be regularly assessed. Pernicious anaemia can be a secondary consequence of gastrectomy as a result of the loss of intrinsic factor (produced by gastric parietal cells) or reduced absorption of vitamin B_{12}, which can be supplemented by intramuscular injection. Megaloblastic anaemia may result from folate deficiency, particularly if dietary intake is poor and malabsorption is present; oral supplementation may be necessary.

Dietary guidance following gastric reconstruction should focus on the need for:

- Small, frequent, regular meals.
- Avoiding large quantities of fluids at meal times.
- Eating a variety of nutrient dense non-bulky, i.e. not high fibre, cereal foods and small amounts of fruit and vegetables.
- Boosting nutrient intake via food enrichment strategies if food intake is compromised.
- Nutritional supplements or micronutrient preparations as indicated.

- Suggesting remedial dietary measures for dumping syndrome or malabsorption if present.

Internet resources

British Society of Gastroenterology   www.bsg.org.uk
Reflux Advice   www.refluxadvice.co.uk

References

Festi D, Scaioli E, Baldi F, Vestito A, Pasqui F, Biase ARD. (2009) Body weight, lifestyle, dietary habits and gastroesophageal reflux disease. *World Journal of Gastroenterology* 15: 1690–1701.

National Institute for Health and Care Excellence (NICE). (2004) *Photodynamic Therapy for High-grade Dysplasia in Barrett's Oesophagus*. London: NICE.

Tytgat GN, McColl K, Tack J, *et al*. (2008) New algorithm for the treatment of gastro-oesophageal reflux disease. *Alimentary Pharmacology & Therapeutics* 27: 249–256.

Yeomans ND. (2011) The ulcer sleuths: The search for the cause of peptic ulcers. *Journal of Gastroenterology and Hepatology* 26: 35–41.

Zong L, Chen P, Chen Y, Shi GG. (2011) Pouch Roux-en-Y vs no pouch Roux-en-Y following total gastrectomy: a meta-analysis based on 12 studies. *Journal of Biomedical Research* 25(2): 90–99.

7.4.4   Gastroparesis

Sarah Wilson

Key points

- Gastroparesis is associated with numerous medical conditions and may be induced by medication.

- Chronic symptoms may lead to serious nutritional consequences, including fluid and electrolyte imbalance and nutritional deficiencies.

- Treatment is supportive and aims to improve symptoms, restore nutritional status and optimise glycaemic control in patients with diabetes.

- Dietary advice may include a reduction in the size, fat and fibre content of meals, as well as texture modification. Enteral or parenteral nutritional support may be indicated if oral intake is inadequate or poorly tolerated.

Gastroparesis is a condition describing disordered motility of the stomach. It is characterised by a delay in gastric emptying in the absence of any obstruction (Bouras & Scolapio, 2004).

Normal gastric motility

Relaxation of the fundus (proximal stomach) allows the stomach to accommodate large volumes of food. Contractions of the antrum (distal stomach) grind food and gastric juices into liquid chyme. Coordinated contractions between the stomach and duodenum pump chyme through the pylorus in tightly controlled spurts. Gastric motility is controlled by smooth muscle lining the gut and interstitial cells of Cajal within smooth muscle, which act as electrical pacemakers to generate contractions.

The rate of gastric emptying is influenced by complex neural and hormonal signals produced in response to meal composition (Karamanolis & Tack, 2006). Receptors in the small intestine detect distension, pH and the products of digestion, such as fatty acids, peptides and amino acids. Gut mucosal cells release various hormones in response to these products of digestion, which either stimulate or inhibit gastric emptying (Camilleri, 2006). This feedback process is regulated by the autonomic and enteric nervous system, as shown in Figure 7.4.3.

SECTION 7

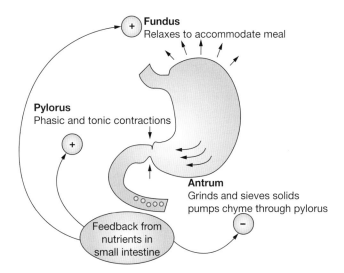

Figure 7.4.3 Motor events during normal gastric emptying (source: Rayner & Horowitz 2005. Reproduced with permission of Macmillan Publishers Ltd)

Causes

It is thought that gastroparesis is primarily caused by neuropathy or myopathy resulting in impaired fundus relaxation, decreased antral contractions, spasm of the pylorus, gastric arrhythmia or a combination of these factors (Tack, 2007). The result is undigested food that remains in the stomach for longer than normal, leading to mild to severe gastrointestinal symptoms. In patients with diabetes, gastroparesis may lead to poor glycaemic control.

Gastroparesis is more common in women and may be acute or chronic depending on the underlying aetiology. The main causes of chronic gastroparesis are idiopathic (unknown), diabetes mellitus and post surgery (Soykan *et al.*, 1998). Conditions associated with gastroparesis include (Parkman *et al.*, 2004; Rayner & Horowitz, 2005):

- Idiopathic.
- Diabetes.
- Surgery affecting the stomach or vagus nerve.
- Critical illness.
- Gastro-oesophageal reflux disease.
- Chronic liver, renal or pancreas disease.
- Cancer, e.g. pancreatic, gastric, oesophageal.
- Connective tissue disorders, e.g. scleroderma.
- Neurological disorders, e.g. Parkinson's disease.
- Conditions affecting the nervous system, e.g. enteric neuropathy.
- Motility disorders, e.g. chronic intestinal pseudo obstruction, constipation.
- Infection, e.g. virus.
- Anorexia nervosa.
- Medication induced.

Chronic gastroparesis may contribute to patient morbidity and severely affect quality of life (Parkman *et al.*, 2004). Severe gastroparesis is associated with multiple hospital admissions and longer length of stay (Kashyap & Farrugia, 2010).

Idiopathic gastroparesis

Idiopathic causes may affect up to a third of patients with gastroparesis and are more common in women (Soykan *et al.*, 1998). Acute onset occurs in 50% of patients with idiopathic gastroparesis (Parkman *et al.*, 2011). It is suspected that viral infection may be responsible for gastroparesis in this subgroup (Bityutskiy *et al.*, 1997).

Diabetic gastroparesis

Gastroparesis affects up to 50% of patients with diabetes mellitus (Horowitz *et al.*, 1996); it is more common in patients with type 1 diabetes. Chronic hyperglycaemia causes damage to the vagus nerve, which regulates gastric emptying. Loss of the interstitial cells of Cajal and neuronal nitric oxide synthase (nNOS) may also play a role in the pathogenesis (Kashyap & Farrugia, 2010). Gastroparesis may worsen glycaemic control as the stomach does not empty regularly, leading to episodes of hyperglycaemia as well as hypoglycaemia. Acute hyperglycaemia may itself slow the rate of gastric emptying (Schvarcz *et al.*, 1997). Poor glycaemic control as a result of gastroparesis may inaccurately imply poor concordance with dietetic advice. Gastroparesis should be suspected if glycaemic control is poor despite reported compliance to diet (Patrick & Epstein, 2008).

Post surgical gastroparesis

Gastroparesis has been reported after gastric resection, Roux-en-Y gastric bypass, Whipple's procedure, fundoplication, oesophagectomy, vagotomy and after heart and lung transplant (Parkman *et al.*, 2004). It is thought to result from damage to the vagus nerve during surgery and may also be induced by certain medications (Parkman *et al.*, 2004):

- Fibre.
- Alcohol.
- Tobacco.
- Marijuana.
- Antacids.
- Opioids.
- Calcium channel blockers.
- Proton pump inhibitors.
- L-dopa.
- Lithium.
- High dose tricyclic antidepressants.
- Anticholinergics.
- Progesterone.
- Ocreotide.

Symptoms

Symptoms of gastroparesis range from asymptomatic to severe and may include:

- Nausea.
- Vomiting.
- Abdominal bloating.
- Early satiety and/or post prandial fullness.
- Abdominal pain.

- Reflux and/or retching.
- Poor glycaemic control.
- Constipation or diarrhoea.

Symptoms of gastroparesis usually occur >1 hour after a meal (Karamanolis & Tack, 2006). More immediate symptoms suggest a psychosomatic or other cause (Bouras & Scolapio, 2004). The Gastroparesis Cardinal Symptom Index (GSCI) is a validated patient questionnaire that can be used to quantify the severity of symptoms (Revicki et al., 2003). However, studies have shown the relationship between severity of symptoms (GSCI scores) and gastric emptying rate is poor, suggesting other factors, such as visceral hypersensitivity, may contribute to symptoms (Cassilly et al., 2008).

Nutritional consequences

Many patients with gastroparesis initially present as overweight or obese; therefore signs of malnutrition may be missed (Bizer et al., 2005). Gastrointestinal discomfort as a result of gastroparesis may lead to anorexia, food aversions and an unbalanced or reduced oral intake. Vomiting may result in oesophagitis, fluid and electrolyte disturbances, pulmonary aspiration and harm dentition (Bouras & Scolapio, 2004). Inadequate oral intake may result in protein energy malnutrition, weight loss and micronutrient deficiencies. Poor oral intake, weight loss and electrolyte losses from vomiting may result in a high risk of refeeding syndrome.

Poor glycaemic control may increase risk of micro- and macro-vascular complications of diabetes. Delayed gastric emptying may result in impaired absorption of medications, affecting the treatment of other medical conditions. Undigested food in the stomach may form into solid masses called bezoars, which can exacerbate symptoms of gastroparesis and cause obstruction (Tack, 2007). Many patients with gastroparesis endure symptoms for many years before receiving an accurate diagnosis and suffer from depression and anxiety (Soykan et al., 1998).

Few studies have investigated the nutritional status of patients with gastroparesis; however, anaemia, dehydration, deficiency of vitamin D, thiamine and zinc, and inadequate oral intake of calories, protein and other micronutrients have been observed (Brown et al., 1999; Ogorek et al., 1991). There is a need for further research in this area and for vigilant nutritional screening due to the potential risk of refeeding syndrome and micronutrient deficiencies.

Nutritional assessment

A detailed nutritional assessment is required to ensure an effective treatment plan.

Anthropometry

Measures include:

- Weight, height, waist circumference (consider ascites, oedema, dehydration).
- Weight history and percentage weight loss if relevant.
- Body mass index (BMI) or mid upper arm circumference (MUAC).
- Calculate nutritional requirements based on need for weight gain or loss or if the underlying aetiology indicates additional stress, e.g. cancer, post surgery.

Biochemistry

The following should be assessed:

- Urea, creatinine, sodium, potassium, magnesium, phosphate and corrected calcium to assess hydration, renal function, electrolyte depletion and risk of refeeding syndrome.
- Blood glucose levels pre and post meals and $HbA1_c$ for patients with diabetes.
- Haemoglobin, ferritin, folate and B_{12} levels to detect anaemia.
- Albumin, transferrin and prealbumin are poor markers of nutritional status in the presence of raised inflammatory markers such as C-reactive protein and erythrocyte sedimentation rate.
- Liver function – may be affected by parenteral nutrition.
- If micronutrient or trace element deficiency is suspected, check 25-hydroxycholecalciferol (vitamin D), zinc, selenium and copper.

Clinical status

The following should be assessed:

- Establish underlying aetiology, e.g. diabetes, post surgery or idiopathic.
- Observations, e.g. temperature, fluid balance.
- Bowel form, frequency and incidence of constipation or diarrhoea. The Bristol Stool chart is helpful to clarify stool form (Lewis & Heaton, 1997).
- Symptom history, type and pattern, duration and frequency. Severity of symptoms can be rated using the GSCI questionnaire (Revicki et al., 2003). A food and symptom diary may help to identify any patterns.
- Any problems with dentition that may affect the patient's ability to chew food.
- If the patient has diabetes, frequency of blood sugar monitoring, insulin injection site (if relevant), incidence and treatment of hypoglycaemia.
- Intake of herbal or sports supplements, laxatives, vitamin and mineral preparations, prescription and non-prescription medications. Note medications that may delay gastric emptying (see Chapter 7.4.3).

Dietary assessment

The following should be assessed:

- Diet history – current intake versus usual intake.
- Previous dietary measures tried.
- Evidence of disordered eating, e.g. binging or self induced vomiting.

SECTION 7

- Percentage of oral intake vomited if relevant.
- Meal pattern.
- Portion sizes.
- Food intolerances and/or allergies.
- Tolerance to different textures – solid, soft, puréed, liquid.
- Dietary balance – proportion of carbohydrate, protein, fat, fruit and vegetables.
- Fibre intake – soluble and insoluble sources.
- Fluid intake – alcohol, carbonated drinks, caffeine, etc..
- Dietary sources of iron, folate, thiamine, calcium, vitamin D and other at risk micronutrients.

Socioeconomic status

The following should be assessed:

- Smoking.
- Illicit drugs use; note those that delay gastric emptying as listed under Post surgical gastroparesis.
- Physical activity.
- History of depression and/or stress.
- Patient's understanding of normal digestion and nutrition.
- Motivation and support.
- Stage of behavioural change and barriers to change.
- Cooking skills and facilities, e.g. equipment to blend food.

Clinical investigation and management

Gastroparesis is diagnosed by demonstrating delayed gastric emptying after other causes are ruled out, such as obstruction by endoscopy or barium studies, and any psychological cause, such as bulimia nervosa or rumination syndrome.

Investigations

Nuclear scintigraphy is the gold standard measure of gastric emptying. Retention of >10% of gastric contents after 4 hours of an isotope labelled test meal indicates abnormal emptying (Tougas *et al.*, 2000). Results must be interpreted carefully as test meals vary between centres and even in normal subjects daily gastric emptying varies by 20% (Patrick & Epstein, 2008). The severity and frequency of abnormal gastric emptying should be considered to determine a clinically significant diagnosis of gastroparesis (Tack, 2007).

Other measures of gastric emptying include the Smart Pill, ^{13}C-octanoic acid breath testing, magnetic resonance imaging and ultrasonography. Manometry studies measure motility patterns in the stomach and duodenum. Different patterns indicate neuropathy or myopathy and may help to determine the underlying aetiology of gastroparesis. Electrogastrography may provide information on gastric dysarthymia (Patrick & Epstein, 2008). Many of these investigations are expensive and available only in a research setting.

Treatment

Treatment aims to optimise management of the underlying cause of gastroparesis, improve glycaemic control in patients with diabetes, reduce symptoms and restore nutrition and hydration.

Medications

Prokinetics are used to accelerate gastric emptying; however, studies have not shown an associated improvement in symptoms (Sturm *et al.*, 1999; Talley, 2003). Antiemetics may help to reduce nausea; some antiemetics need to be taken 30 minutes prior to meals for best effect. Low dose tricyclic antidepressants may relieve symptoms of nausea, vomiting and pain. Some medications delay gastric emptying and should be avoided (see Chapter 7.4.3).

Botox

Botulinum toxin injected into the pylorus to reduce pylorospasms has not shown any benefit in double blind placebo controlled trials (Arts *et al.*, 2007; Friedenberg *et al.*, 2008).

Gastric electrical stimulation

This involves surgical insertion of a gastric pacemaker to stimulate gastric contractions. Studies have shown that gastric electrical stimulation (GES) improves symptoms of nausea and vomiting in some patient groups; however, there is little evidence that the procedure improves gastric emptying rate (Abell *et al.*, 2003; McCallum *et al.*, 2011). The National Institute for Health and Care Excellence (NICE, 2004) has approved the use of GES in specialist units for patients with nausea and vomiting uncontrolled by medications.

Continuous insulin pump

This may improve glycaemic control in patients with diabetes through the more precise use of short acting insulin. Research is being undertaken into the potential benefit in patients with gastroparesis.

Surgery

A venting gastrostomy may relieve symptoms in some patients but be counterproductive in others (Kim & Nelson, 1998; Bouras & Scolapio, 2004). As a last resort, a subtotal gastrectomy may provide symptom relief in refractory patients with postsurgical gastroparesis (Eckhauser *et al.*, 1998).

Psychological measures

Limited evidence has suggested biofeedback and acupuncture may improve symptoms of gastroparesis in some patient groups (Rashed *et al.*, 2002; Wang, 2004).

Nutrition

Dietary modification may improve tolerance to oral intake, although there is little evidence to support this

(Karamanolis & Tack, 2006). Nutritional status should be restored through the provision of fluid, electrolytes, and macro- and micro-nutrients using the safest and best tolerated form of oral, enteral or parenteral support.

There are no controlled trials of nutritional intervention on clinical outcome in patients with gastroparesis (Abell *et al.*, 2006a). The diet currently recommended for patients with gastroparesis is one based on small frequent meals that are low in fat and fibre, and texture modified (Parkman *et al.* 2004). Large, nutrient dense meals may slow gastric emptying due to the time required for the stomach to grind contents down and negative feedback from the small intestine (Hunt & Stubbs, 1975; Camilleri, 2006). Fat in general delays gastric emptying (Cunningham & Read, 1989; Lin *et al.*, 2001). However, in clinical practice, fat is often well tolerated in liquid form and enables the provision of adequate calories (Parish & Yoshida, 2005). Removal of fibre naturally present in food accelerated gastric emptying in one study (Benini *et al.*, 1995). However, in another study, the addition of fibre did not affect gastric emptying rate (Bianchi & Capurso, 2002). Soluble fibre may increase symptoms of bloating (Bianchi & Capurso, 2002). Insoluble fibre may increase risk of bezoar formation (Abell *et al.*, 2006b; Rayner & Horowitz, 2005). Liquids empty faster than solid meals and many patients with gastroparesis have normal liquid emptying times (Read & Houghton, 1989). Homogenised food may also empty faster than solids (Karamanolis & Tack, 2006).

Advice should consider overall dietary balance, fluid and micronutrient intake, as well as glycaemic control in patients with diabetes. Adequate fluid intake should be encouraged to replace losses and prevent constipation. Carbonated drinks may exacerbate symptoms of bloating (Parkman *et al.*, 2004). Excess alcohol and smoking may delay gastric emptying and should be discouraged (Bujanda, 2000; Miller *et al.*, 1989).

Dietetic strategies

As there is a lack of evidence, the following strategies should be tried but adapted to individual patient symptoms:

- Encourage small frequent meals.
- Reduce fat and fibre:
  - Limit fried foods and nutrient dense meals such as takeaways.
  - Fat in liquid form may be well tolerated and a useful source of energy.
  - Reduce intake of very fibrous foods such as stringy fruit and vegetable skins, pips, seeds and high fibre muesli, etc.
- Modify texture:
  - Liquid, puréed, or soft foods may be better tolerated than solid meals.
  - Adapt texture to symptoms, e.g. if symptoms are worse at night, encourage greater intake of liquid calories during the evening.
  - Food fortification may be required to ensure adequate energy intake.
- Optimise glycaemic control:
  - Establish regular meal pattern.
  - Encourage more frequent blood sugar monitoring before and after meals.
  - Consider giving short acting insulin after meals rather than before.
  - Ensure appropriate treatment of hypoglycaemia.
- Other:
  - Consider a multivitamin supplement if diet is inadequate.
  - Patients may benefit from sitting upright during meals.
  - Encourage patients to chew food well.
  - Reduce stress at meal times.

Nutritional support

Patients unable to maintain an adequate oral intake may require enteral or parenteral nutritional support. Oral liquid supplements are often well tolerated, including those containing fat. Patients with diabetes should be offered milk style supplements in preference to juice style supplements as a first line measure. Nasojejunal (NJ) feeding is recommended for patients with vomiting and nausea who are unable to tolerate gastric feeding. Following a successful trial of NJ feeding, jejunostomy placement may maintain hydration and nutrition; however, it is associated with significant complications, including tube displacement and infection (Jones *et al.*, 2003; Fontana & Barnett, 1996). A surgically placed needle–catheter jejunostomy may be preferable to a gastrostomy with a jejunal extension, as the extension tubes often migrate back into the stomach (Karamanolis & Tack, 2006).

Continuous feeding is generally better tolerated than bolus feeding (Abell *et al.*, 2006b). Fibre free feeds may be better tolerated in gastric feeding and in jejunal feeding if small bowel overgrowth or intestinal dysmotility is suspected (Parish & Yoshida, 2005). In studies of gastrostomy fed paediatric patients, whey based formulae decreased gastric empting time; however, there are as yet no studies confirming this effect in adults (Fried *et al.*, 1992).

Parenteral nutrition may be indicated during acute exacerbations of symptoms or for patients with severe intestinal dysmotility who do not tolerate jejunal feeding (Bouras & Scolapio, 2004).

Effective management of patients with gastroparesis requires a multidisciplinary team approach with close liaison between medical and surgical teams, nursing staff, dietitian, psychologist and pharmacist (Abell *et al.*, 2006a).

Internet resources

Gastroparesis and Dysmotilities Association (GPDA) http:// digestivedistress.com

References

Abell TL, McCallum R, Hocking M, *et al*. (2003) Gastric electrical stimulation for medically refractory gastroparesis. *Gastroenterolology* 125: 421–428.

Abell TL, Bernstein RK, Cutts T. (2006a). Treatment of gastroparesis: a multidisciplinary clinical review. *Neurogastroenterology and Motility* 18(4): 263–283.

Abell TL, Malinowski S, Minocha A. (2006b) Nutrition aspects of gastroparesis and therapies for drug-refractory patients. *Nutrition in Clinical Practice* 21: 23–33.

Arts J, Holvoet L, Caenepeel P, *et al*. (2007) Clinical trial: a randomized-controlled crossover study of intra-pyloric injection of botulinum toxin A in gastroparesis. *Alimentary Pharmacology & Therapeutics* 26: 1251–1258.

Benini M, Castellani G, Brighenti F, *et al*. (1995) Gastric emptying of a solid meal is accelerated by the removal of dietary fibre naturally present in food. *Gut* 36(6): 825–830.

Bianchi M, Capurso L. (2002) Effects of guar gum, ispaghula and microcrystalline cellulose on abdominal symptoms, gastric emptying, orocacal transit time and gas production in healthy volunteers. *Digestive and Liver Disease* 34(Suppl 2): S129–133.

Bityutskiy LP, Soykan I, McCallum RW. (1997) Viral gastroparesis: a subgroup of idiopathic gastroparesis – clinical characteristics and long-term outcomes. *American Journal of Gastroenterology* 92: 1501–1504.

Bizer E, Harrell S, Koopman J, *et al*. (2005). Obesity is common in gastroparesis despite nausea, vomiting, and early satiety (abstract). *Gastroenterology* 128: M1895.

Bouras EP, Scolapio JS. (2004) Gastric motility disorders: management that optimizes nutritional status. *Journal of Clinical Gastroenterology* 38: 549–557.

Brown RO, Dickerson RN, Abell TL, Werkman RF, Hak LJ. (1999) A one year experience with a pharmacist-coordinated nutritional support clinic. *American Journal of Health-System Pharmacy* 56: 2324–2327.

Bujanda L. (2000) The effects of alcohol consumption upon the gastrointestinal tract. *American Journal of Gastroenterology* 95(12): 3374–3382.

Camilleri M. (2006) Integrated upper gastrointestinal response to food intake. *Gastroenterology* 131: 640–658.

Cassilly DW, Wang RY, Friedenberg FK, Nelson DB, Maurer AH, Parkman HP. (2008) Symptoms of Gastroparesis: use of the Gastroparesis Cardinal Symptom Index in symptomatic patients referred for gastric emptying scintigraphy. *Digestion* 78: 144–151.

Cunningham KM, Read NW. (1989) The effect of incorporating fat into different components of a meal on gastric emptying and postprandial blood glucose and insulin responses. *British Journal of Nutrition* 61: 285–290.

Eckhauser FE, Conrad M, Knol JA, *et al*. (1998) Safety and long-term durability of completion gastrectomy in 81 patients with postsurgical gastroparesis syndrome. *American Journal of Surgery* 64: 711–717.

Fontana RJ, Barnett JL. (1996) Jejunostomy tube placement in refractory diabetic gastroparesis: a retrospective review. *American Journal of Gastroenterology* 91(10): 2174–2178.

Fried, MD, Khoshoo V, Secker DJ, Gilday DL, Ash JM, Pencharz PB. (1992) Decrease in gastric emptying time and episodes of regurgitation in children with spastic quadriplegia fed a whey-based formula. *Journal of Paediatrics* 120(4): 570–572.

Friedenberg FK, Palit A, Parkman HP, Hanlon A, Nelson DB. (2008) Botulinum toxin A for the treatment of delayed gastric emptying. *American Journal of Gastroenterology* 103: 416–423.

Horowitz M, Wishart JM, Jones KL, Hebbard GS. (1996) Gastric emptying in diabetes: an overview. *Diabetes Medicine* 13: S16–22.

Hunt JN, Stubbs DF. (1975) The volume and energy content of meals as determinants of gastric emptying. *Journal of Physiology* 245(1): 209–225.

Jones MP, Maganti K. (2003) A systematic review of surgical therapy for gastroparesis. *American Journal of Gastrointereology* 98: 2122–2129.

Karamanolis G, Tack J. (2006) Nutrition and motility disorders. *Best Practice and Research Clinical Gastroenterology* 20: 485–505.

Kashyap P, Farrugia G. (2010) Diabetic gastroparesis: what we have learned and had to unlearn in the past 5 yrs. *Gut* 59: 1716–1726.

Kim CH, Nelson DK. (1998) Venting percutaneous gastrostomy in the treatment of refractory idiopathic gastroparesis. *Gastrointestinal Endoscopy* 47(1): 67–70.

Lewis SJ, Heaton KW. (1997) Stool form scale as a useful guide to intestinal transit time. *Scandinavian Journal of Gastroenterology* 32(9): 920–924.

Lin HC, van Citters GW, Heimer F, Bonorris G. (2001) Slowing of gastrointestinal transit by oleic acid: a preliminary report of a novel, nutrient-based treatment in human. *Digestive Diseases and Sciences* 46: 223–229.

McCallum R, Lin Z, Forster J, Roeser K, Hou Q, Sarosiek I. (2011) Gastric electrical stimulation improves outcomes of patients with gastroparesis for up to 10 years. *Clinical Gastroenterology and Hepatology* 9(4): 314–319.e1.

Miller G, Palmer KP, Smith B, *et al*. (1989) Smoking delays gastric emptying of solids. *Gut* 30: 50–53.

National Institute for Health and Care Excellence. (2004) Gastro-electrical stimulation for patients with diabetes. Available from: http://publications.nice.org.uk/gastroelectrical-stimulation-for-gastroparesis-ipg103. Accessed 8 August 2012.

Ogorek CP, Davidson L, Fisher RS, Krevsky B. (1991) Idiopathic gastroparesis is associated with a multiplicity of severe dietary deficiencies. *American Journal of Gastroenterology* 86: 423.

Parkman HP, Hasler WL, Fisher RS. (2004) American Gastroenterological Association technical review on the diagnosis and treatment of gastroparesis. *Gastroenterology* 127(5): 1592–1622.

Parkman HP, Yates K, Hasler WL, *et al*.; National Institute of Diabetes and Digestive and Kidney Diseases Gastroparesis Clinical Research Consortium. (2011) Clinical features of idiopathic gastroparesis vary with sex, body mass, symptom onset, delay in gastric emptying, and gastroparesis severity. *Gastroenterology* 140(1): 101–115.

Parrish CR, Yoshida CM. (2005) Nutrition intervention for the patient with gastroparesis: An update. *Practical Gastroenterology* 29(8): 29–66.

Patrick A, Epstein O. (2008) Review article: gastroparesis. *Alimentary Pharmacology & Therapeutics* 27(9): 724–740.

Rashed H, Cutts T, Luo J, *et al*. (2002). Predictors of response to a behavioral treatment in patients with chronic gastric motility disorders. *Digestive Diseases and Sciences* 47: 1020–1026.

Rayner CK, Horowitz M. (2005) New management approaches for gastroparesis. *Nature Clinical Practice Gastroenterology & Hepatology* 2: 454–462.

Read NW, Houghton LA. (1989) Physiology of gastric emptying and pathophysiology of gastroparesis. *Gastroenterology Clinics of North America* 18: 359–373.

Revicki DA, Rentz AM, Dubois D, *et al*. (2003) Development and validation of a patient- assessed gastroparesis symptoms severity measure: the Gastroparesis Cardinal Symptom Index. *Alimentary Pharmacolgy & Therapeutics* 18: 141–150.

Schvarcz E, Palmer M, Aman J, Horowitz M, Stridsberg M, Berne C. (1997) Physiological hyperglycemia slows gastric emptying in normal subjects and patients with insulin-dependent diabetes mellitus. *Gastroenterology* 113: 60–66.

Soykan I, Sivri B, Sarosiek I, Kierran B, McCallum RW. (1998) Demography, clinical characteristics, psychological profiles, treatment and long-term follow-up of patients with gastroparesis. *Digestive Diseases and Sciences* 43: 2398–2404.

Sturm A, Holtmann G, Goebell H, Gerken G. (1999) Prokinetics in patients with gastroparesis: a systematic analysis. *Digestion* 60(5): 422–427.

SECTION 7

Tack J. (2007) The difficult patient with gastroparesis. *Best Practice and Research Clinical Gastroenterology* 21: 379–391.

Talley NJ. (2003) Diabetic gastropathy and prokinetics. *American Journal of Gastroentereology* 98(2): 264–271.

Tougas G, Eaker EY, Abell TL, *et al.* (2000) Assessment of gastric emptying using a low-fat meal: Establishment of international control values. *American Journal of Gastroenterology* 95: 1456–1462.

Wang L. (2004) Clinical observation on acupuncture treatment in 35 cases of diabetic gastroparesis. *Journal of Traditional Chinese Medicine* 24: 163e5.

7.4.5 Disorders of the pancreas
Mary Phillips

Key points

■ Pancreatic disease presents complex multifactorial nutritional challenges.

■ Enteral feeding with a peptide feed is the feeding regimen of choice in acute pancreatitis, with emphasis on achieving this early in the disease process.

■ Pancreatic cancer and chronic pancreatitis are both associated with progressive malnutrition and patients benefit from early dietetic intervention.

■ Pancreatic surgery is highly complex and pre- and post-operative optimisation of nutritional status is required.

■ Long term micronutrient deficiencies are becoming more apparent, and screening for these is recommended.

■ Probiotics are not recommended in severe acute pancreatitis.

Pancreatic disorders may be benign or malignant, and include acute and chronic pancreatitis and pancreatic cancers. The nutritional consequences of these conditions are diverse and often complicated to manage and therefore present many challenges for dietitians. The pancreas has three main functions that are essential in the digestion and absorption of food and nutrients (Neoptolemos & Bhutani, 2008a,b):

* *Endocrine:*
  ○ Release of insulin and glucagon from islet cells mainly located in the tail of the pancreas.
* *Exocrine:*
  ○ Release of digestive enzymes from acinar cells found mainly in the head of the pancreas.
  ○ Release of bicarbonate to neutralise gastric acid.

Pancreatic enzyme release is stimulated in three phases. The taste and smell of food stimulates an initial release of pancreatic enzymes (cephalic phase). This is followed by the second surge, which is believed to be triggered by gastric distension (gastric phase). The third, and most significant, stimulant of pancreatic enzyme release occurs when the products of digestion are delivered into the duodenum (intestinal phase). This final stage is responsible for the ongoing release of enzymes for 2–3 hours post prandially (Keller & Layer, 2005).

Acute pancreatitis

Acute pancreatitis is an inflammatory condition with an overall mortality of 10–15% (Mann *et al.*, 1994, Corfield *et al*, 1985); most commonly associated with gallstone disease or high alcohol intakes. Other causes include trauma, surgery, hypertriglyceridaemia, endoscopic retrograde cholangiopancreatography (ERCP) and drug reaction. In some patients the cause is unknown (Neoptolemos & Bhutani, 2008a,b). Acute pancreatitis usually presents with severe abdominal pain, caused by the auto activation of enzymes within the gland. In the initial stages the treatment is conservative, consisting of pain relief and organ support where necessary. Keeping the patient nil by mouth reduces pancreatic stimulation.

On admission patients are scored to predict disease severity using one of a number of scoring systems. These include Apache II or RANSON criteria, and more frequently the modified Glasgow (or Imrie) score (Table 7.4.3). Increasingly, C-reactive protein (CRP) is considered an independent marker of severity (UK Working Party on Acute Pancreatitis, 2005). In cases of mild pancreatitis most patients are kept nil by mouth until the pain has resolved; however, in some units oral feeding is started early. Recent studies suggest initiation of early oral diet may reduce length of stay when compared with fasting or clear fluids only (Sathiaraj *et al.*, 2008, Eckerwall *et al.*, 2007). The hospital stay is usually short, but if gallstones are the cause of the pancreatitis, a laparoscopic cholecystectomy should be performed.

Patients with severe acute pancreatitis (SAP) may present with, or develop, multiorgan failure or systemic inflammatory response syndrome (SIRS). These patients require intensive care support and may need multiple interventions with hospital admissions stretching over

Table 7.4.3 Modified Glasgow (or Imrie) severity scoring for acute pancreatitis

Parameter	Indicative level
P (PaO$_2$ – arterial blood gas)	PaO$_2$ < 7.9 kPa
A (Albumin)	<32 g/L
N (Neutrophils)	WCC > 15 mmol/L
C (Calcium)	<2 mmol/L
R (Renal)	Urea > 16 mmol/L
E (Enzymes)	LDH > 600 IU/L or AST > 100 IU/L
A (Age)	>55 years
S (Sugar)	Glucose > 10 mmol/L

A score of ≥3 within 48 hours of admission is predictive of severe disease (Blamey et al., 1984) and an indicator for enteral feeding.
WCC, white cell count; LDH, lactate dehydrogenase; AST, aspartate transaminase.

many weeks or months. Comprehensive nutritional support is indicated and enteral feeding is considered to be the gold standard. However, parenteral nutrition may be needed when enteral nutrition is poorly tolerated, either as a sole source of nutrition or ideally, in addition to slow rate enteral feeding (Neoptolemos & Bhutani, 2008a,b; Sakorafas et al., 2010).

Many complications of pancreatitis are septic in origin and the use of enteral feeding to reduce bacterial translocation has been widely studied (Sakorafas et al., 2010). There are many complications of acute pancreatitis that can influence the delivery and tolerance of enteral feeding, including:

- Hyperglycaemia.
- Malabsorption.
- Weight loss and loss of muscle mass – often dramatic.
- Delayed gastric emptying and high nasogastric (NG) aspirates.
- Continuing high NG aspirates with jejunal feeding.
- Nausea and vomiting.
- Prolonged periods of nil by mouth for multiple procedures.
- Paralytic ileus secondary to electrolyte imbalance.
- Antibiotic related diarrhoea.
- Peripheral oedema.
- Gastrointestinal oedema – diarrhoea, obstruction.
- Ascites.
- Gastric varices.
- Colonic necrosis and faecal peritonitis.

Severe acute pancreatitis is usually treated aggressively with multiorgan support and antibiotics. In some instances, necrosis develops and the necrotic tissue is removed surgically with either an open necrosectomy or preferably, a minimally invasive necrosectomy to reduce the risk of further sepsis. The degree of necrosis and damage arising from inflammation, and the location of such damage, will help predict any long term insufficiency. Extensive disease in the head of the pancreas is more likely to result in long term exocrine insufficiency [requiring pancreatic enzyme replacement therapy (PERT)], whereas disease centred in the tail of the pancreas is more likely to lead to endocrine insufficiency (type 1 diabetes mellitus).

Chronic pancreatitis

Chronic pancreatitis is a progressive inflammatory disease resulting in the destruction of the pancreas. The incidence is between 20 and 200 per 100 000. Chronic pancreatitis is caused by excessive alcohol consumption in 70–90% of cases (Neoptolemos & Bhutani, 2008a,b; Layer & Melle, 2005). In severe cases chronic pancreatitis causes intractable pain and severe malnutrition, leading to multiple admissions for procedures to reduce pain. These include coeliac or endoscopic plexus blocks; thoracic splanchnicectomy; gastric and biliary bypass surgery; ductal drainage procedures or even pancreatic resection. A multidisciplinary team approach is crucial in managing patients with chronic pancreatitis to prevent malnutrition, while managing exocrine insufficiency and optimising pain control.

Patients may be prescribed pancreatic enzymes for pain control, which some studies have suggested provide potential benefit due to a negative feedback mechanism inhibiting cholecystokinin (CCK) release (Hammer, 2010). There is no strong evidence of pain relief benefit provided by PERT, although there may be a benefit from enzymes in tablet rather than the enteric coated form (Khalid & Whitcomb, 2002).

Pancreatic cancer

Pancreatic cancer is the fifth most common cause of cancer death in the UK, with a median survival following diagnosis of 6 months. The high mortality is due to vague early symptoms (including nausea and vomiting, back pain and weight loss), resulting in tumours being diagnosed late, often after they have already metastasised. Early symptoms may include jaundice and new onset diabetes. Unfortunately 85% of patients with pancreatic cancer are identified as having non-resectable tumours at diagnosis, with the most common type of tumour being ductal adenocarcinoma (Neoptolemos & Bhutani, 2008a,b).

Patients who have operable disease and who are fit for surgery are likely to have one of the following procedures:

- Whipple's procedure – removal of the duodenum, head of the pancreas, gallbladder and distal stomach.
- Pylorus preserving pancreaticoduodenectomy (PPPD) – removal of the duodenum, head of the pancreas and gallbladder, but the stomach is left intact.
- Distal pancreatectomy – removal of the tail of the pancreas and usually the spleen.

- Total pancreatectomy – removal of the duodenum, the entire pancreas, gallbladder, usually the spleen, and sometimes the distal stomach.

Postoperatively, patients may experience delayed gastric emptying and/or dumping syndrome (depending on the extent of gastric resection), early satiety, endocrine and exocrine insufficiency, brittle diabetes (following total pancreatectomy) and in the long term vitamin and mineral deficiency.

Treatment options for non-resectable disease include chemotherapy, radiotherapy, palliative surgery (including gastric and biliary bypass), palliative biliary and duodenal stenting, and eventually palliative care (see Chapter 7.15.3).

Nutritional consequences of pancreatic disease

Regardless of whether pancreatic damage has arisen as a result of cancer, acute or chronic pancreatitis, or surgical resection, the nutritional consequences are similar, and can be classified according to their aetiology.

Pain

Pain is a key symptom in both benign and malignant disease, and can play a significant role in the development of malnutrition. Pain may be continuous, but is often associated with eating due to stimulation of the pancreatic secretions following ingestion. Consequently, patients may avoid eating in an attempt to minimise pain. Some patients benefit from soft or liquid based diets, which are thought to result in decreased pancreatic stimulation. (Jacobson *et al.*, 2007).

Endocrine insufficiency

Islet cells, which produce insulin, are predominantly located in the tail of the pancreas. Therefore, pancreatic disease affecting this area or resection of the distal pancreas may result in endocrine insufficiency. In patients with non-resectable malignant disease or chronic pancreatitis, this insufficiency may only become apparent over time. Diabetes caused by pancreatic resection may be brittle, with patients prone to sudden episodes of hypoglycaemia. Insulin is often required and care must be taken to ensure that malnourished patients do not receive inappropriate energy restrictive advice.

Exocrine insufficiency

Malabsorption as a result of exocrine insufficiency causes a variety of symptoms, including steatorrhoea (frequent, pale, loose, floating stools), abdominal bloating and flatulence, unexplained weight loss and micronutrient deficiencies, such as anaemia and fat soluble vitamin deficiency. Malabsorption is managed with PERT. Most patients with pancreatic disease will require PERT with each meal or snack, and with oral nutritional supplements (if prescribed). These enzymes should be given at the beginning of the meal and the dose titrated up until symptoms of malabsorption are under control.

Management
Low fat diets

Exocrine insufficiency has historically been managed through restriction of dietary fat intake. It is now widely accepted that the use of low fat diets will exacerbate malnutrition and therefore fat restriction is only recommended for symptom control in those who do not respond to PERT (Lankisch, 1999). If nutritional support is indicated, patients should receive high energy, high protein advice in conjunction with PERT to manage exocrine insufficiency.

Pancreatic enzyme replacement therapy

The recommendations for the use of PERT are:

- Enzymes should be prescribed for use with all meals, snacks and nutritional supplements.
- Enzymes are most frequently prescribed in capsule form, although tablet, granules or powered forms are also available.
- Capsules should be swallowed whole at the beginning of the meal, with a cold drink to prevent denaturation of the enzyme.
- Where more than one capsule or tablet is prescribed at a time, their ingestion should be spread out through the meal.
- Enzyme activity peaks at 45 minutes and wears off after 2–3 hours, so enzymes should be given regularly with sip feeds consumed over >45 minutes.
- When granules or powdered enzymes are indicated, these products should be mixed with an acidic fruit purée, swallowed immediately without chewing and the mouth rinsed with a cold drink to prevent premature activation of the enzyme and enzymic damage to the oral mucosa (mouth ulcers).
- Where possible, peptide or elemental feeds should be used for enteral feeding; these feed formulae should not require the use of pancreatic enzymes for digestion.

Micronutrient deficiencies

Multiple micronutrient deficiencies have been associated with pancreatic insufficiency in both benign and malignant disease (Armstrong *et al.*, 2007; Dujsikova *et al.*, 2008). The most clinically significant is vitamin D deficiency, which is associated with osteopenia and osteoporosis (Dujsikova *et al.*, 2008). Routine supplementation with a calcium and vitamin D supplement (Armstrong *et al.*, 2007) and regular monitoring of vitamin D and parathyroid hormone (PTH), and DEXA scans are recommended routinely for patients with chronic pancreatitis (Duggan *et al.*, 2010). Case reports have highlighted incidences of vitamin A deficiency night blindness (Livingstone *et al.*, 2003), deficiencies of selenium, zinc and vitamin E. In addition, anaemia has also been reported (Armstrong *et al.*, 2007).

Enteral feeding

Acute pancreatitis

Historically, patients with SAP were kept nil by mouth for considerable periods of time and if patients were fed, it was usually parenterally (Mitchell et al., 2003). Over the last 20 years, however, evidence has shown that enteral feeding is safer and is associated with reduced morbidity and mortality, and best practice is now to establish feeding via the enteral route early in the evolution of disease (Petrov et al., 2009).

This is supported by a recent Cochrane review of randomised control studies comparing enteral and parenteral nutrition in pancreatitis, which concluded that enteral feeding was associated with a trend towards reduced length of stay and significant reduction in the development of multiorgan failure, systemic complications, need for surgical interventions and overall mortality when compared with patients receiving parenteral nutrition (Al-Omran et al., 2010). Although this review included studies involving patients with pancreatitis of any severity, a subgroup analysis of patients with SAP found similar conclusions. These data were supported by three other meta analyses (Petrov & Whelan, 2010; Petrov et al., 2008a; Marik & Zaloga, 2004) and a recent randomised study (Wu et al., 2010).

The European Society for Clinical Nutrition and Metabolism (ESPEN) guidelines concluded that there is strong evidence that enteral feeding in the first 5–7 days of mild pancreatitis is of no benefit but it is indicated in severe disease, even in the presence of complications such as fistula, pseudocyst and ascites, and that a peptide based feed should be used (Meier et al., 2006). Although enteral feeding is acknowledged to be the optimal feeding route for patients with acute pancreatitis, debate remains as to whether gastric or jejunal feeding is most suitable, and how early enteral feeding should be initiated.

A recent systematic review on the safety and tolerance of NG feeding in SAP found that approximately 80% of patients tolerated full feeding (Petrov et al., 2008b). It showed that there was no difference in mortality or feed tolerance between patients receiving NG or nasojejunal (NJ) feeding. However, an adequately powered randomised controlled study is needed to support the routine use of NG feeding in SAP. In practice, many patients present with nausea and vomiting, in which case NJ feeding is the enteral feeding route of choice. Further studies have reviewed the timing of initiation of enteral feeding, and concluded that there was significant reduction in the risk of multiorgan failure, infectious complications and mortality when enteral feeding was started within 48 hours of admission (Petrov et al., 2009).

Patients with SAP do not normally commence oral intake until the abdominal pain has resolved, and enteral feeding should continue until oral intake sufficient to satisfy their requirements can be maintained. Patients will often require supplementary enteral feeding in addition to a good oral intake due to the high nutritional requirements associated with this disease. The earlier ESPEN guidelines set energy requirements for patients with SAP at 25–35 kcal (100150 kJ)/kg in the active stage of the disease (Meier et al., 2002).

Chronic pancreatitis

Up to 10% of patients with chronic pancreatitis have intractable pain and malnutrition that does not respond to oral nutritional support. Enteral feeding is often used in these cases, and jejunal feeding may be helpful in cases of duodenal stenosis, delayed gastric emptying or food avoidance due to pain (Meier et al., 2006). Distal jejunal feeding can help to reduce the pain associated with chronic pancreatitis; this is known as *pancreatic rest* (Lordan et al., 2009).

Postoperative enteral feeding

Many pancreatic centres use jejunal feeding post pancreatic surgery, although route, feed formulation and timing of initiation of enteral feeding varies widely across the UK. A solid evidence base is needed to determine best practice (Phillips et al., 2009).

Novel substrates

Probiotics and immune enhancing products

Initial studies appeared to favour the use of probiotics in acute pancreatitis (Qin et al., 2008; Olah et al., 2002). However, probiotics are currently not recommended in acute pancreatitis following a large multicentred randomised double blind, placebo controlled trial in patients with SAP. Probiotic administration was associated with a significant increase in the incidence of bowel ischaemia and increased mortality in the supplemented group (Bessekink et al., 2008). A recent systematic review on the composition of enteral feeds administered to patients with acute pancreatitis concluded that probiotic and immune enhancing products did not further improve patient outcome, and are therefore not recommended (Olah & Romics, 2010).

Antioxidants

Several studies have examined the use of antioxidants for pain control in chronic pancreatitis. A randomised placebo controlled double blind trial of antioxidant supplements found an increase in the number of pain free days in the supplemented group (Bhardwaj et al., 2009). However, a meta analysis reviewing 22 randomised controlled studies concluded that there was insufficient evidence to support antioxidant therapy (Mohseni Salehi Monfared et al., 2009). Subsequent studies in patients with acute pancreatitis confirm the need for further research (Sateesh et al., 2009).

Eicosapentaenoic acid

Many studies have examined the use of fish oils in managing the dramatic weight loss seen in patients with advanced cancer, particularly pancreatic cancer. Some studies have shown weight gain and improved quality of life when eicosapentaenoic acid (EPA) supplements are used (Fearon *et al.*, 2003) However, a Cochrane review that identified five trials (including a total of 587 patients) concluded there was insufficient data to establish whether oral EPA was more effective than a placebo in improving symptoms in patients with cachexia syndrome (Dewey *et al.*, 2007).

Drug interactions

Octreotide (Sandostatin®) is used to inhibit pancreatic secretions and may be used postoperatively to prevent or treat pancreatic leaks, or to treat neuroendocrine tumours. The product literature states a reduction in pancreatic trypsin release of 76% and in amylase of 84% (Berberat *et al.*, 1999), and similar reduction is also assumed for lipase secretion; the use of octreotide is therefore associated with worsening malabsorption (Witt & Pedersen, 1989).

Lanreotide® or Sandostatin LAR® are long acting versions of octreotide.

References

Al-Omran M, Albalawi ZH, Tashkandi MF, Al-Ansary LA. (2010) Enteral versus Parenteral nutrition for acute pancreatitis. *Cochrane Database of Systematic Reviews* CD002837.

Armstrong T, Strommer L, Ruiz-Jasbon F, *et al.* (2007) Pancreaticoduodenectomy for peri-ampullary neoplasia leads to specific micronutrient deficiencies. *Pancreatology* 7(1): 37–44.

Berberat PO, Freiss H, Uhl W, Buchler MW. (1999) The role of ocreotide in the prevention of complications following pancreatic resection. *Digestion* 60: 15–22.

Bessekink MGH, van Santvoort HC, Buskens E, *et al.* (2008) Probiotic prophylaxis in predicted severe acute pancreatitis: a randomised, double blind, placebo-controlled trial. *Lancet* 371: 651–660.

Bhardwaj P, Garg PK, Maulik SK, Saraya A, Tandon RK, Acharya SK. (2009) A randomised controlled trial of antioxidant supplementation for pain relief in patients with chronic pancreatitis. *Gastroenterology* 136(1): 149–159.

Blamey SL, Imrie CW, O'Neill J, Gilmour WH, Carter DC. (1984) Prognostic factors in acute pancreatitis. *Gut* 25(12): 1340–1346.

Corfield AP, Cooper MJ, Williamson RC. (1985) Acute pancreatitis: a lethal disease of increasing incidence. *Gut* 26: 724–729.

Dewey A, Baughan C, Dean T, Higgins B, Johnson I. (2007) Eicosapentaenoic acid (EPA, an omega 3 fatty acid from fish oils) for the treatment of cancer cachexia. *Cochrane Database of Systematic Reviews* CD004597.

Duggan S, O'Sullivan M, Feehan S, Ridgway P, Conlon K. (2010) Nutrition treatment of deficiency and malnutrition in chronic pancreatitis: a review. *Nutrition in Clinical Practice* 25(4): 362–370.

Dujsikova H, Dite P, Tomandl J, Sevcikova A, Precechtelova M. (2008) Occurrence of metabolic osteopathy in patients with chronic pancreatitis. *Pancreatology* 8(6): 583–536.

Eckerwall GE, Tingstedt BB, Bergenzaun PE, Andersson RG. (2007) Immediate oral feeding with mild acute pancreatitis is safe and may accelerate recovery – a randomised clinical study. *Clinical Nutrition* 26(6): 758–763.

Fearon KCH, von Meyenfeldt MF, Moses AGW, *et al.* (2003) Effect of a protein and energy dense n-3 fatty acid enriched oral supplement on loss of weight and lean tissue in cancer cachexia: a randomised double blind trial. *Gut* 52: 1479–1486.

Hammer HF. (2010) Pancreatic exocrine insufficiency: diagnostic evaluation and replacement therapy with pancreatic enzymes. *Digestive Diseases* 28(2): 339–343.

Jacobson BC, Vander Vliet MB, Hughes MD, Maurer R, McManus K, Banks PA. (2007) A prospective, randomized, trial of clear liquids versus low-fat solid diet as the initial meal in mild acute pancreatitis. *Clinical Gastroenterology & Hepatology* 5(8): 946–951.

Keller J, Layer P. (2005) Human pancreatic exocrine response to nutrients in health and disease. *Gut* 54(Suppl VI): vi1–vi28.

Khalid A, Whitcomb DC. (2002) Conservative treatment of chronic pancreatitis. *European Journal of Gastroenterology* 14(9): 943–949.

Lankisch PG. (1999) What to do when a patient with pancreatic exocrine insufficiency does not respond to pancreatic enzyme substitution: A practical guide. *Digestion* 60: 97–104.

Layer P, Melle U. (2005) Chronic pancreatitis: definition and classification for clinical practice. In: Dominguez-Munoz JE, Malfertheiner P (eds) *Clinical Pancreatology for Practising Gastroenterologists and Surgeons*. Oxford: Blackwell Publishing, Chapter 21.

Livingstone C, Davis J, Marvin V, Morton K. (2003) Vitamin A deficiency presenting as night blindness during pregnancy. *Annals of Clinical Biochemistry* 40: 292–294.

Lordan JT, Phillips M, Chun JY, *et al.* (2009) A safe, effective, and cheap method of achieving pancreatic rest in patients with chronic pancreatitis with refractory symptoms and malnutrition. *Pancreas* 38(6): 689–692.

Mann DV, Hershman MJ, Hittinger R, Glazer G. (1994) Multicentre audit of death from acute pancreatitis. *British Journal of Surgery* 81: 890–893.

Marik PE, Zaloga GP. (2004) Meta-analysis of Parenteral nutrition versus enteral nutrition in patients with acute pancreatitis. *BMJ* 328: 1407–1413.

Meier R, Beglinger C, Layer P, *et al.*, ESPEN Consensus Group. (2002) ESPEN guidelines on nutrition in acute pancreatitis. *Clinical Nutrition* 21(2): 173–183.

Meier R, Ockenga J, Pertkiewicz M, *et al.* (2006) ESPEN guidelines on enteral nutrition. *Pancreas Clinical Nutrition* 25: 275–284.

Mitchell RM, Byrne MF, Baillie J. (2003) Pancreatitis. *Lancet* 361: 1447–1455.

Mohseni Salehi Monfared SS, Vahidi H, Abdolghaffari AH, Nikfar S, Abdollahi M. (2009) Antioxidant therapy in the management of acute, chronic and post-ERCP pancreatitis: a systematic review. *World Journal of Gastroenterology* 15(36): 4481–4490.

Neoptolemos JP, Bhutani MS. (2008a) Acute pancreatitis. In: *Fast Facts: Diseases of the Pancreas and Biliary Tract*. Oxford: Health Press Limited, pp. 62–70.

Neoptolemos JP, Bhutani MS. (2008b) Pancreatic cancer. In: *Fast Facts: Diseases of the Pancreas and Biliary Tract*. Oxford: Health Press Limited, pp. 93–94.

Olah A, Romics L. (2010) Evidence-based use of enteral nutrition in acute pancreatitis. Langenbecks. *Archives of Surgery* 395(4): 309–316.

Olah A, Belagyi T, Issekutz A, Gamal ME, Bengmark S. (2002) Randomised clinical trial of specific lactobacillus and fibre supplement to early enteral nutrition in patients with acute pancreatitis. *British Journal of Surgery* 89(9): 1103–1107.

Petrov M,S Whelan K. (2010) Comparison of complications attributable to enteral and parenteral nutrition in predicted severe acute pancreatitis: a systematic review and meta-analysis. *British Journal of Nutrition* 103(9): 1287–1295.

Petrov MS, van Santvoort HC, Besselink MGH, van der Heijden GJMG, Windsor JA, Gooszen HG. (2008a) Enteral nutrition and the risk of mortality and infectious complications in patients with severe acute pancreatitis: A meta-analysis of randomised trials. *Archives of Surgery* 143(11): 1111–1117.

Petrov MS, Correia MI, Windsor JA. (2008b) Nasogastric tube feeding in predicted severe acute pancreatitis. A systematic review of the literature to determine safety and tolerance. *Journal of the Pancreas* 9(4): 440–448.

Petrov MS, Pylypchuk RD, Uchugina AF. (2009) A systematic review on the timing of artificial nutrition in acute pancreatitis. *British Journal of Nutrition* 101: 787–793.

Phillips M, Lordan JT, Menezes N, Karanjia ND. (2009) Feeding patients following pancreaticoduodenectomy; A UK national survey. *Annals of the Royal College of Surgeons of England* 91(5): 385–388.

Qin HL, Zheng JJ, Tong DN, *et al.* (2008) Effect of *Lactobacillus plantarum*. Enteral feeding on the gut permeability and septic complications in the patients with acute pancreatitis. *European Journal of Clinical Nutrition* 62: 923–930.

Sakorafas GH, Lappas C, Mastoraki A, Delis SG, Safioleas M. (2010) Current trends in the management of infected necrotizing pancreatitis. *Infectious Disorders – Drug Targets* 10(1): 9–14.

Sateesh J, Bhardwaj P, Singh N, Saraya A. (2009) Effect of antioxidant therapy on hospital stay and complications in patients with early acute pancreatitis: a randomised controlled trial. *Tropical Gastroenterology* 30(4): 201–206.

Sathiaraj E, Murthy S, Mansard MJ, Rao GV, Mahukar S, Reddy DN. (2008) Clinical trial: oral feeding with a soft diet compared with clear liquid diet as initial meal in mild acute pancreatitis. *Alimentary Pharmacology & Therapeutics* 28(6): 777–781.

UK Working Party on Acute Pancreatitis. (2005) UK Guidelines for the management of acute pancreatitis. *Gut* 54: 1–9.

Witt K, Pedersen NT. (1989) The long-acting somatostatin analogue SMS 201-995 causes malabsorption. *Scandinavian Journal of Gastroenterology* 24(10): 1248–1252.

Wu XM, Ji KQ, Wang HY, Li GF, Zang B, Chen WM. (2010) Total enteral nutrition in prevention of pancreatic necrotic infection in severe acute pancreatitis. *Pancreas* 39(2): 248–251.

7.4.6   Malabsorption

Helen Truby, Kathryn Hart and Janeane Dart

Key points

■ Malabsorption may be nutrient specific (affecting fat or carbohydrate) or more generalised (impairing the absorption of all or many nutrients). It may be the manifestation of a primary absorptive defect or a symptom of another underlying condition.

■ Tests for malabsorption commonly measure malabsorbed compounds in urine or faeces, absorbed compounds in blood or breath, or the activity of digestive enzymes. Breath tests can also be used to make an indirect assessment of carbohydrate malabsorption.

■ The aims of dietary treatment are replacement of lost fluid and electrolytes, symptom relief and achievement of nutritional adequacy (monitoring and replacing nutrient deficiencies).

Malabsorption has many different causes (Table 7.4.4). Dietary measures can be used to alleviate symptoms and nutritional supplementation may be necessary to correct nutritional depletion or prevent further nutritional deterioration. It is however vital that the underlying cause of the malabsorption is identified and, if possible, treated.

Diagnostic features

Clinical features of malabsorption may include some or all of the following:

- Diarrhoea or change in stool consistency.
- Abdominal distension.
- Flatulence or wind.
- Loss of weight in adults or growth failure in children.
- Hypoproteinaemia (or low albumin).
- Iron deficiency anaemia or low serum ferritin.

Generalised nutrient deficiencies are likely and the risk of specific deficiencies is heightened by disease or resection in particular sites of the gastrointestinal tract, chronic diarrhoea and/or self imposed dietary restriction (Figure 7.4.4). The elderly, infants and young children are particularly at risk of dehydration with loss of fluid and electrolytes during acute episodes of diarrhoea.

Very loose stools, with or without urgency, is the most common presenting feature and the nature of the stool often indicates the type or site of the malabsorption:

- *Fat malabsorption* results in steatorrhoea, where the stool is pale, malodorous, greasy and unformed. Stools are often difficult to flush and may leave a greasy residue in the toilet.
- *Carbohydrate malabsorption* more typically results in diarrhoea that is watery and frothy due to the presence of fermented sugars.
- If more than one nutrient is malabsorbed, e.g. due to loss of absorptive surface or pancreatic insufficiency, this distinction is less clear-cut and for milder forms of malabsorption, no stool abnormalities may be reported, e.g. iron deficiency anaemia is a common presenting feature of adults with untreated coeliac disease.

The term malabsorption is often used to incorporate states that should be more correctly defined as maldigestion. Maldigestion refers to any disruption to the digestive (rather than absorption) phases of food and nutrient processing, specifically those relating to enzyme activity.

Clinical tests

Investigations for malabsorption utilise either measurement of absorbed test substances in the blood or urine,

Table 7.4.4 Common causes of malabsorption

Reason for malabsorption	Common causes
Reduced absorptive capacity	Intestinal resection Short bowel syndrome Villous atrophy, e.g. coeliac disease; tropical sprue Active inflammatory bowel disease Gastro- and jejuno-colic fistulae Infiltration, e.g. amyloid, scleroderma, lymphoma Vascular insufficiency Mucosal damage, e.g. drugs or irradiation, or following surgery or serious gastroenteritic infection Some bariatric surgery procedures: biliopancreatic diversion with duodenal switch procedure, Roux-en-Y gastric bypass
Enzyme deficiencies	Disaccharidase deficiency, e.g. primary alactasia or secondary lactase deficiency Lipase and or proteolytic enzyme deficiency, e.g. pancreatic insufficiency
Intra lumenal factors	High pH in duodenum, e.g. achlorhydria Low pH in duodenum, e.g. Zollinger–Ellison syndrome Bile salt deficiency, e.g. obstructive jaundice
Infection	Deconjugation of bile salts by bacterial colonisation of the small intestine, e.g. blind loop syndrome Competition for nutrients, e.g. parasitic infections Rapid intestinal transit time, e.g. gastroenteritis
Impaired transport mechanisms	Impaired fat transport, e.g. congenital lymphangiectasia, retroperitoneal fibrosis Impaired monosaccharide transport, e.g. congenital primary malabsorption of glucose and galactose, secondary glucose malabsorption following surgery, protein energy malnutrition or gastroenteritis

or quantification of unabsorbed substances in faeces and/or urine.

Fat

Although the 3-day quantification of stool fat has been the standard test for determining fat malabsorption, this test is poorly reproducible, non-diagnostic and unpleasant for the client. More specific tests using a single small stool sample, such as immunoreactive trypsinogen, faecal elastase-1, faecal chymotrypsin and faecal microscopy, are all used as indicators of pancreatic dysfunction. Breath tests for fat malabsorption, including the use of labelled (^{14}C) triolein or a labelled mixed triglyceride fat load may provide an assessment of both lipolysis and absorption in adults, but are not suitable for infants and very young children.

Carbohydrate

The most useful test for the diagnosis of carbohydrate malabsorption is the hydrogen breath test. Normally cells do not produce hydrogen but in the colonic gut flora will do so if a suitable substrate, such as an unabsorbed disaccharide, is present. The hydrogen then produced will be absorbed into blood and can be detected and measured as it is exhaled via the breath. Measurement of breath hydrogen following a test load of lactose (25–50 g) is recommended for the diagnosis of lactose malabsorption, offering similar specificity and sensitivity to alternative methods (mucosal lactase assay and lactose tolerance test), but in a simpler and less invasive way. This test is associated with a false negative rate of up to 25% and a

trial of a lactose free diet may be considered if malabsorption is still suspected despite a negative test result. New criteria have been proposed to reduce the frequency of false negative results (Di Stefano *et al.*, 2004). In infants, unabsorbed lactose in the stool can be clearly identified by paper chromatography or other tests for faecal reducing substances.

The generic methods of breath testing, mucosal enzyme assays (via endoscopic biopsy) and oral tolerance tests can be applied to other disaccharides if specific malabsorption is suspected.

Tests for non-nutrient specific malabsorption

Non-nutrient specific malabsorptive diarrhoea may be caused by generalised loss of absorptive capacity, pancreatic insufficiency or small bowel bacterial overgrowth. Certain bariatric procedures deliberately induce modest (Roux-en-Y gastric bypass) or substantial malabsorption (biliopancreatic diversion with duodenal switch procedure), which then require specific dietetic advice to ensure micronutrient sufficiency (see Chapter 7.13.3). Similarly, malabsorption is often also a key feature of short bowel syndrome, and in these cases the dietitian needs to be actively involved in the management of nutrient, fluid and electrolyte abnormalities and symptom management (see Chapter 7.4.9).

Serological testing (IgA antiendomysial antibodies, antihuman tissue transglutaminase and IgG deamidated gliadin peptide) may be used to assess the likelihood of coeliac disease in symptomatic individuals, with confirmation using the gold standard method of endoscopic jejunal biopsy (see Chapter 7.4.7). No optimal test for

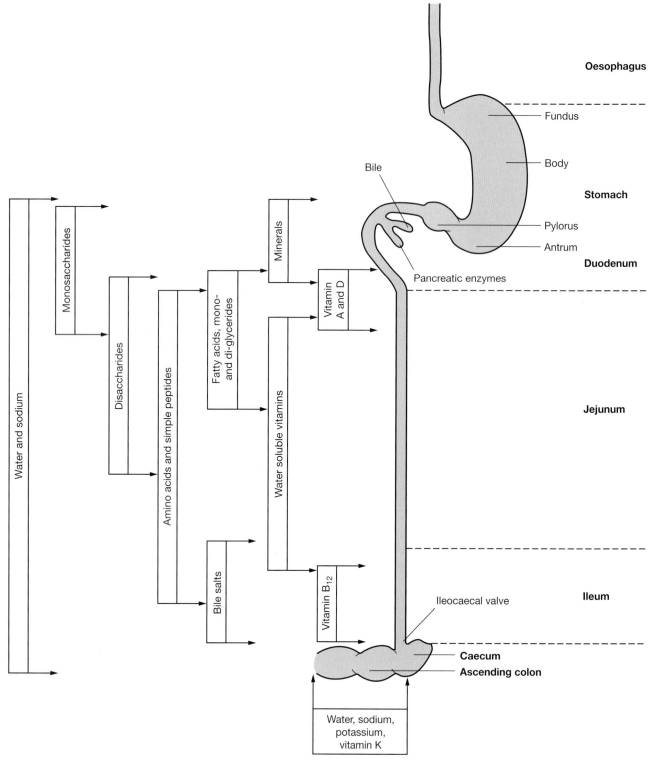

Figure 7.4.4 Principal absorption sites for nutrients

small bowel bacterial overgrowth has been identified. Cultures of small bowel aspirates are recommended, although less sensitive hydrogen breath tests are easier to perform and are more frequently employed. Non-invasive tests for pancreatic insufficiency are limited by the large reserve capacity of the pancreas, which means that 90%

tissue involvement may be required before reductions in pancreatic enzyme secretions are seen. Imaging techniques are used to investigate changes in pancreas structure in severe insufficiency, but faecal elastase remains the first line assessment for malabsorption of suspected pancreatic origin (Thomas *et al.*, 2003).

Dietary treatment

Whatever the cause of malabsorption, the principles of dietary therapy remain consistent:

- Daily replacement of large losses of fluid and electrolytes.
- Dietary treatment of the primary disorder, e.g. removal of gluten in coeliac disease.
- Dietary measures to provide symptom relief.
- Work towards restoring optimal nutritional status, with supplementation for micronutrients and/or trace elements as required.

Specific aspects of particular types of malabsorption are considered below.

Fat malabsorption

The main nutritional significance of the loss of fat is the associated loss of energy and fat soluble vitamins A, D, E and K. Unabsorbed fatty acids may also form complexes with minerals such as calcium and iron, thus inhibiting their absorption. This can increase the risk of long term complications such as iron deficiency anaemia or osteoporosis.

In those with proven chronic malabsorptive states, supplements of fat soluble vitamins will be required to restore losses and prevent further deficiency. In cases of persistent malabsorption, it may be necessary to administer these in a micelleised (water soluble) form or by injection. In children, deficiency of essential fatty acids can occur, necessitating supplementation. Zinc status can also be compromised and measurement of red blood cell zinc can guide the need for supplementation.

Steatorrhoea compromises nutritional status due to energy loss via the stool and may be exacerbated by self selection of low fat foods for symptom relief by the patient. Steatorrhoea due to pancreatic insufficiency can be treated with pancreatic enzymes and clinical practice guidelines exist for both the most common causes, namely cystic fibrosis (see Chapter 7.4.13) and pancreatitis (see Chapter 7.4.5). If despite additional drug therapy (options include the addition of a proton pump inhibitor or acid suppression with an H_2 blocker), the symptoms of steatorrhoea continue to be unacceptable, or are causing electrolyte disturbances or mineral deficiencies, dietary fat intake can be reduced (30% energy), replacing energy via modular carbohydrate supplementation (see Chapter 6.3). Alternatively or additionally, a proportion of long chain triglycerides (LCTs) can be substituted with medium chain triglycerides (MCTs). MCTs are more readily hydrolysed by pancreatic enzymes and about one-third of ingested MCTs can directly enter mucosal cells and be hydrolysed by a mucosal lipolytic system, the medium chain fatty acids then passing into the portal vein.

Intervention studies generally use MCT containing supplements and formulae as pure MCT supplements are often unpleasant and poorly tolerated. If used for cooking, the oil must not be heated above 150–160°C or its palat-ability is further impaired. Medium chain triglycerides can cause osmotic diarrhoea and so divided doses of 1 mL, four times a day [providing 1463–1672 kJ (350–400 kcal)] may be better tolerated.

There is good evidence that in acute pancreatitis, elemental or semi elemental feeds are effective when delivered via a tube placed past the ligament of Treitz; there is less evidence of effectiveness of this approach in mild or moderate pancreatitis, although this is accepted in practice (Pancreatitis Practice Guidance Summary www .pennutrition.com).

Carbohydrate malabsorption

Lactose malabsorption

The enzyme lactase is required for the breakdown of the disaccharide lactose into galactose and glucose, which are absorbed. Varying degrees of deficiency of lactase can lead to lactose remaining within the intestine, causing osmotic diarrhoea. Colonic bacteria further ferment the lactose, resulting in symptoms such as abdominal distension, flatulence and explosive watery diarrhoea, which is often acidic in nature and may cause perianal dermatitis. Lactose intolerance occurs in three main forms.

Congenital alactasia

This is a rare autosomal recessive disorder characterised by complete absence of lactase, and requires total and permanent lactose exclusion. The symptoms of profuse watery diarrhoea appear soon after initial feeding with a lactose containing milk. Breastfeeding is contraindicated and the use of lactose free infant formulae is essential. Paediatric dietetic expertise will be required to ensure that the diet remains lactose free but nutritionally adequate from weaning onwards.

Primary lactase deficiency

A gradual reduction in lactase production (lactase non-persistence) causes symptoms of lactose maldigestion in older children and adults (Enattah et al., 2002). This autosomal recessive trait is particularly common in people whose genetic origins lie in countries where milk consumption after infancy is traditionally rare, i.e. South East Asia, India, the Middle East and parts of Africa. The prevalence may exceed 50% in South America, Africa and Asia, and reaching almost 100% in some Asian countries. Data from the USA suggest a prevalence of between 15% (in white people) and 80% (in black people), whilst European rates range from 2% in Scandinavia to about 70% in Sicily (Sahi, 1994).

In lactase non-persistence, undigested lactose and the products of its bacterial fermentation can cause the gastrointestinal symptoms described earlier, although not everyone with low lactase levels has physical symptoms of lactose intolerance (Iqbal et al., 1996). The clinical effects are dose related and only become marked at high levels of intake, e.g. 50-g loads. Many malabsorbers can tolerate moderate intakes of milk products and complete avoidance of lactose is unnecessary and undesirable due to most dairy foods being nutrient dense. Instead,

SECTION 7

symptoms should be stabilised at a low intake and lactose containing foods then reintroduced in gradually increasing amounts. The individual level of tolerance varies, but most people with low lactase levels can consume 6 g/serving without discomfort (Johnson *et al.*, 1993). In some cases, up to 25 g/day (spread throughout the day) or sufficient dairy products to provide 1500 mg of calcium/day may be well tolerated (Suarez *et al.*, 1997; 1998). Fermented milk products may be better tolerated with both delayed gastric emptying and increased transit time being cited as possible reasons, along with the positive effects of certain probiotic strains of bacteria. Yogurts that contain some microbial beta-galactosidase can result in the beneficial proliferation of colonic flora such as bifidobacteria, which can metabolise lactose, and regular lactose ingestion can actually improve tolerance over time (Hertzler & Savaiano, 1996, de Vrese *et al.*, 2001). Exogenous lactase via drops or tablets can be added to milk to reduce lactose load or ready to drink reduced lactose milks and reduced lactose yoghurts are available.

Symptoms may also be less likely to occur if lactose is consumed with food rather than in isolated liquid form such as a glass of milk between meals (Vesa *et al.*, 1996). There is some evidence that temperature may also be related to tolerance, with warm milk being less well tolerated, but there is individual variation (Peuhkuri *et al.*, 2000).

Since the clinical effects of lactose intolerance are similar to those of irritable bowel syndrome, the possibility of primary lactase deficiency should always be considered, particularly in genetically susceptible groups or in children complaining of recurrent abdominal pain, where more common organic causes have already been excluded. It should also be borne in mind that the prevalence of lactose intolerance may be overestimated, with similar gastrointestinal symptoms resulting from a range of other physiological and psychological factors, including milk aversion (McBean & Miller, 1998; Rosado, 1997; Suarez & Levitt, 1996). In those with irritable bowel syndrome (IBS), tolerance to fermentable carbohydrates (fructose and lactose in particular) may be worth investigating further as they have been demonstrated to elicit IBS symptoms in some individuals (Gibson & Shepherd, 2010). Quantification of fructans and other short chain carbohydrates in grains and cereals is available (Biesiekierski *et al.*, 2011). A clinical pathway for IBS management can be found in Chapter 7.4.10.

Secondary lactase deficiency

This is a common, usually temporary, consequence of damage to the intestinal brush border as a result of severe gastroenteritis, intestinal surgery, chemotherapy, HIV and AIDS, untreated coeliac disease or cow's milk protein intolerance. The condition is characterised by diarrhoea that persists after the primary disorder has been treated and is particularly likely to occur in infants and children. Severe secondary lactose intolerance is sometimes accompanied by secondary sucrose intolerance.

Although transient in nature, it may take weeks rather than days for lactase secretion to be adequately re-established. Most lactase production takes place in the older cells at the tips of the villi rather than in the newer cells at the base. Lactase production is therefore the first of the disaccharidases to be affected by damage to the villi and the last to be restored.

Management depends on the severity of symptoms. In adults and children, avoidance of lactose for a few days will cause symptoms to subside and it can then gradually be reintroduced into the diet with the use of foods such as lactose reduced milk, fermented milk products such as yogurt and hard cheeses. As tolerance improves, the range of lactose containing foods and their level of consumption can be increased. Because the condition is usually resolved within a relatively short timescale, the avoidance of milk and milk based foods, even by children, is unlikely to pose a nutritional problem. However, if lactose (and hence milk) restriction is required for >3–4 weeks, the question of nutritional adequacy in terms of calcium, protein and energy will need to be addressed.

Formula fed infants with secondary lactase deficiency may require a lactose free infant formula as a temporary substitute for cow's milk. Breast milk is usually tolerated but in severe cases, partial or total substitution by a lactose free formula may be necessary. If the secondary lactase intolerance has resulted from an intolerance to cow's milk protein, an alternative milk free, lactose free formula will be required (see Chapter 7.11.2).

Malabsorption of other disaccharides

Primary disaccharidase deficiencies

Congenital disorders such as sucrose–isomaltase deficiency can occur but are rare. Management requires total avoidance of the disaccharide substrate.

Secondary disaccharidase deficiency

Production of enzymes such as sucrase and maltase is less likely to be affected by intestinal damage than lactase, but severe enteropathies or infections, particularly in children, may result in malabsorption of disaccharides, such as sucrose coexisting alongside lactose malabsorption. Temporary avoidance of major sources of sucrose followed by its gradual reintroduction may be necessary.

Monosaccharide malabsorption

Fructose

A natural sweetener with a low glycaemic index, fructose occurs naturally in fruit, vegetables and honey in varying proportions either in the monosaccharide form or bound with sucrose as a disaccharide, such as in sugar cane and sugar beet. In processed foods, high fructose corn syrup (HFCS) has different properties as it is derived from hydrolysed corn starch. There is emerging evidence that excess consumption of fructose and HFCS in particular could be contributing to adiposity, dyslipidaemia, the metabolic syndrome and non-alcoholic fatty liver disease (Elliott *et al.*, 2002; Bantle *et al.*, 2000; Ouyang *et al.*, 2008).

Fructolysis occurs in the small intestine, with fructose being transported to the liver via the GLUT5 mechanism, which does not require insulin. Unabsorbed fructose enters the colon where it is a substrate for bacteria, which produce short chain fatty acids, organic acids and gases. A range of gastrointestinal disturbances such as bloating, abdominal pain, loose stools and flatulence are symptomatic consequences of colonic fermentation byproducts and may become more common in adults as dietary fructose consumption increases (Beyer *et al.*, 2005).

In very young children, apple and pear juices that contain a large proportion of free fructose have been linked to toddler diarrhoea, which resolves when dietary fructose is limited (see Chapter 3.8.12). The breath hydrogen test can be used alongside diet and symptom diaries to gauge individual tolerance to fructose.

Secondary malabsorption of monosaccharides

This may occur in infants following surgery, protein energy malnutrition or gastroenteritis. An initial period of intravenous fluids is often necessary to correct water and electrolyte imbalances. This will be followed by the use of a carbohydrate free formula, during which time there should be careful monitoring for signs of hypoglycaemia. The problem is thought to be one of monosaccharide malabsorption, since disaccharidase activity is normal. The ability to tolerate carbohydrates slowly improves and a monosaccharide such as glucose or fructose may be added to the diet in increasing increments of 1% of normal carbohydrate intake. These children are often underweight and gravely ill, and parenteral nutrition may be life saving if resumption of adequate oral nutrition is delayed. The detailed dietary management of carbohydrate malabsorption in infants and children should be sought in paediatric dietetic textbooks (see Chapter 3.8).

Protein malabsorption

Malabsorption states in which there is a deficiency of enzymes or proenzymes involved in protein digestion, e.g. enterokinase or trypsinogen, are not indications for the dietary restriction of protein. When increased protein losses occur due to an enteropathy or malabsorption, a high protein intake (0.5–1.5 g/kg/day) should be prescribed to allow for the decreased efficiency of absorption. If fat malabsorption is present, foods with a high protein content but which are also low in fat must be selected. Modular protein supplements can be used in conjunction with glucose polymers (Chapter 6.3 and Appendix A10).

Pancreatic enzyme replacement therapy is often a central aspect of management of such malabsorption and maldigestion states that lead to pancreatic insufficiency (Toouli *et al.*, 2010) and more specifically in cystic fibrosis (see Chapter 7.4.13).

Internet resources

Pancreatitis Practice Guidance Summary   www.pennutrition.com

References

Bantle JP, Raatz SK, Thomas W, Georgopoulos A. (2000) Effects of dietary fructose on plasma lipids in healthy subjects. *American Journal of Clinical Nutrition* 72(5): 1128–1134.

Beyer PL; Caviar EM, McCallum RW. (2005) Fructose intake at current levels in the United States may cause gastrointestinal distress in normal adults. *JAMA* 105 (10): 1559–1566.

Biesiekierski JR, Rosella O, Rose R, *et al.* (2011) Quantification of fructans, galacto-oligosaccharides and other short-chain carbohydrates in processed grains and cereals. *Journal of Human Nutrition and Dietetics* 24(2): 154–176.

De Vrese M, Stegelmann A, Richter B, Fenselau S, Laue C, Schrezenmeir J. (2001) Probiotics–compensation for lactase insufficiency. *American Journal of Clinical Nutrition* 73(2Suppl): 421S–429S.

Di Stefano M, Missanelli A, Miceli E, Strocchi A, Corazza GR. (2004) Hydrogen breath test in the diagnosis of lactose malabsorption: Accuracy of new versus conventional criteria. *Journal of Laboratory and Clinical Medicine* 144 (6): 313–318.

Elliott SS, Keim NL, Stern JS, Teff K, Havel PJ. (2002) Fructose, weight gain, and the insulin resistance syndrome. *American Journal of Clinical Nutrition* 76(5): 911–922.

Enattah NS, Sahi T, Savilahti E, Terwilliger JD, Peltonen L, Järvelä I. (2002) Identification of a variant associated with adult-type hypolactasia. *Nature Genetics* 30(2): 233–237.

Gibson PJ, Shepherd SJ. (2010) Evidence-based dietary management of functional gastrointestinal symptoms: The FODMAP approach. *Journal of Gastroenterology and Hepatology* 25(2): 252–258.

Hertzler SR, Savaiano DA. (1996) Colonic adaptation to daily lactose feeding in lactose maldigesters reduces lactose intolerance. *American Journal of Clinical Nutrition* 64: 232–236.

Iqbal TH, Bradley R, Reilly HM, Lewis KO, Cooper BT. (1996) Small intestinal lactase status, frequency of distribution of enzyme activity and milk intake in a multi-ethnic population. *Clinical Nutrition* 15: 297–302.

Johnson AO, Semenya JG, Buchowski MS, Enwonwu CO, Scrimshaw NS. (1993) Adaptation of lactose maldigesters to continued milk intakes. *American Journal of Clinical Nutrition* 58: 879–881.

McBean LD, Miller GD. (1998) Allaying fears and fallacies about lactose intolerance. *Journal of American Dietetic Association* 98: 671–676.

Ouyang X, Cirillo P, Sautin Y, *et al.* (2008) Fructose consumption as a risk factor for non-alcoholic fatty liver disease. *Journal of Hepatology* 48(6): 993–999.

Peuhkuri K, Vapaatalo H, Nevala R, Korpela R. (2000) Temperature of a test solution influenced abdominal symptoms in lactose tolerance tests. *Scandinavian Journal of Clinical Laboratory Investigation* 60(1): 75–80.

Rosado JL. (1997) Lactose digestion and maldigestion: Implications for dietary habits in developing countries. *Nutrition Research Reviews* 10: 137–149.

Sahi T. (1994) Hypolactasia and lactase persistence. Historical review and the terminology. *Scandinavian Journal of Gastroenterology Supplements* 202: 1–6.

Suarez FL, Levitt MD. (1996) Abdominal symptoms and lactose: The discrepancy between patients' claims and the results of blinded trials. *American Journal of Clinical Nutrition* 64: 251–252.

Suarez FL, Savaiano D, Arbisi P, Levitt MD. (1997) Tolerance to the daily ingestion of two cups of milk by individuals claiming lactose intolerance. *American Journal of Clinical Nutrition* 65: 1502–1506.

Suarez FL, Adshead J, Furne JK, Levitt MD. (1998) Lactose maldigestion is not an impediment to the intake of 1500mg calcium daily as dairy products. *American Journal of Clinical Nutrition* 68: 1118–1122.

Thomas PD, Forbes A, Green J, *et al.* (2003) Guidelines for the investigation of chronic diarrhoea, Second edition. *Gut* 52(Suppl V): v1–v15.

SECTION 7

Toouli J, Biankin, AV, Oliver MR, Pearce CB, Wilson JS, Wray NH. (2010) Management of pancreatic exocrine insufficiency: Australasian Pancreatic Club recommendations. *Medical Journal of Australia* 193(8): 461–467.

Vesa TH, Marteau P, Zidi S, Briet F, Pochart P, Rambaud JC. (1996) Digestion and tolerance of lactose from yogurt and different semi-solid fermented dairy products containing Lactobacillus acidophilus and bifidobacteria in lactose maldigestion – is bacterial lactase important? *European Journal of Clinical Nutrition* 50: 730–733.

7.4.7 Coeliac disease

Helen Fraser-Mayall

Key points

- The prevalence of coeliac disease is 1 in 100. It affects people of all ages, although the average age of diagnosis is between 40 and 60 years.

- It is a multisystem disease that affects many organs, not just the gastrointestinal tract.

- Treatment is a lifelong gluten free diet that avoids wheat, rye and barley and their derivatives. Some patients may also be sensitive to oats.

- Dietetic management aims to optimise absorption of nutrients and help prevent or treat complications, e.g. osteoporosis.

- Dietetic advice needs to be tailored to individual needs due to varying degrees of sensitivity to gluten.

- The prevalence of type 1 diabetes and autoimmune thyroid disease is increased in patients with coeliac disease.

Coeliac disease is an inflammatory condition of the small intestinal mucosa that is induced by the ingestion of gluten and which improves clinically and histologically when gluten is excluded from the diet. It is alternatively termed coeliac sprue or gluten sensitive enteropathy. Gluten is often used as a generic term to collectively describe all the cereal proteins that are toxic to individuals with coeliac disease. Wheat, barley and rye have all been shown to cause intestinal inflammation in coeliac patients, but the possible toxicity of oats continues to be debated (British Society of Gastroenterology (BSG), 2010). Coeliac disease can present at any age and has a wide range of clinical manifestations. The average age of diagnosis has risen in the UK to 40–60 years (BSG, 2010).

Traditionally, coeliac disease has been associated mainly with gastrointestinal symptoms, e.g. diarrhoea, abdominal pain and bloating, as chronic inflammation of the small intestine is a feature of the immune response to gluten. However, increasingly non-gastrointestinal features of coeliac disease have been recognised in people presenting with the disease. Some people with coeliac disease have no obvious symptoms (NICE, 2009). Coeliac disease is a multisystem disorder that can affect a variety of organs and can present with non-specific symptoms that may be overlooked in diagnosis (Johnston *et al.*, 1998).

Intolerance to gluten is permanent; the key treatment is lifelong adherence to a gluten free diet that can be difficult to accept and follow. Dietary compliance is associated with severity of symptoms and the more symptomatic, the greater the need for compliance with the gluten free diet (Westman *et al.*, 1999). Persistent problems are most often due to non-compliance, but other reasons are lactose intolerance, pancreatic insufficiency and microscopic colitis (Ahmad *et al.*, 2002). Gluten intolerance can also manifest itself as dermatitis herpetiformis, which appears as a cutaneous rash and may be associated with gastrointestinal symptoms.

Coeliac disease is more prevalent in people with autoimmune conditions such as type 1 diabetes or autoimmune thyroid disease, and in first degree relatives of people with coeliac disease (NICE, 2009). Primary complications of coeliac disease are osteoporosis and malignancy; however, recent work has indicated that the risk of malignancy is not as significant as previously thought (BSG, 2010).

Coeliac disease results from an immune reaction to antigenic fractions within gluten. The responsible fraction of gluten in wheat is gliadin, an alcohol soluble prolamin that is a mixture of proteins, and the different gluten peptides are involved in different ways. Some peptides cause mucosal damage by triggering an immunological pathway that has a rapid effect (innate immune response), whereas others stimulate a different immunological response (adaptive immune response) (Ciccocioppo *et al.*, 2005).

As well as gliadin in wheat, prolamins found in other cereals, e.g. secalin in rye and hordein in barley, also trigger the immunological response leading to coeliac disease. Similar proteins (avenins) are found in oats, but these are not thought to be harmful to the majority people with coeliac disease (see Oats section).

Onset and prevalence

Coeliac disease can develop and be diagnosed at any age. It was historically only associated with childhood, but now only 9% of all coeliac patients are diagnosed under the age of 16 years. This is partly due to the exclusion of gluten in infant formula and partly the increase in diagnosis rate in the adult population (BSG, 2010). Recent evidence suggests introducing gluten between 4 and 7 months while breastfeeding may reduce the risk of coeliac disease and wheat allergy (ESPGHAN, 2008). Current weaning guidelines recommend that the age range at which to begin weaning should not change unless there is strong scientific evidence (BDA, 2013).

The prevalence of coeliac disease has historically been difficult to determine because many cases with coeliac disease do not have specific signs and symptoms. Therefore, the prevalence has been considerably underestimated. In national studies in the UK, the prevalence ranges between 0.8% and 1.9%. This is broadly similar to the prevalences found in other international studies (NICE, 2009). Recognition of this higher prevalence demonstrates the clinical variability of coeliac disease (Leeds et al., 2008). It affects 1 in 100 people in the UK, making it much more common than previously thought. Delayed diagnosis is common, with 13 years being the average time from first reporting of symptoms to diagnosis. Under diagnosis is a big problem and as many as 500 000 people remain undiagnosed in the UK.

The prevalence of coeliac disease is at least 10% in first degree relatives and approximately 2% in second degree relatives (Hogberg et al., 2003). When coeliac disease is inherent in a family, there is a 1 in 10 chance that a new baby will develop the condition. There is limited evidence that the prevalence of coeliac disease is twice as high in females as in males (NICE, 2009). Coeliac disease is associated with a particular HLA genotype, with the HLA DQ heterodimer appearing to confer disease susceptibility. Approximately 95% of people with coeliac disease have been shown to have HLA DQ antigen and studies looking at identical twins have found concordance levels of 75–90% (Greco et al., 2002) (see Chapter 5.1).

Clinical presentation

In children and adults, coeliac disease can present with a broad range of signs and symptoms, the most frequent being:

* Abdominal pain, cramping or distension.
* Chronic or intermittent diarrhoea.
* Faltering growth in children.
* Fatigue.
* Iron deficiency anaemia.
* Nausea or vomiting.
* Weight loss.

Symptoms in children with coeliac disease depend on the age at presentation, and can develop following weaning and the introduction of foods that contain gluten at between 6 months and 2 years (Fasano, 2005). Under the age of 2 years the clinical picture is characterised by a lethargic or irritable child, with loose, pale, offensive smelling stools and a bloated abdomen. In infants, vomiting, anorexia and constipation may be seen. Between the ages of 2 and 16 years coeliac disease presents with gastrointestinal symptoms, nutritional deficiencies, impaired growth and generally failing to thrive. Short stature or growth delay may be picked up during weight and height assessment. Typically a child presents with:

* Loss of appetite.
* Faltering growth.
* Unhappy or clingy behaviour.
* Abnormal stools.
* Abdominal distension.
* Small stature.
* Muscle wasting.

In children with coeliac disease stools become pale, frequent and bulky. Constipation and diarrhoea may be seen and can alternate, and vomiting may also occur. Atypical symptoms may include dental enamel defects, recurrent mouth ulcers, muscle pain and stiffness. Symptoms such as anaemia and short stature are often common and it is therefore important that children are carefully monitored to ensure early diagnosis. In older children, an atypical presentation is more common, with failure to achieve normal growth.

The traditional view of a patient presenting with coeliac disease is one of being underweight. In adults, the clinical picture is very variable (Emami, 2008; Green et al., 2001; Tursi et al., 2001; Gillett et al., 2003; Lo et al., 2003; Vilppula et al., 2008). Although the onset can be acute and cause severe diarrhoea and rapid weight loss, it is usually more insidious with less obvious symptoms resulting from chronic malabsorption such as:

* Tiredness.
* Irritability.
* Depression.
* Breathlessness.
* Anaemia.
* Oedema.
* Abdominal discomfort.
* Mild gastrointestinal upsets.
* Unexplained weight loss.
* Recurrent mouth ulcers.
* Bone and joint disorders, arthralgia or osteoporotic fracture.
* Infertility.
* Dental enamel defects.
* Neurological symptoms.

The nature of these symptoms explains why the condition is not always recognised. Studies of newly diagnosed adult patients have found that fewer than half have symptoms of diarrhoea, and even fewer show signs of weight loss (Green & Jabri, 2003). Dickey & Kearney (2006) suggested that patients with coeliac disease can be of normal weight or overweight at diagnosis. Valletta et al. (2010) found that coeliac disease and obesity could coexist both in children and adolescents.

SECTION 7

The absence of signs of malabsorption can be explained by coeliac disease affecting mainly the proximal small bowel, so there is considerable functional reserve. In the absence of obvious signs of malabsorption, symptoms such as tiredness and anaemia may be attributed to other causes (Hin *et al.*, 1999). Diagnosis is therefore often missed or delayed, particularly in elderly people (Hankey & Holmes, 1994). A common misdiagnosis is irritable bowel syndrome (Shahbazkhani *et al.*, 2003). In adults, anaemia may be a particularly important indicator of coeliac disease. In coeliac patients identified by serological screening (with subsequent confirmatory biopsy), over 80% did not have gastrointestinal symptoms, but over half did have anaemia (Hin *et al.*, 1999). Coeliac disease should therefore be considered in any patient with anaemia or symptoms of tiredness, especially when there is a family history of the disease.

Diagnosis

Biochemistry

Specific circulating antibodies are present in coeliac disease and titres decrease when a gluten free diet is commenced. The National Institute for Health and Care Excellence (NICE, (2009) recommends the use of serological tests for endomysial antibodies (EMAs) and tissue transglutaminase antibodies (TTGAs) in the diagnostic process for coeliac disease. It is essential for patients to continue having a normal gluten containing diet before considering diagnostic tests for coeliac disease. The NICE (2009) guidelines recommend that if the diet has been changed, foods that contain gluten should be eaten in at least one meal every day for at least 6 weeks before testing.

However, immunoglobulin A (IgA) deficiency will produce a false negative result and people with coeliac disease are more likely to be IgA deficient: 2.5% in coeliac disease compared with 0.25% in the general population (Lenhardt *et al.*, 2004). The use of IgG antibody testing is recommended in those deficient in IgA (NICE, 2009). Therefore, a combination of TTG and EMA testing is used. Blood samples are initially tested for IgA TTG antibodies and positive results are then tested using an EMA test. Positive EMA individuals should be referred for duodenal biopsy. Those with only TTG positive results need to be considered for further evaluation, but the majority of these have antibody titres at the lower range compared with those who are also EMA positive (BSG, 2010). While these tests are useful, especially in primary care, a duodenal biopsy is necessary to confirm diagnosis. Where suspicion of coeliac disease is high, a patient should proceed to biopsy regardless of serological test results. They can also be useful as a screening tool to identify silent or undiagnosed cases of coeliac disease in high risk groups, e.g. family history of the disease, type 1 diabetes or autoimmune thyroid disease.

Small bowel histology

Duodenal biopsy should be performed in all patients suspected of having coeliac disease and all those who

merit exclusion of coeliac disease (BSG, 2010). Duodenal biopsy carries minimal risk, and has high positive and negative predictive values. Duodenal biopsies should be taken in those with:

- Positive coeliac antibodies.
- Iron deficiency anaemia.
- Folate deficiency.
- Osteomalacia.
- Malabsorption.
- Abnormal duodenal appearances.
- Significant unexplained weight loss.

Negative coeliac serology should not preclude duodenal biopsy in those who have other indications (Hopper *et al.*, 2007). Visible abnormalities at endoscopy include mucosal pallor, visible vessels, mosaic pattern, micronodular appearance, scalloping and reduction in duodenal folds. These changes have been shown to correlate with degrees of villous atrophy (Niveloni *et al.*, 1998). As with serological testing, it is essential that a gluten containing diet be maintained before a biopsy is carried out.

Marsh classification

The stages of damage to the small bowel seen in coeliac disease are graded by the Marsh (1992) classification:

- Marsh 0: normal mucosa.
- March 1: increased number of intraepithelial lymphocytes.
- Marsh 2: increased lymphocytes and crypt depth.
- Marsh 3: partial or complete villous atrophy – classic coeliac lesion.
- Marsh 4: villous atrophy without lymphocytes: rare and typically unresponsive to diet.

Long term consequences

Malignancy

Coeliac disease is associated with a small increase in the risk of malignant small intestinal lymphomas, mainly non-Hodgkin's lymphoma (West *et al.*, 2004a; Catassi *et al.*, 2005). The risk of lymphoma is reduced by adherence to a strict gluten free diet and after approximately 5 years the risk is likely to have been reduced to the level of the general population (Holmes *et al.*, 1989; Askling *et al.*, 2002). Coeliac disease also increases the risk of small bowel adenocarcinoma (Holmes *et al.*, 1989; Howdle *et al.*, 2003). However, research by Van Heel & West (2006) has suggested a decrease in the risk of breast cancer in people with coeliac disease, although the reasons for this are unclear.

Osteoporosis

Undiagnosed coeliac disease is related to low bone mineral density, osteoporosis and increased risk of fractures (NICE, 2009). Bone metabolism is disturbed and both treated and untreated people with coeliac disease appear to have an increased risk of osteoporosis. Approximately 75% of adults with untreated coeliac disease suffer from osteopenia or osteoporosis (Corazza *et al.*, 2005). Even in people with few symptoms of coeliac disease, bone mineral density can be significantly lower than in the general population. There is reduced bone mineral density, osteopenia or osteoporosis in 20– 50% of patients newly diagnosed with coeliac disease, making it the most common complication of coeliac disease (Bianchi & Bardella, 2002). Risk factors, specifically related to coeliac disease that may reduce bone mineral density and increase the risk of osteoporosis include:

- Late or delayed diagnosis of coeliac disease in adult life.
- Chronic malabsorption of calcium prior to diagnosis.
- Reduced intake of calcium following diagnosis; bread and cereal foods contribute to about 30% of daily calcium intake (Henderson *et al.*, 2003).
- Lapses from the gluten free diet.
- Persistent villous atrophy.
- Lactose intolerance.
- Low BMI.

Many of these may result in chronic malabsorption of foods, with calcium malabsorption leading to greater bone loss. There is a moderate risk of fracture in coeliac disease (Thomason *et al.*, 2003, Ludvigsson *et al.*, 2007). Following a gluten free diet helps to optimise calcium absorption and improve bone mineral density, although it may not restore this to the level found in a non-coeliac population (Corazza *et al.*, 1995, McFarlane *et al.*, 1995; Pazianas *et al.*, 2005). The prevalence of reduced bone density after 1 year of following a gluten free diet is similar to that after 3 years. This suggests that the extent of bone mass gain in the first year of dietary treatment is indicative of overall bone mineral density improvement (Corazza *et al.*, 2005). A calcium rich gluten free diet can achieve better remineralisation (Ciacci *et al.*, 1996) (see Chapter 7.9.1).

Calcium requirements in adults

The BSG (2007) guidelines for osteoporosis in inflammatory bowel disease and coeliac disease recommend 1000– 1500 mg of calcium/day for adults with coeliac disease.

Calcium requirements in children

There are no guidelines recommending a higher requirement for calcium in children with coeliac disease. It is recommended that an individualised calcium rich, gluten free diet is followed that uses reference nutrient intake values (Department of Health, 1991) as a guide (see Appendix A2).

Associated conditions

Type 1 diabetes

The association between coeliac disease and type 1 diabetes mellitus is probably due to a common genetic predisposition. The gene *HLA DQB1* is present in the majority of people with both coeliac disease and type 1 diabetes (Hervonen *et al.*, 2004; Antonio & Gino, 2009). Approxi-

mately 2–10% of people with coeliac disease will also have type 1 diabetes mellitus. Coeliac disease should therefore be suspected in any patient who has type 1 diabetes with gastrointestinal symptoms or unexplained anaemia. Presentation of coeliac disease is often silent in type 1 diabetes and many diabetes centres screen patients for coeliac disease (Saukkonen *et al.*, 1996). There is also evidence to suggest that screening of siblings should be carried out as the incidence of coeliac disease in this group has been found to be 1.3–3.8% (Sumnik *et al.*, 2005). Adherence to the gluten free diet can improve growth parameters in children and long term blood glucose control in people with type 1 diabetes (Saadah *et al.*, 2004).

Autoimmune disorders

The link between coeliac disease and autoimmune thyroid disease is well recognised, with a prevalence of autoimmune thyroid disease of 7% in coeliac disease. Graves' disease (hyperthyroidism) and Hashimoto's thyroiditis (hypothyroidism) are the most common conditions (Ch'ng *et al.*, 2005; Valentino *et al.*, 2002). Screening patients with these thyroid disorders for coeliac disease is strongly recommended (NICE, 2009). Sjögren's syndrome is an autoimmune disorder with a coeliac disease prevalence of 4.5–15% (Luft *et al.*, 2003; Rutherford, 2004).

Abnormal liver function

Elevated transaminase levels can be associated with coeliac disease, with 42% of patients newly diagnosed with coeliac disease found to have raised levels (Duggan & Duggan, 2005), the majority returning to having normal levels after commencement of a gluten free diet. Biliary cirrhosis has been linked with coeliac disease in some (Floreani *et al.*, 2002), but not all, populations (Habior *et al.*, 2003). It is recommended that people with autoimmune liver conditions should be considered for screening of coeliac disease (NICE, 2009).

Down's syndrome

The high prevalence of coeliac disease in people with Down's syndrome (5–6%) (Goldacre *et al.*, 2004; Carnicer *et al.*, 2001) is possibly explained by genetic factors, although the nature of the linkage remains to be determined (Morris *et al.*, 2000).

Dermatitis herpetiformis

Dermatitis herpetiformis is the skin presentation of coeliac disease. It is characterised by a persistent, itchy blistering rash that usually occurs on the knees, elbows, buttocks and back, although it can affect any area of skin. Intestinal biopsy nearly always shows the characteristic flattening of intestinal villi. Gastrointestinal symptoms may be mild and absent; fewer than 10% of people with dermatitis herpetiformis have gastrointestinal symptoms characteristic of coeliac disease (Caproni *et al.*, 2009).

SECTION 7

Another 20% have atypical symptoms, but >60% will have undiagnosed coeliac disease (Coeliac UK). Diagnosis of dermatitis herpetiformis is by biopsy of an unaffected area of skin. The NICE (2009) recommends that people with dermatitis herpetiformis should be screened for coeliac disease.

Dermatitis herpetiformis is less common than coeliac disease, with a UK incidence of about 1 in 10 000; it is more common in men and usually presents at 15–40 years of age, being rare in children. As with coeliac disease, there is an inherited tendency to develop the disease, and there are links with autoimmune thyroid disease and type 1 diabetes (Reunala & Collin, 1997), with both patients with dermatitis herpetiformis and family members being at increased risk of developing these disorders (Hervonen *et al.*, 2004).

The condition is managed by a gluten free diet, but as it can often take several months before the rash improves and nearly 2 years before it disappears completely, a range of medications may need to be prescribed to control the rash, including dapsone.

Patients with dermatitis herpetiformis are affected by the same long term complications at those with coeliac disease, including lymphoma (Hervonen *et al.*, 2005). There is a high prevalence of anaemia, which may be exacerbated if dapsone treatment is used. There is also increased of osteoporosis (Reunala & Collin, 1997). It is therefore important that attention is paid to the overall nutritional content of the diet, particularly in respect of micronutrients, as well as gluten avoidance.

Management

Guidelines for the diagnosis and management of CD are available, including:

- *Children:*
  - British Society of Paediatric Gastroenterology, Hepatology and Nutrition (BSPGHAN, 2006) http://bspghan.org.uk.
- *Adults:*
  - British Society of Gastroenterology (BSG, 2010) www.bsg.org.uk.
  - Primary Care Society of Gastroenterology (PCSG, (2006) www.pcsg.org.uk.
  - Clinical Resource Efficiency Support Team (CREST, (2006) www.gain-ni.org.uk.

The dietitian has a key role to play in supporting patients in the effective management of coeliac disease both in terms of optimising nutrient intake and maintaining quality of life. Diet therapy is essential in the management of patients with coeliac disease.

Dietary management

All newly diagnosed coeliac patients should have a nutritional assessment with a dietitian to establish overall dietary adequacy and associated goals. Following a gluten free diet requires specific education, which should be provided by a dietitian with experience in coeliac disease (BSG, 2010).

Dietary objectives

The dietary objectives are to ensure that people with coeliac disease:

- Exclude all dietary sources of gluten.
- Know which foods and ingredients are naturally free from gluten.
- Substitute gluten containing foods and ingredients with gluten free alternatives to improve dietary acceptability, nutritional adequacy and compliance.
- Consume a balanced diet which helps maintain health and prevent or manage associated diseases, particularly osteoporosis.

The dietitian needs to ensure that the diet is sufficiently energy and nutrient dense to meet increased needs and help restore losses. At diagnosis, iron deficiency is common as well as subclinical deficiencies of other vitamins and minerals, especially folate, vitamin D and calcium. Additional vitamin and mineral supplementation, particularly of iron, may be required for a period of weeks or months in those shown to have deficiencies.

The limited period (typically 20–30 minutes) allocated to an outpatient appointment for a newly diagnosed coeliac patient rarely allows all topics to be discussed. A survey of provision of dietetic services in the UK showed that a quarter of dietetic departments in the UK allocated 1 hour a month per 100 000 per population (Nelson *et al.*, 2007) despite the minimum recommended level of provision of 8 hours per month per 100 000. More hours were allocated where a multidisciplinary team undertook care either in a gastroenterology or specialist coeliac clinic setting. Coeliac review clinics take place both in primary and secondary care, with different healthcare professionals (HCPs) taking the lead. Dietitian led coeliac clinics are evolving in the management of patients with coeliac disease (Wylie *et al.*, 2005), although dietitian led clinics should have support from gastrointestinal physicians (Leeds *et al.*, 2008).

A new patient appointment check list is available from Coeliac UK to assist dietitians in covering the most important issues, such as a simple explanation of the principles of a gluten free diet, provision of written information on gluten containing foods, obtaining gluten free products, symptoms, cross contamination and eating out. Individuals should be encouraged to join Coeliac UK to gain access to the annually updated food and drink directory, gluten free products and manufacturers. Coeliac UK also provides a nationwide support group network and a wide range of information leaflets.

Symptoms of coeliac disease such as bloating and diarrhoea usually improve within a few weeks of commencing a gluten free diet. It often takes >12 months for mucosal damage to the small bowel to be completely repaired and villi return to normal (Dickey *et al.*, 2000), so other symptoms such as anaemia may take longer to improve. A dramatic drop in antibody levels will be seen in the first month following commencement of the diet, but antibodies may still be present 12 months after commencement of the diet. For this reason, positive antibodies or a degree of villous atrophy in the first 12 months following diagnosis do not necessarily suggest that the patient is not adhering to the diet (Midhagen *et al.*, 2004).

Dietary sources of gluten

A typical daily diet contains an estimated 10–20 g of gluten derived from multiple sources and a gluten free diet therefore necessitates the calculated avoidance of many foods (BSG, 2010). Gluten is used here as a generic term to encompass all the proteins derived from wheat (gliadins), rye (secalins) and barley (hordeins). Oats contain the gluten like protein avenins and their place in the gluten free diet is not uniform. Some people may be sensitive to avenins and individual tolerance should be assessed. Wheat flour is a particularly ubiquitous constituent of a modern diet being contained in bread, breakfast cereals, pasta, pizza, pastry, biscuits, cakes and sauces. The presence of gluten in foods made from wheat flour, such as bread, cakes, biscuits, pasta and pastry, is easy to identify. However, gluten is also a hidden component of many manufactured foods and can be present in almost any type of product, e.g. vending machine drinks. These sources are much less apparent and are also difficult to predict since some brands in a product range may contain gluten while others do not. Under European law food labels must now show the presence, or possible presence, of gluten (see Chapter 4.5).

Food labelling

If a food has a gluten containing cereal as an ingredient, this must be stated on the label. Some ingredients that are derived from gluten containing cereals, such as glucose syrup and maltodextrin, are exempt from this labelling as the level of gluten contained in them is below the level that is toxic in coeliac disease (EC 2000; EC 2003; EC 2005). Previously, the standard for gluten free was <200 parts per million (ppm) of gluten. Legislation for labelling of gluten free foods is based on the Codex standard (2008) (used in the UK and Europe); foods labelled as gluten free must contain <20 ppm of gluten, or if labelled as very low gluten, 20–100 ppm (see Chapter 4.5).

Manufactured foods may contain gluten as a result of wheat flour being added as an ingredient, processing aid, binder, filler or a carrier for flavourings and spices. Although wheat flour may only be present in small amounts, this can still be significant in terms of gluten content. Since February 2000, manufacturers are required to state in the ingredients listing the origin of starch or modified starch if this is likely to contain gluten. Other substances derived from wheat, rye, barley (or oats) may be used as an ingredient, e.g. barley malt extract.

Coeliac UK licenses the Crossed Grain symbol (Figure 7.4.5) to a growing number of manufacturers who produce gluten free foods and drinks. It is an internationally recognised symbol and registered trademark. Many food manufacturers and supermarkets use their own symbol to flag up gluten free foods. It is essential that

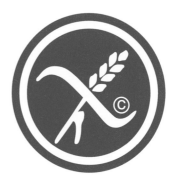

Figure 7.4.5 The Coeliac UK Crossed Grain symbol licensed to manufacturers to indicate a gluten food produce [source: Coeliac UK. Reproduced with permission of Coeliac UK (www.coeliac.org .uk)]

patients check the ingredients list on foods and not just the allergy advice box on the food label.

Contamination

Gluten may also be present due to cross contamination during production but this may not be flagged up on the label (Collin *et al.*, 2004). Contamination with wheat, rye, barley (or oats) can occur during food production or storage. For example, flour particles from foods being made in one area can be suspended in the atmosphere and cross contaminate supposedly gluten free foods being produced in another. Traceability of ingredients and minimising risk of contamination are essential components of quality control on the food industry and the food service sector. It is important that gluten free foods are not contaminated with gluten during storage and preparation.

In the home, practical measures that patients can take to reduce the risk of contamination include:

- Wash surfaces, chopping boards or utensils thoroughly before preparing food or use a separate set of utensils.
- Use a separate toaster for gluten free breads or toaster bags, or foil on a clean grill to make gluten free toast.
- Cook gluten free food in separate dishes.
- Wash hands after handling gluten containing food.
- Serve gluten free food with separate utensils.
- Use separate containers for butter, jams, chutneys, etc., or ensure that a clean knife or spoon is always used to serve them.
- Ensure that gluten free food is not prepared in a floury atmosphere.

Foods and ingredients naturally free from gluten

Most foods that have not been processed, such as fresh meat, fish, eggs, cheese, milk, fruit and vegetables, can be safely included in a gluten free diet (see Table 7.4.5).

Prescription of gluten free products

Gluten free prescribing guidelines were produced for healthcare professionals by the collaboration of Coeliac UK, BDA, BSPGHAN and PCSG (2011). The national

Table 7.4.5 Gluten content categorisation of some foods

	Gluten free	May contain gluten	Gluten containing
Cereals and flours	Manufactured gluten free products Rice (white, brown, wild, rice flour, ground rice) Maize (corn), maize starch, cornmeal, popping corn Polenta Potato flour, potato starch Soya, soya flour Bean flours (chick pea flour, split pea flour) Sago, tapioca, cassava Arrowroot Amaranth Buckwheat Millet Quinoa Sorghum Teff Cornflour	Oats (contain gluten like protein; may cause symptoms in some patients – see text)	Wheat, rye, barley Bulgar wheat, durum wheat Spelt, triticale, kamut Wheat flour (e.g. plain/self raising/strong flour) and other flours derived from rye, barley, spelt, triticale and oats Wheat starch Wheatgerm Wheat bran, oat bran Semolina, couscous Malt and malted barley
Bread, cakes and biscuits	Manufactured gluten free products, e.g. bread, rolls, crispbread, biscuits Pastry, cakes biscuits made with gluten free flours or mixes Rice cakes Cakes made without flour (e.g. macaroons) Gluten free pizza bases		Bread and bread products containing wheat, rye, barley, including croissants, brioche, naan bread, pitta bread, chapattis, parathas, ciabatta, ryebread Ordinary biscuits, crispbread, crackers, matzos, rusks Ordinary cakes and pastries, muffins and scones Pizza, pastry, croutons Batter, pancakes, Yorkshire pudding
Pasta	Manufactured gluten free pasta Corn pasta; rice pasta	Rice noodles	Fresh, dried or canned pasta and noodles
Breakfast cereals	Manufactured gluten free muesli Buckwheat flakes	Cornflakes Rice cereals Porridge oats and oatmeal	Wheat based breakfast cereals Muesli
Fruit, vegetables, pulses and nuts	Fresh, frozen, canned, dried whole or sliced fruit Fresh, frozen, canned vegetables Peas, beans, lentils Plain, roasted, salted nuts	Chips Instant mashed potato Vegetables in sauce Canned fruit pie fillings Canned baked beans Dry roasted nuts	Vegetables and potatoes coated with batter, breadcrumbs or flour Fruit pies, pasties or fruit coated with batter or flour
Milk and dairy products	Whole, semi skimmed, skimmed milk Dried skimmed milk Evaporated and condensed milk Sterilised and UHT milk Soya milk Goat's milk Cream Cheese including cheese spreads and processed cheese	Yogurts and fromage frais Coffee and tea whiteners Artificial cream	Milk with added fibre Yogurt and fromage frais containing muesli or cereals
Meat and meat products	Fresh red meat, poultry, game and offal Meat canned or prepacked in its own juices of jelly Smoked or cured pure meat such as bacon or ham Gluten free sausages Continental sausages that are 100% meat	Beefburgers Canned meat products Meat pastes, pâtés	Any type of meat coated in breadcrumbs or batter Meat pies and puddings Haggis Ordinary sausages and sausage meat Faggots and rissoles
Fish and shellfish	All fresh fish and other seafood Smoked, kippered and dried fish Fish canned in oil or brine Gluten free fish fingers	Fish in sauce Fish pastes and pâtés	Fish/shellfish in batter or breadcrumbs Fish cakes Fish fingers Taramasalata

Table 7.4.5 (Continued)

	Gluten free	May contain gluten	Gluten containing
Eggs	Whole eggs Egg yolk Egg white Meringue (free from flour)	Egg substitutes	Scotch eggs
Desserts and puddings	Jelly Sorbets Milk puddings made with gluten free ingredients Custard powders	Ice cream Instant dessert Mousses	Semolina and macaroni milk puddings Trifle Sponge and suet puddings
Fats and oils	Butter Lard Vegetable oils, margarines and fat spreads Reduced and low fat spreads		Suet
Soups, sauces and seasonings	Salt, peppercorns Tomato purée Garlic, herbs and spices Wine and cider vinegars Pickled vegetables in vinegar Gluten free stuffing mix	Canned and packet soups Packet sauces and sauce mixes 'Cook-in' sauces Bottled sauces and ketchups Stock and stock cubes Gravy browning and mixes Mustard powder Curry powder Mayonnaise, salad cream, salad dressings Pickles and chutneys Tamari (Japanese soy sauce)	Soyu (Chinese soy sauce) Mixed seasonings and spices that specify flour on the label Stuffing and stuffing mixes
Savoury snack foods	Plain potato crisps Home made popcorn Prawn crackers Pappadums	Flavoured crisps and snacks	Snack products made from wheat, rye, barley Pretzels
Preserves and spreads	Sugar, glucose, golden syrup, treacle, molasses Jam, conserves, honey, marmalade Peanut and other nut butters	Mincemeat Lemon curds and cheeses Chocolate or other sweet spreads	
Confectionery	Boiled sweets/jellies	Sweets, chocolate, toffees, etc. Iced lollies Chewing gum	
Beverages	Tea, coffee Fruit juices, fruit squash Mineral water Clear fizzy drinks Cocoa Milk Spirits, wines, liqueurs, cider, sherry, port Complan, Build-up Specialist gluten free beers	Herbal teas Chocolate powders and drinks Milk shakes and mixes Sports and health drinks	Vending machine chocolate drinks Barley waters Cloudy fizzy drinks Malted milk drinks Beer, lager, ale and stout, home brewed beers, low alcohol beers and lagers.
Miscellaneous	Gelatine Bicarbonate of soda, cream of tartar Fresh and dried yeast Tofu Food colourings, essences and flavourings Cake coverings and decorations Marzipan Meat, vegetable and yeast extracts	Baking powder	Ice cream cones and wafers Communion wafers Quorn

guidelines were based on a review of data from the National Diet and Nutrition Survey (NDNS) (Henderson *et al.*, 2003) and provide recommendations that suggest reasonable amounts of gluten free foods that should be prescribed as part of a balanced diet. These guidelines are based on the consumption of 50% of total energy as carbohydrate, with gluten free prescribable foods providing 15% of total energy. Gluten free sources of carbohydrate such as potatoes, rice and breakfast cereals make up the remaining 35% of total energy. Energy requirements of the different sexes and ages are taken into account, as well as variables such as a high activity level, pregnancy and breastfeeding (Holmes *et al.*, 2004). The guidance provides a minimum monthly requirement in unit values that are based on carbohydrate content and cost. The guidance is not mandatory and products are prescribed at the discretion of the general practitioner (GP).

In principle, prescriptions provide equal access to gluten free products. Although, increasingly, gluten free staple products are available in supermarkets, they continue to be significantly more expensive than standard staple foods (Carr, 2011). Gluten free specialist foods have been available on prescription since the late 1960s. In this time the range of products on prescription has increased and the prescribing practices have also become variable, with some people receiving more gluten free food on prescription than others. However, prescriptions may help patient adherence to a gluten free diet.

Products available on prescription

Foods such as gluten free bread, plain biscuits and crackers, pasta and pizza bases are prescribable according to the Advisory Committee on Borderline Substances (ACBS) for people medically diagnosed with coeliac disease or dermatitis herpetiformis. Prescribable gluten free flours and flour mixes are also available for home baking. The types of gluten free foods available are summarised in Table 7.4.6. Further details can be found in the *British National Formulary*, the *Monthly Index of Medical Spe-*

Table 7.4.6 Prescribable and non-prescribable gluten free foods

Type of product	Gluten free products available	Notes
Prescribable gluten free foods		
Bread and rolls	White, brown, wholemeal bread (sliced/unsliced), rolls, baguettes High fibre bread Bread mixes	Some breads and rolls are vacuum packed either fully or partially baked; a few products are available fresh (and can be frozen)
Flour substitutes	Flour mixes (white, brown, high fibre)	Can be used for home baking
Biscuits	Digestives, tea biscuits Crackers/savoury biscuits Crispbread	
Pasta	Fusilli, lasagne, macaroni, penne, rigati, spaghetti, spirals, tagliatelle	
Convenience foods	Pizza bases	
Non-prescribable gluten free foods		
Available from supermarkets, health food stores and by mail order		
Breakfast cereals	Muesli Hot breakfast cereal	
Bread products	Breadsticks Naan bread	
Biscuits	Wafers Pretzels	
Cakes	Madeira cake Ginger cake Fruit cake Rich fruit cake Cake mixes	
Seasonal fare	Mince pies Christmas pudding	
Confectionery	Chocolate bars Cereal bars Ice cream cones	
Convenience	Pizza – frozen and chilled Fish fingers Chicken nuggets Fish cakes	
Miscellaneous	Yorkshire puddings Stuffing mix	

Table 7.4.7 Manufacturers of branded gluten free foods

Manufacturer	Brand names
Bakers Delight Ltd	Bakers Delight
Community Foods	Orgran
General Dietary Ltd	Ener-G
Gluten Free Foods Ltd	Barkat, Glutano, Tritamyl, Warburtons
Heron Quality Foods Ltd	Heron Foods
Innovative Solutions	Pure
Novartis Consumer Health	Bi-Aglut
Nutrition Point Limited	Dietary Specials, Glutafin, Trufree

NB: Manufacturers and product names are liable to change. A full list of all currently available proprietary gluten free foods can be obtained from Coeliac UK.

cialities (MIMS), the Drug Tariff, or obtained directly from the manufacturers (Table 7.4.7). It should be noted that the names of both the producers and products are liable to change. A full list of all currently available proprietary gluten free foods can be obtained from Coeliac UK.

The supply of gluten free foods on prescription by prescribing schemes led by community pharmacists has been demonstrated to reduce costs by 20% (Carr, 2011) due to improved product controls, e.g. the scheme did not recommended prescribing gluten free cake mix or sweet biscuits. These are widely available in supermarkets and are not essential to the gluten free diet, although they may serve an important role in the social aspects of food and quality of life. The scheme also was able to show a considerable saving in GPs time and was preferred by patients. People with coeliac disease and dermatitis herpetiformis are not classified as chronically sick and hence not entitled to free NHS prescriptions (although the usual exemptions apply). A prepayment facility can represent a significant saving.

Gluten free cakes, fancy biscuits, cereal bars, breakfast cereals, chilled and frozen pizzas, chicken nuggets, fish fingers and fish cakes are also available for purchase but not prescribable (Table 7.4.6). They are usually more expensive than standard products, but their use may make the diet more appealing, inclusive and socially acceptable.

Oats

It was initially assumed that oats were toxic due to the observation that patients had continued symptoms whilst ingesting oats. However, many sources of oats are significantly contaminated with wheat flour during processing. Oats can be included in the diet of adults (Janatuinen *et al.*, 2002) and children with coeliac disease (Hogberg *et al.*, 2004) without causing damage to the gastrointestinal tract. In practice however, recommendations on the inclusion of oats in the diet are variable. Hernando *et al.* (2008) suggests uncontaminated oats are tolerated by most people with coeliac disease, while Lundin *et al.* (2003) found that 1 in 20 people were sensitive to uncon-

taminated oats. Further systematic reviews confirmed this (Garsed *et al.*, 2007; Haboubi *et al.*, 2006).

The exclusion of oats in a gluten free diet is still advised by some. Although it is possible that a small minority of coeliac individuals will not tolerate oats, the weight of evidence supports the safety of oats obtained from gluten free manufacturers. The BSG (2010) advises that coeliac individuals can use labelled gluten free oats safely. it also recommends that adults avoid oats for the first 6–12 months after diagnosis with coeliac disease. This is a pragmatic approach to allow for full symptom improvement before oats are introduced. Children should first be established on a strict gluten free diet and introduced to oats once the diet is established, usually after a year. The inclusion of oats in the diet should be considered on an individual basis and progress reviewed regularly.

The addition of oats in the gluten free diet has benefits in terms of improving variety and as a valuable source of fibre, especially soluble fibre. Coeliac UK produces a list of oats and oat products that are free from contamination. It is essential the person with coeliac disease is aware of the contamination risk and only uses products that are known to be safe.

Dietary balance

Lifelong dietary restrictions and an adherence to a gluten free diet can be difficult to accept and follow (Sverker *et al.*, 2005). Nutrient intake may also be compromised due to the essential avoidance of bread and cereals, which are are important sources of carbohydrate, fibre, vitamins and minerals. While gluten avoidance is the principal dietary objective, it should not be overlooked that, once optimal absorption is established on the gluten free diet, people with coeliac disease are just as likely as the general population to develop unrelated health problems such as hypertension, dyslipidaemia, obesity and type 2 diabetes, although the risk of vascular disease may be slightly less (West *et al.*, 2004b). As already mentioned, coeliac disease also conveys its own health risks such as osteoporosis. People therefore need to adopt diet and lifestyle measures that encompass all aspects of health.

Dietetic follow-up

The PCSG (2006) management guidelines recommend that after initial dietetic assessment patients are reviewed after 3 and 6 months, and thereafter annually if otherwise well. The BSG (2002) guidelines recommended regular follow up at 6–12-month intervals. The BSG (2010) guidelines recommend an annual full blood count, assessing vitamin and mineral status.

The follow-up care of patients ranges from patients being seen in specialist clinics (followed up by GPs, gastroenterologists, consultants, dietitians or nurse specialists) to being discharged back to the community without any provision for follow-up. Stucky *et al.*, (2009) concluded that a team approach was ideal, with a clinician and dietitian being necessary to provide the best follow-up care. A dietitian should supervise treatment, including follow-up, because of the potential long term complications (BSG, 2010).

Patients usually return to a follow-up appointment with lots of questions about their diet, lifestyle and experiences of living with coeliac disease. Sverker *et al.* (2005) concluded that the lived experiences of patients with coeliac disease were more varied and profound than expected. It is important to take psychological and social aspects into account and how these may potentially impact on patient compliance.

The following topics should be discussed at a review appointment:

- Gluten content of the diet.
- Calcium intake.
- Dietary compliance.
- Symptomatic improvement.
- Nutritional status.
- Blood test results.
- Gluten free prescriptions.
- Membership of Coeliac UK and use of the food and drink directory.

Ongoing dietetic support is essential both at diagnosis and follow-up to assess and review nutritional status and to review possible nutritional issues or deficiencies. It is essential for good compliance, as well as promoting an overall healthy balanced diet for long term health. An annual dietetic review is important because even experienced coeliac patients may be inadvertently consuming gluten or having an unbalanced diet (McFarlane *et al.*, 1995). Compliance to a gluten free diet is improved by regular dietetic intervention (Pietzak, 2005; Wylie *et al.*, 2005) and patients prefer to see a dietitian for long term follow-up, with a doctor available if needed (Bebb *et al.*, 2006). Serology markers cannot replace a trained dietitian's evaluation in assessment of adherence to the gluten free diet (Leffler *et al.*, 2007).

In addition, weight gain after diagnosis is common and may contribute to morbidity in the long term. Patients may have additional medical conditions, such as diabetes, which also require dietetic input. It is important that the dietitian works collaboratively with a patient to ensure that dietary advice meets an individual's needs. This should be carried out on an ongoing basis in order to improve healthcare with patient centred information and to increase quality of life.

Diet related problems

Poor compliance

Evaluating compliance is a particularly important aspect of a dietary review as the difficulties in following a gluten free diet should not be underestimated. Many patients are tempted to deviate from the dietary constraints in some circumstances, especially if there are no obvious penalties (such as unpleasant symptoms) from doing so. Compliance is particularly likely to be a problem in people found to have silent coeliac disease where the benefits from gluten avoidance will be even less obvious (Westman *et al.*, 1999). Studies indicate that compliance varies greatly in adults, with between 45% and 94% of

patients adhering to the gluten free diet (Holmes & Catassi, 2000).

The dietitian and other healthcare professionals should actively support the individual in developing strategies to effectively manage their own behaviour, e.g. through the use of behaviour change techniques, Dietitians with skills in motivational interviewing can encourage behavioural change and help with dietary adherence (Stucky *et al.*, 2009). Such skills are particularly important in helping older patients, since many patients with coeliac disease are now being diagnosed at a later age. The attitude of healthcare professionals is important, as stated by Silvester & Rashid (2007) '*rather than condemn those individuals with coeliac disease, who struggle with the complete elimination of gluten from their diet, health care professionals must adopt a more enlightened view that looks beyond non compliance as an act of individual failure or defiance to consider social factors that render compliance difficult, even for the well informed and highly motivated patient*'.

The ubiquity of gluten in food may mean that some people inadvertently consume gluten, assuming a food to be gluten free or due to cross contamination within the home, e.g. using the same bread board to slice ordinary and gluten free bread, or eating out, e.g. frying gluten free foods in oil previously used to cook a flour coated product. These aspects should be explored during a dietetic consultation. Catassi *et al.* (2007) established that gluten contamination in gluten free products could not be completely avoided. They showed that changes in the height of the villous lining of the gut occurred at an intake of 50 mg of gluten/day.

Whilst dietitians should remind patients of the reasons for compliance with a gluten free diet, it is important that they also help foster a positive dietary outlook by emphasising the many foods that can be eaten, by encouraging appropriate use of prescribable gluten free foods and by suggesting ways in which particular difficulties can be overcome. Patients should also know where to obtain further advice on queries or problems so that they feel they have a constant source of support.

Some NHS trusts, e.g. Cumbria Partnership NHS Foundation Trust, support coeliac patients by employing coeliac lifestyle advisor–patient experts. Following an initial appointment with a dietitian, a referral can be made to the advisor via the dietitian. Depending on the individual's needs, the advisor may arrange a home visit or provide training to catering and healthcare staff at nursing homes. Topics such as cross contamination, how to obtain locally sourced gluten free products and advise on eating out are discussed.

Continuing symptoms

The most common cause of continuing symptoms or a poor response to the diet is gluten consumption due to contamination, non-compliance or a high level of sensitivity. Another reason for poor response may be secondary lactose intolerance, which is common in those newly diagnosed with coeliac disease. A trouble shooting approach in dietetic management of coeliac patients is needed when patients present with ongoing symptoms. A focused dietary history is essential for the elimination of possible sources of gluten in the form of contamination, oats or foods containing malt extract. Patients who are found to be highly sensitive to gluten will need to use proprietary gluten free foods.

Non-responsive coeliac and refractory coeliac disease

Despite following a strict, gluten free diet, after 1 year an individual may remain clinically unwell; this is defined as refractory coeliac disease. Recent guidelines (Rubio-Tapia et al., 2010) provide useful information on the classification and management of refractory coeliac disease.

Levels of sensitivity to gluten

Some people are more sensitive to the effects of gluten than others and react to levels of gluten that are tolerated by other people with coeliac disease. The revised Codex standard of gluten free foods of 20 ppm will provide safer limits overall. The term gluten free implies no gluten; however, even naturally gluten free cereals, e.g. rice, can contain up to 20 ppm or 20 mg/kg of gluten. This amount of gluten is not usually toxic to people with coeliac disease who can eat unlimited amounts of products with gluten at a level of <20 ppm.

Codex wheat starch

Codex wheat starch is highly processed, which improves the texture and taste of foods, and has a level of gluten within the Codex standard. Products containing this are mainly obtained on prescription (Table 7.4.6). They are labelled as gluten free (<20 ppm) and are suitable for all people with coeliac disease. This means that gluten free foods that contain Codex wheat starch should no longer cause a problem for sensitive patients. The previous level of 200 ppm of gluten in products had an additive effect, and eating large quantities may have led to ongoing symptoms in the more sensitive individuals. Further details of Codex wheat starch can be found at www.coeliac.org.uk/healthcare-professionals/diet-information/codex-wheat-starch.

Coexisting disorders requiring dietary intervention

The presence, or subsequent development, of other disorders, including type 1 diabetes or hyperlipidaemia, requires dietetic input. Weight reducing or vegetarian diets also require individual dietetic consultation to ensure nutritionally adequacy, especially in respect of calcium intake.

Constipation

The gluten free diet may lead to a reduction in the intake of fibre due to reduced consumption of cereals, resulting in constipation. This may be alleviated by the following advice:

- Increasing fibre intake from fruit and vegetables, especially dried fruit, potato skins and pulses (peas, beans and lentils).
- Using higher fibre varieties of prescribable gluten free bread, mixes and crackers, and gluten free muesli.
- Increasing consumption of wholegrain gluten free cereals such as brown rice and buckwheat.
- Increasing fluid consumption.
- Increasing activity level.

Lactose intolerance

Newly diagnosed patients with coeliac disease may also suffer from secondary lactose intolerance as a result of gut inflammation, which results in a lactase deficiency. Lactase is found in the brush border of the small intestine. Symptoms of lactose intolerance are similar to some of the symptoms of coeliac disease, such as bloating, excess wind and diarrhoea. Once established on a gluten free diet, the inflammation subsides and lactose digestion returns to normal. Lactose intolerance is therefore usually temporary. However, it can take up to a couple of years for lactase production to return to. It is essential that during this time dietary advice is given to ensure adequate calcium intake from non-dairy sources (fortified gluten free bread or rolls, soya milk or yoghurt). Supplementation with calcium may be required to ensure adequate intake. Individuals should have their diet assessed and advice should be given on an individual basis. Lactose intolerance should be considered in patients with ongoing symptoms but who are known to be following a gluten free diet. A hydrogen breath test can diagnose lactose intolerance; this is a non-invasive test and has good sensitivity and specificity (Romagnuola, 2002) (see Chapter 7.4.6).

Type 1 diabetes

Dietary management of the combined diseases requires professional guidance from a dietitian. The aim of dietary management is to improve blood glucose control as well as support people with the gluten free diet. Children with coeliac disease and type 1 diabetes mellitus should have their growth and development carefully monitored. Gluten free alternatives to bread, pasta, biscuits and flour have approximately the same glycaemic index (GI) as their gluten containing counterparts (Packer et al., 2000) so should not compromise glycaemic control and can be incorporated into the diet in the same way as normal products. Patients should be encouraged to choose the higher fibre varieties where possible (see Chapter 7.12).

Dietary considerations in particular groups

Weaning

Breastfeeding may be protective and may delay onset of coeliac disease (Kramer & Kakuma, 2002; Hill et al., 2005). A group of researchers in Sweden has suggested that the risk of coeliac disease is reduced in children who are breastfed whilst gluten is gradually introduced into the diet (Ivarsson *et al.*, 2000; 2002). Introducing gluten containing cereals during the first 3 months of life to at risk groups of children has been found to increase the risk of coeliac disease by five times compared to when gluten is introduced between 4 and 6 months (Norris *et al.*, 2005). This study also showed that there was no benefit in delaying the introduction of gluten beyond 6 months. Guidelines regarding the age of introduction of gluten into the diet are the same regardless of family history of coeliac disease. The Food Allergy and Intolerance Specialist Group (FAISG, 2005) advice for infants with an increased risk of coeliac disease is therefore to continue breastfeeding (if possible) until the introduction of solids. Solids should not be introduced before the age of 4 months (preferably 6 months) and gluten should not be included before the age of 6 months.

Children

The North American Society for Pediatric Gastroenterology, Hepatology and Nutrition (NASPGHAN) has produced guidelines on diagnosis and management in children (Hill *et al.*, 2005). It is recommended that children with coeliac disease be monitored with periodic assessments of symptoms, growth (with signs of poor growth investigated), physical examination and adherence to a gluten free diet.

A paediatrician and paediatric dietitian should see children with coeliac disease at least once a year (ideally 6-monthly), with an initial follow-up within the first 3 months of diagnosis. An annual assessment should also be offered that should include a detailed dietary assessment to look for possible nutrient deficiencies, compliance with the diet and the need for any nutritional supplementation. If symptoms recur, then urgent clinical review is required.

In preschool children, it is generally easier if the whole family eats gluten free foods; difficulties at meal times are more likely if a young child sees that everyone else has different foods on their plate. Other children's parties need not be a problem if the situation is discussed with the host parent beforehand and a supply of gluten free food provided (although its consumption by the right child may be harder to police). Food at their own parties should be gluten free. Preschool groups present few problems since the children are usually only allowed to eat food under supervision. Play dough used in such groups is sometimes made from ordinary flour and, although flavourings are usually added to give an unpleasant taste, can occasionally be a source of gluten consumption.

It is important that a coeliac child is not excluded from school activities as well as social events, such as eating out, parties and holidays. Most children adapt surprisingly quickly to the idea that they cannot eat certain foods and are willing to take their own supply of suitable items to eat outside the home. There may however be some situations that pose temptations, e.g. the common practice of swapping snacks in the playground.

Teenagers

Rebellion against the dietary constraints of a gluten free diet is common in adolescence (Fabiani *et al.*, 1996). Studies in teenagers with coeliac disease show that only about 50–65% follow a gluten free diet (Mayer *et al.*, 1991; Kumar *et al.*, 1988). Peer group pressure may lead to consumption of takeaway or fast foods, such as fish and chips, pies, hamburgers or pizzas. Those who become ill after doing so are usually wary of future indiscretions, but others with a higher degree of gluten tolerance may not suffer any immediate symptoms. Teenagers should be reminded that damage to the intestinal mucosa will still occur, but also offered as much positive advice as possible regarding what foods can suitably be eaten when eating out with friends. Parents should also consider that the appetites of teenagers, particularly boys, can be voracious and that dietary indiscretions are more likely to occur when they are hungry; providing plenty of gluten free snacks may help.

Transition to adult services is obviously a critical period and should be addressed in a timely and sympathetic manner to meet the needs of the young person and according to the best practice guidance (Maki & Collin, 1997; Ljungman & Myrdal, 1993).

Adults

The greatest difficulties usually arise when eating away from home, but can be averted to some extent by advance planning. At work, some canteens will, with notice, provide gluten free meals and others will be willing to microwave a preprepared meal supplied by the person with coeliac disease. Hotels and restaurants can be scoped in advance and if necessary sent information about the diet. Many airlines will provide gluten free meals on long distance (not always short haul) flights if sufficient notice is given. Nevertheless, carrying a supply of gluten free rolls, crackers or similar foods is a wise precaution when travelling, on holiday or going to social functions, so that suitable foods are always available.

Pregnancy

Undiagnosed coeliac disease has been associated with reduced fertility and unfavourable pregnancy outcomes, such as an increased risk of miscarriage (Ciacci *et al.*, 1996). However, compliance with a gluten free diet reduces these risks to those of the general population. There are no specific guidelines for pregnant women with coeliac disease. Those who are diagnosed and adhering to a gluten free diet prior to conception should follow the same advice as non-coeliac pregnant women (see Chapter 3.2).

Older people

Older patients will always find it difficult to change the eating habits of a lifetime overnight, but many will do so successfully if given sufficient help in making suitable dietary substitutions. Some will also welcome feeling fitter on a gluten free diet after perhaps years of having had undiagnosed coeliac disease with consequent chronic tiredness and feeling below par.

Gluten avoidance may be more difficult in those dependent on others for meals. Meals on wheels services may not provide gluten free diets, although most will endeavour to provide suitable food choices, e.g. a piece of fruit instead of a pudding, once they understand the nature of the diet. Since the prevalence of coeliac disease among elderly people is increasing as awareness and diagnosis of the condition improves, educating residential and care homes regarding the needs of coeliac patients is particularly important.

Future developments

Despite improvements in the quality of gluten free foods, some patients still find elements of the diet difficult. Therefore, there is interest in dietary supplements (peptidases) that digest gluten in the food prior to its entry into the small intestine; however, further research is required (Tennyson *et al.*, 2009).

Further reading

Baic S, Denby N, Danna K. (2007) *Living Gluten Free for Dummies*. Chichester: John Wiley & Sons.

Coxon K. (2010) *Coeliac Disease, The Essential Guide*. Forward Press.

Gazzola A. (2011) *Coeliac Disease. What You Need to Know*. Sheldon Press.

Howdle P. (2007) *Your Guide to Coeliac Disease*. London: The Royal Society of Medicine.

Internet resources

British Society of Gastroenterology www.bsg.org.uk

British Society for Paediatric Gastroenterology, Hepatology and Nutrition (BSPGHAN) http://bspghan.org.uk

Coeliac Society of Ireland www.coeliac.ie

Coeliac UK www.coeliac.org.uk

    Codex Wheat Starch www.coeliac.org.uk/healthcare-professionals/diet-information/codex-wheat-starch

    EC Directives http://ec.europa.eu/food/food/labellingnutrition/medical/index_en.htm

Gluten-free foods: a prescribing guide www.coeliac.org.uk/document-library/378-gluten-free-foods-a-revised-prescribing-guide/

Nutrition and Diet Resources (NDR) www.ndr-uk.org

Primary Care Society of Gastroenterology (PCSG) www.pcsg.org.uk

Social networking

www.facebook.com/coeliac

www.facebook.com/coeliacuk

www.facebook.com/CoeliacSocIreland

Free from food manufacturers

A number of the larger specialist producers will send welcome packs or samples, as well as provide information and advice on coeliac disease and gluten free diets to both consumers and health professionals:

Coeliac Disease Resource Centre (CDRC) (Dr Schar) www.glutafin.co.uk

Genius Gluten Free www.geniusglutenfree.com

Glutafin Gluten Free (Care Line 0800 988 2470) www.glutafin.co.uk

Juvela (Advice Line 0800 783 1992) www.juvela.co.uk

Small manufacturers and niche products

The Cake Crusader www.thecakecrusader.co.uk

Glu-2-Go (batter mix, flavourings) www.glu2go.co.uk

Green's Gluten Free Beers www.glutenfreebeers.co.uk

Sally's Sizzling Sausage Company www.sallysizzlers.com

Tilquhillie Fine Foods (GF oats, muesli, puddings, cakes) www.tilquhilliefinefoods.com

References

Ahmad S, Abdulkarim MD, Lawrence J, Burgart MD, Jacalyn AJ, Murray MD. (2002) Etiology of non responsive celiac disease: results of a systematic approach. *American Journal of Gastroenterology* 97: 2016–2021.

Antonio Di S, Gino RC. (2009) Coeliac disease. *Lancet* 373: 140–193.

Askling J, Linet M, Gridley G. (2002) Cancer incidence in a population-based cohort of individuals hospitalised with coeliac disease or dermatitis herpetiformis. *Gastroenterology* 123(5): 142–135.

Bebb JR, Lawson A, Knight T, Long RG. (2006) Long-term follow up of coeliac disease – what do coeliac patients want? *Alimentary Pharmacology & Therapeutics* 23: 827–831.

Bianchi ML, Bardella MT. (2002) Bone and celiac disease. *Calcified Tissue International* 71: 465–471.

British Dietetic Association (BDA). (2013) Complementary feeding: introduction of solid food to an infant's diet. Avialble at www.bda.uk.com/policies/WeaningPolicyStatement.pdf. Accessed 12 August 2013.

British Society of Gastroenterology (BSG). (2002) Guidelines for the Management of patients with coeliac disease. Available at www.bsg.org.uk. Accessed 23 April 2012.

British Society of Gastroenterology (BSG). (2007) Guidelines for osteoporosis in inflammatory bowel disease and coeliac disease. Available at www.bsg.org.uk. Accessed 23 April 2012.

British Society of Gastroenterology (BSG). (2010) The management of adults with coeliac disease. Available at www.bsg.org.uk. Accessed 23 April 2012.

British Society of Paediatric Gastroenterology, Hepatology and Nutrition (BSPGHAN). (2006) Guidelines for the diagnosis and Management of coeliac disease in children. Available at http://bspghan.org.uk. Accessed 23 April 2012.

Caproni M, Anigga E, Melani L. (2009) Guidelines for the diagnosis and treatment of dermatitis herpetiformis. *Journal of the European Academy of Dermatology and Venerology* 23: 633–638.

Carnicer J, Farre C, Varea V, Vilar P, Moreno J. Artigas J. (2001) Prevalence of coeliac disease in Down's syndrome. *European Journal of Gastroenterology & Hepatology* 13 (3): 263–267.

Carr L. (2011) Prescribing of gluten free specialist foods. Coeliac UK's Position. *Dietetics Today* 37: 8–9.

Catassi C, Bearzi I, Holmes G. (2005) Association of celiac disease and intestinal lymphomas and other cancers. *Gastroenterology* 128: S79–S86.

Catassi C, Fabiani E, Iacono G, *et al.* (2007) A prospective, double blind, placebo-controlled trial to establish a safe gluten threshold for patients with coeliac disease. *American Journal Clinical Nutrition* 5: 160–166.

Ch'ng CL, Biswas M, Benton A. (2005) Prospective screening for coeliac disease in patients with Graves' hyperthyroidism using anti-gliadin and tissue transglutaminase antibodies. *Clinical Endocrinology* 62(3): 303–306.

SECTION 7

Ciacci C, Cirillo M, Auriemma G, DiDato G, Sabbatini F, Mazzacca G. (1996) Celiac disease and pregnancy outcome. *American Journal of Gastroenterology* 91: 718–722.

Clinical Resource Efficiency Support Team (CREST). (2006) Guidelines for the diagnosis and management of coeliac disease in adults. Available at www.crestni.org.uk.

Ciccocioppo R, Di Sabatino A, Corazza GR. (2005) The immune recognition of gluten in coeliac disease. *Clinical and Experimental Immunology* 140(3): 408–416.

Coeliac UK, BDA, BSPGHAN and PCSG. (2011). Gluten free foods: Revised prescribing guide. Available at www.coeliac.org.uk/sites/files/coeliac/a5_prescribing_guidelines_hires_for_print_and_web_june12.pdf. Accessed 13 August 2013.

Collin P, Thorell L, Kaukinen K, Maki M. (2004) The safe threshold for gluten contamination in gluten-free products. Can trace amounts be accepted in the treatment of coeliac disease? *Alimentary Pharmacology & Therapeutics* 19: 1277–1283.

Corazza GR, Di Sario A, Cecchetti L. (1995) Bone mass and metabolism in patients with celiac disease. *Gastroenterology* 109(1): 122–128.

Corazza GR, Di Stefano M, Maurino E. (2005) Bones in coeliac disease: diagnosis and treatment. *Gastroenterology* 19(3): 453–465.

Department of Health. (1991) *Dietary Reference Values for Food Energy and Nutrients for the United Kingdom*. London: The Stationery Office.

Dickey W, Kearney N. (2006) Overweight in celiac disease: prevalence, clinical characteristics, and effect of a gluten-free diet. *American Journal of Gastroenterology* 101: 2356–2359.

Dickey W, Hughes DF, McMillan, SA. (2000) Disappearance of endomysial antibodies in treated coeliac disease does not indicate histological recovery. *American Journal of Gastroenterology* 95: 712–714.

Duggan JM, Duggan AE. (2005) Systematic review: the liver in coeliac disease. *Alimentary Pharmacology & Therapeutics* 21: 515–518.

Emami MH. (2008) Diagnostic accuracy of IgA anti-tissue transglutaminase in patients suspected of having coeliac disease in Iran. *Journal of Gastrointestinal and Liver Diseases* 17: 141–146.

European Society Paediatric Gastroenterology Hepatology and Nutrition (ESPGHAN). (2008) Complementary feeding: A commentary by the ESPGHAN Committee on Nutrition. Available at www.espghan.org.uk. Accessed 23 April 2012.

Fabiani E, Catassi C, Villari A, *et al.* (1996) Dietary compliance in screening-detected coeliac disease adolescents. *Acta Paediatrica Supplement* 412: 65–67.

Fasano A. (2005) Clinical presentation of coeliac disease in the paediatric population. *Gastroenterology* 128: S68–73.

Floreani A, Betterle C, Baragiotta A, *et al.* (2002) Prevalence of coeliac disease in primary biliary cirrhosis and of antimitochondrial antibodies in adult coeliac disease patients in Italy. *Digestive and Liver Disease* 34: 258–261.

Food Allergy and Intolerance Specialist Group (FAISG), The British Dietetic Association (BDA). (2005) *Consensus Statement. Practical Dietary Prevention Strategies for Infants at Risk of Developing Allergic Diseases*. Birmingham: BDA.

Garsed K, Scott B. (2007) Can oats be taken in a gluten-free diet? A systematic review. *Scandinavian Journal of Gastroenterology* 42: 171–178.

Gillett PM, Drummond H, Goddard C, Shand A, Satsangi, J. (2003) Complications of coeliac disease – how common and can they be prevented? *Gut* 52: A10.

Goldacre MJ, Wotton CJ, Seagroatt V, Yeates D. (2004) Cancers and immune related diseases associated with Down's syndrome: a record linkage study. *Archives of Disease in Childhood* 89: 1014–1017.

Greco L, Romino R, Coto I, *et al.* (2002) The first large population based twin study of coeliac disease. *Gut* 50: 624–628.

Green PHR, Jabri B. (2003) Coeliac disease. *Lancet* 362: 383–392.

Green PHR, Stavropoulos SN, Panagi SG, *et al.* (2001) Characteristics of adult coeliac disease in the USA: results of a national survey. *American Journal of Gastroenterology and Hepatology* 96: 126–131.

Habior A, Lewartowska A, Orlowska J, *et al.* (2003) Association of coeliac disease with primary biliary cirrhosis in Poland. *European Journal of Gastroenterology and Hepatology* 15: 159–164.

Haboubi NY, Taylor S, Jones S. (2006) Coeliac disease and oats: a systematic review. *Postgraduate Medical Journal* 82: 672–678.

Hankey GL, Holmes GKT. (1994) Coeliac disease in the elderly. *Gut* 35: 65–67.

Henderson L, Gregory J, Swan G. (2003) The National Diet and Nutrition Survey 2002. Available at http://food.gov.uk/multimedia/pdfs/ndnsprintedreport.pdf. Accessed 13 August 2013.

Hernando A, Mujico JR, Mena MC, Lombardia M, Mendez E. (2008) Measurement of wheat gluten and barley hordeins in contaminated oats from Europe, the United States and Canada by Sandwich R5 ELISA. *European Journal of Gastroenterology and Hepatology* 20: 545–554.

Hervonen K, Viljamaa M, Collin P. (2004) The occurrence of type 1 diabetes in patients with dermatitis herpetiformis and their first-degree relatives. *British Journal of Dermatology* 150(1): 136–138.

Hervonen K, Vornanen M, Kautiainen H, Collin P, Reunala T. (2005) Lymphoma in patients with dermatitis herpetiformis and their first-degree relatives. *British Journal of Dermatology* 152(1): 82–86.

Hill ID, Dirks MH, Liptak GS, *et al.* (2005) Guidelines for the diagnosis and treatment of celiac disease in children: Recommendations of the North American Society of Pediatric Gastroenterology, Hepatology and Nutrition. *Journal of Pediatric Gastroenterology and Nutrition* 40: 1–19.

Hin H, Bird G, Fisher P, Mahy N, Jewell D. (1999) Coeliac disease in primary care: case finding study. *British Medical Journal* 318: 164–167.

Hogberg L, Faith-Magnusson K, Grodzinsky E, Stenhammer L. (2003) Familial prevalence of coeliac disease: a twenty year follow-up study. *Scandinavian Journal of Gastroenterology* 38(1): 61–65.

Hogberg L, Laurin P, Falth-Magnusson K, *et al.* (2004) Oats to children with newly diagnosed coeliac disease: a randomised double blind study. *Gut* 53: 649–654.

Holmes GK, Catassi C. (2000) *Coeliac Disease*. London: Health Press Limited.

Holmes GKT, Prior P, Lane MR, Pope D, Allan RN. (1989) Malignancy in coeliac disease effect of a gluten free diet. *Gut* 30: 333–338.

Holmes GK, Blow C, Butt S, *et al.* (2004) *Gluten-Free Foods: A Prescribing Guide*. Byfleet: Good Relations Healthcare.

Hopper AD, Cross SS, Hurlstone DP. (2007). Pre endoscopy serological testing for coeliac disease – an evaluated clinical decision tool. *BMJ* 334: 729–732.

Howdle PD, Jalal PK, Holmes GKT, Houlston RS. (2003) *Quarterly Journal of Medicine: An International Journal of Medicine* 96: 345–353.

Ivarsson A, Persson LA, Hernell O. (2000) Short and long term effects of breast feeding on child health. *Advances in Experimental Medicine and Biology* 478: 139–149.

Ivarsson A, Hernell O, Stenlund H, Persson LA. (2002) Breast-feeding protects against celiac disease. *American Journal of Clinical Nutrition* 75: 914–921.

Janatuinen EK, Kemppainen TA, Julkunen RJK, *et al.* (2002) No harm from five year ingestion of oats in coeliac disease. *Gut* 50: 332–335.

Johnston SD, Watson, RG, McMillan SA, Sloan J, Love AH. (1998) Coeliac disease detected by screening is not silent – simply unrecognized. *Quarterly Journal of Medicine* 91(12): 853–860.

Kramer MS, Kakuma R. (2002) *The Optimal Duration of Exclusive Breastfeeding: A Systematic Review*. Geneva: World Health Organisation.

Kumar PJ, Walker-Smith J, Milla P, Harris G, Colyer J, Halliday R. (1988) The teenage celiac: follow up study of 102 patients. *Archives of Diseases in Childhood* 63: 916–920.

Leeds JS, Hopper AD, Sanders DS. (2008) Coeliac disease. *BMJ* 88: 157–170.

Leffler D, George J, Dennis M, Cook EF, Schuppan D, Kelly CP. (2007) A prospective comparative study of five measures of gluten-free diet adherence in adults with CD. *Alimentary Pharmacology & Therapeutics* 26: 1227–1235.

Lenhardt A, Plebani A, Marchetti F. (2004) Role of human-tissue transglutaminase IgG and anti-gliadin IgG antibodies in the diagnosis of coeliac disease in patients with selective immunoglobulin A deficiency. *Digestive & Liver Disease* 36(11): 730–734.

Ljungman G, Myrdal U. (1993). Compliance in teenagers with coeliac disease – a Swedish follow up study. *Acta Paediatrica* 82: 235–238.

Lo W, Sano K, Lebwohl B, Diamond B, Green PHR. (2003) Changing presentation of adult celiac disease. *Digestive Diseases and Sciences* 48: 395–398.

Ludvigsson JF, Michealsson E, Ekbom A, Montgomery SM. (2007) Coeliac disease and the risk of fractures – a general population based cohort study. *Alimentary Pharmacology & Therapeutics* 25: 273–285.

Luft LM, Barr SG, Martin LO. (2003) Autoantibodies to tissue transglutaminase in Sjögren's syndrome and related rheumatic diseases. *Journal of Rheumatology* 30(12): 2613–2619.

Lundin KEA, Nilsen EM, Scott HG, *et al.* (2003) Oats induced villous atrophy in coeliac disease. *Gut* 52: 1649–1652.

Maki M, Collin P. (1997). Coeliac disease. *Lancet* 349: 1755–1759.

Marsh MN. (1992) Gluten, major histocompatibility complex, and the small intestine. A molecular and immunobiologic approach to the spectrum of gluten sensitivity ('celiac sprue'). *Gastroenterology* 102: 330–354.

Mayer M, Greco L, Troncone R, Auricchio S, Marsh MN. (1991). Compliance of adolescents with coeliac disease on a gluten free diet. *Gut* 32: 881–885.

McFarlane XA, Bhalla AK, Reeves DE, Morgan LM, Robertson DA. (1995) Osteoporosis in treated adult coeliac disease. *Gut* 1995a; 36: 710–714.

Midhagen G, Aberg AK, Olcen P, *et al.* (2004) Antibody levels in adult patients with coeliac disease during gluten-free diet: a rapid initial decrease of clinical importance. *Journal of Internal Medicine* 256: 519–524.

Morris MA, Yiannakou JY, King AL, *et al.* (2000) Coeliac disease and Downs syndrome: associations not due to genetic linkage on chromosome 21. *Scandinavian Journal of Gastroenterology* 35(2): 177–180.

National Institute for Health and Care Excellence (NICE). (2009) *Coeliac Disease Recognition and Assessment of Coeliac Disease.* Guideline 86. Available at www.nice.org.uk.

Nelson M, Mendoza M, McGough N. (2007) A survey of provision of dietetic services for coeliac disease in the UK. *Journal of Human Nutrition and Dietetics* 20: 403–411.

Niveloni S, Fiorini A, Dezi R. (1998) Usefulness of videoduodenoscopy and vital dye staining as indicators of mucosal atrophy of coeliac disease: assessment of interobserver agreement. *Gastrointestinal Endoscopy* 47(3): 223–229.

Norris JM, Barriga K, Hoffenberg EJ, *et al.* (2005) Risk of celiac disease autoimmunity and timing of gluten introduction in the diet of infants at increased risk of disease. *Journal of the American Medical Association* 293: 2342–2351.

Packer SC, Dornhurst A, Frost GS. (2000) The glycaemic index of a range of gluten-free foods. *Diabetic Medicine* 17(9): 657–660.

Pazianas M, Butcher GP, Subhani JM. (2005) Calcium absorption and bone mineral density in celiacs after long term treatment with gluten-free diet and adequate calcium intake. *Osteoporosis International* 16(1): 56–63.

Pietzak MM. (2005). Follow-up of patients with celiac disease: Achieving compliance with treatment. *Gastroenterology* 128: S135–S141.

Primary Care Society of Gastroenterology (PCSG). (2006) The management of adults with coeliac disease in primary care. Available at www.pcsg.org.uk.

Reunala T, Collin P. (1997) Diseases associated with dermatitis herpetiformis. *British Journal of Dermatology* 136(3): 315–318.

Romagnuola J. (2002) Using breath tests wisely in a gastroenterology practice: An evidence-based review of indications and pitfalls in interpretation. *American Journal of Gastroenterology* 98: 1113–1126.

Rubio-Tapia A, Murray JA. (2010) Classification and management of refractory coeliac disease. *Gut* 59: 547–557.

Rutherford RM. (2004) Prevalence of coeliac disease in patients with sarcoidosis. *European Journal of Gastroenterology and Hepatology* 16(9): 911–915.

Saadah OI, Zacharin M, O'Callaghan A, Oliver MR, Catto-Smith A. (2004) Effect of gluten-free diet and adherence on growth and diabetic control in diabetics with coeliac disease. *Archives of Disease in Childhood* 89: 871–876.

Saukkonen T, Savilahti E, Reijonen H, Ilonen J, Tuomilehto-Wolf E, Akerblom HK. (1996) Coeliac disease: frequent occurrence after clinical onset of insulin-dependent diabetes mellitus. *Diabetic Medicine* 13: 464–470.

Shahbazkhani B, Forootan M, Merat S. (2003) Coeliac disease presenting with symptoms of irritable bowel syndrome. *Alimentary Pharmacology & Therapeutics* 18(2): 231–235.

Silvester JA, Rashid M. (2007) Long Term follow up of individuals with coeliac disease: An evaluation of current practice guidelines. *Canadian Journal Gastroenterolgy* 21(9): 557–564.

Stucky C, Lowdon J, Howdle P. (2009) Dietitians are better than clinicians in following up coeliac disease. *Proceedings of the Nutrition Society* 68: 249–251.

Sumnik Z, Kolouskova S, Malcova H, *et al.* (2005)High prevalence of coeliac disease in siblings of children with Type 1 diabetes. *European Journal of Paediatrics* 164: 9–12.

Sverker A, Hensing G, Hallert C. (2005) Controlled by food" – lived experiences of coeliac disease. *Journal of Human Nutrition and Dietetics* 1: 171–110.

Tennyson CA, Lewsi KL, Green PHR. (2009) New and developing therapies for celiac disease. *Therapeutic Advances in Gastroenterology* 2: 303–309.

Thomason K, West J, Logan RFA. (2003) Fracture experience of patients with coeliac disease: a population based study. *Gut* 52: 518–522.

Tursi A, Giorgetti G, Brandimarte G, Rubino E, Lombardi D, Gasbarrini G. (2001) Prevalence and clinical presentation of subclinical/silent celiac disease in adults: An analysis on a 12-year observation. *Hepato-Gastroenterology* 48: 462–464.

Valentino R, Savastano S, Tommaselli AP. (2002) Markers of potential coeliac disease in patients with Hashimoto's thyroiditis. *European Journal of Endocrinology* 146: 479–483.

Valletta E, Fornaro M, Cipolli M, Conte S, Bissolo F, Danchielli C. (2010) Celiac disease and obesity: need for nutritional follow-up after diagnosis. *European Journal of Clinical Nutrition* 64: 1371–1372.

Van Heel DA, West J. (2006) Recent advances in coeliac disease. *Gut* 55: 1037–1046.

Vilppula A, Collin P, Maki M. (2008) Undetected coeliac disease in the elderly: a biopsy-proven population–based study. *Digestive and Liver Disease* 40: 809–903.

West J, Logan RFA, Smith CJ, Hubbard R, Card TR. (2004a) Malignancy and mortality in people with coeliac disease: population based cohort study. *British Medical Journal* 329: 716–718.

West J, Logan RFA, Card TR, Smith C, Hubbard R. (2004b) Risk of vascular disease in adults with diagnosed coeliac disease: a population based study. *Alimentary Pharmacology & Therapeutics* 20: 1–7.

Westman E, Ambler GR, Royle M, Peat J, Chan A. (1999) Children with coeliac disease and insulin dependant diabetes mellitus-

growth, diabetes control and dietary intake. *Journal of Pediatric Endocrinology and Metabolism* 12: 433–442.

Wylie C, Geldart S, Winwood P. (2005). Dietitian-led coeliac clinic: A successful change in working practice in modern healthcare. *Gastroenterology Today* 15(1): 11–12.

7.4.8 Inflammatory bowel disease

Derbhla O'Sullivan

Key points

- Malnutrition is common in inflammatory bowel disease (IBD) and good nutrition is crucial for optimal clinical outcome.

- Enteral nutrition (elemental, peptide or polymeric) can be used as a primary treatment or adjunctive treatment to medical and surgical therapies for the treatment of active Crohn's disease or for nutritional support.

- Dietary treatment of Crohn's disease is especially useful in children and in cases where medical therapy is contraindicated.

- People with IBD need considerable dietetic support during relapse of disease and ongoing support during remission.

- Multidisciplinary team work is invaluable for caring for this lifelong relapsing–remitting condition.

Inflammatory bowel disease (IBD) is the collective term to describe Crohn's disease, ulcerative colitis and IBD, including type unclassified (IBDU) (Silverberg *et al.*, 2005). Although these are distinct disorders with differences in their presentation and management, they share a number of common features. Inflammatory bowel disease is a relapsing–remitting inflammatory disorder of unknown aetiology, which can significantly impair quality of life. The lifetime medical costs associated with the care of IBD can be comparable to major chronic diseases such as diabetes mellitus or cancer (IBD Standards, 2009). Nutrition therapy is pivotal in IBD, whether as the primary treatment or in a supportive role.

Prevalence

Both ulcerative colitis and Crohn's disease are diseases of young people with a peak incidence between the ages of 20 and 40 years (Marshall & Hilsden, 2003). With a reported prevalence of 400 per 100 000 (Rubin *et al.*, 2000) there are approximately 240 000 patients with IBD in the UK [ulcerative colitis 243 per 100 000 (146 000 people) in the UK population of 60 million and Crohn's disease 145 per 100 000 (87 000 people)]. There is a South–North gradient to the incidence of IBD in the UK, with rates being highest in Scotland. Compared with the non-Jewish Caucasian population, IBD occurs more frequently in Ashkenazi Jews and at about the same level in families originating from Africa or the Caribbean. For second generation Indian and Pakistani families, the incidence of Crohn's disease is about the same, but is higher for ulcerative colitis (Silverberg *et al.*, 2005).

Causation and risk factors

While there is no evidence that specific immune mediated reactions to food play a role in most patients with either Crohn's disease or ulcerative colitis (Bischoff *et al.*, 2000), it is commonplace for patients with gastrointestinal disorders to believe that something in their diet has caused their condition (Jones *et al.*, 1985). The cause of both Crohn's disease and ulcerative colitis remains unknown, yet is likely to be multifactorial; a combination of genetic predisposition and environmental triggers. There is a genetic predisposition that increases the risk of IBD about 10-fold in first degree relatives of an IBD patient and which probably determines the pattern and severity of the disease in any individual patient. Much research is focused on understanding the role of bacteria in the gut and the many different parts of the immune system's response to external triggers. It seems quite likely that the trigger for the disease varies between individuals (IBD Standards, 2009; NACC, 2007; Stange *et al.*, 2006; 2008).

Smoking is consistently documented to be associated with IBD. Current smokers are more likely to develop Crohn's disease and, following diagnosis, have a poorer prognosis with a significantly higher chance of surgical resection, and (if smoking continues) a greater chance of recurrence at the surgical anastomosis (Mahid *et al.*, 2006; Mowat *et al.*, 2011). Smoking cessation is associated with a 65% reduction in the risk of a relapse in Crohn's disease as compared with continued smokers (Johnson *et al.*, 2005). In contrast, smoking decreases the risk of ulcerative colitis (Mahid *et al.* 2006).

Clinical features

Inflammatory bowel disease results in an uncontrolled inflammatory response in the bowel wall. Crohn's disease most commonly affects the small bowel, often the terminal ileum, although any part of the gastrointestinal tract from the mouth to the anus can be affected. All layers of the intestine are affected and the rectum is often spared. It is characterised by distinct areas of inflammation, often associated with granulomas and deep fissuring ulceration, interspersed with areas of unaffected bowel tissue. Crohn's disease can follow either of two patterns; stricturing disease (narrowing of the intestine causing obstruction) or fistulising disease (where the disease creates holes in the bowel wall that allow the faecal contents to leak out) (IBD Standards, 2009).

Ulcerative colitis causes an area of continuously inflamed mucosa, starting in the rectum and extending up the colon to varying degrees. The intestinal lining becomes red and inflamed, and bleeds readily. It also follows a relapsing–remitting course, although the first presentation is often the most severe.

Both ulcerative colitis and Crohn's disease are associated with an equivalent increased risk of colonic carcinoma (Ekbom et al., 1990a,b; Friedman et al., 2008; Softley et al., 1988). About 5% of patients with IBD affecting the colon are unclassifiable because they have some features of both Crohn's disease and ulcerative colitis. This is now termed as IBDU (Silverberg et al., 2005).

Symptoms and diagnosis

The main presenting symptoms of IBD are abdominal pain, diarrhoea, sometimes with blood and mucus in the stool, and weight loss. Both Crohn's disease and ulcerative colitis can produce symptoms of urgency, profound fatigue and anaemia, with, for some patients, associated inflammation of the joints, skin, liver or eyes. Malnutrition and weight loss are common with patients often altering their eating habits to alleviate symptoms (IBD Standards, 2009). When diagnosed in childhood (about 25% of all cases) the disease is often more severe than if presenting in adulthood, with major consequences on life long morbidity (Van Limbergen et al., 2008). Symptoms can severely affect self esteem and social functioning, particularly among the young and newly diagnosed.

The diagnosis of IBD is confirmed by clinical evaluation and a combination of haematological, endoscopic, histological or imaging based investigations (Mowat et al., 2011; Stange et al. 2006; 2008). Laboratory investigations should include full blood count, urea and electrolytes, liver function tests, erythrocyte sedimentation rate (ESR) or C-reactive protein (CRP), ferritin, transferrin saturation, vitamin B_{12} and folate (Mowat et al., 2011). The most frequent test used to diagnose IBD is a colonoscopy with multiple biopsies. Imaging, e.g. ultrasound, magnetic resonance imaging, computed tomography scanning and barium fluoroscopy, can be helpful in diagnosis and the assessment of disease extent. Faecal calprotectin is also used in some centres to detect colonic inflammation and to help identify functional diarrhoea. Other causes of diarrhoea include irritable bowel syndrome (IBS) and infection and may be present alongside IBD, e.g. after travel abroad.

Several disease indices are available to describe the severity of Crohn's disease and ulcerative colitis. However, the most suitable indices to use in dietetic assessments are ones that include factors that are obtainable by a dietitian and are known locally such as the Harvey Bradshaw Index (HBI) (Harvey & Bradshaw, 1980) and The Simple Clinical Colitis Activity Index (Walmsley et al., 1998). These can be useful in combination with other clinical measures such as blood results to help indicate remission versus active disease.

The HBI is a validated clinical index used for Crohn's disease that is also called the simple index. It is based on five items:

1. General wellbeing (0 = very well, 1 = slightly below par, 2 = poor, 3 = very poor, 4 = terrible).
2. Abdominal pain (0 = none, 1 = mild, 2 = moderate, 3 = severe).
3. Number of stools per day.
4. Abdominal mass (0 = none, 1 = dubious, 2 = definite, 3 = definite and tender).
5. Complications: arthralgia, uveitis, erythema nodosum, aphthous ulcers, pyoderma gangrenosum, anal fissure, new fistula, abscess (score 1 per item).

The first three items are scored for the previous day. A score of 3 or less indicates the disease is in remission. A score of >6 indicates the disease is active and the patient has relapsed.

The Simple Clinical Colitis Activity Index is based on six parameters:

1. Bowel frequency during day (0 = 1–3/day, 1 = 4–6/day, 2 = 7–9/day, 3 = >9/day).
2. Bowel frequency during night (1 = 1–3/night, 2 = 4–6/night).
3. Urgency of defecation (1 = hurry, 2 = immediately, 3 = incontinence).
4. Blood in stool (1 = trace, 2 = occasionally frank, 3 = usually frank).
5. General wellbeing (0 = very well, 1 = slightly below par, 2 = poor, 3 = very poor, 4 = terrible).
6. Extracolonic features (score 1 per manifestation): arthritis, pyoderma gangrenosum, erythema nodosum, uveitis.

A score of <2.5 defines remission (Higgins et al., 2005) and a score of 5 or more defines relapse.

Management

Drug treatment

Drug therapy for IBD is a rapidly evolving field. Antibiotics such as metronidazole and ciprofloxacin have an important role in treating secondary complications in

Table 7.4.8 Common nutritional deficiencies in patients with inflammatory bowel disease (IBD)

Nutritional deficiency	Common causes
Dietary energy	Poor appetite as a result of symptoms or drug side effects Catabolic effects of chronic inflammation Malabsorption (as a result of ileal IBD or following ileal resection)
Protein	Increased nitrogen losses High requirements for tissue repair
Vitamins D and K	Bile salt deficiency
Iron	Poor intake Poor absorption Chronic blood loss (especially in ulcerative colitis)
Folate	Impaired absorption Use of sulphasalazine
Vitamin C	Low consumption of fruit and vegetables
Vitamin B_{12}	Ileal resection Small bowel overgrowth
Calcium	Use of corticosteroids Malabsorption and chronic diarrhoea Avoidance of dairy food
Magnesium and zinc	Malabsorption and chronic diarrhoea Short bowel syndrome
Sodium and potassium	Avoidance of dairy foods Persistent diarrhoea and vomiting

IBD, such as abscess and bacterial overgrowth (Castiglione *et al.*, 2003). However, corticosteroids such as prednisolone, 5-aminosalicylates (e.g. sulfasalazine, mesalazine and osalazine), and immunosuppressive drugs such as azathioprine and mercaptopurine are the mainstay of medical management for inducing and maintaining remission; they suppress the symptomatic effects of IBD. Corticosteroids are the biggest risk factors in postoperative complications (Dignass *et al.*, 2010). Thirty per cent of patients will fail to respond to these drugs or be intolerant of them, and these patients may then be considered for antitumour necrosis factor-alpha biological therapies such as infliximab, or surgery (IBD Standards, 2009).

Surgery

Between 50% and 70% of patients with Crohn's disease will undergo surgery within 5 years of diagnosis. In total ulcerative colitis, lifetime surgery rates are about 20–30%. Of patients who have chronic relapsing ulcerative colitis, about 50% need a colectomy, though rates vary between countries and regions (Carter *et al.*, 2004; IBD Standards, 2009; Oresland, 2006; Roberts, 2007).

The most common forms of surgery for Crohn's disease are removal of the diseased part of the small bowel, with or without part of the colon; and partial or total removal of the colon and/or rectum (proctocolectomy) with formation of a stoma, which may be permanent. For people who have ulcerative colitis, restorative proctocolectomy is the most common operation. This involves removal of the colon and rectum, combined with the fashioning of an ileal pouch. This is made from the terminal ileum and joined to the anus to form a reservoir, which replaces the rectum, thus avoiding a permanent ileostomy (IBD Standards, 2009; Stange *et al.* 2006; 2008; Travis *et al.*, 2008; Parks & Nicholls, 1978).

Nutritional implications

In cases where diarrhoea is prolonged, or bloody and severe, water and salt loss and poor absorption of nutrients may occur, leading to anaemia, dehydration, severe weight loss and nutritional depletion (Table 7.4.8).

Drug treatment may also impact on nutritional status. Prolonged use of corticosteroids may cause growth retardation in children, muscle wasting, diabetes, peptic ulcer, osteoporosis, liver and renal damage. Nausea and diarrhoea are common side effects of aminosalicylates and immunosuppressant drugs. Sulfasalazine is a folic acid antagonist and its long term use can cause megaloblastic anaemia. Folate deficiency is also associated with hyperhomocysteinaemia, which increases the risk of thromboembolic disease in IBD.

Dietary management

The aims of dietary management in IBD include:

- Achieving and maintaining good nutritional status during both active disease and remission.
- Helping to alleviate clinical symptoms in combination with medical and/or surgical treatment.
- Helping to treat clinical complications in combination with medical treatment.

- Achieving remission in Crohn's disease patients, when enteral nutrition is used as a primary treatment or in combination with medical treatment.

Patients report that access to a dietitian is vital (Jones *et al.*, 2009; Prince *et al.*, 2010) and the need for increased dietetic access is recommended (IBD Standards Standard A5, 2009). Malnutrition is present in up to 85% of patients with IBD, and weight loss occurs in up to 80% of patients with Crohn's disease and 18–62% of patients with ulcerative colitis (Gassull & Cabre, 2001; Geerling *et al.*, 1999). All IBD patients should be weighed and their nutritional needs assessed (IBD Standards Standard A10, 2009). Therefore, nutritional intake and dietary advice are important when patients are admitted, when they relapse and during periods of remission. Osteoporosis is common in IBD (Tilg *et al.*, 2007) and the daily recommendation for calcium intake in patients with IBD is 1000 mg (Lewis& Scott, 2007).

Patients should be encouraged to follow as normal a diet as is possible for their clinical state, and which is balanced in terms of overall composition. Most will benefit from relatively small meals of high energy and nutrient density consumed at fairly frequent intervals. At times when appetite is poor, food fortification strategies or supplement use may be necessary (see Chapter 6.3). The importance of adequate fluid intake in the presence of diarrhoea, pyrexia or fistulae should be stressed. Nutritional status should be assessed at regular intervals and the growth of children and young people closely monitored.

Additional dietary manipulations may be needed to help to alleviate the effects of the disease or the consequences of intestinal resection, or to achieve remission in Crohn's disease patients. Some IBD patients may need to avoid specific foods that appear to exacerbate symptoms, but unnecessary food avoidance should be discouraged; the justification for excluding specific foods to help to alleviate symptoms should always be carefully considered. In many patients with IBD, functional symptoms, e.g. abdominal pain, bloating, flatulence and diarrhoea, are more problematic than symptoms due to inflammation that may be attributed to IBS (Camilleri, 2011).

Specific aspects of dietary management of crohn's disease

People with Crohn's disease are at particular risk of nutritional deficiencies because this form of IBD is more likely to:

- Occur in children or young adults whose energy needs are high.
- Result in malabsorption as a result of ileal inflammation or resection.
- Necessitate repeated surgery to treat complications such as strictures or fistulae.

Restoring and maintaining good nutritional status is a treatment priority at all stages of the illness. As far as possible, this should be achieved by means of a diet comprised of ordinary foods which minimises disruption to normal life.

Since appetite tends to be poor in active disease, the diet needs to be of high energy and nutrient density, and various strategies can be deployed to help to achieve this (see Chapter 6.3). Many patients will avoid greasy, spicy or irritant foods in an attempt to minimise symptoms, but the nutritional impact of any food restrictions imposed by the patient should be carefully explored with the patient. If fat malabsorption is resulting in problematic symptoms, fat restriction to tolerance levels may be necessary, but care must be taken to avoid compromising energy intake. Substitution of some long chain triglycerides (LCTs) with medium chain triglycerides (MCTs), or dietary fortification with carbohydrate polymers may be necessary. Additional fat soluble vitamins are also likely to be required and a daily multivitamin supplement may be advisable if food intake remains inadequate or malabsorption is pronounced.

In specific circumstances, protein and energy support is indicated, such as when the absorptive capacity of the gut is reduced in short bowel syndrome or in the perioperative care of patients with significant (>15%) weight loss or low body mass index (National Collaborating Centre for Acute Care, 2006). This may mean parenteral nutrition (PN) including home PN in a minority of Crohn's disease patients with intestinal failure. Approximately 20% of home PN patients in Europe have underlying Crohn's disease, which is about one case per 1.5 million population (Bakker *et al.*, 1999).

Use of enteral nutrition

In Crohn's disease, withdrawal of normal food and replacement with enteral nutrition (EN) or PN can be used to induce remission in some patients (King *et al.*, 1997; Griffiths, 1998; Seo *et al.*, 1999, Goh & O'Morain, 2003). The enteral route has been considered more appropriate if it is working and accessible, as PN is invasive, carries more risks of serious complications and leads to gut atrophy arising from complete bowel rest (Lomer, 2011). The reason why EN is efficacious in treating active CD is unknown. Proposed mechanisms have included improved nutritional status, bowel rest, reduced dietary antigens, a direct immunomodulatory effect via alterations in fat content and reduced gastrointestinal microbial activity (Bannerjee *et al.*, 2004, Gassull, 2004, Lomer *et al.*, 2005, Tsujikawa *et al.*, 2003, Zachos *et al.*, 2007). Enteral nutrition has a role in primary treatment and as adjunctive treatment to medical and surgical therapies for treatment of active Crohn's disease or for nutritional support (Akobeng & Thomas, 2007; Zachos *et al.*, 2007, Mowat *et al.*, 2011). It is used as a primary treatment for active Crohn's disease in children and adolescents (Griffiths *et al.*, 1995; Lochs *et al.*, 2006; Zachos *et al.*, 2007). Enteral nutrition induces disease remission, but also ensures adequate growth and development and avoids side effects from drug therapy (Sandhu *et al.*, 2010). It has been shown to improve mucosal healing in paediatric patients (Beattie *et al.*, 1994; Borrelli *et al.*, 2006; Fell *et al.*, 2000).

In adults with Crohn's disease, the evidence for using EN to induce disease remission is not so strong, and it is less effective than corticosteroids (Griffiths *et al.*, 1995; Zachos *et al.*, 2007). However, it is an alternative therapy to corticosteroids (Lochs *et al.*, 2006) and can be particularly useful where medical therapy is contraindicated, where patients or physicians choose this treatment option (Mowat *et al.*, 2011), or in young adults and in patients with or at risk of malnutrition. There are no known long term health consequences associated with EN.

The different types of EN used in Crohn's disease include elemental (amino acid) formula, peptide (semi elemental) formula and polymeric (whole protein) formula. There is no difference in efficacy between elemental and polymeric diets when used to induce remission in Crohn's disease (Zachos *et al.*, 2007). Palatability and social inconvenience can be limiting; however, their impact can be offset by close support from a dedicated dietetic service (King *et al.*, 1997). Choice of EN can depend on patient preference and local policy; EN is usually prescribed for 2–8 weeks. While the patient is taking exclusive EN, it is normal to exclude all other foods or drink except still water. Close dietetic monitoring is essential and some of the problems that may occur and strategies for dealing with them are summarised in Table 7.4.9. By 10 days there should be a clinical response and patients may even go into disease remission (Giaffer *et al.*, 1990), but longer studies indicate that mucosal healing does not occur until later on and 8 weeks or more may be required (Fell *et al.*, 2000; Lomer, 2011; Yamamoto *et al.*, 2007) (see Chapter 6.4).

Use of diet to maintain remission

Supplementary EN providing 35–50% of energy requirements using either an elemental or polymeric formula has been shown to help in the maintenance of disease remission if provided for up to 12 months (Akobeng & Thomas, 2007). Following a period of food withdrawal with EN, transition to normal foods needs to be made with care. Patients are often apprehensive about which foods to eat and may eliminate certain foods, fearing that they may worsen symptoms and cause a relapse. High fibre diets are not normally indicated as food reintroduction diets (Jones *et al.*, 1985). Exclusion diets are not recognised in national guidelines for Crohn's disease in maintenance of remission. However, diets such as an elimination or LOFFLEX (low fat fibre limited exclusion) diet can be useful following a period of EN (Riordan *et al.*, 1993; Woolner *et al.*, 1998) and can be used as a starting point for food reintroduction by patients who, without dietetic support, may exclude random foods, which may lead to possible nutritional inadequacy.

Riordan *et al.* (1993) reported that following a period of exclusive EN, most patients would relapse shortly after resumption of a normal diet. The elimination diet involved reintroducing a single food each day, and excluding any food that provoked symptoms. The elimination diet was compared against tapered steroids and usual diets/general dietary advice for efficacy of prolonging remission (Riordan *et al.* 1993).

The LOFFLEX diet was developed by Woolner *et al.* (1998) as a method of food reintroduction that was easier and less time consuming than the elimination diet. The LOFFLEX diet was found to have the same efficacy for maintaining remission as the elimination diet. Foods that have been reported by >5% of Crohn's disease patients to cause symptoms are excluded. Patients follow a basic diet for 2–4 weeks and, provided that the patient is still in a state of remission, further food reintroduction

Table 7.4.9 Problems associated with use of formula diets in patients with Crohn's disease

Problem	Cause and/or solution
Loss of weight	May be due to not meeting nutritional requirements in the first few days If weight loss continues into the second week, increase the prescribed quantity of feed Monitor symptoms
Tiredness	Ensure the patient is meeting their requirements for feed and fluid Encourage the patient to rest
Postural hypotension	This often occurs in first few days if fluid intake is inadequate
Hunger	This seldom occurs if an adequate amount of feed is prescribed and consumed Try increasing the frequency and quantity of drinks
Headache	This may be due to caffeine withdrawal or to an inadequate fluid intake
Bad breath	Ensure good oral hygiene Brushing teeth three times a day may help, as may using mouth wash and consuming water after each drink
Green liquid stools	An infrequent, mild side effect
Diarrhoea	This may be osmotic, advise drinking the product slowly or perhaps diluting it with water If given nasogastrically, slow the rate of administration Suggest trying different flavours, consuming from a covered glass with ice and a straw or freezing/warming the drinks
Dislike of drink	Many people will become accustomed to the taste in time

follows. A list of 25 specific foods is given in the LOFFLEX and each food is tested for 4 days. After gradual cessation of the liquid diet, additional drinks are useful throughout the LOFFLEX diet period as snacks or supplements.

Low or reduced fibre diets are often also used in clinical practice because patients find them easier to follow, and they are less limiting and more nutritionally adequate than exclusion or elimination diets. Whatever method is used for food reintroduction, it is important that each patient is given the support they need to make a safe return to normal eating, and if food intolerance is found, that they are given structured advice to ensure that a balanced diet can be consumed.

Use of diet in stricturing Crohn's disease

Patients with stricturing Crohn's disease should be advised to alter and reduce their fibre intake to help prevent the risk of bowel obstruction and reduce associated symptoms (Meier & Gassull, 2004; Woolner et al., 1998). The degree of dietary stricture will be dependent on the nature (inflammatory and/or fibrotic) and extent (tightness and length) of the stricture (Lomer, 2011). Typically, high fibre foods (wholegrains, skins and pips in fruit and vegetables, nuts and seeds) and foods that are difficult to mechanically break down, e.g. gristle, skin on meat or fish, are avoided (Lomer, 2011).

Specific aspects of dietary management of ulcerative colitis

There is no indication for the use of EN to treat ulcerative colitis; however, nutrition is still of primary importance in preventing the detrimental effects of malnutrition (Burke et al., 1997; Gonzalez-Huix et al., 1993).

Management of an acute relapse

Severe attacks can be fatal and require emergency hospital admission with intravenous fluid and electrolyte support, possibly blood transfusion, and steroid administration to induce remission as quickly as possible. If symptoms fail to improve or complications such as haemorrhage or toxic megacolon occur, or if precancerous changes are detected, surgery will be needed; a colectomy is curative.

Low fibre diets are often used for symptom relief while waiting for medical treatment to take effect. If time permits, preoperative nutritional support may be indicated. Peri- and post-operative support to maintain an adequate nutritional state is also very important. In the absence of massive bleeding, perforation, toxic megacolon or obstruction, EN rather than PN should be the mode of choice. Dietary measures to alleviate the effects of colonic resection may be needed.

Patients suffering from a mild or moderate attack, or recovering from a more severe attack, will usually have lost weight and need to increase dietary energy and protein intake. Oral energy supplements may be necessary if this cannot be achieved by use of normal foods alone. Particular attention should be paid to micronutrient requirements and supplements should be given if needed.

Management during remission

Patients in remission should be encouraged to consume a varied, well balanced diet, and unnecessary food exclusions discouraged.

Other aspects of nutrition

Probiotics

Bacteria or yeast generally ingested orally as therapy are termed probiotics. They may be administered as a single organism or a defined mixture, aiming to beneficially alter the microbial ecology of the gut. The agents most studied in IBD are *Escherichia coli* Nissle 1917, VSL#3, *Lactobacillus rhamnosus* GC, *Bifidobacterium* and *Saccharomyces boulardii* (Mowat et al., 2011; Pham et al., 2008). There is evidence for the effectiveness of VSL#3 in preventing pouchitis (Mimura et al., 2004; Gionchetti et al., 2003) and some evidence of benefit in maintenance and treatment of ulcerative colitis (Bibiloni et al., 2005; Miele et al., 2009). Three randomised placebo controlled studies have shown that *E. coli* Nissle 1917 (Mutaflor®) 200 mg daily is equivalent to standard doses of mesalazine in maintaining remission in ulcerative colitis (Schultz, 2008) and therefore may be an option for patients who are unable or unwilling to take mesalazine (Mowat et al., 2011). There is no clear evidence to support any role for probiotics in the maintenance of Crohn's disease either after surgical or medically induced remission (Rolfe et al., 2006).

Food intolerance

The prevalence of IBS-like symptoms in ulcerative colitis patients in remission is about three times higher than in hospital controls (Ansari et al., 2008). Thirty-three per cent of ulcerative colitis patients and 57% of Crohn's disease patients have been reported to have IBS symptoms and IBS-like symptoms. Irritable bowel-like symptoms in IBD patients in long standing remission are two to three times higher than that in the normal population (Simren et al., 2002). The association between symptoms of IBD and diet has received much attention (Crowe, 2001; Jones et al., 1985; Riordan et al., 1993). However, the tools available for measuring and predicting food intolerances remain suboptimal. Traditional allergy testing concentrated on the measurement of IgE mediated responses, but this approach has not proven useful in gastrointestinal food sensitivity (Bruijnzeel-Koomen et al., 1995; Crowe, 2001; Shanahan, 1993). While the role of IgG based testing for food specific antibodies has shown some promise in IBS, research is ongoing (Atkinson et al., 2004; Zar et al., 2005a,b) (see Chapter 7.11.2).

Lactose intolerance

Lactose intolerance can occur in Crohn's disease where ileal damage or resection results in malabsorptive problems (Mishkin, 1997; Von Tirpitz et al., 2002), but there is evidence that IBD patients avoid dairy products more often than necessary (Mishkin, 1997; Banos-Madrid et al., 2004). Lactose intolerance is much less likely to be associated with ulcerative colitis (Mishkin, 1997; Ginard et al., 2003), other than in patients with primary lactose intolerance. In all such patients, lactose intake may need to be limited but rarely needs to be excluded altogether (see Chapter 7.4.6). Consideration of calcium intake should be addressed where dairy foods are limited (see Chapter 7.4.6).

Internet resources

British Society of Gastroenterology   www.bsg.org.uk
Crohn's and Colitis UK   www.nacc.org.uk
Crohn's in Childhood Research Association (CICRA)   www.cicra.org/
CORE (Digestive Disorders Foundation)   www.corecharity.org.uk
NHS Evidence   www.evidence.nhs.uk
The Crohn's and Colitis Foundation of America   www.ccfa.org
UK Clinical Research Network portfolio (gastrointestinal)   http://public.ukcrn.org.uk

References

Akobeng AK, Thomas AG. (2007) Enteral nutrition for maintenance of remission in Crohn's disease. *Cochrane Database of Systematic Reviews* CD005984.

Ansari R, Attari F, Razjouyan H, *et al.* (2008) Ulcerative colitis and irritable bowel syndrome: relationships with quality of life. *European Journal of Gastroenterology and Hepatology* 20: 46–50.

Atkinson W, Sheldon TA, Shaath N, Whorwell PJ. (2004) Food elimination based on IgG antibodies in irritable bowel syndrome: a randomised controlled trial. *Gut* 53: 1459–1464.

Bakker H, Bozzetti F, Staun M, *et al.* (1999) Home parenteral nutrition in adults: a European multicentre survey in 1997. ESPEN-Home Artificial Nutrition Working Group. *Clinical Nutrition* 18: 135–140.

Bannerjee K, Camacho-Hubner C, *et al.* (2004) Anti-inflammatory and growth-stimulating effects precede nutritional restitution during enteral feeding in Crohn's disease. *Journal of Pediatric Gastroenterology and Nutrition* 38: 270–275.

Banos-Madrid R, Salama-Benerroch H, Moran-Sanchez S, Gallardo-Sanchez F, Albadalejo-Merono A, Mercader-Martinez J. (2004) Lactose malabsorption in patients with inflammatory bowel disease without activity; would it be necessary to exclude lactose products in the diet of all patients? *Anales de Medicina Interna* 21: 212–214.

Beattie RM, Schiffrin EJ, Donnet-Hughes A, *et al.* (1994) Polymeric nutrition as the primary therapy in children with small bowel Crohn's disease. *Alimentary Pharmacology & Therapeutics* 8: 609–615.

Bibiloni R, Fedorak RN, Tannock GW, *et al.* (2005) VSL#3 probiotic-mixture induces remission in patients with active ulcerative colitis. *American Journal of Gastroenterology* 100: 1539–1546.

Bischoff SC, Mayer JH, Manns MP. (2000) Allergy and the gut. *International Archives if Allergy and Immunology* 121: 270–283.

Borrelli O, Cordischi L, Cirulli M, *et al.* (2006) Polymeric diet alone versus corticosteroids in the treatment of active pediatric Crohn's disease: a randomized controlled open-label trial. *Clinical Gastroenterology and Hepatology* 4: 744–753.

Bruijnzeel-Koomen C, Ortolani C, Aas K, *et al.*. (1995) Adverse reactions to food. European Academy of Allergology and Clinical Immunology Subcommittee. *Allergy* 50: 623–635.

Burke A, Lichtenstein GR, Rombeau JL. (1997) Nutrition and ulcerative colitis. *Baillieres Clinical Gastroenterology* 11: 153–174.

Camilleri M. (2011) Managing symptoms of irritable bowel syndrome in patients with inflammatory bowel disease. *Gut* 60: 425–428.

Carter MJ, Lobo AJ, Travis SPL. (2004) British Society of Gastroenterology Guidelines for inflammatory bowel disease 2004. *Gut* 53(Suppl V): v1–16.

Castiglione F, Rispo A, Di Girolamo E, *et al.* (2003) Antibiotic treatment of small bowel bacterial overgrowth in patients with Crohn's disease. *Alimentary Pharmacology & Therapeutics* 18: 1107–1112.

Crowe SE. (2001) Gastrointestinal food allergies: do they exist? *Current Gastroenterology Reports* 3: 351–357.

Dignass A, Van AG, Lindsay JO, *et al.* (2010) The second European evidence-based Consensus on the diagnosis and management of Crohn's disease: Current management. *Journal of Crohn's and Colitis* 4: 28–62.

Ekbom A, Helmick C, Zack M, *et al.* (1990a) Ulcerative colitis and colorectal cancer. A population based study. *New England Journal of Medicine* 323: 1228–1233.

Ekbom A, Helmick C, Zack M, *et al.* (1990b) Increased risk of large-bowel cancer in Crohn's disease with colonic involvement. *Lancet* 336: 357–359.

Fell JM, Paintin M, Arnaud-Battandier F, *et al.* (2000) Mucosal healing and a fall in mucosal pro-inflammatory cytokine mRNA induced by a specific oral polymeric diet in paediatric Crohn's disease. *Alimentary Pharmacology &. Therapeutics* 14: 281–289.

Friedman S, Rubin PH, Bodian C, *et al.* (2008) Screening and surveillance colonoscopy in chronic Crohn's colitis: results of surveillance program spanning 25 years. *Clinical Gastroenterology and Hepatology* 6: 993–998.

Gassull MA. (2004) Review article: the role of nutrition in the treatment of inflammatory bowel disease. *Alimentary Pharmacology & Therapeutics* 20(Suppl 4): 79–83.

Gassull MA, Cabre E. (2001) Nutrition in inflammatory bowel disease. *Current Opinion on Clinical Nutrition and Metabolic Care* 4: 561–569.

Geerling BJ, Stockbrugger RW, Brummer RJ. (1999) Nutrition and inflammatory bowel disease: An update. *Scandinavian Journal of Gastroenterology Supplements* 230: 95–105.

Giaffer MH, North G, Holdsworth CD. (1990) Controlled trial of polymeric versus elemental diet in treatment of active Crohn's disease. *Lancet* 335: 816–819.

Ginard D, Riera J, Bonet L, Barranco L, Reyes J, Escarda A, Obrador A. (2003) Lactose malabsorption in ulcerative colitis. A case controlled study. *Gastroenterology and Hepatology* 26: 469–474.

Gionchetti P, Rizzello F, Helwig U, *et al.* (2003) Prophylaxis of pouchitis onset with probiotic therapy: a double-blind, placebo-controlled trial. *Gastroenterology* 124: 1202–1209.

Goh J, O'Morain CA. (2003) Nutrition and adult inflammatory bowel disease. *Alimentary Pharmacological & Therapeutics* 17: 307–320.

Gonzalez-Huix F, Fernandez-Banares F, Esteve-Comas M, *et al.* (1993) Enteral versus parenteral nutrition as adjunct therapy in acute ulcerative colitis. *American Journal of Gastroenterology* 88: 227–232.

Griffiths AM. (1998) Inflammatory bowel disease. *Nutrition* 14: 788–791.

Griffiths AM, Ohlsson A, Sherman PM, *et al.* (1995) Metaanalysis of enteral nutrition as a primary-treatment of active Crohn's disease. *Gastroenterology* 108: 1056–1067.

Harvey RF, Bradshaw MJ. (1980) Measuring Crohn's disease activity. *Lancet* 1: 1134–1135.

Higgins PDR, Schwartz M, Mapili J, Krokos I, Leung J, Zimmermann EM. (2005) Patient defined dichotomous end points for remission and clinical improvement in ulcerative colitis. *Gut* 54(6): 782–788.

IBD Standards Working Group. (2009) Quality care: Service standards for the healthcare of people who have inflammatory bowel disease (IBD). Available at www.ibdstandards.org.uk/uploaded_files/IBDstandards.pdf. Accessed 19 September 2012.

Johnson GJ, Cosnes J, Mansfield JC. (2005) Review article: smoking cessation as primary therapy to modify the course of Crohn's disease. *Alimentary Pharmacology & Therapy* 21: 921–931.

Jones VA, Dickinson RJ, Workman E. (1985) Crohn's disease: Maintenance of remission by diet. *Lancet* 2: 177–180.

Jones R, Hunt C, Stevens R, Dalrymple J, Driscoll R, Sleet S, Blanchard SJ. (2009) Management of common gastrointestinal disorders: quality criteria based on patients' views and practice guidelines. *British Journal of General Practice* 59: 199–208.

King TS, Woolner JT, Hunter JO. (1997) The dietary management of Crohn's disease. *Alimentary Pharmacology & Therapeutics* 11: 17–31.

Lewis NR, Scott BB. (2007) Guidelines for osteoporosis in inflammatory bowel disease and coeliac disease 2007. Available at www.bsg.org.uk/clinical-guidelines/ibd/guidelines-forosteoporosis-in-inflammatory-bowel-disease-and-coeliacdisease.

Lochs H, Dejong C, Hammarqvist F, *et al*. (2006) ESPEN Guidelines on enteral nutrition: Gastroenterology. *Clinical Nutrition* 25: 260–274.

Lomer MCE. (2011) Dietary considerations in IBD. In: Whayman K, Duncan J, O'Connor M(eds) *Inflammatory Bowel Disease Nursing*. London: Quay Books, pp. 139–159.

Lomer MCE, Grainger SL, Ede R, *et al*. (2005) Lack of efficacy of a reduced microparticle diet in a multi-centred trial of patients with active Crohn's disease. *European Journal of Gastroenterology and Hepatology* 17: 377–384.

Mahid SS, Minor KS, Soto RE, *et al*. (2006) Smoking and inflammatory bowel disease: a meta-analysis. *Mayo Clinic Proceedings* 81: 1462–1471.

Marshall JK, Hilsden RJ. (2003) Environment and epidemiology of inflammatory bowel diseases. In: Satsangi J, Sutherland RL (eds) *Inflammatory Bowel Diseases*. London: Elsevier, pp. 17–28.

Meier R, Gassull M. (2004) Consensus recommendations on the effects and benefits of fibre in clinical practice. *Clinical Nutrition* 1(Suppl 1): 73–80.

Miele E, Pascarella F, Giannetti E, *et al*. (2009) Effect of a probiotic preparation (VSL#3) on induction and maintenance of remission in children with ulcerative colitis. *American Journal of Gastroenterology* 104: 437–443.

Mimura T, Rizzello F, Helwig U, *et al*. (2004) Once daily high dose probiotic therapy (VSL#3) for maintaining remission in recurrent or refractory pouchitis. *Gut* 53: 108–114.

Mishkin S. (1997) Dairy sensitivity, lactose malabsorption and elimination diets in inflammatory bowel disease. *American Journal of Clinical Nutrition* 65: 564–567.

Mowat C, Cole A, Windsor A, *et al*. (2011) Guidelines for the management of inflammatory bowel disease in adults. *Gut* 60: 571–607.

NACC. (2007) Unravelling the mystery of Inflammatory Bowel Disease. Available at www.nacc.org.uk/downloads/research/NACC_ResearchReview2001-2006.pdf.

National Collaborating Centre for Acute Care. (2006) *Nutrition Support in Adults. Oral Nutrition Support, Enteral Tube Feeding and Parenteral Nutrition*. London: National Collaborating Centre for Acute Care. Available at www.rcseng.ac.uk. accessed 19 Sept 2012.

Oresland T. (2006) Review article: colon-saving medical therapy vs. colectomy in ulcerative colitis—the case for colectomy. *Alimentary Pharmacology & Therapeutics* 24(Suppl 3): 74–79.

Parks AG, Nicholls RJ. (1978) Proctocolectomy without ileostomy for ulcerative colitis. *BMJ* 2: 85–88.

Pham M, Lemberg DA, Day AS. (2008) Probiotics: sorting the evidence from the myths. *Medical Journal of Australia* 188: 304–308.

Prince A, Moose A, Whelan K, *et al*. (2010) Patients with Crohn's disease and ulcerative colitis have similar food and nutrition problems and share views on research priorities in inflammatory bowel disease. *Journal of Human Nutrition and Dietetics* 23: 460–461.

Riordan AM, Hunter JO, Cowan RE, *et al*. (1993) Treatment of active Crohn's disease by exclusion diet: East Anglian multicentre controlled trial. *Lancet* 342: 1131–1134.

Roberts SE. (2007) Mortality in patients with and without colectomy admitted to hospital for ulcerative colitis and Crohn's disease: record linkage studies. *BMJ* 335: 1033.

Rolfe VE, Fortun PJ, Hawkey CJ, *et al*. (2006) Probiotics for maintenance of remission in Crohn's disease. *Cochrane Database Systematic Reviews* 4: CD004826.

Rubin GP, Hungin AP, Kelly PJ, *et al*. (2000) Inflammatory bowel disease: epidemiology and management in an English general practice population. *Alimentary Pharmacology & Therapeutics* 14: 1553–1559.

Sandhu BK, Fell JM, Beattie RM, Mitton SG, Wilson DC, Jenkins H. (2010) Guidelines for the Management of Inflammatory Bowel Disease in Children in the United Kingdom. *Journal of Pediatric Gastroenterology and Nutrition* 50(Suppl 1): S1–S13.

Seo M, Okada M, Yao T, Furukawa H, Matake H. (1999) The role of total parenteral nutrition in the management of patients with acute attacks of inflammatory bowel disease. *Journal of Clinical Gastroenterology* 29: 270–275.

Schultz M. (2008) Clinical use of *E. coli* Nissle 1917 in inflammatory bowel disease. *Inflammatory Bowel Disease* 14: 1012–1018.

Shanahan F. (1993) Food allergy: fact, fiction, and fatality. *Gastroenterology* 104: 1229–1231.

Silverberg MS, Satsangi J, Ahmad T, *et al*. (2005) Toward an integrated clinical, molecular and serological classification of inflammatory bowel disease: Report of a Working Party of the 2005 Montreal World Congress of Gastroenterology. *Canadian Journal of Gastroenterology* 19(Suppl A): 5–36.

Simren M, Axelsson J, Gillberg R, Abrahamsson H, Svedlund J, Björnsson E. (2002) Quality of life in inflammatory bowel disease in remission: The impact of IBS-like symptoms and associated psychological factors. *American Journal of Gastroenterology* 97: 389–396.

Softley A, Clamp SE, Watkinson G, *et al*. (1988) The natural history of inflammatory bowel disease: has there been a change in the last 20 years? *Scandinavian Journal of Gastroenterology Supplements* 144: 120–123.

Stange EF, Travis SP, Vermeire S, *et al*. for the European Crohn's and Colitis Organisation (ECCO). (2006) European evidence based consensus on the diagnosis and management of Crohn's disease: definitions and diagnosis. *Gut* 55(Suppl 1): i1–15.

Stange EF, Travis SPL, Vermeire S, *et al*. for the European Crohn's and Colitis Organisation (ECCO). (2008) European evidence-based consensus on the diagnosis and management of ulcerative colitis: definitions and diagnosis. *Journal of Crohn's and Colitis* 2: 1–23.

Tilg H, Moschen AR, Kaser A, *et al*. (2007) Gut, inflammation and osteoporosis: Basic and clinical concepts. *Gut* 57: 684–694.

Travis SPL, Stange EF, Lémann M, *et al*. for the European Crohn's and Colitis Organization (ECCO). (2008) European evidence-based consensus on the diagnosis and management of Ulcerative Colitis: current management. *Journal of Crohn's and Colitis* 2: 24–62.

Tsujikawa T, Andoh A, Fujiyama Y. (2003) Enteral and parenteral nutrition therapy for Crohn's disease. *Current Pharmaceutical Design* 9: 323–332.

Van Limbergen J, Russell RK, Drummond HE, *et al*. (2008) Definition of phenotypic characteristics of childhood-onset inflammatory bowel disease. *Gastroenterology* 135(4): 1114–1122.

Von Tirpitz C, Kohn C, Steinkamp M, *et al*. (2002) Lactose intolerance in active Crohn's disease: clinical value of duodenal lactase analysis. *Journal of Clinical Gastroenterology* 31: 49–53.

Walmsley RS, Ayres RCS, Pounder RE, Allan RN. (1998) A simple clinical colitis activity index. *Gut* 43: 29–32.

Woolner JT, Parker TJ, Kirby GA, *et al*. (1998) The development and evaluation of a diet for maintaining remission in Crohn's disease. *Journal of Human Nutrition and Dietetics* 11: 1–11.

Yamamoto T, Nakahigashi M, Saniabadi AR, *et al*. (2007) Impacts of long-term enteral nutrition on clinical and endoscopic disease activities and mucosal cytokines during remission in patients with Crohn's disease: a prospective study. *Inflammatory Bowel Disease* 13: 1493–1501.

Zachos M, Tondeur M, Griffiths AM. (2007) Enteral nutritional therapy for induction of remission in Crohn's disease. *Cochrane Database of Systematic Reviews* CD000542.

Zar S, Mincher L, Benson MJ, Kumar D. (2005a) Food-specific IgG4 antibody-guided exclusion diet improves symptoms and rectal compliance in irritable bowel syndrome. *Scandinavian Journal of Gastroenterology* 40: 800–807.

Zar S, Benson MJ, Kumar D. (2005b) Food-specific serum IgG4 and IgE titers to common food antigens in irritable bowel syndrome. *American Journal of Gastroenterology* 100: 1550–1557.

7.4.9 Intestinal failure and intestinal resection

Alison Culkin

Key points

Intestinal failure

- Type 1 and 2 intestinal failure is common, usually reversible and requires short term parenteral nutrition.

- Type 3 intestinal failure is rare and irreversible and requires home parenteral nutrition.

- Dietary treatment is determined by the type, length and quality of the remaining intestine.

- Patients with a jejunostomy are recommended a diet high in energy, protein, fat and sodium, but restricted in fibre and fluid.

- Patients with a colon in continuity are recommended a diet high in energy, protein and carbohydrate, and moderate in fat to achieve energy balance whilst avoiding steatorrhoea. A reduced oxalate intake is advised to prevent kidney stones.

- Enteral support should be provided in the form of polymeric supplements and feeds usually have sodium added. Elemental formulae provide no benefit over polymeric formulae.

Resection of the large intestine

- Sodium and fluid balance should be closely monitored.

- A well-balanced diet based on the principles of healthy eating should be encouraged without unnecessary food restrictions.

Intestinal failure

The term intestinal failure was first used by Fleming & Remington (1981) to describe patients with *'a reduction of functioning gut mass below the minimal amount necessary for adequate digestion and absorption of nutrients'*. More recently, a group of international experts agreed the following definition, *'Intestinal failure results from obstruction, dysmotility, surgical resection, congenital defect, or disease associated loss of absorption and is characterised by the inability to maintain protein energy, fluid, electrolyte, or micronutrient balance'* (O'Keefe *et al.*, 2006).

Disease diagnosis and classification

The diagnosis and classification of intestinal failure is not yet agreed. The following classifications attempt to combine severity, type and length of nutritional support required (Lal *et al.*, 2006; Carlson *et al.*, 2010):

- *Type I* – self limiting, usually <28 days duration; includes postoperative ileus or small bowel obstruction requiring short term parenteral nutrition (PN).

- *Type 2* – lasting >28 days' duration and includes complex Crohn's disease, trauma, intestinal fistula or abdominal sepsis. These patients are severely ill with major resections of the bowel plus septic, metabolic and nutritional complications requiring multidisciplinary intervention with metabolic and nutritional support to permit recovery.

- *Type 3* – generally irreversible and therefore known as chronic intestinal failure resulting from massive bowel resection, leading to short bowel syndrome, e.g. mesenteric infarct/thrombosis, massive intestinal volvulus, inflammatory bowel disease and chronic radiation enteritis. This group also includes failure of intestinal motility, e.g. chronic idiopathic intestinal pseudo obstruction, visceral myopathy/neuropathy, scleroderma and sclerosing peritonitis. These patients usually require long term home PN (HPN).

Type 1 and 2 are often referred to as acute intestinal failure. Occasionally, in type 2 intestinal failure it is not appropriate to close the abdomen after surgery and the patient is left with an open abdomen (laparostomy). The prevalence of type 1 and 2 is currently unknown, but estimates range from 10 to 15% of patients undergoing intestinal resection and intestinal obstruction. The Association of Surgeons of Great Britain and Ireland has published principles on the surgical management of patients with acute intestinal failure, which include information on the prevention and treatment of type 1 and 2 (Carlson *et al.*, 2010). The introduction of enhanced recovery after surgery (ERAS) programs may reduce the incidence of postoperative ileus in the future (see Chapter 7.17.5).

The incidence of type 3 is also unknown but estimates can be made based on the number of patients requiring HPN in data collected by national surveys, including the British Artificial Nutrition Survey. The latest report estimated a prevalence of seven patients per million population, although it is recognised that this may be an underestimate (Jones *et al.*, 2009).

Nutritional consequences of intestinal failure and short bowel syndrome

Short bowel syndrome (SBS) is a subcategory of intestinal failure and has been defined by O'Keefe *et al.* (2006) as *'Short-bowel syndrome-intestinal failure results from surgical resection, congenital defect or disease-associated loss of absorption and is characterised by the inability to maintain protein-energy, fluid, electrolyte or micronutrient balances when on a conventionally accepted, normal diet'*. The effect of intestinal resection is best understood by considering where nutrients are normally absorbed. Most nutrients are absorbed within the first 100–150 cm of jejunum. Exceptions are vitamin B_{12} and bile salts, which are absorbed at specific receptor sites in the terminal ileum (Figure 7.4.6). Resection of the small

bowel will therefore affect absorption, but the outcome for the patient will depend on the type, length and quality of the remaining small bowel and the presence or absence of a functioning colon. Extensive resection may result in the remaining end of the small intestine being anastomosed to the colon (jejunocolic or ileocolic anastomosis) or ending at a stoma on the abdomen (jejunostomy or ileostomy). The loss of the ileum and some of the jejunum considerably impairs digestive and absorptive function. A residual small bowel length of <200 cm can be deemed as SBS, and can lead to nutritional, fluid and electrolyte depletion if not adequately managed. When the absorptive function of the colon is no longer available, more fluid and electrolytes will be lost. Nightingale *et al.* (1992) have shown that the following lengths of small bowel are inadequate to be managed on diet alone, and parenteral support of some form is required:

- <100 cm of jejunum will need long term intravenous fluid and electrolyte replacement.
- <75 cm of jejunum will need long term PN, fluid and electrolytes.
- <50 cm of jejunum plus colon will need long term PN, fluid and electrolytes.

All patients with SBS have problems with fluid and electrolyte balance, particularly in the immediate postoperative period, with nutrient requirements increased as a result of malabsorption.

Nutritional assessment

It is important that all patients undergoing surgery have their intestinal function assessed on a daily basis. A

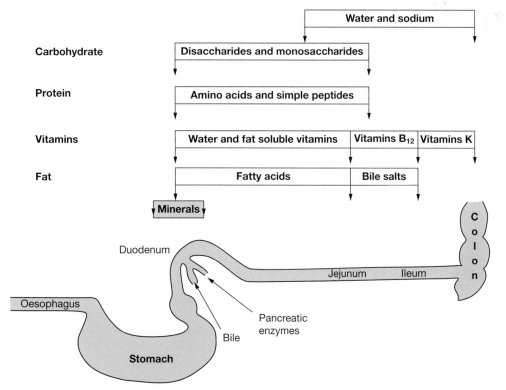

Figure 7.4.6   Sites of nutrient absorption (adapted from Thomas & Bishop 2007, figure 4.11.1, 9. 497. Reproduced with permission of Blackwell Publishing)

dietitian or nutritional support team should assess patients who fail to regain adequate function after day 5 as follows.

Anthropometry

Determine the perioperative nutritional status. Assessment of nutritional status should include weight, body mass index (BMI), percentage weight loss, mid arm circumference (MAC), triceps skinfold thickness TST), mid arm muscle circumference (MAMC) and grip strength. Is there evidence of oedema/ascites? If so, an estimated dry weight should be used to calculate BMI.

Biochemistry

Determine the hydration status of the patient. Do they appear dehydrated or overloaded? The administration of excessive volumes of 0.9% sodium chloride is common and can exacerbate postoperative ileus (Lobo *et al.*, 2002). Routine haematology and biochemistry, including urinary electrolytes, should be monitored. A random urinary sodium is invaluable in assessing hydration status; a value of <20 mmol/L indicates dehydration. Are there any other electrolyte deficiencies, i.e. potassium, magnesium, sodium? Are there micronutrient deficiencies, i.e. folate, iron, selenium, zinc, vitamins D or B_{12}?

Clinical assessment

Determine the underlying cause. What are the chances of resolution? Is the patient septic? Ongoing sepsis will result in increased nutritional requirements and a higher risk of metabolic and infective complications. Assessment of fluid balance is crucial, aiming for an intestinal output of <1500 mL/day and a urine volume of >1000 mL/day.

Dietary assessment

Determine the perioperative nutritional intake and compare with estimated requirements. Is nutritional support required? If a patient has failed or is expected to fail to establish on enteral nutrition (EN), then PN should be considered. An assessment of the adequacy of oral diet once weaned from PN or EN is also of importance.

Economic and social assessment

Postoperative complications cause a prolonged length of hospital stay that results in increased healthcare cost. Factors contributing to reduced quality of life for patients include:

- Infection including intra-abdominal sepsis.
- Inadequate wound, fistula and stoma care, which can result in excoriated skin.
- High intestinal losses leading to dehydration and electrolyte disturbances.
- Poor provision of nutrition resulting in malnutrition.
- Immobility.
- Depression.

All of the above increase the length of rehabilitation during which time the patient is unable to return to work and family life.

Clinical investigations

Computerised tomography (CT) is invaluable to investigate intra-abdominal sepsis along with a contrast study to assess the presence of an anastomotic leak. The management of abdominal sepsis is the most important aspect of care and can predict mortality and morbidity. Before considering reconstructive surgery in a patient with type 2 intestinal failure, it is important that radiological assessment has been completed as this provides a detailed understanding of the postoperative anatomy and the likelihood of parenteral independence (Carlson, 2003).

Clinical management

Fluid and sodium management of short bowel syndrome

The focus of treatment aims to reduce intestinal losses, thereby preventing dehydration and electrolyte disturbances; restricting oral fluid intake and using an oral rehydration solution achieves this. In some patients (known as secretors) intestinal losses of fluid and electrolytes may exceed the amount taken in by mouth, and parenteral replacement will be required. This is particularly likely to occur if the stoma is situated <100 cm along the jejunum (Nightingale *et al.*, 1990). Secretors may be in constant negative fluid and sodium balance. Those who can maintain sodium balance will still lose considerable amounts of sodium from their stoma and these losses will need to be replaced. Patients with an intestinal output of <1500 mL/day can usually maintain their sodium balance by adding extra salt to food, during cooking and by eating salty foods. An oral sodium supplement will be required when losses are greater than this. This should be provided as a glucose electrolyte solution with sodium content of at least 90 mmol/L, known as electrolyte mix (containing 20 g of glucose, 3.5 g of sodium chloride and 2.5 g of sodium bicarbonate). The patient should be encouraged to consume a litre of electrolyte mix, sipping it slowly throughout the day. The mix can be unpalatable and adding a small amount of juice or cordial, chilling and sipping through a straw may enhance its acceptability. Oral fluids with a lower sodium concentration, such as water or tea, should be restricted to <1 L/day as they will increase intestinal losses (Nightingale, 1994). Some patients will not be able to achieve adequate fluid and sodium balance by oral means and will require either subcutaneous or intravenous saline, possibly with additional magnesium, which can be administered at home (Martinez-Riquelme *et al.*, 2005).

Although it is common practice to encourage patients to consume foods and fluids separately, there is no evidence to support this advice. Woolf *et al.* (1987) found that restricting fluid intake around meals did not improve nutrient absorption in stable patients either with or without a colon. However, many patients with a high output stoma or fistula anecdotally report a benefit.

Pharmaceutical management

Other factors such as increased gastric acid production and reduced intestinal transit time exacerbate the problems of dehydration and sodium depletion in patients with SBS (Lennard-Jones, 1994). Gastric antisecretory drugs such as proton pump inhibitors have been shown to reduce intestinal losses by 1.5 kg/24 hours (Nightingale *et al.*, 1991). Patients who fail to absorb oral preparations may benefit from parenteral administration (Jeppesen *et al.*, 1998). Octreotide is a somatostatin analogue that reduces gastric, pancreatic and biliary secretions (Rodrigues *et al.*, 1989). However, its use should be reserved for patients with very high intestinal losses as it is given by a subcutaneous injection, three times daily. If there is no improvement after 3 days, it should be discontinued. Octreotide is frequently used in an attempt to heal a fistula, but this use is not supported by randomised controlled trials (Lloyd *et al.*, 2006). Antidiarrhoeal agents such as loperamide and codeine phosphate benefit patients by decreasing the frequency and weight of intestinal output and prolonging the transit time (Mainguet & Fiasse, 1977). These drugs are usually needed in very high doses and should be taken 30–60 minutes before meals. Cholestyramine, an ion exchange resin used in patients with bile salt malabsorption, is likely to increase bile salt loss, decrease the bile salt pool and further reduce jejunal bile salt concentration, possibly to a level below the micellar concentration. It is therefore not recommended for patients with a colon in continuity except as a possible treatment for hyperoxaluria (Lennard-Jones, 1994). Magnesium deficiency is common and can usually be corrected with an oral magnesium oxide supplement, although this can also result in increased intestinal output. If oral supplements are ineffective, then magnesium sulphate can be added to normal saline and given subcutaneously or intravenously to maintain plasma concentrations (Martinez-Riquelme *et al.*, 2005). Vitamin D concentrations should be measured and replaced if found to be deficient as vitamin D will increase the intestinal and renal absorption of magnesium (Nightingale, 2001).

Nutritional management

The nutritional management of intestinal failure is a dynamic process that involves overlap or transition between diet, EN and PN as the patient's condition changes. The judgement to start nutrition support in type 1 and 2 intestinal failure is often fraught with indecision. The wait and see approach or the presence or absence of bowel sounds is misleading and can result in significant time without adequate nutrition in those who may benefit from PN. Despite the obvious benefits of PN support in patients with type 1 and 2 intestinal failure, a recent report on the use of PN revealed good standards of care in only 19% of UK hospitals. The report highlighted a lack of adequate consideration of EN, delays in the initiation of PN, and inadequate assessment and monitoring, resulting in avoidable metabolic and infective complications [National Confidential Enquiry into Patient Outcome and Death (NCEPOD), 2010)]. It is common for patients who develop an enterocutaneous fistula to be placed nil by mouth and to start PN and octreotide in an attempt to heal the fistula. However, in patients where closure is unlikely to occur spontaneously, an oral diet can be introduced. Patients with intestinal fistulae who have over 75 cm of normal small intestine distal to the fistula may be candidates for fistuloclysis, a technique in which EN is infused into the distal small intestine (Teubner *et al.*, 2004). Further details on this technique can be found on the website of the Intestinal Rehabilitation Unit at Salford Royal Hospital (www.i-rehab.org.uk).

The general principles of nutritional management can be summarised as:

- Immediately post surgery, PN will be required. Close attention should be paid to fluid and electrolyte balance (especially sodium and magnesium as losses may be very high).
- In order to stimulate gut adaptation, enteral intake should be introduced as soon as possible while still continuing some parenteral support. Initially, the patient's oral fluid intake should not exceed 500 mL/day.
- When fluids are tolerated, small meals and snacks can gradually be introduced. Food introduction to patients also likely to need long term PN should aim to find a balance between eating for pleasure and avoiding high intestinal losses. For those likely to be able to manage on diet alone, the aim should be to maximise intake to achieve adequate absorption.
- Parenteral support can be reduced as oral intake increases. However, parenteral fluids and/or oral glucose electrolyte solutions are likely to be needed to meet fluid and sodium requirements until gut adaptation takes place. Additional nutritional support in the form of polymeric supplements or overnight feeding may be required. If the patient is receiving an enteral feed, sodium may need to be added to increase the sodium content to >90 mmol/L. This can be achieved by adding 10–20 mL of 30% sodium chloride (50–100 mmol) to ready to hang feeds; this measure may allow the patient to stop taking oral electrolyte mix during the day.
- As adaptation occurs, gradual transition to a more normal diet can be made, with inadequacies in nutrition or fluid intake being compensated by nutritional support measures if indicated.
- Since restoration of intestinal lactase levels is one of the last adaptive mechanisms to occur, large lactose loads may need to be avoided initially. However, there is no evidence that stable patients, either with or without a colon, benefit from a lactose free diet (Arrigoni *et al.*, 1994). Therefore, foods containing lactose should not be excluded from the diet of short bowel patients as they provide a valuable source of macro- and micro-nutrients.

It is imperative that patients with SBS adhere to an appropriate regimen in order to maximise the remaining intestine and reduce dependence on PN. For over 50 years it has been known that patients who have significant bowel resections need to consume excessive oral nutrients to overcome malabsorption and avoid malnutrition. However, it was not until the 1990s that the exact composition of the diet depending on intestinal anatomy was identified (Nordgaard *et al.*, 1994). Balance studies have shown energy requirements exceeding 2.5 times basal energy expenditure [30–60 kcal (125–250 kJ)/kg/day] and nitrogen intakes of 0.2–0.25 g/kg/day are required to prevent protein energy malnutrition (Woolf *et al.*, 1987; Messing *et al.*, 1991). Recent studies have confirmed these findings and recommendations (Crenn *et al.*, 2004; Estívariz *et al.*; 2008), and the promotion of a hyperphagic diet is now established. This involves the provision of high energy meals and snacks as well as food fortification and nutritional supplements. For patients who have difficulties in achieving recommended oral macronutrient intakes, oral nutritional supplements or enteral feeding may provide additional nutrients. Nocturnal EN is often utilised to maximise absorption by increasing the length of time the bowel is exposed to nutrients. McIntyre *et al.* (1986) compared an elemental versus a polymeric formula and found no significant differences in the percentage of macronutrient absorption. Cosnes *et al.* (1992) compared a semi elemental verses a polymeric formula and demonstrated improved nitrogen absorption on the semi elemental (p = 0.012). No other differences in absorption were shown. The contrasting results in nitrogen absorption are likely to be related to the composition of the formulae investigated. Elemental formula is less palatable, has a higher osmolality and requires larger volumes to meet estimated nutritional requirements in comparison to polymeric formula, and therefore if additional nutritional support is required to maintain or improve nutritional status in patients, then a polymeric formula is recommended. Joly *et al.* (2009) randomised patients to usual diet or usual diet plus continuous enteral feeding using a polymeric formula and found increased absorption of energy, nitrogen and fat with no increase in intestinal output whilst receiving continuous enteral feeding compared to those on diet alone. The continuous method of feeding may improve intestinal absorption to an extent that patients no longer require PN and should, therefore, be a treatment option for all short bowel patients with over 75 cm of small bowel. If a vitamin, mineral or trace element deficiency is demonstrated, an appropriate supplement can be prescribed. If >100 cm of terminal ileum is resected, then the patient will become depleted in vitamin B_{12} and will require replacement via an intramuscular injection every 3 months.

In practice there are two types of patients with SBS and it has become apparent that patients differ in their response to dietary manipulation depending on the presence or absence of a colon, and this determines whether the additional energy requirements should be provided from fat or carbohydrate (Table 7.4.10).

Patients with a jejunostomy

Patients with a jejunostomy have had varying lengths of jejunum, ileum and colon removed. The remaining small bowel is then brought to the surface of the abdomen to create a stoma (jejunostomy) (Figure 7.4.7). Patients have immediate problems postoperatively due to large intesti-

Table 7.4.10 Summary of evidence based recommendations for the dietary treatment for patients with short bowel syndrome

	Jejunocolic anastomosis	Stoma (jejunostomy)
Total energy	30–60 kcal/kg/day (125–250 kJ/kg/day)	30–60 kcal/kg/day (125–250 kJ/kg/day)
Nitrogen	0.2–0.25 g/kg/day	0.2–0.25 g/kg/day
Protein	1.25–1.5 g/kg/day	1.25–1.5 g/kg/day
Fat (% of total energy)	20–30	30–40
MCT (% if total fat)	50	No proven benefit
Carbohydrate (% of total energy)	50–60	40–50
Fibre	Low to moderate	Low
Sodium chloride	Normal	Additions usually required
Enteral nutrition	Polymeric	Polymeric

MCT, medium chain triglyceride.

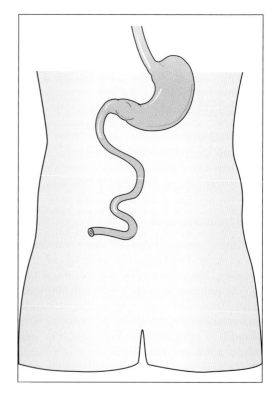

Figure 7.4.7 Jejunostomy (courtesy of Northwest London Hospital Trust, Medical Illustrations Department)

nal losses from the jejunostomy leading to fluid and sodium depletion. Malnutrition will occur if appropriate nutritional support is not instigated. In addition, the patient will also experience a rapid transit time, reducing the potential for nutrient absorption and resulting in subsequent weight loss and malnutrition. Studies of short bowel patients consuming their usual diet indicate that on average <50% of oral fat intake is absorbed. The role of fat restriction has been controversial, with conflicting results from different research groups (Andersson *et al.*, 1974; Hessov *et al.*, 1983; Ovesen *et al.*, 1983; Woolf *et al.*, 1983; McIntyre *et al*, 1986; Crenn *et al.*, 2004). Overall, it appears that there is no significant benefit to patients following a low fat diet and since fat provides a concentrated form of energy and makes the diet palatable in addition to providing essential fatty acids, these patients should therefore be encouraged to have a high intake of fat.

It is often recommended that due to the rapid transit through the intestine, that dietary fibre is limited in patients with SBS. However, only one study has been conducted manipulating the fibre content of the diet of jejunostomy patients. McIntyre *et al.* (1986) conducted a randomised controlled trial in four jejunostomy patients who received diets that were isocaloric and isonitrogenous, but with variable amounts of fat, fibre and carbohydrate over a 2–3-day period; no significant benefit of manipulating the diet was found. Despite a lack of evidence, patients anecdotally report a reduction in intestinal output on a low fibre diet.

Patients with a jejunocolic anastomosis

Patients with a jejunocolic anastomosis have had the ileum and some jejunum resected, and the remaining jejunum anastomosed to the colon (Figure 7.4.8). They experience diarrhoea and/or steatorrhoea with resultant malabsorption, weight loss and malnutrition. The presence of the colon in continuity is advantageous because it enables water and sodium to be absorbed, and results in a slower intestinal transit, aiding nutrient absorption. A comparison of the effects of a diet either high in carbohydrate (60%) and low in fat (20%) or vice versa (20% carbohydrate and 60% fat) found that patients with a colon absorbed a higher percentage of energy on the high carbohydrate, low fat diet, but that no such difference was seen in jejunostomy patients. This suggests that patients with a colon salvage energy as a result of the fermentation of unabsorbed carbohydrate to easily absorbed short chain fatty acids (Nordgaard *et al.*, 1994). Colonic digestion can supply up to 1000 kcal (4.19 kJ)/day in patients with <200 cm of jejunum in continuity (Nordgaard *et al.*, 1996). These patients should be encouraged to take a diet as high in carbohydrate as can be tolerated without causing bloating due to increased gas production. A reduction in fat intake is often helpful as this decreases magnesium and calcium losses, and reduces steatorrhoea/diarrhoea and oxalate absorption (Lennard-Jones, 1994). However, a reduced fat intake will also reduce energy intake and so in practice, a compromise has to be found between including fat for energy and avoiding steatorrhoea. Replacement of long chain triglyceride (LCT) with a medium chain triglyceride (MCT) fat emulsion has been shown to increase energy and fat absorption in patients with a colon (Jeppesen & Mortensen, 1998).

A secondary consequence of steatorrhoea is a greater risk of calcium oxalate renal stones, due to increased colonic oxalate absorption and resultant hyperoxaluria. A low oxalate diet is advisable in these circumstances; will restrict intake of tea, spinach, beetroot, rhubarb, peanuts and chocolate. Avoiding chronic dehydration is another important measure to reduce the risk of renal stones (Nightingale *et al.*, 1992).

In conclusion, short bowel patients need to consume as much as twice the average estimated requirements of energy and protein to compensate for lack of absorptive capacity. Patients with a jejunostomy will benefit from a high fat diet whereas those with a colon should focus on increasing the carbohydrate content of the diet (see Table 7.4.10). Close dietetic supervision of these patients is vital during the early stages and until intestinal adaptation has taken place. Manipulation of the diet and changes in medication should be staged, with several days allowed for each stage and to assess the impact of each change on intestinal output. Each patient is individual and it will need a lot of time and patience to find the combination that best suits. Patients benefit from the support of a multidisciplinary team where there is close liaison between doctors, nurses, dietitians and pharmacists.

Future advances in treatment

Glucagon like peptide 2 (GLP 2), a hormone secreted by the intestine, has been shown to increase the growth of

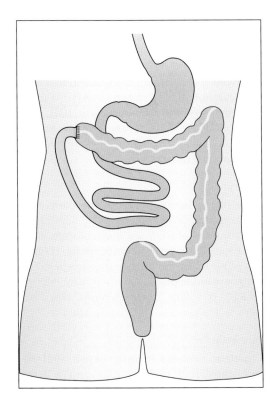

Figure 7.4.8 Jejunocolic anastomosis (courtesy of Northwest London Hospital Trust, Medical Illustrations Department)

SECTION 7

normal cells in the intestine, allowing the intestine to absorb more fluid and nutrients, which may help to reduce dependency on PN. An analogue of GLP 2 is being evaluated and could be a promising therapy for patients with SBS (Jeppesen *et al.*, 2005).

Small bowel transplantation offers an alternative treatment to patients with chronic intestinal failure dependent on HPN. However, although survival is improving, it does not yet match that achieved by HPN and should be reserved for patients with complications of HPN, such as liver disease and poor venous access (Middleton, 2007).

Resection of the large intestine

Disease processes

Resection of the large intestine is usually performed due to inflammatory bowel disease (IBD), cancer of the colon, diverticulitis or the genetic condition familial adenomatous polyposis (FAP).

Disease consequences

Until the early 1980s, resection of the colon and rectum resulted in the creation of a permanent stoma, either an ileostomy (following complete removal of the colon and rectum) or colostomy (after removal of the terminal segment of the colon and rectum). Intestinal effluent is collected in a bag fixed around the stoma onto the skin. These procedures are still performed if disease requires such extensive rectal resection that no functioning muscle tissue in the anal area remains, e.g. as in IBD. A major improvement has occurred with the development of the restorative proctocolectomy, a procedure that involves the creation of a pouch reservoir from a segment of ileum, which is then joined to the anus. The pouch acts as an artificial rectum, thus conserving anal continence and avoiding the need for a stoma. This technique is commonly used to treat patients with ulcerative colitis or FAP and is much more acceptable to patients than a permanent ileostomy.

Ileal pouches derive their names from the number of limbs of ileum used in their fashioning (J pouch, S pouch and W pouch). These surgical procedures, which anastomose different pouch types to the anal canal (the ileal pouch anal anastomosis), share common methodology. Ileal reservoirs can also be constructed without an ileal pouch by anal anastomosis, e.g. the continent ileal reservoir or Kock pouch, but these procedures are now less frequently performed.

Pouch creation is complex and the operation is often done in two stages. First, colectomy (removal of the colon) and proctectomy (removal of diseased rectal mucosa) are performed, leaving the rectal muscular cuff and anal sphincter intact. A pseudo rectum (pouch) is constructed by joining a portion of the terminal ileum to the anal canal and a temporary ileostomy created to divert bowel contents away from the newly formed pouch, allowing it to heal. A further operation then anastomoses the pouch to the intestine and reverses the ileostomy. The

safety, feasibility and short term outcome of performing this operation laparoscopically has demonstrated similar results to open surgery with improvements shown in recovery outcomes (Larson *et al.*, 2006).

Following surgery, problems with stool frequency and/ or consistency are likely to occur, but continence is usually achieved within 10 days and over a period of about 1 year, the pouch gradually adapts with bowel movements becoming less frequent and more solid in consistency (Nicholls & Williams, 2002).

Nutritional consequences

Removal of the colon results in considerable loss of absorptive capacity in respect of fluids and electrolytes, especially sodium. Initially, considerable quantities of both electrolytes and fluid will be lost (between 1200 and 2000 mL/day) and requirement for both will be increased for at least 6–8 weeks. After this time, the ileum appears to adapt and losses decrease, although they still remain in the order of 400–600 mL/day. However, in contrast to those with accompanying ileal resection, the digestive and absorptive capacity of the small intestine remains, so that no major nutritional deficiencies are to be expected, except for vitamin B_{12} and bile acids, which occur in about one-third of patients (Christl & Scheppach, 1997). More recently, concerns have been raised that patients with an ileostomy are chronically dehydrated and have depleted calcium and magnesium stores, putting them at risk of renal impairment, renal stones and bone demineralisation (Ng *et al.*, 2004).

Nutritional assessment

Anthropometry

Determine the perioperative nutritional status. Patients may be malnourished prior to surgery and their nutritional risk will need to be identified and action taken in order to avoid a deterioration in nutritional status and poor surgical outcome (Fulham, 2004). Assessment of nutritional status should include weight, BMI, percentage weight loss, MAC, TST, MAMC and grip strength. Is there evidence of oedema/ascites? If so, an estimated dry weight should be used to calculate the BMI.

Biochemistry

Determine the hydration status of the patient. Do they appear dehydrated or overloaded? The administration of excessive volumes of 0.9% sodium chloride is common and can exacerbate postoperative ileus (Lobo *et al.*, 2002). Are there any electrolyte deficiencies, i.e. potassium, magnesium, sodium. Are there any micronutrient deficiencies, i.e. folate, iron, selenium, zinc, vitamin D or B_{12}.

Clinical assessment

Is the patient septic? Ongoing sepsis will result in increased nutritional requirements and a higher risk of metabolic and infective complications. Assessment of fluid balance is crucial aiming for an intestinal output of <1500 mL/day and a urine volume of >1000 mL/day.

SECTION 7

Dietary assessment

Determine the perioperative nutritional intake and compare this to estimated requirements. Is nutritional support required? If a patient has failed or is expected to fail to establish on EN, then PN should be considered. Assessment should be made of the adequacy of an oral diet once weaned from PN or EN.

Economic and social assessment

Postoperative complications cause a prolonged length of hospital stay that results in increased healthcare cost. Factors contributing to reduced quality of life for patients include:

- Infection including intra-abdominal sepsis.
- Inadequate wound, fistula and stoma care, which can result in excoriated skin.
- High intestinal losses leading to dehydration and electrolyte disturbances.
- Poor provision of nutrition resulting in malnutrition.
- Immobility.
- Depression.

All of the above increase the length of rehabilitation during which the patient is unable to return to work and family life.

Clinical management

Perioperative fasting in gastrointestinal surgery is no longer recommended and early enteral feeding should be encouraged (Fearon *et al.* 2005; Lewis *et al.* 2009). The long term consequences in terms of faecal volume and biochemistry appear to be similar in patients after restorative proctocolectomy with a J pouch (Okamoto *et al.*, 1995) and those with conventional panproctocolectomy and permanent ileostomy. However, due to the kidneys' attempt to conserve water and sodium, both groups of patients are at greater risk of uric acid stones as a result of producing urine that is low in volume and pH, and with a high concentration of calcium and oxalate compared with control subjects (Christie *et al.*, 1996). In addition, J pouch patients may be at increased risk of calcium stones and abnormal bile acid metabolism. Patients with pouches should be advised regarding the possibility of developing pouchitis, inflammation within the pouch, which can occur in up to 50% patients. Symptoms include increased pouch frequency, reduced stool consistency and urgency, and usually respond well to antibiotics. The probiotic VSL#3 may be beneficial in maintaining remission of pouchitis and is recommended by the British Society of Gastroenterology (Mowat *et al.*, 2011) and a Cochrane systematic review (Holubar *et al.*, 2010).

Nutritional management

While the ileum is adapting and the stool or stomal effluent remains liquid, fluid losses should be replaced by the consumption of 1.5–2 L/day of fluid. Additional salt, e.g. up to one teaspoon added to food during the course of

a day, may be necessary in hot weather or if losses are particularly high. As stool frequency and consistency improve, losses will decrease, but it remains important to ensure adequate fluid and sodium provision. An episode of vomiting or diarrhoea can rapidly create an electrolyte imbalance and the provision of extra potassium (via fruit juices) and sodium (via extra salt on food or salty beverages such as soup or meat extracts) is advisable (Pearson, 2008). In severe cases, parenteral saline may be necessary.

It should not be overlooked that many patients will be nutritionally depleted after colorectal surgery, particularly if they suffered chronic ill health beforehand and food intake was poor. If, as in the case of pouch patients, two, or even three, operations are required, this is a further strain on nutritional status. It will also take some time before normal appetite is restored. It is therefore important that patients are encouraged to consume small, frequent, nutrient dense meals and snacks, and that additional oral nutritional support measures are instituted when necessary. Return to normal body composition in ulcerative colitis patients undergoing J pouch has been described (Christie & Hill, 1990; Jensen *et al.*, 2002).

Dietary guidance for ileostomy and pouch patients is similar. People should be encouraged to:

- Adopt a regular meal pattern. Some may need smaller meals at more frequent intervals. Those with pouches may need to avoid eating late at night to avoid nocturnal stool production.
- Eat a varied well balanced diet based on healthy eating principles.
- Consume meals slowly and chew foods well.
- Drink plenty of fluids (1.5–2 L/day) and more in hot weather.
- Consume extra fluid and salt if stool or stoma losses suddenly increase or during episodes of vomiting or fever. Medical advice may be needed if these losses are severe or persistent.

The range of foods consumed can be gradually increased and patients should be encouraged to eat a normal diet based on the principles of healthy eating. No foods are specifically contraindicated for ileostomy or pouch patients, but some foods can cause unpleasant symptoms such as stool odour or flatulence. Blockage with undigested food residues can occur, particularly if the stoma or anastomosis is tight. Occasionally, a low residue diet is required if obstruction regularly occurs. However, in most people this is unnecessary and avoidance of the few specific foods that typically cause the problem is sufficient to prevent it. There is a small amount of evidence (Steenhagen *et al.*, 2006; Chartrand-Lefebvre *et al.*, 1990; Pearson 2002; 2008) on food related problems in ileostomy/pouch patients, including:

- *Poorly digested foods* (most likely to cause blockage) – grapefruit, lettuce, mushrooms, sweet corn, fruit or vegetable skins, lentils, peas, nuts, seeds, tomatoes, coconut, fibrous fruit and vegetables such as celery or pineapple, and Chinese food.

- *Increased stool odour* – onions, garlic, brassica vegetables (Brussel sprouts, cabbage, cauliflower and broccoli), beans, fish and eggs.
- *Increased flatulence/bloating* – baked beans, lentils, peas, onions, garlic, brassica vegetables, fizzy drinks, beer and lager.
- *Increased stool frequency* – beer, spirits, Chinese food, wholewheat cereals, corn, apples, wine, fried and spicy foods, strawberries, potatoes, bread, bananas, fruit, fruit juice and vegetables.
- *Decrease in stool consistency* – beer, wine, fried fish, strawberries, corn, popcorn, spirits, coleslaw, grapefruit, turnips, raspberries and fruit juice.
- *Perianal irritation* – spicy foods, citrus fruit, raw carrot, nuts and seeds.

It appears that the majority of patients with an ileal pouch report that some form of dietary restriction is required to help prevent unpleasant symptoms and that this impacts on quality of life (Coffey *et al.*, 2002). However, it should be remembered that individual tolerance may vary considerably, so patients should be encouraged to discover for themselves on a trial and error basis which foods are best tolerated. Patients should also be warned that foods such as beetroot could change the colour of the stool to such an extent that it can be mistaken for bleeding. Continuing problems with stool frequency may be treated with loperamide. There is no evidence that supplementary fibre in the form of pectin or methylcellulose is helpful in this respect (Thirlby & Kelly, 1997). A recent study investigated the effect of a fermentable oligo-, di- and mono-saccharides and polyols (FODMAP) diet on bowel function in 15 patients without a colon and reported a significant reduction in daily stool frequency. However, this result was limited to those without pouchitis (Croagh *et al.*, 2007).

All patients should receive regular follow-up to ensure that diet related problems are remedied, unnecessary food restrictions avoided and adequate nutritional status maintained.

Drug–nutrient interactions

The following should be noted:

- Proton pump inhibitors – no interaction with food or nutrients demonstrated.
- Loperamide – no interaction with food or nutrients demonstrated. Aim to avoid syrup formulations as these contain sorbitol, which can act as a laxative.
- Octreotide – no information available.
- Colestyramine– no interaction with food or nutrients demonstrated. Other drugs should be taken at least 1 hour before or 4–6 hours after to reduce possible interference with absorption.

Further reading

Birch J (ed). (2008) *Stoma care*. Chichester, Wiley Blackwell.
Braga M, Ljungqvist O, Soeters P, Fearon K, Weimann A, Bozzetti F. (2009) ESPEN Guidelines on Parenteral Nutrition: Surgery. *Clinical Nutrition* 28: 378–386.

Jeppesen PB, Mortensen PB. (2001) Dietary treatment of patients with a short bowel. In: Nightingale JMD (ed) *Intestinal Failure*. London: Greenwich Medical Media Ltd, pp. 393–404.
Langnas AL, Goulet O, Quigley EMM, Tappenden KA. (2008). *Intestinal Failure. Diagnosis, Management and Transplantation*. Oxford: Blackwell Publishing.
Van Gossum A, Cabre E, Hébuterne X, *et al.* (2009) ESPEN Guidelines on Parenteral Nutrition: gastroenterology. *Clinical Nutrition* 28: 415–427.
Williams J (ed). (2002) *The Essentials of Pouch Care Nursing*. London: Whurr Publishers Ltd.

Internet resources

Crohn's and Colitis UK (formerly known as NACC) www.crohnsandcolitis.org.uk
Ileostomy and Internal Pouch Support Group www.iasupport.org.uk
Intestinal Rehabilitation Unit at Salford Royal Hospital www.i-rehab.org.uk
Patients on Intravenous and Nasogastric Nutrition Therapy (PINNT) www.pinnt.com
St Mark's Hospital & Academic Institute www.stmarkshospital.org.uk

References

Arrigoni E, Marteau P, Briet F, Pochart P, Rambaud JC. (1994) Tolerance and absorption of lactose from milk and yogurt during short bowel syndrome in humans. *American Journal of Clinical Nutrition* 60: 926–929.
Andersson H, Isaksson, B, Sjögren B. (1974) Fat-reduced diet in the symptomatic treatment of small bowel disease: Metabolic studies in patients with Crohn's disease and in other patients subjected to ileal resection. *Gut* 15: 351–359.
Carlson GL. (2003) Surgical management of intestinal failure. *Proceedings of the Nutrition Society* 62(3): 711–718.
Carlson G, Gardiner K, McKee R, MacFie J, Vaizey C. (2010) *The Surgical Management of Patients with Acute Intestinal Failure*. London: Association of Surgeons of Great Britain and Ireland. Available at www.asgbi.org.uk/download.cfm?docid=74E316BB-F98D-41D1-854DD3080327CAB0. Accessed 14 June 2012.
Chartrand-Lefebvre C, Heppell J, Davignon I, Dubé S, Pomp A. (1990) Dietary habits after ileal pouch-anal anastomosis. *Canadian Journal of Surgery* 33: 101–105.
Christie PM, Hill GL. (1990). Return to normal body composition after ileoanal J-pouch anastomosis for ulcerative colitis. *Diseases of the Colon and Rectum* 33: 584–586.
Christie PM, Knight GS, Hill GL. (1996) Comparison of relative risks of urinary stone formation after surgery for ulcerative colitis: conventional ileostomy vs. J-pouch. A comparative study. *Diseases of the Colon and Rectum* 39: 50–54.
Christl SU, Scheppach W. (1997) Metabolic consequences of colectomy. *Scandinavian Journal of Gastroenterology Supplement* 222: 20–24.
Coffey JC, Winter DC, Neary P, Murphy A, Redmond HP, Kirwan WO. (2002) Quality of life after ileal pouch-anal anastomosis: an evaluation of diet and other factors using the Cleveland global quality of life instrument. *Diseases of the Colon and Rectum* 45: 30–38.
Cosnes J, Evard D, Beaugerie L, Gendre JP, Le Quintrec Y. (1992) Improvement in protein absorption with a small-peptide-based diet in patients with high jejunostomy. *Nutrition* 8: 406–411.
Crenn P, Morin MC, Joly F, Penven S, Thuillier F, Messing B. (2004) Net digestive absorption and adaptive hyperphagia in adult short bowel patients. *Gut* 53: 1279–1286.
Croagh C, Shepherd SJ, Berryman M, Muir JG, Gibson PR. (2007) Pilot study on the effect of reducing dietary FODMAP intake on bowel function in patients without a colon. *Inflammatory Bowel Disease* 13: 1522–1528.
Estívariz CF, Luo M, Umeakunne K, *et al.* (2008) Nutrient intake from habitual oral diet in patients with severe short bowel syn-

drome living in the south eastern United States. *Nutrition* 24: 330–339.

Fearon KC, Ljungqvist O, Von Meyenfeldt M, *et al*. (2005) Enhanced recovery after surgery: A consensus review of clinical care for patients undergoing colonic resection. *Clinical Nutrition* 24: 466–477.

Fleming CR, Remington M. (1981) Intestinal failure. In: Hill GL (ed) *Nutrition and the Surgical Patient*. New York: Churchill Livingstone, pp. 219–235.

Fulham J. (2004) Improving the nutritional status of colorectal surgical and stoma patients. *British Journal of Nursing* 13: 702–708.

Hessov I, Andersson H, Isaksson B. (1983) Effects of a low-fat diet on mineral absorption in small-bowel disease. *Scandinavian Journal of Gastroenterology* 18: 551–554.

Holubar SD, Cima RR, Sandborn WJ, Pardi DS. (2010) Treatment and prevention of pouchitis after ileal pouch-anal anastomosis for chronic ulcerative colitis. *Cochrane Database of Systematic Reviews* 6: CD001176.

Jensen MB, Houborg KB, Vestergaard P, Kissmeyer-Nielsen P, Mosekilde L, Laurberg S. (2002) Improved physical performance and increased lean tissue and fat mass in patients with ulcerative colitis four to six years after ileoanal anastomosis with a J-pouch. *Diseases of the Colon and Rectum* 45: 1601–1607.

Jeppesen PB, Mortensen PB. (1998) The influence of a preserved colon on the absorption of medium chain fat in patients with small bowel resection. *Gut* 43: 478–483.

Jeppesen PB, Staun M, Tjellesen L, Mortensen PB. (1998) Effect of intravenous ranitidine and omeprazole on intestinal absorption of water, sodium, and macronutrients in patients with intestinal resection. *Gut* 43: 763–769.

Jeppesen PB, Sanguinetti EL, Buchman A, *et al*. (2005) Teduglutide (ALX-0600), a dipeptidase IV resistant glucagon-like peptide 2 analogue, improves intestinal function in short bowel syndrome patients. *Gut* 54: 1224–1231.

Joly F, Dray X, Corcos O, Barbot L, Kapel N, Messing B. (2009) Tube feeding improves intestinal absorption in short bowel syndrome patients. *Gastroenterology* 136: 824–831.

Jones BJM, Baxter JP, Smith T, Petrie A. (2009) Adult home parenteral nutrition (HPN). In: Smith T (ed) *Annual BANS Report*. Redditch: BAPEN, pp. 25–33.

Lal S, Teubner A, Shaffer JL. (2006) Review article: intestinal failure. *Alimentary Pharmacology & Therapeutics* 24: 19–31.

Larson DW, Cima RR, Dozois EJ, *et al*. (2006) Safety, feasibility, and short-term outcomes of laparoscopic ileal-pouch-anal anastomosis: a single institutional case-matched experience. *Annals of Surgery* 243: 667–670.

Lennard-Jones JE. (1994) Review article: practical management of the short bowel. *Alimentary Pharmacology & Therapeutics* 8: 563–577.

Lewis SJ, Andersen HK, Thomas S. (2009) Early enteral nutrition within 24 h of intestinal surgery versus later commencement of feeding: a systematic review and meta-analysis. *Journal of Gastrointestinal Surgery* 13: 569–575.

Lobo DN, Bostock K, Neal KR, Perkins AC, Rowlands BJ, Allison SP. (2002) Effect of salt and water balance on recovery of gastrointestinal function after elective colonic resection: a randomised controlled trial. *Lancet* 359: 1812–1818.

Lloyd DA, Gabe SM, Windsor AC. (2006) Nutrition and management of enterocutaneous fistula. *British Journal of Surgery* 93: 1045–1055.

Mainguet P, Fiasse R. (1977) Double-blind placebo controlled study of loperamide (Imodium) in chronic diarrhoea caused by ileocolic disease or resection. *Gut* 18: 575–579.

Martinez-Riquelme A, Rawlings J, Morley S, Kendall J, Hosking D, Allison S. (2005) Self-administered subcutaneous fluid infusion at home in the management of fluid depletion and hypomagnesaemia in gastro-intestinal disease. *Clinical Nutrition* 24: 158–163.

McIntyre PB, Fitchew M, Lennard-Jones JE. (1986) Patients with a high jejunostomy do not need a special diet. *Gastroenterology* 91: 25–33.

Messing B, Pigot F, Rongier M, Morin MC, Ndeïndoum U, Rambaud JC. (1991) Intestinal absorption of free oral hyperalimentation in the very short bowel syndrome. *Gastroenterology* 100: 1502–1508.

Middleton SJ. (2007) Is intestinal transplantation now an alternative to home parenteral nutrition? *Proceedings of the Nutrition Society* 66: 316–320.

Mowat C, Cole A, Windsor A, *et al*. (2011) Guidelines for the management of inflammatory bowel disease in adults. *Gut* 60: 571–607.

National Confidential Enquiry into Patient Outcome and Death (NCEPOD). (2010) A mixed bag: An enquiry into the care of hospital patients receiving parenteral nutrition. Available at www.ncepod.org.uk/2010report1/downloads/PN_report.pdf. Accessed 14 June 2012.

Ng DHL, Wooton SA, Jackson AA, Stroud MA. (2004) Sodium and mineral status of ileostomy patients. *Clinical Nutrition* 23: 1488.

Nicholls RJ, Williams J. (2002) The ileo-anal pouch. In: Williams J (ed) *The Essentials of Pouch Care Nursing*. London: Whurr Publishers Ltd, pp. 68–98.

Nightingale JMD. (1994) Clinical problems of a short bowel and their treatment. *Proceedings of the Nutrition Society* 53: 373–391.

Nightingale JMD. (2001) Management of a high-output jejunostomy. In: Nightingale JMD (ed) *Intestinal Failure*. London: Greenwich Medical Media Limited, pp. 375–392.

Nightingale JMD, Lennard-Jones JE, Walker ER, Farthing MJG. (1990) Jejunal efflux in short bowel syndrome. *Lancet* 336: 765–768.

Nightingale JMD, Walker ER, Farthing MJG, Lennard-Jones JE. (1991) Effect of omeprazole on intestinal output in the short bowel syndrome. *Alimentary Pharmacology & Therapeutics* 5: 405–412.

Nightingale JMD, Lennard-Jones JE, Gertner DJ, Wood, SR, Bartram CI. (1992) Colonic preservation reduces the need for parenteral therapy, increases incidence of renal stones, but does not change the high prevalence of gall stones in patients with a short bowel. *Gut* 33: 1493–1497.

Nordgaard I, Hansen BS, Mortensen PB. (1994) Colon as a digestive organ in patients with short bowel. *Lancet* 343: 373–376.

Nordgaard I, Hansen BS, Mortensen PB. (1996) Importance of colonic support for energy absorption as small bowel failure proceeds. *American Journal of Clinical Nutrition* 64: 222–231.

Okamoto T, Kusunoki M, Kusuhara K, Yamamura T, Utsunomiya J. (1995) Water and electrolyte balance after ileal J pouch-anal anastomosis in ulcerative colitis and familial adenomatous polyposis. *International Journal of Colorectal Disease* 10: 33–38.

O'Keefe SJ, Buchman AL, Fishbein TM, Jeejeebhoy KN, Jeppesen PB, Shaffer J. (2006) Short bowel syndrome and intestinal failure: consensus definitions and overview. *Clinical Gastroenterology and Hepatology* 4: 6–10.

Ovesen L, Chu R, Howard L. (1983) The influence of dietary fat on jejunostomy output in patients with severe short bowel syndrome. *American Journal of Clinical Nutrition* 38: 270–277.

Pearson M. (2002) Dietary aspects of internal pouches. In: Williams J (ed) *The Essentials of Pouch Care Nursing*. London: Whurr Publishers Ltd, pp. 165–179.

Pearson M. (2008) Nutrition. In: Birch J (ed) *Stoma Care*. Chichester: Wiley Blackwell, pp. 210–232.

Rodrigues CA, Lennard-Jones JE, Thompson DG, Farthing MJG. (1989) The effects of octreotide, soy polysaccharide, codeine and loperamide on nutrient, fluid and electrolyte absorption in the short-bowel syndrome. *Alimentary Pharmacology & Therapeutics* 3: 158–169.

Steenhagen E, de Roos NM, Bouwman CA, van Laarhoven CJ, van Staveren WA. (2006) Sources and severity of self-reported food intolerance after ileal pouch-anal anastomosis. *Journal of the American Dietetic Association* 106: 1459–1462.

Teubner A, Morrison K, Ravishankar HR, Anderson ID, Scott NA, Carlson GL. (2004) Fistuloclysis can successfully replace parenteral feeding in the nutritional support of patients with enterocutaneous fistula. *British Journal of Surgery* 91: 625–631.

Thirlby RC, Kelly R. (1997) Pectin and methylcellulose do not affect intestinal function in patients after ileal pouch-anal anastomosis. *American Journal of Gastroenterology* 92: 99–102.

Woolf GM, Miller C, Kurian R, Jeejeebhoy KN. (1987) Nutritional absorption in short bowel syndrome. Evaluation of fluid, calorie, and divalent cation requirements. *Digestive Diseases and Sciences* 37: 8–15.

Woolf GM, Miller C, Kurian R, Jeejeebhoy KN. (1983) Diet for patients with a short bowel: High fat or high carbohydrate? *Gastroenterology* 84: 823–828.

7.4.10   Irritable bowel syndrome

Yvonne Mckenzie

Key points

■ Irritable bowel syndrome is a common gastrointestinal disorder of medically unexplained symptoms.

■ Management aims to improve the severity and frequency of symptoms and quality of life, and may require a combined lifestyle, dietary and pharmacological approach.

■ A new efficacious treatment is the restriction of short chain carbohydrates (low FODMAP diet). Successful management requires advanced dietetic knowledge, adequate clinical time and resources for patients.

■ Patient empowerment should be supported to enable them to self manage their condition in the long term.

Irritable bowel syndrome (IBS) is a common functional gastrointestinal disorder. The UK prevalence is 10–20%, with a similar incidence worldwide despite differences in lifestyle (Spiller *et al.*, 2007). With functional dyspepsia, IBS accounts for 40–60% of all gastroenterology outpatient referrals (Jones *et al.*, 2000). Irritable bowel disease was first described in 1818 (Thompson, 2006) and since then diagnostic criteria and treatment options have evolved, but the heterogeneity of IBS continues to challenge clinicians. It is no longer a diagnosis of exclusion of organic pathologies, but one of medically unexplained symptoms. Irritable bowel syndrome is chronic, recurring abdominal pain or discomfort associated with disturbed bowel habit in the absence of an organic cause (Longstreth *et al.*, 2006). Until recently, dietetic practice utilised dietary fibre modification and exclusion diets to manage symptoms.

Diagnostic criteria

There are no pathology tests to diagnose IBS, but the National Institute for Health and Care Excellence (NICE, 2009) guidance gives positive, costeffective diagnostic criteria (Box 7.4.1). Red flags or red flag indicators prompt secondary care referral for investigation of more serious pathologies (Table 7.4.11). In research, the more complex Rome III criteria (Drossman, 2006) are used.

Classification

Recognised subtypes of IBS are based on the predominant stool pattern (Longstreth *et al.*, 2006). The Bristol Stool Form Scale (Heaton *et al.*, 1992) is recommended to assess stool consistency (Longstreth *et al.*, 2006) (Table 7.4.12).

Disease processes

The cause of IBS symptoms is only partially understood. A leading hypothesis is enteric nervous system dysfunction, with an individual's emotional and physical wellbeing being relevant to risk (Spiller *et al.*, 2007). Central nervous system interaction may potentially lead to symptoms of dysmotility (pain) and transit (altered bowel habit). Approximately 60% of IBS patients report symptom worsening, especially pain, within 15 minutes or up to 3 hours after eating (Simrén *et al.*, 2001). Motility studies have demonstrated delayed gastric emptying, and exaggerated

---

Box 7.4.1   Positive diagnostic criteria for irritable bowel syndrome and tests to be carried out to exclude other diagnoses (NICE, 2008)

• Abdominal pain or discomfort that is:
  ○ Relieved by defaecation *or*
  ○ Associated with altered bowel frequency or stool form
  and at least two of the following:
  ○ Altered stool passage (straining, urgency, incomplete evacuation)
  ○ Abdominal bloating
  ○ Symptoms made worse by eating
  ○ Passage of mucus
  for at least 6 months.
• Supporting diagnosis: lethargy, nausea, backache and bladder symptoms
• Tests: full blood count (FBC), erythrocyte sedimentation rate (ESR), C-reactive protein (CRP), antibody testing for coeliac disease

Table 7.4.11 Red flag indicators, red flags for referral to secondary care (NICE, 2008) and differential diagnoses for irritable bowel syndrome (IBS)

Red flag indicators and red flags for non-IBS disease	Differential diagnoses for IBS
Unintentional or unexplained weight loss	Bowel infections, e.g. *Giardia lamblia*
Rectal bleeding	Coeliac disease/gluten sensitivity
Family history of bowel or ovarian cancer	Crohn's disease
Change in bowel habit to looser and/or more frequent stools persisting for more than 6 weeks in a person aged over 60 years [NB: US guidelines: from age 50 years regardless of symptoms is used (Brandt *et al.*, 2009)]	Ulcerative colitis Lymphocytic and collagenous colitis Colorectal cancer
Anaemia	Small intestinal bacterial overgrowth
Abdominal and/or rectal masses	Bile acid related diarrhoea
Inflammatory markers for inflammatory bowel disease	Lactose or other carbohydrate intolerance
Symptoms suggesting ovarian cancer	Food hypersensitivity

Table 7.4.12 Irritable bowel syndrome (IBS) subtypes by predominant stool pattern

IBS with	Subtype	Definition	Bristol Stool Form Scale: predominant form
Diarrhoea	IBS-D	Loose (mushy)/watery stools for ≥25% of bowel movements Hard or lumpy stool for ≤25% of bowel movements	Types 6, 7
Constipation	IBS-C	Hard or lumpy stools for ≥25% of bowel movements Loose (mushy)/watery stools for ≤25% of bowel movements	Types 1, 2
Diarrhoea/constipation – mixed	IBS-M	Hard or lumpy stools for ≤25% of bowel movements Loose (mushy)/watery stools for ≤25% of bowel movements	Types 3–5
Unspecified	IBS-U	Insufficient abnormality of stool consistency to meet criteria for IBS-C, IBS-D or IBS-M	Type 3–5

small bowel and colonic responses to eating (Spiller *et al.*, 2007). Gut hypersensitivity, associated with pain, bloating and urgency to evacuate, results from the sensitisation of afferent nerve pathways originating from the gastrointestinal tract. A gut hypersensitivity prevalence of 50–90% in IBS patients has been shown (Azpiroz *et al.*, 2007).

Increasing evidence implicates a low grade inflammatory status (Barbara *et al.*, 2004; Spiller *et al.*, 2000; Walker *et al.*, 2009) and it is noteworthy that IBS like symptoms are often observed in quiescent inflammatory bowel disease. Increased colonic permeability is a suggested mechanism, which exposes the mucosa to abnormal dietary and bacterial challenges that maintain innate immune activation, possibly leading to secondary food hypersensitivity (Park & Camilleri, 2006; Tobin *et al.*, 2008). Stressors, psychological distress, life events and negative coping style may translate into physiological responses that exacerbate symptoms (Mayer *et al.*, 2001; Walker *et al.*, 1993; Whitehead *et al.*, 1992). Improvement may be delayed until such issues resolve (Bennett *et al.*, 1998).

Acute gastroenteritis is the strongest known risk factor for developing IBS (Spiller & Garsed, 2009). The consequential disruption of the intestinal ecosystem may lead to chronic symptoms in 30% of cases after 2–3 years and in 15% of cases after 8 years. Female gender, younger age, prior anxiety and/or depression and fever or weight loss during the acute enteric illness are risk factors for symptom persistence (Marshall *et al.*, 2010). Dysbiosis

(alteration in the gastrointestinal microbiota) exists in all IBS subtypes (Kassinen *et al.*, 2007; Parkes *et al.*, 2012). There is abnormal colonic bacterial fermentation in IBS compared with healthy controls (King *et al.*, 1998). However, a role for small intestinal bacterial overgrowth in IBS remains controversial (Ford *et al.*, 2009).

From twin studies there is a stronger association for environmental rather than genetic contributions to IBS (Spiller *et al.*, 2007), although IBS can cluster within families.

Disease consequences

Irritable bowel syndrome depreciates quality of life and is associated with substantial healthcare costs (Agarwal & Spiegel, 2011). Symptoms vary both within and between individuals. Bloating is the second most bothersome symptom after pain (Ringel *et al.*, 2009); distension may cause the abdominal girth to increase by >10 cm during the day. There are no long term complications of IBS, although an insufficient dietary fibre intake is associated with diverticular disease (Painter, 1985).

Comorbidity with somatic and chronic pain disorders, such as in fibromyalgia, chronic fatigue syndrome, temporomandibular joint disorder, chronic pelvic pain, non-ulcer dyspepsia, biliary dyskinesia, anxiety, depression and migraine, can exacerbate symptoms (Quigley *et al.*, 2009; Spiller *et al.*, 2007). Individuals with IBS have a normal life expectancy (Chang *et al.*, 2010).

SECTION 7

Patient perspective

Many people with IBS suffer in silence due to a lack of awareness of the condition or ineffective treatment, but they should not feel alone with the burden of their diagnosis (Brandt *et al.*, 2009). Misconceptions exist about IBS being caused by dietary habits and colitis, worsening with age, causing malnutrition or developing into cancer (Halpert *et al.*, 2007). Therefore, patient reassurance and management of patient expectations are important once diagnosis is established.

Gastroenterology patients view diet as having an important role to play in their condition and, whilst a large proportion of patients are interested in receiving dietary advice, few expect to receive it in clinic (Adesokan & Neild, 2012). Individuals may self manage symptoms by carrying out food intolerance testing. The European Academy of Allergy and Clinical Immunology task force report (Stapel *et al.*, 2008) concluded that serum IgG4 is irrelevant in the diagnosis of food allergy or intolerance and should not be measured to account for food related symptoms.

Public health aspects

Access to clean public toilets can be a major issue for individuals with IBS. The UKs charity IBS Network supports people with IBS, campaigns on their behalf and offers a *Can't Wait* card scheme for its members, for international use as well as within the UK. Since 1977 the International Foundation for Functional Gastrointestinal Disease (IFFGD) has designated April as the International IBS Awareness month.

Nutritional consequences

Prevalence of perceived food intolerance is higher in IBS than in the general population (Monsbakken *et al.*, 2006), as patients frequently alter what they eat in an attempt to alleviate symptoms (Halpert *et al.*, 2007). However, without sound evidence, individuals should restrain from avoiding certain foods as this can lead to undernutrition, e.g. inadequate calcium intake due to dairy exclusion.

Assessment

Most patients are diagnosed and managed in primary care (Thompson *et al.*, 2000). Guidelines for the diagnosis and management of IBS in primary care (NICE, 2008) highlight the importance of avoiding unnecessary investigations to confirm diagnosis and good communication with the patient, supported by evidence based information. Dietitians should use evidence based IBS guidelines (BDA, 2010). Assessment should follow the ABCDE format.

Anthropometry

Weight, body mass index (BMI) and weight history should be assessed.

Biochemistry

The tests shown in Box 7.4.1 may be carried out. Coeliac disease should been ruled out and screening conducted at a time when the individual has been consuming gluten in more than one meal every day and has been doing so for at least 6 weeks (NICE, 2009). If endomysial antibodies (EMAs) or tissue transglutaminase (tTG) have not been checked, they should be measured prior to changing gluten intake. Other biochemisty, e.g. haematinics, should be normal (see Chapter 7.4.7).

Clinical assessment

Allergies and a family history of gastrointestinal problems, e.g. coeliac disease, inflammatory bowel disease, IBS, as well as any IBS medication or nutritional supplements should be recorded. Recording the IBS symptom profile before and after intervention is essential. There is no widely adopted validated method for measuring IBS symptom outcomes in clinical practice. The IBS Severity Score (IBS-SS) (Francis *et al.*, 1997), the Functional Bowel Disorder Severity Index (FBDSI) (Drossman *et al.*, 1995) and the Gastrointestinal Symptom Rating Scale (GSRS) (Svedlund *et al.*, 1988) are the most widely recognised tools. The Bristol Stool Form Scale (Heaton *et al.*, 1992) aids IBS subtyping. It is important to discuss IBS with the patient to ensure they understand that it is a positive diagnosis.

Faecal calprotectin is a cost effective sensitive marker of intestinal inflammation that is used to differentiate functional symptoms from active IBD in secondary and primary care. Hydrogen breath testing may help to identify which dietary management strategy is most appropriate (see Chapter 7.4.8).

Dietary assessment

Individuals may already have excluded certain foods and their thoughts on how these foods affect their IBS symptoms should be explored. Certain food avoidances may require nutritional intake assessment, e.g. calcium. Food and symptom diaries of an individual's usual diet may be useful. First line assessment is to:

- Identify any food allergies or intolerances – atopy, e.g. asthma and allergic rhinitis, may implicate food allergy in the symptomology.
- Check for regular eating pattern and a good eating lifestyle.
- Check for healthy eating, considering milk and lactose, non-starch polysaccharides (NSPs), fatty foods, fluid, caffeine and alcohol intakes.

Economic and social assessment

An empathic understanding of lifestyle circumstances is important and relevant to treatment options and concordance with dietary intervention, e.g. any stressors affecting a patient's quality of life, including physical activity, work, education and family circumstances.

Management

Clinical management

Options, either singly or in combination, include dietary, pharmacological and behavioural interventions to improve IBS symptoms and quality of life. These should be discussed with each individual to provide the most appropriate care pathway (NICE, 2008), imparting the education they need to self manage their symptoms long term. Self help information covering lifestyle modification should be considered in primary care (NICE, 2008).

Commonly prescribed drugs to manage IBS are:

- *Antispasmodics* – antimuscarinics and smooth muscle relaxants are used to reduce motility, e.g. for meal induced symptoms. Peppermint oil capsules, hyoscine butylbromide and mebeverine provide modest global symptom improvement (Ford *et al.*, 2008; Enck *et al.*, 2010).
- *Bulk forming, osmotic and stimulant laxatives*, e.g. macrogols, ispaghula husk, senna. NICE (2008) discourages lactulose.
- *Antidiarrhoeal agents*, e.g. loperamide.
- *Tricyclic analgesics*, e.g. amitriptyline and nortriptyline (at low doses if first line medication) give insufficient relief. Selective serotonin reuptake inhibitors are also used, but evidence favours the use of tricyclics.

Behavioural interventions and psychological therapy, such as cognitive behaviour therapy, relaxation techniques, psychodynamic interpersonal therapy, may reduce pain and other symptoms and improve quality of life (Spiller *et al.*, 2007). These may be considered for those who have had symptoms for at least 12 months and have not responded to first line treatments (NICE, 2008). Reflexology, acupuncture and aloe vera have shown no benefit and are therefore not recommended (NICE, 2008). Self help organisations, such as IBS Network, can assist individuals to self manage and come to terms with their functional disorder.

Nutritional management

Nutritional management aims to improve the severity and frequency of IBS symptoms and quality of life through dietary and lifestyle modification, whilst supporting dietary adequacy in line with general healthy eating guidelines. The UK evidence based practice guidelines for the dietetic management of IBS in adults (BDA, 2010) are for dietitians' use in the UK healthcare setting. These give graded evidence statements, clinical and research recommendations, and good practice points stemming from five systematic reviews relating to IBS symptom improvement and the role of milk and/or lactose, NSPs, fermentable carbohydrates, probiotics and empirical and elimination diets.

An IBS algorithm (Figure 7.4.9), a logical three line sequence of interventions for successful dietetic management, forms the basis of these guidelines and can be used in clinical practice. The lifestyle and dietary clinical practice recommendations are summarised in Box 7.4.2; for further details see McKenzie *et al.* (2012).

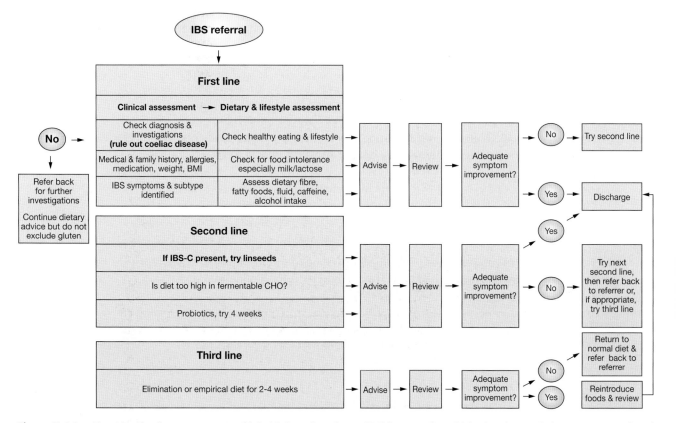

Figure 7.4.9 Algorithm for the management of irritable bowel syndrome (IBS) [source: The British Dietetic Association 2013. Reproduced with permission of the British Dietetic Association (www.bda.uk.com)]
CHO, carbohydrate; BMI, body mass index; IBS-C, irritable bowel syndrome – C

SECTION 7

Box 7.4.2 Clinical practice considerations and evidence based recommendations for irritable bowel syndrome (IBS) [adapted from McKenzie *et al*. (2012)]

First line: Healthy eating and lifestyle management

(a) Encourage a regular meal pattern, take time over meals, sit down to eat, chewing food thoroughly, avoid late night eating, encourage good food variety and ensure nutritional adequacy in line with general healthy eating guidelines

(b) Drink plenty of caffeine free, alcohol free, non-fizzy fluids spread throughout the day, aiming for 1.5–3.0 L/day (35 mL/kg)

(c) Encourage exercise, relaxation and coping strategies for the demands of everyday life

	SIGN 50 Grade of recommendation

Removing milk and dairy products to improve IBS symptoms

(d) In individuals in whom sensitivity to milk is suspected and a lactose hydrogen breath test is not available or appropriate, a trial period of a low lactose diet is recommended. This is particularly useful in individuals with an ethnic background with a high prevalence of primary lactase deficiency	D
(e) Use a low lactose diet to treat individuals with a positive lactose hydrogen breath test	D
(f) In individuals where milk is suspected as a problem food but symptoms do not improve on a low lactose diet, assess other components of milk, e.g. cow's milk protein, as a contributing factor. Recommend a milk free diet or, in some cases, an alternative mammalian milk	D

Non-starch polysaccharides

(g) First line: Avoid using dietary supplementation of wheat bran to treat IBS. Individuals should not be advised to increase their intake of wheat bran above their usual dietary intake	C

Second line: Advanced dietary interventions: linseeds, fermentable carbohydrates; probiotics

(h) For individuals with IBS-C, dietary supplementation of ground linseeds can be recommended for a 3-month trial. Improvements in constipation, abdominal pain and bloating from linseed supplementation may be gradual	D

Fermentable carbohydrates, for all IBS subtypes

(i) For individuals with IBS and suspected or diagnosed fructose malabsorption, assess dietary intake of all short chain fermentable carbohydrates (fructose, fructans, galacto-oligosaccharides and polyols). There is likely to be a benefit in reducing intake	B
(j) For individuals with IBS and abdominal bloating, abdominal pain and/or flatulence, assess dietary intake of fermentable carbohydrates as there may be a benefit in reducing intake	D
(k) There may be individual tolerance levels to fermentable carbohydrates. A planned and systematic challenge of foods high in fermentable carbohydrates will identify which foods can be re-introduced to the diet and what individual tolerance levels are	D

Probiotics, no IBS subtype specified

(l) Probiotics can be considered, ideally, after assessing the effectiveness of restricting intake of fermentable carbohydrates. Advise individuals choosing to try probiotics to select one product at a time and monitor the effects. They should try it for a minimum of 4 weeks at the dose recommended by the manufacturer	B
(m) There is considered to be no associated harm in taking probiotics for individuals with IBS	B

Third line: Elimination and empirical diets

(n) Where food is considered to be a trigger for IBS symptoms, particularly IBS-D, an elimination or empirical diet can be considered	D
(o) The initial phase of an elimination or empirical diet should be followed for 2–4 weeks	D
(p) If there is no symptom improvement within 2–4 weeks of the initial phase of an elimination or empirical diet, and foods consumed within the diet are not suspected to be symptom triggers, specific foods are an unlikely cause of IBS symptoms	D

For mild symptoms first line management may be sufficient. Evidence suggests that in individuals with IBS, a fatty meal induces greater abdominal pain than it does in healthy controls (Simrén et al., 2007) and bloating is exaggerated after lipid infusion (Serra et al., 2002). There are no trials showing that individuals with IBS have greater sensitivity to caffeine or alcohol, and the placebo effect, known to be high in IBS (Kaptchuk et al., 2008; Spiller, 1999), should be borne in mind.

In the UK, lactose intolerance is reported to be present in 10% of people with IBS, but lactose avoidance rarely cures IBS (Spiller et al., 2007). Other currently unknown components of milk may contribute to symptoms (Parker et al., 2001) and suitable alternatives to cow's milk include calcium enriched non-mammalian milks and yoghurt. A recent meta analysis (Ford et al., 2008) was unable to show that dietary fibre was an efficacious treatment for IBS; however, many of the trials lacked good design criteria and used inappropriate placebos.

Successful advanced management relating to fermentable carbohydrates is achieved by providing detailed verbal and written resources on avoidance of the relevant foods, including suitable alternatives to ensure the diet is nutritionally adequate. A dietitian should provide education with advanced training in the necessary knowledge and skills. The required dietetic consultation times may be greater than that currently offered in many NHS outpatient clinics. And initial consultation may last 45–60 minutes, with the second taking 30–45 minutes. If healthcare settings are unable to facilitate dietary education on reducing fermentable carbohydrates, current practice is to follow the NICE guidelines (2008). Following adequate symptom relief after 4–8 weeks, planned and systematic reintroduction of foods high in these carbohydrates verifies individual tolerance to fermentable carbohydrates. This increases dietary variety and supports long term self care.

A diet restricted in short chain carbohydrates [fermentable oligo-, di- and mono-saccharides, and polyols (FODMAPs)] is a recent successful treatment for IBS, with evidence for its effectiveness coming from Australia and the UK (Gibson & Shepherd, 2010; Staudacher et al., 2011). Examples of foods high in FODMAPs include wheat and rye based staples, e.g. bread, pasta, pizza, onion, garlic, pulses, apple, pear, stone fruit, sugar free chewing gum, mammalian milks and yoghurts. Examples of foods low in FODMAPs are oats, potatoes, rice, gluten free bread and pasta, spelt, green leafy vegetables, tomatoes, carrots, most berries, citrus fruit, lactose free milk and yoghurt, and (calcium enriched) plant based milks.

Therapeutic alteration of the gastrointestinal microbiota by probiotics could be beneficial and care should be taken to recommend the exact strain or species that research has shown to be of benefit in treating IBS (Parkes et al., 2010).

Third line dietary intervention is usually unnecessary in IBS management. Dietitians should seek medical advice for any concerns over the management of existing or suspected allergy.

Internet resources

IBS Network   www.ibsnetwork.org
International Foundation for Functional Gastrointestinal Disorders (IFFDG)   www.aboutibs.org/site/about-ibs/april-ibs-awareness-month
UK training on the low FODMAP diet and functional gastrointestinal disorders   www.kcl.ac.uk/fodmaps

Patient resources

BDA IBS Food Fact sheet   www.bda.org.uk
Nutrition and Diet Resources (NDR)   www.ndr-uk.org

References

Adesokan A, Neild P. (2012) Attitudes and expectations of gastroenterology outpatients about the importance of diet and possible relationship to their symptoms. *Frontline Gastroenterology* 3: 278–282.

Agarwal N, Spiegel BM. (2011) The effect of irritable bowel syndrome on health-related quality of life and healthcare expenditures. *Gastroenterology Clinics of North America* 40: 11–19.

Azpiroz F, Bouin M, Camilleri M, et al. (2007) Mechanisms of hypersensitivity in IBS and functional disorders. *Neurogastroenterology and Motility* 19(Suppl 1): 62–88.

Barbara G, Stanghellini V, de Giorgio R, et al. (2004) Activated mast cells in proximity to colonic nerves correlate with abdominal pain in irritable bowel syndrome. *Gastroenterology* 126(3): 693–702.

Bennett EJ, Tennant CC, Piesse C, Badcock CA. (1998) Level of chronic life stress predicts clinical outcome in irritable bowel syndrome. *Gut* 43: 256–261.

Brandt LJ, Chey WD, Foxx-Orenstein AE, et al. (2009) An evidence-based systematic review on the management of irritable bowel syndrome. *American Journal of Gastroenterology* 104: S1–S35.

British Dietetic Association (BDA). (2010) UK evidence-based practice guidelines for the dietetic management of irritable bowel syndrome (IBS) in adults. Available at www.bda.uk.com. Accessed 28 January 2013.

Chang JY, Locke III GR, McNally MA, et al. (2010) Impact of Functional Gastrointestinal Disorders on Survival in the Community. *American Journal of Gastroenterology* 105(4): 822–832.

Drossman DA. (2006) The functional gastrointestinal disorders and the Rome III process. *Gastroenterology* 130: 1377–1390.

Drossman DA, Li Z, Toner BB, et al. (1995) Functional bowel disorders: A multicenter comparison of health status, and development of illness severity index. *Digestive Diseases and Sciences* 40(5): 986–995.

Enck P, Junne F, Klosterhalfen S, Zipfel S, Martens U. (2010) Therapy options in irritable bowel syndrome. *European Journal of Gastroenterology and Hepatology* 22(12): 1402–1411.

Ford AC, Talley NJ, Spiegel BM, et al. (2008) Effect of fibre, antispasmodics, and peppermint oil in the treatment of irritable bowel syndrome: systematic review and meta-analysis. *BMJ* 337: a2313.

Ford AC, Spiegel BM, Talley NJ, Moayyedi P. (2009) Small intestinal bacterial overgrowth in irritable bowel syndrome: systematic review and meta-analysis. *Clinical Gastroenterology and Hepatology* 7: 1279–1286.

Francis CY, Morris J, Whorwell PJ. (1997) The irritable bowel severity scoring system: a simple method of monitoring irritable bowel syndrome and its progress. *Alimentary Pharmacology & Therapeutics* 11(2): 395–402.

Gibson PR, Shepherd SJ. (2010) Evidence-based dietary management of functional gastrointestinal symptoms: The FODMAP approach. *Journal of Gastroenterology and Hepatology* 25: 252–258.

Halpert A, Dalton CB, Palsson O, *et al.* (2007) What patients know about irritable bowel syndrome (IBS) and what they would like to know. National Survey on Patient Educational Needs in IBS and development and validation of the Patient Educational Needs Questionnaire (PEQ). *American Journal of Gastroenterology* 102: 1972–1982.

Heaton KW, Radvan J, Cripps H, Mountford RA, Braddon FE, Hughes AO. (1992) Defecation frequency and timing, and stool form in the general population: a prospective study. *Gut* 3: 818–824.

Jones J, Boorman J, Cann P, *et al.* (2000) British Society of Gastroenterology guidelines for the management of the irritable bowel syndrome. *Gut* 47(Suppl 2): ii1–19.

Kassinen A, Krogius-Kurikka L, Mäkivuokko H, *et al.* (2007) The fecal microbiota of irritable bowel syndrome patients differs significantly from that of healthy subjects. *Gastroenterology* 133: 24–33.

Kaptchuk TJ, Kelley JM, Conboy LA, *et al.* (2008) Components of placebo effect: randomised controlled trial in patients with irritable bowel syndrome. *BMJ* 336: 999–1003.

King TS, Elia M, Hunter JO. (1998) Abnormal colonic fermentation in irritable bowel syndrome. *Lancet* 352: 1187–1189.

Longstreth GF, Thompson WG, Chey WD, Houghton LA, Mearin F, Spiller RC. (2006) Functional bowel disorders. *Gastroenterology* 130: 1480–1491.

Marshall JK, Thabane M, Garg AX, Clark WF, Moayyedi P, Collins SM. (2010) Eight year prognosis of postinfectious irritable bowel syndrome following waterborne bacterial dysentery. *Gut* 59: 605–611.

Mayer AE, Naliboff BD, Chang L, Coutinho SV. (2001) Stress and irritable bowel syndrome. *American Journal of Physiology and. Gastrointestinal Liver Physiology* 280(4): G519–G524.

McKenzie YA, Alder A, Anderson W, *et al.*; on behalf of Gastroenterology Specialist Group of the British Dietetic Association. (2012) British Dietetic Association evidence-based practice guidelines for the dietary management of irritable bowel syndrome in adults. *Journal of Human Nutrition and Dietetics* 25: 260–274.

Monsbakken KW, Vandvik PO, Farup PG. (2006) Perceived food intolerance in subjects with irritable bowel syndrome – etiology, prevalence and consequences. *European Journal of Clinical Nutrition* 60: 667–672.

National Institute for Health and Care Excellence (NICE). (2008) Irritable bowel syndrome in adults: Diagnosis and management of irritable bowel syndrome in primary care. CG61.

National Institute for Health and Care Excellence (NICE). (2009) Coeliac disease: Recognition and assessment of coeliac disease. CG86.

Painter NS. (1985) The cause of diverticular disease of the colon, its symptoms and its complications. Review and hypothesis. *Journal of the Royal College of Surgery Edinburgh* 30(2): 118–122.

Park MI, Camilleri M. (2006) Is there a role of food allergy in irritable bowel syndrome and functional dyspepsia? *A systematic review. Neurogastroenterology and Motility* 18: 595–607.

Parker TJ, Woolner JT, Prevost AT, Tuffnell Q, Shorthouse M, Hunter JO. (2001) Irritable bowel syndrome: is the search for lactose intolerance justified? *European Journal of Gastroenterology and Hepatology* 13: 219–225.

Parkes GC, Sanderson JD, Whelan K. (2010) Treating irritable bowel syndrome with probiotics: the evidence. *Proceedings of the Nutrition Society* 69: 187–194.

Parkes GC, Rayment NB, Hudspith BN, *et al.* (2012) Distinct microbial populations exist in the mucosa-associated microbiota of subgroups of irritable bowel syndrome. *Neurogastroenterology and Motility* 24: 31–39.

Quigley EMM, Fried M, Gwee KA, *et al.* (2009) *Irritable Bowel Syndrome: A Global* Perspective. WGO Global Guidelines. Munich: World Gastroenterology Organization.

Ringel Y, Williams RE, Kalilani L, Cook SF. (2009) Prevalence, characteristics, and impact of bloating symptoms in patients with irritable bowel syndrome. *Clinical Gastroenterology and Hepatology* 7(1): 68–72.

Serra J, Salviola B, Azpiroz F, Malagelada JR. (2002) Lipid-induced intestinal gas retention in irritable bowel syndrome. *Gastroenterology* 123: 700–706.

Simrén M, Månsson A, Langkilde AM, *et al.* (2001) Food-related gastrointestinal symptoms in the irritable bowel syndrome. *Digestion* 48: 20–27.

Simrén M, Agerforz P, Björnsson ES, Abrahamsson H. (2007) Nutrient-dependent enhancement of rectal sensitivity in irritable bowel syndrome (IBS). *Gastroenterology and Motility* 19: 20–29.

Spiller RC. (1999) Problems and challenges in the design of irritable bowel syndrome clinical trials: experience from published trials. *American Journal of Medicine* 107(5 Suppl 1): 91–97.

Spiller RC, Garsed K. (2009) Postinfectious irritable bowel syndrome. *Gastroenterology* 136(6): 1979–1988.

Spiller RC, Jenkins D, Thornley JP, *et al.* (2000) Increased rectal mucosal enteroendocrine cells, T lymphocytes, and increased gut permeability following acute Campylobacter enteritis and in postdysenteric irritable bowel syndrome. *Gut* 47: 804–811.

Spiller R, Aziz Q, Creed F, *et al.* (2007) Guidelines on the irritable bowel syndrome: mechanisms and practical management. *Gut* 56: 1770–1798.

Stapel SO, Asero R, Ballmer-Weber BK, *et al.* (2008) Testing for IgG4 against foods is not recommended as a diagnostic tool: EAACI Task Force Report. *Allergy* 63: 793–796.

Staudacher HM, Whelan K, Irving PM, Lomer MC. (2011) Comparison of symptom response following advice for a diet low in fermentable carbohydrates (FODMAPs) versus standard dietary advice in patients with irritable bowel syndrome. *Journal of Human Nutrition and Dietetics* 24: 487–495.

Svedlund J, Sjodin I, Dotevall G. (1988) GSRS – A clinical rating scale for gastrointestinal symptoms in patients with irritable bowel syndrome and peptic ulcer disease. *Digestive Diseases and Sciences* 93: 129–134.

Thompson WG. (2006) The road to Rome. *Gastroenterology* 130: 1552–1556.

Thompson WG, Heaton KW, Smyth GT, Smyth C. (2000) Irritable bowel syndrome in general practice: prevalence, characteristics and referral. *Gut* 46: 78–82.

Tobin MC, Moparty B, Farhadi A, DeMeo MT, Bansal PJ, Keshavarzian A. (2008) Atopic irritable bowel syndrome: a novel subgroup of irritable bowel syndrome with allergic manifestations. *Annals of Allergy, Asthma, and Immunology* 100(1): 49–53.

Walker EA, Katon WJ, Roy-Byrne PP, Jemelka RP, Russo J. (1993) Histories of sexual victimization in patients with irritable bowel syndrome or inflammatory bowel disease. *American Journal of Psychiatry* 150: 1502–1506.

Walker MM, Talley NJ, Prabhakar M, *et al.* (2009) Duodenal mastocytosis, eosinophilia and intraepithelial lymphocytosis as possible disease markers in the irritable bowel syndrome and functional dyspepsia. *Alimentary Pharmacology & Therapeutics* 29: 765–773.

Whitehead WE, Ceowell MD, Robinson JC, Heller BR, Schuster MM. (1992) Effects of stressful life events on bowel symptoms: subjects with irritable bowel syndrome compared with subjects without bowel dysfunction. *Gut* 33: 825–830.

7.4.11 Disorders of the colon and rectum
Diane Brundrett

Key points

■ Constipation may be a primary disorder associated with inadequate fluid, fibre or activity levels, or a secondary consequence of medication or underlying disease. Management may require a combination of dietary, behavioural and pharmacological strategies.

■ Acute diarrhoea can cause severe dehydration, especially in young children and elderly people. The management of chronic diarrhoea depends on the underlying cause but aims to minimise or restore fluid and nutrient losses.

Diverticulitis (inflammation or inflammation of diverticula in the bowel wall) may necessitate bowel rest and a bland diet during acute phases of the disease. A high fibre intake may be more appropriate for secondary prevention. Disorders of the bowel include constipation, diarrhoea, diverticulitis, irritable bowel syndrome (IBS) and colorectal cancer. Irritable bowel syndrome or disease is a common functional bowel disorder. Management must be tailored to the symptom profile of the individual and may require a combined dietary, pharmacological and lifestyle approach. It is discussed in detail in Chapter 7.4.10. Colorectal cancer is the second most common cause of cancer in the UK. The aetiology is not fully understood but its development is associated with lifestyle, such as smoking, inactivity and dietary factors. The nutritional intervention may involve nutritional support or dietary modification (see Chapter 7.15.3). The nutritional effects and management of colon and rectum resection can be found in Chapter 7.4.9.

Constipation

The prevalence of constipation in North America is estimated to be 12–19% (Higgins & Johanson, 2004). Reported constipation prevalence rates in Europe are similar at 17% (Peppas *et al.*, 2008). However, prevalence rates vary due to varying diagnostic criteria. In England, nearly 16 million prescriptions were dispensed for laxatives in 2010 (NHS Business Services Authority, 2012). Constipation is twice as common in women as men (Higgins & Johanson, 2004) and appears to increase with increasing age, particularly after the age of 65 years. About 40% of pregnant women complain of constipation (Cullen & O'Donoghue, 2007).

The word constipation has a different meanings to different people. While some believe they are constipated if they do not have a daily bowel movement, normal stool elimination may be three times a day or twice a week depending on the person. Constipation is defaecation that is unsatisfactory because of infrequent stools, difficult stool passage or a feeling of incomplete evacuation. Stools can be hard and dry and may be large or small. Constipation is a symptom, not a disease. Factors associated with an increased risk of constipation include a low fluid intake, a low fibre diet and reduced mobility. A high fibre intake is associated with a lower prevalence of constipation (Dukas *et al.*, 2003).

Diagnostic criteria

Diagnosis is confirmed using the Rome III Committee's diagnostic criteria (Longstreth *et al.*, 2006). Criteria must be fulfilled for the last 3 months, with symptom onset at least 6 months prior to diagnosis. The criteria are:

1. Must include two or more of the following:
   - Straining during at least 25% of defaecations.
   - Lumpy or hard stools in at least 25% of defaecations.
   - Sensation of incomplete evacuation for at least 25% of defaecations.
   - Sensation of anorectal obstruction or blockage for at least 25% defaecations.
   - Manual manoeuvres to facilitate at least 25% of defaecations, e.g. digital evacuation, support of the pelvic floor.
   - Fewer than three defaecations per week.
2. Loose stools are rarely present without the use of laxatives.
3. Insufficient criteria for IBS.

The Bristol Stool Chart (Lewis & Heaton, 1997) may aid diagnosis as it correlates well with colonic transit times (Figure 7.4.10).

Disease process

Constipation is a common gastrointestinal complaint that can cause physical and psychosocial problems. The cause of constipation can be multifactorial, but it can be divided into functional (primary) and secondary. Functional constipation is chronic constipation where there is no underlying disease but there is a neurological, psychological or psychosomatic cause. This type of constipation can be further classified into three categories:

• *Normal transit constipation* – stool passes through the colon at a normal rate, but the patient perceives difficulty in emptying their bowels. This condition is most common in young women.

SECTION 7

Bristol Stool Chart

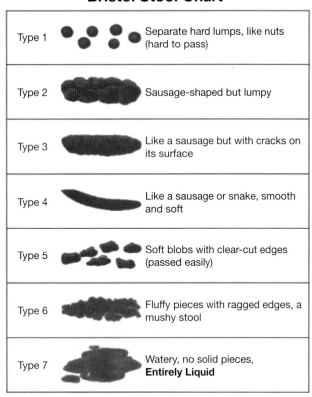

Type 1		Separate hard lumps, like nuts (hard to pass)
Type 2		Sausage-shaped but lumpy
Type 3		Like a sausage but with cracks on its surface
Type 4		Like a sausage or snake, smooth and soft
Type 5		Soft blobs with clear-cut edges (passed easily)
Type 6		Fluffy pieces with ragged edges, a mushy stool
Type 7		Watery, no solid pieces, **Entirely Liquid**

Figure 7.4.10 Bristol stool chart [from Lewis & Heaton (1997) © Informa Health Care]

- *Slow transit constipation* – there are infrequent bowel movements, decreased urgency or straining to have bowels open and an increased colonic transit time.
- *Pelvic floor dysfunction* that is characterised by dysfunction of the pelvic floor or anal sphincter and can follow childbirth.

Those diagnosed with functional constipation may be particularly affected by behavioural or psychological factors. They may regularly ignore the urge to have a bowel movement, feel uncomfortable using toilets outside of their home or have limited access to toilet facilities. Constipation is common in those with a history of depression, anxiety, eating disorders, sexual abuse and physical abuse (Wald *et al.*, 1989; Levy *et al.*, 2006). Changes in routine, such as travel, reduced levels of exercise or mobility, can lead to an alteration in bowel habits.

Secondary constipation is constipation caused by a drug or a medical condition, as shown in Table 7.4.13.

Disease consequences

A population based study in individuals with constipation found a decrement in health related quality of life when compared to subjects without a functional gastrointestinal disorder (Irvine *et al.*, 2002). Chronic constipation can lead to faecal impaction with resulting faecal incontinence, increased risk of urinary tract infections, rectal bleeding and prolapse.

Table 7.4.13 Causes of secondary constipation

Cause	Examples
Endocrine and metabolic diseases	Diabetes (with autonomic myopathy) Hypercalcaemia Hypokalaemia Hyperparathyroidism Hypothyroidism Uraemia Pregnancy
Connective tissue disorders	Amyloidosis Scleroderma
Neurological diseases	Autonomic neuropathy Stroke Hirschsprung's disease Multiple sclerosis Parkinson's disease Spinal cord injuries or tumours
Structural abnormalities	Anal fissures or strictures Haemorrhoids Colonic strictures Inflammatory bowel disease Colorectal cancer Rectal prolapse Volvulus Megacolon or megarectum
Drugs	Opioid analgesics – codeine, morphine, fentanyl Diuretics Iron supplements Antacids Antispasmodics Antidepressants – commonly tricyclic antidepressants Antiepileptics Antipsychotics Calcium supplements Antihistamines Calcium channel blockers

Clinical assessment

When a patient presents complaining of constipation, an evaluation of their medical history and a physical examination may reveal the cause. The decision to do further investigations, such as a colonoscopy or colonic transit studies, will be based on the patient's symptoms, family history and age; laboratory tests are rarely useful. It is important that malignancy is excluded especially in the elderly or if there is a history of blood in the stools or weight loss. The aim of any intervention is to relieve the symptoms and to restore normal bowel habits with minimal side effects.

Nutritional assessment

Anthropometry

Assess the weight and height and calculate body mass index (BMI). Is there a history of weight loss? Constipation is more common in those with a history of an eating disorder.

Table 7.4.14 Oral laxatives used in the management of constipation

Category of laxative	Example	Mode of action
Bulking agents	Ispaghula husk, methylcellulose, sterculia, frangula	Increase the amount of fibre in the diet, increasing the weight and water absorbent properties of the stool Patients must be advised to have a good fluid intake
Stimulant laxatives	Senna, bisacodyl, sodium picosulfate	Increase intestinal motility by stimulation of colonic nerves
Faecal softeners	Liquid paraffin	Soften the stool, but their use is discouraged as has been associated with adverse effects, including anal seepage and irritation
Osmotic laxatives	Lactulose, magnesium salts (e.g. Epsom salts), magrocols (e.g. Movicol)	Act as a softening agent by increasing water absorption in the stool Lactulose may also have a stimulant effect

Biochemistry

Is the patient a poorly controlled diabetic? Is calcium raised or potassium level low? Check thyroid function. Is the patient uraemic? Is the patient dehydrated?

Clinical assessment

Check bowel frequency. Does the patient have a medical diagnosis that may increase their risk of constipation? Is the patient taking any drugs that may cause constipation? Are there any relevant psychosocial factors? Has the patient experienced a reduction in their mobility?

Dietary assessment

Take a diet history and review fibre and fluid intake.

Economic and social assessment

Does the patient express any concerns about lack of income or knowledge to achieve a well balanced diet? Are there any psychosocial factors that may be relevant?

Management

Lifestyle

Advice may be given to set time aside to go to the toilet, especially after meals to make the most of the gastrocolic response. Increased activity levels can help improve bowel habits.

Medication

If possible, adjust any constipating medication. Oral laxatives may be offered if non-pharmacological methods have not been successful. A patient will usually be prescribed a bulk forming laxative initially. If hard stools continue, patients are switched to or have an osmotic laxative added. If stools are soft but difficult to pass, or there is inadequate emptying, a stimulant laxative can be added. Patients with short term constipation should be advised to stop taking the laxatives once the stools have become soft and are easy to pass. For patients with chronic constipation, laxatives should slowly be withdrawn. Laxatives can be continued long term in patients who take a constipating drug that cannot be stopped or

there is a medical cause for the constipation. Further information on the use of oral laxatives is given in Table 7.4.14. Prucalopride is a new drug that may be prescribed for women with chronic constipation who have not had adequate relief of their symptoms using laxatives (NICE, 2010).

Biofeedback

Biofeedback is a bowel training programme run by specialist nurses or physiotherapists, which involves retraining muscles and nerves to coordinate and produce satisfactory effort to empty the bowel. Benefit from biofeedback therapy seems limited to patients with pelvic floor dysfunction (Frattini & Norgueras, 2008).

Surgery

Surgery is considered in a minority of patients and the results of total or partial removal of the colon to improve bowel function are often poor. Even if there is an improvement in bowel habits, quality of life postoperatively can be adversely affected by abdominal pain, postoperative incontinence or diarrhoea (Fitzharris et al., 2003). Kamm et al. (1988) recommend that those with normal transit constipation being considered for surgery have a preoperative psychosocial assessment as it is recognised that many of these patients have psychological issues that can predispose them to a poor surgical outcome.

Nutritional management

Advice should be given to ensure that the individual has regular meals with a well balanced diet containing wholegrains, fruit and vegetables. Adults should aim to eat 18–30 g of fibre/day. Patients should be advised to increase their fibre intake gradually to help minimise bloating and flatulence. Fibre increases the bulk of the stool, which distends the colon and stimulates propulsive activity and colonic transit. The beneficial effects of a higher fibre intake may be seen in a few days or it may take several weeks to be effective. More specific advice about types of dietary fibre may be of benefit to those with chronic constipation. There is evidence to support increasing the soluble fibre intake of the diet for constipation (Suares & Ford, 2011).

The beneficial effects of following a high fibre diet can be enhanced by increasing fluid intake to 1.5–2.0 L/day (Anti *et al.*, 1998). An increased fluid intake is needed with bulking agents and osmotic laxatives. Currently, there is limited evidence available from controlled trials to support the routine use of probiotics in the treatment of constipation (Chmielewska & Szajewska, 2010).

Diarrhoea

Diarrhoea is an alteration of normal bowel movement characterised by an increase in water content, volume or frequency of stools. Diarrhoea is a symptom of which there can be many causes and it can be categorised as follows:

- *Acute diarrhoea* – that lasting <4 weeks.
- *Chronic diarrhoea* – that lasting >4 weeks.
- *Faecal incontinence* – inability to control bowel movements with the involuntary passing of liquid or solid stool.
- *Functional diarrhoea* – continuous or recurrent syndrome characterised by the passage of loose or watery stools without abdominal pain or discomfort.

Diagnostic criteria

There are many definitions of diarrhoea; Table 7.4.15 shows those that are generally accepted. The British Society of Gastroenterology (Thomas *et al.*, 2003) defines diarrhoea as the abnormal passage of three or more loose or liquid stools per day for >4 weeks and or a daily stool weight >200 g/day. However, the Rome III Committee defines it as at least 75% of stools being loose (mushy) or watery and without pain for the last 3 months, and with symptom onset at least 6 months before diagnosis (Long-streth *et al.*, 2006). Use of the Bristol Stool Chart (Figure 7.4.10) can aid diagnosis; stool types 5–7 tending towards diarrhoea.

Disease process

Acute diarrhoea is usually a symptom of a bowel infection (gastroenteritis) that may be caused by a virus, food poisoning, a bacterial infection, consumption of contaminated food or water from a foreign country (traveller's diarrhoea) or antibiotics. *Clostridium difficile* is a common cause of hospital acquired diarrhoea (Baldi *et al.*, 2009). Disruption of the bowel microflora by antibiotics creates an environment in which *C. difficile* can proliferate. Other causes include anxiety, drinking excessive alcohol or caffeine containing fluids, chemotherapy, acute radiation enteritis, intestinal ischaemia and the early presentation of a chronic cause, e.g. the initial presentation of inflammatory bowel disease (IBD). Many drugs can cause diarrhoea, e.g. antacids, nonsteroidal anti-inflammatory drugs, statins, selective serotonin reuptake inhibitors and some chemotherapy agents. Chronic diarrhoea has a broader range of possible causes than acute diarrhoea, as shown in Table 7.4.15.

Table 7.4.15 Causes of chronic diarrhoea

Cause	Example
Irritable bowel syndrome (IBS)	
Chronic infection	Functional disorders such as IBS may follow infection
Small bowel	Coeliac disease Crohn's disease Bile acid malabsorption – resection or disease of the terminal ileum leads to increased levels of bile salts in the colon that can stimulate diarrhoea Lactase deficiency, lactose intolerance Small bowel bacterial overgrowth Mesenteric ischaemia Radiation enteritis Lymphoma
Colonic	Diverticular disease Colon cancer Ulcerative colitis and Crohn's colitis Microscopic colitis
Pancreatic – associated with steatorrhoea	Chronic pancreatitis Pancreatic cancer Cystic fibrosis
Other	Hyperthyroidism Diabetes – may be related to metformin or autonomic neuropathy Laxative use Medication

Disease consequences

Diarrhoea is a common reason for people seeking medical advice. Acute infectious diarrhoea is one of the commonest illnesses worldwide, particularly in developing countries, where it is the primary cause of childhood mortality. Diarrhoea is the second leading cause of death worldwide (Lawler & Wallace, 2003). The prevalence of chronic diarrhoea in an elderly population has been reported to be 7–14% (Talley *et al.*, 1992). The prognosis of chronic diarrhoea will depend on the underlying cause.

Nutritional consequences

Consequences of prolonged diarrhoea include dehydration, malnutrition, weight loss, anaemia and electrolyte imbalances. In children from developing countries, diarrhoea may lead to zinc deficiency, stunted growth and impaired cognitive development (World Gastroenterology Organization, 2008a).

Nutritional assessment

A full nutritional assessment should be conducted.

Anthropometry

Measure weight and height and calculate BMI. Has the patient lost weight? Calculate their percentage weight loss. Consider assessing grip strength, mid arm muscle circumference and triceps skinfold thickness to assess fat mass and muscle mass.

Biochemistry

Acute diarrhoea can rapidly lead to a loss of potassium and sodium. Do the blood results indicate that the patient is dehydrated? Are they iron, folate, vitamin B_{12} or zinc deficient? Does the patient have a raised C-reactive protein (CRP), white cell count (WCC) or erythrocyte sedimentation rate (ESR)?

Clinical assessment

Check bowel frequency and how long the patient has been experiencing symptoms for. Ask about stool consistency and colour. Use of the Bristol Stool Chart (Figure 7.4.10) may help your patient to describe their stools.

Does the patient look or feel dehydrated? Do they report a decreased urine output?

Does the patient have a medical diagnosis that could be the cause of the diarrhoea? Is the patient taking any medications that may cause diarrhoea?

Dietary assessment

Has the patient noticed a change in appetite? Take a diet history and evaluate fibre intake. Does the patient associate any particular foods with causing diarrhoea? Assess the types of fluid and the volume of fluid being drunk.

Economic and social assessment

Is there a history of anxiety? Are there food safety issues that may increase their risk of food poisoning?

Clinical assessment and management

Acute diarrhoea often resolves without complications in a few days, although dehydration can occur if symptoms are severe, especially in children and the elderly. If a bacterial infection is suspected, a stool sample should be sent to confirm whether antibiotic therapy is the appropriate treatment. Initial investigations for chronic diarrhoea will include blood and stool tests, although a detailed history in the assessment of the patient can help to establish whether the symptoms have an organic or functional cause. Symptoms of <3 months' duration, continuous or nocturnal diarrhoea and a significant weight loss are suggestive of an organic disease. Abdominal pain with intermittent diarrhoea and constipation is suggestive of IBS (Longstreth *et al.*, 2006). A diagnosis of overflow diarrhoea, which occurs due to faecal impaction following a period of constipation, should be excluded. Rectal examination, colonoscopy or flexible sigmoidoscopy and biopsy can exclude cancer, microscopic colitis and IBD. Antibody tests and duodenal biopsy may be performed to eliminate coeliac disease. A selenium homocholic acid taurine (SeHCAT) test or a trial of cholestyramine will help to determine if bile acid malabsorption is the cause and a hydrogen breath test can confirm small bowel bacterial overgrowth.

Antidiarrhoeal medication, e.g. loperamide, can relieve symptoms in adults by increasing gastrointestinal transit time, but it is not appropriate when the diarrhoea is caused by a bacterial infection.

Nutritional management

Acute diarrhoea

As episodes of acute diarrhoea are usually brief and self limiting, the focus of advice needs to be on the prevention of dehydration by encouraging a good fluid intake such as water, soft drinks (preferably not fruit juices) and savoury drinks. Oral rehydration solutions (glucose and electrolyte mixtures) increase water absorption by stimulation of sodium glucose transport in the small intestine and should be encouraged if dehydration is apparent. There is little evidence to support fasting as a treatment for acute diarrhoea (Wingate *et al.*, 2001), so if an individual wishes to eat, they should be encouraged to do so.

Babies should be encouraged to continue breast or bottle feeding (see Chapter 3.8). The World Gastroenterology Organization (2008a) recommends the administration of zinc sulphate supplements to children in developing countries suffering from persistent diarrhoea as this has been shown to help reduce the duration and severity of diarrhoeal episodes.

Much work has been done to investigate the role of probiotics in the treatment of diarrhoea. A systematic review (Allen *et al.*, 2010) concluded that probiotics appear to be safe and have beneficial effects in shortening the duration and reducing stool frequency in acute infectious diarrhoea. However, due to the wide variability in study design, more research is needed to develop specific treatment guidelines that can advise on which probiotics to use in different patient groups. In children it has been demonstrated that *Lactobacillus reuteri, Lactobacillus rhamnosus GG* and *Lactobacillus casei* are useful in treating acute infectious diarrhoea (World Gastroenterology Organization, 2008b). Further research is needed to clarify the importance of probiotics in the prevention of acute diarrhoea in adults and children.

A Cochrane systematic review (Pillai & Nelson, 2007) examining the treatment of *C. difficile* infection in adults concluded that there was insufficient evidence to support the use of probiotics in combination with antibiotics. While Hickson *et al.* (2007) have reported that a proprietary yoghurt drink containing probiotics was more effective than placebo in preventing antibiotic associated diarrhoea and *C. difficile* infection, the reliability of these results has been questioned due to the study's exclusion criteria (Wilcox & Sandoe, 2007).

Chronic diarrhoea

Some conditions with diarrhoea as a symptom, such as coeliac disease (see Chapter 7.4.7), lactose intolerance (see Chapter 7.4.6) and intestinal failure (see Chapter 7.4.9) require dietary manipulation as part of their first line treatment. If chronic diarrhoea is thought to have a functional cause, then advising a low fermentable oligo-, di- and mono-saccharides and polyols (FODMAPs) diet can be an effective approach to management of this challenging condition (Gibson & Shepherd, 2010) (see Chapter 7.4.10). There is limited evidence on specific dietary modifications for other causes of chronic diarrhoea that may help to alleviate symptoms and the advice given is probably best described as anecdotal. General advice that may be given includes:

* Explain the importance of maintaining a good fluid intake to help replace intestinal losses. If drinking milk is perceived to worsen the diarrhoea, appropriate advice can be given to exclude it from the diet until symptoms have settled.
* Continue to eat small frequent meals, choosing soft, low fibre foods such as white bread, mashed potato, plainly cooked pasta or rice, white fish, plainly cooked chicken, plain biscuits or crackers and jelly.
* Avoid high fibre foods such as wholegrain breads, whole wheat cereals, nuts and seeds, fruit skins and pith, vegetable skins and stalks, which may increase intestinal transit time and exacerbate symptoms.
* Foods known to aggravate symptoms should be excluded; spicy and greasy foods may stimulate diarrhoea.
* Drinking large volumes of undiluted fruit juice, caffeine containing drinks and alcohol should be discouraged.

If there are concerns about nutritional adequacy, advice on food fortification and oral nutritional supplements may be needed.

Diverticular disease

Diverticular disease is a common condition that occurs when small pouches, called diverticula, form in the wall of the colon. There are three terms used to describe diverticula in the large bowel:

* Diverticulosis – the presence of asymptomatic diverticula.
* Diverticular disease – when diverticula cause symptoms of abdominal pain and diarrhoea.
* Diverticulitis – when diverticula become inflamed or infected and cause severe pain, fever and changes in bowel habit.

Diagnostic criteria

Diverticular disease can be difficult to diagnose from the symptoms alone; these include pain on the left side of the abdomen and a change in bowel habit. A colonoscopy or barium enema may be carried out to confirm the presence of diverticula. When there is a history of diverticular disease, a diagnosis of diverticulitis may be made by physical examination, taking a medical history and carrying out a blood test to look for signs of infection.

Disease processes

Comparisons between different countries show that diverticular disease is more common in those countries with a typical western diet. A diet low in fibre is thought to be a significant risk factor for the development of diverticular disease, as first described by Painter & Burkitt (1971). A low dietary fibre intake leads to constipation and increases the intraluminal pressure in the sigmoid colon, segmentation and herniation of the mucosa through the muscle in areas of weakness.

Disease consequences

The prevalence of diverticular disease increases with age, from under 10% in those under 40 years to 50–66% in those aged over 80 years. Both sexes are equally affected by the condition. About 70% of those with diverticular disease will have one or more episodes of diverticulitis. As diverticular disease is predominantly a disease of the elderly, it will become an increasingly important health burden in the UK as a result of our ageing population. Complications of diverticulitis include the development of abscesses, fistulae, obstruction, diverticular haemorrhage and perforation of the bowel.

Nutritional assessment

Anthropometry

Is the patient underweight, normal weight or overweight? Is there a history of weight loss?

Biochemistry

Has a change in bowel habit resulted in dehydration? Does the patient have a raised CRP, WCC or ESR?

Clinical assessment

Is there a history of abdominal pain or a change in bowel habit?

Dietary assessment

If diverticulitis has been diagnosed, a fluid only diet for 2–3 days may be recommended until symptoms settle. Advise on supplementation with nutritious fluids until a normal diet can be resumed.

If diverticular disease has been diagnosed, a diet history should be taken to assess fibre and fluid intake. Advising on increased fibre intake, particularly from fruit and vegetables, may help to reduce the risk of disease progression.

Economic and social assessment

Does the patient express any concerns about having a lack of income or knowledge to achieve a well balanced diet?

Prevention

Epidemiological studies and the geographical distribution of the disease suggest that a high fibre intake may provide a protective role in the development of diverticular disease (Aldoori *et al.*, 1998). There is some evidence to suggest that vigorous exercise such as jogging or running can help to reduce the risk of developing this condition (Aldoori *et al.*, 1995).

No treatment is routinely offered to those with asymptomatic diverticular disease, but the results of a study by Aldoori *et al.* (1994) suggest that there is a prophylactic benefit from adopting a high fibre diet as a significant inverse relationship between dietary fibre intake and risk of developing clinically evident diverticular disease was found. Cereal fibres were found to be less protective than insoluble fibres from fruit and vegetables. A high fibre diet has also been suggested as beneficial for those with complications and recurrences of diverticulitis (Hyland & Taylor, 1980).

Clinical and nutritional management

Treatment of diverticulitis starts with antibiotics. A fluid only diet may be recommended until symptoms start to improve as digesting solid foods may make symptoms worse. An improvement will generally be seen after 2–3 days and then food can gradually be reintroduced. There is little research on diet and diverticulitis, but avoiding foods that can irritate the bowel, such as fruit and vegetable skins, seeds and nuts, and spicy foods, may be beneficial until symptoms have settled and a normal food intake can be resumed.

Surgery is recommended when it is acknowledged that other medical treatment is not working. Surgery is often undertaken to protect against the risk of peritonitis. Depending on the site and extent of bowel resection, dietary modification may be needed postoperatively (see Chapter 7.4.9).

Possible new treatments for diverticular disease include the use of 5-aminosalicylate compounds (Di Mario *et al.*, 2006) and probiotics. Interest in the role of probiotics in maintaining remission of symptomatic, uncomplicated diverticular disease is growing, but further work is needed

before specific recommendations can be made (Lamiki *et al.*, 2010).

Internet resources

CORE – Fighting Gut and Liver Disease   www.corecharity.org.uk

References

Aldoori WH, Giovannucci EL, Rimm EB, Wing AL, Trichopoulos DV, Willet WC. (1994) A prospective study of diet and the risk of symptomatic diverticular disease in men. *American Journal of Clinical Nutrition* 60: 757–764.

Aldoori WH, Giovannucci EL, Rimm EB. (1995) Prospective study of physical activity and the risk of symptomatic diverticular disease in men. *Gut* 36: 276–282.

Aldoori WH, Giovannucci EL, Rocket HRH, Sampson L, Rimm EB, Willet WC. (1998) A prospective study of dietary fiber types and symptomatic diverticular disease in men. *Journal of Nutrition* 128: 714–719.

Allen SJ, Martinez EG, Gregorio GV, Dans LF. (2010) Probiotics for treating acute infectious diarrhoea. *Cochrane Database of Systematc Reviews* 11: CD003048.

Anti M, Pignataro G, Armuzzi A, *et al.* (1998) Water supplementation enhances the effect of high fibre diet on stool frequency and laxative consumption in adult patients with functional constipation. *Hepatogastroenterology* 45(21): 727–732.

Baldi F, Bianco MA, Nardone G, Pilotto A, Zamparo E. (2009) Focus on acute diarrhoeal disease. *World Journal of Gastroenterology* 15(27): 3341–3348.

Chmielewska A, Szajewska H. (2010) Systematic review of randomized controlled trials: Probiotics for functional constipation. *World Journal of Gastroenterology* 16(1): 69–75.

Cullen G, O'Donoghue D. (2007) Constipation and Pregnancy. *Best Practice & Research Clinical Gastroenterology* 21(5):, 807–818.

Di Mario F, Comparato G, Fanigliulo L, *et al.* (2006) Use of mesalazine in diverticular disease. *Journal of Clinical Gastroenterology* 40(Suppl3): S155–159.

Dukas L, Willet WC, Giovannucci EL. (2003) Association between physical activity, fiber intake, and other lifestyle variables and constipation in a study of women. *American Journal of Gastroenterology* 98(8): 1790–1796.

Fitzharris GP, Garcia-Aguilar, J, Parker SC, *et al.* (2003) Quality of life after subtotal colectomy for slow transit constipation: both quality and quantity count. *Diseases of the Colon and Rectum* 46: 433–440.

Frattini JC, Norgueras JJ. (2008) Slow transit constipation: A review of a colonic functional disorder. *Clinics in Colon and Rectal Surgery* 21(2): 146–152.

Gibson PR, Shepherd SJ. (2010) Evidence-based dietary management of functional gastrointestinal symptoms: The FODMAP approach. *Journal of Gastroenterology and Hepatology* 25(2): 252–258.

Hickson M, D'Souza AL, Muthu N, *et al.* (2007) Use of probiotic Lactobacillus preparation to prevent diarrhoea associated with antibiotics: randomized double blind placebo controlled trial. *BMJ* 335: 80.

Higgins PDR, Johanson JF. (2004) Epidemiology of constipation in North America. A systematic review. *American Journal of Gastroenterology* 99(4): 750–759.

Hyland JMP, Taylor I. (1980) Does a high fibre diet prevent the complications of diverticular disease? *British Journal of Surgery* 67(2): 77–79.

Irvine EJ, Ferrazzi S, Pare P, Thompson WG, Rance L. (2002) Health-related quality of life in functional GI disorders: Focus on constipation resource utilization. *American Journal of Gastroenterology* 97: 1986–1993.

SECTION 7

Kamm MA, Hawley PR, Lennard-Jones JE. (1988) Outcome of colectomy for severe idiopathic constipation. *Gut* 29(7): 969–973.

Lamiki P, Tsuchiya J, Pathak S, *et al.* (2010) Probiotics in diverticular disease of the colon: an open label study. *Journal of Gastrointestinal and Liver Disease* 19(1): 31–36.

Lawler JV, Wallace MR. (2003) Diagnosis and treatment of bacterial diarrhoea. *Current Gastroenterology Reports* 5(1): 287–294.

Levy RL, Olden KW, Naliboff BD, *et al.* (2006) Psychosocial aspects of the functional gastrointestinal disorders. *Gastroenterology* 130: 1447–1458.

Lewis SJ, Heaton KW. (1997) Stool form scale as a useful guide to intestinal transit time. *Scandinavian Journal of Gastroenterology* 32(9): 920–924.

Longstreth GF, Thompson WG, Chey WD, Houghton LA, Mearin F, Spiller RC. (2006) Functional Bowel Disorders. *Gastroenterology* 130: 1480–1491.

National Institute for Health and Care Excellence (NICE). (2010) *Prucalopride for the Treatment of Chronic Constipation in Women.* London: NICE. Available at www.nice.org.uk.

NHS Business Services Authority. (2012) NHS Prescription Services Gastro-Intestinal System National Charts/ Available at www.nhsbsa.nhs.uk/PrescriptionServices. Accessed 16 June 2012.

Painter NS, Burkitt DP. (1971) Diverticular disease of the colon: A deficiency disease of Western civilization. *BMJ* 2: 450–454.

Peppas G, Alexiou VG, Mourtzoukou E, Falagas ME. (2008) Epidemiology of constipation in Europe and Oceania: a systematic review. *Gastroenterology* 8: 5.

Pillai A, Nelson RL. (2007) Probiotics for treatment of Clostridium difficile-associated colitis in adults. *Cochrane Database of Systematic Reviews* 2008(1): CD004611.

Suares NC, Ford AC. (2011) Systematic review: the effects of fibre in the management of chronic idiopathic constipation. *Alimentary Pharmacology & Therapeutics* 33(8): 895–901.

Talley NJ, O'Keefe EA, Zinsmeister AR, Melton LJ. (1992) Prevalence of gastrointestinal symptoms in the elderly: a population based study. *Gastroenterology* 102: 895–901.

Thomas PD, Forbes A, Green J, *et al.* (2003) *Guidelines for the Investigation of Chronic Diarrhea*, 2nd edn. *Gut* 53(Suppl V): v1–v15.

Wald A, Hinds JP, Caruana BJ. (1989) Psychological and physiological characteristics of patients with severe idiopathic constipation. *Gastroenterology* 97(4): 932–937.

Wilcox MH, Sandoe JA. (2007) Probiotics and diarrhoea. Data are not widely applicable. Letter. *BMJ* 335: 171.

Wingate D, Phillips SF, Lewis SJ, *et al.* (2001) Guidelines for adults on self-medication for the treatment of acute diarrhea. *Alimentary Pharmacology & Therapeutics* 15(6): 773–782.

World Gastroenterology Organization (WGO). (2008a) Practice guideline: Acute diarrhoea. Available at www.worldgastroenterology.org. Accessed 28 January 2013.

World Gastroenterology Organization (WGO). (2008b) Practice guideline: Probiotics and prebiotics. Available at www.worldgastroenterology.org. Accessed 28 January 2013.

7.4.12 Liver and biliary disease

Susie Hamlin and Julie Leaper

key points

- Malnutrition is common in cirrhosis in both obese and non-obese individuals.

- Assessment of nutritional status in all patients is essential and should include anthropometric measurements, clinical evaluation and review of dietary intake.

- Nutritional support should be provided to meet high requirements, whilst considering specific nutrient deficiencies.

- Restriction of essential nutrients should be assessed in individual cases and should be avoided unless indicated.

Liver disease refers to any disorder of the liver, including steatosis, fibrosis, hepatitis, cirrhosis or cancer. Liver disease is the fifth largest cause of death in the UK, with an upward trend in mortality compared with other major causes of death (BASL & BSG, 2009).

Anatomy and function of the liver

The liver is the largest solid organ in the body, weighing approximately 1.5 kg in adults and lies in the right upper quadrant of the abdomen, behind the rib cage. The liver has two anatomical lobes with the right lobe being the biggest (Figure 7.4.11). The portal vein provides blood from the splanchnic circulation and carries 75% of the blood entering the liver, which is rich in the end products of digestion. The hepatic artery supplies the liver with oxygen from the systemic circulation. The venous outflow from the liver is via the hepatic vein into the vena cava (Hill, 2009).

Sixty per cent of the liver consists of hepatocytes that are arranged in thin layers, resulting in a larger surface area for exchange of substances with blood. Bile canaliculi are very small channels between adjacent hepatocytes that allow bile, produced in the liver, to pass to the common bile duct. This travels via the cystic duct to the gall bladder for concentration and storage or into the duodenum via the common bile duct. The liver plays an essential role in the function of many processes, including the metabolism of nutrients (Table 7.4.16).

Classification of liver disease

Acute liver injury

Acute liver injury is rare and is found in previously healthy non-cirrhotic individuals who develop deterioration in coagulopathy and altered mental state over <26 weeks. It can be further subdivided into fulminant hepatic failure

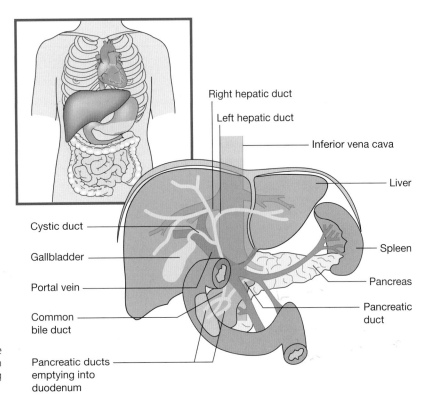

Figure 7.4.11 Anatomy of the liver [source: The British Liver Trust. Reproduced with permission of the British Liver Trust (www.britishlivertrust.org .uk)]

Table 7.4.16 Major functions of the liver

Function	Examples
Digestion	Bile acid production
Carbohydrate metabolism	Maintenance of glucose homeostasis Storage of glycogen Gluconeogenesis Mobilisation of glucose in response to hypoglycaemia
Protein metabolism	Utilisation of amino acids for protein synthesis and gluconeogenesis Deamination of amino acids into urea for excretion Regulation of amino acid supply to peripheral tissues Synthesis of plasma albumin, prothrombin, fibrinogen and clotting factors
Lipids and lipoproteins	Production of triglycerides and lipoprotein formation Synthesis of phospholipids and cholesterol Synthesis and degradation of non-esterified fatty acids Ketogenesis
Vitamins	Storage of vitamins A, B_2, B_3, B_6, B_{12}, K, folate Synthesis of prothrombin and factor VII requiring vitamin K Conversion of tryptophan to nicotinic acid Hydroxylation of vitamin D
Detoxification/deactivation	Oxidation of alcohol $\rightarrow$ acetaldehyde $\rightarrow$ acetate $\rightarrow$ CO_2 + fatty acids + H_2O Deactivation of drugs in the cytochrome P450 system Conjugation of oestrogens, corticosteroids and other steroid hormones for excretion
Excretion	Excretion of porphyrins, drugs, environmental toxins and heavy metals via bile secretion
Immune function	Adaptive immune system – T and B lymphocyte production Innate immune system Cytokine and inflammatory signalling cell production Kupffer cell formation (mononuclear phagocyte system) Tumour necrosis factor alpha (TNF-α) production
Haematological function	Synthesis of haem Regulation of iron metabolism

Table 7.4.17 Common causes of acute liver failure

Cause	Examples
Drugs	Paracetamol
	Tetracycline
	Halothane
	Troglitazone
	Antibiotics
	Non-steroidal anti-inflammatory drugs
Viral infections	Hepatitis viruses A, B and E
	Hepatitis viruses non-A, non-B
	Epstein–Barr virus
	Cytomegalovirus
	Yellow fever virus
	Reye's syndrome
	Herpes simplex
Alcohol	Alcoholic hepatitis
Non-viral infections	Toxoplasmosis
	Leptospira
Bacterial infections	Tuberculosis
	Pyogenic – liver abscess
Protozoal infections	Malaria
	Amoebiasis
Toxins	Amanita phalloides
	Aflatoxin
	Carbon tetrachloride
Other	Acute fatty liver of pregnancy
	Wilson's disease
	Herbal medicines
	Budd–Chiari
	Idiopathic
	HELLP syndrome of pregnancy

Table 7.4.18 Causes of chronic liver disease

Cause	Examples
Alcohol	Alcoholic liver disease
Metabolic syndrome	Non-alcoholic fatty liver disease (NAFLD)
	Non-alcoholic steatohepatitis (NASH)
Infections	Viral hepatitis B and C (most common)
	Viral hepatitis D, E and G
	Schistosomiasis
	Syphilis
Autoimmune	Autoimmune hepatitis
	Primary biliary cirrhosis and coeliac disease often coexists
Biliary tract disease	Primary sclerosing cholangitis and inflammatory bowel disease often coexists
Biliary obstruction	Biliary atresia/neonatal hepatitis
	Congenital biliary cysts
	Secondary biliary cirrhosis as a result of bile duct occlusion by gallstones or strictures
	Cystic fibrosis
Vascular disorders	Budd–Chiari syndrome
	Veno-occlusive disease/portal vein thrombosis
Drugs and toxins	Methotrexate
	Amiodarone
	Isoniazid
Metabolic disorders	Tyrosinaemia
	Wilson's disease
	Haemochromatosis
	Alpha-1-antitrypsin deficiency
	Porphyria
	Glycogen storage diseases
Bacterial infections	Tuberculosis
	Pyogenic – liver abscess
Miscellaneous	Sarcoidosis
	Jejunoileal bypass
	Caroli's syndrome
Cryptogenic	Liver disease of unknown aetiology

(FHF) and subfulminant hepatic failure. Fulminant hepatic failure is diagnosed in patients who develop encephalopathy within 8 weeks of the onset of symptoms of liver disease, with subfulminant hepatic failure described in those who do not develop encephalopathy for up to 26 weeks.

Acute liver injury often affects younger people and has a high morbidity and mortality (Polson & Lee, 2005). The most common cause of FHF in the UK is paracetamol toxicity (Table 7.4.17). Other causes include medication and hepatitis A, B and E, with 17% of cases of unknown cause (Bernal et al., 2010). Prognosis depends, to some extent, on the grade of encephalopathy:

- 20% survival without transplant if grade IV encephalopathy.
- 60% survival without transplant if grade II encephalopathy.

Patients who survive FHF usually make a full recovery (Vaquero et al., 2003).

Chronic liver disease

Hepatocellular damage may occur over several years initially via a build up of fat in the liver (fatty liver), which develops via inflammation and scarring to irreversible cirrhosis. An acute episode may also be superimposed on pre-existing chronic disease (Table 7.4.18).

Compensated cirrhosis occurs where the liver is cirrhotic, but there is no evidence of liver failure and no symptoms have developed. A patient can be asymptomatic with up to 80% of the liver damaged. Decompensated cirrhosis can appear where the liver is cirrhotic and symptoms of liver disease, e.g. ascites, jaundice, varices or encephalopathy, have developed. Decompensation can be part of progressive liver disease or can result from a sudden insult to an already cirrhotic liver.

Diagnostic criteria and classification

Presentation

Patients commonly present with elevated liver enzymes or decompensated liver disease. Many patients are asymp-

Table 7.4.19 Common investigations for liver disease

Test	Abnormality	Interpretation
Hepatitis B surface antigen	Positive	Implies chronic infection
Hepatitis C antibody	Positive	Suggests chronic infection
Alpha-1-antitrypsin level	Low	Investigations in alpha-1-antitrypsin deficiency
Antiendomysial antibodies	Positive	Suggestive of coeliac disease
Ferritin and iron binding studies	Elevated	Suggestive of haemochromatosis
Autoantibodies and immunoglobulins	ASM/ANA positive IgG	Suggestive of autoimmune hepatitis
Full blood count	Macrocytosis	Specific for alcohol excess only if gamma-glutamyltransferase elevated
	Thrombocytopenia	Suggestive of hypersplenism (portal hypertension)

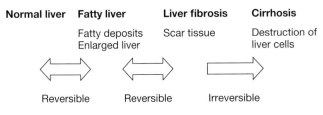

Figure 7.4.12 Stages of liver disease

tomatic until routine blood tests reveal abnormal liver function tests, which require further investigation or become unwell with an episode of decompensation. Many symptoms may be apparent such as malaise, itch and lethargy, which are common in patients with chronic liver disease.

Patient history

Weight, height and abdominal girth will be considered as risk factors for non-alcoholic fatty liver disease (NAFLD) in addition to alcohol history and risk factors for hepatitis C virus such as intravenous drug use. Prescribed and non-prescribed medication and herbal remedies will be investigated. Tattooing and prior medical interventions, surgery and transfusion history are all important information to obtain. To reach a diagnosis, investigations are performed that are relevant to the patient's history. Some common investigations are listed in Table 7.4.19, but this list is by no means exhaustive.

In response to liver injury, e.g. alcohol, NAFLD or chronic hepatitis C infection, fatty liver progresses to fibrosis. If the causative agent is removed, e.g. abstinence from alcohol, weight loss and antiviral treatment, normal hepatocyte structure can be restored at this stage. If the injury is chronic or recurrent, fibrosis can progress to cirrhosis, which is irreversible. The fibrous progression disrupts the architecture of the liver and impairs liver function (Figure 7.4.12).

Cirrhosis is often scored using the Child–Pugh score (sometimes the Child–Turcotte–Pugh score). It is used to determine prognosis as well as the required level of treatment, and is one of the scoring systems used when considering the need for referral for liver transplantation.

Table 7.4.20 Severity of cirrhosis using grading scores – modified Child–Pugh classification for cirrhosis (source: Friedman 2011. Reproduced with permission of Elsevier)

Measure	1 point	2 points	3 points
Total bilirubin [μmol/L (mg/dL)]	<34 (<2)	34–50 (2-3)	>50 (>3)
Serum albumin (g/L)	>35	28–35	<28
Prothrombin time (seconds increased)	1–3	4–6	>6
Ascites	None	Mild	Moderate/severe
Hepatic encephalopathy	None	Grade I–II (or suppressed with medication)	Grade III–IV (or refractory)

Table 7.4.21 Classification of Child–Pugh score (source: Pugh et al. 1973. Transection of the oesophagus for bleeding oesophageal varices. British Journal of Surgery 60: 646–649)

Points	Class
5–6	A
7–9	B
10–15	C

The score employs five clinical measures of liver disease (Table 7.4.20). Each measure is scored 1–3, with 3 indicating most severe derangement. Chronic liver disease is classified into Child–Pugh class A, B or C, using the added score from Table 7.4.21. In primary sclerosing cholangitis (PSC) and primary biliary cirrhosis (PBC), the bilirubin references are altered to reflect the fact that these diseases feature high conjugated bilirubin levels.

Other measures have become more common over the past 10 years in assessing the severity of liver disease, prognosis and need for referral for liver transplantation. The Model for End Stage Liver Disease (MELD) scoring system and the United Kingdom End Stage Liver Disease (UKELD) system are used to predict the mortality among patients on the waiting list for liver transplantation (Malinchoc et al., 2000, Neuberger et al., 2008).

Disease processes

Changes in metabolism

Carbohydrate and fat metabolism was demonstrated by Owen et al. (1983) to be altered in cirrhosis following an overnight fast. Cirrhotic patients develop starvation type metabolism similar to that of a 2–3-day fast in healthy people. This is due to decreased hepatic glycogen stores and reduced glycogenolysis. Fat and protein are metabolised as a short term energy source, which creates an accelerated response to starvation. Altered glucose metabolism is common in chronic liver disease with up to 96% exhibiting impaired glucose tolerance (Hickman & Macdonald, 2007) and up to 35% developing diabetes (Muller et al., 1994). In these patients insulin resistance has been implicated by reduced hepatic degradation and increased secretion of insulin, with elevated plasma levels of insulin alongside normal glucose tolerance (Matos et al., 2002).

Metabolism of protein and amino acids is abnormal, with increased protein catabolism present even in early stages of cirrhosis. Protein deficiency worsens as liver disease develops (Sanchez & Aranda-Michel, 2006). The alterations in amino acid metabolism associated with liver disease are shown by the reduced levels of circulating branched chain amino acids (leucine, isoleucine and valine), increased levels of circulating aromatic amino acids (phenylalanine, tryptophan and tyrosine) and methionine.

Alcoholic liver disease

Alcoholic liver disease is a major cause of liver disease throughout the world and patients often have risk factors for other liver diseases, e.g. NAFLD or chronic viral hepatitis (O'Shea et al., 2010). The risk of developing the disease increases with overall alcohol intake. However, where intakes of alcohol are high and over a long time, 90–100% have fatty liver but only 20–35% develop alcoholic hepatitis and 8–20% develop alcoholic cirrhosis (Barve et al., 2008). Oxidative stress, proinflammatory cytokines and reduced levels of adiponectin, which has anti-inflammatory properties, have been implicated as pathways of injury as a result of alcohol (Tilg et al., 2011). The disease ranges from steatosis (fatty liver) through steatohepatitis to cirrhosis.

Alcoholic hepatitis

Alcoholic hepatitis presents as an acute decompensation of the liver function in a person with a history of alcohol abuse (Sougioultzis et al., 2005). By itself, alcoholic hepatitis does not lead to cirrhosis and is distinct from cir-

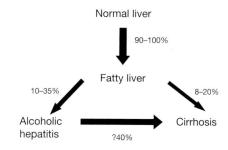

Figure 7.4.13 Progression of alcoholic liver disease in heavy drinkers (source: McCullough & O'Connor 1998. Reproduced with permission of Wiley-Blackwell Publishing)

rhosis caused by long term alcohol consumption. The progression of alcoholic liver disease in heavy drinkers is shown in Figure 7.4.13 (McCullough & O'Connor, 1998). Patients with alcoholic hepatitis usually present with the rapid onset of jaundice, fever, hepatomegaly and anorexia. Symptoms of portal hypertension may also be involved, such as ascites, encephalopathy and variceal bleeding.

There is a significant mortality associated with severe alcoholic hepatitis; Stickel et al. (2003) reported a 28-day mortality of higher than 40% in patients with severe alcoholic hepatitis. Typical age of presentation is between 40 and 60 years, and the female gender is an independent risk factor for alcoholic hepatitis (Lucey et al., 2009). Maddrey's discriminant function is a formula with good correlation and predictive value for 30-day mortality. A value of >32 is indicative of severe alcoholic hepatitis with a 3-month mortality rate of 55% (Sargent, 2005). Other factors that correlate with a poor prognosis are renal impairment, encephalopathy and increased white cell count (Philippe, 2007).

Primary biliary cirrhosis

This is a chronic and progressive autoimmune disease where the bile ducts become inflamed and destroyed, resulting in biliary cirrhosis. The aetiology is largely unknown, although genetic, immune system and environmental factors have been considered (Levy & Lindor, 2003). Up to 95% of those diagnosed are female with average age of onset between 30 and 70 years (Lee & Kaplan, 1998). Symptoms include osteoporosis, pruritus (itching), fatigue and jaundice. Patients with advanced primary biliary cirrhosis and cirrhosis may develop ascites and hepatic encephalopathy. The association between primary biliary cirrhosis and coeliac disease has been investigated extensively and the incidence ranges from 0–11% (Rubio-Tapia & Murray, 2007).

Primary sclerosing cholangitis

This is a chronic progressive disorder characterised by inflammation and fibrosis of the biliary tree, leading to liver cirrhosis, portal hypertension and liver failure (Maggs & Chapman, 2008). It is associated with inflammatory bowel disease in a large number of cases (Weismuller *et al.*, 2008). The aetiology is still unclear, although primary sclerosing cholangitis could be caused by autoimmune, genetic or inflammatory disease. The incidence of hepatic osteodystrophy is between 4% and 10% and should be investigated at new diagnosis (Chapman *et al.*, 2010).

Non-alcoholic fatty liver disease

This is described in detail in the Clinical investigation and management section.

Viral hepatitis

Viral hepatitis is mainly caused by chronic disease, namely hepatitis B virus (HBV) and hepatitis C virus (HCV). Other causes include hepatitis A, D and E virus, but these are not discussed within the scope of this chapter.

Hepatitis B virus

Worldwide, an estimated 2 billion people have been infected with hepatitis B virus (HBV), and >350 million have chronic liver infections (WHO, 2008). Hepatitis B virus may cause an acute illness or develop into a chronic disease, which causes cirrhosis and possibly, liver cancer. It is transmitted by the blood and body fluids of an infected person and can be transmitted from mother to child at the time of birth, within households (non-sexual), between sexual partners and via needle sharing, as well as through occupational and healthcare related incidents (Shepard *et al.*, 2006).

Hepatitis C virus

About 130–170 million people are chronically infected with hepatitis C virus (HCV) and >350 000 people die from HCV related liver diseases each year (WHO, 2011). It causes chronic hepatitis, leading to cirrhosis with increased risk of hepatocellular carcinoma and intrahepatic cholangiocarcinoma (El-Serag *et al.*, 2009). Transmission is usually via infected blood, which can include drug use, blood products prior to HCV screening, tattooing or piercing. Treatment includes the use of pegylated interferon, in combination with ribavirin as preferred treatment (NICE, 2010b). Direct acting antiviral agents are now being developed that may change the drug regimens currently used (Ghany *et al.*, 2011).

Autoimmune hepatitis

Autoimmune hepatitis is a progressive disease of unknown aetiology, which may occur as a result of an environmental trigger in a genetically susceptible person, e.g. virus or drug induced. At least 70% of patients are female, with half younger than 40 years of age; however, onset may range from childhood to the elderly (Makol *et al.*, 2011).

Metabolic liver disease

Wilson's disease

This is an autosomal recessive genetic disorder in which copper accumulates in tissues, resulting in acute or chronic liver disease with neuropsychiatric symptoms. Acute Wilson's disease appears in approximately 5% of patients, with an increased ratio of 3:1 in females; however, the cause for this is uncertain (Taylor & Corbani, 2009). Fulminant Wilson's disease is usually fatal without transplantation (Polson & Lee, 2005).

Chronic Wilson's disease usually presents with hepatitis or cirrhosis and symptoms of hepatomegaly, ascites or jaundice. The progression of disease depends on the effectiveness of chelation treatment.

Haemochromatosis

Haemochromatosis is an autosomal genetic recessive disease characterised by the abnormal accumulation of iron in major organs, leading to accumulation in tissues and primarily the liver, causing cirrhosis (van Bokhoven *et al.*, 2011). Iron deposits can also accumulate in endocrine organs and the heart. Diagnosis can be suspected in middle aged men with cirrhosis, bronzed skin, joint inflammation and diabetes (Pietrangelo, 2006).

Alpha-1-antitrypsin deficiency

This is an autosomal recessive genetic disorder caused by defective production of alpha-1-antitrypsin (AAT), which affects the liver and lungs. There is no treatment other than symptom management and liver transplantation (Fairbanks & Tavill, 2008) (see Chapter 5.1).

Disease consequences

Mortality

Liver disease mortality in the UK is rising at a time when liver death rates are dropping in most of Europe. Ninety-five per cent of all liver disease is largely preventable. The average age of death from liver disease is 59 years (compared with 82–84 years for heart and lung disease or stroke). Government mortality statistics for the UK highlight that deaths from liver disease are showing an upward trend, increasing by 12% in the last 3 years, which is equates to 46 244 deaths. Over the last 10 years people have been presenting with and dying from liver disease at a younger age, with a five-fold increase in the development of cirrhosis in 35–55-year olds. There has been a 32% increase in people under 35 years dying from alcoholic liver disease in England and Wales (British Association for the Study of the Liver & Bristish Society of Gastroenterology, 2009). Deaths from liver disease over the next 20 years are predicted to double (British Liver Trust, 2009). Effective prevention strategies or treatments need to be available for the three main causes of liver disease; alcohol, viral hepatitis and obesity. These decrease the risk of developing cirrhosis, liver cancer and their associated mortality.

Patient perspective

Patients with liver disease may need the support of outside agencies and charities. Some are listed in the additional contacts section at the end of the chapter. The British Liver Trust (2011) stated, '*Patient support groups prove to be an invaluable resource helping to inform, educate and reassure patients. The mutual sharing of factual information and coping strategies can help reduce the fear associated with illness and help people to manage their condition and symptoms more effectively'.*

Public health aspects and prevention

The key risk factors for liver disease in developed countries are NAFLD, alcoholic liver disease and hepatitis C. These risk factors are relevant to a large proportion of the population and are modifiable. Examples of early prevention measures include early identification of HCV infection through screening and its treatment, reduction in heavy drinking, and use of interventions for obesity and the metabolic syndrome. Early prevention and management of these factors also form the basis for treatment.

Alcohol

Alcoholic liver disease is a major health and economic problem in the western world. Alcohol misuse and alcohol related problems, especially binge drinking and alcohol related liver disease, are major public health concerns. There is also an increasing number of people with alcohol related problems who services need to be provided for. In 2006/2007, alcohol misuse cost the UK economy £25.1 billion; £2.7 billion of this was NHS expenditure. In 2008, over 78% of the incurred costs were for hospital based care. The projected cost to the NHS is continuing to rise as >1 in 25 adults are dependent on alcohol, and the UK has one of the highest rates of binge drinking in Europe. This continued rise in alcohol misuse will significantly burden liver services (NICE, 2010a). The National Institute for Health and Care Excellence guidelines describe the problems associated with hazardous drinking behaviour and the difference between alcohol dependence and alcohol use disorders.

However, not everyone who is alcohol dependent goes on to develop liver disease. Risk factors of alcohol induced liver disease include:

- *Alcohol dependence* – liver damage only occurs in approximately 20% of people with alcohol dependence (Stokkeland *et al.*, 2008).
- *Gender* – women are more susceptible to alcohol related liver damage than men, with one study suggesting the risk is almost 50% higher (Corrao *et al.*, 1997).
- *Body mass index* – being overweight or obese increases the risk of alcohol related liver disease (Bellantani *et al.*, 1997).
- *Race* – some studies suggest people of African origin are more susceptible than Caucasians (Stranges *et al.*, 2004).
- *Genetic predisposition* – there is no clear evidence, but the fact that only a minority of heavy drinkers develop liver disease suggests a genetic predisposing factor (Zintzaras *et al.*, 2006).
- *Pattern of drinking* – drinking alcohol only at meal times appears to carry a lower risk of alcohol related

liver disease than other patterns of alcohol consumption (Bellantani *et al.*, 1997).
- *Hepatitis C infection* – there is a strong association between hepatitis C, unlike hepatitis B, and the development of advanced alcoholic liver disease (Mendenhall *et al.*, 1991).

UK government advice

Official UK guidance recommends that men should not regularly drink >3–4 units of alcohol/day and women no >2–3 units/day. Regular drinking is defined as drinking every day or most days of the week. It is also recommended that people do not drink alcohol for 48 hours after a heavy drinking session to enable recovery (see Chapter 4.2).

Pregnant women and women trying to conceive should avoid drinking alcohol. If they do choose to drink alcohol, they are advised to not drink >1–2 units of alcohol once or twice a week and not to get drunk, to minimise the risk to the baby. The National Institute for Health and Care Excellence (2010a) advises women to avoid alcohol in the first 3 months of their pregnancy in particular, because of the increased risk of miscarriage. However, in 2011 the Royal College of Physicians (RCP, 2011) submitted a report to the House of Commons' Science and Technology Committee that aimed to change this advice. The RCP argued that the last systematic review of the evidence by the government was in 1995 and that the current wording of the UK guidelines appears to sanction daily or near daily drinking. The frequency of alcohol consumption is an important risk factor for the development of alcohol dependency and alcoholic liver disease, and the RCP wants increased clarity in the guidance. Someone drinking 4 units/day (the current upper limit for men) would be classed as a hazardous or high risk drinker using the World Health Organization's standard tool for identifying people at risk of alcohol related harm (WHO, 2009).

In addition, the RCP recommended limits for safe drinking by older people in a separate guidance, as they may be particularly vulnerable to harm from alcohol due to biological changes associated with ageing. The current guidelines are based primarily on evidence for younger age groups and there is concern they are not appropriate for older people. The RCP has proposed a change to no more than 21 units/week for men and 14 units/week for women, with some alcohol free days.

Obesity

The Health Survey for England showed that nearly one in four adults and over one in 10 children (aged 2–10 years) are obese. In 2007, the Foresight report predicted that if no action were taken, 60% of men, 50% of women and 25% of children would be obese by 2050. The prevalence of NAFLD is estimated at between 20% and 30% in western adults (Browning *et al.*, 2004; Bedogni *et al.*, 2005) and rises to 90% in extreme obesity (Machado *et al.*, 2006). The rising burden of obesity will clearly have huge implications for the future burden of liver disease. Strategies to reduce obesity will reduce the burden of NAFLD.

Obesity is a major public health priority and the UK government is developing strategies to deal with this issue (see Chapter 4.2). Non-alcoholic fatty liver disease is discussed further in this chapter and obesity management is discussed in Chapter 7.13.2 and Chapter 7.13.3.

Hepatitis C

Alcohol and obesity advice is important in the treatment of hepatitis C (Lieber, 2001; Monto et al., 2010). Obesity can reduce the effectiveness of antiviral treatments; obese patients [body mass index (BMI) >30 kg/m²] should be advised to try to lose weight prior to starting antiviral treatment (Bressler et al., 2003). Key advice to people with hepatitis C is weight maintenance within a healthy BMI to avoid obesity, in particular central obesity, and to follow the appropriate guidance for alcohol intake specific to their stage of disease and past medical history.

Nutritional consequences

Malnutrition is an increasingly recognised complication of liver disease that has been shown to adversely affect outcome (Alberino et al., 2001). Protein energy malnutrition (PEM) is common in chronic liver disease, with a prevalence of up to 20% in compensated cirrhosis (Coltorti et al., 1991) and 75–90% in decompensated cirrhosis (Carvalho & Parise, 2006; DiCecco et al., 1989). For those awaiting transplant, the figure is almost 100% (Figueiredo et al., 2000). Protein energy malnutrition has been shown to have a correlation with the following (Mullen & Weber, 1991; McCullough & Bugianesi, 1997; Plauth et al., 1997; Runyon, 1998):

- Worsening ascites.
- Increased infection rate.
- Worsening encephalopathy.
- Higher rate of variceal bleeding.
- Increased hospital readmissions.
- Increased mortality.

There is a direct correlation between the progression of liver disease and the severity of malnutrition. Patients with cirrhosis develop PEM irrespective of the aetiology of disease (Thuluvath & Triger, 1994), with the incidence similar in alcoholic and non-alcoholic patients (McCullough & Bugianesi, 1997). The reasons patients experience these severe changes to their nutritional status are multifactorial, and are most often seen in patients with chronic liver disease, although they can develop with acute disease that is not resolving.

Reduced nutrient intake

Protein energy malnutrition is exacerbated by reduced nutrient intake and is a result of one or a combination of factors (Saunders et al., 2010; O'Brien & Williams, 2008; Tsiaousi et al., 2008) including:

- Loss of appetite due to the presence of cytokines, e.g. tumour necrosis factor.
- Early satiety, commonly found when ascites results in reduced gastric capacity.
- Unnecessary dietary restrictions further exacerbating the choice and volume of food.
- Nausea and vomiting due to gastroparesis, small bowel dysfunction and bacterial overgrowth.
- High alcohol intakes replacing food energy, or reduced intake due to oesophagitis, gastritis or pancreatitis.
- Altered taste sensation due to deficiency of zinc or magnesium.
- Weakness or fatigue affecting inclination to eat or prepare food.
- Malabsorption, e.g. steatorrhoea.
- Repeated investigations that require prior fasting.

Altered energy expenditure

Debate continues as to whether hypermetabolism contributes to body wasting in cirrhotic patients. The causes of this increase in energy expenditure are unclear and metabolic rates may change frequently over time with complications of liver disease, e.g. infection, gastrointestinal bleeding or development of ascites. Muller et al. (1999) studied 473 clinically stable patients with liver disease and identified 34% of these as hypermetabolic, defined as resting energy expenditure 120% of the expected values. Clinical or biochemical markers of liver disease did not predict increased metabolism, suggesting that it may be caused by extrahepatic events, e.g. systemic inflammatory response. Some patients may compensate for the increased energy expenditure by reducing activity levels, but remain at high risk of malnutrition.

Malabsorption

A number of mechanisms can contribute to malabsorption. Patients with cholestatic liver disease, e.g. primary sclerosing cholangitis and primary biliary cirrhosis, may experience a reduction in the bile salt pool, resulting in fat malabsorption. Those with alcoholic liver disease frequently experience pancreatitis, which leads to malabsorption of fat (Renner et al., 1984) and changes in the structure of the small intestine and brush border enzymes due to alcohol (Bhonchal et al., 2008). Many patients with alcoholic liver disease experience rapid intestinal transit times, increased permeability of the mucosa, and altered salt and water absorption. The administration of medicines, e.g. neomycin, lactulose or cholestyramine, as part of the specific medical management of symptoms may also result in increased bowel movements and reduced absorption of nutrients.

Hepatic osteodystrophy

An important complication of chronic liver disease is osteodystrophy, which includes osteoporosis and osteomalacia. Clinically these patients present with bone pains, backache, reduced height, fractures and scoliosis (Goel & Kar, 2010). The reasons for this are multifactorial, including poor intake and absorption of calcium, altered vitamin D synthesis, malnutrition and steroid use in certain liver conditions.

Osteoporosis

Risk factors for osteoporosis and subsequent fracture irrespective of cirrhosis include a low BMI of $<19\,kg/m^2$, alcohol excess, steroid use, physical inactivity, previous fragility fracture, early maternal hip fracture (<60 years), hypogonadism and premature menopause (<45 years). Cirrhotic patientsfrequently present with increasing age, especially when in the middle decades; these patients often have a low BMI, may have had excessive alcohol intakes and could be receiving steroids (Collier *et al.*, 2002). Foods often advised for nutritional support measures correlate with foods rich in calcium, such as milk, cheese and yoghurts. Dietary intake usually decreases with disease progression. Cirrhotic patents should routinely be supplemented with 800 IU of vitamin D and 1000 mg of calcium (Collier *et al.*, 2002). However, in patients with increased cardiovascular risk, such as those with NAFLD, DEXA scanning may be performed to confirm osteodystrophy prior to commencing supplements (Bolland *et al.*, 2011) (see Chapter 7.9.1s).

Vitamins

Thiamine deficiency is discussed further in the section on Alcoholic liver disease.

There is a high incidence of fat soluble vitamin deficiencies in liver disease, with levels related to the severity of disease (Abbott-Johnson *et al.*, 2011). In primary biliary cirrhosis, vitamin A deficiency is seen in 20% of cases, but is often clinically asymptomatic (Talwalkar & Lindor, 2003). In advanced primary sclerosing cirrhosis, up to 82% of patients will be deficient in vitamin A (Lee & Kaplan, 2002). Malham *et al.* (2011) demonstrated that compromised vitamin D status can be found in 85% of patients with alcoholic liver disease and up to 47% with primary biliary cirrhosis, and that more than standard clinical dose repletion may be required.

Deficiency of vitamin E is rare, but can be seen in chronic cholestatic liver disease. Symptoms include muscle weakness, ataxia and haemolysis, and in advanced primary sclerosing cirrhosis these can be seen in 40–50% of patients (Lee & Kaplan, 2002). Vitamin K requires bile salts for absorption and therefore cholestasis can affect levels in liver disease. Supplementation may be given by intramuscular injections, but should be avoided in patients with low muscle mass or abnormal clotting; therefore, intravenous injection of vitamin K may be preferable.

Minerals

Serum magnesium levels are decreased in liver cirrhosis, which may be attributed to decreased intake or increased excretion (Das *et al.*, 2011). Zinc is discussed in the Nutritional management section.

Nutritional assessment

Detailed nutritional assessment is critical in patients with liver disease in order to provide optimal nutritional support. Some markers of nutritional status used in other clinical areas are not useful in liver disease as symptoms, dietary intake and nutritional status are prone to rapid change. The dietary advice provided must be monitored regularly and alterations made to treatment plans to reflect these changes.

Anthropometry

Weight

Correct interpretation of the weight of fluid in patients with ascites and oedema is vital. Body mass index, percentage weight loss and nutritional requirements must be calculated using dry weights or estimated dry weights. Body mass index can be grossly misleading in interpreting the level of malnutrition if adjustments for dry weight are not made. Dry weight can be estimated from:

Dry weight = wet weight

– estimated weight of ascites or oedema

The amount of ascites and/or oedema can be calculated using Mendenhall's (1992) figures (Table 7.4.22). These figures have limitations and often patients have more fluid than this evidence based estimate advises. Weight histories and dry weight following paracentesis can provide the best estimate of actual flesh weight, with adjustment if necessary for peripheral oedema. Patients may have up to 20–30 L of ascites and therefore 20–30 kg must be taken off the wet weights, as well as further subtraction for peripheral oedema, in order to calculate estimated dry weights.

Upper arm anthropometry

Measurement of mid arm circumference (MAC), triceps skinfold thickness (TSF) and mid arm muscle circumference (MAMC) should be taken to identify fat and muscle stores (see Chapter 2.2). Morgan *et al.* (2006) showed that MAMC and TSF could be used to develop a subjective global assessment tool for patients with cirrhosis where anthropometry showed substantial interobserver agreement.

The ESPEN guidelines (Plauth *et al.*, 2006) recommend simple methods for identifying undernutrition, including anthropometry or handgrip. Mid arm muscle circumference has been shown to detect body cell mass depletion and its effect on adverse outcome in end stage liver disease (Figueiredo *et al.*, 2000).

Table 7.4.22 Estimation of fluid weight in ascites or oedema (source: Mendenhall 1992, pp 363–84. Reproduced with permission of Taylor & Francis)

Severity	Ascites (kg)	Peripheral oedema (kg)
Minimal	2.2	1.0
Moderate	6.0	5.0
Severe	14.0	10.0

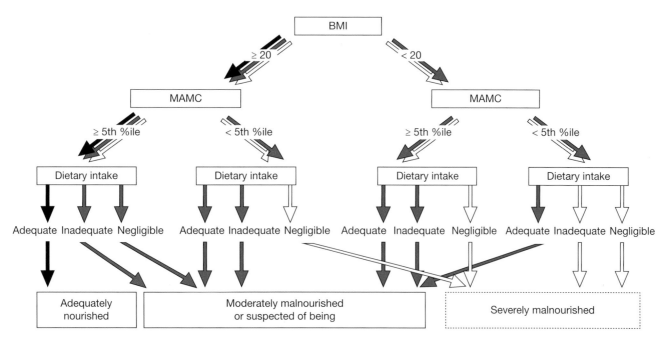

Figure 7.4.14 Royal Free Hospital Global Assessment (RFH-GA) scheme for determining nutritional status in patients with cirrhosis (source: Morgan *et al*. 2006. Reproduced with permission of Nature Publishing Group)
BMI, body mass index; MAMC, mid arm muscle circumference; %ile, percentile

Bioelectrical impedance analysis

Kyle *et al*., (2004) suggested that bioelectrical impedance analysis (BIA) use in the routine assessment of patients with ascites and oedema was not adequately validated. However, Plauth *et al*. (2006) suggested that estimation of body cell mass with BIA could be used despite limitations in patients with ascites. However, BIA is not used routinely in clinical practice.

Grip strength dynamometry

Alvares-da-Silva & Reverbel da Silveira (2005) showed that lower handgrip strength predicted a poorer clinical outcome in patients with cirrhosis, who had higher rates of development of:

* Uncontrolled ascites.
* Hepatic encephalopathy.
* Spontaneous bacterial peritonitis.
* Hepatorenal syndrome.

Changes in measurements can be found over 1–2 weeks and therefore help in monitoring of nutritional advice. Care needs to be taken when interpreting results with encephalopathic patients due to their difficulty following the instructions properly.

Screening tools

Malnutrition Universal Screening Tool

The Malnutrition Universal Screening Tool ('MUST') (Elia, 2003) was developed in order to categorise patients for risk of malnutrition, and has been found to be an easy, quick, reproducible and internally consistent method. Patients with liver disease frequently have fluid overload and therefore dry weights have to be calculated, including percentage dry weight loss, in order to use the tool.

Adequate training is essential to ensure dry weight is calculated accurately in order to use BMI and percentage weight loss in this tool.

Royal Free Hospital Global Assessment

This tool uses dry weight BMI, MAMC and an assessment of nutritional intake to categorise patients into adequately, moderately (or suspected of being so) or severely malnourished.

In 2006, Morgan *et al*. validated the Royal Free Hospital Global Assessment (RFH-GA) tool, which is simple, reproducible and capable of predicting outcome in patients with cirrhosis (Figure 7.4.14). Dietary intakes were assessed as inadequate if the patient's intake failed to meet estimated requirements but were >500 kcal/day, with intakes under 500 kcal/day being categorised as negligible. The category of malnutrition established was found to predict poorer survival in those who were moderately or severely malnourished, and those with decompensated liver disease were more likely to be malnourished than those with compensated liver disease. A BMI of <20 kg/m^2 was associated with poorer survival. The subjective override can be used to change the categorisation by a single category if there has been recent change, e.g. weight loss or steatorrhoea.

Interestingly, the study showed a preferential decrease in fat mass for women compared with muscle mass in men, with this area warranting further research. Further confirmation of the RFH-GA predictive power was found when it was compared with the Child–Pugh and MELD scores (Gunsar *et al*., 2006). Dietitians use this tool as part of the patient assessment at UK liver transplant centres.

Recently, a nutritional prioritising tool for patients with cirrhosis has been developed and validated against the RFH-GA. Initial results suggested that it can identify patients with cirrhosis who are at high risk for malnutrition, although further multicentre validation is required (Arora *et al.*, 2011).

Biochemistry

Careful interpretation of biochemistry is required in liver disease. Hepatic albumin synthesis is decreased in liver disease and therefore using albumin as a marker of nutritional status is unreliable (Campos *et al.*, 2002). Declining albumin and deterioration in liver function tests (LFTs), e.g. bilirubin and alkaline phosphatase, are a better indicator of liver disease or acute phase response rather than nutrition.

Alkaline phosphatase

Alkaline phosphatase (ALP) is present in two major sites in the body, the liver and bones. It is associated with the biliary tract and elevated levels can indicate biliary tract diseases. If glutamyl transpeptidase (GGT) is not elevated in conjunction with ALP, the ALP is most likely of bone origin.

Glutamyl transpeptidase

Glutamyl transpeptidase (GGT) is present in hepatocytes and biliary cells. It is interpreted in conjunction with ALP and elevated levels are associated with the biliary tract diseases. It is sometimes incorrectly interpreted as a sensitive and specific marker of alcohol misuse, but studies have shown that the sensitivities of elevated GGT for alcohol varies between 52% and 94% (Aithal & Ryder, 2005).

Alanine aminotransferase and aspartate transaminase

Alanine aminotransferase (ALT) and aspartate transaminase (AST) are found within hepatocytes and are sensitive markers of hepatocyte injury.

Bilirubin

The bile pigments bilirubin and biliverdin are produced from substances containing haem, e.g. haemoglobin. They are transported in the blood attached to serum albumin (unconjugated bilirubin). In the liver, two glucaronate groups are attached to form conjugated bilirubin, which is excreted into the bile canaliculi. Bacteria in the gut convert bilirubin to stercobilinogen, which then forms stercobilin; stercobilin is responsible for the colour of faeces. When bilirubin is elevated, jaundice develops with the characteristic yellowing of the skin and viscera. Bilirubin is usually elevated with ALP as it is present in the biliary tract. Pale stools and jaundice are indicative of biliary tract disorders.

Albumin

Albumin is one of the many proteins synthesised by the liver and accounts for 65% of serum protein (Martin & Friedman, 2004). Albumin has a half-life of approximately 21 days and therefore serum albumin concentrations are slow to respond to alterations in protein synthesis. The liver normally produces 12–15g of albumin/day and hypoalbuminaemia may be indicative of poor synthetic

function in cirrhosis (Johnson, 1999). As a result, albumin is one of the criteria for the Child–Pugh classification of cirrhosis (Table 7.4.21). Caution is needed in interpreting hypoalbuminaemia as it may not be specific to liver disease. It is also seen in postsurgical patients, acute pancreatitis and chronic inflammatory conditions, or reflects gastrointestinal or glomerular losses in conditions such as nephrotic syndrome.

Clinical assessment

Physical signs of liver disease and potential nutritional issues include (Figure 7.4.15):

* *Muscle wasting* – identified by visceral muscle loss, especially in the upper arms and temples, decreased activities of daily living or fatigue. Subcutaneous fat stores may mask this.
* *Presence of jaundice* – shown by yellow skin, eyes and scratch marks, which increase suspicion of potential fat malabsorption.
* *Encephalopathy* – reversed sleep patterns or confusion affecting meal patterns.
* *Development of ascites and/or oedema* – increased abdominal or peripheral swelling leading to fatigue and early satiety.
* *Spider nevi, red palms or altered nail appearance* (white half moon extends down the nail bed), indicate deteriorating liver disease and cirrhosis).
* *Micronutrient deficiencies* – hair loss, poor skin condition and dentition, night blindness and altered taste may all indicate various vitamin or mineral deficiencies.

Dietary assessment

Food intake can be assessed using a diet history or recall method. Patterns of eating will identify issues with altered sleep patterns and bloating, especially towards the evening. It is important to establish when symptoms such as fatigue, nausea, early satiety or abdominal pain may affect appetite and nutritional intake. Encephalopathic patients may not be able to reliably recall their intake and relatives may help to provide a more accurate history of their intake. Food charts may also be useful where staff can monitor intakes for inpatients and using local hospital systems to identify where accurate reporting is required.

Calculation of requirements

In clinical practice, either the ESPEN guidelines (Plauth *et al.*, 2006) of 35–40 kcal/kg of body weight/day or calculation of basal metabolic rate (BMR) using the Henry (2005) equations (see Chapter 6.1) with added stress and activity factors according to the Parenteral and Enteral Nutrition Group (BDA) guidelines (Todorovic & Micklewright, 2011) are used (Table 7.4.23). It is important for both calculations to use estimated dry weight as previously described. The stress factor chosen should relate to the symptoms present, i.e. if only ascites is present, then a 30% stress factor is appropriate. Patients with multiple

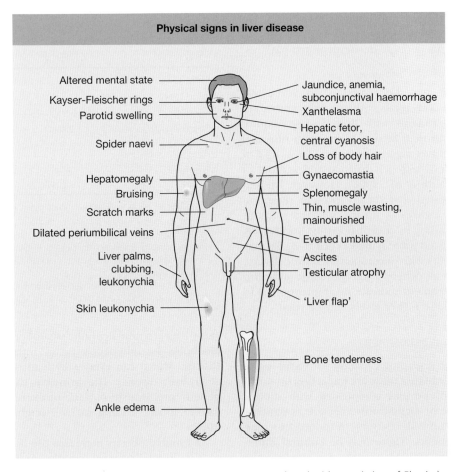

Figure 7.4.15 Signs of liver disease (source: Bacon *et al.* 2006, p 62. Reproduced with permission of Elsevier)

Table 7.4.23 Stress factors for liver disease (Kondrup & Muller, 1997; Hasse, 2001; Plauth *et al.*, 2009)

Compensated liver disease	0–20%
Decompensated liver disease	30–40%
Acute (fulminant) liver failure/ventilated	20–30%
Post transplant (postoperative period)	30%

Table 7.4.24 Nitrogen and protein requirements for liver disease (Plauth *et al.*, 2006)

	Nitrogen (g)	Protein (g)
Compensated liver disease	0.19–0.20	1.2–1.3
Decompensated liver disease (nitrogen balance)	0.20–0.25	1.2–1.5
Acute (fulminant) liver failure	0.20–0.25	1.2–1.5
Post transplant	0.20–0.25	1.2–1.5

symptoms require a 40% stress factor. Nitrogen or protein requirements are shown in Table 7.4.24 (Plauth *et al.*, 2006).

Obesity

There is a lack of evidence regarding energy requirements in patients with liver disease who have a high BMI; however, the following may be used:

- For compensated liver disease, weight loss can be appropriate. Requirements for BMR are estimated using dry weight, omitting stress and activity factors.
- For decompensated liver disease, weight loss, even in those with a high BMI, should not be actively encouraged unless the patient can be closely monitored. Requirements for energy are calculated as described previously, adding stress and activity factors. Energy

intake may be reduced only under close monitoring of protein stores with anthropometry. It should be ensured that 0.5–1 kg/week weight loss is not exceeded and there is clarity between wet and dry weights.

Nitrogen and protein requirements should be adjusted according to BMI (Todorovic & Micklewright, 2011):

- BMI >30 kg/m^2 × 0.75.
- BMI >50 kg/m^2 × 0.65.

These recommendations are a guide for calculation of energy and nitrogen requirements for maintenance of nutritional status. The key element is the monitoring of nutritional status, i.e. weight (if not fluid overloaded),

SECTION 7

upper arm anthropometry and hand grip strength. On monitoring it may become necessary to increase protein requirements upwards in obese decompensated patients.

Requirements for repletion and weight gain

For weight gain it may be necessary to add 400–1000 kcal/day to previous totals with adequate anthropometric monitoring. Patients with liver disease require significantly higher protein intakes to maintain nitrogen balance. Most guidelines suggest an intake of 1.2–1.5 g of protein/day to achieve nitrogen balance and accrual of lean body mass (Plauth *et al.*, 2006). However, Nielsen *et al.* (1995) suggested that dietary protein retention remains efficient at intakes of up to 2 g/kg/day without adverse effects, including in encephalopathy. Kondrup & Muller (1997) suggested protein intakes of 1.5–2 g/kg may be required in patients with decompensated liver disease for nitrogen repletion. Where anthropometric monitoring and careful assessment indicate no improvement in nutritional status, these higher levels may be tried.

Economic and social assessment

Essential information regarding economic or social issues is critical to identify whether these are impacting on nutritional status or will prevent compliance with dietary advice. Finances can be significantly affected, as patients may be chronically unwell, resulting in reduced income and reliance on benefits. There may be cultural differences in the treatment of illness as this may need to take account of dietary beliefs.

Assessment in fulminant hepatic failure

This group of patients may not exhibit PEM to the same extent as those with chronic liver disease. However, it is still essential to assess the presence of fluid overload, jaundice and encephalopathy, which may contribute to a decline in nutritional status in the context of a hypermetabolic state. In patients who are awake and not encephalopathic, a full assessment can be performed as for chronic liver disease. In intensive care settings where patients are sedated, intubated and ventilated due to grade IV encephalopathy, assessment will be more difficult. Weight may need to be estimated or information may be required from relatives.

Clinical investigation and management

Non-alcoholic fatty liver disease

This is closely related to obesity and represents the hepatic manifestation of the metabolic syndrome. The prevalence of NAFLD has risen rapidly in parallel with rising levels of obesity and diabetes, and is now the commonest cause of liver disease in the West (de Alwis & Day, 2008). Though the natural histories of alcoholic liver disease and NAFLD differ, both may finally progress to end stage liver disease. Non-alcoholic fatty liver disease is a spectrum of fatty liver diseases in which there is a build up of fat in liver cells. These range from simple steatosis

Table 7.4.25 International Diabetes Federation waist circumference cut offs for central obesity (source: Alberti *et al.* 2007. Reproduced with permission of Blackwell Publishing)

Country/ethnic group		Waist circumference (as a measure of central obesity)
South Asian/Chinese/ South and Central American/Japanese	Male Female	>90 cm >80 cm
Europids	Male Female	>94 cm >80 cm

In the USA, adult treatment panel (ATP) III values are used for clinical purposes: male >102 cm; female >88 cm.
For ethnic South and Central Americans, use South Asian recommendations until further data are available.
For sub-Saharan Africans, use European data until more specific data are available.
For Eastern Mediterranean and Middle East (Arab) populations, use European data until more specific data are available.

(fatty liver) to non-alcoholic steatohepatitis (NASH). Non-alcoholic steatohepatitis is an inflammatory fibrosing disease, which can eventually lead to cirrhosis and end stage liver disease. The principal causes of NAFLD are genetic predisposition, lack of exercise and increase in calorie intake leading to overweight and obesity (Day, 2002).

Abdominal obesity increases the flux of free fatty acids to the liver. Excessive circulating fatty acids increase insulin resistance and in NAFLD there is no insulin mediated suppression of lipolysis. This increases the risk of NAFLD and is an important parameter to measure when carrying out an assessment (Table 7.4.25). It is estimated that 48–100% of people with NAFLD are asymptomatic. Many have no specific symptoms, such as fatigue and right upper quadrant pain, and NAFLD is often an incidental finding on abnormal LFTs, predominately ALT. Often the ratio of AST to ALT is >1, which differentiates NAFLD from alcohol related fatty liver disease (Day, 2002).

Factors that increase the likelihood of developing NAFLD include:

- Overweight, particularly central obesity.
- High cholesterol or triglyceride levels.
- Type 2 diabetes.
- Insulin resistance.
- Hypertension.

These are all features of the metabolic syndrome, defined as the presence of central obesity with at least two of the following (International Diabetes Federation, 2006):

- Hypertension of 130/85 mmHg or higher, or on treatment.
- Hypertriglyceridaemia – fasting triglyceride of >1.7 mmol/L or current use of fibrates.
- Low high density lipoprotein (HDL) cholesterol of <1.03 mmol/L (male) and <1.29 mmol/L (female).
- Glucose intolerance or known type 2 diabetes mellitus.

Consequently, the presence of NAFLD is also strongly associated with increased cardiovascular risk and its incidence is rising with the increasingly obese UK population. Therefore, it should always be considered important even if the liver is not at the more fibrotic end of the spectrum.

Management

Patients with NAFLD will require treatment of each aspect of the metabolic syndrome and prescription of appropriate medications. If blood cholesterol is high and patients are insulin resistant or hypertensive, dietary advice as well as medical treatment may be necessary.

Secondary non-alcohol fatty liver disease

It is possible for some conditions to lead to the same liver clinical picture as NAFLD; this is known as secondary NAFLD. Secondary NAFLD/NASH is rare in adults and is unrelated to insulin resistance or metabolic syndrome. Causes of secondary NAFLD/NASH include pregnancy related fatty liver disease and intestinal jejunoileal bypass surgery (Adams & Angulo, 2006).

Ascites

Ascites is the most common complication of cirrhosis, and approximately 60% of patients with compensated cirrhosis develop ascites within 10 years (Ginès & Schrier, 2009). The development of ascites in cirrhosis indicates a poor prognosis with mortality of approximately 40% at 1 year and 50% at 2 years (Guevara & Ginès, 2005). Patients with cirrhosis and ascites are at high risk for other liver disease complications, including refractory ascites, spontaneous bacterial peritonitis (SBP), hyponatraemia or hepatorenal syndrome (HRS) (Moore & Aithal, 2006). The absence of these ascites related complications qualify ascites as uncomplicated.

Ascites only occurs when portal hypertension has developed and is related to an inability to excrete an adequate amount of sodium into urine, leading to a positive sodium balance. Hypoalbuminaemia contributes by reducing vascular oncotic pressure, retaining fluid within the vessels and fluid leaks into the peritoneal space. Ascites can be very distressing and patients often suffer from early satiety, reflux and lack of mobility. In addition, paracentesis drains are highly protein losing and peripheral muscle wasting has the potential to be severe without adequate nutritional support. The European Association for the Study of the Liver (EASL, 2010) has graded ascites and given suggestions for treatment. Treating ascites can reduce abdominal pain and discomfort, and may improve appetite, reduce early satiety and allow an increase in food intake. The risk of spontaneous bacterial peritonitis is reduced with a reduction in the ascites and this also reduces stress on the respiratory system and the risk of pleural effusion.

Diuretic resistant ascites and diuretic intractable ascites are collectively known as refractory ascites. Once refractory ascites has developed, the median survival of patients is approximately 6 months and liver transplantation may be considered (Guevara & Ginès, 2005; Moreau *et al.*, 2004).

Management

Sodium restriction

See section on Nutritional management for detailed information.

Diuretics

Diuretics are prescribed when patients present with the first episode of grade 2 (moderate) ascites. Aldosterone antagonists are prescribed initially, and depending on response the dose is increased to a maximum of 400 mg. If there is poor response (<2 kg/week) or if patients develop hyperkalaemia, loop diuretics are added, e.g. furosemide (Angeli *et al.*, 2010).

Aldosterone antagonists such as spironolactone are potassium sparing and weak natrietics. If patients develop hyperkalaemia of >6 mmol/L in the absence of renal failure, this should resolve with the discontinuation of the drug and long term potassium restriction is unlikely to be necessary. Loop diuretics such as furosemide may be used in combination to aldosterone antagonists. These are powerful natrietics and are potassium loosing. The dose is 40 mg, increasing in 40-mg increments to 160 mg/day. If patients develop severe hypokalaemia (<3 mmol/L), loop diuretics need to be discontinued (Angeli *et al.*, 2010). The maximum recommended weight loss during diuretic therapy is 0.5 kg/day in patients without oedema and 1 kg/day in patients with oedema (EASL, 2010).

Fluid restriction

Fluid intake should be restricted only in patients with dilutional hyponatraemia where a serum sodium level of 120–125 mmol/L can occur (Moore & Aithal, 2006). Close liaison with the medical team is necessary regarding the level and length of restriction, which can be relaxed as serum sodium levels normalise. Nutritional support products and nutritious fluids should be prioritised within fluid restrictions if, as is common, the patients are malnourished and suffering from early satiety due to volume of ascites.

Paracentesis

Paracentesis is the therapeutic drainage of ascites from the abdomen using a transabdominal catheter. The volume of ascitic fluid removed may vary from 20 mL for diagnostic purposes to over 20 L to relieve abdominal distension. Large volume paracentesis (LVP) is the first line therapy in patients with large ascites (grade 3 ascites). It is performed together with the administration of albumin (8 g/L of ascitic fluid removed) (Ginès *et al.*, 1996). This is required to maintain circulating blood volume, prevent rapid shifts of body fluid and subsequent hypovolaemic shock, and to prevent circulatory dysfunction after LVP. Serial paracentesis may be the only means of treating refractory ascites. These patients are at risk of high protein losses from repeated drainage of protein rich ascitic fluid. Therefore, dietary intake must include

SECTION 7

sufficient protein to compensate; up to 2.0 g/kg of dry weight can be tolerated with close monitoring and anthropometry (Nielsen *et al.*, 1995).

Transjugular intrahepatic portosystemic shunts

Transjugular intrahepatic portosystemic shunts (TIPS) decompress the portal system with a shunt inserted between the high pressure portal venous area and the low pressure hepatic venous area. This reduces portal pressure and is effective in the control of recurrent ascites. It also beneficially affects renal function and may have beneficial effects on nitrogen balance and body weight (Plauth *et al.*, 2004). A major complication after TIPS insertion is the development of hepatic encephalopathy, which occurs in 30–50% of patients undergoing the procedure (Riggio *et al.*, 2008).

Encephalopathy

Hepatic encephalopathy has been explained as a reversible impairment of cognitive function or altered level of consciousness (Voight & Conn, 1995). The severity of encephalopathy is commonly quantified using the West Haven criteria (Ferenci *et al.*, 2002) (Table 7.4.26). Encephalopathy is usually an acute presentation in a cirrhotic, decompensated patient or a patient with acute liver injury. The common causes of acute encephalopathy are illustrated in Box 7.4.3. The management of encephalopathy secondary to both acute and chronic liver failure involves the treatment and prevention of its precipitants.

Sepsis

Patients with chronic liver disease are more susceptible to infections including spontaneous bacterial peritonitis. Good infection control management, full septic screen when an infection is suspected and the use of antibiotics, if appropriate, is necessary. Preserving the integrity of the gut wall to reduce the risk of bacterial translocation could also help reduce sepsis and can be achieved with small frequent meals or enteral nutrition in cognitively impaired patients (MacFie, 2004).

Constipation

Current treatment of encephalopathy assumes that colonic bacteria produce ammonia and constipation must be avoided in patients with encephalopathy. Patients are prescribed laxatives so they pass two to four soft stools daily. Lactulose is commonly prescribed and has a prebiotic effect in addition to the osmotic laxative effect it exerts.

Poor nutritional intake

Endogenous waste from protein catabolism can precipitate encephalopathy; therefore, periods of fasting should be avoided and aggressive nutritional support is necessary to meet calculated nutritional requirements in this group of patients. Providing adequate protein in malnourished patients with end stage liver disease can improve mental status and preserve lean body mass (Bemeur *et al.*, 2010). Aggressive nutritional support is necessary and is discussed in more detail in the section on Nutritional management.

Wernicke's encephalopathy

The Wernicke–Korsakoff syndrome develops in thiamine deficient people. Thiamine is an essential cofactor in the metabolism of carbohydrate and alcohol. People with excessive or hazardous drinking habits are at high risk of developing Wernicke's encephalopathy. It comprises of a combination of global confusion, eye signs and ataxia. Uncommonly, the patient is drowsy or in a state of stupor, but may also be disorientated, apathetic or have impaired memory. These clinical abnormalities may develop acutely or evolve over several days. It is reversible with thiamine administration.

Korsakoff's psychosis is an amnesic state in which there is profound impairment of memory but relative preservation of other intellectual abilities; confabulation may be a feature. Korsakoff's psychosis generally develops after an acute episode of Wernicke's encephalopathy and is irreversible (NICE, 2010a).

As thiamine requirements are linked to carbohydrate intake, it is very important that intravenous dextrose and excessive carbohydrate from food or enteral nutrition is not given to a thiamine deficient patient without thiamine being administered. In patients who present intoxicated, unconscious or confused, especially those with known

---

Table 7.4.26 West Haven criteria for grading encephalopathy (source: Lockwood *et al.* 2002. Reproduced with permission of Wiley-Blackwell Publishing)

Grade	
1	Trivial lack of awareness; euphoria or anxiety; shortened attention span; impaired performance of addition or subtraction
2	Lethargy or apathy; minimal disorientation for time or place; subtle personality change; inappropriate behavior
3	Somnolence to semi stupor, but responsive to verbal stimuli; confusion; gross disorientation
4	Coma (unresponsive to verbal or noxious stimuli)

Box 7.4.3 Common causes of acute encephalopathy

- Portosystemic shunting – 30–50% incidence post shunting
- Sepsis/infections (including bacterial peritonitis)
- Constipation
- Dehydration caused by vomiting and/or diarrhoea/poor nutritional intake
- Uraemia/azotaemia, e.g. diuretic induced
- Gastrointestinal bleeding/variceal bleeding
- Electrolyte disturbances
- Acid–base disturbances
- Drugs (sedatives, alcohol)

Table **7.4.27** Percentage risk of hepatocellular carcinoma (HCC) development related to cause of cirrhosis (Ryder, 2003)

Cause of cirrhosis	Gender	Percentage risk per year of development of HCC
Hepatitis B	Males and females	3–12
Hepatitis C	Males and Females	3–5
Genetic haemochromatosis	Males and Females	7–9
Alcoholic liver disease	Males	1–4

cirrhosis or alcohol histories, Wernicke's encephalopathy should always be considered a potential diagnosis and treated accordingly. Initially, parenteral thiamine may be required on admission, followed by oral preparations of at least 100 mg/day as per refeeding guidelines and up to 300 mg/day (NICE, 2006).

Hepatocellular carcinoma

Hepatocellular carcinoma (HCC) was previously thought to be a relatively rare cancer but it is becoming increasingly more prominent in the UK with the hepatitis C epidemic. It occurs more frequently in Asia due to the high incidence of hepatitis B, but it is usually detected earlier due to HCC screening programmes in the hepatitis B population. The percentage risk of HCC development related to cirrhosis is shown in Table 7.4.27. The average age in the UK at which HCC develops is 66 years. Treatments offered depend on the size and stage of the tumour (Ryder, 2003).

Management

Surgery

The only proven curative therapies are surgical, either hepatic resection or liver transplantation, and criteria for referral exist (Ryder, 2003). Many patients have established cirrhosis and therefore surgery is often carried out in specialist centres as patients can be at risk of liver decompensation after surgery. Non-surgical treatments are used when surgery is considered inappropriate.

Percutaneous alcohol injections

Alcohol is injected into the tumour to cause tumour necrosis.

Chemoembolisation

Concentrated chemotherapy drugs are delivered via a catheter direct to the tumour site. This avoids any dilutional effect that may occur during standard administration of chemotherapy.

Chemotherapy

Standard chemotherapy regimens show poor response, so they usually only offered in the context of trials.

Radiofrequency ablation

Radiofrequency ablation is a procedure where the hepatocellular tumour is ablated using the heat generated from the high frequency alternating electrical current. A general anaesthetic is not always necessary and therefore it may be performed in day care.

Liver transplantation

There are seven liver transplant centres in the UK and Ireland. The UK has approximately 6000 surviving liver transplant recipients and annually about 600 people with liver disease receive a liver transplant. The post transplant population is growing. Nearly 550 of those 600 patients survive for 1 year after transplant and at least 50% live 20 years. Patients meeting transplant criteria should be offered a transplant only if it is felt they have a >50% probability of survival at 5 years after transplantation with a quality of life that is acceptable to the patient (Neuberger et al., 2008).

Nutritional management

When taking into account the incidence and consequence of PEM and specific micronutrient deficiencies, meeting the patients calculated requirements is pivotal to their management. Close liaison with the multidisciplinary team (MDT) is vital in order to prevent unnecessary dietary restrictions.

Oral nutrition

The pattern of food intake can influence energy balance in liver cirrhosis. Verboeket-van de Venne et al., (1995) showed that after a short term fast of 9 hours, fat is used as an alternative fuel to glucose, which cannot be produced in sufficient quantities due to the depleted glycogen stores in the liver. By giving four to six meals/day, oxidation of carbohydrate was significantly lower than carbohydrate intake, which resulted in a positive balance of carbohydrate. This pattern may also help patients with early satiety caused by reduced volume as ascites increases. Interestingly, Le Cornu et al. (2000) found that nutritional counselling may produce similar outcomes when compared with oral nutritional supplements (ONS) and therefore these simple changes can be very effective.

Owen et al. (1983) established that after an overnight fast, patients with cirrhosis show increased rates of fat oxidation and gluconeogenesis. Whilst glucose oxidation and glycogenolysis are reduced compared with healthy controls, Swart et al. (1989) found that a late evening snack improved nitrogen balance, with Plank et al. (2008) showing that there is an improvement in nutritional status as a result. The late evening snack, which reduces fasting periods overnight, should include 50 g of carbohydrate, and examples of suitable snacks are shown in Box 7.4.4. Thought should be given to inpatient snacks and meal times in order to allow the provision of at least a 50-g carbohydrate snack or supplement in the evening. Tsien et al. (2012) critically reviewed the evidence for provision of a late evening snack, concluding that there

SECTION 7

Box 7.4.4 Examples of 50g carbohydrate snacks

- Two crumpets with 200 mL of milk
- One to one and a half milk based 1.5 kcal/mL supplement (dependent on composition)
- One juice based 1.5 kcal/mL supplement (dependent on composition)
- Two and a half thick slices of bread
- Breakfast cereal (30 g) with milk
- One slice of fruit cake
- Scone with jam and 300 mL of milk
- Five dried dates and 200 mL of milk
- Small square of flapjack and 300 mL of milk

---

is insufficient evidence to recommend a branch chain amino acid (BCAA) enriched supplement in preference to a high carbohydrate supplement. Further randomised adequately powered trials are required that also investigate effect on clinical outcome.

Patients who are unable to meet their nutritional requirements from a normal diet will require ONS (see Chapter 6.3). Standard polymeric supplements can be used according to patient preference and should be prescribed to make up the energy and protein deficit. The use of sip feeds that contain 20g of protein per bottle can be especially useful when trying to meet nutritional requirements. This group of patients may need to use sip feeds long term and therefore it is vital that time is spent establishing flavour and product preferences in order to aid compliance. Fluid restrictions create increased difficulty when trying to meet requirements and close liaison with the MDT is vital (see Ascites section on fluid restrictions). Plauth *et al.* (2006) supported the use of ONS, which can improve nutritional status and survival in severely malnourished patients with alcoholic hepatitis. Close monitoring is essential, both of oral intakes and tolerance as patients can vary quickly from one day to another.

Enteral nutrition

If patients are unable to tolerate an oral diet or fail to achieve adequate requirements orally, a nasogastric (NG) tube should be inserted (see Chapter 6.4). There should be a low threshold for initiation of enteral feeding as patients deteriorate quickly, with the priority being to meet nutritional requirements consistently. Historically, there has been a reluctance to pass NG tubes when varices are present; however, this is not supported by evidence (Plauth *et al.*, 2006). Cabré *et al.* (1990) demonstrated that albumin levels and Child–Pugh scores were improved with enteral nutrition in severely malnourished patients with cirrhosis. In patients with alcoholic liver disease, aggressive enteral nutrition decreased bilirubin levels and improved hepatic encephalopathy (Kearns *et al.*, 1992). Overnight NG feeding decreases the fasting period and helps achieve nutritional requirements in those who are

taking an oral diet and supplements but still not achieving estimated requirements or have deteriorating anthropometric measurements.

For those who are encephalopathic, 24-hour NG feeding should be encouraged in order to avoid protein boluses and minimise fasting periods so as to utilise the nutrition most effectively. Placement of NG tubes can be difficult as increasing confusion leads to tubes becoming dislodged, resulting in suboptimal nutritional intake. The MDT is essential in order to discuss local management of these patients, which may require increased nursing care, secure taping of the tube, fixation devices or even restraints.

A high energy density feed (at least 1.5 kcal/mL) should be used to achieve estimated requirements within smaller volumes for those who have delayed gastric emptying, complain of bloating or require fluid restrictions. Most feeds contain <100 mmol of sodium when meeting requirements and therefore specific low sodium feeds are usually not required. These can also have a low protein to energy ratio that prevents protein requirements from being met. The rate of feed should be built up according to local policy on enteral feeding and within refeeding syndrome guidelines if necessary.

Nasojejunal feeding

There are few specific guidelines regarding the use of nasojejunal (NJ) feeding tubes in liver disease. Wicks *et al.* (1994) identified that in post liver transplant patients NJ feeding was as successful in maintaining nutritional status as parenteral nutrition. In practice, NJ tubes may be used for patients who have poor absorption, indicated by high aspirates, nausea and vomiting, or early satiety caused by ascites and chronic malnutrition. Continuous infusion of enteral feed into the small bowel has the added benefit of avoiding fasting times and therefore optimising carbohydrate oxidation and improvements in nitrogen balance.

Gastrostomy and jejunostomy feeding

The placement of percutaneous endoscopic gastrostomy (PEG) tubes is associated with a higher risk of complications due to ascites or varices, and is contraindicated according to Plauth *et al.* (2006). However, Ponsky *et al.* (1989), cited in Loser *et al.* (2005), suggested that the presence of mild to moderate ascites is not a contraindication for PEG placement due to the absence of increased complications, although altered coagulopathy [international normalised ratio (INR) >1.5] would be an absolute contraindication.

Jejunostomy tubes have been used historically for post liver transplant patients and were placed during surgery. Their use has declined significantly as patients can be adequately fed with NG or NJ tubes. Elective placement of jejunostomy tubes in post transplant patients may be for prolonged feeding with gastric aspirate or vomiting issues.

Parenteral nutrition

Parenteral nutrition (PN) should be reserved for patients for whom there is no enteral feeding route available (Plauth *et al.*, 1997) (see Chapter 6.5). This form of nutritional support is more expensive, and associated with a higher incidence of infections and electrolyte imbalance when compared with enteral nutrition (Sanchez & Aranda-Michel, 2006). Hepatic abnormalities, e.g. hepatic steatosis, intrahepatic cholestasis or elevated liver function tests, can occur in up to 75% of adults receiving PN (Guglielmi *et al.*, 2006). Other causes must be identified first, e.g. sepsis when patients develop a deterioration in their LFTs. Usually only monitoring, or a small reduction in the energy content of the feed (to 25 kcal/kg when including nitrogen energy or to 20 kcal/kg from non-nitrogen sources) is required (Kumpf, 2006).

Guidelines from the ESPEN (Plauth *et al.*, 2009) have further clarified the use of PN in liver disease when clinically indicated. In alcoholic hepatitis and liver cirrhosis intravenous glucose (2–3<t#g/kg/day) should be given when fasting for >12 hours, with thiamine prescribed prior to starting. Parenteral nutrition should be started immediately in moderate to severely malnourished patients, and where fasting will occur for 72 hours or more, water soluble vitamins and trace elements should be included. Energy and protein requirements should be calculated as described in the Enteral assessment section. Monitoring is essential for blood glucose and electrolytes for refeeding syndrome. Plauth *et al.* (2009) also suggested that PN should be started in acute liver failure where patients are unlikely to eat or receive enteral nutrition for 5–7 days. Intravenous glucose should be given (2–3 g/kg/day) to maintain glucose levels or in the case of hyperglycaemia, adequate insulin regimens to maintain normoglycaemia should be prescribed. Blood glucose monitoring continues to be essential, as well as blood ammonia levels in order to adjust PN amino acid content.

For those with ascites or oedema, fluid restriction may be required. These patients would normally also be sodium restricted to 80–100 mmol/L/day.

Studies suggest that the provision of a small amount of enteral nutrition may minimise complications such as sepsis. This may be due to decreasing the risk of bacterial translocation by preventing alterations to the structure and function of the gut (Guglielmi *et al.*, 2006). In long term PN, liver function may be aided by the use of structure lipids, n-3 fatty acids or cyclical feeding (Rubin *et al.*, 2000).

Alcoholic hepatitis

Conventional therapy is based largely on abstinence from alcohol as well as general supportive and symptomatic care. Patients with alcohol related liver disease are often malnourished and this has a detrimental effect on survival. The Veterans Affairs Cooperative study (Mendenhall *et al.*, 1991) found the prevalence of PEM to be 100% in patients with alcoholic hepatitis, the severity of which correlated with the degree of liver dysfunction. Protein energy malnutrition correlated with short and long term mortality, clinical severity of liver disease and biochemical hepatic dysfunction.

A randomised trial by Cabré *et al.* (2000) investigated both the short and long term effects of steroids (prednisolone 40 g/day) or total enteral nutrition (2000 kcal/day) in patients with alcoholic hepatitis. During the 28-day treatment phase, mortality was similar between the groups, but occurred earlier in the total enteral nutrition (TEN) group (median day 7 versus median day 23). Mortality during the 1-year follow-up period was significantly higher in the steroid group and occurred in the immediate weeks after the treatment phase, mainly due to infections. The trial concluded that TEN is no worse than steroid treatment in the short term management of alcoholic hepatitis.

Patients fed after a period of reduced nutritional intake and heavy alcohol use are at risk of developing refeeding syndrome. It is important to ensure vitamin B Co strong and a treatment dose of thiamine are prescribed or intravenous Pabrinex preparation given prior to commencing enteral feeding. The management of refeeding syndrome is discussed further in Chapter 6.4.

Nutritional assessment and goals

All patients with alcoholic hepatitis should be assessed for PEM, as well as vitamin and mineral deficiencies. Those with severe disease should be treated aggressively with enteral nutritional therapy (O'Shea *et al.*, 2010). An energy intake of 35–40 kcal/kg of dry body weight/day and protein intake of 1.2–1.5 g/kg of body weight are recommended (Plauth *et al.*, 2006). Some researchers suggest a higher energy intake of 45 kcal/kg may be necessary (McCullough & O'Connor, 1998), but the key to adequate nutritional support is close monitoring.

Steroid use

Corticosteroids have been studied intensively in alcoholic hepatitis. They are used as anti-inflammatory agents but are associated with side effects, including poor wound healing and susceptibility to infection (Rambaldi *et al.*, 2008). The National Institute for Health and Care Excellence (2010a) recommends the use of steroids in severe alcoholic hepatitis with a Maddrey's discriminant function of 32 or more. Patients should be concurrently prescribed calcium and vitamin D supplements as bone protection with blood glucose monitoring and treatment if elevated.

Fulminant hepatic failure

Stabilisation of metabolic disturbances is essential as alkalosis and acidosis can both occur (Polson & Lee, 2005). Hepatic encephalopathy symptoms may hide those of hypoglycaemia; therefore, continuous glucose infusions and monitoring is critical. Nutritional support is vital with NG or NJ feeding following local guidelines. Current practice in UK specialist liver centres favours high energy, high protein feeds to meet requirements in this highly catabolic group.

Wilson's disease

Initial medical therapy is with chelating agents, e.g. D penacillamine and trientine. Zinc may also be used alone or in combination with a chelating agent. Foods high in copper, including chocolate, liver, nuts, mushrooms and shellfish, are best avoided, especially in the first year of treatment (Roberts & Schilsky, 2008).

Liver transplant nutrition

Initially following a liver transplant, patients are often enterally fed. Long term management involves food safety advice, weight maintenance and lifestyle advice. Some immunosuppression medication can cause hyperkalaemia, but this is often transient and short term low potassium diets may be indicated. If required, further advice can be obtained from specialist transplant centres.

Haemochromatosis

Haemochromatosis cannot be treated with a low iron diet. It is managed by reducing the systemic iron overload through therapeutic phlebotomy to achieve a serum ferritin of <50 μg/L. Patients however are often reluctant to eat foods rich in iron as they feel anxious regarding absorbing iron. Simple advice can be:

- Avoid vitamin and mineral supplements containing iron and vitamin C (ascorbic acid) as vitamin C aids iron absorption.
- Avoid drinking fresh fruit juice with meals due to their high vitamin C content.
- Limit intake of red meat to 70 g cooked weight/day (Scientific Advisory Committee on Nutrition, 2010).
- Do not avoid fruit and vegetables, including green leafy iron rich ones, as phytates and oxalates reduce iron bioavailability.
- Alcohol can accelerate disease progression; therefore, reduced alcohol intake is recommended.
- Calcium and tannins inhibit iron absorption so drinking dairy products and tea with meals may inhibit dietary iron absorption.

Non-alcoholic fatty liver disease

Obesity

Weight reduction improves all risk factors associated with the metabolic syndrome and further reduces the risk for type 2 diabetes (Targher et al., 2007). A reduction of 10% from baseline weight over 6–12 months has been shown to correct aminotransferase levels and decrease hepatomegaly. However, too rapid weight loss can cause worsening steatohepatitis and increase the risk of gall stone disease. Crash diets where weight loss exceeds 1.5 kg/week should be discouraged. Monitoring LFTs may be necessary if patients lose weight rapidly as this may precipitate deterioration in liver function (Day, 2006).

Dietary changes alone are associated with high failure rate at achieving and maintaining weight loss for multifactorial reasons. Dietary intervention should include behaviour modification therapy, cognitive behavioural therapy and the use of support groups. Consensus is lacking as to what diet or lifestyle approach is best for NAFLD and NASH patients, primarily due to insufficient evidence (Zivkovic et al., 2007). Obesity and further strategies for its management are discussed in Chapter 7.13.2.

Non-cirrhotic patients

It is important to assess the stage of liver disease as the advice for a cirrhotic NAFLD (NASH) patient differs from a patient with a fatty liver or fibrosis. At initial assessment, the stage of liver disease, weight, BMI and waist circumference should be obtained and clear goals for weight loss discussed with the patient, with advice to avoid crash dieting or excessive weight loss. Exercise should be encouraged as this improves insulin sensitivity independently of change in weight. (Duncan et al., 2003) Basic principles of weight loss in NAFLD pre cirrhosis are to:

- Aim for a BMI below 25 kg/m².
- Aim for a reduction of 10% from baseline weight over 6–12 months.
- Calorie restriction to achieve a 0.5–1 kg (1–2 lb)/week weight loss.
- Avoid weight loss that exceeds 1.5 kg/week.
- Encourage exercise for 30 minutes/day minimum.
- Encourage weight maintenance through long term lifestyle changes.
- Give food group advice as illustrated in the eatwell plate (see Figure 4.2.2):
  ○ Aim for five portions of fruit and vegetables/day.
  ○ Eat low glycaemic index foods.
  ○ Avoid refined sugars and saturated fats.

Diets high in soluble and insoluble fibre have been shown to improve insulin resistance, and low glycaemic index diets have proved beneficial (Harrison et al., 2002). Excessive carbohydrate intakes should be avoided. In addition, each aspect of the metabolic syndrome should be addressed individually and treated with appropriate medical and dietary therapy as appropriate. Alcohol should be discussed with the patient's doctor.

Hyperlipidaemia

Dyslipidaemia is present in 20–80% of patients with NAFLD. Improvement in lipidaemia also helps in the prevention of coronary heart disease. Diets should be low in saturated and *trans* fat, with proportionally more unsaturated fat. Total fat intake should be advised to be below 35% of daily intake with 15–20% made up of monounsaturates and minimal *trans* fats. n-3 Fatty acids have antiarrhythmic and anti-inflammatory effect and reduce triglycerides. An intake of 450 mg/day (equivalent to the recommended two portions of oily fish/week) is recommended. Fibrates should be used if indicated (Day, 2002).

Hypertension

Hypertension should be treated with antihypertensives as necessary for tight blood pressure control of

<140/80 mmHg, especially in those with impaired fasting glucose or type 2 diabetes mellitus. Management of hypertension is similar to that in other patients: restriction of sodium to a no added salt diet, which is 80–100 mmol of sodium (4.6–5.75 g salt)/day (American Gastroenterological Association, 2002).

Diabetes mellitus or impaired fasting glucose

Type 2 diabetes mellitus is common in patients with NAFLD as it is an element of the metabolic syndrome. Tight glycaemic control is necessary and is achieved by maximising use of oral hypoglycaemic agents or insulin.

Cirrhotic patients

In cirrhosis, despite the appearance of obesity, some patients with advanced liver disease will have PEM, and therefore require a full dietary assessment for evidence of protein malnutrition. Dietary restriction in patients with elevated nutritional requirements risks worsening PEM, and should only be contemplated under careful supervision with regular anthropometric measurement. Calculating nutritional requirements in the obese patient is discussed in the Nutritional assessment section. Protein energy malnutrition is associated with reduced transplant graft and patient survival (Stickel *et al.*, 2008). Weight loss should not be recommended in cirrhotic patients with end stage liver disease due to the risk of PEM. For patients with stable compensated cirrhosis and HCC, it may be appropriate to try and achieve weight loss before proceeding to or whilst waiting for a liver transplant (British Transplant Society, 2011).

Hepatitis C

Hepatitis C affects people differently and can affect appetite, especially if patients have cirrhosis. However, many people have no symptoms at all. If patients are well there is no evidence for any sort of therapeutic diet, vitamin supplements or herbal preparations. Patients should be encouraged to eat a healthy well balanced diet, such as those promoted by the eatwell plate (see Chapter 4.2) and maintain a BMI within a health range.

A rising incidence of NAFLD with increasing obesity and in combination with hepatitis C are intrinsically linked to poorer outcomes in liver disease (EASL, 2011). Weight maintenance is important for many reasons. There is growing evidence that obesity and insulin resistance can accelerate hepatitis C progression and increase the risk of HCC in chronic hepatitis C (Okuda *et al.*, 2002, Lonardo *et al.*, 2004, EASL, 2011). Obesity can also reduce the effectiveness of antiviral treatments, so patients with a BMI of >30 kg/m² should be advised to try to lose weight prior to starting antiviral treatment as this may help the antiviral response (Bressler *et al.*, 2003).

Patients on antiviral treatments

Antiviral treatments are usually prescribed for 6- or 12-month periods with the aim of eradicating the virus. Side effects include poor appetite and weight loss, nausea and vomiting, sore mouth and throat, metallic taste, lethargy and depression.

If patients unintentionally lose >10% of their body weight, it becomes clinically significant and malnutrition risk is heightened (Heymsfield & Matthews, 1994). As first line advice, food fortification advice is appropriate. If weight loss persists, oral nutritional supplements can be prescribed under the ACBS indication for disease related malnutrition and reviewed on a monthly basis. Occasionally, chaotic lifestyles make the use of such products difficult and staggered prescribing may be necessary.

Alcohol

Regular alcohol consumption in hepatitis C leads to accelerated fibrosis progression and possibly reduced response to antiviral therapy. Therefore, intake should be limited, especially if antiviral treatment is to commence (Anand *et al.*, 2006). Alcohol advice depends on the patient and their clinical state and previous alcohol history; medical staff should direct the decision regarding alcohol intakes. If patients are drinking alcohol to excess (hazardous or dependent drinking), thiamine and vitamin B Co strong should be prescribed to reduce the risk of clinically significant complications of B vitamin deficiency, such as neuropathy and Wernicke's encephalopathy (NICE, 2010a).

Telaprevir

Telaprevir (VX-950), marketed under the brand name Incivek, is a pharmaceutical drug for the treatment of hepatitis C. Patients are usually prescribed this for a 12-week period, three times per day. Telaprevir is ineffective if taken on an empty stomach and patients must consume at least 20 g of fat with each dose (Revill *et al.*, 2007). This can be in any form, in standard meals or fatty foods as per patient preference. In theory, the increase in energy from this advice could cause weight gain. However, in reality, patients may have a poor appetite as a side effect of antiviral treatment and, if appropriate, fat supplements such as Calogen (Nutricia) or Fresubin 5cal shot (Fresenius) can be prescribed to be taken at the same as Telaprevir.

Ascites and oedema

The diagnosis and classification has been covered in the section on Clinical investigation and management. By the time patients have developed ascites they have advanced cirrhosis and appetites are so poor nutritional support is often necessary. The volume of abdominal fluid that can build up in ascites can severely limit dietary intake due to feelings of satiety, reflux and constipation, and reduced mobility and ability to shop, cook and prepare meals. As with any dietary modification in liver disease, the priority is to meet nutritional requirements as PEM is common by this stage of liver disease. It is important that nutritional requirements are met whilst keeping sodium intake within the recommended level for the patient's current condition.

Salt reducing advice should be given to patients with Grade 2 (moderate) ascites or above. Salt should be restricted to 4.6–6.9 g (80–120 mmol)/day (EASL, 2010).

SECTION 7

Traditionally, a no added salt diet is advised, which is 80–100 mmol of sodium (4.6–5.75 g salt)/day. The recommendation for the general population is 6 g/day (Cappuccio *et al.*, 2011).

Refractory ascites

Salt should be restricted to 5.2 g/day, which corresponds to 90 mmol/day of sodium. There is no evidence to support the prophylactic use of salt restriction in cirrhotic patients who have never had ascites, nor is bed rest advocated as a treatment of ascites (EASL, 2010). Sodium intakes vary enormously between patients and each patient should be assessed individually. Very often, reducing a few key foods can have a profound impact on daily net sodium intake while maintaining a regular intake. Simple no added salt advice includes the following points:

- No added salt to meals.
- Avoid salty snacks such as crisps (20 mmol of sodium) and soups.
- Encourage high energy high protein snacks with a 50-g carbohydrate rich snack in the evening.

However, if this advice needs to be expanded, assess current dietary intake and reduce the following as required:

- No salt added at the table.
- Only a pinch in cooking.
- Avoid salt substitutes.
- Up to 100 g of cheese/week.
- Up to four slices bread/day.
- Reduce processed foods:
  - Bacon, ham, sausages, paté.
  - Smoked fish and meat tinned in brine.
  - Fish and meat pastes.
  - Tinned and packet soup.
  - Auce mixes, stock cubes, soya sauce, mono sodium glutamate.
  - Tinned vegetables.
  - Bottled sauces and chutneys.
  - Meat and vegetable extracts.
  - Salted nuts and crisps.

Patients can find it helpful to be able to calculate how much salt is in their diet and the following guidance can be helpful. Advise patients to look at food labels and check to see how much salt three is per 100 g. If there is only a figure for sodium on the label, patients should be advised to multiply this by 2.5 to obtain the salt content. Patients can calculate whether food is high, medium or low in salt using the figures:

- High salt – >1.5 g/100 g (0.6 g of sodium).
- Medium salt – 0.3–1.5 g/100 g portion (0.6–1 g of sodium).
- Low salt – 0.3 g/100 g (0.1 g of sodium).

Nutritional support

Most milk type nutritional supplements contain 8–10 mmol of sodium, while juice based supplements have very small amounts. However, milk type sip feeds have considerably higher protein than juice based sip feeds and are often the supplements of choice, especially if patients are undergoing therapeutic paracentesis when protein losses per drain can exceed 90 g of protein.

If artificial enteral feeding is necessary, most standard enteral feeds (1 kcal/mL) are suitable as they contain <40 mmol of sodium/L. High energy and protein feeds are often prescribed (1.5–2 kcal/mL) as they provide more energy and protein in smaller volumes. Tolerance to larger volumes due to early satiety and bloating may be difficult and fluid restrictions need to be considered. Overnight NG feeding allows the patients to be disconnected from the feeding pump during the day and encourages the maintenance of oral intake during the day. Sip feeds, if prescribed in addition to the NG feed, can be flushed down the tube rather than drunk if the patient is struggling to consume them orally.

Hepatic encephalopathy

Protein energy malnutrition is a risk factor for hepatic encephalopathy and low protein diets are not recommended. There is a paucity of evidence that they contribute to any improvement in encephalopathy and may cause harm due to worsening nutritional status (Cordoba *et al.*, 2004; Plauth *et al.*, 2006). Adequate nutrition *per se* counteracts hepatic encephalopathy and should be provided by the enteral route if at all possible.

Nutritional energy and protein requirements should be calculated as discussed in the Nutritional assessment section. Periods of fasting should be minimised as endogenous waste from protein catabolism can precipitate encephalopathy. If patients are eating and drinking, a frequent meal pattern of four to six small meals and snacks should be recommended. Late evening 50-g carbohydrate snacks are crucial as these reduce protein catabolism during overnight fasting and promote a positive nitrogen balance (Tsuchiya *et al.*, 2005; Yamanaka-Okumura *et al.*, 2006).

If enteral feeding is indicated, overnight feeding helps break the overnight fast and maintain a positive nitrogen balance (Owen *et al.*, 1983; Zillikens *et al.*, 1993). If enteral nutrition is the sole source of nutrition, 24-hour enteral feeding may be required to avoid the fasting period until the encephalopathic episode resolves, and then reviewed.

Lactulose is a non-absorbable disaccharide used as a laxative as it inhibits ammonia producing bacteria in the gut wall and acts as an osmotic laxative. The antibiotics rifaximin, neomycin and metronidazole may also be prescribed, and fluid electrolyte imbalances corrected.

Branched chain amino acids

Supplementation with branched chain amino acids (BCAAs) remains under investigation both as a nutritional supplement and as a means to treat hepatic encephalopathy. The BCAAs, especially leucine, appear to have an important anabolic role in protein synthesis and there is an increased requirement for BCAAs with metabolic stress or injury. Studies have shown that BCAAs increase muscle mass and performance (Laviano *et al.*, 2005) and it has been reported that supplementation with oral BCAAs improved energy metabolism in cirrhotic patients (Tsuchiya *et al.*, 2005; Als-Nielsen *et al.*, 2003). They also compete with the serotonin precursor tryptophan for the same amino acid transporter at the blood–brain barrier. Hence, it has been suggested that BCAA supplementation may reduce the brain uptake of tryptophan. Studies have shown levels of BCAAs to be depleted in advanced liver disease and malnutrition (Blonde-Cynober *et al.*, 1999).

The aromatic amino acids (AAAs) are tyrosine, tryptophan and phenylalanine. There is usually homeostasis in the concentration of BCAAs and AAAs. However, amino acid metabolism is altered in liver disease and there is a reduced ratio of BCAAs to AAAs. The increase in AAAs is related to the reduced capacity of the liver to remove them. The proposed cause for hepatic encephalopathy is enhanced passage of AAAs through the blood–brain barrier, resulting in the creation of false neurotransmitters, e.g. octopamine, which cause hepatic encephalopathy symptoms (Dejong *et al.*, 2007). It has been suggested that BCAA supplementation will improve hepatic encephalopathy by improving the ratio of BCAAs to AAAs.

The effect of BCAAs in liver disease has been studied for many years with inconsistent results. A Cochrane review described 11 randomised controlled trials and found that there was no convincing evidence that BCAAs had a significant benefit to patients with hepatic encephalopathy (Als-Nielsen *et al.*, 2003). However, more recently, two large randomised controlled trials (Marchesini *et al.*, 2003; Muto *et al.*, 2005) have shown positive results. Muto *et al.* (2005) concluded that with adequate energy and protein intake long term supplementation with BCAAs in decompensated liver cirrhosis improved event free survival, serum albumin and quality of life.

In 2006, the ESPEN (Plauth *et al.*, 2006) reviewed the additional evidence from the above trials and gave the following recommendations:

- Use BCAA enriched formulae in patients with hepatic encephalopathy arising during enteral nutrition.
- Oral BCAAs can improve clinical outcome in advanced cirrhosis.
- Ensuring an adequate nutrient intake should be the primary goal.
- Long term (12 and 24 months) nutritional supplementation with oral BCAA granules. Oral nutrient supplements are useful in slowing the progression of hepatic failure and prolonging event free survival.

The advised length of treatment varies from 12 to 24 months in most studies and to adopt this into clinical practice, compliance due to palatability is likely to be problematic. Benefits are unlikely to be seen in the inpatient population due to the length of time needed to see effects. Patient selection for the use of BCAAs needs to be carefully evaluated regarding their condition and likely prognosis with advanced cirrhosis.

There is no consensus on the recommended dose of BCAAs to date, although there is a recommendation to take them at night as BCAAs are used as energy during the day but are used for protein synthesis at night (Fukushima *et al.*, 2003). In the UK, BCAAs have not been adopted in the UK liver transplant specialist centres, nor is a palatable product as yet available. However, this is a developing area and specialist centres should be contacted for advice regarding any UK developments.

Probiotics

Probiotics have been studied as a treatment for hepatic encephalopathy given the theory of altered ammonia production causing confusion. However, following a Cochrane review (McGee *et al.*, 2011), the use of probiotics cannot be recommended for patients with hepatic encephalopathy, with further randomised trials needed.

Wernicke's encephalopathy

See the section on Clinical investigation and management.

Diabetes

Conditions in which diabetes mellitus and glucose intolerance are most commonly seen are NAFLD, cirrhosis, acute viral hepatitis, steatohepatitis, chronic autoimmune hepatitis and acute liver injury. Steroid induced diabetes is often seen as steroids are commonly used in some liver diseases and for post transplant rejection.

Maintaining tight blood glucose control and optimising insulin and/or oral hypoglycaemic therapies is of vital importance in liver disease. In non-cirrhotic patients with conditions such as NAFLD, poor glycaemic control is associated with increased cardiovascular risk and increased infection, rates and can predispose to malnutrition in cirrhosis (Musso *et al.*, 2003). Diabetes is associated with mobilisation of adipose tissue, fatty acids and increased protein catabolism, which plays a role in the aetiology of muscle wastage. As a result hyperglycaemia will exacerbate muscle wastage and predispose to PEM. In addition, patients with liver cirrhosis are at increased risk of bacterial and fungal infection and increased blood glucose levels predispose to nosocomial infections. Blood glucose of >11 mmol/L has been shown to cause a 10-fold increase in infection rates (McMillan & Rizza, 1996).

Dietary intervention

Dietary advice should be modified to meet the patient's estimated protein and energy requirements and standard healthy eating diabetic dietary advice should only be used in patients who show no signs or are not at risk of PEM. In cirrhotic malnourished patients, healthy eating advice is inappropriate and simple low refined carbohydrate advice such as given below is adequate. Priority should be given to meeting elevated nutritional requirements, a small, frequent meal pattern inclusion of ONS as necessary, and a 50-g late evening snack. Close liaison with diabetes care teams is often necessary to optimise insulin and oral hypoglycaemic regimens. Simple dietary advice includes:

- Reduce refined carbohydrate, e.g. sugar, sweets, sugary drinks.

- Small frequent meals with snacks between, especially 50-g carbohydrate evening snacks.
- Fruit and vegetables used in moderation as they have low energy density and can result in early satiety.
- ONS as necessary to meet elevated energy and protein requirements.

If parenteral or enteral feeding is indicated, appropriate adjustment to oral hypoglycaemic agents and insulin regimens to optimise glycaemic control needs liaison with medical and diabetes teams as appropriate.

Reactive hypoglycaemia

Symptomatic reactive hypoglycaemia is common. Patients should be advised to avoid fasting and encouraged to eat in a small, frequent meal pattern with adequate quantities of carbohydrate and regular snacks. It is also advisable to have a meal or snack prior to exercising.

Zinc deficiency and liver disease

The liver plays an important role in zinc homeostasis and zinc deficiency in cirrhosis is associated with impaired liver function and regeneration (Grüngreiff, 2002), and alteration in taste perception (Madden et al., 1997). Malnutrition in cirrhotic patients is also likely to contribute to zinc deficiency, especially in alcoholic patients (Poschl et al., 2004). Cirrhosis has been implicated as a cause of zinc deficiency as a result of multiple factors including decreased intestinal absorption which in itself may cause damage to intestinal mucosa (Karayalcin et al., 1988). Additionally, there are increased urinary losses of zinc through diuretics in patients with cirrhosis (Yoshida et al., 2001) and reduced circulating albumin levels, which results in reduced binding of zinc to albumin.

The pathogenesis of hepatic encephalopathy derived from liver failure is likely to be related to zinc deficiency (Romero-Gomez et al., 2001; Yang et al., 2004). Despite mixed results from research, zinc supplementation should be considered for patients with hepatic encephalopathy who do not respond to standard therapy and in whom serum levels have been measured and deficiency established (Blei & Cordoba, 2001; Takuma et al., 2010).

Malabsorption

Malabsorption and maldigestion of gastrointestinal nutrients frequently exists in patients with liver disease; however, the extent to which they occur can vary considerably depending on the underlying disease and the individual. Ulcerative colitis is commonly seen in people with primary sclerosing cirrhosis, and coeliac disease in patients with primary biliary cirrhosis. Additionally, in alcoholic liver disease pancreatic insufficiency is common. Other reasons for malabsorption can include bacterial overgrowth resulting from impaired small bowel motility or the administration of medications such a cholestyramine, lactulose and antibiotics. Malabsorption of fat soluble vitamins is common, especially in cholestatic disease where reduced absorption of carbohydrates, protein, water soluble vitamins and minerals has also been demonstrated (Matos et al., 2002).

Steatorrhoea

This develops if secretion of bile is significantly impaired (cholestasis) and as a result reduced amounts of bile salts reach the duodenum. Bile acids also act as cofactors for digestive lipases, protecting them from the proteolytic effects of other digestive enzymes. Steatorrhoea is a frequent symptom in cholestatic diseases, such as primary biliary cirrhosis where the small intrahepatic bile ducts are progressively destroyed, leading to cholestasis and primary sclerosing cirrhosis in which inflammation and fibrosis of the bile ducts lead to narrowing of the biliary system. Steatorrhoea may be so severe that it compromises the nutritional status of the patient and may be a direct cause of malnutrition (Zaina et al., 2004). Cholestatic disease is frequently associated with a fat soluble vitamin deficiency (Feranchak et al., 2005).

A subjective diagnosis can be made on classic steatorrhoea symptoms such as loose, bulky, greasy, pale, floating stools, with an offensive smell following ingestion of a fat containing food. Oily droplets may appear in the toilet water or on toilet tissue.

The initial dietary assessment of all patients with jaundice, primary biliary cirrhosis and primary sclerosing cirrhosis should include consideration of the potential of steatorrhoea. Even when symptoms are absent, the patient should be advised to observe bowel habits in case steatorrhoea develops in view of the risk of malnutrition.

Fat restriction

If indicated, the aim of dietary treatment is to alleviate symptoms, prevent decline in nutritional status and fat soluble vitamin deficiencies. Fat is an important and palatable source of energy for any patient requiring nutritional support, and for patients with liver disease a reduction in fat intake should only be used if:

- There is objective or subjective evidence of symptoms of steatorrhoea and these distress the patient.
- Symptoms of steatorrhoea are accompanied by weight loss and muscle wasting ascertained by upper arm anthropometry.
- The patient feels very nauseous or has marked indigestion or borborygmus (stomach rumbling) that does not respond to antiemetics or antacids following fat ingestion.

The degree of fat tolerance will vary between patients and needs to be assessed on an individual basis. A detailed diet history from the patient to assess which foods cause symptoms is necessary and advice should be to reduce the intake of these initially. If the patient cannot determine which foods are causing symptoms and the steatorrhoea is severe, then they should initially reduce foods that are high in fat. Steatorrhoea caused by pancreatic exocrine insufficiency can be treated with pancreatic enzyme replacement therapy (see Chapter 7.4.5). Pancreatic enzyme replacement therapy is not indicated in biliary steatorrhoea.

Nutritional support

Meeting the nutritional requirements for energy and protein of patients with steatorrhoea remains a priority to maintain or improve nutritional status. Fat intake should only be reduced to individual tolerance. As fat is such a valuable source of energy, a potential energy deficit from fat restriction has to be replaced with an appropriate replacement energy source:

- *Carbohydrates* – complex carbohydrate intake can be increased in patients with a good appetite. Refined carbohydrates such as sugar, sweets and glucose polymers can be useful in patients without diabetes.
- *Medium chain triglycerides (MCTs)* – water soluble and do not require bile salts for emulsification, e.g. Liquigen and MCT Procal.
- *Oral nutritional supplements* are useful, especially juice based sip feeds that contain only minimal fat and are fortified with fat soluble vitamins. Some high protein supplements are also low in fat and well tolerated.

If enteral feeding is required, consideration should be given to the enteral feed's fat source:

- *MCT based feeds* – provide a greater percentage of fat as MCTs. There are a number of feeds available ranging from 1 to 1.5 kcal/mL.
- *Low fat semi elemental feeds* – indicated where steatorrhoea is severe, but have the disadvantage that a high volume is needed to meet nutritional requirements.

Fat soluble vitamins

Patients with overt symptoms of steatorrhoea or chronic steatorrhoea are at risk of developing deficiencies of the fat soluble vitamins (Floreani *et al.*, 2000). Deficiency should be suspected, levels checked and supplemented if necessary. Patients with steatorrhoea without clinical signs of deficiency may benefit from a multivitamin supplement, including fat soluble vitamins. Absorption will be improved with resolution of steatorrhoea (Kennedy & O'Grady, 2002). Current practice regarding fat soluble vitamin screening and supplementation varies throughout the UK liver centres. It is important that dietitians check with their hospital pharmacy which supplements are available and what dosage is recommended.

Hepatorenal syndrome

Hepatorenal syndrome (HRS) is defined as the occurrence of renal failure in a patient with advanced liver disease in the absence of an identifiable cause of renal failure (Arroyo *et al.*, 1996). Often the precipitating factor is a bacterial infection on the background of vasodilatation in the splanchnic arterial bed and cardiac output that is insufficient for the patient's needs. There are two types of HRS.

Type 1 hepatorenal syndrome

This is a rapidly progressive acute renal failure that frequently develops as a result of a precipitating factor for deterioration of liver function together with deterioration of other organ function. Precipitating factors include sepsis, such as spontaneous bacterial peritonitis (SBP), and acute alcoholic hepatitis, although sometimes the identifiable cause for an episode of decompensation is unclear.

Type 2 hepatorenal syndrome

Type 2 occurs in patients with refractory ascites and there is a steady, but moderate, degree of functional renal failure, often with rapid sodium retention. Patients with type 2 HRS may eventually develop type 1 HRS either spontaneously or following a precipitating event such as SBP (Arroyo *et al.*, 1996).

Management

The renal function can often be improved by using vasoconstrictor drugs such as terlipressin to increase arterial pressure (Salerno *et al.*, 2007). Renal replacement therapy may be necessary when the patient becomes severely fluid overloaded or hyperkalaemic, or develops metabolic acidosis. The prognosis of HRS is poor, with an average median survival time of approximately 3 months (Ginès *et al.*, 1993; Ginès & Schrier, 2009).

Fluid management in patients with HRS is of particular importance and close liaison with the MDT is necessary to determine any fluid limitations. Serum potassium levels should be monitored on a daily basis and diet therapy and nutritional support adjusted as is necessary. Patients may be symptomatic of uraemia and antiemetics may be required. Careful consideration of protein intake is necessary and protein may need to be reduced to 1.0–1.2 g/kg of dry body weight if uraemia is problematic. Energy requirements should be calculated as described in the Nutritional assessment section, with the appropriate stress factors added to basal metabolic rate (see Chapter 7.5.1).

Drug–nutrient interactions

The following should be noted:

- Telaprevir – requires 20 g of fat with dose.
- Neomycin – malabsorption of calcium, iron and potassium.
- Metronidazole – avoid alcohol, consider sodium content.
- Furosemide – malabsorption of calcium, magnesium, potassium and zinc.
- Spironolactone – limit alcohol, risk of hyperkalaemia.

Further reading

Bircher J, Benhamou JP, McIntyre N, Rizzetto M. (1999) *Oxford Textbook of Clinical Hepatology*, 2nd edn. Oxford: Oxford University Press.

Department of Health. (1995) Sensible Drinking. The Report of an Inter-Departmental Working Group. London, Department of Health. London: The Stationery Office..

SECTION 7

Hamlin S, Leaper J. (2009) Nutrition in liver disease. In: Sargent S (ed) *Liver Disease: An Essential Guide for Nurses and Health Care Professionals*. Chichester: Wiley Blackwell, pp. 234–251.

Long RG, Scott BB. (2005) *Gastroenterology and Liver Disease*. London: Elsevier Mosby.

Sargent S. (2009) *Liver Diseases – An essential guide for Nurses and Health Care Professionals*. London: Blackwell Publishing.

Internet resources

BDA Gastroenterology Specialist Group   www.bda.uk.com
British Association for the Study of the Liver   www.basl.org.uk
British Liver Trust   www.britishlivertrust.org.uk
British Society of Gastroenterology   www.bsg.org.uk
Cancer backup   www.cancerbackup.org.uk
Drinkaware   www.drinkaware.co.uk
European Association for the Study of the Liver   www.easl.eu
European Society for Clinical Nutrition and Metabolism   www.espen.org

References

Abbott-Johnson W, Kerlin P, Clague A, Johnson H, Cuneo R. (2011) Relationships between blood levels of fat soluble vitamins and disease etiology and severity in adults awaiting liver transplantation. *Journal of Gastroenterology and Hepatology* 26: 1402–1410.

Adams LA, Angulo P. (2006) Treatment of non-alcoholic fatty liver disease. *Postgraduate Medical Journal* 82: 315–322.

Aithal GR, Ryder S. (2005) Liver disease. In: Long RGS, Scott BB (eds) *Specialist Training in Gastroenterology and Liver Disease*. Edinburgh: Elsevier Mosby, pp. 184–239.

Alberino F, Gatta A, Amodio P, et al. (2001) Nutrition and survival in patients with liver cirrhosis. *Nutrition* 17: 445–450.

Alberti KGMM, Zimmet P, Shaw J. (2007) International Diabetes Federation: a consensus on Type 2 diabetes prevention. *Diabetic Medicine* 24: 451–463.

Als-Nielsen B, Koretz RL, Kjaergard LL, Gluud C. (2003) Branched-chain amino acids for hepatic encephalopathy. *Cochrane Database of Systematic Reviews* 2: CD001939.

Alvares-da-Silva MR, Reverbel da Silveira T. (2005) Comparison between handgrip strength, subjective global assessment, and prognostic nutritional index in assessing malnutrition and predicting clinical outcome in cirrhotic outpatients. *Nutrition* 21: 113–117.

American Gastroenterological Association. (2002) American Gastroenterological Association Medical Position Statement: Nonalcoholic fatty liver disease. *Gastroenterology* 123: 1702–1704.

Anand BS, Currie S, Dieperink E, et al. (2006) Alcohol use and treatment of hepatitis C virus: results of a national multicenter study. *Gastroenterology* 130: 1607–1616.

Angeli P, Fasolato S, Mazza E, et al. (2010) Combined versus sequential diuretic treatment of ascites in non-azotaemic patients with cirrhosis: results of an open randomised clinical trial. *Gut* 59: 98–104.

Arora S, Mattina C, McAnenny C, et al. (2011) The development and validation of a nutritional prioritising tool for use in patients with chronic liver disease. (Abstract – unpublished work, personal communication).

Arroyo V, Ginés P, Gerbes AL, et al. (1996) Definition and diagnostic criteria of refractory ascites and hepatorenal syndrome in cirrhosis. International Ascites Club. *Hepatology* 23: 164–176.

Bacon BR, O'Grady JG, Di Bisceglie AM, Lake JR. (2006) *Comprehensive Clinical Hepatology*, 2nd edn. Elsevier Health Sciences.

Barve A, Khan R, Marsano L, Ravindra KV, McClain C. (2008) Treatment of alcoholic liver disease. *Annals of Hepatology* 7: 5–15.

Bedogni G, Miglioli L, Masutti F, Tiribelli C, Marchesini G, Bellantani S. (2005) Prevalence of and risk factors for nonalcoholic fatty liver disease: the Dionysos nutrition and liver study. *Hepatology* 42: 44–52.

Bellantani S, Saccoccio G, Costa G, et al. (1997) Drinking habits as cofactors of risk for alcohol induced liver damage. *Gut* 41: 845–850.

Bemeur C, Desjardins P, Butterworth RF. (2010) Role of nutrition in the management of hepatic encephalopathy in end-stage liver failure. *Journal of Nutrition and Metabolism*. Article ID 489823, 12 pages.

Bernal W, Auzinger G, Dhawan A, Wendon J. (2010) Acute liver failure. *Lancet* 376: 190–201.

Bhonchal S, Nain CK, Prasad KK, et al. (2008) Functional and morphological alterations in small intestine mucosa of chronic alcoholics. *Journal of Gastroenterology and Hepatology* 23: 43–48.

Blei AT, Cordoba J. (2001) Hepatic encephalopathy. *American Journal of Gastroenterology* 96: 1968–1976.

Blonde-Cynober F, Aussel C, Cynober L. (1999) Abnormalities in branched-chain amino acid metabolism in cirrhosis: influence of hormonal and nutritional factors and directions for future research. *Clinical Nutrition* 18: 5–13.

Bolland MJ, Grey A, Avenell A, Gamble GD, Reid, IR. (2011) Calcium supplements with or without vitamin D and risk of cardiovascular events: reanalysis of the Women's Health Initiative limited access dataset and meta-analysis. *BMJ* 342: 2040.

Bressler BL, Guindi M, Tomlinson G, Heathcote J. (2003) High body mass index is an independent risk factor for nonresponse to antiviral treatment in chronic hepatitis C. *Hepatology* 38: 639–644.

British Association for the Study of the Liver and British Society of Gastroenterology. (2009) The national plan for liver services UK – A time to act: Improving liver health and outcomes in liver disease. London: BASL and BSG. Available at www.bsg.org.uk/sections/liver-news/the-national-plan-for-liver-services-uk-2009.html. Accessed 25 November 2011.

British Liver Trust (2009) *Facts about liver disease*. Available at www.britishlivertrust.org.uk/home/about-us/media-centre/facts-about-liver-disease.aspx. Accessed 2 December 11.

British Liver Trust. (2011) *Welcome!* Available at www.britishlivertrust.org.uk/home/find-support.aspx. Accessed 2 December 11.

British Transplant Society. (2011) British Transplantation Society Guidelines for liver transplantation for patients with non-alcoholic steatohepatitis. British Transplantation Society. Available at: www.bts.org.uk/transplantation/standards-and-guidelines/. Accessed 24 October 2011.

Browning JD, Szczepaniak LS, Dobbins R, et al. (2004) Prevalence of hepatic steatosis in an urban population in the United States: impact of ethnicity. *Hepatology* 40: 1387–1395.

Cabré E, Gonzalez-Huix F, Abad-Lacruz A, et al. (1990) Effect of total enteral nutrition on the short-term outcome of severely malnourished cirrhotics. A randomized controlled trial. *Gastroenterology* 98: 715–720.

Cabré E, Rodriguez-Iglesias P, Caballeria J, et al. (2000) Short- and long-term outcome of severe alcohol-induced hepatitis treated with steroids or enteral nutrition: a multicenter randomized trial. *Hepatology* 32: 36–42.

Campos AC, Matias JE, Coelho JC. (2002) Nutritional aspects of liver transplantation. *Current Opinion in Clinical Nutrition* 5: 297–307.

Cappuccio FP, Capewell S, Lincoln P, McPherson K. (2011) Policy options to reduce population salt intake. *BMJ* 343: d4995.

Carvalho L, Parise ER. (2006) Evaluation of nutritional status of nonhospitalized patients with liver cirrhosis. *Arquivos degastroenterologia* 43: 269–274.

Chapman R, Fevery J, Kalloo A, et al. (2010) Diagnosis and management of primary sclerosing cholangitis. *Hepatology* 51: 660–678.

Collier JD, Ninkovic M, Compston JE. (2002) Guidelines on the management of osteoporosis associated with chronic liver disease. *Gut* 50: i1–9.

Coltorti M, Del Vecchio-Blanco C, Caporaso N, Gallo C, Castellano L. (1991) Liver cirrhosis in Italy. A multicentre study on presenting modalities and the impact on health care resources. National Project on Liver Cirrhosis Group. *Italian Journal of Gastroenterology* 23: 42–48.

Cordoba J, Lopez-Hellin J, Planas M, *et al.* (2004) Normal protein diet for episodic hepatic encephalopathy: results of a randomized study. *Journal of Hepatology* 41: 38–43.

Corrao G, Ferrari P, Zambson A, Torchio P. (1997) Are the recent trends in liver cirrhosis mortality affected by changes in alcohol consumption? Analysis of latency period in European countries. *Journal of Studies on Alcohol* 58: 486–494.

Das B, Chandra P, Thimmaraju K. (2011) Serum magnesium level in patients with liver cirrhosis. *International Journal of Biological Medical Research* 2: 709–711.

Day CP. (2002) Non-alcoholic steatohepatitis (NASH): where are we now and where are we going? *Gut* 50: 585–588.

Day CP. (2006) Non-alcoholic fatty liver disease: current concepts and management strategies. *Clinical Medicine* 6: 19–25.

de Alwis NM, Day CP. (2008) Non-alcoholic fatty liver disease: the mist gradually clears. *Journal of Hepatology* 48: S104–112.

Dejong CHC, Van de Poll HCG, Soeters PB, Jalan R, Old Damink SWM. (2007) Aromatic amino acid metabolism during liver failure. *Journal of Nutrition* 137: 1579S–1585S.

DiCecco SR, Wieners EJ, Wiesner RH, Southorn PA, Plevak DJ, Krom RA. (1989) Assessment of nutritional status of patients with end-stage liver disease undergoing liver transplantation. *Mayo Clinic Proceedings* 64: 95–102.

Duncan GE, Perri MG, Theriaque DW, Hutson AD, Eckel RH, Stacpoole PW. (2003) Exercise training, without weight loss, increases insulin sensitivity and postheparin plasma lipase activity in previously sedentary adults. *Diabetes Care* 26: 557–562.

Elia M. (2003) *Screening for Malnutrition: A Multidisciplinary Responsibility. Development and Use of the Malnutrition Universal Screening Tool ('MUST') for Adults.* Birmingham: BAPEN.

El-Serag HB, Engels EA, Landgren O, *et al.* (2009) Risk of hepatobiliary and pancreatic cancers after hepatitis C virus infection: A population-based study of U.S. veterans. *Hepatology* 49: 116–123.

European Association for the Study of Liver. (2010) EASL clinical practice guidelines on the management of ascites, spontaneous bacterial peritonitis, and hepatorenal syndrome in cirrhosis. *Journal of Hepatology* 53: 397–417.

European Association for the Study of Liver. (2011) EASL Clinical Practice Guidelines: Management of hepatitis C virus infection. *Journal of Hepatology* 55: 245–264.

Fairbanks KD, Tavill AS. (2008) Liver disease in alpha 1-antitrypsin deficiency: a review. *American Journal of Gastroenterology* 103: 2136–2141.

Feranchak AP, Gralla J, King R, *et al.* (2005) Comparison of indices of vitamin A status in children with chronic liver disease. *Hepatology* 42: 782–792.

Ferenci P, Lockwood A, Mullen K, Tarter R, Weissemnborn K, Blei AT; The members of the working party. (2002) Hepatic encephalopathy—definition, nomenclature, diagnosis, and quantification: Final Report of the Working Party at the 11th World Congresses of Gastroenterology, Vienna, 1998. *Hepatology* 35: 716–721.

Figueiredo FA, Dickson ER, Pasha TM, *et al.* (2000) Utility of standard nutritional parameters in detecting body cell mass depletion in patients with end-stage liver disease. *Liver Transplantation* 6: 575–581.

Floreani A, Baragiotta A, Martines D, Naccarato R, D'Odorico A. (2000) Plasma antioxidant levels in chronic cholestatic liver diseases. *Alimentary Pharmacology & Therapeutics* 14: 353–358.

Foresight. (2007) *Tackling Obesities – Future Choices*. London: Foresight. Available at www.idea.gov.uk/idk/core/page.do?pageId =8267926. Accessed 18 February 2011.

Friedman LS, Keefe EB (eds). (2004) *Handbook of Liver Disease*, 2nd edn. Edinburgh: Churchill Livingstone.

Fukushima H, Miwa Y, Ida E, *et al.* (2003) Nocturnal branched-chain amino acid administration improves protein metabolism in patients with liver cirrhosis: comparison with daytime administration. *Journal of Parenteral and Enteral Nutrition* 27: 315–322.

Ghany MG, Nelson DR, Strader DB, Thomas DL, Seeff LB. (2011) An update on treatment of genotype 1 chronic hepatitis C virus infection: 2011 practice guideline by the American Association for the Study of Liver Diseases. *Hepatology* 54: 1433–1444.

Ginès P, Schrier RW. (2009) Renal failure in cirrhosis. *New England Journal of Medicine* 361: 1279–1290.

Ginès P, Quintero E, Arroyo V, *et al.* (1987) Compensated cirrhosis: natural history and prognostic factors. *Hepatology* 7: 122–128.

Ginès A, Escorsell A, Ginès P, *et al.* (1993) Incidence, predictive factors, and prognosis of the hepatorenal syndrome in cirrhosis with ascites. *Gastroenterology* 105: 229–236.

Ginès A, Fernandez-Esparrach G, Monescillo A *et al.* (1996) Randomized trial comparing albumin, dextran 70, and polygeline in cirrhotic patients with ascites treated by paracentesis. *Gastroenterology* 111: 1002–1010.

Goel V, Kar P. (2010) Hepatic osteodystrophy. *Tropical Gastroenterology* 31: 82–86.

Grüngreiff K. (2002) Zinc in liver disease. *Journal of Trace Elements in Experimental Medicine* 15: 67–78.

Guevara M, Ginés P. (2005) Hepatorenal syndrome. *Digestive Diseases* 23: 47–55.

Guglielmi FW, Boggio-Bertinet D, Federico A, *et al.* (2006) Total parenteral nutrition-related gastroenterological complications. *Digestive and Liver Diseases* 38: 623–642.

Gunsar F, Raimondo ML, Jones S, *et al.* (2006) Nutritional status and prognosis in cirrhotic patients. *Alimentary Pharmacology & Therapeutics* 24: 563–572.

Harrison SA, Finck C, Helsinki D, Torgerson S. (2002) Orlistat treatment in obese, non alcoholic steatohepatitis patients: a pilot study. *Hepatology* 36: 406A.

Hasse J (2001) Nutritional assessment and support of organ transplant recipients. *Journal of Parenteral and Enteral Nutrition* 25: 120–131.

Henry CJK. (2005) Basal metabolic rate studies in humans: measurement and development of new equations. *Public Health Nutrition* 8(7A): 1133–1152.

Heymsfield SB, Matthews D. (1994) Body Composition: Research and Clinical Advances—1993 A.S.P.E.N. Research Workshop. *Journal of Parenteral and Enteral Nutrition* 18(2): 91–103.

Hickman IJ, Macdonald GA. (2007) Impact of diabetes on the severity of liver disease. *American Journal of Medicine* 120(10): 829–834.

Hill H. (2009) Anatomy and physiology. In: Sargent S (ed) *Liver Diseases: An Essential Guide for Nurses and Health Care Professionals*. Chichester: Wiley Blackwell, pp. 1–14.

International Diabetes Federation. (2006) The IDF consensus worldwide definition of the metabolic syndrome. Available at www .idf.org/webdata/docs/IDF_Meta_def_final.pdf. Accessed 14 August 2013.

Johnson D. (1999) Special considerations in interpreting liver function tests. *American Family Physician* 59: 2223–2230.

Karayalcin S, Arcasoy A, Uzunalimoglu O. (1988) Zinc plasma levels after oral zinc tolerance test in nonalcoholic cirrhosis. *Digestive Diseases and Sciences* 33: 1096–1102.

Kearns PJ, Young H, Garcia G, *et al.* (1992) Accelerated improvement of alcoholic liver disease with enteral nutrition. *Gastroenterology* 102: 200–205.

Kennedy PTF, O'Grady JG. (2002) Diseases of the liver: Chronic liver disease. *Hospital Pharmacy* 9: 137–143.

Kondrup J, Muller MJ. (1997) Energy and protein requirements of patients with chronic liver disease. *Journal of Hepatology* 27: 239–247.

Kumpf VJ. (2006) Parenteral nutrition-associated liver disease in adult and pediatric patients. *Nutrition in Clinical Practice* 21: 279–290.

Kyle UG, Bosaeus I, De Lorenzo AD, *et al.* (2004) Bioelectrical impedance analysis–part I: review of principles and methods. *Clinical Nutrition* 23: 1226–1243.

Laviano A, Muscaritoli M, Cascino A, *et al.* (2005) Branched-chain amino acids: the best compromise to achieve anabolism? *Current Opinion in Clinical Nutrition* 8: 408–414.

Le Cornu KA, McKiernan FJ, Kapadia SA, Neuberger JM. (2000) A prospective randomized study of preoperative nutritional supplementation in patients awaiting elective orthotopic liver transplantation. *Transplantation* 69: 1364–1369.

Lee YM, Kaplan MM. (1998) Primary biliary cirrhosis. In: Friedman LS, Keeffe EB (eds) *Handbook of Liver Disease*. Edinburgh: Churchill Livingstone, pp. 197–214.

Lee YM, Kaplan, MM. (2002) Management of primary sclerosing cholangitis. *American Journal of Gastroenterology* 97: 528–534.

Levy C, Lindor KD. (2003) Current management of primary biliary cirrhosis and primary sclerosing cholangitis. *Journal of Hepatology* 38: S24–37.

Lieber CS. (2001) Alcohol and hepatitis C. *Alcohol Research & Health* 25: 245–254.

Lonardo A, Adinolfi LE, Loria P, Carulli N, Ruggiero G, Day CP. (2004) Steatosis and hepatitis C virus: Mechanisms and significance for hepatic and extrahepatic disease. *Gastroenterology* 126: 586–597.

Loser C, Aschl G, Hebuterne X, *et al.* (2005) ESPEN guidelines on artificial enteral nutrition–percutaneous endoscopic gastrostomy (PEG). *Clinical Nutrition* 24: 848–861.

Lucey MR, Mathurin P, Morgan TR. (2009) Alcoholic hepatitis. *New England Journal of Medicine* 360: 2758–2769.

MacFie J. (2004) Current status of bacterial translocation as a cause of surgical sepsis. *British Medical Bulletin* 71: 1–11.

Machado M, Marques-Vidal P, Cortez-Pinto H. (2006) Hepatic histology in obese patients undergoing bariatric surgery. *Journal of Hepatology* 45: 600–606.

Madden AM, Bradbury W, Morgan MY. (1997) Taste perception in cirrhosis: its relationship to circulating micronutrients and food preferences. *Hepatology* 26: 40–48.

Maggs JR, Chapman RW. (2008) An update on primary sclerosing cholangitis. *Current Opinion in Gastroenterology* 24: 377–383.

Makol A, Watt KD, Chowdhary VR. (2011) Autoimmune hepatitis: a review of current diagnosis and treatment. *Hepatitis Research and Treatment* 2011: 390916.

Malham M, Jorgensen SP, Ott P, *et al.* (2011) Vitamin D deficiency in cirrhosis relates to liver dysfunction rather than aetiology. *World Journal of Gastroenterology* 17: 922–925.

Malinchoc M, Kamath PS, Gordon FD, Peine CJ, Rank J, ter Borg PC. (2000) A model to predict poor survival in patients undergoing transjugular intrahepatic portosystemic shunts. *Hepatology* 31: 864–871.

Marchesini G, Bianchi G, Merli M, *et al.* (2003) Nutritional supplementation with branched-chain amino acids in advanced cirrhosis: a double-blind, randomized trial. *Gastroenterology* 124: 1792–1801.

Martin P, Friedman LS. (2004) Assessment of liver function and diagnostic studies. In: Friedman LS, Keefe EB (eds) *Handbook of Liver Disease*, 2nd edn. Philadelphia: Churchill Livingstone, pp. 1–14.

Matos C, Porayko MK, Francisco-Ziller N, DiCecco S. (2002) Nutrition and chronic liver disease. *Journal of Clinical Gastroenterology* 35: 391–397.

McCullough AJ, Bugianesi E. (1997) Protein-calorie malnutrition and the etiology of cirrhosis. *American Journal of Gastroenterology* 92: 734–738.

McCullough AJ, O'Connor JFB. (1998) Alcoholic liver disease: Proposed recommendations for the American College of Gastroenterology. *American Journal of Gastroenterology* 93: 2022–2036.

McGee RG, Bakens A, Wiley K, Riordan SM, Webster AC. (2011) Probiotics for patients with hepatic encephalopathy. *Cochrane Database of Systematic Reviews* 11: CD008716.

McMillan MM, Rizza RA. (1996) Nutritional support in hospital patients with diabetes mellitus. *Proceedings of the Mayo Clinic* 71: 587–594.

Mendenhall CL. (1992) Protein-calorie malnutrition in alcoholic liver disease. In: Watson RRW (ed) *Nutrition and Alcohol*. Boca Raton: CRC Press, pp. 363–384.

Mendenhall CL, Seeff L, Diehl AM, *et al.* (1991) Antibodies to hepatitis B virus and hepatitis C virus in alcoholic hepatitis and cirrhosis: their prevalence and clinical relevance. The VA Cooperative Study Group (No. 119). *Hepatology* 14: 581–589.

Monto A, Alonzo J, Watson JJ, Grunfeld C, Wright TL. (2010) Steatosis in chronic hepatitis C: Relative contributions of obesity, diabetes mellitus, and alcohol. *Hepatology* 36: 729–736.

Moore KP, Aithal GP. (2006) Guidelines on the management of ascites in cirrhosis. *Gut* 55 (Suppl 6): 1–12.

Morgan MY, Madden AM, Soulsby CT, Morris RW. (2006) Derivation and validation of a new global method for assessing nutritional status in patients with cirrhosis. *Hepatology* 44: 823–835.

Moreau R, Delegue P, Pessione F, *et al.* (2004) Clinical characteristics and outcome of patients with cirrhosis and refractory ascites. *Liver International* 24: 457–464.

Mullen KD, Weber Jr FL. (1991) Role of nutrition in hepatic encephalopathy. *Seminars in Liver Disease* 11: 292–304.

Muller MJ, Pirlich M, Balks HJ, Selberg O. (1994) Glucose intolerance in liver cirrhosis: role of hepatic and non-hepatic influences. *European Journal of Clinical Chemistry Clinics* 32: 749–758.

Muller MJ, Bottcher J, Selberg O, *et al.* (1999) Hypermetabolism in clinically stable patients with liver cirrhosis. *American Journal of Clinical Nutrition* 69: 1194–1201.

Musso G, Gambino R, De Michieli F, *et al.* (2003) Dietary habits and their relations to insulin resistance and postprandial lipemia in nonalcoholic steatohepatitis. *Hepatology* 37: 909–916.

Muto Y, Sato S, Watanabe A, *et al.* (2005) Effects of oral branched-chain amino acid granules on event-free survival in patients with liver cirrhosis. *Clinical Gastroenterology and Hepatology* 3: 705–713.

National Institute for Health and Care Excellence (NICE). (2006) *Nutrition Support for Adults Oral Nutrition Support, Enteral Tube Feeding and Parenteral Nutrition*. London: NICE.

National Institute for Health and Care Excellence (NICE). (2010a) *Alcohol-Use Disorders*. London: NICE.

National Institute for Health and Care Excellence (NICE). (2010b) *Hepatitis C – Peginterferon Alfa and Ribavirin*. London: NICE.

Neuberger J, Gimson A, Davies M, *et al.* (2008) Selection of patients for liver transplantation and allocation of donated livers in the UK. *Gut* 57: 252–257.

Nielsen K, Kondrup J, Martinsen L, *et al.* (1995) Long-term oral refeeding of patients with cirrhosis of the liver. *British Journal of Nutrition* 74: 557–567.

O'Brien A, Williams R. (2008) Nutrition in end-stage liver disease: principles and practice. *Gastroenterology* 134: 1729–1740.

Okuda M, Li K, Beard MR, *et al.* (2002) Mitochondrial injury, oxidative stress, and antioxidant gene expression are induced by hepatitis C virus core protein. *Gastroenterology* 122: 366–375.

O'Shea RS, Dasarathy S, McCullough AJ (2010) Alcoholic liver disease. *Hepatology* 51: 307–328.

Owen OE, Trapp VE, Reichard GA, *et al.* (1983) Nature and quantity of fuels consumed in patients with alcoholic cirrhosis. *Journal of Clinical Investigation* 72: 1821–1832.

Philippe L. (2007) Acute alcoholic hepatitis. *Hepatitis.org* (online). Available at www.hepatitis.org/hepatalcool_angl.htm. Accessed 30 November 2011.

Pietrangelo A. (2006) Hereditary haemochromatosis. *Annual Reviews in Nutrition* 26: 251–270.

Plank LD, Gane EJ, Peng S, *et al.* (2008) Nocturnal nutritional supplementation improves total body protein status of patients with liver cirrhosis: a randomized 12-month trial. *Hepatology* 48: 557–566.

Plauth M, Merli M, Kondrup J, Weimann A, Ferenci P, Muller MJ. (1997) ESPEN guidelines for nutrition in liver disease and transplantation. *Clinical Nutrition* 16: 43–55.

Plauth M, Schutz T, Buckendahl DP, *et al.* (2004) Weight gain after transjugular intrahepatic portosystemic shunt is associated with improvement in body composition in malnourished patients with cirrhosis and hypermetabolism. *Journal of Hepatology* 40: 228–233.

Plauth M, Cabre E, Riggio O, *et al.* (2006) ESPEN Guidelines on Enteral Nutrition: Liver disease. *Clinical Nutrition* 25: 285–294.

Plauth M, Cabre E, Campillo B, *et al.* (2009) ESPEN Guidelines on Parenteral Nutrition: Hepatology. *Clinical Nutrition* 28: 436–444.

Polson J, Lee WM. (2005) AASLD position paper: the management of acute liver failure. *Hepatology* 41: 1179–1197.

Poschl G, Seitz HK. (2004) Alcohol and cancer. *Alcohol and Alcoholism* 39: 155–165.

Rambaldi A, Saconato HH, Christensen E, Thorlund K, Wetterslev J, Gluud C. (2008) Systematic review: glucocorticosteroids for alcoholic hepatitis–a Cochrane Hepato-Biliary Group systematic review with meta-analyses and trial sequential analyses of randomized clinical trials. *Alimentary Pharmacology & Therapeutics* 27: 1167–1178.

Renner IG, Savage WT, 3rd, Stace NH, Pantoja JL, Schultheis WM, Peters RL. (1984) Pancreatitis associated with alcoholic liver disease. A review of 1022 autopsy cases. *Digestive Diseases and Sciences* 29: 593–599.

Revill P, Serradell N, Bolos J, Rosa E. (2007) Telaprevir. *Drug Future* 32: 788.

Riggio O, Angeloni S, Salvatori FM, *et al.* (2008) Incidence, natural history, and risk factors of hepatic encephalopathy after transjugular intrahepatic portosystemic shunt with polytetrafluoroethylene-covered stent grafts. *American Journal of Gastroenterology* 103: 2738–2746.

Roberts EA, Schilsky ML. (2008) Diagnosis and treatment of Wilson disease: an update. *Hepatology* 47: 2089–20111.

Romero-Gomez M, Boza F, Garcia-Valdecasas MS, Garcia E, Aguilar-Reina J. (2001) Subclinical hepatic encephalopathy predicts the development of overt hepatic encephalopathy. *American Journal of Gastroenterology* 96: 2718–2723.

Royal College of Physicians (RCP). (2011) Science & Technology Select Committee Inquiry on alcohol guidelines. Available at www.rcplondon.ac.uk/policy/reducing-health-harms/alcohol. Accessed 25 October 2011.

Rubin M, Moser A, Vaserberg N, *et al.* (2000) Structured triacylglycerol emulsion, containing both medium- and long-chain fatty acids, in long-term home parenteral nutrition: a double-blind randomized cross-over study. *Nutrition* 16: 95–100.

Rubio-Tapia A, Murray JA. (2007) The liver in celiac disease. *Hepatology* 46: 1650–1658.

Runyon BA. (1998) Management of adult patients with ascites caused by cirrhosis. *Hepatology* 27: 264–272.

Ryder S. (2003). Guidelines for the diagnosis and treatment of hepatocellular carcinoma (HCC) in adults. *Gut* (Suppl III): iii1–iii8.

Salerno F, Gerbes A, Ginés P, Wong F, Arroyo V. (2007) Diagnosis, prevention and treatment of hepatorenal syndrome in cirrhosis. *Gut* 56: 1310–1318.

Sanchez AJ, Aranda-Michel J. (2006) Nutrition for the liver transplant patient. *Liver Transplantion* 12: 1310–1316.

Sargent S. (2005) The aetiology, management and complications of alcoholic hepatitis. *British Journal of Nursing* 14: 556–562.

Saunders J, Brian A, Wright M, Stroud M. (2010) Malnutrition and nutrition support in patients with liver disease. *Frontline Gastroenterology* 1: 105–511.

Scientific Advisory Committee on Nutrition (SACN). (2010). *Iron and Health*. London: The Stationery Office.

Shepard CW, Simard EP, Finelli L, Fiore AE, Bell BP. (2006) Hepatitis B virus infection: epidemiology and vaccination. *Epidemiologic Reviews* 28: 112–125.

Sougioultzis S, Dalakas E, Hayes PC, Plevris JN. (2005) Alcoholic hepatitis: from pathogenesis to treatment. *Current Medical Research and Opinion* 21: 1337–1346.

Stickel F, Hoehn B, Schuppan D, Seitz HK. (2003) Review article: Nutritional therapy in alcoholic liver disease. *Alimentary Pharmacology & Therapeutics* 18: 357–373.

Stickel F, Inderbitzin D, Candinas D. (2008) Role of nutrition in liver transplantation for end-stage chronic liver disease. *Nutrition Reviews* 66: 47–54.

Stokkeland K, Hilm G, Spak F, Franck J, Hultcrantz R. (2008) Different drinking patterns for women and men with alcohol dependence with and without alcoholic cirrhosis. *Alcohol and Alcoholism* 43: 39–45.

Stranges S, Wu T, Dorn JM, *et al.* (2004) Relationship of alcohol drinking pattern to risk of hypertension: a population-based study. *Hypertension* 44: 813–819.

Swart GR, Zillikens MC, van Vuure JK, van den Berg JW. (1989) Effect of a late evening meal on nitrogen balance in patients with cirrhosis of the liver. *BMJ* 299: 1202–1203.

Takuma Y, Nouso K, Makino Y, Hayashi M, Takahashi H. (2010) Clinical trial: oral zinc in hepatic encephalopathy. *Alimentary Pharmacology & Therapeutics* 32: 1080–1090.

Talwalkar JA, Lindor KD. (2003) Primary biliary cirrhosis. *Lancet* 362: 53–61.

Targher G, Bertolini L, Rodella S, *et al.* (2007) Nonalcoholic fatty liver disease is independently associated with an increased incidence of cardiovascular events in type 2 diabetic patients. *Diabetes Care* 30: 2119–2121.

Taylor R, Corbani T. (2009) Metabolic liver disease. In: Sargent S (ed) *Liver Diseases: An Essential Guide for Nurses and Health Care Professionals*. Chichester: John Wiley & Sons.

Thuluvath PJ, Triger DR. (1994) Evaluation of nutritional status by using anthropometry in adults with alcoholic and nonalcoholic liver disease. *American Journal of Clinical Nutrition* 60: 269–273.

Tilg H, Moschen AR, Kaneider NC. (2011) Pathways of liver injury in alcoholic liver disease. *Journal of Hepatology* 55(5):1159–1161.

Todorovic VE, Micklewright A. (2011) *PEN Group: A Pocket Guide to Clinical Nutrition*, 3rd edn. Birmingham: The Parenteral And Enteral Nutrition Group of the BDA.

Tsiaousi ET, Hatzitolios AI, Trygonis SK, Savopoulos CG. (2008) Malnutrition in end stage liver disease: recommendations and nutritional support. *Journal of Gastroenterology and Hepatology* 23: 527–533.

Tsien CD, McCullough AJ, Dasarathy S. (2012) Late evening snack –Exploiting a period of anabolic opportunity in cirrhosis. *Journal of Gastroenterology and Hepatology* 27: 430–431.

Tsuchiya M, Sakaida I, Okamoto M, Okita K. (2005) The effect of a late evening snack in patients with liver cirrhosis. *Hepatology Research* 31: 95–103.

van Bokhoven MA, van Deursen CT, Swinkels DW. (2011) Diagnosis and management of hereditary haemochromatosis. *BMJ* 342: c7251.

Vaquero J, Chung C, Cahill ME, Blei AT. (2003) Pathogenesis of hepatic encephalopathy in acute liver failure. *Seminars in Liver Disease* 23: 259–269.

Verboeket-van de Venne VW, Westerterp KR, van Hoek B, Swart GR. (1995) Energy expenditure and substrate metabolism in patients with cirrhosis of the liver: effects of the pattern of food intake. *Gut* 36: 110–116.

Voight M, Conn H. (1995) Hepatic encephalopathy. In: Kirsch R, Robson S, Trey C (eds) *Diagnosis and Management of Liver Disease*. London: Chapman and Hall Medical, pp. 140–147.

SECTION 7

Weismuller TJ, Wedemeyer J, Kubicka S, Strassburg CP, Manns MP. (2008) The challenges in primary sclerosing cholangitis – aetio-pathogenesis, autoimmunity, management and malignancy. *Journal of Hepatology* 48(Suppl 1): S38–57.

Wicks C, Somasundaram S, Bjarnason I, *et al.* (1994) Comparison of enteral feeding and total parenteral nutrition after liver transplantation. *Lancet* 344: 837–840.

World Health Organization (WHO). (2008) Hepatitis B. Available at www.who.int/mediacentre/factsheets/fs204/en/. Accessed 30 November 2011.

World Health Organization (WHO). (2009) Alcohol and injuries: emergency department studies in an international perspective. Available at www.who.int/substance_abuse/publications/alcohol/en/. Accessed 1 December 2011.

World Health Organization (WHO). (2011) Hepatitis C. Available at www.who.int/mediacentre/factsheets/fs164/en/. Accessed 30 November 2011.

Yamanaka-Okumura H, Nakamura T, Takeuchi H, *et al.* (2006) Effect of late evening snack with rice ball on energy metabolism in liver cirrhosis. *European Journal of Clinical Nutrition* 60: 1067–1072.

Yang SS, Lai YC, Chiang TR, Chen DF, Chen DS. (2004) Role of zinc in subclinical hepatic encephalopathy: comparison with somatosensory-evoked potentials. *Journal of Gastroenterology and Hepatology* 19: 375–379.

Yoshida Y, Higashi T, Nouso K, *et al.* (2001) Effects of zinc deficiency/zinc supplementation on ammonia metabolism in patients with decompensated liver cirrhosis. *Acta Medica Okayama* 55: 349–355.

Zaina FE, Parolin MB, Lopes RW, Coelho JC. (2004) Prevalence of malnutrition in liver transplant candidates. *Transplantation Proceedings* 36: 923–925.

Zillikens MC, van den Berg JW, Wattimena JL, Rietveld T, Swart, GR. (1993) Nocturnal oral glucose supplementation. The effects on protein metabolism in cirrhotic patients and in healthy controls. *Journal of Hepatology* 17: 377–383.

Zintzaras E, Stefanidis I, Santos M, Vidal F. (2006) Do alcohol-metabolizing enzyme gene polymorphisms increase the risk of alcoholism and alcoholic liver disease? *Hepatology* 43: 352–361.

Zivkovic AM, German JB, Sanyal AJ. (2007) Comparative review of diets for the metabolic syndrome: implications for nonalcoholic fatty liver disease. *American Journal of Clinical Nutrition* 86: 285–300.

7.4.13 Cystic fibrosis

Alison Morton

Key points

■ Cystic fibrosis is a multisystem disorder mainly affecting the respiratory and gastrointestinal systems.

■ There is a positive association between nutritional status, lung function and survival.

■ Patients have increased energy requirements, increased energy losses and often poor oral intake.

■ Regular dietetic counselling aims to achieve a good nutritional status by minimising the effects of malabsorption with pancreatic enzyme replacement therapy and optimising nutritional intake.

■ With increased longevity, new nutritional challenges occur, including diabetes, disordered eating, osteoporosis, liver disease, renal disease and transplantation.

The first clear description of cystic fibrosis (CF) was in the late 1930s (Andersen, 1938). Dietary management of CF has changed dramatically over the years and optimising nutrition has been integral to the improved life expectancy of patients. The replacement of the traditional low fat diet with a high fat diet in the 1980s and the introduction of acid resistant pancreatic enzyme replacement therapy (PERT) were milestones in management.

Cystic fibrosis is a complex multisystem disorder. Intestinal malabsorption occurs in approximately 90% of patients. In the past, malnutrition, weight loss and poor growth were considered inevitable consequences of disease progression, leading to impaired respiratory muscle function, immunological impairment and respiratory failure. Achieving and maintaining a normal nutritional status and growth is an integral part of modern CF management.

Prevalence

Cystic fibrosis is the most common autosomal recessively inherited disease in the UK, mainly affecting Caucasian. One in 25 people in the UK are carriers of a CF gene mutation (i.e. 2.3 million people) (Lewis, 2000), leading to an incidence of approximately 1 in 2500 births (Dodge *et al.*, 2007). The incidence in non-Caucasians is much lower, and estimated to be 1 in 20 000 in ethnic Africans and 1 in 100 000 in Oriental populations (Corey *et al.*, 1988). In the UK, approximately 9000 people have CF (Cystic Fibrosis Trust, 2011).

Aetiology

The genetic defect is located on the long arm of chromosome 7 and results in abnormalities in the production and function of a protein called the cystic fibrosis trans-membrane conductance regulator (CFTR). This protein acts as a chloride channel regulating sodium, chloride, bicarbonate and water transport across epithelial cell membranes. The lack of production or reduction of CFTR results in thick mucus secretions that can obstruct small airways, causing fibrosis and bronchiectasis. CFTR is widespread throughout the body and explains why CF is a multisystem condition affecting many organs. The two major systems affected are the respiratory system and the gastrointestinal tract.

Although over 85% of the CF population in the UK share the same genetic defect (p.Phe508del mutation) (Cystic Fibrosis Trust, 2011), >1800 different mutations have been identified (CF Mutation Database, 2011). Different gene mutations result in different levels of disease severity (see Chapter 5.1).

Diagnostic criteria and classification

National newborn screening for CF was introduced in the UK in 2005–2006. Newborn blood spot screening involves a heel prick blood sample being taken from all babies to test for a number of diseases. The screen for CF looks at the concentration of immunoreactive trypsin (IRT), which is raised in neonates with CF. If the IRT is positive, the infant is referred for a sweat test and genetic screening to confirm the diagnosis. An elevated chloride concentration in the sweat test is diagnostic of CF. Cystic fibrosis is usually confirmed by two positive sweat tests or by the identification of two genetic mutations. The gene mutations are determined from a sample of blood or cells from the oral mucosa. Initially, only the four most common mutations are looked for (followed by a 32 mutation panel). Infants presenting with meconium ileus should also have a sweat test and genetic testing.

Most patients are now diagnosed early by newborn screening or following investigation after presenting with meconium ileus. It is important to remember that in people with milder mutations and those born prior to national newborn screening, the diagnosis may be made later in life. Symptoms that are suggestive of CF include:

- Recurrent respiratory symptoms.
- Prolonged diarrhoea and pale, greasy, offensive stools.
- Failure to thrive in children, delayed puberty or under-nutrition in adults.
- Male infertility.
- Pancreatitis.
- Rectal prolapse.

Disease process

As already mentioned, the two major systems affected are the respiratory system and the gastrointestinal tract.

Respiratory function

People with CF have chronic and often severe respiratory infections. The presence of viscid mucus in the lungs increases the risk of colonisation by pathogens. Chronic chest infections cause inflammation and irreversible lung damage, leading to progressive lung disease. Infection and reduction in lung function contribute to the increased energy requirements of these patients. Regular antibiotic therapy, anti-inflammatory drugs and physiotherapy are aimed at preventing lung damage and preserving lung function.

Gastrointestinal function

Abnormal CFTR in the pancreas may cause the exocrine ducts to become obstructed, preventing secretion of pancreatic enzymes and resulting in malabsorption. Approximately 90% of patients in Northern Europe are pancreatic insufficient (Littlewood et al., 2006). Patients with milder mutations are usually pancreatic sufficient. Pancreatic insufficiency results in significant fat malabsorption and steatorrhoea. Clinically relevant symptoms include frequent pale, oily and offensive stools, abdominal pain, poor growth, malnutrition and deficiencies of fat soluble vitamins and essential fatty acids.

Malabsorption in CF is multifactorial with contributory factors including abnormal ion transfer in the gut due to CFTR and altered bile salt composition, motility and transit time (Littlewood et al., 2006). Pancreatic enzyme replacement therapy can be inactivated by increased duodenal acidity due to pancreatic bicarbonate deficiency, which may also result in bile salt precipitation.

Disease consequences

Prognosis

Cystic fibrosis was once a life limiting disease of childhood. Life expectancy, though still reduced, has increased dramatically due to many factors, including specialist centre care, better nutritional support and improved treatment of respiratory infections. Median survival in the UK is currently 34.4 years (Cystic Fibrosis Trust, 2011) and has been predicted to be at least 50 years for children born in 2000 (Dodge et al., 2007). Over half of patients with CF in the UK are 16 years or older (Cystic Fibrosis Trust, 2011).

Impaired energy intake

Poor energy intakes are frequently reported in patients with CF. This may be a consequence of generalised poor appetite worsened by infection related anorexia during pulmonary exacerbations, abdominal pain and gastro-oesophageal reflux. As the disease progresses, patients may find it difficult to maximise oral intake due to dyspnoea, early satiety and dry mouth or taste changes due to oxygen or drug therapy. Behavioural factors, including food refusal, eating behaviour problems, depression and disordered eating, may further limit food intake.

Increased energy expenditure

Energy requirements in CF vary greatly, but are largely related to the extent of lung disease and the frequency and severity of respiratory infections. In addition, some of the medications used to treat respiratory symptoms increase resting energy expenditure.

With increased longevity, new nutritional comorbidities are emerging, including CF related diabetes, renal disease, osteoporosis, arthropathy, pancreatitis, liver disease, renal disease and need for transplantation. Many women with CF also face the nutritional challenge of pregnancy.

Nutritional consequences

Impaired nutrient absorption

Lack of pancreatic enzymes in pancreatic insufficient patients has a devastating effect on nutritional status. Pancreatic enzyme replacement therapy should be started if a patient has two CFTR mutations associated with pancreatic insufficiency. In addition, patients who present with obvious symptoms of malabsorption should commence PERT as soon as diagnosis of CF is made. Pancreatic insufficiency should always be confirmed by measuring faecal pancreatic elastase (FPE) (Borowitz et al., 2009). If clinical symptoms of malabsorption are absent, measurement of FPE to establish pancreatic status should be undertaken and PERT should only be commenced if pancreatic insufficiency is diagnosed (Littlewood et al., 2006; Borowitz et al., 2009). Some patients may have persistent difficulties controlling malabsorption despite optimal PERT, and they experience increased losses of protein, fat and fat soluble nutrients in the stool. The undigested fat may bind other minerals and lead to increased excretion.

Fat soluble vitamins

Biochemical evidence of deficiencies of fat soluble vitamins (vitamins A, D, E and K) is found early in infants diagnosed with CF by newborn screening (Sokol et al., 1989; Neville & Ranganathan, 2009). All pancreatic insufficient patients require daily supplementation with these vitamins. Pancreatic sufficent patients should be individually assessed and advised.

Vitamin A

The major consequence of vitamin A deficiency is ocular, with abnormal dark adaptation (night blindness) and xerophthalmia being reported (Petersen et al., 1968). Asymptomatic conjunctival xerosis with abnormal dark adaptation despite vitamin A supplementation has been reported (Huet et al., 1997). Although such problems are rare, subclinical deficiency may be common and the consequence of this is difficult to assess but may be significant.

Mild or subclinical vitamin A deficiency may also impair the integrity of the respiratory epithelium (McCullough et al., 1999). Loss of ciliated cells and increased mucus secretion make bacteria more likely to adhere to the surface and colonise the lungs (Chandra, 1988; Biesalski & Nohr, 2003). Linking subclinical vitamin A deficiency and lung function is difficult. However, there is a correla-tion between increased number of respiratory exacerbations (Hakim et al., 2007) and reduced/poorer lung function (Aird et al., 2006).

Beta-carotene has antioxidant properties, acting as a free radical scavenger that may prevent or slow oxidative damage in the lung. There is currently insufficient evidence to recommend routine supplementation with beta-carotene.

Vitamin E

Severe vitamin E deficiency is rare in modern CF care, but historically has been associated with neurological degeneration (Sitrin et al., 1987), haemolytic anaemia (Wilfond et al., 1994) and decreased cognitive function (Koscik et al., 2005). Vitamin E is also an important antioxidant, helping to protect the lungs from damage during the inflammatory response to infection.

Vitamin D

Vitamin D is classically considered for its role in calcium absorption, metabolism and bone mineralisation. There is increasing recognition of the non-skeletal roles of vitamin D in muscle function, diabetes, cardiovascular disease, innate immunity and some forms of cancer (Holick & Chen, 2008). Overt vitamin D deficiency in CF is rare, but both rickets and osteomalacia have been reported (Scott et al., 1977; Elkin et al., 2002). Subclinical vitamin D status may be significant in the context of health outcomes rather than overt deficiency (Maqbool & Stallings, 2008). There is a lack of consensus on the optimal vitamin D level in CF to maintain bone health. A level of 20 ng/mL (50 nmol/L) has been recommended in the European Cystic Fibrosis Mineralisation Guidelines (Sermet-Gaudelus et al., 2011), whilst the recommendation from the UK Cystic Fibrosis Trust (2007) and North American CF Bone Health Consensus Statements (Aris et al., 2005) is a minimum level of 30 ng/mL (75 nmol/L).

Low or suboptimal vitamin D levels are common in most paediatric and adult patients with CF despite routine and high dose supplementation (Grey et al., 2008; Green et al., 2010). Although studies do not report a direct link between low vitamin D levels and low bone density, it is likely that low vitamin D levels do play a role in low bone mineral density in CF (Hall et al., 2010).

Vitamin D status may also be linked to lung function, with evidence of a positive association between lung function and serum vitamin D levels in children (Green et al., 2008) and adults (Stephenson et al., 2007) being reported.

Vitamin K

Severe vitamin K deficiency prolongs bleeding time. In CF, vitamin K deficiency has been associated with coagulopathies, including haematomas, intracerebral haemorrhage and severe life threatening bleeds (Hamid & Khan, 2007; McPhail, 2010). Subclinical vitamin K deficiency is common in pancreatic insufficient patients and universal in patients with CF related liver disease (Rashid et al., 1999) from an early age (Conway et al., 2005). This level of deficiency has been linked to reduced bone mineral density (Conway *et al.*, 2005).

Nutritional assessment

Individual assessment is essential to determine the interventions that are both appropriate and acceptable for each patient. Factors that need to be considered include age, clinical condition, nutritional status and history, pancreatic status, nutritional requirements, family circumstances, financial constraints, religious and cultural dietary beliefs, and food preferences and tolerances.

Anthropometry

This should include:

- Accurate measurement of weight, height, body mass index (BMI) (and head circumference in young children) should be undertaken at every clinic visit and plotted on the appropriate percentile chart in children (Sermet-Gaudelus *et al.*, 2011) (see Chapter 3.8).
- Assessment of pubertal stage in peripubertal children until puberty is complete (Sermet-Gaudelus *et al.*, 2011).
- Assessment of bone mineral density and body composition by dual energy X ray absorptiometry should be performed from around 8–10 years of age (Sermet-Gaudelus *et al.*, 2011).

Biochemistry

The following should be assessed:

- Annual assessment of fat soluble vitamin status (A, D, and E) (Borowitz *et al.*, 2009).
  - Assessment of vitamin A status in CF is difficult as both retinol and retinol binding protein (RBP) decrease during the acute phase response to infection; RBP is depressed in plasma zinc deficiency. Vitamin A status should be measured at a time of clinical stability together with RBP, plasma zinc and a positive acute phase protein such as C-reactive protein (CRP) (Stephenson & Gildengorin, 2000).
  - Serum or plasma vitamin E levels are used to assess vitamin E status. Vitamin E circulates in the blood bound to lipoproteins and therefore status is more accurately assessed using vitamin E to total lipid ratio in patients with high or low lipid levels.
  - Plasma 25 hydroxyvitamin D is the conventional marker of status. There should be awareness of seasonal variation in levels.
  - Assessment of vitamin K deficiency is difficult in CF as prothrombin time is not a very sensitive marker of vitamin K status. Protein or prothrombin induced by vitamin K absence or antagonism (PIVKA II) and undercarboxylated osteocalcin are more sensitive markers that are mostly used in research.
- Urea and electrolytes, liver function, full blood count at least annually.
- Annual oral glucose tolerance test.

Annual dietary assessment

The dietary assessment should include:

- Dietary intake including appetite.
- Contribution of oral supplements and enteral tube feeds.
- Knowledge and titration of PERT, including assessment of symptoms of malabsorption.
- Fat soluble vitamin supplementation.
- Use of non-prescribed supplements.
- Control of CF related diabetes.
- Other aspects of food intake, e.g. feeding behaviour problems or body image.

Nutritional management

Nutritional status has important prognostic significance, with a positive association being seen between body weight, height, BMI and survival (Corey *et al.*, 1988; Beker *et al.*, 2001; Stern *et al.*, 2008) and between nutritional status and lung function (Pedreira *et al.*, 2005). A diet that achieves and maintains good nutritional status is required to ensure that growth is optimised, resistance to infection maximised and outcome improved. Current recommendations state children and adolescents should achieve a BMI at or above the 50th percentile, adult females at or above $22 \, \text{kg/m}^2$ and adult males at or above $23 \, \text{kg/m}^2$ (Stallings *et al.*, 2008). Good nutrition education from diagnosis is needed in order to achieve these aims. Optimal PERT is an essential part of this education.

Pancreatic enzyme replacement therapy

The main aims of PERT are to:

- Enable a normal to high fat diet to be eaten.
- Control the signs and symptoms associated with maldigestion and malabsorption.
- Promote and maintain normal nutritional status and growth.
- Achieve optimal fat soluble vitamin and essential fatty acid status.

Types of enzyme preparations

The enteric coated, acid resistant microsphere and mini microsphere preparations are significantly more effective than the traditional powder based and enteric coated tablet formulations in correcting fat malabsorption. The enzymes are protected from inactivation by gastric acid and only release their activity when the pH rises above 5.5 in the duodenum, resulting in improved fat and nitrogen absorption (Littlewood *et al.*, 2006). In the USA, generic and prescribable proprietary PERT are available. Generic products should not be used in CF care (Borowitz *et al.*, 2009).

High strength enzyme preparations

High strength enzyme preparations became available in the mid 1980s. They were developed to improve PERT by reducing the number of capsules taken per meal. In the early 1990s, there were concerns about the safety of some high strength preparations, which were linked with the development of fibrosing colonopathy (colonic strictures), particularly in children (Smyth et al., 1994). As a result, the UK Committee on the Safety of Medicines (CSM, 1995) advised that:

- The total dose of lipase should not usually exceed 10 000 units/kg of body weight/day.
- Pancrease HL® and Nutrizym 22® should *not* be used in children with CF under 15 years.

It has been suggested that fibrosing colonopathy may be more closely related to the amount of methacrylic acid copolymer (MAC) coating in some preparations (Prescott & Bakowski, 1999). Consequently, in the UK the high strength preparations Creon 25000® and Creon 40000®, which do not contain MAC, are used for many adults and some paediatric patients. Changing to Creon 40000® has been shown to reduce total daily lipase dose with improvement in symptoms of malabsorption and an increase in body weight (Littlewood et al., 2011). Patients must receive detailed advice and assessment before they change their enzyme preparation.

Enzyme dosage and administration

To date, there are no studies in infants, children or adults to determine the optimal dose of PERT or whether there is a dose–response association (Stallings et al., 2008; Borowitz et al., 2009). Enzyme therapy is based on historical recommendations and consensus statements published after the reports of fibrosing colonopathy. Enzyme dose should be based on fat intake and taken with all fat containing food and drinks consumed. There is large individual variation in the enzyme dosage required, but it should not usually exceed 10 000 units of lipase/kg/day. In the USA, dosage is calculated as units of lipase/kg/meal (Stallings et al., 2008; Borowitz et al., 2009). The recommendations are:

- Newborn infants – 2000–5000 units of lipase/120 mL of feed and with increasing feed volume, no greater than 2500 units of lipase/kg of body weight/feed.
- Younger than 4 years – 1000 units of lipase/kg of body weight/meal.
- Older than 4 years – 500 units of lipase/kg of body weight/meal, with a recommended maximum of 2500 units of lipase/kg of body weight/meal.

Alternatively, the dose can be based on the fat content of meals and snacks. Australian guidelines recommend doses of 500–1000 units of lipase/g of fat for an infant and 500–4000 units of lipase/g of fat for a child or adult. The lowest effective dose of enzyme should be used (Anthony et al., 1999). Patients requiring >10 000 units of lipase/kg/day need assessment and further investigation.

Individual requirements for pancreatic enzymes depend upon a number of factors including:

- Degree of residual pancreatic function.
- Pharmacological characteristics of the preparation.

- Dissolution characteristics of the preparation – some patients may respond better to one product than another.
- Timing and method of enzyme administration.
- Fat content of the diet.
- Factors affecting pH within the gastrointestinal tract.

It is important to stress to patients that any dose adjustment should be dietetically or medically supervised to avoid inappropriate or excessive enzyme intake.

The method of enzyme administration is important. Microspheres must not be chewed or crushed as this will reduce enzyme efficacy. Microspheres should not be sprinkled on, or mixed with, the whole meal as exposure to hot food or food with a pH of >5.5 reduces efficacy. For infants and young children, microspheres should be mixed with a small amount of expressed breast milk, infant formula or a little semi solid food, e.g. apple purée, and given from a teaspoon with feeds. The capsules should be swallowed whole as early as possible; most children will manage this by 3–4 years of age (Sinaasappel et al., 2002). Enzymes are best given in a divided dose with half before the meal and half during it, though this may vary between individuals and adjustment of the timing of administration may be necessary. Guidelines on PERT are summarised in Box 7.4.5.

> **Box 7.4.5** Guidelines for the use of pancreatic enzyme preparations
>
> Enzymes should be taken with all fat containing meals, snacks and drinks
>
> Enzymes should be taken with every meal, with ideally half the dosage being taken before and half during the meal
>
> If meals last longer than 30 minutes, enzymes should be taken before, during and towards the end of the meal
>
> The dose should be varied according to the fat content of food with extra enzymes taken with higher fat meals and snacks
>
> Enzymes should not be taken with fat free snacks and drinks, e.g. soft drinks, fruit drinks, fruit, glucose polymer supplements, boiled or jelly sweets
>
> Capsules containing enteric coated tablets or microspheres should be swallowed without being chewed (to avoid losing their effectiveness). For young children, or if swallowing is difficult, the capsules should be opened and the contents mixed with a little soft food or fruit purée and administered from a teaspoon. Granules must not be sprinkled over a meal
>
> Under medical/dietetic supervision, the enzyme dose should be increased (e.g. by one to two capsules) if the stools are fatty, loose, offensive or frequent.
>
> Adequate hydration is important, especially with higher strength enzyme preparations
>
> Enzymes should be taken with all fat containing enteral tube feeds; they should not be added to the feed or routinely administered via the feeding tube.

Monitoring the effectiveness

Even with modern PERT, maldigestion and malabsorption may still occur. Factors that may contribute to inadequate PERT include:

- *Patients failing to recognise or report steatorrhoea* – patients tend to become accustomed to what is a normal stool pattern for them and may fail to recognise symptoms of steatorrhoea and that their enzyme dosage needs adjusting.
- *Inadequate education* – knowledge of enzyme titration according to dietary fat intake and timing of administration may be inadequate.
- *Lack of regular dietetic assessment* – regular assessment PERT is essential to achieve an appropriate balance between PERT and food intake (Littlewood *et al.*, 2006).
- *Non-adherence with guidance given* – patients may not take their PERT or adhere to advice given in respect of timing or dosage. People with CF should be encouraged to openly discuss any adherence issues they experience.
- *Other factors*, including low duodenal pH, e.g. due to excessive production of gastric acid or reduced pancreatic bicarbonate, can result in inappropriate release or inactivation of enzymes. Practical considerations such as enzyme storage and stock rotation are also important as enzymes denature over time.

The efficacy of PERT can be assessed by measurement of faecal fat and calculation of the coefficient of fat absorption or stool weight, although these are now mainly used as research tools in the UK. Faecal fat microscopy and steatocrit may also be used. More usually, effectiveness of PERT is monitored by assessment of nutritional status or growth and abdominal symptoms.

Nutritional requirements

Energy

The dietary energy requirements of people with CF are usually higher than those recommended for the general population. This is due to the increased energy expenditure resulting from inflammation and infection, and continuing energy losses due to malabsorption. It has generally been accepted that energy requirements for people with CF are 120–150% of the estimated average requirement for energy. More recently, energy intakes of 110–200% of those of the healthy population have been recommended (Stallings *et al.*, 2008). However, as a result of early diagnosis by newborn screening and the variability of disease expression, individual energy needs will vary greatly.

Protein

Protein requirements have not been well researched but it is generally accepted that the protein intake should be higher than average to compensate for loss of nitrogen in the faeces and sputum.

Fat

Fat restriction to reduce symptoms of steatorrhoea is not necessary with modern PERT. Restricting fat compromises energy intake, fat soluble vitamins and essential fatty status. It is usually recommended that fat provide 35–40% of energy, although in practice studies shows that this is difficult to achieve, with intakes of between 30% and 35% more likely (White *et al.*, 2004). With increasing longevity and a greater variability in clinical condition, consideration needs to be given to dietary composition in relation to long term health. A relatively high fat intake should not solely be achieved by an excessive intake of saturated fat. Fats such as spreads and oils can be derived from monounsaturated sources. Olive oil can be drizzled on food to increase the energy density, instead of deep frying. Patients should be individually assessed and advised, and if overweight or obese, fat restriction would be appropriate. The dietary intake of the n-3 fatty acids should be as recommended for the general population. More research is required to determine the efficacy of intervention with pharmacological doses. The use of medium chain triglyceride oil preparations in cooking is no longer recommended as it is unpalatable and PERT is still needed to aid absorption.

Dietary fibre

The need for an energy dense diet means that the intake of fibre may be low. Recommendations for fibre intake in CF are limited. Further research in this area is needed due to the complexity of the CF gut.

Water soluble vitamins

Routine supplementation is unnecessary; diets should be assessed individually for dietary adequacy. Parenteral vitamin B_{12} may be required following resection of the terminal ileum for meconium ileus (Sinaasappel *et al.*, 2002).

Fat soluble vitamins

Vitamins A, D, E and K should be provided from diagnosis onwards in pancreatic insufficient patients. Vitamin requirements vary, so regimens often combine a multivitamin preparation (or A and D capsules), an additional vitamin E supplement and a vitamin K supplement. To achieve adequate plasma levels of vitamin D, an additional separate vitamin D supplement is usually necessary to avoid vitamin A toxicity. Specific CF vitamin supplements are available, but often still need the addition of extra vitamin D and K.

Annual monitoring of plasma levels is recommended as a minimum for all patients. It is essential that all patients are individually assessed and that doses are adjusted depending on plasma levels. Pancreatic sufficient patients often require vitamin D supplementation to achieve adequate levels. Hypervitaminosis A and E have been reported in patients with CF following lung transplantation (Stephenson *et al.*, 2005) and higher plasma levels have also been found in children and young adults compared with the general population (Huang *et al.*, 2006; Maqbool *et al.*, 2008). Deficiency is the primary concern in patients with CF, but with early diagnosis and improved treatments the consequence of high levels is also of concern.

Current recommendations for fat soluble vitamin supplementation in pancreatic insufficient patients are based on historical data and vary between countries (Sinaasappel *et al.*, 2002; Borowitz *et al.*, 2009; Sermet-Gaudelus *et al.*, 2010). The recommended starting doses per day are:

- *Vitamin A:*
  - Younger than 1 year: 1500 IU (455 μg) (Sermet-Gaudelus *et al.*, 2010).
  - Older than year: 4000–10 000 IU (1200–3000 μg) (Cystic Fibrosis Trust Nutrition Working Group, 2002).
- *Vitamin E:*
  - Younger than 1 year: 10–50 mg.
  - Older than 1 year: 50–100 mg.
  - Adults: 100–200 mg (Cystic Fibrosis Trust Working Group, 2002).
- *Vitamin D:*
  - Younger than 1 year: 1000–2000 IU (25–50 μg).
  - Older than year and adults: 1000–5000 IU (25–125 μg/day) (Sermet-Gaudelus *et al.*, 2011).
- *Vitamin K:*
  - Younger than 2 years: 300 μg/kg rounded to the nearest mg.
  - 2–7 years: 5 mg.
  - Older than 7 years: 10 mg (Cystic Fibrosis Trust, 2007).

Minerals and trace elements

Sodium

Cystic fibrosis results in an abnormally high concentration of sodium excreted in sweat, and sodium losses are increased in conditions causing excessive sweating, e.g. hot climates or extreme physical exertion. In these circumstances salt supplements are recommended.

Iron

Iron deficiency is common and increases with age (von Drygalski & Biller, 2008). It is related to disease severity, malabsorption and loss of iron in the sputum rather than dietary deficiency and there should be awareness of increased iron requirements.

Calcium

Reduced bone mineral density is common in adolescents and adults with CF. Negative calcium balance may be due to malabsorption, increased endogenous faecal losses of calcium (Schulze *et al.*, 2003) and vitamin D insufficiency. Attention to calcium intakes is important and supplementation may be necessary.

To meet the nutritional requirements of people with CF, a staged approach to nutritional intervention is rec-

ommended (Cystic Fibrosis Trust Working Group, 2002; Sinaasappel *et al.*, 2002).

First stage intervention: improving food and energy intake

Increasing meal frequency, choosing energy dense foods and using food fortification measures are the first stage of intervention. In the USA, behavioural intervention in conjunction with nutritional counselling is recommended in children 1–12 years of age to promote weight gain (Stallings *et al.*, 2008).

Second stage intervention: supplements

There should always be an emphasis on the use of normal food rather than supplements, but if intake remains poor despite encouraging a high energy diet, oral dietary supplements are the next stage of intervention. These include modular products, e.g. glucose polymer liquids and powders, fat emulsions or mixed fat and carbohydrate products, or sip feeds supplements. A systematic review (Smyth & Walters, 2000) highlighted the lack of evidence of efficacy for oral energy supplements in CF. However, this does not mean they are not of benefit to individuals.

A multicentre study of short term use of a high fat milk based supplement demonstrated significant weight gain in individuals with CF (Skypala *et al.*, 1998). In contrast, a small study comparing the use of oral supplements with dietary counselling over a 3-month period found no significant change in energy intake or nutritional status in either group (Kalnins *et al.*, 2005). In adults however, supplements have been shown to be effective in significantly increasing energy intakes when compared with diet alone (White *et al.*, 2004). A large, longer term randomised controlled trial of oral supplements in mild to moderately malnourished children with CF found no improvement in nutritional status or other clinical outcomes. It concluded '*oral supplements should not be regarded as an essential part of the management of mildly malnourished children with CF*' (Poustie *et al.*, 2006). However, the study did not consider the use of supplements in adult patients, the short term use in acute situations, in more severely malnourished individuals or those with end stage lung disease, or the impact of energy only supplements.

A CF specialist dietitian should carefully monitor the introduction, use and efficacy of supplements. The type and quantity of supplement recommended depends on the patient's age, preference and requirements. Supplements should be taken in addition to normal food to increase total daily energy intake and should not replace a meal. Ideally, they should be given with a snack between meals, as a drink after meals or later in the evening. Altering the type or flavour of the supplement may help to prevent taste fatigue.

Third stage intervention: enteral tube feeding

Enteral tube feeding is considered when dietary education, behavioural intervention and oral nutritional supplementation fail to improve nutritional status. Enteral tube feeds can be provided via a fine bore nasogastric tube, gastrostomy or, more rarely, jejunostomy. In the UK, approximately 20% of patients are gastrostomy fed and 5% nasogastrically fed (Cystic Fibrosis Trust, 2011). There is no evidence to show which route is most effective; the choice depends largely on patient preference and the likely duration of supplementary feeding. Early reports of enteral tube feeding were limited by methodology, sample size and duration, but weight gain or improved growth was reported. Few studies have assessed efficacy of long term tube feeding in different age groups and a Cochrane Systematic Review reports no randomised controlled trials (Conway et al., 1999).

Earlier intervention is associated with improved outcomes (Walker & Gozal, 1998; Oliver et al., 2004). Gastrostomy feeding in children with mild respiratory compromise was shown to improve weight and height gain during the first year of feeding; this stabilised during the second year but no improvement in respiratory function was reported (Truby et al., 2009). Studies do report stabilisation of lung function (Efrati et al., 2006), but nutritional support may need to be long term in order for there to be significant benefits.

Enteral tube feeds are usually administered overnight and provide 30 – 50% of total energy requirements (Steinkamp & von der Hardt, 1994). Some patients may receive a greater proportion of their energy needs, if oral intake is particularly poor or nutritional requirements are exceptionally high.

Feed formulae

Whole protein, polymeric feeds are usually well tolerated in patients with CF. Adults and older children are usually given energy dense feeds (1.5–2 kcal/mL); however, occasionally a specialist high fat feed formulated for people with pulmonary disease may be used or additional fat added as a fat emulsion to increase fat intake and energy density. This allows smaller volumes of feed to be administered. Young children are usually given paediatric whole protein feeds providing 1.5 kcal/mL. Infants should be given a high energy infant formula.

Low fat elemental feeds are not usually required for patients with CF, although they are still widely used in some countries. It has been hypothesised that they are better absorbed in people with CF, but they are expensive, have a high osmolality and generally a lower energy density than whole protein feeds. Elemental formulae with a high proportion of MCT fat have been shown to improve weight gain even in patients with advanced lung disease (Williams et al., 1999). There remains controversy as to whether these preparations require PERT, with one study showing that their absorption may be equivalent to that of whole protein formulae with enzyme replacement (Erskine et al., 1998). Clinical practice varies and optimum feed type has yet to be established and may vary with clinical situations.

Enzyme administration during enteral tube feeds

Pancreatic enzymes are usually administered orally at the beginning of the feed and sometimes during or at the end of the feed. Enzyme requirements are dependent on the rate of infusion, type and fat content of the feed. As the feed is continuously infused over a long period, lower doses of enzymes are required than would be normally administered with a meal containing the equivalent fat content. Increased gastric lipase production (Balasubramanian et al., 1992) may also help fat digestion from continuously infused feeds. The method of enzyme administration varies between countries and the optimum pattern of enzyme administration remains to be established.

Problems with enteral tube feeding

Complications with tube feeding in CF are rare. Nasogastric tube displacement, although uncommon may occur due to coughing, vomiting or physiotherapy. Nocturnal hyperglycaemia requiring insulin therapy may occur in patients given night time feeds (Smith et al., 1994). Careful monitoring of blood glucose levels are essential when feeds are introduced and periodically thereafter.

Parenteral nutrition

Parenteral nutritional support is not recommended for long term treatment, but may be useful for short term support when enteral tube feeding is contraindicated, e.g. after major gastrointestinal surgery or in severely ill patients awaiting transplantation (Sinaasappel et al., 2002).

Special considerations

Infants

The success of National Newborn Screening Programmes for Cystic Fibrosis depends on the appropriate management of identified infants and improved outcomes. Management of the newborn infant diagnosed through newborn screening is, for many, different from the nutritional management of those diagnosed symptomatically. The focus is on maintaining health by preventing nutritional and respiratory complications (Borowitz et al., 2009; Sermet-Gaudelus et al., 2010). There is a lack of well designed clinical trials to support practice, hence management has developed mainly through clinical experience. In 2009, the North American CF Foundation developed recommendations for management of infants based on a systematic review of the evidence and expert opinion (Borowitz et al., 2009). In 2010, The European Cystic Fibrosis Society Neonatal Screening Group used a modified Delphi Methodology to provide a consensus framework for the management of screened infants (Sermet-Gaudelus et al., 2010).

Most infants will thrive if given breast milk or standard infant formula. Breast feeding should be encouraged. The routine use of hydrolysed formula is not recommended but it may be required for infants who have undergone surgical resection for meconium ileus or those with malabsorption unrelated to CF, e.g. cow's milk protein intolerance (Borowitz et al., 2009; Sermet-Gaudelus et al., 2010).

SECTION 7

If fat malabsorption is adequately controlled, infants will usually thrive on energy intakes of 100–130 kcal/kg of body weight/day. If the infant is failing to thrive despite optimising their milk intake and PERT, energy intakes should be adapted to achieve normal growth. A higher energy infant formula should be prescribed. Alternatively, breast fed infants may be offered top up formula feeds.

All pancreatic insufficient infants should be commenced on PERT at a starting dose of 2000 units of lipase/100 mL of standard formula or breast feed. The dose should be increased if there are symptoms of malabsorption or inadequate weight gain, but the lipase intake should be kept below 10 000 units/kg of body weight/day (Sermet-Gaudelus et al., 2010). Enteric coated microspheres/mini microspheres should be given on a teaspoon with all feeds mixed with a small amount of the infant's milk or a small amount of fruit purée. They should not be added directly to a bottle of feed.

Gastro-oesophageal reflux is common in infants with CF (Heine et al., 1998). Unless treated, this may compromise growth and exacerbate respiratory symptoms. Treatments include thickening feeds, and using a prethickened infant formula and motility stimulants.

All pancreatic insufficient infants should be given fat soluble vitamin supplements in liquid form from diagnosis. Sodium chloride supplementation should be considered for all infants with CF and increased during hot weather or other times of increased salt loss, e.g. diarrhoea (Sermet-Gaudelus et al., 2010).

Weaning foods should be introduced between 4 and 6 months of age, and a normal weaning diet should be established by the end of the first year. The dose of PERT should be adjusted to the fat content of the weaning food. Commercial weaning foods are low in salt and sugar; therefore, dietary advice is essential at this time.

Preconception

There is little evidence upon which to base recommendations for nutritional management of women with CF in the preconceptional period, during pregnancy and post partum. Recommendations are therefore largely based on the recommendations for the non-CF population, but are adapted and modified to incorporate knowledge and understanding of the nutritional requirements of CF. As nutritional status plays an integral role in the preconceptional period and throughout pregnancy, a thorough preconceptional nutritional assessment should be performed (Edenborough et al., 2008). This should include:

- Assessment of weight, height and BMI.
- Dietary assessment and review of PERT, gastrointestinal symptoms and absorption.
- Assessment of glycaemic status by oral glucose tolerance test in the non-diabetic patient or optimising glycaemic control in those with CFRD.
- Increasing awareness of food safety issues.
- Measurement of fasting plasma vitamins A, D and E, and review of vitamin therapy (including non-prescription items).

Care should be taken to avoid excessive intakes of vitamin A because of the risk of teratogenicity. In practice, supplemental vitamin A is usually continued at a dose of <10 000 IU/day and plasma levels are closely monitored (Edenborough et al., 2008).

Pregnancy

Due to increased life expectancy, pregnancy in women with CF is becoming increasingly common. Pregnancy is generally well tolerated although there are increased risks to both mother and child. Prepregnancy lung function and nutritional status are important predictors of foetal and maternal outcome (Lau et al., 2011). Poor foetal outcomes have been associated with a poor prepregnancy weight (BMI <20 kg/m^2) and a forced expiratory volume of <60% predicted values (Lau et al., 2011). A high incidence of gestational diabetes has been reported (Lau et al., 2011). Early participation of the MDT is essential to ensure an optimal outcome.

During pregnancy the primary nutritional aims are to:

- Achieve adequate weight gain – regular monitoring of nutritional status and weight gain is essential to optimise outcomes. Oral nutritional supplements or enteral tube feeding may be required.
- Minimise the impact of pregnancy related problems on food intake. Due to hormonal and mechanical changes in pregnancy, gastro-oesophageal reflux, heartburn, nausea, vomiting and constipation may occur more frequently. These can be more common in women with CF and can reduce food intake. Guidance on ways to alleviate these problems and improve nutrient intake are essential.

Successful breastfeeding in mothers with CF has been achieved (Gilljam et al., 2000). Breast feeding increases maternal nutritional requirements. Individual advice about infant feeding according to the mother's clinical condition and circumstances should be given. Many drugs pass into breast milk and therefore may be contraindicateds during pregnancy and lactation, or are contraindicated during breastfeeding (Edenborough et al., 2008).

Cystic fibrosis related diabetes

Cystic fibrosis related diabetes (CFRD) is the most common comorbidity in people with CF and its prevalence increases with age. Data suggest 2% of children, 19% of adolescents and 40–50% of adults have CFRD (Moran et al., 2009). Few people with CF have normal glucose tolerance and CFRD is part of a spectrum of glucose tolerance abnormalities (Moran et al., 2010). Cystic fibrosis related diabetes shares features of type 1 and type 2 diabetes, but it is a distinct entity.

Cystic fibrosis related diabetes is primarily caused by insulin deficiency due to loss of insulin secreting beta cells within the islets of Langerhans. The causes are multifactorial (Nathan et al., 2010), but obstruction of pancreatic ducts by abnormal, thick secretions causing progressive pancreatic damage is a major factor. In CF there is also an element of insulin resistance (Hardin et al., 2001).

Cystic fibrosis related diabetes mainly occurs in people with the most severe CF mutations that are associated with exocrine pancreatic insufficiency (Adler et al., 2008). The importance of early detection, treatment and optimising control of CFRD cannot be overemphasised as CFRD is associated with deterioration in respiratory function and clinical and nutritional status, and increased morbidity and mortality. The negative impact of diabetes on nutritional decline appears to be more pronounced in those who are still growing during the prediabetic years (White et al., 2009). Optimising control of CFRD is important as microvascular complications are increasingly recognised.

Patients with CFRD should be managed by a specialised multidisciplinary team with expertise in diabetes and CF. Oral diabetic agents are not as effective as insulin in improving nutritional and metabolic outcomes, and therefore insulin is the medical treatment of choice (Moran et al., 2010).

The primary aim of treatment in CFRD is to maintain nutritional status. The maintenance of a diet high in energy, fat, protein and sodium to compensate for losses is important. This is in contrast to the management of type 1 and type 2 diabetes. The diet should also be healthy and well balanced. Some substitution of saturated fat with monounsaturated fat is advisable as long as this does not compromise total energy intake. The use of carbohydrate counting to guide insulin therapy can help to optimise control. If a patient with CFRD is malnourished, overnight enteral feeding with an adjusted insulin regimen can be given. All patients should receive individualised dietary review and advice at the time of the diagnosis of CFRD. Awareness of emerging issues, such as obesity, in some people with CF make this even more important. In a minority of patients, it may be necessary to consider energy restriction.

Cystic fibrosis associated liver disease

Cystic fibrosis associated liver disease (CFLD) occurs in 27–35% of patients and 5–10% will develop multilobular cirrhosis in the first decade of life. Portal hypertension often develops during the second decade and liver failure usually occurs in adulthood (Debray et al., 2011). Liver disease may make it increasingly difficult to meet nutritional requirements. It further exacerbates malnutrition by increasing steatorrhoea, which is often unresponsive to increasing enzyme dosage. Oral intake may be reduced as a result of nausea, early satiety resulting from an enlarged liver and/or spleen and abdominal pain.

Nutritional support is an essential part of treatment of CFLD and optimising nutritional status is the primary goal. Close monitoring is essential, especially if the disease progresses to end stage ascites and encephalopathy. Nasogastric feeding may be required to meet energy requirements. Gastrostomy feeding is not recommended in advanced liver disease because of the risk of a gastric haemorrhage (Debray et al., 2011).

Distal intestinal obstruction syndrome

Distal intestinal obstruction syndrome (DIOS) is caused by the accumulation of viscous mucus and intestinal contents that completely or partially block the intestinal lumen. Incomplete or impending DIOS is common and patients present with a short history of abdominal pain and/or distension and a faecal mass in the ileocaecum. Complete DIOS is less common, but in addition to the features of incomplete DIOS, the patient has a complete intestinal obstruction with vomiting of bilious material and/or fluid levels in the small intestine on abdominal X ray (Columbo et al., 2011).

Risk factors for DIOS include a severe genotype associated with pancreatic insufficiency (though it does occur in pancreatic sufficient patients), a history of meconium ileus at birth, previous episodes of DIOS, poorly controlled fat absorption, dehydration and CFRD (Columbo et al., 2011).

Both DIOS and incomplete DIOS are initially managed medically. Assessment of PERT and absorption should be undertaken, including knowledge of enzyme titration, timing and adherence with therapy. Advice about increasing fluid intake is also important. The role of increasing fibre intake is unclear (van der Doef et al., 2011) and this should only be done with caution.

Lung or heart and lung transplantation

Lung transplantation has become a viable option for CF patients with end stage lung disease. Some may be declined for transplantation based on low weight as poor nutritional status is linked with increased mortality and poorer outcomes. Most patients will have had intensive nutritional input throughout life that makes nutritional management in the pretransplant period challenging or existing interventions more complex. Maximising oral intake can be difficult due to anorexia, dyspnoea, early satiety, dry mouth or taste changes due to oxygen or drug therapy. In addition, exceptionally high energy requirements, metabolic consequences of respiratory failure, presence of CFRD and need for non-invasive ventilation in some can make enteral tube feeding challenging. Some centres may use appetite stimulants at this time.

In the early postoperative period, a clean diet is usually recommended with awareness of food safety issues. Restoring and maintaining optimal nutritional status is a priority. In the long term, other nutritional problems may emerge, e.g. diabetes due to corticosteroids and other forms of immunosuppression, hyperlipideamia, high plasma levels of the fat soluble vitamins, osteoporosis and renal failure.

Cystic fibrosis related low bone mineral density

Reduced bone mineral density is common in adolescents and adults with CF. Bone mineral content (BMC) and bone mineral density (BMD) are usually normal in well nourished children with good lung function, though several cross-sectional studies report low BMC/BMD in some children with CF (Sermet-Gaudelus et al., 2011).

SECTION 7

The aetiology of bone disease in CF is multifactorial. Risk factors include poor nutritional status and reduced lean body mass, vitamins D and K deficiency, poor calcium intake and negative calcium balance, delayed puberty, infection, inflammation, the use of corticosteroids (Sermet-Gaudelus *et al.*, 2011) and abnormal CFTR expression in bone cells (Haworth, 2010).

Bone mineral acquisition in childhood, especially during the pubertal growth spurt in adolescence, is a major determinant of adult bone health. It is therefore essential to implement prevention strategies and from diagnosis to address issues relating to bone health in people with CF. Dietetic management should focus on:

- Optimising weight gain and growth with particular attention to lean body mass.
- Optimising vitamin D and vitamin K status and supplementation protocols.
- Optimising skeletal accretion of calcium by attention to calcium intakes and supplementation where necessary.
- Encouraging appropriate physical activity with the support of the CF specialist physiotherapist.

Drug–nutrient interactions

The following should be noted:

- Vitamin A – hepatotoxic drugs, retinoids, tetracycline antibiotics, warfarin.
- Vitamin E – anticoagulant drugs, ciclosporin, warfarin.
- Vitamin K – warfarin.
- Calcium – bisphosphonates, quinolone antibiotics, tetracycline antibiotics.

Internet resources

Cystic Fibrosis Foundation   www.cff.org
Cystic Fibrosis Medicine   www.cfmedicine.com
Cystic Fibrosis Mutation Database   www.genet.sickkids.on.ca
Cystic Fibrosis Trust   www.cftrust.org.uk
Cystic Fibrosis World Wide   www.cfww.org

References

Adler AI, Shine BSF, Chamnan P, Haworth CS, Bilton D. (2008) Genetic determinants and epidemiology of cystic fibrosis-related diabetes. Results from a British cohort of children and adults. *Diabetes Care* 31: 1789–1794.

Aird FK, Greene SA, Ogston SA, Macdonald TM, Mukhopadhyay S. (2006) Vitamin A and lung function in CF. *Journal of Cystic Fibrosis* 5: 129–131.

Andersen DH. (1938) Cystic fibrosis of the pancreas and its relation to celiac disease: a clinical and pathological study. *American Journal of Diseases in Childhood* 56: 344–399.

Anthony H, Collins CE, Davidson G, *et al.* (1999) Pancreatic enzyme replacement therapy in cystic fibrosis: Australian guidelines. Paediatric Gastroenterological Society and the Dietitians Association of Australia. *Journal of Paediatrics and Child Health* 35: 125–129.

Aris RM, Merkel PA, Bachrach LK, *et al.* (2005) Guide to bone health and disease. *Clinical Endocrinology and Metabolism* 90: 1888–1896.

Balasubramanian K, Zentler-Munro PL, Batten JC, Northfield TC. (1992) Increased intragastric acid-resistant lipase activity and lipolysis in pancreatic steatorrhoea due to cystic fibrosis. *Pancreas* 7: 305–310.

Beker LT, Russek-Cohen E, Fink RJ. (2001) Stature as a prognostic factor in cystic fibrosis survival. *Journal of the American Dietetic Association* 101: 438–442.

Biesalski HK, Nohr D. (2003) Importance of vitamin – A for lung function and development. *Molecular Aspects of Medicine* 24: 431–440.

Borowitz D, Robinson KA, Rosenfeld M, *et al.* (2009). Cystic Fibrosis Foundation evidence-based guidelines for management of infants with cystic fibrosis. *Journal of Pediatrics* 155: S73–93.

Chandra RK. (1988) Increased bacterial binding to respiratory epithelial cells in vitamin A deficiency. *BMJ* 297: 834–835.

Columbo C, Ellemunter H, Houwen R, Munck A, Taylor C, Wilschanski M, on behalf of the ECFS. (2011) Guidelines for the diagnosis and management of distal intestinal obstruction syndrome in cystic fibrosis patients. *Journal of Cystic Fibrosis* 10: S24–S28.

Committee on Safety of Medicines. (1995) *Report of the Pancreatic Enzyme Working Party*. Medicines Control Agency UK.

Conway SP, Morton A, Wolfe S. (1999) Enteral tube feeding for cystic fibrosis. *Cochrane Database of Systematic Reviews* 3: CD001198.

Conway SP, Wolfe SP, Brownlee KG, *et al.* (2005) Vitamin K status among children with cystic fibrosis and its relationship to bone mineral density and bone turnover. *Pediatrics* 115: 1325–1331.

Corey M, McLaughlin FJ, Williams M, Levison H. (1988) A comparison of survival, growth and pulmonary function in patients with cystic fibrosis in Boston and Toronto. *Journal of Clinical Epidemiology* 41: 583–591.

Cystic Fibrosis Trust Nutrition Working Group. (2002) *Nutritional Management of Cystic Fibrosis*. London: Cystic Fibrosis Trust.

Cystic Fibrosis Trust. (2007) *Bone Mineralisation in Cystic Fibrosis*. UK Cystic Fibrosis Trust Bone Mineralisation Working Group. Bromley: Cystic Fibrosis Trust.

Cystic Fibrosis Trust. (2011) *UK CF Registry Annual Data Report 2009*. Bromley: Cystic Fibrosis Trust.

Cystic Fibrosis Mutation Database. (2011) Population variation table. Available at www.gent.sickkids.on.ca. Accessed 19 October 2012.

Debray D, Kelly D, Houwen, R, Strandvik B, Colombo C. (2011) Best practice guidance for the diagnosis and management of cystic fibrosis-associated liver disease. *Journal of Cystic Fibrosis* 10: S29–S36.

Dodge JA, Lewis PA, Stanton M, Wilsher J. (2007) Cystic fibrosis mortality and survival in the UK: 1947–2003. *European Respiratory Journal* 29: 522–526.

Edenborough FP, Borgo G, Knoop C, *et al.* (2008) Guidelines for the management of pregnancy in women with cystic fibrosis. *Journal of Cystic Fibrosis* 7: S2–S32.

Efrati O, Mei-Zahav M, Rivlin J, *et al.* (2006) Long term nutritional rehabilitation by gastrostomy in Israeli patients with cystic fibrosis: clinical outcome in advanced pulmonary disease. *Journal of Pediatric Gastroenterology and Nutrition* 42(2): 222–228.

Elkin SL, Vedi S, Bord S, Garrahan NJ, Hodson ME, Compston JE. (2002) Histomorphometric analysis of bone biopsies from the iliac crest of adults with cystic fibrosis. *American Journal of Respiratory and Critical Care Medicine* 166: 1470–1474.

Erskine JM, Lingard CD, Sontag MG, Accurso FJ. (1998) Enteral nutrition for patients with cystic fibrosis: comparison of a semi-elemental and non elemental formula. *Journal of Pediatrics* 132: 265–269.

Gilljam M, Antoniou M, Shin J, Dupuis A, Corey M, Tullis DE. (2000) Pregnancy in cystic fibrosis. Fetal and maternal outcome. *Chest* 118: 85–91.

Green D, Carson K, Leonard A, *et al.* (2008) Current treatment recommendations for correcting vitamin D deficiency in pediatric patients with cystic fibrosis are inadequate. *Journal of Pediatrics* 153(4): 554–559.

Green DM, Leonard AR, Paranjape SM, Rosenstein BJ, Zeitlin PL, Mogayzel Jr PJ. (2010) Transient effectiveness of vitamin D_2 therapy in pediatric cystic fibrosis patients. *Journal of Cystic Fibrosis* 9: 143–149.

Grey V, Atkinson S, Dury D, *et al*. (2008) Prevalence of low bone mass and deficiencies of vitamin D and K in pediatric patients with cystic fibrosis from 3 Canadian centers. *Pediatrics* 122: 1014–1020.

Hakim F, Kerem E, Rivlin J, *et al*. (2007) Vitamin A and E and pulmonary exacerbations in patients with cystic fibrosis. *Journal of Pediatric Gastroenterology and Nutrition* 45: 347–353.

Hall WB, Sparks AA, Aris RM. (2010) Vitamin D deficiency in cystic fibrosis. *International Journal of Endocrinology* 2010: 218691.

Hamid B, Khan A. (2007) Cerebral hemorrhage as the initial manifestation of cystic fibrosis. *Journal of Child Neurology* 22: 114 2010:218691115.

Hardin DS, LeBlanc A, Marshall, G, Seilheimer DK. (2001) Mechanisms of insulin resistance in cystic fibrosis. *American Journal of Physiology, Endocrinology and Metabolism* 281: 1022–1028.

Haworth CS. (2010) Impact of cystic fibrosis on bone health. *Current Opinion in Pulmonary Medicine* 16: 616–622.

Heine, RG, Button BM, Olinsky A, Phelan PD, Catto-Smith AG. (1998) Gastro-oesophageal reflux in infants under 6 months with cystic fibrosis. *Archive of Diseases in Childhood* 78: 44–48.

Holick MF, Chen TC. (2008) Vitamin D deficiency: a worldwide problem with health consequences. *American Journal of Clinical Nutrition* 87: S1080–S1086.

Huang SH, Schall JI, Zemel BS, Stallings VA. (2006) Vitamin E status in children with cystic fibrosis and pancreatic insufficiency. *Journal of Pediatrics* 148: 556–559.

Huet F, Semama D, Maingueneau C, Charavel A, Nivelon JL. (1997) Vitamin A deficiency and nocturnal vision in teenagers with cystic fibrosis. *European Journal of Pediatrics* 156: 949–951.

Kalnins D, Corey M, Ellis L, Pencharz PB, Tullis E, Durie PR. (2005) Failure of conventional strategies to improve nutritional status in malnourished adolescents and adults with cystic fibrosis. *Journal of Pediatrics* 147: 399–401.

Koscik RL, Lai HC, Laxova A, *et al*. (2005) Preventing early, prolonged vitamin E deficiency: an opportunity for better cognitive outcomes via early diagnosis through neonatal screening. *Journal of Pediatrics* 147: S51–S56.

Lau EMT, Barnes DJ, Moriarty C, *et al*. (2011) Pregnancy outcomes in the current era of cystic fibrosis care: A 15-year experience. *Australian and New Zealand Journal of Obstetrics and Gynaecology* 51: 220–224.

Lewis PA. (2000) The epidemiology of cystic fibrosis. In Hodson ME, Geddes DM (eds) *Cystic Fibrosis*, 2nd edn. London: Arnold, pp. 13–25.

Littlewood JM, Wolfe SP, Conway SP. (2006) Diagnosis and treatment of intestinal malabsorption in cystic fibrosis. *Pediatric Pulmonology* 41: 35–49.

Littlewood JM, Connett GJ, Sander-Struckmeier, S, Henniges F; Creon 40,000 Study Group. (2011) A 2-year post-authorization safety study of high-strength pancreatic enzyme replacement therapy (pancreatin 40,000) in cystic fibrosis. *Expert Opinion in Drug Safety* 10: 197–203.

Maqbool A, Stallings VA. (2008) Update on fat-soluble vitamins in cystic fibrosis. *Current Opinion in Pulmonary Medicine* 14: 574–581.

Maqbool A, Graham-Marr RC, Schall J, Zemel B, Stallings VA. (2008) Vitamin A intake and elevated serum retinol levels in children and young adults with cystic fibrosis. *Journal of Cystic Fibrosis* 7: 137–141.

McCullough FSW, Northrop-Clewes CA, Thurnham DI. (1999) The effect of vitamin A on epithelial integrity. *Proceedings of the Nutrition Society* 58: 289–293.

McPhail GL. (2010) Coagulation disorder as a presentation of cystic fibrosis. *Journal of Emergency Medicine* 38: 320–322.

Moran A, Dunitz J, Nathan B, Saeed A, Holme B, Thomas W. (2009) Cystic fibrosis-related diabetes: Current trends in prevalence, incidence, and mortality. *Diabetes Care* 32: 1626–1631.

Moran A, Brunzell C, Cohen RC, *et al*.; CFRD Guidelines Committee. (2010) Clinical care guidelines for cystic fibrosis-related diabetes. A position statement of the American Diabetes Association and a clinical practice guideline of the Cystic Fibrosis Foundation, endorsed by the Pediatric Endocrine Association. *Diabetes Care* 22: 2697–2708.

Nathan BM, Laguna T, Moran A. (2010) Recent trends in cystic fibrosis-related diabetes. *Current Opinion in Endocrinology, Diabetes and Obesity* 7: 335–341.

Neville LA, Ranganathan SC. (2009) Vitamin D in infants with cystic fibrosis diagnosed by newborn screening. *Journal of Pediatrics and Child Health* 45: 36–41.

Oliver MR, Heine RG, Ng CH, Volders E, Olinsky A. (2004) Factors affecting clinical outcome in gastrostomy-fed children with cystic fibrosis. *Pediatric Pulmonology* 37: 324–329.

Pedreira CC, Robert RG, Dalton V, *et al*. (2005) Association of body composition and lung function in children with cystic fibrosis. *Pediatric Pulmonology* 39: 276–280.

Petersen RA, Petersen VS, Robb RM. (1968) Vitamin A deficiency with xerophthalmia and night blindness in cystic fibrosis. *American Journal of Diseases in Childhood* 116: 662–665.

Poustie VJ, Russell JE, Watling RM, Ashby D, Smyth RL: CALICO Trial Collaborative Group. (2006) Oral protein energy supplements for children with cystic fibrosis; CALICO multicentre randomised controlled trial. *BMJ* 332: 632–636.

Prescott P, Bakowski MT. (1999) Pathogenesis of fibrosing colonopathy: the role of methacrylic acid copolymer. *Pharmacoepidemiological Drug Safety* 8: 377–384.

Rashid M, Durie P, Andrew M, *et al*. (1999) Prevalence of vitamin K deficiency in cystic fibrosis. *American Journal of Clinical Nutrition* 70: 378–382.

Schulze KJ, O'Brien KO, Germain-Lee EL, Baer DJ, Leonard ALR, Rosenstein BJ. (2003) Endogenous fecal losses of calcium compromise calcium balance in pancreatic-insufficient girls with cystic fibrosis. *Journal of Pediatrics* 143: 765–771.

Scott J, Elias E, Moult PJ, Barnes S, Wills MR. (1977) Rickets in adult cystic fibrosis with myopathy, pancreatic insufficiency and proximal tubular dysfunction. *American Journal of Medicine* 63: 488–492.

Sermet-Gaudelus I, Mayell SJ, Southern KW. (2010) Guidelines on the early management of infants diagnosed with cystic fibrosis following newborn screening. *Journal of Cystic Fibrosis* 9: 323–329.

Sermet-Gaudelus I, Bianchi ML, Garabedian M, *et al*. (2011) European cystic fibrosis bone mineralisation guidelines. *Journal of Cystic Fibrosis* 10: S16–S23.

Sinaasappel M, Stern M, Littlewood J, *et al*. (2002) Nutrition in patients with cystic fibrosis: a European Consensus. *Journal of Cystic Fibrosis* 1: 51–75.

Sitrin MD, Lieberman F, Jensen WE, Noronha A, Milburn C, Addington W. (1987) Vitamin E deficiency and neurologic disease in adults with cystic fibrosis. *Annals of Internal Medicine* 107: 51–54.

Skypala IJ, Ashworth FA, Hodson ME, *et al*. (1998) Oral nutritional supplements promote weight gain in cystic fibrosis patients. *Journal of Human Nutrition and Dietetics* 11: 95–104.

Smith DL, Clarke JM, Stableforth DE. (1994) A nocturnal nasogastric feeding programme in cystic fibrosis adults. *Journal of Human Nutrition and Dietetics* 7: 257–262.

Smyth R, Walters S. (2000) Oral calorie supplements for cystic fibrosis. *Cochrane Database of Systematic Reviews* 2: CD000406.

Smyth RL, van Velzen D, Smyth AR, Lloyd DA, Heaf DP. (1994) Strictures of ascending colon in cystic fibrosis and high-strength pancreatic enzymes. *Lancet* 343: 85–86.

Sokol RJ, Reardon MC, Accurso FJ, *et al*. (1989) Fat-soluble-vitamin status during the first year of life in infants with cystic fibrosis identified by screening of newborns. *American Journal of Clinical Nutrition* 50: 1064–1071.

Stallings VA, Stark LJ, Robinson KA, Ferenchak AP, Quinton H, Clinical Practice Guidelines on Growth and Nutrition Subcommittee; Ad Hoc Working Group. (2008) Evidence-based practice recommendations for nutrition-related management of children and adults with cystic fibrosis and pancreatic insufficiency: Results of a systematic review. *Journal of the American Dietetics Association* 108: 832–839.

Steinkamp G, von der Hardt H. (1994) Improvement of nutritional status and lung function after long-term nocturnal gastrostomy feedings in cystic fibrosis. *Journal of Pediatrics* 124: 244–249.

Stephenson CB, Gildengorin G. (2000) Serum retinol, the acute phase response, and the apparent misclassification of vitamin A status in the third National Health and Nutrition Examination Survey. *American Journal of Clinical Nutrition* 72: 1170–1178.

Stephenson A, Brotherwood M, Robert R, *et al*. (2005) Increased vitamin A and E levels in adult cystic fibrosis patients after lung transplantation. *Transplantation* 79: 613–615.

Stephenson A, Brotherwood M, Robert R, Atenafu E, Corey M, Tullis E. (2007) Cholecalciferol significantly increases 25-hydroxyvitamin D concentrations in adults with cystic fibrosis. *American Journal of Clinical Nutrition* 85: 1307–1311.

Stern M, Wiedemann B, Wenzlaff P, on behalf of the German Cystic Fibrosis Quality Assessment Group. (2008) From registry to quality management: the German Cystic Fibrosis Quality Assessment project 1995–2006. *European Respiratory Journal* 31: 29–35.

Truby H, Cowlishaw P, O'NeilC, Wainwright C. (2009) The long term efficacy of gastrostomy feeding in children with cystic fibrosis an anthropometric markers of nutritional status and pulmonary function. *Open Respiratory Medicine* 3: 112–115.

Van der Doef HPJ, Kokke FTM, van der Ent CK, Houwen RHJ. (2011) Intestinal obstruction syndromes in cystic fibrosis: meconium ileus, distal intestinal obstruction syndrome and constipation. *Current Gastroenterology Reports* 13: 265–270.

von Drygalski A, Biller J. (2008) Anemia in cystic fibrosis: Incidence, mechanisms, and association with pulmonary function and vitamin deficiency. *Nutrition in Clinical Practice* 23: 557–563.

Walker SA, Gozal D. (1998) Pulmonary function correlates in the prediction of long-term weight gain in cystic fibrosis patients with gastrostomy tube feedings. *Journal of Pediatric Gastroenterology and Nutrition* 27: 53–56.

White H, Morton AM, Peckham DG, Conway SP. (2004) Dietary intakes in adult patients with cystic fibrosis – do they achieve guidelines? *Journal of Cystic Fibrosis* 3: 1–7.

White H, Pollard K, Etherington C, *et al*. (2009) Nutritional decline in cystic fibrosis related diabetes: The effect of intensive nutritional intervention. *Journal of Cystic Fibrosis* 8: 179–185.

Wilfond BS, Farrell PM, Laxova A, Mischler E. (1994) Severe haemolytic anemia associated with vitamin E deficiency in infants with cystic fibrosis: implications for neonatal screening. *Clinical Pediatrics* 33: 2–7.

Williams SG, Ashworth F, McAlweenie A, Poole S, Hodson ME, Westaby D. (1999) Percutaneous endoscopic gastrostomy feeding in patents with cystic fibrosis. *Gut* 44: 87–90.

7.5.1   Acute and chronic kidney disease

Sue Perry and George Hartley
Additional contributors: Christel Lyell and Nicki Ruddock

Key points

- Nutrition has a central role in the management of acute and chronic kidney disease.

- This includes reduction of cardiovascular disease risk, monitoring of nutritional status and limiting the effects of reduced kidney function.

- Several dietary elements usually require consideration and may change over time.

Nutritional treatment has a central role in the management of both acute and chronic kidney disease. Dietetic interventions to reduce cardiovascular disease risk are important in early chronic kidney disease (CKD). Regular monitoring of nutritional status and limiting the effects of reduced kidney function are important considerations in acute kidney injury, progressive chronic kidney disease and established renal failure. As several dietary elements usually require consideration, an appreciation of both medical and dietetic aspects of care is required in order to produce appropriate and individualised dietetic treatment plans.

Each kidney contains up to 1 million nephrons; each nephron being a filtering unit of tiny blood vessels (glomeruli) attached to a tubule. The glomeruli normally filter approximately 100 mL of plasma/min. The rate at which this takes place is known as the glomerular filtration rate (GFR). The kidney has a number of important functions, including the excretion of waste products, electrolyte homeostasis (including sodium, potassium, calcium and phosphate), regulation of fluid, acid–base balance and metabolic processes; and hormone production, including erythropoietin and renin, and activation of vitamin D.

The glomerular filtration rate is the best index of overall kidney function. In clinical practice, serum creatinine levels are used to monitor renal function as levels rise with decreasing GFR. However, the kidneys have a large functional reserve and serum creatinine levels only rise when at least 50% of kidney function is lost (GFR <60 mL/min). Creatinine is also subject to non-renal influences, which make it insufficiently sensitive to detect moderate CKD on its own. Therefore, an estimate of GFR (eGFR) is made using an equation that corrects for some of the more significant influences, such as age and weight. Serum creatinine also correlates with muscle mass and in those with increased muscle mass, GFR will be underestimated; in those with reduced muscle mass GFR will be overestimated.

Definitions of kidney disease

Chronic kidney disease is defined as either kidney damage (proteinuria, haematuria or anatomical abnormality) or GFR of <60 mL/min/1.73 m^2 present on at least two occasions for 3 or more months (Department of Health, 2004). Established renal failure (ERF) is an irreversible, long term condition for which regular dialysis treatment or transplantation is required if the individual is to survive (Department of Health, 2004). It is also known as end stage renal disease (ESRD) or kidney failure.

Manual of Dietetic Practice, Fifth Edition. Edited by Joan Gandy.
© 2014 The British Dietetic Association. Published 2014 by John Wiley & Sons, Ltd.
Companion Website: www.manualofdieteticpractice.com

Acute kidney injury (AKI) is a sudden decline in kidney function, often occurring over hours or days. Many people make a complete recovery from AKI, but some are left with CKD or even ERF (Department of Health, 2004). It has now replaced the older term acute renal failure.

Chronic kidney disease

Diagnostic criteria and classification

In 2002 a classification system for CKD based on GFR was adopted worldwide (Table 7.5.1). There has been debate about the implications of having a reduced GFR, but the evidence suggests that if eGFR is <60 mL/min, there is an increased risk of mortality. As a normal GFR is approximately 100 mL/min, reduced kidney function can be explained to patients as a percentage of normal function (Table 7.5.1).

Aetiology

There is extensive clinical evidence that diabetes, hypertension and the presence of proteinuria are risk factors for progression of CKD (NICE, 2008a). The most common causes are shown in Table 7.5.2. Despite the wide range of causes of kidney injury, once there is a significant loss of nephrons, the result is a common pathway character-

ised by hypertension, proteinuria and progressive decline in GFR (Metcalfe, 2007). The remaining nephrons develop glomerular hypertension and the GFR increases for each nephron (called hyperfiltration). This causes increased

Table 7.5.1 Stages of chronic kidney disease [source: National Clinical Guideline Centre (NCGC) 2008. Reproduced with permission of the National Clinical Guideline Centre]

Stage*	GFR (mL/min/1.73 m^2)	Description
1	≥90	Normal or increased GFR, with other evidence of kidney damage
2	60–89	Slight decrease in GFR, with other evidence of kidney damage
3A	45–59	Moderate decrease in GFR with or without other evidence of kidney damage
3B	30–44	
4	15–29	Severe decrease in GFR, with or without other evidence of kidney damage
5	<15	Established renal failure

*Use the suffix (p) to denote the presence of protein urea when staging chronic kidney disease.
GFR, glomerular filtration rate.

Table 7.5.2 Common causes of chronic kidney disease (CKD)

Cause	Mechanism	Comments
Diabetic nephropathy	Part of systemic microvascular disease of diabetes The first sign is microalbuminuria, which presents when eGFR is normal	The leading cause of renal failure in the UK Approx. 50% of those with diabetes have proteinuria and reduced kidney function and 75% of these have hypertension
Hypertensive atherosclerosis	Long standing high blood pressure	A common cause of established renal failure
Renal artery stenosis	Often caused by atherosclerosis	May cause hypertension
Heart failure	Age, diabetes and smoking can all cause ischaemic heart disease and renal artery stenosis	Heart failure is frequently found with CKD
Obesity	A risk factor for CKD, acting partly through a link with diabetes and hypertension More likely to develop glomerular hyperfiltration and albuminuria	Obesity often causes hypertension, insulin resistance and CVD There is a strong association between abdominal obesity, metabolic syndrome and CKD
Polycystic kidney disease	Multiple cysts that gradually enlarge	Inherited, often causes established renal failure in middle age
Reflux nephropathy	Reflux of urine from the bladder back up the ureters	Often inherited
Glomerular disease	Many different types of glomerulonephritis May occur in children	Usually diagnosed by renal biopsy Usually proteinuria and/or haematuria.
Nephrotic syndrome	Caused by a wide range of glomerular diseases	Combination of heavy proteinuria, low serum albumin and fluid retention Often severe hyperlipidaemia
Microscopic vasculitis	Inflammation of the small blood vessels	For example, Wegener's granulomatosis
Myeloma	Bence Jones proteins precipitate in kidney tubules	Can cause acute kidney injury or CKD

CVD, cardiovascular disease; eGFR, estimated glomerular filtration rate.

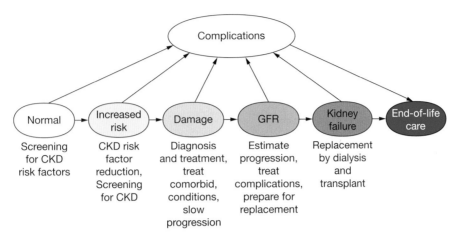

Figure 7.5.1 Overall health approach to chronic kidney disease (CKD) (source: Levey *et al.* 2007. Reproduced with permission of Macmillan Publishers Ltd)

glomerular permeability and excessive protein filtration. In addition, hypertension and hyperlipidaemia stimulate the abnormal production of growth factors and cytokines that, together with the glomerular hypertension, eventually lead to interstitial fibrosis and glomerulosclerosis (Metcalfe, 2007). The rate of decline of kidney function is highly variable and depends on the cause as well as its treatment.

Nephrotic syndrome

This is the term for a group of symptoms, including proteinuria (>3.5 g/day), low blood protein levels (serum albumin <25 g/L), severe hyperlipidaemia and peripheral oedema. A wide range of glomerular diseases causes it and, although relatively rare in adults, it is important as it has serious complications. All patients should be referred to a nephrologist for further investigations, which often includes a renal biopsy (Hull & Goldsmith, 2008).

Disease consequences

The two main outcomes of CKD are loss of kidney function, leading to complications and kidney failure, and the development of cardiovascular disease (CVD) (National Kidney Foundation, 2002). There is a far greater likelihood of death from CVD than from CKD progression through to ERF. The cardiovascular risk is more apparent in younger patients, e.g. a 35-year-old man on dialysis has the same risk of a cardiovascular death as an 80-year old not on dialysis (National Kidney Foundation, 2009a). Although CKD becomes more prevalent with increasing age, people aged over 70 years who have a stable eGFR between 45 and 59 mL/min and no other evidence of kidney damage are unlikely to experience complications related to CKD. The greatest risks are to those who have progressive CKD.

For those who do reach ERF and start renal replacement therapy (RRT), mortality rates are very high. Five-year mortality rates in incident RRT patients are 50–73% for patients aged over 65 years of age (Zoccali *et al.*,

2010). The main cause of death continues to be CVD, although in addition to hypertension and hypercholesterolaemia, the presence of CKD mineral and bone disorders, and anaemia may complicate and accelerate vascular disease (Renal Association, 2010c,d).

Public health aspects and prevention

There has been a recent change in focus in renal medicine from the treatment of patients with ERF to the earlier identification and prevention of CKD. One reason is that CKD is more common than previously thought and is increasing in prevalence in the UK and around the world. The prevalence of CKD (stages 3–5) in the UK is approximately 8.5% (Stevens *et al.*, 2007). Another reason is the significant number of late referrals to nephrology services; currently between 20% and 30% of all referrals. These patients do not have the opportunity for preparation and choice regarding dialysis or conservative management. Late referrals also have a higher morbidity and mortality and a poorer quality of life on dialysis (Renal Association, 2009a). Dialysis treatment is expensive; 1–2% of the total NHS budget is spent on treating patients with ERF, although they comprise only 0.05% of the population (NHS Kidney Care, 2010).

In order to identify and treat patients earlier, Kidney Disease: Improving Global Outcomes (KDIGO) (Levey *et al.*, 2007) and the National Institute for Health and Care Excellence (NICE, 2008a) have recommended an overall health approach (Figure 7.5.1) and an integrated care strategy involving public awareness, professional education, policy influence, and improved care delivery systems, all underpinned by research.

This approach should help to identify those who:

- Have, or are at risk of developing, CKD.
- Need intervention to minimise CVD risk, and what that intervention should be.
- Will develop progressive kidney disease and/or complications of kidney disease. and how they can be managed.
- Need referral for specialist kidney care.

Table 7.5.3 Complications seen in chronic kidney disease (CKD) stages 3–5

Cardiovascular disease	Main cause of death in patients with CKD
Hypertension	Both a cause and a complication of CKD Elevated blood pressure is associated with a faster rate of decline in GFR
Dyslipidaemia	Very prevalent in CKD and is influenced by renal function and degree of proteinuria
Increased risk of diabetic complications	Poor glycaemic control is associated with faster rate of decline in GFR Increased risk of CVD and retinopathy in patients with both diabetes and CKD
CKD mineral and bone disorder	Caused by alterations in the control mechanisms for calcium and phosphorus homeostasis
Protein energy wasting	Serum albumin, dietary protein and energy intake may fall as GFR falls
Metabolic acidosis	Kidneys become unable to remove sufficient H^+ ions and serum bicarbonate levels fall
Hyperkalaemia	Can be life threatening, especially if K^+ >6.5 mmol/L
Fluid (and sodium) retention	Can be a problem, e.g. in nephrotic syndrome
Anaemia	Kidneys become unable to produce sufficient erythropoietin as GFR falls
Gout	Blood urate level rises as GFR falls, leading to increased risk of gout
Depression	As with any chronic disease, CKD may be associated with depression, especially if there are physical symptoms

GFR, glomerular filtration rate; CVD, cardiovascular disease.

Nutritional consequences and complications

Most of the complications seen in CKD have nutritional causes or consequences. They are most often seen in stages 4 and 5, although some may start to develop during stage 3 (Table 7.5.3).

Protein energy wasting

Undernutrition is a major problem in those with CKD stages 4 and 5, and is currently known as protein energy wasting (PEW) (Fouque *et al.*, 2008). It is associated with increased morbidity, greater healthcare requirements and reduced functional ability. Its onset and severity is related to GFR; below 60 mL/min there is a higher prevalence of impaired nutritional status, which ranges from 28% to 48% in patients with CKD stage 4 (Heimburger *et al.*, 2000). Also, from this stage, serum cholesterol and serum albumin levels begin to decline. Low serum albumin is a strong predictor of adverse outcomes. However, the association between albumin and poor survival mainly reflects its associations with inflammation, comorbidity and fluid overload, as well as poor nutrition (Kaysen *et al.*, 2002; Jones, 2001).

Although one cause of protein energy wasting is an inadequate diet, other causes include chronic inflammation, intercurrent catabolic illnesses and metabolic acidosis (Stenvinkel *et al.*, 2000). Several criteria should be considered to diagnose PEW; these are biochemical criteria (including low albumin and/or cholesterol levels), low body weight, weight loss, reduced total body fat, loss of muscle mass and low protein or energy intakes. Additional measures of nutrition and inflammation, e.g. C-reactive protein (CRP), are also helpful (Fouque *et al.*, 2008).

Low protein and energy intakes become more common as GFR falls, particularly when GFR falls below 25 mL/min (Ikizler *et al.*, 1995). Uraemia is common at this stage, causing nausea, lethargy and taste changes, which adversely affect appetite. Metabolic acidosis (low plasma bicarbonate) is also common at this stage, and is associated with increased protein catabolism and reduced synthesis of serum albumin (de Brito-Ashurst *et al.*, 2009).

Patients who are undernourished when they start dialysis are four times as likely to die within 2 years than those who are well nourished. Once dialysis starts, appetite and nutritional status usually improve. However, a gradual but significant decline is often seen in all nutritional markers with increasing years on dialysis (Chumlea *et al.*, 2003). A low percentage of body fat at the start of dialysis and fat loss over time have been found to be independently associated with higher mortality. In particular, a body mass index (BMI) of >23 kg/m² is associated with reduced mortality in dialysis patients and a BMI of <20 kg/m² is associated with the highest mortality rates (Leavey *et al.*, 2001).

Dyslipidaemia

Plasma triglycerides start to increase early in CKD and show the highest concentrations in those with nephrotic syndrome and in those receiving dialysis (NICE, 2008b). However, there is often a reduction of total, high density (HDL) and low density lipoprotein (LDL) cholesterol concentrations when GFR falls below 60 mL/min. Chronic inflammation is a common feature in dialysis patients and may cause PEW and progressive atherosclerotic CVD (Stenvinkel *et al.*, 2002). Surprisingly, on dialysis, obesity, hypercholesterolaemia and hypertension appear to be protective features that are associated with increased survival; this is known as reverse epidemiology. It appears that the adverse effects of PEW and inflammation are more dominant than traditional risk factors (Kalantar-Zadeh *et al.*, 2003). However, being overweight is not an advantage to patients with renal transplants, in

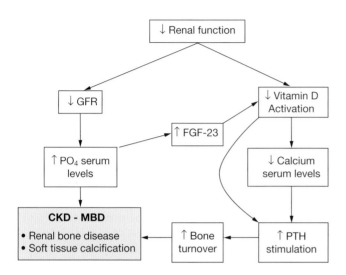

Figure 7.5.2 Bone and mineral metabolism in renal disease
PTH, parathyroid hormone; GRF, glomerular filtration rate; FGF-23, fibroblast growth factor-23; CKD–MBD, chronic kidney disease–mineral and bone disorder

whom obesity and hyperlipidaemia are quite common (Kalantar-Zadeh *et al.*, 2003).

Mineral and bone disorders

As CKD advances and kidney function declines, mineral homeostasis becomes progressively impaired. Hyperphosphataemia develops from CKD stage 4 onwards as the excretion of phosphate can no longer match dietary intake. Serum levels of the phosphate regulating fibroblast growth factor 23 increase as GFR falls. This inhibits the activation of vitamin D by the kidneys (Gutierrez *et al.*, 2005), resulting in low circulating levels and hypocalcaemia. This stimulates parathyroid hormone (PTH) production by the parathyroid gland, a condition known as secondary hyperparathyroidism. Without therapeutic intervention, CKD mineral and bone disorder (CKD–MBD) will develop (Figure 7.5.2). This is a relatively new term that defines the complex syndrome that includes both renal bone disease (renal osteodystrophy) and soft tissue calcification (Kidney Disease: Improving Global Outcomes CKD–MBD Work Group, 2009].

The condition is associated with adverse outcomes. Traditionally, hyperphosphataemia and secondary hyperparathyroidism have been associated with increased morbidity from renal osteodystrophy, skeletal and bone pain, and fractures. However, more recently, it has also been associated with increased mortality in dialysis patients (Block *et al.*, 2004; Covic *et al.*, 2009) and concerns over vascular calcification (especially involving the coronary arteries) have increased. Observational studies show that coronary artery calcification is common and extensive in dialysis patients (Goodman *et al.*, 2000; Guerin *et al.*, 2000) and that it is linked to an increase in cardiovascular mortality rates (London *et al.*, 2003).

Hyperkalaemia

Hyperkalaemia has potentially adverse cardiac effects, causing arrhythmias and cardiac arrest. It can be life threatening, especially if potassium levels are above 6.5 mmol/L. Patients may present with associated muscle weakness and feel generally unwell, or they may be completely asymptomatic. Hyperkalaemia is rarely caused by renal dysfunction alone until GFR has fallen below 30 mL/min (Bakris *et al.*, 2000). Some patients may develop hyperkalaemia as early as CKD stage 3, usually as a result of the side effects of taking medications such as angiotensin converting enzyme (ACE) inhibitors or angiotensin receptor blockers (ARBs). If serum potassium levels are 6.0 mmol/L or above, and other drugs that promote hyperkalaemia have been discontinued, ACE inhibitors or ARBs should be stopped (NICE, 2008). At this point, other causes of raised potassium levels, including diet, should be investigated. These include:

- Potassium sparing diuretics, e.g. spironolactone.
- Metabolic acidosis.
- Uncontrolled diabetes or insulin deficiency.
- Catabolism as a result of trauma or weight loss.
- Constipation.
- Dehydration.
- Sudden decline in residual renal function.
- Blood transfusion.
- Haemolysed blood sample.

Controlling serum potassium is particularly important during haemodialysis.

Fluid and sodium retention

As kidney function deteriorates, the ability to excrete excess sodium is reduced and sodium retention can occur. Serum sodium level is a poor indicator of sodium status, but a better indicator of hydration. Hence, hypernatraemia and hyponatraemia usually indicate dehydration and overhydration respectively. Excess dietary sodium leads to increased thirst, which can compound problems of fluid balance.

Fluid retention is unlikely in early CKD, apart from conditions such as nephrotic syndrome when fluid retention is common. When urine output is reduced and fluid intake exceeds output, fluid accumulates in the body, causing hypertension and oedema. Severe fluid overload, or even mild overload in individuals with heart failure, can result in pulmonary oedema and shortness of breath. Although ankle swelling can indicate fluid overload, patients may have several excess litres of fluid without oedema being clinically apparent. Acute changes in body weight usually represent changes in fluid balance in these patients. Clinical examination of the patient by medical staff or bioelectrical impedance is useful in determining fluid status.

Nutritional assessment

Nutritional monitoring should take place regularly in all patients with progressive CKD from stage 4 onwards, as PEW becomes more frequent. The use of a variety of nutritional markers is recommended (Fouque *et al.*, 2008; Renal Association, 2010b). A full nutritional assessment should include the following.

SECTION 7

Anthropometry

As a minimum, (oedema free) body weight, percentage weight change and BMI should be measured. Careful interpretation of weight change is important; a history of oedema or rapid weight loss or gain may be due to changes in fluid status. Attention should be paid to dry weight for those with oedema or on dialysis. For longitudinal measures, the use of skinfold callipers to assess mid upper arm circumference (MUAC) and triceps skinfold thickness are useful. In haemodialysis patients, high MUAC is a predictor of greater survival, particularly in those with low BMIs (Noori *et al.*, 2010).

Biochemistry

Serum cholesterol, urea, creatinine, eGFR, potassium, phosphate, serum albumin, CRP, urinary protein loss and fluid status should be measured (Renal Association, 2010b; 2011b).

Clinical history

This should include appetite, comorbidities and presence of oedema.

Dietary intake

A 24-hour recall or 3-day food diary should be used to assess dietary protein and energy intake.

Functional assessment

This assesses the ability to conduct the activities of daily living. Measurement of handgrip strength has been found to correlate well with lean body mass (Heimburger *et al.*, 2000).

Subjective global assessment

This has been validated for use in patients with ERF and is linked with adverse outcomes and mortality (Enia *et al.*, 1993). In dialysis patients, the 7-point subjective global assessment may validly distinguish different degrees of PEW associated with increasing risks of mortality (de Mutsert *et al.*, 2009). In addition, social and economic factors should be taken into account, e.g. patients living alone can be at greater nutritional risk.

Ideal body weight (IBW) should be calculated from height and ideal BMI, which would be:

- $20 \, kg/m^2$ for those with an actual BMI of $<20 \, kg/m^2$.
- $25 \, kg/m^2$ for those with a BMI $>25 \, kg/m^2$.
- Actual BMI if $20–25 \, kg/m^2$ (Renal Association, 2010b).

Management stages 1–3

Clinical management

The medical management of CKD mainly consists of interventions to slow the rate of decline in renal function and limit any associated complications, such as CVD. In addition, specific treatments such as immunosuppressive therapy for autoimmune disorders may also be required. The medical management of all patients with CKD stages 1–3 should include reduction of all modifiable cardiovascular risk factors including:

- Strict control of hypertension (blood pressure 140/90 mmHg; 130/80 mmHg in diabetes mellitus).
- Tight glucose control in diabetes (HbA1$_c$ 48–58 mmol/mol).
- Achieving a healthy weight (BMI 20–25 kg/m^2).
- Lipid lowering (total cholesterol <4 mmol/L; LDL <2 mmol/L).
- Smoking cessation if appropriate.
- Regular exercise.
- Limiting alcohol intake (men <3 units/day; women <2 units/day).

Of these, the interventions that have been found to be particularly effective at reducing the progression of CKD are strict blood pressure control, use of ACE inhibitors or ARBs, strict glucose control in diabetes and the use of statins (National Kidney Foundation, 2002).

Uncomplicated CKD stages 1–3 can usually be managed in primary care. Serum creatinine and eGFR should be regularly monitored, as should proteinuria and albuminuria. Most people in this category will not develop ERF during their lifetime and information provided should concentrate on cardiovascular risk reduction. However, those with progressive CKD, such as rapidly declining eGFR (>5 mL/min/year) or significant proteinuria are likely to require nephrology referral.

Hypertension

There is strong evidence that lowering blood pressure reduces cardiovascular risk and progression of CKD (NICE, 2008a). Interventions that inhibit the renin angiotensin aldosterone system activity, such as ACE inhibitors or ARBs, provide cardiovascular and renal protection (together with a reduction in proteinuria) (National Kidney Foundation, 2002). However, they can cause hyperkalaemia.

Hyperlipidaemia

Statins have been found to be safe and effective at reducing cardiovascular mortality. They should be considered for primary prevention in all CKD stages 1–4 and transplant patients with a >20% risk of CVD over 10 years (Renal Association, 2010c).

Alcohol, smoking and exercise

Clients should be encouraged to exercise, achieve a healthy weight and stop smoking to reduce CVD risk (NICE, 2008b; Renal Association, 2010c). A low or moderate alcohol intake is recommended as heavy alcohol intake is linked with hypertension.

Dietetic management

Most of the evidence for dietetic treatment of early CKD comes from research that focused on dietetic interventions to reduce CVD. There is evidence that good glycaemic control in those with diabetes, weight reduction in those with obesity and nutritional support in those with PEW improve patient outcomes. The main aims of dietetic treatment in these patients are to reduce the progression both of CKD and CVD.

Protein

Protein restriction has been found to help alleviate uraemic symptoms and was thought to possibly delay the progression of renal disease (Bennett *et al.*, 1983), although evidence for this is inconclusive (Levey *et al.*, 1996; NICE, 2008a). The risk of developing PEW in patients following low protein diets has led to concern about their use (Kopple *et al.*, 1997). There is insufficient evidence to recommend an optimal protein level, but it is generally considered that dietary protein intake should not be <0.8 g/kg/day (SIGN, 2008).

Energy

Energy requirements are not increased. As many patients with early CKD have diabetes or hypertension and obesity is common, weight management is an important part of the dietetic treatment. Those with a high risk of or with CVD should modify their fat intake and include oily fish once a week in their diet.

Obesity

Weight loss programmes have been shown to reduce proteinuria, blood pressure and rate of renal decline (Navaneethan *et al.*, 2009). Weight reduction also has beneficial effects on associated risk factors, including insulin resistance, diabetes, dyslipidaemia and left ventricular hypertrophy (Abrass, 2004). Patients who may benefit the most from weight loss are those with a BMI of greater 30 kg/m^2, type 2 diabetes or an increased waist circumference (regardless of BMI) (Teta, 2010; Renal Association, 2010b).

Modifications of lifestyle, physical activity and individualised dietary advice tailored to food preferences are initial measures. For sustainable weight loss, a gradual decrease in energy intake by 500–600 kcal/day is recommended. This should be accompanied by close dietetic supervision to avoid exacerbation of uraemic symptoms (Teta, 2010). High protein diets for weight loss may be unsafe for patients with CKD. Protein intake exceeding 20% of total energy is not recommended, because of the potential detrimental effects on kidney function (Friedman, 2004). Pharmacological measures are generally unsafe, except for orlistat, which has been used with some success. Bariatric surgery may help in severe obesity (see Chapter 7.13.3).

Diabetes

Strict glycaemic control has been found to both delay the onset and slow the progression of microvascular complications in type 1 diabetes [Diabetes Control and Complications Trial (DCCT) Research Group, 1993]. In type 2 diabetes, improved glycaemic control appears to provide a similar benefit.

Sodium

Advice to reduce dietary salt intake to <6 g/day has been shown to achieve a modest reduction in blood pressure in those with hypertension and in those with diabetes (Suckling *et al.*, 2010). The Dietary Approach to Stop Hypertension Sodium (DASH) trials showed that increasing fruit and vegetable, wholegrain and fish intake, and a low salt diet combined with lower intakes of fat, saturated fats, sugar and red meat led to lower blood pressures compared with a control group. However, this trial did not include adults with CKD. Due to the potential for increased potassium and phosphate levels, patients with CKD may not be able to adhere to the DASH diet, although the principle of salt reduction is still recommended (SIGN, 2008) (see Chapter 7.14.4).

Given the impact of sodium reduction on blood pressure, the current recommended intake of salt is 6 g (100 mmol of sodium)/day (Renal Association, 2011b). Most dietary sodium consumed is from salt added to processed food and patients may need help in how to interpret the varying information on food labels. A small amount of salt may be used in cooking, but no extra salt should be added at the table. Herbs and spices should be encouraged, but salt substitutes should be avoided due to their potassium content (SIGN, 2008).

Infrequently, some patients with later stages of CKD lose excessive amounts of sodium in the urine. Dietary sodium intake in these individuals should not be restricted as they may become salt and fluid depleted.

Fluid

Most patients do not need to change from the usual recommendation and an adequate fluid intake should be encouraged to promote excretion of waste products. Some may need a higher fluid intake, such as those with kidney stones or those with a salt losing enteropathy. However, those with a tendency to fluid retention, such as those with nephrotic syndrome, may need to limit both their salt and fluid intakes (see CKD stage 5 (haemodialysis) for further information).

Potassium

Dietary potassium should not be restricted only in those with raised serum levels, as many foods containing potassium are required for a healthy balanced diet. Both dietary restrictions and serum potassium levels should be regularly monitored (NICE, 2008) (see CKD stage 4 for further information).

Phosphate

Dietary intake of phosphate is rarely limited at this stage of CKD.

Nephrotic syndrome

Traditionally, high protein diets have been advocated to correct for urinary protein losses. However, studies have demonstrated that a high protein diet was ineffective in correcting hypoalbuminaemia (Mansy *et al.*, 1989). Moreover, the increased protein intake tends to further increase proteinuria, whereas low protein diets (<0.8 g/kg/day) have a slight antiproteinuric effect (Giordano *et al.*, 2001). However, as muscle wasting can be a problem in these patients, a low protein diet is not recommended. In practice, a dietary protein intake of 0.8–1 g/kg of IBW/day is suggested. Dietary management of nephrotic syndrome requires the consideration of the following:

- Obesity – careful assessment is essential due to generalised oedema.
- Lipids, including lipid lowering drugs and a cardioprotective diet.
- A diet containing 100 mmol of sodium (<6 g of salt)/day will help to minimise hypertension and fluid overload.
- Fluid may need to be restricted (together with salt restriction) when gross oedema is present.
- Dietary protein intake should be limited to 0.8–1.0 g/kg of IBW.
- Ensure adequate energy intake during periods of acute deterioration.

Management of stage 4

Clinical management

In addition to the reduction of modifiable cardiovascular risk factors, treatment of renal anaemia, metabolic acidosis and CKD–MBD become an important part of management. Nephrology reviews usually include measurement of eGFR, haemoglobin, calcium, phosphate, potassium, bicarbonate and PTH. Ideally, these patients should be managed in a dedicated clinic by a multidisciplinary team (Renal Association, 2009a).

Patients with progressive CKD should also be offered an appropriate education programme aimed at improving their understanding of their condition and the treatment options; RRT (haemodialysis, peritoneal dialysis or a transplant) or conservative care (NICE, 2008a; Renal Association, 2009a). It can take up to 1 year to prepare fully for RRT, but this programme should enable a planned start using an established access (such as a fistula for haemodialysis or a peritoneal dialysis catheter) or by preemptive renal transplantation.

Renal anaemia

Treatment is with iron and erythropoiesis stimulating agents (ESAs) as required, with regular monitoring of both serum ferritin and haemoglobin levels.

Metabolic acidosis

Sodium bicarbonate supplementation is recommended to correct metabolic acidosis. This may also help to reduce protein catabolism and retard the progression of CKD (de Brito-Ashurst et al., 2009).

Mineral and bone disorder

Management of CKD–MBD involves the correction of biochemistry by limiting dietary phosphate together with the use of various agents, including phosphate binders, vitamin D compounds and calcimimetics. In some cases, surgical removal of the parathyroid glands may be required. It can be difficult to achieve an effective combination of different therapies, and frequent monitoring of blood levels and adjustments may be required. To help achieve adequate phosphate control, phosphate binders may be required in addition to any dietary restriction. These work by limiting the absorption of phosphate from the gastrointestinal tract. Although they are used in patients with CKD stage 4, most of the evidence regarding their effectiveness comes from their use in patients on dialysis. Both calcium carbonate (Slatapolsky et al., 1986) and calcium acetate (Schiller et al., 1989) have been used as phosphate binders. They are inexpensive and, compared to non-calcium containing binders, are relatively well tolerated (Navaneethan et al., 2011), but there are concerns that their use is associated with vascular calcification (Goodman et al., 2000; Guerin et al., 2000; London et al., 2003). Newer agents such as sevelamer hydrochloride/carbonate and lanthanum carbonate are significantly more expensive, but offer the potential advantage of being calcium free. In practice, a mixture of both calcium and non-calcium containing binders are used, but care should be taken to avoid high calcium levels and to limit the intake of calcium from phosphate binders (National Kidney Foundation, 2003).

Alfacalcidol is an active vitamin D analogue that is also used in the management of CKD–MBD. It can be effective at suppressing PTH levels, but it also promotes calcium and phosphate absorption, leading to an increase in their serum levels. Careful biochemical monitoring is therefore required, and its use balanced against other effects (Table 7.5.4). Where PTH levels remain high, tertiary hyperparathyroidism has developed. Treatment involves either a parathyroidectomy or cinacalcet therapy. Cinacalcet is a calcimimetic agent that increases the sensitivity of calcium sensing receptors in the parathyroid gland, thereby inhibiting PTH secretion. It is expensive and NICE

Table 7.5.4 Recommended bone biochemistry levels in chronic kidney disease

	Serum phosphate (mmol/L)	Serum calcium* (mmol/L)	Parathyroid hormone (PTH)
CKD 3–5 patients (not on dialysis)	0.9–1.5	Kept within normal reference range	Consider treatment where levels are progressively increasing and remain persistently higher than upper reference limit
Dialysis patients (stage 5D)	1.1–1.7	2.1–2.5	Between two and nine times upper limit of normal. Marked changes in levels in either direction within range should prompt initiation or change in therapy

*Adjusted for albumin concentration.

(2007) currently recommends that cinacalcet be reserved for individuals in whom surgery is contraindicated.

Dietetic management

The aim is to promote a healthy well balanced diet, taking into account the nutritional treatment of comorbidities. Other factors, particularly the monitoring of both serum electrolyte levels and nutritional status, become more important in order to provide appropriate and timely dietetic advice.

By CKD stage 4, complications such as fluid and electrolyte imbalance, metabolic acidosis, anaemia and uraemia are common. Though these have an adverse effect on nutrition, wellbeing and blood levels can vary greatly between individuals. Some patients experience hyperkalaemia with mild renal impairment, whilst others will maintain normal levels even in advanced disease. Careful review of each patient is required. Dietary recommendations depend on biochemistry, normal dietary intake, comorbidities and nutritional status.

The National Institute for Health and Care Excellence (NICE, 2008a) recommends that where dietary intervention is indicated, the risks and benefits of dietary protein restriction should be discussed within the context of education, detailed dietary assessment and supervision. In addition, those with progressive CKD should be offered dietary advice concerning potassium, phosphate, protein, calorie and salt intake. Any dietary changes also need to consider other dietary restrictions a person might be following. It is important to consider the overall nutritional adequacy of the diet, bearing in mind that a restrictive diet may increase the risk of PEW.

Protein

As with earlier stages of CKD, there is debate as to the optimal level of protein intake. High protein intakes are associated with high phosphate intakes as foods that contain protein usually contain phosphate. Due to the prevalence of hyperphosphataemia, it is advisable to avoid high protein intakes and to aim for a protein intake of 0.75–1.0 g/kg of IBW (SIGN, 2008; Renal Association, 2010b). A higher protein intake may also increase metabolic acidosis. As uraemia becomes more likely at this stage, protein intake may decline and should be regularly monitored.

Energy

Energy expenditure is similar to that of healthy individuals (Monteen et al., 1986). An intake of 35 kcal/kg/day should be adequate for most patients (Kopple et al., 1986), but 30 kcal/kg may be more appropriate in those over 60 years of age when energy expenditure is reduced. However, it is important to ensure an adequate energy intake in order to prevent negative nitrogen balance and weight loss. Careful interpretation of weight change is important, as a history of oedema or rapid weight change may be due to changes in fluid status.

Sodium and fluid

A daily sodium intake of 100 mmol/day (6 g of salt) is recommended at this stage for most patients. However, sodium bicarbonate given to correct acidosis may also contribute significantly to sodium intake. Only patients with resistant oedema (such as those with nephrotic syndrome or heart failure) are likely to need advice regarding both sodium and fluid intake. If required, the fluid allowance is usually between 500 and 1000 mL/day plus the previous day's (24-hour) urine output.

Potassium

Hyperkalaemia becomes increasingly common as GFR falls. Dietetic advice to treat hyperkalaemia can allow ACE inhibitors or ARBs to be continued, facilitating the optimal treatment of hypertension and proteinuria (NICE, 2008a). However, as potassium levels at the lower end of normal are not advisable, it is important to ensure that the diet is not too restrictive. The lowest mortality risk may be between 4.1 and 5.5 mmol/L (Korgaonkar et al., 2010). The aim of a low potassium diet is to control serum potassium levels within an acceptable range whilst encouraging a well balanced diet. The level of potassium restriction should be individualised according to dietary intake, blood levels and medical treatment, but intakes of approximately 1 mmol/kg of IBW may be required. In practice, this involves limiting or avoiding those foods with high potassium content. Non-essential foods should be limited or avoided first, e.g. coffee and chocolate. Fruit, vegetables and potatoes contain significant amounts of potassium, as do meat, fish and milk, but as the latter are important components of most diets, they should not be restricted unnecessarily. Cooking methods may need to be adapted, e.g. boiling potatoes and vegetables lowers their potassium content. There is evidence that some people have been found to have low serum vitamin C levels on a low potassium diet (Pollock et al., 2005). Nowadays, people should be able to consume up to five 80-g portions of fruit and vegetables daily, but should also be provided with appropriate education on limiting or avoiding those that are particularly high sources of potassium, e.g. bananas and dried fruit.

Patients with diabetes should be advised that pure fruit juice, milk or chocolate are not the best treatment for hypoglycaemia when following a low potassium diet. Table 7.5.5 gives an example of a first line low potassium diet that could be used until personalised dietary advice can be provided. The skill of the dietitian is in limiting those foods that are high in potassium and have the least nutritional value, whilst considering patient preference and nutritional adequacy.

Phosphate

Hyperphosphataemia becomes increasingly common when GFR falls below 40 mL/min. A low phosphate diet is an important part of its treatment, although phosphate binders are often required, as discussed earlier. Foods contain phosphate in organic or inorganic forms. Inorganic phosphate is more readily absorbed than organic phosphate, and phytate (found in fibre rich foods) may also reduce phosphate absorption further (Kalantar-Zadeh et al., 2010). Organic phosphate is naturally found in foods that are high in protein, but usually only 40–60%

Table 7.5.5 First line potassium lowering dietary advice [source: The British Dietetic Association 2013. Reproduced with permission of The British Dietetic Association (www.bda.uk.com)]

	Foods high in potassium – reduce intake of the following	Lower potassium alternatives
Fruit	Avocado, bananas, dried fruit, e.g. apricots, currants, dates, figs, prunes, raisins, sultanas	Fruit should be limited to a maximum of three portions/day A portion is 80g or about a handful
Vegetables	Vegetables that have not been boiled, e.g. steamed, stir fried or raw Beetroot (fresh), sundried tomatoes, tomato purée	Two to three small (80g) portions of other vegetables Boil vegetables if possible Limit salads to one small bowl/day
Starchy foods	Jacket/baked potatoes Oven, microwave or retail chips Manufactured potato products, e.g. hash browns, frozen roast potatoes, potato waffles, potato wedges Unboiled sweet potato, cassava, plantain, taro, yam	Boiled potatoes, potatoes that have been par-boiled, then roasted or fried Boiled sweet potatoes, cassava, plantain, taro, yam Have no more than one serving of potato or starchy vegetable/day Pasta, rice, noodles, breads.
Snacks	Potato crisps/snacks, nuts, chocolate, fudge Biscuits and cakes containing lots of nuts, dried fruit or chocolate	Corn or maize based snacks Boiled, chewy and jelly sweets Marshmallows, mints, popcorn Biscuits and cakes not containing dried fruit, nuts or chocolate
Drinks	Coffee, malted milk drinks, (e.g. Horlicks, Ovaltine), drinking chocolate, cocoa, fruit and vegetable juices, smoothies Limit milk to 400mL ($\frac{2}{3}$ pint)/day or 200mL ($\frac{1}{3}$ pint) milk plus one yogurt/day Beer, cider, stout and wine	Tea, herbal tea, squash and cordial, mineral water, flavoured water, fizzy drinks Spirits are generally lower in potassium than other alcoholic drinks Remember to keep within safe limits for alcohol intake
Salt substitutes	Do *not* use salt substitutes, e.g. Lo-salt, So-Lo, Low Sodium salt	Other seasonings, e.g. pepper, herbs, spices

NB: This is initial advice only and should only be used until a registered dietitian can provide personalised dietary advice.

of the phosphate is absorbed from the gastrointestinal tract. Any restriction of dietary phosphate is likely to limit the intake of meat, fish, poultry, eggs and milk. Hence, foods with a high protein to phosphate ratio should be encouraged to ensure that protein intake is not compromised by phosphate restriction (Kalantar-Zadeh *et al.*, 2010). Consideration should be given to the individual's nutritional status, and care taken to ensure an adequate protein intake.

Inorganic phosphates are found in food additives and some highly processed foods and carbonated drinks. As over 90% of inorganic phosphate may be absorbed, their intake should be limited. Encouraging fresh foods rather than processed foods is likely to reduce both phosphate and sodium intake. Table 7.5.6 lists high phosphate foods that may be recommended in first line advice. Current UK guidelines recommend that serum phosphate levels be maintained between 0.9 and 1.50mmol/L for CKD stages 4 and 5 (not on dialysis) (Renal Association, 2011b).

Management of stage 5 (established renal failure)

Clinical management

Once eGFR falls below 15mL/min and uraemia, fluid overload or PEW persist despite medical treatment, RRT should commence if the patient has opted to dialyse. Ideally this should be planned so that dialysis can start with an arteriovenous fistula or peritoneal dialysis cath-

eter. Those patients who have opted not to dialyse should continue to have conservative management of their renal failure. In all cases, regular monitoring of renal function is an essential part of the continuing care of these patients.

Dietetic management

The aims will vary depending on the mode of RRT or if the patient is managed conservatively. There have been more studies in patients on dialysis than in earlier stages of CKD, particularly focusing on the treatment of PEW and CKD–MBD as these are both associated with increased morbidity and mortality. Recently, the heamodialysis population has shown a demographic shift from predominantly undernutrition to overnutrition (Kramer *et al.*, 2006) and this will need to be taken into account when providing dietetic advice.

Management of haemodialysis

Clinical management

Haemodialysis is the main mode of dialysis in most developed countries. In 2007 it was the established mode of dialysis in the UK in about two-thirds of patients (Renal Association, 2009b). In haemodialysis, blood is circulated through a machine that passes it through very small tubes made from a semi permeable membrane. Surrounding these tubes is the dialysate, which consists of sterile water and electrolytes. Blood cells and proteins are too pass

Table 7.5.6 First line advice on foods high in phosphate whose intake should be reduced

Dairy foods	Cheese spread, processed cheese Condensed milk, evaporated milk, milk shakes Malted milk drinks, e.g. Horlicks, Ovaltine Hard cheeses, e.g. cheddar Soft cheeses, e.g. Brie Limit milk to 300 mL (½ pint)/day
Meat, fish and nuts	Offal, e.g. liver, kidney, pâté Herring, kippers, pilchards, sardines, whitebait Crab, fish paste, scampi Nuts and seeds
Cereals and snacks	Chocolate, fudge Cakes, biscuits and cereals containing chocolate, nuts or seeds, e.g. muesli, cereal bars Baking powder, rock cakes and scones
Processed foods and drinks	Food additives containing phosphates or phosphoric acid; check labels on processed foods and carbonated drinks Examples of foods that may have these additives include ham, sausages, breaded chicken, cake mixes, instant sauces and dark carbonated drinks

NB: This is initial advice only on which foods to limit and should only be used until a registered dietitian can provide personalised dietary advice.

through the pores in the membranes, but small molecules such as urea, water and electrolytes pass through into the dialysate. In this way, excess water and uraemic toxins are removed and electrolyte and acid–base balance are restored. However, amino acids, glucose, vitamins and trace elements may also be removed by dialysis. The best access to the patient's blood is via an arteriovenous fistula, though a central venous catheter (usually into the internal jugular vein) can be used when access is needed immediately. Haemodialysis usually takes place three times per week, but several forms of more frequent haemodialysis (such as daily) have recently been evaluated and are associated with improved outcomes (Renal Association, 2009b). It is usually hospital based; although some patients dialyse at home.

Dietetic management

The main aims of the dietetic management of haemodialysis are:

- Regular monitoring of nutritional status in order to be able to prevent or treat PEW.
- Regular monitoring and dietetic advice to help maintain electrolytes within acceptable ranges.
- To help control fluid balance.
- To promote a healthy well balanced diet taking into account nutritional treatment of comorbidities.

Dietetic assessment should be provided at the start of dialysis in order to identify those who require nutritional supplementation as well as those who need fluid removal, and to balance this with advice on any dietary restrictions that may be required. After 6–8 weeks of dialysis, many patients notice an improvement in symptoms and dietary advice may need to change. For stable patients, nutritional changes are likely to be gradual after this. Multidisciplinary working is a vital part of ensuring appropriate treatment for these patients (Renal Association, 2010b).

Regular dietetic monitoring is likely to be beneficial and may lead to both a significant reduction in the proportion of patients with PEW and a significant decrease in phosphate levels (Campbell *et al.*, 2009).

Protein

In haemodialysis, protein requirements are increased, partly due to the loss of amino acids through the dialysis filter and the fact that dialysis itself can increase protein catabolism (Fouque *et al.*, 2007). A safe level of protein intake is likely to be at least 1.1–1.2 g/kg of IBW in order to achieve nitrogen balance (Fouque *et al.*, 2007; Renal Association, 2010b; British Dietetic Association Renal Nutrition Group, 2011). At least 50% of protein should be of high biological value (National Kidney Foundation, 2000). However, high protein intakes of >1.4 g/kg may not improve survival and may be harmful (Shinaberger *et al.*, 2006).

Energy

Energy expenditure does not appear to be increased (Cuppari & Avesani, 2004). Recommended energy intake is 30–35 kcal/kg of IBW/day for all patients depending upon age and physical activity (Renal Association, 2010b). Studies have reported that energy intakes are often lower than this, and may be as low as 20–25 kcal/kg/day (Rocco *et al.*, 2002). It has also been shown that energy intake may be insufficient, particularly on dialysis days. Even if protein intake is adequate, an inadequate energy intake is likely to result in a negative nitrogen balance. When assessing energy intake, a food diary that includes a dialysis day, a non-dialysis day and a weekend day as a minimum or several dietary interviews can be helpful (Fouque *et al.*, 2007).

Obesity

Current evidence suggests that a BMI of >23 kg/m^2 is protective for these patients. However, obese patients on dialysis who are eligible for a kidney transplant should be encouraged to lose weight. Transplants are rarely undertaken in those with a BMI of >35 kg/m^2 as graft survival appears to be decreased in obese patients.

Diabetes

Intensive glucose control in type 2 diabetes may have less of a protective effect against cardiovascular events in these patients (Reaven et al., 2009). Achieving an HbA1$_c$ of <58 mmol/mol in elderly patients with type 2 diabetes may have a modest effect on outcome and needs to be weighed against the risk of hypoglycaemic events. Haemodialysis per se has no significant long term effect on glycaemic control in insulin treated type 2 diabetic patients.

Sodium and fluid

Most patients show a progressive reduction in urine output. For most patients, limiting sodium and fluid intake is required to control blood pressure and to prevent excessive fluid weight gains. In haemodialysis, very high fluid weight gains between dialysis sessions [intradialytic weight gain (IDWG)] are associated with increased mortality risk, particularly cardiovascular risk (Kalantar-Zadeh et al., 2009). However, patients with very little fluid weight gain between dialysis sessions are at highest risk of death as this is associated with poor nutritional status and may reflect poor oral intake (Lopez-Gomez et al., 2005).

It is very difficult to ignore thirst as the overriding stimulus is plasma osmolality, to which serum sodium contributes the most (Tomson, 2001). Patients with poorly controlled diabetes may also be extremely thirsty. Reducing sodium intake suppresses thirst and therefore excessive IDWG. Patients on a low sodium diet (with advice to drink only when thirsty) have been found to gain significantly less weight than those on a standard diet and fluid intake (Rigby-Matthews et al., 1999). A low sodium diet also improves blood pressure control and may result in the withdrawal of antihypertensive treatment (Krautzig et al., 1998). Hence for most patients, the focus should be on limiting salt intake rather than on fluid intake.

When fluid needs to be considered, the current guidelines for fluid intake vary from 500 to 1000 mL in addition to daily urine output in order to achieve an IDWG of 2–2.5 kg or 4–4.5% dry body weight (Fouque et al., 2007). In order to achieve this, drinks and food with a high fluid content (sauces, soup, ice cream, etc.) should be counted as part of a daily fluid allowance. The water content in other foodstuffs such as fruit and vegetables is not counted. Drinking from a full small cup is usually more helpful than using a part filled larger cup or mug. However, any fluid allowance given should be reassessed regularly as residual renal function (urine output) is likely to change. Reducing sodium and fluid in addition to both potassium and phosphate, whilst ensuring that protein and energy intake is adequate, is difficult and a stepwise approach to educate the patient is most important (Fouque et al., 2007).

Potassium

Hyperkalaemia is a common indication for emergency dialysis in patients already on haemodialysis and 3–5% of deaths in dialysis patients have been attributed to hyperkalaemia. The highest mortality rate is when potassium levels exceed 5.6–6.0 mmol/L (Kovesdy et al., 2007). Serum potassium levels (measured at the start of dialysis) should be 4–6 mmol/L (Renal Association, 2009b). Dietetic advice to reduce dietary potassium intake should be provided when serum potassium levels approach 6 mmol/L, but other causes for hyperkalaemia should be investigated and corrected. For these patients, a daily intake of potassium of 50–70 mmol (1950–2730 mg) or 1 mmol/kg of IBW may be required (Fouque et al., 2007).

However, low potassium levels may lead to an increased mortality rate, especially when pre-dialysis levels are lower than 4 mmol/L (Kovesdy et al., 2007). Hypokalaemia towards the end or immediately after dialysis may be corrected by relaxing dietary potassium or by increasing the dialysate potassium concentration. Information regarding dietary advice required for a low potassium diet is described earlier.

Phosphate

The use of a phosphate restricted diet in combination with oral phosphate binders is now well established in the management of hyperphosphataemia and secondary hyperparathyroidism in patients on dialysis. Use of phosphate binders, vitamin D compounds and calcimimetics is described earlier. Limiting phosphate intake to 800–1000 mg (27–32 mmol)/day (adjusted for dietary protein needs) is recommended when serum phosphate levels or PTH are elevated (Fouque et al., 2007). The recommended serum phosphate level is 1.1–1.7 mmol/L (measured at the start of each dialysis session) (Renal Association, 2011b). Low phosphate levels are associated with increased mortality as are high phosphate levels in dialysis patients. Some patients may have PEW and CKD–MBD; the association between low serum phosphate levels and increased mortality rate may be due to a decline in protein intake and worsening PEW (Shinaberger et al., 2008). Dietary advice required for a low phosphate diet is described earlier.

Management of peritoneal dialysis

Clinical management

Peritoneal dialysis is a form of dialysis in which dialysis fluid is introduced into the peritoneal cavity via a peritoneal dialysis catheter in the patient's abdomen, where it draws waste products and excess water out of the blood using the peritoneal membrane as a filter. Most people dialyse every day either by manual exchanges performed four to five times a day [continuous ambulatory peritoneal dialysis (CAPD)] or overnight using a machine [automated peritoneal dialysis (APD)]. The fluid must stay inside the peritoneal cavity for a period of time (a dwell) to allow removal of waste products and fluid. Different dialysis regimens can be prescribed to maximise an individual's dialysis to ensure efficiency.

Dietetic management

The main aims of the dietetic management of peritoneal dialysis are:

- Regular monitoring of nutritional status to prevent or treat PEW.
- Regular monitoring and dietetic advice to help to maintain electrolytes within acceptable ranges.
- To help control fluid balance.
- To promote a healthy well balanced diet taking into account nutritional treatment of comorbidities.

Dietetic assessment should be undertaken at the start of dialysis to make a baseline assessment. Any symptoms of uraemia at this time usually start to recede and appetite improves. As residual renal function is relatively preserved in this patient group and dialysis is performed each day, some diet and fluid restrictions may be more relaxed.

Protein

Protein requirements are increased to compensate for protein losses into the dialysis fluid. The actual amount of protein lost by individuals is variable and is dependent on the properties of their peritoneal membrane and the dialysis regimen. Recommendations for protein requirements for this group have become more conservative over time with increasing evidence to suggest neutral nitrogen balance can be achieved at much lower intakes than previously recommended. Current consensus suggests aiming for a protein intake of 1.2 g of protein/kg of IBW (Renal Association, 2010b) although intakes of between 1.0 and 1.2 g of protein/kg of IBW may be adequate for many individuals with no adverse effect on nutritional status (Dombros *et al.*, 2005, British Dietetic Association Renal Nutrition Group, 2011).

Energy

Energy requirements are 30–35 kcal/kg of IBW, although older, less active patients may achieve neutral energy balance with intakes less than this. Monitoring actual body weight will help to assess if energy intake is appropriate for an individual. Unlike other renal patient groups, energy intake is obtained by the absorption of glucose from the peritoneal dialysis fluid as well as from diet. Glucose acts as an osmotic agent to ultrafiltrate fluid (UF) from the patient, so while it is in contact with the peritoneal membrane, not only does it facilitate fluid removal but it is also absorbed, hence contributing to total energy intake.

The amount of energy obtained from the peritoneal dialysis fluid is dependent on the amount of glucose in the bags (increased in some bags to increase UF) and the characteristics of the individual's peritoneal membrane. In CAPD, approximately 60% of the daily dialysate glucose load is absorbed in those with a normally functioning membrane (Dombros *et al.*, 2005), which can be 300–800 kcal/day. Those using high glucose concentration bags will regularly be absorbing large amounts of energy, which may cause undesirable weight gain.

To minimise glucose absorption (and therefore non-nutritive energy), other bags are available that use alternative osmotic agents, e.g. icodextrin (a non-absorbable glucose polymer) and amino acids. Icodextrin is often used to maximise UF, particularly for longer dwells, and amino acid bags can be indicated in those with poor nutritional intake. These may be useful glucose sparing strategies for those with obesity or diabetes. Glucose absorption from the peritoneal dialysis fluid can make meeting other dietary requirements more difficult as there needs to be a higher concentration of nutrients in the recommended reduced dietary energy intake.

Obesity

The high energy load provided by the treatment can cause weight gain. Central obesity can worsen or develop in some peritoneal dialysis patients, together with an increased risk of hyperlipidaemia and insulin resistance (Renal Association, 2010a). Practically, it can also be difficult to achieve an adequate dialysis dose in those patients with a high body weight. As for haemodialysis, there may be a protective element to having a higher BMI; however, this will affect the individual's suitability for a transplant.

Diabetes

Glycaemic control can become more difficult to manage due to the glucose absorbed from the peritoneal dialysis fluid. This may require an increase in insulin or oral hypoglycaemic drugs (Reaven *et al.*, 2009). Some individuals may have a set dialysis regimen against which diabetes medications can be titrated; however, many patients alter dialysis regimens to address their fluid balance on a day to day basis so tight glycaemic control can become challenging.

Sodium and fluid

The fluid requirement for those on peritoneal dialysis depends on an individual's residual renal function (urine output) and the UF achieved by peritoneal dialysis. Whilst limiting fluid helps prevent fluid overload, an appropriate dialysis regimen individualised to best match the UF potential is the most important predictor of adequate fluid balance. The use of high glucose bags is associated with detrimental changes in peritoneal membrane function, which can occur over time as well as with weight gain and poor glycaemic control in diabetes (Renal Association, 2010b). Limiting sodium and fluid intake helps to minimise the need for their use.

Potassium

Most people who have peritoneal dialysis are able to have a normal potassium intake. For some, the removal of potassium by the dialysis can be so efficient that a high potassium intake is required to maintain normal potassium levels. High serum potassium levels may indicate ineffective dialysis. Monitoring potassium levels will inform what level of potassium in the diet is required.

Constipation

Constipation is associated with peritoneal dialysis catheter malfunction and peritonitis, which can result in peritoneal dialysis failure. Constipation needs to be dealt with in a proactive, preventative manner. Laxatives are often taken regularly, but if changing the diet, fibre should be increased gradually and the potassium and fluid content of the diet should also be considered to ensure that target potassium levels are achieved and fluid overload is prevented (Lee, 2011).

Phosphate

The same dietetic principles apply to patients on peritoneal dialysis as for those on haemodialysis, and the same phosphate levels are recommended.

Protein energy wasting

Although felt to be diminishing, PEW is still prevalent, particularly amongst those with other comorbidities. In peritoneal dialysis, several factors have been found to be associated with PEW. The frequency of gastrointestinal symptoms is high, varying from diarrhoea, constipation, abdominal pain, delayed gastric emptying, and nausea and vomiting (Cano *et al.*, 2007b). Management of these symptoms may help improve appetite and food intake. For those who have fluid in their peritoneal cavity in the day, bloating and a feeling of satiety may also be experienced. Inadequate dialysis has been implicated in contributing to PEW (Churchill *et al.*, 1996; Paniagua *et al.*, 2002) and the level of residual renal function is thought to be directly related to nutritional intake independent of dialysis dose (Caravaca *et al.*, 1999; Wang *et al.*, 2001). The peritoneal membrane characteristics are also associated with PEW and fluid overload caused by poor volume management is also associated with poorer nutritional status (Wang *et al.*, 2003; Cheng *et al.*, 2005). Although some of these factors are difficult to manage or cannot be altered, it is important they are considered when formulating clinical treatment plans to address PEW.

Complications

A serious but uncommon complication of peritoneal dialysis is encapsulating peritoneal sclerosis (EPS). It is characterised by bowel obstruction and marked sclerotic thickening of the peritoneal membrane. Symptoms such as anorexia, nausea, vomiting and weight loss are common. In cases with milder gastrointestinal features, nutritional status may be maintained by ensuring adequate food intake with oral nutritional supplements and antiemetics as required. However, more severe cases may warrant enteral tube feeding if the gastrointestinal tract allows or parenteral feeding when it is impossible to establish adequate nutrition using the gut.

Management of kidney transplantation

Clinical management

Renal transplantation is the most common solid organ transplant procedure and is considered the gold standard for RRT as a successful transplant can lead to the restoration of renal function. Survival following renal transplantation is better than that for age matched individuals remaining on the transplant waiting list (Wolfe *et al.*,

1999). The longer patients receive dialysis, the greater their risk for post transplantation morbidity and mortality.

A transplant is considered to be the first choice for patients who are considered fit for major surgery and for chronic immunosuppression (Renal Association, 2011c). During a kidney transplant, the donor kidney is usually placed in the iliac fossa and the existing kidneys are not removed. Almost all transplants will provoke a powerful immunological rejection response in the recipient, which will destroy renal tissue; therefore immunosuppression is needed to avoid rejection.

Acute rejection generally occurs days to weeks after surgery. Chronic rejection, however, occurs slowly over months or years and leads to progressive loss of renal function. Eventually, as transplant function declines, the patient is likely to suffer symptoms of advancing kidney failure. As with patients with CKD, dietary changes may be required at some stage.

The most frequently used immunosuppressive agents are tacrolimus and ciclosporin. Other immunosuppressives used are mycophenolate mofetil, azathioprine, sirolimus and corticosteroids. Some of their adverse effects have nutritional implications, as shown in Table 7.5.7.

The medical and dietetic management of transplantation can be divided into three main periods and the aims for medical management are:

- *Pretransplant* – to correct or improve complications of ERF in order to optimise outcome.
- *Immediate post transplant phase* – to prevent acute rejection, optimise graft function and minimise infection.
- *Later post transplant phase* (from 3–6 months after surgery) – to preserve good graft function and prevent the long term consequences of immunosuppression, including premature CVD (Renal Association, 2011d).

Dietetic management

The main aims are:

- *Pretransplant phase* – to correct or improve nutritional status and CKD-MBD, and to treat obesity.
- *Immediate post transplant phase* – to monitor nutritional status and ensure adequate protein and energy intake, monitor electrolyte levels and treat as appropriate, and provide food safety advice.
- *Later post transplant phase* – to provide adequate, but not excessive, protein intake and to promote a healthy well balanced diet, taking into account nutritional treatment of comorbidities to reduce CVD risk.

Pretransplant phase

The aim of pretransplant nutritional management is to optimise outcomes in the early and the late transplant period. Ideally, an multidisciplinary team (MDT) approach should be taken, including diet, lifestyle changes and medication to aid in the correction or improvement of PEW, dyslipidaemia, obesity, CKD-MBD and hypertension. The presence of these comorbidities is predictive of related complications in the post transplant period.

Table 7.5.7 Drug–nutrient interactions

Medication	Nutrient interactions	Nutritional implications
ACE inhibitors/ARBs	Enhanced hypotensive effect when given with alcohol	Can cause hyperkalaemia
Potassium sparing diuretics, e.g. spironolactone		Can cause hyperkalaemia
Atorvastatin, simvastatin	Grapefruit juice can increase the plasma concentration of statins	
Ciclosporin, tacrolimus	Grapefruit juice can increase the plasma concentration of these medications	Hyperkalaemia Hypercholesterolaemia
Sirolimus		Hyperlipidaemia Hypokalaemia
Erythropoetin		Correct iron or folate deficiencies before starting Supplemental iron may improve the response
Corticosteroids		Weight gain Glucose intolerance Lipid abnormalities Osteoporosis
Calcium based phosphate binders, e.g. calcium acetate, Calcichew	Interacts with iron tablets. Do *not* take iron tablets within 2 hours of taking these medications	May cause hypercalcaemia
Alfacalcidol, calcitriol		May cause hypercalcaemia
Cinacalcet		May cause hypocalcaemia

ACE inhibitors, angiotensin converting enzyme inhibitors; ARB, angiotensin receptor blocker.

Poor nutritional status during the pretransplant period is associated with higher post transplant morbidity and mortality (Chan *et al.*, 2011). It has been shown that obesity may lead to increased risks post transplant, particularly if the BMI is >35 kg/m² (Holley *et al.*, 1990, Gill *et al.*, 1993, Pischon & Sharma, 2001, Gore *et al.*, 2006). Although studies suggest that moderate obesity does not affect major transplantation outcomes (Johnson *et al.*, 2002; Howard *et al.*, 2002), it is still reasonable to recommend that obese transplant candidates aim to reach a more desirable BMI.

Immediate post transplant phase
A successful kidney transplant enables previous dietary restrictions to be relaxed. However, some patients find it hard to relax their diet and fluid intake.

Protein and energy
In the first 4 weeks after transplantation, a diet providing 1.2–1.3 g of protein/kg of body weight may prevent negative nitrogen balance (Teplan *et al.*, 2009; Chan *et al.*, 2011). An energy intake of 30–35 kcal/kg is advised as it helps to ensure positive nitrogen balance (Teplan *et al.*, 2009, Danovitch, 2005).

Sodium and fluid
A low sodium diet may help those with post transplant hypertension and fluid overload (Danovitch, 2005). As kidney function improves, patients become polyuric and need encouragement to drink lots of fluid. This may be difficult for a patient who has spent years on dialysis trying to reduce their fluid intake; encouragement and reassurance are essential.

Potassium
Hyperkalaemia is associated with ciclosporin and tacrolimus, especially during the immediate post transplant period when dosages are high. This may be exaggerated by graft dysfunction. Treatment may require limitation of dietary potassium.

Phosphate
Hypophosphataemia is very common during the early weeks post transplant due to phosphaturia (Kasiske *et al.*, 2000). Oral phosphate supplementation may be needed where profound hypophosphataemia persists despite a liberal dietary intake. Phosphate binders should be discontinued as renal function improves to avoid severe hypophosphataemia.

Food borne infections
Transplant patients, even those who are not nutritionally compromised, may be susceptible to an increased incidence of infection. During the early post transplant period and in periods of acute illness, the likelihood of food borne infection is high due to significant suppression of the immune system (Chan *et al.*, 2011). Although there is no evidence to support the use of restrictive clean diets, it is prudent to provide general food safety advice to kidney transplant recipients (Chan *et al.*, 2011). Providing education on food safety may help minimise the risk for contamination. This may help to reduce the risks of infection with the following:

- *Listeria monocytogenes* – raw milk, soft cheeses and hot dogs.
- *Nocardia asteroids* – decaying vegetables.

- *Salmonella* – associated with undercooked, contaminated meat, poultry and eggs, as well as raw milk. Raw seafood and raw fruit and vegetables also present an increased risk.
- *Legionella* – contaminated or unsafe water supply (Danovitch, 2005).

Long term dietetic management

Protein

It has been shown that 0.8 g/kg/day of protein intake as well as limiting sodium intake can stabilise long term renal function and maintain an adequate nutritional status in the kidney transplant recipient (Bernardi *et al.*, 2003). High protein intakes should be discouraged because of the dangers of protein induced hyperfiltration. For stable patients, a normal protein intake of 0.8–1.0 g/kg of IBW should be the aim.

Energy

Energy intake and expenditure should be balanced to maintain desirable body weight and to prevent weight gain. For stable transplant patients who require weight reduction, a daily energy intake of 25 kcal/kg of IBW is a reasonable starting point.

Nutritional consequences and complications

Long term immunosuppression is associated with several nutrition related problems; these are obesity, dyslipidaemia, glucose intolerance, hypertension and CKD–MBD.

Obesity

Weight gain and obesity are common. This may be due to several factors, including a feeling of wellbeing after transplantation with increased food intake, improved quality of life (physical and psychological), freedom from dietary restrictions, a sedentary lifestyle, hyperphagia and higher body fat accumulation related to corticosteroids. Obesity is associated with CVD events and mortality (National Kidney Foundation, 2009b). Diet and other behaviour modifications have been shown to help reduce weight over the short term (National Kidney Foundation, 2009b).

Dyslipidaemia

Cardiovascular disease remains the main cause of long term mortality in the transplant population. There is no reason to believe that the management of complications of atherosclerotic CVD is different from that for the general population (National Kidney Foundation, 2009b). A diet in line with the latest lipid management guidelines for the general population is likely to benefit transplant recipients with dyslipidaemia (Chan *et al.*, 2011), although statins are usually required.

New onset diabetes mellitus

This is common and may reflect increased dietary intake, weight gain and the use of immunosuppressive agents, specifically corticosteroids, tacrolimus, sirolimus and, to a lesser extent, ciclosporin. The incidence of new onset diabetes mellitus after transplantation (NODAT) is highest in the first 3 months after transplantation. Its presence is associated with poorer outcomes, including increased graft failure, mortality and CVD (National Kidney Foundation, 2009b]. Diet, weight loss if appropriate and exercise provide the basis for the initial management (Davidson *et al.*, 2003). Oral hypoglycaemic agents or insulin may also be required.

Hypertension

Hypertension is an important risk factor for CVD as well as graft survival. Weight loss and exercise in the obese hypertensive patient may also play an important role in its treatment. Hypertensive patients are likely to benefit from limiting sodium intake to 2–3 g/day (Chan *et al.*, 2011).

CKD–MBD

CKD–MBD is common in transplant recipients. Calcium, phosphate and vitamin D metabolism are influenced by several factors resulting from the earlier period of CKD. Corticosteroids may cause osteoporosis, which may further affect MBD management. Hypercalcaemia is common and is usually due to hyperparathyroidism that persists from the preceding period of CKD (National Kidney Foundation,, 2009a,b]. Hypophosphataemia may persist and dietary phosphate intake should be individualised according to blood levels. A supplement of Vitamin D (or analogue) may also be required.

Management for those receiving conservative management

The number of people who choose not to have dialysis continues to rise, possibly as a result of an ageing population with multiple comorbidities. For these patients, regular review is important and the focus of care is symptom management. The main aims are to provide all aspects of clinical care, with the exception of dialysis, including the management of anaemia, together with ongoing support by the MDT in liaison with community and palliative care services. Little is known about the appropriate level of nutritional intervention for this patient group and there are no documented recommendations. Realistically, an approach that promotes enjoyment of food and mealtimes combined with symptom control would appear prudent.

Nutritional support in protein energy wasting

Early identification of any decline in nutritional status and its proactive management is essential as correcting established malnutrition is difficult. Assessment of oral intake should be part of a full assessment of nutritional status and medical causes should also be identified and treated. Once the appropriate nutritional plan is in place, regular monitoring is essential in order to evaluate the effectiveness of the intervention. The frequency of monitoring will depend on individual needs.

First line dietetic advice should be to fortify the existing diet with additional nutrient dense foods, relax any current dietary limitations (dependent on current bio-chemistry) and provide individualised advice. The use of sugary foods and sweet drinks should be encouraged, when appropriate, and fats are also a useful source of energy. Both mono- (MUFAs) and poly-unsaturated fatty acids (PUFAs) should be encouraged in all patients; however, high fat foods such as pastries, biscuits and cakes should not be discouraged in poor eaters or it will be difficult to meet energy requirements. As cholesterol levels are often lower in CKD stages 4 and 5, it is debatable as to whether a strict cardioprotective diet is as important at this time.

It has not yet been established if provision of nutritional support to patients prior to developing ERF leads to reduced morbidity and mortality, although there is some evidence that it improves nutritional markers in those on haemodialysis. A diet consisting of 45 kcal/kg and 1.5 g of protein/kg/day has been found to promote weight gain and improve albumin levels in malnourished haemodialysis patients (Kuhlmann *et al*., 1999). Oral nutritional supplements should be added if oral intake cannot be improved following dietetic intervention (Renal Association, 2010b). Glucose polymers (powders/liquids) and fat emulsions are ideal for increasing energy in patients with poor appetites who are unable to take adequate energy via normal food. If electrolyte levels are high, renal specific supplements that are low in electrolytes should be considered (Cano *et al*., 2006) (see Chapter 6.3).

Enteral tube feeding should be considered if the nutrient intake remains suboptimal despite oral supplements, although percutaneous endoscopic gastrostomy feeding is difficult in patients on peritoneal dialysis due to complications such as peritonitis. Other types of nutritional support that may be used are:

- *Intraperitoneal amino acids (IPAAs)* – sometimes used in CAPD and provide amino acids via dialysis. It is normal practice to insist that a high energy snack is eaten at the time of infusion, although evidence for this is limited (Jones *et al*., 1998).
- *Intradialytic parenteral nutrition (IDPN)* – a form of parenteral nutrition given via the venous return whilst on haemodialysis. Again, evidence for this is limited (Cano *et al*., 2007a; Bossola *et al*., 2010).

A meta analysis found that both oral and enteral nutritional support improved protein and energy intake, and increased serum albumin in haemodialysis patients (Stratton *et al*., 2005). This view is supported by a further review of the use of oral nutritional supplements and IDPN (Bossola *et al*., 2010). The conclusion was that the long term use of oral nutritional supplements is safe and may be useful in terms of improvement of nutritional parameters such as serum albumin and body weight. However, it remains to be clarified if their use is associated with increased survival. Intradialytic parenteral nutrition was also found to improve serum albumin and body weight, but did not influence survival. Percutaneous endoscopic gastrostomy feeding has been successful in those on haemodialysis, but the numbers of patients in the studies were low. It requires frequent monitoring but can lead to increases in weight and albumin levels; however, levels of phosphate have been found to be low at times (Holley & Kirk, 2002) (see Chapter 6.4).

Considerations for long term dietetic care of patients

Nutritional treatment in these patients can be complex because several nutrients often need to be managed simultaneously, the diet needs to change over time and comorbidities may need to be taken into account. The complexity of a regimen has been one of the most frequently identified barriers to patient compliance (Mitch & Klahr, 1993). Although a stepwise approach to educating the patient is important, giving knowledge alone does not necessarily lead to a change in behaviour. Behavioural change techniques are appropriate for patients with CKD as they can enhance patient motivation by reducing resistance to change. It can be helpful to explain why the diet may differ from a healthy diet and why this is of benefit. It has been found that people with CKD appreciate advice on what they can have to eat rather than lists of what they should avoid (Department of Health, 2004) (see Chapter 1.3).

Priorities may change over time, e.g. a moderate salt intake and cardioprotective diet that is important in early CKD is likely to be a lower priority if there is a greater need for nutritional support, when ensuring a high energy intake and adequate protein may mean foods that are higher in fat, sugar and salt are included in the diet. Cardiovascular death in later stages of CKD is more likely to be due to non-traditional risk factors such as phosphate control. Good glycaemic control is crucial in preventing or delaying the progression of early CKD in those with diabetes, but in ERF, opinion suggests that less strict glycaemic control may be preferable because this may reduce the risk of hypoglycaemia. In early CKD, weight loss is helpful in most obese patients, but on haemodialysis, obese patients currently fare better. As with the dietetic treatment of other chronic diseases, assessing the patient's motivation as well as their dietary understanding is important, together with jointly agreeing goals.

Micronutrients

The metabolism and status of micronutrients is altered in renal failure, but absolute requirements for trace elements have yet to be established. Iron deficiency is common, especially when erythropoietin therapy is used. Unfortunately, oral supplementation is ineffective and parenteral iron is often required. Zinc and selenium levels are also reduced, but routine supplementation is not recommended (Gilmour *et al*., 1998). Deficiencies in vitamin C, thiamine, riboflavin and pyridoxine may occur in individuals who are following a low protein diet. Chronic kidney disease results in a rise in vitamin A levels by up to 20% above baseline, primarily because of an increase in retinol binding protein; however, toxicity is rare because the vitamin is bound to the protein and is

Table 7.5.8 Dietary components and renal disease

	Protein	Energy	Potassium	Phosphate	Sodium and fluid
Significance in renal disease	Sufficient needed to avoid protein energy wasting Lower intake may delay progression of CKD (contentious)	Sufficient required to maintain energy balance and prevent protein energy wasting	Hyperkalaemia may cause cardiac arrhythmias/arrest	Hyperphosphataemia involved with development of CKD–mineral and bone disorder	Excess intake leads to fluid overload and hypertension
Acute kidney injury	≥1.0 g/kg body weight (BW) (see text)	Matched to requirements (see text)	As required (see text)	As required (see text)	As required (see text)
CKD stages 1–3	>0.8 g/kg BW	Aim to achieve ideal weight	Unlimited unless hyperkalaemic	No limitation	100 mmol of sodium (rarely fluid overloaded)
Nephrotic syndrome	0.8–1.0 g/kg ideal body weight (IBW)	30–35 kcal/kg IBW	Not limited unless hyperkalaemic	Not limited unless hyperphosphataemic	100 mmol of sodium + fluid limited if overloaded
CKD stage 4	0.75–1.0 g/kg IBW	30–35 kcal/kg IBW	Unlimited unless hyperkalaemic	Intake usually limited to 27–32 mmol if phosphate or PTH levels raised	100 mmol of sodium +fluid limited if overloaded
Haemodialysis	Minimum 1.1–1.2 g/kg IBW	30–40 kcal/kg IBW	Intake usually limited to approx. 1 mmol/kg BW	Intake usually limited to 27–32 mmol (adjusted for protein needs) – see text	100 mmol of sodium + fluid limitation usually required
Peritoneal dialysis	Minimum 1.0–1.2 g/kg IBW	30–35 kcal/kg of IBW (including glucose absorbed from dialysate)	Not limited unless hyperkalaemic	Intake usually limited to 27–32 mmol (adjusted for protein needs) – see text	100 mmol of sodium + fluid limitation usually required
Transplant	0.8–1 g/kg long term	Aim to maintain desirable weight	Not limited unless hyperkalaemic	Hypophosphataemia is common	80–120 mmol of sodium

Recommended intakes are for daily amounts.
CKD, chronic kidney disease; PTH, parathyroid hormone.

therefore inactive. Studies of vitamin E status in renal failure report contradictory findings. There is no evidence that supplements of vitamin B_{12}, folic acid, biotin, pantothenic acid, vitamins A or E are routinely required to correct deficiencies in any group of patients. High dose supplements of folic acid, pyridoxine and vitamin B_{12} show no benefit on cardiovascular morbidity or mortality and are not recommended.

There is some evidence that patients on low potassium diets can become vitamin C deficient. However, a high intake of vitamin C (2 g/day) is associated with hyperoxalosis and this may result in oxalate containing kidney stones. A lower dose (100 mg/day) does not appear to alter serum oxalate in patients on dialysis (Gilmour et al., 1998).

Abnormal renal metabolism, inadequate intake and/or gastrointestinal absorption and dialysis losses account for vitamin deficiencies amongst dialysis patients (Fouque et al., 2007). The European Society of Parenteral and Enteral Nutrition (ESPEN) has recommended that due to dialysis induced losses, water soluble vitamins should be supplied; folic acid (1 mg/day), pyridoxine (10–20 mg/day) and vitamin C (30–60 mg/day). Haemodialysis does not induce significant trace element losses; however, supplementation of zinc (15 mg/day) and selenium (50–70 mg/day) may be useful in depleted patients (Cano et al., 2006). The provision of water soluble vitamins has been associated with significantly lower mortality rates, but few UK units prescribe these (Fissell et al., 2004). It is currently recommend that haemodialysis patients be prescribed supplements of water soluble vitamins (Renal Association, 2010b). However, there are no recommendations regarding vitamin supplementation for peritoneal dialysis patients. The limited research in this area suggests there may be deficiency of some B vitamins and vitamin C. Individual dietary assessment will help establish if supplementation is necessary. For those with a successful renal transplant, regular supplementation is not needed (Martins et al., 2004). Table 7.5.8 summarises the requirements of the major nutrients to be considered in renal disease.

Acute kidney injury

Acute kidney injury (AKI) describes the disorder where kidney function abruptly deteriorates. It has now replaced

Table 7.5.9 Causes of acute kidney injury

Location	Cause	Example
Prerenal	Reduced intravascular volume	Blood loss, gastroenteritis, diuretics, hypoalbuminaemia, burns
	Cardiac failure	
	Vasodilatation	Sepsis
	Increased resistance to renal blood flow	Renal artery disease Renal vein thrombosis
	Hepatorenal syndrome*	
Renal	Glomerular disease	Primary renal disease or as part of a multisystem disorder (includes any cause of acute glomerulonephritis)
	Intrarenal vascular disease	Vasculitis Atheroembolic disease Haemolytic uraemic syndrome
	Tubulointerstitial disease	Acute tubular necrosis: post ischaemic (prerenal)** Toxic agents: drugs, poisons, X ray contrast Acute interstitial nephritis: infective, infiltration, (e.g. lymphoma), drug reaction
Post renal Obstruction to the flow of urine can be at any level from the intrarenal tubules to the urethra	Intrarenal obstruction	Crystals: uric acid, oxalate, calcium Abnormal proteins, e.g. myeloma
	Ureteric obstruction (needs to be bilateral unless only one functioning kidney)	
	Bladder outflow obstruction	Prostate or bladder tumours, calculi
	Urethral obstruction	Tumours, strictures

*The hepatorenal syndrome is an incompletely understood syndrome in which acute kidney injury occurs in association with liver failure. The liver failure is the primary lesion and renal function generally improves as the hepatic failure recovers.
**Acute tubular necrosis can result from any prerenal cause of renal failure if of sufficient duration and intensity. In hospital this is most commonly seen in the context of sepsis, trauma, major surgery and cardiac failure.

the term acute renal failure. The definition of AKI has changed in recent years, and detection is now mostly based on monitoring creatinine levels, with or without urine output. Criteria such as RIFLE (Bellomo *et al.*, 2004) and AKIN (Mehta *et al.*, 2007) have been used to diagnose AKI. Recently, Kidney Disease: Improving Global Outcomes (KDIGO, 2012) has produced a clinical practice guideline for AKI, which includes a globally acceptable definition by merging aspects of both RIFLE and AKIN and by defining its severity in three stages. This should enable the incidence, management and outcomes of AKI to be compared.

In general terms, AKI differs from CKD in that the decline in renal function is more rapid, taking place over hours or days, and is also potentially reversible. It covers a broad spectrum of conditions and clinical settings. Forms of kidney injury can be mild or severe and the condition of individuals may vary from being mobile around the ward with single organ failure to being cared for in the critical care unit with multiorgan failure. Renal replacement therapy may or may not be required. Causes of AKI are shown in Table 7.5.9. There is an overlap between the first two groups as any prerenal cause can lead to ischaemic damage to the kidney, causing the pathological acute tubular necrosis.

Disease process and consequences

Acute kidney injury is estimated to affect 7% of general hospital admissions (Nash *et al.*, 2002) and up to 20% of critically ill patients (Hegarty *et al.*, 2005). It is more likely to develop in individuals with pre-existing CKD, and is more common in older individuals. Patients may present with a reduced urine volume or with general symptoms such as nausea and vomiting. More serious presentations include pulmonary oedema, pericarditis, confusion or depressed levels of consciousness. It may also be detected incidentally following blood tests performed either routinely or to investigate other complaints.

Mortality rates range from 10% in uncomplicated AKI to 80% in patients with multiorgan failure (Cosentino *et al.*, 1994). Individuals die from their underlying disease and complications, rather than from renal failure. Poor nutritional status is associated with higher mortality rates (Mault *et al.*, 1983), but survival rates improve as nutritional support is increased (Abel *et al.*, 1973; Bartlett *et al.*, 1986; Rainford, 1981).

Management

The medical and nutritional management of the patient with AKI are closely linked and are dependent upon the

Table 7.5.10 Nutritional requirements in acute kidney injury

	Non-catabolic (no RRT)	Non-catabolic (on IHD)	Catabolic (on IHD)	Catabolic (on CRRT)
Protein (g/kg/day)	1.0	1.2	1.5	Up to max of 1.7 in hypercatabolism
Energy	Not affected by acute kidney injury Tailored to individual requirements and clinical state			
Fluid	Usually restricted, unless on CRRT			
Electrolytes	Monitor and adjust intake as required Will vary depending on disease state and type of treatment Solutions used in CRRT contain electrolytes			
Micronutrients	Requirements are not well documented Fat soluble vitamin and antioxidant status is low CRRT has negative effect on balance of some vitamins and trace elements. Consider supplementation – see text			

IHD, intermittent haemodialysis, RRT, renal replacement therapy; CRRT, continuous RRT.

patient's clinical state. Consequently, treatment regimens will need to be tailored to the particular needs of the individual.

Medical management

Unless the patient presents with a life threatening indication for urgent RRT, e.g. pulmonary oedema, severe hyperkalaemia or pericarditis, initial treatment will be aimed at the underlying cause of renal failure. This will involve efforts to preserve renal function, together with investigations to elucidate the cause of renal failure. Since the kidneys are dependent upon an adequate blood supply, measures to restore the circulating blood volumes and blood pressure are important. Other important general measures include aggressive treatment of sepsis and measures to improve cardiac function if impaired. Patients with an intrinsic renal cause for AKI will need further investigation, possibly including a renal biopsy, to ascertain whether any specific therapy is needed. More general management includes withdrawal of potentially nephrotoxic agents from the patient's therapy. Where the patient's urinary tract is obstructed, prompt relief of the obstruction may preserve renal function.

If the cause of AKI cannot be reversed, then it is likely that RRT will become necessary. A number of treatment options are available, and the modality chosen will reflect clinical need together with the facilities available locally. Intermittent haemodialysis, as discussed earlier in CKD, can be used in AKI patients who are stable. Dialysis treatment will usually undertaken on alternate days or in some cases daily. If the patient is oliguric, fluid balance becomes a critical aspect of management since intermittent haemodialysis provides limited opportunity for fluid removal. For individuals with cardiovascular instability, continuous RRT (CRRT) is the most suitable mode of RRT. It provides efficient correction of blood biochemistry and the steady removal of fluid, making it suitable for treating the sickest of patients. Continuous RRT can take a number of different forms, with haemofiltration being commonly employed. This technique involves blood passing across a filter to remove waste products and electrolytes. A

sterile replacement solution infusion maintains fluid balance. Running continuously over the day, CRRT enables large volumes of fluid to be removed.

Dietetic management

The general aim is to maintain nutritional status, whilst limiting the complications of renal failure. Early intervention is preferable since the timescale is much shorter in AKI than in CKD. A patient's nutritional requirements are influenced by a number of factors, and can vary greatly between individuals (Table 7.5.10). Individualised assessment will enable the nutritional prescription to be matched to the patient's needs. It is recommended that a dietitian conducts this assessment (Renal Association, 2011a).

Acute kidney injury has no effect on an individual's energy requirements (Schneeweiss et al., 1990). Even in patients with AKI and multiorgan failure, measured energy requirements are only 20% above resting values (Bouffard et al., 1987). Whilst absolute protein requirements are not well documented, they are influenced by the patient's clinical condition together with any RRT that they may receive.

Common causes of non-catabolic AKI include dehydration, nephrotoxins and urinary obstruction. In these cases, protein turnover rates are not increased and daily intakes of 1.0 g of protein/kg of body weight where RRT is not required, and 1 2 g/kg of body weight where intermittent haemodialysis is used, are recommended (Cano et al., 2006). Oral diet alone or with the addition of nutritionally dense supplementary sip feeds will frequently be sufficient to meet nutritional needs in these patients. If not, artificial nutritional support should be implemented. Wherever possible, this should be provided via the enteral route. Nutritionally dense feeds, with or without a reduced electrolyte content, are useful when the control of fluid balance and/or serum phosphate and potassium levels is an issue.

Fluid and electrolyte intake should be individualised according to blood biochemistry and fluid status. Frequent monitoring of blood biochemistry is essential to guide provision. Indications for potassium, phosphate, sodium and fluid restriction are similar to those in CKD. However, allowing a more liberal phosphate intake may be a better management approach if it helps to promote food intake. In the short term, maintaining a good nutritional intake is more of a priority than achieving serum phosphate control. Dietary restrictions are likely to be required until renal function begins to improve. When this happens, patients may become polyuric. An increased fluid intake (adequate to cover the large urine volumes and insensible losses) should then be maintained. As serum potassium and phosphate levels normalise, any dietary restrictions can be lifted.

Causes of catabolic AKI include sepsis and trauma; protein turnover rates in these patients are increased and negative nitrogen balance results. Patients will frequently have multiorgan failure and be managed in an intensive care unit. They present complex therapeutic challenges and require a broad appreciation of the management of nutrition in critical illness. Such issues are beyond the scope of any discussion, but major considerations in relation to AKI are outlined (see also Chapter 7.17.1).

Artificial nutritional support will usually be required. Where the enteral route cannot be used, parenteral nutrition support should be considered. Energy should be provided as a balance of carbohydrate and fat since patients will have both impaired glucose tolerance and reduced lipid clearance (Druml et al., 1983). Nitrogen should be sourced from a standard mixture of essential and non-essential amino acids (Brown et al., 2010) as some non-essential amino acids become conditionally essential in AKI and critical illness.

During CRRT, care is needed to avoid the potential over provision of energy from hidden sources. The metabolism of glucose and lactate contained in some of the solutions used during CRRT may result in significant energy gains. This area is explored in more detail elsewhere (Hartley, 2011). Continuous RRT also has a negative influence on nutrient balance with significant losses of amino acids (Davenport & Roberts, 1989; Frankenfield et al., 1993; Davies et al., 1991). Protein intakes should be increased to compensate for these losses and the patient's catabolic rate (Brown et al., 2010). A daily protein intake up to a maximum 1.7 g/kg for hypercatabolic individuals on CRRT is currently recommended (Cano et al., 2006; 2009; Renal Association, 2011a). To achieve these high protein intakes in enterally fed patients without excessive energy, protein rich supplements can be added to feeds to increase the nitrogen to calorie ratio.

Continuous RRT allows feed volumes and electrolyte intake to be liberalised; clearance rates are so great that intravenous supplementation with phosphate and other electrolytes may be required. However, technical advances have led to the development of newer solutions that should result in less supplementation being required. Frequent monitoring of blood levels is essential. Micronutrient losses on CRRT may also be significant. Documented daily ultrafiltrate losses include 100 mg of vitamin C (Bellomo & Boyce, 1993), 290 μg of folate (Fortin et al., 1999), 4 mg of thiamine and 0.97 μmol (77 μg) of sele-nium (Berger et al., 2004). These losses are superimposed upon the low antioxidant status reported in AKI (Druml et al., 1998; Story et al., 1999). Since the losses of vitamin C, thiamine and selenium exceed the amounts provided by commonly used parenteral sources and for some of these nutrients in many enteral feeds, selective micronutrient supplementation may be needed. Cases of severe oxalosis have been reported in individuals with AKI receiving daily vitamin C supplements of 500 mg intravenously (Friedman et al., 1983) or 5000 mg orally (Mashour et al., 2000); megadoses of vitamins should be avoided.

Internet resources

British Dietetic Association Renal Nutrition Group www.bda.uk.com
Kidney Patient Guide www.kidneypatientguide.org.uk
National Kidney Foundation (USA) www.kidney.org
National Institute for Health and Care Excellence (NICE)
    Clinical guideline 169 Prevention, detection and management of acute kidney injury up to the point of renal replacement therapy www.nice.org.uk/cg169
    NICE Pathways Chronic Kidney Disease Overview http://pathways.nice.org.uk/pathways/chronic-kidney-disease/chronic-kidney-disease-overview
Renal Association www.renal.org
UK National Kidney Federation www.kidney.org.uk

Useful recipe books for patients

Jackson H, Cassidy A, James G. (2006) *Eating Well with Kidney Failure*. London: Class Publishing.
Jackson H, Green C, James G. (2009) *Eating Well for Kidney Health*. London: Class Publishing.

References

Abel RM, Beck CH, Abbott WM, Ryan JA, Barnett GO, Fischer, M. (1973) Improved survival from acute renal failure after treatment with intravenous essential L-amino acids and glucose. *New England Journal of Medicine* 283(14): 695–699.

Abrass CK. (2004) Overview: obesity: what does it have to do with kidney disease? *Journal of the American Society of Nephrology* 15: 2768–2772.

Bakris GL, Siomos M, Richardson D, et al. (2000) ACE inhibition or angiotensin receptor blockade: Impact on potassium in renal failure. *Kidney International* 58: 2084–2092.

Bartlett RH, Mault JR, Dechert RE, Palmer J, Swartz RD, Port FK. (1986) Continuous arteriovenous hemofiltration: improved survival in surgical acute renal failure? *Surgery* 100(2): 400–408.

Bellomo R, Boyce N. (1993) Acute continuous hemodiafiltration: a prospective study of 110 patients and a review of the literature. *American Journal Kidney Diseases* 21(5): 508–518.

Bellomo R, Ronco C, Kellum JA, Mehta RL, Palevsky P. (2004) Acute renal failure – definition, outcome measures, animal models, fluid therapy and information technology needs: the Second International Consensus Conference of the Acute Dialysis Quality Initiative (ADQI) Group. *Critical Care* 8(4): R204–R212.

Bennett SE, Russell GI, Walls, J. (1983) Low protein diets in uraemia. *BMJ* 287: 1344–1345.

Berger MM, Shenkin A, Revelly JP, et al. (2004) Copper, selenium, zinc, and thiamine balances during continuous venovenous hemodiafiltration in critically ill patients. *American Journal of Clinical Nutrition* 80(2): 410–416.

Bernardi A, Biasia F, Pati T, Piva M, D'Angelo A, Bucciante G. (2003) Long-term protein intake control in kidney transplant recipients:

effect in kidney graft function and in nutritional status. *American Journal of Kidney Disease* 41(3 Suppl 1): S146–152.

Block GA, Klassen PS, Lazarus JM, Ofsthun N, Lowrie EG, Chertow GM. (2004) Mineral metabolism, mortality, and morbidity in maintenance hemodialysis. *Journal of the American Society of Nephrology* 15(8): 2208–2218.

Bossola M, Tazza L, Giungi S, Rosa F, Luciani G. (2010) Artificial nutritional support in chronic hemodialysis patients: A narrative review. *Journal of Renal Nutrition* 20(4): 213–223.

Bouffard Y, Viale JP, Annat G, Delafosse B, Guillaume C, Motin J. (1987) Energy expenditure in the acute renal failure patient mechanically ventilated. *Intensive Care Medicine* 13: 401–404.

British Dietetic Association (BDA) Renal Nutrition Group. (2011) *Evidence Based Dietetic Guidelines: Protein Requirements Of Adults On Haemodialysis And Peritoneal Dialysis*. Birmingham: BDA.

Brown RO, Compher C; American Society for Parenteral and Enteral Nutrition Board of Directors. (2010) A.S.P.E.N. clinical guidelines: nutrition support in adult acute and chronic renal failure. *Journal of Parenteral and Enteral Nutrition* 34(4): 366–377.

Campbell KL, Ash S, Zabel R, McFarlane C, Juffs P, Bauer JD. (2009) Standardised nutrition guidelines by renal dietitians is associated with improved nutrition status. *Journal of Renal Nutrition* 19(2): 136–144.

Cano N, Fiaccadori, E, Tesinsky P, *et al.* (2006) ESPEN guidelines on enteral nutrition: adult renal failure. *Clinical Nutrition* 25: 295–310.

Cano NJM, Fouque D, Roth H, *et al.*; and the French Study Group for Nutrition in Dialysis. (2007a) Intradialytic parenteral nutrition does not improve survival in malnourished hemodialysis patients: a 2-year multicenter, prospective, randomised study. *Journal of the American Society of Nephrology* 18: 2583–2591.

Cano AE, Neil AK, Kang JY, *et al.* (2007b) Gastrointestinal symptoms in patients with end-stage renal disease undergoing treatment by hemodialysis or peritoneal dialysis. *American Journal of Gastroenterology* 102: 1990–1997.

Cano NJ, Aparicio M, Brunori G, *et al.*; ESPEN. (2009) ESPEN Guidelines on Parenteral Nutrition: adult renal failure. *Clinical Nutrition* 28(4): 401–414.

Caravaca F, Arrobas M, Dominguez C. (1999) Influence of residual renal function on dietary protein and calorie intake in patients on incremental peritoneal dialysis. *Peritoneal Dialysis International* 19(4): 350–356.

Chan M, Patwardhan A, Ryan C, *et al.* (2011) Evidence based practice guidelines for the nutritional management of adult kidney transplant recipients. *Journal of Renal Nutrition* 21(1): 47–51.

Cheng LT, Tang W, Wang T. (2005) Strong association between volume status and nutritional status in peritoneal dialysis patients. *American Journal of Kidney Diseases* 45(5): 891–902.

Chumlea WC, Dwyer J, Bergen C, *et al.* (2003) Nutritional status assessed from anthropometric measures in the HEMO study. *Journal of Renal Nutrition* 13: 31–38.

Churchill DN, Taylor DW, Keshaviah PR. (1996) Adequacy of dialysis and nutrition in continuous peritoneal dialysis: Association with clinical outcomes. *Journal of the American Society of Nephrology* 7(2): 198–207.

Cosentino F, Chaff C, Piedmonte M. (1994) Risk factors influencing survival in ICU acute renal failure. *Nephrology, Dialysis & Transplantation* 9(Suppl 4): 179–182.

Covic A, Kothawala P, Bernal M, Robbins S, Chalian A, Goldsmith D. (2009) Systematic review of the evidence underlying the association between mineral metabolism disturbances and risk of all-cause mortality, cardiovascular mortality and cardiovascular events in chronic kidney disease. *Nephrology, Dialysis & Transplantation* 24(5): 1506–1523.

Cuppari L, Avesani C. (2004) Energy requirements in patients with chronic kidney disease. *Journal of Renal Nutrition* 14(3): 121–126.

Danovitch GM. (2005) Handbook of Kidney transplantation, 4th edn. *Nutrition in the Kidney Transplant Recipient*. Philadelphia: Lippincott Williams & Wilkins.

Davenport A, Roberts NB. (1989) Amino acid losses during high-flux hemofiltration in the critically ill patient. *Critical Care Medicine* 17(10): 1010–1014.

Davidson J, Wilkinson A, Dantal J, *et al.* (2003) New-onset diabetes after transplantation: 2003 international consensus guidelines. *Transplantation* 75(10): SS3–SS24.

Davies SP, Reaveley DA, Brown EA, Kox WJ. (1991) Amino acid clearances and daily losses in patients with acute renal failure treated by continuous arteriovenous hemodialysis. *Critical Care* 19(12): 1510–1515.

De Brito-Ashurst I, Varagunam M, Raftery MJ, Yaqoob MM. (2009) Bicarbonate supplementation slows progression of CKD and improves nutritional status. *Journal of the American Society of Nephrology* 20: 2075–2084.

De Mutsert R, Grootendorst DC, Boeschoten EW, *et al.* (2009) Subjective global assessment of nutritional status is strongly associated with mortality in chronic dialysis patients. *American Journal of Clinical Nutrition* 89: 787–793.

Department of Health. (2004) The National Service Framework for Renal Services. Available at http://webarchive.nationalarchives.gov.uk/+/www.dh.gov.uk/en/Healthcare/Longtermconditions/Vascular/Renal/DH_4102636.

Diabetes Control and Complications Trial (DCCT) Research Group. (1993) The effect of intensive treatment of diabetes on the development and progression of long-term complications in insulin-dependent diabetes mellitus. *New England Journal of Medicine* 329: 683–689.

Dombros N, Dratwa M, Feriani M, *et al.* (2005) European best practice guidelines for peritoneal dialysis. 8 Nutrition in peritoneal dialysis. *Nephrology Dialysis Transplantation* 20(9): ix28–ix33.

Druml W, Laggner AN, Kleinberger G, Lenz K. (1983) Lipid metabolism in acute renal failure. *Kidney International* 24(Suppl 16): S-139–S-142.

Druml W, Schwarzenhofer M, Apsner R, Horl WH. (1998) Fat-soluble vitamins in patients with acute renal failure. *Mineral and Electrolyte Metabolism* 24: 220–226.

Enia G, Sicuso C, Alati G, Zoccali C, Pustorino D, Biondo A. (1993) Subjective global assessment of nutrition in dialysis patients. *Nephrology Dialysis Transplantation* 8: 1094–1098.

Fissell RB, Bragg-Gresham JL, Gillespie BW, *et al.* (2004) International variation in vitamin prescribing and association with mortality in the Dialysis Outcomes and Practice Patterns Study (DOPPS). *American Journal of Kidney Diseases* 44(2): 293–299.

Fortin MC, Amyot SL, Geadah D. (1999) Serum concentrations and clearances of folic acid and pyridoxal-5-phosphate during venovenous continuous renal replacement therapy. *Intensive Care Medicine* 25(6): 594–598.

Fouque D, Vennegoor M, Wee PT, *et al.* (2007) ERA–EDTNA European best practice guideline on nutrition. *Nephrology Dialysis Transplantation* 22(Suppl 2): ii45–ii87.

Fouque D, Kalantar-Zadeh K, Kopple J, *et al.* (2008) A proposed nomenclature and diagnostic criteria for protein–energy wasting in acute and chronic kidney disease. *Kidney International* 73: 391–398.

Frankenfield DC, Badellino MM, Reynolds HN, Wiles CE III, Siegel JH, Goodarzi S. (1993) Amino acid loss and plasma concentration during continuous hemodiafiltration. *Journal of Parenteral and Enteral Nutrition* 17(6): 551–561.

Friedman A. (2004) High-protein diets: potential effects on the kidney in renal health and disease. *American Journal of Kidney Diseases* 44(6): 950–962.

Friedman AL, Chesnelof RW, Gilbert FF. (1983) Secondary oxalosis as a complication of parenteral alimentation in ARF. *American Journal Nephrology* 3: 248.

Gill IS, Hodge EE, Novick AC, Steinmuller DR, Garred D. (1993) Impact of obesity on renal transplantation. *Transplant Proceedings* 25: 1047–1048.

Gilmour ER, Hartley GH, Goodship THJ. (1998) Trace elements and vitamins in renal disease. In: Mitch WE, Klahr S (eds) *Handbook of Nutrition and the Kidney*, 3rd edn. New York: Lippincott-Raven, pp. 105–122.

Giordano M, De Feo P, Lucidi P, *et al.* (2001) Effects of dietary protein restriction on fibrinogen and albumin metabolism in nephrotic patients. *Kidney International* 60(1): 235–242.

Goodman, WG, Goldin, J, Kuizon, BD, *et al.* (2000) Coronary-artery calcification in young adults with end-stage renal disease who are undergoing dialysis. *New England Journal of Medicine* 342(20): 1478–1483.

Gore JL, Pham PT, Danovitch GM, *et al.* (2006) Obesity and outcome following renal transplantation. *American Journal of Transplantation* 6: 357–363.

Guerin AP, London GM, Marchais SJ, Metivier F. (2000) Arterial stiffening and vascular calcifications in end-stage renal disease. *Nephrology, Dialysis & Transplantation* 15(7): 1014–1021.

Gutierrez O, Isakova T, Rhee E, *et al.* (2005) Fibroblast growth factor-23 mitigates hyperphosphatemia but accentuates calcitriol deficiency in chronic kidney disease. *Journal of the American Society of Nephrology* 16(7): 2205–2215.

Hartley GH. (2011) Nutrition in kidney disease. In: Todorovic VE, Micklewright A (eds) *A Pocket Guide to Clinical Nutrition*, 4th edn. Birmingham: British Dietetic Association.

Hegarty, J, Middleton, RJ, Krebs, M, *et al.* (2005) Severe acute renal failure in adults: place of care, incidence and outcomes. *Quarterly Journal of Medicine* 98(9): 661–666.

Heimburger O, Quereshi AR, Blaner WS, Bergland L, Stenvinkel P. (2000) Hand-grip muscle strength, lean body mass, and plasma proteins as markers of nutritional status in patients with chronic renal failure close to start of dialysis therapy. *American Journal of Kidney Diseases* 36: 1213–1225.

Holley JL, Kirk J. (2002) Enteral tube feeding in a cohort of chronic hemodialysis patients. *Journal of Renal Nutrition* 12(3): 177–182.

Holley JL, Shapiro R, Lopatin WB, Tzakis AG, Hakala TR, Starzl TE. (1990) Obesity as a risk factor following cadaveric renal transplantation. *Transplantation* 49: 387–389.

Howard RJ, Thai VB, Patton PR, *et al.* (2002) Obesity does not portend a bad outcome for kidney transplant recipients. *Transplantation* 73(1): 53–55.

Hull RP, Goldsmith DJA. (2008) Nephrotic syndrome in adults. *BMJ* 336: 1185–1189.

Ikizler TA, Green JH, Wingard RL, Parker RA, Hakim RM. (1995) Spontaneous dietary protein intake during progression of chronic renal failure. *Journal of the American Society of Nephrology* 6: 1380–1391.

Johnson DW, Isbel NM, Brown AM, *et al.* (2002) The effect of obesity on renal transplant outcomes. *Transplantation* 74(5): 675–681.

Jones CH. (2001) Serum albumin – a marker of fluid overload in dialysis patients? *Journal of Renal Nutrition* 11: 59–56.

Jones M, Hagen T, Boyle CA, *et al.* (1998) Treatment of malnutrition with 1.1% amino acid peritoneal dialysis solution: Results of a multicentre outpatient study. *American Journal of Kidney Diseases* 32(5): 761–769.

Kalantar-Zadeh K, Block G, Humphreys MH, Kopple JD. (2003) Reverse epidemiology of cardiovascular risk factors in maintenance dialysis patients. *Kidney International* 63: 793–808.

Kalantar-Zadeh K, Regidor DL, Kovesdy CP, *et al.* (2009) Fluid retention is associated with cardiovascular mortality in patients undergoing long-term hemodialysis. *Circulation* 119: 671–679.

Kalantar-Zadeh K, Gutekunst L, Mehrotra R, *et al.* (2010) Understanding sources of dietary phosphorus in the treatment of patients with chronic kidney disease. *Clinical Journal of the American Society of Nephrology* 5: 519–530.

Kasiske BL, Vazquez MA, Harmon WE, *et al.* (2000) Recommendations for the outpatient surveillance of renal transplant recipients. American Society of Transplantation. *Journal of the American Society of Nephrology* 11: S1–S86.

Kaysen GA, Dubin JA, Muller H,. Mitch WE, Rosales LM, Levin NW; the Hemo Study Group. (2002) Relationships among inflammation nutrition and physiologic mechanisms establishing albumin levels in hemodialysis patients. *Kidney International* 61: 2240–2249.

Kidney Disease: Improving Global Outcomes (KDIGO) CKD-MBD Work Group. (2009) KDIGO clinical practice guideline for the diagnosis, evaluation, prevention, and treatment of Chronic Kidney Disease-Mineral and Bone Disorder (CKD-MBD). *Kidney International* 76(Suppl 113): S1–S130.

Kidney Disease: Improving Global Outcomes (KDIGO). (2012) Clinical practice guideline for acute kidney injury. *Kidney International Supplements* 2(Suppl. 1): 1–141.

Kopple JD, Monteon FJ, Shaib JK. (1986) Effect of energy intake on nitrogen metabolism in nondialysed patients with chronic renal failure. *Kidney International* 29: 734–742.

Kopple JD, Levey AS, Greene T, *et al.* (1997) Effect of dietary protein restriction on nutritional status in the modification of diet in renal disease study. *Kidney International* 52: 778–791.

Korgaonkar S, Tilea A, Gillespie BB, Kiser, M., *et al.* (2010) Serum potassium and outcomes in CKD: insights from the RRI-CKD Cohort Study. *Clinical Journal of the American Society of Nephrology* 5: 762–769.

Kovesdy CP, Regidor DL, Mehrotra R, *et al.* (2007) Serum and dialysate potassium concentrations and survival in haemodialysis patients. *Clinical Journal of the American Society of Nephrology* 2: 999–1007.

Kramer HJ, Saranathan A, Luke A, *et al.* (2006) Increasing body mass index and obesity in the incident ESRD population. *Journal of the American Society of Nephrology* 17: 1453–1459.

Krautzig S, Janssen U, Koch KM, Granolleras C, Shaldon S. (1998) Dietary salt restriction and reduction of dialysate sodium to control hypertension in maintenance haemodialysis patients. *Nephrology Dialysis Transplantation* 13: 552–553.

Kuhlmann M, Schmidt F, Kohler H. (1999) High protein/energy vs. standard protein/energy nutritional regimen in the treatment of malnourished haemodialysis patients. *Mineral and Electrolyte Metabolism* 25: 306–310.

Leavey SF, McCullough K, Hecking E, Goodkin D, Port FK, Young EW. (2001) Body mass index and mortality in 'healthier' as compared to 'sicker' haemodialysis patients. Results from the dialysis outcomes and practice patterns study (DOPPS). *Nephrology Dialysis Transplantation* 16: 2386–2394.

Lee A. (2011) Constipation in patients on peritoneal dialysis: a literature review. *Renal Society of Australasia Journal* 7(3): 122–129.

Levey AS, Adler S, Caggiula AW, *et al.* (1996) Effects of dietary protein restriction on the progression of moderate renal disease in the Modification of Diet in Renal Disease Study. *Journal of the American Society of Nephrology* 7: 2616–2626.

Levey AS, Atkins R, Coresh J, *et al.* (2007) Chronic kidney disease as a global public health problem: Approaches and initiatives – a position statement from Kidney Disease Improving Global Outcomes CKD as a global public health problem: Approaches and initiatives. *Kidney International* 72: 247–259.

London GM, Guerin AP, Marchais SJ, Metivier F, Pannier B, Adda H. (2003) Arterial media calcification in end-stage renal disease: impact on all-cause and cardiovascular mortality. *Nephrology, Dialysis & Transplantation* 18(9): 1731–1740.

Lopez-Gomez JM, Villaverde M, Jofre, R, Rodriguez-Benitez P, Perez-Garcia R. (2005) Interdialytic weight gain as a marker of blood pressure, nutrition, and survival in hemodialysis patients. *Kidney International* 67(Suppl 93): S63–S68.

Mansy H, Goodship THJ, Tapson JS, Hartley GH, Keavey P, Wilkinson R. (1989) Effect of a high protein diet in patients with the nephrotic syndrome. *Clinical Science* 77(4): 445–451.

Martins C, Pecoits-Filho R, Riella MC. (2004) Nutrition for the post renal transplant recipients. *Transplantation Proceedings* 36: 1650–1654.

Mashour S, Turner JF, Merrell R. (2000) Acute renal failure, oxalosis, and vitamin C supplementation: a case report and review of the literature. *Chest* 118(2): 561–563.

Mault JR, Bartlett RH, Dechert RE, Clark SF, Swartz RD. (1983) Starvation: a major contribution to mortality in acute renal failure. *Transactions of the American Society of Artificial Internal Organs* XXIX: 390–395.

Mehta RL, Kellum JA, Shah SV, et al. (2007) Acute Kidney Injury Network: report of an initiative to improve outcomes in acute kidney injury. *Critical Care* 11(2): R31.

Metcalfe W. (2007) How does early chronic kidney disease progress? *Nephrology Dialysis Transplantation* 22(Suppl 9): ix26–ix30.

Mitch WE, Klahr S. (1993) *Handbook of Nutrition and the Kidney*, 3rd edn. New York: Little, Brown and Company.

Monteen FJ, Laidlaw SA, Kopple JD. (1986) Energy expenditure in patients with chronic renal failure. *Kidney International* 30: 741–747.

Nash K, Hafeez A, Hou S. (2002) Hospital-acquired renal insufficiency. *American Journal Kidney Diseases* 39(5): 930–936.

National Institute for Health and Care Excellence (NICE). (2007) Cinacalcet for the treatment of secondary hyperparathyroidism in patients with end-stage renal disease on maintenance dialysis therapy London: NICE.

National Institute for Health and Care Excellence (NICE). (2008a) Chronic kidney disease: Early identification and management of chronic kidney disease in adults in primary and secondary care. Available at http://www.nice.org.uk/Guidance/CG73. Accessed March 2011.

National Institute for Health and Care Excellence (NICE). (2008b) Clinical guidelines and evidence review for lipid modification: cardiovascular risk assessment and the primary and secondary prevention of cardiovascular disease. Available at www.nice.org .uk/nicemedia/pdf/CG67NICEguideline.pdf. Accessed March 2011.

National Kidney Foundation. (2000) K/DOQI clinical practice guidelines for nutrition in chronic renal failure. *American Journal of Kidney Diseases* 35(Suppl 2): S17–S104.

National Kidney Foundation. (2002) K/DOQI Clinical practice guidelines for chronic kidney disease: evaluation, classification and stratification. *American Journal of Kidney Diseases* 39: S1–S266.

National Kidney Foundation. (2003) K/DOQI clinical practice guidelines for bone metabolism and disease in chronic kidney disease. *American Journal Kidney Diseases* 42(4 Suppl 3): S1–201.

National Kidney Foundation. (2009a) KDIGO clinical practice guideline for the diagnosis, evaluation, prevention, and treatment of chronic kidney disease-mineral and bone disorder (CKD-MBD). *Kidney International* 113: S1–130.

National Kidney Foundation. (2009b) KDIGO clinical practice guideline for the care of kidney transplant recipients. *American Journal of Transplantation* 9(Suppl 3): S131–S155.

Navaneethan SD, Yehnert H, Moustarah F, et al. (2009) Weight loss interventions in chronic kidney disease: a systematic review and meta-analysis. *Clinical Journal of the American Society of Nephrology* 4(10): 1565–1574.

Navaneethan SD, Palmer SC, Vecchio M, Craig JC, Elder GJ, Strippoli GF. (2011) Phosphate binders for preventing and treating bone disease in chronic kidney disease patients. *Cochrane Database of Systematic Reviews* 2: CD006023.

NHS Kidney Care. (2010) Kidney disease: Key facts and figures. Available at www.kidneycare.nhs.uk. Accessed May 2011.

Noori N, Kopple JD, Kovesdy CP, et al. (2010) Mid-arm muscle circumference and quality of life and survival in maintenance haemodialysis patients. *Clinical Journal of the American Society of Nephrology* 5: 683–692.

Paniagua R, Amato D, Vonesh E, Coreea-Rotter R, Ramos A, Moran J, Mujais S; Mexican Collaborative study Group (2002) Effects of increased peritoneal clearances on mortality rates in peritoneal dialysis: ADEMEX, a prospective, randomised, controlled trial. *Journal of the American Society of Nephrology* 13: 1307–1320.

Pischon T, Sharma AM. (2001) Obesity as a risk factor in renal transplant patients. *Nephrology Dialysis Transplantation* 16: 14–17.

Pollock C, Voss D, Hodson E, Crompton C. (2005) Caring for Australasians with Renal Impairment (CARI). The CARI guidelines. Nutrition and growth in kidney disease. *Nephrology* 10(Suppl 5): S177–230.

Rainford DJ. (1981) Nutritional management of acute renal failure. *Acta Chirugica Scandinavica* 507(Suppl): 327–329.

Reaven PD, Moritz TE, Schwenke DC, et al. (2009) Intensive glucose-lowering therapy reduces cardiovascular disease events in Veterans Affairs diabetes trial participants with lower calcified coronary atherosclerosis. *Diabetes* 58(11): 2642–2648.

Renal Association. (2009a) Planning, initiating and withdrawal of renal replacement therapy. Available at www.renal.org/clinical/ GuidelinesSection/RenalReplacementTherapy.aspx. Accessed April 2011.

Renal Association. (2009b) Haemodialysis. Available at www.renal .org/Clinical/GuidelinesSection/Haemodialysis.aspx. Accessed April 2011.

Renal Association. (2010a) Peritoneal dialysis in CKD. Available at www.renal.org/Clinical/GuidelinesSection/PeritonealDialysis.aspx. Accessed May 2011.

Renal Association. (2010b) Nutrition in CKD. Available at www.renal.org/Clinical/GuidelinesSection/NutritionInCKD.aspx. Accessed March 2011.

Renal Association. (2010c). Cardiovascular disease in CKD. (2010). Available at www.renal.org/Clinical/GuidelinesSection/ CardiovascularDiseaseInCKD.aspx. Accessed May 2011.

Renal Association (2010d). CKD-mineral and bone disorders. Available at www.renal.org/Clinical/GuidelinesSection/CKD-MBD.aspx. Accessed May 2011.

Renal Association. (2011a) Clinical practice guidelines – acute kidney injury. Available at www.renal.org/Clinical/Guidelines Section/AcuteKidneyInjury.aspx

Renal Association. (2011b) Detection, monitoring and care of patients with CKD. Available at www.renal.org/Clinical/Guidelines Section/Detection-Monitoring-and-Care-of-Patients-with-CKD .aspx. Accessed March 2011.

Renal Association. (2011c) Assessment of the potential kidney transplant recipient. Available at www.renal.org/Clinical/Guidelines Section/AssessmentforRenalTransplantation.aspx. Accessed June 2011.

Renal Association. (2011d) Post operative care of the kidney transplant recipient. Available at www.renal.org/Clinical/Guidelines Section/Post-operative-Care-Kidney-Transplant-Recipient.aspx. Accessed June 2011.

Rigby-Matthews A, Scriber BH, Ahman S. (1999) Control of interdialytic weight gain does not require fluid restriction in hemodialysis patients. *Journal of the American Society of Nephrology* 10: 267A.

Rocco MV, Paranandi, L, Burrowes, JD, Cockram, DB, Dwyer, JT, Kusek, JW, Leung J, Makoff R, Maroni B, Poole D. (2002). Nutritional status in the HEMO Study cohort at baseline. *American Journal of Kidney Diseases* 39(2): 245–256.

Schiller LR, Santa Ana CA, Sheikh MS, Emmett M, Fordtran JS. (1989) Effect of the time of administration of calcium acetate acetate on phosphorus binding. *New England Journal of Medicine* 320: 1110–1113.

Schneeweiss B, Graninger W, Stockenhuber F, et al. (1990) Energy metabolism in acute and chronic renal failure. *American Journal of Clinical Nutrition* 52: 596–601.

Scottish Intercollegiate Guidelines Network (SIGN). (2008) Diagnosis and management of chronic kidney disease: A national clinical guideline. Available at www.sign.ac.uk/pdf/sign103.pdf. Accessed April 2011.

Shinaberger CS, Kilpatrick RD, Regidor DL, *et al.* (2006) Longitudinal associations between dietary protein intake and survival in hemodialysis patients. *American Journal of Kidney Diseases* 48(1): 37–49.

Shinaberger CS, Greenland S, Kopple JD, *et al.* (2008) Is controlling phosphorus by decreasing dietary protein intake beneficial or harmful in persons with chronic kidney disease? *American Journal of Clinical Nutrition* 88(6): 1511–1518.

Slatapolsky E, Weerts C, Lopez-Hilker S, *et al.* (1986) Calcium carbonate as a phosphate binder in patients with chronic renal failure undergoing dialysis. *New England Journal of Medicine* 315(2): 157–161.

Stenvinkel P, Heimburger O, Lindholm B, Kaysen GA, Bergstrom J. (2000) Are there two types of malnutrition in chronic renal failure? Evidence for relationships between malnutrition, inflammation and atherosclerosis (MIA) syndrome? *Nephrology Dialysis Transplantation* 15: 953–960.

Stenvinkel P, Alvestrand A. (2002), Review articles: Inflammation in end-stage renal disease: sources, consequences, and therapy. *Seminars in Dialysis* 15: 329–337.

Stevens PE, O'Donoghue DJ, de Lusignan S, *et al.* (2007) Chronic kidney disease management in the United Kingdom: NEOERICA project results. *Kidney International* 72: 92–99.

Story DA, Ronco C, Bellomo R. (1999) Trace element and vitamin concentrations and losses in critically ill patients treated with continuous venovenous hemofiltration. *Critical Care Medicine* 27(1): 220–223.

Stratton RJ, Bircher G, Fouque D, *et al.* (2005) Multinutrient oral supplements and tube feeding in maintenance dialysis: A systematic review and meta-analysis. *American Journal of Kidney Diseases* 46: 387–405.

Suckling RJ, He FJ, MacGregor GA. (2010) Altered dietary salt intake for preventing and treating diabetic kidney disease. *Cochrane Database of Systematic Reviews* 12.

Teplan V, Valkovsky I, Teplan V Jnr, Stollova M, Vyhnanek F, Andel M. (2009) Nutritional consequences of renal transplantation. *Journal of Renal Nutrition* 19(1): 95–100.

Teta D. (2010) Weight loss in obese patients with chronic kidney disease: who and how? *Journal of Renal Care* 36(Suppl 1): 163–171.

Tomson C. (2001) Advising dialysis patients to restrict fluid intake without restricting sodium intake is not based on evidence and is a waste of time. *Nephrology Dialysis Transplantation* 16: 1538–1542.

Wang AY, Sea MM, Ip R, *et al.* (2001) Independent effects of residual renal function and dialysis adequacy on actual dietary protein, calorie and other nutrient intake in patients on continuous ambulatory peritoneal dialysis. *Journal of the American Society of Nephrology* 12: 2450–2457.

Wang AY, Sanderson J, Sea MM, *et al.* (2003) Important factors other than dialysis adequacy associated with inadequate dietary protein and energy intakes in patients receiving maintenance peritoneal dialysis. *American Journal of Clinical Nutrition* 77(4): 834–841.

Wolfe RA, Ashby VB, Milford EL. (1999). Comparison of mortality in all patients on dialysis, patients on dialysis awaiting transplantation and recipients of a first cadaveric transplant. *New England Journal of Medicine* 341: 1725–1730.

Zoccali C, Kramer A, Jager, KJ. (2010) Chronic kidney disease and end-stage renal disease—a review produced to contribute to the report 'the status of health in the European union: towards a healthier Europe'. *Nephrology, Dialysis & Transplantation Plus* 3: 213–224.

7.5.2 Renal stones

Karen Thomsett and Sharon Underwood

Key points

- In developed countries 80% of renal stones are composed of calcium salts, usually calcium oxalate.

- Fluid intake is the most important factor in the dietary treatment of stones.

- Intake of calcium, protein and sodium should also be considered in the management of calcium stones.

- Evidence is limited regarding the efficacy of individual dietary components or of multicomponent dietary strategies for preventing stone recurrence.

- There is increasing evidence to show a link between obesity, metabolic syndrome and diabetes with stone formation.

In developed countries most urinary stones are renal stones; bladder stones are less common. Diagnosis is rarely difficult as the condition is painful, ranging from dull loin pain if the stone is in the renal pelvis to agonising colic if it is lodged in the ureter. Urolithiasis refers to stones originating in the urinary system, including the kidneys and bladder. Nephrolithiasis indicates the presence of calculi in the kidneys.

Generally 80% of stones are composed of calcium salts, usually calcium oxalate and less commonly calcium phosphate (Daudon *et al.*, 1995). The remaining 20% are composed of uric acid magnesium ammonium phosphate (struvite) or cystine. Stones with any other composition are very rare (<1% of total occurrence). Until recently, renal stones in developing countries were considered to be different from those in industrialised countries. In developing countries, phosphate and urate stones predominated. However, the epidemiology of renal stones is changing worldwide, with a predominance of calcium oxalate stones (Daudon *et al.*, 2004) (Table 7.5.11).

SECTION 7

Table 7.5.11 Main classifications of kidney stones

Type of stone	Occurrence (%)	Composition
Calcium oxalate ± calcium phosphate	75	Calcium oxalate, calcium phosphate
Struvite (infection stones)	15	Magnesium ammonium phosphate (triple phosphate)
Pure calcium phosphate	5–7	Calcium phosphate
Uric acid	5–8	Uric acid

In the UK, kidney stones affect up to 5% of the population, with a lifetime risk of passing a kidney stone of about 8–10%. The rate doubles if there is a family member with a history of stone disease. The peak age is 20–50 years with a male to female ratio of about 2:1 (Parmar, 2004). Globally, the incidence is increasing across gender, age and race; prevalence appears to have doubled over the past 30 years and is associated with the socioeconomic status of the population. The overweight and obese are more likely to get stones (Romero *et al.*, 2010) and this association is greater in females. Kidney stones are associated with a small, but significant, increase in the risk of chronic and end stage renal disease, with young women being at greater risk (Tonelli *et al.*, 2012). Renal stones recur and the likelihood that another stone occurring within 5–7 years is 50% (Asplin *et al.*, 1996).

Stones result from nucleation; a phase change when dissolved substances become solid. This requires supersaturated urine; the greater the concentration of two ions, the more likely they are to precipitate. The concentration of ions depends on the urinary pH, ionic strength and solute concentration. Both environmental and nutritional factors have been shown to affect stone nucleation and growth by their effects on urinary constituents and pH. Nucleation is followed by retention of the initial nucleus crystal, growth, aggregation and retention (Basavaraj *et al.*, 2007).

Calcium stones

Calcium oxalate is the main component of 80% of kidney stones (Parmar, 2004). Increased urinary calcium (>300 mg/day in men and >250 mg/day in women or >4 mg/kg of body weight/day) leads to precipitation of insoluble calcium salts and inactivates urinary inhibitors. Inhibitors include citrate, magnesium and the organic substances glycosaminoglycans, prothrombin F1 fragment and Tamm–Horsfall glycoprotein. Promoters of stone formation include low urine volume, low urine pH, calcium, sodium and oxalate (Basavaraj *et al.* 2007). Anatomical factors can influence stone formation.

In 80% of cases there is no underlying cause and the stone can be described as idiopathic. In the remaining 20%, the stone is secondary to other renal factors.

Idiopathic calcium stone disease

This is a syndrome of normal plasma calcium and unexplained hypercalciuria, which is distinguished from primary hyperparathyroidism by normal serum calcium levels. There are three subtypes (Paliouras *et al.*, 2012):

- Absorptive hypercalciuria – increased urinary calcium excretion due to increased intestinal absorption.
- Renal leak hypercalciuria – a primary tubular defect leading to decreased calcium reabsorption.
- Resorptive hypercalciuria – a primary increase in bone mineral turnover.

Contributory factors include:

- *Gender* – men are particularly susceptible and account for 85% of cases.
- *Age* – idiopathic calcium stones occur most commonly occur between 20 and 49 years of age; the incidence rises in the fourth decade.
- *Ethnicity* – the risk is highest for Caucasians, followed by Asians and Hispanics, and then Blacks.
- *Low urine volume* – the risk is greater in people who do not drink sufficiently and in those who work in hot climates or conditions, as a result of the increased likelihood of dehydration.
- *Social class* – the incidence is greater in social classes I and II, possibly associated with a higher intake of dietary animal protein.
- *Dietary factors* that have been suggested to be associated include high intakes of calcium, protein, sodium and possibly vitamin D, sucrose and fructose. A low intake of fluid plays a pivotal role in stone formation, and poor intake of fibre, notably phytate, has been linked with stone formation. However, some of these associations remain equivocal.
- *Obesity* – stone formation is positively associated with a higher urinary oxalate (Taylor & Curhan, 2008b).
- *Increased intestinal absorption of calcium* – the cause is unknown but stones may result from either increased synthesis of 1,25 dihydroxycholecalciferol or the presence of calcitriol intestinal receptor sites (Dretler, 1998). Intestinal hyperabsorption of calcium raises serum calcium (remaining within the normal range), which reduces endogenous parathyroid hormone (PTH) production. This leads to decreased renal tubular reabsorption of calcium and higher urinary excretion in order to maintain a normal serum calcium level.
- *Impaired tubular reabsorption of calcium* – secondary hyperparathyroidism stimulates calcitriol synthesis and increases intestinal calcium reabsorption (Pak, 1998).
- *Hyperoxaluria* – increased urinary oxalate excretion (>45 mg/day) significantly increases stone risk. Given the low oxalate content of most common foods, a variable absorption rate and bioavailability (10–100%), and the influence on oxalate absorption and urinary oxalate excretion by other variables, e.g. fluid intake, the impact of dietary oxalate on urinary excretion remains questionable.

- *Hypocitraturia* – citrate binds to calcium anions in the tubular lumen, increasing their solubility and inhibiting the nucleation of calcium oxalate crystals. In addition, citrate also inhibits crystal aggregation and growth. Citrate excretion is regulated by urinary pH with acidosis reducing renal excretion. Dietary factors associated with hypocitraturia include a low intake of fruit and vegetables and high intake of sodium and protein. Some medications have been implicated, notably thiazide diuretics and angiotensin converting enzyme (ACE) inhibitors (Melnick *et al.*, 1998).
- *Acidic urinary pH* promotes the precipitation of calcium phosphate and, to a lesser extent, calcium oxalate.
- *Hyperuricosuria* – total urinary uric acid output is usually normal in stone formers, but the concentration is increased. This is thought to reduce the activity of urinary inhibitors.

Role of diet in idiopathic calcium stone formation

Calcium

For many years it was assumed that a high calcium intake increased the risk of stone formation. However, severe calcium restriction (<400 mg/day) does not reduce the frequency of new stone formation in patients with recurrent urolithiasis and may be detrimental as negative calcium balance and secondary hyperoxaluria can occur (Parmar, 2004). A large prospective study found a 34% lower incidence of stone occurrence amongst men on a high calcium diet (Curhan *et al.*, 1993). However, this study was carried out on healthy subjects and may not be applicable to patients with existing stones. Several more recent studies have shown that an adequate calcium intake is associated with decreased stone formation. Curhan *et al.* (2004) found that in previously non-stone forming younger women, a higher intake of calcium was related to a lower risk of kidney stone formation.

Protein

The influence of excessive protein has become clearer in recent years, but the mechanism remains complex. Following a protein load there is a brief period of metabolic acidosis and, although urinary pH *per se* is not a major risk factor, calcium phosphate and, to a lesser degree, calcium oxalate are less soluble in acid conditions. Dietary protein has been found to increase oxaluria and uricosuria, which are associated with urolithiasis (Borghi *et al.*, 2002).

Sodium

Urinary sodium excretion correlates with urinary calcium excretion (Parmar, 2004). A high sodium diet increases calcium excretion and consequently the risk of stone formation. Hypercalciuric patients may be more sensitive to the calciuric effect of a sodium load. High sodium intake also increases the saturation of monosodium urate, the crystals of which can act as a basis for calcium crystallisation.

Vitamin D

The role of excessive vitamin D intake in stone formation is controversial. There is a correlation between plasma vitamin D and calcium excretion; therefore, patients should be discouraged from self medication multivitamin preparations or fish liver oil capsules containing vitamin D. However, a large epidemiological study found a lower incidence of renal stones in men with a high intake of vitamin D (Curhan *et al.*, 1993). A review by Parivar *et al.*, (1996) found that there was no conclusive evidence linking excessive dietary vitamin D intake or prolonged exposure to sunlight with a higher incidence of urolithiasis. It has been shown that combined calcium and vitamin D supplements can increase the risk of stones (Yalamanchili & Gallagher, 2012). Prospective studies are needed to clarify the relationship between vitamin D and kidney stone formation and whether nutritional vitamin D supplementation increases the risk of stone occurrence.

Fluid

A low fluid intake results in low urinary output with an increase in the concentration of ionic particles and the saturation level of various salts, increasing the likelihood of precipitation.

Fibre

There are conflicting epidemiological studies on the role of fibre intake on urolithiasis risk, largely as a result of the different definitions and analytical methods used to estimate fibre intake. Phytate binds to calcium and exhibits a strong inhibitory effect on urinary crystallisation of calcium salts such as calcium oxalate and calcium phosphate. Until further studies are conducted, no conclusions can be made on any role of fibre in stone formation.

Diagnosis of idiopathic hypercalciuria

A range of tests and assessments are required to establish the likely cause and type of stone.

24-Hour urine collection

An accurate 24-hour urine collection will provide information on the elevated amounts of excretory products. The urine must be collected while consuming the usual diet and fluid intake, and the urine quantity passed measured.

Biochemistry

Serum concentrations of calcium, sodium, oxalate, uric acid, electrolytes and PTH should be measured.

Imaging studies

These include:

- Plain X ray helps identify the composition, size and shape of stones.
- Renal ultrasonography – is frequently used as the first investigation to identify calculi.

SECTION 7

- Computerised tomography is more sensitive and establishes the size, number and position of the stones and the extent of obstruction.
- Plain renal tomography helps identify stones not detected by other means.

Dietary history

A diet history helps to ascertain the past and present intake of all relevant nutrients to establish if hypercalciuria is due to diet or hyperabsorption. Hypercalciuria on a low or normal calcium diet (<700 mg/day) indicates hyperabsorption.

Social history

Patients should be asked about past and present occupations to establish whether their working environment is likely to have caused long periods of dehydration and/or increased insensible losses, e.g. miners, long distance lorry drivers and heavy metal workers. Caucasians who have worked abroad in a hot climate are at similar risk. Prolonged bed rest, e.g. following limb fracture, can also be a contributory cause as this results in mobilisation of calcium from the bones and leads to hypercalciuria. Previous history is important as a stone may have formed in the past and been growing slowly.

Dietary treatment of idiopathic hypercalciuria

The necessity of dietary restrictions to treat idiopathic hypercalciuria and, more importantly, to prevent the recurrence of stones is controversial.

Calcium

Calcium restriction is not indicated in patients with idiopathic hypercalciuria who have normal intestinal absorption of calcium. A decreased calcium intake will result in the preferential absorption of oxalate and increased oxaluria. Increasing dietary calcium decreases urinary oxalate excretion by binding with oxalate in the intestine (Pak et al., 2005) and dietetic advice should take this into account. For example, black tea is a good source of oxalate, but adding milk (containing calcium) decreases oxalate absorption significantly. Dark chocolate increases urinary excretion of oxalate compared with milk chocolate (De O G Mendonca et al., 2003).

Many studies support the theory that increasing calcium intake will beneficially decrease urinary oxalate excretion (Lemann et al., 1996; Coe et al., 1992). Reduced bone mineral content (BMC) has been reported in idiopathic stone formers who have been following a low calcium diet (352 ± 20 mg) for 10 years (±0.7 years) (Fuss et al., 1990a). The reduction in BMC was as pronounced as that observed in hyperparathyroid stone formers. Although comparison with normal subjects showed that idiopathic renal stone formers had lower than average BMC, whether or not they restricted calcium intake, those on a low calcium diet were found to have lower BMC in the distal radius than those on a free diet (Fuss et al., 1990b). This may be due to one or more of the following causes:

- Idiopathic hypercalciuria, if not compensated by an adequate calcium supply, will lead to negative calcium balance.
- Hypophosphataemia in idiopathic renal stone formation is associated with increased resorption and decreased formation of bone.
- Elevated circulating levels of 1,25 dihydroxyvitamin D can induce bone resorption and result in negative calcium balance, especially if associated with a low calcium diet (Fuss et al., 1990a).

The role of calcitriol (1,25 dihydroxycholecalciferol) remains uncertain. Studies have shown that calcitriol potentiates the loss of bone mineral by aggravating the negative calcium balance caused by a low calcium diet (Coe et al., 1992). Calcitriol and its analogues are able to reduce the production of PTH, which explains the failure of serum PTH levels to rise if dietary calcium is low.

Oxalate

The majority of urinary calculi contain oxalate, which suggests that dietary oxalate intake should be reduced. However, approximately 60% of urinary oxalate is endogenous, being produced from the metabolism of glycine, glycolate and hydroxyproline or synthesised from glyoxalate metabolism (Holmes & Assimos, 1998). Normally, in hepatic peroxisomes, glyoxalate is metabolised to glycine and glycolate by alanine glyoxylate aminotransferase (AGT) and glyoxalate reductase hydroxypyruvate reductase (GRHPR), respectively. Inherited defects of these enzymes lead to oxalate hyperproduction. *Oxalobacter fomigenes* (a Gram negative anaerobic enteric bacterium) assists oxalate homeostasis by using oxalate for its biosynthesis and promoting oxalate secretion. Its absence from the intestinal lumen is associated with increased oxalate absorption and oxalate calcium nephrolithiasis (Hatch et al., 2006). Supplementation with ascorbic acid increases urinary oxalate levels and grapefruit juice increases excretion of both oxalate and citrate in the urine (Baxmann et al., 2003).

Total oxalate is found as two main fractions, soluble and insoluble. The soluble oxalate fraction contains oxalic acid and the water soluble salts of sodium and ammonia When bound to calcium, iron and magnesium oxalate become insoluble and absorption is limited. About 30% of ingested oxalate is degraded by anaerobic intestinal microflora, with the rest being absorbed in the small and large intestine. Absorption ranges from 10% to 100% (Grieff et al., 2013).

The effectiveness of dietary restriction of oxalate alone is equivocal; restrictions should be confined to patients who normally have a high consumption of oxalate rich foods and should address other dietary recommendations, including optimising fluid intake, controlling calcium intake and reducing sodium intake (Table 7.5.12).

Body weight

Lemann et al. (1996) showed that weight is a major determinant of urinary oxalate excretion in healthy adults. In addition, Taylor & Curhan, (2008b) showed a relationship

Table 7.5.12 Principal dietary sources of oxalate (Kasidas & Rose, 1980; Harvard School of Public Health, 2007) There are limited data available and much of the information is conflicting. The oxalate content of food varies considerably between plants of the same species, possibly as a result of differences in soil quality, ripeness, climate or method of harvesting and storage, and methods used for analysis.

Food	Oxalic acid content (mg/100 g)
Beetroot – pickled	500
Beetroot – boiled	675
Carob powder	73
Chocolate	117
Cocoa	623
Nuts – most nuts are high in oxalate*	
Almonds	435
Pecans	202
Peanuts	187
Parsley (can be used in small amounts)	100
Rhubarb	600–860
Spinach	600–750
Swiss chard	645
Tea infusion (mg/100 mL) – black tea without milk	55–78
Wheatgerm	269

*Analysis of pistachio and chestnuts show they have very low levels of gastric soluble oxalate and are suitable in moderation (Ritter et al., 2007).
Foods that contain moderate amounts of oxalate and should be taken in limited quantities include berries such as gooseberries, raspberries and strawberries; okra; sweet potato; potato.

between higher weight and higher urinary oxalate. Weight, body mass index (BMI) and urinary creatinine were all positively and independently associated with urinary oxalate. Although the reasons for these associations are unclear, it is likely that endogenous oxalate production increases with body weight. Therefore, modest weight reduction in overweight stone formers may be beneficial. Weight reduction should be supervised as rapid or extreme weight gain or loss may precipitate stone development (Stoller & Bolton, 1995).

Fluid

There is consensus that an oral fluid intake sufficient to produce a urine output of at least 2 L/day (ideally 3–3.5 L of fluid intake) is adequate hydration for stone patients. A high intake of fluid has been shown to be effective when used as the only method of stone prevention (Borghi et al., 1996; Preminger et al., 2007). A review by Kleiner (1999) stressed that dietitians should promote and monitor fluid intake among patients. The importance of extra fluids in hot weather and hot climates should be stressed. Drinking water from a water softener is not recommended as the mineral content, e.g. calcium, is reduced and the sodium is correspondingly increased.

Sodium

A high sodium intake leads to increased urinary sodium and calcium excretion due to inhibition of reabsorption in the proximal tubule and the Loop of Henle. Sodium intake should be reduced to 80–100 mmol/day and dietary intake can be monitored by urinary analysis.

Protein

A high dietary intake of protein can increase the excretion of calcium and uric acid, and decrease the excretion of citrate. Protein restriction to 0.8–1.0 g/kg/day in patients with idiopathic hypercalciuria has been shown to reduce urinary excretion of urea, calcium, uric acid and oxalate, and increase urinary citrate excretion (Giannini et al., 1999). These effects are thought to be due to a reduction in bone resorption and renal loss of calcium due to the decreased exogenous acid load.

Citrate

Citrate is a naturally occurring urinary stone inhibitor that binds calcium in solution to form highly soluble calcium citrate complex. This complex decreases the ionic concentration of calcium and hence the relative saturation of calcium oxalate and calcium phosphate in the urine. However, the benefits from large intakes of citrus fruit and vegetables may be offset by the resultant hyperoxaluria caused by the consequent increased intake of dietary oxalate.

Fish oils

Eicosapentanoic acid (EPA) has been reported to decrease urinary calcium excretion in people with idiopathic hypercalciuria who have erythrocyte ion transport abnormalities and different erythrocyte membrane lipid composition compared with healthy controls (Curhan & Curhan, 1997). There may be a group of patients for whom fish oil supplementation could correct this defect; however, evidence to date is inconclusive. A study by Yasui et al. (2001) showed that a highly purified preparation of EPA reduced urinary calcium in patients with urinary stones. However, a prospective study found no association between the intake of n-3 fatty acids and the risk of kidney stone formation (Taylor et al., 2005). Epidemiological studies demonstrated reduced a incidence of nephrolithiasis associated with consumption of EPA (Dyerberg et al., 1975). Eicosapentanoic acid is believed to have a protective role in the prevention of nephrolithiasis by reducing urinary calcium and oxalate excretion through alteration of prostaglandin metabolism (Ortiz-Alvarado et al., 2012).

Vitamin C

Vitamin C is excreted in urine in its unmetabolised form and as oxalate. There is considerable uncertainty as to the definitive effect of vitamin C on stone formation. In a large study, there was no increased risk associated with high intakes of vitamin C (Curhan et al., 1999). This contrasts with a recent prospective study that showed that the use of ascorbic acid supplements (1000 mg) increased the risk of calcium oxalate stones in men (Thomas et al.,

2013). This may not be generalisable to women who have a reduced risk of stone formation, but dietary advice to avoid supplemental vitamin C is prudent.

Other dietary factors

Cranberry juice

In normal subjects, 500 mL of cranberry juice for 2 weeks has been shown to decrease ioxalate and phosphate excretion, while increasing citrate excretion (McHarg *et al.*, 2003). In addition, there was a decrease in the relative supersaturation of calcium oxalate, which tended to be significantly lower than that induced in the control group given water alone. The authors concluded that cranberry juice had antilithogenic properties and, as such, deserves consideration as a conservative therapeutic protocol in managing calcium oxalate urolithiasis. However, Gettman *et al.* (2005) showed that cranberry juice exerted a mixed effect on urinary stone formation; it increased the risk of calcium oxalate and uric acid stone formation, but decreased the risk of brushite (calcium phosphate) stones. Current advice should be to avoid cranberry juice and its products until further research proves otherwise. It should be noted that cranberry juice is contraindicated in patients taking warfarin (see Chapter 5.3).

Sucrose and fructose

A high sucrose intake has been shown to increase urinary calcium excretion independent of calcium intake, although the mechanism is unknown. A positive association between sucrose intake and new kidney stone formation has been shown in women but not men (Curhan *et al.*, 2004). Taylor & Curhan (2008a) prospectively examined the relationship between fructose and incident stones in women and men, and concluded that fructose intake was independently associated with an increased risk of incident kidney stones. At present, the evidence is insufficient to recommend restriction of sucrose and/or fructose *per se*. However, intake should be addressed in the context of reducing body weight and thus the incidence of the metabolic syndrome and diabetes, which are associated with stone formation.

Non-dietary treatment of idiopathic hypercalciuria

Thiazide or hydrochlorothiazide diuretics appear to act on the renal tubules, causing greater reabsorption of calcium and restoring parathyroid function, intestinal calcium absorption and urinary calcium excretion to normal. Potassium citrate or bicarbonate, given with the thiazide, prevents hypokalaemia and improves the excretion of citrate (Pak, 1994). Potassium phosphate may suppress calcitrol synthesis and thus decrease calcium absorption (Parmar, 2004).

Secondary calcium stone disease

Secondary calcium stone disease usually results from one of the following conditions.

Primary hyperparathyroidism

The treatment of primary hyperparathyroidism is a parathyroidectomy. Parathyroid hormone levels should always be measured when assessing patients with stones. If parathyroidectomy is delayed or unsuccessful, a low calcium diet may be prescribed to lower plasma and urine calcium levels. In some cases, surgical removal of the stone may be required.

Medullary sponge kidney

In medullary sponge kidneys. tiny cysts form in the medulla (the inner part of the kidney) causing a sponge like appearance. These cysts keep urine from flowing freely through the tubules. Hypercalciuria, incomplete distal renal tubular acidosis and hypocitraturia are common. Increasing fluid intake is vital.

Renal tubular acidosis

This is a rare condition, caused by primary or secondary damage to the renal tubules in which acid urine cannot be produced because of a failure of bicarbonate reabsorption; therefore, calcium phosphate stones are formed. Renal tubular acidosis can be treated by alkalis and/or diet to normalise serum bicarbonate and pH. A diet rich in animal protein will increase the urinary acidity, so a reduction in animal protein intake may be helpful. Some patients may choose to make radical changes to their diet and become vegetarian or vegan to reduce their symptoms. They may require advice to ensure a nutritionally balanced diet.

Primary hyperoxaluria

Type 1 primary hyperoxaluria is an autosomal recessive condition that is caused by an inborn error of glyoxylic acid metabolism. Glyoxylic acid is normally transaminated to glycine or glycolic acid, but if the necessary enzymes are absent, oxalic acid will be produced. Two enzyme deficiencies, and hence two forms of primary hyperoxaluria, have been identified: absence of alanine glyoxalate aminotransferase (type 1) and of D-glycerate dehydrogenase (type 2). The majority of cases are type 1. Type 3 currently has no identified enzyme deficiency.

The full biochemistry of oxalic acid and glyoxylic acid metabolism is not known, but in patients with primary hyperoxaluria the production and excretion of oxalic acid is greatly increased. Calcium oxalate is insoluble so renal stones readily occur and in addition, oxalosis (systemic oxalate deposition) in the heart, bones, joints, eyes and other tissues is common. When this occurs the prognosis is very poor.

Treatment of primary hyperoxaluria comprises:

- *Pyridoxine supplements* – the only known effective treatment for primary hyperoxaluria. It is a cofactor in the alanine glycoxylate pathway and reduces oxalate production by inducing enzyme activity (Parmar, 2004). Although not all patients respond to pyridoxine, it remains the main treatment. Magnesium supplementation in conjunction with high dose pyridoxine results in reduced urinary oxalate excretion.
- *Increased fluid intake and increasing urinary volume* to 3 L/24 hours should be encouraged.
- Patients may be advised to follow a *low oxalate diet*, although there is no substantial benefit in the long

term for those with primary hyperoxaluria. A list of foods high in oxalate that should be avoided is shown in Table 7.5.12.

- In those with hypercalciuria, *oral citrate supplements*, given in conjunction with the use of thiazide diuretics is beneficial. Oral phosphate supplements may also be considered.
- *Oxalobacter formigenes* may be given orally as it degrades oxalate.
- *Dialysis* can be used to remove oxalate.
- *Combined liver and kidney, isolated liver or isolated renal transplantation* are options that may have to be considered.

Secondary hyperoxaluria

There are several causes of secondary hyperoxaluria:

- *Iatrogenic* – hyperoxaluria may occur as a result of the treatment used for idiopathic hypercalciuria.
- *Intestinal bypass, bariatric surgery and bowel disease* – enteric hyperoxaluria can result from fat malabsorption by the small bowel from any cause, including resection, e.g. ileostomy formation, intrinsic disease as seen with Crohn's disease, jejunoileal bypass and Roux-en-Y gastric bypass (Lieske *et al.*, 2008). If this results in steatorrhoea, calcium will bind with fatty acids in the gut and be unable to bind with oxalate; as a result, more oxalate will be passively absorbed. Treatment focuses on reducing dietary oxalate to reduce hyperoxaluria, and decreasing intake of fat to reduce steatorrhoea. Medium chain triglyceride oil has no effect on oxalate absorption and therefore can be used to increase energy intake if required. Oral calcium supplements have also been used to precipitate oxalate in the intestinal lumen, and cholestyramine may be used to bind fatty acids, bile acids and oxalate. Oral citrate supplements and a high fluid intake can also be beneficial.
- *Excessive vitamin C intake* (doses >1000 mg) has been implicated as a risk factor for stone formation as a result of ascorbate being metabolised to oxalate, which is then excreted in the urine.
- Vitamin D overdose will cause increased intestinal absorption of calcium.
- Prolonged immobilisation leads to bone reabsorption and consequent hypercalcaemia and hypercalciuria.

Uric acid stones

Uric acid is produced by the biochemical conversion of dietary and endogenous purines. People with diabetes are more prone to forming uric acid stones (Lieske *et al.*, 2006). Factors that lead to uric acid calculi formation include (Pak *et al.*, 2001):

- *Persistently acidic urine* – uric acid stones are associated with obesity, the metabolic syndrome and type 2 diabetes, and such patients have been found to have a lower urinary pH with a decreased rate of ammonium excretion, postulated to be due to renal tubule insulin resistance (Maalouf *et al.*, 2007).

Table 7.5.13 Principal dietary sources of purines (Clifford *et al.*, 1976; Wood, 1996)

Meat sources	Fish sources	Other sources
Liver	Anchovies	Yeast and extracts
Heart	Crab	Beer
Kidney	Fish roes	Asparagus
Sweetbreads	Herring	Cauliflower
Meat extracts, e.g. Oxo	Mackerel	Mushrooms
	Sardines	Beans and peas
	Shrimps	Spinach
	Sprats	
	Whitebait	

- *Hyperuricosuria* (>750 mg/day of uric acid).
- *Low urine volume*.

Treatment

Dietary modification

Weight loss, where applicable, is advocated with encouragement to follow a vegetarian diet that will reduce protein intake and promote urine alkalinity. A high protein intake increases the acid load that the kidneys buffer. Patients with uric acid stone disease have a defect in the production of this buffer, resulting in acidic urine, which increases the amount of less soluble uric acid. Elderly people often have a defect in this buffering process and hence have a higher incidence of uric acid stones (Rodman, 1991). Therefore, it is wise to recommend a decrease in protein consumption for all stone formers; particularly sources of protein that also have high purine content.

Patients should be advised to avoid foods rich in purine (Table 7.5.13). However, the necessity for severe restriction has been superseded by the use of allopurinol, and potassium citrate can be given to increase urinary pH and so prevent precipitation of uric acid (Parmar, 2004).

Fluid intake

As with all types of stones, a high fluid intake, sufficient to produce a daily urine output of at least 2 L is desirable. Patients with chronic diarrhoea or high ileostomy outputs have an increased risk of uric acid stones due to the loss of fluid and alkali that allows uric acid supersaturation. In patients with chronic diarrhoea syndromes, the use of potassium salts to replace alkali can cause intestinal irritation and therefore sodium bicarbonate may be the preferred treatment. The aim is to reach a urine pH of above 6 when uric acid is unlikely to be supersaturated. In patients with an ileostomy, the amount of fluid required to maintain an adequate urine output may result in excessive stoma output; a balance may have to be achieved between the two.

Potassium or sodium citrate

These are used to increase urinary pH to 6–6.5, but are often contraindicated in end stage kidney disease due to a risk of hyperkalaemia and disorders of coagulation.

Allergic reactions, e.g. skin rash, are common. The use of sodium citrate is counter intuitive due to sodium's association with an increased risk of stone formation.

Struvite (infection) stones

These stones contain magnesium ammonium phosphate and calcium phosphate, and are more common in women than men. Recurrent infection of the urinary tract with a urea splitting organism and anatomical predisposition are the main causes. The organisms break down urea, producing ammonia and resulting in more alkaline urine. Magnesium ammonium phosphate and calcium phosphate are extremely insoluble in alkaline conditions and once urinary pH exceeds 7.2, struvite will precipitate spontaneously with a rapid rate of growth. Staghorn, a calcareous cast of the collecting system, is a common feature of this stone type (Moe, 2006).

Treatment

Diet has no role in the treatment of struvite stones.

Surgery

The best treatment of struvite calculi is stone removal. However, bacterial penetration of small residual calculi may still occur and long term antibiotics will be required.

Eradication of the infection

The best prevention for struvite calculi is to eradicate the source of the infection by antimicrobial therapy. After clearance of the struvite calculi, 3 months of oral culture specific antibiotic treatment is recommended.

Urease inhibitor

It has been shown that it is possible to inhibit the action of the urea splitting enzyme urease in the bacteria in the kidney, thus preventing ammonia release, by using aceto-hydroxamic acid (1 g/day). Data on usage for 2 or more years do not show a sufficient significant difference between patients and controls to recommend treatment for all patients. The inhibitor must be given with antibiotics as it has no antibacterial effect. Approximately 20–30% of patients are unable to tolerate acetohydroxamic acid because of side effects, including deep vein thrombosis and haemolytic anaemia (Parmar, 2004).

Cystine stones

Cystine stones occur in a very rare autosomal recessive genetic disorder affecting the renal tubular reabsorption of cystine, arginine and ornithine, and resulting in increased concentration of cystine in the urine (Table 7.5.14). Cystine is relatively insoluble in urine, with a limit of solubility at pH 7.5 and 37°C of 243 mg/L (Coe et al., 2005), so homozygous cystinurics readily precipitate cystine and stone episodes in this population usually occur by 20 years of age. Heterozygotes (asymptomatic carriers) may excrete up to 10 times as much cystine as normal, but do not form cystine stones.

Table 7.5.14 Urinary concentration of cystine

Patient group	Cystine concentration (μmol/L)
Normal	10–100
Heterozygous cystinurics	200–600
Homozygous cystinurics	1400–4200

Treatment

Dilution of urine

The patient should be advised to drink enough fluid to pass at least 3 L of urine/day. A fluid plan should be advised to ensure an adequate regular intake, particularly at bedtime and during the night. This treatment is seen as a very simple way of preventing recurrence of stones but in practice, compliance can be difficult. Salt restriction significantly reduces urinary cystine excretion (Jaeger et al., 1986). Care should be taken that hyponatraemia does not result from very high fluid intake.

Alkalinisation of urine

Urine alkalinisation with citrate increases the solubility of cystine and may decrease stone formation (Anderton, 1998). Potassium citrate is preferred to sodium citrate or sodium bicarbonate if sodium restriction is imposed concurrently. Urine alkalinisation may be used when penicillamine therapy is not well tolerated.

Medication

The sulphydryl group in the chelating agent D-penicillamine reacts with cystine to form a more soluble complex in urine. The treatment carries a high risk of side effects, including rashes, thrombocytopenia, neutropenia, proteinuria and nephrotic syndrome. Alpha-mercaptopropionylglycine (α-MPG) or mercaptamine has been used as an alternative to penacillamine. It has similar side effects but is better tolerated (Lindell et al., 1995). Captopril is used as it forms captopril–cysteine disulphide, which is 200 times more soluble than cystine. However, its effectiveness in the treatment of cystinuria has not been consistently shown (Sloand & Izzo, 1987).

Diet

Salt restriction reduces cystine excretion (Rodriguez et al., 1995) so a no added salt diet (80–100 mmol/day) or lower should be advised. Further dietary treatment is a last resort. Restriction of animal protein is associated with reduction in intake of the cystine precursor methionine as well as cystine, so a diet low in methionine will reduce urinary cystine. However, such a diet is restrictive and difficult to follow because animal protein from meat, fish, cheese, eggs and milk has to be limited to 30 g/day. Additional protein requirements must be met from vegetable protein.

Melamine stones

In 2008, 294 000 infants in China were affected by melamine contaminated infant formula with 5000 hospitalised and six deaths. Melamine was used as a nitrogen bulking agent to artificially increase the apparent protein content. Renal damage was thought to be the result of kidney stones formed from melamine and uric acid or from melamine and its cocrystallising chemical derivative, cyanuric acid (Zheng et al., 2013).

Ketogenic diet

Nephrolithiasis has been observed in children receiving the ketogenic diet. The prevalence ranges from 3% to 10%, in comparison to one in several thousand in the general population. Analysis of the stones shows a varied picture, with uric acid stones predominating (Furth et al., 2000). Major causative factors include hypercalciuria due to increased bone demineralisation with acidosis, hypocitraturia and acidic urine (see Chapter 3.8).

References

Anderton JG. (1998) Cystinuria: an update. Journal of the Royal Society of Medicine 91: 220–221.

Asplin JR, Favus MJ, Coe FL. (1996) Nephrolithiasis. In: Brenner BM (ed) Brenner and Rector's The Kidney, 5th edn. Philadelphia: Saunders.

Basavaraj DR, Biyani CS, Browning AJ, Cartledge JJ. (2007) The role of urinary stone inhibitors and promoters in the pathogenesis of calcium containing stones. EAU-EBU Update Series 5: 126–136.

Baxmann AC, Mendonca CD, Heilberg IP. (2003) Effect of vitamin C supplements on urinary oxalate and pH in calcium stone-forming patients. Kidney International 63: 1066–1071.

Borghi L, Mesci T, Amato F, Briganti A, Novarini A, Giannini A. (1996) Urinary volume, water and recurrences in idiopathic calcium nephrolithiasis: a 5-year randomised prospective study. Journal of Urology 155: 839–843.

Borghi L, Schianchi T, Meschi T, et al. (2002) Comparison of two diets for the prevention of recurrent stones in idiopathic hypercalciuria. New England Journal of Medicine 346: 77–84.

Clifford AJ, Riumullo JA, Young VR, Scrimshaw NS. (1976) Effect of oral purines on serum and urinary uric acid of normal and gouty humans. Journal of Nutrition 106: 428.

Coe FL, Parks JH, Asplin JR. (1992) The pathogenesis and treatment of kidney stones. New England Journal of Medicine 327(16): 1141–1151.

Coe Fl, Evans A, Worcester E. (2005) Kidney Stone Disease. Journal of Clinical Investigations 115(10): 2598–2608.

Curhan GC, Curhan SG. (1997) Diet and urinary stone disease. Current Opinion in Urology 7: 222–225.

Curhan GC, Willett WC, Rimm EB, Stamfer MJ. (1993) A prospective study of dietary calcium and other nutrients and the risk of symptomatic kidney stones. New England Journal of Medicine 328: 833–838.

Curhan GC, Willett WC, Speizer FE, Stampfer MJ. (1999) Intake of vitamin B6 and C and the risk of kidney stones in women. Journal of the American Society of Nephrology 10(4): 840–845.

Curhan GC; Willett WC, Knight EL, Stampfer MJ. (2004) Dietary factors and the risk of incident kidney stones in younger women: Nurses' Health Study II. Archives of Internal Medicine 164(8): 885–891.

Daudon M, Donsimoni R, Hennequin C, et al. (1995) Sex and age-related composition of 10617 calculi analysed by infrared spectroscopy. Urology Research 23: 319–326.

Daudon M, Bounxouei B, Santa Cruz F, et al. (2004) Composition of renalstones currently observed in non-industrialized countries. Progress in Urology 14(6): 1151–1161.

de O G Mendonca C, Martini LA, Baxmann AC, et al. (2003) Effects of an oxalate load on urinary oxalate excretion in calcium stone formers. Journal of Renal Nutrition 13(1): 39–46.

Dretler SP. (1998) The physiologic approach to the medical management of stone disease. Urology Clinics of North America 25(4): 613–623.

Dyerberg J, Bang HO, Hjorne N. (1975) Fatty acid composition of the plasma lipids in Greenland Eskimos. American Journal of Clinical Nutrition 28: 958–966.

Furth SL, Casey JC, Pyzik PL, et al. (2000) Risk factors for urolithiasis in children on the ketogenic diet. Pediatric Nephrology 15(1–2): 125–128.

Fuss M, Pepersack T, Bergman P, Hurard T, Simon J, Corvilain J. (1990a) Low calcium diet in idiopathic urolithiasis: a risk factor for osteopenia as great as in primary hyperparathyroidism. British Journal of Urology 65: 560–563.

Fuss M, Pepersack T, Van Geel J, et al. (1990b) Involvement of low-calcium diet in the reduced bone mineral content of idiopathic renal stone formers. Calcified Tissue International 46: 9–13.

Gettman MT, Ogan K, Brinkley LJ, Adams-Huet B, Pak CY, Pearle MS. (2005) Effect of cranberry juice consumption on urinary risk factors. Journal of Urology 174(2): 590–594.

Giannini S, Nobile M, Sartori L, et al. (1999) Acute effects of moderate dietary protein restriction in patients with idiopathic hypercalciuria and calcium nephrolithiasis. American Journal of Clinical Nutrition 69(2): 267–271.

Grieff M, Bushinsky DA. (2013) Nutritional prevention of kidney stones. In: Kopple JD, Massry SG, Kalantar-Zadeh K (eds) Nutritional Management of Renal Disease, 3rd edn. Academic Press.

Harvard School of Public Health. (2007) Available at https://regepi.bwh.harvard.edu/health/Oxalate/files. Accessed 24 March 2013.

Hatch M, Cornelius J, Allison M, et al. (2006) Oxalobacter sp. reduces urinary oxalate excretion by promoting enteric oxalate secretion. Kidney International 69: 691–698.

Holmes RP, Assimos DG. (1998) Glyoxylate synthesis, and its modulation and influence on oxalate synthesis. Journal of Urology 160: 1617–1624.

Jaeger P, Portmann L, Saunders A, Rosenberg LE, Their SO. (1986) Anticystinuric effects of glutamine and of dietary sodium restriction. New England Journal of Medicine 315: 1120–1103.

Kasidas GP, Rose GA. (1980) Oxalate content of some common foods: determination by an enzymatic method. Journal of Human Nutrition 34: 255–266.

Kleiner SM. (1999) Water: an essential but overlooked nutrient. Journal of the American Dietetic Association 99: 200–206.

Lemann J, Pleuss JA, Worcester EM, Hornick L, Schrab D, Hoffman RG. (1996) Urinary oxalate excretion increases with body size and decreases with increasing dietary calcium intake among healthy adults. Kidney International 49: 200–208.

Lieske JC, de la Vega LS, Gettman MT, et al. (2006) Diabetes mellitus and the risk of urinary tract stones: a population-based case-control study. American Journal of Kidney Disease 48: 897–904.

Lieske JC, Kumar R, Collazo-Clavell ML. (2008) Nephrolithiasis after bariatric surgery for obesity. Seminars in Nephrology 28: 163–173.

Lindell A, Denneberg T, Edholm E, et al. (1995) The effect of sodium intake on cystinuria with and without tiopronin treatment. Nephron 71: 407–415.

Maalouf NM, Cameron MA, Moe OW, Adams-Huet B, Sakhaee K. (2007) Low urine pH: a novel feature of the metabolic syndrome. Clinical Journal of the American Society of Nephrology 2: 883–888.

McHarg T, Rodgers A, Charlton K. (2003) Influence of cranberry juice on the urinary risk factors for calcium oxalate stone formation. BJU International 92: 765–768.

Melnick JZ, Preisig PA, Haynes S, *et al.* (1998) Converting enzyme inhibition causes hypocitraturia independent of acidosis or hypokalemia. *Kidney International* 54: 1670–1674.

Moe OW. (2006) Kidney stones: pathophysiology and medical management. *Lancet* 367: 333–344.

Ortiz-Alvarado O, Miyaoka R, Kriedberg C, *et al.* (2012) Omega-3 fatty acids eicosapentaenoic acid and docosahexaenoic acid in the management of hypercalciuric stone formers. *Urology* 79: 282–286.

Pak CYC. (1994) Citrate and renal calculi: an update. *Mineral and Electrolyte Metabolism* 20: 371–377.

Pak CYC. (1998) Kidney stones. *Lancet* 351: 1797–1801.

Pak CYC, Sakhaee K, Peterson RD, Poindexter JR, Frawley WH. (2001) Biochemical profile of idiopathic uric acid nephrolithiasis. *Kidney International* 60: 757–761.

Pak CYC, Odvina CV, Pearle MS, *et al.* (2005) Effect of dietary modification on urinary stone risk factors. *Kidney International* 68: 2264–2273.

Paliouras C, Tsampikaki E, Alivanis P, Aperis G. (2012) Pathophysiology of nephrolithiasis. *Nephron Reviews* 4: e14, 58–65.

Parivar F, Low RK, Stoller ML. (1996) The influence of diet on urinary stone disease. *Journal of Urology* 155: 432–440.

Parmar MS. (2004) Kidney stones. *BMJ* 328: 1420–1424.

Preminger GM, Tiselius HG, Assimos DG, *et al.* (2007) Guideline for the management of ureteral calculi. *Journal of Urology* 178(6): 2418–2434.

Ritter MMC, Savage GP. (2007) Soluble and insoluble oxalate content of nuts. *Journal of Food Composition and Analysis* 20: 169–174.

Rodman JS. (1991) Management of uric acid in the elderly patient. *Geriatric Nephrology and Urology* 1: 129.

Rodriguez LM, Santos F, Malaga S, Martinez V. (1995) Effect of a low sodium diet on urinary elimination of cystine in cystinuric children. *Nephron* 71: 416–418.

Romero V, Akpinar H, Assimos DG. (2010) Kidney stones: A global picture of prevalence, incidence and associated risk factors. *Reviews in Urology* 12(2–3): e86096.

Sloand JA, Izzo JL Jr. (1987) Captopril reduces urinary cystine excretion in cystinuria. *Archives of Internal Medicine* 147(8): 1409–1412.

Stoller ML, Bolton DM. (1995) Urinary stone disease. In: Tanagho EA, McAninch JW (eds) *Smith's General Urology*. New Jersey: Prentice-Hall International Inc, pp. 276–304.

Taylor EN, Curhan GC. (2008a) Fructose consumption and the risk of kidney stones. *Kidney International* 73: 207–212.

Taylor EN, Curhan GC. (2008b) Determinants of 24hour urinary oxalate excretion. *Clinical Journal of the America Society of Nephrology* 50: 1453–1460.

Taylor EN, Stampfer MJ, Curhan GC. (2005) Fatty acid intake and incident nephrolithiasis. *American Journal of Kidney Disease* 45: 267–274.

Thomas LDK, Elinder C-G, Tiselius H-G, Wolk A, Åkesson A. (2013) Ascorbic acid supplements and kidney stone incidence among men: A prospective study. *JAMA Internal Medicine* 173(5): 386–388.

Tonelli M, Todd Alexander R, Hemmelgarn BR, *et al.* (2012) Kidney stones and kidney function loss: a cohort study. *BMJ* 345: e5287.

Wood AJJ. (1996) The management of gout. *New England Journal of Medicine* 334(7): 445–451.

Yalamanchili V, Gallagher J. (2012) Incidence of hypercalciuria and hypercalcemia during a vitamin D trial in postmenopausal women. *Endocrine Reviews* 33; OR38-1.

Yasui T, Tanaka H, Fujita K, Iguchi M, Kohri K. (2001) Effects of eicosapentaenoic acid on urinary calcium excretion in calcium stone formers. *European Urolology* 39(5): 580–585.

Zheng X, Zhao A, Xie G, *et al.* (2013) Melamine-induced renal toxicity is mediated by the gut microbiota. *Science Translational Medicine* 5(172): 172 ra22.

7.6 Neurological disease

7.6.1 Parkinson's disease
Karen Green

Key points

- Parkinson's disease (PD) is a progressive neurodegenerative disorder and the most common form of parkinsonism.

- Parkinson's disease can have a considerable impact on nutritional intake as a result of both the effects of the disease and side effects of drug treatment.

- Nutritional inadequacies should be identified and corrected as early as possible. Dietetic intervention may be necessary to prevent undesirable weight gain or loss.

- Up to 95% of people with PD will develop swallowing difficulties that need to be addressed promptly by the dietitian and speech and language therapist to prevent weight loss and malnutrition.

Parkinson's disease (PD) is a chronic and relentlessly progressive neurodegenerative disease; it is the primary and most common form of parkinsonism. Parkinsonism is an umbrella term used to cover a range of conditions, which share the main symptoms of slow movement, possible tremor, rigidity and problems with walking [Parkinson's UK (PUK), 2011]. The prevalence of PD in Europe has been estimated at between one in every 800 and one in every 1500 population (von Campenhausen *et al.*, 2005); in the UK, one in every 500 people has PD. This currently equates to approximately 120 000 people in the UK (PUK, 2011). It is characterised by the signs and symptoms listed in Table 7.6.1, which can be remembered by the mnemonic TRAP.

Other motor symptoms include hypomimia (lack of facial expression), dysarthria (speech difficulty), dysphagia, sialorrhoea (excessive secretion of saliva) and poor manual dexterity. Non-motor symptoms include cognitive impairment, depression, dementia, sleep disorders, orthostatic hypotension, fatigue and olfactory dysfunction (loss of taste and smell function). Gastrointestinal dysfunction is receiving increasing attention and recognition as an important clinical component of PD (Pfeiffer,

2011). These symptoms are usually more apparent in the advanced stages of the disease.

Diagnostic criteria and classification

Onset of PD at ages over 50 years is considered to be late onsets PD. Around 5–10% of individuals are diagnosed before the age of 50 years. Parkinson's disease is classified as juvenile onset when diagnosed under the age of 20 years, or early onset when diagnosed between 20 and 50 years of age (Calne, 2001).

Disease process

Part of the disease process develops as cells are destroyed (by an unknown trigger or event) in parts of the brain stem, particularly the crescent shaped cell mass known as the substantia nigra. Nerve cells in the substantia nigra send out fibres to tissue located in both sides of the brain. There the cells release an essential neurotransmitter known as dopamine that helps control movement and coordination (Lang & Lozano, 1998). Loss of dopamine in the corpus stratia is the primary defect in PD, and

Manual of Dietetic Practice, Fifth Edition. Edited by Joan Gandy.
© 2014 The British Dietetic Association. Published 2014 by John Wiley & Sons, Ltd.
Companion Website: www.manualofdieteticpractice.com

SECTION 7

Table 7.6.1 Signs and symptoms of Parkinson's disease (PD)

Feature (TRAP)	Description	Effect
Tremor at rest	Involuntary shaking of the upper and lower limbs, e.g. hands, fingers and legs. Classical PD tremor is the pill rolling tremor	It is most apparent when the affected part is at rest or the person is under stress Although tremor is rarely disabling, it is one of the symptoms that bothers patients most
Rigidity	Muscles remain in a constantly contracted state, causing symptoms such as muscle stiffness, weakness or aching	Patients are less aware of impaired movement but this may be obvious to a carer, e.g. raising the patient's arm results in ratchet-like jerky movements (cogwheel rigidity)
Akinesia	Slowness of movement, which is often the most disabling feature of the disease	Normal activities such as washing and dressing may take hours There may also be slowness in speech and delayed reaction to conversation
Postural instability	Impaired balance and coordination result in general unsteadiness in movement, particularly while turning; and increased risk of falls	Patients often develop a forward lean or sometimes a stooped posture with the head bowed and the shoulders dropped Gait disturbance becomes more obvious; some patients may halt in mid stride, sometimes toppling over as a result, others may shuffle along with knees flexed and ultimately some may be unable to walk unaided

symptoms usually appear when at least 80% of the dopamine is lost. As a result, dopamine deficiency affects the nerves and muscles controlling movement and coordination, and may also be responsible for associated cognitive decline.

Genetics

It has been reported that men are more likely to develop PD than women (Baldereschi *et al.*, 2000). A prospective study showed men were 1.5 times more likely than women to develop PD (Alves *et al.*, 2009). The genetic components of some forms of PD have been identified, and it can be inherited in both a recessive and dominant manner.

Disease consequences

Parkinson's disease is associated with disability, morbidity, institutionalisation, high demand on healthcare input and mortality (Mutch *et al.*, 1986; Shulman *et al.*, 2001; Parashos *et al.*, 2002; Elbaz *et al.*, 2002; Leibson *et al.*, 2006; Aarsland *et al.*, 2009). Due to the progressive nature of the disease, it is generally expected that the signs and symptoms of the disease will become more pronounced each year. The natural history of PD is very variable and it is extremely difficult to accurately predict how, or how quickly, the disease will progress in a specific individual. However, Poewe & Wenning (1996) reported that approximately 80% of people who are diagnosed late will become significantly disabled or die within 10–14 years of diagnosis.

Public health aspects and prevention

Although the cause of PD remains unknown, a number of factors that increase the risk of developing this disease have been identified, including early diet, genetics and environment. Other factors that may prevent or slow

down PD development and progression have also been found, e.g. antioxidants, levodopa and non-steroidal anti-inflammatory drugs (NSAID). Free radicals, unstable and potentially damaging molecules generated by normal chemical reactions in the body, are thought to contribute to nerve cell death, thereby leading to PD (Dexter *et al.*, 1994; Alam *et al.*, 1997). In normal circumstances free radical damage is kept under control by antioxidants that protect cells from this damage. Vitamins E and C, coenzyme Q10 (CoQ10), nicotinamide adenine dinucleotide (NADH) and Ginkgo biloba have been shown to have antioxidant properties and it has been speculated that their supplementation may provide some protection against PD (Beal, 1998; Fariss & Zhang, 2003; Etminan *et al.*, 2005). However, to date, there is limited research to support these claims.

Nutritional consequences

The symptoms associated with PD vary from individual to individual; therefore, each individual will experience varying degrees of nutritional inadequacies as a consequence of the disease. Some of the most commonly reported nutritional consequences of the disease are discussed below.

Weight loss

This is a major feature of the disease, whether it is progressive weight loss or obvious malnutrition. Approximately half of all sufferers will experience unintentional weight loss and about three-quarters will experience eating difficulties of some kind (Cushing *et al.*, 2002; Palhagen *et al.*, 2005). It has been reported that women are more prone to weight loss than men (Durrieu *et al.*, 1992). Weight loss can result from reduced energy intake, which has been attributed to increased lethargy, olfactory dysfunction, dysphagia and gastrointestinal dysfunction. In addition, the decline in cognition can lead to lowered energy intake by affecting interest in food and eating habits. Cognitive impairment in PD can vary depending on which part of the brain is impaired and the timing of onset and progression of the disease (Stennis Watson & Leverenz, 2010). Beyer et al. (1995) found that as the disease progresses, individuals with PD were four times more likely to lose 4.5 kg more than age matched controls. This is mainly attributed to subtle chronic rather than acute bouts of energy imbalance in the form of decreased energy intake (Toth, 1999).

The nutritional effects of poor food intake may also be exacerbated by increased energy expenditure as a result of tremor or rigidity (Levi et al., 1990) although one study found that resting energy expenditure (REE) was 15% lower in PD patients compared with healthy controls due to decreased physical activity (Toth, 1999). However, dyskinesia can use up more energy than the PD patient consumes and this can contribute to severe weight loss, possibly as a result of increased energy consumption by skeletal muscle.

Up to 95% of people with PD will develop swallowing difficulties (Logemann et al,, 1997). This needs to be addressed promptly by both the dietitian and speech and language therapist to prevent and/or treat weight loss and malnutrition as appropriate. The risk of aspiration is often overlooked in people living with PD and as a consequence, pneumonia is a commonly reported cause of death in this group (Robbins et al., 2008; Miller et al., 2009a,b).

The on–off syndrome can occur in patients on long term antiparkinsonian medication, which causes sudden alterations in or loss of functional ability The main feature of the off period is increased muscle tone (rigidity), and of the on period, increased involuntary movements (dyskinesias). Off periods, also known as motor fluctuations, are unpredictable and may last for a few minutes or many hours. Drug adjustment is often titrated in an attempt to overcome this problem; however, at some stage this syndrome affects the patient's ability to prepare meals and, feed themselves, and thereby increases the risk of the patient developing malnutrition, leading to weight loss.

Autonomic failure

Autonomic failure has been found in 47% of patients with PD (Allcock et al., 2004) and the associated symptoms can impact on the maintenance of appropriate nutritional intake. For further details of the mechanism of autonomic failure and its nutritional consequences and dietary management, see Chapter 7.6.3.

Bone health and osteoporosis

Hypovitaminosis D is highly prevalent in people living with PD (Sato et al., 1997; Evatt et al., 2008) and disease severity and bone density have been shown to be correlated (Sato et al., 1997). Patients with PD have been found to have a defect in the renal synthesis of 1,25 dihydroxy vitamin D (1,25 [OH]$_2$D) (Jackson et al., 2007). Some researchers have suggested that people living with PD should be supplemented with 1 alpha hydroxyvitamin D3 (vitamin D3), the more active form of vitamin D,

which can help increase bone density and dramatically lower the risk of fracture in these patients (Boonen et al., 2007). This is essential for patients who are bed bound or immobile. Calcium and vitamin D status should therefore be assessed early in the disease to prevent or decrease the incidence of osteoporosis.

Constipation

This is a commonly reported feature of PD (Cassani et al., 2011), with the number of PD patients experiencing constipation ranging from 20% to 89% (Edwards et al., 1991; Stocchi et al., 2000; Siddiqui et al., 2002; Kaye et al., 2006). It is thought that constipation occurs as a result of:

- Reduced peristalsis causing delayed gut transit time.
- Lack of fibre intake due to difficulties chewing fibrous foods.
- Lack of fibre when following a texture modified diet, e.g. puréed food.
- Lack of fluid intake as a response to problems with urgency and frequency of micturition or incontinence.
- Reduced mobility.
- Side effect of some antiparkinsonian medications.

Weight gain

In contrast to the weight loss that develops as part of this disease itself, weight gain has been noted to occur following deep brain stimulation surgery (DBS) (Tuite et al., 2005). Sauleau et al. (2009) found that 38% of their patient group was overweight, with a body mass index (BMI) of 26–29.9 kg/m^2 6 months post DBS. This was attributed to the improvement in motor control, rather than improvement in energy intake. Weight gain may also occur in individuals treated with dopaminergic agonists, sometimes as a result of impulse control difficulty with compulsive eating (Nirenberg & Waters, 2006). For further information about DBS, see Clinical management later.

Nutritional assessment

Nutritional assessment should include the following aspects.

Anthropometry

Weight, height, BMI and Malnutrition Universal Screening Tool ('MUST') score (or an alternative validated nutritional screening tool) are used to determine nutritional status, and baseline measurements recorded to allow progress to be monitored. Other measurements, e.g. mid upper arm circumference (MUAC), should be considered, although severe rigidity or motor fluctuations may make these impossible.

Biochemistry

There are no specific tests that track the progress of PD; however, during periods of illness in a hospital setting, e.g. aspiration, inflammatory markers will help monitor the clinical status of the patient.

Clinical assessment

Clinical observations will vary depending on the setting in which patients are treated. However, it is worth noting fluid balance (dehydrated or overloaded), bowel movements (frequency and consistency), temperature (apyrexial or pyrexial), swallowing difficulties, motor function (on–off periods) and drug regimens. Consider any comorbidity when devising an individually tailored care plan.

Dietary assessment

Food charts in a hospital setting or food diaries in a community setting are important. There may be difficulties communicating with the patient for various reasons, including on–off periods, speech difficulties or poor memory due to dementia. The appropriateness of the method of nutritional support the individual is currently receiving and their tolerance to the prescribed regimen should be considered. This will help when devising and updating the care plan. Focus should be on total energy intake versus requirements, and any food avoidance or changes to dietary intake should be noted.

Economic and social assessment

Links with carers and community teams who are involved in the patient's care at all levels should be made where appropriate to ensure streamlined holistic care. The focus should be living arrangements, and difficulties with obtaining food, meal preparation and cooking.

Management

Clinical management

Although there is no treatment capable of slowing or stopping the progression of the disease, current treatments can effectively relieve the symptoms, especially in the early years. Many people who are adequately treated notice very little or no progression of symptoms over the first few years. However, within 5–10 years of onset, symptoms will disrupt activities of daily living (ADL). Clinical management is therefore directed at minimising the symptoms and disabilities of the patient.

Drug management

The type of medication used varies between individuals according to the nature and severity of symptoms. Many of the available medications have significant side effects; therefore, the aim of drug therapy is to find a balance between effective symptom control and avoidance of side effects. The following are commonly used drugs in the management of PD:

- Levodopa – Madopar® (co-beneldopa), Sinemet® (co-careldopa), Stalevo® and Duodopa®.

- Dopamine agonists – Ropinolrole®, Cabergoline®, Apomorphine®.
- Selegiline.
- Anticholinergics: Benzhexol®, Orphenadrine®, Benztropine®.
- Amantidine.
- Catechol-O-methyltransferase (COMT) inhibitors – Entacapone®, Tolcapone®.

Levodopa is used to replace or mimic dopamine in the brain and, in conjunction with COMT inhibitors, to limit the conversion of levodopa to dopamine in the peripheral tissues, thereby facilitating a greater proportion of levodopa to cross the blood–brain barrier. Dopamine agonists, which mimic dopamine, are usually the first drugs prescribed for those diagnosed with juvenile onset PD (Uitti *et al.*, 1999). It is also used alongside levodopa. The efficiency of drug therapy tends to diminish with time and the duration of benefit after each dose becomes progressively shorter; this is known as end dose failure.

Surgical procedures

Deep brain stimulation is a surgical procedure used to treat the debilitating symptoms of PD, such as tremor, rigidity, stiffness, slowed movement and walking problems. Currently, the procedure is used only for patients whose symptoms cannot be adequately controlled with medications. It uses a surgically implanted, battery operated medical device, a neurostimulator, which is likened to a heart pacemaker and about the size of a stopwatch. It delivers electrical stimulation to targeted areas in the brain that control movement, blocking the abnormal nerve signals that cause tremor and PD symptoms. Research is ongoing to ascertain the effectiveness of DBS in the longer term.

Nutrition management

Both the treatment and effects of PD may compromise nutritional intake and nutrition management aims to:

- Identify nutritional inadequacies at an early stage.
- Implement measures to correct deficiencies or nutrition related problems.
- Find ways to minimise any practical difficulties associated with eating or swallowing.
- Prevent undesirable weight gain or loss.
- Lessen the impact of drug therapy side effects on dietary intake.
- Regular monitoring of nutritional status throughout the progression of the disease.

No special diet is required for PD in the early stages of the disease; however, it is important to establish and maintain good eating habits throughout the course of the condition (Glynn, 2003). Information should be provided on how to adopt the Healthy Eating Guidelines (Food Standards Agency) (see Chapter 4.2) and incorporated by Parkinson's UK into its booklet *Diet and Parkinson's;* this will help prevent undesirable weight gain.

As the disease progresses, more specific diet therapy may be needed to help overcome problems that affect nutritional intake and status.

Weight loss and poor oral intake

Guidance on how to optimise nutrient intake with nutrient dense foods, food fortification measures or imaginative use of nutritional supplements may be necessary. Other strategies to help overcome problems such as anorexia, sensory impairment and fatigue may also be helpful (see Chapter 6.3). Due to a lack of research on energy requirements in PD, advice is based on best practice and clinical experience. It is not unheard of for patients exceeding 3000 kcal/day to maintain an ideal weight, and others lose weight. Calculating requirements is based on Schofield's equation. Weight gain factors range from 600 to 1000 kcal in addition to basal metabolic rate (BMR) to promote weight gain, if necessary, or 25–35 kcal/kg ideal body weight (NICE, 2006b), especially in underweight patents.

Dysphagia

As stated earlier, this problem needs to be addressed promptly to prevent weight loss and malnutrition. Significant problems with swallowing require expert assessment from a speech and language therapist and guidance regarding food texture modification (see Chapter 7.3). If altered texture diets, e.g. puréed diets, may be nutritionally inadequate and not sufficiently energy dense to meet the patient's nutritional requirements, additional use of energy dense nutritional supplements may be indicated to prevent weight loss. However, these may be contraindicated in patients who require thickened fluids. Prethickened nutritional supplements available on the market include Fresubin Thickened Stage 1 & 2 (1.5 kcal/mL) (Fresenius Kabi) and Nutilis Complete Stage 1 (2.4 kcal/mL) (Nutricia), and would benefit patients with dysphagia and weight loss.

Bone health

Evidence suggests that people living with PD should be routinely supplemented with 1000–1500 mg of calcium (e.g. Calchicew) and 10–15 μg (400–600 IU) of vitamin D (Ad-Cal D3 Forte) daily (Sato et al., 2001). However, more recent research has proposed that these older studies used low cut-offs to define vitamin D deficiency, and that intake should exceed 20 μg (800 IU) of vitamin D to prevent falls and for optimal skeletal health (Bischoff-Ferrari et al., 2006; Knekt et al., 2010). Dietary sources of calcium and vitamin D should also be encouraged if possible. The treating neurologist should know if patients want to increase their vitamin D beyond current guidelines, and agree this with them.

Constipation

Dietary advice is aimed primarily at softening and increasing the bulk of the stool. This should be the first treatment strategy and it usually works in most PD patients.

Fluid

Patients should drink a minimum of 1.2 L (six to eight glasses) of fluid/day as a minimum and in addition to water provided by food. Factors such as physical activity, age and weather can affect this requirement. Fluids that can be suggested are water, cordial fruit juice, prune juice, vegetable juice, tea, coffee, smoothies and drinking yoghurt. People living with PD often have a weaker sense of thirst and, if necessary, should be helped and encouraged to drink at regular intervals throughout the day.

Fibre

Fibre rich foods that are easy to manage, e.g. high fibre breakfast cereals, wholemeal bread, easy to peel fruit (e.g. bananas or satsumas), dried fruit and golden linseeds are suitable. Golden linseeds should be introduced into the diet slowly, e.g. start with 1 teaspoon/day up to maximum of 1 tablespoon/day over a week, and can be added to foods such as breakfast cereal, yoghurts or soups. The use of vegetables, peas, beans and lentils as meal components should be encouraged. The common practice of adding bran to foods should not be encouraged, as this is more likely to create problems than solve them. Advice on increasing fibre (18–24 g/day) and fluid (up to 2.5 L/day) simultaneously should be given to prevent exacerbating symptoms of constipation.

Protein manipulation

Advising advanced PD patients with motor fluctuations to manipulate protein consumption has become very common. This practice in any form, i.e. protein restriction, reduction or redistribution, is not supported by convincing and well designed randomised controlled trials. Most of the evidence comes from small pilot trials. It is well documented that patients who follow a protein restricted diet (PRD) experience an increase in total energy expenditure (Barichella et al., 2007; Cereda et al., 2009), resulting in weight loss over time (Riley & Lang, 1988; Paré et al., 1992; Barichella et al., 2006). The long term adequacy of protein controlled dietary regimens has not been established. Protein requirements are based on more than 0.8 g of protein/kg of ideal body weight (IBW) (Wolfe et al., 2008) or using the dietary reference values. Timing of medications around meal times should be addressed to avoid protein–levopdopa interaction.

In the absence of curative treatment, the management of PD remains largely palliative despite the huge advances that have been achieved in medical knowledge. The National Institute for Health and Care Excellence (NICE, 2006a) advises, *'Palliative care should be applied throughout the course of the disease and not limited to the terminal end of life period'*. Achievement of best quality of life for patients and their carers and families is the goal of palliative care. The palliative stage of the disease is defined by:

- Inability to tolerate dopaminergic therapy.
- Unsuitable for surgery, e.g. DBS.
- Presence of advanced comorbidity (MacMahon & Thomas, 1998).

Medication may be stopped due to lack of drug efficacy and increasing sensitivity to side effects such as hallucinations. Active and aggressive nutritional support may also be withdrawn if it causes discomfort or distress. Regular contact with the palliative care team is advised at this stage and it is very important that there is good, effective and open communication within the multidisciplinary team (see Chapter 7.16).

Drug–nutrient interactions

Levodopa (L-dopa) and protein

Large neutral amino acids in dietary proteins compete with L-dopa for intestinal absorption and transport across the blood–brain barrier. This limits L-dopa's efficacy and is responsible for the occurrence of motor fluctuations. Taking levodopa 45 minutes before meals, with a carbohydrate such as a cracker or a biscuit, can help to stop this happening. Reducing the amount of protein is not advised as it is an important part of a balanced diet.

Internet resources

Department of Health   www.dh.gov.uk
National Service Framework for Long-term (Neurological) Conditions (2005)   www.dh.gov.uk/en/Publicationsandstatistics/ Publications/PublicationsPolicyAndGuidance/DH_4105361
European Parkinson's Disease Association (EPDA)   http://epda.eu .com
National Institute for Health and Care Excellence   www.nice.org.uk
Clinical guideline on the diagnosis and management of Parkinson's disease in primary and secondary care in England and Wales (2006). CG 35. NB: Endorsed in Northern Ireland   www.nice .org.uk/guidance/CG35 Currently under review
Parkinson's UK   www.parkinsons.org.uk
Best practice guideline for dietitians on the management of Parkinson's (2010). Produced by BDA in association with Parkinson's UK   www.parkinsons.org.uk/advice/publications/professionals/ dietitians_best_practice_guide.aspx
The Professional's Guide to Parkinson's Disease (2007) www .parkinsons.org.uk/pdf/B126_Professionalsguide.pdf

References

Aarsland D, Marsh L, Schrag A. (2009) Neuropsychiatric symptoms in Parkinson's disease. *Movement Disorders* 24: 2175–2186.

Alam ZI, Jenner A, Daniel SE, *et al.* (1997) Oxidative DNA damage in the parkinsonian brain: an apparent selective increase in 8-hydroxyguanine levels in substantia nigra. *Journal of Neurochemistry* 69: 1196–1203.

Allcock LM, Ullyart K, Kenny RA, Burn D. (2004) Frequency of orthostatic hypotension in a community based cohort of patients with Parkinson's disease. *Journal of Neurology, Neurosurgery and Psychiatry* 75: 1470–1471.

Alves G, Muller B, Herlofson K, *et al.* (2009) Incidence of Parkinson's disease in Norway: the Norwegian Park West study. *Journal of Neurology, Neurosurgery and Psychiatry* 80: 851–857.

Baldereschi M, Di Carlo A, Rocca WA, *et al.* (2000) Parkinson's disease and parkinsonism in a longitudinal study: two-fold higher incidence in men. ILSA Working Group. Italian Longitudinal Study on Aging. *Neurology* 55: 1358–1363.

Barichella M, Marczewska A, De Notaris R, *et al.* (2006) Special low-protein foods ameliorate post-prandial off in patients with advanced Parkinson's disease. *Movement Disorders* 21: 1682–1687.

Barichella M, Savardi C, Mauri A, *et al.* (2007) Diet with LPP for renal patients increases daily energy expenditure and improves motor function in parkinsonian patients with motor fluctuations. *Nutritional Neuroscience* 10: 129–135.

Beal MF. (1998) Excitotoxicity and nitric oxide in Parkinson's disease pathogenesis. *Annals of Neurology* 44(Suppl 1): S110–S114.

Beyer PL, Palarino MY, Michalek D, Busenbark K, Koller WC. (1995) Weight change and body composition in patients with Parkinson's Disease. *Journal of the American Dietetic Association* 95(9): 979–983.

Bischoff-Ferrari HA, Giovannucci E, Willett WC, Dietrich T, Dawson-Hughes B. (2006) Estimation of optimal serum concentrations of 25-hydroxyvitamin D for multiple health outcomes. *American Journal of Clinical Nutrition* 84(1): 18–28.

Boonen S, Lips P, Bouillon R, Bischoff-Ferrari HA, Vanderschueren D, Haentjens P. (2007) Need for additional calcium to reduce the risk of hip fracture with vitamin D supplementation: Evidence from a comparative meta-analysis of randomised controlled trials. *Journal of Clinical Endocrinology & Metabolism* 92(4): 1415–23.

Calne DB. (2001) Parkinson's disease is not one disease. *Parkinsonism and Related Disorders* 7(1): 3–7.

Cassani E, Privitera G, Pezzoli G, *et al.* (2011) Use of probiotics for the treatment of constipation in Parkinson's disease patients. *Minerva Gastroenterologica e Dietologica* 57(2): 117–121.

Cereda E, Pezzoli G, Barichella M. (2009) The role of an electronic armband in motor function monitoring in patients with Parkinson's disease. *Nutrition* 26(2): 240–242.

Cushing ML, Traviss KA, Calne SM. (2002) Parkinson's disease: Implications for nutritional care. *Canadian Journal of Dietetic Practice and Research* 63(2): 81–87.

Dexter DT, Holley AE, Flitter WD, *et al.* (1994) Increased levels of lipid hydroperoxides in the parkinsonian substantia nigra: an HPLC and ESR study. *Movement Disorders* 9: 92–97.

Durrieu G, Llau ME, Rascol O, Senard JM, Rascol A, Montastruc JL. (1992) Parkinson's disease and weight loss: a study with anthropometric and nutritional assessment. *Clinical Autonomic Research* 2: 153–157.

Edwards LL, Pfeiffer RF, Quigley EMM, Hofman R, Baluff M. (1991) Gastrointestinal symptoms in Parkinson's disease. *Movement Disorders* 6: 151–156.

Elbaz A, Bower JH, Maraganore DM, *et al.* (2002) Risk tables for parkinsonism and Parkinson's disease. *Journal of Clinical Epidemiology* 14: 25–31.

Etminan M, Gill SS, Samii A. (2005) Intake of vitamin E, vitamin C, and carotenoids and the risk of Parkinson's disease: a meta-analysis. *Lancet Neurology* 4: 362–365.

Evatt ML, Delong MR, Khazai N, Rosen A, Triche S, Tangpricha V. (2008) Prevalence of vitamin d insufficiency in patients with Parkinson disease and Alzheimer disease. *Archives of Neurology* 65(10): 1348–1352.

Fariss MW, Zhang JG. (2003) Vitamin E therapy in Parkinson's disease. *Toxicology* 189: 129–146.

Glynn K. (2003) Nutritional issues in Parkinson's disease. *Complete Nutrition* 3(4): 13–16.

Jackson C, Gaugris S, Sen SS, Hosking D. (2007) The effect of cholecalciferol (vitamin D3) on the risk of fall and fracture: a meta-analysis. *Quarterly Journal of Medicine* 100: 185–192.

Kaye J, Gage H, Kimber A, Storey L, Trend P. (2006) Excess burden of constipation in Parkinson's disease: a pilot study. *Movement Disorders* 21: 1270–1273.

Knekt P, Kilkkinen A, Rissanen H, Marniemi J, Sääksjärvi K, Heliövaara M. (2010) Serum vitamin D and the risk of Parkinson disease. *Archives of Neurology* 67(7): 808–811.

Lang AE, Lozano AM. (1998) Parkinson's disease: second of two parts. *New England Journal of Medicine* 339(16): 1130–1143.

Leibson C, Long KH, Maraganore DM, *et al.* (2006) Direct medical costs associated with Parkinson's disease: a population-based study. *Movement Disorders* 21: 1864–1871.

Levi S, Cox M, Lugon M, Hodkinson M, Tomkins A. (1990) Increased energy expenditure in Parkinson's disease. *BMJ* 301: 1256–1257.

Logemann JA, Boshes B, Blonsky ER, Fisher HB. (1997) Speech and swallowing evaluation in the differential diagnosis of neurological disease. *Neurologia Neurocirugia Psiquiatria* 18: 71–78.

MacMahon DG, Thomas S. (1998) Practical approach to quality of life in Parkinson's disease: the nurse's role. *Journal of Neurology* 245: S19–S22.

Miller N, Allcock L, Hildreth AJ, Jones D, Noble E, Burn DJ. (2009) Swallowing problems in Parkinson disease: frequency and clinical correlates. *Journal of Neurology, Neurosurgery and Psychiatry* 80(9): 1047–1049.

Mutch W, Strudwick A, Roy SK, Downie AW. (1986) Parkinson's disease: disability, review, and management. *BMJ Clinical Research Edition* 293: 675–677.

National Institute for Health and Care Excellence (NICE). (2006a) *Parkinson's Disease: National Clinical Guideline for Diagnosis and Management in Primary and Secondary Care.* London: NICE.

National Institute of Health and Care Excellence (NICE). (2006b) Nutrition support in adults: oral nutrition support, enteral tube feeding and parenteral nutrition' (Clinical guideline 32). Available at www.nice.org.uk/CG032.

Nirenberg MJ, Waters C. (2006) Compulsive eating and weight gain related to dopamine agonist use. *Movement Disorders* 21: 524–529.

Palhagen S, Lorefalt B, Carlsson M, *et al.* (2005). Does L-dopa treatment contribute to reduction in body weight in elderly patients with Parkinson's disease? *Acta Neurologica Scandinavica* 111(1): 12–20.

Parashos S, Maraganore DM, O'Brien PC, Rocca WA. (2002) Medical services utilization and prognosis in Parkinson disease: a population-based study. *Mayo Clinic Proceedings* 77: 918–925.

Paré S, Barr SI, Ross SE. (1992) Effect of daytime protein restriction on nutrient intakes of free-living Parkinson's disease patients. *American Journal of Clinical Nutrition* 55: 701–707.

Parkinson's Disease UK. (2011) National Parkinson's audit. Available at www.parkinsons.org.uk/audit. Accessed 5 February 2013.

Pfeiffer RF. (2011) Gastrointestinal dysfunction in Parkinson's disease. *Parkinsonism & Related Disorders* 17(1): 10–15.

Poewe WH, Wenning GK. (1996) The natural history of Parkinson's disease. *Neurology* 47: S146–152.

Riley D, Lang AE. (1988) Practical application of a low protein diet for Parkinson's disease. *Neurology* 38: 1026–1031.

Robbins J, Gensler G, Hind J, *et al.* (2008) Comparison of 2 interventions for liquid aspiration on pneumonia incidence: a randomized trial. *Annals of Internal Medicine* 148(7): 509–518.

Sato Y, Kikuyama M, Oizumi K. (1997) High prevalence of vitamin D deficiency and reduced bone mass in Parkinson's disease. *Neurology* 49(5): 1273–1278.

Sato Y, Kaji M, Tsuru T, Oizumi K. (2001) Risk factors for hip fracture among elderly patients with Parkinson's disease. *Journal of the Neurological Sciences* 182(2): 89–93.

Sauleau P, Leray E, Rouaud T, *et al.* (2009) Comparison of weight gain and energy intake after subthalamic versus pallidal stimulation in Parkinson's disease. *Movement Disorders* 24(14): 2149–2155.

Shulman L, Taback RL, Bean J, Weiner WJ. (2001) Comorbidity of the nonmotor symptoms of Parkinson's disease. *Movement Disorders* 16: 507–510.

Siddiqui MF, Rast S, Lynn MJ, Auchus AP, Pfeiffer RF. (2002) Autonomic dysfunction in Parkinson's disease: a comprehensive symptom survey. *Parkinsonism Related Disorders* 8: 277–284.

Stennis Watson G, Leverenz JB. (2010) Profile of cognitive impairment in Parkinson disease. *Brain Pathology* 20(3): 640–645.

Stocchi F, Badiali D, Vacca L, *et al.* (2000) Anorectal function in multiple system atrophy and Parkinson's disease. *Movement Disorders* 15: 71–76.

Toth MJ. (1999) Energy expenditure in wasting diseases: current concepts and measurement techniques. *Current Opinion in Clinical Nutrition & Metabolic Care* 2(6): 445–451.

Tuite PJ, Maxwell RE, Ikramuddin S, *et al.* (2005) Weight and body mass index in Parkinson's disease patients after deep brain stimulation surgery. *Parkinsonism Related Disorders* 11: 247–252.

Uitti R, Ottman R, Goldman SM, *et al.* (1999) Parkinson's disease. *Neuroscience News* 2: 36–43.

von Campenhausen S, Bornschein B, Wick R, *et al.* (2005) Prevalence and incidence of Parkinson's disease in Europe. *European Neuropsychopharmacology* 15: 473–490.

Wolfe RR, Miller SL, Miller KB. (2008) Optimal protein intake in the elderly. *Clinical Nutrition* 27: 675–684.

7.6.2 Motor neurone disease
Elaine Cawadias and Alan Rio

Key points

- Motor neurone disease (MND) patients require coordinated care from a multidisciplinary team that includes dietetic expertise. Nutritional assessment, guidance and monitoring should commence at the earliest possible stage of the disease.

- Body weight loss of greater than 10% from prediagnosis weight is a clinical indicator for oral nutritional supplementation.

- Clinical indicators for gastrostomy are dysphagia, weight loss and inadequate energy intake; if indicated, it should be started early in the disease course.

- Prior to gastrostomy placement, MND patients require detailed assessment by the multidisciplinary team to assess the benefits and risks.

- Patients with respiratory failure require acclimatisation to non-invasive positive pressure ventilation before gastrostomy.

SECTION 7

Motor neurone disease (MND), also known as amyotrophic lateral sclerosis (ALS), is the name given to a group of closely related disorders characterised by degeneration of the motor neurones in the brain, brain stem and spinal cord. This degeneration leads to weakness and wasting of muscles. Early symptoms of MND include awkwardness in fine finger movement and dexterity, wasting in the limbs, foot drop, neck weakness and stiffness in the fingers. Cramping and fasciculations (muscle twitches) in the forearm, upper arm and shoulder girdle may also appear.

As symptoms progress, hand, arm or leg weakness, together with generalised hyperflexia (increased reflex action), can occur. Abductors, adductors and extensors of fingers and thumb become weak, giving rise to the appearance of the skeletal hand. Over time, upper limb weakness may progress to leave the patient with flail arm syndrome; in some patients, spasticity of the limbs may develop. The disease can also affect the neck, tongue, pharyngeal and laryngeal muscles, leading to dysphagia.

The course of the illness, irrespective of its site of onset and pattern of evolution, is progressive. The disease is quite variable with no two people having the same illness trajectory or experiences. It does not affect the senses, and touch, taste, sight, smell and hearing are all preserved. Cognitive function usually remains intact but there is increasing evidence of a dementia component or frontotemporal dementia (FTD), which may have implications for patient decision making and choices concerning treatment options and interventions. Criteria for the diagnosis of FTD syndromes in ALS have been proposed (Strong et al., 2009).

The progression of the disease can be profound and highly distressing for patients and carers; support and forward planning are key elements of care. As the disease accelerates, physical tasks, speech, swallowing and ultimately breathing may become affected. The course of the disease varies according to the site of onset but prognosis is poor, with survival estimated at 2–5 years from symptom onset. In some patients the disease progression is rapid and survival may only be a matter of months. Death is usually due to ventilatory failure (Victor & Ropper, 2001).

Motor neurone disease can affect any adult at any age, the highest incidence being in the 50–70-year age range, with males affected slightly more frequently than females. The incidence of MND in the UK is approximately 2 per 100 000 and prevalence is about 7 per 100 000. Current estimates suggest that approximately 5000 people in the UK have MND (MNDA, 2000).

The cause of MND is unknown in 90–95% of cases and is termed sporadic. Approximately 5–10% of patients will have the familial form of MND (FALS). A number of genetic mutations have been identified, including SOD1, TDP43 and FUS. About 20% of FALS is caused by the SOD1 mutation, with the remaining known mutations accounting for about 65%. The most common inheritance pattern for FALS is autosomal dominant, with each offspring having a 50% chance of inheriting the gene.

Types

The physical effects of the disease depend on which motor neurones are affected. Neurological lesions may primarily occur in the upper motor neurones (from the brain to the spinal cord, termed bulbar onset and affecting swallowing function), lower motor neurones (from the spinal cord to muscles, termed spinal onset and affecting limbs) or both.

It can be difficult to diagnose MND in the early stages as its initial symptoms may be indistinguishable from those of other neurological disorders. Diagnosis can therefore take up to 18 months due to the complexity of the investigations and the need for an accurate diagnosis. Clinical diagnostic tools include electromyography (EMG), nerve conduction studies (NCS), physical neurological examination, magnetic resonance imaging (MRI) and cerebral spinal fluid protein (Leigh et al., 2003). The El Escorial criteria for ALS/MND are often used, with certainty of diagnosis being termed as clinically possible, probable or definitive (World Federation of Neurology Research Group on Neuromuscular Disease, 1994). Motor neurone disease is broadly classified into the following types, although as the disease progresses they become less distinguishable and may overlap.

Amyotrophic lateral sclerosis

This is the most common form of the disease (about two-thirds of cases), typically occurring between 40 and 70 years of age. It involves both upper and lower motor neurone lesions causing muscle weakness and wasting, spasticity (stiffness), hyperactive reflexes (jerking of limbs) and fasciculations. Bulbar onset ALS is seen in about 20% of cases. Symptoms include changes in speech (articulation, volume) and swallowing (food and/or fluids). Limb onset is more common, with symptoms including foot drop, leg, hand or arm weakness. Most patients with limb onset will eventually develop some bulbar symptoms. Survival time from diagnosis is approximately 2–5 years, though 8–10% survive 10 years (Mitsumoto & Munsat, 2001).

Progressive muscular atrophy

This is a rarer form of the disease, accounting for only about 7.5% of MND cases. It tends to occur at a younger age (often below the age of 50 years) and is much more common in men than women (ratio of 3–4:1). It is predominantly a degeneration of lower motor neurones causing:

- Diminished or absent tendon reflexes.
- Muscle weakness and wasting.
- Fasciculation, often starting in the small muscles of one hand.
- Weight loss.

The 5-year survival time is 72% in patients with onset under the age of 50 years and 40% in those with onset over the age of 50 years.

Table 7.6.2 Multidisciplinary team roles in the management of motor neurone disease

Team member	Role
Dietitian	Nutritional support, texture modification, artificial nutrition and hydration, tube feeding and aftercare, continuing support
Speech and language therapist	Speech and swallow assessment, assisted communication aides, texture modification, postural modification for safe feeding, liaison with team regarding timing of alternative feeding methods
Clinical nurse specialist	Educational role, symptom management control, psychological support, coordinated patient care, liaison with community team, advice on tube feeding aftercare
Occupational therapist	Assessment of functional ability, adaptive aides including cutlery and feeding devices, advice on moving and hoisting, support with adjusting to changing lifestyle
Physiotherapist	Exercise, mobility, head support, neck collar, assisted cough, respiratory care including chest clearance and NIPPV use
District nurse	Continuing support, nursing care, feeding tube care, medication, liaison with palliative care and hospice teams
Pharmacist	Medication, alternative methods of administration, i.e. oral versus tube, solid/crushed/liquid, side effects

NIPPV, non-invasive positive pressure ventilation.

Progressive bulbar palsy

This accounts for about 20–25% of cases of MND, mostly occurring in people between the ages of 50 and 70 years, and it is slightly more common in women than men. Progressive bulbar palsy (PBP) affects the upper motor neurones and causes paralysis of the bulbar muscles that control speech, chewing and swallowing. Therefore, it tends to present in a different way from the above two forms of the disease. There is debate about whether PBP is a subtype of ALS or a separate disease; however, about 25% of patients with PBP will progress to ALS (Swash & Desai, 2000). Early symptoms are:

- Slurred or nasal type speech.
- Tongue atrophy with or without fasciculations.
- Pharyngeal weakness.
- Emotional lability.
- Choking on certain foods.

Progression is often rapid, with median survival time from diagnosis being 2–3 years; such rapid progression may have implications for nutritional support.

Primary lateral sclerosis

This is an extremely rare type of MND but with an unknown prevalence. It affects the corticospinal tracts that travel from the brain and are responsible for movement (upper motor neurones). Any part of the body can be affected in primary lateral sclerosis(PLS) and changes include brisk reflexes, increased muscle tone at rest and spasticity. Age of onset is typically in the 50s and is unrelated to the speed of progression of the disease. Unlike most forms of MND, the lifespan of the PLS patient is essentially normal. However, it may progress to MND ALS after a significant period of time, e.g. more than 25 years post PLS diagnosis.

Management

There is no cure for MND and management is targeted at changes in nutrition, respiration and physical functions, and includes supportive measures such as non-invasive positive pressure ventilation (NIPPV) and gastrostomy feeding. Riluzole, which acts by inhibiting the release of glutamate and protecting cells from glutamate mediated damage, is the only National Institute for Health and Care Excellence (NICE) approved drug for MND. It extends survival by about 3 months, primarily in the early stages of the disease. Unlike some neurodegenerative disorders, there is no remission in MND, although there may be temporary plateaus during which no further deterioration occurs.

Multidisciplinary care is crucial, with forward planning and good communication within the healthcare team being cornerstones of care. For dietitians working with patients with MND, a multidisciplinary team (MDT) approach will greatly assist in the assessment and planning of nutritional care and plays a key role in supporting the patient between the hospital and community (Table 7.6.2). Early dietetic referral is encouraged in guidelines produced by the Motor Neurone Disease Association (MNDA, 2000) and ensures that appropriate nutritional advice and monitoring are integrated into patient care (Rio *et al.*, 2005a). The benefits of integrated patient care provided by a multidisciplinary clinic are improved prognosis and enhanced survival compared with MND patients attending a general neurology clinic (Traynor *et al.*, 2003).

Nutritional management

Motor neurone disease affects each patient differently in terms of disease progression. Nutritional management will therefore depend on the nature of the individual

SECTION 7

symptoms. Patients can experience periods of rapid weight loss leading to profound reduction in mobility, a weakened physical state, respiratory muscle weakness and susceptibility to opportunistic oral infections. Nutritional support has a central role in patient management and dietitians can influence decisions on nutritional care. The Royal College of Nursing's (RCN, 2001) identified three stages of the disease process; diagnostic, palliative and terminal. Patients will not remain in these stages for any set period of time and may progress so rapidly that they may move straight from diagnosis to the terminal stage. The dietitian needs to be empathetic and show a flexible and adaptable approach to patient care.

Nutritional assessment

Malnutrition in patients with MND increases the risk of death by 7.7 fold, with nutritional status acting as an independent prognostic indicator (Desport *et al.*, 1999); malnutrition in ALS resembles marasmus. Approximately 20% of patients with MND will develop malnutrition, even those without swallowing difficulties (Worwood & Leigh, 1998), as progression of the disease is associated with declining muscle and adipose tissue reserves. The incidence of malnutrition depends on the criteria used; a number of studies using a BMI of less than $18.5\,kg/m^2$ as an indicator of malnutrition found that 6–53% of patients were malnourished. Although frequently cited, this marker has a number of drawbacks, most notably lack of sensitivity in this patient group. If reduced energy intake is used, 70–100% are affected (Tandan *et al.*, 1999).

Percentage body weight loss is a useful tool. At the time of diagnosis, each 5% decrease in weight has been associated with a 30% increase in risk of death (Marin *et al.*, 2011). A loss of more than 10% from prediagnosis body weight in a short period of time is a clinical indicator for the introduction of nutritional supplements. The MDT should discuss the need for artificial nutrition and hydration.

Nutritional requirements

No disease specific energy or protein requirements have been set for patients with MND. The Schofield equation is commonly used as the starting point for calculating daily energy requirements. However, reliance on standard equations may lead to either under- or over-feeding (Sherman *et al.*, 2004). Resting metabolic rate (RMR) appears to change over the course of the disease and this should be factored into calculations. Despite a paradoxically low physical activity level, people with ALS are hypermetabolic by about 10% when compared to matched controls (Tandan *et al.*, 1999) and this increases as the disease progresses (Vaisman *et al.*, 2009). Patients may also have defective energy homeostasis, whereby the hypermetabolic state may accelerate the disease (Dupuis *et al.*, 2004). However, in end stage disease with mechanical ventilation, RMR is lower and approximates total calorie expenditure (Siirala *et al.*, 2010).

Nitrogen requirements are calculated using percentage body weight loss and malnourished state. Suggested nitrogen requirements are:

- 0.17 g/kg/day for patients in the early stages of disease.
- 0.2 g/kg/day for patients with body weight loss of 10%.
- 0.25 g/kg/day for malnourished patients and body weight loss of greater than 20%.

Fluid intake should be 30–35 mL/kg of body weight, depending on age. Requirements for vitamins and minerals are not affected by the disease state and, although patients may become severely malnourished, overt deficiencies are rare. Fibre intake should aim to meet the current recommended value (18 g/day).

Dietary guidance

Nutritional education should commence as soon as MND is suspected or diagnosed; dietitians are a vital source of consistent and evidence based dietary advice. The basic principles of nutritional support apply, with emphasis on nutrient dense food and drinks, a wide variety of foods, ease of food preparation, meal planning and adoption of a liberal and unrestricted diet. Initially, nutritional intake may be boosted by food fortification and by the consumption of frequent small meals and snacks. However, prescribable energy supplements may be necessary if dietary intake fails to meet requirements or if 10% of body weight is lost (see Chapter 6.3).

Constipation is a frequent digestive complaint with causes including decreased physical activity, fibre intake and fluid intake due to swallowing difficulties, or increased dependence for toileting, weakness in abdominal or pelvic muscles required to push, medications to control drooling or pain and slow bowel transit time. Management of constipation focuses on the underlying causes, which may include increasing fibre intake or fibre supplements, increasing fluid intake including thickened fluids, promoting good bowel habits and establishing a bowel routine, careful use of stool softeners or laxatives and control of medications (types, dosage, timing). Unresolved constipation can lead to faecal impaction due to poor dietary intake, dehydration or muscle weakness. Symptoms of faecal impaction include bloating, abdominal distension and, on abdominal X ray, stools and gas throughout the small bowel. Faecal impaction is resolved with macrogols, inert polymers of ethylene that sequester fluid in the bowels, at dosage of one to three sachets/day. If this is ineffective, eight sachets in 1 L of water for a maximum of 3 days is recommended.

Dietitians should not forget that even in the most debilitated patient the ability to taste, smell and feel the texture of food remains intact, and eating should be made as pleasurable as possible. Patients may enquire about the use of alternative diets, vitamin supplements and plant extracts, and dietitians can help them make an informed choice based on open discussion of their likely efficacy and cost (Cameron & Rosenfeld, 2002; Rosenfeld & Ellis, 2009) (see Chapter 5.4).

Dysphagia

Approximately 70–80% of patients will develop dysphagia during the course of the disease. A speech and language therapist (SLT) can assess the presence, severity and nature of the dysphagia and advise on safe swallowing strategies, including chin tuck, head position, texture modification and use of food and fluid thickeners. Saliva drooling can be managed with medications such as sublingual atropine, amitriptyline, glycopyrronium, dermal hyoscine patches, botox or low dose radiation treatments.

Patients with severe dysphagia have an increased risk of aspiration pneumonia and may be advised to be nil by mouth (NBM). However, this measure denies terminally ill patients the pleasures associated with eating and drinking. A discussion with the patient and their carers regarding the risks of continuing oral intake is advisable. Some patients may choose to take small amounts of food or fluids of an appropriate texture or consistency for pleasure and quality of life.

Artificial nutrition and hydration

Artificial nutrition and hydration (ANH) is indicated in MND patients who have (Miller *et al.*, 2009):

- Severe dysphagia with risk of aspiration pneumonia or recurring chest infections.
- Malnutrition with weight loss of greater than 10% from the prediagnosis weight.
- Suboptimal energy intake.

The goals of ANH should be to (Heffernan *et al.*, 2004):

- Provide additional energy and protein.
- Stabilise body weight.
- Correct malnutrition.
- Act as a route for hydration and medications.
- While it will not completely eliminate the risk of aspiration, it will decrease the risk (there is still a risk of aspirating saliva and secretions).

The most common method of providing ANH is via gastrostomy, either percutaneous endoscopic gastrostomy (PEG) or percutaneous radiological gastrostomy (PRG). Respiratory status pregastrostomy will help define suitability for PEG or PRG insertion (Leigh *et al.*, 2003).

Current evidence demonstrates that PEG or PRG can be inserted any time during the disease, but that the nutritional benefits diminish as patients enter the terminal phase. Ideally, ANH should be for more than 4–6 weeks and careful patient selection is crucial to avoid early post procedure mortality. Pregastrostomy assessment should consider:

- *Respiratory function* – symptoms of poor respiratory function include morning headache, breathlessness, constant shallow breathing, raised PCO_2 levels and reduced forced vital capacity (FVC). Patients with respiratory failure require acclimatisation to NIPPV before gastrostomy. Single step intervention allows the patient to adapt and their response to be fully evaluated whilst minimising complications.
- *Stage of the disease* – patients in the terminal phase are unlikely to benefit from gastrostomy.
- *Malnutrition* – patients presenting with severe malnutrition may benefit from nasogastric feeding, which should be evaluated before placement.
- *Quality of life* – gastrostomy may reduce quality of life by increasing the burden for both patient and carer, and increasing the number of hospital visits. Alternatively, gastrostomy feeding can increase quality of life by reducing the amount of time spent consuming food and the distressing symptoms associated with dysphagia.

When considering ANH in MND patients, the MDT should evaluate the risk–benefit ratio of the gastrostomy procedure. Gastrostomy insertion is a relatively routine procedure and can be performed any time during the course of the disease. However, PEG insertion in MND patients with respiratory failure or respiratory muscle weakness can be life threatening (Mathus-Vliegen *et al.*, 1994) and the 30-day mortality rate following gastrostomy in MND patients is between 2% and 25% (Forbes *et al.*, 2004). Another study showed a median survival of 185 days post PEG with worse outcomes in patients with weight loss of >10% of healthy body weight and FVC <65% (Chio *et al.*, 1999). The findings of a report into patient outcomes and death in the UK showed a less positive experience for patients having PEG; 43% of patients died within 1 week and 19% of advisers thought PEG a futile procedure (Cullinane *et al.*, 2004). However, it should be noted that the MND component in this study was quite small (7%).

This wide variation in mortality represents differing selection criteria and timing, varying respiratory function and nutritional status of the population and the expertise of the clinician involved. Thorough assessment by the MDT as to fitness for the procedure can help identify those MND patients likely to benefit. Dietitians should be aware that not all patients with MND progress to requiring a gastrostomy. When PEG or PRG appears to be indicated it should be offered early in the course of the disease when respiratory function is good and procedural complications are probably fewer. Early placement also has the advantage of greater nutritional benefit (Table 7.6.3). However, patients choose gastrostomy in their own time and for different reasons. Some patients may want to delay having a gastrostomy for as long as possible, which is understandable. Dietitians have a key educational role in helping patients reach this important decision by offering sensitive and timely information. An early referral allows the dietitian to get to know the patient and their family, enabling a relationship to be developed. Initiating education and discussion early allows for a non-crisis decision making process. Patients may have unfounded concepts of artificial feeding and a brief discussion with the patient can open avenues and opportunities to discuss the practical issues.

SECTION 7

Table 7.6.3 Implications of early and late gastrostomy placement

	Early placement	Late placement
Clinical condition	Disease progression at an early stage	Disease state usually advanced
Respiratory status	Good respiratory function (FVC >50%)	Respiratory function often impaired Patients using NIPPV due to poor respiratory function or advanced disease state
Nutritional status	Minimal weight loss Meal times prolonged but dietary intake may be adequate	Weight loss >10% Dietary intake likely to be limited and the patient malnourished
Dysphagia	Swallow function mildly affected	Swallow function poor
Potential risks of gastrostomy insertion	Perceived to be fewer Procedure related	Respiratory (NIPPV) support needed for procedure Increased risk of mortality Stoma site infection
Benefits	Additional energy and protein intake Weight stabilisation (individual weight gain is variable)	Symptom control, including constipation management and reduced risk of aspiration Improved hydration Alleviates anxiety associated with eating and drinking (tube feeding likely to become the sole source of nutrition) Small weight gain/weight stabilisation May help stabilise respiratory function

FVC, forced ventilatory capacity; NIPPV, non-invasive positive pressure ventilation.

Percutaneous endoscopic gastrostomy

Percutaneous endoscopic gastrostomy is the standard nutritional intervention, although insertion of PEG poses a number of clinical challenges for the healthcare team. Risks associated with the procedure are serious, but relatively uncommon. They include infection at the insertion site, bleeding, temporary diarrhoea, cramping, nausea and vomiting (all major or minor), oesophageal perforation and injury to the bowel (Mitchell *et al.*, 2008). Decreased respiratory function and a high lying stomach may be contraindications.

The survival benefit to MND patients once associated with PEG is now unclear. Early evidence suggested improved survival (Mazzini *et al.*, 1995); however, this has not been demonstrated in other studies. It has been suggested that PEG be used for symptom control and improved quality of life rather than for survival (Chio *et al.*, 1999). On the other hand, a more recent study showed that PEG improves survival in dysphagic ALS patients with few side effects, and the procedure is safe and applicable even to patients with impaired respiratory function (Spataro *et al.*, 2011). This may be a reflection of increased experience of clinicians with this patient population. Whilst FVC is commonly used as a guide to respiratory function, it is not a wholly reliable indicator of survival post PEG. In a group of MND patients with a FVC of less than 50% (Gregory *et al.*, 2002), survival was similar to previously published data for a patient group with a FVC above the 50% threshold. In a small group of patients with advanced MND, PEG was successfully inserted without respiratory complications (Boitano *et al.*, 2001). Whilst a low FVC should not deprive patients of gastrostomy, thorough respiratory, nutritional and medical assessments are needed to reduce the 30-day mortality rate (Rio & Leigh, 2001).

Percutaneous radiological gastrostomy

This technique, often called radiologically inserted gastrostomy (RIG), is an alternative method of gastrostomy insertion done by an interventional radiologist. It is suitable for patients with MND as tube placement does not require oral access; instead tubes are placed directly into the stomach, a technique known as the push technique. This technique is therefore suitable for patients with bulbar symptoms, although this group is required to lie flat during the procedure. Preprocedural oximetry and history of desaturation whilst lying flat should be obtained to prevent unnecessary distress at the time of the procedure.

Preprocedural abdominal X rays should be performed to investigate if the patient has either chronic constipation, also known as faecal impaction, or gas in the abdomen. The presence of one of these factors can lead to problems post PRG insertion, which include pain, discomfort and bowel perforation. Serious complications, including bowel perforation, post PRG insertion occur in approximately 2–5%, which, importantly, are avoidable (Rio *et al.*, 2010). Patients who present with faecal impaction or gas in the bowel require these to be resolved prior to the procedure. The standard medications for treatment of chronic constipation are suitable for this patient group and should be prescribed for a minimum of 5–7 days. A repeat abdominal X ray is advised prior to tube placement to check if constipation has resolved; some patients may require a longer duration of laxative use.

Nutritional care of patients with a gastrostomy

Nutritional care of the MND patient with a gastrostomy is similar to the management of any patient receiving ANH. Some patients may receive all their nutrition or they may choose (where appropriate) to supplement oral intake of food or fluids via the gastrostomy. Intake should provide adequate energy and adequate, but not excessive protein, and meet fluid requirements from the formula and addition water. Considerations in choosing a formula include energy density, protein content, fibre or non-fibre content and special requirements (diabetes and renal disease). Feeding schedules are individualised depending on full or supplemental feedings, lifestyle and method of administration (pump, gravity or syringe).

Nutritional care of patients assessed unsafe for gastrostomy

Patients with advanced disease presenting with respiratory failure and malnutrition will benefit from the input of the palliative care team. Patients may consider enteral feeding as symbolic of their fight against the disease. However, gastrostomy placement at this time may not be advisable due to the limited benefit of nutritional support in a patient close to death. Nutritional support should be carefully considered alongside anticipated goals (Ersek, 2003). Palliation of symptoms and comfort should take priority, whilst quality of life is paramount (see Chapter 7.16).

Nutritional support with nasogastric tube (NGT) feeding is advisable in this group of patients with advanced disease. Fine bore NGTs are the primary and most frequently used route of tube feeding in the acute hospital setting. However, patients may find a NGT cosmetically unappealing and socially intrusive. Treatment with a NGT has a number of advantages:

- Less invasive than PEG or PRG.
- Risk of aspiration is the same as with PEG or PRG.
- Allows immediate delivery of nutrition and hydration.

Feeding via a NGT can be a temporary route for ANH where expectations of extended survival and return to normal body weight are not sought. Importantly, NGT feeding also allows the response to enteral nutrition to be fully evaluated whilst the benefit–risk ratio of PEG or PRG is assessed.

Nutritional requirements should be calculated in the usual way (see Chapter 6.4), but feeds should be administered gradually over several days as per patient tolerance. Risk of aspiration can be reduced by:

- Effective saliva/secretion management.
- Limiting oral intake or placing patients nil by mouth.
- Using a daytime feeding regimen.
- Ensuring patients are sat upright during feeding.

Discharge into the community with a NGT requires the support of the local team, including the GP, district nurse, home enteral nutrition team and palliative care team. Community support of patients with a NGT may vary and information for tube replacement and tube care should be provided in advance of discharge. Dietitians have a key leadership role in the coordination and discharge of these patients.

Management of patients who refuse artificial nutrition and hydration therapy

Not all patients with MND will choose to have a feeding tube. Despite dysphagia, prolonged meal times, aspiration pneumonia and the presence of malnutrition, some patients will choose to maintain oral nutritional intake. Reasons why patients refuse ANH will vary and may include (Cawadias & Carroll-Thomas, 2001):

- Denial of the diagnosis.
- Reluctance to have an invasive procedure.
- Decision to let the disease take its course due to preference, age or comorbidities.
- Unwillingness to accept a milestone has been reached.
- Misperceptions about the procedure and how the gastrostomy can be used.
- Fear of the unknown.
- Dislike of change of lifestyle.
- Belief they will be connected to a feeding pump for lengthy periods.
- Inability to manage equipment due to decreased arm function.
- Lack of social support.

Support from the dietitian is vital for these patients and both the acute and community teams should be involved. The MNDA regional care advisor can also offer input and act as a valuable link with the different care services. Ongoing dietetic input and good communication between team members can help these patients maintain their quality of life and dignity. Some patients may initially refuse tube feeding and then suddenly decide they want to go ahead with a gastrostomy. As stated above, caution should be exercised and thorough assessment of medical fitness for the procedure and likely benefit should be evaluated before a hasty decision is made.

Multidisciplinary team in nutritional care

Working in a small team, dietitians may be challenged by the implications of MND and feel overwhelmed. Discussing quality of life issues and end of life decisions may be unfamiliar territory for many dietitians. Service provision differs greatly across the UK and this includes provision of dietetic and multidisciplinary care. Some areas may provide high standards of care, while in others dietitians may find themselves working in isolation with limited resources (Rio & Cawadias, 2009). Where services are limited, dietitians can encourage good practice by regular patient review, adoption of the MNDA nutrition guidelines, liaison with the speech and language therapist, communication with the patient's GP, consulting with a specialist MND centre dietitian and involving the patient in any decisions that affect their care. Confidence in working with this patient population comes with experience, both in terms of time and number of patients. Some patients may visit tertiary referral centres for review, clinical trials or respiratory management. Liaison with the team dietitian, centre coordinator, clinical nurse specialist or neurologist is highly recommended. Not only will this help in terms of patient care, but it also provides a source of professional support and further information.

Further reading

Motor Neurone Disease Association (MNDA). (2000) *MND Resource File: A Patient and Carer Centred Approach for Health and Social Care Professionals*. Northampton: MNDA.

Internet resources

Amyotrophic Lateral Sclerosis Association   www.alsa.org
Motor Neurone Disease (MND) Association   www.mndassociation.org
World Federation of Neurology – Research Group on Motor Neurone Disease   www.wfnals.org

References

Boitano LJ, Jordan T, Benditt JO. (2001) Noninvasive ventilation allows gastrostomy tube placement in patients with advanced ALS. *Neurology* 56: 413–414.

Cameron A, Rosenfeld J. (2002) Nutritional issues and supplements in amyotrophic lateral sclerosis and other neurodegenerative disorders. *Current Opinion in Clinical Nutrition and Metabolic Care* 5: 631–643.

Cawadias E, Carroll-Thomas S. (2001) Nutritional support in ALS: supporting the decision for oral feeding. Poster presentation. Dietitians of Canada Annual Conference, Winnipeg, Canada.

Chio A, Finocchiaro E, Meineri P, Bottacchi E, Schiffer D. (1999) Safety and factors related to survival after percutaneous endoscopic gastrostomy in ALS. ALS Percutaneous Endoscopic Gastrostomy Study Group. *Neurology* 53(5): 1123–1125.

Cullinane M, Gray AJG, Hargraves CMK, *et al.*. (2004) *Scoping our Practice. The National Confidential Enquiry into Patient Outcome and Death*. London: NCEPOD. Available at www.ncepod.org.uk. Accessed 28 August 2012.

Desport JC, Preux PM, Truong TC, Vallat JM, Sautereau D, Couratier P. (1999) Nutritional status is a prognostic factor for survival in ALS patients. *Neurology* 53(5): 1059–1063.

Dupuis L, Oudart H, Rene F, Gonzalez de Aguilar JL, Loeffler JP. (2004) Evidence for defective energy homeostasis in amyotrophic lateral sclerosis: benefit of a high-energy diet in a transgenic mouse model. *Proceedings of the National Academy of Sciences USA* 101(30): 11159–11164.

Ersek M. (2003) Artificial Nutrition and Hydration: Clinical issues. *Journal of Hospice and Palliative Nursing* 5(4): 221–230.

Forbes RB, Colville S, Swingler RJ; Scottish Motor Neurone Disease Research Group. (2004) Frequency, timing and outcome of gastrostomy tubes for amyotrophic lateral sclerosis/motor neurone disease – a record linkage study from the Scottish Motor Neurone Disease Register. *Journal of Neurology* 251(7): 813–817.

Gregory S, Siderowf A, Golaszewski AL, McCluskey L. (2002) Gastrostomy insertion in ALS patients with low vital capacity: respiratory support and survival. *Neurology* 58(3): 485–487.

Heffernan C, Jenkinson C, Holmes T, *et al.* (2004) Nutritional management in MND/ALS patients: an evidence based review. *Amyotrophic Lateral Sclerosis and Other Motor Neuron Disorders* 5(2): 72–83.

Leigh PN, Abrahams S, Al-Chalabi A, *et al.* (2003) The management of motor neurone disease. *Journal of Neurology, Neurosurgery and Psychiatry* 74: 32–47.

Marin B, Desport JC, Kajeu P, *et al.* (2011) Alteration of nutritional status at diagnosis is a prognostic factor for survival of amyotrophic lateral sclerosis patients. *Journal of Neurology, Neurosurgery and Psychiatry* 82: 628–634.

Mathus-Vliegen LM, Louwerse LS, Merkus MP, Tytgat GN, Vianney de Jong JM. (1994) Percutaneous endoscopic gastrostomy in patients with amyotrophic lateral sclerosis and impaired pulmonary function. *Gastrointestinal Endoscopy* 40(4): 463–469.

Mazzini L, Corra T, Zaccala M, Mora G, Del Piano M, Galante M. (1995) Percutaneous endoscopic gastrostomy and enteral nutrition in amyotrophic lateral sclerosis. *Journal of Neurology* 242(10): 695–698.

Miller RG, Jackson CE, Kasarskis EJ, *et al.* (2009a) Practice parameter update: The care of the patient with amyotrophic lateral sclerosis: Drug, nutritional, and respiratory therapies (an evidence-based review): Report of the Quality Standards Subcommittee of the American Academy of Neurology. *Neurology* 73: 1218–1226.

Miller RG, Jackson CE, Kasarskis EJ, *et al.* (2009b) Practice parameter update: The care of the patient with amyotrophic lateral sclerosis: Multidisciplinary care, symptom management, and cognitive/ behavioral impairment (an evidence-based review): Report of the Quality Standards Subcommittee of the American Academy of Neurology. *Neurology* 73: 1227–1233.

Mitchell SL, Tetroe JM, O'Connor AM. (2008) Making Choices: Long Term Feeding Tube Placement in Elderly Patients. Ottawa: The Ottawa Health Research Institute.

Mitsumoto, H, Munsat TL (eds). (2001) *Amyotrophic Lateral Sclerosis: A Guide for Patients and Families*, 2nd edn. New York: Demos Medical Publishing.

Motor Neurone Disease Association (MNDA). (2000) *MND Resource File: A Patient and Carer Centred Approach for Health and Social Care Professionals*. Northampton: MNDA.

Rio A, Cawadias E. (2007) Nutritional advice and treatment by dietitians to patients with amyotrophic lateral sclerosis/motor neurone disease: a survey of current practice in England, Wales, Northern Ireland and Canada. *Journal of Human Nutrition and Dietetics* 20(1): 3–13.

Rio A, Leigh PN. (2001) Noninvasive ventilation allows gastrostomy tube placement in patients with advanced ALS. *Neurology* 57(7): 1351; discussion 1351–1352.

Rio A, Ampong MA, Johnson J, Willey E, Leigh PN. (2005a) Nutritional care of patients with MND: recent advances in management. *British Journal of Neuroscience Nursing* 1: 38–41.

Rio A, Ellis C, Shaw C, *et al.* (2010) Nutritional factors associated with survival following enteral tube feeding in patients with motor neuronc disease. *Journal of Human Nutrition and Dietetics* 23(4): 408–415.

Rosenfeld J, Ellis A. (2009) Nutrition and dietary supplements in motor neuron disease. *Physical Medicine & Rehabilitation Clinics of North America* 19(3): 573–589.

Royal College of Nursing (RCN); MND Nurse Specialist Working Party. (2001) *Paradigm for Disease Management in Motor Neurone Disease*. London: RCN.

Sherman MS, Pillai A, Jackson A, Heiman-Patterson T. (2004) Standard equations are not accurate in assessing resting energy expenditure in patients with amyotrophic lateral sclerosis. *Journal of Parenteral and Enteral Nutrition* 28(6): 442–446.

Siirala W, Olkkola KT, Noponen T, Vuori A, Aantaa R. (2010) Predictive equations over-estimate the resting energy expenditure in amyotrophic lateral sclerosis patients who are dependent on invasive ventilation support. *Nutrition & Metabolism* 7: 70.

Spataro R, Ficano L, Piccoli F, La Bella V. (2011) PEG in ALS: Effect on survival. *Journal of Neurolgical Sciences* 304(1–2): 44–48.

Strong M, Grace GM, Freedman M, *et al.* (2009) Consensus criteria for the diagnosis of frontotemporal cognitive and behavioural syndromes in amyotrophic lateral sclerosis. *Amyotrophic Lateral Sclerosis* 10: 131–146.

Swash M, Desai J. (2000) Motor neuron disease: Classification and nomenclature. *ALS and Other Motor Neuron Disorders* 1: 105–112.

Tandan R, Hiser JR, Krusinski PB, Poehlamn ET. (1999) Energy requirements in amytrophic lateral sclerosis measured by the doubly labelled water methodology. *Neurology* 52(Suppl 2): A2–A3.

Traynor BJ, Alexander M, Corr B, Frost E, Hardiman O. (2003) Effect of a multidisciplinary amyotrophic lateral sclerosis (ALS) clinic on ALS survival: a population based study, 1996–2000. *Journal of Neurology, Neurosurgery and Psychiatry* 74(9): 1258–1261.

Vaisman N, Lusaus M, Nefussy B, *et al.*. (2009) Do patients with amyotrophic lateral sclerosis (ALS) have increased energy needs? *Journal of the Neurological Sciences* 279: 26.

Victor M, Ropper AH (eds.). (2001) *Adams & Victor's Principles of Neurology*. McGraw Hill Medical Publishing Division Worldwide.

World Federation of Neurology. (1994) Criteria for the diagnosis of amyotrophic lateral sclerosis. *Journal of Neurological Sciences* 124(Suppl): 96–107.

Worwood AM, Leigh PN. (1998) Indicators and prevalence of malnutrition in motor neurone disease. *European Neurology* 40(3): 159–163.

7.6.3 Rare neurological conditions

Suzy Yates and Angeline Brookes

Key points

- Patients with Guillain–Barré syndrome may require enteral tube feeding if ventilation is required. Nutritional intervention should concentrate on weight maintenance and meeting nutritional requirements.

- Patients with myasthenia gravis experience varying degrees of dysphagia due to muscle weakness and fatigue; they may require enteral nutrition support as a temporary measure.

- Autonomic dysfunction is a feature of pure autonomic failure, multiple system atrophy and postural orthostatic tachycardia syndrome. Appropriate education, lifestyle and dietary changes are key components of the management, aiming for improvement in or alleviation of symptoms.

Guillain–Barré syndrome

Guillain–Barré syndrome (GBS) is an autoimmune disease affecting the peripheral nervous system. It is characterised by weakness, pain and in some cases paralysis, which ascends up the body. In the majority of cases, symptoms are confined to the limbs; however, in 25% of cases weakness can spread to the trunk and respiratory muscles, leading to a requirement for artificial ventilation (Hughes & Cornblath, 2005). Some patients are also affected by bulbar (muscles of the mouth and throat responsible for chewing, swallowing and talking) muscle weakness, leading to difficulty with swallowing and speech.

It is caused by the body's immune system attacking either the myelin sheath or axons of the cells of the peripheral nervous system. The inflammation and damage to the peripheral cells leads to the characteristic pain and paralysis. A preceding unrelated virus or illness, such as gastroenteritis caused by *Campylobacter jejuni* or Epstein Barr virus often triggers the immune response (Hadden *et al.*, 2001).

Diagnostic classification

In Europe and North America, the most common (approximately 95%) subtype of GBS is acute inflammatory demyelinating polyradiculoneuropathy (AIDP). The other 5% of GBS patients present with axonal subtypes, where the axon of the nerve cell rather than the myelin sheath is damaged. In South East Asia and South America there is a higher prevalence of the axonal subtypes than in Europe and North America (Hughes & Cornblath, 2005). Miller Fisher syndrome is a variant of GBS; this presents with descending rather than ascending paralysis, paralysis of muscles controlling eye movement and facial and bulbar weakness (Hahn, 1998). Electromyography (EMG) and lumbar puncture are used as diagnostic tests for GBS.

Disease consequences and epidemiology

The worldwide incidence of GBS is 2.3 in 100 000. It occurs in both sexes and at any age. The incidence increases with age and it is more common in men than women (van Doorn *et al.*, 2008). The acute deterioration generally lasts 2–4 weeks, after which the patient's function plateaus at the lowest level. After this, recovery begins and can take many months; 4–15% of patients will die, although mortality rates are lower at specialist centres (Hughes & Cornblath, 2005). Most patients will make a full functional recovery, but 20–30% of patients will have a permanent reduction in their level of function (Bersano *et al.*, 2006; Hughes *et al.*, 2005).

Clinical management

Patients should be monitored for deterioration in respiratory function. Intubation and artificial ventilation will be required if respiratory function is compromised secondary to paralysis of respiratory muscles and the diaphragm. These patients will invariably require alternative nutrition, with enteral feeding being the most preferred route via a nasogastric (NG) tube. Intensive care unit (ICU) admission may also be required for patients whose autonomic function is severely affected (see Autonomic dysfunction section). Both intravenous immunoglobulin (IVIg) and plasma exchange have been shown to be equally effective treatments at accelerating recovery, and are most effective if the course of treatment is administered within the first 2 weeks of symptom onset (van Doorn et al., 2008). Medical treatment will also be required for pain management, and potentially also for the management of autonomic failure or dysfunction (see Chapter 7.17.1).

Nutrition related symptoms and consequences

Weight and muscle loss

Weight and muscle loss can occur in both the acute and recovery stages of GBS, and the causes are multifactorial. In the acute phase, weight loss may be caused by muscle atrophy, secondary to reduced nerve conduction to the muscles, or by a prolonged intensive care unit (ICU) admission.

Hypermetabolism

One study has suggested that, due to the infective and inflammatory response, patients with GBS are hypermetabolic and hypercatabolic, leading to weight loss (Rubenoff et al., 1992). However, no studies have measured energy expenditure using validated methods for a large enough sample of this patient group to establish the extent of the effect on metabolic rate.

Dysphagia

In the acute and recovery stages, dysphagia can be a cause of reduced oral intake, and therefore weight loss. One study showed that in the ICU, 57% of GBS patients present with bulbar weakness (Ng et al., 1995), whilst another study assessing 20 years of GBS admissions to the ICU showed that 79% of patients had bulbar dysfunction (Dhar et al., 2008) (see Chapter 7.3).

Limb weakness, pain and fatigue

In the recovery phase of GBS, the reduced ability to self feed may lead to a reduced intake, and therefore weight loss. Upper limb weakness is characteristic and patients may be unable for find it difficult to complete many activities of daily living, including feeding. Patients will only be able to self feed if function has returned to the upper limbs. Even with some function, neuropathic pain may limit the patient's ability to feed. Ruts et al. (2010) showed that even 1 year after the acute phase, 82% of GBS patients reported pain in their extremities. Fatigue, which is also common in GBS, may affect an individual's ability to engage in feeding activities for the length of time required, thereby limiting the amount of food taken at a meal.

Constipation

Constipation related to gastric dysmotility, or use of pain medications such as opioids or codeine phosphate, can cause a reduction in appetite, and therefore a reduction of food eaten, resulting in weight loss.

Gastric dysmotility

Two-thirds of GBS patients develop an element of autonomic dysfunction. One of the many symptoms related to autonomic dysfunction is gastric dysmotility, which affects 15% of severe GBS patients (Burns, 2008). Gastric dysmotility can affect tolerance of enteral feed, resulting in large aspirates and requiring the use of prokinetics. At worst, dysmotility can develop into an ileus.

Nutritional assessment

The following should be noted when completing a nutritional assessment.

Anthropometry

Anthropometric measurements should consider:

- Weight loss and, if possible, measurements of muscle loss –mid upper arm circumferences.
- In recovery/rehabilitation – reduced mobility may lead to abdominal weight gain; waist circumference measurement may be useful.

Clinical assessment

The clinical assessment should consider:

- Gastric aspirates if enterally fed.
- Monitoring of bowel function, paying particular attention to constipation.
- Bulbar weakness – an assessment from a speech and language therapist (SLT) will be required if there is any element of dysphagia with solids or fluids.
- Upper limb power in patients in the recovery stage. Limb power and strength may affect ability to self feed.
- Fine motor skills – can the patient hold cutlery and lift drinks to their mouth, or do they require assistance to do this?.
- Reports of fatigue from nurses or the patient themselves.
- Presence of pressure ulcers – long ICU admission/ immobility can encourage their development.

Dietary assessment

Dietary assessment should consider:

- Is the food and drink of an appropriate texture and consistency in view of the patient's swallow function?
- During the recovery phase – is the patient following any diet that they feel may help symptoms? (see Balanced eating during recovery section)
- Is the patient meeting their nutritional requirements for energy and protein?
- Is the patient meeting their fluid requirements?

Economic and social assessment

For individuals in the recovery phase, is assistance at meal times and during meal preparation available if required?

Nutritional management

Weight loss and muscle loss

As weight loss is multifactorial in GBS, the individual causes should be considered when managing weight loss. It should be remembered that muscle wasting associated with reduced muscle use is unavoidable, and therefore it may be more appropriate to aim for weight stabilisation as a dietetic goal rather than weight gain.

Hypermetabolism

Few studies have investigated the nutritional requirements of patients with GBS. During the acute phase, when patients require intensive care input, Rubenoff *et al.* (1992) have suggested that patients should be fed 40–45 kcal and 2 g of protein/kg of body weight. These recommendations were based on a small sample, and the study did not consider the potential risks of overfeeding. Therefore, during the acute phase on an ICU, requirements should be calculated as for other critical care patients (see Chapter 7.17.1).

During the recovery phase, weekly weights and anthropometric measurements should be monitored. Provision of nutritional supplements may be required to reduce the rate of weight loss and to encourage weight gain; however, it should be remembered that if the patient is immobile, weight gain may occur as adipose tissue rather than lean body mass (see Chapter 6.3).

Dysphagia

A SLT, who will be able to recommend appropriate texture and consistency of food and drink, should assess patients with bulbar weaknesses. If patients are nil by mouth, NG feeding should be initiated unless there is a contraindication. Similarly, NG feeding will be required if patients are intubated. It can also be used to meet nutritional and fluid requirements in dysphagia (see Chapter 7.3 for further management advice on ensuring adequacy of nutritional intake).

Limb weakness, pain and fatigue

If upper limb weakness is present, assistance should be offered to the patient at meal times. Those providing assistance should be aware of the effect of fatigue, and therefore be aware that meal times can be prolonged and that food may go cold. Small regular meals may be more appropriate than three large meals per day. Pain relief should be appropriately provided for meal times so that the patient feels less pain at this time and can concentrate on achieving adequate intake. Assessment from an occupational therapist can determine whether the patient may benefit from modified cutlery for feeding.

Gastric dysmotility and constipation

If patients are suffering from large aspirates, prokinetics such as metaclopromide or erythromycin should be employed to increase absorption and decrease aspirate volume. Constipation can occur as a result of gastric dysmotility, so the use of enteral feeds containing fibre or higher fibre foods may be required alongside laxatives to maintain adequate gut function (see Chapter 7.4.11). An ileus may occur with autonomic dysfunction: if an ileus persists, parenteral nutrition may be required until it resolves and the patient can tolerate enteral intake (see Chapter 6.5).

Balanced eating during recovery

Once the patient is eating and drinking, and a stable weight is maintained, a balanced diet should be recommended during recovery. There is no evidence to suggest that modified diets speed up recovery or improve function. Some support groups recommend the use of diets high in essential fatty acids (EFAs), postulating that this may improve the integrity of the myelin sheath of nerve cells; however, there is no evidence to suggest that taking large oral doses of EFAs can help regenerate damaged myelin sheaths. Similarly, avoidance of foods or food groups has not been shown to aid recovery, and may lead to an unbalanced diet, compromising nutritional status.

Myasthenia gravis

Myasthenia gravis (MG) is an autoimmune disease affecting the neuromuscular junction. It is caused by antibodies linking to neurotransmitter receptors on the muscle end plate, thus disrupting the flow of neurotransmitters from the neurone to the muscle. In the majority of cases, the antibodies link specifically to the acetylcholine receptors.

The disruption in the pathway leads to painless muscle weakness and fatigue. Approximately 85% of patients present with ocular muscle weakness; most patients with ptosis (drooping of the eyelids) and or diplopia (double vision). Only 17% of patients present with ocular muscle weakness without any further muscle weakness (Grob *et al.*, 2008). Bulbar weakness is also a common symptom in MG and presents as dysarthria (poor speech), dysphagia, dysphonia (problems with voice/pitch), nasal sounding speech and masticatory weakness (weakness in the muscles involved in chewing) (Meriggioli & Sanders, 2009). Half of all patients with MG will present with generalised weakness, affecting ocular, bulbar, limb, neck, facial and respiratory muscles.

Diagnostic classification

There are many classifications used in the diagnosis of MG, but the most widely accepted, internationally used is the Myasthenia Gravis Foundation of America Clinical Classification (Nicolle, 2002), which defines MG patients on the basis of the combination of weaknesses present and their severity.

In order to confirm the diagnosis of MG, blood tests should test for the presence of serum receptor antibodies (either antiacetylcholine receptor antibodies or anti-MuSK antibodies). Electromyogram and nerve conduction tests should also be completed. Cholinesterase inhibitor tests use medications such as edrophonium (Tensilon), which prevent the destruction of acetylcholine. The provision of these medications may temporarily improve muscle weakness, thereby supporting the diagnosis of MG.

Disease consequences and epidemiology

The worldwide prevalence of MG ranges from 1.7 to 10.4 per million. It affects children and adults, with children accounting for 10–15% of cases. From puberty to the age of 40 years, MG is three times more prevalent in women than men. Above the age of 50 years, there are more male patients with MG than women (Meriggioli & Sanders, 2009). Mortality associated with MG is usually related to myasthenic crisis, where weakness affects respiratory muscles, leading to a requirement for intubation and ventilation. Alshekhlee *et al.* (2009) reported mortality rates of 4.5% in patients in myasthenic crisis.

Clinical management

Cholinesterase inhibitors are prescribed as they reduce the breakdown of acetylcholine, thereby increasing circulating levels. This has a beneficial effect on muscle weakness, as there is more acetylcholine available for binding to receptors. Pyridostigmine bromide (Mestinon) is a commonly used cholinesterase inhibitor and needs to be administered every 4–6 hours at varying doses. Side effects can include abdominal cramps, diarrhoea and nausea. An antispasmodic medication such as propantheline is frequently prescribed alongside pyridostigmine to reduce such side effects. Immunosuppressive medications such as prednisolone or azathioprine can be used in conjunction with cholinesterase inhibitors.

Plasma exchange and intravenous immunoglobulin treatment are immune therapies that are used when short term improvement is required, e.g. during myasthenic crisis (Wendell & Levine, 2011). Surgical removal of the thymus gland (a thymectomy) may be performed as it has been implicated in the production of receptor antibodies, although this treatment is only done in patients under the age of 60 years.

Nutrition related consequences

Dysphagia

Dysphagia occurs in 15–40% of MG patients (Llabrés *et al.*, 2005). On initial diagnosis, patients should be made aware of dysphagia as a consequence of the condition, as this can greatly impact on the self management of oral intake during future episodes of crisis or deterioration.

Fatigue

Fatigue can impact on oral intake and the ability to consume sufficient nutrition. It is therefore important to ensure optimal timing of the dose of pyridostigmine with respect to meal times in order to maximise oral intake and minimise effects of fatigue. Pyridostigmine should ideally be taken 30 minutes prior to meal times and at regular intervals throughout the day. Achieving this can

inevitably be problematic in the ward environment; however, educating the nursing staff and advising the medical team on appropriate timings should overcome most issues.

Blood glucose management

Blood glucose should be monitored with the commencement of prednisolone and patients should be advised regarding the potential for weight gain with steroid use.

Nutritional assessment

The following points should be noted when completing a nutritional assessment.

Anthropometry

Weight history (percentage weight loss) and body mass index (BMI) should be assessed, as patients presenting with a history of worsening dysphagia frequently experience weight loss.

Clinical assessment

The following points should be considered:

- Bowel function should be monitored closely due to the side effects of pyridostigmine. An antispasmodic medication such as propantheline should be prescribed if required.
- As already mentioned, pyridostigmine should ideally be administered 30 minutes before meals. Liaison with nursing staff and the medical team may be required.
- The patient's ability to manage medications orally should be reviewed. Does a liquid form of medication need to be considered or can the medications be crushed and added to a dessert of suitable consistency?
- Vital capacity (VC) readings will provide an indication of respiratory function, as decreasing VC indicates a worsening of the disease progress, with swallow function likely to be affected.
- The patient's sense of fatigue should be reviewed. Does the patient notice a difference in fatigue depending on the time of day?

Dietary assessment

The dietary assessment should consider:

- The latest recommendations from the SLT regarding the most appropriate choice of oral intake; close liaison is required throughout the disease progression.
- Current oral intake of food, taking into consideration the potential for variability throughout the day secondary to fatigue.
- Current fluid intake, taking into consideration whether thickened fluids are required, as well as the palatability of such drinks.
  Consideration of artificial nutritional support if the patient is not meeting their nutritional requirements or fluid requirements, is unable to manage medications orally?

Economic and social assessment

It can be helpful to advise patients to limit talking and other distractions at meal times as this can impact further on fatigue and swallow function.

Nutritional management

Tailored nutritional management is required throughout the disease course as severity can vary from person to person, as well as on an individual basis during a myasthenic crisis. Close liaison with the SLT should be encouraged in order to best facilitate the patient's nutritional needs. A texture modified diet will be required if the patient is dysphagic. The nutritional adequacy of the diet should be assessed, especially in the case of progressive dysphagia (see Chapter 7.3). Patients often experience increasing fatigue towards the end of the day and it is not uncommon for the recommendation of a texture modified diet to vary according to individual meal times, e.g. patients may successfully manage a soft/moist diet at lunchtime, but benefit from a puréed meal in the evening.

Recommendations should be made for smaller, more frequent meals, rather than aiming to finish full portions at meal times. Additional snacks between meals should be encouraged, including oral sip feeds and dessert based supplements, to enable the patient to meet their nutritional requirements (see Chapter 6.3).

Nutrition support via a NG tube may be required if there are concerns regarding aspiration risk, dysphagia is severe or respiratory function is compromised, e.g. myasthenic crisis. During myasthenic crisis, patients may require intubation and ventilation, which may warrant an ICU admission. For these patients, requirements should be calculated as for other critical care patients (see Chapter 7.17.1).

Enteral feeding as a result of dysphagia is usually a short term measure, as the establishment of an effective medication regimen should assist in improving swallow function. Compared with other neurological conditions, gastrostomy insertion is typically considered too aggressive in MG, due to its variable course and crisis periods (Cereda *et al.*, 2009).

Autonomic failure (dysautonomias)

The autonomic nervous system (ANS) forms part of the central and peripheral nervous system and is responsible for the involuntary, unconscious function of the internal organs. It affects heart rate, digestion, respiration rate, salivation, perspiration, urination and sexual arousal. Although there are many conditions affected by the ANS, the conditions discussed here are pure autonomic failure (PAF), multiple system (MSA) and postural tachycardia orthostatic syndrome (POTS).

Pure autonomic failure

Diagnostic criteria

Pure autonomic failure is characterised by orthostatic (postural) hypotension. Orthostatic hypotension is defined as a decrease in systolic pressure of at least 20 mmHg or in diastolic pressure of at least 10 mm Hg within 3 minutes of sitting or standing, or during a 60 degree° head up tilt (Kaufmann, 1996). In chronic autonomic failure, hypotension can also occur following the ingestion of food, which can aggravate postural hypotension. This is referred to as post prandial hypotension (Puvi-Rajasingham & Mathias, 1996).

Disease consequences and factors affecting symptoms

Autonomic disease may present in any age group, but neurodegenerative disorders affecting the ANS often occur after the age of 50 years (Mathias, 2003a). Symptoms include feeling dizzy, changes in vision such as blurring and pain across the back of the shoulders or neck (often referred to as coat hanger pain) (Bleasdale-Barr & Mathias, 1998). Feeling muddled or vague and falls or loss of consciousness may also occur as a result of hypotension. The severity of symptoms can vary, with some patients eventually becoming unable to stand upright or sit for prolonged periods. Some patients may later be diagnosed with MSA. Autonomic disease can also cause reduced salivation and dry mouth, resulting in difficulty with dry foods. Dysphagia is unusual in PAF but often occurs in the later stages of MSA, leading to risk of aspiration.

Appropriate education, lifestyle and dietary changes with reconditioning are required to restore mobility and maintain quality of life. Factors that can influence orthostatic hypotension include (Mathias, 2003a):

- Time of day – blood pressure is lower in the mornings, especially on waking.
- Speed of positional change, e.g. standing quickly from a sitting or lying position can result in a drop in blood pressure.
- water ingestion – can raise blood pressure.
- Food ingestion – large meals can result in post prandial hypotension.
- Warm conditions, e.g. hot weather and hot baths can lead to hypotension.
- Straining – constipation should be avoided as straining lowers blood pressure further.

Nutritional assessment

The following should be considered as part of the nutritional assessment.

Anthropometry

The anthropometric assessment should review weight, BMI and any history of weight loss.

Clinical assessment

The clinical assessment should consider:

- Bowel function, aiming to avoid constipation.
- Results of autonomic function tests, e.g. presence of post prandial hypotension.
- Level of mobility (severe deconditioning will result in reduced/minimal mobility).

Dietary assessment

Dietary assessment should:

- Obtain an accurate diet history, with a focus on portion sizes, salt, fluid and sugar intake.
- Assess the current oral fluid intake.
- Assess for recent changes to diet or food avoidance.

Economic and social assessment

The impact on meal preparation should be assessed, e.g. other family members may be following a low sodium diet for hypertension.

Clinical investigation and management

Measurement of lying, sitting and standing blood pressure is essential to determine if orthostatic hypotension is present (pulse rate should also be measured to consider POTS). Autonomic investigations should be undertaken to evaluate the cardiovascular system, including measurements of blood pressure during head up tilt at a 60 degree angle, a liquid meal challenge and modified exercise testing. In addition, a 24-hour blood pressure recording should be completed. Post prandial hypotension is assessed by recording blood pressure whilst the patient is lying flat and on head up tilt prior to the ingestion of a liquid meal consisting of carbohydrate, protein and fat, and again 45 minutes after the meal (Mathias, 2003a).

Management is often focused on the alleviation of symptoms and requires a combination of pharmacological and non-pharmacological approaches. Pharmacological interventions can have a significant effect on blood pressure management. Frequently used medications include fludrocortisone, ephedrine, midodrine, desmopressin (DDAVP) and ocreotide. Ocreotide is given as an injection before meals, which can reduce post-prandial hypotension (Mathias, 2003b).

Nutritional management

The aim of nutritional management is to encourage the improvement or alleviation of symptoms. The advice can appear unconventional; however, due to the severity of symptoms, individuals may benefit from making dietary modifications. There are four main areas where dietary adjustments can assist with symptom control, although the supporting evidence for these is limited.

Avoid large meals

Puvi-Rajasingham & Mathias (1996) have shown that consuming three larger meals per day, rather than six smaller meals per day, resulted in significantly lower blood pressure both after and between meals. Therefore, patients should be encouraged to aim for five to six smaller snacks throughout the day, rather than three large meals.

Increase fluid intake

Although the precise mechanisms are unclear, oral fluids increase seated blood pressure in chronic autonomic failure. Studies have shown that the oral ingestion of 480 mL of water increases seated blood pressure in patients with PAF and MSA (Young & Mathias, 2004a). This effect continues to be consistent on a daily basis

(Deguchi et al., 2007). Studies have also shown that the provision of water via a gastrostomy tube has similar haemodynamic effects to the oral ingestion of water (Young & Mathias, 2004b).

As blood pressure is lower on waking, patients are advised to drink 480–500 mL of (non-sugar containing) fluids before getting out of bed. Patients should be advised to have fluid by the bedside before going to bed. Patients should also aim to avoid fluids 1 hour prior to going to bed to avoid the need to get up during the night, which will increase the risk of falls or hypotension.

Increase salt intake

It is speculated that an increased salt intake may help increase blood pressure in patients with orthostatic hypotension; however, there is no evidence to support this and no guidance to suggest recommended quantities. Advice should be aimed at increasing high salt containing foods in the diet and adding additional salt to food at the table rather than using salt tablets. Salt in water solution should not be recommended.

Reduce intake of sugars and carbohydrates

Studies have shown that restriction of carbohydrates and glucose can reduce the effects of postural hypotension (Jansen & Lipsitz, 1995; Mathias et al., 1991). Symptoms of post prandial hypotension have also been found to be less frequent and severe, and significantly shorter with a low carbohydrate intake (25 g) (Vloet et al., 2001). Advice should be aimed at avoiding food and drinks high in sugar, although there may be improved tolerance towards the end of the day when blood pressure is higher.

Weight loss can occur due to food restriction or dysphagia. Due to the high sugar content of most supplement drinks, it can be difficult to recommend an oral sip feed without worsening symptoms. These should be tried on an individual basis as clinical experience suggests that some patients can successfully tolerate 1.5–2 kcal/mL of oral sip feeds if sipped slowly. Alternatively, a lipid-based supplement such as Calogen (Nutricia) or Fresubin 5 kcal Shot (Fresenius) can be beneficial as an additional source of calories. Food fortification advice concentrating on increasing additional fat sources within the diet can also help to prevent weight loss (see Chapter 6.3). Occasionally, enteral feeding may need to be considered, especially if there are concerns regarding dysphagia.

Multiple system atrophy

Multiple system atrophy (MSA) is a progressive neurodegenerative condition characterised by autonomic failure, parkinsonism (see Chapter 7.6.1) and cerebellar ataxia (poor balance and coordination) (Gilman et al., 2008).

Diagnostic criteria and classification

It can be difficult to distinguish between Parkinson's disease and MSA as features that would be atypical of the former, such as rapid progression and poor response to anti-parkinsonism medication, only become evident over time. Early autonomic involvement of the bladder and cardiovascular system can be indicators of MSA. There is no single clinical feature or investigation that confirms MSA. However, recent diagnostic criteria have been agreed to improve the recognition of patients with early or possible MSA (Wenning & Stefanova, 2009).

The diagnostic criteria for probable MSA, according to the second consensus statement on the diagnosis of MSA (Gilman *et al.*, 2008), are:

- A sporadic, progressive, adult (over 30 years) onset disease characterised by:
  - Autonomic failure involving urinary incontinence (with erectile dysfunction in males) or an orthostatic decrease of blood pressure within 3 minutes of standing by at least 30 mmHg systolic or 15 mmHg diastolic; *and*
  - Poorly levodopa responsive parkinsonism; *or*
  - A cerebellar syndrome (gait ataxia with cerebellar dysarthria, limb ataxia, or cerebellar oculomotor dysfunction).

The incidence is approximately 5 per 100 000 population; however, due to under recognition and misdiagnosis, it is calculated that approximately 10% of patients with parkinsonism have MSA (Bhidayasiri & Ling, 2008).

Disease consequences

The disease affects both men and women, usually in their 50s and 60s, with a disease progression that ultimately leads to death within 8 years from symptom onset. However, some individuals have survived for 15 years or more. There is no specific drug therapy available and treatment is aimed primarily at symptom relief (Swinn, 2005).

Nutritional management

As previously discussed, dietary measures can help with the symptomatic relief of orthostatic hypotension. Constipation should be avoided in these patients, as previously discussed. Patients with MSA can experience speech and swallowing difficulties. Speech can become quieter, monotonous and/or slurred. Texture modified diets and oral sip feeds may need to be considered if fatigue impacts on oral intake or if weight loss occurs (see Chapters 7.3 Chapter 6.3). Enteral tube feeding should be considered if there are concerns regarding risk of aspiration. Approximately 30% of patients will develop a degree of stridor (Wenning & Stefanova, 2009); therefore, a radiologically inserted gastrostomy (RIG) may be considered (see Chapter 6.4).

Postural orthostatic tachycardia syndrome

In addition to MSA and PAF, there is a subgroup of patients who present with a disorder termed orthostatic intolerance/tachycardia. This has been defined as the development of symptoms on standing that are relieved when sitting.

Diagnostic criteria

Postural orthostatic tachycardia syndrome has been defined as '*the presence of orthostatic intolerance symptoms associated with a heart rate increase of 30 beats/minute (or a rate that exceeds 120 beats/minute) within the first 10 minutes of standing or upright tilt*' (Grubb *et al.*, 2006). Reported symptoms can include tachycardia, palpitations, fatigue, headache, nausea and light headedness, and can have a limiting impact on everyday activities. It is important to note that many patients with orthostatic intolerance will not have orthostatic hypotension, or indeed a change in blood pressure. Orthostatic intolerance can be incorrectly classified as chronic anxiety or a panic disorder (Grubb *et al.*, 2006).

Disease consequences

The prevalence of POTS is unknown; however, it is estimated to be 5–10 times as common as orthostatic hypotension, and that 40% of patients with chronic fatigue syndrome have POTS. Low *et al.* (2009) noted a consistent female to male ratio of 5:1, with an average age of onset of 30 years. Patients with POTS present with poor exercise tolerance and physical reconditioning can be severe, especially in patients with prominent fatigue.

The most recognised cause of POTS is associated with the connective tissue disorder joint hypermobility syndrome (JHS). In these patients, blood vessels have abnormally elastic connective tissue, resulting in a reduced ability to constrict that in turn results in compensatory tachycardia. One example is Elhers–Danlos syndrome, an inherited connective tissue disorder.

Nutritional management

Patients are encouraged to maintain a high salt and fluid intake as previously discussed, aiming for 2 L of fluid/day. Occasionally, gastric dysmotility can occur and should be managed on an individual basis according to symptoms.

Internet resources

Multiple System Atrophy Trust   www.msatrust.org.uk
Myasthenia Gravis Association   www.mgauk.org

References

Alshekhlee A, Miles JD, Katirji B, Preston DC, Kaminski HJ. (2009) Incidence and mortality rates of myasthenia gravis and myasthenic crisis in US hospitals. *Neurology* 72: 1548–1544.

Bersano A, Carpo M, Allaria S, Franciotta D, Citterio A, Nobile-Orazio E. (2006) Long term disability and social status change after Guillain-Barré syndrome. *Journal of Neurology* 253: 214–218.

Bleasdale-Barr K, Mathias CJ. (1998) Neck and other muscle pains in autonomic failure: their association with orthostatic hypotension. *Journal of the Royal Society of Medicine* 91: 355–359.

Bhidayasiri R, Ling H. (2008) Multiple system atrophy. *The Neurologist* 14: 224–237.

Burns TM. (2008) Guillain- Barré syndrome. *Seminars in Neurology* 28: 152–167.

Cereda E, Beltramolli D, Pedrolli C, Costa A. (2009) Refractory myasthenia gravis, dysphagia and malnutrition: A case report to suggest disease-specific nutritional issues. *Nutrition* 25: 1067–1072.

Deguchi K, Ikeda K, Sasaki I, *et al.* (2007) Effects of daily water drinking on orthostatic and postprandial hypotension in patients with MSA. *Journal of Neurology* 254: 735–740.

Dhar R, Stitt L, Hahn A. (2008) The morbidity and outcome of patients with Guillain-Barré admitted to the intensive care unit. *Journal of the Neurological Sciences* 264: 121–128.

Gilman S, Wenning GK, Low PA, *et al.*. (2008) Second consensus statement on the diagnosis of multiple system atrophy. *Neurology* 71: 670–676.

Grob D, Brunner N, Namba T, Pagala M. (2008) Lifetime course of myasthenia gravis. *Muscle & Nerve* 37: 141–149.

Grubb BP, Kanjwal Y, Kosinski DJ. (2006) The postural tachycardia syndrome: A concise guide to diagnosis and management. *Journal of Cardiovascular Electrophysiology* 17: 108–112.

Hadden RD, Karch H, Hartung HP *et al.*; The Plasma Exchange/Sandoglobulin Guillain-Barré Syndrome Trial Group. (2001) Preceding infections, immune factors, and outcomes in Guillain-Barré syndrome. *Neurology* 56: 758–765.

Hahn AF. (1998) Guillain-Barré syndrome. *Lancet* 352: 635–641.

Hughes RAC, Cornblath DR. (2005) Guillain- Barré syndrome. *Lancet* 366: 1653–1666.

Hughes RAC, Wijdicks EFM, Benson E, *et al.* (2005) Supportive care for patients with Guillain-Barré syndrome. *Archives of Neurology* 62: 1194–1198.

Jansen R, Lipsitz L. (1995) Postprandial hypotension. Epidemiology, pathophysiology and clinical management. *Annals of Internal Medicine* 122: 286–295.

Kaufmann H. (1996) Consensus statement on the definition of orthostatic hypotension, pure autonomic failure and multiple system atrophy. *Clinical Autonomic Research* 6(2): 125–126.

Llabrés M, Molina-Martinez FJ, Miralles F. (2005) Dysphagia as the sole manifestation of myasthenia gravis. *Journal of Neurology, Neurosurgery and Psychiatry* 76: 1297–1300.

Low PA, Sandroni P, Joyner M, Shen WK. (2009) Postural tachycardia syndrome (POTS). *Journal of Cardiovascular Electrophysiology* 20: 352–358.

Mathias CJ. (2003a) Autonomic diseases: Clinical features and laboratory evaluation. *Journal of Neurology, Neurosurgery & Psychiatry* 74(Suppl III): iii31–iii41.

Mathias CJ. (2003b) Autonomic diseases: Management. *Journal of Neurology, Neurosurgery & Psychiatry* 74(Suppl III): iii42–iii47.

Mathias CJ, Armstrong HE, Shareef M, Bannister R. (1991) The influence of food on postural hypotension in three groups with chronic autonomic failure – clinical and therapeutic implications. *Journal of Neurology, Neurosurgery & Psychiatry* 54: 726–730.

Meriggioli MN, Sanders DB. (2009) Autoimmune myasthenia gravis: emerging clinical and biological heterogeneity. *Lancet Neurology* 8: 475–490.

Ng KK, Howard RS, Fish DR, *et al.* (1995) Management and outcome of severe Guillain-Barré syndrome. *Quarterly Journal of Medicine* 88: 243–250.

Nicolle MW. (2002) Myasthenia gravis. *Neurologist* 8: 2–21.

Puvi-Rajasingham S, Mathias CJ. (1996) Effect of meal size on postprandial blood pressure and on postural hypotension in primary autonomic failure. *Clinical Autonomic Research* 6: 111–114.

Rubenoff RA, Borel CO, Hanley DF. (1992) Hypermetabolism and hypercatabolism in Guillain-Barré syndrome. *Journal of Parenteral and Enteral Nutrition* 16: 464–472.

Ruts L, Drenthen J, Jongen JLM *et al.*,; on behalf of the Dutch GBS Study Group. (2010) Pain in Guillain-Barré syndrome. *Neurology* 75: 1439–1447.

Swinn L. (2005) Multiple system atrophy. In: Swinn L (ed) *Parkinson's Disease: Theory and Practice for Nurses*. London: Whurr Publishers Ltd.

van Doorn PA, Ruts L, Jacobs BC. (2008) Clinical features, pathogenesis, and treatment of Guillain-Barré syndrome. *Lancet Neurology* 7: 939–950.

Vloet LC, Mehagnoul-Schipper DJ, Hoefnagels WH, Jansen RW. (2001) The influence of low, normal and high carbohydrate meals on blood pressure in elderly patients with postprandial hypotension. *Journals of Gerontology Series, Biological Sciences and Medical Sciences* 56: M744–748.

Wendell LC, Levine JM. (2011) Myasthenic crisis. *Neurohospitalist* 1: 16–22.

Wenning GK, Stefanova N. (2009) Recent developments in multiple system atrophy. *Journal of Neurology* 256: 1791–1808.

Young TM, Mathias CJ. (2004a) The effects of water ingestion on orthostatic hypotension in two groups of chronic autonomic failure: MSA and PAF. *Journal of Neurology, Neurosurgery & Psychiatry* 75: 1737–1741.

Young TM, Mathias CJ. (2004b) Pressor effect of water instilled via a gastrostomy tube in pure autonomic failure. *Autonomic Neuroscience: Basic and Clinical* 113: 79–81.

7.6.4 Multiple sclerosis

Catherine Dunn and Maryanne Harrison

Key points

- Multiple sclerosis (MS) is a disease of the central nervous system affecting the brain and spinal cord. Damage to the myelin and axons of nerves can lead to significant neurological disability.

- Multiple sclerosis is the most common neurological disease among young adults with an incidence of approximately 1 in 1000; onset is usually between 20 and 40 years.

- It is an incurable, long term condition. Medications can manage symptoms, e.g. fatigue, bladder dysfunction, pain, spasticity and weakness.

- Nutritional management depends on the symptoms and their severity, and varies from a healthy, balanced diet to nutritional support, including enteral tube feeding and dysphagia management.

- There is no conclusive evidence that dietary modification influences the course of MS; however, n-3 and n-6 polyunsaturated fatty acids may play a role in relapsing–remitting MS. There is mounting evidence that vitamin D is implicated in both development and progression of MS.

Multiple sclerosis (MS) is an immune mediated progressive disease of the central nervous system (CNS). The myelin sheaths around the brain and spinal cord are damaged, affecting the ability of the nerve cells to communicate with each other. It is the most common neurological disease among young adults, with an incidence of approximately 1 in 1000 and an onset usually between the ages of 20 and 40 years. Women are about twice as likely to develop MS as men. Multiple sclerosis is characterised by inflammation, demyelination of the protective myelin coating and nerve axon damage throughout the CNS. Diagnosis can be confirmed using magnetic resonance imaging (MRI). It is a long term condition and can have a wide range of clinical presentations that are dependent on the severity and location of CNS damage. Some people become significantly disabled in a very short time, while others live their entire lives with minimal or no disability.

Diagnostic criteria and classification

There are four recognised clinical courses of MS, identified on the basis of the rate of progression (Chiaravalotti & DeLuca, 2008).

- *Relapsing–remitting* – following diagnosis 80% of patients follow this course. It is characterised by periods of acute attacks followed by full or near full recovery. Relapses may last days or months and vary from mild to very severe; the latter may require hospital admission. During relapses, symptoms are exacerbated and new symptoms may develop.
- *Secondary progressive* – approximately 80% of individuals with relapsing–remitting MS later develop secondary progressive MS (Herndon, 2003). Symptoms gradually worsen with or without occasional relapses or minor remissions. As a result, symptoms and disability become steadily worse.
- *Progressive relapsing* – this has a progressive decline after the onset of the disease with some acute periods of symptom relapse. There may or may not be recovery from these acute periods.
- *Primary progressive* – this affects 10–15% of patients; there is continuous and gradual worsening of the symptoms with no distinct periods of relapse or remission of symptoms.

Disease processes

Very little is known about the mechanism and causes of MS, although immunological, environmental and genetic factors have been implicated. Environmental factors include Epstein–Barr virus infection, smoking and low serum concentrations of vitamin D (Ascherio & Munger, 2007). Although vitamin B_{12} plays a role in myelin formation, no definitive relationship has been identified with vitamin B_{12}, although low or decreased levels have been reported in MS (Farinotti et al., 2009). There is a correlation between sunlight exposure and lack of vitamin D both for occurrence and progression of MS. These are now considered predisposing factors for MS (Esparza et al., 1995; Llorca et al., 2005; Freedman et al., 2000; Ponsonby et al., 2005).

The incidence of MS increases with geographical latitude. There is a strong inverse correlation between distance from the equator and duration and intensity of ultraviolet B (UVB) light from sunlight. In turn, serum vitamin D concentration is closely correlated with exposure to UVB (Viglietta et al., 2004). Populations at high latitudes with a high consumption of vitamin D rich fatty fish have a lower than expected prevalence of MS (Goldberg, 1974; Swank et al., 1952; Westlund, 1970). Risk decreases with migration from high to low latitudes (Gale & Martyn, 1995). Less than optimal blood levels of vitamin D have been linked to an increased incidence of MS (Embry et al., 2000; Munger et al., 2006) and there is also a positive association between low blood vitamin D levels and relapse in MS (Soilu-Hanninen et al., 2005; Mowry et al., 2010).

Diet is a poor source of vitamin D compared with sun exposure. A food serving can provide 40–400 IU (1–40 µg) (Yetley, 2008), whereas whole body exposure to sunlight for 20 minutes for a Caucasian during the summer months will produce at least 10 000 IU (Holick, 1995; 2004; Engelsen et al., 2005). However, under circumstances when the strength of the UVB reaching the earth's surface is reduced, e.g. in winter or at high latitude, or where the effectiveness of UVB in catalysing the synthesis of vitamin D is reduced, e.g. increased skin pigmentation, age, use of sunscreen and living in a built up environment diet can become the primary source of vitamin D. Evidence suggests that although 25 hydroxyvitamin D concentrations in blood above 50 nmol/L have been deemed adequate, a minimum of 75 nmol/L and perhaps more than 90 nmol/L is optimum for many health outcomes. This could be achieved by judicious sun exposure or daily supplementation with 1000–4000 IU of colecalciferol, which would increase 25 hydroxyvitamin D to over 75 nmol/L in most individuals. However, as yet there have been no agreed or recommended levels for patients with MS. Further large randomised controlled trials are needed (Bishoff-Ferrari, 2009; Bishoff–Ferrari et al., 2006; Looker et al., 2008).

Disease consequences

Mortality is only slightly higher in MS patients than in the general population. In itself MS is not fatal; causes of death in those with MS are most commonly associated with respiratory and cardiovascular diseases and infections (Ragonese et al, 2008). However, MS is associated with considerable morbidity and many symptoms that include:

- Difficulties with balance and dizziness.
- Fatigue – an overwhelming sense of tiredness.
- Visual problems such as blurred or double vision.
- Numbness, tingling or pins and needles that can be painful.
- Bladder problems.

- Bowel problems.
- Cognitive problems, including memory and thinking.
- Stiffness or spasms in muscles – sometimes called spasticity.
- Emotional and mood changes.
- Tremor.
- Sexual problems.
- Speech difficulties.
- Swallowing difficulties (dysphagia).

People with MS can present with diverse and multiple symptoms of varying severity related to the location of nervous system damage. There is also consistent evidence that health related quality of life is compromised (Ruddick & Miller, 2008).

Nutritional assessment

Using the ABCDE model, there are some key aspects of the nutritional assessment to consider in MS.

Anthropometry

Specialised weighing scales (wheelchair, sitting scales or hoist scales) will be required for patients unable to stand unsupported.

Biochemistry

Measurement of vitamin D levels is helpful before advising on vitamin D supplementation.

Clinical assessment

Identification of MS subtype, presenting symptoms or disability will inform likely nutritional priorities:

- If positioning in bed or a chair is difficult, pressure areas may be present and these may affect nutritional requirements (see Chapter 7.17.6).
- Bladder dysfunction may make people self limit fluid intake, potentially leading to dehydration.
- Constipation is fairly common in MS, although the neurological basis for this is unclear; however, reduced mobility, reduced fluid intake and other dietary changes may play a part (Chia et al., 1995).

Dietary assessment

The dietary assessment should consider:

- Dysphagia may affect food choices; certain food types and textures may need to be avoided.
- Ability to self feed may be affected by weakness or lack of coordination of arm or hand muscles (ataxia); varying degrees of assistance may be needed to eat and drink.
- Fatigue can be debilitating, leaving the person without energy to shop or prepare food and even to eat a meal.
- Alternative diets, e.g. Swank and Best Bet, may be followed; some of these are extremely restrictive.

- There are no specific guidelines on energy and protein requirements in MS; however, energy requirements are likely to be increased with tremor or spasticity.

Economic and social assessment

Many people with MS require the support of carers to eat and drink; daily routine (such as the timing of visits from carers and their duration) may help or hinder oral intake.

Clinical investigation and management

There is no known cure for MS, although stem cells trials are currently being conducted. Non-curative treatment with medications is common in MS. Drug therapy is aimed at either management of symptoms or treatment of MS itself.

Symptom management

Symptoms such as spasticity, ataxia and tremor, fatigue, pain and bladder, bowel and sexual dysfunction can be treated with medication. For example, spasticity may be managed by medications such as baclofen, botulinum toxin or tizanadine. Where fatigue is impacting on daily life, modafinil and amantadine may be prescribed to increase alertness. As with all medications, side effects may impact on nutritional intake and/or nutritional status. For example, baclofen (which acts as a skeletal muscle relaxant) can induce nausea with possible consequent reduction in food intake. A review by Thompson et al. (2010) provides a comprehensive overview of drugs prescribed for symptoms management in MS, their efficacy and associated side effects.

Disease modifying therapies

Since the early 1990s, an increasing number of drugs have been licensed for the treatment of MS, including beta interferon (Avonex and Rebif), natalizumab (Tysabri) and fingolimod (Gilenya), although the latter has not been approved for use in the UK by the National Institute for Health and Care Excellence (NICE). Fingolimod is taken orally, whereas the others are given via injection or intravenous infusion. All these drugs affect the immune system and are known as disease modifying therapies (DMTs). The evidence for efficacy of DMTs in relapsing–remitting MS is far greater than for primary or secondary progressive MS. Nonetheless, there are ongoing trials to evaluate whether the course of progressive forms of MS can be influenced by DMTs.

Rehabilitation

Multidisciplinary rehabilitation is also an important aspect of MS management. Whilst there is no evidence that multidisciplinary rehabilitation programmes influence level of functional impairment, they can improve the experience of people with MS in relation to activity and participation (Khan et al., 2008).

Nutritional management

As with any long term condition, healthy eating should be an integral part of daily life. The eatwell plate should be used as a tool for empowering individuals to achieve optimum nutrition, especially at the beginning of the pathway following diagnosis (see Chapter 4.2). A low saturated fat intake is strongly recommended and ways to ensure this include the use of low fat dairy products and lean meat. Inclusion of oily fish –two to three times a week to provide n-3 polyunsaturated fatty acids (PUFAs) and frequent use of vegetable oils such as sunflower, corn, safflower, nuts seeds and soya to provide n-6 PUFAs (linoleic acid) is recommended. Emphasis is given to eating at least five portions of fruit and vegetables a day and to the inclusion of dark green leafy vegetables. Wholegrain bread and cereals are encouraged, as is enough fluids to produce pale urine. Caffeine intake should be kept to a minimum. As the disease progresses, other priorities may take precedence, e.g. weight loss or weight gain.

Constipation is common in MS and advice on its prevention by dietary means can be very helpful. Individualised high fibre advice, including the use of golden linseeds and prune juice can lead to reduction or cessation of laxative use.

Obesity

Obesity in MS can occur for a variety of reasons, including reduced activity as a consequence of disability, treatment with steroids, depression leading to comfort eating and excessive intake of high fat and/or high sugar foods. Successful treatment depends on an empathetic approach, facilitating behaviour change. A detailed dietary assessment should be completed and agreed realistic targets set that reduce energy intake (Stuifbergen *et al.*, 2003). Appropriate follow-up, ideally in conjunction with the rest of the multidisciplinary team, can be very successful. Obesity may not be successfully treated in all patients and weight loss may not be a realistic goal for some. It may be that prevention of further weight gain is a better approach in some cases.

Alternative diets

In a study by Schwarz *et al.* (2008), 41% of participants with MS reported having used diet modification at some point. In addition to relatively minor dietary modifications, people with MS may choose to follow a variety of alternative or extreme diets with a view to influencing the course of their disease. Diets that offer hope of improvement of symptoms or a cure are very attractive to many people with MS and therefore will have followers. The Swank and Best Bet diets are two of the best known alternative diets for MS; however, gluten free or low allergen diets may also be followed. There is no substantiated evidence that following an alternative diet will affect the MS disease process. Whilst being mindful that restrictive diets can increase risk of certain nutritional deficiencies, health beliefs of individuals must be respected.

Swank diet

Swank *et al.* (1952) demonstrated a correlation between MS and diet, and devised this diet. A low fat diet was advised because of an apparent association between fat intake and MS. A group of 144 people on the Swank diet were followed for up to 34 years, with good results reported in long term disability. Those who adhered strictly to the diet and who were experiencing mild symptoms had slower disability progression than those who had not adhered strictly to the diet. However, there was no control group in this study and therefore there is a likelihood of a self selection bias arising from the probability that only patients who perceived a benefit from the treatment would continue with it. It is therefore impossible to know whether the good results represent a genuine improvement over the entire population of MS patients.

The principles of the diet are:

- Saturated fat kept to 15 g or less/day.
- No red meat for the first year, then 75 g/week.
- Unsaturated fat kept to 20–50 g/day.
- No processed foods containing saturated fat.
- Dairy products must contain 1% or less butter fat.
- Three eggs per week and no more than one per serving.
- Suggested daily cod liver oil and a multivitamin and mineral supplement.

Best Bet diet

The Best Bet diet is a strict exclusion diet based on the premise that undigested food proteins with a similar structure to the protein in myelin pass across a leaky gut and cross the blood–brain barrier. This triggers an autoimmune attack on myelin, so causing, or worsening, MS. A wide range of food types is restricted, including red meat, dairy products, legumes and grains; therefore, achieving a balanced diet will be a challenge. Over 24 dietary supplements are recommended; thus following the Best Bet diet will also be expensive. At the time of writing, no clinical trials or results in relation to the Best Bet diet have been published in any peer reviewed journal. More information can be found at www.ms-diet.org.

Polyunsaturated fatty acids

Both n-3 and n-6 PUFAs have anti-inflammatory properties and have been considered as potential treatments for MS (Harbige *et al.*, 2007; Mehta *et al.*, 2009). Supplementation with n-3 and n-6 PUFAs has been shown to reduce immune cell activation through a variety of complex pathways. However, clinical trials in humans have not demonstrated definitively that PUFA supplementation can influence disability and rate or severity of relapses in MS, which may be due to limitations in trial design and outcome measure selection (Mehta *et al.*, 2009; Farinotti *et al.*, 2009). The evidence supporting the use of PUFAs in the treatment of relapsing–remitting MS is far stronger than for primary or secondary progressive MS.

The NICE (2003) guidelines advise that a daily intake of 17–23 g of linoleic acid (n-3 PUFA) may reduce the accumulation of disability over time, especially early in the disease process. This recommendation was based on a systematic review of three double blind trials undertaken in the early 1980s (Dworkin *et al.*, 1984). However, since publication of the NICE guidelines there has been debate as to the quality of these trials and whether 17–23 g/day is the optimum dose of linoleic acid is uncertain. Rich sources of linoleic acid include:

- Food oils such as corn, sunflower, safflower, peanut, rapeseed.
- Evening primrose oil (available as a supplement).
- Sunflower spread (full fat).
- Nuts such as walnuts, brazil nuts, peanuts.
- Mayonnaise (full fat).
- Taramasalata.

In two double blind, parallel group studies of n-3 PUFA supplementation [fish oil; combination of eicosapentaenoic acid (EPA) and docosahexaenoic acid (DHA)] versus placebo supplementation, no significant differences were found between the groups in terms of progression of disability (Bates *et al.*, 1989) or relapse rates (Weinstock-Guttman *et al.*, 2005), although there was a non-significant trend toward less disability progression in the former study. In both studies there were methodological problems that may have masked any meaningful treatment effect of n-3 PUFA supplementation, such as both groups being instructed to restrict saturated fat intake. However, given that n-3 and n-6 PUFAs are accepted as being beneficial to overall health, their intake should be encouraged in those with relapsing–remitting MS as part of a varied and balanced diet.

A low intake of saturated fat should also be promoted, as there is significant epidemiological evidence that high intakes of saturated fatty acids are detrimentally associated with MS (Harbige & Sharief, 2007). Naturally, this advice must be implemented using clinical judgement, as the nutritional priorities of people with MS differ. Early in the disease process, when disability may be relatively mild, more attention should be paid to promoting PUFA intake, particularly where people are motivated to make positive lifestyle changes. However, it would not be appropriate to focus on PUFA if disease and disability have progressed, or where malnutrition is the primary concern.

Dysphagia

The prevalence of swallowing disorders in MS is high (30–40%) (Restivo *et al.*, 2011). Dysphagia is significantly more prevalent in those with greater neurological disability (Poorjavad *et al.*, 2010). Consequences of dysphagia can be severe, such as the development of pneumonia from aspiration of food or fluid into the lungs. Dysphagia can lead to significant weight loss and dehydration as a result of the inability to meet nutritional and fluid requirements. With progressive forms of MS and where dysphagia exists, swallowing function may deteriorate over time. Where dysphagia is a feature of MS, nutritional management should ideally be undertaken with input from a speech and language therapist, who can advise on modification of food and fluid textures, positioning for eating and drinking, and swallowing strategies to reduce the risk of aspiration with oral intake. Nutritional support (oral or artificial) will be required where dysphagia is associated with an inability to meet nutritional requirements (see Chapter 7.3).

Malnutrition and nutritional support

The incidence of malnutrition in MS has not been determined. However, it is well recognised that unintentional weight loss and cachexia can occur in MS (Payne, 2001; Habek *et al.*, 2010). Contributory factors include (but are not limited to):

- Dysphagia.
- Fatigue.
- Difficulties in self feeding.
- Cognitive impairment.
- Restrictive alternative diet.

Where malnutrition or a high risk of malnutrition has been identified in someone with MS, nutritional support strategies should be implemented.

Oral nutritional support

A food first approach should be recommended with progression to using prescribed nutritional supplements as required (see Chapter 6.3). Prethickened sip feeds are available should dysphagia mean that thickened fluids are required.

Artificial nutritional support

Use of artificial nutritional support (such as nasogastric or gastrostomy feeding) in people with MS has not been studied extensively. It will only be relevant in a small minority of cases, but can be successful in promoting weight gain. It is acknowledged that enteral tube feeding impacts on people's quality of life (Brotherton & Judd, 2007); therefore, quality of life considerations should always guide decision making around gastrostomy feeding.

Internet resources

Multiple Sclerosis Society   www.mssociety.org.uk
Multiple Sclerosis Trust   www.mstrust.org.uk

Further reading

National Council for Palliative Care (NCPC). (2007) *Artificial Nutrition and Hydration: Guidance in End of Life Care for Adults.* London: NCPC.

References

Ascherio A, Munger KL. (2007) Environmental risk factors for multiple sclerosis Part 1: the role of infection. *Annals of Neurology* 61: 288–299.

Bates D, Cartlidge N, French J, *et al.* (1989). A double-blind controlled trial of long-chain n-3 polyunsaturated fatty acids in the treatment of multiple sclerosis. *Journal of Neurology, Neurosurgery and Psychiatry* 53: 18–22.

Bishoff-Ferrari HA. (2009) Vitamin D: What is an adequate vitamin D level and how much supplementation is necessary? *Best Practice and Research in Clinical Rheumatology* 23: 789–795.

Bishoff-Ferrari HA, Giovannucci E, Willett WC, Dietrich T, Dawson-Hughes B. (2006) Estimation of optimum serum concentrations of 25-hydroxyvitamin D for multiple health outcomes. *American Journal of Clinical Nutrition* 84: 18–28.

Brotherton A, Judd P. (2007) Quality of life in adult enteral tube feeding patients. *Journal of Human Nutrition and Dietetics* 20: 513–522.

Chia Y, Fowler C, Kamm M, Henry M, Lemieux M, Swash M. (1995) Prevalence of bowel dysfunction in patients with multiple sclerosis and bladder dysfunction. *Journal of Neurology* 242: 105–108.

Chiaravalotti N, DeLuca J. (2008) Cognitive impairment in multiple sclerosis. *Lancet Neurology* 7: 1139–1151.

Dworkin RH, Bates D, Millar JH, Paty DW. (1984) Linoleic acid and multiple sclerosis: a reanalysis of three double-blind trials. *Neurology* 34: 1441–1445.

Embry AF, Snowdon IR, Vieth R. (2000) Vitamin D and seasonal fluctuations of gadolinium enhancing MRI lesions in MS. *Annals of Neurology* 48(2): 271–272.

Engelsen O, Brustad M, Aksnes L, Lund E. (2005) Daily duration of vitamin D synthesis in human skin with relation to latitude, total ozone, altitude, ground cover, aerosols and cloud thickness. *Photochemistry and Photobiology* 81: 1287–1290.

Esparza ML, Sasaki S, Kesteloot H. (1995) Nutrition, latitude, and multiple sclerosis mortality: an ecologic study. *American Journal of Epidemiology* 142: 733–737.

Farinotti M, Simi S, Pietrantonj C, et al. (2009) Dietary interventions for multiple sclerosis (review). *The Cochrane Library Issue 1*.

Freedman DM, Dosemeci M, Alavanja MC. (2000) Mortality from multiple sclerosis and exposure to residential and occupational solar radiation: a case control study based on death certificates. *Occupational and Environmental Medicine* 57: 418–421.

Gale CR, Martyn CN. (1995) Migrant studies in multiple sclerosis. *Progress in Neurobiology* 47: 425–428.

Goldberg P. (1974) Multiple sclerosis: vitamin D and calcium as environmental determinants of prevalence (a viewpoint) part 1 sunlight, dietary factors and epidemiology. *International Journal of Environmental Studies* 6: 19–27.

Habek M, Hojsak I, Brinar V. (2010) Nutrition in multiple sclerosis. *Clinical Neurology and Neurosurgery* 112: 616–620.

Harbige L, Sharief M. (2007) Polyunsaturated fatty acids in the pathogenesis and treatment of multiple sclerosis. *British Journal of Nutrition* 98(Suppl 1): s46–s53.

Herndon RM. (2003) *Multiple Sclerosis: Immunology, Pathology and Pathophysiology*. New York: Demos Medical Publishing.

Holick MF. (1995) Environmental factors that influence the cutaneous production of vitamin D. *American Journal of Clinical Nutrition* 61(Suppl): 638s–645s.

Holick MF. (2004) Sunlight and vitamin D for bone health and prevention of autoimmune diseases, cancers, and cardiovascular disease. *American Journal of Clinical Nutrition* 80(6): 1678s–1688s.

Khan F, Turner-Stokes L, Kilpatrick T. (2008) Multidisciplinary rehabilitation for adults with multiple sclerosis (review). *The Cochrane Library Issue 3*.

Llorca J, Guerrero P, Prieto-Salceda D, Dierssen-Sotos T. (2005) Mortality of multiple sclerosis in Spain: demonstration of a North-South gradient. *Neuroepidemiology* 24(3): 135–140.

Looker AC, Pfeiffer CM, Lacher DA, Schleicher RL, Picciano MF, Yetley EA. (2008) Serum 25-hydroxyvitamin D status in the US population:1988–1994 compared with 2000–2004. *American Journal of Clinical Nutrition* 88: 1519–1527.

Mehta L, Dworkin R, Schwid S. (2009) Polyunsaturated fatty acids and their potential therapeutic role in multiple sclerosis. *Nature Clinical Practice Neurology*, 5: 82–92.

Mowry EM, Krup IB, Milazzo M, et al. (2010) Vitamin D status is associated with relapse rate in paediatric onset MS. *Annals of Neurology* 67(5): 618–624.

Munger K, Levin LI, Hollis BW, Howard NS, Ascherio A. (2006) Serum 25-hydroxy vitamin D levels and risk of multiple sclerosis. *JAMA* 296(23): 2832–2838.

National Institute for Health and Care Excellence (NICE). (2003) *Multiple Sclerosis; National Clinical Guidelines for Diagnosis and Management in Primary and Secondary Care*. London: NICE.

Payne A. (2001) Nutrition and diet in the clinical management of multiple sclerosis. *Journal of Human Nutrition and Dietetics* 14: 349–357.

Ponsonby AL, Lucas RM, Van Der Mei IA. (2005) UVR, vitamin D and autoimmune diseases – multiple sclerosis, type 1 diabetes, rheumatoid arthritis. *Photochemistry and Photobiology* 81(6): 1267–1275.

Poorjavad M, Derakhshandeh F, Etemadifar M, Soleymani B, Minegar A, Amir-Hadi M. (2010). Oropharyngeal dysphagia in multiple sclerosis. *Multiple Sclerosis* 16(3): 362–365.

Ragonese P, Aridon P, Salemi G, D'Amelio M, Savettieri G. (2008) Mortality in multiple sclerosis: a review. *European Journal of Neurology* 15: 123–127.

Restivo D, Marchese-Ragona R, Patti F, et al. (2011) Botulinum toxin improves dysphagia associated with multiple sclerosis. *European Journal of Neurology* 18(3): 486–490.

Ruddick R, Miller D. (2008) Health-related quality of life in multiple sclerosis: current evidence, measurement and effect of disease severity and treatment. *CNS Drugs* 22(10): 827–839.

Schwarz S, Knorr C, Geiger H, Flachenecker P. (2008) Complementary and alternative medicine for multiple sclerosis. *Multiple Sclerosis* 14: 1113–1119.

Soilu-Hanninen M, Airas I, Mononen I, Heikkla A, Viljanen M, Hanninen, A. (2005) 25-hydroxy vitamin D levels in serum at the onset of MS. *Multiple Sclerosis* 11(3): 266–271.

Stuifbergen AK, Becker H, Timmerman GM, Kullberg V. (2003) The use of individualised goal setting to facilitate behaviour change in women with multiple sclerosis. *Journal of Neuroscience and Nursing* 35(2): 94–99, 106.

Swank RL, Lerstad O, Strom A, Backer J. (1952) Multiple sclerosis in rural Norway. Its geographic and occupational incidence in relation to nutrition. *New England Journal of Medicine* 246: 721–728.

Thompson A, Toosy A, Ciccarelli O. (2010) Pharmacological management of symptoms in multiple sclerosis: current approaches and future directions. *Lancet Neurology* 9: 1182–1199.

Viglietta V, Baecher-Allan C, Weiner HL, Hafler DA. (2004) Loss of functional suppression by CD4+CD25+ regulatory T cells in patients with multiple sclerosis. *Journal of Experimental Medicine* 199: 971–979.

Weinstock-Guttman B, Baier M, Park Y, et al. (2005) Low fat dietary intervention with omega-3 fatty acid supplementation in multiple sclerosis patients. *Prostaglandins, Leukotrienes and Essential Fatty Acids* 73: 397–404.

Westlund K. (1970) Distribution and mortality and time trend of multiple sclerosis and some other diseases in Norway. *Acta Neurologica Scandinavica* 46: 455–483.

Yetley EA. (2008) Assessing the vitamin D status of the US population. *American Journal of Clinical Nutrition* 88(Suppl): 558s–564s.

SECTION 7

7.6.5 Chronic fatigue syndrome/myalgic encephalomyelitis

Jennifer McIntosh

Key points

■ The World Health Organization classifies chronic fatigue syndrome/myalgic encephalomyelitis as a neurological illness.

■ It is a poorly understood, chronic disabling condition affecting both adults and children with 60–70% reporting irritable bowel syndrome symptoms.

■ Dietary advice recommending small, frequent meals as part of a balanced diet may improve patients' energy levels.

The Chief Medical Officer (Department of Health, 2002) and the Medical Research Council (2003) recommend the use of the term chronic fatigue syndrome/myalgic encephalomyelitis (CFS/ME) rather than chronic fatigue syndrome (CFS), myalgic encephalomyelitis (ME) or post viral fatigue syndrome (PVFS). These were often considered to be separate conditions (Whiting *et al.*, (2001), however, they are now considered to be the same condition. The World Health Organization classifies CFS/ME as a neurological illness, although its aetiology is unknown. Several factors have been suggested, including neurological, endocrine, immunological, genetic, psychiatric and infectious (NICE, 2007).

It is a relatively common clinical condition affecting 0.2–0.4% of the population. It causes profound, often prolonged, illness and disability, and can have a substantial impact on the family and individual. The physical symptoms are as disabling as other chronic condition such as multiple sclerosis, rheumatoid arthritis and congestive heart failure (NICE, 2007; Department of Health, 2002) The symptoms vary and often fluctuate in intensity and severity between individuals but also within the individual. This can make it difficult for family, friends and health professionals to understand the condition.

Diagnostic criteria and classification

There is no diagnostic test for CFS/ME and diagnosis is made on the basis of a recognisable pattern of characteristic symptoms and the exclusion of other known causes. There are several sets of diagnostic criteria but in the UK, NICE (2007) diagnostic criteria are used (Box 7.6.1). Diagnosis is considered if symptoms have persisted for 4 months in an adult or 3 months in a child or young person. In a young child or young person the diagnosis should be made or confirmed by a paediatrician. If the following features are present they should be investigated before a diagnosis of CFS/ME is made:

* Localising or focal neurological signs.
* Significant weight loss.
* Sleep apnoea.
* Clinically significant lymphadenopathy.

Box 7.6.1 Criteria for diagnosis of chronic fatique syndrome/myalgic encephalomyelitis [from NICE (2007, p. 14)]

Fatigue with all of the following features:

* New or a specific onset, i.e. not lifelong
* Persistent and/or recurrent
* Unexplained by other conditions
* Has resulted in a substantial reduction in activity level
* Characterised by post exertional malaise and/or fatigue (typically delayed, e.g. by at least 24 hours, with slow recovery over several days)

And one or more of the following symptoms:

* Difficulty with sleeping, such as insomnia, hypersomnia, unrefreshing sleep, a disturbed sleep–wake cycle
* Muscle and or joint pain that is multisite and without evidence of inflammation
* Headaches.
* Painful lymph nodes without pathological enlargement
* Sore throat
* Cognitive dysfunction, such as difficulty thinking, inability to concentrate, impairment of short term memory, and difficulties with word finding, planning or organising thoughts and information processing

* Signs and symptoms of inflammatory arthritis or connective tissue disease.
* Signs and symptoms of cardiorespiratory disease.

Classification of symptom severity

The severity of CFS/ME can vary enormously and is classified as mild, moderate or severe (NICE, 2007):

* *Mild* – patients are mobile, can care for themselves and do light domestic tasks, but with difficulty. Most are still working or in education, but to do this they

have probably stopped all leisure and social pursuits. They often take days off work or school, or rest at the weekend in order to cope with the rest of the week.
- *Moderate* – patients have reduced mobility and are restricted in all activities of daily living, although they may have peaks and troughs in the level of symptoms and ability to do activities. They have usually stopped work, school or college and need rest periods, often sleeping in the afternoon for 1–2 hours. Sleep at night is generally poor of quality and disturbed.
- *Severe* – patients are unable to do any activity for themselves or can carry out minimal daily tasks only (such as face washing and cleaning teeth). They have severe cognitive difficulties and depend on a wheelchair for mobility. They are often unable to leave the house., or, if they do, this has a severe and prolonged after effect. They may also spend most of their time in bed, and are often extremely sensitive to light and noise.

Prevalence

Chronic fatigue syndrome/myalgic encephalomyelitis affects people of every age, gender, ethnicity and socio-economic group, although it is four times more common in women than in men. The most common age at onset is 40–50 years. It is less common in children than in adults, but children can develop CFS/ME, particularly during adolescence (14–15 years). As already mentioned, the prevalence is estimated to be approximately 0.2–0.4% of the population (Department of Health, 2002; White *et al.*, 2007).

Prognosis

Most patients will show some degree of improvement over time, especially with treatment. A substantial number of patients will pursue a fluctuating course with periods of relative remission and relapse, and a significant minority become severely and perhaps permanently disabled (Cairns & Hotopf, 2005; Department of Health, 2002).

Nutrition problems

Chronic fatigue syndrome/myalgic encephalomyelitis is a chronic condition that impacts on nutritional health in a variety of ways. This can be challenging for the individual, their family and /or carers, and healthcare professionals. Simple tasks such as shopping, and preparing and cooking a meal can prove challenging when energy levels are impaired. Patients often report fluctuating energy levels and therefore may need meals that require minimal preparation and effort to eat. Those who are severely affected may require nutritional support, ranging from nutritional supplements to enteral feeding. The following nutritional problems may occur.

Weight gain

It is generally recognised that a large percentage of patients gain weight, averaging 12–18 kg, due to reduced activity levels, increased eating to boost energy levels, comfort eating, medication and less energy to buy or prepare fresh foods. Weight gain can impact on fatigue and pain, and increase other health risks such as diabetes and heart disease (see Chapter 7.13.1).

Weight loss

This tends to be more common in children and young people, and those with symptoms of nausea. Some patients can be severely underweight, which impacts on fatigue levels. Weight loss is particularly common during the initial onset of CFS/ME (see Chapter 6.2).

Irritable bowel syndrome

Approximately 60–70% of CFS/ME patients (Rao *et al.*, 2009) report irritable bowel syndrome (IBS) symptoms that range from mild to severe in severity (see Chapter 7.4.10).

Nausea

Nausea is more common in children and young people, and can affect the ability to eat. There is some evidence for the presence of delayed gastric emptying (Burnet & Chatterton, 2004). Antiemetics may be useful in some patients (see Chapter 7.4.3).

Food intolerances

Food intolerances are frequently self reported and alterative diets, e.g. the anti-Candida and Stone Age diets, are frequently adopted. Currently, there is no evidence to support the use of these diets and they may also lead to nutritional deficiencies, which further impact on energy levels.

Osteoporosis

Osteoporosis can occur due to lack of exposure to sunlight, especially in those severely affected with CFS/ME. Lack of weight bearing exercise and dietary self restriction can increase the likelihood of osteoporosis (see Chapter 7.9.1).

Fluid

Patients can report either over or under drinking, due to increased thirst as part of the symptoms or forgetting to drink due to change in lifestyle, respectively.

Reactive hypoglycaemia

Patients may report a craving for sweet foods when tired, followed by symptoms similar to reactive hypoglycaemia, although there is no evidence to support this.

Other symptoms that may lead to a restrictive diet include difficult or painful swallowing or sore throat, sensitivity to smell or taste of food and disturbed sleep patterns.

Nutritional assessment

Anthropometry

Weight and height should be monitored to calculate and assess body mass index (BMI).

Biochemistry

The following routine blood tests are used to exclude other possible diagnoses (NICE, 2007):

- Full blood count.
- Creatinine, urea and electrolytes.
- Thyroid and liver function tests.
- Erthyrocyte sedimentation rate and C-reactive protein.
- Glucose.
- Urinalysis.
- Serum calcium.
- Creatine phosphokinase.
- Coeliac screen.

Clinical assessment

A detailed weight history prior to CFS/ME and currently is important. Depending on the reason for referral, potential food allergies and intolerance beliefs should be investigated. If symptoms of IBS or nausea are present, further information should be gathered to aid dietary advice. There should be an awareness of the impact of CFS/ME on concentration and short term memory, and it can be helpful if a carer is present in terms of remembering dietary advice given. It helps to provide written information or summary notes.

Dietary assessment

A detailed diet history should be taken, particularly noting use of nutritional supplements and alcohol and caffeine intake. Good and bad days with regard to food intake should be enquired about.

Economic and social assessment

Patients may be unable to work or work only part time, which impacts on their financial situation. There may be less money for food, which limits dietary choices. It is important to assess support available at home for shopping, food preparation and cooking.

Management

There is no single management approach that has been found to be universally beneficial and currently there is no known cure for CFS/ME. Most patients are managed in primary care, ideally with access, if required, to a specialised team that may include a specialist, physiotherapist, occupational therapist, dietitian and psychologist or cognitive behaviour therapist.

Pharmacological interventions

There is no known pharmacological treatment for CFS/ME and also limited evidence on the overall benefits of pharmacological treatments for CFS/ME. The focus is on symptom control for sleep, mood disturbance, IBS and menstrual problems. Some patients report sensitivity to medications and although there is no evidence for this, lower doses than normal given. The most commonly prescribed drugs include antidepressants and melatonin. Tricyclic antidepressants (amitriptyline or trimipramine) are used at a low dose and may be prescribed for poor sleep or pain. Selective serotonin reuptake inhibitors (SSRIs), (fluoxetine, citalopram and paroxetine) may be used for symptoms of anxiety and are less sedating than tricyclics. Side effects of both can include weight gain, cravings for carbohydrate foods, constipation or diarrhoea (see Chapter 7.10.3). Melatonin is responsible for regulating the body's biological clock and is produced naturally in the pineal gland; deficiency can lead to insomnia. Melatonin may be considered for children and young people with CFS/ME who have sleep difficulties, but only under specialist supervision as it is unlicensed in the UK.

Non-pharmacological interventions

The main interventions recognised as beneficial are cognitive behavioural therapy (CBT), graded exercise therapy (GET) and pacing.

Cognitive behaviour therapy

In CFS/ME CBT aims to reduce the level of symptoms, disability and distress as part of the overall management. A number of randomised controlled trials (Deale *et al.*, 1997; Sharpe *et al.*, 1996; Prins *et al.*, 2001; Rao *et al.*, 2001; Taylor *et al.*, 2004; Cox, 1999; Stulemeijer *et al.*, 2005) have reported beneficial effects with CBT on physical functioning, fatigue and global improvement. Two studies (Cox, 2002; Friedberg & Krupp, 1994) have shown no significant difference. It is recommend that CBT should be offered to people with mild or moderate CFS/ME (NICE, 2007; White *et al.*, 2011).

Graded exercise therapy

Graded exercise therapy relies on negotiations between the healthcare professional and the patient, and involves appropriate physical assessment, mutually agreed and meaningful goal setting and education. Initially, an achievable level of physical activity is agreed, followed by gradual and planned increases that are individually tailored to the patient. A number of randomised controlled trials (Fulcher & White 1997; Wearden *et al.*, 1998; Moss-Morris *et al.*, 2005; Wallman *et al.*, 2004; Powell *et al.*, 2001) have shown significant improvements in fatigue and physical function. Again, NICE (2007) recommends that people with mild or moderate CFS/ME should be offered GET.

Pacing

Pacing is managed by the patient and is defined as '*energy management, with the aim of maximising cognitive and physical activity, while avoiding setbacks/relapses due to overexertion'* (NICE, 2007). The evidence to date to support pacing is equivocal.

Other interventions that patients report are beneficial include activity management, sleep management, rest periods, relaxation, relapse and set back advice, and mindfulness based cognitive therapy (Surawy *et al.*, 2005; Sampalli *et al.*, 2009).

Nutritional management

The evidence base for the use of nutrition in CFS/ME is small and conflicting. Current management programmes are based on the available evidence and clinical experience. Patients have access to a large amount of nutritional information, often via the Internet, which can be conflicting. The National Institute for Health and Care Excellence and others (Baumer, 2005; Morris & Stare, 1993) recommend advising a healthy dietary approach. Although one study has shown that CFS/ME patients tend to lead a healthier lifestyle compared with the general population (Goedendorp *et al.*, 2009), explaining the psychological and physical benefits of dietary advice is important in terms of compliance and understanding. Currently, the following is recommended:

- Eating a balanced diet according to the eatwell plate (see Chapter 4.2).
- Incorporating low glycaemic index foods to improve energy levels, particularly in relation to hypoglycaemic type symptoms.
- Aiming to eat every 3–4 hours, e.g. three meals with the addition of three snacks in between to improve energy levels.
- Reducing caffeine intake if sleep is affected or if it impacts adversely on energy levels or bowel symptoms.
- Encouraging adequate fluid intake.
- Possibly reducing or avoiding alcohol, depending on reported impact on symptoms.
- Practical dietary advice regarding problem solving for reduced energy levels, e.g. ready meals or Internet food shopping.

Weight reduction

Initially, it is helpful to assess the reasons for weight gain, which may include reduced activity, cravings, medication or energy levels. In view of reduced activity levels, weight loss may be slower, e.g. 1–2 kg/month. Dietary advice can then be tailored to the individual situation (see Chapter 7.13.2).

Weight gain

It is important that patients understand that weight gain may be a slow process in view of symptoms of nausea. Dietary advice should be tailored to the individual, e.g. food fortification or frequent, small meals and snacks (see Chapter 6.3).

Nausea

Little and often should be encouraged and standard dietary advice for nausea given. If nausea is severe, antiemetic drugs may be considered (NICE, 2007).

Food allergies and intolerances

There is no evidence that CFS/ME sufferers have a greater incidence of immunoglobulin (IgG) mediated food allergy than the general population. However, some patient perceptions are that food allergies or food intolerances may be the cause. Explaining the difference between food allergy and food intolerance and how they are diagnosed can be helpful. Exclusion diets are not generally recommended for managing CFS/ME; however, they can be helpful for symptom management, especially IBS symptoms. Exclusion diets should only be undertaken under the supervision of a dietitian (see Chapter 7.11.2).

Bowel symptom management

Patients often benefit from strategies employed in the management of IBS, particularly modified dietary fibre. There have been some studies recommending use of probiotics (Lakhan & Kirchgessner, 2010; Rao *et al.*, 2009; Sullivan *et al.*, 2009). Low sugar and low yeast diets are popular; however, Hobday *et al.* (2008) and Morris & Stare (1993) found no benefit when compared with healthy eating.

Nutritional supplements

There is insufficient evidence for the use of nutritional supplements; however, patients still report a high usage. If the diet is inadequate or supplementation is advised, a multivitamin and mineral supplement within the recommended daily amount with an essential fatty acid supplement such as evening primrose oil (up to 1 g/day) and fish oils (1 g/day) is recommended. In those with moderate to severe CFS/ME, especially those who are housebound, it is important to assess dietary intake of vitamin D and if necessary to supplement (5–10 μg/day) this to prevent osteoporosis (NICE, 2007; Berkovitz *et al.*, 2009).

Evidence for the use of supplements is conflicting. Cox *et al.* (1991) showed an improvement in energy, pain, emotional reactions and general health with magnesium. However, all other studies have found no conclusive evidence. Nicotinamide adenine dinucleotide (NADH) is involved in ATP metabolism and was shown by Forsyth *et al.* (1999) to improve quality of life and general health, but Santaella *et al.* (2004) reported no significant difference. Following limited reports of benefit (Werbach, 2000), there is a trend to give 1 g/week of vitamin B_{12} intramuscularly for 12 weeks, then monthly for 1 year or more. This appears to have beneficial effects in some patients, but is not accepted medical practice. Essential fatty acid supplementation studies are also conflicting. One randomised controlled trial reported no improvements, while another slightly larger controlled trial reported an overall beneficial affect (Warren *et al.*, 1999;

Behan *et al.*, 1990); Puri *et al.*, 2004). A recent study (Maes & Leunis, 2008) demonstrated some positive results with essential fatty acids; however, more research is needed in this area. There is no evidence to support the use of coenzyme Q10, vitamin C and B complex supplementation.

Complementary and alternative therapies

There is insufficient evidence that complementary therapies are effective treatments for CFS/ME (NICE, 2007). However, people with CFS/ME may choose these therapies due to the frustration of no conventional cure for CFS/ME being helpful. More evidence is required in this area (see Chapter 5.4).

Further reading

Chambers D, Bagnall AM, Hempel S, Forbes C. (2006) Interventions for the treatment, management and rehabilitation of patients with chronic fatigue syndrome/myalgic encephalomyelitis:an updated systematic review. *Journal of the Royal Society of Medicine* 99: 506–520.

Department of Health CFS/ME Working Group. (2002) *A Report to the Chief Medical Officer of an Independent Working Group*. London: Department of Health, 2002. Available at www.dh.gov.uk.

National Institute for Health and Care Excellence (NICE). (2007) Clinical guideline for the diagnosis and management of CFS/ME. Available at www.nice.org.uk/cg53.

Royal College of Paediatrics and Child Health (RCPCH). (2004) *Evidence Based Guideline for the Management of CFS/ME in Children and Young People*. London: RCPCH. Available at www.rcpch.ac.uk.

Internet resources

British Association for CFS/ME (BACME)   www.bacme.info
Northern CFS/ME Network   www.cfsmenorth.nhs.uk/

References

Baumer JH. (2005) Management of chronic fatigue syndrome/ myalgic encephalopathy (CFS/ME). *Archives of Disease in Childhood Education and Practice Edition* 90: 46–50.

Behan PO, Behan WM, Horrobin D. (1990) Effect of high doses of essential fatty acids on the postviral fatigue syndrome. *Acta Neurologica Scandinavica* 82: 209–216.

Berkovitz S, Ambler G, Jenkins M, Thurgood S. (2009) Serum 25-hydroxy vitamin D levels in chronic fatigue syndrome: a retrospective survey. *International Journal of Vitamin and Nutrition Research* 79(4): 250–254.

Burnet RB, Chatterton BE. (2004) Gastric emptying is slow in chronic fatigue syndrome. *Gastroenterology* 4: 32.

Cairns R, Hotopf M. (2005) A systematic review describing the prognosis of chronic fatigue syndrome. *Occupational Medicine* 55: 20–31.

Cox DL. (1999) *An Evaluation of an Occupational Therapy Inpatient Intervention for Chronic Fatigue Syndrome*. PhD Thesis. London: King's College London.

Cox DL. (2002) Chronic fatigue syndrome: An evaluation of an occupational therapy inpatient intervention. *British Journal of Occupational Therapy* 65: 461–468.

Cox IM, Campbell MJ, Dowson D. (1991) Red blood cell magnesium and chronic fatigue syndrome. *Lancet* 337: 757–760.

Deale A, Chalder T, Marks I, Wessely S. (1997) Cognitive behavior therapy for chronic fatigue syndrome: a randomized controlled trial. *American Journal of Psychiatry* 154: 408–414.

Department of Health CFS/ME Working Group. (2002) *A Report to the Chief Medical Officer of an Independent Working Group*. London: Department of Health, 2002. Available at www.dh.gov.uk. Accessed 7 February 2013.

Forsyth LM, Preuss HG, MacDowell AL, Chiazze L, Birkmayer GD, Bellanti JA. (1999) Therapeutic effects of oral NADH on the symptoms of patients with chronic fatigue. *Annals of Allergy, Asthma and Immunology* 82: 185–191.

Friedberg F, Krupp LB. (1994) A comparison of cognitive behavioral treatment for chronic fatigue syndrome and primary depression. *Clinical Infectious Diseases* 18(Suppl 1): S105–110.

Fulcher KY, White PD. (1997) Randomised controlled trial of graded exercise in patients with the chronic fatigue syndrome. *BMJ* 314: 1647–1652.

Goedendorp MM, Knoop H, Schippers GM, Bleijenberg G. (2009) The lifestyle of patients with chronic fatigue syndrome and the effect on fatigue and functional impairments. *Journal of Human Nutrition and Dietetics* 22: 226–231.

Hobday RA, Thomas S, O'Donovan A, Murphy M, Pinching AJ. (2008) Dietary intervention in chronic fatigue syndrome. *Journal of Human Nutrition and Dietetics* 21: 141–149.

Lakhan SE, Kirchgessner A. (2010) Gut Inflammation in chronic fatigue syndrome. *Nutrition and Metabolism* 7: 79.

Maes M, Leunis JC. (2008) Normalization of leaky gut in chronic fatigue syndrome (CFS) is accompanied by a clinical improvement: effects of age, duration of illness and the translocation of LPS from gram-negative bacteria. *Neuroendocrinology Letters* 29(6): 101–109.

Medical Research Council. (2003) *CFS/ME Research Strategy*. MRC CFS/ME Research Advisory Group (RAG) Report. Available at www.mrc.ac.uk.

Morris DH, Stare FJ. (1993) Unproven diet therapies in the treatment of the chronic fatigue syndrome. *Archives of Family Medicine* 2: 181–186.

Moss-Morris R, Sharon C, Tobin R, Baldi JC. (2005) A randomized controlled graded exercise trial for chronic fatigue syndrome: outcomes and mechanisms of change. *Journal of Health Psychology* 10: 245–259.

National Institute for Health and Care Excellence (NICE). (2007) Clinical guideline for the diagnosis and management of CFS/ME. Available at www.nice.org.uk/cg53.

Powell P, Bentall RP, Nye FJ, Edwards RH. (2001) Randomised controlled trial of patient education to encourage graded exercise in chronic fatigue syndrome. *BMJ* 322: 387–390.

Prins JB, Bleijenberg G, Bazelmans E, *et al.* (2001) Cognitive behaviour therapy for chronic fatigue syndrome: a multicentre randomised controlled trial. *Lancet* 357: 841–847.

Puri BK, Holmes J, Hamilon G. (2004) Eicosapentaenoic acid-rich essential fatty acid supplementation in chronic fatigue associated with symptom remission and structural brain changes. *International Journal of Clinical Practice* 58: 297–299.

Rao AV, Prins JB, Bleijenberg G, *et al.* (2001) Cognitive behaviour therapy for chronic fatigue syndrome: a multicentre randomised controlled trial. *Lancet* 357: 841–847.

Rao AV, Bested AC, Beauline TM, *et al.* (2009) A randomized, double-blind, placebo-controlled pilot study of a probiotic in emotional symptoms of chronic fatigue syndrome. *Gut Pathogens* 1: 1–6.

Sampalli T, Berlasso E, Fox R, Petter M. (2009) A controlled study of the effect of a mindfulness-based stress reduction technique in women with multiple chemical sensitivity, chronic fatigue syndrome and fibromyalgia. *Journal of Multidisciplinary Healthcare* 2: 53–59.

Santaella ML, Font I, Disdier OM. (2004) Comparison of oral nicotinamide adenine dinucleotide (NADH) versus conventional therapy for chronic fatigue syndrome. *Puerto Rico Health Sciences Journal* 23: 89–93.

Sharpe M, Hawton K, Simkin S, *et al*. (1996) Cognitive behaviour therapy for the chronic fatigue syndrome: a randomized controlled trial [see comment]. *BMJ* 312: 22–26.

Stulemeijer M, de Jong LW, Fiselier TJ, Hoogveld SW, Bleijenberg G. (2005) Cognitive behaviour therapy for adolescents with chronic fatigue syndrome: randomised controlled trial. *BMJ* 330: 14.

Sullivan A, Nord CE, Evengard B. (2009) Effect of supplement with lactic-acid producing bacteria on fatigue and physical activity in patients with chronic fatigue syndrome. *Nutrition Journal* 8: 4.

Surawy C, Roberts J, Silver A. (2005) The effect of mindfulness training on mood and measures of fatigue, activity and quality of life in patients with chronic fatigue on a hospital waiting list: a series of exploratory studies. *Behavioural and Cognitive Psychotherapy* 33: 103–109.

Taylor RR, Braveman B, Hammel J. (2004) Developing and evaluating community-based services through participatory action research: two case examples. *American Journal of Occupational Therapy* 58: 73–82.

Wallman KE, Morton AR, Goodman C, Grove R, Guilfoyle AM. (2004) Randomised controlled trial of graded exercise in chronic fatigue syndrome. *Medical Journal of Australia* 180: 444–448.

Warren G, McKendrick M, Peet M. (1999) The role of essential fatty acids in chronic fatigue syndrome: a case-controlled study of red cell membrane essential fatty acids (EFA) and a placebo-controlled treatment study with high dose of EFA. *Acta Neurologica Scandinavica* 99: 112–116.

Wearden AJ, Morriss RK, Mullis R, *et al*. (1988) Randomised, double-blind, placebo-controlled treatment trial of fluoxetine and graded exercise for chronic fatigue syndrome. *British Journal of Psychiatry* 172: 485–492.

Werbach MR. (2000) Nutritional strategies for treating chronic fatigue syndrome. *Alternative Medicine Review* 5(2): 93–108.

Whiting P, Bagnall AM, Sowden AJ, Cornell JE, Mulrow CD, Ramirez G.(2001) Interventions for the treatment and management of chronic fatigue syndrome. *JAMA* 286(11): 1378–1368.

White PD, Sharpe MC, Chalder T, DeCesare JC, Walwyn R. (2007) Protocol for the PACE trial: A randomised controlled trial of adaptive pacing, cognitive behaviour therapy, and graded exercise as supplements to standardised specialist medical care versus standardised specialist medical care alone for patients with the chronic fatigue syndrome/myalgic encephalomyelitis or encephalopathy. *BMC Neurology* 7(6): 1–20.

White PD, Goldsmith KA, Johnson AL, *et al*. (2011) Comparison of adaptive pacing therapy, cognitive behaviour therapy, graded exercise therapy, and specialist medical care for chronic fatigue syndrome (PACE): a randomised trial. *Lancet* 377: 823–836.

7.6.6 Neurorehabilitation

Emma Dresner, Jennie Dunwoody, Katie Richards and Samantha Parry

Key points

■ Neurorehabilitation is dependent upon collaboration, goal setting, outcome measures, communication, coordination and effective leadership.

■ The neurological effects of brain injury can have significant implications in terms of nutritional status and intake.

■ It is essential that dietitians are aware of the extent and nature of these effects.

It is imperative that nutritional assessment is carried out within the confines of a specialist team so that expert opinion on other parameters that impact on food intake can be taken into account.

Rehabilitation is a process of assessment, treatment and management by which the individual (and their family and carers) are supported to achieve their maximum potential for physical, cognitive, social and psychological function, participation in society and quality of living. Patient goals for rehabilitation vary according to the trajectory and stage of their condition. Specialist rehabilitation is the total active care of patients (and their families and/or carers) with a disabling condition by a multidisciplinary team (MDT) that has undergone recognised specialist training in rehabilitation and led or supported by a consultant trained and accredited in rehabilitation medicine. Generally, patients requiring specialist rehabilitation are those with complex disabilities.

Such patients typically present with a diverse mixture of medical, physical, sensory, cognitive, communicative, behavioural and social problems. These patients are likely to require specialist input from a wide range of rehabilitation disciplines as well as specialist medical input. A subgroup of patients will have profound disability; these require help for all aspects of their basic care, as well as specialist interventions, e.g. spasticity management, postural support programmes and highly specialist equipment (Turner-Stokes *et al*., 1998). The principles of neurorehabilitation are that it should be goal orientated and individual specific. The emphasis should always be on the individual's lifestyle and background.

This chapter concentrates on neurorehabilitation of individuals who have an acquired brain injury (ABI), which can be divided into traumatic, e.g. road traffic accidents, assaults and falls, and non-traumatic brain injury, e.g. infection, HIV, stroke and, hypoxic brain damage.

General principles

Phases of rehabilitation

Rehabilitation does not occur solely in a specialist centre or unit. It begins from the minute an individual is admitted to hospital and continues long after their return to

SECTION 7

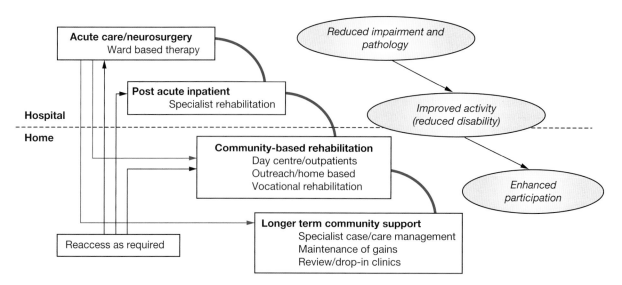

Figure 7.6.1   Phases of rehabilitation (source: National Clinical Guidelines 2013. Reproduced with permission of The Royal College of Physicians)

their community, as shown in Figure 7.6.1. The key to its success is continuity across the phases, leading to seamless care. In an acute hospital or ward, while a patient is waiting to move to a rehabilitation ward or unit, some maintenance interventions are still likely to be needed, such as managing positioning, preventing loss of range of movement, preventing contractures, establishing alternative forms of communication and many others. These interventions are primarily focussed on preventing complications that could magnify later disability.

Guidelines

In 2003, the British Society of Rehabilitation Medicine (BSRM) in collaboration with the Royal College of Physicians (RCP) produced the clinical guidelines for rehabilitation following acquired brain injury (BSRM/RCP, 2003). These guidelines promote interdisciplinary team working towards individual centred goals, with timely interventions to best facilitate cost effective integrated rehabilitation.

More recent guidelines are the BSRM Standards for Rehabilitation Services Mapped to the National Service Framework for Long-Term Conditions (2008) and in 2010 the BSRM, in collaboration with the RCP, joint working party document, Medical Rehabilitation in 2011 and Beyond. This latter report outlined the benefits that rapidly available, ongoing access to high quality rehabilitation services offers patients with disabilities arising from injury or long term conditions. The report is the work of an expert group comprising medical specialists, patients and allied professionals. Following a wide ranging review of the evidence, the group has provided specifications for designing cost effective services that maximise opportunities for recovery.

The neurological rehabilitation team

Following brain injury, rehabilitation from a specialised team should be established as soon as possible. An effec-

tive team works collaboratively to provide integrated care and towards achieving a single set of individual centred goals. The key to the success of neurorehabilitation is collaboration, communication, coordination and leadership. The team comprises a number of healthcare professionals who work closely together in conjunction with the individual and/or carers to assess the individual's needs, devise an individual plan of care and monitor its implementation and progress. The team may include a:

- Dietitian.
- Rehabilitation nurse.
- Physiotherapist.
- Consultant in rehabilitation medicine.
- Speech and language therapist.
- Occupational therapist.
- Music therapist.
- Neuropsychologist.
- Social worker.
- Recreation and leisure facilitator.
- Rehabilitation assistant.

Goal planning

Neurorehabilitation should be goal driven with regular multidisciplinary meetings to discuss, review and set specific, measureable, attainable, relevant and timely (SMART) goals. A standardised set of outcome measures, e.g. the Extended Rehabilitation Complexity Scale, Northwick Park Therapy Dependency Score and Function Assessment Measure, should be used as a marker of outcome within neurorehabilitation (BSRM, 2008).

Consequences of brain injury

Damage to the brain as a result of acquired brain injury can have profound effects on an individual's physical and mental capabilities. The effects depend on the location, nature and extent of the damage. Brain injury can be classified as mild, moderate or severe. In mild cases, patients may be able to return home and even commence paid employment. In more severe cases however, they will be dependent on other people for many aspects of care for the rest of their lives.

Damage to the left hemisphere of the brain is most likely to affect:

- Language.
- Speech.
- Reading and writing ability.

Damage to the right hemisphere is most likely to affect:

- Processing of visual and spatial information.
- Recognition.
- Coordination.

Although damage to brain tissue is irreversible since the body has no ability to regenerate brain cells, in some types of brain injury, particularly stroke, the body does seem able to adapt to some types of damage by rerouting the way in which information is processed, hence enabling the individual in time to recover some or all of an ability, e.g. speech or swallowing. This is termed neuroplasticity.

Nutritional implications of brain injury

The neurological effects of brain injury can have significant implications in terms of nutritional status and intake, and it is essential that dietitians are aware of the extent and nature of these effects in a particular individual before attempting to make nutritional assessment or provide dietary guidance. Dietetic expertise has a vital role in the neurorehabilitation process and a dietitian should be an active member of the specialised team.

Acquired brain injury can significantly alter an individual's nutritional status and mitigating its effects can help an individual cope with the demands of the rehabilitation process. Another key role of the dietitian is to educate other team members about the nutritional implications and management of ABI. To achieve this, it is vital that the dietitian understands the role of other team members.

Effects on the ability to communicate

Aphasia (damage to the language centre in the left hemisphere of the brain) may result in loss of or difficulties with speech (expressive aphasia). The ability to read or even interpret pictures may also be impaired (receptive aphasia). As a result of dysphasia, individuals may be unable to communicate their wishes, e.g. that they are hungry or thirsty, or express their likes and dislikes. Aphasic individuals may also have difficulty in completing a hospital menu card or making sense of dietary information provided in a written or even pictorial form.

Effects on eating behaviour

Behavioural alteration

Behavioural alteration, often resulting from frontal damage, may include:

- Antisocial behaviour, e.g. poor table manners, spitting or throwing food.
- Aggression.
- Physical and/or verbal abuse.
- Disinhibition, e.g. hyperphagia may not be kept in check to the extent it would normally be (Henson et al., 1993).
- Disinterest or apathy.

Mood alteration

Alteration in brain function or sometimes drugs used to treat brain injury may have a direct effect on neurotransmitters and result in short or long term alteration in mood, e.g. depression or withdrawal.

Effects on appetite

Damage to the hypothalamus may result in loss of appetite control, resulting in hyperphagia (Henson et al., 1993) or hyperphagia to particular foods such as a craving for sweet carbohydrate foods. Drug therapy, particularly the use of mood altering drugs, may also affect appetite.

Effects on the physical ability to eat

Ataxia

Ataxia describes tremor or shakiness, usually as a result of damage to the cerebellum, brainstem or pyramid tracts causing poor motor control. It can result in considerable difficulties in getting food to the mouth, possibly to such an extent that the individual has to be fed. Equipment has been devised that enables the ataxic individual to self feed (by creating a resistance against tremor and therefore allowing a smooth transit from plate to mouth), but some individuals find the equipment too large and difficult to use; others feel that it draws attention to their disability and prefer to be discreetly fed by a carer.

Apraxia

Apraxia is the term used to describe disordered purposeful movement. Apraxia is often associated with left hemisphere damage and may appear in a number of forms:

- People with *ideomotor apraxia* may be unable to perform a specific task on request despite understanding the concept and having the physical ability to do so. However, the individual may be able to carry out the task automatically.
- Individuals with *ideational apraxia* may be unable to select the appropriate tool to carry out a particular task, e.g. may try to use a fork as a straw.

Hemiplegia

This results in paralysis of limbs on the side of the body that is opposite to the site of the brain lesion. Other physical consequences may be muscle wasting, limb oedema and slowing of nail growth on the affected side. Hemiplegia is particularly likely to compromise nutritional status

SECTION 7

because energy requirements may be increased as a result of the reduced efficiency of movement and the presence of spasticity (Potempa *et al.*, 1995), and food intake is often limited in both type and amount because of the difficulties of manipulating food with just one hand. Measures such as the use of anti-slip mats and adapted cutlery may be helpful.

Effects on the ability to swallow

Dysphagia is a common consequence of many types of brain injury. Not only may damage to cranial nerves affect the swallowing reflex, but other aspects necessary for the normal swallow, such as the ability to visualise and recognise the food, achieve and maintain an appropriate posture of the head, neck and body and have good lip and tongue movement, may also be affected by brain injury. Abnormal oral reflexes, e.g. tongue thrust and bite reflex, inability to concentrate, fatigue and fear of choking, may further compound a problem. Any loss in swallowing ability is likely to compromise nutritional intake as a result of:

* Insufficient consumption of food (intake of energy and nutrients may be inadequate).
* Limited choice of food (dietary intake may be imbalanced).
* Losses as a result of drooling and leakage of food from the mouth.

Measures that are likely to be needed in dysphagic brain injured individuals are:

* Assessment by the specialist team and appropriate assistance provided, e.g. helping individuals convey food to the back of the mouth to trigger the swallowing reflex.
* Changes in food consistency and texture, which may necessitate either a uniform soft consistency, e.g. puréed foods, or appropriately thickened fluids, depending on the nature of the dysphagia. As altered texture diets are nutritionally dilute, nutritional supplements may be required to meet energy needs.
* Maximisation of sensory input. Foods may become more palatable and easier to swallow if they are served either 'hot' or 'cold', rather than just 'warm' or at room temperature. Chilled foods and drinks are often particularly well accepted. Main meals initially served as hot as possible are more likely to remain at an acceptable temperature throughout what may be a long meal time. Flavourings should be used to make food as appetising as possible.

The management of dysphagia is discussed in detail in Chapter 7.3.

Psychological effects of the injury or disease

As well as physical effects, the psychological consequences of having suffered ABI or having been diagnosed with a serious neurological disorder can affect nutritional intake.

Emotional reactions

Awareness of the nature of the injury or disease and the prospect of permanent or progressive disability is likely to be followed by an emotional reaction similar to that of bereavement and including:

* Shock.
* Emotional lability and depression.
* Realisation (which can result in further depression).
* Adjustment.

Relatives may go through a similar process so both individual and family need support.

Depression may also result from, or be compounded by, chemical changes following the brain injury. Depression can have a profound effect on food intake; individuals may, for a while, simply not want to get better. Physical difficulties with eating or swallowing may be compounded by fatigue and poor concentration. The consequent problems may make people feel frustrated or resentful and consequently irritable, even angry, with carers and health professionals. Alternatively, the inability to cope with what can be a stressful situation can make people withdrawn or tearful.

Social isolation

Embarrassment because eating is accompanied by spillage as a result of tremor, drooling or dribbling, or simply as a result of having to be fed, may make people reluctant to eat with others or in public. As a result, both individuals and their relatives or carers can be very isolated (Osborn & Marshall, 1993). Every effort should be made to help people overcome the problems that cause them most distress and to retain as much independence as possible.

Nutritional management

Table 7.6.4 lists the variety of patients from a nutritional perspective who may present on a neurorehabilitation ward.

Many individuals who have suffered ABI will commence the phase of rehabilitation in a state of undernutrition as a result of the hypercatabolic effects of acute trauma and the likelihood of energy and nitrogen needs not having been met (see Chapter 7.17.2 and Chapter 7.14.5). Undernutrition is particularly likely if the injury was severe (which will result in a greater and more prolonged catabolic response) or the individual was malnourished prior to the injury (as may be the case in some elderly people who have suffered a stroke).

The initial nutritional priority in such individuals is thus to restore nutritional status and maximise ability to participate in therapy sessions. As rehabilitation progresses, this objective gradually changes to helping individuals overcome, or mitigate, their neurological difficulties affecting food intake and ensuring that nutrient intake is adequate. With further recovery but persisting disabilities, the aim may be to prevent weight gain and overnutrition. The ultimate aim is to optimise nutritional

Table 7.6.4 Feeding methods that patients may require on a neurorehabilitation ward

Nil by mouth	All nutrition provided via nasogastric, gastrostomy or jejunal feeding tube
Feeding tube with tastes	Assessed by speech and language therapist as safe to commence trials of oral intake Usually teaspoons with therapist initially, then handed over to nursing staff Majority of nutrition, all fluid and medication via tube
Feeding tube, oral meal and some fluids	Oral intake increasing and commence taking meals during the day Start to reduce volume of nutrition via feeding tube and monitor weight May still need significant amounts of fluid via percutaneous gastrostomy
Feeding tube, oral food and fluid	Managing increased oral intake of food and fluid May start to manage medication orally Continue to reduce nutritional provision via feeding tube Dietitian requests oral intake record charts
Feeding tube water only	Reached a stage where weight can be maintained by oral diet; this may be inclusive of oral nutritional supplements but unable to drink enough to maintain hydration It is not uncommon for patients to be discharged from a rehabilitation setting with a feeding tube for fluids and medication only
Full oral diet	Managing enough food and fluid orally to maintain weight and nutritional status
Healthy eating diet for weight management	Oral intake may reach a stage where unwanted weight increases occur Healthy eating dietary advice will be needed; in extreme cases patients might become hyperphagic as a result of their brain injury

intake in a way that maximises the individual's rehabilitation potential.

Nutritional assessment

Many factors impact upon nutritional intake in the brain injured individual; therefore, it is essential that nutritional assessment is carried out within the confines of a specialist team so that expert opinion on other parameters that impact on food intake (as outlined earlier) can be taken into account.

Factors that need to be considered as part of a nutritional assessment are:

* The cause of the brain injury, its management and likely prognosis.
* The physical and psychological consequences of the injury on:
  o The desire to eat.
  o The ability to eat.
  o The ability to swallow.
  o Bowel function.
  o The ability to carry out everyday tasks.
* The individual's nutritional intake.
* The individual's hydration status.
* The individual's nutritional status and whether this is likely to improve, worsen or remain stable.

The aim is to identify individuals who are:

* Malnourished and in need of nutritional support.
* At risk of malnutrition and whose nutritional status needs to be monitored.
* At risk of dehydration and whose fluid intake and hydration status need to be monitored.
* In need of remedial measures to help alleviate diet related problems.

Multidisciplinary team involvement

Liaison with the other members of the MDT helps to provide a full picture of the individual's overall presenting condition. Each professional will carry out their initial assessment and then come together to discuss the situation and devise achievable interdisciplinary goals that the individual can work towards.

Liaison with other healthcare professionals is key to ensuring all aspects of nutritional care are covered. Dietetic interactions with other members of the MDT may include:

* Close working with the speech and language therapist is essential to be fully aware of the patient's swallow ability.
* Liaising with the occupational therapists to be aware of the patient's physical ability to get food to their own mouth, with or without specialist equipment, or to clarify if they need full assistance.
* Obtaining recommendations from the physiotherapist on posture and positioning to best enable a patient to feed themselves, if able, as well as reducing risk of aspiration.
* Doctors and pharmacists can advise on relevant drug–nutrient interactions. As well as the patient's presenting condition, some of the drugs used may impact on their ability to meet nutritional requirements. They may be on medications that reduce their level of arousal and so they are too tired to eat at meal times or medications may make them feel unwell.

Target weight setting

The use of target weights with this type of patient is a way of ensuring appropriate and timely responses to weight fluctuations. The dietitian should agree on a target weight range with a patient and/or their family or carers on admission to a rehabilitation setting. If this is not possible to do, the target weight should be set in the patient's best interest. Patients in the early stages of rehabilitation and for whom it may still be relatively early post injury may have energy requirements far greater than expected. This may be due to a number of reasons, including autonomic storming, high tone and spasticity or repeated infection.

As time progress, patients may require far less energy as they receive appropriate postural management, medication to manage tone and spasticity, and are sat out in a wheelchair daily. Setting and maintaining target weights are also of great importance when considering a patient's 24-hour postural management. Large fluctuations in weight can cause issues with custom made wheelchairs and splints no longer fitting.

Assessing the extent of nutritional depletion

Weight loss

This is usually the best way of assessing the degree of nutritional depletion in brain injured individuals. Comparison of the individual's weight at the start of rehabilitation with the individual's usual premorbid weight provides a good indication of the extent of energy depletion. This can be calculated as:

$$\% \text{ Usual body weight} = \frac{\text{Current weight (kg)}}{\text{Usual weight (kg)}} \times 100$$

However, measurement of weight is often difficult in severely disabled ABI individuals as appropriate scales may not be available. Hoist or weighbridge type scales can be used to weigh an immobile individual, but such specialist equipment is not always available. When wheelchair or hoist scales are available, then a structured weighing programme can be set up to ensure regular monitoring (see Chapter 7.17.3 for details on alternative weighing scales).

Ascertaining accurate weight trends is invaluable over the period of rehabilitation. It can ensure that nutritional intervention is tailored to the individual. This can often lead to different nutrient provision than first suggested by solely using estimated energy requirements. The weighing programme can enable target weight ranges to be set as the dietitian can be confident that they are working with up to date information. A dietetic or rehabilitation assistant can play a key role in helping to manage the weighing programme and be the liaison between the ward and dietetic department to ensure the patient is weighed in a timely fashion.

Adiposity measurements

These indicate the level of body fat stores, but can be either difficult to measure or inappropriate, in some types of brain injured individuals. Body mass index can only be calculated if measurements of body weight and height are available. As well as practical problems in measuring weight, measurement of height is particularly difficult in brain injured individuals because, even if standing is pos-

sible, they may not be able to stand erect or immobile for long enough. Alternative body measurements such as demispan and knee height, from which height can be derived (see Chapter 2.2), are not always appropriate alternatives since brain injured individuals may be unable to stretch their arms sufficiently for the former measurement or achieve the correct position for the latter. However, it is often possible to obtain an estimate of height directly from the individual or relative.

Skinfold thickness measurements, particularly triceps skinfold thickness, are fraught with problems in many brain injured individuals. In those with hemiplegia, the arm on the affected side may be oedematous, have abnormal muscle wasting and be flaccid or spastic, all of which may distort skinfold measurements. Skinfold measurements at other sites may be affected by poor posture or immobility.

Estimates of muscle mass

Measurements of, for example, mid arm muscle circumference can be useful, but are inappropriate for individuals with limb paralysis (in addition to the likelihood of muscle wasting in the affected arm, there is usually a compensatory increase in muscle mass in the unaffected arm). Immobility will also result in muscle wasting.

Biochemical and haematological indices

Measurements of blood glucose, electrolytes, serum urea and urinary nitrogen are used to monitor the degree of catabolism in the acute post injury phase, but in the rehabilitation phase provide limited information about an individual's nutritional status other than the state of hydration (Labbe, 1986). Haematological indicators may be relevant if anaemia is suspected, and biochemical markers in the rehabilitation setting are likely to be useful in a patient who is undergoing autonomic storming or who has an infection.

Assessing dietary intake

It can be difficult to obtain accurate dietary information from brain injured individuals. Many individuals will have memory and cognitive impairments, and dysphasia (receptive and expressive), which limit their ability to understand or communicate. Behavioural and mood changes may result in hostility or aggression towards the questioner, or alternatively withdrawal and lack of response. It is essential to understand the individual's capabilities as well as limitations and to draw on the expertise and advice from other members of the care team.

The amount and degree of reliability of dietary information that the individual is able to provide will vary considerably and the dietitian will need to be adaptable and innovative to make best use of the relevant circumstances. A skilled dietitian may be able to build up a useful diet history from no more than single word responses to the display of food photographs or food models. The use of specialised computer based packages and technology can be useful for patients with limited communication ability.

One of the most valuable ways of obtaining additional dietary information is by observing meal times. Not only does this give an estimate of the quantity of food and fluid consumed, but it also reveals any physical difficulties associated with eating or swallowing, together with any behavioural problems.

Assessment tools designed to evaluate problems such as food refusal, antisocial behaviour or assistance needed with feeding have been devised for individuals with dementia (Watson 1994a,b; Watson & Deary 1994; VOICES, 1998), but as yet no such assessment tool has been devised for brain injured individuals whose behaviour and care needs are very different. Food and fluid intake charts that are accurately completed can be useful in assessing dietary intake.

Autonomic storming and fluid requirements

Abnormal autonomic function is well recognised after brain injury. This has been variously termed autonomic dysfunction syndrome, or autonomic or sympathetic storming. Features of the syndrome include increases in heart rate, respiratory rate, temperature and blood pressure, with decerebrate or decorticate posturing, increased muscle tone, and profuse sweating. This autonomic storming can greatly increase the nutritional requirements of these patients and also lead to vastly increased fluid requirements due to increased losses from sweating. In order to maintain biochemical markers of dehydration within normal limits, patients often require significantly more than 30–35 mL/kg of fluid/day.

Managing dietary problems

Inadequate food intake is most likely to result from:

- Physical difficulties with eating or swallowing.
- Anorexia (often as a result of depression, anxiety or medication).
- Cognitive issues.
- Frustration or fatigue over the effort involved in eating.
- Intensive therapy.
- Food refusal as a result of behavioural change or because the patient finds it degrading to have to be fed.
- Drug induced side effects such as nausea and vomiting.

Some of these problems may be remedied by quite simple measures, e.g. smaller, more frequent, energy dense meals for those suffering from anorexia or nausea, the use of various aids to help overcome the physical difficulties of getting food to the mouth, assistance with feeding, involvement of patients in meal or menu planning groups, creating a pleasant meal atmosphere or changing the timing of the administration of drugs to lessen their effects on food intake.

Individuals with evidence of malnutrition, or at high risk of malnutrition, will require a greater level of nutritional support via:

- Food enrichment (see Chapter 6.3).
- Use of energy and protein supplements (see Chapter 6.3).
- Enteral feeding (either overnight supplementary or total support, and via the nasogastric or gastrostomy route) (see Chapter 6.4).

The extent, means and route of support will depend on the level of nutritional depletion, the physical and psychological effects of the neurological lesions, whether the condition is relapsing–remitting or chronically progressive, and the preferences of the individual and carers. Specific problems that may have to be addressed are outlined below.

Dehydration

Hydration status is particularly likely to be inadequate in those with poor oral or swallowing abilities. The problem often results from individuals not being encouraged to consume fluids (either in liquid or semi solid form) at regular intervals throughout the day, either because of lack of time by care staff or lack of awareness of the importance of this. In addition to this, the use of medication within this patient group can be a risk factor for dehydration. The potential for increased susceptibility to infection means antibiotics can increase the risk of diarrhoea, as can sorbitol containing supplements. Furthermore, medications used to correct tone, e.g. baclofen, can also have a laxative effect.

Constipation

This is extremely common in neurorehabilitation patients and may result from:

- Inadequate fluid intake.
- Low fibre intake (especially on a modified consistency diet).
- Reduced gut motility (as a result of reduced neurological signals from the brain or muscle wasting in the gastrointestinal tract).
- Reduced mobility of the individual.
- Side effect of medication (such as opiates for pain relief).

Symptoms may be alleviated by increasing consumption of:

- *Fluid* – ideally to about 2 L/day, although some patients may require more, particularly in the early stages following a traumatic brain injury.
- *Fibre rich foods* that are compatible with the individual's eating or swallowing difficulties. Foods such as porridge, wholegrain breakfast cereals, bananas, peeled oranges or satsumas, vegetables with skins, beans, lentils and peas, and prunes and dried fruit may be suitable possibilities. Speech and language therapists should be involved to advise on the suitability of such foods.

All individuals with, or identified as potentially being at risk of, nutritional problems should be regularly monitored and reviewed by the dietitian and other members of the care team.

Involvement of carers

Some relatives or carers might be very involved in the care and management of the patient and may take an interest in the nutritional management. Regular updates on a patient's weight, progress and nutritional intake may be an important part of dietetic input. Providing day in, day out care for someone with serious physical or psychological difficulties is exhausting and emotionally demanding, and people who have this responsibility require considerable support if they are to maintain their own physical and mental health. The needs of carers have been increasingly recognised in recent years and strategies are being put in place to provide better support measures (Department of Health, 1999).

Most units provide support groups or education sessions for carers and direct them to relevant long term support groups, e.g. Headway. Addressing the carer's needs ensures a more holistic approach to neurorehabilitation. The team can play an important part in ensuring that carers know about, and make use of, any available local support services, which could make life easier or help them feel less isolated.

Internet resources

Disabled Living Foundation   www.dlf.org.uk
Headway – the brain injury association   www.headway.org.uk
Royal Association for Disability and Rehabilitation (RADAR)   www.radar.org.uk
The Royal Hospital for Neuro-disability   www.rhn.org.uk
The Royal Hospital for Neuro-disability is a national medical charity, independent from the NHS. It is a hospital and a home that rebuilds the lives of adults affected by severe neurological disability, helping them to achieve the best possible quality of life.

Further reading

Braddom RL. (2004) *Handbook of Physical Medicine and Rehabilitation*. Pennsylvania: Saunders.

British Society of Rehabilitation Medicine (BSRM). (2008) *BSRM Standards for Specialist Rehabilitation Services Mapped on to the NSF for Long Term Conditions*. London: BRSM.

British Society of Rehabilitation Medicine/Job Centre Plus/Royal College of Physicians (BSRM/Job Centre Plus/ RCP). (2004) *Vocational Assessment and Rehabilitation after Acquired Brain Injury – Inter-agency Guidelines*. London: RCP.

Clifton DW Jr (2005). *Physical Rehabilitation's Role in Disability Management*. Missouri: Elsevier Saunders.

Davis S. (2006) *Rehabilitation – The Use of Theories and Models in Practice*. Oxford: Elsevier Churchill Livingstone.

Department of Health (2005). *The National Service Framework for Long-Term Conditions*. London: Department of Health. Available at www.dh.gov.uk. Accessed 25 October 2012.

Gronwall D, Wrightson P, Waddell P. (1998) *Head Injury-The Facts*, 2nd edn. Oxford: Oxford University Press.

Grieve J. (1993) *Neuropsychology for Occupational Therapists*. Oxford: Blackwell Science.

Kumar S. (2000) *Multidisciplinary Approach to Rehabilitation*. Massachusetts: Butterworth-Heinemann.

Laidler P. (1994) *Stroke Rehabilitation: Structure and Strategy*. London: Chapman & Hall.

Muir-Giles G, Clark-Wilson J. (1993) *Brain Injury Rehabilitation – A Neurological Approach*. London: Chapman & Hall.

NHS Confederation. (2005) *Supporting People with Long-Term Conditions*. Briefing no 112. London: NHS Confederation.

Nocan A, Baldwin S. (1998) *Trends in Rehabilitation Policy*. London: King's Fund.

Richards-Hall G. (1994) Chronic dementia – challenges in feeding an individual. *Journal of Gerontological Nursing* 20(4): 21–30.

Robinson J, Turnock S. (1998) *Investing in Rehabilitation*. London: King's Fund.

Rose FD, Johnson DA. (1996) *Brain Injury and After*. Chichester: John Wiley & Sons.

Sinclair A, Dickinson E. (1998) *Effective Practice in Rehabilitation*. London: King's Fund.

Turner-Stokes L, Tonge P, Nyein K, Hunter M, Nielson S, Robinson I. (1998) The Northwick Park Dependency Score (NPDS): a measure of nursing dependency in rehabilitation. *Clinical Rehabilitation* 12(4): 304–318.

References

British Society of Rehabilitation Medicine /Royal College of Physicians (BSRM/RCP). (2003) *Rehabilitation Following Acquired Brain Injury – National Clinical Guidelines*. London: RCP. Available at http://bookshop.rcplondon.ac.uk/contents/43986815-4109-4d28-8ce5-ad647dbdbd38.pdf. Accessed 7 February 2013.

Department of Health. (1999) *Caring about Carers: A National Strategy for Carers*. London: Department of Health. Available at www.dh.gov.uk. Accessed 25 October 2012.

Henson MB, DeCastro JM, Stringer AY, Johnson C. (1993) Food intake by brain injured humans who are in the chronic phase of recovery. *Brain Injury* 7(2): 169–178.

Labbe RF. (1986) Laboratory monitoring of nutritional support. *Archives of Pathology & Laboratory Medicine* 110: 775–776.

Osborn CL, Marshall MJ. (1993) Self feeding performance in nursing home residents. *Journal of Gerontological Nursing* 19(3): 7–14.

Potempa K, Lopez M, Brown LT, Szidon JP, Fogg L, Tinckernell T. (1995) Physiological outcome of aerobic exercise training in hemiparetic stroke individuals. *Stroke* 26(1): 101–105.

Royal College of Physicians/BSRM. (2010) Report of working party. *Medical Rehabilitation in 2011 and Beyond*. London: RCP/BSRM.

Turner-Stokes L, Tonge P, Nyein K, Hunter M, Nielson S, Robinson I. (1998) The Northwick Park Dependency Score (NPDS): a measure of nursing dependency in rehabilitation. *Clinical Rehabilitation* 12(4): 304–318.

VOICES (Voluntary Organisations Involved in Caring in the Elderly Sectors). (1998) *Eating Well for Older People with Dementia*. Herts: VOICES.

Watson R. (1994a) Measuring feeding difficulties in individuals with dementia: developing a scale. *Journal of Advanced Nursing* 19: 257–263.

Watson R. (1994b) Measuring feeding difficulties in individuals with dementia: replication and validation of the Ed Fed Scale #1. *Journal of Advanced Nursing* 19: 850–855.

Watson R, Deary IJ. (1994) Measuring feeding difficulty in individuals with dementia: multivariate analysis of feeding problems, nursing intervention and indicators of feeding difficulty. *Journal of Advanced Nursing* 20: 283–287.

Refsum's disease

Eleanor Baldwin

A Norwegian neurologist, Sigvald Refsum, first described adult Refsum's disease in 1946. He documented four cases from two families, who had been treated between 1937 and 1943. They initially presented with disturbed visual fields and subsequently developed abnormal gait, muscle wasting and paralysis (Refsum, 1946). He first chose the name heredoataxia hemeralopica polyneuritiformis, but later changed the name to heredopathia atactica polyneuritiformis. Fortunately, most of the scientific literature now uses the term adult Refsum's disease (ARD).

It is important when reviewing the literature on Refsum's disease to distinguish between ARD and infantile Refsum's disease (IRD), because they are completely different disorders, with different management strategies and prognosis. Infantile Refsum's disease is the mildest in the spectrum of a group of global disorders of the peroxisomal assembly. As a result, the peroxisome is deficient in multiple enzymes responsible for different metabolic functions. It presents in infancy with severe mental and physical retardation. Adult Refsum's disease is a disorder affecting one metabolic function of the peroxisome and presentation does not usually occur until the second to fifth decade of life with night blindness associated with retinitis pigmentosa and polyneuropathy or other signs.

Diagnostic criteria and classification

Adult Refsum's disease is a rare autosomal recessive disorder of lipid metabolism. Straight chain fatty acids are normally degraded by beta oxidation in the mitochondria. However, fatty acids with a complicated structure including a methyl or other functional group on carbon 3 can only be broken down by alpha or omega oxidation in the peroxisomes. The fatty acid phytanic acid (3, 7, 11, 15 tetra methyl hexadecanoic acid) is a common branched chain fatty acid in the diet that is derived from the microbial degradation of the chlorophyll side chain. Normally, this fatty acid is rapidly degraded by alpha oxidation so that plasma levels are usually less than 10 μmol/L (normal range 0–30 μmol/L). The alternative omega oxidation pathway for phytanic acid has a much lower capacity. Patients with ARD have a mutation in an enzyme in the alpha oxidation pathway that degrades phytanic acid. As a result, patients present with plasma phytanic acid levels ranging from 100 to 6000 μmol/L.

The clinical symptoms of ARD evolve slowly and visual symptoms are usually noticed first. Typically, night blindness occurs in the teens, followed by a reduction in the visual fields associated with retinitis pigmentosa. On questioning, patients describe anosomia (lack of sense of smell). Some will have bony abnormalities such as short third or fourth toes or fingers. Deafness, peripheral neuropathy and cerebellar ataxia develop later. Nerve conduction studies are abnormal, with slowing of conduction velocities, and cataracts are common. When the phytanic acid levels are very high (>1000 μmol/L), icthyosis (rough, hard, scaly, skin), paralysis and cardiac involvement (conduction abnormalities and cardiomyopathy) can occur.

A diagnosis of retinitis pigmentosa in association with any of the above symptoms should arouse suspicion of ARD. Suspected cases of Guillain–Barré syndrome, particularly when they present with acute demylinating polyneuropathy that appears to be familial and recurrent, should be tested for Refsum's disease as Refsum's can mimic Guillain–Barré (Verny *et al.*, 2006). Measurement of plasma phytanic acid and genetic testing will confirm the diagnosis of ARD.

Manual of Dietetic Practice, Fifth Edition. Edited by Joan Gandy.
© 2014 The British Dietetic Association. Published 2014 by John Wiley & Sons, Ltd.
Companion Website: www.manualofdieteticpractice.com

Genetics

Refsum's disease is genetically heterogenous; two Refsum's disease genes, phytanoyl CoA hydroxylase (PAHX) and peroxin 7 (PEX7, the PTS2 receptor), have been identified (Jansen *et al.*, 2004). Peroxin 7 is responsible for importing PAHX into the peroxisome along with a small number of other proteins. A severe deficiency in peroxin 7 function is associated with rhizomelic chondrodysplasia. A further enzyme defect in the alpha oxidation pathway involving alpha methyl acyl CoA racemase (AMACR) can mimic ARD, but levels of pristanic acid are more elevated than those of phytanic acid. Another Refsum like disorder has also recently been identified, called PHARC (polyneuropathy, hearing loss, ataxia, retinitis pigmentosa, cataract) (Fiskerstrand *et al.*, 2010), which involves deficiency in aldehyde. It is caused by mutations in alpha/beta hydrolase 12 (ABDH 12), which is involved in the metabolism of the endocannabinnoid 2 arachidonyl glycerol. This disorder presents with similar symptoms to ARD, but patients do not have anosomia and both plasma phytanic acid level and peroxisomal function are normal.

Metabolism and disease processes

The clinical manifestations of ARD usually begin in adolescence with night blindness and then progressive loss of visual field and diagnosis of retinitis pigmentosa (Reuther *et al.*, 2010). The other clinical manifestations described earlier develop later. Phytanic acid accumulates in the plasma and all fat containing tissues, liver, brain, adipose tissue, etc. The mechanisms that cause these symptoms remain obscure; however, molecular distortion and antimetabolite hypotheses have been put forward (Young *et al.*, 2001; Wierzbicki *et al.*, 2002); modern evidence favours a mechanism based on mitochondrial toxicity. Anecdotally, lifespan appears normal (personal communication). Provided phytanic acid levels are well controlled, the acute complications (cardiac), icthyosis and acute neuropathy do not develop. Retinitis pigmentosa seems to progress as people age and within siblings with the condition there can be significant differences in the clinical severity of symptoms (personal communication).

Management

Treatment of people with ARD follows three approaches:

- *Dietary restriction of phytanic acid* to a level (l<10 mg) at which the omega oxidation pathway has the capacity to manage and gradually reduce the phytanic acid present in the plasma. Case study reports and audits of groups of Refsum's disease patients attending a Refsum's clinic for more than 10 years have demonstrated that Refsum's patients can be successfully managed by diet, without the development of cardiomyopathy or high plasma phytanic acid levels requiring plasmapheresis (Baldwin *et al.*, 2010).

- *Supportive management of symptoms*. Cochlear implants have successfully treated deafness in at least three Refsum's patients (personal communication). Physiotherapy can induce symptomatic improvement in physical strength and emoliants can soothe itchy, scaly skin. Appropriate use of social services for sensory assessments and agencies such as the Royal National Institute for the Blind for advice on living with visual impairment and blindness can help patients to improve their quality of life.

- *Plasmapheresis* should be offered when the plasma phytanic acid levels are very high (1000 μmol/L and above) and acute symptoms such as cardiac abnormalities or acute polyneuropathy are evident, or the clinical condition of the patient is rapidly deteriorating. More than half of phytanic acid in the plasma is localised within very low density (VLDL), low density (LDL) and high density (HDL) lipoprotein particles. Low density lipoprotein and VLDL bound phytanic acid can be effectively eliminated from plasma with extracorporeal LDL apheresis using membrane differential filtration (Straube *et al.*, 2003).

Nutritional assessment

At diagnosis a full dietetic assessment should be made.

Anthropometry

Anthropometric assessment should include:

- Weight.
- Height.
- Body mass index (BMI).
- Weight history.

Dietary assessment

The dietary history should assess intake of foods rich in phytanic acid (Table 7.7.1). Phytanic acid is a type of fat made by some animals (ruminants) when they digest grass. It is also found in fish because they eat algae, or have eaten fish that have eaten algae. The higher the fat content of the food that contains phytanic acid, the higher the phytanic acid content will be, e.g. cheddar cheese will contain more phytanic acid than reduced fat cheddar cheese.

Caffeine intake and recreational drug use should be assessed. Adrenergic substances theoretically increase the plasma phytanic acid levels by increasing lipolysis.

Dietary management

Advice should be given on complete avoidance of foods containing phytanic acid (Table 7.7.1) and appropriate substitutes suggested. The Westminster Diet for ARD is based on the analysis of the phytanic acid component of common foods listed by Brown *et al.* (1993). The absolute level of phytanic acid in, for example, beef and dairy products will depend on the feed the cattle have been

Table 7.7.1 Foods rich in phytanic acid and suitable alternatives that are low in or contain virtually no phytanic acid

Foods	Foods containing phytanic acid – to be avoided	Foods low in phytanic acid
Meat, meat products and meat substitutes	Beef Beef burgers Calves liver and kidneys Cottage pie Duck Goose Lamb Mutton Meat lasagne Rabbit Shepherd's pie	Bacon Bean curd Chicken Chicken liver Turkey Eggs Ham Pork Pork liver and kidneys Pork sausages Quorn Soya meat substitutes, e.g. soya mince, soya sausages, etc. Tofu
Dairy products	Cheese made from cow's, sheep's or goat's milk Milk Cream Cow's milk (full cream or semi skimmed) Goat's milk Sheep's milk Ice cream Yoghurt (full cream or Greek) Butter Ghee	Cheese substitutes made from soya, e.g. Pure soya cheese spread, redwood soya cheeses, Bute island foods soya cheeses Cream substitute (Alpro soya single cream, soya too dairy free spray cream, soya too cooking cream and soya too topping cream) Cow's milk (skimmed only) Soya milk Swedish glace ice cream substitute Yoghurt (fat free or virtually fat free only) Soya yoghurt style puddings Low fat spreads made only from vegetable oil, e.g. Pure range Vegetable ghee
Other fats and oils	Suet	Vegetable suet, lard
Fish	Fish, especially oily fish such as herring, salmon and sardines Shellfish – clams, mussels, octopus, prawns, shrimps. Fish oil	Soya or pulse based fish substitutes such as Redwood foods fish style fingers, fish style steaks, scampi style pieces and Thai style fish cakes
Nuts	Walnuts and peanuts	Very few nuts have been analysed
Alcoholic drinks	Any drinks containing cream, e.g. Bailey's Irish Cream	Any alcoholic drink that does not contain cream
Bread and baked goods	Brioche, croissants, shortcrust pastry Biscuits and cakes made with butter, suet or fish oil	Puff pastry Filo pastry,* e.g. Jus-Rol All bread, biscuits and cakes that do not contain butter, suet or fish oil
Breakfast cereals	Tesco choco snaps	Breakfast cereals that do not contain milk powder (skimmed milk powder is appropriate) Small portions only of cereals containing nuts, e.g. muesli
Confectionery	Milk chocolate	Dark chocolate, carob, chocolate that does not contain milk fat or butter Fat free sweets, e.g. boiled sweets

*Check ingredients label as filo pastry is occasionally made with butter.

given (Lough, 1977). Therefore, the values in Brown *et al.*'s article should be taken as a representation only. The phytanic acid content of a food product will also relate to the overall fat content because phytanic acid is a fatty acid. Therefore, products such as semi skimmed milk will inevitably have a lower phytanic acid content than full cream milk.

Foods known to contain virtually no phytanic acid include:

- Most breakfast cereals (for exceptions see list).
- Safflower oil, corn oil, olive oil, sunflower seed oil.
- Bread, rice, pearl barley, pasta.
- Jelly.
- Honey.
- Tea, coffee.
- Cooked green vegetables, carrots, mushrooms, onions, potatoes and swede.
- Salad vegetables.
- Fruit.

A moderate caffeine intake (200–350 mg/day for adult women and 300–450 mg/day for adult men) should be advised.

A suitable n-3 fatty acid supplement should be encouraged as status in peroxisomal disorders is known to be low (Martinez *et al.*, 2000) and oily fish is excluded in ARD due to its high phytanic acid content (Omacor™ is the only supplement known to have a low phytanic acid content).

Anecdotal reports (Perera *et al.*, 2011) suggest that Orlistat therapy may be beneficial in some patients by reducing absorption of fat and fatty acids, including phytanic acid. However, weight loss must be monitored and rapid weight loss avoided.

Regular dietetic review is recommended to maximise dietary compliance and support people with ARD. The symptoms of ARD can be controlled by diet (Baldwin *et al.*, 2010), but deterioration in vision occurs over time. This can result in practical difficulties in following the diet (cooking, shopping and reading food labels), depression and social isolation, which can also affect body weight. It is also essential to ensure rapid access to advice on nutritional support to avoid deterioration during episodes of intercurrent illness or fasting for unrelated surgery.

During weight loss or fasting

During weight loss or extended periods of fasting, the plasma phytanic acid levels increase exponentially, doubling approximately every 29 hours (Wierzbicki *et al.*, 2003). This is because of the liberation of phytanic acid stored in the liver and adipose tissue. Patients often have a low BMI at diagnosis. Nutritional supplementation to promote weight gain may be required at diagnosis, during periods of intercurrent illness or pre or post surgery. Most nutritional supplements are suitable for use, with the exception of those containing fish oil, full fat milk or full fat dairy products, because these ingredients are rich in phytanic acid. Weight gain can cause a reduction in plasma phytanic acid as some of the phytanic acid will be shunted into adipose tissue deposits. Patients should be advised against weight loss unless the plasma phytanic acid levels are well controlled and their symptoms are stable. Where weight loss is advised, rates should be slow (0.25 kg or less/week) and the plasma phytanic acid levels should be closely monitored in order to detect and avoid deterioration.

Drug–nutrient interactions

The role of the peroxisome in drug metabolism in man is unclear, especially in patients with deficient or abnormal peroxisomal function. However, some lipid lowering drugs (e.g. fibrates) and hypoglycaemic drugs (thiazolidinediones; glitazones) rely on mechanisms associated with increased peroxisomal activity in animals and should be used with caution in people with peroxisomal disorders. The only common drug known to be metabolised through the peroxisome is ibuprofen, which is metabolised through a pathway involving AMACR. Therefore, alternative non-steroidal anti-inflammatory drugs are preferred in people with ARD.

Refsum's Clinic

Chelsea & Westminster NHS Foundation Trust, 369 Fulham Rd, London SW10 9NH. Tel: 020 8746 8178.

Internet resources

Adult Refsum's Disease   www.refsumdisease.org
Information for patients, carers and clinicians – devised by a European Union collaborative project for research into the diagnosis, prognosis and treatment of Refsum disease
Adult Refsum's Disease support network   www.health.groups .yahoo.com/group/refsumsdiscussion
National Information Centre for Metabolic Diseases (CLIMB)   www.climb.org.uk
Royal National Institute for the Blind   www.rnib.org.uk.
The Vegan Society   www.vegansociety.com

References

Baldwin EJ, Gibberd FB, Harley C, Sidey MC, Feher MD, Wierzbicki AS. (2010) The effectiveness of long-term dietary therapy in the treatment of adult Refsum disease. *Journal of Neurology, Neurosurgery and Psychiatry* 81(9): 954–957.

Brown J, *et al.* (1993) Diet and Refsum's disease. The determination of phytanic acid and phytol in certain foods and the application of this knowledge to the choice of suitable convenience foods for patients with Refsum's disease. *Journal of Human Nutrition and Dietetics* 6: 295–305.

Fiskerstrand T, H'mida-Ben Brahim D, Johansson S, *et al.* (2010) Mutations in ABHD12 cause the neurodegenerative disease PHARC: an inborn error of endocannabinoid metabolism. *The American Journal of Human Genetics* 87: 410–417.

Jansen GA, Waterham HR, Wanders RJ. (2004). Molecular basis of Refsum disease: sequence variations in phytanoyl-CoA hydroxylase (PHYH) and the PTS2 receptor (PEX7). *Human Mutations* 23(3): 209–218.

Lough AK. (1977) The phytanic acid content of the lipids of bovine tissues and milk. *Lipids* 12(1): 115–119.

Martinez M, Vázquez E, García-Silva MT, *et al.* (2000) Therapeutic effects of docosahexaenoic acid ethyl ester in patients with generalised peroxisomal disorders. *American Journal of Clinical Nutrition* 71(1): 376S–385S.

Perera NJ, Lewis B, Tran H, Fietz M, Sullivan DR. (2011) Refsum's disease – Use of the intestinal lipase inhibitor, Orlistat, as a novel therapeutic approach to a complex disorder. *Journal of Obesity* p. ii.482021. Epub 2010 Sep 1.

Refsum S. (1946) Heredopathia atacticsa polyneuritiformis: A familial syndrome not hitherto described. A contribution to the clinical study of the hereditary disorders of the nervous system. *Acta Psychiatrica Scandinavica* 21 (Suppl 38): 11–303.

Reuther K, *et al.* (2010). Adult Refsum disease: a form of taporetinal dystrophy accessible to therapy. *Survey Ophthalmology* 55: 531–538.

Straube, R Gackler D, Thiela A, Muselmann L, Kingreen H, Klingel R. (2003) Membrane differential filtration is safe and effective for the long term treatment of Refsum syndrome – an update of treatment modalities and pathophysiological cognition. *Transfusion and Apheresis Science* 29(1): 85–91.

Verny C, Prundean A, Nicolas G, *et al*. (2006) Refsum's disease may mimic familial Guillian Barre syndrome. *Neuromuscular Disorders* 16(11): 805–808.

Wierzbicki AS, Lloyd MD, Schofield CJ, Feher MD, Gibberd FB. (2002) Refsum's disease: a peroxisomal disorder affecting phytanic acid alpha oxidation. *Journal of Neurochemistry* 80: 727–735.

Wierzbicki AS, Mayne PD, Lloyd MD, *et al*. (2003). Metabolism of phytanic acid and 3-methyl-adipic acid excretion in patients with adult Refsum disease. *Journal of Lipid Research* 44: 1481–1488.

Young SP, Johnson AW, Muller DP. (2001). Effects of phytanic acid on the vitamin E status, lipid composition and physical properties of retinal cell membranes: implications for adult Refsum disease. *Clinical Science (London)* 101(6): 697–705.

7.8

Inherited metabolic disorders in adults

Sarah Boocock, Louise Robertson, Avril Micciche, Sarah Adam, Heidi Chan, Charlé Maritz, Sarah Ripley, Hazel Rogozinski, Pat Portnoi and Sarah Donald

Key points

■ Most inherited metabolic disorders (IMDs) require dietetic input as part of their treatment. This may include dietary modification of the amount or type of protein, fat and/or carbohydrate.

■ Many IMDs need an emergency regimen as part of treatment during a metabolic decompensation.

Inherited metabolic disorders (IMDs) are a rare group of genetic diseases where a mutation in a single gene affects the production or degradation of protein, carbohydrate or fat (see Chapter 5.1). There is often an enzyme or transport protein defect that can cause serious illness due to toxin accumulation if not treated. Inherited metabolic disorders can develop at any time, including during adulthood, but usually the later they present, the less severe they are. As medical science improves, more patients with IMDs are now surviving into adulthood, resulting in a need for adult services and a smooth transition from paediatric services. In the UK, the incidence is 1 in 800, but this varies between countries and ethnicity (Sanderson et al., 2006). This chapter outlines the dietetic treatment for adults with the most common IMDs and practical strategies to aid a successful outcome. Chapter 3.8.16 introduces the topic in children.

Phenylketonuria

Phenylketonuria (PKU) is an autosomal, recessive IMD caused by a deficiency of the enzyme phenylalanine hydroxylase (PAH), which catalyses the conversion of phenylalanine into tyrosine. High phenylalanine blood concentrations are neurotoxic during infancy and childhood, leading to irreversible brain damage if not treated from birth. The severity of PKU depends on the amount of residual activity of PAH.

Nutritional management

Dietary treatment is a restricted phenylalanine diet and involves:

- Protein substitute, which contains all the indispensable (essential) amino acids except phenylalanine – 60–80 g

of protein equivalent taken in three to four doses throughout the day.
- Low protein diet and exchanges (one exchange = 1 g of protein = 50 mg of phenylalanine).
- Prescribed low protein foods – bread, pasta, rice, flour, cereals and milk.
- Naturally low protein foods – fruit, vegetables, fats and sugars.

Patients on this PKU diet should be reviewed 6 monthly and those off diet annually (National Society for Phenylketonuria, 2004). Blood phenylalanine concentrations in adults should be monitored at least monthly using dried blood spot analysis [Medical Research Council (MRC), 1993]. Annual biochemical monitoring, including nutritional bloods and particularly vitamin B_{12}, is recommended (Hvas et al., 2006).

For those returning to the PKU diet, a step wise introduction should be used. A baseline measurement of blood phenylalanine should be taken before any dietary changes are made. It is important to identify the patient's or care team's reasons for recommencing the diet, as these can be later used as outcome measures to help ascertain the success of the diet.

Protein substitute should initially be given once a day and slowly increased to the full requirement. Once the full dose of protein substitute is reached, high protein foods can be safely excluded. Cow's milk should be swapped for a lower protein alternative and prescribed low protein foods should be introduced to help lower phenylalanine intake, ensure sufficient energy intake and provide variety. If the desired phenylalanine levels are not achieved, protein exchanges should be considered. A dietary review 3–6 months after restarting the diet can ascertain the benefits of the diet and whether it should be continued in late treated patients (see Late treated PKU section).

Table 7.8.1 Evidence for diet for life in phenylketonuria

Study findings when off diet	Reference
Negative mood reported by both patient and family member	Ten Hoedt et al. (2010)
Reduced quality of life	Bik-Multanowski et al. (2008)
Tremors, brisk tendon reflexes, and impaired co ordination	Cerone et al. (1999)
Lower scores on accuracy and performance speed when off diet for 5 years	Channon et al. (2007)
Phobias, low self esteem, social isolation and lack of autonomy	Brumm et al. (2010)

Diet for life

There is a growing body of evidence to suggest that patients with PKU should stay on diet for life. Table 7.8.1 summarises some of this evidence. Acceptable blood phenylalanine levels in adults vary worldwide with no general consensus. Levels range from <600 μmol/L in the USA and Germany, and <1200–1500 μmol/L in France. In the UK, a blood phenylalanine concentration of between 120 and 700 μmol/L is recommended, aiming for <480 μmol/L for good control (MRC, 1993). The restrictive nature of the PKU diet can make adherence challenging. It is vital to educate patients on the benefits of adhering to the diet, but also to support their decision if they choose not to follow the diet. For women of child bearing age the risks of conceiving off diet must be emphasised (see Maternal phenylketonuria section).

Adult patients can be classified into four groups, each with specific problems and nutritional issues requiring different strategies for care and monitoring (Figure 7.8.1).

Maternal phenylketonuria

Women with PKU must return to a strict diet when planning a pregnancy. High phenylalanine levels are teratogenic for the foetus and raised levels during pregnancy can cause microcephaly, mental retardation, congenital heart disease, spontaneous abortion and low birth weight (<2500 g) (Lenke & Levy, 1980).

Metabolic control must be closely monitored during pregnancy and the target range for phenylalanine should be maintained between 60 and 250 μmol/L (MRC, 1993); however, this range may differ at different centres. Tighter control is necessary as there is a positive amino acid gradient across the placenta, thereby exposing the foetus to higher phenylalanine concentrations than the mother (Cleary & Walter, 2001). Evidence suggests that optimal birth outcomes occur when the phenylalanine level is between 120 and 360 μmol/L by 8–10 weeks of gestation and this is then maintained throughout pregnancy (Koch et al., 2003). Ideally, patients should commence the diet before conception.

Preconception

Patients should have phenylalanine levels within the recommended range for a couple of weeks and feel confi-

dent about the diet before stopping contraception. A baseline blood test should be done before patients start the diet to give an indication of phenylalanine levels while off diet. The appropriate number of protein exchanges to start the diet can be estimated from the off diet level. Patients will be required to monitor this one to two times a week. Folic acid is provided in the amino acid supplements. However, if levels are low before going back on diet, patients may be advised to take a standard 400 μg preparation. Once the diet has been commenced, this can be discontinued provided the amino acid supplement has adequate amounts of folic acid and the serum folate level is within range.

Arachidonic acid (AA) levels appear adequate in PKU patients due to the abundance of linoleic acid in the diet from vegetable oils and spreads (Cleary et al., 2006). However, the conventional dietary sources of docosahexaenoic acid (DHA) such as fish are prohibited in the PKU diet. Evidence suggests that preformed DHA is needed in the diet (Cleary et al., 2006) and that DHA can have beneficial effects on foetal development (SACN & Committee on Toxicity, 2004). It has recently been recommended that pregnant and lactating women should have an intake of at least 200 mg of preformed DHA (Koletzko et al., 2008). Some amino acid supplements may already have added DHA or it can be given separately. Care should be taken to recommend DHA supplements without additional vitamins A and D.

First trimester

A frequent problem during the first trimester is morning sickness. Patients may find it difficult to tolerate the amino acid supplement and energy intake may be compromised due to nausea and vomiting. It may be useful to advise eating little and often, encouraging patients to have plenty of energy dense foods such as sugary, non-caffeinated drinks and to snack on low protein foods every 2–3 hours. This advice will help to prevent the phenylalanine level from increasing. Reducing the volume of supplement at each dose, spreading it out over the day or changing the supplement to tablet form may be useful. Increasing the dose of amino acid supplement to drive the phenylalanine level down is also advisable. Supplementing the diet with products such as glucose polymers will provide important extra energy (see Appendix A10). The phenylalanine level will increase if the patient becomes catabolic, which is detrimental to the foetus.

Second and third trimesters

During the second trimester (16–20 weeks), the phenylalanine tolerance increases as the baby grows rapidly and it may be necessary to increase the exchanges by two to three at a time to keep up with the baby's growth. It is also important to consider whether or not to supplement tyrosine during the pregnancy. Little evidence is available to support this, but it has been speculated that low tyrosine could be a factor in foetal damage in maternal PKU (Rohr et al., 1998). Practice varies but many centres supplement from 16 weeks of gestation onwards or when tyrosine levels are below 40 μmol/L. Tyrosine can

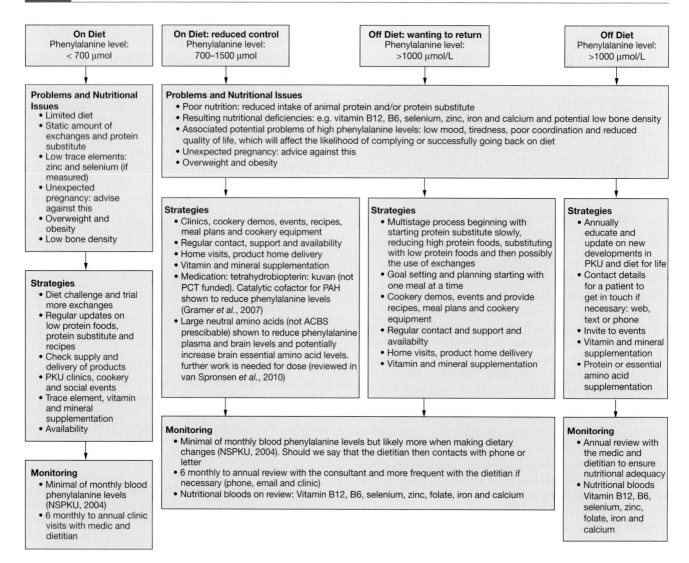

Figure 7.8.1 Challenges and strategies in adult phenylketonuria (PKU)

be supplemented using powder formulations. Aim to provide a total of 8 g of tyrosine/day from the supplement and additional tyrosine powder combined.

Late treated phenylketonuria

Adults with PKU born prior to the late 1960s typically have severe intellectual disabilities and challenging behaviour, as it was not until then that newborn screening for PKU was introduced. Patients were not commenced on diet early in life. These individuals should be considered for dietary treatment, because metabolic control has been shown to progressively improve behaviour in such patients (National Institute of Health, 2000). Phenylalanine concentrations in people with classical PKU are typically >1500 μmol/L pre diet. The desired blood phenylalanine concentration in treated adult PKU patients is 120–480 μmol/L but values up to 700 μmol/L still show benefits (MRC, 1993).

Anecdotal evidence suggests that lowering blood phenylalanine with a phenylalanine restricted diet can improve communication, relationships with carers and social skills, although not all show benefit. A randomised

placebo controlled double blind trial of a phenylalanine restricted diet in adults with late diagnosed PKU concluded that there are potential benefits to quality of life for the individuals and their carers (Lee *et al.*, 2009); while the overall benefit was not high, a positive effect in about three-quarters of the individuals was demonstrated. About 70% of the carers continued with the diet even after the trial had ended. Another study demonstrated that giving a phenylalanine restricted diet to adults with previously untreated PKU led to economic benefits to the UK's NHS and society in general (Brown & Guest, 1999).

Urea cycle disorders

The urea cycle metabolises the hepatic pool of nitrogen and a fault in an enzyme in the pathway results in a urea cycle disorder (UCD) causing hyperammonaemia (Leonard, 2006). Accumulation of ammonia in the brain may lead to damage that can result in coma and death if left untreated (Singh, 2010). Protein aversion is common, leading to disordered eating and a poor quality diet.

Some adults may rely on artificial feeding. There is limited evidence on the long term outcome in adults.

The UCDs are:

- Carbamoyl phosphate synthase deficiency (CPS).
- Ornithine transcarbamoylase deficiency (OTC).
- Citrullinaemia.
- Argininosuccinic aciduria (ASA).
- Arginase deficiency.
- N-acetyl glutamate synthase deficiency (NAGS).
- Ornithine amino transferase deficiency (OAT).

The most prevalent UCD results from OTC deficiency, which is an X linked disorder, while the other disorders are inherited in an autosomal recessive manner. Clinical presentation in adults varies due to residual enzyme activity, genotype and exogenous nitrogen load (Singh, 2007). By restricting nitrogen consumption from protein, ammonia production is limited. Ammonia scavenging drugs such as sodium benzoate and/or sodium phenylbutyrate are used to treat these disorders pharmacologically as they provide an alternative pathway for excretion of excess nitrogen (Scaglia, 2010).

Nutritional management

Long term management is to restrict protein intake whilst maintaining optimal nutritional status with supplementation. The WHO/FAO/UNU (2007) recommends safe protein levels based on actual body weight. Within that daily requirement, part of the protein intake should comprise natural protein, with the remainder from essential amino acid supplement. Protein tolerance is greater in those with higher levels of residual enzyme and when pharmacological doses are high (Singh, 2010). Protein should be evenly distributed throughout the day along with medication.

Energy provision should be sufficient to prevent fluctuations in weight. Sources include naturally low protein foods that are high in energy, specialist low protein prescribable items and high energy, non-protein nutritional supplements. Restricting protein also restricts the intake of certain vitamins and minerals and can therefore lead to significant deficiencies in the long term. Determination of micronutrient levels from diet diary analysis and plasma biochemistry is useful in influencing whether supplementation is required. Often, depletion in vitamin B_{12} and calcium levels is observed and regular monitoring of such nutrients after supplementation is a requisite.

Lean body mass will be broken down to produce arginine if the urea cycle does not produce sufficient quantities. Therefore, arginine becomes an essential nutrient and oral supplementation is necessary (Singh, 2007). L-Arginine can be administered in all the UCDs except in arginase deficiency where it does not become essential.

Treatment when unwell

Metabolic decompensation occurs when the body is in a catabolic state. This is exacerbated by infections, fever, trauma, surgery, intense physical activity and prolonged labour. During such periods, the body requires additional non-protein energy to prevent the breakdown of lean body mass. Withdrawal of protein should be initiated immediately and the oral emergency regimen commenced (see Emergency regimens section). Ammonia scavengers need to be administered orally or intravenously depending on the function of the gastrointestinal tract.

Organic acidaemias

Propionic acidaemia (PA) and methyl malonic acidaemia (MMA) are autosomal recessive disorders whereby isoleucine, valine, methionine, threonine and odd chain fatty acids are not metabolised fully. The deficient enzyme is propionyl-CoA carboxylase in PA, and methyl-malonyl-CoA mutase, which is vitamin B_{12} dependent, in MMA (Yannicelli, 2010). Some MMA patients respond well to vitamin B_{12} supplementation. Isovaleric acidaemia (IVA) affects leucine metabolism, whereas glutaric aciduria type 1 (GA1) affects lysine and tryptophan metabolism.

Nutritional management

This entails a high energy, low protein diet with supplementation of amino acids, except for the propiogenic acids in MMA and PA (Ogier de Baulny et al., 2005). Supplementation of glycine is indicated in IVA and lysine in GA1. L-Carnitine supplementation counteracts urinary losses of acylcarnitine (Ogier de Baulny et al., 2005). Vitamin and mineral replacement are advised to prevent deficiencies. Additional aims of the long term management include prevention of fasting and immediate medical and dietary treatment during illness (see Emergency regimens section).

Disorders of fatty acid oxidation

Fatty acid oxidation disorders (FAODs) are autosomal recessive genetic disorders in the mitochondrial fatty acid oxidation pathway. During increased energy demand, mitochondrial fatty acid oxidation plays an important role in energy homeostasis as it competes with glucose as the primary oxidative substrate (Spiekerkoetter et al., 2010). Fatty acid oxidation disorders vary in severity and can present in infancy or during adolescence and adulthood. During infancy patients typically present with encephalopathy and hypoglycaemia as a result of the accumulation of toxic metabolites or during periods of increased energy demand. Cardiomyopathy is a life threatening complication of acute metabolic decompensation in many patients with FAOD. Patients with a milder phenotype may not present until adulthood and typically present with exercise intolerance and recurrent episodes of rhabdomyolysis (the breakdown of muscle, which leads to the release of muscle fibre contents, myoglobin) and myoglobunuria (Gillingham, 2010).

Fatty acid oxidation consists of four components; the carnitine cycle, beta oxidation cycle, electron transfer path and ketone bodies synthesis (Stanley et al., 2006):

SECTION 7

- *Carnitine cycle defects* – carnitine transport defect (OCTN2), carnitine palmitoyltransferase 1 (CPT-1) deficiency, carnitine/acylcarnitine translocase (TRANS) deficiency and carnitine palmitoyltransferase 2 (CPT-2) deficiency.
- *Beta oxidation defects* – very long chain acyl-CoA dehydrogenase (VLCAD) deficiency, medium chain acyl-CoA dehydrogenase (MCAD) deficiency, short chain acyl-CoA dehydrogenase (SCAD) deficiency, long chain 3-hydroxyacyl-CoA dehydrogenase (LCHAD) deficiency, short chain 3-hydroxyacyl-CoA dehydrogenase (SCHAD) deficiency, medium chain 3 ketoacyl-CoA thiolase (MCKT) deficiency and 2, 4-dienoyl-CoA reductase (DER) deficiency.
- *Electron transport defects* – ETF/ETF DH deficiencies.
- *Ketone synthesis* – HMG-CoA synthase and HMG-CoA lyase.

Nutritional management

Fatty acid oxidation disorders are treated mainly by diet. The primary aim is to reduce fatty acid oxidation by avoiding fasting, limiting dietary fat intake in severe disorders and using the emergency regimen during illness.

Fasting

There are few published data on fasting duration in MCADD, the most common of the FAODs. It is important that prolonged fasting is avoided as fatty acid oxidation rates increase with fasting (Gillingham, 2010). The British Inherited Metabolic Disease Group (BIMDG) set a safe fasting time for older children and teenagers with MCADD as 12 hours (Dixon, 2007a). Generally, fasting for >12 hours should be avoided (Gillingham 2010).

Fats and essential fatty acids

Fat restriction in patients with SCADD and MCADD does not appear to be of any benefit and patients can follow a normal diet. In MCADD this is due to near normal oxidation of medium chain fatty acids (MCFAs) (Dixon, 2007a). Medium chain fatty acids enter the mitochondria without being bound to carnitine, therefore bypassing the step at which fatty acid oxidation is normally regulated (CPT1). Therefore, patients with SCADD or MCADD should never be given medium chain triglycerides (MCTs) as ingestion could lead to a more severe metabolic disturbance than with long chain fats (Gillingham, 2010; Dixon, 2007a).

For long chain fatty acid oxidation defects, dietary long chain fats (LCTs) should be restricted (calculated as a percentage of total energy derived from fat) to minimise fatty acid oxidation (Spiekerkoetter et al., 2010). The safe upper limit for LCT intake has not been established, as this will depend on the severity of the disorder (Dixon, 2007a). Patients on a low fat diet are at an increased risk for essential fatty acid (EFA) deficiency and supplementation with EFAs should be provided. In patients developing exercise induced rhabdomyolysis, enrichment of the diet with MCTs, with or without carbohydrates, prior to exercise may be beneficial (Dixon, 2007b; Spiekerkoetter et al., 2010).

Carnitine therapy

There is clear evidence that treatment with carnitine in patients with primary carnitine transport defect improves cardiac and skeletal muscle function (Spiekerkoetter et al., 2010). Supplementation with L-carnitine in long chain FAODs remains controversial (Gillingham, 2010; Stanley et al., 2006).

Emergency regimen

Intervention with increased fluid and carbohydrates during acute illness is crucial (see the Emergency regimens section).

Homocystinuria

Homocystinuria (HCU) results from a deficiency of the enzyme cystathionine β synthase (CβS), which is involved in the metabolism of the amino acid methionine. CβS is dependent on a cofactor derived from pyridoxine (vitamin B_6) and the biochemical response to pyridoxine distinguishes the two phenotypes of homocystinuria. In the pyridoxine responsive phenotype, pharmacological doses of pyridoxine partially or completely control the biochemical abnormalities, and in the non-pyridoxine responsive phenotype pyridoxine has no effect. The disorder is characterised by the accumulation of homocysteine and methionine in blood. Untreated homocystinuria can lead to developmental delay, ectopia lentis and severe myopia, skeletal abnormalities and thromboembolism (Levy et al., 2002). Newborn screening has led to early diagnosis and effective treatment, and fertility does not appear to be affected.

The biochemical aim of treatment is to control, and if possible normalise, the severe hyperhomocysteinaemia. The clinical aims are to prevent abnormalities in the four organ systems and optimise intelligence in patients diagnosed by newborn screening. In late diagnosed patients, the aim is to prevent life endangering vascular events and manage existing complications (Yap, 2003). Routine measurement of total homocysteine (tHcy) enables treatment effectiveness to be monitored. The aim is to maintain levels at 80–120 μmol/L; in the normal population tHcy levels are 5–15 μmol/L.

Nutritional management

Treatment of non-pyridoxine responsive homocystinuria is through dietary methionine restriction with methionine/protein exchanges (20 mg of methionine = 1 g of protein) and a methionine free amino acid preparation, e.g. XMet Homidon and HCU Cooler. Manufactured low methionine foods are available on prescription, provide variety in an otherwise very limited diet and are a valuable energy source. The protein substitute used should contain cysteine as this amino acid is usually formed from methionine but becomes deficient in HCU due to the metabolic block. The protein substitute should be given in divided doses together with the methionine exchanges at main meals. This prevents excessive rises in plasma homocysteine, ensures a complete range of amino acids and allows protein synthesis. If vitamins and minerals are not contained in the protein substitute, these must be provided separately. Folic acid (5 mg/day) is prescribed to ensure adequate intake for use in the remethylation pathway (Walter *et al.*, 1998). The principal pathway for the metabolism of dietary methionine is through conversion of homocysteine to cysteine.

Betaine

Betaine is a methyl donor that stimulates the methylation of homocysteine and reduces homocysteine levels, but usually results in significantly increased plasma methionine levels. Oral betaine can improve biochemical control in individuals where dietary compliance is poor. However, compliance with betaine can also be an issue. The safety of betaine therapy in pregnancy has not been established, but there have been reports that suggest no adverse maternal or foetal effects (Pierre *et al.*, 2006).

Maternal homocystinuria

Newborn screening has led to early diagnosis and effective treatment. Unlike maternal PKU, no strong evidence of teratogenic effects has been found. Fertility does not appear to be affected; however, the incidence of spontaneous abortion is high and there is evidence of increased risk for thromboembolic complications, especially postpartum. Anticoagulant therapy during pregnancy and 6 weeks postpartum will minimise these risks (Levy *et al.*, 2002).

Maple syrup urine disease

Maple syrup urine disease (MSUD) is characterised by the accumulation of the branched chain amino acids (BCAAs), leucine, isoleucine and valine, and their metabolites, which are neurotoxic and life threatening. Leucine is thought to be one of the main toxic metabolites and is restricted in the diet using leucine exchanges (50 mg of leucine = 0.5 g of protein = one exchange). Essential dietary components also include BCAA free protein substitute, vitamin and mineral supplements and low protein prescribed and natural foods similar to those for PKU. Dietary treatment is life long and aims to maintain plasma BCAAs within safe ranges; leucine 200–400 µmol/L, isoleucine 100–200 µmol/L and valine 100–300 µmol/L. Illness is treated by an emergency regimen that should include the usual protein substitute.

Tyrosinaemia

Type 1 tyrosinaemia results in an increased plasma tyrosine and its metabolites, including succinylacetone, which damage the liver. Treatment is a combination of 2-(2-nitro 4-trifluoromethylbenzoyl)-1, 3-cyclohexanedione (NTBC) and a low tyrosine, low phenylalanine diet, aiming to maintain plasma tyrosine at 200–400/500 µmol/L. A tyro-sine and phenylalanine free protein substitute is given, plus low protein foods (as in PKU). Tyrosine is given as 1-g protein exchanges.

Galactosaemia

Galactosaemia is an autosomal recessive, rare, inherited metabolic condition in which there is an inability to metabolise galactose. It is caused primarily by the deficiency of the enzyme galactose 1 phosphate uridyl transferase (GALT). Patients present initially in the neonatal period with a life threatening liver disease, and after the initial crisis, are managed with a low galactose, lactose free diet. Presentation at an adult clinic usually follows transfer from a paediatric clinic. Occasionally, patients present having been discharged from a clinic earlier in their lives and may not be on diet. As a result of the enzyme deficiency, galactitol and galactonate accumulate in abnormal quantities. Increased galactitol causes cataracts and galactonate is believed to play a role in hepatic and renal toxicity.

Ovarian dysfunction, central nervous system problems, language and speech defects, cataracts and reduced bone mineral density have been reported (Berry & Elas, 2011). Complications are independent of diet and occur even if the diet is started immediately after birth (Waggoner *et al.*, 1990, Schweizer *et al.*, 1993). The cause of these problems is unknown, but may result from endogenous galactose synthesis. Endogenous production is a constant in patients and is not influenced by diet. Adults have been shown to have slower rates of release of endogenous galactose than newborns (Schadewaldt *et al.*, 2004). Most centres measure red blood cell galactose 1 phosphate annually, and aim for levels of <0.60 µmol/g of haemoglobin (<150 µmol/L), but the measurement varies in and between individuals and is probably most useful as a compliance monitor, detecting severe non-compliance (Bosch, 2006).

Nutritional management

Life long dietary restriction of galactose is the only effective treatment for galactosaemia, i.e. following a low galactose diet. Table 7.8.2 summaries the issues associated with this diet. The main source of galactose is lactose; so all lactose is excluded from the diet. There are other sources of galactose, but in the UK these are not restricted and there is no evidence for making the diet stricter. Other countries may have different policies. The following are allowed in the UK:

- *Galactosides* – found in legumes, soya and cocoa. Although galactosides are the main subunit of these oligosaccharides, they are not hydrolysed by the intestinal mucosa.
- *Free and bound galactose* – occurs in small amounts in many fruits and vegetables, but is probably insignificant.
- *Galactose* – can also be found in offal in galactocerebrosides.

Table 7.8.2 Dietary issues in adult galactosaemia

Dietary and monitoring issues	Evidence	References
Need for strict life long dietary restriction	No randomised controlled trials in adults comparing patients on and off diet therefore consensus to maintain a low galactose diet for life. However, an individual with Q188R mutation stopped a strict diet at 3 years, and developed normally.	Lee *et al.* (2003)
Alcohol	No evidence that alcohol intake should be limited	Walter *et al.* (1999)
Bone mineral density (BMD)	Low BMD due to primary ovarian insufficiency	Rubio-Gozalbo *et al.* (2002)
Calcium and vitamin D supplementation	Supplement calcium, vitamin D and other nutrients to ensure long term bone health	MacDonald (2013)
Biochemical monitoring of control	Galactose-1-phosphate measurement varies in and between individuals and is better regarded as a compliance indicator Annual monitoring suggested	Bosch (2006) Walter *et al.* (1999)
Restriction of galactosides, free and bound galactose, galactocerebrosides	Foods containing these are allowed in the UK, but not in some other countries. There is no evidence to suggest that restriction of these foods is harmful	MacDonald *et al.* (2001); Bosch (2011)

Figure 7.8.2 Protected designation of origin (PCO) seal (source: European Commission, Agricultural and Rural Development 2013. Reproduced with permission of the European Commission, Agriculture and Rural Development)

Practicalities of a lactose free diet

Milk, all milk products and derivatives are excluded. This includes all milk (cow's, sheep's, goat's, etc.), yoghurt, most cheese, dairy desserts, butter and cream. Milk derivatives such as whey and casein must also be avoided. Low lactose milk and products are not suitable. All manufactured foods such as biscuits and cakes must be carefully checked. However, as milk is a potential allergen, and all allergens must be clearly labelled, all packaging should carry information on the presence of milk.

In the UK a number of hard mature cheeses are now allowed following extensive analysis. This includes Emmental, Gruyere, Jarlsberg, Italian Parmesan and Grano Padano. Only mature cheddar cheese from the West Country farmhouse Cheesemakers Association is allowed, and can be identified by the red and yellow PDO seal (Protected Designation of Origin), which is shown in Figure 7.8.2.

Calcium requirements for teenagers are particularly high and it is important for both adults and teenagers to have a good intake of calcium, as decreased bone mineralisation in both females and males has been reported

(Panis *et al.*, 2004). A calcium supplemented milk replacement is recommended (such as soya) and a calcium supplement is often necessary. The intake of other nutrients such as vitamin K and vitamin D must be adequate for good bone health. Alcohol is allowed in moderation; there is little information on its adverse effects in galactosaemia.

Diet for life

It is unclear how much tolerance to galactose changes with age. One adult woman with classical galactosaemia who discontinued her diet at 3 years has shown good progress (Lee *et al.*, 2003). However, relaxation of the diet in adults is not recommended.

Maternal galactosaemia

Pregnancy is not common in galactosaemia due to female fertility issues. However, if pregnancy occurs the diet should be followed strictly; outcome appears to be good.

Glycogen storage disorder types I and III

Glycogen storage disorder (GSD) type I is divided into two major subtypes, type Ia and type Ib. Type Ia is characterised by a deficiency in the enzyme glucose 6 phosphatase. Type Ib is characterised by a deficiency in glucose 6 phosphate translocase enzyme. These enzymes function together and are responsible for the breakdown of glycogen stores in order to maintain blood glucose levels within normal range during periods of fasting. Both subtypes phenotypically display glucose 6 phosphatase deficiency, characterised most usually by growth retardation, hypoglycaemia, hepatomegaly and a deranged biochemical profile (Goldberg & Slonim, 1993). Type Ib patients also suffer from chronic neutropenia and functional deficiencies of neutrophils and monocytes (Chou *et al.*, 2002).

Glycogen storage disorder type III is characterised by a deficiency in the glycogen debrancher enzyme (amylase

1,6 glucosidase). This is a key enzyme in the degradation of glycogen, and its deficiency leads to hypoglycaemia and an accumulation of short chain glycogen. Type IIIb is characterised by a deficiency of the debrancher enzyme in the liver only, whereas the majority of patients have type IIIa which is characterised by a more widespread deficiency of the enzyme in both skeletal and cardiac muscle.

Poor metabolic control comprising high plasma concentrations of uric acid, cholesterol, lactate and triglycerides consequently occur when patients are hypoglycaemic, which is frequently. It has been demonstrated that secondary metabolic control is better when the tendency toward hypoglycaemic episodes is decreased (Weinstein & Wolfsdorf, 2002). Long term consequences of GSD type I and III can include hepatic adenomas, hepatocellular carcinoma, progressive renal insufficiency, short stature and hypoglycemic brain damage (Roth, 2009).

The current treatment is dietary therapy to prevent and manage hypoglycaemia, and emergency regimens during periods of illness. In addition, patients with type Ib are also treated with granulocyte colony stimulating factor to restore myeloid function (Chou et al., 2002). Biochemical markers of poor control, such as lactate, cholesterol, uric acid and triglycerides, should be monitored in addition to liver ultrasound. These patients will also need to be monitored for any micronutrient deficiencies. Bone density may also be monitored. It is advisable for this group of patients to have a facility to test blood glucose while adjusting their diet, and cornstarch therapy or an overnight feeding regimen.

Nutritional management

The aim of dietary treatment is to maintain normoglycaemia. The following aspects of the patient's diet need to be taken into consideration.

Percentage of total daily energy from carbohydrate

It is recommended that 65% of total energy comes from carbohydrate sources, 10–15% from protein and 25% from fat (Goldberg & Slonim, 1993).

Meal and snack pattern

Most centres recommend small, frequent carbohydrate containing meals throughout the day with either continuous tube feeding overnight or the use of uncooked cornstarch (Glycosade®) to prevent hypoglycaemia (Mayatepek et al., 2010), with a guideline dose of 0.2–0.25 g of glucose/kg/hour (Dixon, 2007c). Some adult patients remain reliant on continuous overnight feeding

Supplementation with uncooked cornstarch (Glycosade®)

Uncooked cornstarch is digested slowly, providing a steady release of glucose in between meal times and overnight. The amount and timing of administration depends on the patient's weight and tendency towards hypoglycaemia during fasting periods. In most cases it is given every 4–6 hours. A weight based dose is given at bedtime to cover the fasting period overnight. Cornstarch should not be mixed with drinks high in ascorbic or citric acid, nor should it be heated.

Weight maintenance

Importantly, a balance between energy from cornstarch and normal food needs to be achieved in order to maintain weight and prevent micronutrient deficiencies. Patients should be encouraged to engage in physical activities up to individual limits, but to avoid contact sports due to the high risk of bleeding, infection and liver damage (Roth, 2009).

Fructose and galactose restriction

Some centres recommend a restriction in fructose and galactose containing foods, although the degree of restriction of these foods is still debated.

Emergency regimens

These patients should be provided with an emergency regimen during periods of fasting or illness (see Emergency regimens section).

Pregnancy in inherited metabolic disorders

An increasing number of children with IMDs are now surviving into adulthood due to expanding newborn screening programmes and improvements in diagnostic tests and therapeutic interventions (Lee, 2002). Many of these patients are able to integrate into the community, form relationships and have children (Lee, 2006). The main aim of managing a pregnancy in a woman with an IMD is to optimise maternal health by regularly monitoring metabolic markers and evaluating nutritional status at regular intervals.

Preconception

Fertility can be a problem in women with classical galactosaemia (Walter, 2000) due to primary ovarian failure, usually manifesting as secondary amenorrhoea (de Jongh et al., 1999). However, spontaneous pregnancies have been reported (de Jongh et al., 1999; Briones et al., 2001). In women with GSDI, subfertility may be due to oligomenorrhoea secondary to polycystic ovaries (Lee, 2006) and maternal HCU may be associated with a risk of early miscarriage, especially with poor metabolic control (Walter, 2000).

It is essential that all IMD patients are offered genetic counselling at the early stages of planning a pregnancy. The risk of having a child with MCAD is 1 in 10 000, but for adults with the condition the risk is 1 in 100 (Lee, 2006). Preimplantation genetic diagnosis is widely available for X linked IMDs such as OTC and antenatal diagnosis is also available.

Pregnancy

Although there are clear guidelines about managing pregnancy in PKU, little has been published regarding pregnancy in other IMDs, apart from case reports or small

SECTION 7

patient series (Walter, 2000; Langendonk *et al.*, 2012). A major risk for women with IMDs of energy metabolism (MSUD, UCD, FAOD, GA1 and GSD), especially during the first trimester, is metabolic decompensation due to morning sickness and weight loss. This can cause reduced intake of medication or dietary supplements, resulting in poor metabolic control (Lee, 2006). It is essential that women and their local obstetric services have an up to date copy of their oral and intravenous emergency protocol. Nutritional status and metabolic control should be optimised in all women on a restricted diet before conception to improve the outcome of the pregnancy (Lee, 2006).

The teratogenic effects of hyperphenylalaninaemia in maternal PKU have been well documented, yet little is known in pregnancies associated with other IMDs, although normal foetal outcome has been reported (Pierre *et al.*, 2006; Walter, 2000). Some IMDs worsen during pregnancy, such as dyslipidaemia, particularly hypertriglyceridaemia, in lipoprotein lipase deficiency leading to pancreatitis. The risk of thromboembolic complications during pregnancy appears to be increased in women with HCU. Anticoagulation therapy should be included in the management (Pierre *et al.*, 2006).

Labour

Labour and delivery is a period of increased metabolic stress and it is important that a clear delivery protocol is devised beforehand. Women may require additional energy supplementation, usually in the form of intravenous dextrose. Additional complications in labour may include bleeding tendencies due to platelet dysfunction in GSDI, deterioration of underlying organ damage, i.e. cardiomyopathy, in GSDIII and women with mitochondrial respiratory chain disorders may tire more easily during labour and need earlier intervention to shorten labour.

Post partum

The post partum period is a time of considerable risk for metabolic decompensation, especially in IMD of protein metabolism, such as MSUD and OTC deficiency. This could be due to an increased protein load following the involution of the uterus and can typically last up to 6–8 weeks. Women should continue oral or intravenous emergency regimens until they are able to have a normal oral intake post delivery. Women with HCU are at increased risk of venous thrombosis post delivery and aspirin and low dose subcutaneous heparin should be continued throughout. In addition, women who wish to breastfeed should be encouraged to have extra fluids and an increased energy intake.

Emergency regimens

Many inherited metabolic disorders are complicated by episodes of decompensation and potentially encepha-

lopathy, and require an emergency regimen. During episodes of illness, catabolism and a fasting state secondary to poor oral intake can cause the production of metabolites that, in specific disorders, have the potential to be toxic.

Metabolic disorders requiring an emergency regimen during periods of illness are:

* Urea cycle disorders.
* Organic acidaemias.
* Maple syrup urine disease.
* Fatty acid oxidation disorders.
* Glycogen storage disorders.
* Fructose-1, 6-bisphosphatase deficiency.
* Disorders of ketogenesis.

To prevent periods of decompensation, an emergency regimen should be administered. The emergency regimen is a glucose polymer solution (25% carbohydrate) that is given regularly while the usual diet is stopped for 24 hours. Glucose polymers used may include Maxijul, Polycal, Caloreen, Vitajoule and S.O.S 25.

The emergency regimen should be commenced immediately if the patient becomes unwell, e.g. nausea, vomiting, diarrhoea, high temperature or any illness resulting in loss of appetite and inability to take the normal diet. It is important to check regularly that the patient has an up to date emergency regimen, a supply of glucose polymer and knows how to make up the emergency regimen drink.

The aim of an emergency regimen is to provide an exogenous energy source to prevent catabolism, prevent or reduce production of toxic metabolites and prevent hypoglycaemia. The emergency regimen is the same for all disorders; however for some, it may be used in addition to medications and amino acid supplements (such as in MSUD). The emergency regimen is not nutritionally complete, so ideally should not be followed for >24–48 hours and it is advisable that the patient contacts their metabolic team to inform them that the emergency regimen is in use.

The emergency regimen formulation is a 200 mL drink (25% carbohydrate solution) given every 2–3 hours, day and night. It should aim to provide a total fluid volume of 2–2.4 L/24 hours. For patients who are vomiting, taking small sips frequently throughout the day may be easier. If the patient is tube fed, then a 24-hour feeding regimen can be devised that provides 25% carbohydrate. Alternatively, fruit juices and commercial drinks such as Lucozade original (17% carbohydrate) and Ribena (not light) (10% carbohydrate) can be used and extra glucose polymer added to make it up to a 25% carbohydrate solution.

Fat is not routinely used as part of the emergency regimen as it delays gastric emptying, may reduce palatability, is less easy to mix and may be difficult to take if the patient is vomiting. However, fat should never be added to the emergency regimen in fatty acid oxidation disorders. Dioralyte may be used to treat diarrhoea or vomiting; however, it contains very little glucose and is not a replacement for glucose polymer drinks and must be used in conjunction with glucose polymer drinks to provide an adequate concentration of carbohydrate. It may be advisable to provide a lower concentration of carbohydrate solution when the patient has diarrhoea to prevent exacerbating both the diarrhoea and the illness.

The emergency regimen should be started at home upon the first signs of illness. However, if the emergency regimen is not tolerated and the patient continues to vomit, they should attend an accident and emergency (A&E) department immediately as they will need 10% intravenous dextrose and medical management. Over the following 24–48 hours as the patient improves, intravenous fluids can be reduced as oral feeding is increased.

Reintroduction of normal diet

If the emergency regimen is well tolerated, the patient's normal diet or feeds can be reintroduced over 1–2 days. However, for patients usually on low protein diets, their normal diet should be gradually regraded over a period of 1–2 days. It is always beneficial to use their clinical condition as a guide. It is advisable to continue with the emergency regimen drinks until the patient is back to eating normally, clinically improving and receiving their full energy requirements.

A three stage approach to using the emergency regimen (Dixon & Leonard, 1992) is:

- If in doubt that the patient is unwell, give an emergency regimen drink and review their condition every 1–2 hours.
- If there is an improvement after this time, the normal diet can be resumed.
- If the patient's condition has deteriorated, the full emergency regimen should be commenced for 24–48 hours.
- If the emergency regimen is not tolerated, i.e. vomiting or refusing drinks, then the patient should go to A&E for intravenous fluids.

Further reading

Shaw V, Lawson M. (2007) *Clinical Paediatric Dietetics*, 3rd edn. Oxford: Wiley Blackwell.

Internet resources

Association for Glycogen Storage Diseases   www.agsdus.org
British Inherited Metabolic Disease Group   www.bimdg.org.uk
Galactosaemia Support Group   www.galactosaemia.org
National Information Centre for metabolic Diseases   www.climb.org.uk
National Society for Phenylketonuria   www.nspku.org
Nutricia Nutrition   http://nutrition.nutricia.com
Vitaflo UK   www.vitaflo.co.uk

References

Berry G, Elas L. (2011) Introduction to the Maastricht workshop: lessons from the past and new direction in galactosaemia. *Journal of Inherited Metabolic Disorders* 34: 249–255.

Bik-Multanowski M, Didycz B, Mozrzymas R, *et al*. (2008) Quality of life in non-compliant adults with Phenylketonuria after resumption of the diet. *Journal of Inherited Metabolic Diseases* 32(1): 126.

Bosch AM. (2006) Classical galactosaemia revisited. *Journal of Inherited Metabolic Diseases* 29: 515–525.

Bosch AM. (2011) Classic galactosemia: dietary dilemmas. *Journal of Inherited Metabolic Diseases* 34(2): 257–260.

Briones P, Girós M, Martinez V. (2001) Second spontaneous pregnancy in a galactosaemic woman homozygous for the R188R mutation. *Journal of Inherited Metabolic Diseases* 24: 79–80.

Brown MC, Guest JF. (1999) Economic impact of feeding a phenylalanine-restricted diet to adults with previously untreated phenylketonuria. *Journal of Intellectual Disability Research* 43: 30–37.

Brumm VL, Bilder D, Waisbren SE. (2010) Psychiatric symptoms and disorders in phenylketonuria. *Molecular Genetics and Metabolism* 99 (Suppl 1): S59–63.

Cerone R, Schiaffino MC, Di Stefano S, Veneselli E. (1999) Short Communication, Phenylketonuria: diet for life or not? *Acta Paediatrica* 88: 664–666.

Channon S, Goodman G, Zlotowitz S, Mockler C, Lee P. (2007) Effects of dietary management of Phenylketonuria in long-term cognitive outcome. *Archives of Disease in Childhood* 92: 213–218.

Chou JY, Matern D, Mansfield BC, Chen YT. (2002) Type I glycogen storage diseases: disorders of the glucose-6-phosphatase complex. *Current Molecular Medicine* 2(2): 121–143.

Cleary M, Walter J. (2001). Assessment of adult phenylketonuria. *Annals of Clinical Biochemistry* 38: 450–458.

Cleary MA, Feillet F, White FJ, *et al*. (2006) Randomised controlled trial of essential fatty acid supplementation in phenylketonuria. *European Journal of Clinical Nutrition* 60(7): 915–920.

De Jongh S, Vreken P, IJst L, Wanders RJA, Jacobs C, Bakker HD. (1999) Spontaneous pregnancy in a patient with classical galactosaemia. *Journal of Inherited Metabolic Diseases* 22: 754–755.

Dixon M. (2007a) Medium chain acyl CoA dehydrogenase deficiency. Available at www.bimdg.org. Accessed March 2011.

Dixon M. (2007b). Disorders of fatty acid oxidation and ketogenesis. In: Shaw V, Lawson M (eds) *Clinical Paediatric Dietetics*, 3rd edn. Oxford: Blackwell Publishing.

Dixon M. (2007c). Glycogen storage diseases. In: Shaw, Lawson (eds) *Clinical Paediatric Dietetics*, 3rd edn. Oxford: Blackwell Publishing.

Dixon M, Leonard J. (1992) Intercurrent illness in inborn errors of intermediary metabolism. *Archives of Disease in Childhood* 67: 1387–1391.

Gillingham MB. (2010) Nutrition management of patients with inherited disorders of mitochondrial fatty acid oxidation. In: Acosta PB (ed) *Nutrition Management of Patients with Inherited Metabolic Disorders*. Sudbury: Jones and Bartlett Publishers.

Goldberg T, Slonim AE. (1993) Nutrition therapy for hepatic glycogen storage diseases. *Journal of the American Dietetic Association* 93(12):1423–1430.

Gramer G, Burgard P, Garbade SF, Linder M. (2007) Effects and clinical significance of tetrahydrobiopterin supplementation in phenylalanine hydroxylase-deficient hyperphenylalaninaemia. *Journal of Inherited Metabolic Diseases* 30(4): 556–562.

Hvas A, Nexo E, Neilsen J. (2006) Vitamin B12 and Vitamin B6 supplementation is needed amongst adults with phenylketonuria. *Journal of Inherited Metabolic Disorders* 29: 47–53.

Koletzko B, Lien E, Agostoni C, *et al*.; World Association of Perinatal Medicine Dietary Guidelines Working Group. (2008) The roles of long-chain polyunsaturated fatty acids in pregnancy, lactation and infancy: review of current knowledge and consensus recommendations. *Journal of Perinatal Medicine* 36(1): 5–14.

Koch R, Hanley W, Levy H, *et al*. (2003). The Maternal Phenylketonuria International Study: 1984–2002. *Pediatrics* 112: 1523–1529.

Langendonk J, Roos C, Angus L, *et al*. (2012) A series of pregnancies in women with inherited metabolic disease. *Journal of Inherited Metabolic Diseases* 35: 419–424.

Lee PJ. (2002) Growing older: The adult metabolic clinic. *Journal of Inherited Metabolic Diseases* 25: 252–260.

Lee PJ. (2006) Pregnancy issues in inherited metabolic disorders. *Journal of Inherited Metabolic Diseases* 29: 311–316.

Lee PJ, Milburn M, Wendel U, Schadewaldt P. (2003) A woman with untreated galactosaemia. *Lancet* 362: 446.

Lee PJ, Amos A, Robertson, *et al*. (2009) Adults with late diagnosed PKU and severe challenging behaviour: a randomised placebo-controlled trial of a phenylalanine-restricted diet. *Journal of Neurology, Neurosurgery & Psychiatry* 80: 631–663.

Lenke RL, Levy HL. (1980) Maternal phenylketonuria and hyperphenylalaninaemia. *New England Journal of Medicine* 303: 1202–1208.

Leonard JV. (2006) Disorders of the urea cycle and related enzymes In: Fernandes J, Saudubray JM, van den Berghe G, Walter JH. (eds) *Inborn Metabolic Diseases: Diagnosis and Treatment*, 4th edn. Berlin: Springer.

Levy HL, Vargas JE, Waisbren SE, *et al*. (2002) Reproductive fitness in maternal homocystinuria due to cystathionine β-synthase deficiency. *Journal of Inherited Metabolic Diseases* 25: 299–314.

MacDonald A. (2013) *Manual of Clinical Paediatric Dietetics*, 4th edn. Oxford, Blackwell Scientific Publications (in preparation).

MacDonald A, *et al*. (2001) Abstracts, SSIEM 39th Annual Symposium: Prague, Czech Republic, 4–7 September 2001. *Journal of Inherited Metabolic Diseases* 24: Supplement 1.

Mayatepek E, Hoffmann B, Meissner T. (2010) Inborn errors of carbohydrate metabolism. Best practice and research. *Clinical Gastroenterology* 24(5): 607–618.

Medical Research Council (MRC) Working Party on Phenylketonuria. (1993) Recommendations on the dietary management of phenylketonuria. *Archives of Diseases in Childhood* 68: 426–427.

National Institute of Health. (2000) Phenylketonuria: Screening and Management. *NIH Consensus Statement* 17(3): 1–27.

National Society for Phenylketonuria (NSPKU). (2004) *Management of PKU*. NSPKU Pictorial Guide. Available from NSPKU www.nspku.org.

Ogier de Baulny H, Benoist JF, *et al*. (2005) Methylmalonic and propionic acidaemias: Management and outcome. *Journal of Inherited Metabolic Diseases* 28: 415–423.

Panis B, Forget PP, van Kroonenburgh MJ, *et al*. (2004) Bone metabolism in galactosaemia. *Bone* 35(4): 982–987

Pierre G, Gissen P, Chakrapani A, MacDonald A, Preece M, Wright J. (2006) Successful treatment of pyridoxine – unresponsive homocystinuria with betaine in pregnancy. *Journal of Inherited Metabolic Diseases* 29: 688–689.

Rohr FJ, Lobbregt D, Levy HL. (1998) Tyrosine supplementation in the treatment of maternal phenylketonuria. *American Journal of Clinical Nutrition* 67(3): 473–476.

Roth K. (2009) Genetics of glycogen-storage disease type I: treatment and medication. Available at http://emedicine.medscape.com/article/949937-overview. Accessed 1st December 2013.

Rubio-Gozalbo ME, Hamming S, van Kroonenburgh MJ, Bakker JA, Vermeer C, Forget PP. (2002) Bone mineral density in patients with classic galactosaemia. *Archives of Disease in Childhood* 87(1): 57–60.

Sanderson S, Green A, Preece M, Burton H. (2006) The incidence of inherited metabolic disorders in the West Midlands, UK. *Archives of Disease in Childhood* 91(11): 896–899.

SACN & Committee on Toxicity. (2004) Advice on fish consumption: benefits & risks. Available at http://cot.food.gov.uk/cotreports/cotjointreps/sacnfishconsumption. Accessed 20 August 2013.

Scaglia F. (2010). New insights in nutritional management and amino acid supplementation in urea cycle disorders. *Molecular Genetics and Metabolism* 100: S72–S76.

Schadewaldt P, Kamalanathan L, Hammen HW, Wendel U. (2004) Age dependence of endogenous galactose formation in Q188R homozygous galactosaemic patients. *Molecular Genetics and Metabolism* 81(1): 31–44.

Schweizer S, *et al*. (1993) Long-term outcome in 134 patients with galactosaemiae. *European Journal of Pediatrics* 152: 36–43.

Singh RH. (2007). Nutritional management of patients with urea cycle disorders. *Journal of Inherited Metabolic Diseases* 30: 880–887.

Singh RH. (2010). Nutrition management of patients with inherited disorders of urea cycle enzymes. In: Acosta PB (ed) *Nutrition Management of Patients with Inherited Metabolic Disorders*. Jones and Bartlett Publishers, Chapter 11.

Spiekerkoetter U, Bastin J, Gillingham M, Morris A, Wijburg F, Wilcken B. (2010) Current issues regarding treatment of mitochondrial fatty acid oxidation disorders. *Journal of Inherited Metabolic Diseases* 33: 555–561.

Stanley CA, Bennett MJ, Mayatepek E. (2006) Disorders of mitochondrial fatty acid oxidation and related metabolic pathways In: Fernandes J, Saudubray JM, van der Berghe G, Walter JH (eds) *Inborn Metabolic Diseases, Diagnosis and Treatment*. Berlin: Springer: Chapter 13.

Ten Hoedt A, De Sonnerville L, Francois B, *et al*. (2011) High phenylalanine levels directly affect mood and sustained attention in adults with phenylketonuria: a randomised double-blind, placebo-controlled, crossover trail. *Journal of Inherited Metabolic Disease* 34(1): 165–171.

Van Spronsen FJ, de Groot MJ, Hoeksma M, Reijngoud D, van Rijn M. (2010) Large neutral amino acids in the treatment of PKU: from theory to practice. *Journal of Inherited Metabolic Disorders* 33: 671–676

Waggoner DD, Buist NR, Donnell GN. (1990) Long-term prognosis in galactosaemia; results of a survey of 350 cases. *Journal of Inherited Metabolic Diseases* 13: 802–818

Walter JH. (2000) Inborn errors of metabolism and pregnancy. *Journal of Inherited Metabolic Diseases* 23: 229–236.

Walter JH, Wraith JE, White FJ, Bridge C, Till J. (1998) Strategies for the treatment of Cystathionine β-synthase deficiency: the experience of the Willink Biochemical Genetics Unit. *European Journal of Pediatrics* (Suppl 2): S71–S76.

Walter JH, Collins JE, Leonard JV. (1999) Recommendations for the management of galactosaemia: UK Galactosaemia Steering Group. *Archives of Disease in Childhood* 80(1): 93–96.

Weinstein DA, Wolfsdorf JI. (2002) Effect of continuous glucose therapy with uncooked cornstarch on the long-term clinical course of type 1a glycogen storage disease. *European Journal of Pediatrics* 161 (Suppl 1): S35–S39.

WHO/FAO/UNU Expert Consultation. (2007) *Protein and Amino Acid Requirements in Human Nutrition*. WHO Technical Report Series no. 935. Singapore: United Nations University Press.

Yannicelli S. (2010) Nutritional management of patients with inherited disorders of organic acid metabolism. In: Acosta PB (ed) *Nutrition Management of Patients with Inherited Metabolic Disorders*. Sudbury: Jones and Bartlett Publishers, Chapter 8.

Yap S. (2003) Classical homocystinuria: Vascular risk and its prevention. *Journal of Inherited Metabolic Diseases* 26: 259–265.

7.9

Musculoskeletal disorders

7.9.1 Osteoporosis

Jean Redmond and Inez Schoenmakers

Key points

- Osteoporosis is the most common clinical disorder of bone metabolism; it is a major and increasing public health problem.

- To maximise peak bone mass attainment and to minimise age related bone loss, a balanced diet sufficient in calcium, good vitamin D status and regular weight bearing physical activity are essential.

- Low bone mineral density, a high propensity to fall, a low body weight and other comorbidities are risks for osteoporotic fracture.

- A high percentage of hip fracture patients are malnourished on admission to hospital and their nutritional status may decline in the postoperative period.

Osteoporosis is the most common clinical disorder of bone metabolism and primarily affects the elderly population. It is characterised by low bone mass and microarchitectural deterioration of bone tissue with a consequent increase in bone fragility and susceptibility to fractures (World Health Organization, 1994). Osteoporotic fractures are a significant cause of morbidity and mortality, particularly in developed countries (Johnell & Kanis, 2006). Most commonly, these are fractures of the hip, vertebrae and wrist. The incidence of osteoporotic fractures increases with advancing age, and the lifetime risk of any osteoporotic fracture lies within the range of 40–50% in women and 13–22% for men (Johnell & Kanis, 2005). As people live longer and the world's population grows, osteoporosis and fracture incidence will increase. The estimated 1.7 million hip fractures occurring worldwide in 1990 may rise to 6.3 million by 2050 (Cooper *et al.*, 1992), with Asia expecting to see the greatest increases (Cooper *et al.*, 1992; Prentice, 2004).

Fractures are associated with a substantial decline in an individual's functional status, a loss of independence, difficulty with normal daily activities and chronic pain. In particular, hip fractures are associated with significant increases in morbidity and mortality in the elderly (Bentler *et al.*, 2009). These fractures can also cause psychological symptoms (most notably depression and loss of self esteem), associated morbidity and consequent dependency that may influence social roles for patients and their families (National Osteoporosis Foundation, 2010).

The pathogenesis of osteoporosis reflects the complex interaction between genetic, metabolic and environmental factors that determine bone growth, peak bone mass, calcium homeostasis and bone loss. Ageing, physical activity, sex hormone levels and nutritional status influence these factors. The increasing burden of osteoporosis means that modifiable factors such as nutrition have become of public health importance.

Functions and structure of bone and disease process

Bone is a specialised connective tissue, serving three major functions:

- Metabolic – a reserve and buffer of minerals.
- Mechanical – providing structure and muscular attachment for movement.
- Protective – enclosing bone marrow and vital organs.

Metabolic control of calcium

The metabolic function of bone is crucial for calcium homeostasis. The plasma concentration of ionised calcium is strictly maintained, which is essential for the functioning of all body cells (Department of Health, 1998). When ionised calcium concentration falls, the parathyroid hormone (PTH) concentration increases, which inhibits renal calcium excretion and stimulates liberation of calcium from bone. Parathyroid hormone also stimulates the renal synthesis of the active form of vitamin D (calcitriol, $1,25(OH)_2D$) which, in turn, enhances intestinal calcium absorption.

Structure of bone

Macroscopically bone has two components that differ in structure and function; cortical (compact) bone with a dense structure and trabecular (cancellous) bone, consisting of a latticework of bony tissue (trabeculae) (Department of Health, 1998). The adult human skeleton is composed of 80% cortical bone and 20% trabecular bone; different bones have different ratios of cortical to trabecular bone (Clarke, 2008). Cortical bone has mainly mechanical and protective functions, whereas trabecular bone also has a metabolic function in mineral regulation (Department of Health and Human Services, 2004). Bone consists of an extracellular mineralised matrix and a number of cell types, including osteoblasts, osteocytes and osteoclasts, and the cells of its vascular and nervous supply. The matrix consists of mineral salts [mainly hydroxyapatite ($Ca_{10}(PO_4)_6(OH)_2$) crystals] bound to proteins, largely collagen (Department of Health and Human Services, 2004). The osteoblast is the primary bone forming cell which creates the osteoid (prebone tissue), and facilitates calcification. Osteoclasts remove bone tissue and provide for the release of calcium and phosphate ions. The osteocytes respond to changes in strain on bone, thereby driving and regulating the action of osteoblasts and osteoclasts (Ward, 2011).

Bone development, metabolism and the development of osteoporosis

Two processes, modelling and remodelling, mediate change in size and shape of bone during bone growth and in response to mechanical stress (Department of Health and Human Services, 2004). During childhood and adolescence, the process of modelling allows for skeletal growth. Increases in length, i.e. longitudinal growth, occur at the growth plates (Clarke, 2008), while increases in diameter, i.e. radial growth, result from the deposition of new bone on the external surfaces and resorption on the internal surfaces. An increase in the amount of bone tissue occurs until peak bone mass (PBM) is achieved. The majority of bone mass is achieved by the end of longitudinal growth (~18 years) and an additional 5–10% of bone mass is accrued during the third decade of life. Gender and ethnic differences determine PBM, as well as a variation determined by lifestyle factors (Rizzoli & Bonjour, 1999). Achieving a high PBM within an individual's genetic potential is crucial for the prevention of osteoporosis in later life.

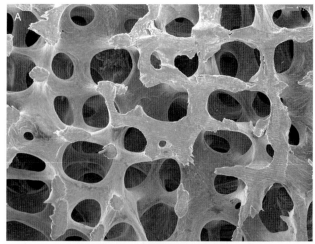

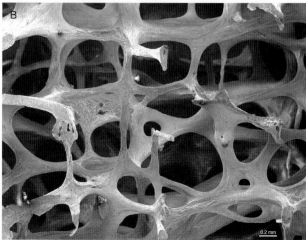

Figure 7.9.1 Comparison of (A) normal and (B) osteoporotic vertebrae, with thinning of the trabeculae (source: T. Arnett, University College London, 2013. Reproduced with permission of T. Arnett)

After skeletal growth is complete, remodelling of bone continues throughout adulthood. In health, remodelling is a coupled process; the amount of bone removed by resorption is replaced by new bone formation. Bone loss occurs when the rate of bone resorption exceeds that of bone formation (Figure 7.9.1), and occurs during menopause and with advancing age (National Osteoporosis Foundation, 2010) (Figure 7.9.2). The lifetime risk of developing osteoporosis is therefore determined by a combination of:

- Attainment of maximal PBM through optimal growth in childhood, adolescence and young adulthood.
- Maintenance of bone mass in middle age.
- Rate of age related bone loss.

Diagnostic criteria and classification

The diagnosis of osteoporosis relies on the quantitative assessment of bone mineral density (BMD) or bone mineral content (BMC), usually by dual energy X ray absorptiometry (DXA) of the axial skeleton (skull, spine, ribs and sternum), with the femoral neck providing the reference site (National Osteoporosis Guideline Group,

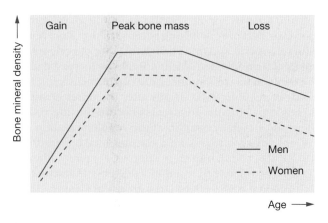

Figure 7.9.2 Age related changes in bone mass throughout life (source: Poole & Compston 2006, figure 5, p. 1252. Reproduced with permission of the *British Medical Journal*)

Table 7.9.1 Classification of bone mass and osteoporosis in adults (WHO, 1994)

Normal	BMD or BMC ≤1 SD below the average value of young adults
Low bone mass or osteopenia	BMD or BMC >1 SD below the young adult average but ≤–2.5 SD
Osteoporosis	BMD or BMC >2.5 SD below the young adult average value
Severe osteoporosis (established osteoporosis)	BMD or BMC >2.5 SD below the young adult average value and presence of one or more fragility fractures

NB: These cut-offs do not apply to children
BMD, bone mineral density; BMC, bone mineral content.

Table 7.9.2 Clinical risk factors used for the assessment of fracture probability [adapted from National Osteoporosis Guideline Group (2010)]

Age
Sex
Low body mass index (≤19 kg/m²)
Previous fragility fracture, particularly of the hip, wrist and spine, including morphometric vertebral fracture
Parental history of hip fracture
Current glucocorticoid treatment (any oral dose for 3 months or longer)
Current smoking
Alcohol intake of ≥3 units/day
Propensity to fall

Specific patient groups at increased risk of osteoporosis
Rheumatoid arthritis
Inflammatory bowel disease (Crohn's disease/ulcerative colitis)
Coeliac disease
Anorexia nervosa
Athletic amenorrhea
Malabsorption syndromes
Untreated hypogonadism in men and women
Prolonged immobility
Organ transplantation
Type I diabetes
Hyperthyroidism and hyperparathyroidism
Chronic liver disease
Chronic obstructive pulmonary disease

Drugs that may influence bone metabolism
Corticosteroids
Thyroxine
Heparin
Loop diuretics, e.g. furosemide, increase urinary excretion of calcium (unlike thiazides which decrease calcium loss)
Proton pump inhibitors (PPIs) interfere with calcium absorption

2010). Categories of the disease are defined in terms of bone mineral mass, as shown in Table 7.9.1 (World Health Organization, 1994). These diagnostic criteria apply to post menopausal women and men aged 50 years and older, but may not apply to premenopausal women and younger men (Lewiecki *et al.*, 2008).

Osteoporosis is associated with an increased risk of fragility fracture, i.e. fractures caused by minimal trauma, such as a fall from a standing position (Prentice *et al.*, 2006). These fractures are most common at the hip, vertebrae and wrist, but osteoporotic fractures can occur elsewhere in the skeleton (Prentice *et al.*, 2006). At present there is no universally accepted policy for population screening in the UK and most other countries to identify individuals with osteoporosis or those at high risk of fracture. Patients are identified opportunistically on the finding of a previous fragility fracture or the presence of significant clinical risk factors, as shown in Table 7.9.2. These factors may act through their association with low BMD or through a BMD independent mechanism (Poole & Compston, 2006; National Osteoporosis Guideline Group, 2010).

The differential diagnosis of osteoporosis is based on the assessment of risk factors and a range of tests. The choice of test depends on the severity of the disease, age at presentation and the presence or absence of fractures

(National Osteoporosis Guideline Group, 2010). Routine investigations to exclude secondary causes of osteoporosis include full blood count and erythrocyte sedimentation rate, liver and renal function tests, bone function tests (calcium, phosphate, vitamin D status, PTH and alkaline phosphatase) and thyroid function tests (Poole & Compston, 2006), and may include assessment of nutrient deficiencies.

The National Institute for Health and Care Excellence (2012) recommends the assessment of the risk of fragility fracture using either FRAX® (FRAX (www.shef.ac.uk/FRAX) or QFracture (www.qfracture.org). FRAX®, the WHO fracture risk assessment tool, can be used for people aged 40–90 years with or without BMD values, and can be applied to men and women from several European countries (National Osteoporosis Guideline Group, 2010). QFracture can be used for people aged between 30 and 84 years without the requirement of BMD values and is validated in UK primary care populations to include ethnic origin and many comorbidities.

Dietary assessment

Dietary assessment through a 24-hour diet history and food frequency questionnaire or through the use of food diaries will indicate if a patient's dietary calcium intake and other nutrients are adequate to meet recommendations.

Nutritional aspects of bone development and osteoporosis

A range of nutrients are involved in bone development and maintenance. Bone formation requires adequate supplies of energy, amino acids, the main bone forming minerals (calcium, phosphorus, magnesium and zinc) and other ions including copper, manganese, carbonate and citrate, and vitamins (C, D, K) that are involved in crystal and collagen formation, cartilage and bone metabolism and/or calcium and phosphate homeostasis (Prentice et al., 2006). Of these, calcium and vitamin D are the most commonly associated with bone health (Shea et al., 2002; Greer & Krebs; 2006; Huncharek et al., 2008).

General recommendations are to consume a calcium intake close to the reference nutrient intake (RNI), optimise vitamin D status through adequate summer sunshine exposure (and dietary supplementation where appropriate), be physically active, have a body weight in the healthy range, restrict salt intake and consume plenty of fruit and vegetables (Department of Health, 1998).

Calcium

The evidence base for the long term effects of dietary calcium intake on bone health through randomised controlled trials is limited and there are knowledge gaps, particularly in children and young adults. In addition, a paradox exists between populations; while a low calcium intake is associated with an increased risk of osteoporosis in older Caucasian subjects, this may not be the case universally (Prentice, 2004). In the UK, the RNI for calcium is derived factorially and is calculated on the basis of the needs for growth and the maintenance of bone mineralisation, and takes into account factors influencing bioavailability of calcium to the skeleton (Department of Health, 1998). The RNI represents a value that is likely to provide for the nutrient needs of 95% of the population. There is no international consensus on calcium recommendations. The recommendation in the UK and European Commission are similar, but may be different from specific EU countries and the USA.

Children

Children need to absorb 70–150 mg of calcium/day for growth and bone mineralisation. Adolescent females and males require at least 250 mg and 300 mg/day, respectively (Department of Health, 1998). Taking into consideration the percentage of calcium absorbed, the RNI and recommended daily amount (RDA) are set between 350 and 1300 mg/day (see Appendix A2). Results from observational and intervention studies indicate that a higher intake of dietary calcium or dairy products, with and without vitamin D, significantly increases total body and lumbar spine BMC in children and reduces the risk of fractures (Goulding et al., 2004; Manias et al., 2006). This may be particularly relevant in individuals with low

calcium intakes, or at specific stages of development. However, data are conflicting because of the 'bone remodelling transient' and/or a change in a rate of bone remodelling occurring when calcium intake is increased above the habitual intake (Prentice, 2004). This may result in an initial increase in BMD shortly after the onset of supplementation, with little additional effect of the intervention thereafter or after cessation of the supplementation. The current advice is to ensure a calcium intake close to the RNI or RDA and that calcium supplementation in healthy children is unlikely to result in a decrease in fracture risk (Winzenberg et al., 2006; Department of Health, 1998).

Young adults

From about age of 35–40 years, bone mineral is lost at an average rate of 0.3–0.4% of bone mass/year. During this time, a healthy balanced diet should be followed, while remaining physically active and maintaining a healthy body weight.

Older age

A phase of rapid bone loss occurs in women during the first 5–10 years after the menopause, after which bone loss occurs at a slower rate (see Chapter 3.1.3). Calcium supplementation has little effect on BMD in women who are within the first 5 years after the menopause (Department of Health, 1998), although calcium may be effective in reducing bone loss during later post menopause (>5 years) (Dawson-Hughes et al., 1990). A meta analysis reported that calcium supplementation as a stand alone intervention has a small, but positive, effect on bone density and a trend toward reduction in vertebral fractures (Shea et al., 2002). Calcium supplementation over 4 years may reduce bone loss from the hip and femoral neck in both men and women with low dairy intakes (McCabe et al., 2004). However, the long-lasting effects of calcium supplementation are not clear. Speculation has also arisen regarding calcium supplementation (but not dietary calcium intake) and an increased risk of cardiovascular disease (Bolland et al., 2011; Li et al., 2012). Observational studies reported that a higher lifetime and current calcium intake are associated with a reduced risk of osteoporosis (Nieves et al., 2008). Men are also affected by age related bone loss. A cross sectional analysis demonstrated that dairy calcium intake was positively associated with total hip and femoral neck BMD in men aged older than 60 years (McCabe et al., 2004).

Dietary sources

Calcium is present in a wide range of foods, although the bioavailability may vary appreciably. Dairy products, such as milk, yoghurt and cheese, are all good sources of bioavailable calcium, and provide more calcium per calorie than any other typical food in a western diet (Heaney, 2000). Fish that is consumed whole with the soft edible bones (such as whitebait, canned sardines or canned salmon) is also a good source of calcium. In some countries there is statutory fortification with calcium, e.g. in the UK, there is a requirement that flour is fortified with calcium, in addition to optional fortification of certain products by the food industry. For those following a vegan diet, pulses, whole grains, nuts and seeds, dried fruit (such as apricots), tofu and green vegetables, such as spinach, broccoli and kale, provide a source of calcium, although the bioavailability is not as high as from dairy products. For those who are unable to consume foods that provide good sources of calcium, e.g. due to milk allergy or because they are vegan, foods that are fortified with calcium or calcium supplements are advisable (see Chapter 3.6). The British Dietetic Association (2005) recommends a point system whereby each point is 50 mg of calcium and at least 14 points daily should be consumed (see Appendix A5). Additional considerations for dietary advice include:

- Low fat dairy products contain similar amounts of calcium as full fat products and may be more suitable for those on a cardioprotective diet.
- Gluten free bread varies in calcium content, and this should be taken into consideration when advising a coeliac patient.
- Soya products are good alternatives to cow's milk for dairy free or vegan diets; calcium enriched options should be advised. However, phytic acid in soya reduces the calcium bioavailability to approximately 75% that of cow's milk.
- Calcium from drinking water is well absorbed, but the contribution of water to nutrient intake is generally not assessed. The calcium content of water varies from region to region (0–300 mg/L) (Department of Health, 1998).

Vitamin D

Vitamin D is essential for the development and maintenance of a healthy skeleton and for muscle function. Classical vitamin D deficiency causes rickets in children and osteomalacia in children and adults; it is associated with increased bone loss in older people. It is also associated with muscle weakness and a propensity to fall (Prentice et al., 2008, Bischoff-Ferrari et al., 2005; 2006; Francis, 2007). Intervention studies have reported conflicting results and may be discordant with observational studies. In addition, data in younger people are scarce (Ross et al., 2010). Meta analyses of vitamin D supplementation trials in older adults investigating the effect on fracture risk and falls have concluded that vitamin D supplementation with >700 IU/day (17.5 μg/day) is needed for a beneficial effect (Bischoff-Ferrari et al., 2005; 2006; Francis, 2007).

Vitamin D status is assessed by the measurement of the plasma concentration of 25(OH)D, which serves as a reservoir for further hydroxylation to the active metabolite $1,25(OH)_2D$. Vitamin D deficiency is defined as a plasma concentration of 25(OH)D of <25 nmol/L in the UK and <40–60 nmol/L in the USA (Department of Health, 2007; Ross et al., 2010,), although other thresholds have been proposed (Prentice et al., 2008; Ross et al., 2010).

There are two forms of vitamin D, D_3 and D_2. Vitamin D_3 can be obtained from the diet and by cutaneous synthesis following exposure to sunlight (Fraser, 2004; Lips, 2007; Prentice, 2008). Very few foods are natural sources of vitamin D_3, but it is available in supplements and used in food fortification (Ovesen et al., 2003). Vitamin D_2 is derived from plant sources, and may be the preferred form for vegans. While vitamin D_3 and D_2 are considered to have the same antirachitic activity, recent studies have shown that vitamin D_3 may increase plasma 25(OH) D more efficiently than vitamin D_2 (Ross et al., 2010; Department of Health, 2007), but this may be overcome by more frequent intake of vitamin D_2.

The proportion of vitamin D that is derived from sun exposure versus diet varies considerably worldwide, across population groups and between individuals, mainly because of wide differences in skin exposure to ultraviolet B (UVB) radiation, cutaneous synthesis, e.g. due to ageing and skin pigmentation, and in food fortification practices and supplement use (Lips, 2007; Fraser, 2004). Older people are vulnerable to vitamin D insufficiency because cutaneous synthesis becomes less efficient, and declining kidney function is associated with impaired synthesis of active forms of vitamin D. Those who are housebound or living in institutions are at risk due to limited opportunities for sun exposure. Limited and unvaried diets are common in elderly people and may exacerbate the problem. If cutaneous synthesis is insufficient, meeting the recommended intakes for vitamin D through the use of supplements may be needed.

In the UK and the USA, the RNI and RDA for vitamin D (see Appendix A2) are based on the requirements for bone health and assume adequate intakes of other nutrients. In the UK, a RNI is not set for people between 4 and 64 years of age because it is assumed that skin synthesis will generally ensure adequacy. Those at risk of inadequate sunlight exposure should ensure sufficient dietary vitamin D or consider supplementation. A RNI of 10 μg (400 IU)/day has been made for pregnant and lactating women, individuals confined indoors and for those in the population aged over 65 years. In contrast, the US RDA assumes a moderate contribution from cutaneous produced vitamin D in the general public; a RDA is formulated for all age groups. The European Union population reference intake is 0–10 μg/day for every age group.

Other nutrients and food groups

Protein and acid–base balance

Protein intake affects bone in several ways as it provides the organic component of the structural matrix of bone, increases the anabolic hormone insulin like growth factor 1 (IGF1), may increase urinary calcium and is reported to increase intestinal calcium absorption (Heaney & Layman, 2008). Amino acid precursors from dietary protein are required to build and maintain bone structure (Darling et al., 2009); an inadequate anabolic drive due to insufficient dietary protein may decrease bone strength (Bonjour, 2005; Heaney & Layman, 2008). Adequate dietary protein is therefore essential for optimal gain of bone mass during childhood and adolescence, and preservation of bone mass with ageing. Elderly patients with hip fracture are often undernourished and one study has shown that those given daily oral nutritional supplements (20 g of protein; 254 kcal) showed improved clinical outcome (Delmi et al., 1990).

In the general population, however, there is inconsistent evidence about the relationship between high and low protein intakes and bone health. The effect of protein may be biphasic, with potentially detrimental effects at high intakes because of its effects on calcium excretion in the urine (Prentice *et al.*, 2006). Dietary protein is a major contributor to endogenous acid production, which is believed to influence the balance between osteoblastic and osteoclastic activity and increase urinary calcium excretion, although, this may be important only when calcium intakes are low. The overall evidence shows that adequate dietary protein has a small but favourable effect (Darling *et al.*, 2009); therefore, dietary protein intakes should be advised within recommendations, particularly for the elderly.

Phosphorus

Approximately 85% of total body phosphorus is found in the skeleton. In western diets, phosphorous intake is usually adequate. The evidence on whether dietary phosphorus intake has any effect on bone health is inconsistent, although a low calcium to phosphorus ratio (molar ratio ≤0.50), has been reported to be detrimental (Kemi *et al.*, 2010).

Potassium and sodium

Although bone does not contain appreciable amounts of potassium and sodium, these nutrients may impact on bone health through a role in maintaining calcium homeostasis. A high potassium diet is believed to reduce urinary calcium excretion. In contrast, a high dietary sodium intake is believed to be associated with increased urinary calcium excretion in the short term, while long term outcomes are less certain (Teucher *et al.*, 2008).

Potassium is ubiquitous in the diet, but is most abundant in green and root vegetables, fruit, legumes and milk/yoghurt. Due to their high potassium and low sodium content, in addition to their contribution to an alkaline environment, a diet rich in fruit and vegetables is thought to be beneficial for bone health (Lin *et al.*, 2003; New, 2004).

Magnesium and zinc

Magnesium is widely distributed in soft and bony tissue; 50–60% of total body magnesium and 30% of total body zinc is found in bone. The exact role of magnesium in bone health is not known, although severe magnesium deficiency may disrupt calcium homeostasis. Zinc deficiency is associated with reduced bone mass and stunted growth, but human studies are lacking (Department of Health, 1998).

Vitamin K

Vitamin K refers to a group of fat soluble compounds and acts as a cofactor for the carboxylation of a protein (osteocalcin) involved in bone formation. The RNI of 1 μg/kg of body weight/day is based on the level that are sufficient to maintain blood coagulation, but this may be suboptimal for adult bone health (Cashman & O'Connor, 2008). Low dietary intake of vitamin K is associated with low

BMD and increased risk of fracture in older women. Supplementation studies with vitamin K1 in postmenopausal women showed a reduction of bone loss or improvement of BMD in some but not all sites (Braam *et al.*, 2003; Bolton-Smith *et al.*, 2007).

Vitamin C

Vitamin C is required for collagen hydroxylation. There are limited studies in this area but cross sectional data suggest a trend to higher BMD with increased vitamin C intake in adolescents and middle aged women, but not in postmenopausal women (Department of Health, 1998).

Other dietary factors

Carbonated drinks

Associations have been found between high consumption of carbonated drinks and low BMD and increased risk of fracture in adolescents (Manias *et al.*, 2006). This was initially attributed to their influence on the acid–base balance (particularly colas containing phosphoric acid), but this has since shown to be modest compared to other foods. It is likely that the associations with high carbonated drink consumption may be partly attributed to confounding environmental factors, the displacement of milk from the diet and/or an effect of caffeine.

Vegetarian and vegan diets

Cross sectional and longitudinal population based studies do not suggest that there is a real BMD difference between vegetarians and omnivores, other than that which may be accounted for by differences in weight and lifestyle (New, 2004). The impact of a vegetarian diet on bone health is however complex to evaluate, since the composition of diets of vegetarians and omnivores may differ considerably with respect to their calcium, protein, alkali, vitamin K and phytoestrogen content. In addition, there may be differences in key lifestyle characteristics, such as levels of physical activity (New, 2004). Veganism is associated with a diet that contains a low level of bioavailable calcium (Sanders, 1999) and low protein intakes, which may be detrimental to bone (see Chapter 3.6).

Lactose intolerance

People with lactose intolerance may have a reduced calcium intake from dairy sources. The limited evidence available suggests that patients with lactose intolerance are not at an increased risk of osteoporosis, provided that their calcium requirements are met (Enattah *et al.*, 2005) through non-dairy sources of calcium or supplements (see Chapter 7.4.6).

Other factors influencing bone health

Body composition

Bone mineral density is influenced by overall body size and weight; a higher lean to fat ratio is associated with a higher BMD in younger women and in men, whilst the reverse is true for older women (Department of Health,

1998). Epidemiological evidence and a meta analysis of 12 prospective, population based cohorts including 60 000 men and women, showed that total number of sustained fractures, osteoporotic fractures and hip fractures are all inversely related to body mass index (BMI) (De Laet et al., 2005). Its association with muscle weakness, nutritional deficiencies of protein or vitamin D, decreased padding over the greater trochanter of the hip, or a greater liability to fall may explain the role of a low BMI as a risk factor for hip fracture (De Laet et al., 2005).

Although a high BMI is associated with a lower risk of fracture in older people, recent evidence suggests a higher risk of fractures such as at the wrist and ankle in obese patients. Obesity should therefore not be regarded as a protective factor for fracture risk. Rather, underweight should be regarded as a significant risk factor (De Laet et al., 2005) and a healthy body weight within the normal range should be encouraged.

Recent weight loss and hip fracture risk

Weight loss, irrespective of current weight, is associated with an increased risk of fracture, and may be greater for those that suffered involuntary weight loss (Ensrud et al., 1997; 2003). In older women the association between weight loss and the rate of bone loss and fracture risk at the hip was found to be independent of other known risk factors (Ensrud et al., 2003). This may be explained by the decline in mechanical load, a decrease in nutritional intake, including calcium and protein, or be linked to alterations in levels of hormonal factors.

Subgroups of the population at particular risk

Several subgroups of the population are vulnerable to the development of osteoporosis. Anorexia nervosa is associated with a lower bone mass and an increased risk of fractures. Amenorrhea is thought to play an important role in the development of osteoporosis; other risk factors include IGF1 deficiency, low androgen levels and hypercortisolaemia (Misra & Klibanski, 2011) (see Chapter 7.10.1).

Inflammatory bowel disease (IBD) is associated with a modest decrease in BMD and an increase in fracture risk related to malabsorption of nutrients and cumulative corticosteroid use. For patients with Crohn's disease and ulcerative colitis, the relative risk of overall fracture is 1.3 and 1.2 and for hip fractures is 1.5 and 1.4, respectively, compared to the general population (Lewis & Scott, 2007). There is also a modest increased risk of fracture in coeliac disease (Lewis & Scott, 2007); BMD is observed to be more reduced in those with severe compared with mild villous atrophy and there is a significant improvement in BMD after introduction of a gluten free diet. Adults with IBD or coeliac disease are recommended to ensure a daily intake of calcium (from dietary sources or supplements) of 1000 mg/day (1200 mg for postmenopausal women and men >55 years) and to be vitamin D replete (Lewis & Scott, 2007) (see Chapter 7.4.7 and Chapter 7.4.8). Chronic liver disease is associated with

increased risk of osteoporosis. Therefore, the proposed guideline for these patients is to consume 1000 mg of calcium/day and 800 IU of vitamin D/day (Collier et al., 2002) (see Chapter 7.4.12).

Patients with rheumatoid arthritis (RA) also exhibit an increased rate of osteoporosis; reduced BMD in these patients relates to their age, postmenopausal status and disease activity, severity and duration (Coulson et al., 2009; Pye et al., 2010). Fracture risk in this patient group is associated with medication use; steroid and prednisone therapy increase and tumour necrosis factor (TNF) inhibitors decrease overall fracture risk. Although the majority of RA patients have one or more risk factors for osteoporosis, the minority receives preventive treatment (Coulson et al., 2009) (see Chapter 7.9.3).

Organ transplantation is associated with an increased risk of osteoporosis and fractures. This may be related to the primary disease requiring organ transplantation or medication use. Before transplantation it is recommended to ensure adequacy of calcium intake and vitamin D status, encourage weight bearing exercises and treat prevalent osteoporosis (Cohen et al., 2004). The most rapid rates of bone loss occur during the early post transplantation period (6–12 months); rapid resumption of weight bearing exercise, supplementary calcium (1000–1500 mg/day in divided doses), at least 400–800 IU of vitamin D/day, in addition to treatment with bisphosphonates or calcitriol is recommended (Cohen et al., 2004).

The presence of chronic obstructive pulmonary disease (COPD) is a risk factor for the development of osteoporosis. Chronic obstructive pulmonary disease may also be associated with other risk factors for osteoporosis, such as poor capability for physical exercise and corticosteroid use. Patients with COPD are also at higher risk of associated comorbidities such as a low BMI and, impaired nutritional status, and are more likely to be tobacco smokers and of high age (Vrieze et al., 2007). Intervention studies specifically designed for patients with COPD are currently lacking and no specific guidelines have yet been established for the treatment of osteoporosis in this group (Lehouck et al., 2010) (see Chapter 7.1).

Management

The aim of the treatment of osteoporosis is to reduce the risk of falls and fractures. Treatment includes pharmacological approaches, lifestyle advice and dietary interventions. Some pharmaceutical interventions also require associated nutritional interventions to optimise the treatment effects and to prevent side effects.

Lifestyle advice

Exercise

Exercise, particularly weight bearing exercise, can help to build bone and increase peak bone mass in youth and help to maintain bone tissue in adults. It may also help to improve posture, balance and muscle power, all of which help to prevent falls. People with osteoporosis are more likely to fracture a bone when they fall, but as they are mostly older patients they are also at a higher risk of falling due to decreased muscle power and poorer balance (National Osteoporosis Foundation, 2010). An individualised exercise programme under the supervision of a specialist should be directed to prevent further bone loss and fractures by weight bearing exercise, and a reduction of the risk of falls by increasing muscle power and balance. Exercise after a fracture aims to relieve pain and to help rehabilitation (National Osteoporosis Foundation, 2010).

Pharmacological treatments

These agents may inhibit bone resorption (antiresorptive) or stimulate bone formation (anabolic). Antiresorptive treatments act to prevent bone loss and slow the bone remodelling cycle, thereby reducing the relative risk of fractures. Anabolic agents stimulate bone formation and reduce bone resorption. In the UK, the following drug therapies for osteoporosis are available (brand names are given in parentheses):

- *Bisphosphonates:*
  - Alendronate (Fosamax).
  - Cyclical etidronate (Didronel PMO).
  - Ibandronate (Bonviva).
  - Risedronate (Actonel).
  - Zoledronic acid (Aclasta).
- *Selective oestrogen modulator (SERM):*
  - Raloxifene (Evista).
  - Human RANK ligand antibody.
  - Denosumab (Prolia).
- *Other:*
  - Hormone replacement therapy (HRT).
  - Calcitonin.
- *Anabolic agents:*
  - Strontium ranelate (Protelos).
  - PTH treatment (Preotact, Forsteo).

Pharmacological treatment strategies often include the recommendations of calcium and vitamin D supplements to ensure adequacy of these nutrients and to maximise benefit or to prevent hypocalcaemia. The recommended dosages can exceed the RNI or RDA for the age group. Patients with a poor kidney function may be prescribed calcitriol (Rocaltrol) or alfacalcidiol, instead of vitamin D. The methods and frequency of administration of these drugs is highly dependent on their mode of action and includes oral, intramuscular and intravenous administrations. They may be also be used in combination or as alternating therapies (Bilezikian, 2008). Oral bisphosphonates must be taken fasted and may be associated with upper gastrointestinal side effects. Compliance to osteoporosis treatment needs to be considered in the evaluation of the patient.

Nutritional care of the hip fracture patient

Fractures of the proximal femur (hip) are a cause of substantial morbidity and mortality in older people (Avenell & Handoll, 2010) and may have long term effects. It has been shown that 9 months after their hip fracture, people still have a poorer quality of life than age and sex matched controls (Cranney et al., 2005), and many fail to return to their previous state of mobility.

Nutrition status of hip fracture patients

Protein energy malnutrition is common among elderly patients hospitalised with an acute hip fracture (Nematy et al., 2006; Bastow et al., 1983; Delmi et al., 1990; Lumbers et al., 2001). Rapid deterioration in nutritional status due to surgery and hospitalisation is common (Corish & Kennedy, 2000; Nematy et al., 2006; Bastow et al., 1983; Delmi et al., 1990; Eneroth et al., 2005). Protein energy malnutrition is associated with an increased risk of complications (Eneroth et al., 2006; Lumbers et al., 1996; Houwing et al., 2003) and there is evidence that nutritional support, particularly when overseen by a specialist dietitian and dietetic assistant, lowers the risk of postoperative complications, particularly in underweight patients (Duncan et al., 2006; Delmi et al., 1990; Eneroth et al., 2005). The European Society for Parenteral and Enteral Nutrition (ESPEN) guidelines (2006) recommend oral nutritional supplements (ONS) for this group (Volkert et al., 2006), but enteral feeding also may be considered. Compliance to ONS is often low. This may have contributed to the conclusion in the recent Cochrane review on nutritional supplementation for hip fracture aftercare that the evidence for the effectiveness of protein and energy feeds is weak (Avenell & Handoll, 2010) (see Chapter 6.3).

Assessment

Nutritional assessment of the hip fracture patient will include the following.

Anthropometry

Current weight, usual weight and percentage weight change, current height (and height as a young adult) or demispan and BMI should be measured. When there are difficulties with obtaining measurements of weight and height, the mid upper arm circumference (MUAC) can be used as an index of malnutrition; this correlates well with BMI in this patient group (Maffulli et al., 1999).

Biochemistry and fluid balance

To estimate metabolic stress the following should be assessed; elevated temperature, raised white cell count, elevated C-reactive protein, raised blood urea and low serum albumin.

Clinical assessment

Symptoms including Glasgow Coma Score (GCS), degree of dysphagia, appetite, anorexia, nausea, taste disturbances, pain, cognitive impairment should be assessed.

Dietary assessment

This should include a diet history and food frequency questionnaire to assess the adequacy of macro- and micro-nutrient intake prior to admission. A 24-hour recall after admission and surgery are important to assess reduced voluntary oral intakes post surgery (Sullivan et al., 2004; Nematy et al., 2006).

Economic and social assessment

This should include social history, family support and discharge plan (home or medium to long term care).

Nutritional management

Patients undergoing orthopaedic surgery have increased metabolic requirements, which are often unrecognised (Eneroth *et al.*, 2006). Estimation of total energy requirements of patients may be calculated by estimating basal metabolic rate (BMR), adding a stress factor of 20% (to account for the increased energy requirements because of surgical correction of the fractured femoral neck) and adding another 10–25% (based on the level of mobility) to allow for rehabilitation, physical activity and diet induced thermogenesis (Nematy *et al.*, 2006) (see Chapter 6.1).

Dietary advice should aim to achieve a high protein, high energy diet in small and frequent portions, potentially with the use of supplements and fortified foods. Monitoring and discharge planning are an important part of the dietetic care of a hip fracture patient.

Further reading

Cauley JA, Chlebowski RT, Wactawski-Wende J, *et al.* (2013) Calcium plus vitamin D supplementation and health outcomes five years after active intervention ended: The Women's Health Initiative. *Journal of Women's Health* 22(11): 915–929.

Department of Health. (1998) *Nutrition and Bone Health with Particular Reference to Calcium and Vitamin D: Report of the Subgroup on Bone Health (Working Group on the Nutritional Status of the Population) of the Committee on Medical Aspects of Food and Nutrition Policy.* London: The Stationery Office.

Department of Health and Human Services (2004) *Bone Health and Osteoporosis: A Report of the Surgeon General.* Rockville: Department of Health and Human Services, Office of the Surgeon General.

Howe TE, Shea B, Dawson LJ, *et al.* (2011) *Exercise for Preventing and Treating Osteoporosis in Postmenopausal Women.* The Cochrane Collaboration. Chichester, John Wiley & Sons, Ltd.

National Osteoporosis Guideline Group (2010) Guideline for the diagnosis and management of osteoporosis. Available at www.shef.ac.uk/NOGG/NOGG_Pocket_Guide_for_Healthcare _Professionals.pdf. Accessed 20 August 2013.

Poole KE, Compston JE. (2006) Osteoporosis and its management. *BM* 1–1256.

Reid IR, Bolland MJ, Grey A. (2013) Effects of vitamin D supplements on bone mineral density: a systematic review and meta-analysis. *Lancet* dx.doi.org/10.1016/S0140-6736(13)61647-5.

Internet resources

American Society for Bone Mineral Research www.asbmr.org
International Osteoporosis Foundation www.iofbonehealth.org
National Osteoporosis Society www.nos.org.uk

Tools for the assessment of fragility fracture

FRAX® www.shef.ac.uk/FRAX
QFracture www.qfracture.org

References

Avenell A, Handoll HH. (2010) Nutritional supplementation for hip fracture aftercare in older people. *Cochrane Database of Systematic Reviews* CD001880.

Bastow MD, Rawlings J, Allison SP. (1983) Benefits of supplementary tube feeding after fractured neck of femur: a randomised controlled trial. *BMJ (Clinical Research Edition)* 287: 1589–1592.

Bentler SE, Liu L, Obrizan M, *et al.* (2009) The aftermath of hip fracture: discharge placement, functional status change, and mortality. *American Journal of Epidemiology* 170: 1290–1299.

Bilezikian JP. (2008) In: Rosen CJ (ed). *Primer on the Metabolic Bone Diseases and Disorders of Mineral Metabolism*, 8th edn. Washington, DC. The American Society of Bone and Mineral Research.

Bischoff-Ferrari HA, Willett WC, Wong JB, Giovannucci E, Dietrich T, Dawson-Hughes B. (2005) Fracture prevention with vitamin D supplementation: a meta-analysis of randomized controlled trials. *JAMA* 293: 2257–2264.

Bischoff-Ferrari HA, Giovannucci E, Willett WC, Dietrich T, Dawson-Hughes B. (2006) Estimation of optimal serum concentrations of 25-hydroxyvitamin D for multiple health outcomes. *American Journal of Clinical Nutrition* 84: 18–28.

Bolland MJ, Grey A, Avenell A, *et al.* (2011) Calcium supplements with or without vitamin D and risk of cardiovascular events: reanalysis of the Women's Health Initiative limited access dataset and meta-analysis. *British Medical Journal* 342: d2040.

Bolton-Smith C, McMurdo ME, Paterson CR, *et al.* (2007) Two-year randomized controlled trial of vitamin K1 (phylloquinone) and vitamin D3 plus calcium on the bone health of older women. *Journal of Bone and Mineral Research* 22: 509–519.

Bonjour JP. (2005) Dietary protein: an essential nutrient for bone health. *Journal of the American College of Nutrition* 24: 526S–36S.

Braam LA, Knapen MH, Geusens P, *et al.* (2003) Vitamin K1 supplementation retards bone loss in postmenopausal women between 50 and 60 years of age. *Calcified Tissue International* 73: 21–26.

Cashman KD, O'Connor E. (2008) Does high vitamin K1 intake protect against bone loss in later life? *Nutrition Reviews* 66: 532–538.

Clarke B. (2008) Normal bone anatomy and physiology. *Clinical Journal of the American Society of Nephrology* 3(Suppl 3): S131–139.

Cohen A, Sambrook P, Shane E. (2004) Management of bone loss after organ transplantation. *Journal of Bone and Mineral Research* 19: 1919–1932.

Collier JD, Ninkovic M, Compston JE. (2002) Guidelines on the management of osteoporosis associated with chronic liver disease. *Gut* 50(Suppl 1): i1–9.

Cooper C, Campion G, Melton LJ 3rd. (1992) Hip fractures in the elderly: a world-wide projection. *Osteoporosis International* 2: 285–289.

Corish CA, Kennedy NP. (2000) Protein-energy undernutrition in hospital in-patients. *British Journal of Nutrition* 83: 575–591.

Coulson KA, Reed G, Gilliam, BE, Kremer JM, Pepmueller PH. (2009) Factors influencing fracture risk, T score, and management of osteoporosis in patients with rheumatoid arthritis in the Consortium of Rheumatology Researchers of North America (CORRONA) registry. *Journal of Clinical Rheumatology* 15: 155–160.

Cranney AB, Coyle D, Hopman WM, Hum V, Power B, Tugwell PS. (2005) Prospective evaluation of preferences and quality of life in women with hip fractures. *Journal of Rheumatology* 32: 2393–2399.

Darling AL, Millward DJ, Torgerson DJ, Hewitt CE, Lanham-New SA. (2009) Dietary protein and bone health: a systematic review and meta-analysis. *American Journal of Clinical Nutrition* 90: 1674–1692.

Dawson-Hughes B, Dallal GE, Krall EA, Sadowski L, Sahyoun N, Tannenbaum S. (1990) A controlled trial of the effect of calcium supplementation on bone density in postmenopausal women. *New England Journal of Medicine* 323: 878–883.

De Laet C, Kanis JA, Oden A, *et al.* (2005) Body mass index as a predictor of fracture risk: a meta-analysis. *Osteoporosis International* 16: 1330–1338.

Delmi M, Rapin CH, Bengoa JM, Delmas PD, Vasey H, Bonjour JP. (1990) Dietary supplementation in elderly patients with fractured neck of the femur. *Lancet* 335: 1013–1016.

Department of Health. (1998) *Nutrition and Bone Health with Particular Reference to Calcium and Vitamin D*: Report of the Subgroup on Bone Health (Working Group on the Nutritional Status of the Population) of the Committee on Medical Aspects of Food and Nutrition Policy. London: The Stationery Office.

Department of Health. (2007) *Update on Vitamin D: Position Statement by the Scientific Advisory Committee on Nutrition*. London: Department of Health.

Department of Health and Human Services. (2004) *Bone Health and Osteoporosis: A report of the Surgeon General*. Rockville: Department of Health and Human Services, Office of the Surgeon General.

Duncan DG, Beck SJ, Hood K, Johansen A. (2006) Using dietetic assistants to improve the outcome of hip fracture: a randomised controlled trial of nutritional support in an acute trauma ward. *Age and Ageing* 35: 148–153.

Enattah N, Pekkarinen T, Valimaki MJ, Loyttyniemi E, Jarvela I. (2005) Genetically defined adult-type hypolactasia and self-reported lactose intolerance as risk factors of osteoporosis in Finnish postmenopausal women. *European Journal of Clinical Nutrition* 59: 1105–1111.

Eneroth M, Olsson U-B, Thorngren K-GR. (2005) Insufficient fluid and energy intake in hospitalised patients with hip fracture. A prospective randomised study of 80 patients. *Clinical Nutrition* 24: 297–303.

Eneroth M, Olsson UB, Thorngren KG. (2006) Nutritional supplementation decreases hip fracture-related complications. *Clinical Orthopaedics and Related Research* 451: 212–217.

Ensrud KE, Cauley J, Lipschutz R, Cummings SR. (1997) Weight change and fractures in older women. Study of Osteoporotic Fractures Research Group. *Archives of Internal Medicine* 157: 857–863.

Ensrud KE, Ewing SK, Stone KL, Cauley JA, Bowman PJ, Cummings SR. (2003) Intentional and unintentional weight loss increase bone loss and hip fracture risk in older women. *Journal of the American Geriatric Society* 51: 1740–1747.

Francis RM. (2007) The vitamin D paradox. *Rheumatology (Oxford)* 46: 1749–1750.

Fraser DR. (2004) Vitamin D-deficiency in Asia. *Journal of Steroid Biochemistry and Molecular Biology* 89–90: 491–495.

Goulding A, Rockell JE, Black RE, Grant AM, Jones IE, Williams SM. (2004) Children who avoid drinking cow's milk are at increased risk for prepubertal bone fractures. *Journal of the American Dietetic Association* 104: 250–253.

Greer FR, Krebs NF. (2006) Optimizing bone health and calcium intakes of infants, children, and adolescents. *Pediatrics* 117: 578–585.

Heaney RP. (2000) Calcium, dairy products and osteoporosis. *Journal of the American College of Nutrition* 19: 83S–99S.

Heaney RP, Layman DK. (2008) Amount and type of protein influences bone health. *American Journal of Clinical Nutrition* 87: 1567S–1570S.

Houwing RH, Rozendaal M, Wouters-Wesseling W, Beulens JW, Buskens E, Haalboom JR. (2003) A randomised, double-blind assessment of the effect of nutritional supplementation on the prevention of pressure ulcers in hip-fracture patients. *Clinical Nutrition* 22: 401–405.

Huncharek M, Muscat J, Kupelnick B. (2008) Impact of dairy products and dietary calcium on bone-mineral content in children: results of a meta-analysis. *Bone* 43: 312–321.

Johnell O, Kanis J. (2005) Epidemiology of osteoporotic fractures. *Osteoporosis International* 16 (Suppl 2): S3–7.

Johnell O, Kanis JA. (2006) An estimate of the worldwide prevalence and disability associated with osteoporotic fractures. *Osteoporosis International* 17: 1726–1733.

Kemi VE, Karkkainen MU, Rita HJ, *et al.* (2010). Low calcium : phosphorus ratio in habitual diets affects serum parathyroid hormone concentration and calcium metabolism in healthy women with adequate calcium intake. *British Journal of Nutrition* 103(4): 561–568.

Lehouck A, Van Remoortel H, Troosters T, Decramer M, Janssens W. (2010) COPD and bone metabolism: a clinical update. *Revue des Maladies Respiratoire* 27: 1231–1242.

Lewiecki EM, Gordon CM, Baim S, *et al.* (2008) International Society for Clinical Densitometry 2007 Adult and Pediatric Official Positions. *Bone* 43: 1115–1121.

Lewis N, Scott B. (2007) *Guidelines for Osteoporosis in Inflammatory Bowel Disease and Coeliac Disease*. British Society of Gastroenterology. Available at www.bsg.org.uk/pdf_word_docs/ost_coe_ibd.pdf. Accessed 1st December 2013.

Li K, Kaaks R, Linseisen J, *et al.* (2012) Associations of dietary calcium intake and calcium supplementation with myocardial infarction and stroke risk and overall cardiovascular mortality in the Heidelberg cohort of the European Prospective Investigation into Cancer and Nutrition study (EPIC-Heidelberg). *Heart* 98: 920–925.

Lin PH, Ginty F, Appel LJ, *et al.* (2003) The DASH diet and sodium reduction improve markers of bone turnover and calcium metabolism in adults. *Journal of Nutrition* 133: 3130–3136.

Lips P. (2007) Vitamin D status and nutrition in Europe and Asia. *Journal of Steroid Biochemistry and Molecular Biology* 103: 620–625.

Lumbers M, Driver LT, Howland RJ, Older MW, Williams CM. (1996) Nutritional status and clinical outcome in elderly female surgical orthopaedic patients. *Clinical Nutrition* 15: 101–107.

Lumbers M, New SA, Gibson S, Murphy MC. (2001) Nutritional status in elderly female hip fracture patients: comparison with an age-matched home living group attending day centres. *British Journal of Nutrition* 85: 733–740.

Maffulli N, Dougall TW, Brown MT, Golden MH. (1999) Nutritional differences in patients with proximal femoral fractures. *Age and Ageing* 28: 458–462.

Manias K, McCabe D, Bishop N. (2006) Fractures and recurrent fractures in children; varying effects of environmental factors as well as bone size and mass. *Bone* 39: 652–657.

McCabe LD, Martin BR, McCabe GP, Johnston CC, Weaver CM, Peacock M. (2004) Dairy intakes affect bone density in the elderly. *American Journal of Clinical Nutrition* 80: 1066–1074.

Misra M, Klibanski A. (2011). Bone health in anorexia nervosa. *Current Opinion in Endocrinology, Diabetes and Obesity* 18(6): 376–382.

National Institute for Health and Care Excellence (NICE). (2012) *Osteoporosis: Fragility Fracture Risk*. NICE Clinical Guideline 146. London: National Clinical Guideline Centre.

National Osteoporosis Foundation. (2010) *Clinician's Guide to Prevention and Treatment of Osteoporosis*. Washington, DC: National Osteoporosis Foundation.

National Osteoporosis Guideline Group. (2010) *Guideline for the Diagnosis and Management of Osteoporosis*. Available at www.shef.ac.uk/NOGG/NOGG_Pocket_Guide_for_Healthcare_Professionals.pdf. Accessed 1st December 2013

Nematy M, Hickson M, Brynes AE, Ruxton CH, Frost GS. (2006) Vulnerable patients with a fractured neck of femur: nutritional status and support in hospital. *Journal of Human Nutrition and Dietetics* 19: 209–218.

New SA. (2004) Do vegetarians have a normal bone mass? *Osteoporosis International* 15: 679–688.

Nieves JW, Barrett-Connor E, Siris ES, Zion M, Barlas S, Chen YT. (2008) Calcium and vitamin D intake influence bone mass, but not short-term fracture risk, in Caucasian postmenopausal women from the National Osteoporosis Risk Assessment (NORA) study. *Osteoporosis International* 19: 673–679.

Ovesen L, Brot C, Jakobsen J. (2003) Food contents and biological activity of 25-hydroxyvitamin D: a vitamin D metabolite to be reckoned with? *Annals of Nutrition and Metabolism* 47: 107–113.

Poole KE, Compston JE. (2006) Osteoporosis and its management. *BMJ* 333: 1251–1256.

Prentice A. (2004) Diet, nutrition and the prevention of osteoporosis. *Public Health Nutrition* 7: 227–243.

Prentice A. (2008) Vitamin D deficiency: a global perspective. *Nutrition Reviews* 66: S153–164.

Prentice A, Goldberg GR, Schoenmakers I. (2008) Vitamin D across the lifecycle: physiology and biomarkers. *American Journal of Clinical Nutrition* 88: 500S–506S.

Prentice A, Schoenmakers I, Laskey MA, De Bono S, Ginty F, Goldberg GR. (2006) Nutrition and bone growth and development. *Proceedings of the Nutrition Society* 65: 348–360.

Pye SR, Adams JE, Ward KA, Bunn DK, Symmons DP, O'Neill TW. (2010) Disease activity and severity in early inflammatory arthritis predict hand cortical bone loss. *Rheumatology (Oxford)* 49: 1943–1948.

Rizzoli R, Bonjour JP. (1999) Determinants of peak bone mass and mechanisms of bone loss. *Osteoporosis International* 9 (Suppl 2): S17–23.

Ross AC, Taylor CL, Yaktine AL, Del Valle HB. (2010) *Dietary Reference Intakes for Calcium and Vitamin D. Committee to Review Dietary Reference Intakes for Vitamin D and Calcium*. Washington, DC: Institute of Medicine.

Sanders TA. (1999) The nutritional adequacy of plant-based diets. *Proceedings of the Nutrition Society* 58: 265–269.

Shea B, Wells G, Cranney A, *et al.* (2002) Meta-analyses of therapies for postmenopausal osteoporosis. VII. Meta-analysis of calcium supplementation for the prevention of postmenopausal osteoporosis. *Endocrine Reviews* 23: 552–559.

Sullivan DH, Nelson CL, Klimberg VS, Bopp MM. (2004) Nightly enteral nutrition support of elderly hip fracture patients: a pilot study. *Journal of the American College of Nutrition* 23: 683–691.

Teucher B, Dainty JR, Spinks CA, *et al.* (2008) Sodium and bone health: impact of moderately high and low salt intakes on calcium metabolism in postmenopausal women. *Journal of Bone and Mineral Research* 23: 1477–1485.

Volkert D, Berner YN, Berry E, *et al.* (2006) ESPEN Guidelines on Enteral Nutrition: Geriatrics. *Clinical Nutrition* 25: 330–360.

Vrieze A, De Greef MH, Wijkstra PJ, Wempe JB. (2007) Low bone mineral density in COPD patients related to worse lung function, low weight and decreased fat-free mass. *Osteoporosis International* 18: 1197–1202.

Ward K. (2011) Musculoskeletal phenotype through the life course: the role of nutrition. *Proceedings of the Nutrition Society* 71: 27–37.

Winzenberg TM, Shaw K, Fryer J, Jones G. (2006) Calcium supplementation for improving bone mineral density in children. *Cochrane Database of Systematic Reviews* CD005119.

World Health Organization (WHO). (1994) Assessment of fracture risk and its application to screening for postmenopausal osteoporosis. Report of a WHO Study Group. *World Health Organization Technical Report Series*. 1994/01/01 ed. Geneva: WHO.

7.9.2 Arthritis

Dorothy J Pattison

Key points

- Early dietary guidance and an exercise programme are effective in reducing symptoms of osteoarthritis and may delay the need for joint replacement.

- Glucosamine or chondroitin products are not recommended for the treatment of osteoarthritis.

- Fish oil supplements rich in n-3 polyunsaturated fatty acids have been found to ameliorate pain and symptoms of rheumatoid arthritis.

- Specific food avoidance cannot be recommended for rheumatoid arthritis; patient experiences should not be ignored and dietary assessment and advice should be given accordingly.

- People with rheumatoid arthritis are at high risk of comorbidities including cardiovascular disease and osteoporosis.

The term arthritis refers to a number of different conditions that can affect the joints at any stage of life. Two key features of arthritis are joint pain and inflammation leading to tenderness, swelling and stiffness. Arthritis can be divided into inflammatory, non-inflammatory and connective tissue arthritis groups. Inflammatory arthritis may be acute, e.g. septic arthritis, or chronic, e.g. rheumatoid arthritis (RA), or acute on chronic, e.g. gout. The most common non-inflammatory arthritis is osteoarthritis (OA). Connective tissue diseases, as the name suggests, are inflammatory conditions affecting the connective tissues (tendons, ligaments, dermis), e.g. systemic lupus erythematosus (SLE) and fibromyalgia. Osteoarthritis and RA are the most prevalent forms of arthritis presenting to rheumatology clinics in the UK.

This chapter will discuss the dietary management of OA, RA and associated comorbidities. The dietary management of gout and osteoporosis are dealt with in Chapter 7.9.3 and Chapter 7.9.1, respectively.

Osteoarthritis

Osteoarthritis refers to a clinical syndrome of joint pain accompanied by varying degrees of functional limitation and reduced quality of life. It is the most common form of arthritis and one of the leading causes of pain and disability worldwide. Osteoarthritis usually affects the distal two joints of the fingers and the base of the thumb as well as the knees, hips and spine. Risk factors for OA include age, gender, obesity, trauma and genetics. The primary site for OA is the cartilage at the ends of bones in a joint. Surface cartilage breaks down and erodes until the bones become exposed and damaged, causing pain, swelling and reduced movement. Osteoarthritis is a metabolically

SECTION 7

active repair process that takes place in all joint tissues and involves localised loss of cartilage and remodelling of bone. Injuries may trigger the need for the joint tissues to repair. In some people, either because of devastating injury or an error in the ability to repair, the process cannot compensate, resulting in continuing tissue damage and eventual symptomatic OA. Joint failure can be minimal or complete depending on its severity. Although pain, swelling, stiffness and a reduction in physical activity are all typical outcomes of OA, structural changes in the joint can occur without accompanying symptoms.

Clinical management

The majority of published evidence relates to the management of knee OA, although many patients have multiple joint involvement (NICE, 2008). Treatment primarily consists of alleviating pain, using analgesics, e.g. paracetamol, sometimes in combination with a low dose non-steroidal anti-inflammatory drug (NSAID). Topical application of a NSAID preparation may also provide relief. An injection of corticosteroids directly into the joint is sometimes used to relieve severe local pain and inflammation. If pain becomes debilitating, joint replacement surgery is a successful procedure used to improve the quality of life (NICE, 2008). Physiotherapy and occupational therapy interventions have a major focus on self management education and have integral, evidence based roles in disease management.

Dietary management

Dietary intervention for OA includes the management of obesity, in particular prior to joint replacement surgery, and the management of related comorbidities.

Obesity

Every step taken increases the load on the hip or knee joint by three to five times body weight; therefore, the physical stresses imposed on the joints by excessive body weight are considerable (Aspden, 2011). Since OA primarily affects load bearing joints, obesity can worsen symptoms and may accelerate joint degradation. Many patients with OA are already overweight at the time of diagnosis and others become increasingly overweight as a result of reduced physical activity and/or inappropriate dietary intake. Weight reduction or maintenance of an ideal body weight or preventing progression to obesity is an integral part of management. Clinical trials have demonstrated that weight reduction in combination with increased physical activity can improve symptoms such as pain and stiffness, primarily in knee OA (Huang *et al.*, 2000; Messier *et al.*, 2004).

It is generally accepted that obesity predisposes to OA. However, OA in the joints of the hand, primarily nodal OA affecting middle aged women, has been shown to occur more frequently in obese people, which cannot be attributed to the effect of increased physical load. Recent research into the causes of OA and its progression has focussed on the biological activity of adipose tissue OA.

It is believed that a reduction in adipose tissue, rather than body weight alone, is responsible for improvement in symptoms (Aspden, 2011). Toda *et al.* (1998) found that reducing fat mass gave greater symptomatic relief than could be explained by the reduction in body weight alone. A UK study confirmed that metabolic factors such as hypertension, hypercholesterolaemia and blood glucose levels are associated with OA independent of obesity, indicating that important systemic and metabolic components are involved in the aetiology of OA (Hart *et al.*, 1995). Weight loss can ameliorate symptoms and delay the need for joint replacement (Niu *et al.*, 2009). Therefore, dietary modification may be indicated in cases where hyperlipidaemia and other factors of the metabolic syndrome are present.

Nutrition and surgery

Some patients requiring surgical joint replacement may be at increased risk of nutritional depletion. This may be particularly relevant in the frail and elderly, especially if functional loss has already limited dietary intake preoperatively. Lower levels of haemoglobin, ferritin, albumin and protein intakes have been demonstrated in OA and RA patients 10 days after joint replacement surgery compared to preoperative levels (Haugen *et al.*, 1999). Improved postoperative recovery has been shown in elderly patients (decreased hospital length of stay) undergoing hip replacement and given perioperative nutritional supplements as part of a rapid recovery programme for lower extremity arthroplasty patients (Berend *et al.*, 2004).

Dietary supplements

Glucosamine and chondroitin

Glucosamine is found naturally in the body; it plays an important role in the synthesis of glycosaminoglycans and glycoproteins. These are important for ligaments, tendons, cartilage and the synovial fluid of joints. It has been suggested that the way in which these joint structures are built and maintained contributes to the development and the progression of OA. Studies in animals have found that glucosamine can both delay degradation and repair damaged cartilage. However, results from randomised controlled trials (RCTs) on the effectiveness of chondroitin and glucosamine are conflicting. Trials that reported sizeable effects on joint pain were often of poor quality and/or small sample size, whereas larger, methodologically robust trials generally found only small or no effect (NICE, 2008). A meta analysis of 20 studies of glucosamine in the management of OA of the knee and hip using a preparation of glucosamine sulphate (1500 mg/ day) in patients with symptomatic OA failed to show benefit in terms of pain and function (Towheed *et al.*, 2005). A more recent meta analysis of RCTs of glucosamine, chondroitin or a combination of both in patients with hip or knee OA found no clinically relevant effect of either supplement alone or in combination on perceived joint pain or minimal joint space width (Wandel *et al.*, 2010). Both meta analyses reported that glucosamine and chondroitin were safe.

Herbal and other dietary supplements

Some pharmacological treatments for OA are ineffective in some patients and some, such as NSAIDs, often have serious side effects. Thus, patients frequently turn to complementary/alternative medicines.

Whilst many manufacturers of dietary supplements claim that their product will reduce symptoms or even alter the course of disease, there is only weak scientific evidence to support the use of nutritional supplements in the management of OA. Most types of supplements promoted for the treatment of OA are unlikely to cause harm, but some plant based remedies can be toxic.

Long *et al.* (2001) conducted a systematic review of herbal medicines and plant extracts (administered orally or topically) in OA. Twelve RCTs and two systematic reviews were included. There was no compelling or only weak evidence, i.e. at least one RCT) for significant clinically relevant benefits for six oral preparations; promising evidence, i.e. at least two RCTs with favourable outcomes, for Devil's claw (*Harpagophytum procumbens*) and avocado soyabean unsaponifiables (ASU); and moderately strong evidence, i.e. three RCTs or more, for phytodor (Long *et al.*, 2001). As yet, there is no convincing evidence that fish oil supplementation confers clinical benefit in the management of OA.

Rheumatoid arthritis

Rheumatoid arthritis is an inflammatory disease that largely affects the synovial joints. Synovial joints are moveable and contain synovial fluid; they are predominant in limbs where mobility is important. Rheumatoid arthritis typically affects the small joints of the hands and the feet, usually symmetrically. It is a systemic disease and so can affect several organs, including the heart, lungs and eyes. The prevalence of RA in the UK is around 400 000 (Wiles *et al.*, 1999), with approximately 12 000 people developing the disease per year (Symmons *et al.*, 2002). Rheumatoid arthritis occurs three times more frequently in women than men and can develop at any stage of life, with a peak age of incidence in the UK for both genders between 50 and 60 years. Drug treatment aims to relieve symptoms and to modify the disease process, thus preventing structural damage and progressive functional loss. Approximately one-third of people stop work because of the disease within 2 years of onset (Young *et al.*, 2002). Clearly, RA is costly to the UK economy and to individuals (NICE, 2009).

Clinical management

Current drug treatment includes the use of paracetamol and/or codeine for pain relief. Non-steroidal anti-inflammatory drugs (ibuprofen, naproxen and diclofenac) are taken to relieve pain and reduce joint swelling. More recently, COX 2 inhibitors have been developed, e.g. celecoxib and etoricoxib, which relieve pain and stiffness as well as reducing inflammation. Traditional NSAIDs can increase the risk of stomach problems, e.g. peptic ulceration, whereas COX 2 inhibitors carry a lower risk of such problems, but are associated with a greater risk of cardiovascular complications. These drugs do not act on the progression of RA.

National clinical guidelines for the management of RA recommend early introduction of the traditional second line disease modifying antirheumatic drugs (DMARDs), primarily the immunosuppressant drugs methotrexate and sulphasalazine, and also hydroxychloroquine and leflunomide. Corticosteroids are used to provide rapid relief of symptoms such as pain, stiffness and joint swelling. They are used on a short term basis due to the associated side effects of weight gain, muscle weakness and loss of bone mass (NICE, 2009).

In the last two decades, the concerted effort to identify the main immune modulators of RA at a cellular level, including cytokines and TNF, has resulted in the development of biological agents that block their activity. These specifically designed immunological proteins inhibit the inflammatory pathways that cause RA, and include agents such as etanercept, infliximab, adalumimab and rituximab.

Physical therapy

Tiredness and fatigue are major problems experienced by people with RA. Patients should be encouraged to keep active within their capabilities, but to rest sufficiently and have a nutritionally adequate and healthy eating pattern as part of the management of RA. Physical therapies include physiotherapy, occupational therapy and podiatry, and predominately aim to control pain, minimise joint stiffness and limit joint damage, to facilitate the best possible function and health related quality of life, with the least adverse treatment effects.

Diet

Several studies have shown poor eating patterns and nutritionally inadequate diets in people with RA (Morgan *et al.*, 1997; Stone *et al.*, 1997; Goff & Basari, 1999). There are various explanations for these consistent findings:

- The pain and fatigue associated with RA can considerably impair appetite, particularly during acute flare ups, a characteristic of the condition.
- Joint pain and deformity have adverse effects on mobility, functional ability and manual dexterity. Consequently, shopping, food preparation, cooking and even eating can become difficult, complex and tiring.
- Medications taken to control the disease can cause nausea and anorexia or interact with nutrients, e.g. methotrexate blocks the action of folic acid and patients require folate supplements.
- Popular diets and alternative lifestyle regimens are widely available to people with RA, but they are generally based on personal experiences, not scientifically proven and are very likely to compromise nutrient intake.

If pain and disability cause feeding problems, a rheumatology occupational therapist can assess the patient, if necessary in their home, and advise on adapted eating utensils and home modifications to improve ability in the kitchen and maintain a desirable nutritional status.

Dietary supplements

Antioxidants

Epidemiological studies assessing dietary intake prior to the onset of inflammatory arthritis, particularly RA, have identified low dietary intakes of antioxidant nutrients such as vitamin C and beta cryptoxanthin in adults who developed inflammatory arthritis compared with those who did not (Pattison *et al.*, 2004a; 2005). Heliövaara *et al.* (1994) found lower serum levels of antioxidants in healthy individuals who went on to develop RA than in those who did not develop RA. However, it is unclear if the serum levels of antioxidants are low due to poor dietary intake prior to the onset of RA or are depleted via activity in the body's endogenous immune defence system.

A recent systematic review of studies of antioxidants, vitamins A, C and E, and selenium supplements in RA, osteoarthritis or other inflammatory conditions, concluded that there is no robust evidence to show antioxidant supplements confer any symptomatic benefit in the management of the above conditions (Canter *et al.*, 2007). This is not to say that individual patients obtain symptomatic improvement with these supplements, but in recommended doses they do no harm.

Fatty acids

The polyunsaturated fatty acids (PUFAs), n-6 and n-3 are precursors of inflammatory mediators, including prostaglandins and leucotrienes. There are different series of prostaglandins and leucotrienes with various pro- or anti-inflammatory properties. Prostaglandins of the two series, e.g. PG2 and PGI2, are the most potent inflammatory prostaglandins and originate from the n-6 PUFA arachidonic acid, whereas the n-3 PUFAs are metabolised to less inflammatory eicosanoids.

The potential benefits of changing the combination of fats in the diet of people with RA have been of interest to rheumatologists and researchers for many years, particularly increasing the intake of long chain n-3 PUFAs found in fish oils, eicosapentaenoic acid (EPA) and docosahexaenoic acid (DHA) (Adam, 1995). The most likely mechanism through which n-3 PUFAs act as anti-inflammatory agents is by competing with arachidonic acid for incorporation into inflammatory cell membranes and for metabolism by the enzymes of eicosanoids synthesis, thus reducing the production of the two series prostaglandins and four series leucotrienes (Calder, 2006) (Figure 7.9.3). n-3 PUFAs have other anti-inflammatory effects, independent from altered eicosanoids production, such as a decrease in the production of proinflammatory cytokines, e.g. interleukin 1β and 1α (IL1β, IL1α), TNF, and of reactive oxygen species. Eicosapentaenoic acid is also the

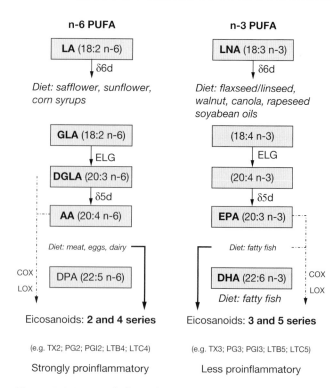

Figure 7.9.3   Metabolism of n-6 and n-3 fatty acids

precursor of the less inflammatory series three prostaglandins and series five leucotrienes (Calder, 2006).

There is strong evidence for the clinical efficacy of n-3 PUFAs in RA. Several reviews of trials of fish oil have found benefit from supplementation. A meta analysis by Fortin *et al.* (1995) concluded that dietary fish oil supplements for 3 months significantly reduce tender joint count and duration of early morning stiffness. A more recent meta analysis of 17 RCTs assessed the pain relieving effects of n-3 PUFAs in RA and in joint pain secondary to inflammatory bowel disease (Goldberg & Katz, 2007). Outcome measures included patient assessed pain, physician assessed pain, duration of morning stiffness, number of painful and/or tender joints, Ritchie articular index and NSAID consumption. Supplementation for 3–4 months significantly reduced patient reported joint pain, minutes of morning stiffness, number of painful and/or tender joints and NSAID consumption. The authors concluded that n-3 PUFAs were a useful adjunctive treatment for the joint pain associated with RA. Galarraga *et al.* (2008) undertook a randomised, double blind placebo controlled study to determine whether long chain n-3 rich cod liver oil could reduce the daily NSAID requirement of patients with RA by at least 30% without worsening of their disease activity. Patients in the treatment group received 10 g of fish oil supplement/day, containing 2.2 g of n-3 PUFAs (1.5 g of EPA + 700 mg of DHA), for 9 months. Compared with 10% in the placebo group, 40% of patients in the treatment group were able to reduce NSAID consumption by 30%. The key message from this study was that fish oil supplementation should be considered in RA patients to help reduce NSAID intake in order to attenuate the associated risk of gastrointestinal and cardiovascular adverse events (Galarraga *et al.*, 2008).

Research has demonstrated an increase in the benefits gained from increasing n-3 PUFA intake if there is a simultaneous reduction in the dietary intake of n-6 PUFAs, thus increasing the ratio of n-3 PUFAs to n-6 PUFAs (Adam *et al.*, 2003). Consequently, altering dietary PUFA composition in favour of an increase in n-3 fatty acid intake could reduce or modify the inflammatory process and potentially dampen down disease activity. It is of some relevance then that over the last 100 years or so the western diet has become rich in n-6 PUFAs, whilst at the same time the consumption of n-3 PUFAs has greatly decreased (Simpoulous, 2009).

Food intolerance and exclusion diets

The withdrawal of food in patients with RA results in decreased production of the chemical mediators of inflammation; on the reintroduction of foodstuffs, the symptoms return (Buchanan *et al.*, 1991). Similarly, trials of elemental diets in RA patients have provided little objective evidence of benefit, with only temporary improvement in symptoms (Kavanaghi *et al.*, 1995).

Food intolerances have been demonstrated in some RA patients. Commonly reported intolerances include milk, corn, wheat and azo dyes, but there is no evidence that prevalence is greater than in the general population (Buchanan *et al.*, 1991; van de Laar & van der Korst, 1992). However, many patients self impose food restrictions to gain self empowerment in the management of their condition. Goff & Basari (1999) have reported that 67% of RA patients avoided a certain food or a number of foods, most commonly citrus fruit, tomatoes, vinegars, pickles, dairy products, red meat and alcohol. Clearly, the greater the number of foods avoided, particularly dairy products, then the greater the risk of nutritional imbalance or even deficiency.

Other supplements

As in many people with chronic diseases, the use of alternative and complementary dietary therapies is popular in patients with RA; supplement use is particularly common. A survey of patients with RA found that half of the respondents took some form of dietary supplement, the most common being cod liver oil. Other supplements frequently mentioned included evening primrose oil, iron, garlic, apple cider vinegar, vitamin C, selenium, B vitamins, calcium, general multivitamins and antioxidant supplements (Goff & Basari, 1999). None of the above supplements is supported by strong evidence of clinical efficacy in symptomatic RA. A systematic review of extract of New Zealand green lipped mussel found little evidence of efficacy in the management of RA (Cobb & Ernst, 2006). The results of a Cochrane review of herbal interventions compared with placebo in RA found seven studies that indicated benefits of gamma-linoleic acid (GLA) supplementation from evening primrose oil, borage seed oil or blackcurrant seed oil. Gamma-linoleic acid supplementation resulted in reduced pain intensity and improved disability, but an increase in adverse events, mainly gastrointestinal (Cameron *et al.*, 2011).

Vegetarian and vegan diets

A systematic review identified a small number of studies in which periods of fasting were followed by a vegetarian diet for up to 4 months' duration. The pooled analysis found improvement in symptoms of RA, such as duration of morning stiffness, number of tender and swollen joints, and pain (Müller *et al.*, 2001). However, the results could be confounded by the period of fasting prior to the vegetarian diet, which may have dampened inflammatory activity. Strict vegan diets comprising uncooked foods rich in lactobacilli have been reported by patients to improve symptoms, but these studies have not been substantiated by more objective measures of disease activity (Nenonen *et al.*, 1998).

Although symptomatic improvements are experienced after fasting and/or an elemental diet or vegetarian diet, the reasons for this are unclear. Possible explanations may be:

- The elimination of foods to which the patient is allergic or intolerant, e.g. a gluten free, vegan diet regimen given to patients with active RA reduced IgG antibody levels against gliadin, compared to the non-vegan diet controls (Hafström *et al.*, 2001).
- Inflammatory activity is attenuated by caloric restriction or reduction in gut involvement, but the effects could be a result of a coincidental remission (part of the course of the condition), weight loss or a placebo effect (Kavanaghi *et al.*, 1995).

Comorbidities

Cardiovascular disease

Patients with RA are at an increased risk of cardiovascular disease (CVD), especially ischaemic heart disease (IHD) and heart failure, and over 50% of premature deaths in RA are due to CVD (Symmons & Gabriel, 2011). Recent studies suggest that CVD mortality and morbidity in RA are of similar magnitude to those seen in people with type 2 diabetes mellitus (van Halm *et al.*, 2009). It may be that the increase in CVD observed in RA is due to the traditional risk factors for CVD (see Chapter 7.14.1) being more frequent in individuals with RA than in the general population, or they have an additional deleterious effect. Alternatively, some of the excess CVD risk might be explained by the adverse impact of the inflammation and immune changes of RA on blood vessel walls (Symmons & Gabriel, 2011).

Although hyperlipidaemia is less frequent in RA than the general population, a meta analysis confirmed that dyslipidaemia might affect up to half of all patients with RA, principally low levels of high density lipoprotein (HDL) cholesterol (Steiner & Urowitz, 2009). Further studies are required to assess the value of dietary modification for dyslipidaemia and obesity. However, until more is known, the best strategy is to manage risk factors as for the general population, along with aggressive treatment of disease activity. Further work is needed to establish whether using lower targets for cholesterol and blood pressure management will be of benefit in terms of CVD risk (Peters *et al.*, 2010).

Osteoporosis

Patients with RA and other forms of inflammatory arthritis are at an elevated risk of developing osteoporosis. This may be due to adverse effects on bone metabolism from the increased production of proinflammatory cytokines or the increasing loss of bone mass caused by corticosteroid treatment. Lack of weight bearing exercise, insufficient sunlight exposure and poor dietary intake are all detrimental to bone health (see Chapter 7.9.1).

Healthy eating

Despite folklore a specific diet for arthritis has never been proven. As with all patients, a full dietary assessment will identify dietary inadequacies and their causes. In the absence of a specific intervention for RA, dietary advice should focus on achieving optimal nutritional status through a nutritionally balanced diet.

However, there is evidence to support the role of n-3 fatty acids in the amelioration of inflammation and RA symptoms, as well as some epidemiological evidence for a role for antioxidants in reducing the risk of inflammatory arthritis (Cerhan *et al.*, 2003; Pattison *et al.*, 2004a; 2005). Although conflicting results have been reported, high red meat consumption may have a role in increasing the risk of developing RA (Grant, 2000, Pattison *et al.*, 2004b; Benito-Garcia *et al.*, 2007). The Mediterranean type diet has received a growing amount of attention in recent years because of its association with healthy populations living within the Mediterranean basin. Two studies of very different designs have investigated the effect of a diet based on the characteristics of a Mediterranean diet in people with RA (Sköldstam *et al.*, 2003; McKellar *et al.*, 2007). In a small randomised, controlled, parallel study, RA patients followed a modified Mediterranean diet for three months. Participants reported a significant reduction in disease activity, functional ability and improved vitality compared with those who followed the control diet (Sköldstam *et al.*, 2003). Despite an increase in reported consumption of antioxidant rich foods in the Mediterranean diet group, the levels of plasma antioxidants and urinary malondialdehyde (MDA), a marker of oxidative stress, did not change. However, the plasma levels of vitamin C, retinol and uric acid were inversely correlated to variables related to RA disease activity (Hagfors *et al.*, 2003). In a community based project in socially deprived areas, a 6-week educational programme with an emphasis on cooking and eating a Mediterranean type diet was studied. Women in the intervention group reported a healthier dietary intake and showed significant improvement in patient global assessment at 6 months, pain score at 3–6 months, duration of early morning stiffness at 6 months and Health Assessment Questionnaire (HAQ) score at 3 months (McKellar *et al.*, 2007).

Other forms of arthritis and arthralgia

Vitamin D and joint pain

Recently, there has been increased interest in the role of vitamin D in musculoskeletal conditions as the measurement of vitamin D levels is now readily available. In a recent study, 70% of consecutive new patients to general rheumatology clinics had vitamin D deficiency (defined as ≤53 nmol/L) and 26% had severe deficiency (defined as ≤25 nmol/L) (Haroon *et al.*, 2011). In patients diagnosed with OA and inflammatory joint disease, 62% and 69%, respectively, were deficient in vitamin D.

Osteomalacia is a bone disease caused by chronic and severe calcium, vitamin D or phosphate depletion of any cause. Bone pain, muscle weakness, tenderness and difficulty walking are common manifestations. In past years the most common causes of osteomalacia were malabsorption or prolonged lack of exposure to sunlight. However, nutritional deficiency is now a more common issue.

The multidisciplinary rheumatology team

People with arthritis and other musculoskeletal conditions need a wide range of high quality support and treatment, ranging from simple advice to highly specialised treatments. Multidisciplinary services are central to the management of arthritis, including a need for rapid referral to other specialists. The multidisciplinary team usually includes a rheumatologist, nurse specialist, physiotherapist, occupational therapist, dietitian, podiatrist, health psychologist, social worker and pharmacist. While full time roles are not warranted for all specialists, clearly defined access to all should be available. The multidisciplinary team has been shown to be effective in optimising management of patients with arthritis (Vliet Vlieland & Hazes, 1997).

Internet resources

Arthritis Care www.arthritiscare.org.uk
Arthritis Research UK (formerly Arthritis Research Campaign) www.arthritisresearchuk.org
British Health Professionals in Rheumatology www.rheumatology.org.uk/bhpr
Disabled Living Foundation www.dlf.org.uk
National Rheumatoid Arthritis Society www.nras.org.uk

References

Adam O. (1995) Anti-inflammatory diet in rheumatic diseases. *European Journal of Clinical Nutrition* 49: 703–717.

Adam O, Beringer C, Kless T, *et al.* (2003) Anti-inflammatory effects of a low arachidonic acid diet and fish oil in patients with rheumatoid arthritis. *Rheumatology International* 23: 27–36.

Aspden RM. (2011) Obesity punches above its weight in osteoarthritis. *Nature Reviews Rheumatology* 7: 65–68.

Benito-Garcia E, Feskanich D, Hu FB, *et al.* (2007) Protein, iron, and meat consumption and risk for rheumatoid arthritis: a prospective cohort study. *Arthritis Research & Therapy* 9: R16.

Berend KR, Lombardi AV, Mallory TH. (2004) Rapid recovery protocol for peri-operative care of total hip and total knee arthroplasty patients. *Surgical Technology International* 13: 239–247.

Buchanan HM, Preston PM, Buchanan WW. (1991) Is diet important in rheumatoid arthritis? *British Journal of Rheumatology* 30: 125–134.

Calder PC. (2006) n-3 Polyunsaturated fatty acids, inflammation, and inflammatory diseases. *American Journal of Clinical Nutrition* 83: 1505S–1519S.

Cameron M, Gagnier JJ, Chrubasik S. (2011) Herbal therapy for treating rheumatoid arthritis. *Cochrane Database of Systematic Reviews* 2: CD002948.

Canter PH, Wider B, Ernst E. (2007) The antioxidant vitamins A, C, E and selenium in the treatment of arthritis: s systematic review of randomised controlled trials. *Rheumatology (Oxford)* 46: 1223–1233.

Cerhan JR, Saag KG, Merlino LA, *et al.* (2003) Antioxidant micronutrients and risk of rheumatoid arthritis in a cohort of older women. *American Journal of Epidemiology* 157: 345–354.

Cobb CS, Ernst E. (2006) Systematic review of marine nutriceutical supplement in clinical trials for arthritis: the effectiveness of the New Zealand green-lipped mussel Perna canaliculus. *Clinical Rheumatology* 25: 275–284.

Fortin PR. Lew RA, Liang MH, *et al.* (1995) Validation of a meta-analysis: the effects of fish oil in rheumatoid arthritis. *Journal of Clinical Epidemiology* 48: 1379–1390.

Galarraga B, Ho M, Youssef HM, *et al.* (2008) Cod liver oil (*n-3* fatty acids) as an non-steroidal anti-inflammatory drug sparing agent in rheumatoid arthritis. *Rheumatology* 47: 665–669.

Goff LM, Basari M. (1999) An assessment of the diets of people with rheumatoid arthritis. *Journal of Human Nutrition and Dietetics* 12: 93–101.

Goldberg RJ, Katz J. (2007) A meta-analysis of the analgesic effects of omega-3 polyunsaturated fatty acid supplementation for inflammatory joint pain. *Pain* 129: 210–223.

Grant WB. (2000) The role of red meat in the expression of rheumatoid arthritis. *British Journal of Nutrition* 84: 589–595.

Hafström I, Ringertz B, Spångberg A, *et al.* (2001) A vegan diet free of gluten improves the signs and symptoms of rheumatoid arthritis: the effects on arthritis correlate with a reduction in antibodies to food antigen. *Rheumatology (Oxford)* 40: 1175–1179.

Hagfors L, Leanderson P, Sköldstam L, *et al.* (2003) Antioxidant intake, plasma antioxidants and oxidative stress in a randomized, controlled, parallel, Mediterranean dietary intervention study on patients with rheumatoid arthritis. *Nutrition Journal* 2: 5.

Haroon M, Bond U, Quillinan N *et al.* (2011) The prevalence of vitamin D deficiency in consecutive new patients seen over a 6-month period in general rheumatology clinics. *Clinical Rheumatology* 30: 789–794.

Hart DJ, Doyle DV, Spector TD. (1995) Association between metabolic factors and knee osteoarthritis in women: the Chingford Study. *Journal of Rheumatology* 22: 1118–1123.

Haugen M, Homme KA, Reigstad A, *et al.* (1999) Assessment of nutritional status in patients with rheumatoid arthritis and osteoarthritis undergoing joint replacement surgery. *Arthritis Care and Research* 12: 26–32.

Heliövaara M, Knekt P, Aho K, *et al.* (1994) Serum antioxidants and risk of rheumatoid arthritis. *Annals of the Rheumatic Diseases* 53: 51–53.

Huang MH, Chen CH, Chen TW, *et al.* (2000) The effects of weight reduction on the rehabilitation of patients with knee osteoarthritis and obesity. *Arthritis Care and Research* 13: 398–405.

Kavanaghi R, Workman E, Nash P, *et al.* (1995) The effects of elemental diet and subsequent food reintroduction on rheumatoid arthritis. *British Journal of Rheumatology* 34: 270–273.

Long L, Soeken K, Ernst E. (2001) Herbal medicines for the treatment of osteoarthritis: a systematic review. *Rheumatology* 40: 779–793.

McKellar G, Morrison E, McEntegart A, *et al.* (2007) A pilot study of a Mediterranean-type diet intervention in female patients with rheumatoid arthritis living in areas of social deprivation in Glasgow. *Annals of the Rheumatic Diseases* 66: 1239–1243.

Messier SP, Loeser RF, Miller GD, *et al.* (2004) Exercise and dietary weight loss in overweight and obese older adults with knee osteoarthritis: the Arthritis, Diet, and Activity Promotion Trial. *Arthritis & Rheumatism* 50: 1501–1510.

Morgan SL, Anderson AM, Hood SM, *et al.* (1997) Nutrient intake patterns, body mass index and vitamin levels in patients with rheumatoid arthritis. *Arthritis Care and Research* 10: 9–17.

Müller H, de Toledo FW, Resch KL. (2001) Fasting followed by vegetarian diet in patients with rheumatoid arthritis: a systematic review. *Scandinavian Journal of Rheumatology* 30: 1–10.

National Institute for Health and Care Excellence (NICE). (2008) *Osteoarthritis: The Care and Management of Osteoarthritis in Adults*. NICE Clinical Guideline 59. London: Royal College of Physicians.

National Institute for Health and Care Excellence (NICE). (2009) *Rheumatoid Arthritis: The Management of Rheumatoid Arthritis in Adults*. NICE Clinical Guideline 79. London: Royal College of Physicians.

Nenonen MT, Helve TA, Rauma AL, *et al.* (1998) Uncooked, lactobacilli-rich, vegan food and rheumatoid arthritis. *British Journal of Rheumatology* 37: 274–281.

Niu J, Zhang YQ, Torner J, *et al.* (2009) Is obesity a risk factor for progressive radiographic knee osteoarthritis? *Arthritis Rheumatism* 61: 329–335.

Pattison DJ, Silman AJ, Goodson NJ *et al.* (2004a) Vitamin C and the risk of developing inflammatory polyarthritis: prospective nested case-control study. *Annals of the Rheumatic Diseases* 63: 843–847.

Pattison DJ, Symmons DPM, Lunt M, *et al.* (2004b) Dietary risk factors for the development of inflammatory polyarthritis: evidence for a role of red meat consumption. *Arthritis & Rheumatism* 50: 3804–3812.

Pattison DJ, Symmons DPM, Lunt M, *et al.* (2005) Dietary β-cryptoxanthin and inflammatory polyarthritis: results from a population-based prospective study. *American Journal of Clinical Nutrition* 82: 451–455.

Peters MJL, Symmons DPM, McCarey D, *et al.* (2010) EULAR evidence-based recommendations for cardiovascular risk management in patients with rheumatoid arthritis and other form of inflammatory arthritis. *Annals of the Rheumatic Diseases* 69: 325–331.

Simpoulous AP. (2009) Omega-6/omega-3 essential fatty acids: Biological effects. In: Simpoulous AP, Bazan NG (eds) *Omega-3 Fatty Acids, the Brain and Retina. World Review of Nutrition and Dietetics* 99: 1–16.

Sköldstam L, Hagfors L, Johansson G. (2003) An experimental study of a Mediterranean diet intervention for patients with rheumatoid arthritis. *Annals of the Rheumatic Diseases* 62: 208–214.

Steiner G, Urowitz MB. (2009) Lipid profiles in patients with rheumatoid arthritis: mechanisms and the impact of treatment. *Seminars in Arthritis & Rheumatism* 38: 372–381.

Stone J, Doube A, Dudson D, *et al.* (1997) Inadequate calcium, folic acid, vitamin E, zinc and selenium intake in rheumatoid arthritis patients: results of a dietary survey. *Seminars in Arthritis & Rheumatism* 27: 180–185.

Symmons DPM, Gabriel SE. (2011) Epidemiology of CVD in rheumatic disease, with a focus on RA and SLE. *Nature Reviews in Rheumatology* 7: 399–408.

Symmons D, Turner G, Webb R, *et al.* (2002) The prevalence of rheumatoid arthritis in the United Kingdom: new estimates for a new century. *Rheumatology* 41(7): 793–800.

Toda Y, Toda T, Takemura S, *et al.* (1998) Change in body fat, but not body weight or metabolic correlates of obesity, is related to symptomatic relief of obese patients with knee osteoarthritis after a weight control program. *Journal of Rheumatology* 25: 2181–2186.

Towheed TE, Maxwell L, Anastassiades TP *et al.* (2005) Glucosamine therapy for treating osteoarthritis. *Cochrane Database of Systematic Reviews* 2: CD002946.

SECTION 7

van de Laar MA, van der Korst JK. (1992) Food intolerance in rheumatoid arthritis. I. A double-blind, controlled trial of the clinical effects of the elimination of milk allergens and azo dyes. *Annals of the Rheumatic Diseases* 51: 298–302.

van Halm VP, Peters MJ, Voskuyl AE, *et al.* (2009) Rheumatoid arthritis versus diabetes as a risk factor for cardiovascular disease: a cross-sectional study, the CARRE Investigation. *Annals of the Rheumatic Diseases* 68: 1395–1400.

Vliet Vlieland TP, Hazes JM. (1997) Efficacy of multidisciplinary team care programs in rheumatoid arthritis. *Seminars in Arthritis and Rheumatism* 27: 110–122.

Wandel S, Jüni P, Tendal B, *et al.* (2010) Effects of glucosamine, chondroitin, or placebo in patients with osteoarthritis of hip or knee: network meta-analysis. *BMJ* 341: c4675.

Wiles N, Symmons DPM, Harrison B, *et al.* (1999) Estimating the incidence of rheumatoid arthritis – Trying to hit a moving target? *Arthritis & Rheumatism* 42(7): 1339–1346.

Young A, Dixey J, Kulinskaya E, *et al.* (2002) Which patients stop working because of rheumatoid arthritis? Results of five years' follow up in 732 patients from the Early RA Study (ERAS). *Annals of the Rheumatic Diseases* 61: 335–340.

7.9.3 Gout

Joan Gandy

Key points

■ Gout is the most common form of inflammatory arthritis and is associated with poor quality of life.

■ Risk factors that are associated with the increase in gout prevalence include offal, seafood, alcohol and fructose corn syrup.

■ Other risk factors include obesity, hypertension and other features of the metabolic syndrome.

■ Recommendations for the management include weight management, healthy eating, exercise and staying well with avoidance of dietary risk factors such as offal.

Gout is the most common form of inflammatory arthritis in men (Roddy & Doherty, 2010) and is associated with poor quality of life (Roddy *et al.*, 2007). It is caused by uric acid crystallising as monosodium urate (MSU) in joints, and sometimes other tissues, causing inflammation, swelling and severe pain; often experienced as excruciating attacks of pain. The metatarsal phalangeal joint (the joint between the big toe and ball of the foot) is most commonly affected. Gout is associated with high plasma levels of uric acid, hyperuricacidaemia, over a long period. It is present in most gout sufferers; however, high levels do not lead to gout in everyone and levels can be normal during an attack (Campion *et al.*, 1987; Zhang *et al.*, 2006a). For gout to occur there is usually sustained hyperuricacidaemia, MSU crystal formation and inflammation caused by interaction between MSU and inflammatory processes. The upper limit for urate is 0.42 mmol/L for men and 0.36 mmol/L for premenopausal women.

In humans uric acid is the end product of purine metabolism. Purines are the bases guanine and adenine, which with thymine and cystosine form the genetic code material of RNA and DNA. Hyperuricacidaemia is caused by one of the following mechanisms, or a combination of them:

- Increased endogenous production of uric acid.
- Decreased renal excretion of uric acid.
- Increased dietary intake of purine.

Prevalence

The incidence of gout in the UK is 2.68 per 1000 person years (4.42 in men and 1.32 in women) (Soriano *et al.*, 2011). Prevalence varies between countries and populations, with New Zealand Maoris having a particularly high prevalence of 6.4%. This variation is probably due to genetic, environmental and dietary factors. Gout is uncommon in premenopausal women as oestrogen increases uric acid excretion. Prevalence increases in men and women with age, with mean ages of onset of 60.1 and 67.7 years, respectively.

Diagnosis

Severe pain, swelling and erythema (redness) over a joint are strongly suggestive, but not diagnostic, of gout. A clinical diagnosis should be confirmed by demonstration of MSU crystals in the synovial fluid of the joint (Zhang *et al.*, 2006a). In chronic gout, large crystal deposits may form on joints (tophi) and joints may become eroded (Schumacher, 2008). Risk factors for gout and associated conditions should also be assessed.

Risk factors and associated conditions

Hyeruricacidaemia, age and genetic factors influence the risk of developing gout. Other risk factors for gout include:

- Dietary factors.
- Alcohol consumption.
- Metabolic syndrome and its components.
- Diuretic use.
- Renal disease.

Dietary factors

An association between diet and gout has been recognised anecdotally for many years. This has now been confirmed in large well designed epidemiological studies, such as the Health Professionals Follow-up Study (HPFS), which followed over 50000 men for 10 years. Consumption of seafood and meat was associated with relative risks for gout of 1.51 and 1.41, respectively (Choi *et al.*, 2004a). There was no association with purine rich vegetables. Low fat dairy products were protective as was coffee consumption (Choi *et al.*, 2007a). The relative risk (RR) of gout for participants drinking two or more sugar sweetened soft drinks was 1.85; the RR was similar for fructose consumption, although there was no increased risk associated with the consumption of diet soft drinks (Choi & Curhan, 2008).

It has been suggested that vitamin C may be protective and a further analysis of the HPFS (Choi *et al.*, 2009) showed a RR of developing gout of 0.55 in participants who consumed >1500 mg of dietary vitamin C/day compared with those consuming <250 mg/day.

It is important to remember that these are associations that are suggestive of links between diet and the risk of developing gout. Well designed, randomised trials are needed to confirm the role of dietary factors in the prevention and treatment of gout.

Alcohol

Alcohol consumption has a graded relationship. The type of alcoholic drink influenced the risk of developing gout, with the highest risk being amongst beer drinkers, followed by spirit drinkers (Choi *et al.*, 2004b). While the amount of alcohol consumed was important, the high amount of purines in beer may also have influenced the results. Data from the Framingham Heart Study showed that women who were heavy drinkers had a three-fold higher risk of developing gout than abstinent or light drinkers (Bhole *et al.*, 2010). Heavy drinking men were twice as likely to develop gout as abstinent or light drinking men. A dose dependent relationship between the amount of alcohol consumed in the 48 hours before an acute attack and an attack has also been shown (Zhang *et al.*, 2006b).

Metabolic syndrome

There is an association between gout and the metabolic syndrome and its individual components; obesity, hypertension, type 2 diabetes and dyslipidaemia. In the National Health and Nutrition Examination Study, the prevalence of metabolic syndrome amongst patients with gout was 62.8% compared with 25.4% in the age and gender matched group without gout (Choi *et al.*, 2007b). In a large analysis of over 170000 gout patients, Primatesta *et al.* (2011) reported that more than half (58.1%) had one or more of the comorbidities of metabolic syndrome; diabetes (15.1%), dyslipidaemia (27.0%) and hypertension (36.1%) were the most common. The presence of these comorbidities was associated with increased risk of an acute attack, with women being particularly vulnerable. Gout is associated with an increased risk of myocardial infarction (Kuo *et al.*, 2013), heart failure and cardiac associated mortality (Krishnan, 2012). Lifestyle and dietetic management of the components of metabolic syndrome is becoming increasingly important.

Diuretic use

There is an association between the use of diuretics and gout, although this relationship is confounded by the reason for the use of the diuretics, e.g. hypertension, which may also increase the risk of gout (Choi *et al.*, 2005; Mikuls *et al.*, 2005). There is some evidence to suggest that diuretic use may be associated with acute gout attacks (Hunter *et al.*, 2006).

Renal disease

Chronic renal disease greatly increases the risk of gout (Mikuls *et al.*, 2005), as does dialysis and transplantation.

Clinical management

Acute episodes of gout are managed with non-steroidal anti-inflammatory drugs (NSAIDs) or colchicine. Once the acute phase has subsided, the condition can be kept under control with long term drug treatment:

- Allopurinol – a xanthine oxidase inhibitor that reduces uric acid production.
- Febuxostrate – a xanthine oxidase inhibitor. The National Institute for Health and Care Excellence (2008) recommends its use when allopurinol is contraindicated.
- Uricosuric drugs, e.g. probenecid or sulfinpyrazone, increase urinary uric acid excretion.

Dietary and lifestyle management

There is a paucity of evidence from large, well designed studies to support the use of dietary modifications in the management of gout. Recommendations for the dietary and lifestyle management of gout are mainly based on epidemiological and observational studies, and expert opinion (Jordan *et al.*, 2007; Zhang *et al.*, 2006a). In 2012 the American College of Rheumatology published guidelines for the management of gout and in which it also considered reducing risk factors for comorbidities, including the metabolic syndrome and its components, insulin resistance, type 2 diabetes (see Chapter 7.12), dyslipidaemia (see Chapter 7.14.3), hypertension (see Chapter 7.14.4) and obesity (see Chapter 7.13.2) (Khanna *et al.*, 2012). The recommendations are summarised in Table

Table 7.9.3 General health, diet and lifestyle recommendations for patients with gout [modified from Khanna *et al.* (2012)]

Weight loss for obese/overweight patients to achieve a BMI that promotes general health
Healthy overall diet
Exercise (achieve physical fitness)
Smoking cessation
Stay well hydrated

Avoid	Limit	Encourage
Organ meats (offal) high in purines, e.g. liver, kidney, sweetbreads	Serving sizes of: Beef, lamb, pork Seafood with high purine content, e.g. sardines, shellfish, anchovies, fish roe, mackerel, sprats, whitebait	Low fat or non-fat dairy products
High fructose corn syrup sweetened fizzy drinks, other beverages or foods	Serving of naturally sweetened fruit juice Table sugar, sweetened beverages and desserts Table salt Sauces, gravies Meat and yeast extracts Quorn	Vegetables*
Alcohol >2 units/day in men and >1 unit/day in women in all gout patients Any alcohol during periods of frequent gout attacks or poorly controlled advanced gout	Alcohol, particularly beer, but also wine and spirits in all gout patients	

*Some vegetables are moderate sources of purines, e.g. asparagus, cauliflower and spinach; however, there is no convincing evidence to recommend their avoidance.

7.9.3. The evidence for restricting purines comes mainly from epidemiological studies such as the HPFS. However, a recent case crossover study of 633 participants with gout showed that acute purine intake increased the risk of an attack five-fold. The restriction of purines is also supported by expert guidelines (Jordan *et al.*, 2007; Khanna *et al.*, 2012).

Given the comorbidities associated with gout, including the metabolic syndrome and cardiac morbidities, dietetic management is likely to become increasingly important in this form of arthritis.

Internet resources

American College of Rheumatology www.rheumatology.org
Arthritis Care www.arthritiscare.org.uk
Arthritis Research UK www.arthritisresearchuk.org
British Society for Rheumatology www.rheumatology.org.uk
European League Against Rheumatism www.eular.org
UK Gout Society www.ukgoutsociety.org

References

Bhole V, de Vera M, Rahman MM, Krishnan E, Choi H. (2010) Epidemiology of gout in women: fifty-two-year follow up of a prospective cohort. *Arthritis & Rheumatism* 62: 1069–1076.
Campion EW, Glynn RJ, DeLabry LO. (1987) Asymptomatic hyperuricemia. Risks and consequences in the Normative Aging Study. *American Journal of Medicine* 82(3): 421–426.
Choi HK, Curhan G. (2008) Soft drinks, fructose consumption, and the risk of gout in men: prospective cohort study. *BMJ* 336: 309–312.
Choi HK, Atkinson K, Karlson EW, Willett W, Curhan G. (2004a) Purine-rich foods, dairy and protein intake, and the risk of gout in men. *New England Journal of Medicine* 350: 1093–1103.
Choi HK, Atkinson K, Karlson EW, Willett W, Curhan G. (2004b) Alcohol intake and risk of incident gout in men: a prospective study. *Lancet* 363: 1277–1281.
Choi HK, Atkinson K, Karlson EW, Curhan G. (2005) Obesity, weight change, hypertension, diuretic use, and risk of gout in men: the health professionals follow-up study. *Archives of Internal Medicine* 165: 742–748.
Choi HK, Willett W, Curhan G. (2007a) Coffee consumption and risk of incident gout in men: a prospective study. *Arthritis & Rheumatism* 56: 2049–2055.
Choi HK, Ford ES, Li C, Curhan G. (2007b) Prevalence of the metabolic syndrome in patients with gout: the Third National Health and Nutrition Examination Survey. *Arthritis & Rheumatism* 57: 109–115.
Choi HK, Gao X, Curhan G. (2009) Vitamin C intake and the risk of gout in men: a prospective study. *Archives of Internal Medicine* 169: 502–507.
Hunter DJ, York M, Chaisson CE, Woods R, Niu J, Zhang Y. (2006) Recent diuretic use and the risk of recurrent gout attacks: the online case-crossover gout study. *Journal of Rheumatology* 33(7): 1341–1345.
Jordan KM, Cameron JS, Snaith M, *et al*; British Society for Rheumatology and British Health Professionals in Rheumatology Standards, Guidelines and Audit Working Group (SGAWG). (2007) British Society for Rheumatology and British Health Professionals in Rheumatology guideline for the management of gout. *Rheumatology* 46(8): 1372–1374.
Khanna D, Fitzgerald JD, Khanna PP, *et al.* (2012) American College of RheumatologyGuidelines for Management of Gout. Part 1: Systematic Nonpharmacologic and Pharmacologic Therapeutic Approaches to Hyperuricemia. *Arthritis Care & Research* 64: 1431–1446.
Krishnan E. (2012) Gout and the risk for incident heart failure and systolic dysfunction. *BMJ Open* 2: e000282.
Kuo CF, Yu KH, See LC, *et al.* (2013) Risk of myocardial infarction among patients with gout: a nationwide population-based study. *Rheumatology* 52(1): 111–117.

Mikuls TR, Farrar JT, Bilker WB, Fernandes S, Schumacher HR Jr, Saag KG. (2005) Gout epidemiology: results from the UK General Practice Research Database, 1990–1999. *Annals of Rheumatic Diseases* 64: 267–272.

National Institute for Health and Care Excellence (NICE). (2008) Febuxostat for the management of hyperuricaemia in people with gout (TA164). Available at http://guidance.nice.org.uk/TA164/Guidance. Accessed 5 March 2013.

Primatesta P, Plana E, Rotherbacher D. (2011) Gout treatment and comorbidities: a retrospective cohort study in a large US managed care population. *BMC Musculoskeletal Disorders* 12: 103–109.

Roddy E, Doherty M. (2010) Epidemiology of gout. *Arthritis Research and Therapy* 12(6): 223.

Roddy E, Zhang W, Doherty M. (2007) The changing epidemiology of gout. *Nature Clinical Practice in Rheumatology* 3(8): 443–449.

Schumacher HR Jr. (2008) The pathogenesis of gout. *Cleveland Clinic Journal of Medicine* 75 (5): S2–4.

Soriano LC, Rothenbacher D, Choi HK, Rodríguez LAG. (2011) Contemporary epidemiology of gout in the UK general population. *Arthritis Research & Therapy* 13: R39.

Zhang W, Doherty M, Pascual E, *et al.* (2006a) EULAR evidence based recommendations for gout. Part I: Diagnosis. Report of a task force of the Standing Committee for International Clinical Studies Including Therapeutics (ESCISIT). *Annals of Rheumatic Diseases* 65(10): 1301–1311.

Zhang Y, Woods R, Chaisson CE, Neogi T, Niu J, McAlindon TE, Hunter D. (2006b) Alcohol consumption as a trigger of recurrent gout attacks. *American Journal of Medicine* 119: 800–808.

7.10.1 Eating disorders

Kate Williams

Key points

■ Dietitians in all areas of clinical practice should be alert to signs of undiagnosed disordered eating and be able to offer guidance on further investigation and support.

■ Dietitians working in the field of eating disorders management should be part of a multidisciplinary team, and have appropriate support and supervision.

Eating disorders are syndromes in which abnormalities of eating behaviour, which are driven by psychological factors, are severe and persistent enough to impair health and nutrition; interfere with social eating; and give rise to distress in the sufferer and those close to them. In all areas of clinical practice, dietitians discuss with their patients the detail of eating behaviour, so are often able to identify disordered eating. Although some people with eating disorders may go to great lengths to conceal them, many may welcome the opportunity to raise their concerns and begin to get help. It is important for dietitians to enable patients to talk honestly about their eating, identify possible eating disorders and offer support to get the help they need. Disordered eating may severely interfere with the dietetic treatment of other conditions, so dietitians need to be alert to the possibility of disordered eating in all areas of clinical practice in order to achieve good outcomes of treatment.

As changing eating behaviour and improving nutrition are central to recovery from eating disorders, dietitians can make important contributions to the care and treatment of people with these conditions. There are few areas of dietetic practice that demand more skill in engaging and motivating patients, and communicating with colleagues. A warm, empathic and non-judgemental therapeutic relationship can empower a patient to discuss anxiety and distress about eating, and use help and support. For a guide to developing and using these skills, see Gable (2007). For detailed reviews of the contribution of the dietitian to the management of eating disorders, see Hart *et al*. (2011), American Dietetic Association (ADA) (2011), Garrett *et al*. (2005) and Herrin (2003).

Background and historical perspective

In anorexia nervosa the central feature is deliberate and persistent restriction of food intake. It, or at least a condition with very similar features, has been described for hundreds, possibly thousands, of years (Vandereycken & van Deth, 1994; Brumberg, 1988; Grimm, 1996). Anorexia nervosa was first named in the medical literature in the late 19th century by Gull (1874; 1888) and Lasègue (1873). Strikingly, these descriptions do not refer to the fear of fatness as an essential feature; this seems to have emerged in western cultures during the 20th century, alongside increasing social valuation of thinness, especially in women (Bruch, 1973). The condition may present differently in some individuals, especially those from non-western cultures (Nasser, 1997).

Bulimia nervosa is a condition in which there is a cycle of restriction of food intake, followed by binge eating and extreme efforts to compensate for the feared fattening effects of the binge, commonly by repeated restriction of eating, vomiting, excessive use of laxatives or over exercising. Russell first described it in the medical literature

---

in 1979. He characterised it initially as a development of anorexia nervosa (Russell, 1979). It quickly became clear that it might arise without any previous episodes of anorexia. The change from restricting anorexia to bulimia nervosa is not unusual (Fairburn & Harrison, 2003) and people with eating disorders may display different symptoms at different times. Partial syndromes are a common presentation.

In 1992 Spitzer *et al.* proposed diagnostic criteria for binge eating disorder, in which the individual regularly binge eats, but does not compensate for the binges. The binge eating is distinguished from normal occasional overeating by its persistence and frequency, and the psychological distress associated with it. It is generally associated with obesity, which may be severe.

Diagnostic criteria and classification

Two published sets of diagnostic criteria for eating disorders are in use; the International Classification of Diseases, published by the World Health Organization, and the Diagnostic and Statistical Manual of Mental Disorders (DSM), published by the American Psychiatric Association (1994). These documents set out criteria for the diagnosis of the major disorders, anorexia nervosa and bulimia nervosa, and for some partial syndromes (Table 7.10.1). DSM IV also proposes diagnostic criteria for binge eating disorder for research purposes (Box 7.10.1). These strict definitions allow the identification of the disorders for research and other purposes, but in clinical practice dietitians may encounter many people with disordered eating who do not exactly meet any of these criteria, but need help to recover. The next revision of DSM (DSM V) is likely to include diagnostic criteria for binge eating disorder as one of the eating disorders not otherwise specified (EDNOS).

Features and processes of eating disorders

It can be difficult to understand disorders that provoke behaviour that seems very abnormal and damaging. It may be helpful for the practitioner seeking to develop an empathic relationship with a person with an eating disorder to have some awareness of the way the disorders develop and become entrenched.

Anorexia nervosa

The central feature of anorexia nervosa is restriction of food intake severely enough to keep body mass index below $17.5\,kg/m^2$ and often much lower, with the resulting constellation of features of starvation. This is accompanied by a conviction that the restriction of food intake is appropriate for the individual, usually because they feel the need to reduce their weight.

It is known that there are genetic predisposing factors (Bulik *et al.*, 2007; Gorwood *et al.*, 2003). Some personality traits and thinking styles are known to increase vulnerability to developing anorexia nervosa. A tendency to perfectionism, rule bound and rigid thinking, and attention to detail at the expense of a broader and more flexible approach can predispose to the disorder (Treasure *et al.*, 2010). Distressing experiences in early life such as emotional or physical neglect, or physical or sexual abuse add to the risk. A very usual trigger in western cultures is dieting, which is tried by the great majority of adolescent girls and many boys. Well publicised diets offer many detailed rules, and may seem gratifying to a person with a perfectionistic, rigid and detail focussed approach. In vulnerable individuals, dieting may become entrenched because of anxiety about breaking self imposed rules, and perfectionism and self criticism driving continually increasing efforts. The pursuit of weight loss can seem rewarding and offer a distraction from persistent emotional distress, becoming increasingly extreme and fixed behaviour. Any increase in food intake may result in rapid weight gain because of repletion of glycogen stores with associated water, and so add to the belief that breaking the rules of the diet will result in uncontrollable weight increase.

From this experience develops a profound fear of fatness and weight gain, and body image distortion, although other anxieties may predominate in some individuals. In many individuals, the increasing hunger and food craving lead to binge eating, with anxiety driven attempts to compensate for the binge with purging or exercise (Fairburn & Harrison, 2003). The behaviour may become very fixed because it begins at a time of rapid brain development, and the malnutrition itself may interfere with this process, in particular the maturation of emotional regulation, so that the person may find it difficult to counter the anxiety and other emotions that drive the abnormal behaviour (Treasure *et al.*, 2010; Harrison *et al.*, 2009).

Bulimia nervosa

The major feature of bulimia nervosa is a cycle of restriction of eating, which may be very severe, followed by food craving and uncontrolled excessive eating. This raises anxiety about the possible weight increase the binge might cause, provoking attempts to compensate, most commonly by self induced vomiting, excessive use of laxatives or excessive exercise, and further restriction of eating. This binge–starve cycle is driven by over valuation of thinness, and attempts to lose weight as a means to improve low self esteem. Low mood can deprive the individual of the motivation to change (Ruhsing *et al.*, 2003). Predisposing factors include poor impulse control and, like in anorexia nervosa, distressing early experience increases risk. Attempts to diet, commonly beginning in the early teenage years, may be unsuccessful in response to hunger and food craving, setting up the binge–starve cycle (Figure 7.10.1). It is possible that binge eaters have an increased drive to seek rewarding behaviour, and that the binge–starve cycle can become entrenched as food deprivation increases the reward of eating, so the drive to binge becomes increasingly

SECTION 7

Table 7.10.1 Diagnostic criteria for eating disorders

ICD-10 (World Health Organization, 1992)	DSM-IV (American Psychiatric Association, 1994)
Anorexia nervosa For a definite diagnosis, all the following are required: a) Body weight is maintained at least 15% below that expected (either lost or never achieved) or BMI ≤17.5 or less. Prepubertal patients may fail to make the expected weight gain during the period of growth b) The weight loss is self induced by avoidance of 'fattening foods'. One or more of the following may also be present: self induced vomiting; self induced purging; excessive exercise; use of appetite suppressants and/or diuretics c) There is body image distortion in the form of a specific psychopathology whereby a dread of fatness persists as an intrusive, overvalued idea and the patient imposes a low weight threshold on him/herself d) A widespread endocrine disorder involving the hypothalamic–pituitary–gonadal axis is manifest in women as amenorrhoea and in men as a loss of sexual interest and potency. (An apparent exception is the persistence of vaginal bleeds in anorexic women who are receiving hormonal replacement therapy, most commonly taken as the contraceptive pill.) There may also be elevated levels of growth hormone, raised levels of cortisol, changes in the peripheral metabolism of the thyroid gland, and abnormalities of insulin secretion e) If onset is prepubertal, the sequence of pubertal events is delayed or even arrested (growth ceases; in girls the breasts do not develop and there is primary amenorrhoea; in boys the genitals remain juvenile). With recovery, puberty is often completed normally, but menarche is late	A. A refusal to maintain body weight at or above a minimally normal weight for age and height, e.g. weight loss leading to maintenance of body weight <85% of that expected; or failure to make expected weight gain during a period of growth, leading to a body weight <85% of that expected) B. Intense fear of gaining weight or becoming fat, even though underweight C. Disturbance in the way in which one's body weight or shape is experienced, undue influence of body weight or shape on self evaluation, or denial of the seriousness of the current low body weight D. In postmenarcheal females, amenorrhoea, i.e. the absence of at least three consecutive menstrual cycles. (A woman is considered to have amenorrhea if her periods occur only following hormone, e.g. oestrogen, administration) Type of anorexia nervosa is also specified as: **Restricting type:** during the current episode of anorexia nervosa, the person has not regularly engaged in binge eating or purging behaviour, i.e. self induced vomiting or the misuse of laxatives, diuretics or enemas) **Binge eating/purging type:** during the current episode of anorexia nervosa, the person has regularly engaged in binge eating or purging behaviour, i.e. self induced vomiting or the misuse of laxatives, diuretics or enemas)
Bulimia nervosa For a definite diagnosis, all of the following are required: a) There is persistent preoccupation with eating, and an irresistible craving for food; the patient succumbs to episodes of overeating in which large amounts of food are consumed in short periods of time b) The patient attempts to counteract the 'fattening' effects of food by one or more of the following: self induced vomiting; purgative abuse; alternating periods of starvation; use of drugs such as appetite suppressants, thyroid preparations or diuretics. When bulimia occurs in diabetic patients, they may choose to neglect their insulin treatment c) The psychopathology consists of a morbid dread of fatness, and the patient sets her/himself a sharply defined weight threshold, well below the premorbid weight that constitutes the optimum or healthy weight in the opinion of the physician. There is often, but not always, a history of an earlier episode of anorexia nervosa, the interval between the two disorders ranging from a few months to several years. This earlier episode may have been fully expressed, or may have assumed a minor cryptic form with a moderate loss of weight and/or a transient phase of amenorrhoea	A. Recurrent episodes of binge eating. An episode of binge eating is characterised by both of the following: 1. Eating in a discrete period of time, (e.g. within 2 hours, an amount of food that is definitely larger than most people would eat during a similar period of time and under similar circumstances 2. A sense of lack of control over eating during the episode, e.g. a feeling that one cannot stop eating or control what or how much one is eating B. Recurrent inappropriate compensatory behaviour in order to prevent weight gain, such as self induced vomiting; misuse of laxatives, diuretics, enemas or other medications; fasting or excessive exercise C. The binge eating and inappropriate compensatory behaviours both occur on average at least twice a week for 3 months D. Self evaluation is unduly influenced by body shape and weight E. The disturbance does not occur exclusively during episodes of anorexia nervosa

powerful (Davis *et al.*, 2008; Thanos *et al.*, 2008; Wang *et al.*, 2011).

Partial and mixed syndromes, including binge eating disorder

In any individual, the symptoms of an eating disorder may change over time, so that they move from one diagnostic category to another (Fairburn & Harrison, 2003). In clini-

cal practice, the most commonly occurring eating disorders are partial syndromes that do not fully meet diagnostic criteria for anorexia nervosa or bulimia nervosa. Management strategies can be agreed on the basis of the most damaging or distressing symptoms. Binge eating disorder is characterised by repeated episodes of binge eating, without significant compensatory behaviours other than repeated attempts at dieting (Spitzer *et al.*, 1992). Levels of concern about weight and shape are

Box 7.10.1 Research criteria for binge eating disorder (American Psychiatric Association 1994)

A. Recurrent episodes of binge eating. Binge eating is characterised by two of the following:
  • Eating in a discrete period of time, e.g. 2 hours, an amount of food that is definitely larger than most people would eat during a similar period of time and in the same circumstances
  • A sense of lack of control over eating during the episode, e.g. a feeling that one cannot stop eating or control how much one is eating
B. The binge eating episodes are associated with three or more of the following:
  • Eating much more rapidly than normal
  • Eating until feeling uncomfortably full
  • Eating large amounts of food when not feeling physical hunger
  • Eating alone because of being embarrassed by how much one is eating
  • Feeling disgusted with oneself, depressed or very guilty after overeating
C. Marked distress regarding binge eating is present
D. The binge eating occurs on average at least 2 days per week for 6 months
E. The binge eating is not associated with the regular use of inappropriate compensatory behaviours, e.g. purging, fasting, excessive exercise, and does not occur exclusively during the course of anorexia nervosa or bulimia nervosa

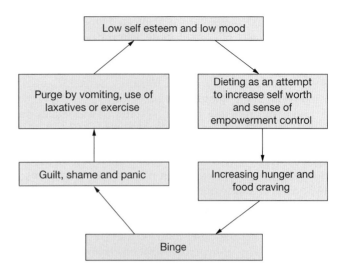

Figure 7.10.1 Binge–starve cycle in bulimia nervosa

cultural norms. Anorexia has long been recognised as having the highest mortality of any mental disorders (Harris & Barraclough, 1998), and Hoek's review (2006) of more recent evidence confirms this. Significant causes of death include suicide and cardiac complications. There are concerns about the risk of death resulting from inappropriate refeeding practice (Royal College Psychiatrists, 2010). For bulimia nervosa, Hoek & Hoeken (2003) and Hoek (2006) found an incidence at about 1% among young women. Over whole populations, they found incidence rates of at least 8 per 100 000 person years for anorexia nervosa and 12 for bulimia nervosa.

Prevention

Prevention of eating disorders presents a complex challenge. It is clear that protection of children from abuse and neglect is helpful in the prevention of eating disorders and other mental health problems. Direct interventions aimed at preventing eating disorders in vulnerable populations have been counter productive (Carter et al., 1997; Mann et al., 1997). There is continuing controversy about the part played by cultural influences. In their general practice, dietitians should emphasise eating to support general health and nutrition, rather than focussing too narrowly on control of body weight (ADA, 2011).

Medical and nutritional effects of eating disorders

Anorexia nervosa

Much of the information about the physical and psychological effects of starvation in otherwise healthy individuals comes from the classic work of Keys et al. (1950), known as the Minnesota Experiment, in which healthy male volunteers ate approximately half of their energy requirement for a 12-week period (Keys et al., 1950; Kalm & Semba, 2005). Starvation results in general malnutrition, affecting all tissues and organs (Mitchell & Crow, 2006). The main tissue loss is adipose tissue and muscle

similar to those in the other eating disorders, and higher than in obese people without binge eating disorder (Wilfley et al., 2003). Childhood obesity, negative early experience and low self esteem are predisposing factors (Fairburn et al., 1998).

Epidemiology and public health aspects

Incidence and prevalence

Researchers considering incidence and prevalence of eating disorders often urge caution, and suggest that published figures may be underestimates for a number of reasons, including secrecy about symptoms and reluctance to seek treatment (Rooney et al., 1995; Hudson et al., 2007; Hoek & Hoeken, 2003; Hoek, 2006). For example, Keski-Rahkonen (2007) found that in a community sample, half of the cases of anorexia nervosa had not been detected by healthcare services.

Hoek & Hoeken (2003) and Hoek (2006) reviewed the literature on incidence and prevalence, and found that the highest incidence of anorexia nervosa was at age 15–19 years, and in Europe and the USA prevalence of anorexia in that age group was around 0.3%. The female to male ratio was more than 10 to 1. Outside western societies, the prevalence is lower, but there is some evidence that it is increasing with the spread of western mass. Internal organs are not affected until the more advanced stages of malnutrition, when liver, heart and brain reduce in mass, with resulting loss of function (Treasure *et al.*, 2010; Winston & Stafford, 2000; Casiero & Frishman, 2006), and gut function is compromised (Robinson, 2000; Robinson *et al.*, 1988).

Endocrine function can be severely disturbed as an adaptation to starvation, affecting the thyroid and adrenal glands and the gonads via the hypothalamus and pituitary axis (Lawson & Klibanski, 2008; Connan *et al.*, 2000). Suppression of thyroid function results in bradycardia, hypotension and hypothermia, with subjective cold sensitivity and poor sleep. The reduction in fat mass reduces leptin secretion, while cortisol secretion is increased. The tendency to central deposition of adipose tissue that is usually a feature of hypercortisolaemia is absent because adipose tissue is depleted, but during recovery a common cause of distress is central distribution of the repleting fat mass (Lawson & Klibanski, 2008). Suppression of sex hormones results in amenorrhoea in women, and a range of other effects. These endocrine changes underlie the increased risk of osteoporosis that accompanies the nutritional deficit. The development of the illness during adolescence, when bone density should be increasing rapidly, adds further to the risk (Teng, 2011). This is a major physical complication of anorexia nervosa, and may not completely reverse with recovery of endocrine function, healthy body weight and good nutrition (Serpell & Treasure, 1997; Zipfel *et al.*, 2000; Teng, 2011).

The effects on the gut can make increasing food intake uncomfortable and add to its aversiveness. The direct effects of persistent vomiting may damage teeth and the soft tissues of the mouth. Iron and riboflavin deficiency can cause glossitis and angular cheilosis, making eating uncomfortable (Newton & Travess, 2000; Frydrych *et al.*, 2005). Peristalsis is slow, causing delayed gastric emptying (Robinson *et al.*, 1988), bloating and constipation.

The volunteers in the Minnesota Experiment also showed increases in depression, preoccupation with food to the exclusion of other interests, obsessive and bizarre eating behaviour, and social isolation (Keys *et al.*, 1950). These psychological effects are all seen in anorexia nervosa.

Bulimia nervosa

Bulimia nervosa can result in erratic body weight. Vomiting and laxative use can cause disturbances in blood electrolytes, in particular low potassium (Fairburn & Harrison, 2003). Bingeing and vomiting can cause damage to the gastrointestinal tract (Ruhsing *et al.*, 2003; Mitchell & Crow, 2006), including gastro-oesophageal reflux, and acid erosion of the teeth (Frydrych *et al.*, 2005).

Binge eating disorder

This disorder is often associated with obesity, which may be extreme, and a history of weight cycling, with many attempts to reduce body weight, often including a variety of commercial diets and medication. The physical com-

plications and excess mortality relate generally to the associated obesity (Bulik & Reichborn-Kjennerud, 2003; Wilfley *et al.*, 2003). People with any eating disorder may find it very difficult to regulate their food intake appropriately. They may experience abnormalities of normal physiological sensations of hunger and satiety (Treasure *et al.*, 2012), and during the development of the disorder may have overridden them by persistent restriction or repeated binge eating, having lost the ability to respond normally. There are changes in the production of gut hormones associated with physiological appetite control, which may further serve to entrench the abnormal eating (Prince *et al.*, 2010). Erratic and distorted food choice and meal pattern may further impair physiological appetite regulation. Persistently abnormal eating may have prevented the learning needed for development of normal eating, or abolished previously learned behaviour. Avoidance of social eating, or the anxiety associated with it, may make it impossible to use social benchmarking to judge appropriate food intake. Eating, or not eating, may be almost entirely in response to emotional cues. As the individual becomes more socially isolated, particularly avoiding social eating, social and learned eating cues may be lost, leaving eating behaviour driven primarily by emotional cues.

Management

Eating disorders have physical, psychological and social features that may all need expert management. It is therefore essential that the resources of a multidisciplinary team are available, and that dietitians do not work alone (NICE, 2004; ADA, 2011). Good communication among the members of the multidisciplinary team is therefore a high priority. There is also a particular need for good communication and effective working partnerships between specialist dietitians in eating disorders and those in acute medical or intensive care services, to which patients with anorexia nervosa may be admitted (Royal College of Psychiatrists, 2010). The dietitian can make a valuable contribution to the team by improving the nutritional knowledge of all team members (Cordery & Waller, 2006) and raising awareness of the risk of refeeding syndrome (Hearing, 2004).

Ambivalence about recovery and fluctuating motivation challenge everyone involved in the work towards recovery. Skills in counselling and motivation enhancement are needed for help and support to be effective (Treasure & Schmidt, 2001). Throughout the treatment process, a collaborative and motivational approach can support behaviour change and recovery (Feld *et al.*, 2001). Recovery from an eating disorder can be a difficult and complex process. This can present challenges to practitioners, so good support and governance are essential. Dietitians working in this area should seek appropriate supervision. Skilled supervision can help dietitians with the development and productive use of their skills, effective collaboration among colleagues, maintenance of professional and personal boundaries, and managing what can be a distressing experience (BDA, 2008; ADA, 2011).

Major elements of treatment include psychotherapy, medication to help manage depression and anxiety, and development of social skills and skills to support managing eating, such as shopping and cooking. The dietitian can contribute by managing nutritional risk, supporting nutritional rehabilitation and providing education on food and nutrition.

Identification in dietetic clinical practice

In general dietetic practice, indications of disordered eating may be apparent before a formal diagnosis is made, or at a level of severity and frequency that do not meet diagnostic criteria, but nevertheless cause distress, damage health and nutrition, and impair dietetic management. It is therefore important that dietitians are alert to signs and symptoms of disordered eating, and are able to manage them, or refer for more specialist support. It is perhaps not surprising that disordered eating arises in situations where anxiety about eating and nutrition is high, e.g. in the management of obesity (de Zwaan, 2001) and diabetes (Fairburn et al., 1991).

Routine dietetic assessment may expose signs that might indicate disordered eating. Anthropometry may reveal reluctance to be weighed, underweight in the absence of known physical cause or obesity associated with a history of weight cycling. Biochemical indicators include low blood potassium, which may result from persistent vomiting or laxative abuse, or low sodium because of water loading to suppress hunger or falsify weight. Diet history may show erratic eating; restriction of amount and variety of food; rigidity and inappropriate rules about eating and food choice; binge eating or other presentations of uncontrolled overeating such as grazing or night eating; deranged eating pattern; and high anxiety about eating. The SCOFF (Morgan et al., 1999) and ESP tools (Cotton et al., 2003) (Table 7.10.2) are very brief questionnaires designed and validated for use in primary care to help identify disordered eating. Dietitians can use them, or selected questions from them, to help confirm concerns about the presence of an eating disorder, and to encourage their patients to talk about their eating and agree appropriate management.

Dietetic assessment

Although people with eating disorders may present with a great variety of dietetic problems, from severe underweight and malnutrition to severe obesity and weight cycling, the assessment process can be similar for all eating disorders. The aims of assessment are to begin to develop a trusting and productive therapeutic relationship that will support recovery; to develop and maintain motivation to change (Herrin, 2003; Gable 2007, ADA 2011); and to gather the information needed to make a dietetic diagnosis and negotiate a treatment plan (BDA, 2009).

The structure of the process is similar to any dietetic assessment, but may require more time than average because of the ambivalence and anxiety of the patient, and the complexity of the history. It may be helpful to use more than one session to complete the process. Much information may come from previous medical assessment, e.g. diagnoses, results of blood tests and information on medication. However, the most important element is the conversation with the patient, and usually also family members if the patient is living with them, and especially if they are under 18 years of age. The way in which this conversation is conducted will be led to some extent by the patient, but the information needed falls into the standard dietetic assessment framework.

Anthropometry

This includes:

- Weight, height and body mass index (BMI).
- For people under 18 years old, height, weight and BMI centiles. Expected weight for height and for expected height may also be useful.

Being weighed can be distressing for a person with an eating disorder, so clear explanation of the need for body weight should be given, and permission should be sought and recorded carefully.

Biochemistry

This includes:

- *Electrolytes* – low levels of sodium, potassium and magnesium in the context of low body weight may indicate chronic low intake. Low potassium may result from use of laxatives or self induced vomiting. Low sodium is most likely to be due to excessive water intake to suppress hunger or falsify body weight.
- *Iron status* – haemoglobin may be low if food intake has been severely restricted for a long period, but may be protected by reduced iron loss with amenorrhoea. Much more commonly, low ferritin indicates low iron stores.
- *White cell count* – overall white cell count, or one or more elements of total white cells, may be low in chronic semi starvation.

Table 7.10.2 Screening questions for eating disorders

SCOFF (Morgan et al., 1999)	ESP (Cotton et al., 2003)
Do you make yourself **S**ick because you feel uncomfortably full? Do you worry you have lost **C**ontrol over how much you eat? Have you recently lost more than **O**ne stone in a 3-month period? Do you believe yourself to be **F**at when others say you are too thin? Would you say that **F**ood dominates your life?	Are you satisfied with your eating patterns? Do you ever eat in secret? Does your weight affect the way you feel about yourself? Have any members of your family suffered with an eating disorder? Do you currently suffer with or have you ever suffered in the past with an eating disorder?

- *Urea* – be low in chronic severe restriction of food intake.

Low levels of urea, electrolytes and other biochemical indicators may be masked by dehydration, resulting in false normal results (Caragaro *et al.*, 2005), so care should be taken to interpret blood test results alongside indicators of hydration, such as blood pressure.

Clinical assessment

This includes:

- *Eating disorder diagnosis* and other diagnoses of both physical and psychological disorders.
- *Endocrine function* – indicators include amenorrhoea, hypotension with postural drop, bradycardia, hypothermia and subjective feeling of cold, and poor sleep.
- *Low bone mineral density* – DEXA scan to measure bone density is recommended for people with a history of low weight for 6 months or longer (NICE, 2004).
- *Psychological effects* such as low or labile mood, irritability, impaired memory or concentration.
- *Medication*.

Dietetic assessment

This includes:

- *Detailed history of weight and eating.* It is helpful to take a history at least from the beginning of the eating disorder symptoms, and sometimes from infancy, to consider early feeding difficulties. The history should seek to identify periods of low or high weight, and the degree of abnormality, weight cycling and instability, and any times when weight has been normal and stable. This can help to develop a shared understanding of the way eating, body weight, psychological factors and life events relate to each other.
- *Current diet and disordered eating symptoms:*
  - Restriction of amount and variety of foods eaten, foods avoided, foods that are acceptable.
  - Meal pattern, timing and frequency of eating, and variability of meal pattern.
  - Irrational or exaggerated rules and beliefs about eating.
  - Binge eating, grazing or other uncontrolled overeating; foods used for binge eating.
  - Purging and compensatory behaviour, such as vomiting, laxative use and excessive exercise.
  - Emotional responses to food and eating, such as anxiety or disgust.
  - Social context of eating.
  - Fluid intake, which may be restricted or excessive.
  - Alcohol intake.
  - Nutritional supplements such as vitamins.
- *Impaired appetite regulation and subjective ability to control food intake.*

Economic and social assessment

This includes:

- *Education or employment* – these may help to structure the day and eating pattern, or impede routine if there are changing work shifts or an erratic timetable. Education or employment may be important motivators, or worsen anxiety, distress and low self esteem.
- *Finance* – persistent severe binge eating may generate debt. Worries about money may add to stress associated with buying and using food.
- *Social support* – it is useful to identify family members and friends who can support recovery.
- *Household information* – facilities for food preparation, sharing meals with other members of the household.

Feelings

Assessment of motivation and concerns is essential to begin the process of change. The assessment process can help identify the stage of change (Prochaska & DiClemente, 1983), concerns raised by the eating disorders and reasons for recovery. These will inform the priorities for change in eating behaviour, identify barriers to change and motivators for change, and form a basis for the treatment plan.

Dietetic treatment of eating disorders

Aims and priorities for treatment should be negotiated collaboratively by the dietitian and the sufferer, and carers when appropriate, especially when the sufferer is a child or adolescent. Modest steps towards the treatment aims can then be planned in the form of SMART (specific, measurable, achievable, relevant and time limited) goals. This process should proceed alongside psychological treatment to support changes in thinking and behaviour. Treatment outcomes are likely to include several domains, as shown in Table 7.10.3.

Anorexia nervosa

Evidence for the effectiveness of dietetic interventions is limited, but there is agreement in published guidance that dietetic care is an essential element of management (Hart *et al.*, 2011). Treatment may be provided in a hospital inpatient setting, day care or outpatient service. Regular weight monitoring and medical monitoring are essential at each stage of treatment, to ensure that appropriate management is in place for any problems that arise.

Treatment is in three distinct phases; medical stabilisation and management of refeeding syndrome risk, nutrition rehabilitation and increasing responsibility for normal and healthy eating, and finally, maintenance and relapse prevention.

Phase 1: stabilisation

The early stage of refeeding carries risk, especially if the anorexia is severe, and is uncomfortable and distressing.

Table 7.10.3 Treatment outcomes for eating disorders

Treatment domain	Outcome
Biochemical	Normalised blood urea and electrolytes Normalised white cell count Normalised iron status (haemoglobin and ferritin)
Psychological	Reduced anxiety about eating and weight More stable mood Increased motivation to prevent relapse
Behaviour change domain	Reduced restriction of eating Abolition of binge eating Abolition of purging Healthier food choices Normal fluid intake
Physical domain	Healthy body mass index In children and adolescents, normal growth, or catch-up growth as appropriate Improved bone mineral density
Symptom change domain	Reduced reflux, bloating, constipation Normal sleep Abolished faintness, giddiness Normal body temperature control Normal menstruation
Patient focused domain	Achievement of aims for employment or education Avoiding hospital admission Independent living Improved personal relationships Improved social eating Appropriate physical activity

Gradual increases in food intake, with good information, clear explanations and consistent support can help manage increased anxiety. It may be difficult to strike the optimal balance between keeping food intake low to prevent refeeding syndrome and increasing it quickly enough to reduce the risks imposed by the malnutrition (Royal College Psychiatrists, 2010).

The evidence on the management of refeeding syndrome comes largely from critical care, where patients are acutely ill or physically traumatised (NICE, 2006a), and so are catabolic (see Chapter 7.17.1). People with anorexia nervosa are generally not critically ill, but are severely starved, so rapidly become anabolic with refeeding. This difference in response to increasing food intake may affect the risk of refeeding syndrome, but evidence is lacking. However, there is a clear risk of refeeding syndrome in anorexia nervosa (Birmingham *et al.*, 1996; Fisher *et al.*, 2000), so some caution is needed, and close monitoring is essential. This may be particularly challenging in non-specialist settings such as medical wards or intensive care units, where the Royal College of Psychiatrists (2010) guidance may be especially useful. The consensus is that feeding can safely be begun at about 80 kJ (20 kcal)/kg of body weight/24 hours (Royal College

Psychiatrists, 2010), using a tube feeding formula or food.

To prevent Wernicke–Korsakoff syndrome, prophylactic thiamine should be given daily, following guidance given by NICE (2006a) for the prevention of refeeding syndrome. There is likely to be a general deficiency of micronutrients, so multivitamins and minerals should be given to correct deficiencies and as part of global nutritional rehabilitation (Rock & Vasantharajan, 1995; Setnick, 2010; Hadigan *et al.*, 2000). Total fluid should be controlled, as cardiac capacity may be limited by loss of cardiac muscle mass, and rapid increase in blood volume may risk cardiac failure (Winston & Stafford, 2000). Weight gain may be rapid during the first 7–10 days of refeeding because of rehydration and, sometimes, temporary fluid retention, especially if persistent vomiting or laxative abuse are stopped. Explanation of the effect and reassurance that it is self limiting may be helpful.

Tube feeding

Where tube feeding is the preferred route, bolus feeding is generally easier to manage, as it allows the patient to be mobile, and it is easier to supervise the delivery of the feed and so prevent sabotage. Because the overall volume initially is low, bolus volume can be relatively low, which helps to prevent bloating and discomfort. Six boluses of 100–150 mL/day will allow delivery of an adequate volume of feed for a person of 25–45 kg. At first, an isotonic formula is preferable, as it does not cause osmotic movement of water into the gut, which may be uncomfortable and create a pseudo-dumping syndrome, with faintness due to fall in blood pressure. As feed volume is increased, a higher density feed may help prevent feelings of bloating (Gentile *et al.*, 2010).

Oral feeding

Initially, care should be taken to limit carbohydrate and ensure a high intake of potassium and phosphate, as blood levels can fall rapidly as part of refeeding syndrome (NICE, 2006a). This can be achieved by giving a high proportion of intake as cow's milk as a source of phosphate, and fruit juice as a source of potassium. It may be more comfortable to give fruit juice diluted with water, especially if the mouth is sore. Small meals with a modest amount of food choice can help manage anxiety. Too much choice may be overwhelming.

It should be possible to accommodate vegetarian diets without difficulty. Avoidance of meat and fish is culturally common, and required by some religions, and there is no reason to challenge such a choice at this stage. If vegetarianism has developed as part of the eating disorder pathology, it may be addressed later in treatment. Vegan diets, with no animal products, present some risks as these diets tend to have low energy density, so the patient is faced with a relatively large volume of food. The high fibre content may be uncomfortable and possibly increase the risk of gastric dilatation or rupture (Saul *et al.*, 1981). If a vegan diet is to be used, food provision should be planned to provide adequate phosphate (most easily by using a soya milk with added phosphate) and to minimise volume and fibre. Monitoring of blood and physical condition should be vigilant, and treatment adjusted according to results.

Phase 2: nutritional rehabilitation

The National Institute for Health and Care Excellence (2004) recommends weight gain at a rate of about 0.5 kg/week for outpatients and 0.5–1.0 kg/week for inpatients, who can be supported and monitored more intensively. Individual variation on this may be negotiated, e.g. for patients with a very long history or if reduction of other symptoms such as purging are to be given priority. Setting and reviewing SMART goals can establish the aims. The aims during this stage are:

- To recover weight, ideally to a healthy weight that will restore normal endocrine function and so reduce the risk of osteoporosis.
- To restore optimal nutritional status and normalise blood indicators of poor nutrition.
- To replete body stores of nutrients.
- To increase confidence and knowledge to support ability to eat normally and independently, as appropriate for age and social circumstances.
- Reduction of physical symptoms of malnutrition.
- Reduction of anxiety about eating and preoccupation with food.
- Reduction of abnormal eating behaviour.
- Abolition of purging.

These goals must be aimed for alongside psychological work to reduce eating disorder psychopathology and symptoms. Strategies to achieve these aims may include:

- Careful calculation of energy intake to achieve weight gain at the agreed rate.
- Multivitamin and mineral supplementation.
- Negotiated meal plans to support regular eating, increasing amount and variety of food, and normalising meal pattern.
- A portion exchange system to develop flexibility.
- Planning eating to prevent anxiety associated with eating, especially when making decisions under pressure.
- Education on healthy, normal eating and body weight.
- Information about specific nutritional deficiencies such as low iron status.
- Education on natural appetite control and support to improve it.
- Practising eating, shopping and cooking with support as appropriate for the person's age, circumstances and

lifestyle, to improve confidence, independence and flexibility.

Phase 3: maintenance of improvement and relapse prevention

There is a risk of relapse of anorexia. People recovering need help to identify possible situations that may increase risk of relapse, and to develop strategies to prevent relapse, and to identify it quickly and reverse it. Some risk situations may involve particular kinds of eating, and the dietitian can help to anticipate and plan for these. Difficulties can arise in some social situations such as celebrations or unexpected eating; periods of religious fasting; and situations where the choice of food may be very limited, such as travelling or staying with friends. Planning for these situations can help to reduce risk. Skills in meal planning and good knowledge of healthy, normal eating can be helpful, in particular learning and practising appropriate use of foods that may be perceived as unhealthy; usually high fat and high sugar foods.

Bulimia nervosa

The main element of treatment for bulimia nervosa is cognitive behavioural therapy (CBT) (NICE, 2004). Dietetic intervention may be helpful alongside this for patients who are finding stabilising eating particularly difficult, or who have poor knowledge or confidence to feed themselves in a healthy way, or who have particular nutritional problems such as iron deficiency anaemia. As part of the CBT, patients will be encouraged to self monitor eating and purging by keeping a diary; this will also usually be used to record all food and fluid intake (Table 7.10.4). The CBT approach asks for recording of the situation, thoughts and feelings before the eating episode (antecedents); the date and time of eating and drinking, and details of type and amount of foods and fluids consumed or avoided (behaviour), and a subjective rating of whether this was a meal, snack or binge; and the thoughts, feelings and events after it (consequences). Learning this ABC approach can be helpful in showing the way dietary restriction leads to hunger and food craving, the powerful impulse to eat and the events or feelings that may then trigger binge eating.

The aims of treatment include:

- Abolition of binge eating and purging.
- Reduction of restriction of amount and variety of food.
- Establishment of regular, stable eating that is healthy and socially normal for the individual.
- Improvement in appetite regulation.
- Stabilisation of body weight in the healthy range.

Table 7.10.4 Example of headings for a self-monitoring diary

Date	Time	Food and drink	Antecedents	Behaviour (meal, snack or binge)	Consequences

- Increased confidence and reduced anxiety about eating.

There may also be a need to manage other influences on appetite, such as the use of alcohol or cannabis.

Strategies to reduce hunger and the drive to binge include:

- Improve understanding of the ways that restriction of food intake drives uncontrolled eating, in particular physiological hunger, which may not be recognised, and the hyper reward of eating when food deprived.
- Ensure adequate calorie intake to maintain weight, or increase it at an agreed rate if underweight. It may be reassuring to explain how this is calculated.
- Education to improve understanding of the factors that affect body weight, in particular the effects of shifts of glycogen and fluid.
- Regular, frequent meals and snacks, normally beginning with at least six eating episodes/day. This helps to prevent excessive hunger, which may increase the drive to binge, and also avoids feelings of fullness, which may provoke an impulse to vomit.
- Using the foods least likely to provoke bingeing or purging. This usually means not using high fat or high sugar foods at first.
- Using foods most likely to reduce hunger. Low energy density, high fibre and low glycaemic index foods may be helpful.
- Identifying times when the risk of binge eating is high, and replacing the binge with regular small snacks.
- Managing shopping and storage of food to have the planned food available, and avoid having binge food easily accessible.
- Planning meals to ensure they are available on time, and to prevent anxiety associated with making decisions quickly.
- Encouraging the use of alternative activities to deal with emotional distress. Activities that are distracting, calming and enjoyable, such as creative activities, social contact and relaxation exercises, may be especially effective.

Strategies to reduce purging and minimise harm include:

- Improved understanding of body weight regulation and the factors that influence it.
- Initially, keeping meals and snacks small, to prevent a feeling of fullness that may provoke vomiting or laxative use.
- Initially, encouraging the use of alternatives to specific foods that the individual finds difficult to tolerate, often high fat, high sugar foods. Excessively strict rules are not helpful.
- Plan activities to follow each meal and snack, as a distraction and to help reduce anxiety.
- Eating with other people may be helpful.
- Planned, appropriate exercise may help improve tolerance of regular eating.
- Stabilise fluid balance with regular fluid intake, and management of dehydrating factors such as vomiting, laxative use, alcohol and excessive caffeine intake.

- Advice on protecting teeth if vomiting does occur. Rinsing with water helps to remove acid from the mouth.
- If blood potassium is low because of vomiting or laxative use, advice on food sources of potassium, while implementing strategies to reduce purging.

As treatment progresses, the variety of foods can be increased. Difficult foods can be reintroduced in a safe context to reduce associated anxiety. Foods such as chocolate or crisps can be taken after a meal to prevent between meal hunger adding to the risk of uncontrolled eating. It may help to choose a single serving package, to control the amount, and to try it in a public place, where binge eating will be difficult. Individuals may be able to plan the safest situation for themselves. Success in using challenging foods in an appropriate way can help to develop confidence to tackle further goals.

Binge eating disorder

There are many similarities between binge eating disorder and bulimia nervosa. As with bulimia nervosa, CBT is commonly used to help people to overcome binge eating, along with diary keeping to help link thoughts, feelings and events to binge eating, and to develop strategies to deal with them.

People with binge eating disorder are generally obese and anxious to reduce their weight. Abolition of binge eating alone generally has little impact on weight. Excessive restriction of food will maintain hunger, so it may be difficult to achieve weight loss while binge eating is active and therefore some individuals may find it easier to reduce binge eating before beginning weight reduction. It may be possible to support patients to begin weight reduction while they are reducing their binge eating behaviour by restoring regular, stable eating while maintaining a modest deficit in energy intake of about 1.7–2 MJ (400–500 kcal)/day, and ideally gradually increasing physical activity as appropriate for the individual.

As eating is stabilised, binge eating reduced and confidence increased, a larger energy deficit may be tolerated, and obesity management strategies, including medication, can be applied by following NICE (2006b) guidance. As obesity is often extreme, bariatric surgery may be appropriate. It is not clear whether binge eating worsens outcome of bariatric surgery (Niego *et al.*, 2007; Bocchieri-Ricciardi *et al.*, 2006). In practice, the waiting time for bariatric surgery may be lengthy, and the time may be well spent in reducing eating pathology and body weight, and supporting the individual to improve the knowledge and confidence to manage their eating post surgery.

Internet resources

B-eat   www.b-eat.co.uk
   The leading charity and support group for eating disorders.
Institute of Psychiatry   www.iop.kcl.ac.uk
   Eating disorders research resource   www.iop.kcl.ac.uk/sites/edu
Royal College of Psychiatrists   www.rcpsych.ac.uk
   Eating disorders resources   www.rcpsych.ac.uk/
      mentalhealthinfoforall/problems/eatingdisorders.aspx

References

American Dietetic Association. (2011) Position of the American Dietetic Association: nutrition intervention in the treatment of eating disorders. *Journal of the American Dietetic Association* 111(8): 1236–1241.

American Psychiatric Association. (1994) *Diagnostic and Statistical Manual of Mental Disorders*, 4th edn (DSM-IV). Washington, DC: American Psychiatric Association.

Birmingham CL, Alothman AF, Goldner EM. (1996) Anorexia nervosa: refeeding and hypophosphataemia. *International Journal of Eating Disorders* 20(2): 211–213.

Bocchieri-Ricciardi LE, Chen EY, Munoz D, *et al.* (2006) Pre-surgery binge eating status: effect on eating behavior and weight outcome after gastric bypass. *Obesity Surgery* 16: 1198–1204.

British Dietetic Association (BDA). (2008) *Practice Supervision Guidelines*. Birmingham: BDA.

British Dietetic Association (BDA). (2009) *Nutrition and Dietetic Care Process*. Birmingham: BDA.

Bruch H. (1973) *Eating Disorders; Obesity, Anorexia Nervosa and the Person Within*. New York: Basic Books.

Brumberg JJ. (1988) *Fasting Girls; The History of Anorexia Nervosa*. New York: Plume.

Bulik CM, Reichborn-Kjennerud T. (2003) Medical morbidity in binge eating disorder. *International Journal of Eating Disorders* 34 (Suppl): 39–48.

Bulik CM, Slof-Op't Landt MCT, van Furth EF, Sullivan PF. (2007) The genetics of anorexia nervosa. *Annual Review of Nutrition* 27: 263–275.

Caragaro I, Di-Pascoli L, Favaro A, Nardi M, Santonastaso P. (2005) Sodium depletion and hemoconcentration – overlooked complications in patients with anorexia nervosa? *Nutrition* 21(4): 438–445.

Carter JC, Stewart A Dunn VJ, Fairburn CG. (1997) Primary prevention of eating disorders: might it do more harm than good? *International Journal of Eating Disorders* 22(2): 167–172.

Casiero D, Frishman WH. (2006) Cardiovascular complications of eating disorder. *Cardiology in Review* 14(5): 227–231.

Connan F, Lightman S, Treasure J. (2000) Biochemical and endocrine complications. *European Eating Disorders Review* 8(2): 144–157.

Cordery H, Waller G. (2006) Nutritional knowledge of healthcare professionals working in eating disorders. *European Eating Disorders Review* 14(6): 462–467.

Cotton M-A, Ball C, Robinson P. (2003) Four simple questions can help screen for eating disorders. *Journal of General Internal Medicine* 18(1): 53–56.

Davis C, Levitan RD, Kaplan AS, *et al.* (2008) Reward sensitivity and the D2 dopamine receptor gene; a case control study of binge eating disorder. *Progress in Neuro-Psychopharmacology and Biological Psychiatry* 32: 620–628.

De Zwaan M. (2001) Binge eating disorder and obesity. *International Journal of Obesity and Related Disorders* 25 (Suppl 1): S51–55.

Fairburn CG, Harrison PJ (2003) Eating disorders. *Lancet* 361: 407–416.

Fairburn CG, Peveler RC, Davies B, Mann JI, Mayou RA. (1991) Eating disorders in young adults with insulin dependent diabetes mellitus: a controlled study. *BMJ* 303: 17–20.

Fairburn CG, Doll HA, Welch SL, Hay PJ, Davies BA, O'Conner ME. (1998) Risk factors for binge eating disorders: a community-based, case-control study *Archives of General Psychiatry* 55(5): 425–432.

Feld R, Woodside DB, Kaplan AS, Olmsted FP, Carter JC. (2001) Pretreatment motivational enhancement therapy for eating disorders; a pilot study. *International Journal of Eating Disorders* 29(4): 393–400.

Fisher M, Simpser E, Schneider E. (2000) Hypophosphatemia secondary to oral refeeding in anorexia nervosa study. *International Journal of Eating Disorders* 28(2): 181–187.

Frydrych AM, Davies GR; McDermott BM. (2005) Eating disorders and oral health: a review of the literature. *Australian Dental Journal* 50(1): 6–15.

Gable J. (2007) *Counselling Skills for Dietitians*, 2nd edn. Oxford: Blackwell.

Garrett A, Cockfield A, Philpot U, Passman L, Hoyle A. (2005) *A Briefing Paper for Dietitians Working with Patients with Eating Disorders*. Birmingham: Mental Health Group of the British Dietetic Association.

Gentile MG, Pastorelli P, Ciceri R, Manna GM, Collimedaglia S. (2010) Specialised refeeding treatment fir anorexia nervosa patients suffering from extreme undernutrition. *Clinical Nutrition* 29: 627–632.

Gorwood P, Kipman A, Foulon C. (2003) The human genetics of anorexia nervosa. *European Journal of Pharmacology* 480: 163–170.

Grimm VE. (1996) *From Feasting to Fasting: Attitudes to Food in Late Antiquity*. London: Routledge.

Gull WW. (1874) Anorexia nervosa (apepsia hysterica, anorexia hysterica). *Transactions of the Clinical Society of London* 7: 22–28.

Gull WW. (1888) Clinical notes, anorexia nervosa. *Lancet* 1: 516–517.

Hadigan CM, Anderson EJ, Miller KK, *et al.* (2000) Assessment of macronutrient and micronutrient intake in women with anorexia nervosa. *International Journal of Eating Disorders* 28(3): 284–292.

Harris EC, Barraclough B. (1998) Excess mortality of mental disorder. *British Journal of Psychiatry* 173: 11–53.

Harrison A, Sullivan S, Tchanturia K, Treasure J. (2009) Emotion recognition and regulation in anorexia nervosa. *Clinical Psychology and Psychotherapy* 16: 348–356.

Hart S, Russell J, Abraham S. (2011) Nutrition and dietetic practice in eating disorder management *Journal of Human Nutrition and Dietetics* 24(2): 144–153.

Hearing SD. (2004) Refeeding syndrome. *BMJ* 328: 908–909

Herrin M. (2003) *Nutrition Counselling in the Treatment of Eating Disorders*. New York: Brunner-Routledge.

Hoek HW. (2006) Incidence, prevalence and mortality of anorexia nervosa and other eating disorders. *Current Opinion in Psychiatry* 19(4): 389–394.

Hoek HW, van Hoeken D. (2003) Review of the prevalence and incidence of eating disorders. *International Journal of Eating Disorders* 34: 383–396.

Hudson JI, Hiripi E Harrison GP, Kessler RC. (2007) The prevalence and correlates of eating disorders in the National Comorbidity Survey Replication. *Biological Psychiatry* 61(3): 348–358.

Kalm LM, Semba RD. (2005) They starved so that others be better fed: remembering Ancel Keys and the Minnesota Experiment. *Journal of Nutrition* 135(6): 1347–1352.

Keski-Rahkonen A, Hoek HW, Susser ES, *et al.* (2007) Epidemiology and course of anorexia nervosa in the community. *American Journal of Psychiatry* 164(8): 1259–1265.

Keys A, Brozek J, Henschel A, Mickelsen O, Taylor HL. (1950) *The Biology of Human Starvation*. Minneapolis: University of Minneapolis Press.

Lasègue EC. (1873) De l'anorexie hystérique. *Archives Générales de Médecine* 1: 385–403.

Lawson EA, Klibanski A. (2008) Endocrine abnormalities in anorexia nervosa *Nature Clinical Practice* 4(7): 407–414.

Mann T, Nolen-Hoeksema S, Huang K, Burgard D, Wright A, Hanson K (1997) Are two interventions worse than none? Joint primary and secondary prevention of eating disorders in college females. *Health Psychology* 16(3): 215–225.

Mitchell JE, Crow S. (2006) Medical complications of anorexia nervosa and bulimia nervosa. *Current Opinion in Psychiatry* 19(4): 438–443.

Morgan JF, Reid F, Lacey JH. (1999) The SCOFF questionnaire: assessment of a new screening tool for eating disorders. *BMJ* 319: 1467–1468.

Nasser M. (1997) *Culture and Weight Consciousness*. London: Routledge.

National Institute for Health and Care Excellence (NICE). (2004) *Nutrition Support in Adults*. National Clinical Practice Guideline No. 9. London: NICE.

National Institute for Health and Care Excellence (NICE). (2006a) *Eating Disorders*. National Clinical Practice Guideline No. 32. London: NICE.

National Institute for Health and Care Excellence (NICE). (2006b) *Obesity*. National Clinical Practice Guideline No. 43. London: NICE.

Newton JT, Travess HC. (2000) Oral complications. *European Eating Disorders Review* 8(2): 83–87.

Niego SH, Koffman MD, Weiss JJ, Geliebter A. (2007) Binge eating in the bariatric surgery population: a review of the literature. *International Journal of Eating Disorders* 40: 349–359.

Prochaska JO, DiClemente CC. (1983) Stages and processes of self-change of smoking: Toward an integrative model of change. *Journal of Consulting and Clinical Psychology* 51(3): 390–395.

Prince AC, Brooks SJ, Stahl D, Treasure J. (2010) Systematic review and meta-analysis of the baseline concentrations and physiologic responses of gut hormones to food in eating disorders. *Journal of Clinical Endocrinology and Metabolism* 95: 3057–3062.

Robinson PH. (2000) Review article: recognition and treatment of eating disorders in primary and secondary care. *Alimentary Pharmacology and Therapeutics* 14(4): 367–377.

Robinson PH, Clarke M, Barrett J. (1988) Determinants of delayed gastric emptying in anorexia nervosa and bulimia nervosa. *Gut* 29: 458–464.

Rock C, Vasantharajan S. (1995) Vitamin status of eating disorders patients: relationship to clinical indices and effect of treatment. *International Journal of Eating Disorders* 18: 257–262.

Rooney B, McLelland L, Crisp AH, Sedgwick PM. (1995) The incidence and prevalence of anorexia nervosa in three suburban health districts in south west London, UK. *International Journal of Eating Disorders* 18(4): 299–307.

Royal College of Psychiatrists (RCP). (2010) *CR162 MARSIPAN: Management of Really Sick Patients with Anorexia Nervosa*. London: RCP.

Ruhsing JM, Jones LE, Carney CP. (2003) Bulimia nervosa: A primary care review. *Journal of Clinical Psychiatry* 5: 217–224.

Russell GFM. (1979) Bulimia nervosa: an ominous variant of anorexia nervosa *Psychological Medicine* 9: 429–448.

Saul SH, Dekker A, Watson CG. (1981) Acute gastric dilatation with infarction and perforation: Report of fatal outcome in patient with anorexia nervosa. *Gut* 22: 978–983.

Serpell L, Treasure J. (1997) Osteoporosis – a serious health risk in chronic anorexia nervosa. *European Eating Disorders Review* 5(3): 149–157.

Setnick J. (2010) Micronutrient deficiencies and supplementation in anorexia and bulimia nervosa. *Nutrition in Clinical Practice* 25(2): 137–142.

Spitzer RL, Devlin M, Walsh BT, *et al*. (1992) Binge eating disorder: a multisite field trial of the diagnostic criteria. *International Journal of Eating Disorders* 11: 191–203.

Teng K. (2011) Premenopausal osteoporosis, an overlooked consequence of anorexia nervosa. *Cleveland Clinic Journal of Medicine* 78(1): 50–58.

Thanos, PK, Michaelides M, Piyis YK, Wang GL, Volkow ND. (2008) Food restriction markedly increases dopamine D2 receptor in a rat model of obesity. *Synapse* 62(1): 50–61.

Treasure J, Schmidt U. (2001) Ready willing and able to change: motivational aspects of the assessment and treatment of eating disorders. *European Eating Disorders Review* 9(1): 4–18.

Treasure J, Claudino AM, Zucker N. (2010) Eating disorders. *Lancet* 375: 583–593.

Treasure J, Cardi V, Kan C. (2012) Eating in eating disorders. *European Eating Disorders Review* 20(1): e42–49.

Vandereycken W, van Deth R. (1994) *From Fasting Saints to Anorexic Girls: The History of Self-Starvation*. London: Athlone.

Wang G-J, Geliebter A, Volkow ND, *et al*. (2011) Enhanced striatal dopamine release during food stimulation in binge eating disorder. *Obesity* 19(8): 1601–1608.

Wilfley D, Schwartz MB, Spurrell EB, Fairburn CG. (2003) Using the eating disorder examination to identify the specific psychopathology of binge eating disorder. *International Journal of Eating Disorders* 27(3): 259–269.

Winston AP, Stafford PJ. (2000) Cardiovascular effects on anorexia nervosa. *European Eating Disorders Review* 8(2): 117–125.

World Health Organization (WHO). (1992) *The International Classification of Diseases*, 10th edn. (ICD-10) Geneva: WHO.

Zipfel S, Herzog W, Beumont PJ, Russell J. (2000) Osteoporosis. *European Eating Disorders Review* 8: 108–116.

7.10.2 Dementias

Phil Addicott and Annette Dunne

Key points

■ The prevalence of dementia increases with age. As the population ages, it is estimated that by 2021 over 1 million people in the UK will suffer from dementia.

■ Dementia is a progressive degenerative condition with a multifactorial aetiology; there is no effective cure. It is characterised by a decline in memory and the ability to think, communicate and understand, and changes in mood and behaviour.

■ Early nutritional assessment and regular monitoring to encourage adequate food and fluid is important. The food should be nutrient and energy dense, according to individual preferences.

■ Independence should be encouraged for as long as possible.

■ Carers should be valued and supported and involved in decisions that influence the patient.

Dementia is the collective term for conditions resulting from destructive pathological change in brain tissue that cause progressive loss of intellectual function. They are defined by their cognitive and neuropsychological characteristics. Memory decline is the core feature of most disorders, many of which also have impairment of visual spatial skills, language and executive functions. Dementia is characterised by:

- Progressive decline in the ability to remember, learn, understand, communicate and reason.
- Gradual loss of skills including those needed for everyday activities.
- Changes in personality or behaviour.

The behavioural and psychological symptoms in dementia can be summarised as psychosis, depression, anxiety, wandering, restlessness, agitation and aggression. In time, people may lose the ability to care for themselves and become totally dependent on the help of others. In some cases, the decline may be rapid; in others it may occur over a long period of time. Dementia is not in itself fatal and many sufferers can remain in good physical health for years. Eventually, the effects of the disease lead to increasing weakness, and death normally results from infections such as pneumonia or gradual organ failure.

In 2007 the Alzheimer's Society estimated that there are approximately 750 000 people with dementia in the UK, but that this figure is expected to rise to nearly 1 million by 2021. It is anticipated that the prevalence of dementia will increase as the population ages. Dementia usually occurs after the age of 40 years and the incidence increases sharply with age, doubling every 5 years above the age of 40 years. Above the age of 65 years, 4–5 people per 100 are affected. The risk is 1 in 5 over 80 years. The number of people in the UK with younger onset dementia is currently estimated at over 16 000.

A considerable amount of research is being carried out into possible links between diet and dementia. It has been suggested that the risk of Alzheimer's disease increases as levels of homocysteine rise and that this may be related to low plasma levels of folate, vitamins B_{12} and B_6 (Luchsinger *et al.*, 2008). Screening for folate and vitamin B_{12} and B_6 deficiency should be considered as part of nutritional assessment in elderly patients. The evidence for the benefits of supplementation of these micronutrients on cognitive function that is already impaired is controversial. A meta analysis (Wald *et al.*, 2010) found no effect on cognitive function, but recommended further research on the effects of long term supplementation of folate and B vitamins on incidence of dementia.

Research into the role of cholesterol in dementia is ongoing and there have been numerous papers examining the potential benefit of statin medication. Haag *et al.* (2009) examined data from the Rotterdam study and found that statin usage was associated with a reduced risk of developing Alzheimer's disease. However, other studies have not found any beneficial effect on cognitive function (Feldman *et al.*, 2010) and statins have not been found

to be effective at preventing Alzheimer's (McGuinness & Passmore, 2010). Despite speculation, there is no reliable evidence that ginko, ginseng or coffee have a protective effect, nor that environmental aluminium or eating meat are risk factors for dementia.

Types of dementia

Alzheimer's disease

This was first identified by Alois Alzheimer in 1907 and is the most common form of dementia, accounting for 50–60% of cases (Alzheimer's Society, 2007). Dementia results from the loss of neurones from the cortical areas of the brain, resulting in reduced production of acetylcholine and other neurotransmitters. Therefore, there is impaired transmission of messages connected with thought and memory. The brain atrophies and decreases in weight, and microscopic examination reveals large numbers of neurofibrillary tangles (nerve cells become bunched together) and neuritic plaques (deposits of amyloid protein and other cellular debris).

The cause of Alzheimer's disease is unknown, but there appear to be genetic links, specifically with genetic polymorphisms. The best established is the e4 allele apolipoprotein E (*APoE4*) gene on chromosome 19. Normally present in approximately 12% of the population, it is found in 40% of people with Alzheimer's disease (Bayer & Reban, 2004). There is a greater incidence of Alzheimer's disease in women, which may be associated with a variant on the *PCDH11X* gene on the X chromosome (Carrasquillo *et al.*, 2008) (see Chapter 5.1).

Vascular dementia

This term applies to a number of different types of dementia caused by stroke, small vessel disease or dementia associated with diseases of the blood vessels supplying the brain with oxygen. A major consideration is whether the disease is primarily one of the large arteries, e.g. causing multiple infarcts, or one of the smaller perforating arteries, causing small vessel disease. Vascular dementia affects people in different ways and causes communication problems, stroke like symptoms and acute confusion (Brown & Hillam, 2004).

Multiinfarct dementia

Multiinfarct dementia (MID) is the most common type of vascular dementia and is secondary to two or more strokes. It arises from several small lesions or infarcts in the brain that lead to increased areas of brain damage causing symptoms of confusion, which gradually progress to dementia. Unlike Alzheimer's disease, mental decline in MID is likely to start more abruptly and symptoms tend to worsen in a stepwise manner following each attack. Brain damage also tends to occur in localised areas rather than being widespread as in Alzheimer's. Therefore, some mental abilities, or the patient's personality, may remain relatively unaffected, although short term memory loss is nearly always pronounced. Sufferers are more likely to be aware of their condition and often anxious and/or depressed as a result (Bayer & Reban, 2004).

Small vessel disease

This is also known as subcortical vascular dementia or, in a severe form, Binswanger's disease, which is often associated with uncontrolled hypertension. Small vessel disease dementia is caused by damage to small blood vessels deep in the brain. The symptoms develop more gradually and are often accompanied by walking problems (Bayer & Reban, 2004).

Frontotemporal dementia

Frontotemporal dementia is characterised by degenerative atrophy and spongiform change of the frontal lobes and/or the temporal cortex situated laterally on each side of the brain. Presentation is typically before 65 years with about an 8-year survival span. Pick's disease is a type of frontotemporal dementia with widespread scarring, but without spongiform changes. Clinical presentation generally involves early behavioural problems, e.g. disinhibition, lack of hygiene, inappropriate sexual behaviour and repetitive performance of an action. Eating habits may also change; cramming sweet foods is not unusual. In addition, personality changes such as insensitive rudeness or the lack of emotional warmth can be very distressing for partners and carers. However memory is often preserved (Brown & Hillam, 2004).

Creutzfeldt–Jakob disease

Creutzfeldt–Jakob disease (CJD) is a very rare dementia that results in the production of an abnormal prion protein in the brain causing progressive dementia and fatal brain disease. It usually has a long latency period, but once symptoms appear the condition tends to progress rapidly, often causing death within a matter of months (Cousens *et al.*, 1997).

Dementia with Lewy bodies

Often associated with Parkinson's disease, dementia with Lewy bodies is characterised by the presence of small spherical protein containing structures (Lewy bodies) in brain tissue. In Parkinson's, Lewy bodies are characteristically found localised in the brain stem; however, in dementia with Lewy bodies, the Lewy bodies are more widely distributed in the cells of the cortex and subcortex. Clinical features include fluctuating cognitive function, visual hallucinations and the spontaneous motor features of parkinsonism (Brown & Hillam, 2004) (see Chapter 7.6.1).

Other causes of dementia

These include:

- *Huntington's disease* – a genetically determined progressive neurodegenerative disorder resulting in movement disturbances, depression and dementia.
- *Down's syndrome* – dementia is more common in middle aged people with Down's syndrome than in the rest of the population (Janicki & Dalton, 2000).
- *Wernicke–Korsakoff syndrome* – caused by thiamine deficiency, usually as a result of alcohol abuse, and can lead to dementia type symptoms.
- *Pugilistic brain injury* – repeated blows to the head, e.g. from boxing, can cause brain damage, resulting in symptoms of dementia. The symptoms may not become apparent until 30 or 40 years after the end of the boxer's career. The number of fights and length of career seem to be more important than the number of knock outs (Bayer & Reban, 2004).

Diagnosis and medical management

Diagnosis of dementia should only be made after a comprehensive assessment, which should include a clinical cognitive assessment that is then repeated at intervals to assess levels of decline, e.g. Mini Mental State Examination (MMSE). A basic dementia screen should include biochemistry, thyroid function, vitamin B_{12} and folate levels (NICE, 2006). Some subtypes of dementia have broadly agreed criteria for diagnosis based on clinical symptoms, e.g. dementia with Lewy bodies. Structural imaging, e.g. magnetic resonance imaging, should be used to exclude other possible cerebral pathologies and to help establish the subtype diagnosis (NICE, 2006).

Early diagnosis of dementia is important because in some cases it may be possible to prevent it worsening. It is particularly important that people with evidence of vascular dementia receive indicated treatment, e.g. antihypertensive medication, which may reduce the risk of further infarctive damage. Diet and lifestyle measures, e.g. not smoking, eating a healthy balanced diet, losing weight, exercising and reducing salt and alcohol intake are also important.

Medication

At present there is no cure for dementia. Drug treatments have been developed for Alzheimer's disease that can improve symptoms, or temporarily slow down their progression, in some people. There are two types of drugs used to treat Alzheimer's disease, cholinesterase inhibitors and glutamate blockers. Cholinesterase inhibitors increase acetylcholine concentrations, which increase communication between the nerve cells that use acetylcholine as a chemical messenger. This may in turn temporarily improve, or stabilise, the symptoms of Alzheimer's disease, particularly in the earlier stages. Cholinesterase inhibitors licensed in the UK are donepezil hydrochloride (Aricept), rivastigmine (Exelon) and galantamine (Reminyl). Glutamate is released in excessive amounts when brain cells are damaged by Alzheimer's disease, which causes brain cells to be damaged further. Memantine (Ebixa) can protect brain cells by blocking the release of excess glutamate.

The National Institute for Health and Care Excellence (NICE) amended its guidance in 2011 to recommend donepezil, galantamine and rivastigmine as options for managing mild as well as moderate Alzheimer's disease. Memantine is now recommended as an option for managing moderate Alzheimer's disease for people who cannot take cholinesterase inhibitors and as an option for managing severe Alzheimer's disease. These drugs are well tolerated; however, the most frequent side effects include nausea and vomiting, diarrhoea, stomach cramps, headaches, fatigue and loss of appetite; such side effects are likely to have a negative effect on nutritional status.

Nutritional implications

The effects of dementia on food and fluid intake, and therefore nutritional status, are considerable. The behavioural, emotional and physical changes that take place as dementia progresses can all impact on eating habits and food and drink intake (Alzheimer's Society, 2007).

Dietary behaviour

This is dependent on the type of dementia and the individual; each person will experience dementia in a different way. However, a typical pattern is that in the initial stages the individual may experience difficulty in shopping, cooking and storing food; forgetting to eat or forgetting they have eaten, eating spoiled foods and changes in food choices may be noted. As the dementia advances, sufferers may find it more difficult to open their mouth and chew and may pool food in the mouth but not swallow. The ability to eat independently may be lost, non-foods may be eaten, patients may refuse food and become aphasic and therefore unable to express pain, e.g. dental pain, or to ask for food or fluids. They may encounter chewing and swallowing difficulties or become depressed.

As a result of these problems weight loss is common in patients with progressing dementia, which is nearly always a consequence of an inadequate energy intake rather than the disease itself (Prentice et al., 1989). A more recent systematic review (Hanson et al., 2011) found that high energy supplements and other oral feeding options, such as assisted feeding and modified foods, can help people with dementia to gain weight.

Increased energy requirements

In some cases the energy deficit may be exacerbated by increased energy requirements due to excessive walking or pacing up and down. A classic study by Rheaume et al. (1987) showed that patients who wander required an additional energy intake to maintain their nutritional status. Pharmacological interventions for excessive pacing can result in a poor nutritional intake due to over sedation. Exercise and music therapy have been shown to be the most acceptable non-pharmacological interventions to reduce wandering in dementia (Robinson et al., 2006).

Dehydration

Inadequate oral fluid intake and subsequent dehydration is a common problem and is implicated in many of the most common ailments of people with dementia, such as constipation, urinary tract infection, electrolyte imbalance and increased dizziness and confusion, leading to falls, all of which can have a negative effect on nutritional intake. The Royal College of Nursing (2007) Hydration Best Practice Toolkit provides practical advice for healthcare staff in England and Wales on how to minimise the risk and potential harm that dehydration can cause.

Dysphagia

Dysphagia is a common problem in dementia and can be indicated by repeated chest infections, coughing at meal times or a prolonged oral stage (continuous chewing). Providing good nutrition for patients with dementia and dysphagia can be extremely challenging and requires a multidisciplinary approach. Patients require prompt assessment by a speech and language therapist who can advise on appropriate texture modifications of food and consistency of fluids with the aim of reducing risk of aspiration pneumonia (Kindell, 2002). Dysphagia can occur at the early stages of dementia (see Chapter 7.3).

Nutritional assessment

Patients with dementia are vulnerable to developing malnutrition and it is essential that an environment appropriate and validated nutritional screening tool be routinely used. Patients should be weighed at regular intervals. Calculation of nutritional requirements should include factors for stress or weight gain, and mobility and diet induced thermogenesis. (see Chapter 6.1 and 6.2). Food and fluid charts need to be accurately completed for patients identified as being high risk of malnutrition. However, if food and fluid charts are not available, assessment of food intake usually depends on a combination of obtaining information from relatives or care staff and observing actual practice at meal times. Note should be taken of any carers' reports of weight loss; loose fitting clothing may be an indicator of a problem with nutrient intake (Bayer & Reban, 2004).

Features that increase the likelihood of inadequate nutritional intake are:

- Sensory impairment, e.g. smell or taste.
- Poor or missing dentition.
- Constipation or loose stools.
- Food refusal due to depression, paranoia or confusion.
- Poor mental state and challenging behaviour.
- Physical difficulties in chewing or swallowing provided food.
- Inappropriate meal time environment and inability to eat independently.
- Medications resulting in side effects of dry mouth and altered taste or, in particular, heavy sedation, e.g. antidepressants and antipsychotics.

It is also important to check the nutritional adequacy of the food being offered. Texture modified food, e.g. fork mashable or puréed food, may need fortification in order to provide sufficient nutrition (see Chapter 6.3). The frequency with which food is offered and the time available for assisting people are important. In institutions there may be short intervals between meals and long gaps when nothing is offered, as well as limited time to encourage and assist patients to eat and drink.

Dietary management

A number of strategies can be employed to optimise nutritional intake. These will vary according to the individual circumstances and stage of the disease, and perhaps additional clinical problems, e.g. over sedation, diabetes or depression.

People who live alone in their own homes should be encouraged to:

- Engage with health and social care services and be reassured in regard to the benefits of accepting help, such as a package of care.
- Keep a store of foods that do not require cooking and can be opened easily, i.e. not canned or heavily packaged food. Suitable foods include bread, breakfast cereals, milk, cheese, sliced ham and bananas.
- Keep a good supply of cold drinks if preparation of hot drinks is a problem.
- Make use of meal delivery services and/or meals provided in day care or luncheon clubs.
- Be involved in food preparation for as long as possible and be aware of food fortification ideas.
- Sit with relatives or carers to promote the social side of eating and so that the relative or carer can act as an example or model for the confused or forgetful person.
- People with dementia, their relatives and carers, and the professionals who support them need access to reliable resources, e.g. Nutrition in the Community Settings (Welsh Assembly Government, 2011).

Guidance for care staff in institutions should emphasise the following:

- Importance of nutritional screening and the role of good nutrition in preventing weight loss, malnutrition and the prevention of pressure sores.
- Develop a high protein and energy menu that includes rich sources of fibre, calcium, folate and vitamins D, B_{12} and B_6.
- Importance of being able to provide, when required, appealing and nutritionally good, texture modified meals, and be able to accurately thicken fluids to the recommended consistency.
- Develop a finger food menu for patients who are too distracted to sit through a meal.
- Need for specialist feeding aids, e.g. adaptive cutlery, deep lipped plates, non-slip place mats, wide neck and large handled mugs, and clothing protection where necessary.

- Benefit of investing in training, e.g. how to safely assist patients to eat or importance of hydration.
- Importance of adequate fluid consumption.
- Need to recognise individual variation in terms of nutrient needs and personal likes and dislikes.
- Benefits of nutritional supplements for those with inadequate nutritional intake and weight loss.
- The importance of a robust protected meal time policy and a calm and appropriate meal time environment.

Advice to carers should focus on the need to:

- Offer small nutritious meals and drinks at regular intervals. Not only does this help meet nutritional and fluid needs, but the routine of a regular meal pattern also provides comfort and reassurance to many people with dementia.
- Provide a variety of foods that the person likes and allow more time for the meal than is usual.
- Avoid assisting people to eat when they are not fully alert or if they are lying down or anxious.
- Help maintain the person's independence by providing foods they can manage themselves. Deep lipped plates, non-slip place mats, adapted utensils or finger foods may be helpful.
- Distracted or wandersome patients may do better with finger foods, e.g. chips, sandwiches, biscuits, etc. (avoid giving to patients with swallowing difficulties).
- Make the most of good times of the day (usually breakfast and lunchtime) to provide foods that are good sources of nutrients and energy.
- Provide regular fluids in a wide necked mug or cup; avoid filling to the brim to avoid spillages. Avoid giving drinks via straws or in spouted beakers as they are not dignified and may increase risk of aspiration as they direct fluids to the back of the mouth and decrease oral control. Fluids can also be given as soup, sauces or jelly (Kindell, 2002).

Meal time environment

Meal times should be given priority in the daily routine of people with dementia. The eating environment needs to be calm and relaxed. People with dementia should be advised that the meal time is about to start after being offered the opportunity to use the toilet and reminded or assisted with hand washing. In some cases people with dementia can help lay the table, which can be a good source of social contact and stimulation (Kindell, 2002). People with dementia may struggle to concentrate at meal times if there are other distractions; therefore, televisions should be switched off, as should loud music, but calm quiet music can help reduce agitation (Cohan-Mansfield et al., 2009).

The Social Care Institute for Excellence (SCIE, 2011) recommends that people with dementia be allowed to sit and eat in a place where they feel comfortable. Carers should describe the food they are offering and ensure that the food is presented colourfully and attractively. The area in which a person with dementia eats should be bright and well lit so they can see the food easily. Images of food can also be used for reminiscence activities; this can help stimulate discussion and interest in food and meal times by helping the person to reconnect with familiar foods from their past.

Eating assistance strategies

Relatives or carers may be able to provide advice on the level of support typically required. The following strategies may be helpful in overcoming poor dietary intake related to dementia:

- Involve the person with dementia with meal preparation for as long as possible, e.g. putting out napkins or cutlery; talking about food preferences can be a useful prompt.
- Overemphasising tidy eating habits should be avoided. Serving one familiar food at a time may help overcome confusion. Cutting food into smaller pieces (before the plate is taken to the patient) may be helpful (Bayer & Reban, 2004).
- If a person with dementia become distracted during the meal or passively sits in front of their meal without eating, gentle verbal prompts can be useful.
- Hand over hand assistance can be useful for people who are having difficulty coordinating cutlery, i.e. gently place the utensil in the person's hand and use your hand to guide them to start eating. Often once started, they will be able to carry on independently.
- Take into account individual food preferences but consider that due to taste changes people may prefer sweeter foods or foods with stronger flavours.
- Food should be presented attractively and be colourful; avoid serving white foods on a white plate. Take care that foods and drinks are not too hot.
- If self feeding is more erratic, specialist feeding aids, e.g. weighted cutlery, deep lipped plates and non-slip place mats, may help; eventually the person may need to be fed for at least part of their meal.
- Some people with dementia become sensitive to foods of mixed textures, e.g. minestrone or cornflakes in milk, and may spit them out; if so, a softer single texture food may be appropriate (Kindell, 2002).
- If a person walks away from an unfinished meal, be wary of assuming that the person has finished or dislikes the food. They may need some verbal prompts to come back to the table, or gesturing to the empty chair can show the person what is meant. If the person refuses to settle, they may benefit from finger foods (Kindell, 2002).
- Dementia sufferers with dysphagia should be positioned upright to reduce risk of aspiration; texture modified foods may need to be fortified in order to provide adequate nutrition and nutritional intake should be maximised when the desire to eat is higher.
- If fortifying foods and beverages proves insufficient, nutritional supplements will need to be prescribed. If a patient requires thickened fluids, consider using a prethickened supplement drink.

In the final stages of the illness, a multidisciplinary best interest meeting may be needed in order to make decisions concerning the use of enteral feeding or intravenous hydration for people who lack capacity to make this particular decision themselves. If known, the views of the patient must be considered as well as the opinions of relatives or carers. For more information, refer to the Mental Capacity Act (2005) (see Chapter 3.7). Each individual case should be reviewed on its individual merits.

Needs of carers

It is estimated that 600 000 people in the UK act as the primary carers for people with dementia (Alzheimer's Society, 2007). Caring can be an overwhelming experience and the costs of caring are significant. Many carers face financial hardship as they are often forced to give up work and pay high care bills from limited income or private savings. However, the needs of those who care for dementia sufferers in the domestic setting have been increasingly recognised. Under UK legislation, the Carers and Disabled Children Act (2000), carers aged 16 years or over who provide a regular and substantial amount of care for someone aged 18 years or over have the right to an assessment of their needs as a carer. In addition, the Carers (Equal Opportunities) Act (2005) places a duty on local authorities to ensure that all carers know that they are entitled to an assessment of their needs, which must consider their outside interests (work, study or leisure). Under the Employment Act (2007) carers have a statutory right to ask employers for flexible working conditions if they are caring for an adult who is a relative or lives at the same address.

Those carrying out the assessment should seek to identify any psychological distress and psychosocial impact on the carer. Care plans for carers should include tailored interventions and practical support, including access to respite and short break services that meets the needs of both the carer and the person with dementia (NICE, 2006).

Health professionals should work closely with the relatives/carers of someone with dementia because the latter:

- Know the persons best and are more likely to be able to identify or interpret any needs and problems.
- May be aware of relevant medical history, e.g. diabetes, gastrointestinal problems or dysphagia.
- Will be aware of the person's dietary preferences and recent body weight history.
- Have to implement any guidance given by health professionals.

When talking to relatives or carers, it is important to consider that caring for someone with dementia is extremely demanding, both physically and emotionally. Carers may feel:

- Unappreciated as that they are giving a lot for little return.

- Resentful that their lives are dominated by this situation.
- Guilty that they feel like this.
- Impatient and angry, which is often a sign of stress.
- Depressed and bereft at the loss of the person they once knew and whose company they will be unable to enjoy again.
- Isolated, particularly if they are trying to cope alone.
- Frightened of the difficulties ahead.

Carers need to be provided with information about what dementia is and the best way of caring for a person with dementia. This can increase their confidence, decrease levels of stress and improve the care they provide for the person with dementia (Alzheimer's Society, 2007). Information such as the comprehensive booklet entitled *Who Cares* (Department of Health, 2007) provides information and support for carers of people with dementia.

Drug–nutrient interactions

Donepezil, galantamine, rivastigmine and memantine are well tolerated; however, the most frequent side effects include nausea and vomiting, diarrhoea, stomach cramps and headaches, fatigue and loss of appetite.

Antipsychotic drugs may also be taken and may also impact on nutritional status (see Chapter 7.10.3).

Internet resources

Alzheimer's Society   www.alzheimers.org.uk
Alzheimer's Research UK   www.alzheimersresearchuk.org
Department of Health
   Who Cares   www.dh.gov.uk/prod_consum_dh/groups/dh_digital
      assets/@dh/@en/documents/digitalasset/dh_078091.pdf
Her Majesty's Government Legislation   www.legislation.gov.uk
   Carers and Disabled Children Act (2000)
   Carers (Equal Opportunities) Act (2005)
   Mental Capacity Act (2005)
   Employment Act (2007)
National Institute for Health and Care Excellence (NICE)
   Dementia, supporting people with dementia and their carers in health and social care   http://guidance.nice.org.uk/CG42/NICEGuidance/pdf/English).
Voluntary Organisations Involved in Caring in the Elderly Sectors (VOICES)
   Eating Well for Older People with Dementia   www.cwt.org.uk/publications.html#dementia

References

Alzheimer's Society. (2007) *Dementia UK, A Report into the Prevalence and Cost of Dementia*; prepared by the Personal Social Services Research Unit (PSSRU) at the London School of Economics and the Institute of Psychiatry at King's College London, for the Alzheimer's Society. London: The Alzheimer's Society.

Bayer A, Reban J. (2004) *Alzheimer's Disease and Related Conditions*. Czech Republic: MEDEA Press.

Brown, J, Hillam J. (2004) *Dementia – Your Questions Answered*. London: Churchill Livingstone.

Carrasquillo MM, Zou F, Pankratz S, *et al*. (2008) Genetic variation in PCDH11X is associated with susceptibility to late-onset Alzheimer's disease. *Nature Genetics* 41: 192–198.

Cohen-Mansfield J, Dakheel-Ali M, Marx M. (2009) Engagement in persons with dementia: the concept and its measurement. *American Journal of Geriatric Psychiatry* 17(4): 299–307.

Cousens SN, Zeidler M, Esmonde TF, *et al*. (1997) Sporadic Creutzfeld-Jacob disease in the UK: analysis of epidemiology surveillance data 1970–96. *BMJ* 315: 389–395.

Department of Health (2007). Who Cares. Available at www.dh.gov.uk/prod_consum_dh/groups/dh_digitalassets/@dh/@en/documents/digitalasset/dh_078091.pdf.

Feldman HH, Doody RS, Kivipelto M, *et al*. (2010) Randomized controlled trial of atorvastatin in mild to moderate Alzheimer disease – LEADe. *Neurology* 74: 956–964.

Haag MDM, Hofman A, Koudstaal PJ, Stricker BHC, Breteler MMB. (2009) Statins are associated with a reduced risk of Alzheimer disease regardless of lipophilicity – The Rotterdam Study. *Journal of Neurology Neurosurgery & Psychiatry* 80: 13–17.

Hanson LC, Ersek M, Gilliam R, Carey TS. (2011) Oral feeding options for people with dementia: A systematic review. *Journal of American Geriatrics* 59(3): 463–472.

Janicki MP, Dalton AJ. (2000) Prevalence of dementia and impact on intellectual disability service. *Mental Retardation* 38(3): 276–288.

Kindell J. (2002) *Feeding and Swallowing Disorders in Dementia*. Oxon: Speechmark Publishing Ltd.

Luchsinger JA, Tang M, Miller J, Green R, Mayeux R. (2008) Higher folate intake is related to lower risk of Alzheimer's disease in the elderly. *Journal of Nutrition, Health & Aging* 12(9): 648–650.

McGuinness B, Passmore P. (2010) Can statins prevent or help treat Alzheimer's disease? *Journal of Alzheimer's Disease* 20: 925–933.

National Institute for Health and Care Excellence (NICE) (2006; amended 2011) *Dementia: Supporting People with Dementia and their Carers in Health and Social Care*. Available at http://guidance.nice.org.uk/CG42. Accessed 28 July 2011.

Prentice AM, Leavesley K, Murgatroyd PR, *et al*. (1989) Is severe wasting in elderly mental patients caused by an excessive energy requirement? *Age and Aging* 18: 158–167.

Rheaume Y, Riley M, Volicer L. (1987) Meeting the nutritional needs of Alzheimer's patients who pace constantly. *Journal of Nutrition for the Elderly* 7: 43–52.

Robinson L, Hutchings D, Dickinson HO, *et al*. (2006) Effectiveness and acceptability of non-pharmacological interventions to reduce wandering in dementia: a systematic review. *International Journal of Geriatric Psychiatry* 22(1): 9–22.

Royal College of Nursing. (2007) Hydration Best Practice Toolkit. Available at www.rcn.org.uk/newsevents/campaigns/nutritionnow/tools_and_resources/hydration. Accessed 28 June 2011.

Social Care Institute of Excellence (SCIE). (2011) Eating well for people with dementia. Available at www.scie.org.uk/publications/dementia/eating/environment.asp. Accessed 8 August 2011.

Welsh Assembly Government (WAF). (2011) *Nutrition in Community Settings – A Pathway and Resource Pack for Health and Social Care Professionals, the Third Sector, Care Home Staff, Relatives and Carers*. Cardiff: WAF.

Wald DS, Kasturiratne A, Simmonds M. (2010) Effect of folic acid, with or without other B vitamins, on cognitive decline: Meta-analysis of randomized trials. *American Journal of Medicine* 123(6): 522–527.

7.10.3 Nutrition and mental health
Ursula Philpot

Key points

■ Emerging evidence suggests that nutrition may have a role in mental health.

■ The number of dietitians working in mental health is limited, but it is a growing area within the profession.

■ Dietitians may be managed by non-dietetic personnel; therefore, they must be prepared to articulate their key skills and be clear about their professional boundaries, duties, roles and responsibilities.

■ People with a severe mental illness are at greater risk of developing cancer, coronary heart disease, diabetes and obesity related illnesses than the general population.

■ Some medications used to treat mental illness have side effects, including weight gain, hyperglycaemia and gastrointestinal problems.

Mental health is defined by the World Health Organization (WHO) as *'a state of wellbeing in which an individual realizes his or her own abilities, can cope with normal stresses of life, can work productively and is able to make a contribution to his or her community'*. Approximately one in four people in Britain has the diagnosis of a mental disorder or mental illness (McManus *et al.*, 2009). This is defined as a psychological or behavioural pattern associated with distress or a disability that is not a part of normal development or culture. Mental health disorders are experienced as problems with emotions (affect), behaviours, thoughts (cognitions) or perceptions. The disorders can significantly affect all areas of someone's life, from problems with day to day functioning through to those with relationships, work and quality of life. The most common mental health disorders in the UK are depression, eating disorders and anxiety disorders. The recognition and understanding of mental health conditions have changed over time, although there are still variations in the definition, assessment and classification of mental disorders. The ICD 10 Classification of Mental and Behavioural Disorders (World Health Organisation, 1992), and the DSM IV Classification of Mental Disorders (American Psychiatric Association, 1994) are widely accepted guidelines on diagnosis.

There are growing numbers of dietitians working in mental health settings in the UK, but the numbers per population varies greatly across regions. Common areas of employment include eating disorders, intensive care units, secure units, autism, older adults and dementia care, learning disabilities, forensic services and healthy living teams.

Causes of mental distress

There are many opinions about what causes mental distress. One belief is that personality is shaped by both life experiences and genetics. This means that some people may become more vulnerable to mental health problems than others through a combination of upbringing and life events, combined with genetic factors. The following are a range of possible causes of mental distress.

Difficult family background

Growing up in an environment where feelings are not validated or spoken about, feeling uncared for or scared by a parent, or having been or being abused in some way can affect the development of children and leave them insecure and vulnerable to mental distress. However, being too overprotected as a child is also a risk factor.

Hidden feelings

If children are punished for getting angry, crying or laughing too loudly, they learn that they should not feel strong emotions. This leaves them feeling bad and out of control when emotions are experienced; thus leading to behaviours that try to suppress emotions, such as eating disorders, or drug or alcohol misuse.

Stressful life events

These may be traumatic events, such as the death of someone close, or longer term struggles, such as being the victim of some form of harassment or oppression.

Biochemistry

Biochemistry can affect mood, e.g. a stressful or frightening situation will trigger the body's fight or flight response and drive the body to produce adrenaline (epinephrine). If physical activity does not use all the adrenaline produced, the body remains tense and the mind stays over active.

Genetics

There is a genetic component to the risk factors for the development of disorders such as bipolar disorder, schizophrenia or eating disorders. This may be either direct or through personality traits, such as perfectionism, which may have a genetic basis.

Common mental health disorders seen by dietitians

The most common mental health disorders that require dietetic input are:

- Schizophrenia.
- Depression.
- Alzheimer's disease.
- Obsessive compulsive disorder (OCD).
- Anxiety or panic and phobias.
- Drug and alcohol problems.
- Personality disorders.
- Eating disorders (see Chapter 7.10.1).
- Post traumatic stress disorder (PTSD).
- Learning disabilities (see Chapter 3.7).
- Bipolar disorder.

Schizophrenia

Schizophrenia is a mental illness that can severely interfere with abilities to perform everyday tasks and activities, caused by confusion and withdrawal. Symptoms can include hearing voices and seeing things that other people cannot.

Depression

Depression is the most common psychiatric illness and is increasing in prevalence worldwide (McManus et al., 2009). Depression is characterised by dysphoric mood (feeling sad, hopeless, miserable or low) and sometimes mania caused by euphoric mood (elated, happy, excited, irritable or high). Depression is thought to result from an imbalance of the neurotransmitters that carry messages between brain cells. This can be disturbed by many factors, such as the effects of stress, trauma, relationship breakdown or hormonal changes, or as a side effect of some types of medication such as tranquillisers, steroids, antihypertensive and antihyperthyroid drugs. Genetic influences on brain function may make some people more susceptible to depression (Tsuang et al., 2004).

Personality disorders

The term personality disorder refers to a diagnostic category of psychiatric disorders characterised by a chronic, inflexible and maladaptive pattern of relating to the world. This maladaptive pattern is evident in the way a person thinks, feels and behaves, which may lead to personal problems that induce extreme anxiety, distress and depression. The most noticeable feature of these disorders is their negative effect on interpersonal relationships. People diagnosed with personality disorder may also be very inflexible, i.e. they may have a narrow range of attitudes, behaviours and coping mechanisms that they cannot change easily or at all. They may not understand why they need to change, as they do not feel they have a

problem. Their behaviours can result in maladaptive coping skills, such as self harm, substance misuse and eating disorders.

People with personality disorders may find it difficult to:

- Make or keep relationships.
- Get on with people at work.
- Get on with friends and family.
- Keep out of trouble.
- Control their feelings or behaviour.

Disordered eating

Eating disorders are considered in Chapter 7.10.1. However, dietitians working in mental health settings will see a large number of service users with eating disorders not otherwise specified (EDNOS) and/or a range of disordered eating symptoms such as food restriction, binge eating, vomiting and laxative misuse. This may be part of a dual diagnosis with other disorders such as depression, OCD and personality disorders. In line with NICE (2006) guidance, EDNOS should be treated along the same lines as the eating disorder it most resembles. With all disordered eating, a psychologically based multidisciplinary team (MDT) approach is best practice. It is important to have an understanding of the psychological function of the eating behaviour in order to treat it successfully.

Treatment services in mental health

Mental health services are based in hospitals and the community. Psychotherapy (talking therapies) and psychiatric medication are two of the major treatment options, as are social interventions, peer support and self help. Patients are usually referred to as service users. The majority of service users enter treatment voluntarily, but for some it may be involuntary. Service users may be detained under the Mental Health Act according to specific sections; this is colloquially known as being sectioned. Some specialist services cannot be offered in a local mental health service. These are often provided on a regional basis, are known as out of area placements and are tertiary services. Examples include eating disorder, high secure, personality disorder, forensic and alcohol detoxification units. Treatment services are provided by various mental health professionals.

Psychiatrists

Psychiatrists are medically trained doctors specialising in mental health. They are responsible for arranging admission and discharge of service users for diagnosis and prescription of medication.

Clinical psychologists

Clinical psychologists assess and treat service users with a variety of psychological therapies. Dietitians and psychologists often work together, especially in the treatment of eating disorders. Psychologists can offer advice on the different approaches to use to support dietary change.

Occupational therapists

Occupational therapists are often very experienced in working with groups and are involved in teaching life skills and activities, including shopping, cooking and budgeting. There is often close collaboration with dietitians and occupational therapists, e.g. when working on healthy lifestyle groups.

Pharmacists

The specialist pharmacist in psychiatry is a valuable resource for information on drugs used in psychiatric medicine, particularly in relation to side effects such as weight gain.

Psychiatric nurses

Psychiatric nurses offer support to people and the families of people who have mental health problems. They assess and develop care plans, give medication and some psychotherapy, either formally [via training in techniques such as cognitive behaviour therapy (CBT)] or informally.

Social workers

Social workers offer support for rehabilitation with regard to housing, benefits, and family work. They also assess the mental state of service users in order to determine whether sectioning under the Mental Health Act is appropriate.

Physiotherapists

Physiotherapists support service users to effect physical, cognitive and behavioural change through the use of exercise, relaxation therapy, stress management, electrical modalities and manual skills.

Counsellors or psychotherapists

These offer a range of talking therapies. Counsellors or psychotherapists are trained practitioners who work with people over the short or long term to help them bring about effective change or enhance their wellbeing.

Allied health professionals

Allied health professionals are often the minority professions within mental health settings, although numbers are growing. They may have more generic roles within mental health settings, e.g. occupational therapists as well as nursing staff will often act as a key workers for a clients with various disorders. However, because dietitians do not undertake compulsory placements in mental health settings as part of preregistration training, they are not currently insured to undertake care coordinator or key worker roles in the same way.

As the number of dietitians is limited, they must carefully consider their duty of care to ensure they identify not only those service users most at risk, but also those most likely to benefit from dietetic input, i.e. ensuring they do the most good (or least harm) to the highest number of people within a case load population. This often involves working with carers and ward staff to ensure the basics, such as screening tools, staff training and the hospital menus, are right, rather than seeing a high number of direct clinical cases. A professional who is not a dietitian commonly manages dietitians; therefore an individual dietitian may represent their profession alone within the service. Dietitians must therefore be prepared to articulate their key skills to the team and be clear about their professional boundaries, duties, roles and responsibilities within the team.

Community mental health teams

Most service users with a mental health problem do not need to see a psychiatrist. The general practitioner (GP) is responsible for first line support, including assessment, medication and referrals to a counsellor or psychotherapist. However, if problems are more complicated or serious, the GP will refer the service user to a community mental health team (CMHT). This is a community based team made up of a MDT. Usually, one member of the MDT, such as a social worker or nurse, becomes the key worker for the service user.

Key worker

The key worker's role is to assess the service user's specific difficulties, discuss any plans for treatment and offer counselling, information and advice. The key worker is responsible for keeping in touch with other health professionals who are involved with the service user to ensure coordinated care. All treatments are documented in the care plan, which should list the key problem, what needs to be done and who should be doing what. The service user is always involved in putting together the care plan and will usually be offered a copy of this. Dietitians should ensure that dietetic care plans follow this example, fully involving the service user in joint care planning, and where possible, offering the service user a copy of all correspondence.

Care programme approach

If service users are going to be under the care of the CMHT or specialist services team for a long period, they may be put on the care programme approach (CPA). The key worker acts as the primary link between the client and the healthcare team, organising regular meetings and updates. The CPA is normally implemented by a MDT and aims to:

- Assess health and social needs.
- Draw up a care plan in conjunction with the service user and carers, together with health, local authority and voluntary sector workers.

- Monitor the quality and effectiveness of care.
- Review progress at regular intervals.

Common psychological treatments

Psychological therapies, sometimes referred to as talking treatments, counselling or psychotherapy, are a core treatment for mental illness. Psychological therapy encompasses a broad range of treatments, including talking therapies of different models and different forms of delivery, e.g. individual, family and group). The most appropriate treatment may vary according to the person's age, situation, diagnosis and personal preference. Therapy can either be used on its own or combined with medication. There is considerable evidence in support of the effectiveness of psychological therapies across a range of problems and settings. The National Institute for Health and Care Excellence (www.nice.org.uk)recommends psychological therapies for mild and moderate depression and anxiety, OCD, bipolar disorder, PTSD, eating disorders and schizophrenia. Therapy can help towards reducing distress, symptoms and risk of harm to self or others.

Dietitians need a broad understanding of these treatments to ensure they can work within the psychological approach taken by the team. For example, if a CBT model is used, then aligning dietetic treatment and education to use some CBT based techniques will ensure a consistent and evidenced based approach for the service user and team. Dietitians working within specific treatment teams and modalities will need further training in these specific psychological therapies (see Chapter 1.3).

Cognitive behavioural therapy

This therapy focuses on the here and now to identify maladaptive thinking (cognitions – ideas, mental images, beliefs and attitudes). It recognises that events in the past have shaped the way that an individual currently thinks and behaves, with a particular focus on thought patterns and behaviours learned in childhood. However, CBT does not dwell on the past, but aims to find solutions to change current thoughts and behaviours. Cognitive behavioural therapy has a strong evidence base for phobias, anxiety, depression, OCD and bulimia nervosa, for which it is often delivered within eight to 16 sessions.

Psychodynamic therapy

Psychodynamic therapy (or psychoanalytic psychotherapy) is the general name for therapeutic approaches that try to get the service user to bring to the surface their true feelings, so that they can experience them and understand them. This is often a longer term therapy delivered over a number of years.

Brief or solution focused therapy

This differs from other modes of therapy in that it focuses on a specific problem and provides a direct intervention for this. It is solution based rather than problem oriented. It is less concerned with how a problem arose and more focused on the current factors sustaining it and preventing change.

Systemic and family therapy

This seeks to address how people operate in a family system and not at an individual level, as is usually the focus of other forms of therapy. It looks at people in relationships, dealing with the interactions of groups, their patterns and dynamics. It includes family therapy and marriage counselling.

Didactical behavioural therapy

This therapy is a type of CBT. Its main goal is to teach the service user skills to cope with stress, regulate emotions and improve relationships with others. Didactical behaviour therapy (DBT) is designed for use by people who have urges to harm themselves, such as those who self injure, or who have suicidal thoughts and feelings, but has also been adapted for other conditions where the service user exhibits self destructive behaviours, such as eating disorders and substance abuse.

Interpersonal therapy

This therapy has an evidence base for effective treatment of many psychological conditions, including depression and eating disorders. It is based on the principle that there is a relationship between the way people communicate and interact with others and their mental health.

Standards and policy

There is a large number of policy documents, guidelines and best practice guidance that need to be considered by dietitians working within mental health settings. These change frequently and may vary locally. Some current examples include:

- NICE guidance
  - Prevention, identification, assessment and management of overweight and obesity in adults and children (NICE, 2006).
  - Type 2 diabetes (NICE, 2008).
  - Prevention of cardiovascular disease (NICE, 2010).
- Care Quality Commission (QCC):
  - Standard 5: Meeting Nutritional Needs.
- National Patient Safety Agency (NPSA):
  - Ten High Impact Nursing Standards.
- Council of Europe Resolution:
  - Food and Nutritional Care in Hospitals.
- Essence of Care:
  - Benchmarks for Food and Drink; Best Practice Indicators.
- Patient Environmental Action Team (PEAT) Assessment Criteria.

In Scotland the Mental Health (Care and Treatment) Scotland Act (2003) and Food in Hospitals and Food Fluid

Nutrition Standards governed by Health Improvement Scotland (HIS), formerly known as Quality Improvement Scotland (QIS), are key.

Nutrition in mental health

Evidence from epidemiological studies suggests that nutrition may have an emerging role in mental health. For example, some epidemiological evidence suggests that sugar intake can be positively correlated with the incidence of depression (Weissman *et al.*, 1996; Westover & Marangell, 2002). Unipolar and bipolar depression have been inversely correlated with seafood consumption (Hibbeln, 1998; Noaghiul & Hibbeln, 2003). Peet (2004) suggested that recent increased consumption of processed foods, sugar, *trans*, saturated and n-6 fatty acids, and reductions in fibre, folate and n-3 fatty acids may be partly responsible for increases in mood disorders. The topic of food and mood is an area of emerging interest and with a growing evidence base. However, dietitians need to assert caution when interpreting studies that involve food and mood, as criticisms of papers in this area include low numbers of subjects, poor methodology and assumptions about cause and effect. No single food can cure mental health conditions, but some evidence about particular nutrients and their possible role in mental health are discussed below.

Nutrition supplementation

There is emerging evidence that certain nutritional supplements may play a role in the treatment of mental health conditions, especially considering the high incidence of poor dietary intakes in individuals with these conditions. Dietitians should ensure that those on inadequate diets receive adequate vitamin, mineral and n-3 supplementation if this is not achieved through diet.

Tryptophan

A Cochrane review (Shaw *et al.*, 2002) examined two double blind randomised controlled trials involving a total of 64 service users. They found that tryptophan was better than a placebo at alleviating depression, but the evidence was inadequate to make recommendations other than to ensure adequate protein intake.

Omega 3 Fatty acids

A meta analysis by Ross *et al.* (2007) found that trials of service users with major depressive disorder and bipolar disorder provided evidence that n-3 fatty acids reduce symptoms of depression, with suggestions that ecosapentaenoic acid (EPA) may be better than docosahexaenoic acid (DHA) for treatment of mood disorders. In a more recent systematic review, Appleton *et al.* (2010) concluded that although trial evidence of the effects of n-3 fatty acids on depressed mood has increased, it remains difficult to summarise the evidence because of considerable differences between trials. However, the evidence available does provide some support of a benefit in individuals with diagnosed depressive illness. Therefore, supplementation of n-3, fatty acids, particularly EPA, should be considered.

Folate

A review by Taylor (2004) of three studies involving 151 service users concluded that folate may play a role as an adjunctive treatment for depression, but whether this applies only to those with existing folate deficiencies or to all is unclear. Further research is needed.

Zinc

There is evidence from epidemiological studies that low levels of zinc are associated with depression, but good quality clinical trials that explore the link between zinc supplementation and depression are sparse. A recent systematic review by Lai *et al.* (2012) found only four trials that met their inclusion criteria and they were unable to pool the results of these studies due to their substantial heterogeneity, i.e. the trials were too different from one another to be grouped together in a meta analysis. They found that in the studies that investigated treating depression with zinc supplementation and antidepressants, zinc significantly lowered depressive symptom scores of depressed service users. The authors concluded that the *'evidence suggests potential benefits of zinc supplementation as a stand-alone intervention or as an adjunct to conventional antidepressant drug therapy for depression. However, there are methodological limitations in existing studies and so further well designed, adequately powered research is required'*.

Carbohydrate

In a review of the evidence on carbohydrate and mood, Benton & Nabb (2003) suggested that in many individuals poor mood stimulates the eating of palatable high carbohydrate, high fat foods that stimulate the release of endorphins, which help to self regulate mood. Individual differences in the ability to control or respond to blood glucose levels leave some people vulnerable to binging.

Excess caffeine

Self medication through the misuse of high caffeine drinks and coffee is common, and contributes significant extra energy. Caffeine can cause insomnia, nervousness and restlessness, stomach irritation, nausea, and increased heart and respiration rate. Larger doses might cause headache, anxiety, agitation, chest pain and ringing in the ears, which can exacerbate conditions such as anxiety.

Physical health implications of mental illness

The main nutritional problems as a result of medication, disease state and lifestyle choice are cardiovascular disease (CVD), dyslipidaemia, high blood pressure, constipation, metabolic syndrome, type 2 diabetes and obesity. Common weight related health problems include raised lipids, raised blood glucose, raised blood pressure, diabetes, breathing difficulties, sleep apnoea, poor skin condition and constipation. People with serious mental illness (SMI) such as schizophrenia and bipolar disorder have higher risks of certain physical conditions. For example, they have two to four times the rate of cardio-vascular disease (CVD), two to four times the rate of respiratory diseases and five times the rate of type 2 diabetes than other people (Kupfer, 2005). The reason for this is unknown, but it is likely to be in due to a combination of medication, lifestyle and the disease state itself. A study measuring diet, exercise and obesity in community based men and women with schizophrenia found that none were consuming five or more portions of fruits or vegetables a day and their diets were high in fat and low in fibre compared to the general population, with more than one-third considered physically inactive (Brown *et al.*, 1999). McCreadie (2003) and Compton *et al.*, (2006) support these findings with data showing higher body weight, less physical activity and lower fibre and higher saturated fat intakes in sufferers of schizophrenia. Carbonated drink consumption is often excessive (Lien *et al.*, 2006).

Weight gain and serious mental illness

Weight gain can result as a side effect of medication and the adoption of an unhealthy lifestyle, such as insufficient physical activity and unhealthy dietary preferences, with excess calories consumed through high fat meal choices, excessive portions, snacks, carbonated drinks and takeaways (Brown *et al.*, 1999). The latter may be due to boredom as a result of low occupational activity, increased thirst as a side effect of medication or the perceived positive impact on mood by consumption of caffeine and sugar. Weight gain caused by boredom, especially when service users have long period of residential care and are on restricted access, can be challenging to change. Service users who are on restricted access cannot access foods other than those provided by the wards. Some service users on restricted access can go as far as the vending machines or the hospital shop, which generally promotes the purchasing of foods as part of a daily routine. Long stay service users report that they get bored with menus that remain the same on 3–4 week cycles and chose to order takeaways, especially if menus do not reflect service users' preferences for good quality meat, and spicy foods (Service User Led Audit Group, 2011).

Dieting or weight cycling is also related to depression, with repeated diet failure and episodes of binge eating affecting mood. The use of food as a coping strategy for emotion regulation has the potential to cause overweight or obesity in those experiencing negative mood. Depression also predicts attrition from weight loss programmes, as it can prevent people from engaging in the meal planning and physical activity necessary to lose weight (Markowitw *et al.*, 2008).

Lack of knowledge or skills around meal planning and cooking can also severely limit food choice. Occupational therapy support with improving skills and confidence in the life skills required for everyday living, such as cooking, ironing, cleaning, planning and budgeting, can improve these factors. Joint work between occupational therapists and dietitians can considerably improve service users' occupational skills and healthy eating.

Weight loss

There is a risk of undernutrition in people with some forms of mental illness, particularly if chronic psychotic illness is associated with problems such as low income, poor housing, eating disorders or substance misuse. Malnutrition can also result as an effect of food phobia or paranoid episodes, where there is a belief that food is contaminated in some way. Some people presenting with deterioration in their mental illness may refuse to eat food available on the ward, perhaps from fear that the food is contaminated or poisoned. Usually food that is still packaged will be accepted, but their diet may remain limited and nutritionally unbalanced until medications have improved their condition.

Depressive illness often results in weight loss. This may be a result of taste changes leading to loss of appetite, low motivation for self care so that the patient does not bother to eat, or a preoccupation with other problems so that eating becomes a low priority event, or a combination of these. Similarly, people suffering with anxiety are often too preoccupied to eat or may complain of food getting stuck in their throat.

Unstable diabetes

Erratic meal patterns, binge eating, non-compliance with medication, excessive carbonated drink consumption and excessive sugar consumption are all common causes of unstable diabetes in mental health settings. A holistic care plan should involve the dietitian, the diabetes care team, key worker and the service user and carer.

Nutritional consequences of medication

A high majority of service users with SMI use medications long term. These types of medications are associated with weight gain, constipation, thirst and increased appetite. Increasing weight impacts on motivation and mobilisation, as well as increasing the risk of other health problems such as metabolic syndrome and CVD. Possible effects of commonly used psychotropic drugs on nutrition are shown in Table 7.10.5.

Psychotropic medication

Psychiatric medications used to treat mental disorders are called psychotropic or psychotherapeutic medications. These medications treat the symptoms of mental disorders. They cannot cure the disorder, but they make people feel better so they can function. Medications work differently for different people. Some people only need them for a short time, e.g. a person with depression may feel much better after taking a medication for a few months, and may never need it again. People with SMI may need to take medication for a much longer time. Psychotropic medication works by affecting the brain's neurotransmitters. Neurotransmitters are chemicals that

SECTION 7

Table 7.10.5 Possible effects of commonly used psychotropic drugs on nutrition

Drug type	Examples	Licensed uses	Potential nutritional side effects
Antidepressants			
Tricyclics	Amitriptyline Imipramine Lofepramine Dosulepin Doxepin	Moderate to severe depression, particularly where sedation is required	Dry mouth, blood sugar changes, constipation or (rarely) diarrhoea, nausea and vomiting, epigastric distress, increased appetite and weight gain, SIADH leading to hyponatraemia, anorexia (rarely)
Selective serotonin reuptake inhibitors (SSRIs)*	Citalopram Fluoxetine Fluvoxamine Paroxetine Sertraline Escitalopram	Moderate to severe depression Bulimia nervosa Obsessive compulsive disorder Panic disorder Generalised anxiety disorder Post traumatic stress disorder Social phobia	Anorexia, nausea and vomiting, weight loss/gain, dry mouth, dyspepsia, diarrhoea, taste disturbances, abdominal pain SIADH
Monoamine oxidase inhibitors (MAOIs)	Isocarboxazid Phenelzine Tranylcypromine Moclobemide (reversible MAOI)	Moderate to severe depression Atypical depression Depression with phobic symptoms	Nausea and vomiting, dry mouth, constipation, increased appetite and weight gain, potentiation of action of insulin or oral hypoglycaemic with lowered blood glucose, hypertensive crisis if foods containing tyramine are ingested. NB: This is much less likely with the newer reversible inhibitors of monoamine oxidase (RIMA), such as moclobemide
Presynaptic alpha 2 antagonists	Mirtazapine	Moderate to severe depression	Weight gain, increased appetite
Selective inhibitors of noradrenaline (norepinephrine) reuptake	Reboxetine	Moderate to severe depression	Dry mouth, constipation, lack of appetite, nausea, lowering of plasma potassium concentration following prolonged administration in elderly people
Serotonin and noradrenaline (norepinephrine) reuptake inhibitors (SNRIs)	Venlafaxine Duloxetine	Moderate to severe depression	Constipation, abdominal pain, nausea, vomiting, dry mouth, anorexia, weight changes, diarrhoea, dyspepsia, taste disturbances, increase in serum cholesterol during long term treatment, SIADH
Antipsychotics			
Phenothiazines*	Chlorpromazine Fluphenazine Trifluoperazine	Psychoses Schizophrenia Mania Severe anxiety	Dry mouth, constipation, photosensitivity leading to sun avoidance and low vitamin D levels, appetite increase and weight gain, reduced response to hypoglycaemic agents causing elevated blood glucose
Butyrophenones	Haloperidol	Psychoses Mania Schizophrenia	Nausea, dyspepsia, loss of appetite (less effect on appetite than phenothiazines), dry mouth, constipation
Thioxanthines	Flupentixol Zuclopenthixol	Psychoses Schizophrenia	Increased appetite and weight gain (less commonly weight loss) May affect diabetic control
Substituted benzamides	Pimozide Sulpiride	Psychoses Schizophrenia	Nausea, dyspepsia, abdominal pain, constipation, dry mouth, changes in body weight, glycosuria
Atypical antipsychotics*	Clozapine Olanzapine Quetiapine Risperidone Amisulpride Aripiprazole Ziprasidone (not currently available in the UK)	Psychoses Schizophrenia Mania	Increased appetite and weight gain (likelihood of weight gain greatest with clozapine and then in decreasing order as listed), hyperglycaemia and/or development or exacerbation of diabetes, elevated triglyceride levels, constipation, dry mouth and hypersalivation, impairment of intestinal peristalsis, dysphagia
Hypnotics and anxiolytics			
Benzodiazepines	Diazepam Chlordiazepoxide Lorazepam	Short term anxiety Alcohol withdrawal	Nausea, vomiting, diarrhoea or constipation, appetite and weight changes, dry mouth, metallic taste, dysphagia. These symptoms have been reported both before and up to 6 weeks after withdrawal

Table 7.10.5 (*Continued*)

Drug type	Examples	Licensed uses	Potential nutritional side effects
	Temazepam Nitrazepam	Short term sleep disturbance	As above
Non-benzodiazepine hypnotics	Zopiclone Zolpidem Zaleplon	Short term sleep disturbance	Metallic taste changes, nausea, vomiting, dry mouth
Mood stabilisers			
Lithium salts	Lithium carbonate Lithium citrate	Treatment of mania and hypomania Prophylactic treatment of recurrent affective disorders	Early side effects: Nausea, metallic taste, increased thirst, polyuria, loose stools Later side effects: Weight gain, mild oedema, polyuria, metallic taste, possible hypothyroidism, hyperglycaemia, toxic effects (can result from sodium depletion), loss of appetite, vomiting, diarrhoea
Anticonvulsants			
Benzodiazepines	Clonazepam Clobazam	All forms of epileptic seizure	As for benzodiazepines
Barbiturates	Phenobarbitone Primidone (80% of its activity is phenobarbitone)	Grand mal and focal seizures	Decreased vitamin D levels, decreased folate levels, (rarely) gastrointestinal upsets
Other antiepileptics	Carbamazepine	Temporal lobe, tonic/clonic and partial seizures. (Mood regulation as an alternative to lithium) Neuropathic pain	Mimics action of ADH on kidney, causing water retention, nausea, loss of appetite, vomiting, diarrhoea or constipation (high dose), dry mouth, lowered plasma sodium levels
	Sodium valproate	All types of seizures (mania – valproic acid)	Nausea and vomiting, anorexia, gastric irritation or increased appetite and weight gain, diarrhoea
	Phenytoin	Tonic/clonic seizures Following head injury or surgery	Early side effects: Nausea and vomiting Later side effects: Decreased absorption of vitamin D leading to osteomalacia, increased turnover and decreased absorption of folic acid leading to megaloblastic anaemia, gum hyperplasia and soreness, tooth decay
	Lamotrigine	Partial seizures Primary and secondary generalised tonic/clonic seizures Myoclonic seizures Lennox–Gastaut syndrome	Nausea, vomiting, diarrhoea Possibility of interference with folate metabolism during long term therapy
	Gabapentin Pregabalin	Adjunctive treatment of partial seizures Neuropathic pain	Diarrhoea, dry mouth, dyspepsia, nausea and vomiting, weight gain Constipation, flatulence, blood glucose fluctuations in service users with diabetes
	Levetiracetam	Adjunctive treatment of partial seizures	Anorexia, diarrhoea, dyspepsia, nausea
	Topiramate	Generalised tonic/clonic seizures Partial seizures Adjunct in Lennox–Gastaut Migraine prophylaxis	Weight loss, nausea, anorexia, diarrhoea, dry mouth, taste perversion, metabolic acidosis (?)

*Not all drugs licensed for all indications.
SIADH, syndrome of inappropriate antidiuretic hormone secretion; ADH, antidiuretic hormone.

communicate information throughout the brain and the body, by relaying signals between nerve cells. There are three main types of neurotransmitters:

- Gamma amino butyric acid (GABA).
- Acetylcholine (Ach).
- Bioactive amines:
  - Noradrenaline (norepinephrine).
  - Adrenaline (epinephrine).
  - Dopamine.
  - Serotonin (5HT).
  - Histamine (H1).

The bioactive amines are monoamines, meaning they have a single amino acid group. Monoamines are metabolised by the enzyme monoamine oxidase (MAO) in the nerve synapses. This can result in low concentrations of the neurotransmitters that result in disease. Most people with psychosis (schizophrenia) have unnaturally high levels of dopamine; therefore, the treatment is to lower the monoamine (dopamine) levels. Most antipsychotics (neuroleptics) involve predominately blocking or lowering dopamine levels.

The antidepressant medication monoamine oxidase inhibitor (MAOI) inhibits the breakdown of noradrenaline and adrenaline. This leads to a build up in the synapse and thereby improves mood. These drugs have drug–nutrient interactions that service users must be aware of (Table 7.10.5). Newer antidepressants, selective serotonin reuptake inhibitors (SSRIs), e.g. Prozac, increase the amount of serotonin (and to some extent noradrenaline) in the synaptic gap, which correlates with an increase in mood.

Weight gain

The possible mechanisms for weight gain associated with this medication include:

- Blocking or lowering of ACh peripherally causes dry mouth and increased thirst. This may lead to an increase in the consumption of sugary drinks.
- Drugs that lower serotonin and histamine stimulate appetite and carbohydrate cravings. This may lead to an increase in total energy intake.
- Blocking dopamine, especially the D2 receptors, may increase appetite.
- Lithium may cause weight gain by fluid retention (due to its effect on sodium balance) and by reducing thyroxine levels (which results in a decreased metabolic rate and therefore a decreased energy output).

Therefore drugs that block ACh, serotonin and histamine will have the greatest effect on body weight. Drugs that blocks all three of these will provoke the greatest weight gain, e.g. clozapine, olanzapine and quetiapine.

Antidepressants

In a comprehensive review of antidepressants and weight gain, Zimmermann *et al.* (2003) showed that traditional tricyclic antidepressants, such as amitriptyline, clomipramine, imipramine and lofepramine, caused marked

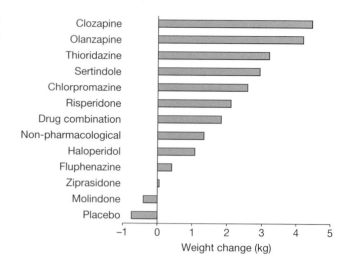

Figure 7.10.2 Effect of 10 weeks of treatment with antipsychotic medication on weight (source: Zimmerman *et al.* 2003. Reproduced with permission of Elsevier Publishing)

weight gain (Figure 7.10.2). The newer form of antidepressants (SSRIs), such as citalopram, paroxetine, fluoxetine and sertraline, may induce weight loss during the first few weeks and may prevent weight gain long term. They are commonly used to treat conditions such as bulimia, panic disorder, OCD and depression. Weight gain with mood stabilisers, such as lithium, can range from 5 to 15 kg over 1–2 years (Baptista, 1999).

Antipsychotic medication

Antipsychotic medications are an important treatment option for many individuals with schizophrenia. A study comparing the effects of older and newer antipsychotics for treating service users with schizophrenia showed that both newer and older types of antipsychotics were associated with weight gain and, of the newer antipsychotics, clozapine appeared to have the greatest potential to induce weight gain (Allison *et al.*, 2003) (Figure 7.10.2).

Parsons *et al.* (2009) and Norvik *et al.* (2009) reported that newer antipsychotic medications, such as olanzapine and quetiapine, also commonly cause dramatic and long term weight gain; with rapid gains of 30 kg over months and that continued over the 3 years of the study. Thakore (2005) found a three-fold increase in intra-abdominal fat stores and associated hypercholesterolaemia with antipsychotic drug use. These side effects can reduce compliance and increase risk of relapse. Whilst alternative medications may have less of an impact on weight, there may be a reluctance to change medications in those people whose mental health problem is well controlled. The concern is that there may be a relapse in control whilst the former drug is reduced and before introducing the new one, and for the consequences if the new drug is not as effective.

Constipation

Constipation is a common side effect of medication and can be severe and even fatal in some cases. Dehydration or an inappropriate diet can compound this.

Polydipsia and hyponatraemia

Polydipsia is associated with some disorders and types of drug treatment, and may result in water intoxication if renal function is impaired (Crammer, 1991). Some service users experience increased thirst sensation as a side effect of antipsychotic medication and consequently drink excessive amounts of fluid, putting themselves at risk of hyponatraemia. The consumption of large quantities of strong coffee or other caffeine rich drinks may make the situation worse. Treatment may necessitate withdrawal of antidepressants, but if continued use of antidepressants is unavoidable, sodium and fluid restriction may be necessary. Dehydration may exacerbate problems such as constipation or urinary incontinence secondary to urinary tract infections.

Additional nutritional problems for inpatient communities

Meal times

Many service users do not get up early and therefore start their day later. The evening meal is often fixed around 5 PM, which means that people are hungry again by 8–9 PM. Access to supper varies but is often limited to toast and cereals; this can promote the purchase of takeaways. Meals times can be a very stressful time for service users and there are many security issues for staff to deal with. There can be difficulties in managing paranoid service users in the same communal eating space as others, sometimes necessitating a staggered approach to meals, which requires different sittings in a short space of time.

Surveyed service users reported that they would prefer staff to sit and eat with them at meal times rather than be there just for observation; giving opportunity to build better relationships with staff and change culture at meal times, thus making them a more normalised and social event (Service User Led Audit Group, 2011). The (CQC) make protected meal times a measurable standard for all mental health trusts.

Takeaways

In the 2011 Service User Led Audit in the north of England, service users gave a number of reasons why takeaways were important to them. Hospital food was perceived as bland; therefore, takeaways were one way that people could have what they considered to be a 'decent meal'. Service users also viewed getting takeaways as a social experience that gives them some control over how and when they eat. It also provided an opportunity for people to eat together, often with staff and friends, in a way that normalised eating. This highlights the importance of service user input into food choice for the menus and dining arrangements. Takeaways in some hospitals have been successfully limited to Fridays or Saturdays and staff place the service users' orders. Hospitals have a duty of care to provide high quality food that meets service users' preferences, nutritional health needs and provides adequate choice (CQC Standard, Outcome 5).

The legal position

In the case of service users who are detained in long stay units, the law states that the hospital is considered the usual residence and therefore a home to service users. However, because of the nature of the residence, e.g. service users cannot access any alternative environment or food provisions, it is reasonable that there may be a case for restricting or adjusting environmental factors, including food type or amount, to support the goal of treating or preventing morbidity or mortality, e.g. to control blood sugars or to prevent weight gain and coronary heart disease in service users identified as high risk. Any restrictions that are placed on service users' food provision must be both justified and reasonable, e.g. not disproportionate to the goal of treatment. In order for this to be legal, there must be a transparent and meaningful consultation with the service users before any such restrictions are applied. All options should be explored in full, and careful consideration given to the type and severity of food restriction needed for treatment, which should be balanced against the service users' right to enjoy a normal diet. Therefore, dietitians should ensure all these steps are followed and all actions and discussions fully documented to ensure legal challenges from service users are avoided.

Management of nutritional issues

Nutrition screening

All service users admitted as inpatients should be screened for nutrition related problems, and those identified as high risk should have a nutritional care plan in place that is reviewed at regular intervals by an appropriately qualified professional (CQC, outcome 5). The Malnutrition Universal Screening Tool ('MUST') has not been validated for mental health settings, and is inappropriate for many of these as selective eating, food phobias or deliberate weight loss, and disordered eating are not easily identified. Therefore, a number of hospitals have adapted 'MUST' or developed their own screening tool, which has then been validated for use through measurements of specificity and sensitivity locally.

Service user led groups

These are often called nutrition steering groups, and may be attended by a nutrition link from each ward. These groups can help to educate and give opportunities to expand choices and experience through activates such as 'come dine with me' groups and themed food nights. Some trusts have catering groups or service user partnership groups, where service user representatives from each ward attend meetings to provide suggestions, comments, compliments, and feedback on menus and quality of the food. Service users also give suggestions for new menus; however, dietitians need to keep in mind the various policies around food in hospitals that each trust needs to adhere to.

Menu and snack choices

Other successful strategies include ensuring the menus are carefully planned to give healthy choices, e.g. all recipes including traditionally higher calorie choices, such as chips and curry, are given a healthy eating makeover aiming for high taste and lower fat. Foods such as snacks may be rated, e.g. red, amber and green (RAG rated), offering service users an informed choice. Stocking non-food items such as puzzle books and magazines in vending machines rather than food, stocking only caffeine and sugar free drinks and limiting shop sold items to small portion sizes are some ways in which hospitals have successfully started to promote healthier eating.

Weight management

A holistic care package should address the psychiatric features of SMI and any physical health consequences (NICE, 2009). A systemic review on interventions to control body weight in service users with schizophrenia suggested that, although weight loss may be difficult, positive effects are possible (Faulkner et al., 2003). In addition, the authors also recommend a combined intervention of diet and exercise as a part of the behavioural modification programme for weight maintenance. The effect of an educational programme on weight gain induced by antipsychotics was examined in an intervention study (Littrell et al., 2003). It was found that after the 6-month intervention, the intervention group did not gain weight (–0.06 lb) compared with the control group, which gained 9.57 lb. This was attributed to a difference in the knowledge about healthy eating habits and lifestyle changes acquired as a part of the educational programme.

Many service users do not find commercial or community based slimming groups useful due to the rapid pace of change expected, misunderstandings around the impact of the medication they are taking, and social and interpersonal difficulties experienced in group settings. In addition, the incidence of disordered eating is high (Hudson et al., 2007). Therefore, many service users will not benefit from the traditional energy balance approach where the focus is on restricting energy, and educational approaches may inadvertently reinforce beliefs about good and bad foods. Instead the focus should be on regular meals and managing carbohydrate load through the day.

Research suggests that service users can successfully lose weight through targeted individualised plans supported by regular dietetic contact (Skouroliakou et al., 2009) or more commonly through service user led weight management groups. A typical 8–10-week programme includes topics such as healthy eating principles, self esteem, activity, meal planning and demonstrations, activity scheduling, motivation, quizzes and evaluation (Chen et al., 2009). Goals were set by the individual and the pace of change was slow, with focus on single changes such as changing to diet drinks and semi skimmed milk, using sweeteners in drinks, frying less and increasing consumption of fruit or vegetables. Service users were self weighed at each session and peer support and suggestions offered. Results at 12 months were typically in the region of a 3-kg weight loss (Gabriele et al., 2009; Chen et al., 2009). Holt et al. (2009) also showed a consistent average weight loss of 0.34–0.07 kg/week (average 3.0 kg/12 months) over 8 years. Weight loss strongly correlated with the number of session attended, with 61 sessions being the average. Weight loss correlated with decreases in CVD risk factors such as blood pressure.

Promoting physical activity

It has been widely acknowledged that being more active contributes significantly to improved health and wellbeing, reducing the likelihood of developing heart disease and obesity, and mental health problems (MIND, 2007). In addition to the physical health benefits of exercise, an increase in physical activity has been linked to improvements in mental health. Collective evidence shows that exercise improves mental health and wellbeing, reduces depression, anxiety and negative symptoms, and improves self esteem and cognitive functioning (Callaghan, 2004). There is accumulating evidence to suggest that increased physical activity may also be an effective treatment for depression (Saxena et al., 2005). It may also alleviate some of the negative symptoms of schizophrenia in addition to anxiety and depression (Faulkner & Biddle, 1999). There is now substantial evidence to support the need for physical activity interventions in service users with serious mental illness (Richardson et al., 2005).

Further reading

Care Programme Approach. Available at www.dh.gov.uk/en/Publicationsandstatistics/Publications/DH_083650.

Internet resources

MIND www.mind.org.uk
Mental Health Foundation www.mentalhealth.org.uk
SANE www.sane.org.uk

References

Appleton K, Rogers P, Ness A. (2010). Updated systematic review and meta-analysis of the effects of n-3 long-chain polyunsaturated fatty acids on depressed mood. *American Journal of Clinical Nutrition* 91(3): 757–770.

Allison DB, Mackell JA, McDonnell DD. (2003) The impact of weight gain on quality of life among persons with schizophrenia. *Psychiatry Services* 54(4): 565–567.

American Psychiatric Association. (1994) *Diagnostic and Statistical Manual of Mental Disorders*, 4th edn (DSM-IV). Washington, DC: American Psychiatric Association.

Baptista T. (1999) Body weight gain induced by antipsychotic drugs: mechanisms and management. *Acta Psychiatrica Scandinavica* 100(1): 3–16.

Benton D, Nabb S. (2003) Carbohydrate, memory and mood. *Nutrition Reviews* 61: S61–S67.

Brown S, Birtwistle J, Roe L, Thompson C. (1999). The unhealthy lifestyle of people with schizophrenia. *Psychological Medicine* 29(3): 697–701.

Callaghan P. (2004).Exercise: a neglected intervention in mental health. *Journal of Psychiatric and Mental Health Nursing* 11: 476–483.

Chen C-K, Chen Y-C, Huang Y-S. (2009) Effects of a 10-week weight control program on obese service users with schizophrenia or schizoaffective disorder: A 12-month follow up. *Psychiatry and Clinical Neurosciences* 63(1): 17–22.

Compton M, Daumit G, Benjamin G, Druss M. (2006) Cigarette smoking and overweight/obesity among individuals with serious mental illnesses: A preventive perspective. *Harvard Review of Psychiatry* 14(4): 212–222

Crammer JL. (1991) Drinking, "thirst and water intoxication". *British Journal of Psychiatry* 159: 83–89

Faulkner G, Biddle S. (1999) Exercise as an adjunct treatment for schizophrenia: A review of the literature. *Journal of Mental Health* 8(5): 441–457.

Faulkner G, Soundy A, Lloyd K. (2003) Schizophrenia and weight management: a systematic review of interventions to control weight. *Acta Psychiatrica Scandinavica* 108: 324–332.

Gabriele J, Dubbert P, Reeves R. (2009)Efficacy of behavioural interventions in managing atypical antipsychotic weight gain. *Obesity Reviews* 10: 442–455.

Hibbeln JR. (1998) Fish consumption and major depression. *Lancet* 351: 1213.

Holt RIG, Pendlebury J, Wildgust J, Buche C. (2009) Intentional weight loss in overweight and obese service users with severe mental illness: 8-year experience of a behavioural treatment program. *Journal of Clinical Psychiatry* 71(6): 800–805.

Hudson J, Hiripib E, Pope G, Kessler R. (2007) The prevalence and correlates of eating disorders in the National Comorbidity Survey. *Biological Psychiatry* 61(3): 348–335.

Kupfer DJ. (2005) The increasing medical burden in bipolar disorder. *JAMA* 293(20): 2528–2530.

Lai J, Moxey A, Nowak G, Vashum K, Bailey K, McEvoy M. (2012) The efficacy of zinc supplementation in depression: Systematic review of Randomized controlled trials. *Journal of Affective Disorders* 136(1–2): e31–39.

Lien L, Lien N, Heyerdahl S, Thoresen M, Bjertness E. (2006) Consumption of soft drinks and hyperactivity, mental distress, and conduct problems among adolescents. *American Journal of Public Health* 96(10): 1815–1820.

Littrell K, Hlligoss N, Krishner C, Petty R, Johnson C. (2003) The effects of an educational intervention on anti-psychotic induced weight gain. *Journal of Nursing Scholarship* 35: 237–241.

Markowitw S, Friedman MA, Arent SM. (2008) Understanding the relationship between obesity and depression; Causal mechanisms and implications for treatment. *Clinical Psychology, Science and Practice* 15(1): 1–20.

McCreadie RG (2003) Scottish Schizophrenia Lifestyle Group. Diet, smoking, and cardiovascular risk in people with schizophrenia: Descriptive study. *British Journal of Psychiatry* 183: 534–539.

McManus S, Meltzer H, Brugha T, *et al.* (2009) Adult psychiatric morbidity in England, 2007. The NHS Information Centre for Health and Social Care. Available at https://catalogue.ic.nhs.uk/publications/mental-health/surveys/adul-psyc-morb-res-hou-sur-eng-2007/adul-psyc-morb-res-hou-sur-eng-2007-rep.pdf. Accessed 9 September 2013.

MIND. (2007) *Ecotherapy Report – the Green Agenda for Mental Health*. London: MIND.

National Institute for Health and Care Excellence (NICE). (2006) Obesity: the prevention, identification, assessment and management of overweight and obesity in adults and children (CG43). Available at www.nice.org.uk/cg043. Accessed 28 August 2013.

National Institute for Health and Care Excellence (NICE). (2008) Type 2 diabetes (CG66). Available at www.nice.org.uk/CG66. Accessed 28 August 2013.

National Institute for Health and Care Excellence (NICE). (2009) *Core Interventions in the Treatment and Management of Schizophrenia in Primary and Secondary Care*. National Clinical Practice Guidelines Number 82. London: NICE.

National Institute for Health and Care Excellence (NICE). (2010) Prevention of cardiovascular disease (PH25). Available at www.nice.org.uk/PH25. Accessed 28 August 2013.

Noaghiul S, Hibbeln JR. (2003) Cross-national comparison of seafood consumption and rates of bipolar disorder. *American Journal of Psychiatry* 160: 2222–2226.

Norvik D, Suarez D, Vieta E, Nabar D. (2009) Recovery in outservice user settings a 36 months result from The Schizophrenia Outservice Users Health Outcomes Study. *Schizophrenia Research* 108(1–3): 223–230.

Parsons B, Allison D, Loebel A, *et al.* (2009) Weight effects associated with antipsychotics: a comprehensive database analysis. *Schizophrenia Research* 110(1–3): 103–110.

Peet M. (2004) International variations in the outcome of schizophrenia and the prevalence of depression in relation to national dietary practices: an ecological analysis. *British Journal of Psychiatry* 184: 404–408.

Richardson C, Faulkner G, McDevitt J, Skrinar G, Hutchinson D, Piette J. (2005) Integrating physical activity into mental health services for persons with serious mental illness. *Psychiatry Services* 56: 324–331.

Ross B, Seguin J, Sieswerda L. (2007) Omega 3 fatty acid as treatment for mental illness; which disorder and which fatty acid. *Lipids in Health and Disease* 18(6): 21.

Saxena S, Van Ommeren M, Armstrong T. (2005) Mental health benefits of physical activity. *Journal of Mental Health* 14(5): 445–451.

Shaw K, Turner J, Del Mar C. (2002) Tryptophan and 5-hydroxytryptophan for depression *Cochrane Database of Systematic Reviews* 1: CD003198.

Service User Led Audit Involvement Strategy Group – Yorkshire and Humber. (2011). *The Whole Dining Experience*. Available at www.yhscg.nhs.uk/secure-services/the-whole-dining-experience.htm. Accessed 9 September 2013.

Skouroliakou M, Giannopoulou I, Kostara C, Hannon J. (2009) Effects of nutritional intervention on body weight and body composition of obese psychiatric service users taking olanzapine. *Nutrition* 25(7–8): 729–735.

Taylor M. (2004) Folate for depressive disorders: Systematic review and meta-analysis of randomized controlled trials. *Journal of Psychopharmacology* 18(2): 251–256.

Thakore H. (2005) Metabolic syndrome and schizophrenia. *British Journal of Psychiatry* 186: 445–456.

Tsuang MT, Bar JL, Stone WS, Faraone SV. (2004) Gene–environment interactions in mental disorders. *World Psychiatry* 3(2): 73–83.

Weissman MM, Bland RC, Canino GJ, *et al.* (1996) Cross-national epidemiology of major depression and bipolar disorder. *JAMA* 276: 293–299.

Westover AN, Marangell LB. (2002) A cross-national relationship between sugar consumption and depression? *Depression and Anxiety* 16: 118–120.

Zimmermann U, Kraus T, Himmerich H, Schuld A, Pollmächer T. (2003) Epidemiology, implications and mechanisms underlying drug-induced weight gain in psychiatric service users. *Journal of Psychiatric Research* 37(3): 193–220.

SECTION 7

7.11

Immunology and immune disease

7.11.1 Nutrition and immunity
Elaine Gardner

Key points

- The immune system is a complex series of processes that interact as the body's defence system.

- Nutrients play a major role in the functioning of a healthy immune system.

- Any challenge to optimum nutritional status has an impact on the immune system.

- The immune system is linked to the pathogenesis of many everyday illnesses and diseases.

- Supplementation with nutrients may have a role in the treatment of illnesses and chronic diseases (through their impact on the immune system), as well as correcting deficiencies.

The immune system is complex and should be viewed as a range of tissues, cells and their products. This defence mechanism guards against invasion by foreign microorganisms and molecules, so protecting against illnesses and communicable diseases. A balance between destruction of foreign cells and avoidance of self destruction is necessary, and the body's ability to distinguish and identify cells and molecules that are part of its self and those that are non-self is fundamental. Further details of the structure and functioning of the immune system can be found in Sompayrac (2011).

Nutrients and the function of a healthy immune system

Adequate intakes are required for the immune system to develop and function correctly. A deficiency can negatively influence the body's defences and impair the their ability to combat infections.

Energy and protein

Infection increases energy requirement due to an increase in the basal metabolic rate. There is an increased need for protein and energy for increased production of cytokines, B and T lymphocytes, macrophages and other leucocytes and their products, e.g. immunoglobulins. If anorexia is present, and protein and energy demands are not met, fat is mobilised. Cytokine and other hormonal responses inhibit the efficient use of fats and the body relies on protein breakdown. The intake of macronutrients is crucial and influences the immune response. If requirements are not met, especially of methoinine and cysteine, wasting will occur as mobilised amino acids are prioritised for the synthesis of proteins related to the immune response.

Arginine

Nitric oxide is synthesised from arginine and is important in immune systems since the inhibition of nitric oxide production increases the body's susceptibility to infectious agents. Nitric oxide production is induced in macrophages and supplementation of arginine benefits the immune response by increasing macrophage activity (Stechmiller et al., 2005). It also plays a role in cell death in infected or tumour cells; it is suggested that this benefits wound healing by increasing collagen synthesis. In older people arginine supplements may enhance the immune response (Moriguti et al., 2005). However, arginine supplementation during an inflammatory state could be detrimental due to the overwhelming production of nitric oxide (Calder, 2007).

Manual of Dietetic Practice, Fifth Edition. Edited by Joan Gandy.
© 2014 The British Dietetic Association. Published 2014 by John Wiley & Sons, Ltd.
Companion Website: www.manualofdieteticpractice.com

Fatty acids

Fatty acids are important in the function of the immune system because they are structural components of cell membranes. The fluidity of membranes (which is affected by the chain length and saturation of incorporated fatty acids) is important for cell surface structures such as receptors, which are crucial in immune functioning. Polyunsaturated fatty acids (PUFAs) have a direct effect on the function of immune cells as they are converted to tissue hormones, e.g. prostaglandins. n-6 and n-3 PUFAs compete in prostaglandin formation, resulting in the production of different prostaglandins. n-3 PUFAs suppress the production of n-6 PUFA derived prostaglandin (Calder, 2006). Prostaglandins derived from n-6 PUFA appear to have strong regulatory functions for a variety of immune cells whose function is dependent on their concentration, with high level suppressing some immune cell functions (Galli & Calder, 2009). Diets rich in n-3 PUFAs tend to inhibit the immune response, whereas n-6 PUFA rich diets tend to promote immune responses, which lead to inflammation (Galli & Calder, 2009). This has implications in the treatment of patients with inflammatory conditions such as rheumatoid arthritis and ulcerative colitis.

Micronutrients

Tables 7.11.1 and 7.11.2 summarise the roles of micronutrients in the immune system. The tables should be viewed with caution as much of the evidence is derived from studies in low income countries, animals and *in vitro*. Micronutrients influence the effectiveness of the immune system and at least an adequate intake is required for the effective functioning of the body's defence mechanisms (Table 7.11.3).

Iron

Iron is essential for the growth, survival and replication of microorganisms and viruses. At the start of an infection, extracellular iron (and to a lesser extent zinc) shifts into the intercellular compartment; this shift is believed to make iron unavailable to some pathogens and so limits their potential growth (Weinberg, 2009). Supplementation with iron has the potential to increase pathogenic replication and its subsequent consequences. This has implications especially with regards to malaria infected children from developing countries, who are often anaemic, and pregnant women from these areas requiring iron containing supplements. Guidance on iron supplementation in malaria endemic areas can be found in a Cochrane review (Ojukwu *et al.*, 2009) and World Health Organization (WHO Secretariat, 2007) consultation document. There is no evidence to suggest that iron supplementation has adverse effects on infectious disease incidence or morbidity in the UK. There may, however, be possible adverse effects on individuals with HIV and children at risk of diarrhoea (SACN, 2010).

Antioxidants

The immune system is particularly at risk from oxidative stress, as many of the cells of the immune system produce reactive oxygen species during their normal functioning. Antioxidant defences have evolved to protect organisms against the damaging effects of free radicals. These defences include molecules that directly remove free radicals, e.g. vitamin E, beta-carotene, vitamin C, and antioxidant enzymes, e.g. glutathione and superoxide dismutase, which have trace metals components, e.g. manganese, copper, zinc and selenium. There is also an interaction between PUFAs and antioxidants, e.g. n-3 PUFAs and vitamin E.

The immune system and disease

Food allergy

The production of IgG or IgE antibodies in response to an allergen may be established before birth and in early childhood (through reprogramming of the immune response), and is dependent on the body's balance between types of T helper cells (Th1 or Th2 cells). Genes can increase or decrease susceptibility to allergies, and early exposure (or lack of exposure) to environmental factors, such as infectious diseases and microbial infections, may influence whether susceptible individuals become atopic (see Chapter 7.11.2).

Atherosclerosis

Atherosclerosis is an inflammatory disease of the arteries resulting in the deposition of plaques (Samson *et al.*, 2012). n-3 PUFAs may block the production of cytokines that promote inflammation and so inhibit the development of atherosclerosis. Vitamin E may help prevent oxidation of low density lipoproteins (Hansson & Hermansson, 2011) (see Chapter 7.14.1 and Chapter 7.14.2).

Autoimmune disease

Autoimmune disease occurs when there is a breakdown in the self preservation mechanism and a level of self destruction by the immune system. A genetic predisposition, lymphocytes with receptors that can recognise the self antigen and environmental factors, e.g. microbial infection, that lead to the breakdown of tolerance mechanisms, which are designed to eliminate self reactive lymphocytes, are all necessary for autoimmune disease to occur. Examples of autoimmune disease are type 1 diabetes mellitus, multiple sclerosis, coeliac disease, Crohn's disease and rheumatoid arthritis.

Cancer

Cancer cells arise when there is malfunction of systems that promote cell growth and those that protect against excessive cell growth in a cell. A weakened immune system can increase the risk of haematological and virus

Table 7.11.1 Vitamins and the immune system

Vitamin	Importance for the immune system	Effect of deficiency on immune system	Possible effects of supplementation
Retinol carotenoids	Differentiation of epithelial cells Development of lymphocytes ↑ Specific lymphocyte subgroups Enhances activity of NK cells Stimulates production of cytokines Activates phagocytic cells	↓ Physical barriers and impairs mucosal immunity ↓ Total number of lymphocytes ↓ Lymphocyte function Altered cytokine networks Altered antibody responses to antigens Impaired antibody production ↓ Phagocytic activity of neutrophils No alteration of neutrophil numbers (in absence of infection) ↓ Number and activity of NK cells Impaired growth, activation and function of B lymphocytes	May be beneficial for individuals with compromised immune systems Does not stimulate immune responses of healthy adults with adequate intakes In elderly, enhances NK cell activity, but no effect on T-cell mediated immunity *Conclusion: little value in well nourished populations*
Vitamin D	Immune system regulator (Lips, 2006) Stimulates production of antimicrobial peptides (including those in epithelial cells of the respiratory tract) Role in production of TNF	? ↑ Immune response to flu virus ? Predisposes children to respiratory infections ↑ Susceptibility to infections due to impaired localised innate immunity and defects in cellular immune response	↑ Subgroups of T cells in women at low doses ? ↓ Incidence of viral respiratory infections (Cannell *et al.*, 2006) *Conclusion: none confirmed*
Vitamin E	Powerful antioxidant ? Reduces prostaglandin synthesis ? Prevents oxidation of PUFA in cell membranes Effects on cytokine production	Impairs B and T cell immunity (Pekmezci, 2011) ↓ Lymphocyte proliferation responses ↑ Serum IgM concentrations, but impaired antibody production Impaired function of phagocytes	? Enhances immune functions (at doses higher than recommended levels) in elderly people (↑ antibody production; ↓ incidence of infections) ? Reduces exercise induced muscle damage and that associated with antiretroviral drugs *Conclusion: may improve immune status, particularly in elderly, but conflicting results on decreased respiratory tract infections*
Vitamin C	Stimulant of leucocyte functions, especially neutrophil and monocyte movement (important in phagocytosis and lymphocyte functions) Antioxidant protection at inflammatory sites, preventing oxidant mediated tissue dammage ? Regulation of inflammatory response	Impaired lymphocyte proliferation of T cells Impaired inflammatory response Impaired function of phagocytes	Enhances neutrophil chemotaxis In reponse to infection, enhances T lymphocyte proliferation (↑ cytokine production, ↑ synthesis of immunoglobulins) *Conclusion: no consistent effect on incidence of colds, but possible modest effect in decreasing duration and severity*
Vitamin B$_6$	Required for synthesis and metabolism of amino acids, and so for the formation of many immune cells and substances ↑ Production of interleukins	Modifies and impairs antibody production Modifies T cell activity Lymphocyte growth and maturation altered	Correction of deficiency rectifies effects on the immune status *Conclusion: no additional benefit to healthy adults*
Folate	Important in protein synthesis	Affects cell mediated immunity by reducing proportion of circulating T lymphocytes, leading to ↓ resistance to infections	? In elderly, improves immune function by altering age related ↓ in NK cell activity *Conclusion: possible protection against infections in elderly, but conflicting results with suggested mechanisms*
Vitamin B$_{12}$	Interactions with folate mechanism Regulatory agent for cellular immunity	Alterations in immunoglobulin secretion and antibody response ↓ Number of lymphocytes Suppresses NK cell activity	Reverses deficiency effects *Conclusion: no additional benefit to healthy adults*

NK, natural killer; TNF, tumour necrosis factor; PUFA, polyunsaturated fatty acid.

Table 7.11.2 Minerals, trace elements and the immune system

Mineral/trace element	Importance for the immune system	Effect of deficiency on immune system	Possible effects of supplementation
Iron (Munoz et al., 2007)	Proliferation of lymphocytes Part of iron metalloenzymes involved in oxidative processes	Intracellular killing of pathogens impaired Slight ↓ in macrophage cytotoxicity ↓ T lymphocyte count Absence of normal immune response to a particular antigen or allergen ↓ T cell function ↓ Innate immune response Altered balance between pro- and anti-inflammatory cytokines	May favour infectious pathogens by providing them with a supply of iron for growth and replication (SACN, 2010) ? Effect on morbidity and mortality from infections is uncertain *Conclusion: no evidence to suggest that in the UK this has adverse effects on infectious disease incidence or morbidity. Possibly adverse effects on individuals with HIV and children at risk of diarrhoea*
Zinc (Prasad, 2008; Prasad et al., 2007; Ibs & Rink, 2004)	Cofactor for substances that modulate cytokine release and thus essential for highly proliferating cells Helps to maintain skin and mucosal membrane integrity Antiviral effect Regulates activation of acute phase response	↓ B and T lymphocyte proliferation and imbalance in T cell subpopulations Defects in cell mediated immunity demonstrated by a depression in delayed hypersensitivity responses ↑ Susceptibility to infections ↓ Number of mature T cells and ↑ in immature T cells Damages protective barrier of the skin, respiratory and gut linings and impaired wound healing Impairs innate immunity (impaired chemotaxis by neutrophils and macrophages, ↓ NK cell activity)	↑ Cellular components of innate immunity, antibody responses and number of cytotoxic cells ↓ Induced apoptosis of macrophages and T cells Reversal of T cell reduced responses when deficiency corrected High levels cause impairment in immunity (in phagocytic cell and lymphocyte function) *Conclusion: zinc has a major role in the immune system at all levels and deficiency manifests with increased susceptibility to infectious agents. Zinc supplementation may help reduce the incidence of infections, especially in the elderly*
Selenium (Beckett et al., 2004)	Component of selenoproteins with some enzymes that exert antioxidant activity (involved in the removal of excess potentially damaging radicals) Essential for both cellmediated and humoral immunity Stimulates lymphocytes and NK cells Interactions with vitamin E	Compromises neutrophil chemotaxis and macrophage function and subsequent killing of phagocytosed bacteria ↑ Oxidative damage in immune cell membranes ↓ Resistance to viruses Impaired antibody production ? ↑ Risk of developing some cancers	↑ Cytotoxic action against virus infected cells Eradication of Keshan disease Improved immune system function *Conclusion: correction of deficiency rectifies effects on the immune status. Possible role in cancer prevention and therapeutic effect on some inflammatory diseases*
Copper	Cofactor in copper dependent enzymes that are important in antioxidant defence (diminishes damage to lipids, proteins and DNA)	↓ Number of circulating neutrophils Affects synthesis and secretion of cytokines In animals, impairments in immune function (↓ thymus weight, ↓ production of antibodies, ↓ activity of NK cells, ↓ antimicrobial activity of phagocytes)	? Correction of deficiency rectifies effects on the immune status (phagocytic index returns to normal values) ? Immunosuppressive at high levels *Conclusion: further clinical trials needed.*
Magnesium	Component of enzymes and needed for normal functioning	↑ Thymus cell proliferation ↑ Levels of interleukins and TNF ↓ Levels acute phase proteins and complement Influences cytotoxicity of T cells and functioning of adhesion molecules	Conflicting results on improvement of asthma symptoms *Conclusion: additional studies warranted*
Manganese	Component of enzymes and needed for normal functioning Antioxidant activity	↓ Lymphocyte antioxidant enzyme activity In animals, ↓antibody synthesis and secretion	?Antibody production improved, but only to certain level (in large amounts inhibition of production occurs) Can cause secondary iron deficiency leading to iron deficiency induced immune system abnormalities *Conclusion: none confirmed*

NK, natural killer; TNF, tumour necrosis factor.

Table 7.11.3 Summary of nutrient requirements for the functioning of the immune system (Maggini et al., 2007)

Body's defence system	Nutrients required
Skin barrier function	Vitamins A, C and E Zinc
Synergistic working to support protective activities in immune cells (cellular immunity)	Vitamins A, B_6, B_{12}, C, D and E Folic acid Iron Zinc Copper Selenium Manganese Magnesium PUFA Methionine Cysteine
Antibody production	
B cell proliferation	Vitamin B_6 Selenium Copper Zinc Glutamine
Promotion of humoral immunity	Vitamins A, D and E Arginine
Indirect action on protein synthesis and/or cell growth	Vitamin B_{12} Folic acid Magnesium Manganese

PUFA, polyunsaturated fatty acid.

associated cancers, but there is disagreement as to whether this applies to solid tumours. Macrophages and natural killer (NK) cells are able to destroy cancer cells that occur in the tissues, but require activation. Unless there is inflammation present, activation does not occur until a tumour becomes large and dying cancer cells activate the macrophages that enlist help from NK cells from the blood. Zinc, selenium, vitamins A and C and PUFAs have been postulated to be involved in ensuring a healthy immune system against cancer (Valdes-Ramos & Benites-Arciniega, 2007). A summary of the relationship between gut flora, immunity and colon cancer can be found in Greer & O'Keefe (2011).

Coeliac disease and gluten sensitivity

Coeliac disease derives from a mechanism that is triggered by the adaptive response of the immune system, whereas gluten sensitivity is connected to the action of the innate immune system and does not involve the function of the intestinal barrier (Sapone et al., 2010; 2011) (see Chapter 7.4.7).

Critical illness and surgery

Following surgical trauma or during critical illness an excessive inflammatory response can be induced that can be followed by an immune suppressed state, which increases susceptibility to infection. Some nutrients, including some amino acids, antioxidant vitamins and minerals, phytochemicals, long chain n-3 fatty acids and nucleotides may be able to influence the immune system (immunonutrition) by improving cell mediated responses. Research is being undertaken on their use in artificial nutritional regimens. Mizcock (2010) and Calder (2007) have reviewed individual nutrients and the rationale for their role in the immune system in critical illness.

Gut health

The gut associated lymphoid tissue secretes antibodies to inhibit the colonisation of pathogens and to prevent the entry of harmful antigens into the blood from the digestive tract. Indigenous bacteria also contribute to the protection at the mucosal surfaces by creating a barrier effect (colonisation resistance). When the balance of the organisms is disrupted, local immune systems may be impaired. Probiotics, prebiotics and synbiotics that rebalance gut bacteria may indirectly produce immune effects. The actions of probiotic bacteria depend on the strain, but they impact on the immune system by:

- Competing with pathogenic bacteria for receptors on the epithelial wall of the gut and for nutrients that are in limited supply.
- Counteracting the increase in gut permeability that occurs after exposure to viruses or foreign antigens.
- Stimulating the immune response to specific antigens.
- Enhancing phagocytosis.

The impact of probiotics on the immune system is reviewed by Rutherford-Markwick & Gill (2004) (see Chapter 5.2).

Soluble dietary fibre has an influence on the immune system. When it is fermented, short chain fatty acids are produced, which are involved in numerous physiological processes, including those directly relating to the intestinal immune function. Gut health and immunity has been reviewed by Scholz-Ahrens et al. (2007), Roy et al. (2006) and Wong et al. (2006).

HIV and AIDS

The human immunodeficiency virus 1 (HIV-1) slowly overwhelms and destroys the immune system, leading to profound immune suppression. It establishes an infection that can be latent and undetectable by the killer T cells for periods of time and then develops so the killer T cells or antibodies no longer recognise the virus (Sompayrac, 2011). As a result it has a high mutation rate and is successful because it preferentially infects and disables the immune system (particularly helper T cells, macrophages and dendritic cells) that would normally defend against it (see Chapter 11.3).

Undernutrition

In any infection, the nutritional status of the host critically determines the outcome of infection. Malnutrition

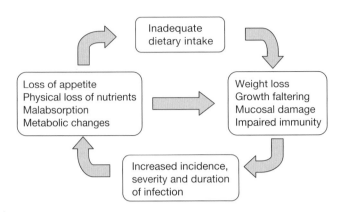

Figure 7.11.1 Cycle of undernutrition and infection [source: Tomkins & Watson 1989. Reproduced with permission of the UN Standing Committee on Nutrition (UNSCN)]

compromises immunity, which increases susceptibility to infection and disease. The general effects of undernutrition on the immune system are:

- Diminished T cell help in immune responses.
- Delayed antibody responses.
- Depressed mucosal antibody in response to mucosal infections.
- Impaired complement activation.
- Decreased lysozyme levels in leucocytes.
- Impaired activity of opsonin (a serum that attaches to bacteria to make them more attractive to phagocytes and thus more likely to be engulfed and destroyed).
- Thymic atrophy (the primary site of T cell development).

Infection has detrimental effects on nutritional status, which can lead to a perpetuating cycle of undernutrition and infection (Figure 7.11.1).

In low income countries, where protein energy malnutrition is more common, the impact of the undernutrition and infection cycle is devastating, resulting in growth retardation in children (and *in utero*) and increased rates of infections and parasite infestations, morbidity and mortality. A full review of the impact of this cycle on the immune system in low income countries can be found in Shetty (2010), Schaible & Kaufmann (2007) and Solomons (2007).

In high income countries, undernutrition is still seen within some societal groups, such as the elderly, who are at risk from the cycle of undernutrition and infection, which results in (subclinical) nutritional deficiencies, loss of weight, poor appetite, poor wound healing, as well as increased rates of infections (see Chapter 6.2).

The immune system in neonates

Cunningham-Rundles *et al.* (2009) reviewed the development of the neonatal immune response, particularly with regard to the effects of micronutrients, and concluded that nutrients mould the developing immune system and that, post birth, the interactions between dietary micro-

nutrients and microbial and environmental antigens define patterns of host defence in later life.

The immune system in the elderly

With ageing the immune system changes and the ability to respond to infections and develop immunity after vaccinations progressively deteriorate (immunosenescence). As a result, there is an increased susceptibility to infections, cancers and autoimmune diseases in the elderly. Innate immunity dysfunction may be due to increased production of proinflammatory cytokines (which may be linked to the development of diabetes, osteoporosis and atherosclerosis due to their inflammatory pathogenesis), a decline in phagocytic capacity and depressed NK cell cytotoxicity.

Changes in the adaptive immune system are two-fold. Humoral immunity is compromised due to the decreased production of immunoglobulin producing B lymphocytes and the loss of immunoglobulin diversity and affinity, leading to less well adapted antibody responses in older people. Age associated changes related to the thymus lead to a reduction in the functional size of the thymus that decreases T cell output and diversity, which may leave the elderly more susceptible to new pathogens.

A number of studies have looked at the effect of vitamin B_6, vitamin E, zinc and multi micronutrients supplementation, but the identification and levels of micronutrients necessary to slow down the immune ageing process are still to be determined. In those elderly that are undernourished, the decrease in immune functions is highly correlated with the intensity of the nutritional deficit and this causes a secondary immune deficiency (in addition to the primary deficiency caused by ageing *per se*). Refeeding may reverse secondary immune changes in the undernourished. Shetty (2010), Aw *et al.* (2007) and Lesourd (2006) have reviewed immune function in the elderly.

Exercise

Exercise has an impact on the immune system. Acute and chronic exercise alters the number and function of neutrophils, monocytes and NK cells of the innate immune system. Lymphocytosis is observed during and immediately after exercise, proportional to the exercise density and duration, with the number of T cells falling below pre-exercise levels during the early stages of recovery, before returning to resting values normally within 24 hours after the last bout of exercise. Acute bouts of moderate exercise have little impact on mucosal immunity, but there may be a link between moderate, regular exercise and a healthy immune system. However, prolonged exercise and intensive training provoke a response that has been linked to increased risk of upper tract respiratory infections during heavy training. This is linked to the elevated circulating stress hormones cortisol and adrenaline (epinephrine), which raise blood pressure and cholesterol levels and suppress the immune system. It is believed that the combined effects of small changes in the immune system may compromise resistance to minor illnesses, especially in elite athletes (Walsh *et al.*, 2011b). The protective effect of exercise against chronic inflammation associated diseases, such as type 2 diabetes and cardiovascular disease, has been attributed to the anti-inflammatory effect of regular exercise. It has been suggested that this may be mediated via both the reduction of visceral fat mass and the establishment of an anti-inflammatory environment with each bout of exercise (Walsh *et al.*, 2011a). These authors concluded '*non-athletes, engaging in moderate physical activity programmes do not require nutritional supplements* [to maintain immune function], *and can obtain all needed nutrients from a healthy and balanced diet*'. The mechanisms and controversies related to exercise and immunology are reviewed by Walsh *et al.* (2011a,b) (see Chapter 4.3).

Further reading

Gredel S. (2011) *Nutrition and Immunity in Man*, 2nd edn. ILSI Europe Concise Monographs. Available from www.ilsi.org/Europe/Publications/Nutrition%20and%20Immunity.pdf. Accessed 10 July 2012.

Hemila H, Chalker E, Douglas B. (2007) Vitamin C for preventing and treating the common cold. *Cochrane Database of Systematic Reviews* 3: CD000980.

Tompkins A, Watson F. (1989) *Malnutrition and Infection: A Review*. Nutrition Policy Paper No. 5. ACC/SCN State of the Art Series. Geneva: United Nations.

Vina J, Gomez-Cabrera MC, Borras C. (2007) Fostering antioxidant defenses: upregulation of antioxidant genes or antioxidant supplementation? *British Journal of Nutrition* 98(Suppl 1): S36–S40.

Wintergerst ES, Maggini S, Hornig DH. (2007) Contribution of selected vitamins and trace elements to immune function. *Annals of Nutrition and Metabolism* 51(4): 301–323.

References

Aw D, Silva AB, Palmer DB. (2007) Immunosesescence: emerging challenges for an aging population. *Immunology* 120: 435–446.

Beckett GJ, Arthur JR, Miller AM, McKenzie RC. (2004) Selenium. In: Hughes DA, Darlington LG, Bendich A (eds). *Diet and Human Immune Function*. Humana Press.

Calder P. (2006) n-3 Polyunsaturated fatty acids, inflammation and inflammatory diseases. *American Journal of Clinical Nutrition* 83: 1505S–1519S.

Calder P. (2007) Immunonutrition in surgical and critically ill patients. *British Journal of Nutrition* 98(Suppl 1): S133–S139.

Cannell JJ, Vieth R, Umhau JC, *et al.* (2006) Epidemic influenza and vitamin D. *Epidemiology and Infection* 134(6): 1129–1140.

Cunningham-Rundles S, Lin H, Ho-Lin D, Dnistrian A, Cassileth BR, Perlman JM. (2009) Role of nutrients in the development of neonatal immune response. *Nutrition Reviews* 67(Suppl 2): S152–S163.

Galli C, Calder PC. (2009) Effects of fat and fatty acid intake on inflammatory and immune responses: a critical review. *Annals of Nutrition and Metabolism* 55: 123–139.

Greer JB, O'Keefe SJ. (2011) Microbial induction of immunity, inflammation and cancer. *Frontiers in Physiology* 1: 168–179.

Hansson GK, Hermansson A. (2011) The immune system in atherosclerosis. *Nature Immunology* 12(3): 204–212.

Ibs KH, Rink L. (2004) Zinc. In: Hughes DA, Darlington LG, Bendich A (eds) *Diet and Human Immune Function*. Humana Press.

Lesourd B. (2006) Nutritional factors and immunological aging. *Proceedings of the Nutrition Society* 65: 319–325.

Lips P. (2006) Vitamin D physiology. *Progress in Biophysiology and Molecular Biology* 92(1): 4–8.

Maggini S, Wintergerst ES, Beveridge S, Hornig DH. (2007) Selected vitamins and trace elements support immune function by strengthening epithelial barriers and cellular and humoral immune responses. *British Journal of Nutrition* 98(Suppl 1): S29–S35.

Mizcock BA. (2010) Immunonutrition and critical illness: an update. *Nutrition* 7–8: 701–707.

Moriguti JC, Ferriolli E, Donadi EA, Marchini JS. (2005) Effects of arginine supplementation on the humoral and innate immune response of older people. *European Journal of Clinical Nutrition* 59(12): 1362–1366.

Munoz C, Rios E, Olivos J, Brunser O, Olivares M. (2007) Iron, copper and immunocompetence. *British Journal of Nutrition* 98 (Suppl 1): S24–S28.

Ojukwu JU, Okebe JU, Yahav D, Paul M. (2009) Oral iron supplementation for preventing or treating anaemia among children in malaria-endemic areas. *Cochrane Database of Systematic Reviews* 3: CD006589.

Pekmezci D. (2011) Vitamin E and immunity. *Vitamins and Hormones* 86: 179–215.

Prasad AS. (2008) Zinc in human health: effect of zinc on immune cells. *Molecular Medicine* 14(5–6): 353–357.

Prasad AS, Beck FW, Boa B, *et al.* (2007) Zinc supplementation decreases incidence of infections in the elderly: effect of zinc on generation of cytokines and oxidative stress. *American Journal of Clinical Nutrition* 85(3): 837–844.

Roy CC, Kien CL, Bouthillier L, Levy E. (2006) Short-chain fatty acids: ready for prime time? *Nutrition in Clinical Practice* 21(4): 351–366.

Rutherford-Markwick KJ, Gill HS. (2004) Probiotics and immunomodulation. In: Hughes DA, Darlington LG, Bendich A (eds) *Diet and Human Immune Function*. Humana Press.

Samson S, Mundkur L, Kakkar VV. (2012) Immune response to lipoproteins in atherosclerosis. *Cholesterol* 2012: 571846.

Scientific Advisory Committee on Nutrition (SACN). (2010) *Iron and Health*. London: The Stationery Office.

Sapone A, Lammers K, Mazzarella G. *et al.* (2010) Differential mucosal IL-17 expression in two gliadin-induced disorders: Gluten sensitivity and autoimmune enteropathy celiac disease. *International Archives of Immunology* 152: 75–80.

Sapone A, Lammers KM, Casolaro V, *et al.* (2011) Divergence of gut permeability and mucosal gene expression in two gluten-associated conditions: celiac disease and gluten sensitivity. *BMC Medicine* 9: 23.

Schaible UE, Kaufmann SH. (2007) Malnutrition and infection: Complex mechanisms and global impacts. *PloS Medicine* 4(5): 806–812.

Scholz-Ahrens KE, Ade P, Marten B, *et al.* (2007) Prebiotics, probiotics and synbiotics affect mineral absorption, bone mineral content and bone structure. *Journal of Nutrition* 137 (3 Suppl 2): 838S–46S.

Shetty P. (2010) *Nutrition, Immunity and Infection*. Wallingford, CABI Organisation.

Solomons NW. (2007) Malnutrition and infection: an update. *British Journal of Nutrition* 98 (Suppl 1): S5–S10.

Sompayrac LM. (2011) *How the Immune System Works*, 3rd edn. Oxford: Wiley Blackwell.

Stechmiller JK, Langkamp-Henken B, Childress B, *et al.* (2005) Arginine supplementation does not enhance serum nitric oxide levels in elderly nursing home residents with pressure ulcers. *Biological Research for Nursing* 6(4): 289–299.

Valdes-Ramos R, Benites-Arciniega AD. (2007) Nutrition and immunity in cancer. *British Journal of Nutrition* 98(Suppl 1): S127–S132.

Walsh NP, Gleeson M, Shephard RJ, *et al.* (2011a) Position statement. Part one: Immune function and exercise. *Exercise Immunology Review* 17: 6–63.

Walsh NP, Gleeson M, Pyne DB, *et al*. (2011b) Position statement. Part two: Maintaining immune health. *Exercise Immunology Review* 17: 64–103.

Weinberg ED. (2009) Iron availability and infection. *Biochimica et Biophysica Acta* 1790: 600–605.

Wong JM, de Souza R, Kendall CW, Emam A, Jenkins DJ. (2006) Colonic health: fermentation and short chain fatty acids. *Journal of Clinical Gastroenterology* 40(3): 235–243.

World Health Organization (WHO) Secretariat, on behalf of the participants to the consultation. (2007) Conclusions and recommendations of the WHO consultation on prevention and control of iron deficiency in infants and young children in malaria-endemic areas. *Food and Nutrition Bulletin* 28(Suppl 4): S621–627.

7.11.2 Food hypersensitivity

Isabel Skypala, Carina Venter and Tanya Wright

Key points

■ Food hypersensitivity is an umbrella term referring to any reaction caused by food that is specific to an individual.

■ It affects 8% of children and 3.7% of adults.

■ Validated diagnostic tests exist for IgE mediated food allergy, lactose intolerance and coeliac disease; often diagnosis may only be achieved through strict and total exclusion of the suspect food, noting the effect on symptoms, followed by a period of reintroduction to see if symptoms are reproducible.

■ Management is mainly through the exclusion of the culprit foods, the level of which depends on the type and severity of food hypersensitivity and the food involved.

■ Food hypersensitivity can have deleterious effects on quality of life; it is therefore essential that the correct diagnosis is made.

■ Children with food hypersensitivity need regular reassessment to determine potential resolution of the allergy, but also to check nutritional status, dietary compliance and coping strategies.

Data from hospital admissions suggest that there has been a substantial rise in the number of patients attending hospital for food allergic events (Gupta *et al*., 2007). Correct diagnosis and management is vital in order to avoid severe or even fatal reactions to food and any nutritional consequences of unnecessary or unsupervised food avoidance, which will also affect quality of life. This chapter will cover the diagnosis and management of these adverse food reactions, usually termed food hypersensitivity (FHS) (Johansson *et al*., 2004).

There is great disparity between perceived and actual prevalence; UK studies reported a 7.2% rate of parental reported food allergy compared with an actual rate of 4% in 12-month-old infants, and a 37% parentally reported rate in 3-year-old children compared with an actual rate of 6% (Venter *et al*., 2007b). This pattern is repeated in adolescents; true allergy was found in only 1.0% of British 15-year olds and 1.7% of Danish young adults, despite a respective reported incidence of 18.7% and 19.6% (Pereira *et al*., 2005; Osterballe *et al*., 2009). The prevalence of self reported allergy amongst US adults was 9.1%, although only 5.3% had a doctor diagnosed food allergy (Vierk *et al*., 2007).

Food allergy is most common in early childhood, with prevalence rates in infants and children varying from 2.3% in Denmark (Osterballe *et al*., 2005) to 8% in the USA (Bock, 1987). The most recently reported prevalence in the UK is 6% (Venter *et al*., 2007b), with the study authors reporting that there was no significant difference between these data on the cumulative incidence of food allergy in children and those published by Bock in the USA 20 years previously. Adults generally have a lower prevalence of food allergy than children; reported prevalence, based on an oral food challenge, ranged from 1.8% in the UK (Young *et al*., 1994), and 2.4–3.7% in Europe (Jansen *et al*., 1994; Zuberbier *et al*., 2004).

Diagnostic criteria and classification

Adverse food reactions and food hypersensitivity are umbrella terms referring to any untoward reaction following the ingestion of a food (or food additive). Adverse reactions to food can be divided into toxic and non-toxic reactions (Bruijnzeel-Koomen *et al*., 1995). Toxic reactions are dose related and can affect any individual exposed to toxic compounds, which may be naturally occurring in foods or added during food preparation, e.g. scombroid fish poisoning or aflatoxins in peanuts.

The nomenclature of non-toxic reactions has been further defined by two European Academy of Allergy and Clinical Immunology (EAACI) task forces (Johansson *et al*., 2001; 2004) as food hypersensitivity (Figure 7.11.2); published guidelines in the USA contain a similar classification (Boyce *et al*., 2010). Where immunological

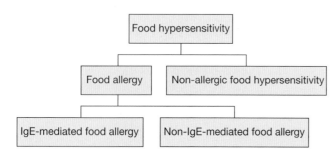

Figure 7.11.2 Proposed nomenclature for food hypersensitivity [European Academy of Allergy and Clinical Immunology Nomenclature Task Force Position Statement (Johansson *et al.*, 2004)]

mechanisms are involved, food hypersensitivity is defined as food allergy. The term immunoglobulin E (IgE) mediated food allergy is preferred when the involvement of food specific IgE antibodies has been demonstrated. Symptoms may be of rapid onset (IgE mediated, e.g. urticaria or anaphylaxis), but can also develop more slowly (non-IgE mediated, e.g. eczema, diarrhoea, vomiting and constipation) or may even be a mixture of both. Severe, generalised allergic reactions to food are classified as anaphylaxis. All other reactions, previously often referred to as food intolerance are classed as non-allergic or non-immune mediated food hypersensitivity. Such reactions may be due to non-immune mediated histamine release, pharmacological effects or enzyme deficiencies. They can be acute and severe (although rarely life threatening), but are more usually chronic and diffuse, and therefore often difficult to diagnose.

The main difference between food allergy and non-allergic FHS is that a protein interacting with the immune system causes food allergy, while non-allergic FHS is caused by other substances in food without immune system involvement. Both the European and US guidelines define coeliac disease as an immune mediated condition, and lactose intolerance as a non-immune mediated condition. The term food hypersensitivity will be used in this chapter according to the above EAACI definition (Figure 7.11.2).

Reactions to food may also be psychologically rather than physically based, i.e. they result from the emotional response to the thought of eating a particular food, and are termed food aversion. Food aversion is not classified as FHS and not discussed further in this chapter, but should always be considered when investigations of FHS are being made.

Food hypersensitivity mechanisms

Immune mediated food allergy

Food allergy results from a faulty and exaggerated response of the immune system following exposure to a foreign protein (allergen). The immune system can normally distinguish allergens that need to be destroyed, e.g. bacterial pathogens, from those that do not, e.g. food proteins, and can mount an appropriate response to protect the body from infection and damage. In addition,

the mucosal lining of the gastrointestinal tract provides a physical barrier to prevent large molecules such as proteins from entering the body.

Everyone is born with an innate immunity, but it is the cells of adaptive immunity that are involved in immune mediated FHS. The main protagonists are the T cell lymphocytes, which recognise and destroy allergens by producing cytotoxic substances or triggering inflammatory responses. When an allergen is encountered, naive T cells develop into either T helper 1 (Th1) or Th2 cells, depending on the presence of specific mediator proteins. The other cells involved in adaptive immunity are the B cell lymphocytes, which create antibodies (classes of immunoglobulin) to carry out further defensive reactions.

The immune system learns to do this in the early months of life, a process known as developing tolerance. If this learning process is faulty, an abnormal response to food proteins can occur, particularly to those that are encountered in early life when the immune system is still immature. Ingestion of the allergen triggers the production of inappropriately high titres of antibodies and/or altered T cell reactivity with consequent systemic effects.

IgE mediated food allergy

Food allergy is most common in atopic individuals. Atopy is defined as a predisposition to become sensitised and produce IgE antibodies to environmental proteins (Johansson *et al.*, 2004). It is clinically defined by a positive skin prick test and/or elevated allergen specific IgE to one or more common environmental allergens. IgE mediated allergy represents the clinical manifestation of an atopic predisposition and in addition to IgE mediated food allergy includes such disorders as asthma and rhinitis.

Classic IgE mediated food allergic reactions, such as those involved in peanut allergy, generally involve the production of Th2 cells. During the first exposure to a food allergen, Th2 cells stimulate B cells to switch from producing immunoglobulin M to immunoglobulin E (IgE), which is specific to that food protein. The IgE antibodies attach themselves to the surfaces of mast cells and blood basophils via a receptor (Maggi *et al.*, 1992; Sutton & Gould, 1993); a process known as sensitisation. The area on a food allergen that provokes the immune response is known as the epitope (Chapman *et al.*, 2006). Epitopes can be linear (sequential) or conformational. Linear epitopes are composed of short sequences of amino acids, most of which lie on the surface of the protein but which can also be hidden within the protein molecule, only becoming exposed when the protein is digested (thus being more likely to trigger delayed reactions). Conformational epitopes depend on the three dimensional structure of the protein because they are composed of amino acids from different parts of the protein sequence, brought together by folding. Due to their structural differences, linear epitopes are not usually affected by heat or proteolysis, whereas conformational epitope structures may be lost when a protein unfolds during cooking or digestion (Lin & Sampson, 2009). Those who experience a resolution of food allergy in childhood or adolescence are more likely to be sensitised to conformational epitopes (Vila *et al.*, 2001; Jarvinen *et al.*, 2007). Epitopes from different food proteins can have a degree of amino acid sequence similarity, known as homology, which enables an IgE antibody specific to one allergen to bind with another structurally similar allergen epitope. Homologous epitopes are common in food allergy, and account for the cross reactivity between different foods and also between foods and pollens.

Many people may become sensitised to an allergen, but only a percentage will experience food allergic symptoms on subsequent exposure to that protein. Symptoms occur when the IgE antibody recognises the allergen and the allergen epitope attaches to the binding site of the antibody. Should the allergen succeed in binding to two IgE antibodies, cross linking them, the membrane of the mast cell perforates and preformed mediators, e.g. histamine and leucotrienes, are released. These mediators are responsible for classic IgE mediated food allergic symptoms; rapid onset sneeze, itch, red facial flush, hives and angioedema.

Non-IgE mediated food allergy

Non-IgE mediated allergy usually involves T cells (particularly the Th1 subset) and other inflammatory cells, e.g. macrophages and eosionophils. T cells become sensitised on initial exposure; subsequent contact with the allergen enables the epitope to combine with the sensitised T cells, which release cytokines, leading to chronic inflammation. Such reactions are usually delayed, although in some cases, patients may show a mixed pathology with both IgE mediated and cell mediated causes.

Figure 7.11.3 summarises the immune process involved in IgE and non IgE mediated allergic reactions.

Non-allergic food hypersensitivity

Non-allergic food hypersensitivity encompasses a wide range of conditions, and therefore has a diverse set of triggers.

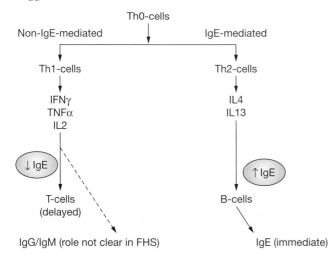

Figure 7.11.3 Food allergy – IgE and non-IgE mediated reactions
Th, T helper; IFN, interferon, TNF, tumour necrosis factor; IL, interleukin; FHS, food hypersensitivity

Mast cell activation

Mast cells can be directly activated by non-immunological mechanisms, with the subsequent release of histamine and other mediators provoking symptoms such as vomiting, diarrhoea and rashes. These symptoms can be severe and in some cases, hypotension and anaphylactoid reactions can occur. The main distinguishing feature from true allergy is that significant amounts of the offending food may be needed to cause a reaction, with symptom severity related to the amount ingested (in contrast to an immunologically mediated reaction where a massive effect can result from minute exposure). However, for practical purposes, this type of FHS is managed in the same way as food allergy. Shellfish and strawberries can both trigger such reactions.

Pharmacological reactions

Many foods and beverages contain substances that are pharmacologically active. Large intakes of, or undue sensitivity to, these substances can result in symptoms such as tremor, sweating, palpitations, headache or migraine, or psychological effects such as insomnia or anxiety. The most common triggers of pharmacological reactions are food additives and naturally occurring substances in foods, including biogenic amines, salicylates, caffeine, theobromines, benzoates, glutamates, nickel and alcohol.

Enzyme deficiencies

Partial or total deficiency of one or more enzymes in the digestive tract, e.g. lactase and disaccharidase deficiency, may result in symptoms of malabsorption when foods containing certain components are consumed.

Symptoms

Symptoms most commonly associated with FHS can broadly be divided into skin, gastrointestinal tract, respiratory system and systemic reactions (Table 7.11.4). These may occur within minutes, hours or days of ingestion.

IgE mediated food allergy

Symptoms suggestive of classic IgE mediated food allergy are acute, typical and may involve more than one organ. They may include one or more of the following: itching (pruritus), urticarial rash (hives), flushing, swelling, nausea, vomiting, abdominal pain, diarrhoea, asthma, rhinitis, tachycardia, hypotension, throat tightness, bronchospasm, shortness of breath, collapse and anaphylaxis. Anaphylaxis is a severe life threatening generalised or systemic hypersensitivity reaction that often includes multiple organ failure, hypotension and shock (Johansson *et al.*, 2001). In adults, mild oropharyngeal symptoms are the most common symptoms. They usually manifest as a condition known as oral allergy syndrome (OAS) (Amlot *et al.*, 1987), which is most often used as a diagnostic term for individuals with food allergy due to homologous epitopes in plant proteins that cause cross reactivity between pollen antibodies and plant food allergens

Table 7.11.4 Symptoms experienced with food hypersensitivity

Target organ	Symptoms
Skin	Pallor
	Erythema
	Pruritus
	Urticaria
	Angio-oedema
	Eczema
	Dermatitis herpetiformis
Gastrointestinal tract	Oral allergy syndrome
	Food protein enteropathy syndrome
	Gastro-oesophageal reflux
	Allergic eosinophilic gastroenteritis/ oesophagitis
	Oral itch, throat itch, lip swelling
	Diarrhoea, nausea, vomiting
	Abdominal pain
	Enteropathy
	Proctocolitis
	Enterocolitis
	Coeliac disease
	Constipation
Respiratory tract	Heiner's syndrome
	Rhinorrhoea
	Asthma
Multisystem	Hypotension
	Anaphylaxis
	Exercised induced anaphylaxis
Controversial symptoms	Otitis media
	Hyperactivity
	Migraine/abdominal migraine
	Enuresis
Other	Irritability
	Listless with other symptoms

(Kondo & Urisu, 2009). The most common form of OAS involves pollen antibodies and is often called pollen food allergy or pollen food syndrome (PFS), to distinguish it from other forms of OAS (Holmann & Burks, 2008). It characteristically manifests in the form of mild to moderate pruritus of the palate, lips, tongue and throat, often accompanied by angio-oedema, numbness or tingling. The onset of IgE mediated food allergic symptoms are usually reported soon after ingesting the offending food, typically within 30 minutes of eating. Those with PFS usually report more rapid onset, most often on biting or chewing the foods (Skypala *et al.*, 2011).

Non IgE mediated food allergy

Both immediate and delayed onset reactions can occur in non-IgE mediated food allergy (Hill *et al.*, 1988). Symptoms may be more diffuse and often less easy to identify (or distinguish from non-allergic FHS). Non-IgE mediated food allergy commonly manifests in skin and gastrointestinal symptoms with mixed patterns of IgE and non-IgE mediated symptoms. There may be differences between children and adults. For example eosinophilic oesophagitis usually presents in children as abdominal pain and

vomiting, but in adolescents and adults, the most common presenting symptoms are dysphagia and food impaction (Noel *et al.*, 2004).

Non-allergic food hypersensitivity

Non-allergic FHS can manifest with similar symptoms to both IgE mediated or non-IgE mediated food allergy. Reactions are usually dose dependent and, although some reactions are delayed, others can occur immediately or within an hour of ingestion. Anaphylactic reactions are not seen with non-allergic FHS.

Triggers of food hypersensitivity reactions

Milk, eggs, peanuts, wheat, soya, tree nuts, fish and shellfish are all common childhood allergens (Bock, 1987). However, shellfish, fish, peanuts, tree nuts, fruit and vegetables are the usual triggers of adult onset IgE mediated FHS (Skypala, 2011). Milk is the food most commonly reported to provoke FHS reactions worldwide (Zuberbier *et al.*, 2004; Kanny *et al.*, 2001; Vierk *et al.*, 2007). More information on individual foods is detailed in the Management section.

Links to other conditions

Rhinitis

Allergic rhinitis is directly linked to food allergy due to the close homology between plant food proteins and pollen proteins. Schäfer *et al.* (2001) found that 73% of subjects reporting adverse food reactions also had allergic rhinitis. This may explain why PFS is the most prevalent food allergy in adults, affecting as it does people with concomitant seasonal allergic rhinitis (Katelaris, 2010). One-quarter of the UK population suffers from allergic rhinitis (Bauchau *et al.*, 2004), one-quarter of whom are likely to be allergic to tree pollen (Royal College of Physicians, 2003). It is known that two-thirds of those with tree pollen allergy are likely to have PFS (Skypala *et al.*, 2011). The incidence of reported allergic rhinitis has trebled in the last three decades in the UK (Gupta *et al.*, 2007). Ziska & Beggs (2012) suggest that climate change and increasing atmospheric carbon dioxide concentrations are likely to affect the severity and prevalence of allergic diseases linked to aeroallergen exposure in the future.

Asthma

Approximately 5.2 million people in the UK suffer from asthma, with about 20% being children (Asthma UK, 2004). Although IgE mediated reactions to foods can involve symptoms of both the upper and lower respiratory tract, asthma is not commonly exacerbated by FHS, except for occupational asthma in relation to food such as wheat flour (baker's asthma). There is a relationship between asthma, allergic rhinitis and food allergy in school age children (Penard-Morand *et al.*, 2005); and having a food allergy is independently associated with life threatening asthma in children (Roberts *et al.*, 2003). Asthmatic adults, who have multiple food allergies or fish allergy, may have an increased risk of hospitalisation and use of oral steroids (Berns *et al.*, 2007). The association between asthma and food allergy persists into old age. Food allergic patients with asthma are more likely to suffer from fatal or near fatal food anaphylaxis. This highlights the need for all asthmatics with food allergy to have a robust food allergy management plan (Colver *et al.*, 2005).

Eczema

Eczema is associated with food allergy, allergic rhinitis and asthma (Burks, 2003). Many children with food allergy also have eczema, and many with adult onset food allergy had eczema as children. Eczema may be exacerbated by food allergic reactions within 2 hours of consuming the relevant food allergen, but more commonly the onset is delayed. It is considered that over 90% of atopic eczema in infants is caused by milk, egg, peanut and soya (Hill *et al.*, 2008), although egg is the most common offender. Other foods such as wheat, tree nuts and seafood may be responsible for reactions in older children and adults (Burks, 2003). However, it has also been shown that some eczematous reactions in those who have pollen food cross reactive allergy could be due to late phase reactions to cooked foods known to provoke symptoms when raw (Bohle *et al.*, 2006).

Gastrointestinal disease

Food hypersensitivity has been linked to a number of diseases of the gastrointestinal tract (see Chapters 7.4) (Lomer, 2009).

Migraine

A close association between migraine and allergic disease has been shown in a number of studies (Aamodt *et al.*, 2007), although it has been suggested that dietary restrictions are not beneficial in most migraine sufferers (Holzhammer & Wober, 2006). A summary of the effects of diet on migraine can be found in Luscombe & Thurgood (2009).

Hyperactivity and behavioural disorders

A meta analysis found a significant effect of artificial food colours on behaviour in hyperactive children (Schab & Trinh, 2004). A study investigating the effect of oral challenges with artificial food colourings and benzoates on hyperactivity in 3-year-old children found behaviour changes when assessed by parentally kept behaviour diaries (Bateman *et al.*, 2004). A follow-up study involving 3- and 8-year-old children taking two different additive mixes suggested that artificial colours or sodium benzoate preservative (or both) in the diet increased hyperactivity (McCann *et al.*, 2007).

Chronic disorders

People with chronic fatigue syndrome/myalgic encephalomyelitis (CFS/ME) often report experiencing FHS (NICE, 2007), although research evidence suggests that IgE mediated allergy is no more common in people with CFS/ME than in the normal population (Kowal-Krzysztof *et al.*, 2002) (see Chapter 7.6.5). Further information can be found in Luscombe & Thurgood (2009).

Disease consequences

Food hypersensitivity can have severe consequences; those diagnosed with food allergy may need to carry adrenaline (epinephrine) in case of a severe reaction that can happen unexpectedly at any time. Food accounts for 33–61% of all causes of anaphylaxis, with over a third of reactions treated as emergencies and most often due to peanuts, tree nuts, fish or shellfish (Pumphrey & Stanworth, 1996; Mullins, 2003). Although mortality is low and only 25% of all fatal anaphylaxis due to food, age range data for fatalities following anaphylaxis suggest that an increasing number of severe reactions to food are suffered by a greater number of younger people, including teenagers and children (Pumphrey, 2000). Morbidity is high and living with a food allergy has been shown to have a well defined effect on quality of life. Childhood food allergy has a significant impact on general health perception, emotional impact on the parent and limitation on family activities (Sicherer *et al.*, 2001b). Parents find shopping for foods for children on restricted diets very difficult, time consuming and confusing, particularly when products which would not be expected to contain nuts have a warning on the label (Food Standards Agency 2009). Results from validated health related quality of life (HRQL) questionnaires found that adolescents and adults with food allergy report more pain, poorer overall health, more limitations on social activity and less vitality when compared with the general population (Flokstra-de Blok *et al.*, 2010). Those who have reintroduced foods back into their diet following a negative oral food challenge report a general improvement in their social life (Eigenmann *et al.*, 2006). The need to fit in with peers may lead some adolescents and young adults with food allergy to take risks, knowingly and purposefully ingesting potentially unsafe foods and not always carrying medication (Sampson *et al.*, 2006).

Prevention

Genotype, exposure to allergens and development of the immune response are involved in the development of allergic disease. Infants born to families with a history of atopy are more at risk of developing allergic diseases than those born to non-atopic families with genetic influences (Kjellman, 1977). Despite a large body of published research, the role that the maternal diet during pregnancy and breastfeeding plays in the development of allergic disease is still unknown; the same is true for feeding and weaning practices.

Maternal food intake in pregnancy

Maternal dietary intake has been extensively researched. The effect of dietary exclusion, or the intake of dietary fats, fruit and vegetables and fatty acids/fatty fish and fish oil supplements during pregnancy and lactation have all been studied. None of these studies has led to any recommendations of dietary changes during pregnancy in order to prevent allergic disease. Similarly, studies examining probiotic supplementation during pregnancy and/or the infant's first 6 months of life in high risk families have been inconclusive.

Vitamin D

Vitamin D has important affects on immune function (Cantorna et al., 2004). Observational studies (Camargo et al., 2007; Devereux et al., 2007; Miyake et al., 2010; Erkkola et al., 2009) support the hypothesis that vitamin D intake in pregnancy may prevent the infant from developing wheeze, asthma and rhinitis in later childhood; the effect on eczema is not completely clear. However, Hypponen et al. (2004) reported that the prevalence of atopy, allergic rhinitis and asthma in adults was higher in those who had received vitamin D supplementation regularly during the first year of life. This paradox may be due to a threshold effect, with both low and high serum vitamin D levels affecting the development of allergic disease (Hypponen et al., 2009). Supplementation during early life was provided at much higher levels than reported in the observational studies during pregnancy.

Antioxidant intake

High maternal dietary intakes of antioxidants, specifically vitamin E, during pregnancy were associated with a decreased response to allergens, which may influence the foetal immune system and affect the risk of childhood atopy (Devereux et al., 2006). The strongest benefit appears to be from maternal vitamin E intake during pregnancy, which was associated with a reduction of wheeze/asthma at in offspring at the ages of 1, 2 and 5 years (Martindale et al., 2005; Litonjua et al., 2006).

Vitamin C could also have a pro-oxidant effect, which may have a negative impact on allergy risk. Thus, a low maternal intake of vitamin C coupled with a high intake of saturated fats during breastfeeding could increase the risk of infant allergies (Hoppu et al., 2000). A higher concentration of vitamin C in the breast milk of atopic mothers was associated with a reduced risk of eczema and a positive skin prick test at 12 months; dietary intake rather than supplements determined the concentration of vitamin C in breast milk (Hoppu et al., 2005).

Breastfeeding and maternal diet whilst breastfeeding

Two systematic reviews (Mimouni et al., 2002; Gdalevich et al., 2001) concluded that exclusive breastfeeding might have some protective effect on the development of allergic disease, which is greater when there is a family history of atopic disease. However, up to one-third of infants with a cow's milk allergy will develop it despite exclusive breastfeeding, probably due to the cow's milk protein in breast milk. Therefore, whether breastfeeding protects against allergic disease needs further research.

Intervention studies in high risk infants

A number of randomised controlled trials in high risk infants have investigated the effect of different dietary allergy prevention programmes during pregnancy, breastfeeding or both. A review by the EAACI concluded that there is no evidence for maternal dietary intervention during pregnancy or lactation in the prevention of allergic disease (Muraro et al., 2004). A systematic review showed that maternal allergen avoidance during pregnancy may be associated with a higher risk of preterm birth and a possible adverse effect on birth weight. Dietary interventions during lactation only did not show any adverse nutritional effects (Kramer et al., 2006).

Use of infant formulae

In an attempt to avoid exposure to milk protein early in life, hydrolysed formulae (extensive or partial) have been investigated as replacement or supplement to breast milk. Studies (von Berg et al., 2003; 2007; 2008) have compared standard cow's milk formula, extensively hydrolysed casein (eHF C), extensively hydrolysed whey (eHF W) and partially hydrolysed whey (pHF W). At 1 year, fewer allergic manifestations were found in the infants receiving eHF C than cow's milk formula, and also less eczema in pHF W and eHF C fed infants than those receiving cow's milk formula. Results from other studies suggest that protein hydrolysates reduce allergic manifestations during the high risk infant's first few years as either a replacement or supplement to breast milk. The nutritional adequacy of these formulae is sufficient for the needs of infants (Hernell & Lonnerdal, 2003), but could lead to insufficient weight gain (Isolauri et al., 1998).

Reviews regarding dietary allergy prevention have been published by the American Academy of Pediatrics (Greer et al., 2008), EAACI (Host et al., 2008) and the European Society for Paediatric Allergology and Clinical Immunology Committee on Hypoallergenic Formulas and the European Society for Paediatric Gastroenterology, Hepatology and Nutrition Committee on Nutrition (Host et al., 1999). The recommendations from these reviews are summarised in Table 7.11.5.

Infant weaning practices

The Department of Health (2009a) and other UK health departments state the introduction of complementary foods should start around 6 months of age. There are some foods that should be avoided before 6 months as they may cause allergies or make the baby ill, namely wheat based foods and other foods containing gluten, eggs, fish, liver, shellfish, nuts, peanut and peanut products, seeds, cow's milk and soft and unpasteurised cheeses. For high risk infants, the following information has been adapted from the British Dietetic Association's

Table 7.11.5 Allergy prevention advice

	AAP position statement	ESPACI/ESPGHAN (1999)	EAACI (2008)
Who is at risk?	If both parents or parent and sibling have documented allergic disease	If have one affected parent or one affected sibling	If have one first degree relative with documented allergic disease
Breastfeeding recommendations	Exclusive breastfeeding up to 6 months	Exclusive breastfeeding 4–6 months	Exclusive breastfeeding, preferably for 6 months but for at least 4 months
Alternatives if breastfeeding not possible or insufficient	Use an eHF, but a pHF could be considered	Use formula with proven reduced allergenicity	Use an eHF until 4 months of age. A pHF may have an effect, although it seems to be less effective than eHF

AAP, American Academy of Pediatrics; ESPACI, European Society of Pediatric Allergology and Clinical Immunology; ESPGHAN, European Society for Pediatric Gastroenterology, Hepatology and Nutrition; EAACI, European Academy of Allergology and Clinical Immunology; eHF, extensively hydrolysed formula; pHF, partially hydrolysed formula.

Food Allergy and Intolerance Specialist Group (2012) position statement on allergy prevention for high risk infants.

Time to wean

The introduction of complimentary food from about 6 months is desirable, but if weaning takes place earlier, it should never occur before 17 weeks (Agostoni *et al.*, 2008). By 6 months weaning should commence and the appropriate textures (Department of Health, 2009a; British Dietetic Association, 2013) and variety of flavours should be introduced to desensitise the child's palate (Mason *et al.*, 2005). Weaning should commence with what are traditionally considered to be low allergenic weaning foods such as rice, potatoes, root and green vegetables, apple, pear, banana and stone fruit given individually or in combination (Martindale *et al.*, 2005). The importance of continuing to breastfeed whilst solids are introduced is being further researched as some research has shown that continuing to breastfeed whilst solids are introduced reduces the risk of reactions to food (Ivarsson *et al.*, 2002; Poole *et al.*, 2006).

Introduction of allergenic foods

A European Union (EU) directive (2007) lists 14 foods or food additives identified as being the source of the majority of adverse food reactions. These are peanuts, tree nuts, sesame seed, mustard seed, cow's milk, eggs, fish, crustaceans, soya, wheat, celery, lupin, molluscs and sulphites. There is no need to delay the introduction of the foods on this list beyond 6 months (Zutavern *et al.*, 2008; Filipiak *et al.*, 2007). It is advisable to introduce these foods in categories, e.g. introduce wheat as one category by giving pasta, bread and other suitable wheat based products over a 2–3-day period (Maier *et al.*, 2008). Introduction should start with a small amount and no more than one new allergenic food at a time, and allow at least 3 days between each new food group in order to enable easy identification of any resulting reactions. The food categories include wheat, well cooked egg, cow's milk (as part of the diet rather than the sole source of nutrition), fish, shellfish and soya products, followed by the other major allergenic foods, should they form a part of the family diet. Peanuts can be introduced into the diet of high risk infants after discussion with a GP, health visitor or medical specialist that it is safe to do so (Department of Health, 2009b).

Nutritional consequences

The avoidance of major food groups by patients with adverse reactions to foods, prior to diagnosis can have a deleterious effect on nutritional status (Fox *et al.*, 2004; Noimark & Cox, 2008). Children with FHS may be substantially affected by the removal of one or more food groups due to the requirements of normal growth and development. Flammarion *et al.* (2011) report that despite energy, protein and calcium intakes being similar, children with food allergy had weight for age and height for age Z scores lower than controls. Adults are most likely to be at nutritional risk if they are avoiding milk or wheat due to confirmed FHS or a self imposed elimination diet, or multiple foods due to OAS or of salicylates or vasoactive amines (des Roches *et al.*, 2006). Milk avoidance is especially common in patients with asthma (Wuthrich *et al.*, 2005); such individuals may be at greater risk of poor bone density if calcium intakes are not optimal, especially in those prescribed regular corticosteroids (Kershaw, 2009). Those who avoid one or more foods for some time prior to referral could be at greater risk of a suboptimal nutritional intake. Vieira *et al.* (2010) found that on referral the infants with suspected cow's milk allergy already had low weight for age and low height for age Z scores. Adults newly diagnosed with coeliac disease may present with nutritional deficiencies such as anaemia (low iron), vitamin B_{12} or folate, and so should receive a nutritional assessment in order to determine any deficiency (McGough *et al.*, 2009). Deficiencies in micronutrients in the elderly, especially zinc, iron and vitamin D, may contribute to the development of allergies (Diesner *et al.*, 2011). There is a growing appreciation of the importance of vitamin D in the development of tolerance, immune system defences and epithelial barrier integrity. Vassallo & Camargo (2010) suggest that, concurrent with the increase in FHS, there is an epidemic of

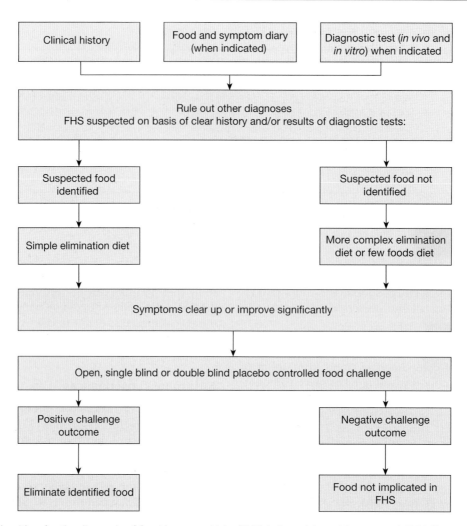

Figure 7.11.4   Algorithm for the diagnosis of food hypersensitivity (FHS) [adapted from Muraro *et al.* (2004)]

vitamin D deficiency caused by decreased sunlight/ultraviolet B (UVB) exposure.

Diagnosis

The first step in the diagnostic pathway is the ascertainment of the problem through the taking of an allergy focussed diet and clinical history, followed by appropriate tests, including the gold standard of the oral food challenge. The correct diagnosis of FHS is complex, and a definitive diagnosis may be difficult to achieve due to the paucity of validated tests and unavailability of oral food challenge facilities. Failure to diagnose FHS, due to negative test results, could risk further potentially severe or even fatal reactions or ongoing chronic disease. Alternatively, a diagnosis achieved on the basis of positive non-validated tests can result in unnecessary restrictions on lifestyle and possible disease from nutrient restriction. A robust diagnostic process is key since <50% of patients reporting reactions to foods are diagnosed with FHS (Seitz *et al.*, 2008). Venter *et al.* (2006a,b; Pereira *et al.*, 2005) have demonstrated that only 12–21% of children and adolescents reporting food allergy were diagnosed with food allergy confirmed by double blind placebo con-

trolled food challenge (DBPCFC). Diagnosis in children is now the subject of NICE (2012) guidance. The dietitian plays a key role in ensuring that a thorough clinical history and relevant tests have been undertaken, so that consideration may be given to the requirement for an elimination diet or supervised oral food challenge in order to confirm or refute a diagnosis. An algorithm of FHS diagnosis is shown in Figure 7.11.4.

Clinical history

Taking a detailed dietary and medical history, together with a physical examination, are essential first steps in the diagnosis of FHS. The information may vary depending on the age of the patient, but the following information should be elicited:

- Current daily dietary intake and pattern, including those foods currently being avoided and those included in the diet.
- Detailed history of any known food reactions, including food eaten, length of time between consumption and symptoms.
- Symptom type and affected organs.

- Suspected food triggers and the quantity likely to elicit a reaction.
- Other known allergies.
- Family history of allergy.

This information will enable the formation of a working diagnosis, inform decisions on diagnostic testing or food elimination and provide useful information for performing a food challenge should this be required. Cross reactions, inaccurate recollection of events and the involvement of multiple foods or the presence of cofactors can confound the clinical history. Therefore, as a supplement to taking a verbal history, diet and symptom diaries may help to identify problem foods, but their efficacy has not been formally assessed. There is little robust evidence to support the role of clinical history in FHS diagnosis, but its use is supported by experts in the field, provided it is not used as a sole diagnostic tool (Boyce *et al.*, 2010). However, validated diagnostic questionnaires have been shown to be effective in the diagnosis of some types of FHS such as OAS (Skypala *et al.*, 2011).

Diagnostic tests

An oral food challenge is considered the definitive test for those with a history of immediate adverse foods reactions in order to establish or exclude a diagnosis of food allergy. However, it is helpful to know whether the presence and level of specific IgE antibodies, bound to mast cells in the skin or circulating in the blood, correlate with clinical history to a sufficient degree to be diagnostic. A negative test suggests that the reaction is less likely to be IgE mediated, but it cannot rule out a diagnosis of FHS.

Skin prick tests

Skin prick tests (SPTs) measure specific IgEs attached to mast cells in the skin and provide an easy method to screen patients of all ages with suspected IgE mediated sensitivity to foods. The skin is pricked through a drop of food extract reagent and any resultant wheal measured against the results of a positive (histamine) and negative (saline or diluent) control. The positive control gives an indication of skin reactivity and the negative control can identify patients with dermatographism (skin reactions to any contact, including the prick with a lancet and not necessarily the allergen applied). In general, allergens eliciting a wheal of 3 mm or greater in diameter than the negative control are considered positive (Bindslev-Jensen *et al.*, 2004). However, some recommend the use of a cut-off of 2 mm in children, especially those younger than 6 months. Skin prick tests have a negative predictive value (NPV) of 95% or more (Sampson, 2004) and are therefore extremely useful in ruling out IgE mediated food allergy. However, since 5% of those with a negative test may have a food allergy, negative results should be verified by other tests such as specific IgE testing or an oral food challenge, especially if severe symptoms have been reported. The predictive value of a positive test is low; only 50–60% of those with positive tests will have a positive oral food challenge (Bock *et al.*, 1988). The reason for this is that a positive test could indicate sensitisation to a food and needs to be of a convincing wheal size and linked to a positive clinical history for that food before it can be considered diagnostic.

Most SPTs are undertaken using purified allergen extracts; however, the allergen content of such extracts can be variable, making them unreliable for certain foods (Akkerdaas *et al.*, 2003). Fresh foods can be used in place of reagents, a procedure known as prick to prick testing (PPT), and may give a more accurate result (Rancé *et al.*, 1997), even though they lack standardisation.

Specific ige tests

Specific IgE tests quantify the level of circulating IgE antibodies specific to a particular food. As with SPTs, the presence of specific IgE in the blood indicates sensitisation but not necessarily clinical allergy. Specific IgE tests are often referred to as radio allergosorbant (RAST) tests, although the technology used now measures fluorescent enzyme labelled IgE (CAP RAST FEIA) and is usually called an immunoassay. Specific IgE is measured as kilo units of allergen per litre (kU_A/L; a test is classed as positive if the result is $>0.34\,kU_A/L$. Some laboratories still grade results 0–6, where 0 is $<0.34\,kU_A/L$. The negative predictive value of immunoassays are similar to those for SPTs, but negative tests need to be interpreted with the history as undetectable serum food specific IgE levels might occur in 10–25% of clinical reactions, depending on the food involved (Ives & Hourihane, 2002).

Guidelines suggest that SPTs and specific IgE estimation are interchangeable and either can be used to good effect with clinical history, However, a positive SPT may not always be confirmed by a corresponding positive serum specific IgE result; research suggests there is a correlation between the wheal size of SPTs and specific IgE levels in children but not in adults (Pongracic *et al.*, 2007). Skin prick tests are often a first line test due to their ease of use, low cost and immediate results. However, specific IgE blood tests may be more universally available, especially in primary care, and are useful for patients with severe eczema, those who have dermatographism or cannot discontinue antihistamines.

Several studies have examined the predictive value of SPT wheal diameters and specific IgE levels, but there is some variance in the results, which appears to suggest they may be specific to particular populations [see Venter *et al.* (2009) for further information). Whilst SPTs and specific IgE tests are good first line tests for the diagnosis of IgE mediated food allergy, they are not useful in the diagnosis of delayed type/non-IgE mediated food allergy or non-allergic FHS due to the absence of the involvement of IgE antibodies in these conditions.

Diagnosis using individual allergens

A major advance in the diagnosis of FHS has been the sequencing of allergens and allergen epitopes, which has demonstrated that certain allergens or epitopes are linked to allergen severity and the likelihood of resolution (Vila *et al.*, 2001; Jarvinen *et al.*, 2007; Ando *et al.*, 2008). This technology can also aid diagnosis to foods which currently have a poor positive predictive value, e.g. soya and wheat (Palosuo *et al.*, 1999; Ballmer-Webber *et al.*, 2007). They can also be used to differentiate between a primary allergy to peanuts or tree nuts and symptoms caused by cross reactions to tree and grass pollen in adults. Although early results are promising, this technology is not available to all practitioners involved in the diagnosis of FHS. It also does not overcome the common difficulty of sensitisation without clinical symptoms, which is widespread in populations and can make positive test results difficult to interpret (Ott *et al.*, 2008; Scala *et al.*, 2010; Ebo *et al.*, 2009).

Atopy patch tests

Atopy patch testing involves food allergens being applied to a healthy area of the patient's skin and the effects evaluated 48–72 hours later. Patch tests are usually used to determine the cause of delayed allergic reactions such as contact dermatitis, e.g. to nickel. It has been suggested that combining the patch test with specific IgE estimation improves the sensitivity and specificity of SPTs and specific IgE test, especially to foods with a poor PPV such as wheat (Niggemann & Beyer, 2005; Allen *et al.*, 2006). However, specialist evaluation is needed to distinguish between allergic reactions and simple irritant ones.

Other tests

Principal amongst the commercial tests are those measuring IgG antibodies. A European position paper published in 2008 stated that this test is not recommended as a diagnostic tool (Stapel *et al.*, 2008): a stance subsequently supported in the USA (Bock, 2010). Similarly, other tests including the leucocyte cytotoxic test, hair analysis, bioresonance diagnostics, auto homologous immune therapy, kinesiology, iridology, sublingual provocative food testing, homeopathic remedies and electro dermal testing (including electro acupuncture and Vega testing), are not valid diagnostic tests for any type of FHS (Niggemann & Grüber, 2004).

Diagnostic exclusion diets

For many patients diagnosis can only be made by means of a combination of clinical history and dietary investigations (diagnostic exclusion diets). A successful elimination diet will improve or resolve the symptoms. There are four types of diagnostic exclusion diets (Grimshaw, 2006).

Single exclusion diet

This excludes all sources of a single food, e.g. milk, as identified from the patient's dietary history.

Multiple food exclusion diet

This excludes a number of foods at the same time, most commonly milk and egg for eczema (Isolauri & Turjanmaa, 1996), and milk, egg and wheat for eosinophilic diseases (Spergel *et al.*, 2002). The major food allergens (peanuts, tree nuts, sesame seed, mustard seed, cow's milk, eggs, fish, shellfish, soya, wheat, celery, lupin, molluscs and sulphites) (European Union, 2006) are usually the first foods to be avoided during a multiple food exclusion diet. The number and combination of foods avoided will depend on the symptoms, and often reflect clinical practices rather than research. Pork, bacon, liver and offal, maize/corn, citrus fruit, berries, potatoes, tomatoes, onions, herbs and spices, chocolate, food colours and food preservatives may also be excluded.

Few foods (oligoallergenic) diet

This includes only a few foods that are known to rarely cause allergic symptoms in the population and are not regularly eaten by the patient. It generally includes two meats (lamb and turkey), two starches (rice and corn), two fruits (pears and nectarines), two vegetables (sweet potato and butternut squash) and only water as a drink (Ventner, 2007). Sometimes a less restrictive few foods diet may be used, particularly if it will improve patient compliance (Table 7.11.6).

Elemental and protein hydrolysate formula diets

Amino acid based formulae are used in infants and young children; elemental feeds are used in older children and adults. These drinks can be used in infants and children in the diagnosis of a range of diseases. In adults these diets are often used in the diagnosis of severe allergic symptoms or in patients suffering from a range of reported food intolerances to establish if food consumption does play a role in their symptoms (Ventner, 2007).

For all exclusion diets, dietetic expertise is key in ensuring patients are educated regarding food avoidance, label reading, suitable alternatives and a healthy balanced diet, despite the dietary restrictions. Non-dietary sources of substances that can provoke reactions may also need to be excluded, but this is very individual and may not always be necessary. Patients should keep a food and symptom diary whilst on the diet in order to monitor both adherence to the dietary advice and any changes in symptoms.

Oral provocation tests

If symptoms improve, dietary exclusion needs to be followed by the reintroduction of the food either during a food challenge (hospital or home) or a reintroduction plan at home. Patients with a history of immediate symptoms or a positive SPT/specific IgE test should be challenged in a hospital setting. All other patients can undergo a food challenge at home or a food reintroduction plan but only if there is no risk of the patient developing immediate severe symptoms (Venter *et al.*, 2009; Allen *et al.*, 2009).

Many clinicians argue that a food challenge is risky and perhaps should not be performed; however, no fatal reactions during a food challenge have been reported in the USA since 1976 (Nowak-Wegrzyn *et al.*, 2009). Zijlstra *et al.* (2009) reported that the high anxiety levels shown by parents of children with suspected nut allergy were significantly reduced after challenge, even in the group with a positive outcome.

Table 7.11.6 Less restrictive few foods diet (Vikerstaff Joneja, 1998)

Meat and alternatives

Lamb
Turkey
Chicken

Acceptable grains and flours

Potato flour, rice flour, cornflour,
arrowroot, sago, tapioca, millet, buckwheat

Starchy foods

Rice (white), pudding rice, rice noodles, rice cakes – plain, Rice Krispies
Cornflour, corn flakes, maize flour, polenta – (not sweetcorn)
Potatoes (no skin) – cooked in any way as long as permitted margarines or oils are used in their preparation
'Kettles' potato chips, only lightly salted flavour
Oven chips or micro chips with no preservatives added

Baking aids

Cream of tartar, sodium bicarbonate, pectin

Fruit

Pears
Nectarines
Peaches
Mango
Fruit should be washed thoroughly and peeled before it is eaten
Tinned fruit in syrup or fruit sorbet made from the allowed fruit is acceptable, but make sure that no preservatives or colourings have been added

Adding extra calories to food

Sugar, golden syrup

Vegetables

Carrots
Parsnip
Greens – only broccoli, marrows and courgettes
Swede
French beans
Squash
Sweet potatoes

No other foods are allowed at all

This includes sweets, chewing gum, popcorn or corn snacks, fizzy drinks or squashes (and alcoholic drinks)
This also means no milk or any dairy products.
No vinegar or bottled sauces are allowed

Milk substitutes

Rice milk with added calcium

Suitable gluten and wheat free products that may be purchased from your pharmacy

Ener-G   Rice loaf
Ener-G   Rice pasta
Glutano   Gluten free pasta
Glutano   Crispbread
Trufree   Cake mix
Trufree   Pastry mix
Dr. Schar Mix A – Cake mix
Dr. Schar Mix C – Flour mix for cooking

Fats and oils

Margarine made from vegetable oil, e.g. Pure, Granose vegetable margarine, Vitaquelle or Vitaseig
Supermarket's own brand of milk free/soya free margarines.
Soya margarines are not allowed
Any oil, e.g. sunflower, olive, rape seed, vegetable, will be suitable.

Basic instructions

- You will have started by following the *observation phase* for 7 days, recording foods and drinks normally taken and symptoms experienced on your normal diet.
- During the observation phase you will have time to plan and shop ahead. It will be necessary to have plenty of appropriate foods to hand.
- The menu is simple – without spices, butter or condiments.
- Do not start at Christmas or around birthdays.
- Use as many fresh food sources as possible.
- Frozen food is the next best alternative.
- You may initially feel worse, but your symptoms should improve within 3–4 days.

This diet should always be followed under the supervision of your dietitian

Flavourings

Sea salt and pepper in moderation
Herbs – mint, parsley, sage, thyme, basil, oregano, rosemary
We do not recommend using a lot of herbs, just a little bit of your favourites

Foods will be reintroduced one at a time after a * day period
Please do not hesitate to contact the dietitian on: *

Drinks

7-Up (non diet) limit to 1–2 cans/day
Water (filtered if possible)
Juices from allowed fruit but make sure that they do not contain any colourings or preservatives

*Number of days and contact details to be supplied by local practitioners.

Box 7.11.1   Example of a one day open challenge procedure for immediate type symptoms (Venter *et al.*, 2009)

Cow's milk
For infants <6 months: use any cow's milk formula
All other children and adults: use skimmed cow's milk

Place 1 drop of cow's milk on lower oral mucosa of the patient
10 minutes' observation
If no reaction, proceed to:

0.5 mL of cow's milk to be drunk	15 minutes' observation
1 mL of cow's milk to be drunk	15 minutes' observation
2 mL of cow's milk to be drunk	15 minutes' observation
5 mL of cow's milk to be drunk	15 minutes' observation
10 mL of cow's milk to be drunk	15 minutes' observation
15 mL of cow's milk to be drunk	15 minutes' observation
25 mL of cow's milk to be drunk	15 minutes' observation
40 mL of cow's milk to be drunk	2 hours' observation

For adults and children:

100–200 mL of cow's milk to be drunk (can use cow's milk formula for children <1 year) or 100–200 mL of yoghurt	2 hours' observation

---

Food challenges should be performed in the following circumstances (Nowak-Wegrzyn *et al.*, 2009):

- Where there is a strong suspicion of allergy, but history or tests do not support the suspicion, or when no other tests are available.
- To demonstrate food tolerance when there is sensitisation to a food that has not been eaten before, cross reactivity is suspected or food processing might enable consumption, e.g. fruit and vegetables that may be tolerated in cooked form in the pollen food allergy syndrome. Also used to ascertain tolerance in cases where there is either no sensitisation to the food but the family is anxious about introducing it at home (usually when another sibling has an allergy or intolerance) or there has been resolution of delayed symptoms on avoidance of a number of allergens, i.e. there is a need to identify the culprit foods.
- To monitor sensitisation/therapy strategies, such as oral sublingual therapy or drug trials; and the management of food allergies or intolerances in cases where the SPT or specific IgE levels have reduced to such an extent that tolerance is highly possible or accidental ingestion of the allergen without any clinical reaction.
- To determine the tolerance level to a food.

Reasons for deferring a food challenge include the following (Nowak-Wegrzyn *et al.*, 2009):

- High likelihood of reacting to the food as predicted by a food reaction history, such as a recent accidental ingestion provoking a reaction, increasing levels or high predictive levels of food specific IgE antibody and the patient's age.
- High risk of anaphylaxis, such as a recent convincing anaphylactic reaction to the food or unstable asthma.
- Cmedical conditions and medications that may interfere with treatment of allergic reactions, e.g. cardiovascular disease, pregnancy or treatment with beta-blockers, and medical conditions that may preclude interpretation of the OFC, e.g. uncontrolled eczema and severe allergic rhinitis.
- Infant or young child is unlikely to cooperate with the challenge, unless special arrangements can be made to provide a longer time to complete the feeding and to provide an adequate observation period.

Food challenges

There are three types of food challenges:

Open food challenges

Both the patient and the clinician performing the challenge know the ingredients of the challenge food, e.g. peanut flapjack used for a peanut challenge (Box 7.11.1).

Single blind placebo controlled food challenges

The challenge, e.g. liquidised egg mixed with a fruit purée or compote, is administered without the patient knowing which dose is active and which is placebo, i.e. the patient is blind but the healthcare professional is not This type of food challenge is particularly useful when dealing with highly anxious children or adults who have major concerns about ingesting the particular food.

Double blind placebo controlled food challenges

During this challenge neither the patient nor the investigator knows when the active or the placebo challenge is performed. This rules out measurement and reporting bias from the observer and the psychological effect from the patient.

The open food challenge is the challenge of choice in most cases when dealing with adults or children suffering from objective symptoms e.g. urticaria, angioedema etc.

(Venter *et al.*, 2007a). Blinded challenges are preferable when dealing with adults or children reporting subjective symptoms (abdominal pain, nausea, headache) or symptoms that are difficult to assess due to the nature of the disease, e.g. eczema.

For research purposes, a double blind placebo controlled food challenge (DBPCFC) is still the preferred method of choice (Bock *et al.*, 1988; Bindslev-Jensen *et al.*, 2004; Sampson *et al.*, 2012) as it is considered the gold standard for diagnosing FHS. This type of challenge is rarely used in clinical practice in the UK as it is costly and labour intensive. For a detailed discussion regarding oral food challenges in cases of chronic urticaria, recurrent angioedema and non-allergic asthma, see Reese *et al.* (2009).

Step wise approach in the planning of a food challenge
History
This should consider:

- Age and age of onset help determine how difficult it may be to perform the food challenge and also the possible food causing the symptoms.
- Food type, e.g. raw or cooked egg, and quantity causing symptoms (helps prevent false negative food challenges).
- Symptoms – speed of onset, type, duration and reproducibility of reactions.
- A thorough description of the most recent reaction – helps when designing challenges.
- Cofactors – whether a combination of foods, or the trigger food taken together with exercise, alcohol or drugs, is necessary to reproduce the reaction.
- List of tolerated foods – these could be used as a placebo or vehicle to mask the challenge food.

Factors to consider when planning a challenge

In any challenge, the food used should mimic the history as closely as possible.

Dose and time intervals for immediate symptoms

The total amount of food given in the challenge is generally based on a normal daily portion of food that is likely to be consumed by the patient and divided into 5–10 doses of increasing size. Some clinicians prefer to start the challenge with a labial rub of the lip (Rancé & Dutau, 1999), but that is not practice everywhere. There is no recommended starting dose that should be used for all patients or challenges, but it should be small enough to minimise the risk of severe reactions (Bindslev-Jensen *et al.*, 2004). The dose may be doubled every 15–30 minutes or increased logarithmically, as guided by the patient's history (Sampson *et al.*, 2012). The timing between each dose should be sufficient to allow symptoms to develop. Recent published guidelines on DBPCFC recommend a top blinded dose of 2 g of food protein, although for some foods such as fish this may need to be higher (Sampson *et al.*, 2012). The food challenge should provide a final sufficient dose of the allergenic food to rule out food allergy, i.e. normal daily intake adjusted for

age (Bindslev-Jensen *et al.*, 2004). A challenge duration of at least 2 hours is needed.

Dose and time intervals for delayed symptoms

The dose of food given in the challenge is generally based on a normal daily portion of food that is likely to be consumed by the patient – as indicated by the patient history or based on age appropriate national food survey data (Bindslev-Jensen *et al.*, 2004). However, some studies have used gradually increasing dosages after day one of the challenge. A challenge period of 1–4 weeks may be required to reach the full daily dose or one that triggers symptoms (Majamaa *et al.*, 1999a,b).

In the UK, normal daily consumption can be calculated by reference to the National Diet and Nutritional Survey (see Chapter 4.2). Detailed information is discussed in Venter *et al.* (2009), which may be useful for dietitians.

Blinding/masking

When performing a DBPCFC, the challenge food should be sufficiently blinded so that the active and placebo challenges are identical regarding taste, appearance, smell, viscosity, texture, structure and volume (Bindslev-Jensen *et al.*, 2004; Vlieg-Boerstra *et al.*, 2004; Sampson *et al.*, 2012). This is less necessary when challenging young children. Cooking, canning and roasting can have different effects on the allergenicity of different foods and any form of processing used for the challenge food, particularly the fat content of the vehicle (Grimshaw *et al.*, 2003), could potentially influence the challenge outcome.

For validated recipes suitable for DBPCFC, see Vlieg-Boerstra *et al.* (2004), van Odijk *et al.* (2005), Palmer *et al.* (2005), Devenney *et al.* (2006) and Vassilopoulou *et al.* (2010).

Patient information prior to the food challenge

Patients should be well informed prior to the challenge/reintroduction at home regarding food avoidance, challenge procedure and which medications should not be used. Detailed information regarding this aspect of the food challenge can found in Venter *et al.* (2009) and Ball (2005).

Safety procedures required to set up and carry out supervised food challenges

Both high and low risk food challenges have the potential to induce anaphylaxis and therefore should be medically supervised with a suitably trained nurse/dietitian providing the challenge doses according to a written protocol. The food challenge setting should be equipped with a crash trolley, emergency drugs and all other safety measures in place. Detailed information regarding this aspect of the food challenge can be found in Venter *et al.* (2009), Ball (2005) and Sampson *et al.* (2012).

Food reintroduction

Food reintroduction at home after a period of exclusion may be used in the diagnosis of non-IgE mediated food allergy or delayed non-allergic FHS. The main differences between a gradual food reintroduction plan and a home

Box 7.11.2   Instructions for standard reintroduction of food (Venter *et al.*, 2007a; Vickerstaff Joneja *et al.*, 2001)

Day 1
Breakfast
Eat a small quantity (quarter of your usual portion) of the test food
If no adverse reactions have been experienced, proceed as follows:
   Wait 4 hours before eating the test food again
Lunch
Eat double the quantity of test food eaten in the morning, i.e. half your normal portion
If no adverse reactions have been experienced, proceed as follows:
   Wait 4 hours before eating the test food again
Evening meal
Eat double the amount of food eaten at lunch time. This should be equal to your normal portion.

Days 2–4
Eat the amounts of the test food that you would normally, e.g. if you eat bread three times/day, you need to try it three times/day. However, if you test a particular cereal, which you normally would eat only once a day, then try it only once a day at breakfast
Any adverse reactions may be due to a delayed reaction to the foods you have eaten in the last 2–3 days
If there is no reaction after 3 days, discontinue testing this food and consider the food safe to eat from now on

See also Ball (2005)

food challenge are that the latter involves control over the food consumed with regard to portion size and blinding. The foods and amounts used for reintroduction regimens vary from centre to centre and are often adjusted for individual cases (Box 7.11.2).

Interpreting food challenge and food reintroduction outcome

During supervised food challenges the patient should be constantly monitored and all signs, symptoms and clinical observations should be recorded on a clinical observation chart. During home challenges or food reintroduction at home, patients or their carers should keep a strict food and symptoms diary.

Open food challenge/food reintroduction is considered negative in the absence of any subjective or objective clinical reaction. It is recommended that a challenge should be stopped and considered positive if a clear, clinical reaction is shown (Table 7.11.7). In the case of a questionable (subjective) reaction, a repeat dose can be given after waiting an additional 10–20 minutes to see if it elicits a more definitive allergic reaction (Niggemann, 2010). However, clinicians need to be prepared in case this extra dose precipitates a severe allergic reaction.

The more organ systems involved in a clinical reaction, the easier it is to make the decision of a positive challenge. It is recommended that a challenge can be considered positive if severe, reproducible or persisting symptoms are experienced (Niggemann, 2010). In children, a mood change (becoming very quiet), ear picking, tongue rubbing, e.g. scratching food out of the mouth, or neck scratching are often the precursors of a positive challenge (Table 7.11.8). The results of a food challenge/reintroduction could be falsely negative when diseases such as eczema, chronic urticaria or functional bowel disorders are in remission or falsely positive when they are active. Allergic reactions to inhalant allergens can also affect the challenge outcome.

False negative challenges could be caused by use of medication prior to challenge, too small challenge dose, too short a challenge period or observation time, or the absence of cofactors such as alcohol or exercise. False positive challenges could be caused by food eaten by mistake prior to the food challenge or cross contamination from too many food challenges on the ward. Other factors that can affect challenges include drugs, hormonal factors and concomitant illnesses (Werfel *et al.*, 2009).

For DBPCFCs, the challenge is considered negative if no symptoms are experienced during the active food challenge or if symptoms are experienced during the placebo phase of the DBPCFC. When symptoms are experienced during both the active and placebo phase of a DBPCFC, the challenge needs to be repeated. Symptoms developing only during the active phase of the challenges indicates a positive food challenge (Niggemann, 2010; Niggemann *et al.*, 2005; Niggemann & Beyer, 2007).

Management strategies after both positive and negative outcomes

Once the challenge and reintroduction of food is completed, sufficient after care should be provided for the patient or their carers to ensure that:

- *After a positive challenge* – the allergenic food is avoided, emergency medication is prescribed if needed and appropriate training is given to administer the medication, e.g. the use of adrenaline (epinephrine) auto injectors, and dietetic advice is given to ensure a balanced diet is maintained despite dietary restrictions.
- *After a negative challenge* – the challenge food is reintroduced into the diet and regularly consumed in order to prevent any nutritional deficiencies or resensitisation.

In some cases, i.e. some primary care settings, these tests may not be available or it may take a long time to obtain results. However, the history could give a good indication of the type and time of onset of symptoms, which should assist healthcare professionals to decide if symptoms are IgE or non-IgE mediated reactions, taking into account that eczema could initially present with delayed symptoms (Flinterman *et al.*, 2006), and then may turn into a presentation of immediate, more severe symptoms.

Table 7.11.7 Subjective and objective symptoms during food challenge (Niggemann, 2010)

	Possible problems with interpretation
Subjective symptoms	
Nausea	All difficult to interpret due to the subjective nature of the symptoms
Stinging/burning of tongue or mouth	
Itching	
Heart palpitations	
Sleeplessness	
Irritability	
Excitement	
General change of behaviour/sense of impending doom	Highly predictive of a positive challenge
Diarrhoea	Could be caused by stress
Abdominal pain and cramps	Could be caused by stress, but also a sign of impending anaphylaxis
Objective symptoms	
Flushing	Difficult to interpret if subsides very quickly
Urticaria	Could be contact urticaria if only around the mouth. Generalised urticaria (in the absence of chronic urticaria) is almost always a sign of a positive challenge
Slight worsening of eczema	Difficult to interpret/could be contact related. However, scored index increase of >15 points is very indicative of positive reactions – may need to wait 48 hours for assessment
Vomiting	Could be caused by food aversion – may need to ensure that vomiting occurs more than once and is severe in nature for a positive result
Cardiovascular symptoms – especially a drop in blood pressure	Almost always a sign of a positive challenge
Respiratory symptoms	Could be aero allergen related/generally uncontrolled symptoms. However, stridor, wheeze, watery rhinitis, redness of eyes and nose, and tears are almost always signs of a positive reaction
Dyspnoea/difficulty breathing	Could be aero allergen related but is often a sign of a positive challenge

Table 7.11.8 Criteria for major and minor criteria for outcome of challenge

Major criteria	Minor criteria
≥3 hives	Eczematous pruritic rash (worsening to ≥10 SCORAD points)*
≥1 site of angio-oedema	
Wheezing	1–2 hives
Dyspnoea	≥1 of sneezing, congestion or rhinorrhoea
Stridor	
Dysphonia	Conjunctivitis
Aphonia	≥1 of nausea, vomiting or diarrhoea for <20 minutes
Severe persistent abdominal symptoms for ≥30 minutes, e.g. abdominal pain/stillness, vomiting, nausea or diarrhoea	A change in behaviour, e.g. irritability, drowsiness, decreased activity, anxiety, distress
Hypotension for age	

- Positive food challenge: presence of ≥1 major criteria or ≥2 minor criteria.
- Negative food challenge: absence of a major or minor criteria.

*Worsening of eczema alone is not a stopping criterion during the challenge. However, if a worsening of eczema to >10 SCORAD points is observed at the end of the active arm of the double blind placebo controlled food challenges (DBPCFC) with no worsening of eczema with the placebo challenge, the diagnosis of cow's milk allergy will be given.

Dietary management

At present, the only means of treatment is avoidance of the problem food, although a number of studies have examined the efficacy of food specific immunotherapy. This technique promotes tolerance to a food through the administration of daily oral doses of the food in increasing amounts until a maintenance dose is reached. It has been successfully used to treat some common food allergies, but cannot yet be recommended in routine practice (Fisher et al., 2011).

Dietary avoidance issues

The dietary management of food hypersensitivity can be complex; unexpected ingredients are often present in a wide range of manufactured foods, and there may be poor comprehension of the dietary requirement and adherence issues. The restriction of food choices can increase the risk of overall dietary imbalance, especially if the problem food is a major contributor to nutrient intake. Help is required to determine the level of avoidance required, and to develop an individualised meal plan and advice on a whole range of lifestyle issues, such as shopping, eating at school or in the workplace, socialising and eating out, holidays abroad and even on occasion on intimate issues such as kissing (Wright, 2006, Skypala & Venter, 2009). All children and adults with moderate to severe food allergy should also have an action plan for dietary management and drug prophylaxis. This has been shown to be effective in reducing the number of accidental exposures resulting in symptoms (Clark & Ewan, 2008; Ewan & Clark, 2005).

The patient's tolerance level or degree of avoidance required will mainly be determined by the type of FHS the patient is suffering from. Most people with IgE mediated food allergy need to completely avoid a trigger food – even in trace amounts. People with non-IgE mediated allergy or non-immune mediated FHS may be able to include small amounts of the food in their diet with no adverse effects. It is currently unknown whether allowing patients to eat small amounts of the trigger food if tolerated on a regular basis has an adverse effect on the development of tolerance or conversely induces further tolerance. Some patients will already be aware of their own tolerance levels; it is therefore important to ask open questions to establish whether or not this is the case.

From a nutritional view, avoidance of a single food or type of food, such as citrus fruit, will be of little significance if nutritionally similar foods, e.g. other fruit and vegetables, can be eaten instead. However, if food avoidance necessitates excluding a major food group, the nutritional impact will be considerable. Even if the food being excluded is not in itself nutritionally significant for most people, e.g. soya or nuts, it may be widely present in manufactured foods, resulting in a subsequent effect on overall dietary balance. Patients who exclude other foods because of, for example, cultural reasons, e.g. excluding nuts and milk in a vegetarian, or they are fussy eaters will also need special consideration if their usual staple foods are being excluded.

Some types of FHS resolve over time; both milk and egg allergies commonly remit in most people by the teenage years. Some forms of non-allergic FHS in adults may be transient, such as secondary lactose intolerance. The necessity for dietary exclusion should be reviewed at intervals so that dietary restrictions are not imposed for longer than necessary due to their major impact on diet and lifestyle.

Food labelling

European food labelling law

The Labelling Directive (2000/13/EC) and its later amendments is the only European Union legislation that refers to allergenic foods. It requires manufacturers to declare all ingredients present in prepackaged foods sold in the European Union, with a few exceptions. It has been amended a number of times (see Chapter 4.5). The most important amendments are listed here.

Directive 2003/89/EC

This lists allergenic foods that must always be labelled when present in a product (Commission Directive, 2003). These include:

- Cereals containing gluten, i.e. wheat, rye, barley, oats, spelt, kamut or their hybridised strains, and products thereof.
- Crustaceans and products thereof.
- Eggs and products thereof.
- Fish and products thereof.
- Peanuts and products thereof.
- Soyabeans and products thereof.
- Milk and products thereof, including lactose.
- Nuts, i.e. almond (*Amygdalus communis L.*), hazelnut (*Corylus avellana*), walnut (*Juglans regia*), cashew (*Anacardium occidentale*), Pecan nut [*Carya illinoiesis (Wangenh.) K. Koch*], Brazil nut (*Bertholletia excelsa*), pistachio nut (*Pistacia vera*), macadamia nut, Queensland nut (*Macadamia ternifolia*) and products thereof.
- Celery and products thereof.
- Mustard and products thereof.
- Sesame seeds and products thereof.
- Sulphur dioxide and sulphites at concentrations of >10 mg/kg or 10 mg/L expressed as SO_2.

All ingredients have to be clearly labelled so that the product from which they are derived is easily recognisable, e.g. milk cannot be listed as caseinate without the word milk being listed next to it.

Directive 2006/142/EC

This lists two further allergenic foods that must be labelled, namely lupin and products thereof, and molluscs and products thereof (Commission Directive, 2006).

Directive 2007/68/EC

This lists those products derived from these foods for which allergen labelling is not required.

The European Food Safety Authority (EFSA; www.efsa.europa.eu) provides more detailed information on food allergen labelling. In the UK the full directives are available from the Food Standards Agency (FSA) (www.food.gov.uk/safereating/allergyintol/label/).

May contain labelling

Manufacturers often use phrases such as 'may contain nut traces', 'made on a production line using soya or milk' or 'produced on a line handling egg' to show that there could be accidental traces of another food in a manufactured product from the production process. If the ingredient is purposeful, even if it is in a trace amount, it has to be listed in the ingredients list. However, there is no legal requirement to state on the label that a food might contain accidental traces of a food. This labelling is completely voluntary and therefore not legally binding, but many manufacturers choose to label their products in this way. Where labels contain this information, patients should be advised to still check the full ingredients listing and not just rely on the allergen advice panel for allergen identification.

Major food triggers

Milk

Cows' milk is a leading cause of food allergy, especially in infants and children. About 2.5% of children suffer from cow's milk allergy with rates ranging from 1.1–7.5% (Bock, 1987; Eggesbo et al., 2001; Gerrard et al., 1973; Hide & Guyer, 1983; Host & Halken, 1990; Schrander et al., 1993). Almost 90% of children will react to other mammalian milks (Bellioni-Businco et al., 1999), such as goat's or sheep's milk. The prognosis of cow's milk allergy is good; remission rates vary, but about 90% of children will grow out of milk allergy by adulthood (Host, 1994; Skripak et al., 2007).

IgE mediated milk allergy in adults is rare, and most adults who report symptoms to milk will not usually have specific IgE antibodies to milk (Zuberbier et al., 2004). Lactose intolerance is the commonest form of non-immune mediated FHS involving milk, but patients also often cite milk as a cause of irritable bowel syndrome symptoms (Monsbakken et al., 2006) and respiratory symptoms (Wuthrich et al., 2005).

IgE mediated cow's milk allergy

IgE mediated cow's milk protein allergy is characterised by acute and rapid onset symptoms, including urticaria, angio-oedema, rhinitis, gastrointestinal upset, vomiting, respiratory distress or anaphylaxis. These reactions are commonly associated with a family history of atopy and usually develop early in infancy when the permeability of the gastrointestinal mucosa is greatest, and soon after exposure to cow's milk in the form of infant formula (Host & Halken 1990) or during early weaning with dairy foods. Symptoms can occasionally present in an exclusively breastfed infant because the mother is taking cow's milk (or derivatives) in her diet and the protein fractions pass through the breast milk causing symptoms in the infant. To determine whether this is the case, all traces of cow's milk and derivatives should be excluded from the mother's diet for approximately 2 weeks. If the symptoms resolve, then this diet should be adhered to for the duration of breastfeeding.

Non-IgE mediated cow's milk allergy

Non-IgE mediated cow's milk allergy is characterised by a delayed reaction following cow's milk protein ingestion. Symptoms typically occur within a few hours and sometimes after 2–3 days, and often include eczema, reflux, abdominal pains, constipation, diarrhoea, bloating and gas.

Non-immune mediated cow's milk hypersensitivity

The most common form of non-immune reactions to cow's milk is to the milk sugar lactose.

Milk avoidance carries a high risk of nutritional deficiencies (particularly energy and calcium), which can cause delayed growth in infants and children, but only if the diet is not managed well. For this reason, it is important that the need for milk exclusion is clearly established. The correct management of cow's milk allergy in breast-fed infants is by complete avoidance of cow's milk protein from the infant's diet if weaned and sometimes in the breastfeeding mother's diet. In part or non-breastfed infants younger than 12 months, a nutritionally complete substitute formula is required. There are a number of available formulae for infants who cannot tolerate whole cow's milk protein or lactose and a dietitian should advise on the most suitable choice, as shown in Table 7.11.9.

Guidance when choosing a formula milk

The choice of formula milk will depend on the infant's requirements, taste preference, degree of hydrolysis required, indications for an amino acid formula, parental preference, clinician experience and many other clinical and non-clinical factors. There are European and world guidance (Fiocchi et al., 2010), algorithms (Vandenplas et al., 2007) and recommendations (Du Toit et al., 2010) to enable the clinician to make the most suitable choice tailored to the individual infant's specific requirements. The clinician may need to prescribe an alternative formula if the infant refuses or reacts to the initial formula recommended. It is essential that infants tolerate sufficient volume of a nutritionally complete cow's milk substitute (Table 7.11.9) to meet their nutritional requirements for growth and development.

Goat's, sheep's and other mammalian milks should not be used as an alternative to cow's milk due to a high degree of cross reactivity resulting in poor tolerance. Furthermore, these milks have a low folate content and can be microbiologically unsafe (Department of Health, 1994). Non-prescribable, non-formula milks made from soya, rice, hemp, potato nut, coconut, pea or oat are not recommended for infants under 1 year old unless all other options have been exhausted and the alternative is no milk at all. When used in cooking they can increase the nutritional content of the diet because they encourage the consumption of a variety of other foods.

Due to inorganic arsenic being a natural component of rice milks, they are not recommended for children younger than 4.5 years (FSA, 2009). When they are used, daily intake should not exceed 200 mL. If used, any of these milks should be enriched with calcium. Products based on soya can be used after 6 months of age; these include soya yogurts, deserts, cream cheeses, hard cheeses and cream. These products can also be used on cereal and in cooking to make sauces, soups, scones, cakes and rice pudding to help to add variety, nutrition and taste to the diet. Oat cream is another useful product. These are available in supermarkets and health food stores or online. Once solid food is introduced into the diet, care has to be taken that it remains free of cow's milk protein, not only from obvious sources such as dairy products but also from its less obvious presence in many manufactured foods. Tables 7.11.10 and 7.11.11 give advice for general avoidance on the exclusion of cow's milk from the diet.

Reintroduction of milk

Cow's milk allergy is often transient and therefore is often challenged every 6–12 months until tolerance is

Table 7.11.9   Nutritionally complete milk substitutes for use in cow's milk hypersensitivity

Type of milk hypersensitivity	Product type*	Product name (manufacturer)
Used for IgE and non-IgE mediated cow's milk allergy	Soya based** Do not use before 6 months unless no other choice, e.g. vegan or refusal of all other suitable formula	Infasoy (Cow & Gate) Wysoy (SMA)
	Casein based hydrolysed cow's milk	Nutramigen Lipil 1 and 2 (MJN) Pregestimil (with MCT oils) (MJN)
	Whey based hydrolysed cow's milk	Pepti Junior (Cow & Gate) Pepti 1 and 2 (Aptamil)
	Amino acid	Neocate LCP (SHS) Neocate Advance and Neocate Active if over 12 months (SHS) Nutramigen AA (MJN)
Lactose intolerance only	NB: *Some of the above products may also be suitable for lactose intolerance; check prescribing indications*	
	Usually contain whole cow's milk protein	Enfamil Lactofree (MJN) SMA LF (SMA)

*The choice of product depends on the age of the child, the level of sensitivity to milk and the presence of coexisting allergies. Check compositional details and prescribing indications for suitability. Choice may also be dictated by the infant's palate.
**Infants under the age of 6 months should not use a soya formula as the first choice due to their phyto-oestrogen content and the risk of becoming sensitised to soya. It can be used if other formulae are either not suitable, not acceptable or not tolerated by the infant, or if the mother is vegan. See www.bda.uk.com for the BDA Paediatric Group Position Statement on the use of soya protein for Infants.
Further details of products currently available and their prescribing indications can be found in the *British National Formulary (BNF)* or the *Monthly Index of Medical Specialities (MIMS)* or obtained directly from the manufacturers. Further information is also available to dietitians in the *Special Foods for Children* booklet compiled by the Dietetic Department, Children's Hospital, Birmingham.
MCT, medium chain triglyceride.

Table 7.11.10   General guidance for milk exclusion

Exclude	Examples of foods to exclude	Notes
Cow's milk	Liquid whole, semi skimmed or skimmed milk Evaporated or condensed milk Dried full fat or skimmed milk powder Fresh and UHT	Goat's, sheep's and other mammalian milk should not be used as an alternative to cow's milk. They are also unsuitable for people requiring total exclusion of lactose or galactose
Dairy products	Butter Margarine or fat spreads containing milk derivatives Cheese and cheese spreads Yogurt Fromage frais Creme fraiche Cream Ice cream	Butter and some hard cheeses may be tolerated by people with mild lactose intolerance
Milk or milk derivatives in manufactured foods	May be described on ingredients lists as: milk, milk solids, non-fat milk solids, milk protein; skimmed milk, skimmed milk powder Casein or caseinates Whey; whey solids; buttermilk *Lactose, milk sugar, whey sugar, whey syrup sweetener. Within the European Union the presence of milk must be *clearly* labelled	Lactose in flavourings and medications may be a problem in some severely allergic patients

*It may not be necessary to exclude lactose and other milk sugars in all cases of cow's milk allergy but, for practical purposes, their presence is usually taken as indicative of the presence of milk, and foods containing them are excluded.

Table 7.11.11   Types of manufactured foods that may contain milk or milk derivatives

Food type	Foods to check
Cereals	Bread and rolls Breakfast cereals Cakes Biscuits and crackers Pizza Pasta (both fresh and tinned)
Fruit and vegetables	Vegetables canned in sauce Instant potato Baked beans Battered or breadcrumbed vegetables and potato products
Meat, fish and alternatives	Meat and fish products, e.g. beef burgers, fish fingers, sausages, ready meals
Other savoury items	Canned and packet soups Instant gravies Sauces/ketchups Crisps and savoury snack foods
Desserts	Instant desserts Dairy desserts Ice cream Custards
Confectionery	Chocolate Toffee Fudge Caramel
Fats and spreads	Margarines and fat spreads
Beverages	Instant drinking chocolate Malted milk drinks Coffee whiteners Pineapple and coconut juice drink

NB: This list is far from exhaustive and all food labels must be checked carefully and checked every time as ingredients do change.

Most of these products can also be milk free if you shop around or use 'free from lists' to locate them.

demonstrated. Most cow's milk allergy will resolve by the age of 5 years. If previous reactions have been severe, then reintroduction should only happen under medical supervision in a hospital setting. In practice, milk reintroduction sometimes happens inadvertently with the child already consuming foods containing small amounts of cow's milk. A clear dietary history can highlight if this has been the case.

If a child passes a milk challenge but then refuses milk and dairy foods due to anxiety or dislike of the taste, parents will need guidance on ways to incorporate hidden milk into the diet, such as in rice pudding, white sauce, scones, creamy soups, risotto, etc. In the rare cases where milk allergy persists into adulthood, a permanent exclusion of cow's milk is necessary.

Lactose intolerant disorders

Lactose intolerance results from an impaired ability to either absorb lactose or its component monosaccharides, resulting in symptoms of malabsorption. If lactose needs to be excluded, food avoidance measures are almost the same as for exclusion of cow's milk protein (see earlier). The main differences with lactose exclusion regimens are that low lactose cow's milk products can often be included. Some foods are naturally very low in lactose, whereas others are manufactured specifically for this purpose. There are also formula milks available that are clinically free from lactose. If total and prolonged (or permanent) lactose exclusion is required, the diet will require careful management to ensure it is varied, nutritious and tastes good. The management of lactose intolerance is discussed in more detail in Chapters 7.4.6.

Congenital disorders of monosaccharide metabolism

Details of these disorders can be found in Chapter 3.8.6 and Chapter 7.8.

Peanuts and tree nuts

Peanuts and tree nuts are the most common foods to cause severe IgE mediated reactions. Between 1999 and 2006, 18 of the 44 deaths from food allergy were caused by tree nuts or peanuts (Pumphrey & Gowland, 2007). Food allergic patients who also have asthma are more likely to have severe reactions to foods, especially to peanuts (Sicherer *et al.*, 2001a). Peanut and tree nut allergies most commonly present in childhood; only 8–10% of cases are diagnosed in adolescence or adulthood (Mullins *et al.*, 2009; Ewan, 1996). Unlike milk and egg allergy, nut allergy rarely resolves. Over 90% of tree nut allergic and 80% of peanut allergic children will remain sensitised and symptomatic into their adult years (Skolnick *et al.*, 2001; Fleischer *et al.*, 2005). However, a proportion of tree nut allergy in adults will develop as a result of cross reacting allergic determinants in foods and pollens causing PFS (Skypala *et al.*, 2011).

It has been estimated that 0.5–1% of the population are likely to develop a peanut or tree nut allergy (Hourihane *et al.*, 1997a), with the prevalence of reported reactions ranging from 0% to 7.3% for any nut (Zuidmeer *et al.*, 2008). The prevalence has continued to rise in some countries; USA telephone survey data suggested that the prevalence had doubled every 5 years, rising from 0.4% in 1997 to 1.4% in 2008 (Sicherer *et al.*, 2010). This is mirrored in Australia (Mullins *et al.*, 2009), but differs from UK data from the 2001/2002 birth cohort showing a 1.2% prevalence compared with 1.4% in 1994/1996 (Venter *et al.*, 2010). Published data on the prevalence of peanut allergy solely in adults are sparse, although Vierk *et al.* (2007) reported that the doctor diagnosed prevalence of peanut allergy was 0.3% in US adults in 2007. The way peanuts are prepared can affect their allergenicity, which explains why peanut allergy is common in the USA, UK and Australia, but uncommon in China where peanuts are boiled rather than roasted (Maleki *et al.*, 2000). A large study in the UK is ongoing to determine whether early introduction of peanuts is more or less likely to provoke peanut allergy (Du Toit *et al.*, 2008). It is for this reason that in 2009 the Department of Health revised its advice to pregnant and breastfeeding women about eating peanuts, and also about eating peanuts in the first few years of life (Department of Health, 2009b).

Peanut shares similar allergen epitopes with tree nuts, especially hazelnut, Brazil nut, almond and also some seeds (de Leon *et al*., 2003). Peanut allergic individuals have a 25–40% risk of developing a coallergy to tree nuts (Sicherer & Sampson, 2000; Bock, 2007). Tree nut allergy prevalence is increasing, with US telephone survey data suggesting it is currently 1.1%, compared with 0.2% in 1997 (Sicherer *et al*., 2010). Whereas walnut was the commonest tree nut provoking allergic reactions in this study, a UK study showed Brazil, almond and hazelnut to be the most common triggers of tree nut allergy (Ewan, 1996), with cashew nut allergy being predominant in Australia (Hill *et al*., 1997). Cashew nut allergy can cause severe reactions (Davoren & Peake, 2005); children with a cashew nut allergy were more likely to experience anaphylaxis than case matched children with a peanut allergy (Clark *et al*., 2007).

Peanut and tree nut allergic individuals are usually advised to avoid all nuts because of the risk of contamination; coexisting allergies to other nuts may not have been identified and are difficult to distinguish (Ferdman & Church, 2006). Adults with PFS to one nut may be able to tolerate other nuts on an individual basis, but the diagnosis of PFS must be confirmed to ensure no primary allergy to nuts exists. Avoidance can be problematic with many manufactured food products containing peanuts or nuts or derivatives (see European food law labelling section). In addition, they are used widely in both the food and cosmetic industries. Peanuts can sensitise via inhalation and the skin, as well as orally; therefore, exposure can also occur via peanut particles in the air or direct contact with peanut containing foods or some topical creams or ointments. In addition, peanut allergens are robust and cannot be removed from surfaces wiped with water alone or with antibacterial wipes (Perry *et al*., 2004). It has been estimated that 5–12% of accidental exposures causing reaction are due to kissing (Eriksson *et al*., 2003), possibly due to the longevity of some of the allergens involved (Maloney *et al*., 2006). Up to 25% of patients may experience an accidental ingestion per year and 66% experience more than five accidental exposures in a lifetime (Sicherer *et al*., 2001a); thus many nut allergic individuals carry adrenaline (epinephrine). Those that do so should know how and when to use it, and this information should be included in a regularly updated management plan. Most reactions occur when eating out, so stringent measures to reduce the risks should be taken to avoid this. For more information on eating out when suffering from a FHS, see Wright (2006).

Refined peanut oil is not allergenic (Hourihane *et al*., 1997a,b), but other nut oils, e.g. walnut, hazelnut, almond and unrefined or cold pressed peanut oil, may contain traces of allergens and should be avoided. Unrefined peanut oil is most likely to be used in Thai, Chinese, Indonesian or Indian cuisine; other nuts oils may be used in salad dressings or garnishes. Food companies have to declare both refined and unrefined peanut oil on food labels. Dietary sources of tree nuts and peanuts are summarised in Table 7.11.12. Peanut allergy sufferers have a greater risk of accidental exposure. Pumphrey & Gowland (2007) reported that 54% of recorded anaphylaxis fatalities between 1999 and 2006 occurred when eating restaurant or takeaway food. Thai, Indonesian, Asian and Chinese cuisines use peanuts and other nuts regularly in dishes. Chefs may often change ingredients or add additional items to dishes on an *ad hoc* basis.

Travelling with a peanut or tree nut allergy can be problematic. Many airlines stopped serving peanuts due to concerns about airborne peanut particles, but this is not universal and it is important that patients notify the airline of their concerns. Translation sheets for restaurants abroad, which give details of the problem, are useful as a list of food ingredients to look out for when travelling. Some brands of products that are nut free in the UK may not be nut free when produced and purchased in other countries (even if they have the same brand name), e.g. some infant formulae or vitamin D preparations may contain peanut. Learning the word for peanut or nuts in the relevant language, wearing medic alert identification and always carrying rescue medication are strongly recommended. Support groups, such as the Anaphylaxis Campaign and Allergy UK, can provide useful advice on all of these issues.

Soya and other legumes

After peanuts, soyabean allergy is the most common legume allergy worldwide (Bernhisel-Broadbent & Sampson, 1989), the prevalence being approximately 0.4%, although this depends on local eating habits and exposure (Zuidmeer *et al*., 2008). Soya allergy is usually a transient allergy of infancy and childhood (Sicherer *et al*., 2000). Savage *et al*. (2010) reported that 50% of their population had a resolution of their soya allergy by the age of 7 years. Only 6.5% of children with a peanut allergy are allergic to soya, although the majority of soya allergic children cannot tolerate peanuts (Bernhisel-Broadbent & Sampson, 1989). Although soya milk was thought to commonly affect children with cow's milk allergy, Zeiger *et al*. (1999) reported that only 14% of a cohort of cow's milk allergic patients were diagnosed allergic to soya. Soya allergy most commonly manifests in older children and adults due to cross reactions between homologous epitopes in soyabeans and birch pollen provoking reactions, which may be severe (Mittag *et al*., 2004; Kleine-Tebbe *et al*., 2002). It is possible that up to 30% of adults with a peanut allergy have cross reactivity to other legumes (Ballmer-Webber *et al*., 2007), although this sensitisation may not be clinically relevant. Soya beans can provoke a range of symptoms including anaphylaxis; inhalation of soyabean dust can also provoke bronchospasm.

Soyabeans are ubiquitous, especially in processed foods, and commonly used as a binding agent, meat extender or replacement for meat in vegetarian dishes. Soya products can be divided up into whole bean products, hull products, protein products and oil products,

Table 7.11.12 Guidance for peanut and tree nut avoidance

Exclude	Examples	Notes
Peanuts and tree nuts	Peanut Brazil Walnut Hazelnut Almond Cashew Pistachio Pecans Macadamia	Some of these may be described as: Mixed nuts Ground nuts Monkey nuts Earth nuts Goober nuts Nutmeg, coconut, pine nut and palm nut are not classified as nuts
Spreads	Peanut butter and other nut spreads	Almond paste used in curries often contains peanuts
Sweets	Praline Noisette	Usually made from hazelnuts but mixed nuts can be used
Desserts and dessert topping	Marzipan Frangipan Amaretto products Macaroons Bakewell tarts Almond essence	Contain almonds but cheaper brands may contain peanut flour as an extender
Sweet paste or ice cream	Marron, e.g. marron glacé	Made from chestnuts but other nuts may be included
Sauces	Worcester sauce Satay sauce Korma sauce Pesto sauce	Contains walnuts Contains peanuts Contains almonds and sometimes peanut paste Made from pine nuts, but could contain other nuts
Hydrolysed vegetable protein	Hydrolysed vegetable protein	Usually from soya or wheat but can be derived from peanut, but this should be labelled clearly on prepacked manufactured foods in the European Union
Cheese	Nut containing or nut coated cheeses	Nut cheeses sold on deli counters can contaminate other products
Oils	Cold pressed gourmet oils, also called unrefined oils Peanut oil Arachis oil Groundnut oil Walnut oil Almond oil Hazelnut oil	Refined oils present in manufactured foods or sold as cooking oils are free from nut protein but still have to be declared on food labels

Manufactured foods containing traces of peanuts or nuts	This can include almost any food but particularly:
	  Cakes, biscuits and pastries
	  Ice cream, desserts and dessert toppings
	  Chocolate bars
	  Cereal bars and confectionery
	  Savoury snack foods
	  Breakfast cereals, especially muesli or nut mixtures
	  Products containing hydrolysed vegetable protein
	  Oriental/Asian food
	  Sauces and salad dressings
	  Mixed salads
	  Wild rice
		All manufactured foods should be considered a source of peanuts/nuts until it is known that this is not the case

and are therefore present in a huge range of products (Table 7.11.13). Refined soyabean oil and soya lecithin (E322) are safe for soya allergic patients to consume, although case reports suggest some individuals may still react to soya lecithin (Dueñas-Laita *et al.*, 2009; Awazuhara *et al.*, 1998; Palm *et al.*, 1999). The allergen associated with PFS reactions, Gly m 4, is unlikely to be present in products derived from roasted soyabeans or highly fermented products such as miso or soya sauce, but is found in soya milk and dietary powders such as body building powders (Mittag *et al.*, 2004). Soya sauce is a highly fermented product containing high levels of histamine and can provoke oral symptoms in some people (Sugiura & Sugiura, 2010).

Allergy to other legumes such as chickpeas and lentils has not been extensively studied in the UK, although in

Table 7.11.13 Soya containing foods (L'Hocine & Boye, 2007)

Whole bean products	Soya sprouts, edamame, soya milk, tofu, miso, natto, yuba, tempeh, soya sauce, soya nuts, soyanut butter, soya cereals, soya cheese, soya milk, soya ice cream/yoghurt/desserts
Hull products	Bread, bakery products, snack bars
Protein products	Soya flour, protein concentrate, protein isolate, textured soya Baby foods, infant formulae, bread, biscuits, pancakes, pastry, crackers, snack foods, noodles, pizza, breakfast cereals, soya milk, ice cream, soya yoghurt and cheese, sausages, tinned meat and fish, soups and gravy, beef burgers, salad dressing, stock cubes, sauces
Oil products	Refined oil, lecithin Cooking oil, salad oil, margarine, salad dressing, mayonnaise, coffee whiteners, chocolate, sweets, pastry filling, cheese dips, emulsifying agents, dietary supplements and body building agents
Emerging products	Isoflavones, functional foods, medications

Table 7.11.14 Sesame products

Alternative names	Foods containing sesame	
Ajonjoli	Falafel	Halva
Benne/benne seed	Burger buns	Hummus
Gomasio	Bread sticks	Tahini
Gingelly	Pastries	Salad dressing
Sesamum indicum	Pretzels	Soups
Sim sim	Bagels	Sauces
Oleum	Biscuits	Noodles
Teel	Rice cakes	Samosa
Till	Crackers	Dips
	Sandwiches	Aqua Libra

India and Spain they are a significant issue (Kumar *et al.*, 2010; Martínez San Ireneo *et al.*, 2008). Lupin is another legume not permitted for use in the UK, but it can be found in gluten free products and also in products containing wheat flour from other continental countries. Allergy to lupin has been reported (Peeters *et al.*, 2007), but the prevalence is low. Amongst those patients referred to specialist allergy services, the estimated prevalence of actual lupin allergy was only 0.3–0.8% (de Jong *et al.*, 2010).

Seeds

Sesame allergy was first reported in 1993 and is now one of the top 10 allergens in the UK and the most common seed allergy worldwide (Gangur *et al.*, 2005; Kägi & Wüthrich, 1993; Dias *et al.*, 2008). The reported prevalence in children ranges from 0.18% (Dalal *et al.*, 2002) to 0.42% (Sporik & Hill, 1996). However, data from the French national allergy data bank showed that around 2% of children and 5% of adults who reported reactions to foods were affected by sesame allergy (Lemerdy *et al.*, 2003). It only remits in about 20% of cases (Cohen *et al.*, 2007). Diagnosis can be difficult; a negative SPT and specific IgE tests to sesame occur in people who develop symptoms on oral food challenge, possibly due to the presence of allergens called oleosins, proteins found in oil bodies present in the seed (Leduc *et al.*, 2006). Other confounding factors for diagnosis are that white sesame seeds contain more protein than the black seeds (Fremont *et al.*, 2002), roasting or frying confers a reduction in allergenicity of the seeds as opposed to boiling (Lee *et al.*, 2009) and sesame oil appears to provoke the most severe reactions (Chiu & Haydik, 1991).

Sesame cross reacts with tree nuts, peanuts, poppy seeds, kiwi and rye (Vocks *et al.*, 1993), with sensitisation linked to a high prevalence of sensitisation to tree nuts (Stutius *et al.*, 2010). Sesame and its derivatives can often be present under a variety of different names, as shown in Table 7.11.14. Unlike peanuts and tree nuts, restaurant staff may not be aware of which dishes contain sesame, a common ingredient in vegetarian dishes and also Thai, Indonesian, Japanese, Chinese, Middle Eastern, Greek and Turkish food. Sesame allergic patients also need to avoid sesame oil, which is a common addition to cooked food also and found in pharmaceutical products and cosmetics, listed using the Latin name *Sesamum indicum*.

The only other significant seed allergy is due to mustard seed, which affects an estimated 1.1% of children and 0.84% of adults, and may cause severe reactions in very small amounts (Morisset *et al.*, 2003). Mustard is a common ingredient in many preprepared foods and sauces, and needs to be considered if there are multiple reactions to foods that do not seem to have common food ingredients.

Fish and shellfish

Reactions to fish and shellfish can be induced both by IgE mediated mechanisms and non-allergic triggers, such as histamine or scombroid poisoning. Seafood is one of the most common causes of food allergy in adults; a telephone survey in the USA estimated the prevalence of seafood (fish, shellfish) as 2.3% (95% CI, 2–2.5%) for any seafood allergy, 2% for shellfish, 0.4% for fish and 0.2% for fish/shellfish (Sicherer *et al.*, 2004). The most frequently reported symptoms are oral itching and vomiting (Hebling *et al.*, 1996), but seafood often provokes severe food allergic reactions. Crustaceans are responsible for 10% of all cases of anaphylaxis to foods in France and 8% of fatal anaphylaxis in the UK (Moneret-Vautrin & Morisset, 2005; Pumphrey, 2000). Seafood allergy is thought to be lifelong (Daul *et al.*, 1990), although there have been no large studies on resolution.

Seafood contains highly cross reactive allergens that cause sensitisation or symptoms through consumption, but also through inhalation due to aerosolisation during cooking (James & Crespo, 2007). Parvalbumin is the dominant allergen in finned fish (Hansen *et al.*, 1997), with beta-parvalbumin being the most potent (Griesmeier *et al.*, 2010). Crustaceans (prawns, shrimps, crayfish, crabs and lobsters) and molluscs (bivalves such as clams, oysters, mussels and scallops, and snails, octopus, squid and cuttlefish) also share a common allergenic protein called invertebrate tropomyosin. The presence of pan allergens means there is strong interspecies cross reactivity between fresh and salt water fish, and also between crustaceans and molluscs, but there is no cross reactivity between shellfish and vertebrate fish (Chapman *et al.*, 2006). However, IgE mediated allergy to one type of fish, mollusc or crustacean does not necessarily indicate avoidance of all fish, molluscs or crustaceans. Fish allergens may be denatured by extreme heat, such as that used in canning fish, but most fish allergic individuals will not tolerate fish cooked under normal conditions (Bernhisel-Broadbent *et al.*, 1992). In contrast, allergens from shellfish, which include crustaceans and molluscs, are not thermo labile and remain potent allergens after cooking. Lehrer *et al.* (2007) demonstrated shrimp allergenic activity in oil used to cook shrimp.

Most seafood is an obvious component of a meal; less obvious sources can include fish stock, Worcestershire sauce, caviar, aspic, buffet food, Asian cuisine, fish oil supplements and other health foods such as green lipped mussels. Seafood can also provoke adverse food reactions due to the presence of natural toxins, either present in live fish or scombroid poisoning where the toxin is produced in the flesh of caught fish. Scombroid poisoning produces symptoms of flushing, sweating, urticaria, gastrointestinal symptoms, palpitations and bronchospasm within an hour of consumption, which in severe cases may be confused with anaphylaxis (Attaran & Probst, 2000). These symptoms are due to the bacterial breakdown of histidine into histamine; tuna, mackerel, skipjack, bonito, herring, sardines, marlin and anchovies all contain natural levels of histidine (Fritz & Baldwin, 2003).

Egg

Approximately 1.3–3.2% of children are reported to have egg allergy (Bock, 1987), which usually resolves in childhood (de Boissieu & Dupont, 2006), although the age at acquired tolerance varies in different population groups (Potamianou-Taprantzi *et al.*, 2002). Newly diagnosed egg allergy can occur in adults due to bird egg syndrome; hypersensitivity to bird allergens precipitating a cross reaction to the egg yolk allergen alpha livetin (Szépfalusi *et al.*, 1994). Asthma is a comorbidity associated with egg allergy (Tariq *et al.*, 2000).

Cooking reduces the allergenicity of eggs by 70% (Ford & Taylor, 1982), and the majority of egg allergic children are likely to be able to tolerate cooked egg (Kemp, 2007). Persistent egg allergy is associated with sensitisation to the linear epitopes of the egg allergen Gal d 1 (ovomucoid), which is not degraded by heat, unlike the other main egg allergen Gal d 2 (ovalbumin) (Jarvinen *et al.*, 2007). There may be a wide variation in the type of egg containing foods that those with an egg allergy can tolerate. Table 7.11.15 shows the type of foods that can be classified as containing well cooked egg, loosely cooked egg and raw egg. Egg can be a less obvious ingredient of foods such as pasta, biscuits, ice cream, egg glazes, sweets and desserts, so labels should always be carefully scrutinised for its presence.

Table 7.11.15 Classification of egg containing foods

Well cooked egg	Lightly cooked egg	Raw egg
Cakes	Scrambled egg	Fresh mayonnaise
Biscuits	Boiled egg	Fresh mousse and shop bought mousse that contains egg
Dried egg pasta	Fried egg	
Pancakes and Yorkshire pudding	Omelette	Fresh ice cream
Egg in sausages, both vegetarian and meat varieties, and also in other processed meats such as burgers	Egg fried rice	Sorbet
	Meringues	Royal icing (both fresh and powdered icing sugar)
	Some marshmallows	
	Lemon curd	Home made marzipan
Prepared meat dishes	Quiche	Raw egg in cake mix and other dishes awaiting cooking (children of all ages love to taste or lick the spoon!)
Well cooked fresh egg pasta	Poached egg	
Quorn	Pancakes	
Sponges and sponge fingers	Egg in batter	
Chocolate bars that contain nougat or dried egg, e.g. Milky Way, Mars bar or Creme egg	Egg in breadcrumbs, e.g. on fish fingers and chicken nuggets	Egg glaze on pastry
	Hollandaise sauce	Horseradish sauce
Some soft centred chocolates	Quiche and flans (fruity and savoury)	Tartar sauce
Soft fruit chews	Egg custard and egg custard tarts	Cheese containing egg white in the form of lysozyme
Egg in some gravy granules	Crème caramel	Mayonnaise
Dried egg noodles	Crème brulée	Salad cream
Waffles	Real (egg) custard	
Commercial marzipan	Tempura batter	
	Yorkshire pudding – some patients who can eat well cooked egg can tolerate this, but it depends on how well cooked they are and if they contain any uncooked batter inside	

Lecithin used in food manufacture is more likely to be derived from soya than egg, but if this is not specified, the origin needs to be checked with the manufacturer. Even if derived from egg, most patients with an egg allergy will tolerate egg lecithin (E322), but reactions have been reported in the past (Palm *et al.*, 1999).

Fruit and vegetables

The most widespread group of foods provoking food allergic reactions in adolescents and adults is fruit, and to a lesser extent, vegetables (Osterballe *et al.*, 2009; Vierk *et al.*, 2007). These reactions are most frequently due to similarity or homology between plant food allergens and specific IgE antibodies of pollen, latex and plant foods provoking the characteristic symptoms of PFS (Amlot *et al.*, 1987). The prevalence of PFS varies according to pollen sensitisation rates, and the pollens involved, with up to two-thirds of those sensitised to birch tree pollen likely to develop PFS (Skypala *et al.*, 2011). The main trigger foods for PFS vary depending on the pollen involved, but most regularly include tree nuts, apples and stone fruit such as peaches and cherries (Table 7.11.16) (Katelaris, 2010). Celery is one of the most common foods to cause oral allergy syndrome in adults in European countries, but is not a major allergen in the UK. The allergy normally involves the celery root (celeriac) rather than the stalk of the plant and can result in anaphylaxis, often to small amounts (Vieths *et al.*, 2002). Unlike other PFS reactions, cooked celery and celery spice are as likely to cause a reaction in sensitive people as raw celery (Ballmer-Weber *et al.*, 2002). Another less prevalent manifestation of oral allergy syndrome is caused by antibodies to natural rubber latex (*Hevea brasilienisis*) cross reacting with various fruit and vegetables; 30–50% of those allergic to natural latex rubber will have associated hypersensitivity reactions to plant foods (Wagner & Breiteneder, 2002).

Symptoms of PFS are generally mild, probably because the allergens involved are extremely labile; however, fruit and vegetables can provoke severe reactions (Ross *et al.*,

2008). These reactions usually involve different allergens to those involved in PFS, including a group known as lipid transfer protein (LTP) allergens. Unlike the allergens involved in PFS, LTP allergens are resistant to proteolysis, pH change and thermal treatments, enabling them to be primary sensitisers (Fernández–Rivas *et al.*, 2006). However, like PFS, allergy involving LTP allergens is due to cross reactivity; those sensitised to peach LTP are more likely to have clinical cross reactivity to other foods containing LTP (Asero *et al.*, 2004). Sensitisation to these allergens is highly prevalent in southern Europe, with limited data showing that they could be relevant in Northern Europeans (Salcedo *et al.*, 2004; Flinterman *et al.*, 2008).

Wheat

Wheat allergy is usually a transient, but important, allergy of childhood, with a reported prevalence of 0.4% in children in the USA (Sicherer & Sampson, 2006; Venter *et al.*, 2006a; Pereira *et al.*, 2005). Almost all children with a wheat allergy achieve tolerance by adolescence (Keet *et al.*, 2009), but despite this 0.5–0.9% of adults report reactions to wheat (Schäfer *et al.*, 2001; Young *et al.*, 1994; Vierk *et al.*, 2007). In adults the most common manifestation is as a trigger of a condition known as food dependent, exercise induced anaphylaxis (FDEIA) (Beaudouin *et al.*, 2006; Dohi *et al.*, 1991). Those affected by this condition can tolerate wheat except when it is consumed within 2 hours of exercising. Anaphylaxis can be induced by exercise alone, but it is possible that 80% of all cases food could be a cofactor (Yang *et al.*, 2008). Shellfish, tomatoes, celery, peanuts, maize, soya, strawberries and cheese have also been implicated as triggers of FDEIA (Shadick *et al.*, 1999; Romano *et al.*, 2001).

Presenting symptoms to wheat are often cutaneous, such as atopic dermatitis and urticaria, but laryngeal oedema and anaphylaxis may occur as the first manifestation (Pourpak *et al.*, 2004). Non-IgE mediated symptoms may be chronic (diffuse gastrointestinal symptoms), with the role of T cells and their cytokines demonstrated in wheat related gastrointestinal symptoms (Latcham *et al.*, 2003). The algorithm for food hypersensitivity classifies coeliac disease as a non-IgE mediated food allergy; and wheat is one of the cereals containing gluten (alcohol soluble prolamins) that can cause this condition (see Chapter 7.4.7). However, in adults wheat is most often reported to provoke gastrointestinal symptoms, most notably in those with irritable bowel disease, although the mechanism is unknown (Monsbakken *et al.*, 2006). Rice, maize, barley and oats can all provoke allergic reactions, but are not common triggers of FHS in the UK, although they should not be ruled out, especially as corn or barley may be minor ingredients in many foods. Although it is not a cereal, buckwheat is often used to replace flour; buckwheat noodles are a common cause of reactions in Korea (Yang *et al.*, 2008) and buckwheat in the form of galettes (pancakes) is becoming a common allergen in France and should be considered in cases of unexplained reactions.

Table 7.11.16	Cross reacting plant food allergens
Birch pollen	Apple, pear, cherry, peach, nectarine, apricot, plum, kiwi, hazelnut, other nuts, almond, celery, carrot, potato
Birch/mugwort	Celery, carrot, spices, sunflower seed, honey
Grass	Melon, watermelon, orange, tomato, potato, peanut, Swiss chard
Ragweed	Watermelon and other melons, banana, courgette, cucumber
Plane tree	Hazelnut, peach, apple, melon, kiwi, peanuts, maize, chickpea, lettuce, green beans
Latex	Avocado pear, chestnut, banana, passion fruit, kiwi fruit, papaya, mango, tomato, pepper, potato, celery

Wheat allergy (IgE mediated) may require total wheat exclusion. Partial exclusion may be sufficient in some non-IgE mediated food allergy or non-allergic food hypersensitivity forms of wheat hypersensitivity; the threshold of sensitivity varies and some people can obtain symptom relief by significant reduction of wheat intake. In the UK, wheat is a major component of most cereal foods and a common ingredient in many manufactured foods, ranging from sausages to ice cream. Wheat exclusion therefore has considerable impact on food choice and nutrient intake. In children, wheat may be an additional allergen excluded alongside milk and/or egg, which increases nutritional risks for calcium deficiency and makes the diet very limited unless a good range of substitutes are introduced. Additionally, a wheat free diet can result in a reduction of dietary fibre and B vitamins.

An excellent range of commercially produced wheat free (and gluten free) products, including bread, biscuits, pastries, pasta and ready meals are available. Some gluten free and wheat products are available on prescription. These are not prescribable for wheat FHS, but usually only for people with coeliac disease who can tolerate wheat starch as it is present in many proprietary gluten free foods. Gluten free products are not suitable for people with wheat allergy unless they are specifically labelled as wheat free. Dietary guidance for wheat exclusion is summarised in Table 7.11.17.

Other triggers

Food additives

Approximately 4.9% of the UK population cite food additives as a trigger of food allergy (Young et al., 1994),

although the true prevalence ranges from 0.1% to 0.4% (Young et al., 1987; Osterballe et al., 2005). Problems are most commonly reported in children (Pereira et al., 2005) and studies suggest artificial colours and the benzoate preservatives can increase hyperactivity in children (McCann et al., 2007). In adults, those with chronic idiopathic urticaria or asthma seem to be more susceptible to reactions to food colours, benzoates and the metabisulphite preservatives (Di Lorenzo et al., 2005). Although it is usually the azo dyes, in particular tartrazine (E102) and sunset yellow (E110), which are considered by the public to be the most likely to be implicated in adverse food reactions. A move towards the use of natural colourings has led to an increase in the use of carmine or cochineal, which being derived from insects can provoke IgE mediated food allergy. Of all the food additives, reactions to sulphites have been the best characterised and are the only food additives required by law to be declared on food labels (see Chapter 4.5). Sulphites are used universally to inhibit the enzymatic and non-enzymatic reactions that control browning (Taylor et al., 2003). They are primarily added to wine, cider, vinegar, pectin, clear or light coloured fruit juices, lime and lemon juice and dried foods such as dried fruit and dried onions (E220–E228). Food hypersensitivity involving sulphites is more likely to affect asthmatic patients, especially those with steroid dependent asthma (Bush et al., 1986). However, following the reduction in the levels of sulphite additives permitted to be added to foods by the US Food and Drug Administration, a significant drop in the number of adverse reactions reported to be linked with sulphite consumption was noted (Timbo et al., 2004). Normal symptoms in sulphite sensitive individuals include the

Table 7.11.17 Dietary guidance for wheat exclusion

Cereal foods that must be excluded	Other foods that may need to be excluded	Cereal foods that can be included
All types of bread, including rolls, malt bread, chapatti, pitta, naan, paratha, croissants, soda bread and fancy breads Some gluten free breads Breakfast cereals unless derived solely from oat, rice and/or maize (corn) Cakes, biscuits and crackers Flour and all foods containing wheat, e.g. pastry, pies, batters, pancakes, sauces Bran Pasta Semolina, couscous Pizza Proprietary gluten free foods containing wheat starch Whole wheat or wheat grains Wheat flour Wheat starch (or modified starch) Wheat bran Wheat germ Wheat binder Wheat gluten Wheat thickener Cereal filler Rusk Breadcrumbs or bread	Manufactured foods containing any of the following ingredients: Modified starch (mostly from maize derived) Wheat germ oil Wheat thickener Raising agent containing wheat starch Hydrolysed wheat protein Spelt Oats* Rye* Barley* Triticale*	Rice and rice flour Corn (maize) and cornflour (polenta) Millet Arrowroot Buckwheat Sago and sago flour Tapioca Quinoa Proprietary gluten free, wheat free foods (NB: only prescribable for coeliac disease, not wheat intolerance *per se*)

*Some patients may have a cross sensitisation with these grains.

development of flushing, nasal and sinus symptoms, bronchospasm and occasional gastrointestinal upset, which usually develop 30–45 minutes after eating a high sulphite food, although they can develop much sooner than this. Like many other types of FHS, sulphite intolerance is dose dependent; whilst a small number of people are sensitive to small amounts, most report symptoms after consuming a dose of >20 mg (see Appendix A5).

Pharmacological food reactions

Reactions to biogenic amines, salicylates and other naturally occurring components of food are poorly researched and understood. It has been proposed that there is no relation between the oral ingestion of biogenic amines and FHS reactions (Jansen et al., 2003). However, a more recent review concluded that histamine intolerance is probably underestimated (Maintz & Novak, 2007). Dietary histamine is degraded by the enzyme diamine oxidase, a lack of which may precipitate symptoms similar to those elicited by an IgE mediated food allergic reaction (Malone & Metcalfe, 1986). Like most pharmacological reactions, a histamine response is dose dependent; most people will react to a large dose but those who are especially sensitive may respond to levels as low as 2.5 mg (Malone & Metcalfe, 1986). Foods rich in biogenic amines include strong cheeses, especially Parmesan cheese and blue cheeses such as Roquefort, red wine, spinach, aubergines, yeast extract and scombroid fish such as tuna and mackerel (Fritz & Baldwin, 2003). Salicylates are signalling molecules usually present in plant foods in the form of salicylic acid. It is unknown whether naturally occurring salicylic acid in foods can provoke a response in individuals with a hypersensitivity to another form of salicylic acid, acetyl salicylate (aspirin). The efficacy of the avoidance of dietary salicylate has been refuted (Dahlén et al., 1994), although others have suggested salicylate intolerance could be relevant in a percentage of people with a pre-existing intolerance to non-steroidal anti-inflammatory drugs who also have diseases of the lower gastrointestinal tract (Raithel et al., 2005). The issue is compounded by the variance of the salicylate content of foods due to varietal differences and growing conditions (Baxter et al., 2001). Dietary advice on salicylate avoidance is further complicated due to large discrepancies in the amounts of salicylate attributed by different studies to specific foods (Swain et al., 1985; Venema et al., 1996; Scotter et al., 2007). The benefits of salicylate avoidance need to be weighed against the fact that a diet high in natural salicylates may be beneficial for the prevention of cancer and heart disease.

Other pharmacological reactions include those reported to dietary methylxanthines, such as caffeine in coffee, cola and chocolate, and theobromine in chocolate. These substances can provoke symptoms such as anxiety and disordered sleep in sensitive individuals (Mathew & Wilson, 1990; Pollak & Bright, 2003), although both coffee and cola drinks have also been reported to trigger urticaria and anaphylaxis (Infante et al., 2003, Fernandez-Nieto et al., 2002). Despite chocolate being the most commonly reported food to provoke symptoms in the prevalence study of Young et al. (1994), allergy to chocolate bars is unlikely due to extensive processing of the cocoa beans (Zak & Keeney, 1976), although it has been proposed that the availability of chocolate containing pieces of roasted or raw cacao nut could lead to an increase in reported reactions (Chapman et al., 2006).

Reactions to alcohol are most commonly due to a deficiency of the enzyme alcohol dehydrogenise, which predominantly affects people of Asian ethnicity (Agarwal et al., 1981). However, alcoholic drinks can provoke FHS reactions or act as a cofactor in precipitating or exacerbating these reactions. The alcoholic drink most commonly reported to cause symptoms is red wine (Linneberg et al., 2008). Rarely, but occasionally, these reactions are due to the pure alcohol itself (Ehlers et al., 2002), but more common precipitants are the biogenic amines or added sodium metabisulphite (Fritz & Baldwin, 2003; Vally & Thompson, 2001). The LTP allergens in barley, wheat and grapes have also been reported to trigger severe IgE mediated allergic responses to beer and wine (Asero et al., 2001; Herzinger et al., 2004; Kalogeromitros et al., 2005).

Further reading

Arshad SH. (2002) *Allergy: An Illustrated Colour Text*. London: Churchill Livingstone.
Ball H. (2005) *Food Challenges for Children – A Practical Guide*. Leicester: Nutrition and Dietetic Department, Leicester Royal Infirmary.
Skypala IJ, Venter C. (2009) *Food Hypersensitivity*. Oxford: Wiley Blackwell.
Wright T. (2006). *Food Allergies*. Class Publishing.

Internet resources

Allergy UK   www.allergyuk.org
Anaphylaxis Campaign   www.anaphylaxis.org.uk
Asthma UK   www.asthma.org.uk
British Dietetic Association   www.bda.uk.com
Food Allergy and Intolerance Specialist Group (2012) Allergy Consensus Statement
    Policy Statement (2013) Complementary feeding: Introduction of solid food to an infant's diet
        British Society for Allergy and Clinical Immunology (BSACI) www.bsaci.org
Department of Health   www.dh.gov.uk
    Introducing your baby to solid food in Birth to Five
Learning Early About Peanut Allergy (LEAP)   www.leapstudy.co.uk
Medic Alert Foundation (medical alert bracelets)   www.medicalert.or.uk
Migraine Trust   www.migrainetrust.org
National Eczema Society   www.eczema.org

References

Aamodt AH, Lars JS, Langhammer L, Knut H, Zwart JA. (2007) Is Headache related to Asthma, hay fever and chronic bronchitis? The head-hunt study. *Headache* 47: 204–221.
Agarwal DP, Harada S, Goedde HW. (1981) Racial differences in biological sensitivity to ethanol: the role of alcohol dehydrogenase and aldehyde dehydrogenase isozymes. *Alcoholism: Clinical and Experimental Research* 5: 12–16.

Agostoni C, Decsi T, Fewtrell M, *et al.* (2008) Complementary feeding: a commentary by the ESPGHAN Committee on Nutrition. *Journal of Pediatric Gastroenterology and Nutrition* 46: 99–110.

Akkerdaas JH, Wensing M, Knulst AC, *et al.* (2003) How accurate and safe is the diagnosis of Hazelnut allergy by means of commercial skin prick test reagents? *International Archives of Allergy and Immunology* 132: 132–140.

Allen KJ, Hill DJ, Heine RG. (2006) Food allergy in childhood. *Medical Journal of Australia* 185: 394–400.

Allen KJ, Davidson GP, Day AS, *et al.* (2009) Management of cows' milk protein allergy in infants and young children: an expert panel perspective. *Journal of Paediatric and Child Health* 45: 481–486.

Amlot PL, Kemeny DM, Zachary C, Parkes P, Lessof MH. (1987) Oral allergy syndrome (OAS): symptoms of IgE-mediated hypersensitivity to foods. *Clinical Allergy* 17: 33–42.

Ando H, Movérare R, Kondo Y, *et al.* (2008) Utility of ovomucoid-specific IgE concentrations in predicting symptomatic egg allergy. *Journal of Allergy and Clinical Immunology* 122: 583–588.

Asero R, Mistrello G, Roncarolo D, Amato S, van-Ree R. (2001) A case of allergy to beer showing cross-reactivity between lipid transfer proteins. *Annals of Allergy, Asthma and Immunology* 87: 65–67.

Asero R, Mistrello G, Roncarolo D, Amato S. (2004) Relationship between peach lipid transfer protein specific IgE levels and hypersensitivity to non-Rosaceae vegetable foods in patients allergic to lipid transfer protein. *Annals of Allergy, Asthma and Immunology* 92: 268–272.

Asthma UK. (2004) Where do we stand?: Asthma in the UK today. Available at www.asthmauk.org.uk.

Attaran RR, Probst F. (2000) Histamine fish poisoning: a common but frequently misdiagnosed condition. *Emergency Medicine Journal* 19: 474–475.

Awazuhara H, Kawai H, Baba M, Matsui T, Komiyama A. (1998) Antigenicity of the proteins in soy lecithin and soy oil in soybean allergy. *Clinical and Experimental Allergy* 28: 1559–1564.

Ball HB. (2005) *Food Challenges for Children, A Practical Guide.* Enderby: Leicestershire Nutrition and Dietetic Service.

Ballmer-Weber BK, Hoffmann A, Wuthrich B, *et al.* (2002) Influence of food processing on the allergenicity of celery: DBPCFC with celery spice and cooked celery in patients with celery allergy. *Allergy* 57: 228–235.

Ballmer-Webber B, Holzhauser T, Scibia J, *et al.* (2007) Clinical characteristics of soybean allergy in Europe: A double-blind, placebo-controlled food challenge study. *Journal of Allergy and Clinical Immunology* 119: 1489–1496.

Bateman B, Warner JO, Hutchinson E, *et al.* (2004) The effects of a double blind, placebo controlled, artificial food colourings and benzoate preservative challenge on hyperactivity in a general population sample of preschool children. *Archives of Disease in Childhood* 89: 506–511.

Bauchau V, Durham SR. (2004) Prevalence and rate of diagnosis of allergic rhinitis in Europe. *European Respiratory Journal* 24: 758–764.

Baxter GJ, Graham AB, Lawrence JR, Wiles D, Paterson JR. (2001) Salicylic acid in soups prepared from organically and non-organically grown vegetables. *European Journal of Nutrition* 40: 289–292.

Beaudouin E, Renaudin JM, Morisset M, Codreanu F, Kanny G, Moneret-Vautrin DA. (2006) Food-dependent, exercise-induced anaphylaxis – update and current data. *Allergy and Immunology Paris.* 38: 45–51.

Bellioni-Businco B, Paganelli R, Lucenti P, Giampietro PG, Perborn H, Businco L. (1999) Allergenicity of goat's milk in children with cows' milk allergy. *Journal of Allergy Clinical Immunology* 103: 1191–1194.

Bernhisel-Broadbent J, Sampson HA. (1989) Cross allergenicity in the Legume botanical family in children with food hypersensitivity. *Journal of Allergy and Clinical Immunology* 83: 435–440.

Bernhisel-Broadbent J, Scanlon SM, Sampson HA. (1992) Fish hypersensitivity. In vitro and oral challenge results in fish-allergic patients. *Journal of Allergy and Clinical Immunology* 89: 730–737.

Berns SH, Halm EA, Sampson HA, Sicherer SH, Busse PJ, Wisnivesky JP. (2007) Food allergy as a risk factor for asthma morbidity in adults. *Journal of Asthma* 44: 377–381.

Bindslev-Jensen C, Ballmer-Webber BK, Bengtsson U, *et al*; European Academy of Allergology and Clinical Immunology. (2004) Standardisation of food challenges in patients with immediate reactions to foods – position paper from the European Academy of Allergology and Clinical Immunology. *Allergy* 59: 690–697.

Bock SA. (1987) Prospective appraisal of complaints of adverse reactions to foods in children during the first 3 years of life. *Pediatrics* 79: 683–688.

Bock SA. (2010) AAAAI support of the EAACI Position Paper on IgG4. *Journal of Allergy and Clinical Immunology* 125: 1410.

Bock SA, Sampson HA, Atkins FM, *et al.* (1988) Double-blind, placebo-controlled food challenge (DBPCFC) as an office procedure: a manual. *Journal of Allergy and Clinical Immunology* 82(6): 986–997.

Bock SA, Munoz-Furlong A, Sampson HA. (2007) Further fatalities caused by anaphylactic reactions to food, 2001–2006. *Journal of Allergy and Clinical Immunology* 119: 1016–1018.

Bohle B, Zwölfer B, Heratizadeh A, *et al.* (2006) Cooking birch pollen-related food: Divergent consequences for IgE- and T cell-mediated reactivity in vitro and in vivo. *Journal of Allergy and Clinical Immunology* 118: 242–249.

Boyce JA, Assa'ad A, Burks WA, *et al.* (2010) Guidelines for the Diagnosis and Management of Food Allergy in the United States: Summary of the NIAID-Sponsored Expert Panel Report. *Journal of Allergy and Clinical Immunology* 126: S1–S58.

British Dietetic Association (2013) (Policy Statement) Complementary feeding: Introduction of solid food to an infant's diet. Available at www.bda.uk.com/policies/WeaningPolicyStatement.pdf. Accessed 28 August 2013.

British Dietetic Association's Food Allergy and Intolerance Specialist Group (2012) Cow's milk free diet for infants and children. Available at www.bda.uk.com and for BDA members. at http://members.bda.uk.com/groups/faisg/info_sheets/FAISG_Milk_FreeChildren.pdf. Accessed 28 August 2013.

Bruijnzeel-Koomen C, Ortolani C, Aas K, *et al.* (1995) Adverse reactions to foods. *Allergy* 50: 623–635.

Burks W. (2003) Skin manifestations of food allergy. *Pediatrics* 111: 1617–1624.

Bush RK, Taylor SL, Holden K, Nordlee JA, Busse WW. (1986) The prevalence of sensitivity to sulfiting agents in asthmatics. *American Journal of Medicine* 81: 816–820.

Camargo CA Jr, Rifas-Shiman SL, Litonjua AA, *et al.* (2007) Maternal intake of vitamin D during pregnancy and risk of recurrent wheeze in children at 3 y of age. *American Journal of Clinical Nutrition* 85: 788–795.

Cantorna MT, Zhu Y, Froicu M, Wittke A. (2004) Vitamin D status, 1,25-dihydroxyvitamin D3, and the immune system. *American Journal of Clinical Nutrition* 80: 1717S–1720S.

Chapman JA, Bernstein IL, Lee RE, *et al.* (2006) Food allergy: a practice parameter. *Annals of Allergy, Asthma and Immunology* 96: S1–S68.

Chiu JT, Haydik IB. (1991) Sesame seed oil anaphylaxis. *Journal of Allergy and Clinical Immunology* 88: 414–415.

Clark AT, Ewan PW. (2008) Good prognosis, clinical features, and circumstances of peanut and tree nut reactions in children treated by a specialist allergy center. *Journal of Allergy and Clinical Immunology* 122: 286–289.

Clark AT, Anagnostou K, Ewan PW. (2007) Cashew nut causes more severe reactions than peanut: case matched comparison in 141 children. *Allergy* 62: 913–916.

Cohen A, Goldberg M, Levy B, Leshno M, Katz Y. (2007) Sesame food allergy and sensitization in children: the natural history and long-term follow-up. *Pediatric Allergy and Immunology* 18: 217–223.

Colver AF, Nevantaus H, Macdougall CF, Cant AJ. (2005) Severe food-allergic reactions in children across the UK and Ireland 1998–2000. *Acta Paediatrica* 94: 689–695.

Dahlén B, Boréus LO, Anderson P, Andersson R, Zetterström O. (1994) Plasma acetylsalicylic acid and salicylic acid levels during aspirin provocation in aspirin-sensitive subjects. *Allergy* 49: 43–49.

Dalal I, Binson R, Reifen Z, *et al.* (2002) Food allergy is a matter of geography after all: sesame as a major cause of severe IgE-mediated food allergic reactions among infants and young children in Israel. *Allergy* 57: 362–365.

Daul CB, Morgan JE, Lehrer SB. (1990) The natural history of shrimp-specific immunity. *Journal of Allergy and Clinical Immunology* 86: 88–93.

Davoren M, Peake J. (2005) Cashew nut allergy is associated with a high risk of anaphylaxis. *Archives of Disease in Childhood* 90: 1084–1085.

de Boissieu D, Dupont C. (2006) Natural course of sensitization to hen's egg in children not previously exposed to egg ingestion. *European Annals of Allergy and Clinical Immunology* 38: 113–117.

de Jong NW, van Maaren MS, Vlieg-Boersta BJ, Dubois AE, de Groot H, Gerth van Wijk R. (2010) Sensitization to lupine flour: is it clinically relevant? *Clinical and Experimental Allergy* 40: 1571–1577.

de Leon MP, Glaspole IN, Drew AC, Rolland JM, O'Hehir RE, Suphioglu C. (2003) Immunological analysis of allergenic cross-reactivity between peanut and tree nuts. *Clinical and Experimental Allergy* 33: 1273–1280.

Department of Health. (1994) *Report on Health and Social Subjects No 45. Weaning and the Weaning Diet*. London: HMSO.

Department of Health. (2009a) Introducing your baby to solid food in Birth to Five. Available at www.dh.gov.uk/prod_consum_dh/groups/dh_digitalassets/documents/digitalasset/dh_107668.pdf.

Department of Health. (2009b) UK Government advice on peanut consumption during early life and allergy risk. Available at www.food.gov.uk/safereating/allergyintol/peanutspregnancy.

des Roches A, Paradis L, Paradis J, Singer S. (2006) Food allergy as a new risk factor for scurvy. *Allergy* 61: 1487–1488.

Devenney I, Norrman G, Oldaeus G, Stromberg L, Falth-Magnusson K. (2006) A new model for low-dose food challenge in children with allergy to milk or egg. *Acta Paediatrica* 95: 1133–1139.

Devereux G, Turner SW, Craig LC, *et al.* (2006) Low maternal vitamin E intake during pregnancy is associated with asthma in 5-year-old children. *American Journal of Respiratory and Critical Care Medicine* 174: 499–507.

Devereux G, Litonjua AA, Turner SW, *et al.* (2007) Maternal vitamin D intake during pregnancy and early childhood wheezing. *American Journal of Clinical Nutrition* 85: 853–859.

Di Lorenzo G, Pacor ML, Mansueto P, *et al.* (2005) Food additive-induced urticaria: a survey of 838 patients with recurrent chronic idiopathic urticaria. *International Archives of Allergy and Immunology* 138: 235–242.

Dias RP, Summerfield A, Khakoo GA. (2008) Food hypersensitivity among Caucasian and non-Caucasian children. *Pediatric Allergy and Immunology* 19: 86–89.

Diesner SC, Untersmayr E, Pietschmann P, Jensen-Jarolim E. (2011) Food allergy: only a pediatric disease? *Gerontology* 57: 28–32.

Dohi M, Suko M, Sugiyama H *et al.* (1991) Food-dependant, exercise-induced anaphylaxis: a study on 11 Japanese cases. *Journal of Allergy and Clinical Immunology* 87: 34–40.

Du Toit G, Katz Y, Sasieni P, *et al.* (2008) Early consumption of peanuts in infancy is associated with a low prevalence of peanut allergy. *Journal of Allergy and Clinical Immunology* 122: 984–991.

Du Toit G, Meyer R, Shah N, *et al.* (2010) Identifying and managing cows' milk protein allergy. *Archives of Disease in Childhood Educational Practice Edition* 95: 134–144.

Dueñas-Laita A, Pineda F, Armentia A. (2009) Hypersensitivity to generic drugs with soybean oil. *New England Journal of Medicine* 361: 1317–1318.

Ebo DG, Bridts CH, Verweji MM, *et al.* (2009) Sensitization profiles in birch pollen-allergic patients with and without oral allergy syndrome to apple: lessons from multiplexed component-resolved allergy diagnosis. *Clinical and Experimental Allergy* 40: 339–347.

Eggesbo M, Botten G, Halvorsen R, Magnus P. (2001) The prevalence of CMA/CMPI in young children: the validity of parentally perceived reactions in a population-based study. *Allergy* 56(5): 393–402.

Ehlers I, Hipler UC, Zuberbier T, Worm M. (2002) Ethanol as a cause of hypersensitivity reactions to alcoholic beverages. *Clinical and Experimental Allergy* 32: 1231–1235.

Eigenmann PA, Caubert JC, Zemore SA. (2006) Continuing food-avoidance diets after negative food challenges. *Pediatric Allergy and Immunology* 17: 601–601.

Eriksson NE, Moller C, Werner S, Magnusson J, Bengtsson U. (2003) The hazards of kissing when you are food allergic. *Journal of Investigational Allergology and Clinical Immunology* 13: 149–154.

Erkkola M, Kaila M, Nwaru BI, *et al.* (2009) Maternal vitamin D intake during pregnancy is inversely associated with asthma and allergic rhinitis in 5-year-old children. *Clinical and Experimental Allergy* 39: 875–882.

European Commission Directive (2003) Directive 2003/89/EC of the European Parliament and of the Council of 10 November 2003 amending Directive 2000/13/EC as regards indication of the ingredients present in foodstuffs. *OJL* 308: 15–18.

European Commission Directive (2006) 2006/142/EC of 22 December 2006 amending Annex IIIa of Directive 2000/13/EC of the European Parliament and of the Council listing the ingredients which must under all circumstances appear on the labelling of foodstuffs. *OJL* 368: 110–111.

European Union. (2006) Directive 2006/142/EC of the European Parliament amendmend of Annex IIIA [Article 6(3a), (10) and (11)]. *Official Journal of the European Union* L368: 110.

European Union. (2007) Directive 2007/68/EC of the European Parliament amendmend of Directive 2000/13/EC. *Official Journal of the European Union* L310: 11.

Ewan PW. (1996) Clinical study of peanut and nut allergy in 62 consecutive patients: new features and associations. *BMJ* 312: 1074–1078.

Ewan PW, Clark AT. (2005) Efficacy of a management plan based on severity assessment in longitudinal and case-controlled studies of 747 children with nut allergy: proposal for good practice. *Clinical and Experimental Allergy* 35: 751–756.

Ferdman RM, Church JA. (2006) Mixed-up nuts: identification of peanuts and tree nuts by children. *Annals of Allergy, Asthma and Immunology* 97: 73–77.

Fernandez-Nieto M, Sastre J, Quirce S. (2002) Urticaria caused by cola drink. *Allergy* 57: 967.

Fernández–Rivas M, Bolhaar S, González-Moncebo E, *et al.* (2006) Apple allergy across Europe: How allergen sensitization profiles determine the clinical expression of allergies to plant foods. *Journal of Allergy and Clinical Immunology* 118: 481–488.

Filipiak B, Zutavern A, Koletzko S, *et al.* (2007) Solid food introduction in relation to eczema: results from a four-year prospective birth cohort study. *Journal of Pediatrics* 151: 352–358.

Fiocchi A, Schünemann HJ, Brozek J, *et al.* (2010) Diagnosis and Rationale for Action Against Cows' Milk Allergy (DRACMA): a summary report. *Journal of Allergy and Clinical Immunology* 126: 1119–1128.

Fisher HR, Toit GD, Lack G. (2011) Specific oral tolerance induction in food allergic children: is oral desensitisation more effective than allergen avoidance?: A meta-analysis of published RCTs. *Archives of Disease in Childhood* 96: 259–264.

SECTION 7

Flammarion S, Santos C, Guimber D, *et al.* (2011) Diet and nutritional status of children with food allergies. *Pediatric Allergy and Immunology* 22: 161–165.

Fleischer D, Conover-Walker M, Matsui E, Wood R. (2005) The natural history of tree nut allergy. *Journal of Allergy and Clinical Immunology* 116: 1087–1093.

Flinterman AE, Knulst A, Meijer Y, Bruijnzeel-Koomen C, Pasmans SG. (2006) Acute allergic reactions in children with AEDS after prolonged cows' milk elimination diets. *Allergy* 61: 370–374.

Flinterman AE, Akkerdaas JH, den Hartog Jager CF, *et al.* (2008) Lipid transfer protein–linked hazelnut allergy in children from a non-Mediterranean birch-endemic area. *Journal of Allergy and Clinical Immunology* 121: 423–428.

Flokstra-de Blok BM, Dubois AE, Vlieg-Boerstra BJ, *et al.* (2010) Health-related quality of life of food allergic patients: comparison with the general population and other diseases. *Allergy* 65: 238–244.

Food Standards Agency (FSA). (2009) Nut allergy labelling – Report of research into the consumer response. Food Standards Agency. Available at www.food.gov.uk/news/newsarchive/2009/may/arsenicinriceresearch.

Ford RP, Taylor B. (1982) Natural history of egg hypersensitivity. *Archives of Disease in Childhood* 57: 649–652.

Fox AR, Du Toit G, Lang A, Lack G. (2004) Food allergy as a risk factor for nutritional rickets. *Pediatric Allergy and Immunology* 15: 566–569.

Fremont S, Zitouni N, Kanny G, *et al.* (2002) Allergenicity of some isoforms of white sesame proteins. *Clinical and Experimental Allergy* 32: 1211–1215.

Fritz SB, Baldwin JL. (2003) Pharmacologic food reactions. In: Metcalfe DD, Sampson HJ, Simon RA, eds. *Food Allergy: Adverse Reactions to Foods and Food Additives*. Oxford: Blackwell Publishing Ltd, pp. 324–341.

Gangur V, Kelly C, Navuluri L. (2005) Sesame allergy: a growing food allergy of global proportions? *Annals of Allergy, Asthma and Immunology* 95: 4–11.

Gdalevich M, Mimouni D, David M, Mimouni M. (2001) Breast-feeding and the onset of atopic dermatitis in childhood: a systematic review and meta-analysis of prospective studies. *Journal of the American Academy of Dermatology* 45: 520–527.

Gerrard JW, MacKenzie JW, Goluboff N, Garson JZ, Maningas CS. (1973) Cow's milk allergy: prevalence and manifestations in an unselected series of newborns. *Acta Paediatrica Scandinavica Supplements* 234: 1–21.

Greer FR, Sicherer SH, Burks AW. (2008) Effects of early nutritional interventions on the development of atopic disease in infants and children: the role of maternal dietary restriction, breastfeeding, timing of introduction of complementary foods, and hydrolyzed formulas. *Pediatrics* 121: 183–191.

Griesmeier U, Vázquez-Cortés S, Bublin M, *et al.* (2010) Expression levels of parvalbumins determine allergenicity of fish species. *Allergy* 65: 191–198.

Grimshaw KE. (2006) Dietary management of food allergy in children. *Proceedings of the Nutrition Society* 65: 412–417.

Grimshaw KE, King RM, Nordlee JA, Hefle SL, Warner JO, Hourihane JO. (2003) Presentation of allergen in different food preparations affects the nature of the allergic reaction–a case series. *Clinical and Experimental Allergy and Immunology* 33: 1581–1585.

Gupta R, Sheikh A, Strachan DP, Anderson HR. (2007) Time trends in allergic disorders in the UK. *Thorax* 62: 91–96.

Hansen TK, Bindslev-Jensen C, Skov PS, Poulsen LK. (1997) Codfish allergy in adults: IgE cross-reactivity among fish species. *Annals of Allergy, Asthma and Immunology* 78: 187–194.

Hebling A, McCants ML, Musmand JJ, Schwartz HJ, Lehrer SB. (1996) Immunopathogenesis of fish allergy: identification of fish-allergic adults by skin test and radioallergosorbent test. *Annals of Allergy, Asthma and Immunology* 77: 48–54.

Hernell O, Lonnerdal B. (2003) Nutritional evaluation of protein hydrolysate formulas in healthy term infants: plasma amino acids, hematology, and trace elements. *American Journal of Clinical Nutrition* 78: 296–301.

Herzinger T, Kick G, Ludolph-Hauser D, Przybilla B. (2004) Anaphylaxis to wheat beer. *Annals of Allergy, Asthma and Immunology* 92: 673–675.

Hide DW, Guyer BM. (1983) Cows milk intolerance in Isle of Wight infants. *British Journal of Clinical Practice* 37(9): 285–287.

Hill DJ, Duke AM, Hosking CS, Hudson IL. (1988) Clinical manifestations of cows' milk allergy in childhood. II. The diagnostic value of skin tests and RAST. *Clinical Allergy* 18: 481–490.

Hill DJ, Hosking CS, Yu Zhie C, *et al.* (1997) The frequency of food allergy in Australia and Asia. *Environmental Toxicology and Pharmacology* 4: 101–110.

Hill DJ, Hosking CS, de Benedictis FM, Oranje AP, Diepgen TL, Bauchau V. (2008) Confirmation of the association between high levels of immunoglobulin E food sensitization and eczema in infancy: an international study. *Clinical and Experimental Allergy* 38: 161–168.

Holmann A, Burks W. (2008) Pollen food syndrome: update on the allergens. *Current Allergy and Asthma Reports* 8: 413–417.

Holzhammer J, Wober C. (2006) Alimentary trigger factors that provoke migraine and tension-type headache. *Schmerz* 20: 151–159.

Hoppu U, Kalliomäki M, Isolauri E. (2000) Maternal diet rich in saturated fat during breastfeeding is associated with atopic sensitization of the infant. European *Journal of Clinical Nutrition* 54(9): 702–705.

Hoppu U, Rinne M, Salo-Vaananen P, Lampi AM, Piironen V, Isolauri E. (2005) Vitamin C in breast milk may reduce the risk of atopy in the infant. *European Journal of Clinical Nutrition* 59: 123–128.

Host A. (1994) Cows' milk protein allergy and intolerance in infancy. Some clinical, epidemiological and immunological aspects. *Pediatric Allergy and Immunology* 5: 1–36.

Host A, Halken S. (1990) A prospective study of cow milk allergy in Danish infants during the first 3 years of life. Clinical course in relation to clinical and immunological type of hypersensitivity reaction. *Allergy* 45(8): 587–596.

Host A, Koletzko B, Dreborg S, *et al.* (1999) Dietary products used in infants for treatment and prevention of food allergy. Joint Statement of the European Society for Paediatric Allergology and Clinical Immunology (ESPACI) Committee on Hypoallergenic Formulas and the European Society for Paediatric Gastroenterology, Hepatology and Nutrition (ESPGHAN) Committee on Nutrition. *Archives of Diseases in Childhood* 81: 80–84.

Host A, Halken S, Muraro A, *et al.* (2008) Dietary prevention of allergic diseases in infants and small children. *Pediatric Allergy and Immunology* 19: 1–4.

Hourihane JO, Kilburn SA, Dean P, Warner JO. (1997a) Clinical characteristics of peanut allergy. *Clinical and Experimental Allergy* 27: 634–639.

Hourihane JO'B, Bedwani SJ, Dean TP, Warner JO. (1997b) Randomised, double blind, crossover challenge study of allergenicity of peanut oils in subjects allergic to peanuts. *BMJ* 314: 1084.

Hypponen E, Sovio U, Wjst M, *et al.* (2004) Infant vitamin d supplementation and allergic conditions in adulthood: northern Finland birth cohort 1966. *Annals of the New York Academy of Science* 1037: 84–95.

Hypponen E, Berry DJ, Wjst M, Power C. (2009) Serum 25-hydroxyvitamin D and IgE – a significant but nonlinear relationship. *Allergy* 64: 613–620.

Infante S. Baeza ML, De Barrio M, Rubio M, Herrero T. (2003) Anaphylaxis due to caffeine. *Allergy* 58: 681–682.

Isolauri E, Turjanmaa K. (1996) Combined skin prick and patch testing enhances identification of food allergy in infants with atopic dermatitis. *Journal of Allergy and Clinical Immunology* 97: 9–15.

Isolauri E, Sutas Y, Salo MK, Isosomppi R, Kaila M. (1998) Elimination diet in cows' milk allergy: risk for impaired growth in young children. *Journal of Pediatrics* 132: 1004–1009.

Ivarsson A, Hernell O, Stenlund H, Persson LA. (2002) Breast-feeding protects against celiac disease. *American Journal of Clinical Nutrition* 75: 914–921.

Ives AJ, Hourihane JO'B. (2002) Evidence-based diagnosis of food allergy. *Current Paediatrics* 12: 357–364.

James JM, Crespo JF. (2007) Allergic reactions to foods by inhalation. *Current Allergy and Asthma Reports* 7: 167–174.

Jansen JJ, Kardinaal AF, Huijbers G, Vleg-Boerstra BJ, Martens BP, Ockhuizen T. (1994) Prevalence of food allergy and intolerance in the adult Dutch populations. *Journal of Allergy and Clinical Immunology* 93: 446–456.

Jansen SC, van-Dusseldorp M, Bottema KC, Dubois AEJ. (2003) Intolerance to dietary biogenic amines: a review. *Annals of Allergy, Asthma and Immunology* 91: 233–240.

Jarvinen KM, Beyer K, Vila L, Bardina L, Mishoe M, Sampson HA. (2007) Specificity of IgE antibodies to sequential epitopes of hen's egg ovomucoid as a marker for persistence of egg allergy. *Allergy* 62: 758–765.

Johansson SGO, Hourihane JO'B, Bousquet J, *et al.* (2001) A revised nomenclature for allergy. An EAACI position statement from the EAACI nomenclature task force. *Allergy* 56: 813–874.

Johansson SGO, Bieber T, Dhal R, *et al.* (2004) Revised nomenclature for allergy for global use: Report of the nomenclature review committee of the World Allergy Organization, October 2003. *Journal of Allergy and Clinical Immunology* 113: 832–836.

Kägi MK, Wüthrich B. (1993) Falafel burger anaphylaxis due to sesame seed allergy. *Annals of Allergy* 71: 127–129.

Kalogeromitros DC, Makris MP, Gregoriou SG, *et al.* (2005) Grape anaphylaxis: a study of 11 adult onset cases. *Allergy and Asthma Proceedings* 26: 53–58.

Kanny G, Moneret-Vautrin DA, Flabbee J, Beaudouin E, Morisset M, Thevenin F. (2001) Population study of food allergy in France. *Journal of Allergy and Clinical Immunology* 108: 133–140.

Katelaris HC. (2010) Food allergy and oral allergy or pollen-food syndrome. *Current Opinion in Allergy and Clinical Immunology* 10: 246–251.

Keet CA, Matsui EC, Dhillon G, Lenehan P, Paterakis M, Wood RA. (2009) The atural history of wheat allergy. *Annals of Allergy, Asthma and Immunology* 102: 410–415.

Kemp A. (2007) Egg allergy. *Pediatric Allergy and Immunology* 18: 696–702.

Kershaw R. (2009) Nutritional consequences of avoidance and practical approaches to nutritional management. In: Skypala IJ, Venter C (eds) *Food Hypersensitivity*. Oxford: Wiley Blackwell.

Kjellman NI. (1977) Atopic disease in seven-year-old children. Incidence in relation to family history. *Acta Paediatrica Scandinavica* 66: 465–471.

Kleine-Tebbe J, Wangorsch A, Vogel L, Crowell D, Haustein U, Veiths S. (2002) Severe oral allergy syndrome and anaphylactic reactions caused by a Bet v 1-related PR-10 protein in soybean, SAM22. *Journal of Allergy and Clinical Immunology* 110: 797–804

Kondo Y, Urisu A. (2009) Oral allergy syndrome. *Allergology International* 58(4):485–91.

Kowal-Krzysztof C, Schacterele-Richard-S, Schur-Peter-H, Komaroff-Anthony-L, DuBuske-Lawrence-M. (2002) Prevalence of allergen-specific IgE among patients with chronic fatigue syndrome. *Allergy and Asthma Proceedings* 23: 35–39.

Kramer MS, Kakuma R. (2006) Maternal dietary antigen avoidance during pregnancy or lactation, or both, for preventing or treating atopic disease in the child. *Cochrane Database of Systematic Reviews* 3: CD000133.

Kumar R, Kumari D, Srivastava P, *et al.* (2010) Identification of IgE-Mediated Food Allergy and Allergens in Older Children and Adults with Asthma and Allergic Rhinitis. *Indian Journal of Chest Disease and Allied Sciences* 52: 217–224.

Latcham F, Merino F, Lang A, *et al.* (2003) A consistent pattern of minor immunodeficiency and subtle enteropathy in children with multiple food allergy. *Journal of Pediatrics* 143: 39–47.

Leduc V, Moneret-Vautrin DA, Tzen JT, Morisset M, Guerin L, Kanny G. (2006) Identification of oleosins as major allergens in sesame seed allergic patients. *Allergy* 61: 349–356.

Lee KE, Hong JY, Son SM, *et al.* (2009) Differences between raw and variously cooked sesame seeds on the allergenicity. *Pediatric Allergy and Respiratory Disease* 19: 56–62.

Lehrer SB, Kim L, Rice T, Saidu J, Bell J, Martin R. (2007) Transfer of shrimp allergens to other foods through cooking oil. *Journal of Allergy and Clinical Immunology* 119: S112.

Lemerdy P, Moneret-Vautrin DA, Rance F, Kanny G, Parisot L. (2003) Prevalence of food allergies in paediatric and adult populations. *CICBAA Databank Alim- Inter* 8: 5–7.

L'Hocine L, Boye JI. (2007) Allergenicity of soybean: new developments in identification of allergenic. proteins, cross-reactivities and hypoallergenization technologies. *Critical Reviews in Food Science and Nutrition* 47: 127–143.

Lin J, Sampson HA. (2009) The role of immunoglobulin E-binding epitopes in the characterization of food allergy. *Current Opinion in Allergy and Clinical Immunology* 9: 357–363.

Linneberg A, Berg ND, Gonzalez-Quintela A, Vidal C, Elberling J. (2008) Prevalence of self-reported hypersensitivity symptoms following intake of alcoholic drinks. *Clinical and Experimental Allergy* 38: 145–151.

Litonjua AA, Rifas-Shiman SL, Ly NP, *et al.* (2006) Maternal antioxidant intake in pregnancy and wheezing illnesses in children at 2 y of age. *American Journal of Clinical Nutrition* 84: 903–911.

Lomer M. (2009) The role of food hypersensitivity in gastrointestinal disorders. In: Skypala IJ, Venter C (eds) *Food Hypersensitivity*. Oxford: Wiley Blackwell.

Luscombe S, Thurgood S. (2009) The role of food hypersensitivity in neurological disorders. In: Skypala IJ, Venter C (eds) *Food Hypersensitivity*. Oxford: Wiley Blackwell.

Maggi I, Parronchi P, Manetti R, *et al.* (1992) Reciprocal regulatory effects of IFNγ and IL-4 on the in vitro development of human Th1 and Th2 clones. *Journal of Immunology* 148: 2142–2147.

Maier AS, Chabanet C, Schaal B, Leathwood PD, Issanchou SN. (2008) Breastfeeding and experience with variety early in weaning increase infants' acceptance of new foods for up to two months. *Clinical Nutrition* 27: 849–857.

Maintz L, Novak N. (2007) Histamine and histamine intolerance. *American Journal of Clinical Nutrition* 85: 1185–1196.

Majamaa H, Moisio P, Holm K, Kautiainen H, Turjanmaa K. (1999a) Cows' milk allergy: diagnostic accuracy of skin prick and patch tests and specific IgE. *Allergy* 54: 346–351.

Majamaa H, Moisio P, Holm K, Turjanmaa K. (1999b) Wheat allergy: diagnostic accuracy of skin prick and patch tests and specific IgE. *Allergy* 54: 851–856.

Maleki SJ, Chung SY, Champagne ET, Raufman JP. (2000) The effects of roasting on the allergenic properties of peanut proteins. *Journal of Allergy and Clinical Immunology* 106: 763–768.

Malone MH, Metcalfe DD. (1986) Histamine in foods: its possible role in non-allergic adverse reactions to ingestants. *Allergy and Asthma Proceedings* 7: 241–245.

Maloney JM, Chapman MD, Sicherer SH (2006) Peanut allergen exposure through saliva: assessment and interventions to reduce exposure. *Journal of Allergy and Clinical Immunology* 118: 719–724.

Martindale S, McNeill G, Devereux G, Campbell D, Russell G, Seaton A. (2005) Antioxidant intake in pregnancy in relation to wheeze and eczema in the first two years of life. *American Journal of Respiratory and Critical Care Medicine* 171(2): 121–128.

Martínez San Ireneo M, Ibáñez MD, Sánchez JJ, Carnés J, Fernández-Caldas E. (2008) Clinical features of legume allergy in children from a Mediterranean area. *Annals of Allergy, Asthma and Immunology* 101: 179–184.

Mason SJ, Harris G, Blissett J. (2005) Tube feeding in infancy: implications for the development of normal eating and drinking skills. *Dysphagia* 20: 46–61.

Mathew RJ, Wilson WH. (1990) Behavioral and cerebrovascular effects of caffeine in patients with anxiety disorders. *Acta Psychiatrica Scandinavica* 82: 17–22.

McCann D, Barrett A, Cooper A, *et al.* (2007) Food additives and hyperactive behaviour in 3-year-old and 8/9-year-old children in the community: a randomised, double-blinded, placebo-controlled trial. *Lancet* 370: 1560–1567.

McGough N, Merrikin E, Kirk E. (2009) Food hypersensitivity involving cereals: coeliac disease. In: Skypala IJ, Venter C (eds) *Food Hypersensitivity*. Oxford: Wiley Blackwell.

Mimouni BA, Mimouni D, Mimouni M, Gdalevich M. (2002) Does breastfeeding protect against allergic rhinitis during childhood? A meta-analysis of prospective studies. *Acta Paediatrica* 91: 275–279.

Mittag D, Akkerdass J, Ballmer-Weber B, *et al.* (2004) Ara h 8, a Bet v 1-homologous allergen from peanut, is a major allergen in patients with combined birch pollen and peanut allergy. *Journal of Allergy and Clinical Immunology* 114: 1410–1417.

Miyake Y, Sasaki S, Tanaka K, Hirota Y. (2010) Dairy food, calcium and vitamin D intake in pregnancy, and wheeze and eczema in infants. *European Respiratory Journal* 35, 1228–1234.

Moneret-Vautrin DA, Morisset M. (2005) Adult food allergy. *Current Allergy and Asthma Report* 5: 80–85.

Monsbakken KW, Vandvik PO, Farup PG. (2006) Perceived food intolerance in subjects with irritable bowel syndrome – aetiology, prevalence and consequences. *European Journal of Clinical Nutrition* 60: 667–672.

Morisset M, Moneret-Vautrin D, Maadi F, *et al.* (2003) Prospective study of mustard allergy: first study with double-blind placebo-controlled food challenge trials (24 cases). *Allergy* 58, 295–299.

Mullins RJ. (2003) Anaphylaxis: risk factors for recurrence. *Clinical and Experimental Allergy* 33: 1033–1040.

Mullins RJ, Dear KB, Tang ML. (2009) Characteristics of childhood peanut allergy in the Australian Capital Territory, 1995 to 2007. *Journal of Allergy and Clinical Immunology* 123: 689–693.

Muraro A, Dreborg S, Halken S, *et al.* (2004) Dietary prevention of allergic diseases in infants and small children. Part III: Critical review of published peer-reviewed observational and interventional studies and final recommendations. *Pediatric Allergy and Immunology* 15: 291–307.

National Institute for Health and Care Excellence (NICE). (2007) Guideline 53: Chronic fatigue syndrome/myalgic encephalomyelitis (or encephalopathy). Diagnosis and management of CFS/ME in adults and children. Available at http://guidance.nice.org.uk/CG116.

Niggemann B. (2010) When is an oral food challenge positive? *Allergy* 65: 2–6.

Niggemann B, Beyer K. (2005) Diagnostic pitfalls in food allergy in children. *Allergy* 60: 104–107.

Niggemann B, Beyer K. (2007) Pitfalls in double-blind, placebo-controlled oral food challenges. *Allergy* 62: 729–732.

Niggemann B, Grüber C. (2004) Unproven diagnostic procedures in IgE-mediated allergic diseases. *Allergy* 59: 806–808.

Niggemann B, Rolinck-Werninghaus C, Mehl A, Binder C, Ziegert M, Beyer K. (2005) Controlled oral food challenges in children–when indicated, when superfluous? *Allergy* 60: 865–870.

Noel RJ, Putnam PE, Rothenberg ME. (2004) Eosinophilic esophagitis. *New England Journal of Medicine* 351: 940–941.

Noimark L, Cox HE. (2008) Nutritional problems related to food allergy in childhood. *Pediatric Allergy and Immunology* 19: 188–195.

Nowak-Wegrzyn A, Assa'ad AH, Bahna SL, Bock SA, Sicherer SH, Teuber SS. (2009) Work Group report: oral food challenge testing. *Journal of Allergy and Clinical Immunology* 123: S365–S383.

Osterballe M, Hansen TK, Mortz CG, Host A, Bindslev-Jensen C. (2005) The prevalence of food hypersensitivity in an unselected population of children and adults. *Pediatric Allergy and Immunology* 16(7): 567–573.

Osterballe M, Mortz CG, Hansen TK, Andersen KE, Bindslev-Jensen C. (2009) The prevalence of food hypersensitivity in young adults. *Pediatric Allergy and Immunology* 20: 686–689.

Ott H, Baron JM, Heise R, *et al.* (2008) Clinical usefulness of microarray-based IgE detection in children with suspected food allergy. *Allergy* 63: 1521–1528.

Palm M, Moneret-Vautrin DA, Kanny G, Denery-Papini S, Frémont S. (1999) Food allergy to egg and soy lecithins. *Allergy* 54: 1116–1117.

Palmer DJ, Gold MS, Makrides M. (2005) Effect of cooked and raw egg consumption on ovalbumin content of human milk: a randomized, double-blind, cross-over trial. *Clinical and Experimental Allergy* 35: 173–178.

Palosuo K, Alenius H, Varjonen E, *et al.* (1999) A novel wheat gliadin as a cause of exercise-induced anaphylaxis. *Journal of Allergy and Clinical Immunology* 103: 912–917.

Peeters KA, Nordlee JA, Penninks AH, *et al.* (2007) Lupine allergy: Not simply cross-reactivity with peanut or soy. *Journal of Allergy and Clinical Immunology* 120: 647–653.

Penard-Morand C, Raherison C, Kopferschmitt C, *et al.* (2005) Prevalence of food allergy and its relationship to asthma and allergic rhinitis in schoolchildren. *Allergy* 60: 1165–1171.

Pereira B, Venter C, Grundy J, Clayton CB, Arshad SH, Dean T. (2005) Prevalence of sensitization to food allergens, reported adverse reaction to foods, food avoidance, and food hypersensitivity among teenagers. *Journal of Allergy and Clinical Immunology* 116: 884–892.

Perry TT, Conover-Walker MK, Pomés A, Chapman MD, Wood RA. (2004) Distribution of peanut allergen in the environment. *Journal of Allergy and Clinical Immunology* 113: 973–976.

Pollak CP, Bright D. (2003) Caffeine consumption and weekly sleep patterns in US seventh-, eighth-, and ninth-Ggaders. *Pediatrics* 111: 42–46.

Pongracic JA, Ouyang F, Kim JS, Caruso D, Wang H, Wang X. (2007) Associations between prick skin tests and allergen specific IgE in children and adults. *Journal of Allergy and Clinical Immunology* 119: S121.

Poole JA, Barriga K, Leung DY, I. (2006) Timing of initial exposure to cereal grains and the risk of wheat allergy. *Pediatrics* 117: 2175–2182.

Potamianou-Taprantzi P, Zanikou S, Psarros P, Syrigou E., Manoussakis M, Saxoni-Papageorgiou P. (2002) Relationship between egg-specific serum IgE concentration and the outcome of specific provocation to egg allergic children. *Allergy* 57: 79.

Pourpak Z, Mansouri M, Mesdaghi M, Kazemnejad A, Farhoudi A. (2004) Wheat allergy: clinical and laboratory findings. *International Archives of Allergy and Immunology* 133: 168–173.

Pumphrey RS. (2000) Lessons for management of anaphylaxis from a study of fatal reactions. *Clinical and Experimental Allergy* 30: 1144–1150.

Pumphrey RS, Gowland MH. (2007) Further fatal allergic reactions to food in the United Kingdom, 1999–2006. *Journal of Allergy and Clinical Immunology* 119: 1018–1019.

Pumphrey RS, Stanworth SJ. (1996) The clinical spectrum of anaphylaxis in north-west England. *Clinical and Experimental Allergy* 26: 1364–1370.

Raithel M, Baenkler HW, Naegel A, *et al.* (2005) Significance of salicylate intolerance in diseases of the lower gastrointestinal tract. *Journal of Physiology and Pharmacology* 56: 89–102.

Rancé F, Dutau G. (1999) Peanut hypersensitivity in children. *Pediatric Pulmonology Supplements* 18: 165–167.

Rancé F, Juchet A, Brémont F, Dutau G. (1997) Correlations between skin prick tests using commercial extracts and fresh foods, specific IgE, and food challenges. *Allergy* 32: 1031–1035.

Reese I, Zuberbier T, Bunselmeyer B, *et al.* (2009) Diagnostic approach for suspected pseudoallergic reaction to food ingredients. *Journal Der Deutschen Dermatologischen Gesellschaft* 7: 70–77.

Roberts G, Patel N, Levi-Schaffer F, Habibi P, Lack G. (2003) Food allergy as a risk factor for life-threatening asthma in childhood: a case-controlled study. *Journal of Allergy and Clinical Immunology* 112: 168–174.

Romano A, Di Fonso M, Guiffreda F, *et al.* (2001) Food-dependent exercise-induced anaphylaxis: clinical and laboratory findings in 54 subjects. *International Archives in Allergy and Immunology* 125: 264–272.

Ross MP, Ferguson M, Street D, Klontz K, Schroeder T, Luccioli S. (2008) Analysis of food-allergic and anaphylactic events in the National Electronic Injury Surveillance System. *Journal of Allergy and Clinical Immunology* 121: 166–171.

Royal College of Physicians. (2003) *Allergy: The Unmet Needs.* Report of a working party. London: RCP.

Salcedo G, Sanchez-Monge R, Diaz-Perales A, Garcia-Casado G, Barber D. (2004) Plant non-specific lipid transfer proteins as food and pollen allergens. *Clinical and Experimental Allergy* 34: 1336–1341.

Sampson HA. (2004) Update on food allergy. *Journal of Allergy and Clinical Immunology* 113: 805–819.

Sampson MA, Munoz-Furlong Anne, Sicherer SH. (2006) Risk-taking and coping strategies of adolescents and young adults with food allergy. *Journal of Allergy and Clinical Immunology* 117: 1440–1445.

Sampson HA, Gerth van Wijk R, Bindslev-Jensen C, *et al.* (2012) Standardizing double-blind, placebo-controlled oral food challenges: American Academy of Allergy, Asthma & Immunology-European Academy of Allergy and Clinical Immunology PRACTALL consensus report. *Journal of Allergy and Clinical Immunology* 130: 1260–1274.

Savage JH, Kaeding AJ, Matsui EC, Wood RA. (2010) The natural history of soy allergy. *Journal of Allergy and Clinical Immunology* 125: 683–636.

Scala E, Alessandri C, Bernardi ML, *et al.* (2010) Cross-sectional survey on immunoglobulin E reactivity in 23 077 subjects using an allergenic molecule-based microarray detection system. *Clinical and Experimental Allergy* 40: 911–921.

Schab DW, Trinh NT. (2004) Do artificial food colours promote hyperactivity in children with hyperactive syndromes? A meta-analysis of double-blind placebo-controlled trials. *Developmental and Behavioural Pediatrics* 25: 423–434.

Schäfer T, Böhler E, Ruhdorfer S, *et al.* (2001) Epidemiology of food allergy/food intolerance in adults: associations with other manifestations of atopy. *Allergy* 56: 1172–1179.

Schrander JJ, van den Bogart JP, Forget PP, Schrander-Stumpel CT, Kuijten RH, Kester AD. (1993) Cow's milk protein intolerance in infants under 1 year of age: a prospective epidemiological study. *European Journal of Pediatrics* 152(8): 640–644.

Scotter MJ, Roberts DPT, Wilson LA, Howard FAC, Davis J, Mansell N. (2007) Free salicylic acid and acetyl salicylic acid content of foods using gas chromatography-mass spectrometry. *Food Chemistry* 105: 273–279.

Seitz CS, Pfeuffer P, Raith P, Bröcker E-B, Trautmann A. (2008) Food allergy in adults: An over- or underrated problem? *Deutsches Arzteblatt International* 105: 715–723.

Shadick NA, Laing MH, Partridge AJ, *et al.* (1999) The natural history of food-dependant exercise-induced anaphylaxis: Survey results from 10-year follow-up study. *Journal of Allergy and Clinical Immunology* 104: 123–127.

Sicherer SH, Sampson HA. (2000) Peanut and tree nut allergy. *Current Opinion in Pediatrics* 12: 567–573.

Sicherer SH, Sampson HA. (2006) 9. Food allergy. *Journal of Allergy and Clinical Immunology* 117(2 Suppl Mini-Primer): S470–475.

Sicherer S, Sampson H, Burks A. (2000) Peanut and soy allergy: a clinical and therapeutic dilemma. *Allergy* 55: 515–521.

Sicherer SH, Furlong TJ, Munoz Furlong A, Burks AW, Sampson HA. (2001a) A voluntary registry for peanut and tree nut allergy: characteristics of the first 5149 registrants. *Journal of Allergy and Clinical Immunology* 108: 128–132.

Sicherer SH, Noone SA, Muñoz-Furlong A. (2001b) The impact of childhood food allergy on quality of life. *Annals of Allergy, Asthma and Immunology* 87: 461–464.

Sicherer SH, Munoz-Furlong A, Sampson HA. (2004) Prevalence of seafood allergy in the United States determined by a random telephone survey. *Journal of Allergy and Clinical Immunology* 114: 159–165.

Sicherer SH, Muñoz-Furlong A, Godbold JH, Sampson HA. (2010) US prevalence of self-reported peanut, tree nut, and sesame allergy: 11-year follow-up. *Journal of Allergy and Clinical Immunology* 125: 1322–1326.

Skolnick HS, Conover-Walker MK, Koerner CB, Sampson HA, Wesley Burks W, Wood RA. (2001) The natural history of peanut allergy. *Journal of Allergy and Clinical Immunology* 107: 367–374.

Skripak JM, Matsui EC, Mudd K, Wood RA. (2007) The natural history of IgE-mediated cows' milk allergy. *Journal of Allergy and Clinical Immunology* 120: 1172–1177.

Skypala I. (2011) Adverse food reactions – an emerging issue for adults. *Journal of the American Dietetic Association* 111: 1877–1891.

Skypala IJ, Venter C. (2009) *Food Hypersensitivity.* Oxford: Wiley Blackwell.

Wright T. (2006). *Food Allergies.* Class Publishing.

Skypala IJ, Calderon MA, Leeds AR, Emery P, Till SJ, Durham SR. (2011) Development and validation of a structured questionnaire for the diagnosis of oral allergy syndrome in subjects with seasonal allergic rhinitis during the UK birch pollen season. *Clinical and Experimental Allergy* 41: 1001–1011.

Spergel JM, Beausoleil JL, Mascarenhas M, Liacouras CA. (2002) The use of skin prick tests and patch tests to identify causative foods in eosinophilic esophagitis. *Journal of Allergy and Clinical Immunology* 109: 363–368.

Sporik R, Hill D. (1996) Allergy to peanut, nuts and sesame seed in Australian children. *BMJ* 313: 1477–1478.

Stapel S, Asero R, Ballmer-Webber B, *et al.* (2008) Testing for IgG4 against foods is not recommended as a diagnostic tool: EAACI Task Force Report. *Allergy* 63: 793–796.

Stutius LM, Sheehan WJ, Rangsithienchai P, *et al.* (2010) Characterizing the relationship between sesame, coconut, and nut allergy in children. *Pediatric Allergy and Immunology* 21: 1114–1118.

Sugiura K, Sugiura M. (2010) Soy sauce allergy. *Journal of the European Academy of Dermatology and Venereology* 24: 852–855.

Sutton BJ, Gould HJ. (1993) The human IgE network. *Nature* 366: 421–428.

Swain AR, Dutton SP, Truswell AS. (1985) Salicylates in foods. *Journal of the American Dietetic Association* 85: 950–960.

Szépfalusi Z, Ebner C, Pandjaitana R, *et al.* (1994) Egg yolk α-livetin (chicken serum albumin) is a cross-reactive allergen in the bird-egg syndrome. *Journal of Allergy and Clinical Immunology* 93: 932–942.

Tariq SM, Matthews SM, Hakin EA, Arshad SH. (2000) Egg allergy in infancy predicts respiratory allergic disease by 4 years of age. *Pediatric Allergy and Immunology* 11: 162–167.

Taylor SL, Bush RK, Nordlee JA. Sulfites. (2003) Sulfites. In: Metcalfe DD, Sampson HJ, Simon RA (eds) *Food Allergy: Adverse Reactions to Foods and Food Additives.* 324–341. Oxford: Blackwell Publishing Ltd, pp. 324–341.

Timbo B, Koehler KM, Wolyniak C, Klontz KC. (2004) Sulfites – a food and drug administration review of recalls and reported adverse events. *Journal of Food Protection* 67: 1086–1091.

Vally H, Thompson PJ. (2001) Role of sulfite additives in wine induced asthma: single dose and cumulative dose studies. *Thorax* 56: 763–769.

van Odijk J, Ahlstedt S, Bengtsson U, Borres MP, Hulthen L. (2005) Double-blind placebo-controlled challenges for peanut allergy the efficiency of blinding procedures and the allergenic activity of peanut availability in the recipes. *Allergy* 60: 602–605.

Vandenplas Y, Koletzko S, Isolauri E, *et al*. (2007) Guidelines for the diagnosis and management of cows' milk protein allergy in infants. *Archives of Disease in Childhood* 92: 902–908.

Vassallo MF, Camargo CA Jr. (2010) Potential mechanisms for the hypothesized link between sunshine, vitamin D, and food allergy in children. *Journal of Allergy and Clinical Immunology* 126: 217–222.

Vassilopoulou E, Douladiris N, Sakellariou A, *et al*. (2010) Evaluation and standardisation of different matrices used for double-blind placebo-controlled food challenges to fish. *Journal of Human Nutrition and Dietetics* 23: 544–549.

Venema DP, Hollmann PCH, Janssen PLTMK. (1996) Determination of acetylsalicylic and salicylic acid in foods, using HPLC with fluorescence detection. *Journal of Agriculture, Food and Chemistry* 44: 1762–1767.

Ventner C. (2007) Food hypersensitivity. In: Thomas B, Bishop J (eds) *Manual of Dietetic Practice*, 4th edn. Oxford: Blackwell Publishing.

Venter C, Pereira B, Grundy J, Clayton CB, Arshad SH, Dean T. (2006a) Prevalence of sensitization reported and objectively assessed food hypersensitivity amongst six year old children: a population-based study. *Pediatric Allergy and Immunology* 17: 356–363.

Venter C, Pereira B, Grundy J, *et al*. (2006b) Incidence of parentally reported and clinically diagnosed food hypersensitivity in the first year of life. *Journal of Allergy and Clinical Immunology* 117: 1118–1124.

Venter C, Pereira B, Voigt K, *et al*. (2007a) Comparison of open and double-blind placebo-controlled food challenges in diagnosis of food hypersensitivity amongst children. *Journal of Human Nutrition and Dietetics* 20: 565–579.

Venter C, Pereira B, Voigt K, *et al*. (2007b) Prevalence and cumulative incidence of food hypersensitivity in the first three years of life. *Allergy* 63: 354–359.

Venter C, Vlieg-Boerstra B, Carling A. (2009) The diagnosis of food hypersensitivity . In: Skypala IJ, Venter C (eds) *Food Hypersensitivity*. Oxford: Wiley Blackwell.

Venter C, Hasan Arshad S, Grundy J, *et al*. (2010) Time trends in the prevalence of peanut allergy: three cohorts of children from the same geographical location in the UK. *Allergy* 65: 103–108.

Vickerstaff Joneja J. (1988) *Dietary Management of Food Allergies and Intolerances*, 2nd edn. Vancouver: JA Hall.

Vickerstaff Joneja JM, Carmona-Silva C. (2001) Outcome of a histamine-restricted diet based on chart audit. *Journal of Nutritional and Environmental Medicine* 11: 249–262.

Vieira MC, Morais MB, Spolidoro JV, *et al*. (2010) A survey on clinical presentation and nutritional status of infants with suspected cow' milk allergy. *BMC Pediatrics* 23 10–25.

Vierk KA, Koehler KM, Fein SB, Street DA. (2007) Prevalence of self-reported food allergy in American adults and use of food labels. *Journal of Allergy and Clinical Immunology* 119: 1504–1510.

Vieths S, Luttkopf D, Reindl J, Anliker MD, Wuthrich B, Ballmer-Weber BK. (2002) Allergens in celery and zucchini. *Allergy* 57: 100–105.

Vila L, Beyer K, Järvinen KM, Chatchatee P, Bardina L, Sampson HA. (2001) Role of conformational and linear epitopes in the achievement of tolerance in cows' milk allergy. *Clinical and Experimental Allergy* 31: 1599–1606.

Vlieg-Boerstra BJ, Bijleveld CM, van der HS, *et al*. (2004) Development and validation of challenge materials for double-blind, placebo-controlled food challenges in children. *Journal of Allergy and Clinical Immunology* 113: 341–346.

Vocks E, Borga A, Szliska C, *et al*. (1993) Common allergenic structures in hazelnut, rye grain, sesame seeds, kiwi, and poppy seeds. *Allergy* 48: 168–172.

von Berg A, Koletzko S, Grubl A, *et al*. (2003) The effect of hydrolyzed cows' milk formula for allergy prevention in the first year of life: The German Infant Nutritional Intervention Study, a randomized double-blind trial. *Journal of Allergy and Clinical Immunology* 111: 533–534.

von Berg A, Koletzko S, Filipiak-Pittroff B, *et al*. (2007) Certain hydrolyzed formulas reduce the incidence of atopic dermatitis but not that of asthma: three-year results of the German Infant Nutritional Intervention Study. *Journal of Allergy and Clinical Immunology* 119: 718–725.

von Berg A, Filipiak-Pittroff B, Kramer U, *et al*. (2008) Preventive effect of hydrolyzed infant formulas persists until age 6 years: long-term results from the German Infant Nutritional Intervention Study (GINI). *Journal of Allergy and Clinical Immunology* 121: 1442–1447.

Wagner S, Breiteneder H. (2002) The latex-fruit syndrome. *Biochemical Society Transactions* 30: 935–940.

Werfel T, Erdmann S, Fuchs T, *et al*. (2009) Approach to suspected food allergy in atopic dermatitis. Guideline of the Task Force on Food Allergy of the German Society of Allergology and Clinical Immunology (DGAKI) and the Medical Association of German Allergologists (ADA) and the German Society of Pediatric Allergology (GPA). *Journal Der Deutschen Dermatologischen Gesellschaft* 7: 265–271.

Wright T. (2006). Food allergies. Class Publishing.

Wuthrich B, Schmid A, Walther B, Seiber R. (2005) Milk consumption does not lead to mucus production or occurrence of asthma. *Journal of the American College of Nutrition* 24: 547S–555S.

Yang Mk, Lee SH, Kim TW, *et al*. (2008) Epidemiologic and clinical features of anaphylaxis in Korea. *Annals of Allergy, Asthma and Immunology* 100: 31–36.

Young E, Patel S, Stoneham M, Rona R, Wilkinson JD. (1987) The prevalence of reaction to food additives in a survey population. *Journal of the Royal College of Physicians London* 21: 241–247.

Young E, Stoneham MD, Petuckevitch A, Barton J, Rana R. (1994) A population study of food intolerance. *Lancet* 343: 1127–1130.

Zak DL, Keeney PG. (1976) Changes in cocoa proteins during ripening of fruit, fermentation and further processing of cocoa beans. *Journal of Agriculture, Food and Chemistry* 24: 483–486.

Zeiger RS, Sampson HA, Bock SA, *et al*. (1999) Soy allergy in infants and children with IgE-associated cows' milk allergy. *Journal of Pediatrics* 134: 614–622.

Zijlstra WT, Flinterman AE, Soeters L, *et al*. (2009) Parental anxiety before and after food challenges in children with suspected peanut and hazelnut allergy. *Pediatric Allergy and Immunology* 21: e439–445.

Ziska LH, Beggs PJ. (2012) Anthropogenic climate change and allergen exposure: The role of plant biology. *Journal of Allergy and Clinical Immunology* 129: 27–32.

Zuberbier T, Edenharter G, Worm M, *et al*. (2004) Prevalence of adverse reactions to food in Germany – a population study. *Allergy* 59: 338–345.

Zuidmeer L, Goldhahn K, Rona RJ, *et al*. (2008) The prevalence of plant food allergies: A systematic review. *Journal of Allergy and Clinical Immunology* 121: 1210–1218.

Zutavern A, Brockow I, Schaaf B, *et al*. (2008) Timing of solid food introduction in relation to eczema, asthma, allergic rhinitis, and food and inhalant sensitization at the age of 6 years: results from the prospective birth cohort study LISA. *Pediatrics* 121: e44–e52.

7.11.3   HIV and AIDS
Karen Klassen

Key points

■ Good nutritional status is important for a healthy immune system.

■ Human immunodeficiency virus (HIV) disease can present with a variety of nutritional problems.

■ Nutritional interventions for people with HIV infection can include management of weight loss, micronutrient deficiencies, gastrointestinal complaints and metabolic diseases, such as dyslipidaemia, insulin resistance and osteoporosis.

The nutritional status of patients with human immunodeficiency virus (HIV) infection remains an important part of the medical management of HIV care worldwide. Both over- and under-nutrition can have important consequences for the health and wellbeing of patients. Although weight loss is much less common since effective antiretroviral therapy (ART) has been available, it is still highly prevalent, and even small amounts of unintentional weight loss may increase the risk of morbidity and mortality in this population. In juxtaposition to this is the rapidly increasing occurrence of obesity and metabolic complications. The combination of HIV infection, ART and lifestyle factors are contributing to the increased risk of cardiovascular disease and events, diabetes and osteoporosis. Nutrition intervention is the first line in the management for all these problems and is therefore crucial for both prevention and treatment in the HIV setting.

Some of the aims of dietetic intervention and nutritional care of patients with HIV infection are:

• Maintaining or achieving a healthy weight for the individual.
• Promoting a well balanced diet in order to optimise macro- and micro-nutrient status.
• Preventing or managing malnutrition and opportunistic infections.
• Preventing food borne illness.
• Improving and supporting quality of life.
• Increasing nutrition self management skills for people living with HIV disease and/or their carers.
• Decreasing hospitalisations, emergency room visits, morbidity and mortality, and cost of care.
• Decreasing or delaying invasive or expensive treatments by providing early, appropriate nutrition interventions.
• Improving tolerance and adherence to medications.
• Preventing or managing metabolic and morphological comorbidities.

The HIV virus was isolated and identified as responsible for acquired immune deficiency syndrome (AIDS) in 1983. HIV infection does not immediately cause AIDS; however, it grows in CD4 T cells, a subset of lymphocytes, and causes them to decrease in most instances, although the rate of decline will vary among individuals. The first antiretroviral medicine for HIV was zidovudine (also known as AZT) and it became available in 1987. Since that time, the development and availability of other ART has been rapidly evolving.

In 2009, it was estimated that 33.3 million people around the world were living with HIV infection. Just over half of all adults living with HIV are women, and 2.6 million children are living with HIV, but a further 16.6 million have been orphaned due to AIDS. According to the Joint United Nations Programme on HIV/AIDS (UNAIDS, 2010), as of 2010, the overall growth of the global AIDS epidemic appears to have stabilised. It was thought to have peaked in 1999, and since then, the overall number of new infections has decreased. Although the rate of new HIV infections has decreased, sub Saharan Africa still bears an inordinate share of the global HIV burden, with 22.5 million (68% of the global total) people there living with HIV infection in 2009.

In the UK, as a direct result of reduced mortality and improved life expectancy with HIV (May *et al.*, 2011), the number of HIV positive people is increasing, and by 2012 it is estimated that 100 000 people will be living with HIV. By 2015, 50% of people living with HIV in the UK will be over the age of 50 years (Health Protection Agency, 2010). While this number is relatively low, it has increased substantially since the 1990s. New diagnoses among men who have sex with men (MSM) remains high. More than half (51%) of HIV diagnosed individuals accessing HIV care in 2009 were infected via heterosexual sex (12 290 men and 21 020 women), of whom 66% were black African and 21% were white (Table 7.11.18). Of those individuals who attended clinics for HIV care, 43% were MSM and 88% of these were white. A small proportion of individuals were infected through injecting drugs (2%, 1550) and mother to child transmission (2%, 1380).

Diagnosis and disease classification

Diagnosis of HIV is based on detecting anti-HIV antibodies in the serum. The enzyme linked immunoabsorbent antibody (ELISA) test, also known as enzyme immunoassay (EIA), was the first HIV test to be widely used; other HIV tests are now available. Most people will

Table 7.11.18 Ethnicity of HIV infected individuals seen for care in the UK

Ethnicity	2000	2009
White	66.5%	52.0%
Black Caribbean	2.5%	3.0%
Black African	23.3%	36.2%
Asian/Oriental	2.4%	3.0%
Other/mixed	6.4%	5.9%

Table 7.11.19 CDC classification system for HIV infected adults and adolescents

CD4 cell category	Clinical category		
	A Asymptomatic, acute HIV or PGL	B* Symptomatic conditions, not A or C	C# AIDS indicator conditions
≥500 cells/μL	A1	B1	C1
200–499 cells/μL	A2	B2	C2
<200 cells/μL	A3	B3	C3

Patients in shadedd categories are considered to have AIDS. PGL persistent generalised lymphadenopathy; CDC, USA Centers for Disease Control.

develop detectable levels of antibodies within 3 months of acquiring HIV. If an HIV test is positive, the most common secondary tests are CD4 T cell count and viral load. The CD4 T cell count is a reliable indicator of the risk of acquiring opportunistic infections and is monitored over time. Viral load is the amount of virus in the peripheral blood and is used as a surrogate marker of viral replication rate. These are also used as markers to evaluate the effectiveness of ART. These markers are strongly associated with clinical response; however, they should be interpreted along with an individual's clinical condition (Gazzard et al., 2008).

HIV disease staging and classification systems have been developed by the Centers for Disease Control (CDC) in the USA (Castro et al., 1993) and the World Health Organization (WHO, 2007). These staging systems are used to track and monitor the HIV epidemic, as well as provide clinicians and patients with information about HIV disease stage and clinical management. The WHO system can be used in resource constrained settings, which may not have access to CD4 cell counts or other laboratory parameters. The CDC disease staging system was developed in 1986 and most recently revised in 1993, and it assesses the severity of HIV disease by CD4 cell count and the presence of specific HIV related conditions (Table 7.11.19).

Category B symptomatic conditions

These are symptomatic conditions occurring in an HIV infected adolescent or adult that meet at least one of the following criteria; including, but are not limited to, the following:

- Bacillary angiomatosis.
- Oropharyngeal candidiasis (thrush).
- Vulvovaginal candidiasis, persistent or resistant.
- Pelvic inflammatory disease (PID).
- Cervical dysplasia (moderate or severe) or cervical carcinoma in situ.
- Hairy leucoplakia, oral.
- Herpes zoster (shingles), involving two or more episodes or at least one dermatome.
- Idiopathic thrombocytopenic purpura.
- Constitutional symptoms, such as fever (>38.5°C) or diarrhoea lasting >1 month.
- Peripheral neuropathy.

Category C AIDS indicator conditions

- Bacterial pneumonia, recurrent (two or more episodes in 12 months).
- Candidiasis of the bronchi, trachea or lungs.
- Candidiasis, oesophageal.
- Cervical carcinoma, invasive, confirmed by biopsy.
- Coccidioidomycosis, disseminated or extrapulmonary.
- Cryptococcosis, extrapulmonary.
- Cryptosporidiosis, chronic intestinal (>1 month in duration).
- Cytomegalovirus disease (other than the liver, spleen or nodes).
- Encephalopathy, HIV related.
- Herpes simplex: chronic ulcers (>1 month in duration), or bronchitis, pneumonitis or esophagitis.
- Histoplasmosis, disseminated or extrapulmonary.
- Isosporiasis, chronic intestinal (>1 month duration).
- Kaposi sarcoma.
- Lymphoma, Burkitt's, immunoblastic or primary central nervous system.
- Mycobacterium avium complex (MAC) or Mycobacterium kansasii, disseminated or extrapulmonary.
- Mycobacterium tuberculosis, pulmonary or extrapulmonary.
- Mycobacterium, other species or unidentified species, disseminated or extrapulmonary.
- Pneumocystis jiroveci (formerly carinii) pneumonia (PCP).
- Progressive multifocal leucoencephalopathy (PML).
- Salmonella septicaemia, recurrent (non-typhoid).
- Toxoplasmosis of brain.
- Wasting syndrome caused by HIV (involuntary weight loss of >10% of baseline body weight) associated with either chronic diarrhoea (two or more loose stools/day for ≥1 month) or chronic weakness and documented fever for 1 month or longer.

Clinical investigation and management

There is no cure for HIV itself but treatment is available. Life expectancy in people treated for HIV infection has increased following the availability and widespread use of ART; however, it still appears to be shorter than that of the general population in the UK (May *et al.*, 2011). If treatment is started early and taken correctly, overall health and life expectancy are greatly improved. However, in the UK, half of adults are diagnosed with HIV at a late stage of infection (CD4 counts <350 cells/mm³ within 3 months of diagnosis). People diagnosed soon after infection may not need to start treatment straight away, depending on their clinical condition and/or CD4 cell counts. Treatment options have improved greatly over recent years; complex regimens with many side effects are being replaced with just one or two pills once or twice a day. Someone who is diagnosed now will have a different experience from someone who has been living with HIV for some time and gone through many different treatment options. Some people suffer side effects with ART, including nausea, diarrhoea, fatigue and headaches, especially in the first few weeks after starting treatment. Other side effects can include metabolic diseases (covered later in this chapter), peripheral neuropathy, lactic acidosis, pancreatitis, mitochondrial toxicity and hepatotoxicity. In some cases, treatment causes changes in body shape, depression and mental health issues. Other people find they are able to lead a very healthy life with HIV and may not suffer the same side effects. As well as managing medications and its side effects, social care, peer support and counselling are all important forms of support for people with HIV.

The British HIV Association has developed guidelines (Table 7.11.20) on treating HIV infection (Gazzard *et al.*, 2008), which provide the rationale for the treatment with antiretroviral drugs as follows:

Table 7.11.20 Recommendations for when to initiate therapy

Presentation	When to treat
Primary HIV infection	Treatment in clinical trial Or when there is neurological involvement Or when CD4 <200 cells/mL for >3 months Or AIDS defining illness
Established HIV infection	
CD4 <200 cells/mL	Treat
CD4 201–350 cells/mL	Treat as soon as possible when patient ready
CD4 351–500 cells/mL	Treat in specific situations with higher risk of clinical events – see text
CD4 >500 cells/mL	Consider enrolment into 'when to start' trial
AIDS diagnosis	Treat (except for tuberculosis when CD4 >350 cells/mL)

- Preservation of specific anti-HIV immune responses that would otherwise be lost, and which are associated with long term non-progression in untreated individuals.
- Reduction in morbidity associated with high viraemia and CD4 depletion during acute infection.
- Reduction in the risk of onward transmission of HIV.

There are currently seven different classes of antiretroviral drugs, each targeting the virus at different stages of its life cycle (Figure 7.11.5). The drug classes are:

- Nucleoside reverse transcriptase inhibitors (NsRTIs).
- Nucleotide reverse transcriptase inhibitor (NtRTI).
- Non-nucleoside reverse transcriptase inhibitors (NNRTIs).
- Protease inhibitors (PIs).
- Fusion inhibitor.
- CCR5 antagonist.
- Integrase inhibitor.

For further reading on the pharmacology and use of ART, see Chen *et al.* (2007).

Public health aspects and prevention

Transmission

The HIV virus is found in the blood and other body fluids, such as semen, vaginal fluid and breast milk; the virus does not survive for long outside the body. The most common form of transmission is through sexual contact, but it can also be transmitted through sharing needles and mother to child transmission via breastfeeding or during delivery.

Stigma

AIDS related stigma and discrimination refer to prejudice, negative attitudes, abuse and maltreatment directed at people living with HIV/AIDS (AVERT). Examples of this are being shunned by family, peers and the wider community; poor treatment in healthcare and education settings; an erosion of rights; and psychological damage. These can negatively affect the success of HIV testing and treatment.

Although the awareness and understanding of HIV have improved in the UK over the past decade, stigma and discrimination still exist and can come from family, friends and healthcare workers. The National AIDS Trust surveyed HIV positive people and found that one in three reported had experienced discrimination in the UK. As a healthcare professional, it is essential to understand how HIV is transmitted, to use universal precautions with all patients [as it is estimated that one-quarter of people infected with HIV in the UK are unaware of their diagnosis (Health Protection Agency, 2010)] and to demonstrate non-judgemental attitudes towards all patients.

Nutritional assessment

Nutritional assessment of patients living with HIV infection may vary depending on the reason for referral and

Stages of HIV replication
1. HIV enters a CD4 cell.
2. HIV is a retrovirus, meaning that its genetic information is stored on single-stranded RNA instead of the double-stranded DNA found in most organisms.
3. HIV DNA enters the nucleus of the CD4 cell and inserts itself into the cell's DNA. HIV DNA then instructs the cell to make many copies of the original virus.
4. New virus particles are assembled and leave the cell, ready to infect other CD4 cells.

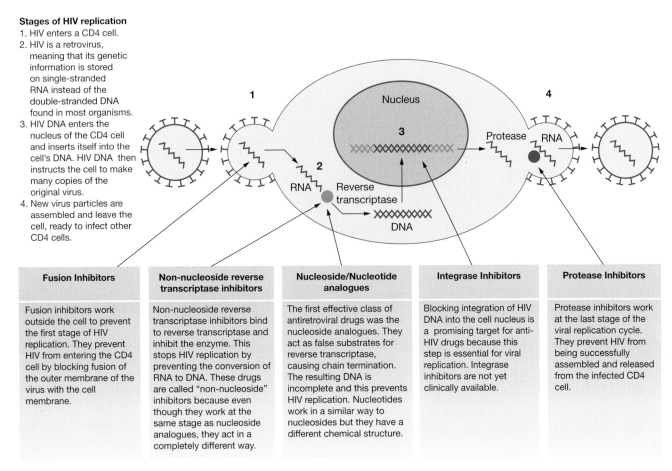

Fusion Inhibitors	Non-nucleoside reverse transcriptase inhibitors	Nucleoside/Nucleotide analogues	Integrase Inhibitors	Protease Inhibitors
Fusion inhibitors work outside the cell to prevent the first stage of HIV replication. They prevent HIV from entering the CD4 cell by blocking fusion of the outer membrane of the virus with the cell membrane.	Non-nucleoside reverse transcriptase inhibitors bind to reverse transcriptase and inhibit the enzyme. This stops HIV replication by preventing the conversion of RNA to DNA. These drugs are called "non-nucleoside" inhibitors because even though they work at the same stage as nucleoside analogues, they act in a completely different way.	The first effective class of antiretroviral drugs was the nucleoside analogues. They act as false substrates for reverse transcriptase, causing chain termination. The resulting DNA is incomplete and this prevents HIV replication. Nucleotides work in a similar way to nucleosides but they have a different chemical structure.	Blocking integration of HIV DNA into the cell nucleus is a promising target for anti-HIV drugs because this step is essential for viral replication. Integrase inhibitors are not yet clinically available.	Protease inhibitors work at the last stage of the viral replication cycle. They prevent HIV from being successfully assembled and released from the infected CD4 cell.

Figure 7.11.5   Actions of drugs that target HIV replication (source: Boehringer Ingelheim 2009. Reproduced with permission of Boehringer Ingelheim Pty Ltd, Germany)

the individual's clinical condition. This section will highlight aspects of nutritional assessment that are specific to working with patients with HIV.

Anthropometry and related tests

Routine nutritional assessment includes anthropometric measurements, and several HIV guidance documents recommend these at the time of starting ART and annually thereafter (Asboe et al., 2011; Lundgren et al., 2008). Using a variety of anthropometric measurements (Table 7.11.21) is helpful in order to adequately assess fat distribution changes and muscle mass loss. Fat free mass (FFM) and fat mass are generally lower in people with HIV (Fields-Gardner et al., 2010). Studies evaluating anthropometry with gold standard measurements have found that anthropometry measurements correlated well with magnetic resonance imaging (MRI) (Scherzer et al., 2008). Furthermore, they found that simple anthropometric measurements, such as mid arm muscle circumference and mid thigh muscle circumference, were associated with health risk indicators almost as strongly as MRI based measures.

In addition to anthropometric measurements, physical examination can provide additional evidence of nutritional status.

Signs of malnutrition can be:

- Easily plucked or falling out hair.
- Poor skin pallor or turgor, or dry, flaky, scaly skin.
- Scooped or cracking nails.
- Muscle wasting and weakness (can be visually determined by looking at the following muscles: temporalis, deltoids, biceps, quadriceps).
- Loss of fat stores can be easily seen by looking at the fat pads under the eyes and by pinching (lightly) the skin behind the triceps.

Biochemical and haematological tests

Biochemistry and haematology assessment will depend on the patient's clinical condition and varies widely as patients with HIV present with a variety of clinical needs (Table 7.11.22).

Clinical assessment

Clinical assessment will include:

- Current medications (including side effects) and medication history.
- Use of supplements, vitamins, herbs and over the counter medicines.

Table 7.11.21 Anthropometric and related assessments of individuals with HIV infection

Measurements	Indication of
Anthropometric	
Weight	Overall nutritional status; however, must be interpreted in individuals with caution and with a view to evaluating other aspects of body composition
Body mass index	Good marker of nutritional status in populations; can determine if overweight, obese or underweight; interpret with caution in individuals
Waist circumference	A good correlate of visceral fat and an indicator of metabolic syndrome
Mid upper arm circumference	Reflection of muscle and subcutaneous fat stores; can compare with reference values and evaluate changes over time
Triceps skinfold	Subcutaneous fat stores; can compare against reference values and serial changes in an individual
Mid arm muscle circumference	A good marker of lean body mass; useful in assessing changes in individuals
Hip circumference	On its own can reflect buttock muscle and fat stores and can be monitored serially in individuals
Waist to hip ratio	Use with reference values, but interpret in light of potential fat loss from lipoatrophy
Other skinfold measurements	Can be used to assess overall subcutaneous fat and estimate total body fat percentage
Other measurements	
Bioelectrical impedance analysis	Low phase angles have been shown to be of prognostic relevance in HIV infected patients (Kyle et al., 2004); however, are not sensitive to detect changes in body shape, nor should be used to evaluate fat atrophy (Schwenk et al., 2001). Can measure body cell mass, which is a component of some definitions of HIV related wasting (see Table 7.11.23)
Handgrip strength	A measure of muscle strength; correlates well with nutritional status; however interpret with caution as limited reference values, and consider factors such as mood, mobility and peripheral neuropathy

- Current medical status (opportunistic infections and comorbid conditions) and medical history.
- Blood pressure.
- Appetite, nausea, vomiting, early satiety, chewing and swallowing difficulties (note dentition).
- Bowel history (including frequency and consistency) and other changes in gastrointestinal function.
- Use risk calculators to calculate 10-year risk of cardiovascular disease (e.g. www.patient.co.uk/doctor/Primary-Cardiovascular-Risk-Calculator.htm) or 10-year risk of fracture (www.shef.ac.uk/FRAX/).

Dietary assessment

The dietary assessment should include:

- A record of dietary intake and food patterns:
  - Depending on the reason for referral, a variety of dietary history tools may be employed, e.g. 24-hour recall, food frequency questionnaire and usual intake pattern.
  - A recall of usual intake in 24 hours is also a good way to check medication adherence.
- Food allergies and intolerances.
- Other lifestyle factors should be included as a part of the dietary assessment:
  - Alcohol intake.
  - Smoking (history and frequency).
  - Substance abuse (history and frequency.
  - Eating out.
  - Erratic meal patterns.
- Nutritional knowledge.

Economic and social assessment

Patients living with HIV infection come from wide socio-economic and ethnic backgrounds, and individual assessment is crucial. Common characteristics to consider include:

- *Psychosocial factors* – depression, substance abuse, dementia and other psychiatric problems that may impede appetite or the ability to prepare meals.
- *Educational factors* – consider basic understanding of bodily functions and key nutritional principles.
- *Living environment* – homelessness, bed and breakfast rooms, access to a stove or refrigerator. Asking patients about their living environment and available cooking and food storage equipment is important for providing the appropriate nutritional advice.
- *Financial factors* – poverty is a common problem and can be cyclical. Major drivers of poverty among people with HIV include:
  - Immigration system.
  - Insufficient benefits.
  - Poor physical or mental health.
  - Unemployment.
  - Inadequate housing.
  - Responsibility for children.

  The Terence Higgins Trust and National AIDS Trust (www.nat.org.uk/Media%20library/Files/Policy/2011/HIV&Poverty.pdf) provide support to many people with HIV living in poverty.
- *Functional status* – the ability to shop and prepare food. Other comorbidities and/or side effects, such as

Table 7.11.22   Laboratory markers used in patients with hiv infection

	Use to assess
Plasma markers	
Urea	Hydration status, renal function (usually measured in an inpatient setting)
Creatinine	Renal function (also useful to calculate estimated glomerular filtration rate) (Labarga et al., 2010))
Potassium	Can be low in poor nutritional states and high in chronic renal disease
Phosphate	Measure of phosphate intake; however, hypophosphataemia is very common in people with HIV infection (Assadi, 2010) and needs to be interpreted in view of dietary intake, malabsorption, vitamin D deficiency and, importantly, tubular renal losses most commonly due to antiretroviral therapy and hyperparathyroidism. A fractional excretion of phosphate will help to determine the cause of hypophosphataemia
Liver function tests (LFTs)	Increased LFTs can be an indicator of liver function, especially considering the high prevalence of coinfection with hepatitis B and C; however, if only alkaline phosphatase is raised, it may be due to increased bone turnover and/or vitamin D deficiency
CD4 T cell count	See text
Viral load	See text
Albumin	Indicator of visceral protein status and related to inflammatory states, e.g. difficult to assess in cases of liver disease and acute infection. It is also an indicator of disease state and mortality. Can be low in malabsorption and states of protein loss
Vitamin B_{12}, folate	Low in macrocytic anaemia, can be related to low dietary intakes or other causes
Ferritin transferrin saturation, total iron binding capacity, etc.	Low in microcytic anaemic, can be related to low dietary intakes or other causes
Zinc, selenium	Need to be interpreted with caution in inflammatory states (see Micronutrients section)
Calcium	Plasma levels are bound to plasma proteins (such as albumin) and are tightly regulated, so are not a good reflector of dietary calcium intake
Vitamin D, parathyroid hormone (PTH)	Vitamin D deficiency is common in HIV as it is in many other individuals. Vitamin D deficiency or dietary calcium deficiency can result in secondary hyperparathyroidism
Other fat soluble vitamins	Can be useful to measure in patients with fat malabsorption
Hormones: testosterone, oestradiol, thyroid	Measured to rule out secondary causes of wasting and low bone mineral density
Fasting lipids (total cholesterol, HDL, LDL, triglycerides)	Use local reference values and national guidelines for target levels
Fasting glucose	Increased fasting or random glucose should warrant an oral glucose tolerance test to rule out diabetes, impaired glucose tolerance or impaired fasting glucose. It has been suggested that fasting insulin and glucose should be routinely measured, and HOMA-IR calculated, particularly in those at highest risk, such as those with metabolic syndrome, obesity, lipodystrophy or a longer exposure to antiretrovirals (Gianotti et al., 2011).
Urine markers	
Protein:creatinine	Reflects renal protein loss and is more sensitive than a dipstick test. Should be measured annually in all patients on ART
Fractional excretion of phosphate (FePi)	FePi = (urine phosphate × serum creatinine × 100)/(serum phosphate × urine creatinine). This should be done fasting and can be used to determine whether hypophosphataemia is a result of renal losses or inadequate dietary intake/reduced gastrointestinal absorption
Faecal markers	
1-alpha antitrypsin	A protein synthesised in the liver that is neither actively secreted nor absorbed. Use with serum levels to determine clearance in order to help diagnose protein losing enteropathy if indicated (Umar & DiBaise, 2010)
Pancreatic elastase	Used to determine exocrine pancreatic function that may result in fat malabsorption and diarrhoea

peripheral neuropathy and severe weight loss, will affect energy levels and ability to prepare food and carry shopping bags. In addition to social services, some HIV charities can provide assistance and support to patients with these conditions.

- *Cultural factors* – dietary restrictions and habits. Becoming acquainted with food habits common in various cultures and religions will assist in providing appropriate nutritional advice. For example, some Somalian, Ethiopian and Eritrean patients may be

Orthodox Christian and may restrict meat during the Lenten season. For some, this will decrease ferritin stores and they may require iron supplementation during this time period. As well as religious restrictions, recent immigrants to the UK may find foods they are familiar with difficult to access. Knowledge of foods commonly consumed will enable the practitioner to advise on appropriate substitutes as well recipe modifications when necessary (see Chapter 3.5).

Energy and protein requirements

Energy requirements are likely to increase by 10% to maintain body weight and physical activity in asymptomatic HIV infected adults not on ART. During symptomatic HIV, and subsequently during AIDS, energy requirements increase by approximately 20–30% to maintain adult body weight (World Health Organization, 2003). Although studies of energy expenditure have not shown an increase in overall total energy expenditure (TEE) in patients with HIV related wasting, this may have been the result of individuals compensating by reducing activity related energy expenditure (AEE). Therefore, weight loss may have resulted from reduced dietary intake (Macallan et al., 1995). Reviews of energy expenditure in HIV have concluded that it appears that resting energy expenditure (REE) is higher (but not always TEE) in HIV infected patients not on ART (Fields-Gardner et al., 2010; Chang et al., 2007), and a meta analysis confirmed this (Batterham, 2005). Factors associated with altered REE appear to be viral load, CD4, use of ART, body composition, hormones and proinflammatory cytokines, as well as other opportunistic infections.

Protein requirements have not been specifically addressed in studies of HIV adults. They may have higher requirements to maintain lean body mass, and general recommendations are 1.2–1.5 g/kg of body weight/day (Ockenga et al., 2006). Protein requirements should take into consideration stage of HIV disease and presence of other infections or comorbidities.

Nutritional problems and their management

It is well known that nutritional deficiencies are commonly associated with an impaired immune response (see Chapter 7.11.1); therefore, malnutrition in patients living with HIV has serious consequences. Adults living with HIV can present with a variety of nutritional problems throughout the course of HIV infection. Furthermore, patients requiring dietetic intervention are often critically unwell, have multiple medical diagnoses and mental health issues, as well as issues surrounding confidentiality, stigma and ART adherence that require a specialist team approach. The complexity of these patients requires input from a specialist dietitian trained in the area of HIV, who plays an active role in the multidisciplinary team (MDT).

The different stages of HIV infection as well as opportunistic infections, comorbidities and metabolic side effects of antiretroviral therapy can all lead to various nutritional problems. Ideally, all patients with HIV infection should have access to a registered dietitian for nutritional advice. Table 7.11.23 shows which patients with HIV in the inpatient and outpatient settings require a referral to an HIV specialist dietitian, and a summary of the possible outcomes from the referral.

Medication side effects

Side effects are most commonly seen in people who have recently started antiretroviral therapy; however, they can also occur due to the HIV infection itself, other opportunistic and comorbid conditions, or other medications. The most common side effects are:

- Nausea.
- Vomiting.
- Diarrhoea.
- Taste changes.
- Dry mouth.
- Flatulence.

Dietetic interventions for these side effects can be found in other chapters of this book.

Wasting and weight loss

Weight loss remains a problem for many people with HIV infection, even those on ART. In a longitudinal cohort of 466 patients followed from 1995 to 2005, the prevalence of wasting and weight loss was 38% (Tang et al., 2005). Several studies have shown that weight or muscle mass loss, even a 5% loss of usual weight, increases the risk of mortality (Tang et al., 2005; Scherzer et al., 2011). Furthermore, HIV wasting disease is defined as an AIDS defining illness (Centers for Disease Control, 1987) that is common in states of severe immunodeficiency (Polsky et al., 2001; Mangili et al., 2006). Many clinicians and researchers in the area felt that the Centers for Disease Control definition of an AIDS defining illness did not fully capture all patients with HIV wasting; therefore, other definitions have been proposed (Table 7.11.24).

In cases of weight loss despite adequate highly active ART (HAART), special consideration has to be given to other factors such as depression, gastrointestinal disease, anorexia, self neglect, e.g. drug users, or dry mouth/lack of saliva caused by medication (Grinspoon et al., 2003).

Aetiology

Weight loss can be due to one or a combination of several factors, depending on the patient's immune function and clinical condition (Figure 7.11.6):

- *Reduced food intake* – this can be due to a poor appetite, dysphagia or nausea.
- *Malabsorption* – can arise from other opportunistic infections, such as *Mycobacterium* spp., *Cryptosporidium*, pancreatic dysfunction or HIV enteropathy (Knox et al., 2000).
- *Hypermetabolism* – resting energy expenditure (REE) is increased in patients not on ART and is positively correlated with viral load and C-reactive protein level

Table 7.11.23 Dietetic interventions and outcomes for treating nutritional problems in patients with HIV infection

Patients requiring a dietetic referral	Dietetic interventions and outcomes of referral
All patients with HIV	Healthy eating principles that ensure adequate nutrition and promote a healthy immune system to reduce infections and prevent development of metabolic comorbidities
Immunocompromised (e.g. CD4+ cell count <200 cells/mL)	Food and water safety counselling to reduce the risk of developing food and water borne illnesses
Pregnant women	Antenatal and postnatal nutrition and breastfeeding education (see Chapter 3.8.2) Improving micronutrient deficiency (including iron) and constipation
Poor dietary intake due to disease or side effects of treatment	Nutrition strategies for symptom management, e.g. anorexia, early satiety, swallowing problems, thrush, nausea and vomiting, diarrhoea, food intolerances Outcomes may be improved diarrhoea and improved dietary intake ensuring adequacy of macro- and micro-nutrients (prevention of weight loss and loss of lean body mass, which is known to increase mortality)
Patients taking antiretrovirals or other medications relating to opportunistic infections or comorbidities	Identifying food–medication interactions and strategies to ensure optimal medication efficacy and provide adherence support
Loss of >5% of usual weight	Alternative feeding methods, e.g. oral supplementation, tube feeding and parenteral nutrition Outcomes may be reduced risk of infections, mortality, hospital admissions (if an outpatient) and length of stay (if inpatient), and improve patient experience (quality of life and energy levels)
Dyslipidaemia and/or lipodystrophy and/or obesity and/or diabetes and/or insulin resistance	Strategies for treatment of body fat changes and altered metabolism (in collaboration with the clinician) include exercise, lipidlowering medications, dietary modifications, glycaemic control, hormonal normalisation and anabolic medications Outcomes may be prevention of cardiovascular disease events, reduced hospital admissions and improved quality of life (obesity related)
Bone disease (osteoporosis, osteopaenia, osteomalacia)	Assessment of dietary and lifestyle factors influencing bone mineral density (dietary protein, calcium, phosphorus and vitamin D; exercise, risk of falls, smoking, alcohol) and advice on altering these as needed Advising on vitamin D ± calcium supplementation Outcomes may include prevention of falls, fractures and hospital admissions
Allergies/intolerances or patients following special diets/taking excess supplementation	Evaluation of nutrition information, special diets, vitamin or mineral or other dietary supplementation, and other nutrition practices Prevention of toxic effects of hypervitaminosis, improved patient experience/wellbeing; ensuring nutritional adequacy, prevention of interactions with ART or other medications
Patients requiring weight loss or gain of lean body tissue	Additional activities and therapies that support good nutrition, e.g. physical exercise, medications for symptom management, chronic disease management, etc., including referral to appropriate exercise facilities See outcomes for dyslipidaemia
Alteration in bowel habit	Assessment of impact on quality of life and diet, dietary advice to improve symptoms (constipation/diarrhoea), discussion with patient about lifestyle factors;.liaising with specialist gastroenterology team/dietitian, communication with GP if supplements or medicines are required Outcomes may be improved quality of life, prevention of nutritional deficiencies and enhanced medication absorption

ART, antiretroviral therapy.

Table 7.11.24 Definitions of HIV related wasting

CDC (Centers for Disease Control, 1987)	Consensus panel (Wanke et al., 2004)	NFHL (Wanke et al., 2000)
Involuntary weight loss of >10% of baseline body weight + either chronic diarrhoea or chronic weakness and documented fever in the absence of concurrent illness or condition	10% unintentional weight loss over 12 months Or 7.5% unintentional weight loss over 6 months Or 5% unintentional weight loss over 3 months Or in men: BCM <35% of total BW with BMI <27 kg/m^2 Or in women: BCM <23% of total BW with BMI <27 kg/m^2 In either men or women, regardless of BCM: BMI <20 kg/m^2	Unintentional loss of >10% of body weight Or BMI <20 kg/m^2 Or Unintentional loss of >5% of body weight in 6 months and persisting for at least 1 year

BW, body weight; BMI, body mass index; BCM, body cell mass.

SECTION 7

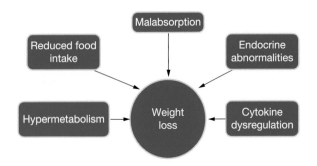

Figure 7.11.6 Potential causes of weight loss in HIV infected individuals

(Chang *et al.*, 2007). Opportunistic infections can also increase energy requirements.

- *Endocrine abnormalities* – altered regulation of anabolic and adipocyte hormones has also been implicated in causing increased REE. Altered regulation of other hormonal axes involved in energy homeostasis could potentially result from chronic immune activation.
- *Cytokine dysregulation* – increased REE is associated with catabolic cytokines interleukin (IL) 1b and tumour necrosis factor alpha (TNFα) abnormalities.

Dietetic treatment

The primary treatment for weight loss and HIV related wasting is treatment of the underlying condition that is leading to the weight loss. However, this is not always apparent and may take some time to diagnose. Therefore, to prevent further weight loss and to restore nutritional status, dietetic therapy is of paramount importance. Evaluating current dietary intake and calculating energy deficits is the first step in the nutritional management of someone who presents with weight loss. As hypermetabolism is one of the potential causes of weight loss, using indirect methods of measuring energy expenditure may help determine metabolic stress, which may be arising from opportunistic infections and other underlying conditions in addition to HIV disease itself. In the absence of objective measurements, anthropometric measurements should be closely monitored to determine effectiveness of nutritional intervention (see Chapter 6.1).

Several studies have shown that dietary counselling with oral nutritional supplements (providing 40–50 kcal/kg; 1.6 g of protein/kg) achieved increases in dietary intake and lean body mass. When resistance exercise training was added, an even greater increase in physical functioning was achieved (Shevitz *et al.*, 2005; Rabeneck *et al.*, 1998). Another study evaluated resistance training and intramuscular testosterone injections in eugonadal men with AIDS wasting and these combined interventions increased muscle attenuation (Fairfield *et al.*, 2001). Other randomised controlled trials (RCTs) of nutritional supplements demonstrated an improvement in both energy and protein intake for patients given macronutrient supplements, compared with patients given placebos

or no supplements, but no uniform improvements in weight, fat mass or fat free mass were found (Grobler *et al.*, 2013). Most studies investigating the role of nutritional supplementation have not included HIV outcomes or mortality, although one trial found an increase in CD4+ cell counts associated with nutritional supplementation (Fields-Gardner *et al.*, 2010).

There is limited evidence regarding mode of artificial nutritional support. Enteral nutritional support is often used as supplementary intake in patients with HIV. For long term artificial nutritional support, gastrostomy feeding is feasible in HIV patients and should be considered as an option. Parenteral nutrition should be used only in patients who are unable to feed enterally (Ockenga *et al.*, 2006).

Diarrhoea and malabsorption are common causes of weight loss and poor nutritional status in patients with HIV. Furthermore, malabsorption in the absence of clinical symptoms has been found to be common in adults with HIV(Knox *et al.*, 2000). Medium chain triglycerides (MCTs) have been used in several studies in patients with HIV and diarrhoea. Use of MCTs results in fewer stools, decreased stool fat and weight, and increased weight gain and fat absorption (Wanke *et al.*, 1996). Several other nutritional interventions for diarrhoea in patients with HIV have been evaluated; however, these were all very small studies and from which conclusions could not be drawn. One study looking at vitamin A and beta-carotene supplements found that they decreased gut permeability and reduced the risk of severe watery diarrhoea. Other studies have looked at elemental diets, probiotics, pancreatic enzymes, calcium carbonate, glutamine and the BRAT diet [bananas, rice, apple sauce, weak tea and toast (American Dietetic Assocation Evidence Analysis Library, 2008)]. Other dietary strategies will depend on the cause and severity of diarrhoea.

Pharmacological agents used to treat HIV wasting have included megestrol acetate, oxandrolone and dronabinol (Grinspoon *et al.*, 2003).

Metabolic complications with nutritional consequences and/or causes

Metabolic complications in people living with HIV can arise from uncontrolled HIV replication, coinfections or as a side effect of some ART medicines. These complications include dyslipidaemias, altered glucose metabolism, bone problems, altered body fat metabolism characterised by changes in body composition, and lactic acidaemia. The majority of antiretroviral medicines used to treat HIV interfere with viral genetic material. Many human metabolic processes are operationally similar to those of HIV viral replication, so it is not surprising that the side effects of ART include metabolic complications. As the population living with HIV ages, the prevalence of metabolic diseases will continue to increase. Helpful guidelines for the management of HIV related comorbidities are produced by the European Clinical AIDS Society (European AIDS Clinical Society).

Dyslipidaemia

Dyslipidaemia can occur from HIV infection or from ART. The following may occur in isolation or in combination, leading to an increased risk of cardiovascular disease:

* Hypertriglyceridaemia.
* Raised total or low density lipoprotein (LDL) cholesterol.
* Decreased high density lipoprotein (HDL) cholesterol.

Observational studies have reported that people living with HIV infection generally consume diets higher in total fat, saturated fat and dietary cholesterol, which has been related to dyslipidaemia (Shah *et al.*, 2005; Hadigan *et al.*, 2001).

Dietetic treatment

As there are several possible causes for dyslipidaemia in HIV infected individuals, evaluating the effect of dietary interventions is a complex task. Some studies have evaluated those with isolated dyslipidaemia, and others those with dyslipidaemia in the presence of lipodystrophy. Dietary advice has also varied between studies. Low fat dietary interventions have been investigated with various findings (Leyes *et al.*, 2008). In adults with HIV and dyslipidaemia, a retrospective review of dietary counselling found that total cholesterol decreased significantly by 13% (Woods *et al.*, 2009; Batterham *et al.*, 2003). Compliance with the dietary advice given was assessed in one trial; only 58 (36%) and 32 (45%) patients reported a good compliance with the prescribed diet at 3 and 6 months, and those with good compliance had a significant reduction in total cholesterol and triglyceride levels, as well as weight loss (Barrios *et al.*, 2002). n-3 Supplements have been shown in several trials to reduce triglycerides (De Truchis *et al.*, 2007), and when combined with dietary advice to reduce saturated fat, had an even greater effect and lowered the risk of lipohypertrophy (Woods *et al.*, 2009). Overall, there appears to be good evidence that a combination of exercise, low saturated fat, high fibre and decreased alcohol consumption all improved dyslipidaemia.

Altered glucose metabolism

Insulin resistance is the initial detectable step in the development of type 2 diabetes mellitus; in patients with HIV, it may be accompanied by abdominal adiposity, reduced limb fat and a buffalo hump. Traditional risk factors such as genetic predisposition, increased body mass index (BMI), smoking and increasing age, as well as HIV related factors such as mitochondrial dysfunction and elevated proinflammatory cytokines, all play a role in the development of diabetes mellitus (Paik & Kotler, 2011). Furthermore, patients on ART are more likely to develop glucose intolerance and diabetes mellitus than controls.

Care should be taken when using $HbA1_C$ as a surrogate measure for glycaemic control in HIV patients as ART use may result in this measure underestimating glycaemia by up to 20%, particularly in patients using the nucleoside

reverse transciptase inhibitors (NRTIs) such as abacavir (Kim *et al.*, 2009). The goals for diabetes mellitus treatment are the same as in uninfected individuals. The European AIDS Clinical Society and Paik & Kotler (2011) provide further information on management considerations.

Lipodystrophy (fat redistribution)

Lipodystrophy syndrome (LDS), also referred to as fat redistribution syndrome, describes body shape changes and metabolic disorders seen in some patients with HIV infection. Although the aetiology is likely multifactorial, most believe it occurs as a result of certain ART medications. Individual and viral factors such as duration of HIV disease, duration of ART, age, BMI, gender and ethnicity all seem to play a role in the development of lipodystrophy (Wohl & Brown, 2008). Limited evidence supports a relationship between low fibre or high glycaemic index (GI) and increased risk of fat deposition (Hendricks *et al.*, 2003).

Fat redistribution can occur in an individual in several ways:

* Lipoatrophy – the loss of subcutaneous fat tissue, most commonly in the legs, arms, buttocks and/or face.
* Fat accumulation (sometimes called lipohypertrophy) – the accumulation of adipose tissue in the intra-abdominal space (Figure 7.11.7), the dorsocervical

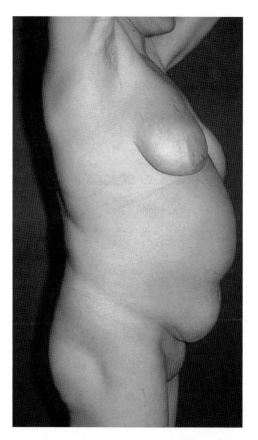

Figure 7.11.7   HIV infected woman with lipodystrophy [source: AIDS Images Library. Reproduced with permission of AIDS Image Library (www.aids-images.ch)]

regions (known commonly as the buffalo hump) and the breasts.

Dietetic management

There have been few RCTs studying lifestyle interventions in the treatment of lipodystrophy; therefore, much of the advice given in clinical practice is based on observational data and case series reports. There is no effective treatment for lipoatrophy using nutrition or lifestyle interventions. However, resistance exercises may improve the appearance of limbs by bulking up muscles to compensate for the loss of fat. Lipoatrophy is managed by switching ART regimens, and several other interventional treatments have b been evaluated, but with limited effectiveness to date (Wohl & Brown, 2008). For facial fat tissue loss, polylactic acid has been reported to produce lasting changes in dermal thickness of the cheeks and is available for patients receiving care in the NHS in the UK (NICE, 2012).

Limited evidence from observational studies shows that a low fibre diet leads to an increased risk of developing lipohypertrophy (Hendricks *et al.*, 2003). A combination of diet and exercise in interventional trials has shown small improvements in abdominal girth and blood pressure, but limited effect on lipids (Engelson *et al.*, 2006;, Driscoll *et al.*, 2004). Furthermore, a combination of both aerobic and resistance training appears be the most beneficial exercise intervention in patients with HIV associated lipodystrophy (Yarasheski & Roubenoff, 2001).

Bone problems

Three main bone diseases have been described in the HIV setting:

*   Osteopaenia and osteoporosis (decreased bone mineral density).
*   Osteomalacia (softening of the bones or demineralisation from severe vitamin D or phosphate deficiency).
*   Avascular necrosis.

The most commonly found and studied of these is reduced bone mineral density (BMD). Factors associated with low BMD in HIV infected patients are both traditional (i.e. well known in all populations to influence BMD) and HIV related:

*   Low weight, BMI.
*   Duration of HIV infection.
*   Older age.
*   Smoking.
*   Non-black/white ethnicity.
*   Corticosteroid exposure.
*   Postmenopausal women.
*   Viral load levels.
*   ART exposure (most commonly, tenofovir and protease inhibitors).

Other risk factors also commonly found in patients with HIV include hypogonadism, vitamin D deficiency and secondary hyperparathyroidism, opiate use and various other medical conditions (McComsey *et al.*, 2010). Lifestyle factors influencing BMD include dietary calcium intake and exercise (North American Menopause Society, 2010). These have not been well explored in patients with HIV infection (see Chapter 7.9.1).

Micronutrient deficiencies

Micronutrient deficiencies are commonly seen in patients with HIV not on ART (Lanzillotti & Tang, 2005). They are also common in countries with poor overall nutritional status in the developing world. The micronutrients most commonly studied in patients with HIV are shown in Table 7.11.25.

Table 7.11.25 Observational studies of micronutrient deficiencies in relation to HIV disease

Micronutrient	Observational findings in HIV
Vitamin A	Low vitamin A levels have been associated with quicker progression of HIV disease and mortality in adults (Semba *et al.*, 1995, Tang *et al.*, 1993)
Vitamin D	Low vitamin D has been associated with HIV disease progression (Viard *et al.*, 2011; Mehta *et al.*, 2010). In the general population, vitamin D deficiency has been associated with cardiovascular disease, diabetes, immune functioning and mortality (Melamed *et al.*, 2008)
Zinc	Serum zinc levels have been linked to HIV disease progression, decreased CD4+ cell counts, and increased mortality (Baum *et al.*, 1997; 2003). An association was seen between people who took over the counter zinc supplements and a more rapid progression to AIDS and mortality (Tang *et al.*, 1993; 1996). This may be because adults with more advanced or symptomatic HIV disease are more likely to take more supplements (Bormann *et al.*, 2009)
Selenium	Low levels have been linked with progression of HIV disease (Baum *et al.*, 1997)
Calcium	Several studies have found that a high percentage of HIV infected individuals have inadequate dietary calcium intake (Arpadi *et al.*, 2009; Bonjoch *et al.*, 2010; Jacobson *et al.*, 2008). An increased dietary calcium intake has been associated with greater bone mineral density in HIV (McComsey *et al.*, 2007)
Iron	Iron deficiency is common, especially in women and in developing countries, and dietary iron appears to be a contributing factor (Castro & Goldani, 2009; Shet *et al.*, 2012)
Phosphate	Hypophosphataemia is commonly seen in patients with HIV regardless of ART use (Day *et al.*, 2005). It is thought that use of tenofovir contributes to renal tubular losses of phosphate; however, vitamin D deficiency, malabsorption and use of antacids can also be contributing factors (Assadi, 2010).

ART, antiretroviral therapy.

Table 7.11.26   Interventional studies of micronutrients in people living with HIV/AIDS

Micronutrient	Findings from randomised controlled trials (RCTs)
Vitamin A	No trials reviewed (Irlam et al., 2010) showed a reduction in disease progression in adults with vitamin A supplementation. In children, vitamin A supplementation showed a reduction in mortality and moderate evidence for morbidity and growth benefits
Vitamin D	Limited RCTs have been done in adults or children. The doses used in trials thus far have been inadequate to achieve optimal repletion of vitamin D stores. One trial found that vitamin D_3 supplementation decreased the risk of developing diabetes (Guaraldi et al., 2011). No risks have been seen to date (Wejse et al., 2009, Arpadi et al., 2009)
Zinc	No benefit of zinc supplements have been seen in pregnant women, furthermore, zinc inhibits iron absorption so mitigates increases in haemoglobin levels, which are often low in pregnancy. In drug users in Florida, those who took the dietary reference intake (DRI) of zinc as a supplement, had a decrease in immunological failure (defined as CD4+ <200 cells/mm^3) and less diarrhoea, compared to those taking placebo (Baum et al., 2010). In children, supplementation reduced risk and progression of diarrhoea in several studies (in Africa), but not prophylactically (Irlam et al., 2010)
Selenium	Reduced diarrhoeal morbidity in pregnant women in Tanzania, and reduced viral load in two separate small trials in American adults (with high drop out rates) (Irlam et al., 2010)
Calcium	Calcium with vitamin D supplements have been given in the control arm of several trials investigating the role of bisphosphonates in treating osteoporosis. These studies found that there was a trend for bone mineral density increases, albeit non-significantly, in those receiving calcium supplements only; however, this was significantly less than in those on bisphosphonates (Mondy et al., 2005, McComsey et al., 2007)
Iron and phosphate	To date, no RCTs have evaluated the influence of diet on iron or phosphate stores in patients with HIV infection. Iron supplements have been given in conjunction with multivitamins to women with hepatitis C (Semba et al., 2007) and improved iron stores and anaemia. The results from this trial cannot be generalised to the HIV infected population as a whole due to the narrow inclusion criteria and short duration
Other	Multi micronutrient formulations have shown a reduction in mortality in patients with a CD4 of <100 cells/mm^3 in Thailand (Jiamton et al., 2003), an increase in CD4 in the US (Kaiser et al., 2006) and an improvement in benefits to mothers and offspring in Tanzania (Fawzi et al., 2004)

It has been suggested that there has been a link with numerous micronutrient deficiencies in patients with HIV. However, trials of micronutrient supplements, especially individual supplements, in patients with HIV have not demonstrated consistent benefits. Micronutrient supplementation in clinical practice should be based on the individual's micronutrient levels in conjunction with available evidence from both the general and HIV specific population (Table 7.11.26).

Obesity

Exercise and dietary interventions have been investigated in HIV positive patients presenting with general obesity or metabolic syndrome. A randomised study of intensive lifestyle intervention, comprised of weekly one on one counselling sessions focusing on reducing saturated fats, increasing fibre and walking, evaluated 34 HIV positive subjects with metabolic syndrome. At 6 months, subjects assigned to the lifestyle intervention group showed a 2.6 cm decrease in waist circumference, as well as significant improvements in systolic blood pressure and HbA1$_C$, but not lipid levels, fasting glucose or insulin resistance (Engelson et al., 2006; Fitch et al., 2006). Dietary advice for the obese should be based on standard dietetic practice and tailored to the individual with HIV (see Chapter 7.13.2).

Food and water safety

General food safety advice may benefit all individuals with HIV; however, those who are severely immunocompromised, e.g. with a CD4+ cell count of <200 cells/mm^3, may benefit from more targeted advice. Salmonellosis has been estimated to be nearly 20 times more common, and often five times more bacteraemic, in AIDS patients compared to patients without AIDS (Hayes et al., 2003). Other microorganisms such as *Giardia lamblia*, *Entamoeba histolytica*, *Cryptosporidium*, *Salmonella*, *Shigella*, *Listeria*, *Yersinia* and *Campylobacter* spp. have been identified as the cause of enteric infections in HIV infected patients and have also been recognised as causing food and water borne diseases. Preventative measures should include food and water safety advice.

Water safety advice is important as *Cryptosporidium* has been isolated from tap water. Cryptosporidiosis can be prevented by boiling tap water, using an appropriate filter or using sterile water. Bottled water or domestic water filters are not necessarily free from *Cryptosporidium* cysts, and therefore should not be recommended in place of boiled water or appropriate filters (Hunter & Nichols, 2002).

Drug–nutrient interactions

Some of the older antiretroviral drugs came with strict food requirements; however, new formulations and new medicines mean that food requirements and timing are less of a concern today in the UK. With the exception of didanosine (ddI), all of the NRTIs/nucleotide reverse transcriptase inhibitors (NtRTIs) may be taken either with food or on an empty stomach. Many people find that taking NRTIs/NtRTIs with food helps reduce side effects such as nausea. It is advised to take efavirenz [an nonnucleoside reverse transcriptase inhibitor (NNRTI)] on an empty stomach to reduce side effects. Most protease inhibitors work better when taken with food; however, the new formulation of lopinavir/ritonavir and fosamprenavir have no food restrictions. Current information on antiretrovirals and food restrictions is available at www.aidsmap.com/resources/Antiretroviral-drugs-chart/page/1412453/.

Further reading

Hendricks KM, Dong KR, Gerrior JL (eds). (2009) *Nutrition Management of HIV and AIDS*. Chicago: American Dietetic Association.
Pribram V (ed). (2010) *Nutrition and HIV*. Oxford: Wiley Blackwell.

Internet resources

Academy of Nutrition & Dietetics
   HIV/AIDS Nutrition Evidence Analysis Project www .adaevidencelibrary.com/topic.cfm?cat=1404
AVERTing HIV & AIDS www.avert.org
British HIV Association www.bhiva.org.uk
Dietitians working in HIV/AIDS www.dhiva.org.uk
European AIDS Clinical Society www.europeanaidsclinicalsociety.org
National AIDS Manual (nam – aidsmap) www.aidsmap.com
   Antiretroviral drugs chart www.aidsmap.com/resources/Antiretroviral-drugs-chart/page/1412453/
National AIDS Trust www.nat.org.uk
HIV and poverty www.nat.org.uk/media/Files/Policy/2011/Poverty%20and%20HIV%202006-2009.pdf

References

American Dietetic Assocation Evidence Analysis Library. (2008) Dietary treatment of diarrhea/malabsorption in people with HIV infection. Available at www.adaevidencelibrary.com/evidence .cfm?evidence_summary_id=250872. Accessed 11 July 2011.
Arpadi S, McMahon D, Abrams E, *et al.* (2009) Effect of bimonthly supplementation with oral cholecalciferol on serum 25-hydroxyvitamin D concentrations in HIV-infected children and adolescents. *Pediatrics* 123: e121–126.
Asboe D, Aitken C, Boffito M, *et al.* (2011) *Routine Investigation and Monitoring of Adult HIV-1-Infected Individuals*. British HIV Association.
Assadi F. (2010) Hypophosphatemia: An evidence-based problem-solving approach to clinical cases. *Iran Journal of Kidney Disease* 4: 195–201.
Barrios A, Blanco F, García-Benayas T, *et al.* (2002) Effect of dietary intervention on highly active antiretroviral therapy-related dyslipemia. *AIDS* 16, 2079–81.
Batterham MJ. (2005) Investigating heterogeneity in studies of resting energy expenditure in persons with HIV/AIDS: a meta-analysis. *American Journal of Clinical Nutrition* 81: 702–713.
Batterham MJ, Brown D, Workman C. (2003) Modifying dietary fat intake can reduce serum cholesterol in HIV-associated hypercholesterolemia. *AIDS* 17: 1414–1416.
Baum MK, Shor-Posner G, Lai S, *et al.* (1997) High risk of HIV-related mortality is associated with selenium deficiency. *Journal of Acquired Immune Deficiency Syndrome and Human Retrovirology* 15(5): 370–374.
Baum MK, ,Campa A, Lai S, Lai H, Page JB. (2003) Zinc status in human immunodeficiency virus type 1 infection and illicit drug use. *Clinical Infectious Diseases* 37(S2):S117–123.
Baum MK, Lai S, Sales S, Page JB, Campa A. (2010) Randomized, controlled clinical trial of zinc supplementation to prevent immunological failure in HIV-infected adults. *Clinical Infectious Diseases* 50: 1653–1660.
Bonjoch A, Figueras M, Estany C, *et al.* (2010) High prevalence of and progression to low bone mineral density in HIV-infected patients: a longitudinal cohort study. *AIDS* 24: 2827–2833.
Bormann JE, Uphold CR, Maynard C. (2009) Predictors of complementary/alternative medicine use and intensity of use among men with HIV infection from two geographic areas in the United States. *The Journal of the Association of Nurses in AIDS Care* 20: 468–480.
Castro L, Goldani LZ. (2009) Iron, folate and vitamin B12 parameters in HIV-1 infected patients with anaemia in southern Brazil. *Tropical Doctor* 39: 83–85.
Castro KG, Ward JW, Slutsker L, Buehler JW, Jaffe HW, Berkelman RL. (1993) 1993 revised classification system for HIV infection and expanded surveillance case definition for AIDS among adolescents and adults. *Morbidity and Mortality Weekly Reports: Recommendations and Reports* 41:RR-17. Available at www.cdc.gov/mmwr/preview/mmwrhtml/00018871.htm. Accessed 30 August 2012.
Centers for Disease Control (CDC). (1987) Revision of the CDC surveillance case definition for acquired immunodeficiency syndrome. Council of State and Territorial Epidemiologists; AIDS Program, Center for Infectious Diseases. *MMWR Morbity & Mortality Weekly Report* 36(Suppl 1): 1S–15S.
Chang E, Sekhar R, Patel S, Balasubramanyam A. (2007) Dysregulated energy expenditure in HIV-infected patients: a mechanistic review. *Clinical Infectious Diseases* 44: 1509–1517.
Chen LF, Hoy J, Lewin SR. (2007) Ten years of highly active antiretroviral therapy for HIV infection. *Medical Journal of Australia* 186: 146–151.
Day SL, Leake Date HA, Bannister A, Hankins M, Fisher M. (2005) Serum hypophosphatemia in tenofovir disoproxil fumarate recipients is multifactorial in origin, questioning the utility of its monitoring in clinical practice. *Journal of Acquired Immune Deficiency Syndrome* 38: 301–304.
De Truchis P, Kirstetter M, Perier A. *et al.* (2007) Reduction in triglyceride level with N-3 polyunsaturated fatty acids in HIV-infected patients taking potent antiretroviral therapy: a randomized prospective study. *Journal of Acquired Immune Deficiency Syndrome* 44: 278–285.
Driscoll SD, Meininger GE, Lareau MT, *et al.* (2004) Effects of exercise training and metformin on body composition and cardiovascular indices in HIV-infected patients. *AIDS* 18: 465–473.
Engelson ES, Agin D, Kenya S, *et al.* (2006) Body composition and metabolic effects of a diet and exercise weight loss regimen on obese, HIV-infected women. *Metabolism* 55: 1327–1336.
Fairfield WP, Treat M, Rosenthal DI, *et al.* (2001) Effects of testosterone and exercise on muscle leanness in eugonadal men with AIDS wasting. *Journal of Applied Physiology* 90: 2166–2171.
Fawzi WW, Msamanga GI, Spiegelman D, *et al.* (2004) A randomized trial of multivitamin supplements and HIV disease progression and mortality. *New England Journal of Medicine* 351: 23–32.
Fields-Gardner C, Campa A, American Dietetics Association. (2010) Position of the American Dietetic Association: Nutrition Intervention and Human Immunodeficiency Virus Infection. *Journal of the American Dietetics Association* 110: 1105–1119.
Fitch KV, Anderson EJ, Hubbard JL, *et al.* (2006) Effects of a lifestyle modification program in HIV-infected patients with the metabolic syndrome. *AIDS* 20: 1843–50.

Gazzard BG, Anderson J, Babiker A, *et al.* (2008) British HIV Association Guidelines for the treatment of HIV-1-infected adults with antiretroviral therapy 2008. *HIV Medicine* 9: 563–608.

Gianotti N, Visco F, Galli L, *et al.* (2011) Detecting impaired glucose tolerance or type 2 diabetes mellitus by means of an oral glucose tolerance test in HIV-infected patients. *HIV Medicine* 12: 109–117.

Grinspoon S, Mulligan K, Department of Health and Human Services Working Group on the Prevention and Treatment of Wasting and Weight Loss. (2003) Weight loss and wasting in patients infected with human immunodeficiency virus. *Clinical Infectious Diseases* 36: S69–78.

Grobler L, Siegfried N, Visser ME, Mahlungulu SSN, Volmink J. (2013) Nutritional interventions for reducing morbidity and mortality in people with HIV. *Cochrane Database of Systematic Reviews* 2: CD004536.

Guaraldi G, Orlando G, Carli F. (2011) Vitamin D3 supplementation decreases the risk of diabetes mellitus among patients with HIV infection. 18th Conference on Retroviruses and Opportunistic Infections, 2011, Boston. Poster 827.

Hadigan C, Jeste S, Anderson EJ, Tsay R, Cyr H, Grinspoon S. (2001) Modifiable dietary habits and their relation to metabolic abnormalities in men and women with human immunodeficiency virus infection and fat redistribution. *Clinical Infectious Diseases* 33: 710–717.

Hayes C, Elliot E, Krales E, Downer G. (2003) Food and water safety for persons infected with human immunodeficiency virus. *Clinical Infectious Diseases* 36: S106–109.

Health Protection Agency. (2010) HIV in the United Kingdom: 2010 report. Available at www.hpa.org.uk/Publications/Infectious Diseases/HIVAndSTIs/1011HIVUK2010Report/. Accessed 10 July 2011.

Hendricks KM, Dong KR, Tang AM, *et al.* (2003) High-fiber diet in HIV-positive men is associated with lower risk of developing fat deposition. *American Journal of Clinical Nutrition* 78: 790–795.

Hunter PR, Nichols G. (2002) Epidemiology and clinical features of Cryptosporidium infection in immunocompromised patients. *Clinical Microbiology Reviews* 15: 145–154.

Irlam JH, Visser MM, Rollins NN, Siegfried N. (2010) Micronutrient supplementation in children and adults with HIV infection. *Cochrane Database of Systematic Reviews* 12: CD003650.

Jacobson DL, Spiegelan D, Knox TK, Wilson IB. (2008) Evolution and predictors of change in total bone mineral density over time in HIV-infected men and women in the nutrition for healthy living study. *JAIDS – Journal of Acquired Immune Deficiency Syndromes* 49: 298–308.

Jiamton S, Pepin J, Suttent R, *et al.* (2003) A randomized trial of the impact of multiple micronutrient supplementation on mortality among HIV-infected individuals living in Bangkok. *AIDS* 17: 2461–2469.

Joint United Nations Programme on HIV/AIDS. (2010) Global Report: UNAIDS report on the global AIDS epidemic: 2010. Available at www.unaids.org/en/media/unaids/contentassets/dataimport/pub/report/2009/jc1700_epi_update_2009_en.pdf. Accessed 14 August 2011.

Kaiser JD, Campa AM, Ondercin JP, Leoung GS, Pless RF, Baum MK. (2006) Micronutrient supplementation increases CD4 count in HIV-infected individuals on highly active antiretroviral therapy: a prospective, double-blinded, placebo-controlled trial. *Journal of Acquired Immune Deficiency Syndrome* 42: 523–528.

Kim PS, Woods C, Georgoff P, *et al.* (2009) A1C underestimates glycemia in HIV infection. *Diabetes Care* 32: 1591–1593.

Knox TA, Spiegelman D, Skinner SC, Gorbach S. (2000) Diarrhea and abnormalities of gastrointestinal function in a cohort of men and women with HIV infection. *American Journal of Gastroenterology* 95: 3482–3489.

Kyle UG, Bosaeus I, De Lorenzo AD, *et al.*, ESPEN. (2004) Bioelectrical impedance analysis-part II: utilization in clinical practice. *Clinical Nutrition* 23: 1430–1453.

Labarga P, Albalate M, Barreiro P. (2010) Glomerular filtration (GF) determined by creatinine clearance (CCR) in 24 hours urine and cockcroft & gault (cg) and modification of diet in renal disease (MDRD) equations in a large cohort of HIV plus patients. *Retrovirology* 7: 39.

Lanzillotti JS, Tang AM. (2005) Micronutrients and HIV disease: a review pre- and post-HAART. *Nutrition in Clinical Care* 8: 16–23.

Leyes P, Martínez E, Forga MET. (2008) Use of diet, nutritional supplements and exercise in HIV-infected patients receiving combination antiretroviral therapies: a systematic review. *Antiviral Therapy* 13: 149–159.

Lundgren JD, Battegay M, Behrens G, *et al.* (2008) European AIDS Clinical Society (EACS) guidelines on the prevention and management of metabolic diseases in HIV. *HIV Medicine* 9: 72–81.

Macallan DC, Noble C, Baldwin C, *et al.* (1995) Energy expenditure and wasting in human immunodeficiency virus infection. *New England Journal of Medicine* 333: 83–88.

Mangili A, Murman DH, Zampini AM, Wanke CA. (2006) Nutrition and HIV infection: review of weight loss and wasting in the era of highly active antiretroviral therapy from the nutrition for healthy living cohort. *Clinical Infectious Diseases* 42: 836–842.

May M, Gompels M, Delpech V, *et al.* (2011) Impact of late diagnosis and treatment on life expectancy in people with HIV-1: UK Collaborative HIV Cohort (UK CHIC) Study. *BMJ* 343: d6016.

McComsey GA, Kendall MA, Tebas P, *et al.* (2007) Alendronate with calcium and vitamin D supplementation is safe and effective for the treatment of decreased bone mineral density in HIV. *AIDS* 21 2473–2482.

McComsey G, Tebas P, Shane E. (2010) Bone disease in HIV infection: a practical review and recommendations for HIV care providers. *Clinical Infectious Diseases* 51: 937–946.

Mehta S, Giovannucci E, Mugusi FM, *et al.* (2010) Vitamin D status of HIV-infected women and its association with HIV disease progression, anemia, and mortality. *PLoS ONE* 5(1): e8770.

Melamed M, Michos E, Post W, Astor B. (2008) 25-hydroxyvitamin D levels and the risk of mortality in the general population. *Archives of Internal Medicine* 168: 1629–1637.

Mondy K, Powderly WG, Claxton SA, *et al.* (2005) Alendronate, vitamin D, and calcium for the treatment of osteopenia/osteoporosis associated with HIV infection. *Journal of Acquired Immune Deficiency Syndrome* 38: 426–431.

National Institute for Health and Care Excellence (NICE). (2012) Interventional procedure overview of deep dermal injection of non-absorbable gel polymer for HIV-related lipoatrophy. Available at www.nice.org.uk/nicemedia/live/11293/42589/42589.pdf. Accessed 30 August 2013.

North American Menopause Society. (2010) Management of osteoporosis in postmenopausal women: 2010 position statement of The North American Menopause Society. *Menopause* 17: 25–54.

Ockenga J, Grimble R, Jonkers-Schuitema C, *et al.* (2006) ESPEN Guidelines on Enteral Nutrition: Wasting in HIV and other chronic infectious diseases. *Clinical Nutrition* 25: 319–329.

Paik IJ, Kotler DP. (2011) The prevalence and pathogenesis of diabetes mellitus in treated HIV-infection. *Best Practice in Research and Clinical Endocrinology and Metabolism* 25: 469–478.

Polsky B, Kotler D, Steinhart C. (2001) HIV-associated wasting in the HAART era: guidelines for assessment, diagnosis, and treatment. *AIDS Patient Care and STDS* 15: 411–423.

Rabeneck L, Palmer A, Knowles JB, *et al.* (1998) A randomized controlled trial evaluating nutrition counseling with or without oral supplementation in malnourished HIV-infected patients. *Journal of the American Dietetic Association* 98: 434–438.

Scherzer R, Shen W, Bacchetti P, *et al.* (2008) Simple anthropometric measures correlate with metabolic risk indicators as strongly as magnetic resonance imaging-measured adipose tissue depots in both HIV-infected and control subjects. *American Journal of Clinical Nutrition* 87: 1809–1817.

Scherzer R, Heymsfield SB, Lee D, *et al*. (2011) Decreased limb muscle and increased central adiposity are associated with 5-year all-cause mortality in HIV infection. *AIDS* 25: 1405–1414.

Schwenk A, Breuer P, Kremer G, Ward L. (2001) Clinical assessment of HIV-associated lipodystrophy syndrome: bioelectrical impedance analysis, anthropometry and clinical scores. *Clinical Nutrition* 20: 243–249.

Semba RD, Caiaffa WT, Graham NM, Cohn S, Vlahov D. (1995) Vitamin A deficiency and wasting as predictors of mortality in human immunodeficiency virus-infected injection drug users. *Journal of Infectious Diseases* 171(5): 1196–1202.

Semba RD, Kumwenda J, Zijlstra E, *et al*. (2007) Micronutrient supplements and mortality of HIV-infected adults with pulmonary TB: a controlled clinical trial. *International Journal of Tuberculosis and Lung Disease* 11: 854–859.

Shah M, Tierney K, Adams-Huet B, *et al*. (2005) The role of diet, exercise and smoking in dyslipidaemia in HIV-infected patients with lipodystrophy. *HIV Medicine* 6: 291–298.

Shet A, Arumugam K, Rajagopalan N, *et al*. (2012) The prevalence and etiology of anemia among HIV-infected children in India. *European Journal of Pediatrics* 171(3): 531–540.

Shevitz AH, Wilson IB, McDermott AY., *et al*. (2005) A comparison of the clinical and cost-effectiveness of 3 intervention strategies for AIDS wasting. *Journal of Acquired Immune Deficiency Syndrome* 38: 399–406.

Tang AM, Graham NM, Kirby AJ, McCall LD, Willett WC, Saah AJ. (1993) Dietary micronutrient intake and risk of progression to acquired immunodeficiency syndrome (AIDS) in human deficiency virus type 1 (HIV-1)-infected homosexual men. *American Journal of Epidemiology* 138: 937–951.

Tang AM, Graham NMH, Saah AJ. (1996) Effects of micronutrient intake on survival in human immunodeficiency virus type 1 infection. *American Journal of Epidemiology* 143: 1244–1256.

Tang AM, Jacobson DL, Spiegelman D, Knox TA, Wanke C. (2005) Increasing risk of 5% or greater unintentional weight loss in a cohort of HIV-infected patients, 1995 to 2003. *Journal of Acquired Immune Deficiency Syndrome* 40: 70–76.

Umar SB, Dibaise JK. (2010) Protein-losing enteropathy: case illustrations and clinical review. *American Journal of Gastroenterology* 105: 43–49; quiz 50.

Viard JP, Souberbielle JC, Kirk O, *et al*. (2011) Vitamin D and clinical disease progression in HIV infection: results from the EuroSIDA study. *AIDS* 25: 1305–1315.

Wanke CA, Pleskow D, Degirolami PC, *et al*. (1996) A medium chain triglyceride-based diet in patients with HIV and chronic diarrhea reduces diarrhea and malabsorption: a prospective, controlled trial. *Nutrition* 12: 766–771.

Wanke CA, Silva M, Knox TA, Forrester J, Spiegelman D, Gorbach SL. (2000) Weight loss and wasting remain common complications in individuals infected with human immunodeficiency virus in the era of highly active antiretroviral therapy. *Clinical Infectious Diseases* 31: 803–805.

Wanke C, Kotler D, Committee HWCC. (2004) Collaborative recommendations: the approach to diagnosis and treatment of HIV wasting. *Journal of Acquired Immune Deficiency Syndrome* 37 (Suppl 5): S284–288.

Wejse C, Gomes V, Rabna P, *et al*. (2009) Vitamin D as supplementary treatment for tuberculosis: a double-blind, randomized, placebo-controlled trial. *American Journal of Respiratory and Critical Care Medicine* 179: 843–850.

Wohl DA, Brown TT. (2008) Management of morphologic changes associated with antiretroviral use in HIV-infected patients. *Journal of Acquired Immune Deficiency Syndrome* 49(Suppl 2): S93–S100.

Woods MN, Wanke CA, Ling PR, *et al*. (2009) Effect of a dietary intervention and n-3 fatty acid supplementation on measures of serum lipid and insulin sensitivity in persons with HIV. *American Journal of Clinical Nutrition* 90: 1566–1578.

World Health Organization. (2003) Nutrient requirements for people living with HIV/AIDS: report of a technical consultation. Available at www.who.int/nutrition/publications/Content_nutrient_requirements.pdf. Accessed 10 July 2011.

World Health Organization. (2007) WHO case definitions of HIV for surveillance and revised clinical staging and immunological classification of HIV-related disease in adults and children. Available at www.who.int/hiv/pub/guidelines/HIVstaging150307.pdf. Accessed 15 uly 2011].

Yarasheski KE, Roubenoff R. (2001) Exercise treatment for HIV-associated metabolic and anthropomorphic complications. *Exercise and Sport Science Reviews* 29: 170–174.

7.12

Diabetes mellitus

Pam Dyson

Key points

- Diabetes is one of the most common non-communicable diseases, has high rates of both morbidity and mortality, and affects over 285 million people globally.

- There are two main types of diabetes; type 1 and type 2.

- Lifestyle interventions, including diet and physical activity, are fundamental to diabetes management, and evidence is accumulating for the most effective strategies.

- The key to successful management is tailoring lifestyle advice to the individual.

Diabetes mellitus (DM) is a metabolic disorder characterised by chronic hyperglycaemia resulting from defects in insulin secretion, insulin action or both (WHO, 2006). It is a one of the most common non-communicable diseases worldwide, and is a leading cause of morbidity and premature death. The global prevalence of diabetes has been estimated by the International Diabetes Federation (IDF, 2009) at 285 million in 2010 (6.6% of world population) and is projected to increase to 439 million (7.8%) by 2030, of whom over 75% will live in lower and middle income countries. Diabetes UK, the leading charity for people with diabetes in the UK, has estimated that 2.8 million adults (4.3%) in the UK had a diagnosis of diabetes in 2010, based on data from the Qualities and Outcomes Framework (QOF) (NHS, 2010a). However, this may be an underestimate; an alternative study reported that the prevalence of diabetes in adults in the UK was already 3.1 million (7.4%) by 2010, and this was projected to rise to 4.6 million (9.5%) by 2030 (Holman *et al.*, 2011).

Diabetes is a disease with high rates of morbidity and mortality (Zimmet *et al.*, 2001). It is associated with macrovascular complications [cardiovascular disease (CVD), stroke, peripheral vascular disease) leading to heart attacks, hemiplegia and amputations, and microvascular complications (neuropathy, retinopathy, nephropathy] causing foot ulcers, blindness and kidney failure (EURODIAB IDDM Complications Study Group, 1994; Turner & Holman, 1995). Apart from the effects of diabetes in terms of health and quality of life, it imposes a financial burden on societies. In the UK in 2009, treatment of diabetes and its associated complications accounted for 10% of the total NHS budget, approximately £9 billion (NHS, 2010b).

Historical perspective

The symptoms of diabetes were described in an Egyptian papyrus in approximately 1500 BC, and the disease was first given the name of *diabetes* (literally meaning a siphon) by the Greek physician Aretaeus, who lived and practised during the second century AD. Although described by other eminent physicians, including Avicenna (980–1037 AD) and Galen (129–210 AD), diabetes was largely unreported and untreated until the 18th century. Eventually, it was identified that the large volumes of urine associated with untreated diabetes contained sugar and the term *diabetes mellitus* was coined by Cullen to distinguish the condition from that of diabetes insipidus (Tattersall, 2009). The discovery of the presence of sugar in the urine led to the development of dietary treatments and two schools of thought developed; one insisting on dietary replacement of sugar lost in the urine (high carbohydrate) and the other on dietary restriction (low carbohydrate). Bouchardat reported improvements in symptoms as a result of severe food shortages during the Paris siege of 1870 and promoted dietary restriction. All physicians, including the Italian physician Catoni, whose dietary restrictions were so severe that he kept his patients under lock and key to ensure compliance, soon adopted this approach. Restricted diets were promoted by Allan in the US and relaxed only slightly with the introduction of insulin in 1921–1922, when Lawrence introduced the Lawrence line diet. Over the past century, the

SECTION 7

development of new agents to treat diabetes, and growing evidence of the effect of dietary therapy has led to many changes in the nutritional recommendations for diabetes.

Diagnostic criteria and classification

Diagnostic criteria

The diagnostic criteria for diabetes have been developed and revised by the World Health Organization (WHO, 2006), and use the occurrence of diabetes specific complications to derive diagnostic cut-off points for diabetes. A diagnosis of diabetes can be made under any of the following circumstances:

- Fasting plasma glucose of 7.0 mmol/L (126 mg/dL) or greater.
- 2-hour glucose of 11.1 mmol/L (200 mg/d:) or greater after ingestion of a 75-g oral glucose load [oral glucose tolerance test (OGTT)].
- Gylcated haemoglobin (HbA1c) of >48 mmol/mol (6.5%).

Glycaemia can be assessed by a simple blood test measuring levels of HbA1c. The WHO (2011) now recommends that this test may be used in the diagnosis of diabetes, provided that stringent quality assurance tests are in place and that assays are standardised to international reference values.

In addition, both impaired glucose tolerance (IGT) and increased fasting glucose (IFG) have been identified as risk factors for developing diabetes, and IGT is also a risk factor for CVD. The diagnostic criteria for IGT and IFG are:

- *IGT* – fasting plasma glucose of <7.0 mmol/dL (126 mg/dL) and 2-hour plasma glucose of 7.8 mmol/L or greater and <11.1 mmol/L (140 and 200 mg/dL) after OGTT.
- *IFG* – fasting plasma glucose of 6.1–6.9 mmol/L (110–125 mg/dL) and (if measured) 2-hour glucose of <7.8 mmol/L (142 mg/dL).

Classification

There are two broad types of diabetes, namely type 1 and type 2.

Type 1 diabetes

Type 1 diabetes is an autoimmune disease characterised by destruction of the insulin producing cells of the pancreas. Its cause is unknown, although genetic factors and certain viruses may play a part. Type 1 diabetes usually presents in children and young adults, although it can be diagnosed at any age. Type 1 diabetes accounts for approximately 10–20% of diabetes and is treated with a combination of insulin replacement by injection or pump therapy and lifestyle modification.

Type 2 diabetes

Type 2 diabetes is most frequently diagnosed in middle aged or elderly people, and is caused by a combination of impaired insulin secretion and resistance to the action of insulin. Type 2 diabetes has a strong genetic component, but is also associated with lifestyle factors; it is more common in societies with high levels of obesity and low levels of physical activity. Although type 2 diabetes is traditionally diagnosed in people over the age of 40 years, it is being increasingly diagnosed in obese children and adolescents, and as many as 1400 children may have type 2 diabetes in the UK (Lobstein & Leach, 2004). Approximately 86% of people with type 2 diabetes are overweight or obese (Haslam, 2011). Type 2 diabetes accounts for approximately 80–90% of diabetes and is treated with a combination of diet, physical activity, oral medications and, increasingly, injectable therapies including insulin.

Other types of diabetes

There are other types of diabetes that are neither type 1 nor type 2, namely:

- *Maturity onset diabetes of the young (MODY)* – a hereditary form of diabetes caused by gene mutations that affect insulin production.
- *Gestational diabetes* – caused by increased insulin demand during pregnancy. It may resolve after birth of the child, but carries an increased risk of type 2 diabetes in later life.
- *Secondary diabetes* – occurs after surgical removal of the pancreas, as a result of pancreatitis, or can be induced by drugs, usually high doses of steroids.

Disease processes

Diabetes is a condition in which the body is unable to utilise the glucose in the blood for energy due to complete or relative lack of insulin, insulin resistance (a condition where the body does not respond adequately to insulin) or a combination of both. Insulin is produced and secreted in the beta cells of the islets of Langerhans in the pancreas; type 1 diabetes is characterised by complete beta cell failure, leading to absolute insulin deficiency, and type 2 diabetes is characterised by progressive beta cell failure and is usually associated with peripheral insulin resistance. Complete or relative lack of insulin results in raised blood glucose levels and the diagnosis of diabetes.

Glucose is the body's primary energy source and is provided by foods containing carbohydrate. Carbohydrate is found in starchy foods such as bread, potatoes, rice and pasta; sugary foods such as sweets, chocolate and cakes; and as natural sugars in milk and fruit. After eating, any excess glucose is first stored in the liver and muscle as glycogen, which is released into the blood stream as blood glucose levels fall. Once glycogen stores are filled, further excess glucose is converted to fat and stored in adipose tissue.

Insulin is the hormone responsible for regulating blood glucose levels and is automatically released as blood glucose levels rise following carbohydrate intake. Insulin facilitates entry of glucose into muscle and adipose tissue cells to be utilised as energy. Lack of insulin leads directly to increased blood glucose levels and the symptoms of diabetes, which are polyuria, polydipsia, fatigue, weight loss and increased susceptibility to infections.

Symptoms

Blood glucose levels above about 12 mmol/L exceed the renal threshold and glucose begins to appear in the urine. The kidneys can only excrete glucose when it is accompanied by fluid, and this extra fluid causes excessive urine production (polyuria) leading to excessive thirst (polydipsia). Lack of insulin means that the body's cells are unable to utilise glucose for energy, and despite high circulating glucose levels, the body has to rely on its stores of fat for energy. The lack of available glucose causes fatigue and weight loss. In the absence of any insulin, people with type 1 diabetes rely entirely on fat and its byproducts, ketones, for energy. Small amounts of ketones can be used for energy, but large amounts cause acidity in the body and result in diabetic ketoacidosis (DKA), a life threatening condition.

Disease consequences

It is challenging to assess mortality and morbidity rates for people with diabetes as many countries do not have diabetes registers or a system of death certification. Where death certificates do exist, diabetes is often not noted as a cause of death and, as a result, available statistics frequently underestimate mortality.

Mortality

A statistical modelling approach used by the IDF (2009) estimated that in 2010, 4 million deaths in the 20–79 year age group (accounting for 6.8% of all deaths globally) were caused by diabetes. Diabetes is associated with premature mortality from a variety of causes including vascular disease, cancer, infectious diseases, intentional self harm, external causes and degenerative disorders (The Emerging Risk Factor Collaboration, 2011). Diabetes doubles the risk of vascular disease, which is the cause of death for nearly 60% of people with diabetes (The Emerging Risk Factor Collaboration, 2010), and people with diabetes are also 25% more likely to die of cancer. Hyperglycaemia is directly associated with risk of death, with levels of >5.6 mmol/L linked with increased risk. On average, a 50-year-old adult with diabetes and without vascular disease, will die 6 years earlier than a counterpart without diabetes.

Morbidity

One of the most important features of diabetes is the association of sustained hyperglycaemia with long term tissue damage and, as a result, morbidity rates are high. Half of all people with type 2 diabetes have already developed a diabetes associated complication by the time of diagnosis (UKPDS Group, 1991).

Macrovascular disease

Macrovascular or CVD affects the large blood vessels and is the most common complication associated with DM. It is associated with premature mortality and poses a disproportionate risk for premenopausal women (Koerbel & Korytkowski, 2003) and ethnic minority groups with DM (Oldroyd et al., 2005). Risk factors for CVD in people with diabetes include hyperglycaemia, hypertension, dyslipidaemia, overweight and obesity, tobacco use, high fat diet and physical inactivity. Management of CVD risk for people with diabetes is multifactorial and studies have shown significant benefits of risk factor control for both type 1 and 2 diabetes, with the exception of glycaemic control in those with type 2 diabetes where controversy remains (DCCT Study Group, 1993; UKPDS Group, 1998a,b). A review of recent studies that have failed to show a significant reduction in CVD events with intensive glycaemic control in people with type 2 diabetes concluded that individual targets for glycaemia may be appropriate, and that management of blood pressure and lipids, smoking cessation and healthy lifestyles are a priority for CVD risk management (Skyler et al., 2009).

Microvascular disease

Microvascular disease affects the small blood vessels, especially in the eye, kidney and nerves. Diabetes is the most common cause of blindness in people of working age in the UK and is also the most common cause of lower limb amputations and end stage renal disease (ESRD) (Diabetes UK, 2010).

Diabetic retinopathy

This describes narrowing or blockage of the blood vessels at the back of the eye and is caused by high blood glucose levels, high blood pressure or a combination of both. It can be divided into early, reversible (background) retinopathy and the more developed stages that require treatment and may result in blindness. It affects 10–65% of people with diabetes globally (International Diabetes Federation, 2009) and the prevalence is related to the duration of diabetes. In the UK, it is estimated that 25% of people with diabetes will develop retinopathy after 5 years (NHS Choices, 2011).

Diabetic nephropathy

This affects the blood vessels in the kidney and the first sign is the presence of small amounts of protein in the urine (microalbuminuria). Microalbuminuria may be present for many years without progression, but can lead to increased protein loss and eventually ESRD requiring dialysis or transplant. Globally, between 5% and 30% of people with diabetes develop nephropathy and figures for the UK suggest that 30% of people with type 2 diabetes will develop kidney disease (Stratton et al., 2000).

Diabetic neuropathy

Diabetic neuropathy describes the nerve damage associated with high blood glucose levels and can affect sensory nerves (resulting in loss of sensation or increased pain sensation), autonomic nerves (leading to warmer, swollen feet or dry, cracked skin) and motor nerves (leading to muscle atrophy and deformities in the shape of the foot). Nerve damage is often associated with peripheral circulatory damage and can lead to foot ulcers, progressing to gangrene and requiring amputation. Peripheral neuropathy is estimated to affect between 15% and 55% of people with diabetes worldwide.

Sexual dysfunction

Erectile dysfunction and female sexual dysfunction are more common in people with diabetes. Erectile dysfunction affects between 35% and 90% of men with diabetes and is associated with increasing age, duration of diabetes, hyperglycaemia, hypertension, hyperlipidaemia, sedentary lifestyle and smoking (Malavige & Levy, 2009). Female sexual dysfunction was reported by 33% of women with diabetes in one study, but it does not appear to be associated with diabetes related factors (Nowosielski et al., 2011).

Depression

People with diabetes appear to have a two-fold increased risk of depression (Anderson et al., 2011), and this is true for both type 1 (Barnard et al., 2006) and type 2 diabetes (Ali et al., 2006). The presence of depression is associated with a reduced quality of life in people with diabetes (Schram et al., 2009).

There is strong evidence that intensive glycaemic control and management of cardiovascular risk factors can reduce both morbidity and mortality associated with diabetes (DCCT Study Group, 1993; UKPDS Group, 1998a,b). There is also evidence that improvements in care have reduced the risk of complications for people with type 1 diabetes over the past 30 years. However, even those receiving intensive treatment still show relatively high levels of complications, with over one-fifth developing proliferative retinopathy and 9% developing nephropathy and CVD (Nathan et al., 2009).

Public health aspects and prevention

There is no evidence for strategies to prevent type 1 diabetes as the aetiology remains unclear, but there is strong evidence from studies in different ethnic groups that type 2 diabetes can be prevented in high risk individuals by lifestyle and pharmacological interventions (Paulweber et al., 2010). Lifestyle interventions show the greatest effect, with reductions of 28–59% in the risk of diabetes following implementation (Walker et al., 2010), and evidence of a legacy effect with lower incidence of diabetes at 7–20 years after intervention (Knowler et al., 2009; Li et al., 2008; Lindstrom et al., 2006). Evidence based European guidelines for diabetes prevention and Diabetes UK lifestyle specific guidelines have recently been published and are summarised below (Paulweber et al., 2010; Dyson et al., 2011).

Components of lifestyle interventions for type 2 diabetes prevention

Weight reduction

Weight reduction in overweight or obese individuals is the dominant factor for diabetes prevention, with weight losses of 5–7% significantly lowering risk; with a 16% reduction in risk is associated with each kilogram lost (Hamman et al., 2006). Although the majority of studies have promoted reduced fat, high fibre diets with a moderate reduction in energy intake, there is emerging evidence that alternative dietary strategies, including the Mediterranean diet and low carbohydrate diets, are effective for weight loss and diabetes risk reduction (Walker et al., 2010).

Physical activity

Increased physical activity reduces the risk of diabetes, and at least 30 minutes/day of moderate activity is recommended.

Diet

Studies have shown that diets high in fibre ($\geq 15\,g/1000\,kcal$), reduced in total fat ($\leq 35\%$ of total energy) and saturated and *trans* fat ($<10\%$ of total energy) can induce weight loss and reduce risk. There are no randomised controlled trials of different dietary strategies to identify the most effective diet for type 2 diabetes prevention.

Despite the strong evidence from randomised controlled trials for the efficacy of diabetes prevention programmes, there is little evidence of translation into the area of public health and diabetes prevalence continues to rise around the world.

Nutritional assessment

Anthropometry

Body weight and body mass index (BMI) should be monitored regularly in people with diabetes, especially those with type 2 diabetes as they are prone to weight gain. Obesity increases the risk of diabetes related complications, especially CVD. Waist circumference predicts both type 2 diabetes and CVD (Yusuf et al., 2004). Waist circumference cut-off points differ according to ethnicity and gender (see Appendix A7).

Biochemistry

Glycated haemoglobin (HbA1$_c$) measures long term glycaemic control (>12 weeks) and should be measured at least once a year. It is now expressed in mmol/mol rather than as a percentage. A conversion table can be found in Appendix A9. Lipid profiles [serum total cholesterol, high density lipoprotein (HDL) and low density lipoprotein (LDL) cholesterol, and triglycerides levels) are measured to assess cardiovascular risk. Microalbuminuria is an indicator of early stage kidney disease; it should be measured annually. In addition, blood creatinine measurements can be used to calculate estimated glomerular filtration rate, which provides an assessment of overall excretory kidney function.

Clinical examination

Blood pressure assesses cardiovascular risk and should be measured at regular intervals and at least once a year. Retinal screening involves dilation of the eyes and a retinal photograph, and is designed to measure diabetic eye disease. In the UK, there is a system in place to ensure that all people with diabetes have a retinal photograph annually. Foot examination assesses skin, blood and nerve supply to the legs and feet, and should be part of the annual review. Injection sites should be examined in people injecting medication to monitor for hyperlipotrophy – hard lumps under the skin caused by repeated injections into the same site, which affect insulin absorption.

Dietary assessment

There is some discussion about the usefulness of diet histories (including the most widely used 24-hour recall) in managing chronic diseases such as diabetes. Many dietitians feel that it is impossible to give people advice about a healthy diet for diabetes unless they have some idea of the individual's usual diet, but there is no evidence that taking a diet history improves diabetes control and strong evidence that up to 67% of people underreport intake, especially of snack foods; BMI is a strong determinant of underreporting (Poslusna et al., 2009). Dietary assessment can be used to evaluate an individual's wishes and willingness to change in the following areas:

- Meal patterns and usual lifestyle – this is often called a typical day and gives additional information about work and physical activity.
- Likes and dislikes, including usual food choices, and attitudes and beliefs about different foods.
- Perceptions and beliefs about food related specifically to health.

Economic and social factors

Factors such as socioeconomic circumstances, ethnic group and occupation will have an effect on the individual's willingness and ability to manage their diabetes.

Clinical management

The aims of management of diabetes are to maintain blood glucose levels as near to the normal range as possible in order to minimise both the short term (hypoglycaemia and diabetic ketoacidosis) and long term (macrovascular and microvascular) complications associated with hyper- and hypo-glycaemia.

Targets for glycaemic control

Internationally, it is generally agreed that for most people the target for HbA1$_c$ level is 53 mmol/mol (7.0%) or less.

In the UK, targets for people with type 2 diabetes and people with type 1 diabetes and diabetes related complications are set lower at <48 mmol/mol (6.5%) (NICE, 2004; 2008a). Targets for self monitored blood glucose levels (SMBGs) in the UK are:

- *Children with type 1 diabetes* (NICE, 2004):
  - Before meals – 4–8 mmol/L.
  - 2 hours post prandial – <10 mmol/L.
- *Adults with type 1 diabetes* (NICE, 2004):
  - Before meals – 4–7 mmol/L.
  - 2 hours post prandial – <9 mmol/L.
- *Type 2 diabetes* (NICE, 2008a):
  - Before meals – 4–7 mmol/L.
  - 2 hours post prandial – <8.5 mmol/L.

Targets for risk reduction of comorbidities

Targets for risk factor reduction in the UK are:

- *Adults with type 1 diabetes* (NICE, 2004):
  - Blood pressure – <135/85 mmHg (in the high risk, aim for <130/80 mmHg).
  - LDL cholesterol – <2.6 mmol/L.
  - Triglycerides – 2.3 mmol/L.
- *Individuals with type 2 diabetes* (NICE, 2008a):
  - Blood pressure – <140/80 mmHg (in the high risk, aim for <130/80 mmHg).
  - No specific targets for lipid levels (aim for the lowest possible).

Pharmaceutical management

Type 1 diabetes

Type 1 diabetes is managed by insulin replacement; there are many different insulins available and the type, dose and regimen depends upon the lifestyle of the individual. Until the 1980s, insulin was only available by extraction and purification from the pancreas of cattle and pigs. This animal insulin is still in use but has been largely replaced by human insulin that is engineered genetically in laboratories. Newer analogue insulin has been introduced over the past few years in an attempt to replicate the action of naturally produced insulin in the body. Insulin can be divided into:

- *Rapid acting analogue insulin* with an onset of action within 5–10 minutes, peaking at 90 minutes and lasting for 3 hours. This type of insulin is commonly taken with meals and can be injected at the time of, or after, eating.
- *Short acting insulin* begins working within 30 minutes, peaks at 2 hours and lasts for 4–8 hours. Like rapid acting insulin, it is usually taken with meals, but is injected 20–30 minutes before eating.
- *Medium and long acting insulins* are usually taken once or twice a day and provide background insulin over 24 hours. They have an onset of action within 90 minutes, peak between 4 and 12 hours and last for 12–24 hours.

- Long acting analogue insulin is promoted as having a flat profile, with no peak action and lasts for 18–24 hours. It is usually taken once a day, often at bedtime.
- Mixed insulin consists of premixed short acting insulin with medium or long acting insulin and is usually taken twice a day, usually before breakfast and before the evening meal. It has an onset of action within 30 minutes, peaks at 2–8 hours and lasts for 16–20 hours.
- Mixed analogue insulin is a mixture of rapid acting and long acting analogue insulin with an onset of action within 5–10 minutes, peaking at 90 minutes and lasting for 16–10 hours.

The majority of people with type 1 diabetes in developed countries are encouraged to use multiple daily injection regimens (known as MDI or basal bolus), typically consisting of one injection of long acting insulin and three (or more) injections of rapid or short acting insulin with meals. This intensive insulin regimen has been shown to be associated with improved glycaemic control and allows for dietary flexibility (DCCT Study Group, 1993; DAFNE Study Group, 2002). The traditional regimen of mixed insulin injected twice daily, usually before breakfast and before the evening meal, is less common and is associated with increased hypoglycaemia in those who do not have regular meals.

Insulin is administered by syringe and needles, pen injection devices or pumps [continuous subcutaneous insulin infusion (CSII)]. Pump therapy consists of a portable pump that delivers rapid acting insulin through a cannula, providing background insulin and a bolus of insulin when food is eaten. Pump therapy is becoming more common; in the UK in 2010 approximately 4% (9750 people) of people with type 1 diabetes were using pump therapy, and guidance has been issued stating that pumps are suitable for those with disabling hypoglycaemia or who have failed to reach an HbA1$_c$ of 69 mmol/mol or less despite MDI therapy (NICE, 2008b).

Type 2 diabetes

Type 2 diabetes is managed clinically with a combination of tablets and injectable therapies, including insulin. In the UK, algorithms have been produced recommending a treatment cascade for those with type 2 diabetes, beginning with a trial of lifestyle measures including structured education (NICE, 2008a). Medication includes:

- *Metformin* is recommended as a first line therapy. It belongs to the biguanide class of drugs and its main action is to increase insulin sensitivity and reduce hepatic gluconeogenesis. It does not cause weight gain or hypoglycaemia and may be associated with a reduced risk of CVD. Around 10% of patients do not respond to metformin and approximately 5–10% of patients a year will need another agent in addition. If maximum tolerated doses of metformin fail to achieve target glucose levels, a second agent is commonly added in.
- *Sulphonylureas* are the recommended second line agent and act directly on the pancreas to stimulate insulin production. They are associated with a weight gain of approximately 3 kg and can cause hypoglycaemia.
- *Metiglinides* are short acting agents that are used to control post prandial rises in glucose. They are taken before main meals and stimulate insulin production for that meal. Essentially, they may be viewed as a short acting sulphonylurea and have similar side effects.
- *Thiazoladinediones* (also known as glitazones) have been used only relatively recently since 1997. They are taken once daily, starting with a low dose, and take up to 3 months to have their maximum effect. Their action is to reduce insulin resistance and they produce a lowering of blood glucose levels comparable to metformin or sulphonylureas. Side effects include weight gain and fluid retention. Glitazones tend to be given as second or third line therapy, partly because of the 10–12 weeks it takes for them to have effect.
- *Acarbose* is an alpha glucosidase inhibitor that reduces the rate of carbohydrate digestion, thus controlling post prandial blood glucose rises. This agent has unpleasant side effects of flatulence, abdominal pain, bloating and diarrhoea. As its effect is moderate compared with the other agents available, it is rarely prescribed in the UK.
- *Incretin agonists* are injectable therapies that mimic the action of naturally produced gut hormones and act by stimulating glucose dependent insulin secretion from the pancreas, reducing glucagon secretion, inhibiting gastric emptying and thus promoting satiety and reducing weight. The most common side effects are nausea and vomiting.
- *Gliptins* prevent rapid degradation of the enzyme dipeptidyl peptidase 4 (DPP 4) and so increase concentrations of endogenous, naturally occurring incretin hormones. They are weight neutral and the most frequent side effect is nausea.

In addition to blood glucose management, people with diabetes frequently take agents to reduce blood pressure (antihypertensives) and blood lipid levels (statins), and may need further agents to treat any diabetes related complication.

Surgical treatment of diabetes

Bariatric surgery is increasingly used as a treatment for obesity in people with type 2 diabetes, with a recent IDF statement calling for surgery to be an accepted treatment option for people with type 2 diabetes and a BMI of 35 kg/m^2 or greater. Surgery can induce diabetes remission, with rates of 72% reported over 2-year follow-up (Dixon et al., 2011) (see Chapter 7.13.3).

Other surgical procedures to treat type 1 diabetes include islet and pancreatic transplants. Both these procedures can restore endogenous insulin secretion, but are only available to a few people because of a shortage of donors and because immunosuppressive drugs have side effects that may outweigh the benefits.

Lifestyle management

Lifestyle therapy, including diet and physical activity, is an integral part of effective management of diabetes and has a vital role in helping people with diabetes achieve and maintain optimal glycaemic control and reduce the risk of long term tissue damage (Bantle *et al.*, 2008). There is evidence that intensive treatment of type 1 diabetes, especially with diet, improves outcomes (Delahanty, 1998) and that dietary change, weight loss and increased physical activity are of benefit to people with type 2 diabetes (Look Ahead Research Group, 2010; Pi-Sunyer *et al.*, 2007), although there are few well designed studies investigating the most effective approach (Nield *et al.*, 2007).

Physical activity

The benefits of increased physical activity for people with type 2 diabetes are clear and include improved glycaemic control and reductions in cardiovascular risk, including positive effects on lipids and blood pressure. Long term studies have shown that these benefits translate into a reduction in cardiovascular events and improvements in mortality and quality of life (Colberg *et al.*, 2010). Physical activity does not appear to have a direct effect on BMI in people with type 2 diabetes, although there is evidence of reduction in visceral adipose tissue (Thomas *et al.*, 2006).

The benefits of physical activity for people with type 1 diabetes are less clear. Although physical activity improves cardiovascular risk and may have a positive effect on quality of life, there is no evidence of improvement in glycaemic control in people with type 1 diabetes (Zinman *et al.*, 2003).

It is recommended that people with diabetes take at least 150 minutes of moderate activity each week. Physical activity guidelines are usually made in terms of daily activity, the most common recommendation being that moderate activity should be taken on at least 5 days each week for 30 minutes. Moderate activity is defined as any activity that raises the heart and breathing rate, but does not induce breathlessness, causes a feeling of warmth or promotes light sweating. For many people, brisk walking is sufficient.

Physical activity generally lowers blood glucose in people with diabetes and may increase the risk of hypoglycaemia in those taking insulin or sulphonylureas. For many people with type 2 diabetes not treated with insulin, the effects of physical activity are beneficial and do not require any adjustment to medication or dietary intake. People with type 1 diabetes require more active management to prevent hypoglycaemia. Management of activity can be facilitated by SMBG and may require adjustment of medication and/or increased carbohydrate intake.

Before activity people with diabetes treated with sulphonylureas or insulin are advised to test their blood glucose levels, aiming for levels within the range of 6–13 mmol/L. If levels are <6 mmol/L, an additional 15–30 g high glycaemic index (GI) carbohydrate should be taken. Examples of high GI carbohydrates include isotonic sports drinks, made up squash, bananas, jelly beans and fruit pastilles. People with type 1 diabetes showing levels of >13 mmol/L should delay activity and test for the presence of ketones as they may be at increased risk of ketoacidosis.

During activity additional high GI carbohydrate may be necessary, depending upon the duration and intensity of exercise. As a rough guide, for any exercise session that lasts >60 minutes, 30–60 g/hour of high GI carbohydrate may be needed.

After prolonged or strenuous activity, the effect of exercise can be assessed by testing blood glucose levels. Consuming high GI carbohydrates within an hour of activity will replenish liver and muscle glycogen stores, and those with type 1 diabetes may need to reduce the post activity insulin dose.

Alcohol

Epidemiological studies have shown that moderate alcohol intake (1–3 units/day) in people with diabetes is associated with improved glycaemic control and reduced CVD and all cause mortality. The guidelines for alcohol intake for people with diabetes do not differ from those for the general population, but there are additional factors for consideration.

Hypoglycaemia is a well documented side effect of alcohol in people with type 1 diabetes, and can occur at relatively low levels of intake and up to 12 hours after ingestion. There is no evidence for the most effective treatment to prevent hypoglycaemia, but pragmatic advice includes recommending insulin dose adjustment, additional carbohydrate or a combination of the two according to individual need.

The amount of carbohydrate in alcoholic drinks can vary greatly with some (dry wines, spirits) containing little or no carbohydrate and some (sweet liqueurs, alcopops) containing significant amounts. Consumption of alcoholic drinks containing carbohydrate raises blood glucose levels and can cause hyperglycaemia. People treated with insulin may take extra to cover the carbohydrate in drinks, but this may exacerbate hypoglycaemia.

There are some medical conditions where alcohol is contraindicated, including hypertension, hypertriglyceridaemia, some neuropathies and retinopathy. As with the general population, alcohol should be avoided during pregnancy and when planning to drive.

Nutritional management

Aims of dietary treatment

Nutritional therapy is an integral part of diabetes self management and treatment. The aims of dietary treatment of diabetes are complementary to those of medical management and have been summarised by Diabetes UK as (Dyson *et al.*, 2011):

- Supporting self management to reduce the risk of type 2 diabetes and the comorbidities associated with diabetes.
- Promoting healthy lifestyles and quality of life.

- Providing flexibility and meeting the needs of all individuals, including those with comorbidities such as coeliac disease and cystic fibrosis (Lindstrom *et al.*, 2006).

Many countries have published nutritional recommendations for diabetes (Dyson *et al.*, 2011; Bantle *et al.*, 2008; Canadian Diabetes Association, 2008; Ha & Lean, 1998) and these have been subject to change over time as evidence emerges for effective dietary treatment of diabetes. Until recently, the majority of nutritional recommendations were based on the consensus of recognised experts in the field, but the recent guidelines from the American Diabetes Association (ADA) and Diabetes UK have moved towards evidence based recommendations. Recent recommendations have been made in terms of topic areas rather than nutrients and stress the importance of tailoring nutritional advice for each individual, taking into account personal and cultural preferences, beliefs, lifestyle and willingness and ability to change.

Education models

Structured education for people with diabetes in the UK is now recommended for all individuals at the time of diagnosis, with regular (at least annual) review (NICE, 2011). Nutritional management should be included as an integrated component of structured education, and there is strong evidence of clinical effectiveness, cost effectiveness and improved quality of life for both type 1 and type 2 diabetes (Dyson *et al.*, 2011). Structured education can be delivered in groups or to individuals. There are four key components to structured education:

- A structured, written curriculum, including philosophy and theoretical principles.
- Trained educators.
- Quality assurance.
- Audit and evaluation of both biomedical and quality of life outcomes.

More detailed criteria for education programmes include the recommendations that all programmes should be patient centred and incorporate individual assessment. They should be reliable, valid, relevant and comprehensive; theory driven and evidence based; flexible and able to cope with diversity and to utilise different teaching techniques; resource effective with supporting materials; written down (including philosophy, aims and objective, timetables and detailed content); and subject to robust audit and evaluation. Although these criteria apply more to structured education in groups, the principles can be applied to all education.

Education delivery

The traditional model of delivering education is the one to one interview between the healthcare professional and the person with diabetes, and is often based upon dietary histories and prescriptive advice. These didactic based approaches have been shown to produce modest improvements in outcomes, but patient education has been shown to be more effective if it also has a behavioural element. Innovative approaches may be needed to deliver education to people with diabetes. Patients with chronic disease, including diabetes, state that they would like information in as many formats as possible and as early as possible after diagnosis, and a variety of techniques including picture charts, video techniques, computer packages, text messaging, email and phone applications can be used (Corben & Rosen, 2005).

Glycaemic control

Carbohydrate is the nutrient that has most effect on blood glucose levels after eating, and is a major nutritional consideration for people with diabetes. All carbohydrate foods are digested to glucose and appear in the blood between 10 minutes and 2 hours or more after eating, and both the amount and type will affect post prandial levels. There is no evidence for an optimal amount of carbohydrate for achieving and maintaining glycaemic control in people with diabetes, and for people with type 1 diabetes the emphasis is on matching insulin to carbohydrate on a meal by meal basis. This process is commonly called carbohydrate counting and insulin adjustment. It requires those with type 1 diabetes to calculate the amount of carbohydrate in each meal and snack, and to inject a matching amount of insulin. There is no evidence supporting the use of carbohydrate counting for people with type 2 diabetes. People with type 1 diabetes treated with fixed doses of insulin, and those with type 2 diabetes are advised to monitor carbohydrate intake by a variety of means, including exchanges, portions or experience based estimation.

Carbohydrate assessment

Carbohydrate awareness is the process of identifying carbohydrate containing foods and is the first step in the process of carbohydrate estimation. Carbohydrate awareness can be facilitated with a variety of teaching aids, including food lists, picture charts, food photographs and food models.

Carbohydrate budgets or portions can be facilitated by a variety of strategies. Traditionally, carbohydrate was restricted in people with diabetes by the use of the exchange system (one exchange contained 10 g of carbohydrate, e.g. ⅔ slice bread, ⅓ pint milk, two plain biscuits), where diets were prescribed with a limited allowance of exchanges at each meal or snack. The modern use of budgets or portions encourages consistent amounts of carbohydrate at each specific meal from day to day, but does not necessarily prescribe a limited amount of carbohydrate. Teaching aids for promoting consistent portion sizes include using household measurements (spoonfuls, cupfuls and units), visual estimation with reference to food photographs, comparing portion size to hand size, e.g. a fist sized portion of starchy food such as rice, potato or pasta, and exchanges lists.

Carbohydrate counting, used by people with type 1 diabetes, is the most accurate method of carbohydrate assessment. The amount of carbohydrate in individual meals and snacks is usually calculated to the nearest 5–10 g, or expressed as carbohydrate portions (CPs), with each portion containing 10 g carbohydrate. Strategies include the use of household measures, exchange or portion lists and visual estimation using food photographs or phone applications. Nutritional labels on packaged foods can provide useful information. It can be helpful to weigh individual foods such as breakfast cereals, rice and pasta where there is no recognised portion size, and food tables are then necessary for carbohydrate calculation.

Type of carbohydrate

The most significant predictor of post prandial blood glucose levels is the amount of carbohydrate eaten, but the type of carbohydrate does have some effect. Relevant concepts are those of GI, sugar and dietary fibre. The GI has been widely promoted for dietary management of diabetes and both the ADA and Diabetes UK recommend a low GI diet. Low GI diets can significantly improve glycaemic control and reduce hypoglycaemia in people with diabetes (Thomas & Elliott, 2009). The GI is a scale that ranks carbohydrate foods by how much they raise blood glucose levels compared with a reference food (usually white bread or glucose). High GI foods cause large fluctuations in glucose and insulin levels, and low GI foods cause smaller fluctuations. It is measured in the laboratory by feeding samples of food containing 50 g of carbohydrate to volunteers and testing blood glucose levels at 15-minute intervals for 2–3 hours. The results are plotted on a graph and the area under the curve (AUC) is compared with a reference food using the formula:

$$\frac{\text{AUC for test food}}{\text{AUC for reference food}} \times 100 = \text{GI value for test food}$$

The GI of the test food is then expressed as a number compared with the reference food. The average results from 10 volunteers are required for each food tested. Table 7.12.1 shows GI ranking by derived values and Table 7.12.2 examples of low, medium and high GI foods. The disadvantages of low GI diets in practice are that this strategy may reinstate a prescriptive approach to dietary advice, other factors may affect the GI of foods, e.g. adding organic acids such as lemon juice or vinegar to a food lowers its GI, and it takes little account of the amount of carbohydrate eaten. This last point is addressed by the concept of glycaemic load (GL).

The GL reflects the amount and quality of carbohydrate eaten and can be expressed by the formula:

$$\frac{\text{GI}}{100} \times \text{Net carbohydrate}$$

$$(\text{total carbohydrate} - \text{dietary fibre}) = \text{GL}$$

Recommendations for the GL of foods and a guideline total daily value are shown in Table 7.12.3.

Table 7.12.1 Glycaemic index values and ranking

Glycaemic index value	Glycaemic ranking
0–55	Low
56–69	Medium
70 or more	High

Table 7.12.2 Examples of low, medium and high glycaemic index (GI) foods

Food	Low GI (<55)	Medium GI (56–69)	High GI (>70)
Bread	Multigrain, stone ground wholemeal, granary and rye		All other wholemeal, brown and white bread, including French and naan bread
Breakfast cereals	High bran cereal, muesli and porridge made with stone ground oats	Other bran cereals, including bran flakes and those with dried fruit	All other corn and wheat based cereals, including wholewheat and sugar coated cereals
Potatoes	Sweet potatoes, yams	New potatoes	Old potatoes – boiled, mashed, baked, roast and chips
Pasta and rice	*Al dente* pasta and egg noodles	Basmati rice, rice noodles	White and brown rice, rice pasta
Vegetables	Pulses, peas, beans and legumes		
Fruit	Apples, pears, stone fruit (peaches, plums, cherries), citrus fruit (oranges, tangerines) and berries	Tropical fruit (bananas, pineapples, mangoes)	
Dairy products	Full fat, semi skimmed and skimmed milk, yogurt	Ice cream	
Cakes and biscuits	Plain sponge cake, fruit and malt breads	Plain biscuits, crackers	Doughnuts, scones
Savoury snacks	Maize or corn chips	Crisps	Extruded potato snacks, pretzels

SECTION 7

Table 7.12.3 Recommendations for low, medium and high glycaemic load (GL)

GL ranking	GL value	Daily GL
Low	10 or less	79 or less
Medium	11–19	80–119
High	20 or more	120 or more

Although GL is a tool for assessing the overall effect of carbohydrates on blood glucose levels, it is complicated to use in practice and is not recommended as a management strategy for people with diabetes.

Sugar was traditionally restricted in people with diabetes as it was commonly assumed that the sugar (sucrose) content of food related directly to blood glucose levels. Traditionally, table sugar (sucrose) has been restricted for people with diabetes and the original nutritional recommendations from the British Diabetic Association (now known as Diabetes UK) in 1992 stated that no more than 25 g of sucrose should be consumed daily. In terms of glycaemic control, sucrose has no more effect on blood glucose levels than isocaloric amounts of starchy carbohydrate and most recommendations do not now impose a rigid restriction on sugar. Apart from sucrose and glycaemic control, there has been some recent research showing that high intakes of sugar sweetened beverages are associated with the development of obesity, type 2 diabetes and CVD (Malik *et al.*, 2010), and that the general advice for healthy eating (<10% of total energy from sugar) should be applied to all individuals.

Dietary fibre is promoted for its cardioprotective effects, but there is little evidence for its effect on glycaemic control in people with diabetes. Some studies report improved glycaemic control, but these use large amounts of fibre (40–50 g/day) with little evidence supporting smaller amounts. The recommendation for the general population for fibre should be applied to people with diabetes (Franz *et al.*, 2010).

Diabetes complications

Cardiovascular disease

People with diabetes have a two-fold increased risk of CVD and it is the leading cause of death (The Emerging Risk Factor Collaboration , 2010). As these people are at high risk, nutrition recommendations are similar to those for people with established heart disease. The aims of nutritional guidelines for CVD are to reduce risk by improving blood lipid profiles and reducing blood pressure by dietary factors such as fat, plant stannols and sterols, salt, dietary fibre and alcohol.

Fat

High fat intakes, especially of saturated fat, are associated with increased lipid levels and risk of heart disease, and current recommendations from both the ADA and Diabetes UK are that people with diabetes reduce saturated fat and replace this with unsaturated fat, particularly monounsaturated fat. There is no strong evidence to support a specific amount of fat in the diet; current guidelines reflect this and have not formulated recommendations for exact proportions of energy derived from fat, but do recommend individual flexibility. There is little evidence for guidelines about *trans* fat intake in people with diabetes, and the guidelines for the general population should be adopted (see Chapter 4.2).

High intakes of oily fish (salmon, trout, herring, mackerel and sardines) are associated with reduced rates of CVD and should be consumed at least twice weekly. There remains controversy about the use of fish oil supplements for people with diabetes, with some evidence of reduction in triglyceride levels in those with hypertriglyceridaemia. Diabetes UK recommends that fish oil supplementation may have therapeutic benefits for this subgroup.

Plant stanols and sterols

Studies have shown that plant sterols and stanols included in manufactured foods such as margarine, yogurt and yogurt drinks can significantly lower cholesterol levels by at least 10% (Thompson & Grundy, 2005). These products can be recommended, but they are only effective at doses of 2 g/day or greater, and they are more expensive than regular products.

Salt

Salt intakes are significantly associated with blood pressure, and studies show that salt reduction lowers blood pressure. The daily average intake of salt in the UK is 8.6 g/day, and most guidelines recommend reductions to 5–6 g/day, effectively reducing consumption by a third. Reductions in salt intake can be achieved by avoiding or reducing salt used in cooking or added at the table, and by avoiding obviously salty foods such as savoury snacks, but the majority of salt (75%) in the western diet comes from processed foods, and effective salt reduction will require intervention from the food industry.

Dietary fibre

Although there is contradictory evidence for dietary fibre in terms of glycaemic control, high intakes of fibre and especially soluble fibre are associated with reductions in total cholesterol and LDL cholesterol levels. Guidelines for people with diabetes recommend adopting the dietary reference values (DRVs) for the general population.

Physical activity, alcohol and weight management

These are all key factors for cardiovascular risk reduction and are discussed fully elsewhere.

Dietary strategies

Dietary strategies to reduce CVD combine some of the individual elements associated with risk reduction, and include the Mediterranean and DASH (Dietary Approaches to Stop Hypertension) diets. These diets recommend reducing saturated fat and substituting fish and olive oil for red meat and butter, and increasing vegetable, fruit and wholegrain intake. The combined effects of these diets have a greater effect on blood pressure than those achieved by the individual components, and significantly reduce cardiovascular risk (see Chapter 7.14.4).

Microvascular disease

The most important predictor of both development and progression of microvascular disease is glycaemic control. All nutritional strategies to maintain or improve blood glucose levels in people with diabetes can be applied to those with microvascular disease. There is very little good quality evidence for specific nutritional management of diabetes related microvascular disease apart from that of glycaemic control.

Hypoglycaemia

People with diabetes treated with insulin, sulphoylureas or metiglinides are at risk of hypoglycaemia and this risk increases with duration of diabetes. Hypoglycaemia is defined as a blood glucose level of <4 mmol/L, and people with diabetes can be advised to 'make 4 the floor', meaning they should treat any level below 4 mmol/L as soon as possible. People without diabetes do not experience hypoglycaemia due to a homeostatic response as blood glucose levels fall; glucose stored in the liver is released into the blood stream by the action of the counter regulatory hormones glucagon, adrenaline (epinephrine) and cortisol. Although this process does occur in people with diabetes, it may by over ridden by the presence of excess insulin and there is evidence of attenuated hormonal response related to duration of diabetes. The causes of hypoglycaemia include:

* Missing or delaying a meal or snack.
* Eating less carbohydrate than normal.
* Increased physical activity or exercise.
* Drinking alcohol.
* Taking excessive amounts of insulin or tablets.

The first symptoms of hypoglycaemia are caused by adrenaline (epinephrine) release and include sweating, shaking, increased heart rate, hunger or nausea, anxiety, irritability, tiredness and headache. As hypoglycaemia progresses, lack of glucose to the brain can cause confusion, lack of coordination, slurred speech, drowsiness and aggression, and eventually convulsions and coma. Hypoglycaemia is rarely fatal, although deaths have been reported following excessive alcohol consumption.

Treatment of hypoglycaemia aims to raise blood glucose levels to the normal range as quickly as possible, avoiding over treating and associated hyperglycaemia and preventing reoccurrence of hypoglycaemia. Glucose is the preferred treatment for hypoglycaemia and advice for treatment follows the rule of 15:

* 15–20 g of glucose taken as soon as possible.
* If glucose levels do not rise above 4 mmol/L after 15 minutes, repeat treatment.
* A follow-up snack containing 15–20 g of carbohydrate may be necessary to reduce the risk of further hypoglycaemia.

Isolated incidences of hypoglycaemia should follow the above guidelines, but repeated hypoglycaemic episodes need further investigation, as prevention is better than cure. Advice for prevention involves identifying the cause and taking steps to prevent reoccurrence by adjusting insulin dose or carbohydrate intake. General advice includes avoiding missing meals, always carrying glucose, testing blood glucose levels before driving and avoiding drinking alcohol on an empty stomach.

Hypoglycaemia unawareness is a condition in which people no longer recognise the symptoms of hypoglycaemia. It is more prevalent in people with type 1 diabetes and is associated with duration of diabetes and intensive management. Symptoms may be restored after a period of maintaining glucose at higher levels and this should be done under medical supervision.

Other nutritional considerations

Protein

In the past, recommendations for protein for people with diabetes have advised that protein intakes should be restricted to the lower end of normal intake as there were concerns about the effect of high protein intake on kidney function and the development of nephropathy. There is insufficient evidence to support protein restriction to prevent the development of diabetic nephropathy, and a systematic review has concluded that there is little evidence to support protein restriction as a management strategy for established diabetic kidney disease (Robertson et al., 2007). Current guidelines recommend that protein intakes for the general population should be adopted for people with diabetes.

Vitamins and minerals

Recent research has investigated the role of vitamin D in diabetes and CVD prevention, and the association between thiamine reduction and the risk of kidney disease and heart disease in people with diabetes. There is, as yet, no firm evidence to support the use of vitamin supplements in people with diabetes.

Chromium, magnesium and zinc are all utilised in carbohydrate metabolism and have been the focus of studies in diabetes. Studies report conflicting results for a benefit of supplementation in terms of glycaemic control, The current advice from Diabetes UK is that there is insufficient evidence to recommend any vitamin or mineral supplement for people with diabetes.

Functional foods

Food such as chilli, karela (bitter gourd) and spices (cinnamon and fenugreek) have been shown to lower blood glucose levels, and are frequently used in traditional medicine. Although they have hypoglycaemic effects, these are unpredictable and they are not currently recommended.

Weight management

Weight loss can improve glycaemic control and reduce cardiovascular risk and all cause mortality in people with type 2 diabetes (Aucott *et al.*, 2004), although there is little evidence for its effect in people with type 1 diabetes. Strategies used to promote weight reduction in people with diabetes include physical activity and dietary, behavioural, pharmacological and surgical interventions.

Dietary interventions

Dietary interventions for weight loss in people with type 2 diabetes have been widely researched, but many of these studies have methodological flaws and were short term, so it is difficult to draw firm conclusions for clinical practice. Different dietary strategies have been used, including low fat diets, low calorie diets, low carbohydrate diets, very low calorie liquid diets, meal replacements and commercial slimming clubs. Regardless of the type of diet used, dietary interventions for obesity have small but significant effects on body weight and improve glycaemic control (Aucott *et al.*, 2004). However, there is no evidence for the most effective diet for inducing weight loss in people with diabetes, and the advice from Diabetes UK is that those with diabetes can adopt any strategy that is recommended for people without diabetes (see Chapter 7.13.2).

Physical activity

Physical activity is not an effective strategy for weight loss for people with diabetes when used in isolation (Boule *et al.*, 2001), but a combination of diet and physical activity is more effective for weight loss than either strategy alone (Shaw *et al.*, 2006). There are very few studies investigating the effects of different types and intensity of physical activity in weight loss and guidelines cannot be formulated for the relative benefits of aerobic or resistance training.

Behavioural therapy

Many different psychological techniques have been used to promote weight loss, including behavioural and cognitive therapy, group therapy, psychodynamic therapy and humanistic therapy. All behavioural interventions have been shown to promote significant weight loss, and adding dietary or physical activity interventions to these increases weight loss (Dyson, 2010). Although the majority of studies do not include people with diabetes, the evidence suggests that behavioural therapy as an adjunct would improve weight loss in people with diabetes (see Chapter 1.3).

Pharmacological and surgical interventions

There is evidence of significant weight loss with both pharmacological and surgical interventions for people with diabetes, although in the UK only one pharmaceutical agent (orlistat) is available (NICE, 2006). Dietary advice is part of the educational package that should be offered to those who adopt these interventions for weight loss.

Considerations for particular groups

Children and adolescents

The aims of dietary treatment of diabetes in children and adolescents are similar to those for adults, with an addi-tional emphasis on providing sufficient energy and nutrients for optimal growth. The International Society for Pediatric and Adolescent Diabetes (ISPAD) has published clinical practice consensus guidelines and the broad approach is that of child centred, individualised care based upon healthy eating recommendations suitable for the whole family (Smart *et al.*, 2009). A multidisciplinary team approach is recommended, with a specialist paediatric dietitian providing education and support to the child, the family, the school and other carers (see Chapter 3.8.8).

Teenagers often have poor glycaemic control and although this may be partly due to lifestyle factors, increased insulin resistance accompanies the adolescent growth spurt, which contributes to higher glucose levels. Body weight changes rapidly during adolescence and both excessive weight gain or weight loss may occur. Inappropriate weight gain requires review and advice about dietary intake, insulin dose and physical activity. Weight loss may be associated with insulin omission in order to control weight and/or an eating disorder. Erratic lifestyles, rebellion and peer pressure can all affect diabetes control and may need specialist psychological input.

A summary of nutritional recommendations is shown in Table 7.12.4.

Energy balance

Childhood and adolescence are times of rapid growth and it can be challenging to meet increased energy demands for optimal growth while maintaining target blood glucose levels. Children with diabetes tend to be heavier than those without diabetes; this may be due to over insulinisation and is associated with snacking to prevent hypoglycaemia. Energy intake can vary greatly from day to day, especially in young children, and dietary advice should be flexible, adaptable and reviewed regularly.

Table 7.12.4 Nutritional recommendations for children and adolescents with diabetes (Smart *et al.*, 2009)

Nutrient	Recommendation
Carbohydrate	50–55% of energy intake
Sucrose	Up to 10% of total energy intake
Dietary fibre	2.8–3.4 g/MJ
Total fat	30–35% of total energy intake
Saturated fat + trans fatty acids	<10% of total energy intake
Polyunsaturated fat	<10% of total energy intake
Monounsaturated fat	10–20% of total energy intake
Protein	10–15% of total energy intake
Salt	<6 g of sodium chloride daily
Vitamins and antioxidants	Encourage natural sources
Diabetic foods	None

Carbohydrates

These should not be restricted in children as this may affect growth. Sugar may provide up to 10% of energy, although excessive consumption in the form of sugar sweetened beverages has been linked to weight gain in children. Denying children all foods containing sugar can have psychological effects and is not recommended. Education about carbohydrate foods is regarded as necessary and the approach recommended is that of the ADA, with three levels of carbohydrate counting (Gillespie *et al.*, 1998).

Fat, protein, vitamin and minerals

Recommendations for these nutrients are no different from those for the general population and are in line with guidelines for promoting health.

Education models

Education models for the delivery of dietary education for children have been developed and include food pyramids and plate models that are designed to promote optimal glycaemic control and reduce the risk of cardiovascular disease. As there are no studies showing that one method is better that another, and there is no international consensus for the most effective tool, it is recommended that appropriate education models should be adapted to the needs of the individual child and family.

Physical activity

This should be promoted for children and adolescents, but it is the commonest cause of hypoglycaemia and needs careful planning on an individual basis. For most children, extra carbohydrate is needed for activity and this is especially true of unplanned activity. Children taking part in regular training sessions or competitive sport will need specialist advice from a paediatric dietitian.

Type 2 diabetes

Type 2 diabetes was formerly unknown in children, but its prevalence is increasing as obesity rates rise. Most children and adolescents with diabetes are obese and will require lifestyle management. There is little evidence for the most effective strategies for management, but recommendations for adults can be adapted for children and should include guidelines for weight reduction, increased physical activity and avoiding energy dense foods and sugar sweetened beverages (Flint & Arslanian, 2011).

Pregnant and lactating women

Women with diabetes who become pregnant are at greater risk of miscarriage, congenital malformation, stillbirth and neonatal death. They should be offered preconception care and advice, and this should be continued during pregnancy. Dietary advice should be offered as part of the education package for women with diabetes and those who develop gestational diabetes (NICE, 2008c).

Preconception care includes advice about establishing optimum glycaemic control and body weight before pregnancy and, in those attempting pregnancy, taking 5 mg of folic acid/day until the 12th week of pregnancy to reduce the risk of neural tube defects (see Chapter 3.2).

Antenatal advice should include standard education about food safety and healthy eating for pregnancy. A multidisciplinary team including a specialist dietitian should provide the education. Glycaemic control is of paramount importance during pregnancy and guidelines recommend that blood glucose levels as near to the normal ranges as possible should be maintained. Insulin resistance increase during pregnancy and women should be advised to increase insulin doses in order to control glucose levels. Body weight monitoring during pregnancy is not recommended by the National Institute for Health and Care Excellence in the UK, although other authorities have issued guidelines and recommend weight gains close to those suggested by prepregnancy weight (Institute of Medicine, 2009; Kitzmiller *et al.*, 2008).

Postnatal care includes support and advice about breastfeeding, which should be encouraged in all women. Insulin requirements are reduced following delivery and breastfeeding may induce hypoglycaemia. Women with diabetes can manage blood glucose levels during breastfeeding by frequent blood glucose tests and a combination of insulin reductions and increased carbohydrate intake. Women with gestational diabetes are at greater risk of type 2 diabetes in the future and may benefit from dietary advice to reduce future risk, especially if they are overweight.

Older adults

Older people with diabetes show reduced physical function, health status and impaired cognitive function compared with those without diabetes (Sinclair *et al.*, 2008), and there is some evidence of poorer nutritional status both in hospital and the general community. The guidelines for management of glycaemia and cardiovascular risk are the same as those for adults, but in the older person with comorbidities, functional dependence or limited life expectancy the targets should be relaxed with the emphasis on avoidance of both symptomatic hyperglycaemia and hypoglycaemia. Nutritional assessment and support for the older person with diabetes who is malnourished should be available (see Chapter 10).

Related comorbidities

Coeliac disease, like type 1 diabetes, is an autoimmune condition and the two are often associated. Approximately 2% of adults and 10% of children with type 1 diabetes have diagnosed coeliac disease and many more may remain undiagnosed. Coeliac UK has produced guidelines for the dietary management of diabetes and coeliac disease in the UK, and recommend individualised advice from a specialist dietitian (see Chapter 7.4.7).

Cystic fibrosis related diabetes (CFRD) is a unique type of diabetes with features of both type 1 and type 2 diabetes and occurs in 40–50% of adults with cystic fibrosis (CF). Insulin is used to treat CFRD and the aim of treatment is to maintain both body weight and blood glucose levels as near to the normal range as possible. Most people with CF are advised to eat an energy dense diet to maintain a healthy body weight and this advice continues to apply to those with CFRD, where the emphasis is on dose adjustment of insulin to match foods eaten rather than dietary restriction.

Disorders of the pancreas, including acute and chronic pancreatitis and cancer of the pancreas, can affect insulin production and may be associated with diabetes. All these conditions are also associated with malabsorption and malnutrition and the support of a specialist dietitian is essential.

Both HIV and AIDS are associated with insulin resistance and increase the risk of developing type 2 diabetes by a factor of four. Diabetes pharmaceutical agents are of limited use in HIV due to interactions with antiretroviral medications, and the main options for treatment are diet and physical activity.

Eating disorders such as anorexia nervosa and bulimia are 2.4 times more common in adolescent girls with type 1 diabetes. The deliberate omission of insulin to aid weight loss, termed diabulimia by the media, has serious health consequences in terms of the development of DKA and diabetes associated complications. Eating disorders in people with type 1 diabetes affect physical and emotional health and cause impaired metabolic control. All members of the diabetes team should be alert to the possibility of eating disorders and insulin dose manipulation, and urgent referral to eating disorder units may be necessary.

Nutrition support

There is very little evidence available for the role of nutrition support in people with diabetes, but the general recommendation is to follow local protocols and guidelines for those without diabetes. Many feeds and supplements are glucose based and will exacerbate hyperglycaemia, and this should be managed by adequate diabetes medication rather than dietary restriction. Diabetes specific formulae (providing energy derived from monounsaturated fat and fructose) have been shown to help glycaemic control, but these are expensive and are not available in the UK.

Palliative care

In common with guidelines for people without diabetes, end of life care for people with diabetes should ensure non-intrusive dietary and management regimens tailored to individual need. The main emphasis is to avoid symptoms of hyperglycaemia and hypoglycaemia as the risk of long term cardiovascular and microvascular complications is not relevant. In line with changes in dietary intake, adjustment of medication may be required.

External agency residents

People in hospitals, prisons, care homes and boarding schools are not in charge of their own nutrition and often have restricted food choice. It is recommended that people with diabetes, their carers and associated staff have sufficient education and/or training to enable healthy food choices where possible. All food provided should include snacks and meals that allow food choices that are in line with dietary recommendations for diabetes. In addition, all residents with diabetes should have access to a registered dietitian and a nutritional care plan for each individual should be developed.

Fasting

Fasting is a significant part of many religions and, although people with diabetes are often exempt, many will choose to respect fasts. Little evidence is available to formulate guidelines, and consideration should be given to the timing and doses of medication, and the carbohydrate and energy density of foods taken when a fast is broken.

Further reading (evidence based nutrition guidelines)

Bantle JP, Wylie-Rosett J, Albright AL, (2008). Nutrition recommendations and interventions for diabetes: a position statement of the American Diabetes Association. *Diabetes Care* 31(Suppl 1): S61–78.

Canadian Diabetes Association. (2008) Canadian Diabetes Association 2008 clinical practice guidelines for the prevention and management of diabetes in Canada. *Canadian Journal of Diabetes* 32 (Suppl 1): S1–201.

Diabetes UK. (2011) Evidence-based nutrition guidelines for the prevention and management of diabetes. Available at www.diabetes.org.uk/Documents/Reports/Nutritional_guidelines.31.05.11.pdf.

Franz MJ, Powers MA, Leontos C, *et al.* (2010) The evidence for medical nutrition therapy for type 1 and type 2 diabetes in adults. *Journal of the American Dietetic Association* 110(12): 1852–1889.

Internet resources

American Diabetes Association (ADA)   www.diabetes.org
Carbohydrate counting   www.carbsandcals.com/about-us
Carbs & Cals   www.carbsandcals.com
   This is a series of books, apps and other resources for managing diabetes.
Diabetes Education and Self-Management for Ongoing and Newly Diagnosed Diabetes (DESMOND)   www.desmond-project.org.uk
Diabetes UK   www.diabetes.org.uk
Dose Adjustment for Normal Eating (DAFNE)   www.dafne.uk.com
European Association for the Study of Diabetes (EASD)   www.easd.org
Glycaemic index   www.glycemicindex.com
International Diabetes Federation (IDF)   www.idf.org
Managing diabetes and sport   www.runsweet.com
National Institute for Health and Care Excellence   www.nice.org.uk
   Numerous Guidelines, pathways, quality standards and technical appraisals are available.
UK Diabetes Education Network   www.diabetes-education.net
X-PERT programme   www.xperthealth.org.uk

References

Ali S, Stone MA, Peters JL, Davies MJ, Khunti K. (2006) The prevalence of co-morbid depression in adults with Type 2 diabetes: a systematic review and meta-analysis. *Diabetes Medicine* 23(11): 1165–1173.

Anderson RJ, Freedland KE, Clouse RE, Lustman PJ. (2011) The prevalence of co-morbid depression in adults with diabetes: a meta-analysis. *Diabetes Care* 24(6): 1069–1078.

Aucott L, Poobalan A, Smith WC, et al. (2004) Weight loss in obese diabetic and non-diabetic individuals and long-term diabetes outcomes – a systemtic review. Diabetes, Obesity and Metabolism 6(2): 85–94.

Bantle JP, Wylie-Rosett J, Albright AL, et al. (2008) Nutrition recommendations and interventions for diabetes: a position statement of the American Diabetes Association. Diabetes Care 31(Suppl 1): S61–78.

Barnard KD, Skinner TC, Peveler R. (2006) The prevalence of co-morbid depressin in adults with Type 1 diabetes: a systematic literature review. Diabetes Medicine 23(4): 445–448.

Boule NG, Haddad E, Kenny GP, Wells GA, Sigal RJ. (2001) Effects of exercise on glycemic control and body mass in type 2 diabetes mellitus: a meta-analysis of controlled clinical trials. JAMA 286(10): 1218–1227.

Canadian Diabetes Association. (2008) Canadian Diabetes Association 2008 clinical practice guidelines for the prevention and management of diabetes in Canada. Canadian Journal of Diabetes 32(Suppl 1): S1–201.

Colberg SR, Sigal RJ, Fernhall B, et al., American College of Sports Medicine, American Diabetes Association. (2010) Exercise and type 2 diabetes: the American College of Sports Medicine and the American Diabetes Association: joint position statement. Diabetes Care 33(12): 147–167.

Corben S, Rosen R. (2005) Self-Management for Long-Term Conditions. London: King's Fund.

DCCT Study Group. (1993) The effect of intensive treatment of diabetes on the development and progression of long-term complications in insulin-dependent diabetes mellitus. The Diabetes Control and Complications Trial Research Group. New England Journal of Medicine 329(14): 977–986.

DAFNE Study Group. (2002) Training in flexible, intensive insulin management to enable dietary freedom in people with type 1 diabetes: dose adjustment for normal eating (DAFNE) randomised controlled trial. BMJ 325: 746.

Delahanty LM. (1998) Clinical significance of medical nutrition therapy in achieving diabetes outcomes and the importance of the process. Journal of the American Dietetic Association 98(1): 28–30.

Diabetes UK. (2010) Diabetes in the UK 2010: Key statistics on diabetes. London: Diabetes UK.

Dixon JD, Zimmet P, Alberti KG on behalf of the IDF Taskforce on Epidemiology and Prevention. (2011) Bariatric surgery: An IDF statement for obese Type 2 diabetes. Diabetic Medicine 28(6): 628–642.

Dyson PA. (2010) The therapeutics of lifesyle management on obesity. Diabetes, Obesity and Metabolism 12: 941–946.

Dyson PA, Kelly T, Deakin T, et al. on behalf of Diabetes UK Nutrition Working Group. (2011) Diabetes UK evidence-based nutrition guidelines for the prevention and management of diabetes. Diabetes Medicine 28(11): 1282–1288.

EURODIAB IDDM Complications Study Group. (1994) Microvascular and acute complications in IDDM patients: the EURODIAB IDDM complications study. Diabetologia 37(3): 278–285.

Flint A, Arslanian S. (2011) Treatment of Type 2 diabetes in youth. Diabetes Care 34(Suppl 2): S177–183.

Franz MJ, Powers MA, Leontos C, et al. (2010) The evidence for medical nutrition therapy for type 1 and type 2 diabetes in adults. Journal of the American Dietetic Association 110(12): 1852–1889.

Gillespie SJ, Kulkarni K, Daly AE. (1998) Using carbohydrate counting in diabetes clinical practice. Journal of the American Dietetic Association 98: 897–905.

Ha TK, Lean ME. (1998) Recommendations for the nutritional management of patients with diabetes mellitus. European Journal of Clinical Nutrition 52(7): 467–481.

Hamman RF, Wing RR, Edelstein SL, et al. (2006) Effect of weight loss with lifestyle intervention on risk of diabetes. Diabetes Care 29(9): 2102–2107.

Haslam D. (2011) UK findings on overweight, obesity and weight gain from PANORAMA, a pan-European cross-sectional study of patients with Type 2 diabetes. Diabetes Medicine 28(Suppl 1): 111–112.

Holman N, Forouhi NG, Goyder E, Wild SH. (2011) The Association of Public Health Observatories (APHO) Diabetes Prevalence Model: estimates of total diabetes prevalence for England, 2010–2030. Diabetes Medicine 28(5): 575–582.

Institute of Medicine. (2009) Weight Gain During Pregnancy: Re-examing the Fuidelines. Washington, DC: The National Academies Press.

International Diabetes Federation (IDF). (2009) Diabetes Atlas, 4th edn. IDF.

Kitzmiller JL, Block JM, Brown FM, et al. (2008) Managing pre-existing diabetes for pregancy: summary of evidence and consensus recommendations for care. Diabetes Care 31(5): 1060–1079.

Koerbel G, Korytkowski M. (2003) Coronary heart disease in women with diabetes. Diabetes Spectrum 16(3): 148–153.

Knowler WC, Fowler SE, Hamman RF, et al. (2009) 10-year follow-up of diabetes incidence and weight loss in the Diabetes Prevention Program Outcomes Study. Lancet 374: 1677–1686.

Li G, Zhang P, Wang J, et al. (2008)The long-term effect of lifestyle interventions to prevent diabetes in the China Da Qing Diabetes Prevention Study: a 20-year follow-up study. Lancet 371: 1783–1789.

Lindstrom J, Ilanne-Parikka P, Peltonen M, et al. (2006) Sustained reduction in the incidence of type 2 diabetes by lifestyle intervention: follow-up of the Finnish Diabetes Prevention Study. Lancet 368: 1673–1679.

Lobstein T, Leach R. (2004) Diabetes may be undetected in many children in the UK. BMJ 328: 1261–1262.

Look AHEAD Research Group. (2010) Long-term effects of a lifestyle intervention on weight and cardiovascular risk factors in individuals with type 2 diabetes mellitus: four-year results of the Look AHEAD trial. Archives of Internal Medicine 170(17): 1566–1575.

Malavige LS, Levy JC. (2009) Erectile dysfunction in diabetes mellitus. Journal of Sexual Medicine 6(5): 1232–1247.

Malik VS, Popkin BM, Bray GA, Despres JP, Hu FB. (2010) Sugar-sweetened beverages, obesity, type 2 diabetes mellitus and cardiovascular disease. Circulation 121(11): 1356–1364.

Nathan DM, Zinman B, Cleary PA, et al. (2009) Modern-day clinical course of type 1 diabetes mellitus after 30 years' duration: the diabetes control and complications trial/epidemiology of diabetes interventions and complications and Pittsburgh epidemiology of diabetes complications experience (1983–2005). Archives of Internal Medicine 169(14): 1307–1316.

National Institute for Health and Care Excellence (NICE). (2004) Diagnosis and Management of Type 1 Diabetes in Children, Young People and Adults. London: NICE, 2004.

National Institute for Health and Care Excellence (NICE). (2006) Obesity: The Prevention, Identification, Assessment and Management of Overweight and Obesity in Adults and Children. London: NICE.

National Institute for Health and Care Excellence (NICE). (2008a) Type 2 Diabetes: The Management of Type 2 Diabetes (Update). London: NICE.

National Institute for Health and Care Excellence (NICE). (2008b) Continuous Subcutaneous Insulin Infusion for the Treatment of Diabetes. London: NICE.

National Institute for Health and Care Excellence (NICE). (2008c) Diabetes in Pregnancy. London: NICE.

National Institute for Health and Care Excellence (NICE). (2011) Diabetes in Adults: Quality Standards. London: NICE.

NHS. (2010a) Quality and Outcomes Framework. Online GP Practice Results Database. London: National Health Service.

NHS. (2010b) Prescribing for diabetes in England 2004/05 to 2009/10. National Health Service, London.

NHS Choices. (2011) Diabetic retinopathy. London: NHS.

SECTION 7

Nield L, Moore HJ, Hooper L, *et al.* (2007) Dietary advice for treatment of type 2 diabetes mellitus in adults. *Cochrane Database of Systematic Reviews* 3: CD004097.

Nowosielski K, Skrzypulec-Plinta V. (2011) Mediators of sexual function in women with diabetes. *Journal of Sexual Medicine* 8(9): 2532–2555.

Oldroyd J, Banerjee M, Heald A, Cruikshank K. (2005) Diabetes and ethnic minorities. *Postgraduate Medical Journal* 81(958): 486–490.

Paulweber B, Valensi P, Lindstrom J, *et al.* (2010) A European evidence-based guideline for the prevention of Type 2 diabetes. *Hormone and Metabolism Research* 41(Suppl 1): S3–36.

Pi-Sunyer X, Blackburn G, Brancati FL, Bray GA, Bright R, Clark JM. (2007) Reduction in weight and cardiovascular disease risk factors in individuals with type 2 diabetes: one-year results of the look AHEAD trial. *Diabetes Care* 30(6): 1374–1383.

Poslusna K, Ruprich J, de Vries J, Jakubikova M, van't Veer P. (2009) Misreporting of energy and micronutrient intake estimated by food records and 24 hour recalls, control and adjustment methods in practice. *British Journal of Nutrition* 101(Suppl 2): S73–85.

Robertson LM, Waugh N, Robertson A. (2007) Protein restriction for diabetic renal disease. *Cochrane Database of Systematic Reviews* CD002181.

Schram MT, Baan CA, Pouwer F. (2009) Depression and quality of life in patients with diabetes: a systematic review from the European depression in diabetes (EDID) research consortium. *Current Diabetes Reviews* 5(2): 112–119.

Shaw K, Gennat H, O'Rourke P, Del Mar C. (2006) Exercise for overweight or obesity. *Cochrane Database of Systematic Reviews* 4: CD003817.

Sinclair AJ, Conroy SP, Bayer AJ. (2008) Impact of diabetes on physical function in older people. *Diabetes Care* 31(2): 233–235.

Skyler JS, Bergenstal R, Bonow RO, *et al.*, American Diabetes Association, American College of Cardiology Foundation, American Heart Association. (2009) Intensive glycemic control and the prevention of cardiovascular events: implications of the ACCORD, ADVANCE and VA diabetes trials: a position statement of the American Diabetes Association and a scientific statement of the American College of Cardiology Foundation and the American Heart Association. *Diabetes Care* 32(1): 187–192.

Smart CE, Aslander-van Vliet E, Waldron S. (2009) Nutritional management in children and adolescents with diabetes. *Pediatric Diabetes* 10 (Suppl 12): 100–117.

Stratton IM, Adler AI, Neil HA, *et al.* (2000) Association of glycaemic with macrovascular and microvascular complicatons of Type 2 diabetes (UKPDS 35): prospective observational study. *BMJ* 321: 405–412.

Tattersall R. (2009) *Diabetes: the Biography*. Oxford: Oxford University Press.

The Emerging Risk Factor Collaboration. (2011) Diabetes mellitus: Fasting glucose and risk of cause-specific death. *New England Journal of Medicine* 364(9): 829–841.

The Emerging Risk Factor Collaboration. (2010 Diabetes Mellitus, fasting blood glucose concentrations and risk of vascular disease: a collaborative meta-analysis of 102 prospective studies. *Lancet* 375: 2215–2222.

Thomas D, Elliott EJ. (2009) Low glycaemic index, or low glycaemic load, diets for diabetes mellitus. *Cochrane Database of Systematic Reviews* 1: CD006296.

Thomas D, Elliott EJ, Naughton GA. (2006) Exercise for type 2 diabetes mellitus. *Cochrane Database of Systematic Reviews* 3: CD002968.

Thompson GR, Grundy SM. (2005) History and development of plant sterol and stanol esters for cholesterol-lowering purposes. *American Journal of Cardiology* 96 (Suppl): 3D–9D.

Turner RC, Holman RR. (1995) Lessons from UK prospective diabetes study. *Diabetes Research and Clinical Practice* 28(Suppl 1): S151–157.

UKPDS Group. (1991) UK Prospective Diabetes Study VII: Study design progress and performance. *Diabetologia* 34: 877–890.

UKPDS Group. (1998a) Tight blood pressure control and risk of macrovascular and microvascular complications in type 2 diabetes: UKPDS 38. UK Prospective Diabetes Study Group. *BMJ* 317: 703–713.

UKPDS Group. (1998b) Intensive blood-glucose control with sulphonylureas or insulin compared with conventional treatment and risk of complications in patients with type 2 diabetes (UKPDS 33). UK Prospective Diabetes Study (UKPDS) Group. *Lancet* 352: 837–853.

Walker KZ, O'Dea K, Gomez M, Girgis S, Colagiuri R. (2010) Diet and exercise in the prevention of diabetes. *Journal of Human Nutrition and Dietetics* 23(4): 344–352.

World Health Organization (WHO). (2006) *Definition and Diagnosis of Diabetes Mellitus and Intermediate Hyperglycaemia*. Geneva: WHO.

World Health Organization (WHO). (2011) *Use of Glycated Haemoglobin (HbA1c) in the Diagnosis of Diabetes Mellitus*. Geneva: WHO.

Yusuf S, Hawken S, Ounpuu S, *et al.* INTERHEART Study Investigators. (2004) Effect of potentially modifiable risk factors associated with myocardial infarction in 52 countries (the INTERHEART study): case control study. *Lancet* 364: 937–952.

Zimmet P, Alberti KG, Shaw J. (2001) Global and societal implications of the diabetes epidemic. *Nature* 414: 82–87.

Zinman B, Ruderman N, Campaigne BN, Devlin JT, Schneider SH for the American Diabetes Association. (2003) Physical activity/exercise and diabetes mellitus. *Diabetes Care* 26(Suppl 1): S73–77.

7.13

Obesity

7.13.1 General aspects and prevention
Linda Hindle

Key points

- Obesity in the UK has trebled in 20 years; about a quarter of adults are obese, and almost a third of children are either overweight or obese.

- Obesity is a serious health risk; it reduces life expectancy and is associated with significant physical morbidity, especially diabetes, and reduced quality of life.

- It is caused by a combination of sedentary lifestyles and poor dietary habits superimposed on a latent genetic susceptibility to weight gain.

- Preventing obesity requires action at all levels, from individual and family counselling, through local initiatives in schools and workplaces to government policies to support and facilitate healthier choices. Environmental changes have the greatest potential to reverse the rising prevalence of obesity.

- Dietitians have a role in obesity management and prevention as a part of their posts, but also as advocates for health in their communities.

Obesity is an excess of body fat to the point that it seriously endangers health. It is defined in terms of body mass index (BMI), which is a measure of relative weight for height and a proxy measure for excess fat, defined as:

$$BMI = weight~(kg)/height~(m)^2$$

(measured in indoor clothing and without shoes)

The World Health Organization (WHO, 1998) classification of obesity in adults is shown in Table 7.13.1.

Obesity in children and adolescents is normally defined in clinical practice as a sex and age specific BMI plotted at or above the 98th percentile based on 1990 BMI data percentile classification charts (SIGN, 2010; NICE, 2006). When population data are collected, children are defined as obese if their BMI is at or above the 95th percentile of the reference curve for age (see Chapter 7.13.4).

However, BMI is an imperfect index because it does not measure body composition and fails to discriminate between lean and fat tissue (Prentice & Jebb, 2001). Thus, individuals with a particularly well developed muscula-

ture may be classified as obese using the BMI alone. In recent years there has been growing interest in the use of waist circumference as an alternative classification system (Lean *et al.*, 1995; McCarthy *et al.*, 2003). This provides a guide to the extent of the abdominal fat stores and a more sensitive measure of long term health risks. This measure may be more appropriate for Asian communities (World Health Organization Expert Consultation, 2004). Current recommended cut-off points for waist circumference for adult Caucasians and Asians are shown in Appendix A7. Table 7.13.2 shows waist measurements in adults as a predictor of health risk; age/gender specific charts are available for children. However, in childhood current recommendations are that waist measurements should not be used for diagnosis purposes, but may be useful in the clinical situation to monitor progress (NICE, 2006; SIGN, 2010).

It may be preferable to make more specific measurements of body fatness. The development of techniques such as bioelectrical impedance analysis has made this a practical reality for clinical practice. Table 7.13.3 gives

Table 7.13.1 Classification of body mass index (BMI) and risk of comorbidities in adults (WHO, 1998; WHO Expert Consultation, 2004)

Classification	BMI (kg/m²)	BMI (kg/m²) Asian origin	Risk of comorbidities
Underweight	<18.5	<18.5	Low (but risk of other clinical problems increased)
Normal range	18.5–24.9	18.5–22.9	Average
Overweight	25.0–29.9	23–27.4	Increased risk
Obese class I	30.0–34.9	27.5–32.4	Moderate
Obese class II	35.0–39.9	32.5–37.4	Severe
Obese class III	>40.0	>37.5	Morbid obesity

Table 7.13.2 Waist measurements in adults as a predictor of health risk (WHO, 2008)

	Men	Asian men	Women	Asian women
Waist circumference (cm)				
Increased risk	≥94		≥80	
Substantially increased risk	≥102	≥90	≥88	≥80
Waist to hip ratio				
Increased risk	≥0.9		≥0.85	

Table 7.13.3 Healthy body fat ranges extrapolated from body mass index cut-offs in adults (Gallagher et al., 2000)

	African American (%)	Asian (%)	Caucasian (%)
Underweight	<20	<25	21
Healthy	20–32	25–35	21–33
Overweight	32–38	35–40	33–39
Obese	>38	>40	>39

useful reference ranges for adults, which broadly correspond to the traditional BMI cut-offs for Caucasian adults. Body fatness centile charts for children are available, although there is still debate about their use in children.

Prevalence

Obesity is the most common nutritional disorder in the world. Globally, there are >1.5 billion overweight adults; at least 500 million of these are obese (Finucane et al., 2011). A systematic review of the economic burden of obesity worldwide concluded that obesity accounted for 0.7–2.8% of a country's total healthcare costs, and that obese individuals had medical costs 30% higher than

normal weight people (Withrow & Alter, 2011). Total healthcare costs attributable to obesity and overweight are projected to double every decade and to account for 16–18% of total US healthcare expenditure by 2030 (Wang, 2008). In the UK the proportion of adults categorised as obese increased from 13% in 1993 to 22% in 2009 for men and from 16% in 1993 to 24% in 2009 for women [Health and Social Care Information Centre (HSCIC), 2010]. By 2050 obesity is predicted to affect 60% of adult men, 50% of adult women and 25% of children (Foresight, 2007).

The prevalences of obesity and overweight rise with age from a relatively low level in the 16–24 year age group to a peak at 65–74 years, after which there is a modest decline. There is also a clear social class gradient in adult obesity, especially in women, where more than twice as many women in social class IV and V are obese relative to professional women in social class I (HSCIC, 2010). There are differences in both the prevalence and impact of obesity between ethnic groups, with Asian populations at an increased risk of obesity related comorbidities at a lower BMI (World Health Organization Expert Consultation, 2004).

There are particular concerns about the rate of increase in overweight and obesity among children and young people, which has approximately trebled in the last 20 years. In the UK, data from the National Child Measurement Programme (NCMP) indicated that 10.5% of boys and 9.2% of girls (all children 9.8%) aged 4–5 years and 20.4% of boys and 17% of girls (all children 18.7%) aged 10–11 years were classified as obese according to the British 1990 population monitoring definition of obesity (≥95th centile) (NCMP, 2009/10). Children are more likely to become obese if they have obese parents. Obese children are more likely to become obese adults than their peers and the degree of obesity tends to increase with age. This suggests that the burden of obesity will increase markedly in the future unless there is effective action to tackle excess weight gain (Wang, 2011).

Impact of obesity on health

Obesity is an independent risk factor for premature death, but it is also strongly associated, probably causally, with a number of other serious medical conditions (Table 7.13.4). Overall, obese people are two to three times more likely to die prematurely than their lean counterparts and, on average, obesity reduces life expectancy by about 9 years (Calle et al., 1999). The morbidity associated with obesity can be broadly divided into metabolic, mechanical and psychosocial disorders (Bray, 1985). Insulin resistance, hyperlipidaemia and hypertension are strongly associated with excess weight, especially in the abdominal region, and characterised by an increased waist circumference. The clustering of these risk factors is described as the metabolic syndrome and strongly predicts an increased risk of cardiovascular disease (CVD) and diabetes. The increase in the risk of developing type 2 diabetes with excess weight is particularly striking (Diabetes Prevention Program Research Group, 2002). It is

Table 7.13.4 Health risks of obesity (WHO, 1998)

Greatly increased (relative risk >3)*	Moderately increased (relative risk 2–3)*	Slightly increased (relative risk 1–2)*
Type 2 diabetes Gallbladder disease Dyslipidaemia Insulin resistance Breathlessness Sleep apnoea Metabolic syndrome	Cardiovascular diseases Hypertension Osteoarthritis (knees) Hyperuricaemia and gout	Certain cancers, including colon, kidney, prostate (men), postmenopausal breast and endometrial (women) Reproductive hormone abnormalities Polycystic ovary syndrome Impaired fertility Low back pain due to obesity Increased anaesthetic risk Foetal defects associated with maternal obesity

*All relative risk estimates are approximate.

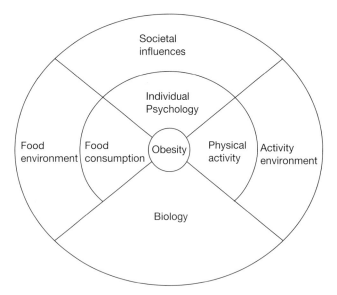

Figure 7.13.1 Factors affecting obesity – a simplified Foresight systems map [from Foresight (2007)]

also important to recognise that regardless of baseline weight, further weight gain increases the risk further.

In recent years the links between obesity and cancer have been recognised and, after smoking, excess weight is the most important modifiable risk factor to reduce the risk of cancer. Obesity is particularly associated with post menopausal breast cancer, colon cancer and cancers of the reproductive system (Calle *et al.*, 2003). Other conditions such as stroke, fatty liver, gallstones and reproductive problems, including polycystic ovarian syndrome and infertility, are all increased in obese subjects.

Mechanical problems, including osteoarthritis, chronic low back pain and breathlessness, are rarely life threatening, but contribute to decreased mobility, reduced work productivity and impaired quality of life. Sleep apnoea is a particular problem for many obese patients. The health risks of obesity in young adults are particularly marked and there is a tendency for the relative risk to increase with age.

Studies are beginning to show that the early origins of many of these conditions, especially metabolic diseases, can be seen among obese children. There is an increasing prevalence of type 2 diabetes in paediatric practice. Evidence that overweight in childhood is a risk factor independent of adult weight is limited. However, since there is tracking of childhood weight into adulthood, the health concerns for obese children are substantial (Lobstein *et al.*, 2004).

There is also an association between obesity and decreased psychological wellbeing, but this is not a simple relationship (Stunkard & Sobel, 1995). Obesity does not cause psychological problems, but the social stigma attached to excess weight can leave many obese people, especially children or those with morbid obesity, with significant psychological morbidity, including depression and low self esteem. In some cases this may contribute to a downward spiral of increasing weight and declining psychosocial functioning. Dietitians are not isolated from prevailing cultural attitudes towards obese people, and establishing an empathic, non-judgemental relationship with an obese patient makes an important contribution towards effective therapy.

Obesity is a serious health risk. There is good evidence that losing even small amounts of weight can decrease the occurrence or severity of risk factors for disease, e.g. insulin resistance and dyslipidaemia, etc., but there is only limited evidence as yet from long term prospective studies with hard outcomes on overall impact, such as incidence of diabetes or reduced mortality. Nonetheless, the decrease in obesity related morbidity with weight loss of even 5–10% among obese people (15–20% in those with a BMI >35 kg/m²) brings significant benefits to the individual, including reductions in medication for other diseases, and improvements in physical functioning and quality of life (SIGN, 2010).

Aetiology

Obesity occurs as a consequence of a long term excess energy consumption relative to an individual's energy use, leading to an accumulation of excess fat. The causes of this imbalance can be traced to a number of factors, including specific genetic traits, which may convey a metabolic predisposition, behavioural factors and environmental circumstances (Jebb, 1997). The Foresight report (2007) referred to a complex web of societal and biological factors that have, in recent decades, exposed inherent human vulnerability to weight gain; in a complex full system obesity map, over 100 variables directly or indirectly influence energy balance. A simplified model divided the Foresight map into seven interrelated themes, as shown in Figure 7.13.1. The themes were:

- *Biology* – the influence of genetics and ill health.
- *Activity environment* – the influence of the environment on an individual's activity behaviour.
- *Physical activity* – the type, frequency and intensity of activities an individual carries out.
- *Societal influences* – the impact of society, e.g. the influence of the media, education, peer pressure or culture.
- *Individual psychology*.
- *Food environment* – the influence of the food environment on an individual's food choices.
- *Food consumption* – the quality, quantity (portion sizes) and frequency (snacking patterns) of an individual's diet.

Genetics and metabolism

There are some diseases in which obesity is a major feature; the most significant of these are the Prader–Willi and Bardet–Biedel syndromes. A further group of patients may develop obesity as a consequence of an endocrine disorder, e.g. hypothyroidism or Cushing's syndrome. These patients represent a tiny proportion of all cases of obesity and usually present with additional symptoms that can be readily identified and usually successfully treated. In children, short stature for age and weight is an indication that further medical tests may be required (SIGN, 2010).

There has been growing interest in the impact of genetics on the development of obesity. Single gene defects have been identified in rare disorders associated with severe obesity, including defects in the *ob* gene, resulting in congenital leptin deficiency, mutations in the leptin receptor, defective POMC (pro opiomelaninocortin) processing and mutations in the MC4 receptor gene (Farooqi & O'Rahilly, 2005). Individuals with these monogenetic disorders have a powerful drive to eat and in them conventional management alone is rarely successful in achieving weight loss. However, once the specific mechanism driving food intake is identified, it becomes a potential target for specific therapeutic interventions. For example, recombinant leptin therapy in children with mutations in the *leptin* gene has resulted in substantial weight loss (Farooqi et al., 1999).

A much greater proportion of the population is likely to exhibit polymorphisms in other genes that have a significant but less dramatic effect on body weight, e.g. mutations in uncoupling proteins, the β3 adrenergic receptor or PPARγ (Hainer et al., 2008). These genes may influence a wide range of metabolic and behavioural characteristics that together determine an individual's susceptibility to obesity. Whether this genetic predisposition becomes apparent may depend on the environmental and behavioural choices of the individual.

There has been extensive research into putative metabolic differences between individuals that may account for differences in susceptibility to obesity. Previous suggestions that obese persons have a markedly lower metabolic rate than lean individuals have been categorically refuted, since increases in weight are associated with increased energy needs (Prentice & Poppitt, 1996). However, this does not preclude differences between individuals in the preobese period. Studies in Pima Indians have shown that a relatively low metabolic rate is associated with an increased risk of future weight gain (Ravussin et al., 1988). Similarly, some studies of post obese subjects have shown minor differences in energy expenditure compared with age and weight matched never obese controls (Astrup et al., 1999). However, these studies are thwarted by difficulties in accounting for subtle differences in body composition. Defects in diet induced thermogenesis and impairments in fat oxidation have also been suggested as metabolic defects that may increase the risk of obesity, but the net effects on energy expenditure are extremely small (Astrup et al., 1996).

In recent years increasing attention has been given to the metabolic control of appetite. A hierarchy of mechanisms, including orosensory, gastrointestinal and neuroendocrine factors control food intake (Blundell & Tremblay, 1995). Defects in any part of these complex pathways may lead to a dysregulation of appetite. This is an area of much current research, particularly given the finding that most of the monogenic obesity syndromes are characterised by metabolic defects in the appetite control system rather than in energy expenditure.

It is only in recent years that it has been acknowledged that behavioural traits may have a genetic basis. However, voluntary behaviour has the potential to override a genetic and metabolic susceptibility to obesity by increasing energy expenditure through voluntary exercise and decreasing energy intake through dietary restraint.

Activity

Physical activity is considered to be protective against the development of obesity. In prospective studies, individuals who maintain a high level of activity gain significantly less weight than inactive people (Coakley et al., 1998). There appears to be a stronger association between sedentary behaviours or physical inactivity and obesity [World Cancer Research Fund (WCRF), 2009]. Television viewing in particular has been linked to the development of obesity because of the combination of sedentary behaviour and snacking on energy dense foods (Reilly et al., 2005).

Studies of exercise as part of a weight loss programme have generally shown little or no increase in weight loss with increased activity, but there is a reduced risk of weight regain (Pavlou et al., 1989). Together these data suggest that physical activity may help to attenuate the rate of weight gain rather than accelerating weight loss. Physical activity recommendations to prevent obesity advocate 45–60 minutes of moderate to intense physical activity daily (Department of Health, 2004; Saris et al., 2003). Increases in physical activity offer additional health benefits and reduce the risk of premature death from CVD and some cancers, as well as reducing the risk of type 2 diabetes.

Table 7.13.5 Evidence for factors that might promote or protect against overweight and weight gain (WHO/FAO, 2003b; Swinburn et al., 2005)

Evidence	Decreases risk	No relationship	Increases risk
Convincing	Regular physical activity High dietary fibre/NSP intake		Sedentary lifestyle High intake of energy dense foods
Probable	Home and school environments that support healthy food choices for children Breastfeeding		Heavy marketing of energy dense foods and fast food outlets Adverse social and economic conditions (developed countries, especially for women) High sugar drinks
Possible	Low glycaemic index foods	Dietary protein content	Large portion sizes High proportion of food prepared outside the home (western countries) 'Rigid restraint/periodic disinhibition' eating patterns
Insufficient	Increased eating frequency		Alcohol

NSP, non-starch polysaccharide.

Diet

A number of dietary factors that may protect against, or conversely promote, the risk of obesity have been identified (WCRF, 2009; WHO/FAO, 2003) (Table 7.13.5). In recent years there has been a tendency to move away from the study of specific foods or nutrients and towards more general dietary patterns. Two of the strongest risk factors for obesity are energy density and portion size.

A series of controlled experimental studies has clearly shown that an increase in the energy density of food increases energy intake through a mechanism described as passive over consumption (Prentice & Poppitt, 1996). This reflects the fact that energy dense diets contain more energy per unit weight and so, if portion size is unaltered, the energy consumed will be greater on energy dense diets. Such diets tend to be high in fat and/or added sugars and low in foods such as fruit and vegetables, which add bulk yet little energy. Energy dense diets fail to stimulate the body's satiety system in proportion to their energy content and hence facilitate over consumption. The energy density theory helps to explain the success of low fat (low energy dense) diets in treating obesity, at least in the short term. However, in the longer term, there are issues relating to compliance and the possible adaptation of the appetite control mechanisms such that long term weight loss is limited unless additional strategies are employed to restrict intake (Bray & Popkin, 1998).

The scientific basis of the energy density theory confines its applicability to solid food. Beverages have a quite different impact on the body's innate appetite control system and liquid calories are much less satiating than the equivalent energy as food. Energy rich drinks, including sugar rich soft drinks and alcoholic beverages, may pose a specific risk factor for obesity due to their low satiating properties (Jebb, 2005).

Portion size also has powerful effects on spontaneous energy intake (Rolls, 2003). A series of studies has now demonstrated that people tend to consume more when offered larger portions, but that the sense of fullness is unaltered and subjects fail to compensate at the next eating occasion. In this way a small energy excess may accumulate incrementally. There is no evidence linking increased frequency of eating with obesity.

Understanding the importance of these dietary habits in the risk of developing obesity helps to tailor strategies for weight loss, which may include a focus on the type of food consumed in order to reduce energy density, an increase or decrease in certain foods, education on appropriate portion sizes and the development of a structured eating plan.

Environmental factors

At a global level, the marked increase in obesity that accompanies urbanisation and economic development provides strong evidence that environmental factors *per se* play a strong part in the aetiology of obesity or unleash a latent genetic predisposition to obesity (Prentice *et al.*, 2005). There is a growing body of research investigating the impact of the built environment on the risk of obesity (Foresight, 2007). Over the last 50 years technology has altered the way people live their lives in developed countries; labour saving devices, cars and internet shopping have reduced our activity level at the same time as we have become surrounded by relatively inexpensive, ready to eat, high calorie foods offered with incentives such as buy one get one free or supersize offers. The Foresight report termed the interplay of these factors as the obesogenic environment, which is defined as the total sum of influences in the environment on promoting obesity in individuals and populations.

Geographical analyses of, for example, the greater density of fast food outlets in poorer neighbourhoods than wealthier districts, is focussing attention on the social and cultural determinants of health inequalities. In today's world it can reasonably be argued that weight gain is a natural response in humans endowed with an

SECTION 7

ancient metabolism designed to withstand famine rather than feast (Prentice, 1997).

Prevention

Prevention of obesity is the key, long term public health goal. This includes the primary prevention of weight gain in lean subjects, secondary prevention of further weight gain in those who are obese, or tertiary prevention through maintenance strategies to avoid weight regain following successful weight loss. There is the greatest population level gain from preventing the development of obesity in the first place, rather than treating obesity once it has occurred, although all of the above are needed. The Foresight (2007) report highlighted the long term, large scale commitment needed to successfully tackle the obesity epidemic, and noted the similarities between this and tackling climate change, both requiring whole societal change with cross government action and long term commitment.

There are important differences between the medical and public health views of the obesity problem and these differences have implications for solutions (Jeffrey, 2002). The medical perspective considers obesity to be an individual level variable; individuals are obese because their body fatness is high compared with population norms and biological ideals. This is caused by differences in individual susceptibility to obesity related to differences in genetics, behaviour, psychology and metabolism. Interventions therefore aim to modify these susceptibilities in the individual as well as helping the individual to cope with an environment that promotes a high energy diet and minimal activity. Population approaches to prevent obesity from this perspective seek to industrialise interventions by scaling them up to wider audiences at lower unit costs.

A review of obesity prevention initiatives in adults and children found most had a focus on educational messages encouraging increased physical activity and a more healthier diet, and concluded that overall the outcomes were modestly positive with the strongest results seen in programmes for children that have high physical activity components (Linde & Jeffrey, 2010). However, the authors noted that the overall effects seen in these studies are considerably smaller than the rate of increase in population obesity, so this approach alone will be ineffective at reversing the rising prevalence of obesity. The solution is more complex than just helping individuals to change their diet and become more active, although these are part of the solution. Policy makers need to weigh the relative benefit of effective interventions reaching a modest number of people against the less effective interventions reaching wider populations (Gortmaker et al., 2011).

Public health models of obesity prevention focus on factors outside of the individual and consider the environment where people live. Thus, the priority to tackle obesity is changing the environment. There has been little research into effective ways of achieving this and therefore options to change the environment are being devel-

oped based on strategies that have been successful in other areas of public health, particularly tobacco control.

It has been argued that obesity prevention interventions should be universal across entire societies, including people of every age and regardless of risk factors, given that there are too little data available on effective ways to identify and manage an individual's obesity risks to justify a population strategy that would devote resources to sorting people by risk or readiness (Linde & Jeffrey, 2010). However, there are specific times in the life course that have greatest potential to impact on obesity (NICE, 2006), including maternity when there is the opportunity to affect the future health risk of the child and the mother; early childhood when there is a high level of parental control and eating, and activity patterns and preferences are being established; and school age when there are opportunities through schools to regulate eating and activity, and to influence the family through the school. Evidence from a growing number of studies has indicated that treating obesity before puberty may have more long lasting effects on relative weight than providing similar treatment after puberty or in adulthood (Jeffrey, 2002).

Specific evidence relating to successful strategies for the prevention of obesity is limited. The paucity of well conducted studies partly reflects the scale and complexity necessary to conduct such studies, especially those involving complex interventions. The Australian Assessing Cost Effectiveness (ACE) in Obesity and ACE Prevention studies have assimilated a broad range of evidence for the prevention of obesity (Vos et al., 2010; Carter et al., 2009). These studies appraise both prevention and treatment interventions in children and adults. Interventions were assessed for comparative effectiveness and cost effectiveness. Of 20 interventions, eight were found to be both health improving and cost saving, and a further three were cost effective (Table 7.13.6). The conclusion from the ACE studies is that policy approaches generally show greater cost effectiveness than health promotion or clinical interventions. No one intervention, however effective, will be sufficient to reverse the obesity epidemic in isolation. Solutions need to be multifaceted, with initiatives throughout governments and across several sectors. Interventions that might have quite small effects when assessed in isolation may still constitute important components of an overall strategy (Gortmaker et al., 2011). Swinburn et al. (2005) proposed a model for obesity prevention using an investment portfolio approach. In this way a strategy is developed incorporating a range of options of varying likelihood of success and varying potential health returns on the investment necessary to deliver the intervention. This proposed approach can be incorporated into a structured planning framework to prevent obesity (Gill et al., 2005). This begins by building the case for action, identifying contributory factors and the points for intervention, defining opportunities for action, evaluating potential interventions and then selecting a portfolio of policies, programmes and appropriate actions. The Institute of Medicine (2010) developed a systems approach framework for obesity prevention in

Table 7.13.6 Cost effectiveness results for selected interventions evaluated in Australia (source: Gortmaker 1991, p. 841. Reproduced with permission of Elsevier)

Intervention type	Target population (years)	Strength of evidence*	DALYs saved
10% unhealthy food and beverage tax (Sacks et al., 2011)**	Adults	4	559 000
Front of pack traffic light nutritional labelling (Sacks et al., 2011)**	Adults	5	45 100
Reduction of junk food advertising to children[†]	Children (0–14 years)	2	37 000
School based education programme to reduce television viewing[†]	Children (8–10 years)	3	8600
Multifaceted school based programme including nutrition and physical activity[†]	Children (6 years)	3	8000
School based education programme to reduce sugar sweetened drink consumption[†]	Children (7–11 years)	3	5300
Family based targeted programme for obese children[†]	Obese children (10–11 years)	1	2700
Multifaceted targeted school based programme[†]	Overweight and obese children (7–10 years)	3	270
Gastric banding adolescents (Ananthapavan et al., 2010)[†]	Severely obese adolescents (14–19 years)	1	12 300
Family based GP mediated programme (Moodie et al., 2008)[†]	Overweight/obese children (5–9 years)	3	510
Gastric banding in adults**	Adults with a BMI over 35 kg/m²	1	140 000

*This classification (1 = strongest; 5 = weakest) is based on criteria adopted in ACE Prevention (Vos et al., 2010). 1 = sufficient evidence of effectiveness; 2 = likely to be effective; 3 = limited evidence of effectiveness; 4 = may be effective; 5 = inconclusive or inadequate evidence.
**Interventions drawn from ACE-Prevention study (Vos et al., 2010).
[†]Interventions drawn from ACE-Obesity study (Carter et al., 2009).
DALY, disability adjusted life years; BMI, body mass index.

the USA that proposed a comprehensive plan with integrated actions throughout society; a coordinated approach to communications; interventions across all demographics; and use of diverse intervention combining initiatives focused on health promotion, the environment and addressing social norms. It recognised the need for long term plans and investment in research, and highlighted that obesity must be considered alongside other societal challenges, such as climate change and poverty reduction, because of the common causes and solutions.

Many community dietitians will be involved in obesity prevention programmes, possibly including intersectoral initiatives and broader environmental policies. However, all dietitians should be vigilant to the potential opportunities for health promotion in their everyday work as well as their role as advocates for health outside their direct clinical practice (see Chapter 4.2).

Further reading

Foresight Report. (2007) *Tackling Obesity: Future Choices*. Available at www.bis.gov.uk.
National Heart Forum. (2008) *Healthy Weight; Healthy Lives: A Toolkit for Developing Local Strategies*. Available at www.ukhealthforum.org.uk.

Internet resources

Association for the Study of Obesity   www.aso.org.uk
International Association for the Study of Obesity   www.iaso.org
International Obesity Task Force   www.iaso.org/iotf
National Obesity Forum   www.nationalobesityforum.org.uk
National Obesity Observatory   www.noo.org.uk
Obesity Learning Centre   www.obesitylearningcentre-nhf.org.uk
World Health Organization   www.who.int/topics/obesity/en

References

Ananthapavan J, Moodie M, Haby M, Carter R. (2010) Assessing cost-effectiveness in obesity: laparoscopic adjustable gastric banding for severely obese adolescents. *Surgery for Obesity and Related Disorders* 6: 377–385.
Astrup A, Buemann B, Toubro S, Raben A. (1996) Defects in substrate oxidation involved in the predisposition to obesity. *Proceedings of the Nutrition Society* 55: 817–828.
Astrup A, Gotzsche PC, van-de-Werken K, et al. (1999) Meta-analysis of resting metabolic rate in formerly obese subjects. *American Journal of Clinical Nutrition* 69: 1117–1122.
Blundell JE, Tremblay A. (1995) Appetite control and energy (fuel) balance. *Nutrition Research Reviews* 8: 225–242.
Bray G. (1985) Complications of obesity. *Annals of Internal Medicine* 103: 1052–1062.
Bray GA, Popkin BA. (1998) Dietary fat intake does affect obesity. *American Journal of Clinical Nutrition* 68: 1157–1173.

Calle EE, Thun MJ, Petrelli JM, Rodriguez C, Heath CW. (1999) Body mass index and mortality in a prospective cohort of U.S. adults. *New England Journal of Medicine* 341: 1097–1105.

Calle EE, Rodriguez C, Walker-Thurmond K, Thun MJ. (2003) Overweight, obesity, and mortality from cancer in a prospectively studied cohort of U.S. adults. *New England Journal of Medicine* 348(17): 1625–1638.

Carter R, Moodie M, Markwick A, *et al.* (2009) Assessing cost-effectiveness in obesity (ACE-obesity): an overview of the ACE approach, economic methods and cost results. *BMC Public Health* 9: 419.

Coakley EH, Rimm EB, Colditz G, Kawachi I, Willett W. (1998) Predictors of weight change in men: Results from The Health Professionals Follow-Up Study. *International Journal of Obesity* 22: 89–96.

Department of Health. (2004) *At Least Five a Week. A Report from the Chief Medical Officer*. London: Department of Health.

Diabetes Prevention Program Research Group. (2002) Reduction in the incidence of type 2 diabetes with lifestyle intervention or metformin. *New England Journal of Medicine* 346(6): 393–404.

Farooqi S, O'Rahilly S. (2005) Monogenic obesity in humans. *Annual Review of Medicine* 56: 443–458.

Farooqi S, Jebb SA, Cook G, *et al.* (1999) Recombinant leptin induces weight loss in human congenital leptin deficiency. *New England Journal of Medicine* 341: 879–884.

Finucane MM, Stevens GA, Cowan MJ, *et al.*, for the Global Burden of Metabolic Risk Factors of Chronic Diseases Collaborating Group (Body Mass Index). (2011) National, regional, and global trends in body-mass index since 1980: systematic analysis of health examination surveys and epidemiological studies with 960 country-years and 9·1 million participants. *Lancet* 377: 557–567.

Foresight. (2007) Foresight trends and drivers of obesity. A literature review for the foresight project on obesity. Available at www.foresight.gov.uk/obesity/outputs/Literature_Review/Literature_Review.pdf.

Gallagher D, Heymsfield SB, Moonseong H, Jebb SA, Murgatroyd PR, Yoichi S. (2000) Healthy percentage body fat ranges: an approach for developing guidelines on body mass index. *American Journal of Clinical Nutrition* 72: 694–701.

Gill T, King L, Cateron I. (2005) Obesity prevention: necessary and possible. A structured approach for effective planning. *Proceedings of the Nutrition Society* 64: 255–261.

Gortmaker SL, Swinburn BA, Levy D, *et al.* (2011) Changing the future of obesity: science, policy, and action. *Lancet* 378: 838–847.

Hainer V, Zamrazilova H, Spaloval J, *et al.* (2008) Role of hereditary factors in weight loss and its maintenance. *Physiology Research* 57(Suppl. 1): S1–S1.

Health and Social Care Information Centre. (2010) Health Survey for England. *Statistics on Obesity, Physical Activity and Diet: England, 2010. 2009 data*. London: The Health and Social Care Information Centre, 2010. Available at www.ic.nhs.uk/webfiles/publications/opad10/Statistics_on_Obesity_Physical_Activity_and_Diet_England_2010.pdf

Institute of Medicine. (2010) *Bridging the evidence gap in obesity prevention: a framework to inform decision making*. Washington, DC: The National Academy Press.

Jebb SA. (1997) Aetiology of obesity. *British Medical Bulletin* 53: 264–285.

Jebb SA. (2005) Dietary strategies for the prevention of obesity. *Proceedings of the Nutrition Society* 64(2): 217–227.

Jeffrey RW. (2002) Public health approaches to the management of obesity. In: Fairburn CG, Brownell KD (eds) *Eating Disorders and Obesity*. New York: Guildford Press, pp. 613–618.

Lean MJ, Han TS, Morrison CE. (1995) Waist circumference as a measure for indicating need for weight management. *BMJ* 311: 158–161.

Linde JA, Jeffrey RW. (2010) Population approaches to obesity prevention. In: Crawford D, Jeffrey RW, Ball K, Brug J (eds) *Obesity Epidemiology*. New York: Oxford University Press, pp. 208–221.

Lobstein T, Baur L, Uauy R. (2004) Obesity in children and young people: a crisis in public health. *Obesity Reviews* 5(Suppl 1): 4–104.

McCarthy HD, Ellis SM, Cole TJ. (2003) Central overweight and obesity in British youth aged 11–16 years: cross sectional surveys of waist circumference. *BMJ* 326: 624.

Moodie M, Haby M, Wake M, Gold L, Carter R. (2008) Cost-effectiveness of a family-based GP-mediated intervention targeting overweight and moderately obese children. *Economics & Human Biology* 6: 363–376.

National Institute for Health and Care Excellence (NICE) (2006). Obesity: the prevention, identification, assessment and management of overweight and obesity in adults and children. Available at www.nice.gov.uk. Accessed 5 September 2012.

Pavlou KN, Krey S, Steffee WP. (1989) Exercise as an adjunct to weight loss and maintenance in moderately obese subjects. *American Journal of Clinical Nutrition* 49: 1115–1123.

Prentice AM. (1997) Obesity – the inevitable penalty of civilisation? *British Medical Bulletin* 53: 229–237.

Prentice AM, Poppitt SD. (1996) Importance of energy density and macronutrients in the regulation of energy intake. *International Journal of Obesity* 20(Suppl 2): S18–S23.

Prentice AM, Jebb SA. (2001) Beyond body mass index. *Obesity Reviews* 2(3): 141.

Prentice AM, Rayco-Solon P, Moore S. (2005) Insights from the developing world: thrifty genotypes and thrifty phenotypes. *Proceedings of the Nutrition Society* 64: 153–161.

Ravussin E, Lillioja S, Knowler WC, *et al.* (1988) Reduced rate of energy expenditure as a risk factor for body weight gain. *New England Journal of Medicine* 318 (8): 467–472.

Reilly JJ, Armstrong J, Dorosty AR, *et al.* (2005) Early life risk factors for obesity in childhood: cohort study. *BMJ* 330: 1357.

Rolls BJ. (2003) The supersizing of America: Portion size and the obesity epidemic. *Nutrition Today* 38(2): 42–53.

Sacks G, Veerman L, Moodie M, Swinburn B. (2011) Traffic-light nutrition labelling and 'junk-food' tax: a modelled comparison of cost-effectiveness for obesity prevention. *International Journal of Obesity (London)* 35: 1001–1009.

Saris WH, Blair SN, van Baak MA, *et al.* (2003) How much physical activity is enough to prevent unhealthy weight gain? Outcome of the IASO 1st Stock Conference and consensus statement. *Obesity Reviews* 4(2): 101–114.

Scottish Intercollegiate Guidelines Network (SIGN). (2010) *Management of Obesity. A National Clinical Guideline*. Guideline 115. Edinburgh: Royal College of Physicians, 2010.

Stunkard AJ, Sobel J. (1995) Psychological consequences of obesity. In Brownell KD, Fairburn CG (Eds.) *Eating Disorders and Obesity: A Comprehensive Handbook*. London: Guilford Press, pp. 417–430.

Swinburn B, Gill T, Kumanyika S. (2005) Obesity prevention: a proposed framework for translating evidence into action. *Obesity Reviews* 6: 23–33.

Vos T, Carter R, Barendregt J, *et al.*, (2010) Assessing Cost-Effectiveness in Prevention (ACE – Prevention). Available at www.sph.uq.edu.au/docs/BODCE/ACE-P/ACE-Prevention_final_report.pdf. Accessed 18 April 2011.

Wang YC, McPherson K, Marsh T, Gortmaker SL, Brown M. (2011) *Health and Economic Burden of the Projected Obesity Trends in the USA and the UK*. Lancet 378: 815–825.

Wang YC, Beydoun MA, Liang L, Caballero B, Kumanyika SK. (2008) Will all Americans become overweight or obese? Estimating the progression and cost of the US obesity epidemic. *Obesity (Silver Spring)* 16: 2323–2330.

Withrow D, Alter DA. (2011) The economic burden of obesity worldwide: a systematic review of the direct costs of obesity. *Obesity Reviews* 12: 131–141.

World Cancer Research Fund (WCRF), American Institute for Cancer Research (AICR). (2009) *Food, Nutrition, Physical Activity and the Prevention of Cancer: a Global Perspective*. London: WCRF/Washington DC: AICR. Available at www.dietandcancerreport.org/ Last accessed 15th February 2013.

World Health Organization (WHO). (1998) *Obesity. Preventing and Managing the Global Epidemic*. Geneva: WHO, 1998.

World Health Organization (WHO). (2003a) *Global Strategies on Diet, Physical Activity and Health*. Geneva: WHO.

World Health Organization/FAO. (2003b) *Diet, Nutrition and the Prevention of Chronic Diseases*. WHO Technical Report Series 916. Geneva: WHO.

World Health Organization (WHO). (2008) Waist circumference and waist-hip ratio. Report of a WHO expert consultation. Available at www.who.int. Accessed 16 February 2013.

World Health Organization Expert Consultation. (2004) Appropriate body mass index for Asian Populations and its implications for policy and intervention strategies. *Lancet* 363: 157–164.

7.13.2 Management of obesity and overweight in adults

Catherine Hankey

Key points

- Moderate weight loss, usually 5–10% of body weight, is the most realistic target for weight management programmes.

- Clinical guidelines advocate structured approaches to weight management using multicomponent interventions for weight loss and weight maintenance components.

- Diet composition can affect compliance with dietary advice, but the effectiveness of approaches depends on the generation of an energy deficit below requirements and learning the behaviours to sustain it.

- Physical activity assists weight maintenance, but alone has little effectiveness for weight loss.

- Weight loss usually slows after 12 weeks, when weight maintenance becomes the target; more than one cycle of weight loss and maintenance are often required to achieve clinically important weight change.

- Medication and surgical approaches are valuable for some patients.

The prevalence of adult overweight and obesity in the UK and worldwide remains at epidemic proportions, and is still increasing (Berghofer *et al.*, 2008). This increased prevalence is reflected in increased body mass index (BMI) across all ages, with older adults increasingly affected. Individuals with a BMI of >35 kg/m² present particular management challenges. The scale of increase in this group, often considered to have severe and complicated obesity, is increasing internationally (WHO, 1998). In Scotland, the incidence of a BMI of >35 kg/m² is 5% and 11% for men and women, respectively.

This increased prevalence has direct effects on particular areas of healthcare. One pertinent example is the increased obesity incidence in women of child bearing age. Pregnancies associated with excessive weight gain and postnatal weight retention are more frequent in those at social disadvantage (Heslehurst *et al.*, 2010) and present particular management challenges.

Obesity incurs considerable additional healthcare and other costs. This is illustrated by the example of drug prescribing in primary care for the obese; this has almost doubled for the majority of drug categories (Counterweight Project Team, 2005). Health economic evaluations have warned of the enormous financial costs that will result from no action to challenge the relentless rise in obesity (Walker, 2003).

Approaches to challenge the international increases in body weight comprise of prevention, which whilst an attractive option (King *et al.*, 2011), does not meet the needs of over three-quarter of adults who are already obese, and weight management. Effective and clinically important weight management is defined as weight loss of 5–10% of body weight for those with a BMI below 35 kg/m², or 15–20% for those whose BMI exceeds 35 kg/m², and followed by weight maintenance for a period of at least a year (SIGN, 2010). The Scottish Intercollegiate Guidelines Network (SIGN) stated that a weight loss of >15% would be required to show health benefits in adults whose BMI is >35 kg/m² or for those with comorbid conditions, such as type 2 diabetes, with a BMI of 30 kg/m². The health benefits of moderate weight loss include improved physical symptoms and biochemical indices, such as plasma lipid profiles, as well as reductions in blood pressure, plasma insulin and glucose. Other benefits include decreases in degenerative joint pain and improved gynaecological health.

Effective weight management needs to be a structured process with clear assessment and management approaches. Often, weight loss is thought of as the only element of weight management, but a weight maintenance phase is required, and is arguably equally important in consolidating weight loss. It is in this context, rather than the target of achieving a BMI in the healthy reference range, that the different strategies for weight management in adults will be discussed. Surgical approaches for weight management, whilst important, are specific and fundamentally different from the others, and are considered separately in Chapter 7.13.3.

Assessment of overweight and obesity

Body mass index

Body mass index is the most widely accepted way to interpret body weight in terms of health risk. A BMI of 18.5–24.9 kg/m^2 is healthy and of 25.1–29.9 kg/m^2 is overweight (WHO, 1998). A BMI of 30 kg/m^2 is considered obese, and in excess of 40 kg/m^2 morbidly obese. Cut-offs differ according to ethnicity, and are lower for South Asian and oriental adults (WHO, 2004). Overall raised BMI has a very broad, often non-specific effect on wellbeing, making people feel less well and less energetic. Poorer general health and poor wellbeing scores reflect this. Reduced physical health and quality of life associated with obesity can contribute to impaired mental wellbeing (Hassan et al., 2003).

Waist circumference and waist to hip ratio

A BMI does not consider body shape and the increased likelihood of negative health effects that are associated with abdominal obesity. This can be illustrated by the case of two women, who, while of the same BMI, age and ethnicity, have large differences in body shape. They are highly likely to show very different health risks. To quantify these differences, measures of body shape have been developed and examined in the context of health risk.

Waist circumference is a simple measurement that can indicate the need for weight management (Lean et al., 1995); those with a larger waist circumference are at greater health risk (Han et al., 1995). The target values for waist circumference have been divided into three zones; green, amber (action level 1) and red (action level 2), as shown in Table 7.13.7. A healthy waist measurement, reflecting low health risk, will be in the green zone; one reflecting moderate health risk in the amber zone (action level 1); and one reflecting high risk in the red zone (action level 2).

Waist circumference should be measured midway between the lowest rib and the iliac crest. Careful identification of the waist using these landmarks will ensure that waist measures can be replicated easily, which is especially important as part of a programme of weight

management. Practitioners can advise patients of where their waist measurement sits in terms of health risk, and they can then monitor themselves. A rule of thumb is that a 1-cm decrease in waist measurement is associated with close to a 0.5 kg of weight loss.

Waist to hip ratio (WHR) is another measure of body shape that has been used to classify health risks, but has been largely superseded by waist circumference measurements. Its value should be considered with caution as there are difficulties in measuring WHR and the errors are greater in women than men (Wing et al., 1992). Furthermore, interventions that reduce body weight will reduce BMI and waist and hip circumferences, but produce small or no changes in the WHR. The limitations of using WHR as a measure of body shape are demonstrated using the example of the INTERHEART case control study. It showed a graded and worldwide significant association with one of the many consequences of obesity, myocardial infarction risk (Yusuf et al., 2005). However, the study provided no evidence that WHR was a better predictor than waist circumference alone for other forms of cardiovascular disease, such as sudden death and stroke. Other metabolic consequences of obesity, such as diabetes, infertility or cancer, were not reported.

Dietetic approaches to weight loss

The accepted target for success or good compliance with weight loss regimens is now between 5% and 20% of body weight, with the outdated target of a BMI within the healthy reference range having been discarded. These targets should be considered in the context of populations living in an obesogenic setting, such as the UK, which favours body weight increases steadily across adulthood. This rate has been estimated at between 0.5 and 1 kg annually (Heitmann & Garby, 1999). For those in receipt of medication prescribed for the treatment of long term chronic disease, unintentional weight gain occurs frequently, and can reach up to 10 kg over 52 weeks (Leslie et al., 2007). Simply arresting or slowing the almost inevitable weight gain in adulthood can therefore be considered a therapeutic success. However, the health benefits can be considerable from clinically important weight loss either in early adulthood, particularly in younger people, through to older people. The effectiveness of a reduced energy regimen in self directed slimming is almost impossible to gauge. However, one estimate indicated that a 10% decrease in overweight was achieved by only 10% of the population attempting to lose weight (Perri et al., 1992). It is against estimates of this nature that the success of weight loss programmes is currently being judged. Most conventional professional dietetic approaches use one to one interviews, which are inherently expensive in terms of staff time, whilst group based approaches are mainly, but not entirely, used by commercial organisations.

Evaluation of studies examining different approaches to achieve intentional weight loss can be carried out using data from those who completed the study (completers analysis) or from all those who entered the study [inten-

Table 7.13.7 Action levels for waist circumference

	Green zone (normal)	Amber zone (action level 1)*	Red zone (action level 2)**
Women	<80 cm	80–87 cm	≥88 cm
	<32 inches	32–35 inches	≥35 inches
Men	<94 cm	94–101 cm	≥102 cm
	<37 inches	37–40 inches	≥40 inches

*Action level – increasing health risks.
**Action level 2 – high health risks, seek advice to lose weight.

tion to treat analysis (ITT)]. Arguably, data should be analysed using both approaches to determine the best case scenario (the completers analysis), as well as an insight into the initial treatment intent, not the treatment eventually administered. Intention to treat analysis should minimise the risks of misleading interpretation of effectiveness that can arise in any intervention research, and provides insight into how generalisable the intervention can be in usual care. It is useful in counteracting the effects of the high attrition rates usually observed in weight management studies, some predictors of which are raised BMI, low aerobic fitness and socioeconomic status (Roumen *et al.*, 2011); however, a consistent set of predictors has not been identified (Moroshko *et al.*, 2011).

All approaches designed to achieve intentional weight loss are dependent on the maintenance of an energy deficit between energy intake and expenditure. The most commonly used approaches to achieve such energy imbalance include dietary change to reduce energy intake and increased physical activity to increase expenditure.

Energy deficit approach

Conventional dietary restriction for many years was with the 1000 kcal (4.2 MJ) diet, but compliance as measured by body weight changes was recognised to be poor. The value of moving away from severe energy restriction was endorsed by Frost *et al.* (1991) who confirmed in their audit of two dietetic weight management approaches, that greater energy restriction did not lead to a greater weight loss in free living subjects. Patients were allocated to either a 1200-kcal regimen, or an individualised prescription based on the Lean & James formula (1986) together with a daily energy deficit close to 600 kcal below estimated energy expenditure. The prescriptions recognised that the heavier a person becomes the greater their energy requirements. In addition to body weight, age and gender also influence the individuals' energy requirements. A mean prescription of 1700 kcal/day over 3 months produced a 5.0 kg weight loss, compared with a 3.0 kg loss achieved with a standard 1100 kcal/day approach (Frost *et al.*, 1991). Formal evaluation of the energy deficit approach for 12 weeks versus a blanket generalised low calorie (1500 kcal/day) approach using a randomised controlled design has been carried out (Leslie *et al.*, 2002). Weight loss did not differ between the treatments (4.3 kg with the energy deficit approach versus 4.9 kg with the generalised low calorie diet). Target weight losses, calculated using estimated energy requirements, and assuming total compliance with each approach were 7.0 and 13.0 kg, respectively. The weight losses achieved using the energy deficit approach were closer to those predicted than they were for the generalised low calorie approach, confirming the findings of Frost *et al.* This moderate energy deficit approach is currently being used as part of a national study of weight management in primary care (McCombie *et al.*, 2012). The energy deficit approach for weight management is advocated in UK national weight management programmes (NICE, 2006; SIGN, 2010).

Differing macronutrient composition

Increased protein/low carbohydrate diets

There are consistent findings from metabolic studies and epidemiological observations that high carbohydrate/low fat diets assist weight loss and prevent regain. Increased protein/low carbohydrate diets, whilst opposing current public health advice, achieve weight loss by using the positive effects of protein on controlling appetite (Weigle *et al.*, 2005).

High protein/low carbohydrate dietary advice is not new; the Atkins diet has generated huge international interest since launch in 1972 and has been republished (Atkins, 1998). The dietary principles of the high protein/low carbohydrate diet are to achieve weight loss, weight maintenance and good health by limiting carbohydrate intake to between 20 and 30 g/day, whilst consuming unprocessed foods rich in protein and fat in unlimited quantities. Foods to be eaten freely are red meat, fish, poultry, eggs and fats. Foods that are severely restricted are most fruit, some vegetables, rice, pasta and other grain products. Initial weight loss with a high protein/low carbohydrate diet is mostly due to glycogen losses (Eisenstein *et al.*, 2002). The satiating effects of protein also encourage weight loss, as was shown in a 26-week randomised controlled trial (RCT) of overweight and obese subjects (Foster *et al.*, 2003). Dietary advice was to consume either a high carbohydrate or a high protein/low carbohydrate diet *ad libitum*. A significantly greater weight loss (−8.9 versus −5.1 kg) was achieved with the high protein/low carbohydrate approach. Efficacy and safety of low carbohydrate diets were considered in a systematic review (Bravata *et al.*, 2003), which concluded that there was insufficient evidence to make recommendations for or against this approach. Three further robust studies of longer duration were subsequently published, allowing more conclusive findings. Two 1-year studies (Eisenstein *et al.*, 2002; Brinkworth *et al.*, 2004) and a 2-year study (Foster *et al.*, 2010) compared low and high carbohydrate diets. The studies reported no differences in weight loss according to dietary treatment (−4.1% versus −2.9% and −4.4% vs −2.5%, respectively for the 1-year studies), and at 2 years weight loss for all participants was 7 kg (7%). Two further systematic reviews compared low carbohydrate (<30 g/day) and low fat diets (<30% of energy/day) and confirmed that both are effective at 12 months in achieving modest weight loss (Hession *et al.*, 2009, Nordmann *et al.*, 2006). Mean weight losses were mostly clinically important at 6 months, with a 4.1 kg difference in favour of the raised protein approach. However, at 1 year this difference had decreased to <2 kg, indicating small and probably unimportant differences between the groups. The attrition rate was 36% overall in the studies included in the review (and is usually around 30% in studies of weight management), although the authors indicated this was significantly lower in the low carbohydrate groups, although the actual numbers were unreported.

Although no studies have reported any actual negative health effects of a low carbohydrate diet in terms of cardiovascular risk factors, questions remain as to the long term health effects of this approach. This approach is at odds with international dietary guidelines and may be detrimental to renal function and bone health, and increase cancer risk, especially in those with existing obesity related disease (Harper & Astrup, 2004). At present there appears to be no advantage in following a low carbohydrate diet in terms of weight loss.

Low glycaemic index

Glycaemic index (GI) is defined as the incremental positive area under the blood glucose curve following 50 g of carbohydrate from a test food divided by the incremental area following 50 g of a reference food (glucose) (Jenkins et al., 1981). Lentils, pasta and apples are examples of low GI foods, and high GI foods include cornflakes, rice and white bread. It has been proposed that a low GI diet would have beneficial effects on appetite by reducing energy intake and thus inducing an energy deficit and encouraging weight loss. However, a review of studies in this area found weight loss was no greater with a low GI compared with a high GI diet (−1.5 kg versus −1.6 kg) and that effects on satiety did not differ (Raben, 2002). A systematic review (Thomas et al., 2007) confirmed these findings, and indicated that there was insufficient evidence to justify a role for a low GI diet in weight management. The weighted mean difference reported between a low GI and a comparator diet was −1.1 kg (95% CI −2.0 to −0.2). However, the relatively few studies were short term and included participants who were not obese, making interpretation difficult.

Very low calorie diet regimens

Very low calorie diets (VLCDs) provide preprepared meals, usually in the form of liquid drinks but they occasionally allow a daily meal based on food. The term is used when energy provision from the entire regimen is <800 kcal/day (National Task Force on the Prevention and Treatment of Obesity, 1993). This national committee concluded that supervision by a physician and the selection of patients with a BMI of >30 kg/m^2 should provide appropriate and adequate safeguards to VLCD use; to date these recommendations remain valid. The recommended VLCD composition includes 1 g of protein/kg of ideal body weight/day to minimise muscle breakdown.

Cholelithiasis has been shown to be the most frequent clinical complication associated with the use of VLCDs, with a reported 10% incidence of clinically recognisable symptoms of gallstones after 16 weeks of VLCD therapy (Yang et al., 1992). The potential dangers with VLCDs are increased with prolonged use and if the person has underlying heart disease. A 12–20-week period is acceptable (National Task Force on the Prevention and Treatment of Obesity, 1993). Publicity concerning VLCD regimens and their advocation by celebrities generated interest for a systematic review and meta analysis (Tsai & Wadden, 2005). Studies compared the use of VLCDs for intentional weight loss with low calorie diets (LCDs) comprised of conventional food over the long and short term. Participants had a BMI of 35–40 kg/m^2, with and without type 2 diabetes. Short term weight loss at 13 weeks was 16% and 10% of body weight in the VLCD and LCD participants, respectively. However, over the longer term, these statistical and clinically important differences observed in favour of VLCDs were lost. After a mean 1.9 years, weight losses were 6.3% and 5.0% respectively. Interestingly, attrition was similar for both treatments, at close to 23%. In practice, VLCD compliance is rarely complete, with patients tending to revert to their usual diet and lifestyle, using VLCDs only sporadically. However, the use of VLCD regimens can be justified in certain situations where quick weight loss is required, e.g. before surgery. Furthermore, it may be that a VLCD approach could be used in those who are obese with a chronic condition, the obvious one being type 2 diabetes. Short term use could be of value if it illustrates to the participant that they are able to lose weight, thus opening the door to other food based weight management programmes more suitable for use over the longer term.

Physical activity strategies to weight loss

The established health benefits of physical activity include reduced blood pressure, improved lipids [especially high density lipoprotein (HDL) cholesterol and triglyceride concentrations] and increased insulin sensitivity. The potential mechanisms linking exercise with weight loss include enhanced resting metabolic rate, preservation of lean tissue, increased total daily energy expenditure and post exercise oxygen consumption (Hill et al., 1994). The influences of physical activity on hunger and satiety are conflicting, with both increases and decreases being reported. A J shaped relationship with appetite involving a paradoxical increase in appetite with complete inactivity has been suggested.

When physical activity or exercise alone is used in the treatment of obesity, weight losses are modest and average 2–3 kg (King & Tribble, 1991). When compared with no intervention, in this case waiting list controls, physical activity achieved greater weight loss, but much less than achieved with dietary interventions (NICE, 2006). However, evidence does exist that exercise alone can produce larger reductions in weight when it is of sufficient frequency, intensity and duration, and there appears to be a dose–response relationship between level of exercise and degree of weight lost. Given the limited ability and desire of overweight and obese adults to exercise, it seems that energy restriction rather than physical activity should remain the focus of the weight loss element in weight management.

A combination of diet and exercise generally produces greater weight losses than diet alone (Skender et al., 1996). One study randomised dieters to an exercise or no exercise group and found that the exercise group lost an average of 10.9 kg during the 12-week intervention period compared with an average of 6.6 kg in the diet only group (Svendsen et al., 1994). Subjects in the exercise group had improved plasma lipids, although weight loss was no different. The National Institute for Health and Care Excellence (2006) reviewed the evidence to answer the question *'does physical activity, 45 minutes three times per week, combined with a 600 kcal energy deficit diet lead to additional weight loss in comparison to diet alone?'* Median weight loss across three studies was 5.6 kg with diet and activity, compared with 4.10 kg for diet alone. A meta analysis examined the same issue, this time considering long term (2-year) effectiveness of diet plus exercise interventions versus diet alone (Wu *et al.*, 2009). At 2 years there was a 1.1 kg or 0.5 kg/m² difference in favour of interventions that harnessed activity and diet. Interestingly, the authors indicated that for both interventions partial weight regain was evident. However, there are often issues when reviewing this topic as dose and duration of physical activity often differ between interventions.

Physical activity may be of most value in the treatment of obesity by encouraging weight maintenance. Fogelholm *et al.* (2000) randomly allocated those who had successfully lost weight to either a moderate or higher intensity walk programme or control. The moderate activity programme was as effective as the higher intensity one in preventing the 2.6 kg regain in the inactive control subjects.

Behaviour modifications in weight management

Behaviour modification has been described as a process that identifies unproductive habits, which are then replaced with adaptive behaviour patterns. A review of the use of behavioural approaches to change health behaviours can be found in Chapter 1.3. Behaviour therapy in weight management addresses two main aims. First, a reduction in the food energy consumed and second, an increase in physical activity and thus total energy expenditure to facilitate weight loss. The most widely used approaches for behaviour modification have been summarised by Avenell *et al.* (2006). These comprise reflective approaches that encourage the individual to reflect on their own actions, self monitoring food intake to identify eating behaviour cues before introducing control methods, stimulus control, changing eating patterns and revising weight loss expectations in line with realistic and clinically important targets. Together with education in nutrition and strategies to manage lapses, self monitoring has been considered vital to the success of these approaches as subjects then contribute to and define a programme of care with which they feel most comfortable. Cognitive approaches are often used in parallel with behavioural methods to combat barriers to weight loss that exists within the patient's framework of beliefs. The administration of behaviour therapy can be either through group teaching or individual counselling.

Wadden (2005) reviewed the results of treatments that included behaviour therapy for weight reduction in the years 1974–2002. Forty-two weight reduction studies were published in four behavioural journals over this period and the rates of weight loss were between 0.4 and 0.5 kg/week across all treatments. This encouraging finding must be tempered by the quality of studies as a recent meta analysis reported that behavioural studies of weight management have in the main been of poor methodological quality, with few following a randomised controlled design or being of a long duration (Ostman *et al.*, 2004). The Scottish Intercollegiate Guidelines Network (SIGN, 2010) reviewed the effectiveness of such approaches and found no studies that showed behaviour modification alone to be effective in inducing weight loss. In reported three small studies whose focus was on behaviour and did include a dietary element, weight loss was 3.8 kg compared with 0.5 kg for a passive intervention (self help). In clinical practice, behavioural skills are important to improve communication between professionals and patients, and encourage maximum patient participation. It is likely that some elements of behavioural approaches are already in use in dietetic practice and that together with dietary advice they contribute towards effective weight management.

Multicomponent weight loss interventions

In the UK clinical guidelines for weight management (NICE, 2006; SIGN, 2010) advocate the use of multicomponent weight loss programmes, comprising three elements; diet, exercise/physical activity and behaviour therapy. This approach has undergone recent thorough investigation (Loveman *et al.*, 2011) in a systematic review that assessed both the clinical and cost effectiveness of multicomponent weight management programmes over the long term in overweight and obese adults. The included studies, largely non-UK based, were diverse in nature and hence meta analysis was precluded. Weight loss was moderate across all studies, although in general weight change appeared to be greater in the intervention groups than comparator groups. Those studies incorporating a longer term follow-up observed weight regain in a majority of subjects. Differences in study design prevented the drawing of firm conclusions concerning the effectiveness of multicomponent weight management. Assessment of cost effectiveness, which is increasingly relevant to justify implementation of all interventions, was also problematic. A preliminary cost effectiveness assessment was carried out with two studies, despite each having limitations, namely a duration of only 36 months, use of prescription antiobesity drugs in some participants and follow-up of <18 months. Each study used a lifetime chronic disease model approach to evaluate the effect of changes in an individual's weight. The models included the costs and benefits from avoiding chronic illnesses such as coronary heart disease and diabetes. Other models are broader and include a wider range of chronic diseases. However, both studies concluded that the long term multicomponent interventions were cost effective, with estimates varying between –£473 and £7200 (US$12 640). As used in cost effectiveness studies, this was expressed as quality adjusted life years gained. The authors cautiously suggested that long term multicomponent weight management interventions in general promoted weight loss in overweight or obese adults, but emphasised that small weight changes and regain were common. Some evidence suggested that multicomponent intervention may be cost effective, but this finding was by no means conclusive. No UK based RCTs were included in the review, a research need was expressed to evaluate the effects of long term multicomponent weight management interventions in a UK setting.

It is unlikely, if not unknown, for any study to draw firm and final conclusions in any research area. However, there are two US based studies following randomised designs that seem to provide robust conclusive findings in relation to dietary composition and follow-up at 2 years. Sacks *et al.* (2009) recognised the possible advantages of different dietary composition in weight loss diets. Using a factorial model, adults were randomised to one of four diets varying in macronutrient composition, but all regimens incorporated an energy deficit of 750 kcal/day. Weight loss was 6 kg at 6 months. Participants were then followed up for 2 years. Attrition was low at 20% and, despite weight regain, losses of 4 kg were maintained, with about 15% of participants maintaining a weight loss of >10%. The authors concluded that the reduced calorie diet, irrespective of macronutrient focus, could lead to clinically meaningful weight loss. Another 2-year study, set this time within primary care, illustrated how behavioural weight loss counselling could best be delivered by using lifestyle coaches (Wadden *et al.*, 2011). All participants were prescribed identical goals for diet and physical activity, but were provided with different levels of support to achieve them. Dietary advice to achieve an energy intake of between 1200 and 1500 kcal was given to participants weighing <113.4 kg, and for up to 1800 kcal if weight was greater. All were advised to exercise for up to 180 minutes/week and given a pedometer. Usual care comprised quarterly visits that included 5–7 minutes reviewing weight change. Brief lifestyle counselling included an additional 15 minutes/month with an auxiliary healthcare provider, while enhanced counselling support offered the option of further tools. This allowed participants to choose the medications orlistat or sibutramine (no longer licensed for use) after 6 months or meal replacement products. Enhanced care attempted to mimic practice in primary care, providing participants with the opportunity to influence their care, guided by practice staff, by choosing one or more of these additional tools. At 2 years usual care achieved weight losses of 1.7 kg, lifestyle counselling 2.9 kg and enhanced support 4.6 kg. Initial weight loss was at least 5% in 21%, 26% and 34% of participants of the three groups, respectively. The enhanced support option was significantly more effective than the other interventions in achieving clinically important weight loss. These two studies effectively illustrate the short and long term effectiveness of weight management approaches.

Weight management in different settings

Group versus individual therapy

Group therapy offers obvious and important benefits for decreasing cost and improving professional resource management (Bitzen *et al.*, 1988; Chenoweth, 1990). Whilst the group environment is undoubtedly unsuitable for some shy or reluctant socialisers, for those agreeable to this approach it allows additional harnessing of structure and peer support not accessible to the subject undergoing individual one to one dietary counselling. Commercial organisations utilise group settings for their sessions. The effectiveness of these was considered earlier. However, other programmes such as Counterweight also offer group based treatments, when these are possible, within the primary care setting.

The Australian Gutbuster waist loss programme was a group programme designed for men who were recruited to a 6-week course and then followed for a year. The programme involved advice on exercise, dietary fat and alcohol intake. Average waist circumference losses of 4% were achieved and lifestyle advice led to lowered fat and alcohol intakes. A more advanced programme that included six additional fortnightly sessions saw falls in waist circumference of 10% (Egger *et al.*, 1996). In contrast to the majority of group based interventions, this approach showed the value of group programmes for weight management in men.

There may be cost benefits from using group approaches to weight management, but this is not entirely clear, as the class number may be small. A recent systematic review (Paul-Ebhohimhen & Avenell, 2009) included RCTs, but not those examining commercial weight treatments. At 12 months a weight difference of 1.4 kg was seen between group versus individual approaches. Subanalyses indicated that financial incentives within group treatments increased weight loss. Subsequent examination by these authors indicated that financial incentives themselves were not a useful tool to maximise weight loss.

The Counterweight programme (an example of weight management in primary care)

Primary care has been advocated by clinical guidelines as a suitable but underutilised setting for weight management. Counterweight is a unique nationwide programme, originally set only in primary care, that harnesses the best evidence based approaches for weight management (Counterweight Project Team, 2008). Primary care staff, including practice nurses, health trainers or healthcare support workers, attend an 8-hour training course, and are subsequently mentored to agreed competency levels by Counterweight specialists. Approaches for delivery are largely one to one, although groups are used where appropriate. Lifestyle change focuses on both diet and physical activity, with key behaviour change strategies underpinning the intervention. The overall aim is for patients to develop skills to manage weight in the long term. Dietary change is based on either the 600-kcal energy deficit approach or on individualised goal setting. As with any weight management approach, the intensity of the intervention can affect both the main outcome, weight change, and the cost and utility of the programme. Counterweight participants receive six appointments over 3 months, delivered on a group or one to one basis, then follow up sessions every 3 months for a year, and then annually (Counterweight Project Team, 2004a,b). This level of intensity probably reflects realistic implementation resource availability within the NHS. As the project harnesses current evidence, there is no requirement to prove its effectiveness in terms of biochemical measures and/or experimental design, such as a RCT. A continuous improvement model to develop the model was employed (Petticrew et al., 2012), and the 5-year outcome data were the starting point for this (Counterweight Project Team, 2008). These data indicate that mean weight loss was 3.0 kg at 12 months (% CI −3.5 to −2.3 kg) and at 24 months was 2.3 kg (95% CI −3.2 to −1.4). Clinically beneficial weight loss of >5% was achieved in 30.7% of the attending population at 12 months and in 31.9% at 24 months. Counterweight achieves and maintains clinically important weight loss.

A multidisciplinary weight management service (a secondary care specialist centre in Glasgow)

The management of obesity by healthcare professionals (dietitians, doctors, nurses, physiotherapists and psychologists) is generally fragmented and each professional group has developed management programmes largely independently of each other. Dietitians offer both inpatient and outpatient services in most general hospitals and in the community. There is little evidence that input to dietetic weight management from specialist health professionals occurs regularly. Practice nurses offer weight management advice to many overweight clients, although this appears to be on an *ad hoc* basis (Hoppe & Ogden, 1997). Physician led obesity clinics are found in only a few UK NHS centres. A specialist weight management service using a multidisciplinary team based approach bringing together dietitians, psychologists, physiotherapists, physicians and surgeons was advocated by SIGN (1996). Greater Glasgow Health Board piloted this innovative service and 3 month outcome data have been published (Morrison et al., 2012). This first phase evaluation indicated that 72.4% of all referrals participated in the programme, with 37.5% completing phase 1 (12 weeks). Of these 809 completers, 35% achieved a clinically important weight loss of 5 kg or more. These data have indicated some approaches to potentially improve service effectiveness. Further longer term data are eagerly awaited from this unique service.

Although multidisciplinary working is widely advocated to take on the task of weight management, there still appears to be reluctance amongst many health professionals. A survey of GPs, practice nurses and dietitians found all three groups of professionals felt underskilled to effectively manage both obesity and overweight (Hankey et al., 2004). Similar findings were reported in a survey of secondary care consultants (Leslie et al., 2005). In both studies dietitians were identified as the professional group most likely to take on weight management, but were considered too scarce to assume a major role. It is unlikely that the views of these health professionals have altered since these studies were completed,

and in fact it is likely that resources are scarcer given the current financial climate. However, in order to evaluate these assertions, it is proposed to return to the Scottish dietetic profession and seek their views on obesity and weight management once more, which will be especially valuable given the recent publication of the revised SIGN (2010) obesity guideline.

Community pharmacy (a possible setting for community based weight management)

The sheer number of adults who are overweight or obese means use of as wide a range as possible of potential opportunities to deliver weight management are justified. Community pharmacists occupy a position of trust and are easily accessible to many. Recent evidence evaluating the effectiveness of community pharmacists in terms of weight management has been systematically reviewed (Gordon et al., 2011). The review indicated that only scant research data exist within this field, and certainly a dearth of robust studies of up to 12 months' duration. Whilst RCTs would appear inappropriate in this setting, further investigation into the clinical and cost effectiveness of weight management in pharmacies is justified.

Commercial slimming organisations

A number of commercial slimming organisations operate in the UK and offer a regular service to those seeking assistance with weight management. Slimming groups are accessible, convenient and relatively inexpensive, and currently their role in the UK is expanding, with partnerships with the NHS becoming established (Stubbs et al., 2011). The 12-week treatment data appear promising, with a 4.0 kg weight loss and 1.5 kg/m^2 reduction in BMI, but further data concerning both attrition rates and information on longer term weight change (at least 1 year), are required to justify the value of this programme (Stubbs et al., 2001).

In addition to this audit, a number of studies have formally examined the effectiveness of commercial approaches. Dansinger et al. (2005) in their randomised study comparing commercial organisations with other dietary approaches showed that at 1 year weight loss with the commercial organisation Weight Watchers was similar to that with other approaches tested at 3.0 kg. Another comparison between a commercial slimming organisation and a self help group found a 4 kg weight loss at 1 year with the commercial programme and a 1 kg weight loss with self help (Heshka et al., 2003). A review (Tsai & Wadden, 2005) of published evidence from commercial and self help groups concurred with these findings. Best results were a 3.2% weight loss at 2 years for Weight Watchers. The effectiveness of a primary care referral to a commercial provider for weight loss treatment was evaluated using a randomised controlled design (Jebb et al., 2011). Participants were randomly allocated to usual care or to receive the commercial programme for 12 months. The attrition rates were similar for both arms of the study at 46% and 39%, respectively. However, the weight loss after 12 months in the commercial setting was more than double that of usual care (5.06 kg versus 2.25 kg). This finding is encouraging and in excess of that achieved in any other study. The intensity of the commercial intervention, either two or three appointments/month, may have strongly influenced the weight loss, favouring success. Uncertainty remains as to the cost effectiveness of such an intervention, and whether the level of intensity applied in this study could be justified and replicated in usual care. The findings of an audit of the same commercial programme contrast with the study findings, indicating that provision of 12 sessions within an NHS referral scheme, delivered over a 12-week period, showed a lower median weight change when all referrals were considered (−2.8 kg/3.1%) and an attrition rate of 46% (Ahern et al., 2011).

The Internet

The Internet appears to offer promise as a tool to facilitate weight management, and in theory this could be at low cost. To date there are relatively few studies of Internet delivered intervention, but in general these show moderate weight loss and some positive effects on weight maintenance. The setting itself is restricted to those who are computer literate and have access to the Internet. These interventions can be either commercial or delivered through national health care routes. McConnan et al. (2007) examined the effect of a combination of dietary and physical activity advice, along with behaviour therapy, in an NHS setting. Patients were randomised to receive usual care or the Internet delivered intervention. Weight loss did not differ between the treatments and was <2 kg. In contrast, two other internet based approaches were compared in a 12-month study, and showed weight losses of 8.3 kg (SD 7.9<kg) and 4.3 kg (SD 6.2 kg), respectively. The higher weight loss was seen with the structured behavioural intervention compared to a self help approach (Gold et al., 2007). Internet based delivery certainly appears to offer promise, alongside challenges, such as determining outcome to a remotely delivered intervention, and further evaluation is justified.

Antiobesity medication

There is only one antiobesity medication available for prescription by physicians for the management of obesity and comorbid conditions, although a number of others are under development. There were two others, an appetite adjuster, sibutramine, and a selective endocannabinoid receptor blocker, rimonabant. Both were removed from use in response to negative health events possibly related to their use. The medication still available for use, orlistat (tetrahydrolipostatin), induces malabsorption (antinutrients). Other medications under development for weight management operate through appetite suppression (or satiety promotion), or by thermogenesis to increase energy expenditure. Importantly, for dietetic practice, the only medication available for use in obesity

per se should be taken in combination with a programme of diet, exercise and behaviour therapy.

Malabsorption

Lipase inhibition induces partial malabsorption of dietary fat by inhibition of triglyceride hydrolysis. The chemically synthesised hydrogenated derivative of lipostatin (orlistat) is a potent inhibitor of gastric, pancreatic and carboxylester lipase. Beales & Kopelman (1994) have suggested that the principles by which the medication operates are sound, although there are possible risks, possibly correctable, of fat soluble vitamins A, D, E and K depletion. Predictable side effects from malabsorption, altered bowel habit, and also bacterial overgrowth of the small bowel have led to around a 37% patient withdrawal from therapy (Sjostrom et al., 1998). A low fat/low energy diet reduces symptoms and maximises weight loss, which at 1 year was 10.2% in the controls versus 6.1% in those receiving medication. At 2 years the difference in weight loss due to orlistat was 3.6 kg. About 20% of patients who took part in studies of orlistat lost at least 10% of body weight, which was twice the number on placebo. This medication is now available in the UK with medical prescription as an over the counter product. The success of this initiative is unknown; however it is sold at a dosage of approximately half its prescription dosage, and is expensive.

Hypoglycaemic agents for diabetes and obesity

Although not classified as an antiobesity agent as such, and only appropriate for use in the management of type 2 diabetes, the glucagon like peptide 1 (GLP 1) receptor agonist does reduce body weight close to clinically important levels. Liraglutide has been licensed for use since 2009 and shows a beneficial effect on both body weight (−3 kg at 26 weeks) (Buse et al., 2009) and diabetic control (a reduction of 1.5% in HbA1$_c$). The medication is administered subcutaneously once daily, and its mode of actions are to improve blood glucose control, mediated by increased insulin secretion, delay gastric emptying and suppress post prandial glucagon secretion.

Maintenance of weight loss

A formal description of weight maintenance is valuable and of particular importance when judging the effectiveness of weight management interventions. Long term weight maintenance has been defined as a change of <3% of body weight (Stevens et al., 2006). A common failing in almost all conventional approaches for weight loss is leaving weight maintenance to chance, so that regain is usual and most often almost complete. Many researchers have found that weight loss is relatively easy to achieve, but that weight maintenance is more challenging. There are a number of follow-up studies that have examined long term weight loss after treatment, but they are not technically addressing weight maintenance. A meta analysis in overweight and obese adults examined long term weight loss after diet and exercise (Curioni & Lourenco, 2005). The findings showed inclusion of physical activity and diet together led to a 20% greater sustained weight loss of 6.7 versus 4.5 kg for diet alone after 1 year. However, in both groups almost half the initial weight loss was regained after 1 year. Douketis *et al.* (2005) confirmed the conclusions of this review that all dietary approaches achieve moderate weight loss, with the exception of surgery, after 2–4 year follow-up. In a bid to challenge the perception that almost no one succeeds in long term weight maintenance, Wing & Hill (2001) identified the characteristics of successful weight losers within the national weight control registry of successful long term weight maintainers. These individuals were defined as 10% weight losers who sustained this loss for a least 1 year, but at 5 years mean weight loss was 30 kg. Common characteristics of maintainers in the registry were the consumption of a low fat diet, a high level of physical activity and regularly weighing themselves and taking responsibility for monitoring their own weight.

The European wide multicentre Diogenes study (Larsen *et al.*, 2010) examined dietary composition in the context of preventing weight regain post weight loss. Adults from eight European countries were randomly assigned to one of five *ad libitum* diets to prevent weight regain over a 26-week period; a low protein/low GI diet, a low protein/high GI diet, a high protein/low GI diet, a high protein/high GI diet, or a control diet. A mean weight loss of 11 kg was seen using a very low calorie diet, and only the low protein/high GI diet was associated with clinically important weight regain (+1.7 kg). Although successful weight maintenance strategies have yet to be defined, there are many reflective papers that consider the factors that prevent weight gain (Swinburn & Egger, 2002).

Conclusions

There is a range of clinical approaches for the achievement of weight loss. The outcome in the majority of these interventions is moderate weight loss, which has been acknowledged to confer health benefits. Long term weight maintenance, dependent on effective weight maintenance strategies, is increasingly recognised as a key element. The moderate energy deficit approach has been shown to lead to a weight loss of close to 5.0 kg over 12 weeks, and has been used within longer term studies and also the Counterweight programme. The value of this approach may lie with an emphasis on eating conventional foods and the introduction of regular meal patterns. The effect of diet composition on weight loss is minimal, although the consumption of a high carbohydrate diet in the longer term should be advocated to reduce the risk of long term chronic disease. Physical activity in addition to dietary intervention can offer opportunities for improved maintenance of weight loss, although physical activity programmes alone result in minimal weight losses. Very low calorie diet approaches are valuable in inducing short term weight loss of up to 10–15 kg, either presurgically or in a setting where subsequent dietary management is proposed. Medical supervision is required, together with

a minimum BMI of 30 kg/m^2 and long term management in these cases.

A wide range of treatments for overweight have been tested, and the majority achieve a modest (5–10%) weight loss, which is sufficient to improve clinical outcomes for type 2 diabetes, plasma lipids, hypertension and other risk factors for ischaemic heart disease. This weight loss is usually achieved over 12 weeks, after which it is difficult for many to achieve further loss. Greater weight loss is usually possible for patients with surgery.

Particular weight management challenges are presented by emerging sectors of the overweight and obese populations. These include the severe and complicated groups, those who are obese and pregnant and likely to retain weight gained in pregnancy, and older people for whom physical activity may be particularly challenging; there are likely to be others.

Weight maintenance following weight loss is crucial to sustain the health benefits of weight losses seen with any of the approaches described for weight management. However, effective approaches for the achievement of weight maintenance have yet to be defined and tested. Many health professionals can contribute to effective weight management programmes; however, given the scale of the problem, the role of the dietitian is perhaps greater in terms of training others to enable them to challenge the epidemic of overweight and obesity.

Further reading

Satter N, Lean M (2009). *ABC of Obesity*. Oxford: Wiley Blackwell.

Internet resources

Association for the Study of Obesity   www.aso.org.uk
Counterweight   www.counterweight.org
Dietitians in Obesity Management   www.domuk.org
International Obesity Task Force   www.iotf.org
SCOPE programme   www.iotf.org/media/scoperelease.htm

References

Ahern AL, Olson AD, Aston LM, Jebb SA. (2011) Weight watchers on prescription: an observational study of weight change among adults referred to weight watchers by the NHS. *BMC Public Health* 11: 434.

Atkins RC. (1998) *Dr Atkins's New Diet Revolution*. New York: Simon and Schuster.

Avenell A, Sattar N, Lean MEJ. (2006) ABC of obesity. Management: Part I – behaviour change, diet and activity. *BMJ* 333: 740–743.

Beales PL, Kopelman PG. (1994) Options for the management of obesity. *Pharmoeconomics* 5(Suppl 1): 18–32.

Berghofer A, Pischon T, Reinhold T, Apovian CM, Sharma AM, Willich SN. (2008) Obesity prevalence from a European perspective: a systematic review. *BMC Public Health* 8: 200 (abstract).

Bitzen PO, Melander A, Schersten B, Svensson M. (1988) Efficacy of dietary regulation in primary health care patients with hyperglycaemia detected by screening. *Diabetic Medicine* 5: 634–639.

Bravata DM, Sanders L, Huang J, *et al.* (2003) Efficacy and safety of low-carbohydrate diets: a systematic review. *JAMA* 289(14): 1837–1850.

Brinkworth GD, Noakes M, Keogh JB, Luscombe ND, Wittert GA, Clifton PM. (2004) Long-term effects of a high-protein, low-carbohydrate diet on weight control and cardiovascular risk markers in obese hyperinsulinemic subjects. *International Journal of Obesity* 28(5): 661–670.

Buse JB, Rosenstock J, Sesti G, *et al.* (2009) Liraglutide once a day versus Exenatide twice a day for type 2 diabetes: a 26-week randomised, parallel-group, multinational, open-label trial (lead-6). *Lancet* 374: 39–47.

Chenoweth DA. (1990) Health promotion programs examined through cost effectiveness analysis. *Occupational Health and Safety* 59: 40–41

Counterweight Project Team. (2004a) A new evidence based model for weight-management in primary care: the Counterweight Programme. *Journal of Human Nutrition and Dietetics* 17: 191–208.

Counterweight Project Team. (2004b) Current approaches to obesity management in UK Primary Care: the Counterweight Programme. *Journal of Human Nutrition and Dietetics* 17: 183–190.

Counterweight Project Team. (2005) The impact of obesity on drug prescribing in primary care. *British Journal of General Practice* 55: 743–749.

Counterweight Project Team. (2008) Evaluation of the Counterweight Programme for obesity management in primary care: a starting point for continuous improvement. *British Journal of General Practice* 58: 548–554.

Curioni CC, Lourenco PM. (2005) Long-term weight loss after diet and exercise: A systemic review. *International Journal of Obesity* 29(10): 1168–1174.

Dansinger ML, Gleason JA, Griffith JL, Selker HP, Schaefer EJ. (2005) Comparison of the Atkins, Ornish, Weight Watchers, and Zone diets for weight loss and heart disease risk reduction: a randomized trial. *JAMA* 293(1): 43–53.

Douketis JD, Macie C, Thabane L, Williamson DF. (2005) Systematic review of long-term weight loss studies in obese adults: clinical significance and applicability to clinical practice. *International Journal of Obesity* 29(10): 1153–1167.

Egger G, Bolton A, O'Neill M, Freeman D. (1996) Effectiveness of an abdominal obesity reduction programme in men: the GutBuster "waist loss" programme. *International Journal of Obesity* 20(3): 227–231.

Eisenstein J, Roberts SB, Dallal G, Saltzman E. (2002) High-protein weight-loss diets: are they safe and do they work? A review of the experimental and epidemiologic data. *Nutrition Reviews* 60 (7 part 1): 189–200.

Fogelholm M, Kukkonen-Harjula K, Nenonen A, Pasanen M. (2000) Effects of walking training on weight maintenance after a very-low-energy diet in premenopausal obese women: a randomized controlled trial. *Archives of Internal Medicine* 160(14): 2177–2184.

Foster GD, Wyatt HR, Hill JO, *et al.* (2003) A randomized trial of a low-carbohydrate diet for obesity. *New England Journal of Medicine* 348(21): 2082–2090.

Foster GD, Wyatt HR, Hill JO, *et al.* (2010) Weight and metabolic outcomes after 2 years on a low carbohydrate versus low fat diet: a randomised trial. *Annals Internal Medicine* 153: 147–157.

Frost G, Masters K, King C, *et al.* (1991) A new method of energy prescription to improve weight loss. *Journal of Human Nutrition and Dietetics* 4: 369–374.

Gold BC, Burke S, Pintauro S, Buzzell P, Harvey-Berino J. (2007) Weight loss on the web: A pilot study comparing a structured behavioural intervention to a commercial program. *Obesity* 15(1): 155–164.

Gordon J, Watson M, Avenell A. (2011) Lightening the load? A systematic review of community pharmacy-based weight management interventions. *Obesity Reviews* 12(11): 897–911.

Han TS, van Leer EM, Seidell JC, Lean MEJ. (1995) Waist circumference action levels in the identification of cardiovascular risk factors: prevalence study in a random sample. *BMJ* 311: 1401–1405.

Hankey CR, Eley S, Leslie WS, Hunter CM, Lean MEJ. (2004) Eating habits, beliefs, attitudes and knowledge among health professionals regarding the links between obesity, nutrition and health. *Public Health Nutrition* 7(2): 337–343.

Harper A, Astrup A. (2004) Can we advise our obese patients to follow the Atkins diet? *Obesity Reviews* 5(2): 93–94.

Hassan MK, Joshi AV, Madhavan SS, Amonkar MM. (2003) Obesity and health-related quality of life: a cross-sectional analysis of the US population. *International Journal of Obesity* 27: 1227–1232.

Heitmann BL, Garby L. (1999) Patterns of long-term weight changes in overweight developing Danish men and women aged between 30 and 60 years. *International Journal of Obesity* 23: 1074–1078.

Heshka S, Anderson JW, Atkinson RL, *et al.* (2003) Weight loss with self-help compared with a structured commercial program: a randomized trial. *JAMA* 289(14): 1792–1798.

Heslehurst N, Rankin J, Wilkinson JR, Summerbell CD. (2010) A nationally representative study of maternal obesity in England, UK: trends in incidence and demographic inequalities in 619 323 births, 1989–2007. *International Journal of Obesity* 34: 420–428.

Hession M, Rolland C, Kulkarni U, Wise A, Broom J. (2009) Systematic review of randomised controlled trials of low-carbohydrate vs. low-fat/low calorie diets in the management of obesity and its comorbidities. *Obesity Reviews* 10: 36–50.

Hill JO, Drougas HJ, Peters JC. (1994) Physical activity, fitness and moderate obesity. In: Bouchard C, Shephard RJ, Stephens T (eds) *Physical Activity, Fitness and Health: International Proceedings and Consensus Statement 1992*. Champaign: Human Kinetics Publishers, pp. 684–691.

Hoppe R, Ogden J. (1997) Practice nurses' beliefs about obesity and weight related interventions in primary care. *International Journal of Obesity* 21: 141–146.

Jebb SA, Ahern AL, Olson AD, *et al.* (2011) Primary care referral to a commercial provider for weight loss treatment versus standard care: a randomised controlled trial. *Lancet* 378: 1485–1492.

Jenkins DJ, Wolever TM, Taylor RH, *et al.* (1981) Glycemic index of foods: a physiological basis for carbohydrate exchange. *American Journal of Clinical Nutrition* 34(3): 362–366.

King AC, Tribble DL. (1991) The role of exercise in weight regulation in nonathletes. *Sports Medicine* 11: 331–349.

King L, Gill T, Allender S, Swinburn BA. (2011) Best practice principles for community-based obesity prevention: development, content and application, *Obesity Reviews* 12(5): 329–338.

Larsen TM, Dalskov SM, van Baak M, *et al.* (2010) Diets with high or low protein content and glycemic index for weight-loss maintenance. *New England Journal of Medicine* 363(22): 2102–2113.

Lean MEJ, James WPT. (1986) Prescription of diabetic diets in the 1980s. *Lancet* 1: 723–725.

Lean MEJ, Han TS, Morrison CE. (1995) Waist circumference indicates the need for weight management. *BMJ* 311: 158–161.

Leslie WS, Lean MEJ, Baillie HM, Hankey CR. (2002) Weight management: a comparison of existing dietary approaches in a work-site setting. *International Journal of Obesity* 26: 1469–1475.

Leslie WS, Hankey CR, McCombie L, Lean MEJ. (2005) Weight management: a survey of current practice in secondary care NHS settings in 2004. *Journal of Evaluation in Clinical Practice* 11(5): 462–467.

Leslie WS, Hankey, CR, Lean MEJ. (2007) Weight gain as an adverse effect of some commonly prescribed drugs: a systematic review. *Quarterly Journal of Medicine* 100: 395–404.

Loveman E, Frampton GK, Shepherd J, *et al.* (2011) The clinical effectiveness and cost-effectiveness of long-term weight management schemes for adults: a systematic review. *Health Technology Assessment* 15(2): 1–182.

McConnan A, Kirk SF, Cockroft JE, *et al.* (2007) The Internet for weight control in an obese sample: results of a randomised controlled trial. *BMC Health Service Research* 7: 206 (Abstract)

McCombie L, Lean MEJ, Haslem D. (2012) Effective UK weight management services for adults. *Clinical Obesity* 2: 96–102.

Moroshko L, Brennan L, O'Brien P. (2011) Predictors of dropout in weight loss interventions: a systematic review of the literature. *Obesity Reviews* 12: 912–934.

Morrison DS, Boyle S, Morrison C, Allardice G, Greenlaw N., Forde L. (2012) Evaluation of the first phase of a specialist weight management programme in the UK National Health Service: prospective cohort study. *Public Health Nutrition* 15(1): 28–38.

National Task Force on the Prevention and Treatment of Obesity. (1993) Very low calorie diets. *JAMA* 270: 967–974.

National Institute for Health and Care Excellence (NICE). (2006) *Obesity – Guidance on the Prevention, Identification, Assessment and Management of Overweight and Obesity in Adults and Children*. Clinical Guideline 43. London: NICE.

Nordmann AJ, Nordmann A, Briel M, *et al.* (2006) Effects of low-carbohydrate vs low-fat diets on weight loss and cardiovascular risk factors, a meta-analysis of randomised controlled trials. *Archives of Internal Medicine* 166: 285–293.

Ostman J, Britton M, Jonsson E. (2004) *Treating and Preventing Obesity: An Evidence Based Review*. Wiley-VCH.

Paul-Ebhohimhen V, Avenell A. (2009) A systematic review of the effectiveness of group versus individual treatments for adult obesity. *Obesity Facts* 2(1): 17–24.

Perri MG, Nezu AM, Viegner BJ. (1992) *Improving the Long Term Management of Obesity*. New York: Wiley Bioscience.

Petticrew M, Zaid M, Jones DJ. (2012) To RCT or not to RCT: deciding when 'more evidence is needed' for public health policy and practice. *Journal of Epidemiology and Community Health* 66(5): 391–396.

Raben A. (2002) Should obese patients be counselled to follow a low-glycaemic index diet? No. *Obesity Reviews* 3(4): 245–256.

Roumen C, Feskens EJM, Corpeleijn, *et al.* (2011) Predictors of lifestyle intervention outcome and dropout: the SLIM study. *European Journal of Clinical Nutrition* 65: 1141–1147.

Sacks FM, Bray GA, Carey VJ, *et al.* (2009) Comparison of weight loss diets with different compositions of fat, protein and carbohydrates. *New England Journal of Medicine* 360: 859–873.

Scottish Intercollegiate Guidelines Network (SIGN). (2010) *Management of Obesity – A National Clinical Guideline*. No 115. Edinburgh: SIGN.

Sjostrom L, Rissanen A, Andersen T, *et al.* (1998) Randomised placebo-controlled trial of orlistat for weight loss and prevention of weight regain in obese patients. European Multicentre Orlistat Study Group. *Lancet* 352: 167–172.

Skender ML, Goodrick GK, Del-Junco DJ, Reeves RS, Darnell L, Gotto AM. (1996) Comparison of 2-year weight loss trends in behavioural treatments for obesity: diet, exercise and combination interventions. *Journal of the American Dietetic Association* 4: 342–346.

Stevens J, Truesdale KP, McClain JE, Cai J. (2006) The definition of weight maintenance. *International Journal of Obesity* 30: 391–399.

Stubbs J, Pallister C, Whybrow S, Avery A, Lavin J. (2011) Weight outcomes audit for 34,271 adults referred to a primary care/commercial weight management partnership scheme. *Obesity Facts* 4: 113–120.

Svendsen OL, Hassager C, Christiansen C. (1994) Six months' follow-up on exercise added to a short-term diet in overweight postmenopausal women–effects on body composition, resting metabolic rate, cardiovascular risk factors and bone. *International Journal of Obesity* 18(10): 692–698.

Swinburn W, Egger G. (2002) Preventive strategies against weight gain and obesity. *Obesity Reviews* 3(4): 289–301.

Tsai AG, Wadden TA. (2005) Systematic review: an evaluation of major commercial weight loss programs in the United States. *Annals of Internal Medicine* 142(1): 56–66.

Thomas D, Elliott EJ, Baur L. (2007) Low glycaemic index or low glycaemic load diets for overweight and obesity. *Cochrane Database of Systematic Reviews* 3: CD005105. (updated 2009).

Wadden T. (2005) Randomized trial of lifestyle modification and pharmacotherapy for obesity. *New England Journal of Medicine* 353(20): 2111–2120.

Wadden TA, Volger S, Sarwer D, Vetter ML, Tsai AG. (2011) A two-year randomized trial of obesity treatment in primary care practice. *New England Journal of Medicine* 365: 1969–1979.

Walker A. (2003) *The Cost of Doing Nothing – The Economics of Obesity in Scotland*. Glasgow: The University.

Weigle DS, Breen PA, Matthys CC, *et al.* (2005) A high-protein diet induces sustained reductions in appetite, ad libitum caloric intake, and body weight despite compensatory changes in diurnal plasma leptin andghrelin concentrations. *American Journal of Clinical Nutrition* 82: 41–48.

Wing RR, Hill JO. (2001) Successful weight loss maintenance. *Annual Review of Nutrition* 21: 323–341.

Wing RR, Jeffery RW, Burton LR, *et al.* (1992) Change in waist-hip ratio with weight loss, and its association with cardiovascular risk factors. *American Journal of Clinical Nutrition* 55: 1086–1092.

World Health Organization (WHO). (1995) Technical Report Series 854. *Physical Status: The Use and Interpretation of Anthropometry*. Report of a WHO Expert Committee. Geneva: WHO.

World Health Organization (WHO) International Obesity Task Force (IOTF). (1998) *Obesity: Preventing and Managing the Global Epidemic*. Report of a WHO Consultation on Obesity, Geneva 3–5 June 1997. Geneva: WHO.

World Health Organization Expert Consultation. (2004) Appropriate body-mass index for Asian populations and its implications for policy and intervention strategies. *Lancet* 363: 157–163.

Wu T, Gao X, Chem M, van Dam RM. (2009) Long-term effectiveness of diet-plus-exercise interventions vs. diet-only interventions for weight loss: a meta-analysis. *Obesity Reviews* 10: 313–323.

Yang H, Petersen GM, Roth MP, Schoenfield LJ, Marks JW. (1992) Risk factors for gallstone formation during rapid loss of weight. *Digestive Diseases & Sciences* 37: 912–918.

Yusuf S, Hawken S, Ôunpuu S, *et al.*, on behalf of the INTERHEART study investigators (2005). Obesity and the risk of myocardial infarction in 27 000 participants from 52 countries: a case control study. *Lancet* 366: 1640–1649.

7.13.3 Bariatric surgery

Gail Pinnock and Mary O'Kane

Key points

■ Bariatric surgery is an effective long term treatment of obesity.

■ Following surgery, clients show significant improvement in comorbidities.

■ Clients are at possible risk of micronutrient deficiencies following surgery.

■ Long term dietetic support is essential.

The weight loss associated with diet, medication and lifestyle change is not always sufficient to improve health of obese clients, and it is now recognised that surgery should be considered, especially in the morbidly obese (NICE, 2006). Bariatric surgery (obesity, weight loss or metabolic surgery) is currently the most effective long term treatment of morbid obesity (Schweitzer *et al.*, 2006; Shah *et al.*, 2006). Maximum weight loss following bariatric surgery varies depending on the procedure (See Table 7.13.8) (Das *et al.*, 2003). The benefits of surgery are well established, with resolution of comorbidities occurring in a significant number of cases (Karlsson *et al.*, 2007; Smith *et al.*, 2008).

Recent data compiled from the National Bariatric Surgery Registry (NBSR, 2011) show average excess weight loss of 58% 1 year after surgery and remission of type 2 diabetes in 85.5% of cases 2 years post surgery. Therefore, it has been suggested, especially in the USA, that surgery be considered as a primary treatment for those with a body mass index (BMI) of >30 kg/m^2 and type 2 diabetes.

There was a nine-fold increase in bariatric surgical procedures between 2003 and 2008 (O'Neill, 2010), with over 7000 undertaken within the NHS in 2009–2010 (NHS, 2011). There are no reliable data on procedures carried out in the private sector.

Table 7.13.8 Bariatric surgery procedures

Procedure	Mechanism of action	Excess weight loss (%)	Impact on nutrition	Supplementation recommended
Intragastric balloon	Restrictive	10	Reduced intake	Multivitamin and mineral supplement
Adjustable gastric band (AGB)	Restrictive, no malabsorption	50	Reduced intake Effect on satiety	Multivitamin and mineral supplement
Sleeve gastrectomy	Restrictive, no malabsorption	50–60	Reduced intake Effect on satiety	Multivitamin and mineral supplement. May also need calcium supplement, vitamin D and vitamin B$_{12}$ injections
Roux-en-Y gastric bypass (RYGB)	Restrictive, possible malabsorption	65–68	Reduced intake Effect on satiety Calcium, iron and vitamin B$_{12}$ absorption affected May experience dumping syndrome	Protein (60–80 g/day) Multivitamin and mineral supplement, calcium supplement, vitamin D, vitamin B$_{12}$ injections
Long limb gastric bypass	Restrictive and malabsorptive, may experience steatorrhoea affecting absorption	65–68	Reduced intake Effect on satiety Macronutrient malabsorption possible Calcium, iron and vitamin B$_{12}$ absorption affected May experience dumping syndrome	Protein (60–80 g/day, may need 80–100 g/day if malabsorbing) Multivitamin and mineral supplement, calcium supplement, vitamin D and vitamin B$_{12}$ injections
Duodenal switch (biliopancreatic diversion with duodenal switch) (DS)	Restrictive and malabsorptive, steatorrhoea affecting absorption	>70	Reduced intake Effect on satiety Macronutrient malabsorption possible Calcium, iron and vitamin B$_{12}$, fat soluble vitamin absorption affected	High protein (80–100 g/day), low fat diet Multivitamin and mineral supplement, high doses of fat soluble vitamins, calcium supplement, vitamin B$_{12}$ injections

Clinical guidelines

In the UK NICE (2006)guidance (recommends surgery as a treatment option if all the following criteria are met:

- BMI >40 kg/m².
- BMI >35 kg/m² with significant disease, e.g. type 2 diabetes, high blood pressure, obstructive sleep apnoea, that could be improved with weight loss.
- Appropriate non-surgical measures have been tried but failed to achieve or maintain adequate, clinically beneficial weight loss for >6 months.
- Has been receiving or will receive intensive management in a specialist obesity service.
- Generally fit for anaesthesia and surgery.
- Commits to need for long term follow-up.

Surgery can be considered as a first line treatment option for those with a BMI of >50 kg/m². However individual NHS trusts may impose their own criteria in addition to those of NICE (2006).

Each treatment centre is required to have a multidisciplinary team (MDT) that can effectively select and manage these complex patients (NICE, 2006). A comprehensive assessment in which the benefits of surgery can be balanced against the risks is essential to enable the patient to make an informed choice in consultation with the MDT. For some patients, the risks may be too great and surgery declined.

Surgical procedures

Bariatric surgery works by gastric restriction, malabsorption or a combination of these; most surgery is performed laparoscopically to shorten the recovery time. The choice of surgical procedure depends on several factors, including the MDT decision, the patient's comorbidities and patient preference. Details of the surgical procedures are shown in Table 7.13.8 and Figure 7.13.2, Figure 7.13.3, Figure 7.13.4, Figure 7.13.5 and Figure 7.13.6).

Roux-en-Y gastric bypass (RYGB) is the most frequently performed procedure, followed by sleeve and adjustable gastric band (AGB) (Burton & Brown, 2011). Duodenal switch is rarely used because of a greater risk of malnutrition and then only for patients with considerable weight to lose; it may be done as a two stage procedure. The intragastric balloon is placed endoscopically into the stomach and then inflated with saline. It is a short term measure, viable for 6 months, and therefore outside NICE guidance.

Novel, less invasive techniques are being developed, although they are not yet in common use in the UK.

Gut hormones

The gastric bypass, sleeve gastrectomy, long limb bypass and duodenal switch affect some gut hormones, including ghrelin, glucagon like peptide 1 and peptide YY, involved in glucose regulation and appetite control, although the mechanism has not yet been elucidated (Rosen & Pomp, 2009). This results in improvements in

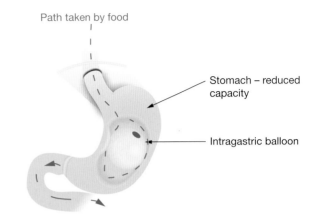

Figure 7.13.2 Intragastric balloon (source: The National Bariatric Surgery Registry: First Registry Report 2010. Reproduced with permission of Dentrite Clinical Systems Ltd)

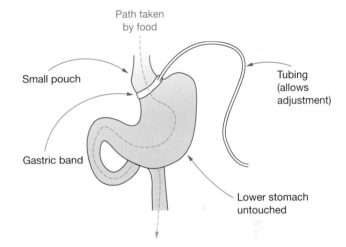

Figure 7.13.3 Adjustable gastric band (source: The National Bariatric Surgery Registry: First Registry Report 2010. Reproduced with permission of Dentrite Clinical Systems Ltd)

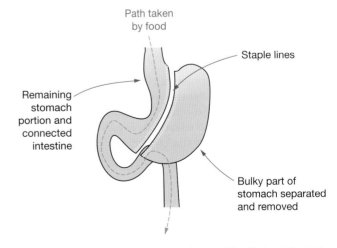

Figure 7.13.4 Sleeve gastrectomy (source: The National Bariatric Surgery Registry: First Registry Report 2010. Reproduced with permission of Dentrite Clinical Systems Ltd)

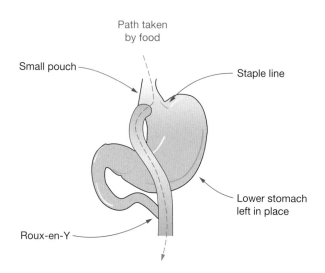

Path taken
by food

Small pouch

Staple line

Lower stomach
left in place

Roux-en-Y

Figure 7.13.5 Roux-en-Y gastric bypass (source: The National Bariatric Surgery Registry: First Registry Report 2010. Reproduced with permission of Dentrite Clinical Systems Ltd)

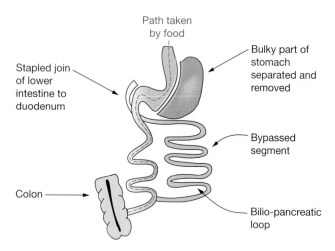

Path taken
by food

Bulky part of
stomach
separated and
removed

Stapled join
of lower
intestine to
duodenum

Bypassed
segment

Colon

Bilio-pancreatic
loop

Figure 7.13.6 Duodenal switch (source: The National Bariatric Surgery Registry: First Registry Report 2010. Reproduced with permission of Dentrite Clinical Systems Ltd)

diabetes control and reduced appetite; however, appetite eventually returns. The exact mechanism has not yet been fully elucidated.

Excess weight loss following surgery

Weight loss following surgery is expressed as excess weight loss (the amount of weight above a BMI of 25 kg/m²). The fastest rate of loss is in the first year, whilst maximum loss is usually achieved in 18 months to 2 years. Unless permanent lifestyle and dietary changes are made, weight regain may occur.

Surgical complications

Mortality rates vary depending on the procedure, but are lower when this is carried out by experienced surgeons in specialist high volume centres, where it is a relatively safe intervention. Complications include anastomotic leaks, bleeding, infection, strictures and obstructions or

incisional hernias (Mechanick *et al.*, 2008). In some situations the dietitian will be required to provide nutritional support. Careful consideration will have been given to the risks and benefits of surgery before the decision to proceed.

Long term complications

The benefits of surgery of improvements in glycaemic control, hypertension, sleep apnoea and hyperlipidaemia are well established (Karlsson *et al.*, 2007; Smith *et al.*, 2008). However, long term problems have been reported, such as nutritional deficiencies (Pournaras & le Roux, 2009; Slater *et al.*, 2004) (Table 7.13.9), metabolic bone disease, renal stones, anastomotic ulcers, strictures and obstructions (Mechanick *et al.*, 2008).

Role of the dietitian

The dietitian is an essential and respected member of the MDT (NICE, 2006), who is involved in the presurgical assessment and preparation, through to post surgical and long term nutritional support and follow-up.

Presurgical assessment

The presurgical dietetic assessment covers the following:

* Weight and dieting history.
* Dietary assessment, including eating behaviours and recognised eating disorders.
* Psychological issues – beliefs, behaviours, motivation, support mechanisms.
* Alcohol and smoking.
* Assessment of the patient's understanding of the impact of surgery on diet and lifestyle.
* Physical activity.
* Current medical history, including comorbidities.
* Past medical history, including past surgery.
* Medication.

Preparation

Once the patient is accepted for surgery, the dietitian continues to work with them, developing coping strategies to enable them to manage the changes needed post surgery. Patients are also encouraged to follow a liver shrinkage diet for 7–14 days before surgery (Fris, 2004). This may be liquid or food based and low in energy and carbohydrate, which reduces the size of the liver, making surgery easier.

Post surgery

After surgery, the dietitian is usually the first point of contact for patients with problems or queries. Typical issues include regurgitation, vomiting, food intolerances, vitamin and mineral supplementation and changes in bowel habit. If persistent vomiting occurs, thiamine deficiency may develop extremely quickly and urgent supplementation, followed by surgical review, is essential.

Table 7.13.9 Incidence of micronutrient deficiencies in bariatric surgery

Vitamin mineral deficiency	Presurgery	Adjustable gastric band	Sleeve gastrectomy	Gastric bypass	Biliopancreatic diversion ± duodenal switch
Thiamine	Uncommon	Uncommon unless protracted vomiting occurs	Uncommon unless protracted vomiting occurs	Uncommon unless protracted vomiting occurs	Uncommon unless protracted vomiting occurs
B₁₂	10–13%	Uncommon	Uncommon	12–33%	Uncommon
Folate	Uncommon	Uncommon	Uncommon	Uncommon	Uncommon
Iron	9–16% of adult women	Uncommon	May occur	20–49%	May occur
Vitamin A	Uncommon	Rare	Rare	Rare but may occur	50% at 1 year 70% at 4 years
Vitamin D and calcium	60–70% (vitamin D)	May occur	May occur	Common Increased risk of metabolic bone disease with low vitamin D, hypocalcaemia and secondary hyperparathyroidism	Very common Increased risk of metabolic bone disease with low vitamin D, hypocalcaemia and secondary hyperparathyroidism
Zinc	Uncommon	Uncommon	Uncommon	May occur	Common
Selenium	Uncommon	Uncommon	Uncommon	May occur	Common
Protein	Uncommon	May occur	May occur	May occur	May occur

A consensus statement for supplementation, gathered from a recent audit of good practice, will shortly be released by BOMSS (see BOMSS website for details).

Short term management

The patient progresses from liquids to puréed foods and then onto normal textured foods. The dietitian must ensure that patients meet their fluid and protein requirements. Diet information is available from the British Obesity and Metabolic Surgery Society (BOMSS) (www.bomss.org.uk).

It is crucial that patients establish new eating behaviours, such as eating slowly, stopping as soon as they feel full and chewing food well. They must also avoid eating and drinking at the same time; initially, this is because the small stomach makes it difficult and subsequently because fluid pushes food through quickly, enabling them to eat more, which slows the rate of weight loss. Patients often struggle with textures such as bread, roast or grilled meat and fibrous vegetables. To compensate, patients may resort to a sloppy, poor quality diet. Unfortunately, foods such as chocolate and crisps tend to be well tolerated.

Long term management

The patient must be encouraged to have a balanced, low fat diet. Reduced stomach capacity can result in grazing throughout the day and a regular meal pattern is necessary to avoid this. To minimise the risk of nutritional deficiencies, patients are advised to take a multivitamin and mineral supplement long term (Aills *et al.*, 2008); problems may occur with non-compliance. Regular blood tests should be carried out and supplementation adjusted as needed. Protein malnutrition may occur after any of the procedures because of food intolerances (especially meat) and alternative sources of protein should be suggested. Following a restrictive and malabsorptive procedure, patients should be encouraged to consume 60–100 g of protein/day. Patients who experience dumping syndrome and related symptoms of hypoglycaemia will need additional support.

Patients need continued dietetic support throughout the weight loss phase to encourage permanent dietary and lifestyle changes. This is equally important in helping with long term weight maintenance.

Women of childbearing age are discouraged from becoming pregnant within the first 12–18 months of surgery. Thereafter, they should be reminded of the importance of nutrition preconception. They may need to change their vitamin supplement to one that does not contain vitamin A; however, those who have had a duodenal switch may need to continue to take high doses of fat soluble vitamins throughout pregnancy.

Internet resources

British Obesity and Metabolic Surgery Society   www.bomss.org.uk
British Obesity Surgery Patient Association (BOSPA)   www.bospa.org
Dietitians in Obesity Management UK (DOMUK)   www.domuk.org

References

Aills L, Blankenship J, Buffington C, Furtado M, Parrott J. (2008) ASMBS Allied Health nutritional guidelines for the surgical weight loss patient. *Surgery for Obesity and Related Diseases* 4: S73–S108.

Burton PR, Brown WA. (2011) The mechanism of weight loss with laparoscopic adjustable gastric banding: induction of satiety not

SECTION 7

restriction. *International Journal of Obesity* 35(Suppl 3): S26–30.

Das SK, Roberts SB, Kehayias JJ, *et al*. (2003) Body composition assessment in extreme obesity and after massive weight loss induced by gastric bypass surgery. *American Journal of Physiology, Endocrinology and Metabolism* 284: E1080–1088.

Fris RJ. (2004) Preoperative low energy diet diminishes liver size. *Obesity Surgery* 14: 1165–1170.

Karlsson J, Taft C, Rydén A, Sjöström L, Sullivan M. (2007) Ten-year trends in health related quality of life after surgical and conventional treatment for severe obesity: the SOS intervention study. *International Journal of Obesity* 31: 1248–1261.

Mechanick JI, Kushner RF, Sugerman HJ, *et al*. (2008) AACE, TOS and ASMBS; medical guidelines for clinical practice for the perioperative nutritional metabolic and non-surgical support of the bariatric patient. *Surgery for Obesity and Related Disease* 4: S109–S184.

National Bariatric Surgery Registry. (2011) *First Registry Report to 2010*. Oxfordshire: Dendrite Clinical Systems.

National Institute for Health and Care Excellence (NICE) (2006) *Obesity: Guidance of the Prevention, Identification, Assessment and Management of Overweight and Obesity in Adults and Children*. London: NICE. www.nice.org.uk/Guidance/CG43). Accessed 2 May 2012.

NHS The Health and Social Care Information Centre. (2011) Statistics on obesity, physical activity and diet: England 2011. Available at www.ic.nhs.uk. Accessed 3 May 2012.

O'Neill P (Office of Health Economics). (2010) *Shedding the Pounds: Obesity Management, NICE Guidance and Bariatric Surgery in England*. Available at www.ohe.org. Accessed 31 August 2013.

Pournaras DJ, le Roux CW. (2009) After bariatric surgery, what vitamins should be measured and what supplements should be given? *Clinical Endocrinology* 71(3): 322–325.

Rosen DJ, Pomp A. (2009). Gastrointestinal hormones and their relationship to bariatric surgery. *Bariatric Times* 04: 17 (April 2009). Available at http://bariatrictimes.com/2009/04/17/. Accessed 3 May 2012.

Schweitzer M, Lidor A, Magnuson T. (2006) Bariatric surgery, health and treatment strategies in obesity. *Advances Psychosomatic Medicine* 27: 53–60.

Shah M, Simha V, Garg A. (2006). Long term impact of bariatric surgery on body weight, co-morbidities and nutritional status. *Journal of Clinical Endocrinology and Metabolism* 91(11): 4223–4231.

Slater GH, Ren CJ, Siegel N, *et al*. (2004). Serum fat-soluble vitamin deficiency and abnormal calcium metabolism after malabsorptive bariatric surgery. *Journal of Gastrointestinal Surgery* 8(1): 48–55.

Smith B, Hinojosa MW, Reavis KM, *et al*. (2008). Remission of diabetes after laparoscopic gastric bypass. *American Surgeon* 74: 948–952.

7.13.4 Childhood obesity

Laura Stewart and Jenny Gillespie

Key points

- Obesity is the most common childhood nutritional disorder worldwide and therefore is an important area for dietitians.

- Managing childhood obesity is challenging due to the need to engage the child or young person, parents or carers and the whole family.

- The consequences of childhood obesity are seen in childhood, adolescence and later in adult life.

- Interventions should be family based, with at least one of the parents involved.

- Changes in diet, physical activity and sedentary behaviours (television watching, computer use and playing video games) should be targeted equally.

- It is important to ensure that normal growth occurs when dietary intake is restricted.

Obesity is the most common childhood nutritional disorder in the world (World Health Organization, 2003; Lobstein *et al*., 2004) and therefore is an important area for dietitians. Managing childhood obesity is challenging due to the need to engage not only with the child or young person but also with their parents and the entire family.

Dietitians may see overweight and obese children individually in a clinical setting or as a group, e.g. in the community (Stewart *et al*., 2005; Sacher *et al*., 2010; Rudolf *et al*., 2006; Edwards *et al*., 2006). This chapter explores the knowledge and skills a dietitian new to this area requires to deliver a childhood weight management programme in either situation (Sahota *et al*., 2010). Dietitians working in childhood obesity need to have an appreciation not only of the complex behavioural issues that need to be explored, but also of the causes and the consequences of childhood obesity.

The prevalence of childhood obesity in the UK dramatically increased over a short number of years during the early 1990s (Reilly & Dorosty, 1999; Chinn & Rona, 2001). Due to the complex manner in which data on child weight are collected, it is difficult to give prevalence figures across the UK in age bands. The National Obesity Observatory (www.noo.org.uk) gives up to date information on prevalence figures for the four UK home countries as well as international comparisons.

Aetiology

Since excess weight gain occurs in a state of positive energy balance, the aetiology of obesity is multifactorial, involving an interaction of the modern obesogenic environment and family lifestyle choices. Increased intakes of energy dense foods (particularly fast foods and snacks), more time spent watching television and playing computer games with a coincidental decrease in the amount of physical activity undertaken by children have all been advocated as the causes of the childhood obesity epidemic (Mulvihill & Quigley, 203; House of Commons Health Committee, 2004; Prentice & Jebb, 1995).

Non-lifestyle related causes

A child or adolescent who is obese but also short for stature should have been seen or be referred to a paediatric endocrinologist for further investigation to exclude possible underlying rare endocrine causes of their obesity, such as hypothyroidism, growth hormone deficiency, Cushing's syndrome and pseudohypoparathyroidism (SIGN, 2010; Han et al., 2010). Young children, particularly those under 2 years who have had a rapid weight gain, are severely obese and appear to be hyperphagic, may have a rare genetic cause to their obesity and referral to a paediatrician for further investigations would be advisable (Han et al., 2010). There are also a number of syndromes that are associated with obesity, such as Prader–Willi syndrome, Down's syndrome and Fragile X.

Definition

Body mass index (BMI) is generally recognised as the most appropriate measure for diagnosing childhood obesity and overweight (Lobstein et al., 2004; SIGN, 2010). It is calculated as for adults as weight (kg)/height (m)^2; however it is only meaningful when it is plotted correctly on age and sex specific centile charts (UK 1990 data). UK BMI centile charts with UK 1990 data are available from Harlow printing (www.healthforallchildren.co.uk) and all dietitians working with obese children should use these charts for diagnosis and monitoring of management (SIGN, 2010; NICE, 2006; Cole et al., 1995; Reilly, 2010; Reilly et al., 2010) (see Chapter 3.8.2). There is a debate about the most appropriate centile cut-off points for defining childhood overweight and obesity. However, in the UK, both the National Institute for Health and Care Excellence (2006) and Scottish Intercollegiate Guidance Network (2010) recommended the use of the 98th centile on the BMI charts to define obesity and the 91st centile to define overweight for clinical use. For epidemiological studies the 95th centile and 85th centiles should be used to define obesity and overweight, respectively (see Chapter 3.8.2).

Consequences

The consequences of childhood obesity have been reported in childhood, adolescence and later in adult life.

Clustering of cardiovascular risk factors, such as high blood pressure, dyslipidaemia, abnormalities in left ventricular mass and/or function, abnormalities in endothelial function, and hyperinsulinaemia and/or insulin resistance, have been reported in children and adolescents. There is evidence that these cardiovascular risk factors are seen in adults who were obese in childhood or adolescence (Han et al., 2010; Reilly, 2005; Reilly et al., 2003). Type 2 diabetes, a disease previously only seen in older adults, is now being reported in adolescents (Han et al., 2010; Drake et al., 2002; Sinha et al., 2002). In girls, psychological problems in relation to low self esteem and behavioural problems, as well as longer term social and economic consequences of achieving a lower income have been reported (Drake et al., 2002; Sinha et al., 2002).

There is good evidence to suggest that obesity in childhood and adolescence does persist, often referred to as tracking into adulthood. The risk of tracking into adulthood can be compounded by parental obesity, the level of obesity and obesity in adolescence (Reilly, 2005; Reilly et al., 2003; Whitaker et al., 2010). Therefore, it is important to treat childhood obesity as early as possible and involving the parents/carers is considered to be important.

Assessment

At the first session with the child, the dietitian needs to obtain baseline measurements of weight and height and to plot these on centile charts. Body mass index should be calculated and then plotted at the correct age on the appropriate centile chart for sex. Although taking the waist measurement can be difficult in obese children, it is a useful tool in monitoring progress in the clinic; however, there are no agreed cut-off points for defining those at health risk (Reilly et al., 2010).

A diet history is useful to elicit information on the family diet and eating pattern; however, it is very important that this does not become a barrier to effective communication. Often the typical day model or a lifestyle diary is utilised as they are seen as more client centred and child friendly information collection methods. The typical day and lifestyle diary are also more effective for ascertaining information on the levels of physical activity that the child normally undertakes, as well as screen time. However dietary information is extracted, the number of takeaway meals the child and family have, the amount and types of snacks the child eats and the amount of pocket money that the child has to spend must be considered. Other details such as age of onset of obesity, eating patterns and family dynamics are most helpful.

Management

Management should encompass the following points:

- It should only be commenced when the parents are ready and willing to make lifestyle changes.

- It should be family based, with at least one of the parents involved.
- Lifestyle changes in diet, physical activity and sedentary behaviours, e.g. screen time – television watching, computer use and playing video games, should be targeted equally.
- Weight maintenance is an acceptable goal of treatment; with height increasing and the BMI decreasing over time (SIGN, 2010; NICE, 2006).

Qualitative studies have identified barriers in the initial access to and subsequent continuation of child weight management programmes, particularly those linked to stigma and difficulty in recognition of the child's overweight status by parents and even in some cases by healthcare professionals (Reid, 2009; Parry *et al.*, 2008; Towns & D'Auria, 2009). It is important for dietitians to be aware of this challenge and of the need to undertake appropriate training of gate keepers in both recognising overweight in children and discussing unhealthy weight in a non-judgemental manner with parents or carers (Stewart, 2008; Chadwick *et al.*, 2008).

Rapport

Childhood weight management clinics have previously reported a high drop out rate (Stewart *et al.*, 2004; Denzer *et al.*, 2004) and dietitians therefore need to carefully consider their manner and approach with the child and family. Successful treatment of obesity demands a sustained commitment and effort from the whole family, and the dietitian must endeavour to maintain a positive attitude and help motivate the child and family towards weight control. The role of the dietitian, whether seeing children and their families individually, in community groups or as part of a multidisciplinary team, is to educate the child and family on the necessary lifestyle changes and to help facilitate behavioural change. It is important that this is done in a positive, enthusiastic, non-judgemental and sensitive manner. Indeed, the development of rapport between the dietitian, child and family has emerged as an important element for families in considering an intervention to be successful (Sahota *et al.*, 2010; Stewart *et al.*, 2008). The whole family should be encouraged to attend sessions and to make necessary lifestyle changes. The dietitian needs to work with the parents/carers to ensure that they are on board with ownership and responsibility in supporting the child and family lifestyle changes. Parents and carers should be encouraged to be positive role models to the child and the family on making the necessary lifestyle changes and to give concrete, timely praise to the child when the child makes positive behaviour changes. It should also be emphasised that the healthy lifestyle messages need to be conveyed to both parents, other family members, teachers and other carers.

Some dietitians may work with individual children and their families or hold group sessions. Where group sessions are used, it is not uncommon to hold some separate sessions for the children and parents. Indeed, most parents appreciate the opportunity to discuss problems they have encountered with other parents, and with the dietitian without the child present. Those dietitians working with individual children and their families should also consider seeing the parents separately from the child as this can lead to important information being revealed that parents would not wish to discuss in front of the child (Stewart *et al.*, 2005).

Consideration needs to be given to the most appropriate model of seeing and interacting with different age groups. Although not based on evidence, there are suggestions that for preschool and lower primary school age children the intervention should be targeted directly at the parent or carer; for upper primary aged children jointly at the child and parent or carer; and for teenagers directly at the adolescent with the parent in a supporting role.

Behavioural modification

The NICE (2006) and SIGN (2010) guidelines suggested that the use of behavioural change tools in the management of childhood obesity are essential (SIGN, 2010; NICE, 2006). Most of these techniques are employed within lifestyle change programmes to assist the client in raising their awareness of lifestyle, focusing on the aspects of their lifestyles which require change, and developing strategies to implement and monitor those changes.

In a review of the use of behavioural change tools in childhood obesity Sahota *et al.* (2010) concluded that using a package of tools was more effective than any one particular tool. Table 7.13.10 summarises the tools a dietitian would be expected to deploy, along with supporting parents to role model and give concrete praise. Tools for problem solving, goal setting, modelling and self monitoring should all be used to help increase self efficacy and positive reinforcement for change (Newman *et al.*, 204; Elder *et al.*, 1999). Behavioural change is a process and the dietitian's role is to facilitate change by helping the child and parent or carer make small steps using SMART (specific, measurable, achievable, realistic, timed) goals (Rollnick *et al.*, 1999).

Diet

The main drive of dietary change is to reduce the total energy intake in the child's diet. Calorie counting is not normally used with children and the dietitian needs to ensure that they can convey the necessary information about dietary energy reduction effectively to the child and family. In a review of the dietary interventions, Collins *et al.* (2006) showed that no one type of dietary manipulation was more effective than another in childhood obesity. Children and their families should be encouraged to reduce the total amount of energy consumed by decreasing foods high in sugar and fat and replacing them with foods lower in energy, such as fruit and vegetables. It is also important to ensure that portion sizes of all foods are appropriate for age; the most commonly used models are the UK eatwell plate and traffic light scheme (Collins *et al.*, 2006).

Table 7.13.10 Brief description of behavioural change techniques (source: Stewart *et al.*, 2008, table 2, p. 466. Reproduced with permission of Wiley-Blackwell Publishing)

Goal setting	Goals for necessary changes in diet, physical activity levels and screen time are agreed between child, parent and dietitian. Goals should be SMART – specific/small, measurable, achievable, recorded and timed
Contracting	The signing of a 'contract' between the child, parent and dietitian establishes a commitment to achieving the goals in the allotted time period
Rewards for reaching goals	The parent agrees to give a reward to the child for achieving the agreed lifestyle change goals. This is a positive reinforcement for the setting and attainment of goals. The reward should be small, inexpensive and non-food or screen time. The parent should also be encouraged to use praise
Self monitoring	Recording targeted lifestyles, i.e. diet, physical activity and screen time. This enhances motivation by increasing self awareness of lifestyle behaviours and allows the child and parent to monitor progress towards set goals
Environmental/ stimulus control	Encouraging changes in the environment to help to: • Reduce the cues that encourage the behaviours requiring change, such as the parent not buying certain foods or the child not walking past a certain shop on the way home from school • Promote new healthier behaviours or routines
Problem solving	Helping the child and family to identify possible 'high risk' situations that may make it difficult to stick to their goals, e.g. holidays, parties and wet weather, as well as identifying barriers to change and developing possible solutions to these barriers. This could be done as a paper exercise or as simulation and role play
Preventing relapse	Near the end of the programme it is important to discuss and offer strategies to help avoid relapse into old behaviours. These include planning ahead for difficult situations and continuing with or returning to goal setting and self monitoring

It is important to ensure that normal growth occurs when dietary intake is restricted. Plotting weight and height on UK growth charts as well as BMI is useful to ensure appropriate growth monitoring, as well as regular nutritional assessment and comparison with appropriate age and sex nutrient requirements. Adequate, but not excessive, quantities of protein, vitamins and minerals for age need to be consumed. Very occasionally a child who dislikes certain foods and does not consume a nutritionally adequate diet may need a supplement of vitamins or minerals (particularly iron and calcium). Written information, including a list of unrestricted foods and foods to be controlled, should be given to the parents and child. Many parents find food labelling confusing and appreciate advice and help with understanding what to look for in and how to read labels on packets.

The problem of foods eaten outside of the home and beyond the parents' influence, and where necessary solutions, should be explored. Suggesting that money previously spent on sweets, chocolate, etc. be used for other items of the child's choice, e.g. games, books and clothing, is sometimes useful, particularly for indulgent grandparents.

Physical activity

Children should be encouraged to increase their overall activity levels to 60 minutes of moderate to vigorous activity each day (SIGN, 2010). Many overweight and obese children dislike team sports and physical education at school and it is therefore important to help the child and family find local activities that they may enjoy and are not embarrassed to take part in. Research has shown that increasing lifestyle activities, such as walking and taking the stairs rather than lift, can be particularly effective in controlling weight on a long term basis (Epstein *et al.*, 1985). Working together with local community groups and leisure partners can be helpful in supporting children and their families to increase their levels of activity and make it enjoyable.

Screen time

Current recommendations are that the amount of time children spend watching television, playing video games and using computers should be no more than 2 hours/day or an average of 14 hours over a week (SIGN, 2010; Epstein *et al.*, 2000; Gortmaker *et al.*, 1996). Some children and parents do find this change particularly difficult and the dietitian needs to help with setting SMART goals to reduce screen time over time.

Outcomes

Weight maintenance in combination with increasing height growth is an acceptable goal of treatment, as this will lead to BMI decreasing over time. For older adolescents, particular those in the very severe BMI range, weight loss may be required and a weight loss of 0.5–1.0 kg/month could be advised (SIGN, 2010). There is emerging evidence to suggest a range of a decrease in BMI standard deviation (SD) scores of between –0.25 (Ford *et al.*, 2010) and –0.5 (Reinehr & Andler, 2004) may lead to an improvement in insulin resistance, dyslipidaemia and cardiovascular risk factors.

Radical therapies

In general, slimming foods, drinks as a replacement for a meal and extreme restrictive diets that exclude food groups are not considered appropriate for this age group.

Both the NICE (2006) and SIGN (2010) guidelines recommended that antiobesity drug therapy could be considered for prescription to obese adolescents who are attending a specialist weight management clinic. In addition, SIGN (2006) recommended that antiobesity drugs should only be prescribed for adolescents with severe obesity (BMI >99.6th percentile) and with comorbidities. Currently, orlistat is the only antiobesity drug available for use in the UK. It is recommended that adolescent patients are regularly reviewed throughout the period of use, with careful monitoring for side effects (NICE, 2006).

Although bariatric surgery in children and adolescents is uncommon in the UK, both guidelines suggest that it could be considered for weight loss in post pubertal adolescents with very severe obesity and comorbidities; importantly, surgery should only be undertaken in a centre of excellence in adult bariatric surgery (SIGN, 2010; NICE, 2006). Since long term side effects of bariatric surgery in adolescents are unknown, it is highly desirable that follow-up should be for life.

Prevention

The increasing prevalence of childhood obesity demonstrates the clear need for a range of management options. It has been recognised that prevention strategies that target all children, including those who fall into the healthy weight range, must also be considered. There are strong arguments towards prevention as a useful approach, particularly on a cost basis, as it is considered to be cheaper to prevent rather that treat obesity (Barlow & Expert Committee, 2007). There is evidence to suggest that children involved in prevention interventions can change their behaviour, although the effectiveness of such interventions is still poorly understood (Summerbell et al., 2009). Dietitians, particularly those working in the area of public health nutrition, have a key role to play in prevention strategies, including the planning, development, delivery and evaluation of interventions that take place in a range of settings and at all ages, from birth through to adolescence. Prevention programmes that take place in schools and also target parents would appear to be an effective route (Gortmaker et al., 1999).

Government policies, such as England's Healthy Weight, Healthy Lives (Department of Health, 2008) or Scotland's Preventing Overweight and Obesity – A Route Map Towards Healthy Weight (The Scottish Government, 2010) drive most health promotion activity related to childhood obesity prevention. Initiatives tend to be educational or health promoting in nature and encourage healthy weight through promotion of healthier food choices and/or increased physical activity. Several countries now have examples of such programmes, including national guidance on the nutritional content of school meals, school walking buses and family based community physical activity programmes.

Social marketing is an emerging approach to obesity prevention. Government, business, health, education and others come together in a society wide movement with the aim to empower whole communities, families and individuals to make positive behavioural changes linked to a healthy lifestyle. French et al. (2010) describe social marketing as the systematic application of marketing, alongside other concepts and techniques to achieve specific behavioural goals for a social good. Current examples of UK social marketing campaigns relevant to childhood obesity include Change4Life in England & Wales, Take Life On One Step At a Time in Scotland and Get A Life-Get Active in Northern Ireland (see Chapter 4.2).

Internet resources

National Institute for Health and Care Excellence (NICE) www.nice.org.uk
  Obesity – guidance on the prevention, identification, assessment and management of overweight and obesity in adults and children (CG43, 2006)
National Obesity Observatory www.noo.org.uk
SIGN www.sign.ac.uk
  Management of obesity (SIGN 115, 2010)

Social networking campaigns

Change4Life (England & Wales) www.nhs.uk/change4life
Take Life On One Step At a Time (Scotland) www.takelifeon.co.uk
Get A Life-Get Active (Northern Ireland) www.getalifegetactive.com

References

Barlow SE, and the Expert Committee. (2007) Expert Committee recommendations regarding the prevention, assessment and treatment of child and adolescent overweight and obesity: Summary report. *Pediatrics* 120: S164–S192.

Chadwick P, Sacher PM, Swain C. (2008) Talking to families about overweight children. *British Journal of School Nursing* 3(6): 271–276.

Chinn S, Rona RJ. (2001) Prevalence and trends in overweight and obesity in three cross sectional studies of British children, 1974–94. *BMJ* 322: 24–26.

Cole TJ, Freeman JV, Preece MA. (1995) Body mass index reference curves for the UK, 1990. *Archives of Disease in Childhood* 73: 25–29.

Collins CE, Warren J, McCoy P, et al. (2006) Measuring effectiveness of dietetic interventions in child obesity: A systematic review of randomized trials. *Archives of Pediatric and Adolescent Medicine* 160(9): 906–922.

Denzer C, Reithofer E, Wabitsch M, et al. (2004) The outcome of childhood obesity management depends highly upon patient compliance. *European Journal of Pediatrics* 163: 99–104.

Department of Health. (2008) *Healthy Weight, Healthy Lives. Across Government Strategy for England*. HM Government.

Drake AJ, Smith A, Betts PR, et al. (2002) Type 2 diabetes in obese white children. *Archives of Disease in Childhood* 86(3): 207–208.

Edwards C, Nicholls D, Croker H, Van Zyl S, Viner R, Wardle J. (2006) Family-based behavioural treatment of obesity: acceptability and effectiveness in the UK. *European Journal of Clinical Nutrition* 60: 587–592.

Elder JP, Ayala GX, Harris S. (1999) Theories and intervention approaches to health-behavior change in primary care. *American Journal of Preventive Medicine* 17(4): 275–284.

Epstein LH, Wing RR, Valoski AM. (1985) Childhood obesity. *Pediatric Clinics of North America* 32(2): 363–379.

Epstein LH, Paluch RA, Gordy CC, et al. (2000) Decreasing sedentary behaviors in treating pediatric obesity. *Archives of Pediatric and Adolescent Medicine* 154: 220–226.

Ford AL, Hunt LP, Cooper A, *et al*. (2010) What reduction in BMI SDS is required in obese adolescents to improve body composition and cardiometabolic health? *Archives of Disease in Childhood* 95: 256–261.

French F, Blair-Stevens C, McVey D, *et al*. (2010) *Social marketing and public health theory and practice*. Oxford: Oxford University Press, 2010.

Gortmaker SL, Must A, Sobol AM, *et al*. (1996) Television viewing as a cause of increasing obesity among children in the United States, 1986–1990. *Archives of Pediatric and Adolescent Medicine* 150(4): 356–362.

Gortmaker SL, Peterson K, Wiecha J, *et al*. (1999) Reducing obesity via a school based interdisciplinary intervention among youth: Planet Health. *Archives of Pediatric and Adolescent Medicine* 151: 409–418.

Han JC, Lawlor DA, Kimm SYS. (2010) Childhood obesity. *Lancet* 375: 1737–1748.

House of Commons Health Committee. (2004) *Obesity Third Report of Session 2003–04*, Volume 1. London: The Stationery Office Limited.

Lobstein T, Baur L, Uauy R, for the IASO International Obesity Task Force. (2004) Obesity in children and young people: a crisis in public health. *Obesity Review* 5 (Suppl 1): 4–85.

Mulvihill C, Quigley R. (2003) *The Management of Obesity and Overweight: An Analysis of Reviews of Diet, Physical Activity and Behavioural Approaches. Evidence Briefing*. NHS Health Development Agency.

National Institute for Health and Care Excellence (NICE). (2006) *Obesity Guidance on the Prevention, Identification, Assessment and Management of Overweight and Obesity in Adults and Children*. NICE clinical guidelines 43. London: NICE.

Newman S, Steed L, Mulligan K. (2004) Self-management interventions for chronic illness. *Lancet* 364: 1523–1537.

Parry L, Netuveli G, Saxena S. (2008) A systematic review of parental perception of overweight status in children. *Journal of Ambulatory Care Management* 31(3): 253–268.

Prentice AM, Jebb SA. (1995) Obesity in Britain: gluttony or sloth? *BMJ* 311: 437–439.

Reid M. (2009) *Debrief of a study to identify and explore parental, young people's and health professionals' attitudes, awareness and knowledge of child healthy weight*. 2008/2009 RE036. Edinburgh: NHS Health Scotland.

Reilly JJ. (2005) Descriptive epidemiology and health consequences of childhood obesity. *Best Practice and Research Clinical Endocrinology and Metabolism* 19(3): 327–341.

Reilly JJ. (2010) Assessment of obesity in children and adolescents: synthesis of recent systematic reviews and clinical guidelines. *Journal of Human Nutrition and Dietetics* 23: 205–211.

Reilly JJ, Dorosty AR. (1999) Epidemic of obesity in UK children. *Lancet* 354: 1874–1875.

Reilly JJ, Methven E, McDowell ZC, *et al*. (2003) Health consequences of obesity. *Archives of Disease in Childhood* 88: 748–752.

Reilly JJ, Kelly J, Wilson DC. (2010) Accuracy of simple clinical and epidemiological definitions of childhood obesity: Systematic review and evidence appraisal. *Obesity Review* 11(9): 645–655.

Reinehr T, Andler W. (2004) Changes in the atherogenic risk factor profile according to degree of weight loss. *Archives of Disease in Childhood* 89: 419–422.

Rollnick S, Mason P, Butler C. (1999) *Health Behavior Change. A Guide for Practitioners*. Edinburgh: Churchill Livingstone.

Rudolf MCJ, Christie D, McElhone S, *et al*. (2006) WATCH IT: a community based programme for obese children and adolescents. *Archives of Disease in Childhood* 91: 736–739.

Sacher PM, Kalotourou M, Chadwick P, *et al*. (2010) Randomised controlled trial of the MEND program: a family community intervention for childhood obesity. *Obesity* 18(S2): S1–S7.

Sahota P, Wordley J, Woodward J. (2010) *Health Behaviour Change Models and Approaches for Families and Young People to Support HEAT 3: Child Healthy Weight Programmes*. Edinburgh: NHS Health Scotland.

Scottish Intercollegiate Guideline Network (SIGN). (2010) *Management of Obesity: A National Clinical Guideline*. 115. Edinburgh: SIGN.

Sinha R, Fisch G, Teague B, *et al*. (2002) Prevalence of impaired glucose tolerance among children and adolescents with marked obesity. *New England Journal of Medicine* 346(11): 802–810.

Stewart L. (2008) Recognizing childhood obesity: The role of the school nurse. *British Journal of the School Nursing* 3(7): 323–326.

Stewart L, Deane M, Wilson DC. (2004) Failure of routine management of obese children: an audit of dietetic intervention. *Archives of Disease in Childhood* 89(Suppl 1): A13–16.

Stewart L, Houghton J, Hughes AR, *et al*. (2005) Dietetic management of pediatric overweight: Development of a practical and evidence-based behavioral approach. *Journal of the American Dietetic Association* 105: 1810–1815.

Stewart L, Chapple J, Hughes AR, *et al*. (2008) The use of behavioural change techniques in the treatment of paediatric obesity: qualitative evaluation of parental perspectives on treatment. *Journal of Human Nutrition and Dietetics* 21(5): 464–473.

Summerbell CD, Waters E, Edmunds L, *et al*. (2009) Interventions for preventing obesity in children. *Cochrane Database of Systematic Reviews* 3: CD001871.

The Scottish Government. (2010) *Preventing Overweight and Obesity in Scotland. A Route Map Towards a Healthy Weight*. Edinburgh: The Scottish Government.

Towns N, D'Auria J. (2009) Parental perceptions of their child's overweight: an integrative review of the literature. *Journal of Pediatric Nursing* 24(2): 115–130.

Whitaker KL, Jarvis MJ, Beeken RJ, *et al*. (2010) Comparing maternal and paternal intergenerational transmission of obesity risk in a large population-based sample. *American Journal of Clinical Nutrition* 91: 1560–1567.

World Health Organization. (2003) *Diet, Nutrition and the Prevention of Chronic Diseases*. WHO TRS 916. Geneva: WHO/FAO.

Cardiovascular disease

7.14.1 General aspects
Catherine Hames

Key points

- Cardiovascular disease (CVD) encompasses coronary heart disease (CHD), stroke and peripheral vascular disease.

- Cardiovascular risk assessment should be used to assess overall risk and to stratify for treatment need.

- Those with existing CVD should be treated preferentially to those who are healthy but have a raised CVD risk.

- A cardioprotective diet is the first line of dietary support for those with, or at risk of, CVD. Risk factors may require additional treatment if dietary support and other lifestyle changes are insufficient to reduce them to acceptable levels.

- The cardioprotective diet includes moderate intakes of fish, including oily fish, reducing saturated fat and replacing it with monounsaturated or polyunsaturated fats, plenty of fruit and vegetables, legumes and nuts, a regular meal pattern, moderate alcohol intake if desired, limited intake of salt and processed foods, and modest intake of lean meat and meat products.

The aetiology of cardiovascular disease (CVD) is multifactorial and strongly associated with risk factors such as hypertension, dyslipidaemia, smoking, lack of physical activity and diabetes mellitus. Cardiovascular disease and its risk factors have similarities in their aetiology and dietary management.

Prevalence and costs

Cardiovascular disease is the most common cause of death in the UK and the major cause of premature death [British Heart Foundation (BHF), 2010]. In 2009, 180 000 people in the UK died of CVD, which was one in three of all deaths. It accounted for more than 45 000 premature deaths, with more than one in four deaths in men and one in five deaths in women before the age of 75 years. Death rates from CVD are highest in Scotland and the North of England, and lowest in the South of England. It is thought that this may be partly attributable to the socioeconomic differences in the populations within these areas. South Asian people living in the UK, who includes immigrants from India, Pakistan, Bangladesh and Sri Lanka have a 50% greater risk of premature death from CHD and stroke (BHF, 2010). Data from England and Wales show African-Caribbean people have a lower than average risk of CHD, but a three-fold higher risk of stroke.

Death rates in the UK continue to remain relatively high in comparison with some other Western European Countries, despite death rates from CVD falling in the UK at one of the fastest rates in Europe (BHF, 2010).

The National Service Framework launched in 2000 had aimed to reduce CVD by 40% by 2010; this target was met 5 years early (Department of Health, 2000). This is in line with the overall reduction in risk since the 1970s after the introduction of statin drugs (reducing blood cholesterol levels), improved screening, prevention and post cardiac event treatments, and an increase in smoking cessation (BHF, 2010).

Coronary heart disease (CHD) is the major cause of mortality in patients presenting with stroke, diabetes and renal disease. Patients receiving renal replacement therapy are 16–19 times more likely to develop CHD than matched controls, with the rate for people with diabetic nephropathy being even greater (Wheeler, 1997; Holt & Goldsmith, 2010). Men with diabetes have over three times the risk of cardiovascular mortality than men without diabetes (Khaw *et al.*, 2001). Those with diabetes and renal disease should be regarded as being at increased risk of CVD, regardless of other risk factors, e.g. dyslipidaemia, hypertension or obesity.

As well as the human cost, CVD has an economic cost for the UK. In 2006 CVD cost the UK health system £14.4

billion. Of this cost, 73% was attributed to hospital care and 20% to medication.

Aetiology

Cardiovascular diseases are interrelated; their causation is due to atherosclerosis, developing slowly over many years and/or thrombosis (blood clots) developing suddenly and causing an acute episode, such as a myocardial infarct or stroke. The incidence of CVD is related to modifiable risk factors, such as dyslipidaemia and hypertension, which in turn can be linked to lifestyle factors, e.g. high saturated fat intake, smoking and lack of physical activity. Therefore, improving lifestyle factors can lead to a reduction in cardiovascular events (De Backer et al., 2003; Wood et al., 2008). The aetiology of atherosclerosis and thrombosis are discussed further in Chapter 7.14.2.

Absolute risk assessment

The risk of CVD is calculated by assessing the combined risk of a number of modifiable and non-modifiable risk factors. In the past, someone's CVD risk was dependent on assessment and treatment of one or two individual risk factors (such as cholesterol level or blood pressure), largely as a result of the NHS being organised into specialist areas. It is now appreciated that a more holistic view of risk factor assessment is essential. As a result, cardiovascular risk assessment is becoming more sophisticated, using lifestyle and risk data to give an overall measure of the risk of a cardiovascular event or death over a set time period. There are a number of risk equations that input information on sex, age, systolic blood pressure, total cholesterol [or total cholesterol to high density lipoprotein (HDL) ratio], diabetes and smoking behaviour to predict 10-year risk of fatal cardiovascular events.

Until 2010 the risk estimation score in the UK was calculated using the American Framingham equations (NICE, 2010). The Framingham equation was developed based on a historic American cohort dating from the 1940s (Anderson et al., 1991). As a result, Framingham equations can overestimate risk by up to 50% in contemporary North European populations. This overestimation is more often seen in people living in more affluent areas. In contrast, it may underestimate risk in higher risk populations, such as those that are more socially deprived. A further disadvantage is that the equation does not take into account family history, with respect to premature death from CHD, ethnicity or social deprivation (NICE, 2010).

In addition to the Framingham risk equations, the National Institute for Health and Care Excellence (NICE, 2010) and Scottish Intercollegiate Guidelines Network (SIGN, 2007) have recommended the use of the following risk assessment tools scores, which have the advantage of including other variables such as social deprivation and family history:

- ASSIGN (developed using a Scottish cohort) (Woodward et al., 2007).

- QRISK (using data from UK general practice databases) (Hippisley-Cox et al., 2007).

In addition, the SCORE risk equation and relative risk chart (Conroy et al., 2003) are recommended by the European Society of Cardiology (Perk et al. 2012). These are thought to give a more accurate estimate of risk due to the large European dataset used. Lastly, the Joint British Societies 2 (JBS2, 2005) guidelines recommend an adjusted Framingham equation. This guidance is currently under review; the new guidelines (JBS3) will use lifetime risk based on adjustments of the current published risk equation and be available at www.jbs3risk.com.

Due to the numbers of risk scores available and variability in the scores used in different regions of the UK, there is a need to establish which score is most applicable to the UK. Current guidance suggests that those with a 10-year risk of CVD of >20% should be considered as high risk (NICE, 2010; JBS2, 2005; ESC, 2007). However, it should be remembered that these equations can only provide an estimate of risk and clinical judgement should always be applied to improve the accuracy of the assessment.

It should be noted that the equations calculate absolute risk (also known as total or global risk), which is defined as the percentage chance of an individual developing a CVD event over a given period of time, e.g. a 10-year risk of 20%. NB: Risk equations should not be used for people with pre-existing CVD.

Prevention

It has been estimated that more than half of deaths and disability from heart disease and stroke could be prevented by modifications to lifestyle, such as diet, activity and smoking (Iqbal et al., 2008). All current guidelines agree that when treating people with elevated risk of CVD the lifestyle factor priorities are (in no particular order of priority):

- Smoking cessation.
- Increased physical activity.
- Management of blood pressure.
- Management of lipids.
- Management of diabetes.
- Healthy food choices.
- Weight management and limiting central obesity.

It is important that dietitians treat the whole person, rather than simply providing dietary themselves or referring the individual for advice on other lifestyle factors. Further details can be found for coronary heart disease in Chapter 7.14.2, for dyslipidaemia in Chapter 7.14.3), for hypertension in Chapter7.14.4), for stroke in Chapter 7.14.5), for diabetes in Chapter 7.12), for management of obesity and overweight in adults in Chapter 7.13.2) and for renal disease in Chapter 7.5.

Despite a reduction in mortality rates from CVD in the UK, the European wide Eurospire III survey showed that the majority of patients with CHD surveyed were still not achieving the recommended lifestyle, blood pressure and lipid targets, despite an increase in medications and screening (Kotseva *et al.*, 2009). In England, health checks have been introduced to identify individuals at risk of developing heart disease, stroke, kidney disease or diabetes, with the focus on preventing these diseases (NHS, 2009). Each screening includes the measurement of cholesterol (total cholesterol and HDL cholesterol), blood pressure and body mass index (BMI), and these are then used to calculate CVD risk. Health checks (www .healthcheck.nhs.uk) are offered to those aged 40–74 years who have not been diagnosed with hypertension, atrial fibrillation, transient ischaemic attacks, hypercholesterolaemia, heart failure or peripheral arterial disease. Eligible people are invited to attend every 5 years. It is estimated that this scheme could prevent 1600 strokes and heart attacks, prevent 4000 people from developing diabetes and detect 20 000 people with diabetes or chronic kidney disease each year (Department of Health, 2008).

Further to this, NICE (2010) has produced guidance on the prevention of CVD that outlines recommendations to improve risk factors at a population level. These guidelines target food and drink providers, marketing, media, the family support sector, national non-governmental organisations, e.g. charities, and farming associations.

The cardioprotective diet

The cardioprotective diet is the first line of dietary advice in protection against the main CVDs. It can be used in primary or secondary prevention and in conjunction with specific dietary advice given on individually relevant risk factors (diabetes, renal disease, dyslipidaemia, hypertension, overweight). This diet should be encouraged in those with an increased risk of CVD, not only in those with established risk factors such as dyslipidaemia or obesity.

Effectivenesst

The cardioprotective diet stems from the Mediterranean diet. The value of eating a Mediterranean style diet came into focus in the late 1950s when men living in Crete, parts of Greece and southern Italy were shown to have the least likelihood of developing CHD (Willett *et al.*, 1995). The premature death rate from heart attack for Greek men was 90% lower than that of American men, with Greek men enjoying the longest life expectancy in the world. However, this is no longer true today, as the traditional Greek diet has become increasingly westernised. Therefore, the focus has been on the benefits of the traditional Mediterranean diet prior to the 1960s. Several elements of this diet have been proposed as being especially protective, and there is now some experimental evidence from randomised controlled trials to support its protective role in high risk populations. The cardioprotective diet is very similar to the proposed cancer protective diet and so may confer other health benefits over those seen in CVD (WCRF, 2007).

Influence on cardiovascular disease

The cardioprotective diet exerts its effects on CVD by altering a wide range of risk factors in a positive way. These may include effects on:

* Blood pressure, lipid oxidation and inflammation (reducing injury to coronary arteries).
* Lipid profile, homocysteine levels and insulin resistance (reducing fibrous plaque formation).
* Platelet aggregation, clotting factors and arrhythmias (reducing the occurrence of thrombosis leading to heart attack and stroke).

The effects of the diet on the cardiovascular system and its benefits alongside statins are summarised in Chapter 7.14.2. Chapter 7.14.3 discusses the effects of diet on blood lipids.

A selection of the guidelines that have been developed in CVD management over the last 5 years is:

* Lipid modification: Cardiovascular risk assessment and the modification of blood lipids for the primary and secondary prevention of cardiovascular disease. NICE CG 67 (2008, revised March 2010).
* Risk Estimation and the prevention of Cardiovascular Disease – A National Clinical Guideline. SIGN 97 (2007).
* Secondary prevention in primary and secondary care for patients following a myocardial infarction. ESC guideline (2007).
* Dietetic guidelines on food and nutrition in the secondary prevention of cardiovascular disease (Mead *et al.*, 2006).
* Diet and Lifestyle Recommendations – A Scientific Statement From the American Heart Association Nutrition Committee (American Heart Association Nutrition Committee , 2006).
* JBS2: Joint British Societies' guidelines on practice prevention of cardiovascular disease in clinical practice. Prepared by the British Cardiac Society, British Hypertension Society, Diabetes UK, HEART UK, Primary Care Cardiovascular Society and The Stroke Association (2005).

From these guidelines and additional information the main elements of the cardioprotective diet have been summarised as discussed below.

Fats

Saturated fat

It is recommended that saturated fatty acids should contribute <10% of total dietary energy. A recent systematic review by Hooper *et al.* (2012) concluded that replacing saturated fat with unsaturated fat might reduce the risk of vascular disease and CHD. However, they concluded that it was unclear if monounsaturated (MUFAs) or polyunsaturated fats (PUFAs) have any further benefit. The

Table 7.14.1 Main sources of saturated, unsaturated and *trans* saturated fats in the diet

Saturated fat	*Trans* saturated fats	Polyunsaturated fat	Monounsaturated fat
Butter, lard, ghee, dripping Fatty meats – beef, lamb, corned beef, sausages, beef burgers, streaky bacon Dairy products – full fat milk, cream, full fat yoghurt, cheese Pies, cakes, biscuits, chocolate and pastry products Coconut	Baked products Cakes, biscuits, pastries Convenience foods, e.g. takeaways, ready meals	Oils – sunflower, soya, linseed, sesame seed, fish Margarines Soyabeans	Olive oil, rapeseed oil, peanut oil (ground nut) Almonds, walnuts, peanuts, avocados

cardioprotective diet was shown to be more effective if followed for 2 years or more. Replacing saturated fat with carbohydrate (starchy) foods did not confer any clear health effects. In addition, they concluded that it was not clear if healthy people benefitted as much as those at risk of CHD or who had CHD.

Practical tips for reducing saturated fat and replacing them with unsaturated fats include:

- Remove fat from meats and avoid processed meats.
- Remove skin from poultry.
- Avoid deep fried snacks and dishes.
- Replace butter, ghee and lard with a vegetable oil such as olive or rapeseed oil; replace full fat dairy products with low fat alternatives or soya products.
- Replace high fat snacks such as crisps, chocolates and biscuits with fruit and nuts.
- Read food labels – aim for <1.5g of saturates/100g.

Trans *saturated fats*

It is recommended that *trans* saturated fats should contribute <2% of total dietary energy. *Trans* fatty acids are produced in the hydrogenation of vegetable oils that are used in the production of margarine and shortening. *Trans* fats can also be formed by subjecting PUFAs to high temperatures (220°C). It has now been demonstrated that *trans* fatty acids raise low density lipoprotein (LDL) cholesterol whilst lowering HDL (Ascherio & Willett, 1997). If possible, saturated and *trans* saturated fats should be replaced with unsaturated fatty acids (MUFAs and PUFAs. Table 7.14.1 lists some of the main sources of saturated, unsaturated and *trans* saturated fats in the diet.

Omega-3 fatty acids

n-3 Fatty acids are the long chain PUFAs, eicosapentaenoic acid (EPA) and docosahexaenoic acid (DHA). They do not have a cholesterol lowering effect; however, they are thought to be protective by improving endothelial function and have anti-inflammatory and antithrombotic effects. In primary prevention, the advice for the general population is to consume one portion of white fish, e.g. haddock and cod, and one portion of oily fish/week, where a portion equals 140g. In secondary prevention,

Table 7.14.2 Fish sources of n-3 fatty acids. High sources per average serving are above the dashed line

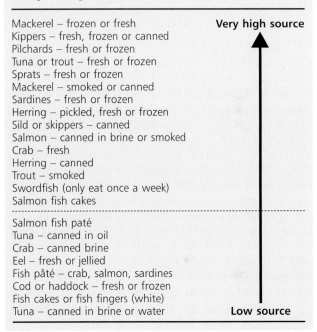

individuals should aim for –two to four portions (total 300g) of oily fish/week. If patients are unable to manage to consume oily fish, a fish body oil supplement may be recommended (NICE, 2007).

A systematic review, Hooper *et al.* (2006) concluded that it was not clear whether dietary or supplemental n-3 fats alter total deaths or cardiovascular events in people at risk or with CVD. Therefore, further research is required in this area. However, the evidence did not suggest that people at high risk should stop including n-3 in their diets; this is an area of growing research to ascertain the exact benefits. Table 7.14.2 shows the highest and lowest fish sources of n-3.

Vegetarian sources of the essential precursor fatty acid alpha-linolenic acid (ALA) include nuts, seeds, dark green vegetables, rapeseed oil, wholegrain cereals and soya products; however, conversion from the ALA to the active EPA and DHA by humans appears poor, especially in men (2–10%).

SECTION 7

Table 7.14.3 Suggested population intakes of oily fish (SACN/COT, 2004)

Population group	Suggested lower limit	Suggested higher limit
Women of reproductive age and girls	One portion of oily fish/week	Two portions of oily fish/week
Pregnant and lactating women	One portion of oily fish/week (but avoid marlin, swordfish, shark and tuna)	Two portions of oily fish/week (but avoid marlin, swordfish, shark and tuna)
Women past reproductive age, boys and men	One portion of oily fish/week	Four portions of oily fish/week

Safety of oily fish and fish oils

Concern has been expressed over the relatively high levels of dioxins and polychlorinated biphenyls (PCBs) present in fish and fish oils (MAFF, 1999). The Scientific Advisory Committee on Nutrition (SACN)and the Committee on Toxicity (COT) issued a joint report in 2004 addressing these issues and suggesting healthy and maximal fish intakes for various population groups (SACN/COT, 2004). Their recommendations for the population are reproduced in Table 7.14.3. Dietitians should also note that levels of dioxins and PCBs are higher in fish liver oil supplements (cod or halibut liver oils) than in fish body oils (MAFF, 1999). Therefore, if fish oil supplementation is indicated, fish body oil rather than fish liver oil (which also contains less n-3 fat) should be recommended.

Salt

It is recommended that the adult population should decrease their salt intake to 6 g/day (2.4 g of sodium/day); this is the equivalent of one level teaspoon (SACN, 2003). The current intake in the UK is estimated to be 8.1 g/day (Sadler *et al.*, 2012); public health initiatives are currently aiming to reduce salt consumption to 3 g/day by 2025 (NICE, 2010). However, a recent systematic review (Taylor *et al.*, 2011) concluded that the benefit of reducing salt intake on clinically significant CVD events was not entirely proven in normotensive and hypertensive people, and that further randomised controlled trials were needed, especially on possible harmful effects of salt restriction in heart failure. They estimated that the benefits of salt restriction were *'consistent with the predicted small effects on clinical events attributable to the small blood pressure reduction achieved'*.

Examples of some common sources of salt in the diet include:

- Ready meals.
- Tinned and packet soups.
- Breads and breakfast cereals.
- Dehydrated meals.
- Processed meats such as bacon and sausages.

- Cooking and pasta sauces.
- Cheese.
- Stock cubes.
- Savoury snacks.

Practical advice to lower salt intake includes:

- Discourage adding salt when cooking or at the table.
- Discourage consumption of food with high salt content.
- Encourage the use of alternatives such as herbs and spices.
- Look for food containing <0.3 g of salt/100 g.

Stanols and sterols

Stanols and sterols are known to lower LDL cholesterol by interfering with biliary and dietary cholesterol absorption from the gut. Sterols and stanols are naturally occurring in the diet; however, a dose of 1.5–2.4 g of stanol/sterol esters/day (20–30 g of margarine or one yoghurt drink) is seen as an optimal intake. They have been shown to lower cholesterol by at least 10% (Thompson & Grundy, 2005). They have been granted a health claims title by the European Food Safety Authority (2010) with no known long term adverse effects (see Chapter 4.5 and Chapter 5.2). To obtain beneficial effects, supplemented foods should be used for at least 2–3 weeks. Currently, stanols and sterols are not recommended by NICE (2010) for primary prevention due to a lack of studies with clinical end points.

Fruit and vegetables

The recommendation is a minimum of 400 g (five portions)/day, with one portion being equal to 80 g of fresh fruit or vegetables (around 3 tablespoons), 30 g of dried fruit or 150 mL of unsweetened fruit or vegetable juice (this should only be taken once per day) (www.nhs.uk/LiveWell/5ADAY). All fruit and vegetables should be encouraged whether tinned, fresh, frozen or juiced. Fruit and vegetables contribute to soluble fibre and antioxidants, giving them a protective effect. They are also rich in folic acid. Fruit and vegetables have a relatively low energy and therefore aid weight management.

Nuts

Nuts are recommended as part of a cardioprotective diet, with almonds, walnuts and pecans seen to be most beneficial.

Soluble fibre

The high viscosity of soluble fibre reduces cholesterol levels by interfering with cholesterol absorption in the gut. Soluble fibre can be found in oats and other wholegrains, beans, pulses, fruit and vegetables, with a recommended intake of 15–20 g/day (Brown *et al.*, 1999). Wholegrain foods, which can include wholemeal breads, wholegrain breakfast cereals, wholegrain pasta and brown rice, should be encouraged to prevent constipation and help with weight control. Epidemiological evidence has suggested that high intakes of wholegrains have a protective effect on CHD risk, reducing the risk of both CVD

Table 7.14.4 Comparison of traditional high fat, low fat and cardioprotective diets

	High fat diet	Low fat/calorie diet	Cardioprotective diet
Meal plan	Refined cereal (such as cornflakes) with whole milk Coffee with full cream milk Two slices of white bread with butter, processed ham and mayonnaise, full fat yoghurt and a packet of crisps Two chocolate coated biscuits Fried fish and chips with a sprinkling of salt Fruit pie and ice cream	Refined cereal (cornflakes) Skimmed milk Black coffee Two slices of white bread, low fat spread, processed ham and low fat mayonnaise. Packet of 'lite' crisps and a low fat yoghurt Three salted rice cakes Breaded cod and oven chips, peas, with a sprinkle of salt Low fat ice cream	Porridge oats made with skimmed milk/soya milk and a chopped banana Glass of fruit juice Coffee Two slices of wholemeal bread with olive based spread, turkey and salad, apple and a low fat yoghurt Handful of almonds Salmon fillet with new potatoes (flavoured with mint), carrots and peas Stewed fruit and low fat yoghurt
Energy (kcals)	2310	1434	1470
Total fat (g)	135.0	46.1	45.5
Saturated fat (g)	48.0	10.9	7.4

and diabetes by up to 30%. However, this evidence has come mostly from observational studies. Large intervention trials with sufficient power would be required to determine a causal link (Peacock *et al.*, 2010).

Carbohydrates

The current recommendation is that carbohydrate should form 50–55% of total dietary energy (Department of Health, 1991); refined carbohydrates should be avoided. There is limited evidence that low glycaemia index (GI) food reduces CVD (Mead *et al.*, 2006). However, low GI diets may be beneficial in those with diabetes or metabolic syndrome and those with high triglycerides (see Chapter 7.12).

Soya protein

The recommendation is that 15–25 g (one to three servings)/day should be taken in exchange for other protein sources such as meats and dairy. Examples of products include soya milk, yoghurts, desserts, spreads, tofu, etc. Soya protein has been shown to lower LDL cholesterol by interfering with liver LDL cholesterol synthesis, and slightly to raise HDL cholesterol (Jenkins *et al.*, 2006; Harland & Haffner, 2008).

Dietary cholesterol

The recommendation is that no more than 300 mg/day should be consumed. It is known that dietary cholesterol can increase blood cholesterol levels; however within the UK, it is thought that dietary cholesterol is unlikely to have any significant impact on blood cholesterol levels (Leeds & Gray, 2001). Shell fish, eggs and offal are rich in cholesterol but are not high in saturated fat and so can be used as healthy alternatives to fatty meats in the diet. However, limiting dietary cholesterol may be required for those patients with inherited high cholesterol (familial hypercholesterolaemia (see Chapter 7.14.3).

Folic acid

Elevated levels of homocysteine have been linked with CVD (Bazzano *et al.*, 2006) with high levels thought to be a predictor for CVD. Folic acid and B vitamins (especially B_{12} and B_6) intakes have been shown to lower homocysteine levels, but supplemented vitamins did not appear to affect cardiovascular events. It is recommended that dietary folate intake should exceed 400 µg/day to prevent elevated homocysteine levels. Promotion of food high in vitamins B_{12}, B_6, folate and riboflavin should be encouraged in a healthy diet.

There is no benefit from vitamin E or garlic supplementation in reducing CVD incidence.

Practical aspects

Practical dietary details are given in Table 7.14.4. The low fat diet will allow weight loss (similar to the cardioprotective diet) but will not provide the protective effects. The low fat diet contains no fruit and vegetables, is lacking in fibre, n-3 fatty acids and is higher in salt.

Cardioprotective dietary advice should always be set in the context of healthy eating guidance, such as the eatwell plate (see Chapter 4.2), to ensure the overall diet is balanced. Over focus on one nutrient (such as saturated fat reduction) can risk compromising the intake of others (such as iron and calcium) if dietary advice is not comprehensive. Other dietary therapeutic objectives, e.g. maintenance of careful glycaemic control in the management of diabetes, may also be relevant.

For frail or elderly people, who are at risk of being nutritionally compromised, especially if appetite and food intake are poor, oily fish, fruit and vegetables can be encouraged, but dietary fat content and composition only altered if this can be achieved with no loss of enjoyment or reduction in dietary energy density (see Chapter 3.3).

Specific considerations

Alcohol

The role of alcohol in the cardioprotective diet remains unclear because of the lack of intervention studies to establish its benefits, but there is clear evidence of the hazards of excessive intakes. Epidemiological evidence suggests that for those at medium or high cardiovascular risk, a modest amount of alcohol is protective (Rimm *et al.*, 1996; Burger *et al.*, 2004; NICE, 2007). The benefits for those at low risk, e.g. young women, are more doubtful. For those at increased cardiovascular risk, a regular intake of 1–2 units/day of any alcohol probably confers maximal protection without adverse effects on triglycerides or blood pressure.

Gout

Some people at high cardiovascular risk will also have gout and may need to avoid high intakes of purines (see Chapter 7.9.3). As oily fish is rich in purines, increasing consumption is contraindicated. In these circumstances, fish oil capsules, which do not contain purines, should be advocated.

Lifestyle

The cardioprotective diet should always be discussed in the context of a healthy lifestyle and reference should be made to activity and exercise levels, smoking cessation and continued use of prescribed medication. More information on these aspects of lifestyle can be obtained from local cardiac rehabilitation programmes or the British Heart Foundation and British Association of Prevention and Cardiac Rehabilitation (BAPCR).

Dietetic participation in cardiac rehabilitation helps to ensure consistency in the delivery of health messages. It also allows dietitians to reinforce the lifestyle messages given by the team and ensures the team remains well informed on dietary issues. The recommendations for physical activity are:

- *Primary prevention* – all patients should be encouraged to increase physical activity to 30 minutes/day at moderate intensity for most days of the week.
- *Secondary prevention* – regular exercise building up to 20–30 minutes/day to the point of slight breathlessness; it is important to encourage cardiac rehabilitation.

Weight and waist circumference

Patients should aim for a healthy weight (BMI 18.5–25 kg/m^2) and waist circumference (<102 cm in European men, <90 cm in Asian men, <88 cm in European women and <80 cm in Asian women) (see Appendix A7).

Acceptability

Patients are often apprehensive about the perceived restrictions of a cardioprotective diet and may be visibly relieved when the positive changes are described and encouraged. The approach to the patient should be determined by the stages of change model (see Chapter 1.3). Those who have never contemplated change will need a different approach from those who have already started to make changes, or have previously made changes but slipped back.

Whilst many people enjoy the cardioprotective diet there are also some who find particular elements of it very difficult. Many people struggle to increase their fruit, veg-

etables and oily fish intakes, whilst reducing and/or modifying their fat intake. Practical advice should be offered to promote dietary change, and giving examples of advocated foods will likely improve adherence, e.g. providing examples of oily fish recipes. Dietary advice should always be tailored to an individual's likes and dislikes.

The cardioprotective diet, like exercise and non-smoking, is protective as long as it is continued. To have eaten well or been fit last year is not helpful now. To help people maintain their healthier habits, regular review is advisable. This may involve dietetic review in a central location or the community, including delegation to other community staff (who must be trained, updated and provided with appropriate support materials).

Motivation can also be boosted by involving the whole family (Wood *et al.*, 2008). Where this occurs, the sense of isolation is reduced and the whole family group (who may also be at increased genetic or lifestyle risk of CHD) reap the benefits of risk reduction (Cousins *et al.*, 1992).

Monitoring and outcomes

Appropriate factors to monitor are shown in Table 7.14.5. It is important to remember that the benefits from dietary

Table 7.14.5 Possible factors to consider for monitoring and evaluation purposes in cardiovascular disease

Domain	Factors
Diet	Portions of oily fish/week
	Portions of fruit and vegetables/day
	Appropriate fat spread
	Appropriate milk
	Appropriate fats in cooking
	Units of alcohol taken/day or week
	Level of fat intake
	Level of salt intake
Emotional	Acceptability of diet
	Barriers to change
	Stages of change
Lifestyle	Smoking
	Exercise levels
	Lipid reduction medication
	Hypertension medication
Risk levels	Waist circumference
	Body mass index
	Weight change
	Total cholesterol
	Triglycerides
	HDL cholesterol
	LDL cholesterol
	Cholesterol to HDL ratio
	Blood pressure (systolic, diastolic)
	Factors relevant to diabetic or renal control
Outcomes	Myocardial infarction
	Angina frequency
	Stroke
	Coronary artery bypass graft
	Angioplasty
	Hospital admissions
	Death

HDL, high density lipoprotein; LDL, low density lipoprotein.

change depend on the extent to which other lifestyle changes have been achieved. These two aspects therefore need to be considered in conjunction in order to assess the effectiveness of risk reduction measures.

Updating the evidence

The UK Heart Health and Thoracic Dietitians Specialist Group regularly update their guidelines on the secondary prevention of CVD by including all relevant systematic reviews of the effect of diet on CVD and risk factors in people with CVD; the most recent is Mead *et al.* (2006).

Further reading

Guidelines

American Heart Association Nutrition Committee, Lichtenstein AH, Appel LJ, *et al.* (2006) Diet and Lifestyle Recommendations Revision 2006:. – A Scientific Statement from the American Heart Association Nutrition Committee. *Circulation* 114(1): 82–96. Errata 114(23): e629 and 114(1): e27.

European Society of Cardiology, Woods DA, Giannuzzi P. (2007) European guidelines on Cardiovascular Prevention in clinical practice. *European Journal of Cardiovascular Prevention and Rehabilitation* 14(Suppl 2): S1–113.

Joint British Societies (JBS). (2005) Joint British Societies' guidelines on practice prevention of cardiovascular disease in clinical HEART UK, Primary Care Cardiovascular Society, The Stroke Association. Prepared by: British Cardiac Society, British Hypertension Society, Diabetes UK, 2005.079988. *Heart* 91: 1–52.

National Institute for Health and Care Excellence (NICE). (2007) Secondary prevention in primary and secondary care for patients following a myocardial infarction. CG48. Available at www.nice.org.uk.

National Institute for Health and Care Excellence (NICE). (2008, revised March 2010). Lipid modification: Cardiovascular risk assessment and the modification of blood lipids for the primary and secondary prevention of cardiovascular disease. CG67. Available at www.nice.org.uk.

Mead A, Atkinson G, Albin D, *et al.* (2006) Dietetic guidelines on food and nutrition in the secondary prevention of cardiovascular disease – evidence from systematic reviews of randomized controlled trials (second update). *Journal of Human Nutrition and Dietetics* 19: 401–419.

Scottish Intercollegiate Guidelines Network (SIGN). (2007) Risk Estimation and the prevention of Cardiovascular Disease – A National Clinical Guideline. SIGN 97. Available at www.sign.ac.uk.

Historic studies of interest

Bucher HC, Hengstler P, Schindler C, Meier G. (2002) N-3 polyunsaturated fatty acids in coronary heart disease: a meta-analysis of randomized controlled trials. *American Journal of Medicine* 112: 298–304.

Burr ML, Fehily AM, Gilbert JF, *et al.* (1989) Effects of changes in fat, fish, and fibre intakes on death and myocardial reinfarction: diet and reinfarction trial (DART). *Lancet* 2: 757–761.

Burr ML, Ashfield-Watt PA, Dunstan FD, *et al.* (2003) Lack of benefit of dietary advice to men with angina: results of a controlled trial. *European Journal of Clinical Nutrition* 57(2): 193–200.

De Lorgeril M, Renaud S, Mamelle N, *et al.* (1994) Mediterranean alpha-linolenic acid-rich diet in secondary prevention of coronary heart disease. *Lancet* 343: 1454–1459.

GISSI-Prevenzione Investigators. (1999) Dietary supplementation with n-3 polyunsaturated fatty acids and vitamin E after myocardial infarction: results of the GISSI-Prevenzione trial. *Lancet* 354: 447–455.

Singh RB, Rastogi SS, Verma R, *et al.* (1992) Randomised controlled trial of cardioprotective diet in patients with recent acute myocardial infarction: results of one year follow up. *BMJ* 304: 1015–1019.

Department of Health, Committee on Medical Aspects of Food Policy. (1994) *Nutritional Aspects of Cardiovascular Disease*. Reports on Health and Social Subjects, 46. London: HMSO.

Internet resources

American Heart Association   www.heart.org
American Stroke Association   www.strokeassociation.org
British Cardiovascular Society   www.bcs.com
British Heart Foundation   www.bhf.org.uk
British Association for Cardiovascular Prevention and Rehabilitation   www.bacpr.com
European Heart Network   www.ehnheart.org
Foundation for Circulatory Health   www.ffch.org
Heart UK   www.heartuk.org.uk
The Stroke Association (UK)   www.stroke.org.uk
   UK Heart Health and Thoracic Dietitians members of the British Dietetic Association can access resources via   www.bda.uk.com

Risk scoring tools

QRisk (UK)   www.qrisk.org
Assign Score (Scotland)   http://assign-score.com

References

American Heart Association Nutrition Committee, Lichtenstein AH, Appel LJ, *et al.* (2006) Diet and Lifestyle Recommendations Revision 2006: – A Scientific Statement from the American Heart Association Nutrition Committee. *Circulation* 114 (1): 82–96. Errata 114(23): e629 and 114(1): e27.

Anderson KM, Odell PM, Wilson PWF, Kannel WB. (1991) Cardiovascular-disease risk profiles. *American Heart Journal* 121: 293–298.

Ascherio A, Willett WC. (1997) Health effects of *trans* fatty acids. *American Journal of Clinical Nutrition* 66(4): 1006S–1010S.

Bazzano LA, Reynolds K, Holder KN, He J. (2006) Effect of folic acid supplementation on risk of cardiovascular diseases: a meta-analysis of randomized controlled trials. *JAMA* 296(22): 2720–2726.

British Heart Foundation. (2010) Coronary heart disease statistics. Available at the British Heart Foundation Statistics Website www.heartstats.org. Accessed 20 February 2013.

Brown L, Rosner B, Willett W, Sacks F. (1999) Cholesterol lowering effects of dietary fibre: A meta-analysis. *Americal Journal of Clinical Nutrition* 69: 30–42.

Burger M, Bronstrup A, Pietrzik K. (2004) Derivation of tolerable upper alcohol intake levels in Germany: a systematic review of risks and benefits of moderate alcohol consumption. *Preventive Medicine* 39: 111–127.

Conroy RM, Pyörälä K, Fitzgerald AP, *et al.* (2003) Estimation of ten-year risk of fatal cardiovascular disease in Europe: the SCORE project. *European Heart Journal* 24: 987–1003.

Cousins JH, Rubovits DS, Duncan JK, Reeves RS, Ramirez AG, Foreyt JP. (1992) Family versus individually oriented intervention for weight loss in Mexican American women. *Public Health Reports* 107: 549–555.

De Backer G, Ambrosioni E, Borch-Johnsen K, *et al.*, for the Third Joint Task Force of the European and other Societies. (2003) European guidelines on cardiovascular disease prevention in clinical practice. *New European Journal of Cardiovascular Prevention and Rehabilitation* 10 (Suppl 1): S1–S78. Available at www.escardio.org/knowledge/guidelines/CVD_Prevention_in_Clinical_Practice.htm.

Department of Health. (1991) *Report on Health and Social Subjects 41 Dietary Reference Values for Food Energy and Nutrients for the United Kingdom.* Report of the Panel on Dietary Reference Values of the Committee on Medical Aspects of Food Policy. London: HMSO.

Department of Health, Committee on Medical Aspects of Food Policy. (1994) *Nutritional Aspects of Cardiovascular Disease.* Reports on Health and Social Subjects, 46. London: HMSO.

Department of Health. (2000) Coronary heart disease: national service framework for coronary heart disease - modern standards and service models. Available at http://www.gov.uk/government/publications/quality-standards-for-coronary-heart-disease-care. Accessed 2 December 2013.

Department of Health. (2008) Putting Prevention First – Vascular Checks: Risk Assessment and Management. London: Department of Health.

European Food Safety Authority. (2010) Health claims. Available at http://ec.europa.eu/food/food/labellingnutrition/claims/community_register/authorised_health_claims_en.htm. Accessed 20 February 2013.

European Society of Cardiology, Woods DA, Giannuzzi P. (2007) European guidelines on Cardiovascular Prevention in clinical practice. *European Journal of Cardiovascular Prevention and Rehabilitation* 14 (Suppl 2): S1–113.

Harland JI, Haffner TA. (2008) Systematic review, meta-analysis and regression of randomised controlled trials reporting an association between an intake of circa 25 g soya protein per day and blood cholesterol. *Atherosclerosis* 200: 13–27.

Hippisley-Cox J, Coupland C, Vinogradova Y, Robson J, May M, Brindle P. (2007) Derivation and validation of QRISK, a new cardiovascular disease risk score for the United Kingdom: prospective open cohort study. *BMJ* 335: 136.

Holt S, Goldsmith D. (2010) *Clinical Practice Guidelines Cardiovascular Disease in CKD,* 5th edn. 2008–2010 Final Draft (26.5.10) incorporating feedback on the module from RA Members. UK Renal Association.

Hooper L, Thompson RL, Harrison RA, *et al.* (2006) Risks and benefits of omega 3 fats for mortality, cardiovascular disease, and cancer: systematic review. *BMJ* 332: 752.

Hooper L, Summerbell CD, Thompson R, *et al.* (2012) Reduced or modified dietary fat for preventing cardiovascular disease. The Cochrane Collaboration. J Wiley & Sons Ltd. Available at http://onlinelibrary.wiley.com Accessed 20 February 2013.

Iqbal R, Anand S, Ounpuu S, *et al.*; INTERHEART Study Investigators. (2008) Dietary patterns and the risk of acute myocardial infarction in 52 countries: results of the INTERHEART study. *Circulation* 118: 1929–1937.

Jenkins DJ, Kendall CW, Faulkner DA, *et al.* (2006) Assessment of the longer-term effects of a dietary portfolio of cholesterol-lowering foods in hypercholesterolemia. *American Journal of Clinical Nutrition* 83(3): 582–591.

Joint British Societies. (2005) JBS 2: Joint British Societies' guidelines on prevention of cardiovascular disease in clinical practice. *Heart* 91(Suppl 5): v1–v52.

Khaw K-T, Wareham N, Luben R, *et al.* (2001) Glycated haemoglobin, diabetes, and mortality in men in Norfolk cohort of European Prospective Investigation of Cancer and Nutrition (EPIC-Norfolk). *BMJ* 322: 15–18.

Kotseva K, Wood D, De Backer G, *et al.* (2009) EUROASPIRE III: a survey on the lifestyle, risk factors and use of cardioprotective drug therapies in coronary patients from 22 European countries. *European Journal of Cardiovascular Prevention and Rehabilitation* 16: 121–137.

Leeds AR, Gray J. (2001) *Dietary Cholesterol as a Cardiac Risk Factor: Myth or Reality?* Huntingdon: Smith-Gordon & Co Ltd.

MAFF. (1999) Dioxins and PCBs in UK and imported marine fish. Food Surveillance Information Sheet no 184. Available at: http://archive.food.gov.uk.

Mead A, Atkinson G, Albin D, *et al.* (2006). Dietetic guidelines on food and nutrition in the secondary prevention of cardiovascular disease – evidence from systematic reviews of randomized controlled trials (second update). *Journal of Human Nutrition and Dietetics* 19: 401–419.

National Institute for Health and Care Excellence (NICE). (2007) Secondary prevention in primary and secondary care for patients following a myocardial infarction. CG48. Available at www.nice.org.uk.

National Institute for Health and Care Excellence (NICE). (2010). Lipid modification: Cardiovascular risk assessment and the modification of blood lipids for the primary and secondary prevention of cardiovascular disease. CG67. Available at www.nice.org.uk.

NHS. (2009) NHS health checks. Available at www.healthcheck.nhs.uk.

Peacock E, Stanley J, Calder PC, *et al.* (2010) UK Food Standards Agency Workshop Report: carbohydrate and cardiovascular risk. *British Journal of Nutrition* 103: 1688–1694.

Perk J, De Backer G, Gohlke H, *et al.* (2012) European guidelines on cardiovascular disease prevention in clinical practice (version 2012). *European Heart Journal* 33(13): 1635–1701.

Rimm EB, Klatsky A, Grobbee D, Stampfer MJ. (1996) Review of moderate alcohol consumption and reduced risk of coronary heart disease: is the effect due to beer, wine or spirits? *BMJ* 312: 731–736.

Sadler K, Nicholson S, Steer T, *et al.* (2012) National Diet and Nutrition Survey – Assessment of dietary sodium in adults (aged 19 to 64 years) in England, 2011. Available at www.dh.gov.uk. Accessed 20 February 2013.

Scientific Advisory Committee on Nutrition (SACN). (2003) *Salt and Health.* London: HMSO

Scientific Advisory Committee on Nutrition (SACN) and the Committee on Toxicity (COT). (2004) Advice on fish consumption: benefits and risks. Available at http://cot.food.gov.uk/cotreports/cotjointreps/sacnfishconsumption. Accessed 2 September 2013.

Taylor RS, Ashton KE, Moxham T, Hooper L, Ebrahim S. (2011) Reduced dietary salt for the prevention of cardiovascular disease. *Cochrane Database of Systematic Reviews* 7:CD009217.

Thompson GR, Grundy SM. (2005) History and development of plant sterol and stanol esters for cholesterol-lowering purposes. *American Journal of Cardiology* 96 (Suppl): 3D–9D.

Wheeler DC. (1997) Cardiovascular risk factors in patients with chronic renal failure. *Journal of Renal Nutrition* 7: 182–186.

Willett WC, Sacks F, Trichopoulou A, *et al.* (1995) Mediterranean diet pyramid: a cultural model for healthy eating. *American Journal of Clinical Nutrition* 61: 1402S–1406S.

Wood DA, Kotseva K, Connolly S, *et al.* (2008) Nurse-coordinated multidisciplinary, family-based cardiovascular disease prevention programme (EUROACTION) for patients with coronary heart disease and asymptomatic individuals at high risk of cardiovascular disease: a paired, cluster-randomised controlled trial. *Lancet* 371: 1999–2012.

Woodward M, Brindle P, Tunstall-Pedoe H; SIGN group on risk estimation. (2007) Adding social deprivation and family history to cardiovascular risk assessment: the ASSIGN score from the Scottish Heart Health Extended Cohort (SHHEC). *Heart* 93(2): 172–176.

World Cancer Research Fund (WCRF). (2007) *Food, Nutrition and the Prevention of Cancer: a Global Perspective.* Washington: American Institute for Cancer Research.

7.14.2 Coronary heart disease

Julie Hinchliffe and Jane Green

Key points

■ Dietitians have a multifaceted role in primary and secondary coronary heart disease prevention.

■ They should be able to advise on public health policy and strategy with key stakeholders, including multiagency work to enhance the local food economy.

■ Food projects using principles of community development, and developing and evaluating local programmes to facilitate healthier eating must be supported.

■ Training other healthcare professionals to deliver consistent key cardioprotective messages is an essential role for dietitians.

■ Dietitians are involved in cardiac rehabilitation programmes for groups and individuals at risk of, or with existing, heart disease.

■ Surgical patients and people with heart failure or cardiac cachexia may require nutritional support.

Coronary heart disease (CHD) is the most common manifestation of cardiovascular disease (CVD). A broad overview of CVD and the cardioprotective diet is given in Chapter 7.14.1. This chapter focuses on the aetiology and management of CHD, and the role of the dietitian in its prevention. Chronic heart failure (CHF) is also discussed, as CHD is the most common cause of this clinical syndrome.

Coronary heart disease can present clinically in a number of different ways, which may include:

• Stable angina – chest pain that is controlled, except on exertion.
• Acute coronary syndrome – myocardial infarction (heart attack) and unstable angina.
• Sudden death, with or without a history of angina, or infarction due to inherited cardiomyopathies or arrhythmias.
• Heart failure as a consequence of CHD of which cachexia is a sign of the end stage of the disease.

Acute coronary syndrome (ACS) is the umbrella term that encompasses:

• *ST elevated myocardial infarction (STEMI)* – the lumen of the artery is blocked by the volume of thrombus, resulting in acute ST elevation (an abnormality of the electrocardiogram), i.e. a traditional heart attack where oxygen supply is cut off, causing death to an area of the heart muscle (Table 7.14.6).
• *Non-ST elevated myocardial infarction (NSTEMI)* – the lumen of the artery is narrowed by the volume of the thrombus or blocks the artery only temporarily, resulting in a shortage of blood supply to the heart muscle that is less severe than in STEMI or intermittent. There is often some damage to the heart muscle, as evidenced by a rise in the cardiac specific serum biomarkers such as troponin.
• *Unstable angina* – new onset chest pain or discomfort, or abrupt deterioration in previously stable angina,

with chest pain or discomfort occurring frequently and with little or no exertion, and often with prolonged episodes. This often presents in a comparable way to acute myocardial infarction (MI), but without biomarker evidence of myocardial necrosis (NICE, 2010a).

Table 7.14.6 Investigative procedures for coronary heart disease

Investigation	Description
Electrocardiogram (ECG)	Monitors the progressive electrical stimulation of the heart muscle. An ECG provides a graph of the heartbeat. Portions of the graph are labelled PQRST (e.g. ST elevation describes a rise in a particular portion of this graph which indicates ischaemia)
Exercise stress testing	ECG recorded whilst the patient is exercising and having symptoms. It can assess whether pain on exertion is due to heart disease
24-hour ECG recording or Holter monitoring	Monitoring during everyday activity including that which produces symptoms
Echocardiography	Ultrasound is used to provide a picture of the heart. It can also be used to measure the speed of blood flow
Electrophysiology studies	Used to study arrhythmia
Angiogram	Radio-opaque fluid is infused into the heart and major vessels. It reveals the outline of the lumen of the coronary arteries and hence the extent of atheromatous disease. It is used in the process of decision making about coronary artery bypass grafting and angioplasty

Table 7.14.7 Risk factors for coronary heart disease (CHD)

Type	Risk factor	Comments
Unmodifiable	Age	Risk increases with age
	Gender	Due to the protective effects of oestrogen, premenopausal women have a lower prevalence of CHD than men of the same age, although this difference can disappear in some circumstances, e.g. coexistence of diabetes
	Genotype	Family history of CHD is strongly associated with increased risk, probably due in part to genetic differences in lipid metabolism or somatotype, e.g. propensity to central or peripheral fat distribution. CHD risk is also enhanced in certain racial groups
	Ethnicity	The risk of CHD is higher in the South Asian population. This includes those of Indian, Pakistani, Bangladeshi and Sri Lankan origin
	Socioeconomic status	The risk of CHD is higher in the lowest socioeconomic groups and lowest in the highest socioeconomic group. In all socioeconomic groups, cardiovascular disease has improved substantially over the past two decades, but the gap between poorer and more affluent sections of society has widened as the rate of improvement has been fastest in the more affluent groups
Modifiable	Smoking	Increases oxidative stress
	Diet	See text
	Physical activity	Physical activity positively influences adiposity, insulin resistance, lipid profile (increases HDL cholesterol) and reduces hypertension
	Hypertension	Increases risk of stroke, induces endothelial dysfunction and contributes to the instability of atherosclerotic plaque
	Lipid profile	Uptake of cholesterol by macrophages causes endothelial damage and is the core of the atherosclerotic plaque; higher LDL – carry cholesterol to be deposited in artery walls; lower HDL – carry excess cholesterol to liver for excretion; higher triglyceride level is inversely related to HDL and is also an independent risk factor. Lipids also influence thrombogenesis
	Abdominal obesity	Effect on CHD is due to consequences in terms of blood pressure, diabetes and cholesterol levels. A high waist measurement is a prerequisite risk factor for the diagnosis of metabolic syndrome (IDF 2005)
	Insulin resistance	Risk marker for cardiovascular disease. Insulin resistance and abdominal obesity are important causative factors in metabolic syndrome
	Psychosocial stress	Depression and social isolation or lack of quality support (SIGN, 2007a). The way that a person deals with stress can encourage less healthy behaviours, e.g. smoking, drinking too much alcohol and overeating

HDL, high density lipoprotein; LDL, low density lipoprotein.

Diagnosis will be based on a combination of presenting symptoms, e.g. chest discomfort, and investigations such as cardiac markers, e.g. troponins, and electrocardiograph changes, e.g. ST segment elevation. There will also be consideration of the patient's individual risk factors for CHD (Table 7.14.7).

Coronary heart disease is the most common cause of death in the UK, causing over 88 000 deaths a year (BHF, 2010a). About one in five men and one in eight women die from the disease. A reduction in mortality from CHD has been shown in most developed countries with the exception of some Eastern European countries. Russia and the Ukraine have the highest mortality from CHD in Europe for both men and women. However, UK death rates compare less favourably with some other Western European countries, with only Ireland and Germany having a higher death rate than the UK (BHF, 2010a). Deaths from CHD also vary across the UK (BHF, 2010a):

- Highest in Scotland and the North of England and lowest in the South of England.

- Highest in the lowest socioeconomic group and lowest in the highest socioeconomic group.
- Higher in the South Asian community (BHF, 2010b).

Dietary factors may contribute to these differences, e.g. variation of fruit and vegetable consumption, but primarily these regional, socioeconomic and ethnic differences reflect health inequalities (see Chapter 4.2, Chapter 3.4 and Chapter 3.5).

Whilst mortality rates are reducing, morbidity rates are not falling as more people survive cardiac events and are living with CHD. This may be a reflection of advances in treatment, such as medications and revascularisation, and reductions in major risk factors such as smoking (BHF, 2010a). The current prevalence of CHD in the UK is estimated to be 2.7 million, of which 1.6 million are men and over 1 million are women (BHF, 2010a).

Pathogenesis

The pathogenesis of CHD is a complex interaction of a number of processes. Both atherosclerosis and thrombosis are fundamental to the development of the disease and each is affected by diet. These two processes are described separately for ease of understanding, but in reality they are interlinked.

Atherosclerosis

The first step in the development of atherosclerosis is injury to arterial endothelium (the metabolically active lining of the artery). In areas of damage, macrophages ingest low density lipoprotein (LDL) and other athero-genic particles to form foam cells. When the macrophages die, the lipid remains in the arterial wall, accumulating over time to form a lipid core or pool (Figure 7.14.1). The formation of this fatty streak is the first stage in plaque development.

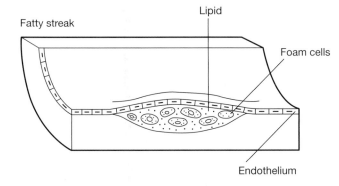

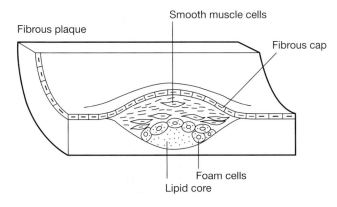

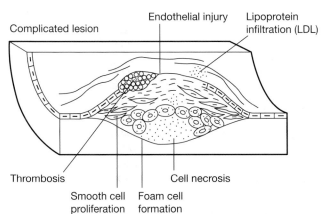

Figure 7.14.1 Stages of atherosclerosis (source: Thomas & Bishop 2007, figure 4.20.1, p. 605. Reproduced with permission of Wiley-Blackwell Publishing)

Subsequent proliferation of smooth muscle cells and development of collagen strands, minor thrombi and cal-cification in this area of lipid accumulation then result in the formation of atherosclerotic plaque. As the plaque grows, it protrudes into the lumen of the artery. The plaques are covered by a fibrous cap, which can rupture. If this happens, it triggers platelet aggregation and the formation of a blood clot.

The narrowing of the lumen of the coronary arteries as a result of plaque development can lead to an inadequate oxygen supply to the myocardium (heart muscle) at times of increased workload to the heart such as physical exer-tion. This is the cause of stable angina. Severe narrowing of the blood vessel leads to unstable angina or NSTEMI. Complete occlusion of the blood vessel by a thrombus (clot) will cut off the supply of oxygen to a section of the myocardium (heart muscle), resulting in a STEMI.

A description of lipoprotein metabolism and its influ-ence on atherogenesis is given in Chapter 7.14.3. More detailed discussion of this subject can be found in the Cardiovascular Disease Report by the British Nutrition Foundation (BNF, 2005).

Thrombosis

Damage to the endothelium at the micro level, or to the cap of a plaque at the macro level, can trigger platelet activation and coagulation. As well as being a cause of acute coronary events, thrombosis is an integral part of plaque development as thrombi can become incorpo-rated into the structure. The repair system is complex because the clot needs to be assembled at the site of damage and then removed when the repair is complete. Over 50 different chemicals are involved in the process, all of which are present in plasma all of the time. A shift in the balance of their activation determines whether the anticoagulants or procoagulants dominate. A brief summary of the coagulation process (Simmons, 1997) is:

- *Stage 1 – vasoconstriction.* In smaller vessels this is caused by release of thromboxane A_2 and serotonin from platelets. Thromboxane also activates other platelets.
- *Stage 2 – platelet plug formation.* Platelets become sticky when activated and form plugs that can cause minute ruptures in small blood vessels. They also release active compounds such as growth factors, which promote smooth muscle cell proliferation, a stage in the process of atherosclerosis.
- *Stage 3 – clot formation.* Platelet aggregation com-bines with the extrinsic and intrinsic pathways to produce a clot (Figure 7.14.2). Prothrombin activator catalyses the split of prothrombin to form thrombin. This in turn causes the polymerisation of fibrinogen to form fibrin threads. These form a mesh, which entrap platelets, plasma and blood cells to form the blood clot; this retracts, expressing the serum.
- *Stage 4 – fibrinolysis.* Plasminogen is activated to produce plasmin, a proteolytic enzyme that digests the fibrin threads. Raised levels of plasminogen activator

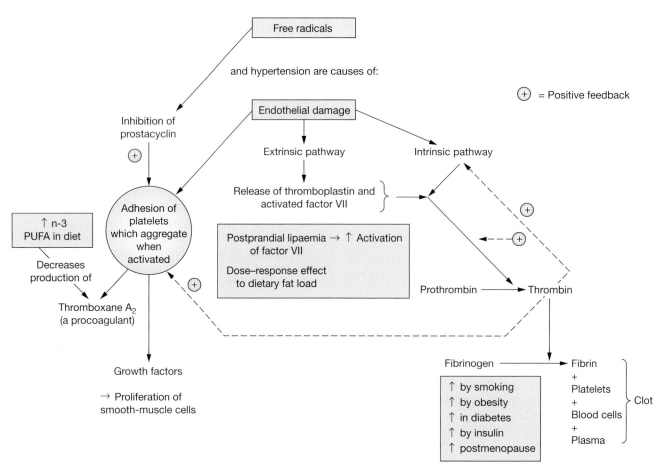

Figure 7.14.2 Diet and haemostasis (source: Thomas & Bishop 2007, figure 4.20.2, p. 606. Reproduced with permission of Wiley-Blackwell Publishing)

inhibitor (PAI-1) which binds with the plasmin and so inhibits the process of clot breakdown, is a known risk factor for CHD.

Blood coagulation is a complex autocatalytic process; more detailed discussions on this subject can be found in the Cardiovascular Disease Report (BNF, 2005).

Risk factors

There is no single cause of CHD and many factors can contribute to its development. Epidemiological studies and clinical trials have identified many of the major risk factors for CHD; these include physical and biochemical parameters as well as features of lifestyle and behaviour. Some risk factors (such as genetic influences) are unmodifiable, but many are potentially modifiable and hence are the focus of disease prevention. Table 7.14.7 summarises conventional risk factors detailed by the Scottish Intercollegiate Guidelines Network (SIGN, 2007a) and Joint British Societies (JBS2, 2005).

Reducing CHD risk requires multifactorial risk assessment and management. Correcting one risk factor alone may have little impact on CHD risk if other risk factors are ignored, e.g. correcting raised cholesterol will be less beneficial if that person continues to smoke and be hypertensive. The benefits of diet and lifestyle change must also

be considered in this context and it is vital that dietitians take a broad perspective of CHD risk that encompasses all contributory factors. The use of global or absolute risk assessment is discussed later in this chapter. From an international perspective, similar approaches to prevention are based on similar principles; the INTERHEART Study highlighted that modifiable risk factors, e.g. diet, account for >90% of the risk of MI worldwide (Yusuf *et al.*, 2004).

Role of diet in the development of coronary heart disease

Many dietary factors may impact on the pathogenesis of CHD, although the significance of some of them remains to be determined (see Chapter 7.14.1). A detailed review of the subject can be found in the Committee on Medical Aspects of Food Policy (COMA) report Nutritional Aspects of Cardiovascular Disease (Department of Health, 1994) and the Cardiovascular Disease Report (BNF, 2005). The key influences are briefly summarised below.

Diet and endothelial dysfunction

A high intake of saturated fat increases LDL cholesterol and reduces HDL cholesterol, causing endothelial damage, which is the first step in the development of atherosclerosis and can trigger thrombosis. The composition and concentration of the lipoprotein fractions, and hence their atherogenic capacity, are affected by diet. This is described in more detail in Chapter 7.14.3.

Diet and thrombogenesis

Many dietary factors influence haemostasis, such as:

- *Dietary fat (quantity and type)* (see Figure 7.14.2) – an increase in the total intake of fat causes postprandial activation of factor VII (FVII) and suppresses fibrinolysis (clot breakdown). Saturated fats increase platelet activity, whereas polyunsaturates have the opposite effect. n-3 Fatty acids attenuate thromboxane A_2 synthesis and thereby suppress platelet activation. (The anticoagulant effect of aspirin is also achieved by inhibition of thromboxane A_2 production.)
- *Energy balance* – non-rapid weight loss improves fibrinolytic activity.
- Alcohol consumption – regular alcohol consumption reduces fibrinogen and FVII concentrations, but heavy drinking reduces fibrinolytic activity.

Diet and oxidative stress

Free radicals are implicated in the processes of both atherosclerosis and thrombosis via:

- Damage to the endothelium.
- Inhibition of prostacyclin and hence increase in platelet activation and aggregation.
- Oxidation of LDL and other atherogenic lipoproteins, leading to their preferential uptake by macrophages to form foam cells.

Epidemiological data suggest that consumption of fruit and vegetables has a protective effect against CHD, but randomised controlled trials using antioxidant vitamin supplements contradict this (Mead *et al.*, 2006). The European Prospective Investigation into Cancer and Nutrition (EPIC) – Heart study (Crowe *et al.*, 2011), a large observational study, showed that consumption of at least eight portions of fruit and vegetables a day gave a 22% lower risk of fatal ischaemic heart disease (IHD) compared with those consuming fewer than three portions a day. A one-portion (80 g) increment in fruit and vegetable intake was associated with a 4% lower risk of fatal IHD. The mechanism by which fruit and vegetables reduce CHD risk at a population level is not yet fully understood and more research is required. The National Institute for Health and Care Excellence (NICE, 2007) recommends a Mediterranean style diet and advises against taking antioxidant supplements (vitamin E and/or C) or folic acid to reduce cardiovascular risk.

Diet and inflammation related factors

Inflammation underlies atherosclerosis and current evidence suggests that anti-inflammatory dietary components, such as n-3 fatty acids, and dietary antioxidants may have a role in reducing injury to the coronary arteries, but more research is required.

Diet and homocysteine

Hyperhomocysteinaemia has been suggested to increase the risk of fibrous plaque formation, thrombosis and arterial injury. Despite epidemiological evidence of an association between these factors, it is not yet clear whether reduction of homocysteine levels by means of folic acid and other B vitamins will reduce CHD events (Mead *et al.*, 2006).

Indirect dietary influences

Indirect dietary influences on CHD development include obesity and its consequences, such as hypertension, hypertriglyceridaemia or type 2 diabetes.

Management

Coronary heart disease management has been shaped by the National Service Framework (NSF) for CHD (Department of Health, 2000) and more recently, the cardiac rehabilitation commissioning pack (Department of Health, 2010a). Alongside this, numerous guidelines have been produced to influence clinical care and the types of investigative procedures used (Table 7.14.8). Other national guidelines explicitly state the need for professional dietetic advice (Joint British Societies, 2005; British Association for Cardiac Rehabilitation, 2007); reviews are currently underway. Providing evidenced based dietary information to all people who have CHD will save more lives than concentrating dietary advice on just those in need of weight management or lipid reduction. The practice of prioritising dietetic time in secondary prevention to those with raised lipids is out of date since the advent of statin therapy (NICE, 2007; 2011).

Overall, the dietary management of CHD depends on the extent to which the disease has progressed and the way in which it is being clinically treated. In the early stages, the main priority will be to achieve change to a cardioprotective diet (see Chapter 7.14.1) in conjunction with other lifestyle risk reduction measures, e.g. increased physical activity. Following a major coronary event, this objective remains the same, but will need to be achieved as part of the stepwise process of cardiac rehabilitation (see later). Invasive surgical procedures may temporarily alter dietetic priorities in favour of nutritional repletion. The development of heart failure or cachexia may necessitate permanent change in these priorities. Understanding the medical and surgical management of CHD in terms of their physical and psychological consequences, e.g. on nutritional status or patient motivation, can help determine what these priorities should be.

Medical management

Medical treatment of CHD depends largely on its manifestation.

Table 7.14.8 Summary of recent coronary heart disease guidance

Society/institute	Guidance
Joint British Societies (JBS)	Guidelines on the prevention of cardiovascular disease in clinical practice (JBS, 2005) (currently being revised)
British Association for Cardiac Rehabilitation (BACR) (Now known as BACPR: British Association for Cardiac Prevention & Rehabilitation)	Standards and core components for cardiac rehabilitation (BACR, 2007) (currently being revised)
Scottish Intercollegiate Guidelines Network (SIGN)	Heart disease guidelines (SIGN, 2007a,b,c)
National Institute for Health and Care Excellence (NICE)	Myocardial infarction: secondary prevention (NICE, 2007)
	Lipid modification: cardiovascular risk assessment and the modification of blood lipids for the primary and secondary prevention of cardiovascular disease (NICE, 2008; reissued 2010c)
	Unstable angina and NSTEMI: the early management of unstable angina and NSTEMI. CG 94 (2010a)
	Stable angina CG126 (NICE, 2011)
	Chronic heart failure: management of chronic heart failure in adults in primary and secondary care (NICE, 2010b)
European Society of Cardiology (ESC)	Guidelines for the diagnosis and treatment of acute and chronic heart failure (ESC, 2008)
	Guidelines for the management of acute coronary syndromes in patients presenting without persistent ST segment elevation (Hamm et al., 2011)

STEMI, ST elevation myocardial infarction; NSTEMI, non-ST elevation myocardial infarction.

Myocardial infarction – STEMI (Hamm et al., 2011)

Medical treatment includes:

- Consideration of immediate primary percutaneous coronary. intervention (PPCI) and revascularisation of the culprit lesion (see later).
- Initiation of appropriate pharmacological therapies for secondary prevention (see later).
- Assessment of left ventricular function.
- Management of cardiovascular risk factors.
- Referral to cardiac rehabilitation services.

Myocardial infarction – NSTEMI and unstable angina (NICE, 2010a)

Medical treatments include:

- Consideration for elective coronary angioplasty.
- Assessment of left ventricular function – recommended for all MI patients and to be considered in the management of unstable angina patients.
- Management of cardiovascular risk factors.
- Initiation of appropriate pharmacological therapies for secondary prevention (see later) and to improve angina symptom control as appropriate.
- Referral to cardiac rehabilitation services as appropriate.

National guidelines, e.g. Hamm *et al.* (2011), NICE (2010a) and SIGN (2007b) have identified four main prophylactic drug groups for the secondary prevention of CHD:

- *Antiplatelet drugs* – aspirin blocks the production of thromboxane, which is one of the chemicals responsi-

ble for platelet agglutination. The benefits of long term use of low dose aspirin in secondary prevention are well documented. For patients with a hypersensitivity to aspirin, clopidogrel monotherapy should be considered as an alternative.

- *Statins* – reduce plasma lipid levels (see Chapter 7.14.3).
- *Beta-blockers* – block the stimulating action of noradrenaline (norepinephrine), thus reducing the force and speed of myocardial contraction. The increase in diastolic interval allows for better coronary perfusion during exercise and a reduction in myocardial oxygen demand. They are used in the treatment of MI, angina, heart failure, arrhythmias and hypertension.
- *Angiotensin converting enzyme (ACE) inhibitors* – have a vasodilatory action through the decreased formation of angiotensin II and increase in protective bradykinin. The main indications for ACE inhibitor therapy include prophylaxis of cardiovascular events, hypertension and all grades of heart failure. Angiotensin II receptor antagonists [also referred to as angiotensin receptor blockers (ARBs)] are used when patients are intolerant to ACE inhibitors. Other vasodilators are nitrates, e.g. glyceryl trinitrate (GTN) spray for symptomatic relief of angina, and calcium channel blockers. Both work by inhibiting smooth muscle contraction in the vessel walls.

If patients do not tolerate oily fish consumption as part of a cardioprotective diet, NICE recommends 1 g/day of n-3 fatty acid ethyl esters for up to 4 years post MI. n-3 Fatty acid supplementation should not be routinely initiated for patients who had an MI >3 months earlier (NICE,

2007). In addition, NICE makes lifestyle recommendations about physical activity, smoking cessation and alcohol consumption. NICE (2011) states there is no evidence that vitamins or fish oil help stable angina.

Surgical management

Following an angiogram (see Table 7.14.6) patients may be referred for an angioplasty and coronary artery bypass graft (CABG).

Angioplasty – percutaneous coronary Intervention

A balloon is introduced and inflated at the site where blood flow through the arterial lumen has been significantly reduced as a result of atherosclerotic plaque. Once in position, the balloon is inflated to increase the size of the arterial lumen. In some cases a small stent (a mesh tube that can be expanded to hold the artery open) is inserted. The term primary percutaneous coronary intervention (PPCI), also known as primary angioplasty, is used for the prompt restoration of flow in STEMI.

Coronary artery bypass graft

In this surgical procedure, one or more diseased coronary arteries are bypassed. Blood vessels (usually taken from the leg) are grafted onto the existing coronary arteries to bypass the occluded section. Access to the heart is gained via the sternum, which is broken in the process. Coronary artery bypass graft (CABG) is a major surgical procedure with all the metabolic and nutritional consequences that this implies (see Chapter 7.17.5). It should also be borne in mind that if patients are advised by the surgical team to lose weight prior to the procedure, some will undergo surgery in a nutritionally depleted state as a result of inappropriate crash dieting. If weight management is still an issue post CABG, patients should be informed that the sternum wound takes about 6 weeks to heal and therefore weight reduction should not be attempted during this time period. For planned CABG prehabilitation, a combination of nurse counselling and a brief cognitive behavioural intervention (Heart OP Programme) has been found to reduce depression and cardiac misconceptions and improve physical functioning before CABG surgery (Furze, 2009).

Cardiac rehabilitation

The Department of Health (2010a) cardiac rehabilitation commissioning pack sets explicit standards for the provision of effective cardiac rehabilitation for high priority patients with CHD. These include NSTEMI, STEMI and unstable angina patients, including all those undergoing reperfusion, e.g. CABG, PCI or PPCI, and newly diagnosed chronic heart failure patients or those with a step change in clinical presentation. Furthermore, the pack recommends extension of services once high priority patient cardiac rehabilitation services have been successfully implemented to include heart transplant patients, patients who have undergone surgery to implant a cardioverter defibrillator or heart valve replacement for reasons other than ACS or heart failure. The pack recommends a seamless pathway involving six stages (Table 7.14.9), with the dietitian influencing the management of each stage. There is no evidence that cardiac rehabilitation is clinically or cost effective for managing stable angina (NICE, 2011).

Stage 1

Initial advice on lifestyle, including diet, is usually given by the ward staff (hence training of other healthcare professionals is an important role of the cardiac rehabilitation dietitian), but the ability of both patients and their families to assimilate information will be severely impaired by anxiety and stress in coming to terms with the diagnosis. In particular, patients receiving immediate PPCI have a very short stay in hospital and should receive stop gap information to ensure they are aware of their local cardiac rehabilitation programme.

Table 7.14.9 Role of the dietitian in cardiac rehabilitation (CR)

Stages	Service delivered by:	Description (Department of Health, 2010a)	Time scale	Role of the dietitian (Mead et al., 2006; Fox et al., 2004)
1	Acute services	Acute event in hospital	2–5 days as inpatient	Training CR staff or practice nurse to deliver consistent key cardioprotective dietary messages
2 and 3	Acute services and primary care	Telephone/home visit initial assessment completed and introduces CR core components Devise individual care plan based on patient risk factors and motivation	5–10 working days from receipt of referral/discharge from hospital	Ensuring dietary resources are up to date Referral criteria to dietitian is not based on lipid levels, but identifies patients struggling with the cardioprotective diet
4	Acute services and primary care	Hospital rehabilitation service – high risk patients Community based rehabilitation service – low risk patients Multidisciplinary approach	8–12 weeks	Deliver group sessions and/or individual consultations to achieve and sustain effective secondary prevention within multidisciplinary care
5 and 6	Primary care	Nurse led coronary heart disease clinics by practice nurses Community exercise classes	Week 12 and beyond	

Following major cardiac surgery, the immediate dietary objectives (to restore recent energy and nutrient losses) may be quite different from the longer term aims (e.g. to reduce fat intake). Some patients may require oral nutritional support measures and hence healthy heart food choices from the hospital menu may not be appropriate at this stage. Good communication between dietetic and nursing and medical staff is essential to ensure that the nutritional objectives are understood and that patients are given food that is appropriate for their nutritional needs.

Stage 2

The cardiac rehabilitation specialist nurse completes an initial assessment with the patient and introduces the core components of cardiac rehabilitation:

- *Lifestyle* – diet, exercise and, if appropriate, weight management and smoking cessation.
- *Risk factor management* – cholesterol, blood pressure and, if diabetic, glucose management.
- *Cardioprotective drug therapy* – rate, rhythm and thrombotic risk management and fluid status can be modified by non-medical prescribing cardiac specialist nurses.
- *Psychosocial wellbeing* – an anxiety and depression screening tool will be used to identify high risk clients to be referred to psychological specialists if needed and available.

Stage 3

A care plan is devised, realistic goals are set from the initial assessment and the patient is enrolled onto a cardiac rehabilitation programme that meets their needs; this may include home based cardiac rehabilitation programmes, e.g. the Heart Manual (Lewin *et al.*, 1992), or a formal cardiac rehabilitation exercise programme. There is usually very little direct dietetic contact during this phase.

Stage 4

A formal cardiac rehabilitation outpatient programme typically lasts for 6 weeks, with twice weekly supervised exercise sessions followed by group education. Community based programmes are becoming more common to improve access and increase participation by women and ethnic minority groups, whose uptake of hospital cardiac rehabilitation programmes is low. Dietetic input depends on the capacity of the service, but usually a dietitian will see the patient in group sessions and/or individually depending on availability of local resources (BHF, 2011). The patient's partner or carer should also be involved since they have an important role in helping the patient implement and maintain the diet and lifestyle measures necessary for secondary prevention.

Dietitians, as part of a multidisciplinary team approach to cardiac rehabilitation, can support patients to achieve and sustain effective secondary prevention (Fox *et al.*, 2004). However, the EUROASPIRE II survey (Kotseva *et al.*, 2004) found that only a third of patients attended the cardiac rehabilitation programme, and those that did

still did not achieve lifestyle and risk factor targets. The EUROACTION trial in eight European countries demonstrated that a multidisciplinary, family based programme improved lifestyle and reduced cardiovascular risk. The results showed that patients in the intervention group reduced their consumption of saturated fat; three quarters of patients and their partners achieved the recommended fruit and vegetable consumption, compared to just over a third of usual care patients, and twice as many in the former group met the recommended weekly intake of oily fish (Wood *et al.*, 2008).

Stages 5 and 6

At the patient's final discharge assessment from the cardiac rehabilitation programme they are signposted to lifestyle maintenance programmes to encourage them to continue to exercise, e.g. local heart care support group or community exercise classes. The patient is referred back to the care of their general practitioner (GP). The NSF for CHD (Department of Health, 2000) advocated the use of disease registers in primary care to provide long term follow-up for CHD patients. The General Medical Council's Good Medical Practice Guide (2006) encourages primary care teams to implement evidenced based care. For CHD this is realised in the Quality Outcome Framework (BMA/NHS Employers, 2011) with clinics run by practice nurses attended by patients for an annual review. Patients may be referred to a dietitian during this phase if they are still struggling to incorporate a cardioprotective diet into their lifestyle.

Chronic heart failure

Chronic heart failure (CHF) is a complex clinical syndrome caused by a reduction in the heart's ability to pump blood around the body. Whilst the most common cause is CHD, other causes include hypertension, valvular heart disease, cardiomyopathy, atrial fibrillation and alcohol abuse. Prevalence of CHF increases sharply with age to about 7% in men and women over 75 years (NHS IC, 2010). Patients with CHF often have a poor quality of life with high mortality rates (10–50% depending on severity). They have a worse prognosis than patients with breast and prostate cancer (NHS IC, 2010), and CHF has become one of the most common causes of hospital admissions. Due to the ageing population and improved survival in patients who develop CVD disease, such as MI, hospital admissions and the number of people diagnosed with CHF are expected to rise.

To address these issues, the NSF for CHD, Standard 11 (Department of Health, 2000) set out a service delivery agenda, and NICE (2010b) has produced clinical guidelines to improve CHF management. Specialist CHF services are currently being developed as it has been shown that they can reduce hospital admissions/mortality rates and improve symptoms (NHS IC, 2010).

The physical effects of CHF include:

- Inadequate cardiac output.
- Fluid imbalance.

Table 7.14.10 New York Heart Association functional classification of heart failure (Dickstein *et al.*, 2008)

Classification	Symptoms	Comments
Class I	Impaired left ventricular failure, but no symptoms, e.g. fatigue or breathlessness	No limitations to activities of daily living
Class II	Comfortable at rest but ordinary physical activity results in fatigue, palpitation or dyspnoea	Mild – slight limitations
Class III	Comfortable at rest but less than ordinary activity results in fatigue, palpitations or dyspnoea	Moderate – marked limitations
Class IV	Symptoms at rest. If any physical activity is undertaken, discomfort is increased	Severe – inability to carry out any activities of daily living without discomfort

- Pulmonary and other oedema.
- Dyspnoea.
- Fatigue.

Echocardiogram is now the gold standard for diagnosis in those patients with a medical history of MI. For patients with no previous history of MI, an echocardiogram is only needed if the B type natriuretic peptide (BNP) test is positive (NICE, 2010b). Heart failure is a progressive condition and is classified into four stages according to the severity of symptoms (Table 7.14.10).

Medical management

In CHF the main treatment objectives are to:

- Prevent progressive damage to the mycocardium.
- Prevent or reverse further enlargement of the heart.
- Improve quality of life through symptom management.
- Prolong life (Opie & Gersh, 2009).

The main cause of CHF is left ventricular systolic dysfunction (LVSD), for which the recommendations for pharmacological management can include the following (NICE, 2010b, Dickstein *et al.*, 2008):

- Angiotensin converting enzyme (ACE) inhibitors are recommended as first line treatment. These can prolong life expectancy, delay progression and improve symptoms. ARBs may be used where ACE inhibitors are not tolerated.
- Beta-blockers are used in controlled heart failure alongside ACE inhibitors and have been proven to reduce mortality in low doses.
- Diuretics are used routinely for the relief of congestive symptoms and fluid retention (peripheral and pulmonary oedema); the removal of fluid and reduction in

blood volume reduces the workload of the heart. This can result in rapid improvement in dyspnoea and improve exercise tolerance.

Other agents such as aldosterone antagonists and digoxin may be considered in addition to the above treatment. Warfarin is recommended in patients with CHF and permanent, persistent or paroxysmal atrial fibrillation without contraindications to anticoagulation, with the aim of reducing the risk of thromboembolic complications including stroke.

Surgical management

Although medical management is the mainstay of treatment, some patients will benefit from invasive procedures (NICE, 2010b; Dickstein *et al.*, 2008) such as:

- Mechanical support cardiac resynchronisation therapy (CRT) with pacemaker function – recommended to reduce morbidity in patients in New York Heart Association (NYHA) classes III–IV who are symptomatic despite optimal medical therapy.
- Heart transplantation, however shortage of donor organs means that many potential recipients are unable to benefit from this.

Dietetic management

Many guidelines for CHF management (SIGN, 2007c; NICE, 2010b; Dickstein *et al.*, 2008) highlight the benefits of lifestyle changes, including dietary manipulation. However, there are no specific evidence based nutritional guidelines and more research is required. The therapeutic aims of dietary management are to:

- Maintain adequate energy intake to prevent obesity, malnutrition and cachexia.
- Reduce the workload for the heart by weight management, and sodium and fluid restriction.
- Provide a nutritionally adequate diet.
- Protect against further heart disease.

Dietetic management in CHF will therefore address the following:

- *Obesity* – should be avoided as it increases cardiac workload. Planned weight loss in CHF should be gradual as rapid weight loss can result in undesirable muscle loss and also increase the risk of inadequate or poor nutritional intake. Hence, weight reduction should not be routinely recommended in moderate to severe CHF (Dickstein *et al.*, 2008).
- *Malnutrition* – the combination of reduced nutritional intake and increased requirements place the CHF patient at risk of malnutrition (Gibbs *et al.*, 2000). Energy intake needs to be sufficient to meet nutritional needs and prevent deterioration in nutritional status. However, weight gain from increased fat stores should be avoided. Gain in adiposity should be distinguished from short term fluctuations in body weight caused by changes in fluid balance (see Chapter 2.2).

- *Cachexia* – see later.
- *Sodium restriction* – sodium and water retention, leading to expansion of extracellular fluid volume, are important components of CHF syndrome. Therefore, it is of little or no benefit to restrict fluid intake if patients who continue to use unlimited amounts of salt. Restricting salt is more relevant in advanced CHF. Severe salt restriction (<2, g/day) is rarely necessary. Where salt restriction needs to be considered, it should be at a no added salt level (see Chapter 6.6). Salt substitutes should be avoided as these are rich in potassium and may lead to hyperkalaemia, especially if patients are on ACE inhibitors and /or spironolactone. Salt restriction can affect food palatability and possibly compromise intake of energy and essential nutrients.
- *Fluid restriction* – an excessive amount of fluid should be avoided as it negates the positive effects of diuretics and induces hyponatraemia. Patients with advanced CHF, with or without hyponatraemia, may need to restrict their fluid intake. There is no evidence based calculation for the level of fluid restriction such as exists for patients with renal failure. In practice, a restriction of 1.5–2 L/day is often advised. Daily weighing is advised for CHF patients to detect sudden or unexpected weight gains (>2 kg in 3 days), which would indicate the need for adjustment of diuretic dose.
- *Maintaining nutritional adequacy* – particular attention should be paid to micronutrient intake since the use of diuretic and other drugs may result in significant urinary losses of potassium and water soluble vitamins. Since appetite is often poor, the diet may need to be relatively nutrient dense and meal frequency may need to be increased. Social factors such as support for food purchasing and preparation, particularly if the patient lives alone, should not be overlooked. Alcohol should only be consumed in moderation, and completely avoided if CHF has been caused by alcohol abuse.
- *Protect against further heart disease* – the key cardio-protective dietary messages should be incorporated (see Chapter 7.14.1). Research study results using 1 g of n-3 fatty acid supplementation in CHF patients are promising, but further studies are needed prior to routine recommendation (GISSI, 2008).

Cardiac cachexia

Chronic heart failure can lead to cardiac cachexia. This complex condition affects many body systems (Anker & Coats, 1999). There is a loss of skeletal and heart muscle, and fat and bone tissue. There are neurohormonal and immunological changes, and impaired functioning. Many of the common symptoms, e.g. anorexia and fatigue, are similar to the cachexia of cancer and chronic infection (see Chapter 7.15.9). Cardiac cachexia has a poor prognosis (50% mortality rate within 18 months of diagnosis), with the amount of weight lost being a strong predictor of mortality. The incidence of cachexia with CHF is not exactly known, but may be about 9% and up to 68% for hospitalised patients.

Dietary management

Nutritional support is required to address anorexia that is exacerbated by:

- Dyspnoea – this increases fatigue during eating, and swallowing exacerbates the symptoms of dyspnoea.
- Oedema.
- Palatability of food, e.g. salt restriction, ACE inhibitors impairing taste.
- Drug reactions, e.g. aspirin, digoxin and ACE inhibitors all cause anorexia.
- Metabolic disturbances, e.g. hyponatraemia or renal failure.
- Depression.

The level of sodium and fluid restriction, and micronutrient needs should be discussed with the referring clinician. Overall, a multidisciplinary team approach is key to ensure that weight loss is minimised as part of the need to address quality of life issues during palliative care. It is now recommended that patients with two or more of the following indicators should be registered on the Gold Standards Framework register:

- CHF NYHA III–IV – shortness of breath at rest or on minimal exertion.
- Patients thought to be in the last year of life by the care team.
- Repeated hospital admissions with symptoms of heart failure.
- Difficult physical or psychological symptoms despite optimal medical treatment.

A discussion with the patient and carer about palliative end of life care should be approached by the care team to ensure an appropriate care plan and support are implemented (see Chapter 7.16; RCGP, 2008).

Dietitians are gradually becoming more involved in the management of heart failure cardiac cachexia, and at an earlier stage, but this is variable across the country. Since the number of hospital admissions this condition is increasing, it is likely that its management will adopt a rising profile in the clinical dietetic caseload. Current research is investigating the use of anabolics, anti-inflammatory drugs, appetite stimulants and nutritional supplements, which will strengthen the evidence base for dietetic practice in this area.

Public health prevention strategies

The multifactorial nature of CHD is reflected in public health strategy. Addressing health inequalities is an important issue as poor quality diet can result in inequalities in people's health. Poor diet can account for 30% of life years lost in early death/disability from diet related diseases such as CHD (National Heart Forum, 2004). Key documents to date that have shaped primary CHD prevention within the public health arena are outlined in Table 7.14.11 (see Chapter 4.2).

The evidence base for dietary aspects of primary CHD prevention is well known (Department of Health,

Table 7.14.11 Key UK public health documents that influence primary coronary heart disease (CHD) prevention

Key documents	Comments
Saving Lives: Our Healthier Nation (Department of Health, 1999)	National policy on public health, e.g. reducing death rate from CHD, stroke and related disease in people under 75 years of age by at least 40% by 2010
Healthy Lives, Healthy People (DH 2010b)	Updated Public Health Strategy to promote health and aim to create wellness service
Our Health and Wellbeing Today (Department of Health, 2010c)	Summary of evidence setting out the nation's health in 2010
Prevention of cardiovascular disease at population level (NICE, 2010b)	Department of Health commissioned NICE to produce public health guidance on prevention of cardiovascular disease (CVD) at population level. CVD includes stroke and peripheral arterial disease
Coronary heart disease: National Service Framework (NSF) for CHD – modern standards and service models (Department of Health, 2000)	Strategy to modernise CHD services. Standard 1 highlights that the NHS needs to work with partner agencies to address CHD prevention in the population
Coronary Heart Disease Ten Years On – Improving Heart Care (Department of Health, 2007)	Report of progress in CHD outcomes and prevention
CHD: Guidance for implementing the preventative aspects of the NSF (HDA, 2001)	Guidance on best practice to support healthier lifestyles: • Reduce smoking • Promote healthy eating • Promote physical activity • Reduce overweight and obesity
Tackling Health Inequalities. A programme for Action (Department of Health, 2003). Securing Good Health for the Whole Population (Wanless, 2004).	Highlights the need to address access issues, especially hard to reach groups. Services and initiatives need to narrow the health gap, not widen it further, as low income and minority ethnic groups are disproportionately affected by CHD
Tackling Health Inequalities: 10 years on. (Department of Health, 2009)	Update from publication of Acheson report 1998 leading to strategic review of health inequalities in 2008
England	
Choosing Health – making healthier choices easier (Department of Health, 2004)	Considers wider determinants and barriers to choosing a healthy lifestyle and inequalities, etc.
Choosing a Better Diet: a food and health action plan (Department of Health, 2005) www.dh.gov.uk	Government plans to improve nutrition and health
Scotland	
Eating for health – meeting the challenge: Co-ordinated action, improved communication and leadership for Scottish Food and Health policy (Scottish Executive, 2004) www.scotland.gov.uk	A strategic framework for food and health
Healthy Eating Active Living (HEAL) (Scottish Government, 2008)	An action plan to improve diet, increase physical activity and tackle obesity
Preventing Overweight and Obesity in Scotland. A route map towards healthy weight (Scottish Government, 2010)	Target areas – energy consumption, energy expenditure, early years, working lives
Wales	
Food and Well Being – Reducing Inequalities through a Nutrition Strategy for Wales. (Welsh Assembly Government, 2003) www.wales.gov.uk	Addresses widening gap in health between the most and least deprived communities
Northern Ireland	
Investing for Health (Department of Health, Social Services and Public Safety, 2003) www.dhsspsni.gov.uk	Plans to improve the health of all people and reduce health inequalities.
Developing New Public Health Strategy for Northern Ireland – Update September 2011 www.dhsspsni.gov.uk	An updated review of Investing in Health

SECTION 7

1994) and implemented in practice via the eatwell plate model.

Drug–nutrient interactions (SIGN, 2007)

Cranberry juice should be avoided in patients prescribed warfarin as this may increase drug potency. St John's wort should be avoided in patients with CHF as this supplement can interact with warfarin, digoxin, eplenerone and selective serotonin reuptake inhibitors.

Internet resources

American Heart Association   www.amhrt.org
British Heart Foundation   www.bhf.org.uk
   British Heart Foundation Heart Statistics   www.heartstats.org
EUROACTION   www.escardio.org/Policy/Pages/EuroAction.aspx
Foundation for Circulatory Health   www.ffch.org
Heart Improvement Programme, NHS   www.heart.nhs.uk
HEART UK   www.improvement.nhs.uk/heart
National Heart Forum   www.heartforum.org.uk
National Institute for Health and Care Effectiveness   www.nice.org.uk
Scottish Intercollegiate Guidelines Network   www.sign.ac.uk
Sustain   www.sustainweb.org
The Heart Manual   www.theheartmanual.com

References

Anker SD, Coats AJS. (1999) Cardiac cachexia: A syndrome with impaired survival and immune and neuroendocrine activation *Chest* 115: 836–847.

British Association for Cardiac Rehabilitation (BACR). (2007) *Standards and Core Components for Cardiac Rehabilitation*. London: BACR.

British Heart Foundation (BHF). (2010a) *Statistics database. Coronary Heart Disease Statistics*. London: BHF.

British Heart Foundation (BHF). (2010b) *Statistics database. Ethnic Differences in Cardiovascular Disease*. London: BHF.

British Heart Foundation (BHF). (2011) *The National Audit of Cardiac Rehabilitation (NACR) Annual Statistics Report 2011*. London: BHF.

British Medical Association (BMA)/ NHS Employers. (2011) *Quality & Outcomes Framework guidance for general medical services (GMS) contract 2011/2012*. London: BMA.

British Nutrition Foundation (BNF). (2005) *Cardiovascular Disease: Diet, Nutrition and Emerging Risk Factors*. Oxford: Blackwell Science.

Crowe FL, Roddam AW, Key TJ, et al.; European Prospective Investigation into Cancer and Nutrition (EPIC)-Heart Study Collaborators. (2011) Fruit and vegetable intake and mortality from ischaemic heart disease: results from the European Prospective Investigation into Cancer and Nutrition (EPIC) – Heart study. *European Heart Journal* 32(10): 1182–1183.

Department of Health, Committee on Medical Aspects of Food Policy. (1994) *Nutritional Aspects of Cardiovascular Disease*. Reports on Health and Social Subjects 46. London: HMSO.

Department of Health. (1999) *Saving Lives: Our Healthier Nation*. London: The Stationery Office.

Department of Health. (2000) *National Service Framework for Coronary Heart Disease*. London: Department of Health.

Department of Health. (2003) *Tackling Health Inequalities. A programme for Action*. London: Department of Health.

Department of Health. (2004) *Choosing Health – making healthier choices easier*. London: Department of Health.

Department of Health. (2005) *Choosing a Better Diet: a food and health action plan*. London: Department of Health.

Department of Health. (2007) *Coronary Heart Disease Ten Years On – improving heart care*. London: Department of Health.

Department of Health. (2009) *Tackling Health Inequalities: 10 years on (report 2009)*. London: Department of Health.

Department of Health. (2010a). *Strategic Commissioning Development Unit (SCDU) CHD & the need for cardiac rehab*. London: Department of Health.

Department of Health. (2010b) *Healthy Lives Healthy People*. London: Department of Health.

Department of Health. (2010c) *Our Health and Wellbeing Today*. London: Department of Health.

Department of Health, Social Services and Public Safety. (2003) *Investing for Health*. Northern Ireland: Department of Health, Social Services and Public Safety.

Dickstein K, Cohen-Solal A, Filippatos G, et al., ESC Committee for Practice Guidelines (CPG). (2008) ESC Guidelines for the diagnosis and treatment of acute and chronic heart failure 2008: the Task Force for the Diagnosis and Treatment of Acute and Chronic Heart Failure 2008 of the European Society of Cardiology. Developed in collaboration with the Heart Failure Association of the ESC (HFA) and endorsed by the European Society of Intensive Care Medicine (ESICM).. *European Heart Journal* 29: 2388–2442.

Fox K, Barber K, Muir L, et al. (2004) Development, implementation and audit of a cardiac prevention and rehabilitation programme for patients with coronary artery disease. *European Heart Journal Supplements* 2004; 6 (Suppl J): J53–58.

Furze G, Dumville JC, Miles JN, Irvine K, Thompson DR, Lewin RJ. (2009) "Prehabilitation" prior to CABG surgery improves physical functioning and depression. *International Journal of Cardiology* 132(1): 51–58.

General Medical Council (GMC). (2006) "Good Practice Guide" Standard for good clinical practice: para 3. London: GMC.

Gibbs CR, Jackson G, Lip GYH. (2000) ABC of heart failure: Non-drug management. *BMJ* 320: 366–369.

GISSI – HF Investigators. (2008) Effect of omega-3 polyunsaturated fatty acids in patients with chronic heart failure (the GISSI-HF trial): a randomised double blind placebo controlled trial. *Lancet* 372: 1223–1230.

Hamm CW, Bassand JP, Agewall S, et al.; ESC Committee for Practice Guidelines. (2011) ESC Guidelines for the management of acute coronary syndromes in patients presenting without persistent ST-segment elevation: The Task force for the management of ACS in patients without persistent ST-segment elevation of the European Society of Cardiology (ESC). *European Heart Journal* 32(23): 2999–3054.

Health Development Agency (HDA). *Coronary Heart Disease: Guidance for implementing the preventative aspects of the NSF*. London: HDA, 2001.

International Diabetes Federation (IDF). The International Diabetes Federation consensus worldwide definition of the metabolic syndrome, 2005. (Available at www.idf.org).

Joint British Societies. (2005) JBS2: Joint British Societies' guidelines on prevention of cardiovascular disease in clinical practice. *Heart* 91: (Suppl 5): v1–v52.

Kotseva K, Wood DA, De Bacquer D, et al. (2004) Cardiac rehabilitation for coronary patients: lifestyle, risk factor and therapeutic management. Results from the EUROASPIRE II Survey. *European Heart Journal Supplements* 6 (Suppl J): J17–J26.

Lewin B, Robertson IH, Cay EL, Irving JB, Campbell M. (1992) Effects of self-help post myocardial infarction rehabilitation on psychological adjustment and use of health services. *Lancet* 339: 1036–1040.

Mead A, Atkinson G, Albin D, et al. (2006). Dietetic guidelines on food and nutrition in the secondary prevention of cardiovascular disease – evidence from systematic reviews of randomized controlled trials (second update). *Journal of Human Nutrition and Dietetics* 19: 401–419.

National Heart Forum (NHF). (2004) *Nutrition and Food Poverty: A Toolkit for Those Involved in Developing or Implementing A Local Nutrition Strategy*. London: NHF.

National Institute for Health and Care Excellence (NICE). (2007) *Myocardial Infarction: Secondary Prevention – Secondary Prevention in Primary and Secondary Care*. Clinical Guideline 48. London: NICE.

National Institute for Health and Care Excellence (NICE). (2010a) *Unstable Angina & NSTEMI: The Early Management of Unstable Angina & NSTEMI*. CG94. London: NICE.

National Institute for Health and Care Excellence (NICE). (2010b) *Chronic Heart Failure: Management of Chronic Heart Failure in Adults in Primary and Secondary Care*. CG108. London: NICE.

National Institute for Health and Care Excellence (NICE). (2010c) *Prevention of Cardiovascular Disease at Population Level*. NICE Public Health guidance 25, London: NICE.

National Institute for Health and Care Excellence (NICE). (2011) *Stable Angina*. Clinical Guideline 126. London: NICE.

NHS IC (The NHS Information Centre for Health & Social Care). (2010) *National Heart Failure Audit*. London: Department of Health.

Opie LH, Gersh BJ. (2009) *Drugs for the Heart,* 7th edn. Philadelphia: Saunders Elsevier.

Royal College of General Practitioners (RCGP). (2008) *Prognostic Indicator Guidance Paper. National Gold Standards Framework Centre England*. London: RCGP.

Scottish Executive. (2004) *Eating for Health - Meeting the Challenge: Co-ordinated Action, Improved Communication and Leadership for Scottish Food and Health policy*. Edinburgh: Scottish Executive.

Scottish Government. (2008) *Healthy Eating Active Living (HEAL)*. Edinburgh: Scottish Government.8

Scottish Government. (2010) *Preventing Overweight and Obesity in Scotland. A Route Map Towards Healthy Weight*. Edinburgh: Scottish Government.

Scottish Intercollegiate Guidelines Network (SIGN). (2007a) *Risk Estimation and the Prevention of Cardiovascular Disease*. A National Clinical Guideline. Publication No 97. Edinburgh: SIGN.

Scottish Intercollegiate Guidelines Network (SIGN). (2007b) *Acute Coronary Syndromes*. A National Clinical Guideline. Publication No 93. Edinburgh: SIGN.

Scottish Intercollegiate Guidelines Network (SIGN). (2007c) *Management of Chronic Heart failure*. A National Clinical Guideline. Publication No 95. Edinburgh: SIGN.

Simmons A. (1997) *Hematology – A Combined Theoretical and Technical Approach*, 2nd edn. London: Butterworth-Heineman.

Thomas B, Bishop J (eds). (2007) *Manual of Dietetic Practice*, 4th edn. Oxford: Blackwell Scientific.

Wales Assembly Government. (2003) *Food and Well Being: Reducing inequalities through a nutrition strategy for Wales*. Cardiff: Welsh Assembly Government.

Wanless D. (2004) *Securing Good Health for the Whole Population*. London: HMSO.

Wood DA, Kotseva K, Connolly S, *et al.*; EUROACTION Study Group. (2008) Nurse-co-ordinated multidisciplinary, family based cardiovascular disease prevention programme. (EUROACTION) for patients with coronary heart disease and asymptomatic individuals at high risk of cardiovascular disease: a paired, cluster-randomised controlled trial. *Lancet* 371: 1999–2012.

Yusuf S, Hawken S, Ounpuu S, *et al.*; INTERHEART Study Investigators. (2004) Effect of potentially modifiable risk factors associated with myocardial infarction in 52 countries (the INTERHEART study): case-control study. *Lancet* 364: 937–952.

7.14.3 Dyslipidaemia

Linda Main

Key points

- Dyslipidaemia should not be treated in isolation but in conjunction with the assessment of cardiovascular disease risk.

- Dietary treatment and advice is still relevant despite statin therapy.

- There is a greater emphasis on increasing high density lipoprotein (HDL) cholesterol levels (by lifestyle as well as dietary means), as well as reduction in low density lipoprotein (LDL) cholesterol.

- Advances in statin therapy mean that a combination treatments are used to aggressively achieve target lipid levels.

Dyslipidaemia refers to the presence of high levels of lipids (cholesterol or triglycerides) or lipoproteins, the compounds in which they are transported in the blood. The clinical significance of dyslipidaemia depends upon a number of risk factors (including lipid levels) that contribute to total risk. Dyslipidaemia is associated with atherosclerosis – the process by which arteries become occluded, which in turn results in or contributes to a number of chronic conditions, including coronary heart disease, stroke and peripheral vascular disease.

Lipid metabolism

Cholesterol

Cholesterol is an essential part of the structure of all cell membranes, and a precursor of bile acids (needed for fat digestion and absorption), steroid hormones and vitamin D. Excess cholesterol can accumulate in blood vessels walls (atheroma), ultimately causing a restriction or inter-ruption in the circulation; this process is called atherosclerosis. Depending upon where the restriction in blood flow occurs, it can result in angina, heart attack, stroke or claudication (pain on walking), and can contribute to other conditions such as erectile dysfunction and Alzheimer's disease. Populations with low levels of blood cholesterol have low levels of coronary heart disease (CHD) and those with high levels of cholesterol have high levels of CHD (Department of Health, 1994) (see Chapter 7.14.2). Approximately 20% of cholesterol is derived from the diet and the remainder is synthesised in the body. Cholesterol is produced in a multistage process mainly in the liver, although most tissues have the ability to make cholesterol.

Triglycerides

Triglycerides are the major storage form of fats and major source of energy in the diet. Many tissues have the ability

SECTION 7

to synthesise triglycerides, including the gut, liver, muscle and adipose tissue (Durrington, 2007).

Lipid fractions (lipoproteins)

All lipids (cholesterol, phospholipids and triglycerides) are insoluble in water (hydrophobic) and therefore have to be transported in the blood as compounds called lipoproteins. Lipoproteins are classified according to their density and size. The composition, interplay and metabolism of lipoproteins are complex and beyond the scope of this chapter; however, the principal features are:

- Lipoproteins are globular complexes of lipids and proteins.
- The definitions of low density lipoprotein (LDL), very low density lipoprotein (VLDL) and high density lipoprotein (HDL) are artificial cut-off points.
- Each lipoprotein has a number of components that are metabolically active and constantly in flux, both in the circulation and within tissue fluids. They exchange components with each other.
- Lipoproteins interact with receptors and enzymes located on the surface of cells.

The main lipoprotein fractions are chlyomicrons, LDL, VLDL and HDL.

Chlyomicrons (from exogenous production)

Chylomicrons are the largest of the particles; they are rich in triglyceride (80–95%) with relatively small amounts of cholesterol (3–7%), phospholipid (3–6%) and protein (1–2%) (Durrington, 2007). They enter the circulation from the gut via the lymphatic system, taking triglycerides and cholesterol from digestion and newly synthesised cholesterol from the gut into the body. Lipoprotein lipase, present on the vascular endothelium of tissues (especially those with a high requirement for triglycerides, i.e. muscle, adipose and lactating breast tissue), releases triglycerides from the core of the chylomicron. Triglycerides are converted into fatty acids and monoglycerides, which are then taken up by the tissues. Over time the chylomicron becomes depleted of triglyceride and is removed from the circulation by the liver.

Very low density lipoproteins (from endogenous production)

Smaller and denser than chylomicrons, VLDLs are rich in triglyceride (59%) and contain about 10–15% cholesterol and 15% phospholipid; they account for around 10–15% of total serum cholesterol (Durrington, 2007). They are produced by the liver with the aim of supplying the tissues with triglycerides. Like chylomicrons, VLDLs become depleted of triglyceride over time under the influence of lipoprotein lipase.

Low density lipoproteins (from endogenous production)

Remnant VLDLs (triglyceride 10%, cholesterol 37%, phospholipid 22%, protein 20–22%) are known as LDL. Being smaller they are able to cross the vascular endothelium and enter the tissues where they are the major supplier of cholesterol for membrane repair and growth, and in the specialised tissues for hormone and vitamin D synthesis. Low density lipoprotein cholesterol accounts for 60–70% of total serum cholesterol. The size of LDL particles varies and this is significant as smaller, denser LDL particles are more atherogenic than larger ones. This form of cholesterol is the major target of cholesterol lowering treatments.

High density lipoproteins (from endogenous production)

High density lipoprotein is composed of 20% cholesterol, 48% protein, 3% triglyceride and 27% phospholipid. These are the smallest lipoproteins and HDL cholesterol accounts for 20–30% of circulating cholesterol. The role of HDL is to collect excess cholesterol from the tissues and return it to the liver where it can be removed from the circulation by conversion to cholesterol rich bile acids that are excreted into the gut. This process is essential to prevent the build-up of surplus cholesterol in the tissues. The levels of HDL are thought to be important in preventing the formation of atheroma and are inversely correlated with CHD risk. The exact role of HDL now appears more complex than originally thought and is the subject of much ongoing debate.

Intermediate density lipoproteins

Intermediate density lipoproteins (IDL) are short lived intermediaries between VLDL and LDL.

Apolipoproteins

Apolipoproteins bind to lipids within the lipoproteins and are classified as A, B, C, etc. with further subclassifications (AI, AII etc.). They are sometimes referred to as Apo A, Apo B, etc. The principal apolipoprotein of HDL is apolipoprotein A and of LDL is apolipoprotein B. Apolipoprotein B is found in all adults but levels vary widely. The level appears to be genetically determined and is higher in adults descendant from African and Indian populations (Durrington, 2007). Europeans with a family history of early heart disease often have higher levels of apolipoprotein A.

Cardiovascular risk

Cholesterol

Raised blood cholesterol level is the single greatest risk factor for CHD and a main risk factor for cardiovascular disease (CVD) (HEARTUK, 2007). Cardiovascular disease is the leading cause of deaths worldwide (WHO, 2008), causing 27% and 32% of deaths in men and women, respectively, during 2004. Raised cholesterol is estimated to cause 18% of global cerebrovascular disease and 56% of global CHD (WHO, 2002). Reducing total cholesterol level reduces cardiovascular risk. On a population basis, a 1 mmol/L reduction in LDL cholesterol is associated with a 12% reduction in all cause mortality, a 19% reduction in coronary mortality and a 21% reduction in vascular events [myocardial infarction (MI), coronary revascularisation and stroke] over 5 years [Cholesterol Treatment Trialists' Collaboration (CTTC), 2005].

Blood cholesterol concentrations (including LDL and HDL levels) are only one of many risk factors that influence the development of CHD, and so cannot predict individual CHD risk alone. A raised level poses a greater threat to an individual at high CHD risk than to someone at low risk. Similarly, the benefits from cholesterol reduction in a particular individual will be affected by other risk factors, e.g. smoking, hypertension, overweight or being physically inactive. It is now recognised that effective prevention of CVD requires multifactorial risk assessment and intervention (see Chapter 7.14.1). For this reason, blood lipid measurements must always be considered in the context of other risk factors and not in isolation. Emphasis is placed on the reduction in LDL cholesterol as this is considered the most atherogenic particle. Conversely, HDL cholesterol reflects cholesterol removal and high levels are therefore believed to be protective.

Triglyceride

Circulating triglycerides are present mainly in VLDL, which is made in the liver (endogenous production), and chylomicrons, which are produced by the gut following digestion (exogenous production). Until fairly recently it was believed that observed associations between blood triglyceride concentration and CHD risk simply reflected the more powerful predictive value of low HDL cholesterol levels (NB: low HDL and high VLDL triglyceride usually coexist). However, a number of studies have indicated a significant and independent association between serum triglyceride concentrations and the incidence of major coronary events (Stampfer et al., 1996; Assmann et al., 1996). A meta analysis that controlled for HDL cholesterol suggested that for every 1 mmol/L rise in serum triglyceride concentration, the relative risk of CHD increased by 14% in men and 37% in women (Hokanson & Austin, 1996). Kannel & Ramachandran (2009) reviewed the role of triglycerides in the aetiology of CVD and concluded that raised fasting or non-fasting triglycerides merit consideration as a prominent CVD risk factor because of their association with insulin resistance, highly atherogenic small LDL particles, low HDL cholesterol and the metabolic syndrome. At present no clear evidence exists from intervention trials to demonstrate that lowering triglyceride levels (independent of other risk factors) reduces major CVD events (Kannel & Ramachandran, 2009).

Genetic predisposition

Plasma concentrations of total cholesterol, LDL cholesterol, HDL cholesterol and triglycerides are heritable risk factors for CVD. So far 95 different genes involved in lipid metabolism have been identified and together these explain 25–30% of the genetic variance for each lipoprotein (Teslovich et al., 2010) Consumer genetic testing may in the future be available as a more accurate method of identifying those at high CVD risk who would benefit from early treatment.

Diet and lifestyle

Many aspects of diet and lifestyle affect blood lipids and can contribute to dyslipidaemia. Diet should be central to the treatment of dyslipidaemia, either as a first line treatment or alongside drug therapy. Metabolic studies have demonstrated a cholesterol lowering effect from diet in the range of 5–35% dependent upon the baseline diet and the extent of dietary changes made (Jenkins et al., 2002; 2003b; 2011). For most people 5–20% cholesterol reduction is more realistic, as shown by free living studies (Jenkins et al., 2006; 2011).

Fat

Following a fat containing meal, blood triglyceride levels rise, triglyceride rich chylomicrons enter the bloodstream and VLDL triglyceride production by the liver will temporarily cease. The amount of fat consumed will determine the rise in triglyceride levels. Sustained reduction of both the total amount of fat in the diet and particularly of saturated fat can reduce total and LDL cholesterol. In populations that consume a western diet, replacing 1% of energy from saturated fat with polyunsaturated fats can reduce CHD incidence by 2–3% (Astrup et al., 2011). Most lipid guidelines recommend a maximum of 10% energy from saturated fat, but may not refer to the replacement energy source (NICE, 2010a, Joint British Societies, 2005). Cholesterol levels can be reduced by substituting saturated fatty acids with unsaturated fatty acids (NICE, 2010a; Hooper et al., 2001a,b; FAO/WHO, 2008,; Astrup et al., 2011). Evidence currently suggests that polyunsaturated fats may have a greater impact on reducing LDL cholesterol than monounsaturated fatty acids (Astrup et al., 2011; FAO/WHO, 2008). While restriction of saturated fat intake is crucial, reduction in the total quantity of dietary fat may not always be necessary. However, despite the fact that the energy restriction of a low fat diet can promote weight loss, low fat diets can increase plasma triglyceride and lower HDL concentrations (Katan et al., 1997). Substituting saturated fat with unsaturated alternatives may also make lipid lowering more palatable and improve compliance. Individual saturated fatty acids have different effects on blood cholesterol levels. Lauric (C12.0), myristic (C14.0) and palmitic acid (C16.0) all increase LDL cholesterol, but stearic acid (C18.0) does not (FAO/WHO, 2008).

Trans fatty acids

Industrially, trans fatty acids are produced by partial hydrogenation of vegetable and marine oils to produce hardened fats such as margarines, cooking fats and shortenings. They have been shown to increase total and LDL cholesterol levels, but unlike saturated fats they also lower HDL cholesterol (SACN, 2007; FAO/WHO, 2008). A 1% energy decrease in trans fats is estimated to reduce the risk of CHD by 12.5% (Oomen et al., 2001). In the UK, the food and catering industries have made significant efforts to remove industrially produced trans fats from the food chain. Trans fatty acids should contribute no more than 2% of food energy (SACN, 2007) and are currently estimated to provide 0.8% of food energy (Bates et al., 2010), although some groups may have a higher intake.

Trans fatty acids from ruminant sources are low in most diets (FAO/WHO, 2008) and there is insufficient evidence to discriminate between the health effects of ruminant and industrially produced trans fats (SACN, 2007). Recent guidance from NICE (2010b) called for additional measures to monitor intakes in population subgroups and for action to reduce intakes through industrial food preparation.

Omega 3 fatty acids

The n-3 fatty acids eicosapentanoic acid (EPA) and docosa-hexanoic acid (DHA) at doses of 2–4 g/day (in purified supplemental form) have been shown to reduce fasting and postprandial blood triglyceride levels (Roche & Gibney, 2000; Castro et al., 2005). A dose of 1 g/day of EPA and DHA (or three portions of oily fish/week) is recommended following a heart attack or MI as this reduces the risk of a second event (NICE, 2007). n-3 Fatty acids from fish or vegetable oils do not have a significant effect on cholesterol levels (Hooper et al., 2004).

Cholesterol

Approximately 30–60% of dietary cholesterol is absorbed (Durrington, 2007) and contributes approximately 20% of the total circulating cholesterol. Most dietary cholesterol comes from foods that are rich in saturated fat, e.g. full fat dairy foods and fatty meats, and reducing saturated fat intake will therefore reduce dietary cholesterol. However, some foods rich in cholesterol are low in saturated fat, including egg yolk, liver and shellfish (prawns, crabs, lobster, squid, octopus and cuttlefish); molluscs (cockles, mussels, oysters, scallops and clams) are very low in cholesterol.

Dietary guidelines for prevention of CVD recommend a restriction of cholesterol intake to between 200 and 300 mg/day (NICE, 2010b; NIH, 2002). Mean daily intakes of cholesterol in the UK NDNS were 304 mg for men and 213 mg for women (Henderson et al., 2003). Restriction of dietary cholesterol over and above that found in foods high in saturated fat is unlikely to have a significant influence on blood cholesterol for most individuals (Leeds & Gray, 2001; Durrington, 2007). However, some individuals with inherited forms of raised cholesterol may benefit from additional restriction.

Carbohydrate

Carbohydrate intake has no direct effect on blood cholesterol levels; however, energy consumed from carbohydrates is inversely proportional to the energy derived from fat in the diet. Therefore, an increase in the proportion of energy derived from carbohydrate is often encouraged as a means of reducing the proportion of saturated fat in the diet. Increasing the total amount of dietary carbohydrate consumed, particularly if energy intake is excessive, can elevate endogenous production of triglyc-

eride by the liver as VLDL (Durrington, 2007). The quality of carbohydrate consumed is particularly important as rapidly absorbed refined carbohydrates can exacerbate hypertriglyceridaemia. Patients with raised triglycerides should be encouraged to choose wholegrains and carbohydrates with a low glycaemic index. Replacing fat energy with carbohydrate energy is associated with a decrease in HDL cholesterol of the order of 1 mmol/L per every 10% of energy from dietary fat that is replaced (Durrington, 2007).

Soluble fibre

Water soluble fibre (psyllium, guar, oat bran and pectin) reduces total and LDL cholesterol (Anderson & Hanna, 1999; Brown et al., 1999; Truswell, 2002; Castro et al., 2005), whereas insoluble fibre has no effect. An increase in soluble fibre intake of 5–10 g/day can reduce LDL cholesterol by 5%. In the USA, the Adult Treatment Panel III guidelines recommend a daily intake of 5--10 g of viscous (soluble) fibres (NIH, 2002). In the UK, cereals are the most practical source of soluble fibre (especially whole oats and barley), followed by nuts and legumes. Some fruit and vegetables (okra, aubergine, citrus fruit, apples, bananas, cabbage, carrots, avocado and dried fruit) are good sources.

Obesity

Overweight and obesity are associated with elevated LDL cholesterol, hypertriglyceridaemia and decreased HDL cholesterol (Hecker et al., 1999). Visceral obesity exaggerates lipid changes as a consequence of insulin resistance (Chan et al., 2004; Carmena et al., 2001). For every 1% above desirable body mass index (BMI), the risk of CHD increases by 3.3% for women and 3.6% for men (Anderson & Konz, 2001). Reviews of weight loss studies predict a drop in cholesterol of 0.23 mmol/L for every sustained 10 kg weight loss in obese and severely obese individuals (Poobalan et al., 2004). Reductions in total cholesterol, LDL cholesterol and triglycerides of 1–1.3%, 0.7% and 1.6–1.9%, respectively, per kilogram of weight lost have also been reported (Anderson & Konz, 2001; Aucott et al., 2011). A modest, sustained weight loss of 5–10% of body weight can therefore confer significant benefit (Aronne & Isoldi, 2007). Weight loss that is achieved through exercise is more effective at raising HDL levels than energy intake restriction (Rashid & Genest, 2007) (see Chapter 7.13.1).

Alcohol

Alcohol is a common cause of hypertriglyceridaemia and can also exacerbate existing hypertriglyceridaemia (Durrington, 2007). Complete alcohol avoidance over a month should bring about a significant reduction in triglyceride level and lifelong abstinence may be necessary. Moderate alcohol consumption produces a small increase in serum HDL cholesterol (0.03–0.05 mmol/L) regardless of its source and epidemiological studies have demonstrated a reduction in CHD incidence (Durrington, 2007). The effect is insufficient to justify alcohol intake in those who currently abstain.

Plant sterols and stanols

Plant sterols are chemically similar to cholesterol and perform similar functions in plants (see Chapter 5.2). They are found naturally in vegetable oils, nuts, seeds and grains, with a typical diet containing 146–405 mg, although vegetarian intakes are significantly higher (Cassidy & Dalais, 2003). Both plant sterols and their hydrogenated form (stanols) decrease the absorption of dietary cholesterol and biliary cholesterol by displacing cholesterol within micelles. The unabsorbed cholesterol is eliminated in the faeces along with virtually all the plant sterols and stanols. This inhibition of cholesterol absorption results in a compensatory increase in cholesterol synthesis; however, the overall effect is a reduction in circulating LDL cholesterol of up to 10% within a 2–3-week period.

The effect is dose responsive, with an optimal intake of 2.0–2.5 g/day, but no significant additional effect on cholesterol reduction above 3.0 g/day (Katan *et al.*, 2003; Hallikainen *et al.*, 2000). The health claim '*Plant sterols and plant stanol esters have been shown to lower/reduce blood cholesterol. High cholesterol is a risk factor in the development of coronary heart disease,*' has been approved for fortified foods (fat spreads, yoghurts, milks, cheese) (EFSA, 2010). Since plant sterols and stanols work by mixing with foods within the gut, fortified foods should be taken at meal times.

Plant sterols and stanols can also reduce the absorption of fat soluble vitamins; however, this can easily be compensated for by a diet rich in fruit and vegetables. Foods fortified with sterols/stanols are not recommended in individuals without hypercholesterolaemia or in pregnant and breastfeeding women unless medically advised. Plant sterols are contraindicated in sitosterolanaemia, a very rare metabolic lipid condition estimated to affect only 80–100 people in the world.

Soya protein

Soya is low in saturated fat and cholesterol, is a good source of high quality vegetable protein, dietary fibre, vitamins, minerals and phytonutrients, and has a low glycaemic index. A number of systematic reviews have demonstrated that soya protein can reduce LDL cholesterol (Reynolds *et al.*, 2006; Harland & Haffner, 2008; Zhan & Ho, 2005, Anderson *et al.*, 1995) via two separate mechanisms. First, soya protein is thought to interfere with LDL cholesterol synthesis; second, the inclusion of soya protein alternatives in the diet can result in the displacement of both saturated fat and cholesterol from animal proteins. Together these effects have been estimated to lower LDLcholesterol by up to 10.3% (4.3% intrinsic and 6.0% displacement) (Jenkins *et al.*, 2010). A recent systematic review and meta analysis of 39 studies has shown that even modest intakes of soya proteins (15–25 g) can result in significant reductions in

cholesterol of approximately 6% (Harland & Haffner, 2008).

Nuts

Tree nuts (almond, Brazil, beechnut, cashew, hazelnut, macadamia, pecan, pistachio and walnut) and peanuts (a legume) are rich in energy, with approximately 75% of the energy from fat (predominately monounsaturated). The saturated fat contents are relatively low (approximately 10% of energy) and should not discourage consumption. Epidemiological studies have associated the frequency of nut consumption with a reduced risk of CVD. A pooled analysis of studies identified a dose–response effect with a 35% risk reduction for CHD for those eating the most nuts (Kris-Etherton *et al.*, 2008). Studies of almonds, peanuts, pecans and walnuts have shown a LDL cholesterol lowering effect of 2–19% (Mukuddem-Petersen *et al.*, 2005). The ability of nuts to lower cholesterol may only be partly explained by their favourable lipid profile (Mukuddem-Petersen *et al.*, 2005, Ros *et al.*, 2010, Nash & Nash, 2008). Concerns over the potential of nuts to cause weight gain could be misplaced as several studies have failed to identify weight gain as a consequence of regular consumption (St-Onge, 2005; Higgs, 2005).

Physical activity

Regular physical activity has beneficial effects on lipid metabolism in overweight and obese individuals, and these are independent of weight loss (Shaw *et al.*, 2006). Increasing aerobic activity has been shown to improve lipid profiles in overweight children and teenagers (Kelley & Kelley, 2007a), adults (Durstine *et al.*, 2001) and older adults (Kelley *et al.*, 2005). Beneficial effects have been shown in both primary (Karmisholt *et al.*, 2005) and secondary (Kelley *et al.*, 2006) prevention and in people with diabetes (Kelley & Kelley, 2007b).

Smoking

Smoking suppresses levels of HDL cholesterol and increases LDL oxidation.

Dietary regimens

Mediterranean diet

The Mediterranean diet describes a pattern of eating that is high in monounsaturated fatty acids (from olives and olive oil), rich in fruit, vegetables, whole grain cereals, low fat dairy products, fish, poultry, nuts and pulses with moderate alcohol consumption and is relatively low in red meat. This dietary pattern was first described in the 7 Countries Study when differences in mean age, blood pressure, serum cholesterol and smoking habits were shown to explain 80% of variance of death from CHD in a 15-year observational study of over 11,000 middle aged men (Keys *et al.*, 1986). Adherence to a Mediterranean style diet is consistent with a reduced prevalence and progression of metabolic syndrome, and favourable improvements in components of metabolic syndrome, e.g. HDL cholesterol, triglycerides, blood pressure, blood glucose and waist circumference (Kastorini *et al.*, 2010).

Portfolio diet

A number of individual dietary components have been shown to have an additive cholesterol lowering effect. The portfolio diet combines specific daily quantities of these (14–23 g of almonds, 1 g of plant sterols, 22.5 g of soya protein and 10 g of soluble fibre per 4.2 MJ (1000 kcal), together with a low saturated fat diet (<7% energy), low dietary cholesterol (<200 mg) and 5–10 portions of fruit, vegetables and pulses (Jenkins *et al.*, 2006). Reductions in cholesterol of up to 35% have been demonstrated in metabolic studies (Jenkins *et al.*, 2003a). In free living populations, average cholesterol reductions of 12–14% were observed. The percentage cholesterol reduction was linked to the degree of adherence to the diet (Jenkins *et al.*, 2006; 2011), with one-third achieving a >20% reduction in LDL cholesterol at 1 year (Jenkins *et al.*, 2006).

Ultimate Cholesterol Lowering Plan

The Ultimate Cholesterol Lowering Plan (UCLP) combines a step by step approach to cholesterol lowering with motivational interviewing techniques. It is a modified portfolio diet that encourages patient compliance through discussion, patient choice and commitment to a range of small dietary changes. The baseline diet (<10% of energy from saturated fat; five portions of fruit and vegetables, one of pulses and two of fish, one of which is oily) can be enhanced by including one or more of the four cholesterol lowering food types (15–25 g of soya protein, 1.5–2.4 g of plant sterols/stanols, 30 g of nuts and 15–20 g of soluble fibre).

Diagnosis, classification and management

Blood biochemistry

A full lipid profile, using venous blood serum, is necessary to aid diagnosis and management of lipid disorders. This should include the follow serum measurements:

- Total cholesterol (mmol/L).
- HDL cholesterol (mmol/L).
- LDL cholesterol (mmol/L) (by Friedwall calculation) or non-HDL cholesterol.
- Total to HDL cholesterol ratio (by calculation).
- Triglycerides – levels are raised following a meal so measurements should be made in a fasting state.
- Apolipoproteins – depending on the clinical circumstances.

Cholesterol targets are shown in Table 7.14.12.

Screening is often carried out at events, in primary care and pharmacies; however, this relies on trained staff using regularly calibrated portable point of care testing equipment and capillary samples of blood. Therefore, screening is only helpful to highlight those who may be at higher risk of dyslipidaemia and a full fasting lipid profile is still

Table 7.14.12 Cholesterol targets (NICE, 2010a; Joint British Societies, 2005)

	Individuals at low risk	Secondary prevention or individuals at high risk* of cardiovascular disease (CVD)
Total serum cholesterol	<5 mmol/L	<4 mmol/L (or a 25% reduction)
LDL cholesterol	<3 mmol/L	<2 mmol/L (or a 30% reduction)
HDL cholesterol		>1.0 mmol/L (men) >1.2 mmol/L (women)

*Individuals with CVD, diabetes, other atherosclerotic disease or an absolute risk of CVD of 20% or more over 10 years.

required to aid diagnosis and management. Home testing kits are not recommended due to their variable results.

Monitoring

Small variations in cholesterol and triglyceride resulting from changes in diet can be difficult to demonstrate due to the variability in many factors including:

- Normal variation in testing of approximately 7% (i.e. a mean total cholesterol of 6.5 mmol/L can fluctuate by ± 0.5 mmol/L).
- Menstrual cycle (cholesterol and triglycerides peak mid cycle).
- Seasonal variations (highest in winter and lowest in summer, perhaps reflecting changes in diet and body weight).
- Interlaboratory variations.
- Illness or trauma (can reduce cholesterol and raise triglycerides).

Clinical features

Dyslipidaemia is usually symptomless and can therefore go undiagnosed; a heart attack may be the first symptom. Specific signs and symptoms usually only occur if the increase in lipid level is severe over a prolonged period. Very high cholesterol levels may result in:

- *Xanthomata* – small soft deposits of cholesterol, sometimes seen as a uniform thickening of the Achilles tendon or as nodules in the tendons of the fingers (tendon xanthomata). Palmar xanthomata may be seen as yellow lines in the creases in the palm of the hand. Tuberose xanthomata occur in the form of masses around the elbows or knees.
- *Corneal arcus* – a white ring visible around the iris of the eye.
- *Xanthelasma* – small soft yellow deposits of cholesterol and other fatty substances found in the skin, often on the eyelids.

Very high triglyceride levels may result in:

- *Small yellow papules with a faint red halo* – often found on the skin of the buttocks, thighs and elbows.

Table 7.14.13 Fredrickson classification of dyslipidaemia

Phenotype: Fredrickson type	I	IIa	IIb	III	IV	V
Increased lipid fraction	Chylomicrons	LDL	LDL and VLDL	IDL	Triglycerides	VLDL and chylomicrons

LDL, low density lipoprotein; VLDL, very low density lipoprotein, IDL, intermediate density lipoprotein.

Table 7.14.14 Aetiological classifications of dyslipidaemia

Elevated cholesterol	Familial hypercholesterolaemia (FH) – single gene alteration Polygenic hypercholesterolaemia – influenced by several genes
Elevated triglycerides	Familial lipoprotein lipase deficiency (familial hypertriglyceridaemia) – single gene Polygenic hypertriglyceridaemia – influenced by several genes
Elevated cholesterol and triglycerides	Familial combined hyperlipidaemia (FCH) Familial dyslipoproteinaemia (broad beta disease) is an additional but rare type

- *Lipaemia retinalis* – plasma lipids visible in the retinal veins and arteries.
- *Acute pancreatitis* – sudden onset inflammation of the pancreas.
- *Hepatosplenomegaly* – enlargement of the liver and spleen.

Classification of primary (familial) dyslipidaemia

The classification and definitions of dyslipidaemia vary. Historically, primary disorders of lipid metabolism were categorised on the basis of the type of lipoprotein fraction that is raised (Frederickson classification), as shown in Table 7.14.13. While this is still used occasionally, a method of classification based on aetiology (genetic cause and the type of lipid raised) is recommended (Table 7.14.14).

Elevated cholesterol

Familial hypercholesterolaemia

Familial hypercholesterolaemia (FH) has a prevalence of 1 in 500 people and is caused by an autosomal dominant gene. It dramatically increases the risk of premature CHD before the age of 50 years (and may be as early as 20–40 years), accounting for 5–10% of early CHD deaths (Holmes *et al.*, 2011). If untreated, sufferers are eight times more like to die from CHD, but when treated early they will have a normal lifespan (Holmes *et al.*, 2011). It is usual for LDL cholesterol levels to be raised from birth and these are two to three times higher than normal.

Carriers of this gene have fewer LDL receptors, which normally take LDL out of the blood, on the surface of liver cells, or their functionality is reduced. Most people have heterozygous FH but one in a million have a more severe form (homozygous or compound heterozygous FH). In the latter cases, plasma cholesterol levels may be as high as 20–30 mmol/L.

Familial hypercholesterolaemia is often accompanied by xanthomata and corneal arcus in undiagnosed individuals. Diagnosis of FH relies on the Simon Broome criteria and/or genetic testing (NICE, 2008). Children from affected parents should be tested early, ideally between 2 and 9 years of age. Treatment with a statin can be started as early as childhood, although some patients are not responsive to statins.

Polygenic hypercholesterolaemia

Polygenic hypercholesterolaemia is common and is characterised by raised total and LDL cholesterol levels (with normal HDL cholesterol and triglyceride levels). Clinical signs such as xanthomas are rare and LDL cholesterol is elevated to a lesser extent. Polygenic hypercholesterolaemia results from several genetic factors and their interaction with environmental, largely nutritional, factors (see Chapter 5.1). Treatment is based on overall cardiovascular risk.

Elevated triglycerides

Familial lipoprotein lipase deficiency

Familial lipoprotein lipase deficiency (LPLD) has a prevalence of 1 in 1 000 000. Severe hypertriglyceridaemia results from a congenital deficiency (autosomal recessive) of the lipoprotein lipase gene and is characterised by the presence of chylomicrons in fasting plasma. Levels of triglycerides are raised from childhood, but the condition may not be picked up until adulthood. Symptoms include recurrent abdominal pain, eruptive xanthomata and attacks of acute pancreatitis. Most medications have only modest benefits. The main treatment is a low fat diet (20–40 g/day) but occasionally restrictions to 10 g of fat or less may be required. Medium chain triglycerides (MCTs) should be consumed with caution as they can exacerbate triglyceride levels (Durrington, 2007). At very low fat intakes, supplements of essential fatty acids and fat soluble vitamins are required. Sufferers are at risk of developing type 1 diabetes.

Polygenic hypertriglyceridaemia

This is a group of disorders in which a genetic disposition interacts with environmental factors such as diet; the prevalence is 1 in 100. Plasma triglycerides are elevated with a normal to slightly elevated cholesterol. Reduction

SECTION 7

of body weight is a key element of management; fish oils may also be prescribed.

Severe polygenic hypertriglyceridaemia (chylomicronaemia syndrome)

This is characterised by a gross accumulation of triglyceride rich VLDL and chylomicrons, and has a prevalence of 1 in 50–100 000; cholesterol is moderately elevated. Uncontrolled diabetes mellitus is often the precipitating factor in those who already have the genetic predisposition.

Elevated cholesterol and triglycerides

Familial combined hyperlipidaemia

Familial combined hyperlipidaemia (FCH) is a common disorder (prevalence 1 in 100) characterised by raised levels of VLDL triglyceride and LDL cholesterol, and low HDL cholesterol. The condition is associated with an increased risk of CHD and is usually diagnosed in adulthood. Environmental factors appear to play a significant role in its expression as people with FCH are often hypertensive and overweight, and may be insulin resistant, have diabetes or gout.

Familial dysbetalipoproteinaemia (broad beta disease, remnant removal disease, floating beta disease, Fredrickson type III)

This is a rare polygenic disorder (prevalence is <1 in 5000) in which abnormal IDL accumulates. This results in the accumulation of broad beta-lipoprotein that carries roughly equal amounts of cholesterol and triglyceride. Intermittent claudication and CHD are equally common symptoms (Durrington & Sniderman, 2005).

Secondary (acquired) dyslipidaemias

Secondary dyslipidaemias can mimic primary dyslipidaemias and have similar consequences, resulting in increased risk of premature CVD or (in the case of high levels of triglycerides) pancreatitis (Table 7.14.15). Treatment of

Table 7.14.15 Conditions and drugs commonly associated with changes in lipid levels (Durrington & Sniderman, 2005)

Condition	Raised cholesterol	Raised triglycerides	Reduced HDL
Obesity	X	X	
Excess alcohol intake		X	
Diabetes, metabolic syndrome		X	X
Hypothyroid	X	X	
Anorexia nervosa	X		
Pituitary disease		X	
Cushing's syndrome	X		
Pregnancy	X	X	
Renal disease – nephrotic syndrome	X		
Renal disease – renal failure		X	
Cholestasis	X		
Cholelithiasis, hepatocellular disease		X	
Pancreatitis		X	
Immune disorders – myeloma, macroglobulinaemia, lupus	X	X	
Hyperuricaemia, gout		X	
Drugs			
Beta-blockers		X	
Thiazide diuretics	X	X	
Microsomal enzyme inducing agents (phenytoin, phenobarbitone, griseofulvin)	X		
Retinoic acid derivatives		X	
HIV antiretroviral therapy	X	X	
Oestrogen		X	
Progesterone	X		
Anabolic steroids	X		X
Amiodarone (antiarrhythmic agent)	X		
Antipsychotic drugs, e.g. olanzapine, clozapine	X		

HDL, high density lipoprotein.

the underlying condition or discontinuation of the offending drugs usually leads to an improvement in the dyslipidaemia. Specific lipid lowering therapy may be required in certain circumstances.

Diabetes and metabolic syndrome

Patients with metabolic syndrome and diabetes are at increased CHD risk with insulin resistance resulting in increased lipid levels. Dyslipidaemia in diabetes and metabolic syndrome is characterised by raised triglycerides, low HDL cholesterol and increased small dense LDL particles. Dyslipidaemia is often present in type I diabetes but HDL levels may be increased or normal (Durrington & Sniderman, 2005).

Drug treatment

Lipid lowering drugs are being increasingly used in the treatment of dyslipidaemia, in patients with established CHD or those at significant risk of developing CHD. They include statins, fibrates and cholesterol absorption inhibitors.

Statins (HMG CoA reductase inhibitors)

Statins are now routinely prescribed for the management of dyslipidaemia and have been shown to significantly reduce the risk of vascular events in those at high risk (Durrington & Sniderman, 2005). Statin therapy is considered cost effective once the absolute risk of CVD exceeds 20% over a 10-year period (equivalent to a CHD risk of 15% or more over 10 years) (NICE, 2010b). Statins reduce LDL cholesterol levels by up to 60% by blocking the enzyme (HMG CoA reductase) in the cholesterol production pathway in the liver. Reduced endogenous cholesterol production causes the liver to take up more cholesterol from the blood by activating the LDL receptor genes. This increases the number of LDL receptors on the surface of the liver, which in turn increases uptake and consequently lowers LDL cholesterol levels. A reduction in blood cholesterol levels occur after 4–6 weeks and longer periods are needed to reduce tissue levels. Statins also help to stabilise atheroma, improve endothelial function and have anti-inflammatory, antioxidant and antithrombotic effects. They can increase HDL cholesterol by about 5% and moderately lower triglycerides.

Statins are generally well tolerated and relatively free of side effects. Occasionally, side effects such as muscle related pain (myopathy) have been reported at higher statin doses. This is usually related to an increase in the muscle enzyme creatinine kinase (CK); elevations of CK (over 10 times normal) should be investigated.

In the UK, atorvastatin, simvastatin, pravastatin, fluvastatin and rosuvastatin are available. Clients taking simvastatin or atorvastatin need to avoid or restrict their intake of grapefruit juice, respectively, as it reduces metabolism and therefore potentiates their effects.

Fibrates

These drugs, e.g. bezafibrate and gemfibrozil, are generally used for mixed dyslipidaemias, and are often used in conjunction with statins in diabetic patients where serum triglycerides are significantly raised. They are effective in reducing triglycerides (by reducing VLDL), improving LDL quality and increasing HDL cholesterol.

Cholesterol absorption inhibitors

Cholesterol absorption inhibitors, e.g. ezetimibe, act at the brush border of the small intestine and prevent the absorption of cholesterol; their cholesterol lowering ability is approximately 18% (Reckless & Morrell, 2005). They are often prescribed when statins are not tolerated or alongside a lower statin dose.

Other drug treatments

Other classes of lipid lowering drugs available include:

- *Nicotinic acid (niacin)* – inhibits triglyceride breakdown and the release of free fatty acids from adipose tissue. It is used to treat hypertriglyceridaemia and mixed dyslipidaemias.
- *Resins or bile acid sequestrants (cholestyramine, colestipol)* – used widely to treat hypercholesterolaemia before statins are prescribed, but were poorly tolerated. A non-absorbed lipid lowering polymer (olesevelam) is better tolerated.
- *Omacor (EPA and DHA)* – has beneficial effects on serum triglyceride levels, but may be poorly tolerated at the high dosage required (2–4 g).
- *Fish oil* – can be prescribed, but >10 mL is needed to provide sufficient EPA and DHA to lower triglycerides. This amount can lead to unacceptable intakes of other fatty acids and dioxins, as well as unpleasant fish odours.

Low density lipoprotein apheresis

Apheresis involves whole blood undergoing a procedure via an external machine, in a manner similar to renal dialysis, on a regular basis so that LDL cholesterol is extracted. It may be used where cholesterol levels remain high or are resistant to statins; however, this technique is not widely available in the UK.

Dietary treatment

A summary of dietary advice for the management of dyslipidaemias is shown in Table 7.14.16. Table 7.14.17 summarises the evidence for the use of dietary interventions.

Drug–nutrient interactions

Grapefruit juice reduces the metabolism of simvastatin and atorvastatin, and therefore potentiates their effects.

Table 7.14.16 Summary of dietary advice for the management of dyslipidaemia

Raised total and LDL cholesterol (with normal HDL cholesterol and triglyceride levels)	Moderately raised triglyceride levels (with normal total, LDL and HDL cholesterol levels)	Raised total and LDL cholesterol and raised triglyceride levels	Low HDL cholesterol
Reduce saturated fat intake Partial substitution of saturated with polyunsaturated and monounsaturated fats, to a level of energy intake appropriate for body weight Encourage the consumption of foods that actively lower cholesterol Moderate intake of dietary cholesterol only if excessive and in familial hypercholesterolaemia if failing to achieve target levels	If obese, weight loss is the overriding treatment priority Energy reduction should come from a reduction in saturated and total fat, and refined carbohydrate, and activity should be increased Remaining carbohydrates should be from more complex sources, especially those with a low glycaemic index Encourage oily fish Reduce or avoid alcohol intake	If obese, weight loss is the overriding treatment priority Reduce saturated and total fat intake Partial substitution with polyunsaturated and monounsaturated fats to a level of energy intake appropriate for body weight Encourage the consumption of foods that actively lower cholesterol Replace high intakes of refined carbohydrates with more complex sources of carbohydrate, especially those with a low glycaemic index Reduce or avoid alcohol Moderate intake of dietary cholesterol if excessive	Modest alcohol intake (1–3 units/day) is acceptable Ensure that total fat intake is not reduced too low, i.e. that some saturated fats are replaced with monounsaturated fats If polyunsaturated fat intake is high, partially substitute with monounsaturates Stop smoking (this depresses HDL cholesterol) Encourage physical activity

Table 7.14.17 Current scientific evidence to support dietary recommendations for total fat and fatty acid intake in adults (FAO/WHO, 2008)

	Convincing	Probable	Possible
Total fat		No relation with CHD events or fatal CHD	
Saturated fatty acids (SFAs)	Increases LDL and TC:HDL ratio when compared to PUFA and MUFA		Increases risk of diabetes
Monounsaturated fatty acids (MUFAs)	Decreases LDL and TC:HDL ratio when substituted for SFA		Reduces risk of metabolic syndrome
Total polyunsaturated fatty acids (PUFAs)	Decreases LDL and TC:HDL ratio when substituted for SFA Reduces risk of CHD events		Reduces risk of metabolic syndrome Increases lipid oxidation with high consumption especially if vitamin E intake is low
n-6 PUFA	Decreases LDL and TC:HDL ratio when substituted for SFA Reduces risk of CHD events	Reduces risk of metabolic syndrome	
n-3 PUFA	Reduces risk of CHD events (DHA and EPA)		Decreases risk of total CHD events and stroke
Trans fats	Lowers HDL and increases TC:HDL ratio in comparison to SFA, MUFA and PUFA Increases risk of CHD events	Increases risk of metabolic syndrome Increases risk of fatal CHD and sudden cardiac death	

CHD, coronary heart disease; TC, triglyceride; HDL, high density lipoprotein; DHA, docosahexaenoic acid; EPA, eicosapentaenoic acid.

Internet resources

HEART UK – The Cholesterol Charity   www.heartuk.org.uk
British Heart Foundation   www.bhf.org.uk

References

Anderson J, Hanna T. (1999) Impact of nondigestible carbohydrates on serum lipoproteins and risk for cardiovascular disease *Journal of Nutrition* 129: 1457S–1466S.

Anderson J, Konz E. (2001) Obesity and disease management: effects of weight loss on comorbid conditions. *Obesity Research* 9: 326S–334S.

Anderson J, Johnstone B, Cook-Newell M. (1995) Meta-analysis of the effects of soy protein intake on serum lipids. *New England Journal of Medicine* 333: 276–282.

Aronne L, Isoldi K. (2007) Overweight and obesity: key components of cardiometabolic risk. *Clinical Cornerstone* 8: 29–37.

Assmann G, Schulte H, Eckardstein AV. (1996) Hypertriglyceridemia and elevated lipoprotein (a) are risk factors for major coronary events in middle-aged men. *American Journal of Cardiology* 77: 1179–1184.

Astrup A, Dyerberg J, Elwood P, et al. (2011) The role of reducing intakes of saturated fat in the prevention of cardiovascular disease: where does the evidence stand in 2010. *Americal Journal of Clinical Nutrition* 93: 684–688.

Aucott L, Gray D, Rothnie H, Thapa, M, Waweru C. (2011) Effects of lifestyle interventions and long-term weight loss on lipid outcomes – a systematic review. *Obesity Reviews* 12(5): e412–425.

Bates B, Lennox A, Swan G. (2010) *National Diet and Nutrition Survey: Headline results from Year 1 of the rolling programme (2008/2009)*. London: Food Standards Agency.

Brown L, Rosner B, Willett W, Sacks F. (1999) Cholesterol lowering effects of dietary fibre: A meta-analysis. *Americal Journal of Clinical Nutrition* 69: 30–42.

Carmena R, Ascaso J, Real J. (2001) Impact of obesity in primary hyperlipidemias. *Nutrition Metabolism and Cardiovascular Diseases* 11: 354–359.

Cassidy A, Dalais F. (2003) *Nutrition and Metabolism – Phytochemicals,* Oxford: Blackwell Science

Castro IA, Barroso LP, Sinnecker P. (2005) Functional foods for coronary heart disease risk reduction: a meta-analysis using a multivariate approach. *American Journal Clinical Nutrition* 82(1): 32–40.

Chan D, Barrett H, Watts G. (2004) Dyslipidemia in visceral obesity: mechanisms, implications, and therapy. *American Journal of Cardiovascular Drugs* 4: 227–246.

CTTC. (2005) Efficacy and safety of cholesterol-lowering treatment: prospective meta-analysis of dats from 90,056 participants 1n 14 randomised trials of statins. *Lancet* 366: 1267–1278.

Department of Health (COMA). (1994) *Nutritional Aspects of Cardiovascular Disease*. London: HMSO.

Durrington PN. (2007) *Hyperlipidaemia: Diagnosis and Management*, 3rd edn. London: Hodder Arnold.

Durrington P, Sniderman A. (2005) *Hyperlipidaemia*. Oxford: Health Press Limited.

Durstine J, Grandjean P, Davis P, Ferguson M, Alderson N, Du Bose K. (2001) Blood lipid and lipoprotein adaptations to exercise: a quantitative analysis. *Sports Medicine* 31: 1033–1062.

EFSA. (2010) Commission Regulation (EU) No 384/2010. *Official Journal of the European Union* 53.

FAO/WHO. (2008) *Interim Summary of Conclusions and Dietary Recommendation on Total Fat and Fatty Acids* – From the joint FAO/WHO Expert Consultation on Fats and Fatty Acids in Human Nutrition 10–14 November 2008. Geneva: WHO.

Hallikainen MA, Sarkkinen ES, Gylling H, Erkkila AT, Uusitupa MI. (2000) Comparison of the effects of plant sterol ester and plant stanol ester-enriched margarines in lowering serum cholesterol concentrations in hypercholesterolaemic subjects on a low fat diet. *European Journal Clinical Nutrition* 54(9): 715–725.

Harland J, Haffner T. (2008) Systematic review, meta-analysis and regression of randomised controlled trials reporting an association between an intake circa 25g soy protein per day and blood cholesterol. *Atherosclerosis* 200: 13–27.

HEARTUK. (2007) *Cholesterol and the Ageing Population*. Available at http://heartuk.org.uk/images/uploads/aboutuspdfs/Cholesterol CrisisReport_070219.pdf. Accessed 2 September 2013.

Hecker K, Pm KE, Zhao G, Coval S, St-Jeor S. (1999) Impact of body weight and weight loss on cardiovascular risk factors. *Current Atherosclerosis Reports* 1: 236–242.

Henderson L, Gregory J, Irving K, Swan G. (2003) *The National Diet and Nutrition Survey: adults aged 19–64 years: Energy, protein, carbohydrate, fat and alcohol intake.* Food Standards Agency, D. O. H., Office for National Statistics, Medical Research Council Human Nutrition Research. London: The Stationery Office.

Higgs J. (2005) The potential role of peanuts in the prevention of obesity. *Nutrition and Food Science* 35: 353–358.

Hokanson J, Austin M. (1996) Plasma triglyceride level is a risk factor for cardiovascular disease independent of high density lipoprotein cholesterol level: a meta analysis of population based prospective studies. *Journal of Cardiovascular Risk* 3: 213–219.

Holmes MV, Harrison S, Talmud PJ, Hingorani AD, Humphries SE. (2011) Utility of genetic determinants of lipids and cardiovascular events in assessing risk. *Nature Reviews Cardioliology* 8: 207–221.

Hooper L, Summerbell CD, Higgins JP, et al. (2001a) Dietary fat intake and prevention of cardiovascular disease: systematic review. *BMJ* 322 757–763.

Hooper L, Summerbell CD, Higgins JP, et al. (2001b) Reduced or modified dietary fat for preventing cardiovascular disease. *Cochrane Database of Systematic Reviews* 3: CD003305.

Hooper L, Thompson RL, Harrison RA, et al. (2004) Omega 3 fats for the treatment and prevention of cardiovascular disease *Cochrane Database of Systematic Reviews* 4: CD003177.

Joint British Societies. (2005) JBS2: Joint British Societies' guidelines on prevention of cardiovascular disease in clinical practice. *Heart* 91: (Suppl 5): v1–v52.

Jenkins D, Kendall C, Marchie A, et al. (2002) Dose response of almonds on coronary heart disease risk factors: Blood lipids, low density lipoproteins, lipoprotein(a), homocysteine and pulmonary nitric oxide: A randomised, controlled, crossover trial. *Circulation* 106: 1327–1332.

Jenkins D, Kendall C, Marchie A, Al E. (2003a) The effect of combining plant sterols, soy protein, viscous fibers, and almonds in treating hypercholesterolemia. *Metabolism* 52: 1478–1483.

Jenkins D, Kendall C, Marchie A, et al. (2003b) Effects of dietary portfolio of cholestetrol-lowering foods vs lovastatin on serum lipids and C-reactive protein. *JAMA* 290: 502–510.

Jenkins D, Kendall C, Faulkner D, et al. (2006) Assessment of the longer-term effects of a dietary portfolio of cholesterol-lowering foods in hypercholesterolaemia. *Americal Journal of Clinical Nutrition* 83: 582–591.

Jenkins D, Mirrahimi A, Srichaikul K, et al. (2010) Soy protein reduces serum cholesterol by both intrinsic and food displacement mechanisms. *Journal of Nutrition* 140(12): 2302S–2311S.

Jenkins DJA, Jones PJ, Lamarche B, Al E. (2011) Effect of a dietary portfolio of cholesterol lowering foods given at 2 levels of intensity of dietary advice on serum lipids in hyperlipidaemia *JAMA* 306: 831–839.

Kannel WB, Ramachandran VS. (2009) Triglycerides as vascular risk factors: new epidemiologic insights for current opinion in cardiology. *Current Opinion Cardiology* 24: 345–350.

Karmisholt K, Gyntelberg F, Gøtzche P. (2005) Physical activity for primary prevention of disease. Systematic reviews of randomised clinical trials. *Danish Medical Bulletin* 52(2): 86–89.

Kastorini CM, Milionis HK, Esposito K, Giugliano D, Goudevenos JA, Panagiotakos DB. (2010). The effect of Mediterranean diet on metabolic syndrome and its components: A meta-analysis of 50 studies and 534,906 Individuals. *Journal of the American College of Cardiology* 57: 1299–1313.

Katan MB, Grundy SM, Willett WC. (1997) Should a low-fat, high-carbohydrate diet be recommended for everyone? Beyond low-fat diets. *New England Journal of Medicine* 337: 563–566.

Katan MB, Grundy SM, Jones P, Law M, Miettinen T, Paoletti R; Stresa Workshop Participants. (2003) Efficacy and safety of plant stanols and sterols in the management of blood cholesterol levels. *Mayo Clinic Proceedings* 78(8): 965–978.

Kelley G, Kelley K. (2007a) Aerobic exercise and lipids and lipoproteins in children and adolescents: a meta-analysis of randomized controlled trials. *Atherosclerosis* 191: 447–453.

Kelley G, Kelley K. (2007b) Effects of aerobic exercise on lipids and lipoproteins in adults with type 2 diabetes: a meta-analysis of randomized-controlled trials. *Public Health* 121: 643–655.

Kelley G, Kelley K, Tran Z. (2005) Exercise, lipids, and lipoproteins in older adults: a meta-analysis. *Preventative Cardiology* 8: 206–214.

Kelley G, Kelley K, Franklin B. (2006) Aerobic exercise and lipids and lipoproteins in patients with cardiovascular disease: a meta-analysis of randomized controlled trials. *Journal of Cardiopulmonary Rehabilitation and Prevention* 26: 131–139.

Keys A, Menotti A, Karvonen M, Al E. (1986) The diet and 15-year death rate in the seven countries study. *American Journal of Epidemiology* 124: 903–915.

Kris-Etherton P, Hu F, Ros E, Sabate J. (2008) The role of tree nuts and peanuts in the prevention of coronary heart disease: Multiple potential mechanisms. *Journal of Nutrition* 138: 1746S.

Leeds A, Gray J. (2001) *Dietary Cholesterol as a Cardiac Risk Factor.* Huntingdon: Smith-Gordon & Co Ltd.

Mukuddem-Petersen J, Oosthuizen W, Jerling J. (2005) A systematic review of the effects of nuts on lipid profiles in humans. *Journal of Nutrition* 135: 2082–2089.

Nash S, Nash D. (2008) Nuts as part of a healthy cardiovascular diet. *Current Atherosclerosis Reports* 10: 529–535.

National Institute for Health and Care Excellence (NICE). (2007) MI secondary prevention. Avaiable at www.nice.org.uk.

National Institute for Health and Care Excellence (NICE). (2008) Familial hypercholesterolaemia CG71. Avaiable at www.nice.org.uk

National Institute for Health and Care Excellence (NICE). (2010a). Lipid modification. Avaiable at www.nice.org.uk

National Institute for Health and Care Excellence (NICE). (2010b) Prevention of cardiovascular disease at population level. Avaiable at www.nice.org.uk.

National Institutes of Health (NIH). (2002) *Third report of the National Cholesterol Education Program (NCEP) Expert Panel on Detection, Evaluation and treatment of High Blood Cholesterol in Adults (Adult Treatment Panel III).* Bethesda: NIH.

Oomen C, Ocke M, Feskens E, Erp-Baart M, Kok F, Kromhout D. (2001) Association between trans fatty acid intake and 10 year risk of coronary heart disease in Zutphen Elderly Study: A prospective population based study. *Lancet* 357: 746–751.

Poobalan A, Aucott L, Smith W, *et al.* (2004) Effects of weight loss in overweight/obese individuals and long-term lipid outcomes–a systematic review. *Obesity Reviews* 5: 43–50.

Rashid S, Genest J. (2007) Effect of obesity on high-density lipoprotein metabolism. *Obesity* 15: 2875–2888.

Reckless J, Morrell J. (2005) *Lipid Disorders – Your Questions Answered.* London: Churchill Livingstone.

Reynolds K, Chin A, Leees K, Nguyen A, Bujnowski D, He J. (2006) A Meta-analysis of the effect of soy protein supplementation on serum lipids. *American Journal of Cardiology* 98: 633–640.

Roche HM, Gibney MJ. (2000) Effect of long-chain n-3 polyunsaturated fatty acids on fasting and postprandial triacylglycerol metabolism. *American Journal of Clinical Nutrition* 71(S1): 232S–237S.

Ros E, Tapsell L, Sabate J. (2010) Nuts and berries for heart health. *Current Atherosclerosis Reports* 12: 397–406.

Scientific Advisory Committee on Nutrition (SACN). (2007) *Update on Trans Fatty Acids and Health: Position Statement by the Scientific Advisory Committee on Nutrition.* SACN.

Shaw K, Gennat H, O'Rourke P, elMar C. (2006) Exercise for Overweight or Obesity. *Cochrane Database of Systematic Reviews* 3: CD003817.

St-Onge M. (2005) Dietary fats, teas, dairy, and nuts: potential functional foods for weight control. *Americal Journal of Clinical Nutrition* 81: 7–15.

Stampfer M, Krauss R, Ma J, *et al.* (1996) A prospective study of triglyceride level, low-density lipoprotein particle diameter, and risk of myocardial infarction. *JAMA* 276: 882–888.

Teslovich TM, Musunuru K, Smith AV, Al E. (2010) Biological, clinical and population relevance of 95 loci for blood lipids. *Nature* 466: 707–713.

Truswell AS. (2002) Cereal grains and coronary heart disease. *European Journal of Clinical Nutrition* 56 (1): 1–14.

World Health Organization (WHO). (2002) *Reducing Risks Promoting Healthy Lives.* Geneva: WHO.

World Health Organization (WHO). (2008) *The Global Burden of Disease: 2004 Update.* Geneva: WHO.

Zhan S, Ho S. (2005) Meta-analysis of the effects of soy protein containing isoflavones on lipid profile. *Americal Journal of Clinical Nutrition* 81: 397–408.

7.14.4 Hypertension

Karin Harnden

Key points

- Hypertension is a major risk factor for cardiovascular disease; it greatly increases the risk of premature death from coronary heart disease and stroke.

- Over 29% of the adult UK population has hypertension or is on antihypertensive medication.

- Obesity, physical inactivity, high salt intake and excessive alcohol consumption are major contributory factors to the development of hypertension.

- Hypertension should be treated in the context of overall cardiovascular risk.

- Diet and lifestyle modification is an integral part of the management of all hypertensive patients, whether on drug therapy or not.

Hypertension (high blood pressure) is a major risk factor for stroke, myocardial infarction (MI), heart failure, chronic kidney disease, peripheral vascular disease, cognitive decline and premature death (NICE, 2011). Globally, about 51% of strokes and 45% of cases of coronary heart disease (CHD) are estimated to be attributable to high systolic blood pressure (WHO, 2009). In people with diabetes, hypertension significantly increases the risk of both cardiovascular and microvascular complications, particularly diabetic nephropathy. Hypertension is one of the most important preventable causes of premature morbidity and mortality worldwide (NICE, 2011). Hypertension is responsible for 13% of global mortality (WHO, 2009).

Definition

Blood pressure is a measurement of the force exerted by the blood circulating in the arteries. The force with which the heart pumps blood, the diameter of the blood vessels and the volume of circulating blood influence blood pressure. When taking a blood pressure reading two figures are recorded:

- Systolic pressure (SBP) – the force during contraction of the heart ventricles.
- Diastolic pressure (DBP) – the blood pressure during relaxation of the heart ventricles.

The pressures are measured in millimetres of mercury (mmHg) and expressed as systolic/diastolic. Readings vary from day to day, and repeated measurements on two or more separate occasions are necessary to establish the usual blood pressure for an individual. Twenty-four hour ambulatory blood pressure monitoring (ABPM) is increasingly being used to confirm the diagnosis of hypertension.

Definitions of normal and abnormal blood pressure are summarised in the British Hypertension Society Guidelines (Williams et al., 2004) and updated in the National Institute for Health and Care Excellence (NICE, 2011) guidelines on the clinical management of primary hypertension in adults, as shown in Table 7.14.18. Similar guidance has been produced by European and WHO expert committees (Mancia et al., 2007; Subcommittee, 1999). In healthy adults, optimal systolic blood pressure is considered to be below 120 mmHg and diastolic pressure below 80 mmHg (120/80). Hypertension is usually symptomless and often only discovered as a result of routine health screening or when overt signs of cardiovascular disease (CVD) develop.

Prevalence

Based on the criteria of SBP >140 mmHg and/or DBP >90 mmHg, in 2009 32.0% of men and 26.9% of women in England were hypertensive or on hypertensive medication (Health Survey for England, 2009). Prevalence rose steeply with age so that by the age of 75 years, 73.3% of men and 64.3% of women had high blood pressure. Prevalence was higher among men than women at all ages, except in the 65–75 year age group. The prevalence of hypertension in childhood is increasing (Din-Dzietham et al., 2007). Raised blood pressure levels in childhood are associated with higher levels in adulthood (Chen & Wang, 2008).

There are genetic influences on blood pressure and the susceptibility to hypertension, and these may be particularly marked in some minority ethnic groups, particularly people of African-Caribbean origin (Agyemang & Bhopal, 2003). In the UK, the two main minority ethnic groups are African Caribbean and South Asian. Khan & Beevers (2005) found the prevalence of hypertension to be 2.6 times higher in the African-Caribbean population and 1.8 times higher in South Asians than in the white population. Mortality due to hypertensive complications in England and Wales is 3.5 times higher in the African-Caribbean population and 1.5 times higher in Asians than the national average (Raleigh, 1997).

Prognostic significance

Hypertension, smoking and raised blood cholesterol are the three main modifiable risk factors for CHD, and hypertension is the single biggest risk factor for stroke. People with hypertension are three times more likely to develop heart disease and stroke, and twice as likely to die from these diseases as people with normal levels (SACN, 2003). The increased risk of cardiovascular events is associated with both SBP and DBP. The risk increases progressively throughout the range of usual blood pressure, starting at about 115/75 mm/Hg (Chobanian et al., 2003; Lewington et al., 2002; Klag et al., 1996). Meta analysis of prospective data from one million adults has shown that each 20 mmHg increase in usual SBP or 10 mmHg increase in DBP doubles the risk of death from CVD (Lewington et al., 2002).

Reducing blood pressure, particularly SBP, significantly reduces the risk of coronary heart disease and stroke (Wang et al., 2005; Turnbull, 2003; Neal et al., 2000). Reducing blood pressure by 10 mmHg can reduce stroke by 41% and CHD events by 22% (Law et al., 2009). In people with diabetes, treatment of hypertension also reduces the risk of diabetic microvascular complications as well as CVD (UKPDS, 1998).

Risk factors

Hypertension occurs when the vessels through which the blood flows become too narrow, or the volume of circulating blood becomes too high. Raised blood pressure increases the workload on the heart and can damage the endothelial lining of blood vessels. It also increases the

Table 7.14.18 Blood pressure (BP) classification (Williams et al., 2004; NICE, 2011)

Category	Systolic BP (mmHg)	Diastolic BP (mmHg)
Optimal blood pressure	<120	<80
Normal blood pressure	<130	<85
High normal blood pressure	130–139	85–89
Stage 1 Hypertension	140–159	90–99
Stage 2 Hypertension	160–179	100–109
Severe Hypertension	≥180	≥110

Ambulatory blood pressure measurement (ABPM) daytime average of >135/85 mmHg but <150/95 mmHg also required in the diagnosis of stage 1 hypertension (NICE, 2011).

SECTION 7

infiltration of blood components such as lipids into the arterial wall, exacerbating endothelial damage, enhancing atherosclerotic deposition and ultimately increasing cardiovascular risk.

Primary hypertension accounts for approximately 90% of cases. The remaining 10% of cases are secondary to a specific cause such as renal or liver disease, cardiac failure and pregnancy. The pathogenesis of primary hypertension remains unknown and probably results from the interaction of a number of factors, including the effects of the ageing process on renal function and peripheral resistance, genetic susceptibility and environmental influences, such as smoking, stress, diet and lifestyle. The most significant diet and lifestyle influences are considered to be (Williams et al., 2004):

- Overweight and obesity.
- Excess salt intake.
- Excess alcohol intake.

Obesity

Obesity is well established as a risk factor for hypertension. The Framingham study found that hypertension is twice as likely in obese subjects (Hubert *et al.*, 1983). Blood pressures increased with increasing body mass index (BMI); SBP increased by 4 mmHg for each 4.5 kg increase in body weight (Higgins *et al.*, 1988). The Nurses' Health Study found that the incidence of hypertension was up to six times higher in those with a BMI of >29 kg/m^2 compared with those with a BMI of <22 kg/m^2 (Manson *et al.*, 1995). A more recent study showed that over half those with hypertension were obese (Ford *et al.*, 2008). Weight gain with age significantly contributes to the rise in hypertension with age (Burt *et al.*, 1995; Vokonas *et al.*, 1988; Yang *et al.*, 2007). Raised blood pressure is particularly linked to central adiposity and this association is more marked in men than women (Strazzullo, 2002; Poirier *et al.*, 2005; Benetou *et al.*, 2004; Canoy *et al.*, 2004).

Salt

Sodium, taken as dietary salt, is a major cause of raised blood pressure and the age related rise. Evidence comes from a variety of sources, including epidemiological, migration, intervention, treatment, animal and genetic studies (Sacks *et al.*, 1988; 2001;Elliott, 1991; Elliott *et al.*, 2007; Cutler *et al.*, 1997; Midgley *et al.*, 1996; Graudal *et al.*, 1998; He & MacGregor, 2010). The relationship between salt and blood pressure is direct and dose related (Denton *et al.*, 1995; Ezzati *et al.*, 2002; Sacks *et al.*, 2001). A recent meta analysis concluded that high dietary salt intake is associated with an increase in stoke and cardiovascular events; a 5-g higher daily salt intake is associated with a 23% increased risk of stroke and a 17% increased risk of total CVD (Strazzullo *et al.*, 2009).

Alcohol

Many epidemiological studies have shown a direct and linear association between alcohol consumption and increased blood pressure, particularly with regular heavy consumption of alcohol or binge drinking (Puddey *et al.*, 1999; Klatsky *et al.*, 1977; Xin *et al.*, 2001). High levels of alcohol consumption are associated with a high risk of stroke, particularly for binge drinkers (Wannamethee & Shaper, 1996).

Management

Antihypertensive therapy can result in reductions in stroke, MI and heart failure of between 20% and 50% (Neal *et al.*, 2000). The management of hypertension has changed in recent years and blood pressure levels alone no longer determine treatment. Risk models should be used to predict likelihood of developing CHD or stroke over 10 years, taking into account gender, age, family history, diabetic status, smoking status, total cholesterol, high density lipoprotein (HDL) cholesterol and blood pressure (NICE, 2010). The NICE guidelines (2011) are:

- Pharmacological treatment should be initiated with SBP of ≥160 mmHg or DBP of ≥100 mmHg and a daytime average ABPM of >150/95 (stage 2 hypertension).
- When SBP is between 140 and 159 mmHg and/or DBP is 90–99 mmHg, pharmacological treatment (stage 1 hypertension) should be decided on the basis of established CVD, diabetes, target organ damage,(e.g. kidney, or an estimated CVD risk of >20% over 10 years.
- People with high normal blood pressure (130–139/85–89 mmHg) should be given diet and lifestyle advice and reassessed annually.

For most patients, optimal goals for blood pressure treatment are ≤140 mmHg SBP and ≤85 mmHg DBP. For patients with diabetes, renal impairment or established CVD, a lower target of ≤130/80 mmHg is recommended.

Drug treatment

Classes of drugs that may be used include:

- *Thiazide diuretics* – inhibit sodium reabsorption from the distal tubules of the kidney, so increasing fluid loss and reducing blood volume.
- *Beta-blockers* – reduce the stimulating action of noradrenaline (noradrenaline) by blocking beta-adrenoreceptors in the heart and peripheral vasculature. Beta-blockers lower blood pressure primarily by reducing the force and rate of cardiac output.
- *Calcium channel blockers* – inhibit smooth muscle contraction in blood vessel walls.
- *Angiotensin converting enzyme (ACE) inhibitors* – reduce the production of the vasoconstrictor angiotensin II.
- *Angiotensin II receptor antagonists* – alternatives for people who cannot tolerate ACE inhibitors.
- *Alpha-blockers* – block alpha-adrenoreceptors and have vasodilatory effects.

Many of the drugs used to treat hypertension are also used in the management of CVD; therefore, the choice of drug will be influenced by the nature of any clinical symptoms present as well as other factors such as age and renal function. Most people require more than one blood pressure lowering hypertensive drug in order to achieve optimal levels of control.

Diet and lifestyle

Guidelines on the management of hypertension emphasise the importance of diet and lifestyle changes (NICE, 2011). All people with high blood pressure should be given diet and lifestyle advice. If implemented, such measures have been shown to avoid the need for drug treatment or reduce the dosage of antihypertensive drugs required (Appel *et al.*, 1997; Whelton *et al.*, 1998). Diet and lifestyle measures may be the only form of treatment needed in people with stage 1 hypertension who have no other evidence of CVD. The effectiveness of lifestyle measures alone should be evaluated for up to 6 months.

People with borderline or high normal blood pressure should also be encouraged to adopt protective diet and lifestyle measures. These can reduce the age associated rise in blood pressure and hence delay or prevent the need for antihypertensive drugs in the future. Dietary advice should be given in the context of general cardio-protection and tailored to individual risk factors and nutritional priorities. Diet and lifestyle measures that should be strongly recommended to people with hypertension are given in Table 7.14.19.

Weight management

Weight loss, whether by dietary means or physical activity, can result in clinically significant reductions in blood pressure. A meta analysis (Neter *et al.*, 2003) concluded that a reduction in weight by energy restriction and/or increased physical activity of 1 kg would result in a fall in both SBP and DBP of 1 mmHg. The blood pressure lower-ing effect of weight loss persists over longer periods, particularly if it is maintained (Harsha & Bray, 2008). Weight loss decreases blood pressure in both hypertensive and normotensive obese subjects, although the effect is greatest in hypertensive subjects (Staessen *et al.*, 1988).

Salt intake

A number of trials have shown the blood pressure lowering effects of salt restriction. A meta analysis by He & MacGregor (2002) of trials of more than 1-month duration showed that a reduction of 6 g of dietary salt lowered blood pressure by 7/4 mmHg in hypertensive individuals and by 4/2 mmHg in those who were normotensive; the reduction was dose responsive. The reduction in blood pressure in response to sodium restriction has been shown to be even more striking in patients with resistant (i.e. does not respond to medication) hypertension (Pimenta *et al.*, 2009). Dose–response trials have clearly demonstrated that the lower the salt intake, the lower the blood pressure (Sacks *et al.*, 2001; MacGregor *et al.*, 1989). Also, salt reduction blunts the age related rise in blood pressure (Sacks *et al.*, 2001). The fall in blood pressure with salt restriction is greatest in those of African origin, older people and those with hypertension (Vollmer *et al.*, 2001). This may partly be due to the diminished responsiveness of the renin angiotensive system in these individuals (He *et al.*, 1998).

Salt reduction can enhance the action of antihypertensive medication and reduce the need for drug therapy (Whelton *et al.*, 1998; MacGregor *et al.*, 1987). It is also additive to other dietary treatments, such as the Dietary Approaches to Stop Hypertension (DASH) diet (see later) (Sacks *et al.*, 2001) and weight reduction (Whelton *et al.*, 1998; The Trials of Hypertension Prevention Collaborative Research Group, 1997). Evidence that a reduction of salt intake has long term beneficial effects on cardiovascular outcomes has come from the 10–15 year follow-up of the Trial of Hypertension Prevention. The group that reduced their original salt intake by 25–30% (from an average of 10 g/ day) had a 25% lower incidence of cardiovascular events (Cook *et al.*, 2007). A reduction of dietary salt from 10 g to 5 g/day would be expected to decrease stroke rate by 23% and CVD by 17% (Strazzullo *et al.*, 2009; Cook *et al.*, 2007; Karppanen & Mervaala, 2006).

The World Health Organization (WHO/FSA, 2010) encourages population sodium reduction strategies and has set a worldwide target for salt intake of no more than 5 g/day. A number of countries have salt reduction programmes and one of the most successful is the UK's programme. In 1994 the Committee on Medical Aspects of Nutrition (COMA) recommended a daily maximum salt intake of 6 g (Department of Health, 1994). A comprehensive review by the Scientific Advisory Committee on Nutrition (SACN, 2003) concluded that evidence for an adverse association between salt and blood pressure had strengthened, and endorsed the COMA recommendation. The National Diet and Nutrition Survey 2000/1 (Hoare *et al.*, 2004) assessed the UK average daily salt consumption to be 9.5 g, with 80% from processed foods and food eaten outside the home. The initial target was to encourage

Table 7.14.19 Lifestyle modifications to prevent and manage hypertension

Lifestyle modification	Approximate systolic blood pressure lowering (mmHg) (Aronow *et al.* 2011)
Lose weight if overweight or obese	5–20/10 kg weight loss
Reduce sodium intake to <6 g of salt/day	2–8
Limit alcohol consumption to <3 units/day for men and <2 units/day for women Less advisable if overweight Binge drinking must be avoided	2–4
Take regular aerobic physical exercise Ideally for >30 minutes/day on at least 5 days/week	4–9
Consume at least five portions/ day of fruit and vegetables	
DASH diet	8–14

manufacturers to reduce salt content of processed foods on a voluntary basis. This has been successful, as the salt content of most of these foods has been reduced by 20–30%. The Food Standards Agency and Consensus Action on Salt and Health (a group of scientific experts aiming to reduce the UK salt intake) have conducted salt awareness campaigns and promoted front of pack food labelling to provide clear indications of salt content. By 2008 the average daily salt consumption in the UK had fallen to 8.5 g (Bates et al., 2010). The NICE guidance (2010) on the prevention of CVD at the population level has set a target of UK daily salt consumption at <6 g for adults by 2015 with a further reduction to 3 g/day by 2025. Children younger than 11 years should consume substantially less than adults.

Potassium

High levels of potassium in the diet are associated with lower blood pressures (Intersalt Cooperative Research Group, 1988; Tunstall-Pedoe, 1999; Cappuccio & MacGregor, 1991; Whelton et al., 1997; Geleijnse et al., 2003; Dickinson et al., 2006a). The blood pressure lowering effect of potassium is greater in those of African origin, in the presence of a high salt intake and in individuals with hypertension. Meta analyses do not support the use of potassium supplements (Dickinson et al., 2006a). Increasing dietary potassium is recommended as treatment for high blood pressure, especially when a reduction in salt intake is not achieved (Whitworth & WHO, 2003; Williams et al., 2004; European Society of Hypertension, 2003). At least five portions of fruit and vegetable should be eaten per day. Most healthy individuals can tolerate an increase in dietary potassium but care should be taken in those with certain conditions, e.g. chronic kidney disease.

Calcium and magnesium

Dietary calcium intake may have a small inverse effect on blood pressure, but studies are inconsistent (Cappuccio et al., 1995). There is insufficient evidence to advocate calcium supplementation (Dickinson et al., 2006b). A recent meta analysis showed that there is an inverse association between risk of elevated blood pressure and intake of low fat dairy foods, as well as with milk and yoghurt (Ralston et al., 2012). The evidence linking dietary magnesium with a positive effect on blood pressure is inconsistent (Burgess et al., 1999; Ma et al., 1995; Mizushima et al., 1998) and dietary supplementation is currently not advised (Dickinson et al., 2006c).

Alcohol

In a meta analysis of 15 randomised controlled trials, Xin et al. (2001) found that reducing alcohol intake lowered SBP and DBP by an average of 3.3 and 2.0 mmHg, respectively. The effect was dose related with larger reductions in alcohol intake producing greater reductions in blood pressure. The effects of intervention were also greater in those with higher baseline blood pressure. Alcohol in small amounts has been shown to have cardioprotective properties and should be allowed in moderation (Power et al., 1998). Alcohol should be restricted to no more than 21 units/week in men and 14 units/week in women, with binge drinking being discouraged (Williams et al., 2004). Alcohol should be taken with food as this seems to lessen the blood pressure raising effects (Stranges et al., 2004).

Other dietary components

A number of other dietary components have been implicated in lowering blood pressure, although the evidence base is not strong enough for these to be incorporated into management guidelines. These include cocoa (Desch et al., 2010), dietary fibre (Whelton et al., 2005), fish oil (Appel et al., 1993), protein (Altorf-van der Kuil et al., 2010) and vitamin D (Geleijnse, 2011). There may be a U shaped relation between coffee and blood pressure levels. Coffee has been reported to lower blood pressure in both abstainers and in those with high coffee intake, and to slightly raise blood pressure (by about 2/1 mmHg) in those with medium (five cups/day) intake (Geleijnse, 2008). Liquorice consumption may raise blood pressure even at levels as low as 50 g/ day for 2 weeks (Sigurjonsdottir et al., 2001).

Physical activity

As well as the benefits of physical activity in terms of energy balance and obesity, aerobic exercise may have direct hypotensive effects. A meta analysis of 54 randomised controlled trials found that aerobic exercise reduced SBP by an average of 3.8 mmHg, and DBP by 2.6 mmHg (Whelton et al., 2002). These effects occurred in both normotensive and hypertensive individuals, and also in overweight and normal weight individuals. Aerobic exercise (brisk walking, jogging or cycling) three to five times/week can reduce SBP and DBP by 3 mmHg (NICE, 2011). However, the effect is variable, and only 30% of subjects have a reduction in SBP of 10 mmHg or more.

Isometric exercise, such as heavy weight lifting, is not recommended for hypertensive patients. However, in a recent, small meta analysis of five trials, isometric exercise of <1 hour/week lowered SBP by 10.4 mmHg and DBP by 6.7 mmHg (Owen et al., 2010). Heavy physical exercise should not be recommended in severe or poorly controlled hypertension until pharmacological therapy is effective.

Multiple lifestyle interventions

In practice, advice is given to alter a number of factors to lower blood pressure. The additive effect of two or more lifestyle interventions will be less than the sum of each of the interventions applied separately (Appel et al., 1997). A number of trials have incorporated multiple lifestyle interventions; the most widely studied and promoted are the DASH trials. The initial DASH diet was high in fruit and vegetables, low fat dairy foods, wholegrain cereals, nuts and seeds, with foods rich in saturated fat and refined sugar being restricted. Thus, the DASH dietary pattern increases intakes of potassium, calcium, magnesium, fibre and protein, while lowering saturated fat. When compared with a typical US diet, the DASH diet significantly lowered SBP and DBP in hypertensive and normotensive individuals by 11.4 and 5.5 mmHg and 3.5 and 2.1 mmHg, respectively (Appel *et al*., 1997). This reduction was achieved within 2 weeks and maintained for the remaining 6 weeks of the study. These dramatic effects were repeated in the DASH sodium trial (Sacks *et al*., 2001), which demonstrated that restriction of dietary sodium had an additive effect on lowering blood pressure. The PREMIER trial demonstrated that the DASH diet is effective in lowering blood pressure over a longer time period and when subjects self select their food (Appel *et al*., 2003). More recently, the ENCORE study showed that the addition of exercise and weight loss advice to the DASH diet for 4 months resulted in even greater blood pressure reductions (Blumenthal *et al*., 2010); there was a 16.1/9.9 mmHg reduction in blood pressure with DASH and weight management, and a 11.2/7.5 mmHg reduction with the DASH diet alone. In USA (Chobanian *et al*., 2003) and Canadian (Hackam *et al*., 2010) national guidelines, the DASH diet is recommended for the treatment of hypertension. Harnden *et al*. (2010) have studied the use of the DASH diet in the UK.

Blood pressure response to dietary manipulation is modulated by genotype, particularly the sensitivity to sodium intake and response to the DASH diet (Svetkey *et al*., 2011). Clear identification of the genotypes involved will have implications for focusing dietary advice.

Prevention

Reducing the prevalence of obesity and reducing salt intake would have the greatest impact on the prevalence of hypertension in the UK population; however, this will not be easy to achieve. Levels of obesity are currently increasing rather than decreasing, and the rising prevalence of childhood obesity heralds many future health problems. Designing and implementing public health strategies that lead to sustained lifestyle modifications to help prevent hypertension is an essential part of the overall strategy to meet national targets for the reduction of CHD and stroke.

Further reading

Medical Research Council, Human Nutrition Research. (2005) Why 6g? A summary of the scientific evidence for the salt intake target. Available at www.mrc.ac.uk/Utilities/Documentrecord/index.htm?d=MRC003362.

National Institute for Health and Care Excellence (NICE). (2011) Hypertension – the clinical management of primary hypertension in adults in primary care. CG127. Available at www.nice.org.uk.

Scientific Advisory Committee on Nutrition (SACN). (2003) Salt and health. Available at www.sacn.gov.uk/pdfs/sacn_salt_final.pdf.

Internet resources

British Hypertension Society   www.bhsoc.org
Blood Pressure Association   www.bpassoc.org.uk
Consensus Action on Salt and Health (CASH)   www.actiononsalt.org.uk
World Action on Salt and Health (WASH)   www.worldactiononsalt.com

References

Agyemang C, Bhopal R. (2003) Is the blood pressure of people from African origin adults in the UK higher or lower than that in European origin white people? A review of cross-sectional data. *Journal of Human Hypertension* 17: 523–534.

Altorf-Van der Kuil W, Engberink MF, Van Rooij FJ, *et al*. (2010) Dietary protein and risk of hypertension in a Dutch older population: the Rotterdam study. *Journal of Hypertension* 28: 2394–2400.

Appel LJ, Miller ER 3rd, Seidler AJ, Whelton PK. (1993) Does supplementation of diet with 'fish oil' reduce blood pressure? A meta-analysis of controlled clinical trials. *Archives of Internal Medicine* 153: 1429–1438.

Appel LJ, Moore TJ, Obarzanek E, *et al*. (1997) A clinical trial of the effects of dietary patterns on blood pressure. DASH Collaborative Research Group. *New England Journal of Medicine* 336: 1117–1124.

Appel LJ, Champagne CM, Harsha DW, *et al*. (2003) Effects of comprehensive lifestyle modification on blood pressure control: main results of the PREMIER clinical trial. *JAMA* 289: 2083–2093.

Aronow WS, Fleg JL, Pepine CJ, *et al*. (2011) ACCF/AHA 2011 Expert Consensus Document on Hypertension in the Elderly A Report of the American College of Cardiology Foundation Task Force on Clinical Expert Consensus Documents Developed in Collaboration With the American Academy of Neurology, American Geriatrics Society, American Society for Preventive Cardiology, American Society of Hypertension, American Society of Nephrology, Association of Black Cardiologists, and European Society of Hypertension. *Journal of the American College of Cardiology* 57: 2037–2114.

Bates B, Lennox A, Swan G. (2010) *The National Diet and Nutrition Survey: Headline results from Year 1 of the Rolling Programme (2008/2009)*. London: Food Standards Agency.

Benetou V, Bamia C, Trichopoulos D, Mountokalakis T, Psaltopoulou T, Trichopoulou A. (2004) The association of body mass index and waist circumference with blood pressure depends on age and gender: a study of 10 928 non-smoking adults in the Greek EPIC cohort. *European Journal of Epidemiolgy* 19: 803–809.

Blumenthal JA, Babyak MA, Hinderliter A, *et al*. (2010) Effects of the DASH diet alone and in combination with exercise and weight loss on blood pressure and cardiovascular biomarkers in men and women with high blood pressure: the ENCORE study. *Archives of Internal Medicine* 170: 126–135.

Burgess E, Lewanczuk R, Bolli P, *et al*. (1999) Lifestyle modifications to prevent and control hypertension. 6. Recommendations on potassium, magnesium and calcium. Canadian Hypertension Society, Canadian Coalition for High Blood Pressure Prevention and Control, Laboratory Centre for Disease Control at Health Canada, Heart and Stroke Foundation of Canada. *CMAJ* 160: S35–45.

Burt VL, Whelton P, Roccella EJ, *et al*. (1995) Prevalence of hypertension in the US adult population. Results from the Third National Health and Nutrition Examination Survey, 1988–1991. *Hypertension* 25: 305–313.

Canoy D, Luben R, Welch A, *et al*. (2004) Fat distribution, body mass index and blood pressure in 22 090 men and women in the Norfolk cohort of the European Prospective Investigation into Cancer and Nutrition (EPIC-Norfolk) study. *Journal of Hypertension* 22: 2067–2074.

Cappuccio FP, MacGregor GA. (1991) Does potassium supplementation lower blood pressure? A meta-analysis of published trials. *Journal of Hypertension* 9: 465–73.

Cappuccio FP, Elliott P, Allender PS, Pryer J, Follman DA, Cutler JA. (1995) Epidemiologic association between dietary calcium intake and blood pressure: a meta-analysis of published data. *American Journal of Epidemiolgy* 142: 935–945.

Chen X, Wang Y. (2008) Tracking of blood pressure from childhood to adulthood: a systematic review and meta-regression analysis. *Circulation* 117: 3171–3180.

SECTION 7

Chobanian AV, Bakris GL, Black HR, *et al.* (2003) The Seventh Report of the Joint National Committee on Prevention, Detection, Evaluation, and Treatment of High Blood Pressure: the JNC 7 report. *JAMA* 289: 2560–2572.

Cook NR, Cutler JA, Obarzanek E, *et al.* (2007) Long term effects of dietary sodium reduction on cardiovascular disease outcomes: observational follow-up of the trials of hypertension prevention (TOHP). *BMJ* 334: 885–888.

Cutler JA, Follmann D, Allender PS. (1997) Randomized trials of sodium reduction: an overview. *American Journal of Clinical Nutrition* 65: 643S–651S.

Denton D, Weisinger R, Mundy NI, *et al.* (1995) The effect of increased salt intake on blood pressure of chimpanzees. *Nature Medicine* 1: 1009–1016.

Department of Health. (1994). Report of the Cardiovascular Review Group of the Committee on Medical Aspects of Food Policy (COMA). Nutritional aspects of Cardiovascular Disease. Available at www.nice.org.uk/niceMedia/documents/nutritioncardiodisease.pdf.

Desch S, Schmidt J, Kobler D, *et al.* (2010) Effect of cocoa products on blood pressure: systematic review and meta-analysis. *American Journal of Hypertension* 23: 97–103.

Dickinson HO, Nicolson D, Campbell F, Beyer FR, Mason J. (2006a) Potassium supplementation for the management of primary hypertension in adults. *Cochrane Database of Systematic Reviews* 3: CD004641.

Dickinson HO, Nicolson D, Cook JV, *et al.* (2006b) Calcium supplementation for the management of primary hypertension in adults. *Cochrane Database of Systematic Reviews* 2: CD004639.

Dickinson HO, Nicolson D, Campbell F, *et al.* (2006c) Magnesium supplementation for the management of primary hypertension in adults. *Cochrane Database of Systematic Reviews* 3: CD004640.

Din-Dzietham R, Liu Y, Bielo MV, SHAMSA F. (2007) High blood pressure trends in children and adolescents in national surveys, 1963 to 2002. *Circulation* 116: 1488–1496.

Elliott P. (1991) Observational studies of salt and blood pressure. *Hypertension* 17: I3–18.

Elliott P, Walker LL, Little MP, *et al.* (2007) Change in salt intake affects blood pressure of chimpanzees: implications for human populations. *Circulation* 116: 1563–1568.

Ezzati M, Lopez AD, Rodgers A, Vander Hoorn S, Murray CJ. (2002) Selected major risk factors and global and regional burden of disease. *Lancet* 360: 1347–1360.

European Hypertension Society. (2003) Guidelines for the management of arterial hypertension. *Journal of Hypertension* 21: 1011–1053.

Ford ES, Zhao G, Li C, Pearson WS, Mokdad AH. (2008) Trends in obesity and abdominal obesity among hypertensive and nonhypertensive adults in the United States. *American Journal of Hypertension* 21: 1124–1128.

Geleijnse JM. (2008) Habitual coffee consumption and blood pressure: an epidemiological perspective. *Vascular Health Risk and Management* 4: 963–970.

Geleijnse JM. (2011) Vitamin D and the prevention of hypertension and cardiovascular diseases: a review of the current evidence. *American Journal of Hypertension* 24: 253–262.

Geleijnse JM, Kok FJ, Grobbee DE. (2003) Blood pressure response to changes in sodium and potassium intake: a metaregression analysis of randomised trials. *Journal of Human Hypertension* 17: 471–480.

Graudal NA, Galloe AM, Garred P. (1998) Effects of sodium restriction on blood pressure, renin, aldosterone, catecholamines, cholesterols, and triglyceride: a meta-analysis. *JAMA* 279: 1383–1391.

Hackam DG, Khan NA, Hemmelgarn BR, *et al.* (2010) The 2010 Canadian Hypertension Education Program recommendations for the management of hypertension: part 2 - therapy. *Canadian Journal of Cardiology* 26: 249–258.

Harnden KE, Frayn KN, Hodson L. (2010) Dietary Approaches to Stop Hypertension (DASH) diet: applicability and acceptability to a UK population. *Journal of Human Nutrition and Dietetics* 23: 3–10.

Harsha DW, Bray GA. (2008) Weight loss and blood pressure control (Pro). *Hypertension* 51: 1420–1405; discussion 1425.

He FJ, MacGregor GA. (2002) Effect of modest salt reduction on blood pressure: a meta-analysis of randomized trials. Implications for public health. *Journal of Human Hypertension* 16: 761–770.

He FJ, MacGregor GA (2010) Reducing population salt intake worldwide: from evidence to implementation. *Progress in Cardiovascular Disease* 52: 363–382.

He FJ, Markandu ND, Sagnella GA, MacGregor GA. (1998) Importance of the renin system in determining blood pressure fall with salt restriction in black and white hypertensives. *Hypertension* 32: 820–824.

Health survey for England. (2009) Vol 1 Health and Lifestyles (NHS The Information Centre). Available at www.ic.nhs.uk/webfiles/publications/003_Health_Lifestyles/hse009report/HSE_09_volume1.pdf.

Higgins M, Kannel W, Garrison R, Pinsky J, Stokes J 3rd. (1988) Hazards of obesity – the Framingham experience. *Acta Medica Scandinavica Supplement* 723: 23–36.

Hoare J, Henderson L, Bates CJ, *et al.* (2004) *National Diet and Nutrition Survey.* London: The Stationery Office.

Hubert HB, Feinleib M, McNamara PM, Castelli WP. (1983) Obesity as an independent risk factor for cardiovascular disease: a 26-year follow-up of participants in the Framingham Heart Study. *Circulation* 67: 968–977.

Intersalt Cooperative Research Group. (1988) Intersalt: an international study of electrolyte excretion and blood pressure. Results for 24 hour urinary sodium and potassium excretion. *BMJ* 297: 319–328.

Karppanen H, Mervaala E. (2006) Sodium intake and hypertension. *Progress in Cardiovascular Disease* 49: 59–75.

Khan JM, Beevers DG. (2005) Management of hypertension in ethnic minorities. *Heart* 91: 1105–1109.

Klag MJ, Whelton PK, Randall BL, *et al.* (1996) Blood pressure and end-stage renal disease in men. *New England Journal of Medicine* 334: 13–18.

Klatsky AL, Friedman GD, Siegelaub AB, Gerard MJ. (1977) Alcohol consumption and blood pressure Kaiser-Permanente Multiphasic Health Examination data. *New England Journal of Medicine* 296: 1194–1200.

Law MR, Morris JK, Wald NJ. (2009) Use of blood pressure lowering drugs in the prevention of cardiovascular disease: meta-analysis of 147 randomised trials in the context of expectations from prospective epidemiological studies. *BMJ,* 338: b1665.

Lewington S, Clarke R, Qizilbash N, Peto R, Collins R. (2002) Age-specific relevance of usual blood pressure to vascular mortality: a meta-analysis of individual data for one million adults in 61 prospective studies. *Lancet* 360: 1903–1913.

Ma J, Folsom AR, Melnick SL, *et al.* (1995) Associations of serum and dietary magnesium with cardiovascular disease, hypertension, diabetes, insulin, and carotid arterial wall thickness: the ARIC study. Atherosclerosis Risk in Communities Study. *Journal of Clinical Epidemiology* 48: 927–940.

MacGregor GA, Markandu ND, Singer DR, Cappuccio FP, Shore AC, Sagnella GA. (1987) Moderate sodium restriction with angiotensin converting enzyme inhibitor in essential hypertension: a double blind study. *BMJ (Clinical Research Edition)* 294: 531–534.

MacGregor GA, Markandu ND, Sagnella GA, Singer DR, Cappuccio FP. (1989) Double-blind study of three sodium intakes and long-term effects of sodium restriction in essential hypertension. *Lancet* 2: 1244–1247.

Mancia G, De Backer G, Dominiczak A, *et al.*, The Task Force for the Management of Arterial Hypertension of the European Society of Hypertension & The Task Force for the Management of Arterial Hypertension of the European Society of Cardioloyg 2007. (2007) Guidelines for the management of arterial hypertension: The Task Force for the Management of Arterial Hypertension of the European Society of Hypertension (ESH) and of the European Society of Cardiology (ESC). *European Heart Journal* 28: 1462–1536.

Manson JE, Willett WC, Stampfer MJ, *et al.* (1995) Body weight and mortality among women. *New England Journal of Medicine* 333: 677–685.

Midgley JP, Matthew AG, Greenwood CM, Logan AG. (1996) Effect of reduced dietary sodium on blood pressure: a meta-analysis of randomized controlled trials. *JAMA* 275: 1590–1597.

Mizushima S, Cappuccio FP, Nichols R, Elliott P. (1998) Dietary magnesium intake and blood pressure: a qualitative overview of the observational studies. *Journal of Human Hypertension* 12: 447–453.

Neal B, MacMahon S, Chapman N. (2000) Effects of ACE inhibitors, calcium antagonists, and other blood-pressure-lowering drugs: results of prospectively designed overviews of randomised trials. Blood Pressure Lowering Treatment Trialists' Collaboration. *Lancet* 356: 1955–1964.

Neter JE, Stam BE, Kk FJ, Grobble DE, Geleijnse JM. (2003) Influence of weight reduction on blood pressure: a meta-analysis of randomized controlled trials. *Hypertension* 42: 878–884.

National Institute for Health and Care Excellence (NICE). (2010) Guidance on the prevention of cardiovascular disease at the population level. Available at http://guidance.nice.org.uk/PH25.

National Institute for Health and Care1 Excellence (NICE). (2011) Hypertension – the clinical management of primary hypertension in adults in primary care. CG127. Available at www.nice.org.uk.

Owen A, Wiles J, Swaine I. (2010) Effect of isometric exercise on resting blood pressure: a meta analysis. *Journal of Human Hypertension* 24: 796–800.

Pimenta E, Gaddam KK, Oparl S, Aban I, Husain S, Dell'Italia LJ, Calhoun DA. (2009) Effects of dietary sodium reduction on blood pressure in subjects with resistant hypertension: results from a randomized trial. *Hypertension* 54: 475–481.

Poirier P, Lemieux I, Maurice P, *et al.* (2005) Impact of waist circumference on the relationship between blood pressure and insulin: the Quebec Health Survey. *Hypertension* 45: 363–367.

Power C, Rodgers B, Hope S. (1998) U-shaped relation for alcohol consumption and health in early adulthood and implications for mortality. *Lancet* 352: 877.

Puddey IB, Rakic V, Dimmitt SB, Beilin LJ. (1999) Influence of pattern of drinking on cardiovascular disease and cardiovascular risk factors – a review. *Addiction* 94: 649–663.

Raleigh VS. (1997) Diabetes and hypertension in Britain's ethnic minorities: implications for the future of renal services. *BMJ*, 314: 209–213.

Ralston RA, Lee JH, Truby H, Palermo CE, Walker KZ. (2012) A systematic review and meta-analysis of elevated blood pressure and consumption of dairy foods. *Journal of Human Hypertension* 26(1): 3–13.

Sacks FM, Svetkey LP, Vollmer WM, *et al.* (2001). Effects on blood pressure of reduced dietary sodium and the Dietary Approaches to Stop Hypertension (DASH) diet. DASH-Sodium Collaborative Research Group. *New England Journal of Medicine* 344: 3–10.

Scientific Advisory Committee on Nutrition (SACN). (2003) Salt and health. Available at www.sacn.gov.uk/pdfs/sacn_salt_final.pdf.

Sigurjonsdottir HA, Franzson L, Manhem K, Ragnarsson J, Sigurdsson G, Wallerstedt S. (2001) Liquorice-induced rise in blood pressure: a linear dose-response relationship. *Journal of Human Hypertension* 15: 549–552.

Staessen J, Fagard R, Amery A. (1988) The relationship between body weight and blood pressure. *Journal of Human Hypertension* 2: 207–217.

Stranges S, Wu T, Dorn JM, Freudheim JL, *et al.* (2004) Relationship of alcohol drinking pattern to risk of hypertension: a population-based study. *Hypertension* 44: 813–819.

Strazzullo P. (2002) Salt-sensitivity, hypertension and cardiovascular ageing: broadening our view without missing the point. *Journal of Hypertension* 20: 561–563.

Strazzullo P, D'Elia L, Kandala NB, Cappuccio FP. (2009) Salt intake, stroke, and cardiovascular disease: meta-analysis of prospective studies. *BMJ* 339: b4567.

Subcommittee G. (1999) 1999 World Health Organization-International Society of Hypertension Guidelines for the management of hypertension. *Journal of Hypertension* 17: 151–183.

Svetkey LP, Harris EL, Martin E, *et al.* (2011) Modulation of the BP response to diet by genes in the renin-angiotensin system and the adrenergic nervous system. *American Journal of Hypertension* 24: 209–217.

The Trials of Hypertension Prevention Collaborative Research Group. (1997). Effects of weight loss and sodium reduction intervention on blood pressure and hypertension incidence in overweight people with high-normal blood pressure. The Trials of Hypertension Prevention, phase II. *Archives of Internal Medicine* 157: 657–667.

Tunstall-Pedoe H. (1999) Does dietary potassium lower blood pressure and protect against coronary heart disease and death? Findings from the Scottish Heart Health Study? *Seminars in Nephrology* 19: 500–502.

Turnbull F. (2003) Effects of different blood-pressure-lowering regimens on major cardiovascular events: results of prospectively-designed overviews of randomised trials. *Lancet* 362: 1527–1535.

UK Prospective Diabetes Study Group (UKPDS) (1998) Tight blood pressure control and risk of macrovascular and microvascular complications in type 2 diabetes: UKPDS 38. *BMJ* 317: 703–713.

Vokonas PS, Kannel WB, Cupples LA. (1988) Epidemiology and risk of hypertension in the elderly: the Framingham Study. *Journal of Hypertension Supplements* 6: S3–9.

Vollmer WM, Sacks FM, Ard J, *et al.* (2001) Effects of diet and sodium intake on blood pressure: subgroup analysis of the DASH-sodium trial. *Annals of Internal Medicine* 135: 1019–1028.

Wang JG, Staessen JA, Franklin SS, Fagard R, Gueyffier F. (2005) Systolic and diastolic blood pressure lowering as determinants of cardiovascular outcome. *Hypertension* 45: 907–913.

Wannamethee SG, Shaper AG. (1996) Patterns of alcohol intake and risk of stroke in middle-aged British men. *Stroke* 27: 1033–1039.

Whelton PK, He J, Cutler JA, *et al.* (1997) Effects of oral potassium on blood pressure. Meta-analysis of randomized controlled clinical trials. *JAMA* 277: 1624–1632.

Whelton PK, Apel LJ, Esperland MA, *et al.* (1998) Sodium reduction and weight loss in the treatment of hypertension in older persons: a randomized controlled trial of nonpharmacologic interventions in the elderly (TONE). TONE Collaborative Research Group. *JAMA* 279: 839–846.

Whelton SP, Chin A, Xin X, He J. (2002) Effect of aerobic exercise on blood pressure: a meta-analysis of randomized, controlled trials. *Annals of Internal Medicine* 136: 493–503.

Whelton SP, Hyre AD, Pedersen B, Yi Y, Whelton PK, He J. (2005) Effect of dietary fiber intake on blood pressure: a meta-analysis of randomized, controlled clinical trials. *Journal of Hypertension* 23: 475–481.

Whitworth JA; World Health Organization, International Society of Hypertension Writing Group. (2003) World Health Organization (WHO)/International Society of Hypertension (ISH) statement on management of hypertension. *Journal of Hypertension* 21: 1983–1992.

Williams B, Poulter NR, Brown MJ, *et al.* (2004) Guidelines for management of hypertension: report of the fourth working party of the British Hypertension Society, 2004-BHS IV. *Journal of Human Hypertension* 18: 139–185.

World Health Organization (WHO). (2009) Global Health Risks. Mortality and burden of disease attributable to selected major risks 2009. Available at www.WHO.int/healthinfo/global_burden_disease/GlobalHealthRisks_report_full.pdf.

World Health Organization (WHO)/Food Standards Agency (FSA) (2010) Creating an enabling environment for population-based salt reduction strategies. Available at http://whqlibdoc.who.int/publications/2010/9789241500777_eng.pdf.

Xin X, He J, Frontini MG, Ogden LG, Motsamai OI, Whelton PK. (2001) Effects of alcohol reduction on blood pressure: a meta-analysis of randomized controlled trials. *Hypertension* 38: 1112–1117.

Yang G, Xiang YB, Zheng W, *et al.* (2007) Body weight and weight change in relation to blood pressure in normotensive men. *Journal of Human Hypertension* 21: 45–52.

7.14.5 Stroke

Fiona Jenkins

Key points

- Stroke is a major cause of morbidity and mortality in the UK.

- Malnutrition in stroke patients is associated with poor long term outcomes.

- Multidisciplinary management of stroke in designated units has been shown to improve long term survival and functional state.

- Nutritional concerns following a stroke can be broadly divided into two streams; risk of malnutrition in the acute phase and the need to provide secondary prevention advice.

- The neurological impairments of stroke can significantly impact on nutritional status and malnutrition can have a negative knock-on effect in terms of slowed recovery and capacity for rehabilitation.

Stroke is the third most common cause of death in the UK (Wolfe *et al.*, 1996) causing over 60 000 deaths each year (Allender *et al.*, 2006). Each year in the UK, over 130 000 people have a stroke (Carroll *et al.*, 2001) and a further 65 000 people will have their first transient ischaemic attack (TIA) (Scarborough *et al.*, 2009). More than 900 000 people in England are living with the effects of stroke; approximately half of these are left dependent on others for everyday living [National Audit Office (NAO), 2005]. The Stroke Association in Scotland estimates that that there are 110 000 stroke survivors in Scotland living with the effects of stroke. At least 450 000 people are severely disabled as a result of stroke in England (NAO, 2005). Most strokes occur in people older than 65 years, but they can occur at any age. The mean age of men presenting with stroke is 72.6 years and of women was 78.8 years, with 49% of people who had a stroke being male and 51% female (Royal College of Physicians, 2010).

The Intercollegiate Stroke Working Party (RCP, 2008) estimated the economic impact of stroke on the English economy to be £7 billion/year, made up from:

- Direct costs to the NHS – £2.8 billion/year.
- Informal care – £2.4 billion/year.
- Lost productivity and disability costs – £1.8 billion/year.

Diagnostic criteria and classification

Strokes and TIAs are acute neurological events, presumed to be vascular in origin, that are caused by cerebral ischaemia, cerebral infarction or cerebral haemorrhage. Symptoms and signs are usually focal and can present as a sudden visual loss in a quarter or a half of the visual field, or visual loss in one eye. Other signs that may be present include numbness, weakness or paralysis, slurred speech and visual disturbances that all develop rapidly. People with ischaemic stroke or TIA do not usually present with a headache.

When a stroke is diagnosed, the signs and symptoms remain beyond 24 hours. In a TIA, the symptoms and signs resolve within 24 hours; they can remain for a few hours but often resolve within minutes. Those with ongoing symptoms should be managed and treated on the assumption that they have had a stroke. The FAST (Face, Arm, Speech, Time) awareness campaign was launched in 2009 by the Department of Health to improve the recognition of the symptoms of stroke and TIA (www.nhs.uk/actfast).

Classification

Strokes are classified by their main causes. Nationally, the most common cause is ischaemic or infarct, occurring in 88% of cases, with the remaining 12% being primary intracerebral haemorrhage (RCP, 2010).

Ischaemic strokes

Ischaemic strokes are caused when a blood vessel in the brain becomes blocked and the cells in the part of the brain served by the affected blood vessel die from lack of oxygen and nutrients. There are two main types of ischaemic stroke:

- *Thrombolytic ischaemic stroke* – caused by the interruption of blood flow to a part of the brain due to the slow formation of a blood clot along the lumen of an artery. Such blood clots (thrombi) usually interrupt blood flow through arteries in the brain, causing damage.

- *Embolic ischaemic stroke* – part of the fatty material from an atherosclerotic plaque or a clot in a larger artery or the heart breaks off and becomes trapped in a narrower artery in the brain. Other causes of emboli are septic and air emboli. Embolic strokes are common complications of arterial fibrillation and atherosclerosis in the carotid arteries.

Haemorrhagic strokes

There are two main types of haemorrhagic stroke:

- *Intracerebral haemorrhagic stroke* – there is bleeding from a blood vessel within the brain. The main cause is high blood pressure.
- *Subarachnoid haemorrhagic stroke* – there is bleeding from a blood vessel between the surface of the brain and the arachnoid tissues that cover the brain.

Disease consequences

Immediate prognosis

The inpatient death rate for people admitted with a stroke was 24% in 2005 (NAO, 2005). The 30-day mortality rate showed a reduction from 20% in 2008 to 17% in 2010 (RCP, 2010). The risk of stroke recurring within 30 days of an ischaemic stroke was found to depend on the cause of the stroke and varied from 20% in the case of large vessel cervical or intracranial atherersclerosis with stenosis to about 1% for lacunar stroke (caused by a blockage of a small non-branching end artery deep in the brain).

Long term prognosis

Hardie *et al.* (2003) have shown that having survived 30 days after a stroke, the risk of dying in the next 10 years of a recurrent stroke was about 25%; this compared with 35% from a cardiovascular event (excluding stroke). The median survival time for people after an ischaemic stroke 6 months previously was shown to be longer in those who were previously independent in activities of daily living (Slot *et al.*, 2008). It must be remembered, however, that around half of stroke survivors are left dependant on others for everyday activities (NAO, 2005).

Diagnosis and treatment

Strokes are usually diagnosed from symptoms and the presence of risk factors. Brain imaging is important to determine whether an ischaemic or haemorrhagic stroke has occurred, as this will determine the treatment. One of the greatest advances in stroke improvement has been pharmacological. In the last decade, the use of a thrombolytic agent within the first few hours has been shown to significantly reduce the destruction of brain tissue in many cases. This consequently reduces the degree of long term disability and improves clinical outcome.

Following a cerebral infarction, the cells in the infarct core begin to die through lack of oxygen and as they do so, they release substances that damage the surrounding area. This zone of secondary damage is potentially salvable and is known as the penumbra. The rapid destruction of the primary clot with the use of a thrombolytic agent results in the thrombus dissolving and the restoration of blood flow to the cerebral tissue that has not been irreversibly damaged, thereby preventing further evolution of the stroke and deterioration of brain tissue. Recombinant plasminogen activator (alteplase) is the only agent currently licensed in the UK for use in acute stroke. The main limitation with thrombolysis is the very short time available in which to perform the necessary tests and administer the drug. Alteplase is currently only licensed to be given within 3 hours of confirmed onset of symptoms (although in some areas this is being extended). During this time a brain scan needs to be performed and analysed; blood samples need to be analysed and results checked; and a safe environment identified in which to give the drug, which is not without complications.

In order to provide the drug in a timely manner, it is essential that there is a strict protocol involving many different organisations. The safe introduction of a thrombolytic service is only possible by promoting the rapid recognition of stroke symptoms in the community, prompt transport of patients to the acute setting and smooth efficient working within the different departments to enable early investigation, stabilisation and treatment. This high focus on stroke is essential not only for patients who receive a thrombolytic agent, but for all stroke patients. The rapid assessment of patients will facilitate all patients with a working diagnosis of stroke being transferred into the stroke care pathway. This will ensure that patients are able to access the multidisciplinary stroke specialist management found in designated units. These have been shown to improve long term survival and functional state (Department of Health, 2007). Thrombolysis should be given in accordance with the National Institute for Health and Care Excellence guidelines (NICE, 2008).

If the patient presents with a TIA and all neurological deficits have been resolved, diffusion weighted magnetic resonance imaging (MRI) or carotid imaging, bloods and electrocardiograph (ECG) should be requested and there should be referral to vascular surgeons as required. It is also important to ensure secondary prevention measures are in place (NICE, 2008), including discussion of individual risk factors. In some areas this timely access to stroke specialist assessment and imaging has been achieved via a number of different systems, including telemedicine, partnership on call rota systems across a number of organisations and the hub and spoke system. In the latter one hospital across a locality provides 24/7 hyperacute care, including thrombolysis, and the patient is then transferred to local hospitals or services for acute care and rehabilitation.

Multidisciplinary management of stroke in designated units has been shown to improve long term survival and functional state (Department of Health, 2007). Patient centred goals, treatment and therapy plans agreed with the patient and developed in partnership with the multi-disciplinary team (MDT) will facilitate the rehabilitation of the patients post stroke. Close working within the MDT will increase the understanding of the impact of where the damage to the brain has occurred and the consequences of this with respect to the neurological impairments. For example:

- People with damage to the right side of the brain are more likely to:
  - Have perception problems – finding it difficult to recognise people, objects or their own body (visual agnosia).
  - Have spatial problems – finding it difficult to judge depth size, distance or position in space.
  - Exhibit impulsive behaviour.
  - Have left sided weakness or paralysis.
- People with damage to the left side of the brain are more likely to:
  - Have language problems.
  - Exhibit tearfulness and outbursts of anger.
  - Have right sided weakness or paralysis.

People with damage to the cerebella are likely to have problems with balance and swallowing.

Stroke can affect the patient in a number of ways and the MDT should work together to assess the impact on the individual patient, agree goals with the patient to address these and develop treatment/therapy plans to enable recovery, introduction of coping strategies or adaptations as required.

Nutritional consequences and management

Dysphagia is present in 64–90% of conscious patients in the acute phase of their stroke, with aspiration confirmed in 22–24% of cases (Mann *et al.*, 1999). Of stroke survivors, 15–20% will have significant dysphagia 1 week post stroke (Smithard *et al.*, 1997), and 1 month post stroke 2% will have persisting swallowing problems. Dysphagia can also lead to respiratory infection or pneumonia (Doggett *et al.*, 2001), undernutrition and dehydration (Whelan, 2001; Kidd *et al.*, 1995; Smithard *et al.*, 1997).

Up to 29% of patients recover their swallow and resume full oral nutrition, although this process may take up to 31 months (ESPEN, 2006). During this period of time it is important to utilise the skills of the dietitian and speech and language therapist to support the recovery and ensure that adequate intake of nutrition and fluids is maintained; considering the role of enteral nutrition and texture modification. Raising awareness of nutritional risk with all MDT members will support the recognition of malnutrition in a timely way that will enable its effective management.

Malnutrition is present in approximately 15% of cases with stroke admitted to hospital and this increases to 30% over the first week of recovery following a stroke (RCP, 2004). Gariballa *et al.* (1998) identified that malnutrition is common and worsens within the first 2 weeks after stroke and this affects outcome. Malnutrition will impact on the patient's ability to participate in rehabilitation due to its impact on fatigue, strength and concentration, thus affecting recovery and long term outcomes.

Table 7.14.20 shows the potential complications or consequences following a stroke, the impact these may have on nutritional intake and how the dietitian can work with the patient and the other members of the MDT to reduce the impact.

Stroke quality markers

Stroke quality markers (QM) were developed as part of the National Stroke Strategy (Department of Health, 2007) as a means of raising the quality of stroke prevention, treatment, care and support, and to provide guidelines to measure the quality of stroke services. The following describes how these relate to the role of the dietitian.

QM1 Awareness raising

As part of their specialist role, staff working with stroke should be able to recognise the symptoms of stroke and know that the person should be treated as an emergency. They must ensure that this knowledge is passed on to other colleagues and members of the general public. Dietitians have a key role in primary prevention through public health nutrition.

QM2 Managing risk

Dietitians can help manage the risk of stroke by promoting healthy living by being able to assess and give information about smoking, diet, weight, alcohol and family history. Their role in secondary prevention is to provide advice with respect to diet and lifestyle, and to train other professionals. Dietitians have a key role in reducing the risk of further strokes and improving the management of conditions such as hyperlipidaemia, diabetes and hypertension as recommended in the RCP guidelines, British Hypertension Society Guidelines and Diabetes UK (see Chapters 7.14.3, Chapter 7.12 and Chapter 7.14.4). This can be delivered one to one, in group sessions, or by training other healthcare professionals to disseminate the information.

QM3 Information, advice and support

Dietitians should provide individual, specialised dietary advice and signposting to other services. . In addition they should facilitate training other healthcare professionals, both in nutritional screening and the first line management of malnutrition. It is important that dietitians offer expert advice in team discussions around the ethics of artificial nutrition.

QM6 (TIA and minor stroke) Treatment

Dietitians provide information and advice for people who have had a stroke or TIA, as highlighted in QM2, and manage other risk factors such as diabetes, hypertension and hyperlipidaemia or ischaemic heart disease.

QM8 Assessment

Patients diagnosed with stroke should receive early multidisciplinary assessment, including swallow assessment as this can impact on nutritional status, and nutritional screening to highlight those at nutritional risk and who require treatment. This includes patients who may be at risk of refeeding syndrome and treat accordingly.

By raising awareness of the impact of malnutrition on patient recovery it has been recognised for many years that malnutrition impacts on recovery of hospital inpatients. Patients with acute stroke often already exhibit a poor nutritional status on hospital admission, which negatively impacts on outcome and costs: length of hospital stay is extended; rehabilitation is delayed; and survival reduced (King's Fund, 1992; Age Concern, 2006; Axelsson *et al.*, 1988; ESPEN, 2006). Dietitians can then undertake a more comprehensive assessment of a patient's nutritional status by assessing oral nutritional intake from food and fluids, thereby assessing nutritional adequacy.

Table 7.14.20 Complications and nutritional consequences of stroke, and their management

Complication and consequence of stroke	Potential nutritional impact	Dietetic and multidisciplinary team actions to reduce impact	MDT partnership working to facilitate implementation of actions
Neurological problems Balance, movement, tone, sensation	Can limit ability to self feed	Ensure appropriate seating/ positioning Adapted utensils Provide support at meal times	Physiotherapist Occupational therapist
Pain Neuropathic, shoulder pain and subluxation, musculoskeletal	Reduced appetite	Optimum pain control Use of appropriate moving and handling techniques	Medical team Nursing team Physiotherapist Occupational therapist
Mood and social interaction problems Depression, anxiety, emotionalism, disinhibition, aggression	Reduced participation in activities such as eating and drinking Reduced appetite	Complete mood assessment and ensure management plan is implemented as required	Occupational therapist Medical team psychologist Care management/social worker
Cognitive impairments Attention and concentration Memory Disturbance of spatial awareness – neglect Disturbance of perception – visual agnosia Apraxia – loss of the conceptual ability to organise activity to achieve a goal Planning, organising, initiating and monitoring behaviour, i.e. disturbances of executive functioning	Easily distracted when eating Forget to eat or what they have eaten Difficulty analysing the position of the plate Cannot recognise or define food on the plate Difficulties with self feeding or recognising cutlery Difficulty matching objects and action Food may be thrown around or played with rather than consumed	Reduce distractions as far as possible Keep food diary, written or pictorial Consider the position of the plate. Monitor and support meal times Consider adapted cutlery, plate and/or guards Errorless/kinaesthetic learning at meal times Behaviour modification techniques	Occupational therapist Psychologist Speech and language therapist Nursing team Assistants
Speech and communication difficulties Aphasia, dysarthria, apraxia of speech Acquired dyslexia	Difficulties filling out a menu or ordering food Difficulty requesting drinks Difficulty communicating thirst, hunger, food preferences	Use supported or facilitated communication, e.g. pictures, slowing down Reduce distractions Liaise with family regarding preferences	Speech and language therapist Nursing team
Visual impairments and hemianopias	Not all food will be seen, therefore not all food will be eaten	Consider where the food is positioned Support practice scanning especially at meal times	Occupational therapist Nursing team Assistants
Bladder and bowel problems Urinary incontinence, faecal incontinence, constipation	Reduced intake of fluids Reduced appetite	Monitor food and fluid intake, adapting as appropriate Support physical activity as much as possible Continence management plan developed	Nursing Physiotherapist Occupational therapist Assistants

(Continued)

Table 7.14.20 (*Continued*)

Complication and consequence of stroke	Potential nutritional impact	Dietetic and multidisciplinary team actions to reduce impact	MDT partnership working to facilitate implementation of actions
Swallowing and nutritional problems Oral health, malnutrition, dehydration	Poor appetite. Reduced food and drink intake (sore mouth) Reduced intake of fluids (distaste for thickened drinks) Reduced overall intake of food and drink (texture modification) Increased risk of aspiration pneumonia as a result of poor oral hygiene Difficulties in taking prescribed medication	Early multidisciplinary assessment including swallow assessment and nutritional screening to highlight those at nutritional risk and who require treatment Undertake a nutritional assessment Consider the need to achieve nutritional requirements via tube feeding, food fortification or supplementation Monitoring patients and adapting advice as required. If long term tube feeding is required, consider percutaneous endoscopic gastrostomy insertion Advise as to how to meet nutritional requirements on a texture modified diet Provide prompts to clear residue in the oral cavity and pharynx if appropriate Work with the pharmacist and medical staff to ensure that medication is prescribed in an appropriate form Reduce distractions and consider presentation of modified texture food and fluids	Speech and language therapist Nursing staff Dysphagia trained professional Pharmacist Medical staff
Sexual dysfunction	Low mood and appetite	Pharmacological interventions, counselling, advice	Occupational therapist Physiotherapist Nurse
Difficulties with activities of daily living Personal, social and vocational	Difficulties in the preparation of food and drink Reduced opportunities to purchase food and drink and go shopping Enteral feeding regimen could prevent normal activities being resumed	Assessment and treatment for remediation and adaptation as appropriate Review feeding regimen to ensure it does not adversely impact personal, social vocational activities, consider bolus feeding/overnight feeding	Occupational therapist Assistants Care management/social worker

MDT, multidisciplinary team.

QM9 (stroke) Treatment

Dietitians oversee the implementation and monitoring of nutritional screening processes and the actions arising from screening, incorporating a multidisciplinary approach to the management of dysphagia. This will ensure that patient receives in-depth assessment and appropriate treatment (Logemann, 1994). Dysphagia is a frequent and potentially serious complication of stroke (Smithard *et al.*, 1997) and in some cases may be the sole or overriding symptom (Celifarco *et al.*, 1990). All stroke patients should have access to dietetic services and be screened for their nutritional status. This includes ensuring patients have their swallow screened within 4 hours of admission and have an ongoing management plan for the provision of adequate nutrition (NICE, 2010). There is mounting evidence, including from the FOOD Trial (Dennis, 2006) and evidence based guidelines, such as the dysphagia guidelines from the Scottish Intercollegiate Guideline Network (SIGN, 2004) and the adult nutritional support guidelines from NICE (2006) that in those patients for whom oral food and fluids are unsafe, alternative nutrition considered. If this plan includes the requirement for tube feeding, this needs to be initiated within 24 hours of admission (RCP, 2008). Dietitians advise patients on achieving nutritional requirements via tube feeding, food fortification or supplementation, monitor patients and adapt advice as required, and advise staff, patients and carers on how to meet nutritional requirements on a texture modified diet. They also provide specialist diabetes education, especially to people who may have been undiagnosed until their admission onto the stroke unit.

QM10 High quality specialist rehabilitation

This includes rehabilitation of nutritional intake and swallowing by reviewing, monitoring and advising as clients return to oral feeding and weaning off artificial nutritional support. It may be useful to consider bolus feeding or overnight feeding to encourage patients to start eating and drinking during the day. It is also important to recognise the impact of therapy on nutritional requirements, taking into account the timing of therapy and nutritional support, the increased energy expenditure and the possible fatigue due to the therapy and the stroke. This is also the opportunity to provide secondary prevention dietary advice.

QM11 End of life care

This includes issues around oral and enteral feeding. There needs to be discussion within the MDT and with family/carers of issues at the end of life, possibly including restricting intake to keeping the mouth moist and clean, rather than other interventions.

QM12 Seamless transfer of care

This concerns the facilitation of seamless transfer of care by ensuring good communication and handover of information between colleagues working in different areas, e.g. from hospital to community, possibly across geographical boundaries.

This is especially important for those discharged from hospital on home enteral feeding in order to .facilitate a safe seamless discharge. It is important to start discharge planning as soon as possible if a patient is going home on home enteral feeding. Howard & Bowen (2001) reported that for successful management of home enteral tube feeding (HETF), access to a dietitian was required to enable suitability of the feeding regimen to be monitored in the context of nutritional status. Similarly, Sayce *et al.* (2000) reported fewer feeding related complications when this was implemented. This was due in part to frequent monitoring by the dietitian. A study to assess HETF in everyday life (Liley & Manthorpe, 2003) showed that patients formed close relationships with the coordinating dietitian, with the process of HETF permitting practical and emotional support to coexist.

QM13 Long term care and support

Dietitians should provide advice and support to help individuals live as independently as possible; this includes individuals on long term enteral feeding regimens and those with comorbidities such as diabetes.

QM14 Assessment and review

This should be a multidisciplinary review, which includes nutritional assessment.

QM17 Networks

Dietitians should be actively involved in any local, national or virtual stroke specific groups or neurodietitian groups, which will support sharing good practice, the provision of evidence based practice and clinical reasoning, and therefore the provision of high quality stroke care.

QM18 Leadership and skills

Nutrition and dietetic staff working within stroke care should have specialised skills and stroke expertise, as well as being a source of expert knowledge for others. Dietitians, like other members of the MDT, have a role in leading developments in stroke care at both local and national level, as well as providing professional support and leadership within the team.

QM19 Workforce review and development

Staffing levels for a 10 bedded unit vary between 0.3 and 0.5 whole time equivalent (WTE), with the requirement for an assistant, whether a specific dietetic assistant or stroke rehabilitation assistant, being equivalent to approximately 0.3 WTE (NAO, 2007).

QM20 Research and audit

Dietitians need to be involved in research and audit to influence the development of high quality services and measure how well their service is performing. One area to consider for research is the metabolic consequences of stroke. Dietitians are encouraged to use the British Dietetic Association (BDA) nutrition and dietetic stroke audit tool to evaluate their services and drive forward service improvements.

Stroke prevention

Risk factors

To prevent stroke or reduce the risk of further stroke it is important to moderate the risk factors where possible. These include:

- Smoking.
- Hypertension.
- Obesity.
- High cholesterol levels.
- Family history of heart disease or diabetes.
- Atrial fibrillation (which can be caused by high blood pressure, mitral valve disease, cardiomyopathy, pericarditis, hyperthyroidism, excessive alcohol intake and high caffeine intake).

The results of the national sentinel audit (RCP, 2010) gave the profile of risk factors for all strokes as:

- Vascular risk factors were present in 81% of patients.
- TIA occurred in 29% of patients.
- Hypertension was present in 57% of patients.
- Atrial fibrillation was present in 27% of patients.
- 21% of patients were on anticoagulants.
- 17% of patients were smokers.
- 8% of patients were documented as having excess alcohol consumption.

The most important causal risk factor for stroke is high blood pressure, causing about 50% of ischaemic strokes (Hankey & Warlow, 1994).

The main cause of haemorrhagic stroke is high blood pressure, the risks for which include:

- Overweight and obesity.
- Drinking excessive amounts of alcohol.
- Smoking.
- Sedentary life style.
- Stress, which may cause a temporary rise in blood pressure.
- Sometimes as the result of a traumatic head injury.

Ethnicity

Compared with the Caucasian population, African-Caribbean people are twice as likely to have a stroke. Their first stroke is also likely to occur at a younger age (Stewart *et al.*, 1999). The African-Caribbean and South Asian communities have particularly high rates of hypertension (Cappuccio *et al.*, 1997; Lane & Lip, 2001). In addition, there is variation in smoking between ethnicities that will influence risk.

Primary and secondary prevention

Measures to prevent stroke include following a healthy diet, particularly reducing salt intake and increasing fruit and vegetable intake. The result of a meta analysis of cohort studies (He *et al.*, 2006) supported the recommendation to consume more than five portions of fruit and vegetables per day. Moderating blood pressure through reducing salt intake and maintaining a healthy weight, and increasing exercise and the intake of n-3 fats through consumption of – one to two portions of oily fish per week are recommended.

Public health measures

Dietitians are working in public health projects and programmes across the community to promote a healthier lifestyle and in the longer term reduce stroke (See Chapter 4.2). It is important to address the risk factors for cardiovascular disease (CVD) both at population and individual level, working in partnership with a number of organisations including:

- Local and national government departments.
- Caterers.
- Food and drink producers.
- Food and drink retailers.
- Marketing and media industries.
- The farming sector.
- National as well as non-governmental organisations.

The NICE (2010) public health guidance on prevention of CVD is a national framework for action to address these issues. It includes the following aims:

- To reduce the population level consumption of salt, recognising that high levels of salt in the diet are linked to high blood pressure. Its recommendations include aiming for a maximum intake of 6g/day per adult by 2015 and 3g by 2025. More low salt products should be made available and low salt products should be sold more cheaply than their higher salt equivalents.
- To substantially reduce the population level consumption of saturated fats, as aiming for an average intake of 6–7% of total energy would greatly reduce CVD and deaths from CVD. This could be supported by ensuring it is viable for manufacturers and caterers to produce foods that are substantially lower in saturated fats.
- To ensure all groups of the population are protected from the harmful effects of industrially produced *trans* fatty acids (IPTFAs) by producing recommendations that include the development of UK validated guidelines and information for the food service sector and local government on removing IPTFAs from the food preparation process.
- To protect children from marketing and promotions in order to reduce the likelihood of them establishing poor eating and drinking practices. Its recommendations include the development of a comprehensive, agreed set of principles for food and beverage marketing aimed at young people based on a child's right to a healthy diet.
- To ensure dealings with government agencies and commercial sector are transparent to support public health agenda.
- To enable consumers to make informed choices by providing clear product labelling.

Drug–nutrient interactions

A number of drugs are used to prevent a stroke. Their main actions include reducing blood pressure, reducing the risk of developing blood clots and reducing lipid levels. These include statins and warfarin, which have known interactions with some foods:

- *Grapefruit and statins:*
  - Grapefruit juice can slow the breakdown of some medications. This causes an increase in the amount of the drug in the blood stream, which increases its effect. It is not clear how long this effect lasts or if it relates to grapefruit or grapefruit juice. This reaction is not associated with other juices.
  - Drinking grapefruit juice should be avoided when taking simvastatin. However, when taking another statin, such as atorvastatin, then grapefruit juice (or the grapefruit) can be taken in small quantities.

- *Fruit, vegetables, fruit juices and warfarin:*
  - Cranberry juice can increase the effect of warfarin, so should be avoided to reduce the risk of bleeding.
  - Foods high in vitamin K, e.g., brussels sprouts, broccoli and liver can stop warfarin form working. It is advised that these should not necessarily be avoided, but large quantities should only be eaten infrequently. This will have a more consistent impact on warfarin levels.

Further reading

Royal College of Physicians (RCP). (2006) Profession specific audit. Available at www.rcplondon.ac.uk.

Internet resources

British Heart Foundation www.bhf.org.uk
British Hypertension Society www.bhsoc.org
Blood Pressure Association www.bpassoc.org.uk
Diabetes UK www.diabetes.org.uk
Foundation for Circulatory Health www.ffch.org
NHS Improvement www.improvement.nhs.uk
NHS – The Fast Campaign www.nhs.uk/actfast
National Institute for Health and Care Excellence www.nice.org.uk
Public Health Guidance www.guidance.nice.org.uk/PHG
NICE guidelines
Stroke: Diagnosis and initial management of acute stroke and transient ischaemic attack (TIA) CG68
Royal College of Physicians www.rcplondon.ac.uk
National Sentinel Stroke Audits www.rcplondon.ac.uk/resources/national-sentinel-stroke-audit
Stroke Association www.stroke.org.uk

References

Age Concern. (2006) Hungry to be Heard. Available at www.ageuk.org.uk/documents/en-gb/hungry_to_be_heard_inf.pdf?dtrk=true.Accessed 12 July 2012.

Allender S, Peto V, Scarborough P, Boxer A, Rayner M. (2006) *Coronary Heart Disease Statistics.* London: British Heart Foundation.

Axelsson K, Asplund K, Norberg A, Alafuzoff I. (1988). Nutritional status in patients with acute stroke. *Acta Medica Scandinavica* 224(3): 217–224.

Cappuccio FP, Cook DG, Atkinson RW, Strazzullo P. (1997) Prevalence, detection and management of cardiovascular risk. *Heart* 78: 555–663.

Carroll K, Murad S, Eliahoo J, Majeed A. (2001) Stroke incidence and risk factors in a population - based prospective cohort study. *Health Statistics Quarterly* 12: 1–9.

Celifarco A, Gerard G, Faegenburg D, Burakoff R. (1990) Dysphagia as the sole manifestation of bilateral strokes. *American Journal of Gastroenterology* 85(5): 610–613.

Dennis M. (2006) FOOD: a multicentre randomised trial evaluating feeding policies in patients admitted to hospital with a recent stroke. *Health Technology Assessment* 10(2): 1–120.

Department of Health. (2007) National Stroke Strategy HD/Vascular Programme/stroke. Available at www.dh.gov.uk.

Doggett DL, Tappe KA, Mitchell MD, Chapell R, Coates V, Turkelson CM. (2001) Prevention of pneumonia in elderly stroke patients by systematic diagnosis and treatment of dysphagia: and evidence-based comprehensive analysis of the literature. *Dysphagia* 16: 279–295.

ESPEN. (2006) ESPEN Guidelines on Enteral Nutrition: Cardiology and Pulmonology. *Clinical Nutrition* 25(2): 311–318.

Gariballa SE, Parker SG, Taub N, Castleden CM. (1998) Influence of nutritional status on clinical outcome after acute stroke. *American Journal of Clinical Nutrition* 68(2): 275–281.

Hardie K, Hankey GJ, Jamrozik K, et al. (2003) Ten-year survival after first-ever stroke in the Perth community stroke study. *Stroke* 34(8): 1842–1846

Hankey GJ, Warlow CP. (1994) *Transient Ischaemic Attacks of the Brain and Eye.* London: Saunders Press.

He FJ, Nowson CA, MacGregor GA. (2006) Fruit and vegetable consumption and stroke: meta-analysis of cohort studies. *Lancet* 367: 323.

Howard P, Bowen N. (2001) The challenges of innovation in the organisation of home enteral tube feeding. *Journal of Human Nutrition and Dietetics* 14: 3–11.

Kidd D, Lawson J, Nesbitt R, MacMahon J. (1995) The natural history and clinical consequences of aspiration in acute stroke. *Quarterly Journal of Medicine* 88: 409–413.

King's Fund. (1992) A positive approach to nutrition as treatment. *Available at* www.bapen.org.uk/pdfs/bapen_pubs/pub_kings_fund.pdf. Accessed 12 July 2012.

Lane DA, Lip GYH. (2001) Ethnic differences in hypertension and blood pressure control in the UK. *Quarterly Journal of Medicine* 94(7): 391–396.

Liley A, Manthorpe J. (2003) The impact of home enteral tube feeding in everyday life: a qualitative study. *Health and Social Care in the Community* 11(5): 415–422.

Logemann JA. (1994) Multidisciplinary management of dysphagia. *Acta Oto-Rhinio-Laryngologica Belgica* 48(2): 235–238.

Mann G, Hankey GJ, Caeron D. (1999) Swallowing functions after stroke: prognosis and prognostic factors at 6 months. *Stroke* 30(4): 744–748.

National Audit Office (NAO). (2005) *Reducing Brain Damage: Faster access to better stroke care.* London: Department of Health.

National Audit Office (NAO). (2007) Joining forces to deliver improved stroke care. Available at www.nao.org.uk/wp-content/uploads/2005/11/0607_stroke.pdf. Accessed 2 September 2013.

National Institute for Health and Care Excellence (NICE). (2006) Nutrition support in adults: oral nutrition support, enteral tube feeding and parenteral nutrition. Available at www.nice.org.uk. Accessed 12 July 2012.

National Institute for Health and Care Excellence (NICE). (2008) NICE Guideline CG68 on Stroke. Available at www.nice.org.uk. Accessed 12 July 2012.

National Institute for Health and Care Excellence (NICE). (2010) Stroke Quality Standards obtained from nutrition. Available at www.nice.org.uk. Accessed 12 July 2012.

Royal College of Physicians. (2004) *National Clinical Guidelines for Stroke,* 2nd edn. London: RCP. Available at www.rcplondon.ac.uk. Accessed 12 July 2012.

Royal College of Physicians (RCP). (2008) *Nutrition and Dietetics Concise Guide for Stroke.* London: RCP.

Royal College of Physicians (RCP). (2010) *The National Sentinel Stroke Audit.* London: RCP.

Sayce HA, Rowe PA, McGonigle RJS. (2000) Percutaneous endoscopic gastrostomy feeding in haemodialysis out-patients. *Journal of Human Nutrition and Dietetics* 13(5): 333–341.

Scarborough P, Peto V, Bhatnagar P, et al. (2009) *Stroke Statistics.* London: British Heart Foundation and Stroke Association.

Scottish Intercollegiate Guidelines Network (SIGN). (2004) Dysphagia guidelines: Management of patients with stroke: Identification and management of dysphagia. Available at www.sign.ac.uk/pdf/sign119.pdf. Accessed 12 July 2012.

Slot KB, Berge E, Dorman P, et al. (2008) Impact of functional status at six months on long term survival in patients with ischaemic stroke: prospective cohort studies. *BMJ* 336: 376–379.

Smithard DG, O'Neill PA, England RE, *et al.* (1997) The natural history of dysphagia following a stroke. *Dysphagia* 12(4): 188–193.

Stewart J, Dundas R, Rudd AG, Wolfe CDA. (1999) Ethnic differences in incidence of stroke: Prospective study with stroke register. *BMJ* 318(7): 967–971.

Whelan K. (2001) Inadequate fluid intake in dysphagic acute stroke. *Clinical Nutrition* 20(5): 423–428.

Wolfe C, Rudd T, Beech R. (1996) *The Burden of Stroke, Stroke Services and Research.* London: The Stroke Association.

7.15

Cancer

17.15.1 General aspects
Clare Shaw

Key points

- Diet is both a causative or protective environmental factor that may influence cancer development.
- Development of cancer may increase the individual's risk of becoming malnourished due to disease or treatment effects.
- Weight loss may increase morbidity and mortality associated with cancer treatment.
- Appropriate nutritional advice and/or artificial nutrition support should be an integral part of the cancer patient's treatment plan.

Cancer has been recognised as a disease for hundreds of years; it was mentioned in ancient Egyptian text. A third of the UK population will be diagnosed with cancer during their lifetime, but as treatments have been developed survival rates have increased significantly. The term *cancer* describes a wide range of malignant tumours that affect virtually every organ and tissue in the body. Cancer is a major cause of mortality and morbidity throughout the world. In Britain, approximately 309 500 new cases occur every year [Cancer Research UK (CRUK), 2011a].

In the UK, the most common cancer sites are the breast, lung, large bowel and prostate, which account for over 50% of cancer diagnoses (CRUK, 2011b). Cancer is generally a disease of increasing age with 64% of cancers occurring in those aged over 65 years. Worldwide survival rates vary greatly; this is largely dependent upon access to diagnostic and treatment services. Although incidence rates of some of the less common cancers are increasing, overall mortality rates from cancer in middle aged people are falling due to improvements in treatment (CRUK, 2012). Many cancers are also treatable if detected at an early stage and increasingly people are living with cancer; it is now recognised as a chronic disease. In the UK, for example, there are approximately 2 million cancer survivors (Maddams *et al.*, 2009). The number of people surviving has improved and for all cancers combined 5-year survival has reached 50% (CRUK, 2011c).

Definition of cancer

Cancer is essentially a consequence of genetic mutations within a cell, which result in the production and prolifera-tion of abnormal cells. This can occur when healthy cells are damaged and undergo replication that is outside the usual control. Some of these genetic mutations are inherited, but most simply occur and accumulate over time as the result of lifestyle and environmental factors. The development of cancer is a complex, multistage process that can be summarised as:

1. *Initiation* – exposure to substances or influences (mutagens) that are capable of initiating genetic mutations. Any DNA damage caused may or may not lead to cancer.
2. *Promotion* – under the influence of promoters, damaged DNA begins to be expressed, resulting in cellular changes. Promoters thus enhance tumour development following exposure to mutagens.
3. *Progression* – a complex process leading to the development of malignant cells that have the capacity to invade other tissues.

A carcinogen is the term for a substance that may influence one or more of these stages. Only a few carcinogens can affect all three.

Cancers spread by invading surrounding tissue until they reach a blood or lymph vessel. Small groups of cells may then break off from the original tumour and be carried to other parts of the body where they may settle and grow. The new cancers that develop are called secondary cancers or metastases. Cancer is therefore not a single disease but a group of diseases; there are over 200 different types of cancer arising from different cells of the body.

Manual of Dietetic Practice, Fifth Edition. Edited by Joan Gandy.
© 2014 The British Dietetic Association. Published 2014 by John Wiley & Sons, Ltd.
Companion Website: www.manualofdieteticpractice.com

Development of cancer

Much remains to be learned about the complex interplay of factors that lead to cancer development, particularly hereditary influences. About 5% of cancer cases are thought to result from inherited genetic mutations, e.g. the *BRCA1* and *BRCA2* genes in breast cancer, but even the aetiology of this form of cancer is not straightforward; not everyone with a cancer predisposing genotype develops the disease (see Chapter 5.1). Ninety-five per cent of cancer cases are defined as sporadic, meaning that it is the unpredictable consequence of a combination of genetics, environment and chance. Since little can be done to alter the influence of genetics and chance, efforts to prevent cancer have to focus on identifying and minimising the risk from factors that are modifiable, i.e. environmental influences. The main environmental factors implicated in the causation of cancer are:

- *Tobacco* – more than a quarter of all cancer deaths in the UK are thought to be tobacco related. Cigarette smoking causes nine in 10 cases of lung cancer and increases the risk of many other types of cancers, particularly those in tissues most exposed to tobacco carcinogens, i.e. cancers of the head and neck, oesophagus, stomach, kidney and bladder.
- *Diet* – can have either harmful or protective influences on cancer development depending on its composition in terms of foods, nutrients and food contaminants (see later).
- *Infection* – certain viruses can cause genetic mutations that may result in cancer development, e.g. the Epstein – Barr virus is associated with some types of lymphatic cancer and human papilloma virus appears to be closely linked with cancer of the cervix. Infection with *Helicobacter pylori* is thought to be a major factor in the development of gastric cancer.
- *Industrial pollutants* – exposure to toxic substances such as asbestos or vinyl chloride can rapidly lead to cancer. This is more of a problem in less developed parts of the world where environmental safety controls are often poor.
- *Ionising radiation* – over exposure to X rays, nuclear emissions or some other sources of radioactivity increases the risk of leukaemia.
- *Sunlight* – most skin cancers are caused by the action of radiation from sunlight on the skin.

Diet and causation of cancer

Although there is a common underlying aetiology, different factors influence the development of each type of cancer. For this reason, relationships between diet and cancer are complex and variable; dietary factors may be involved in the initiation of tumour growth (carcinogens), the promotion of growth or be protective against the development of cancer. It is thought that about half of cancer related deaths are preventable, many of them by diet and lifestyle measures.

It has long been known that many components of the diet have carcinogenic potential. Some of these result from food contamination, e.g. aflatoxin, a potent carcinogen causing liver cancer that is produced by a mould that can grow on grain stored under inappropriate conditions. Other carcinogens such as alkaloids, benzene derivatives or N-nitroso compounds occur naturally in foods or are created during cooking or preservation processes. Alcohol may act as a carcinogen, e.g. when in contact with the tissues of the head, neck or oesophagus.

Diet may have a role to play in the promotion of tumour growth by encouraging replication of cells. This action may be caused by dietary components such as alcohol, or a high fat or high energy diet. Diet and body weight may also influence the growth of cancer cells through the promotion of hormones in the body, e.g. oestrogens in the promotion of breast cancer.

The human body has many defence systems to protect it from potentially harmful agents in its environment – both dietary and non-dietary – and to a large extent can withstand their continuous onslaught. However, the body's ability to do so depends on factors such as immune competence, integrity of mucosal barriers and levels of detoxifying enzymes, all of which are affected by diet. It is therefore not unreasonable to expect that diet is likely to be one of the factors enhancing or diminishing the risk of cancer.

In 1981 Doll & Peto suggested that about one-third of cancers in westernised countries may be attributable to dietary factors, and that as many as 70% of cancers in sites such as the large bowel, breast and prostate may be preventable by dietary modification. The evidence for this has since been comprehensively reviewed in a major report from the World Cancer Research Fund (WCRF) in conjunction with the American Institute for Cancer Research (AICR) (WCRF/AICR, 2007). The report confirmed that there are many links between diet and cancer, both causal and protective. The relationships are complex and, given the quality of the available evidence, difficult to ascertain. The effect on reducing cancer risk if dietary recommendations (Table 7.15.1) are followed is unclear, although a study of 29 564 women showed that following –six to nine of the WCRF recommendations over a 17-year period resulted in a 22% reduction in cancer risk compared with women who did not follow any recommendations (Cerhan *et al.*, 2004).

Nature of the evidence for relationships between diet and cancer

Most of the suggested associations between diet and cancer in humans are based on data from epidemiological studies, which comprised the following types of study (see Chapter 1.1, Research section):

- *Cross sectional studies* compare differences in diet and cancer prevalence, either between or within populations. These observations can provide valuable pointers but are not in themselves evidence of cause and effect as many other relevant factors, e.g. socioeconomic, demographic, genetic, cultural and environmental factors, will also differ.

Table 7.15.1 Dietary recommendations for cancer prevention [based on the World Cancer Research Fund (WCRF) report on Food, Nutrition, Physical Activity and the Prevention of Cancer: a Global Perspective (WCRF/AICR, 2007]

Recommendation	Public health goals	Justification
Be as lean as possible within the normal range of body weight	Median adult body mass index (BMI) to be 21–23 kg/m² depending on the normal range for different populations Level of overweight/obesity to be no more than the current level, or preferably lower, in 10 years	Maintenance of a healthy weight throughout life may be one of the most important ways to protect against cancer
Be physically active as part of everyday life	The proportion of the population that is sedentary to be halved every 10 years Average physical activity levels >1.6	Most populations, and people living in industrialised and urban settings, have habitual levels of activity below levels to which humans are adapted
Limit consumption of energy dense foods Avoid sugary drinks	Average energy density of diets to be lowered towards 125 kcal/100 g Population average consumption of sugary drinks to be halved every 10 years	Consumption of energy dense foods and sugary drinks in increasing worldwide and is probably contributing to the global increase in obesity
Eat mostly foods of plant origin	Population average consumption of non-starchy vegetables and of fruit to be at least 600 g (21 oz)/day Relatively unprocessed cereals (grains) and/or pulses (legumes), and other foods that are a natural source of dietary fibre, to contribute to a population average of at least 25 g/day of non-starch polysaccharide	An integrated approach to the evidence shows that most diets that are protective against cancer are mainly made up from foods of plant origin
Limit intake of red meat and avoid processed meat	Population average consumption of red meat to be no more than 300 g (11 oz)/week, very little if any of which to be processed	An integrated approach to the evidence also shows that many foods of animal origin are nourishing and healthy if consumed in modest amounts
Limit alcoholic drinks	Proportion of the population drinking no more than the recommended limits to be reduced by one-third every 10 years	The evidence on cancer justifies a recommendation not to drink alcoholic drinks. Other evidence shows that a modest amount of alcoholic drinks is likely to reduce the risk of coronary heart disease
Limit consumption of salt Avoid mouldy cereals (grains) or pulses (legumes)	Population average consumption of salt from all sources to be <5 g (2 g of sodium/day) Proportion of the population consuming >6 g of salt (2.4 g of sodium)/day to be halved every 10 years Minimise exposure to aflatoxins from mouldy cereals (grains) or pulses (legumes)	The strongest evidence on methods of food preservation, processing and preparation shows that salt and salt preserved foods are probably a cause of stomach cancer, and that foods contaminated with aflatoxins are a cause of liver cancer
Aim to meet nutritional needs through diet alone	Maximise the proportion of the population achieving nutritional adequacy without dietary supplements	The evidence shows that high dose nutrient supplements can be protective or can cause cancer. The studies that demonstrate such effects do not relate to widespread use amongst the general population, in whom the balance of the risks and benefits cannot confidently be predicted. A general recommendation to consume supplements for cancer prevention may have unexpected adverse effects. Increasing the consumption of the relevant nutrients through usual diet is preferred
Mothers to breastfeed: children to be breastfed	The majority of mothers to breastfeed exclusively for 6 months	The evidence on cancer as well as other diseases shows that sustained, exclusive breastfeeding is protective for the mother as well as the child
Cancer survivors: follow the recommendations for cancer prevention	All cancer survivors to receive nutritional care from an appropriately trained professional. If unable to do so, and unless otherwise advised, aim to follow the recommendations for diet, health weight, and physical activity	Subject to the qualifications made in the WCRF report

- *Case control studies* look for differences between the diet of people with a particular type of cancer and that of carefully matched healthy controls. This has the advantage of creating more homogeneous study populations, but at the same time, such homogeneity in terms of age, social class, occupation, etc. also means that dietary differences between the two groups are likely to be small, or not readily detectable given the limitations of dietary assessment methodology. Alternatively, if dietary differences are observed, it is difficult to know whether they existed in the early stages of cancer development, perhaps many years before, or whether they are a consequence of having the disease. Any attempt to get round this problem by retrospective dietary assessment is fraught with difficulties; most people cannot remember with any accuracy what they ate 5 or 10 years previously.

- *Prospective (cohort) studies* followed people until cancer develops, thus enabling dietary comparison between those who do with those who do not develop the disease, and are particularly informative. However, they are also the most difficult and costly studies to carry out, requiring large numbers of subjects to be monitored for 10–20 years or more. The European Prospective Intervention into Cancer and Nutrition (EPIC) is a major study of this type, investigating the effect of diet, lifestyle, and genetic and environmental factors on the incidence of different forms of cancer.
- *Intervention trials* evaluate the effects of dietary change in a randomised, controlled prospective trial and can provide the clearest evidence of dietary benefit or risk. However, for reasons of cost, they are unlikely to be carried out on a sufficiently large scale, or for long enough, to evaluate the effect of major dietary manipulations, e.g. encouraging a high consumption of fruit and vegetables, on a disease such as cancer.

Animal studies are a valuable supplement to human studies to help explain the mechanisms of carcinogenesis and provide pointers to dietary influences on those mechanisms. However, animal studies ultimately cannot predict dietary risk in free living human populations where many other factors will operate.

Complexity of the relationship between diet and cancer

The interrelationship between diet and the development of cancer is complex and multifactorial. The relationships between diet and cancer are hard to unravel because of the great variability of both the disease and the dietary influences on it. Different cancers are influenced by diet to a different extent. Although all cancers stem from DNA damage, the causes and effects of that damage are very variable. Some cancers, e.g. colorectal and breast, may be strongly linked with diet and body composition; others e.g. leukaemia, have no relationships with diet at all.

Some dietary factors, e.g. non-starch polysaccharide, may be protective against one type of cancer but have no influence at all on another. Also, observed dietary relationships do not always operate in the same direction; energy intake is positively associated with the development of some cancers, e.g. breast and endometrial, but negatively with others, e.g. stomach and oesophageal. A dietary influence may be heightened or diminished by non-dietary factors, e.g. a dietary component may only become a risk factor in certain circumstances, such as a person smoking. The risk or benefit from one dietary component may be affected by the presence or absence of other dietary components, e.g. the level of risk from meat may depend on the level of consumption of protective fruit and vegetables. For these reasons, attempts to assess whether one particular dietary component is beneficial, harmful or neutral in effect are fraught with difficulty and open to misinterpretation. Few dietary risk factors operate in isolation and it seems increasingly likely that it is the combination of harmful and protective influences from both dietary and non-dietary sources that determines the level of cancer risk. The relationships between diet and cancer are therefore based on judgement as to what the research evidence means, as reviewed by the WCRF (2007).

Diet and cancer care

Nutrition is an important aspect of the care of the person with cancer from diagnosis onwards. Many aspects of cancer can affect nutritional status, and impaired nutritional status can in turn affect the response to treatment, the amount of treatment required and the quality of life (NICE, 2004; Henry, 2011). Dietitians working in oncology have a vital role in ensuring that nutritional aspects of patient management are an integral component of multidisciplinary care and that all cancer patients receive the dietetic support they need. The National Institute for Health and Care Excellence (NICE, 2004) recommends that dietitians working in oncology are basic or advanced level practitioners, who have knowledge of the impact of the disease and treatment, and the complex needs of such patients to be able to provide the high level of care required. This criterion is subject to peer review in the NHS (NCAT, 2008). Dietitians need to work in close collaboration with other team members to meet patient needs.

Nutritional implications of cancer

People with cancer are at high risk of nutritional depletion because of the physical and psychological effects of both the disease and its treatment for the following reasons:

- A prolonged catabolic response to the presence of a tumour may occur in some cancer patients, resulting in muscle wasting and weight loss (Laviano *et al.*, 2011).
- Physical symptoms, e.g. pain, dysphagia, vomiting and diarrhoea, may impair food intake or nutrient absorption, or increase nutrient losses.
- The psychological effects of being diagnosed with cancer can result in anxiety and/or depression and impair appetite.
- Cancer treatments often result in pronounced and debilitating side effects. Gastrointestinal consequences such as anorexia, nausea, vomiting, diarrhoea, bloating, pain or cramping inevitably have an adverse effect on nutritional intake, and additional problems such as taste changes, dysphagia, infections and fistulae may further compromise nutritional status.

The risk of weight loss and undernutrition is therefore high. About 40% of cancer patients have been found to have significant protein energy malnutrition (Ravasco *et al.*, 2003; Bozzetti & SCRINIO Working Group, 2009) and in some high risk groups, such as head and neck cancer patients, up to 80% may have some degree of malnutrition. The adverse consequences of this in terms of postoperative recovery time, prevalence of complications and prognosis are well documented (see Chapter 6.2). In cancer patients, undernutrition may also have implications for cancer treatment because chemotherapy dosages are based on body weight and underweight patients may not be given optimum dosages (Andreyev *et al.*, 1998). A patient with muscle wasting is also less likely to be able to withstand the side effects of treatment and will develop more toxicity (Prado *et al.*, 2009).

Preventing and correcting nutritional depletion in order to maintain physical strength and quality of life for as long as possible are therefore important objectives in the care of the cancer patient. The ways in which this is achieved will vary according to the individual clinical circumstances, but primarily comprise:

- Ensuring nutritional and hydration needs are met in an acceptable and appropriate way for each individual throughout the course of the disease.
- Restoring any nutritional inadequacies that occur.
- Minimising the nutritional consequences of the symptoms and side effects of treatment.
- Instituting additional nutritional support measures if dietary intake is inadequate.
- Reviewing the effectiveness of nutritional interventions and adjusting them as necessary.

Close interaction with other members of the multidisciplinary team is essential if these objectives are to be achieved effectively (NICE, 2004; Fearon, 2008).

General aspects of the dietary care of cancer patients

Dietary care of cancer patients may range from offering healthy eating guidance for people who have successfully recovered from treatment, to the provision of total artificial nutritional support for those who are critically ill or unable to manage their full nutritional requirements. In practice, most people will require varying degrees of nutritional intervention throughout the treatment and progression of the disease. It is important to consider the whole treatment plan for the cancer patient as this may involve many weeks or months of a range of different treatments. Assessment of individual needs and problems is therefore the cornerstone of dietary management and should consider:

- *Current nutritional intake* – whether this is sufficient to meet nutritional needs.
- *Current nutritional problems* – the extent to which food and fluid intake is impaired by the physical or psychological effects of the disease or its treatment.
- *Degree of any nutritional depletion* – although to some extent compounded by the cancer process itself, the extent and rapidity of recent weight loss is an important indicator of nutritional depletion (see

Chapter 2.2). Other markers of nutritional status such as anaemia or poor immune function may also be indicative when considered in conjunction with dietary intake.
- *Likelihood of further (or future) nutritional depletion* – surgery will incur significant metabolic costs as a result of pre- and peri-operative starvation and postoperative trauma. Radiotherapy and chemotherapy often result in general disinclination to eat, as well as causing specific problems with eating or swallowing, or exacerbating pre-existing problems. The risk of nutritional depletion is particularly high in those who are already in a malnourished state.
- *Nutritional implications of specific types of cancer*, e.g. malabsorption resulting from pancreatic cancer, *consequences of surgical procedures*, e.g. dumping syndrome following gastric resection, and *consequences of treatment*, e.g. diarrhoea or steatorrhoea following pelvic radiotherapy. These are discussed in more detail in other chapters.

Even if no nutritional problems are identified, the importance of good nutrition should still be stressed and people encouraged to continue to meet their needs via a healthy well balanced diet. If nutritional intake is inadequate, the dietetic objectives are to:

- Increase energy and nutrient intake to meet nutritional requirements in ways that are acceptable to the patient.
- Tackle general and specific problems inhibiting food and fluid intake.
- Identify when further nutritional support measures are necessary in the context of current and future planned anticancer treatment.

In many people, energy, nutrient and fluid intake can be increased by relatively simple dietary measures which increase the frequency and the energy/nutrient density of foods and beverages consumed (see Chapter 6.3). Food enrichment measures, e.g. the addition of milk powder to milk, and adding cheese, butter or cream to foods, can also be an effective way of boosting nutrient intake. Remedial measures to help alleviate treatment side effects affecting food intake, such as mucositis, taste changes, nausea, vomiting or diarrhoea, should also be suggested (see Chapter 6.3 and the later specific cancer chapters). Adequate symptom control is also paramount for these patients.

If oral intake remains inadequate, additional supplementation in the form of sip feeds or other supplements may need to be considered. Artificial nutritional support (enteral and parenteral nutrition) may be necessary following some types of surgery or cancer treatment or in those with severe or worsening malnutrition (see Chapter 6.4 and Chapter 6.5). If the cancer progresses, then palliative measures may become the primary consideration (see Chapter 7.16).

Some oral nutritional supplements are specifically aimed at patients with cancer cachexia. They contain n-3 fatty acids, which due to their anti-inflammatory properties aim to reduce the metabolic element of cancer cachexia whilst also providing additional energy and protein as a drink. A randomised trial in patients with pancreatic cancer failed to show that eicosapentaenoic acid (EPA) supplemented drinks were any better at slowing down weight loss than conventional high energy, high protein drinks (Fearon *et al.* 2003). Poor compliance with n-3 fatty acid supplemented drinks was a factor in the study. Additional studies in different patient groups have also failed to confirm any benefit, although the principles supporting a reduction in the inflammatory reaction produced by cancer are attractive in the management of cachexia (Murphy *et al.*, 2011).

At all stages of the disease, the dietitian has a crucial role in identifying when additional support measures are appropriate and what form these should take in order to optimise nutritional status without impairing quality the life. Social factors must also be considered in assessing nutritional needs. Those who live alone are particularly vulnerable to malnutrition when they are unwell, in pain and find it an effort to shop, cook and eat. People should be encouraged to make use of any help offered by friends and neighbours or other support services available in their community.

It is essential to provide written guidance for patients and carers, together with contact details of a dietitian or another member of the healthcare team. Patients often feel unwell at the time they talk to a dietitian and may find it difficult to remember the advice given, or later think of other questions they wanted to ask. Providing appropriate dietetic support and guidance not only helps patients feel physically better, but often also psychologically better equipped to cope with what is inevitably a traumatic phase in their lives.

Maintaining nutritional status may improve tolerance to treatment in terms of less medication needed for symptom control, a shorter period of chemotherapy induced nausea and vomiting, better tolerance of chemotherapy and fewer treatment delays (Bozzetti, 2001). All cancer patients should therefore be encouraged to regard eating well as an important component of medical care, and a positive step they can take to help maintain their health. Some patients may be at increased risk of gaining weight with treatment, e.g. breast cancer patients, and therefore may require advice on weight maintenance.

Specific aspects of dietary management during cancer treatment

Treatment for cancer usually involves surgery, radiotherapy or chemotherapy (including hormonal treatment), and sometimes a combination of all three.

Surgery

A high proportion of patients undergoing curative treatment will have surgery at some point in their treatment. Surgical removal of a tumour has a number of nutritional implications:

- Preparation for surgery involves a period of nil by mouth.

- Surgery incurs a significant metabolic cost as a result of the response to trauma.
- In all cases, there will be some delay before normal feeding is resumed. If the surgery is major or involves any part of the gastrointestinal tract, there may be considerable delay before feeding is possible via an enteral route. Surgery to the mouth, throat or digestive tract may result in prolonged problems with oral feeding (see Chapter 7.15.2).
- Surgery may result in temporary or permanent side effects that affect food intake, digestion or absorption, e.g. dumping syndrome, intestinal failure, ileostomy.

In addition, some cancer patients will undergo surgery in an already malnourished state and be particularly at risk of severe nutritional depletion. All the above factors need to be taken into account when nutritional care is being planned and may influence the following:

- Whether preoperative nutritional support is indicated, whether this is feasible and, if so, what form it should take. This may include the consideration of immunonutrition, which has been demonstrated to reduce postoperative infection in upper gastrointestinal cancer patients (Gianotti *et al.*, 2002).
- Whether peri- and post-surgical nutritional support is likely to be needed, either at an early stage or if there are delays in resumption of oral feeding or complications.
- Whether support should be total or partial.
- The extent to which the oral route will be accessible.
- Whether support is likely to be short or long term.

Practical aspects of pre- or post-operative nutritional support can be found in Chapter 6.4 and Chapter 7.17.5. As recovery progresses, every effort should be made to restore and maintain good nutritional status, if necessary by means of oral support to optimise nutritional intake. Some patients will require specific guidance to alleviate the postsurgical consequences of gastric or intestinal resection, such as dumping or intestinal failure. Arrangements should be made to ensure that after discharge from hospital the progress of any nutritionally vulnerable patient, particularly in terms of body weight and dietary intake, is monitored at either the primary or secondary care level.

Radiotherapy

This involves the use of ionising radiation within a treatment field to destroy cancer cells. Radiotherapy damages tissue because energy dissipated from ionising radiation generates a series of biochemical events inside the cell. Free radicals are formed and these disrupt DNA, preventing replication, transcription and protein synthesis. When given in combination with chemotherapy, the risk to healthy tissues may be enhanced. Individual radiation treatments, known as fractions, are usually given once daily, sometimes more often (known as hyperfractionated) or less often (hypofractionated); the radiation dose is measured in Gray (Gy). The length of treatment can vary from a single fraction to a 7-week course of five fractions/week. Radical treatment is given with curative intent, whilst palliative treatment is usually given for symptom control, e.g. pain or shortness of breath. Common general side effects of radiotherapy include:

- Anorexia.
- Nausea.
- Fatigue.
- Reduced mood, often related to physical symptoms.

Combinations of these, together with travelling for treatment each day, can have a devastating effect on food intake. Some people will find the fatigue makes shopping, food preparation and eating particularly difficult.

The site at which the radiotherapy is targeted will determine the severity of side effects. Specific side effects of radiotherapy to particular areas of the body can further impair food intake. Radiation to the head and neck often affects the ability to eat or swallow; radiation to the pelvic area often results in abdominal cramps and diarrhoea. If steps are not taken to alleviate them, the nutritional consequences can be severe. The side effects of radiotherapy may also change during the course of treatment, e.g. patients initially experiencing dry mouth may develop a sore mouth at a later stage. Regular dietetic assessment of this patient group is therefore essential to ensure that appropriate and timely advice is given as patients may experience progressive dysphagia. The effects in particular diagnoses are considered in the following chapters. As patients proceed with radiotherapy treatment, there is a high risk of worsening morbidity and quality of life. Patients undergoing radiotherapy should have regular nutrition screening and identification of any difficulties with eating identified at an early stage in order for these to be addressed.

Chemotherapy

Chemotherapy has a systemic effect; the aim is to destroy cancer cells but normal tissue will also be affected. The consequences, and hence side effects, are worst in rapidly dividing tissues such as the lining of the mouth and gastrointestinal tract. Chemotherapy may be given with other targeted therapies, e.g. drugs that affect the growth of cancer cells by different actions. These include monoclonal antibodies that target vascular epidermal growth factor (VEGF), thereby preventing it from stimulating the growth of new blood vessels. Chemotherapy can be administered as oral tablets, a bolus, continuous infusion or combinations of these.

The number of cytotoxic drugs used to treat cancer is continually increasing and each drug has different side effects. When drugs are used in combination, the aim is to increase toxicity to the cancer cells while minimising the side effects. Nevertheless, side effects are common and those that may affect appetite and food intake include:

- Nausea and vomiting.
- Taste changes.
- Stomatitis.

- Mucositis (resulting in sore or painful mouth).
- Oesophagitis.
- Diarrhoea.
- Constipation.
- Neutropenia.

In addition to the impact on nutritional status, cytotoxic drugs may also influence certain nutrients as a result of drug–nutrient interactions. For example, methotrexate is a folate antagonist so its use may need to be accompanied by folinic acid rescue; the administration of folinic acid to speed recovery from methotrexate induced mucositis or myelosuppression. Pyridoxine is used to treat palmar plantar erythrodysesthesia (a painful condition affecting the hands and feet) caused by capecitabine or 5-flurouracil chemotherapy.

Good symptom management is essential to minimise the impact on nutritional intake and nutritional status. Dietary measures that may help alleviate effects of chemotherapy, such as nausea, taste changes or sore mouth, are described in Chapter 6.3, and these should be available to patients undergoing treatment to ensure that their dietary intake and quality of life is maximised.

Endocrine therapies

Hormonal manipulation is used in the treatment of hormone sensitive cancers, e.g. breast and prostate. Cells may vary in their sensitivity to hormones such as oestrogens and progesterones, and sensitivity can be determined by the presence of cellular receptors (oestrogen receptor and progesterone receptor). Treatment interventions may include surgery, e.g. oophorectomy, or more commonly medication that blocks hormone action. For example, some endocrine therapies will block at the receptor level (receptor antagonist) or block part of the process of hormone manufacture, e.g. aromatise inhibitors or luteinising hormone releasing hormone agonists. Endocrine therapies can influence mood and cause a decrease in appetite however, in some patients weight gain may occur after diagnosis (Harvie & Howell, 2005; Parry, 2011).

Monitoring progress of cancer patients

Nutritional assessment should be an integral part of patient monitoring following cancer treatment. Some patients with complex nutritional problems will need ongoing specialist dietetic follow-up. It is essential that all members of the healthcare team are aware of the need to look for and identify emerging nutritional problems so that they can be rectified at an early stage. Appropriate guidance should be given for identified problems or patients referred for dietetic assessment and advice. Patients who are unable to maintain an adequate dietary intake may need nutritional supplementation or artificial nutritional support.

Enteral feeding may be indicated for patients with severe anorexia, dysphagia or mucositis or who have become nutritionally debilitated. In the short term, this is usually achieved by nasogastric or nasojejunal tube, sometimes on an overnight basis. In the long term (for 4 weeks or more), it is more likely to be via gastrostomy or jejunostomy. Parenteral nutrition should only be used when use of the gastrointestinal route is contraindicated, usually for reasons such as bowel obstruction, uncontrollable vomiting or severe malabsorption.

Post recovery dietary guidance

Cancer patients are usually anxious to consume a diet that minimises the chance of disease progression or recurrence. Some may be tempted to follow one of the complementary or alternative dietary regimens promoted for cancer patients (see Chapter 5.4). People should be assured that current evidence suggests that a diet based on the principles of healthy eating, i.e. a well balanced diet relatively high in starch and fibre and low in fat, will offer the most protection. Particular emphasis should be placed on the importance of plentiful consumption of fruit and vegetables and wholegrain cereal foods. In the UK, the NHS Choices website provides appropriate up to date information on healthy eating (see Chapter 4.2) and the WCRF provides dietary guidance for cancer survivors who are able to eat well and have a normal body weight. However, this advice does not apply to patients who have eating difficulties or are losing weight. Dietary guidance for cancer protection is summarised in Table 7.15.1.

Some patients may choose to take vitamin and mineral supplements with the aim of influencing cancer growth or risk of recurrence. Some studies have indicated that such high dose supplements may increase risk, e.g. beta-carotene in lung cancer, or decrease risk, e.g. calcium in colorectal cancer, of disease or recurrence. Studies can be difficult to interpret with conclusions being dependent on the particular dose given, dietary intake, chemical form of the supplement and the combination of any other drugs or nutrients. At present there is insufficient evidence to recommend the use of vitamin or mineral supplements as an adjunct to conventional therapy apart from their use to ensure an adequate dietary intake or to correct a detected deficiency. High doses of vitamins are to be avoided as they may interact with medication, including chemotherapy.

Palliative care

Sometimes cancer cannot be cured and treatment becomes palliative, i.e. focusing on the relief of symptoms rather than treating their cause. As the disease progresses, eating and swallowing difficulties become increasingly likely. The patient's food intake is often a great concern to relatives and carers, and can even be a source of conflict. Patients become increasingly cachectic (see Chapter 7.15.9) and the extent to which nutritional and hydration support should be used to sustain life may eventually need to be discussed. The nutritional care of people who are terminally ill is discussed in Chapter 7.16. Some of the ethical issues involved are discussed in Chapter 1.1.

Alternative diets

Many people with cancer are tempted to try unconventional remedies, including alternative and complementary diets, in the hope of cure or remission (Downer et al., 1994). Alternative diets claim to treat or cure cancer; they are followed instead of conventional cancer treatment. Complementary diets constitute any unusual or unorthodox change to a normal diet and claim to benefit people with cancer; they are followed in association with accepted cancer treatments.

The rationale for trying these diets is understandable; faced with the prospect of a life threatening condition, people will try anything that they think might improve their chances of survival. Patients may also use complementary and alternative therapies to address the emotional and spiritual aspects of the disease and to boost their immune system (Parker et al., 2010). No randomised controlled trials have been carried out to evaluate the benefit of such diets and many healthcare professionals remain sceptical about their value (Cassileth et al., 1991). In addition, cancer patients may not be aware of the potential risks of using complementary and alternative medicines or may not always inform their doctor of their use (Werneke et al., 2004), often because the healthcare professional does not ask the patient if they are taking such therapies. Alternatively, patients may choose to make lifestyle changes with the aim of managing the negative impact that cancer treatment can have on health related quality of life (Ashing-Giwa et al., 2010). These lifestyle changes include eating a healthier diet, increasing exercise, use of complementary or alternative medicine and stress reduction.

The problem with many alternative and complementary diets (see Table 7.15.2) is that they are more likely to worsen nutritional status than improve it. Such diets tend to share a number of common features such as:

- Being vegetarian or vegan.
- Containing large amounts of raw food.
- Advocating the use of organic foods.
- Being low in fat.
- Being low in sugar or sugar free.
- Being low in salt.
- Restricting intake or avoiding dairy products.
- Avoiding processed foods and beverages containing caffeine.
- Encouraging the use of vitamin and mineral supplements.

As a result, these diets often have a low energy density due to their high bulky fibrous food content and low content of fat and carbohydrate. People may therefore find it difficult to eat enough to meet their needs, particularly if they have eating or swallowing problems associated with the disease or its treatment. Restrictions on food choice may cause dietary imbalances. Use of mega doses of vitamins and minerals can create other nutritional distortions and may even be hazardous. Safe upper limits for vitamins and minerals are described in the Food Standards Agency report on this subject (EVM, 2003).

Table 7.15.2 Examples of alternative and complementary dietary regimens used by cancer patients

Dietary regimen	Philosophy	Main dietary principles
The Bristol Cancer Centre Diet (complementary)	The Centre believes that, as part of an holistic approach, diet and nutritional supplements can be important and may well have an influence on recovery by enhancing the effectiveness and reducing side effects of cancer treatment, improving wellbeing and in some cases prolonging survival	Wholefoods Fresh fruit and vegetables Organically grown foods Whole grains Organic poultry, eggs, game and fish in moderation Beans and pulses Freshly made fruit and vegetable juices Supplements of vitamin C, beta-carotene, vitamin B complex, selenium, zinc
Macrobiotics (complementary)	Foods are classified as Yin foods, representing feminine, dark and negative principles, and Yang foods, representing masculine, light and positive principles. The aim is to balance these for each individual in order to obtain a healthy mind and body	Mainly based on cereal grains Vegetables, sea vegetables and fruit Bean and bean products Nuts and seeds Fish Soup made with vegetables, beans and grains Sea vegetables seasoned with sea salt, soy sauce or miso
Dairy free diets (complementary)	Milk and dairy foods promote the growth of cancer, particularly breast and prostate cancer	Soya foods, including soya milk, are substituted for dairy foods Increase consumption of fruit and vegetables (preferably organic) Avoid processed foods, including meats, oils, refined starchy foods, alcohol and fizzy drinks
Gerson therapy (alternative)	Aim is to stimulate the body's own defence system to overcome cancer. Both the nutritional and detoxification parts of the therapy are required	Vegan Fresh fruit and vegetables Freshly made fruit and vegetable juices Supplements of digestive enzymes, niacin, liver capsules, iodine, thyroid extract, potassium compound and vitamin B_{12} injections Coffee enemas

Such regimens may also be expensive, unpalatable and time consuming to prepare. Patients accept this because they have high expectations of their success, but may then suffer feelings of anger and frustration if these are subsequently not met. They may also feel guilty if they have to abandon the diet for any reason. While there is no evidence that these regimens offer any benefit over conventional therapies, and in some instances make matters worse, some cancer patients do claim to feel better on these regimens (Werneke *et al.*, 2004; Cassileth & Deng, 2004). The reason for this is unclear, but may be associated with *doing something positive* to take control of the disease and treatment, and also because of the often excellent psychological support offered along with dietary advice as part of holistic therapy.

It is important that dietitians are aware that patients may be tempted to try, or are already following, alternative or complementary diets. In this situation, the role of the dietitian is to explore whether the patient would like to discuss their dietary intake and change any aspect of their diet:

- If patients ask whether they should try a particular alternative diet, encourage them to find out all they can about the regimen and openly discuss the potential benefits and hazards.

- If the patient wants to try one of these diets, encourage them to follow it for a short period of time, such as a month, and then return for further assessment and discussion.

- If an alternative diet is already being followed, discuss any obvious dietary shortcomings and suggest positive measures that the patient can take to improve nutritional intake. Some patients may be prepared to compromise and will incorporate some aspects of their alternative regimen into a better balanced nutritional programme.

- If alternative or complementary medicines are being taken, refer to the pharmacy to check the supplement, dosage and any possible interaction with conventional medicines that are being prescribed (Werneke *et al.*, 2004).

Ultimately, the patient is responsible for making the decision to follow a complementary or alternative dietary regimen. However, it is the responsibility of the dietitian to ensure that the patient has been given sufficient balanced information and advice on which to base that decision. In order to do this, it is important that dietitians keep up to date with the types of diets being suggested for cancer and their nutritional implications. The progress and dietary intake of patients following alternative diets should be monitored in order to try and ensure that good nutritional status is maintained.

Drug–nutrient interactions

Drug–nutrient interactions may occur with chemotherapeutic agents, drugs used to manage symptoms and additional medication that is being taken to manage comorbidities. These interactions can potentially occur with food, nutritional supplements and herbal preparations. Patients should be encouraged to discuss all additional over the counter supplements with a pharmacist before consuming them to check for any potential adverse reactions.

Further reading

Alpha-Tocopherol, Beta-Carotene Cancer Prevention Study Group (ATBC). (1994) The effect of vitamin E and beta-carotene on the incidence of lung cancer and other cancers in male smokers. *New England Journal of Medicine* 330: 1029–1035.

Brown JK, Byers T, Doyle C, *et al.*; American Cancer Society. (2003) Nutrition and physical activity during and after cancer treatment: An America Cancer Society guide for informed choices. *CA: A Cancer Journal for Clinicians* 53: 268–291.

Cassileth BR, Lucarelli CD. (2003) *Herb-Drug Interactions in Oncology.* Hamilton, Canada: BC Decker.

Cerhan JR, Potter JD, Gilmore JME, *et al.* (2004) Adherence to the AICR cancer prevention recommendations and subsequent morbidity and mortality in the Iowa Women's Health Study Cohort. *Cancer Epidemiology Biomarkers and Prevention* 13(7): 1114–1120.

Department of Health. (1998) Report of the Working Group on Diet and Cancer of the Committee on Medical Aspects of Food and Nutrition Policy. *Nutritional Aspects of the Development of Cancer.* Report on Health and Social Subjects 48. London: Stationery Office.

Department of Health. (2000) *The NHS Cancer Plan: A plan for investment, a plan for reform.* London: Department of Health.

Shaw C (ed). (2011) *Nutrition and Cancer.* Oxford: Wiley Blackwell.

Internet resources

Cancer Research UK   www.cancerresearchuk.org
Macmillan Cancer Support   www.macmillan.org.uk
NHS Choices   www.nhs.uk/livewell/healthy-eating
World Cancer Research Fund   www.wcrf-uk.org

References

Andreyev HJ, Norman AR, Oates J, Cunningham D. (1998) Why do patients with weight loss have a worse outcome when undergoing chemotherapy for gastrointestinal malignancies? *European Journal of Cancer* 34(4): 503–509.

Ashing-Giwa KT, Lim J-W and Gonzalez P. (2010) Exploring the relationship between physical well-being and healthy lifestyle change among European and Latina-American breast and cervical cancer survivors. *Psycho-Oncology* 19: 1161–1170.

Bozzetti F. (2001) Nutrition support in patients with cancer. In: Payne-James J, Grimble G, Silk D (eds) *Artificial Nutrition Support in Clinical Practice.* London: Greenwich Medical Media, pp. 639–680.

Bozzetti F; SCRINIO Working Group. (2009) Screening the nutritional status in oncology: a preliminary report on 1000 patients. *Support Care in Cancer* 17: 279–284.

Cancer Research UK. (2006) Cancer Mortality Statistics. www.cancerresearchuk.org/cancer-info/cancerstats/mortality/. Accessed 2 December 2013.

Cancer Research UK (CRUK). (2011a) Incidence of all cancers. Available at www.cancerresearchuk.org/cancer-info/cancerstats. Accessed 2 December 2013.

Cancer Research UK (CRUK). (2011b) Common cancers. Available at www.cancerresearchuk.org/cancer-info/cancerstats. Accessed 22 February 2013.

Cancer Research UK. (2011c) Cancer survival statistics. Available at www.cancerresearchuk.org/cancer-info/cancerstats. Accessed 2nd December 2013.

Cassileth BR, Deng G. (2004) Complementary and alternative therapies for cancer. *Oncologist* 9(1): 80–89.

Cassileth BR, Lusk EJ, Guerry D, *et al.* (1991) Survival and quality of life among patients receiving unproven as compared with conventional cancer therapy. *New England Journal of Medicine* 324: 1180–1185.

Cerhan JR, Potter JD, Gilmore JME, *et al.* (2004) Adherence to the AICR cancer prevention recommendations and subsequent morbidity and mortality in the Iowa Women's Health Study Cohort. *Cancer Epidemiology Biomarkers and Prevention* 13(7): 1114–1120.

Doll R, Peto R. (1981) The causes of cancer; quantitative estimates of avoidable risks of cancer in the United States today. *Journal of the National Cancer Institute* 66: 1192–1308.

Downer SM, Cody MM, McCluskey P. (1994). Pursuit and practice of complementary therapies by cancer patients receiving conventional treatment. *BMJ* 309: 86–89.

Expert Group on Vitamins and Minerals (EVM). (2003) *Safe Upper Levels for Vitamins and Minerals.* London: Food and Standards Agency. Available at www.food.gov.uk.

Fearon KCH. (2008). Cancer cachexia: Developing multimodal therapy for a multidimensional problem. *European Journal of Cancer* 44(8): 1124–1132.

Fearon KCH, von Meyenfeldt MR, Moses AGW, *et al.* (2003) Effect of a protein and energy dense n-3 fatty acid enriched oral supplement on loss of weight and lean tissue in cancer cachexia: a randomised double blind trial. *Gut* 52: 1479–1486.

Gianotti L, Braga M, Nespoli L, Radaelli L, Beneduce A, Di Carlo VA. (2002) Randomized controlled trial of preoperative oral supplementation with a specialized diet in patients with gastrointestinal cancer. *Gastroenterology* 122: 1763–1770.

Harvie M, Howell A. (2005) The need for lifestyle interventions amongst post menopausal women with early breast cancer. *Women's Health* 1(2): 205–223.

Henry L. (2011) Effect of malnutrition on cancer patients. In: Shaw C (ed) *Nutrition and Cancer.* Oxford: Wiley Blackwell.

Laviano A, Preziosa I, Fanelli FR. (2011) Cancer and nutritional status. In: Shaw C (ed) *Nutrition and Cancer.* Oxford: Wiley Blackwell.

Maddams J, Brewster D, Gavin A, *et al.* (2009) Cancer prevalence in the United Kingdom: estimates for 2008. *British Journal of Cancer* 101(3): 541–547.

Murphy RA, Mourtzakis M, Chu QSC, Baracos VE, Reiman R, Mazurak VC. (2011) Nutritional intervention with fish oil provides a benefit over standard of care for patients with weight and skeletal muscle mass in patients with non small cell lung cancer receiving chemotherapy. *Cancer* 117: 1775–1782.

National Cancer Action Team (NCAT). (2008) Manual for Cancer Services 2008: Rehabilitation Measures. Available at http://ncat.nhs.uk/sites/default/files/Gateway_11008_DEC_rehab_20081117_0.pdf. Accessed 23 August 2011.

National Institute for Health and Care Excellence (NICE). (2004) *Improving Supportive and Palliative Care for Adults with Cancer: The Manual.* London: NICE.

Parker PA, Cohen L, Bekele BN, Hough H, Lee RT, Fisch M. (2010) Complementary and alternative medicine (CAM) use among cancer patients in community oncology settings. *Journal of Clinical Oncology* 28(15): (Suppl 1): 0732–183X.

Parry B. (2011) Nutrition and breast cancer. In: Shaw C (ed) *Nutrition and Cancer*. Oxford: Wiley Blackwell, pp. 334–362.

Prado CMM, Baracos VE, McCargar LJ, *et al.* (2009). Sarcopenia as a determinant of chemotherapy toxicity and time to tumor progression in metastatic breast cancer patients receiving capecitabine treatment. *Clinical Cancer Research* 15(8): 2920–2926.

Ravasco P, Monteiro-Grillo I, Vidal PM, Camilo ME. (2003) Nutritional deterioration in cancer: The role of disease and diet. *Clinical Oncology* 15(8): 443–450.

Werneke U, Earl J, Seydel C, Horn O, Crichton P, Fannon D. (2004) Potential health risks of complementary alternative medicines in cancer patients. *British Journal of Cancer* 90: 408–413.

World Cancer Research Fund/American Institute for Cancer Research (WCRF/AICR). (2007) *Food, Nutrition, Physical Activity and the Prevention of Cancer: a Global Perspective*. Washington, DC: World Cancer Research Fund.

7.15.2 Head and neck cancer

Bella Talwar

Key points

- The dietitian is a key member of the head and neck cancer care team, providing nutritional assessment, advice and support from diagnosis onwards.

- Early referral is crucial to provide nutritional support tailored to the patient's needs. Appropriate and timely intervention aims to overcome the physical, social and psychological challenges.

- Prophylactic tube placement is recommended if oral intake is inadequate, not possible or likely to be restricted during treatment and rehabilitation over a prolonged period of time. Appropriate decision making around prophylactic tube feeding should be discussed at diagnosis as part of the treatment management plan.

- Multifactorial high risk selection criteria for enteral tube feeding, including patient demographics, tumour site and staging, treatment modalities, placement technique and associated morbidity, should be considered on an individual basis.

Cancers of the head and neck are the sixth most common cancers worldwide and constitute 5% of malignancies in the UK (Quinn *et al.*, 2001). The majority of these cancers arise from the surface layers of the upper aerodigestive tract and include a variety of histological types of which squamous cell carcinomas make up 95% of cancers (Argiris *et al.*, 2008). The mouth, lip and tongue (oral cavity), the upper part of the throat and respiratory system (pharynx), and the voice box (larynx) represent 90% of head and neck malignant tumours. Cancers of the salivary glands, nose, sinuses, middle ear and those that originate in the nerve and bone of the head and neck are relatively rare (NICE, 2004).

The age distribution of newly diagnosed patients is in the fifth to seventh decade of life, but it is increasing in the middle aged adult population, and the 3:1 ratio for the prevalence in men and women is decreasing (NICE, 2004).

Tobacco exposure and high alcohol consumption are the two strongest aetiological factors, both independently and synergistically, in the development of primary and secondary head and neck cancers (Marron *et al.*, 2010). Certain tumour sites are associated with specific risk factors. The chewing of beetle nut is linked to cancers of the oral cavity (Proia *et al.*, 2006). Epstein–Barr virus is associated with nasopharyngeal cancers in individuals of oriental origin. Human papilloma virus (HPV 16) is an increasingly recognised causative factor in oropharyngeal and oral cancer, particularly in individuals who are non-smokers or non-drinkers, and in people aged 30–50 years (BAO-HNS, 2011).

The aims of treatment are to eliminate the disease and achieve long term survival. However, the 5year mortality rate from head and neck cancer has not improved significantly over the last 40 years, despite advances in diagnostic tools and treatment modalities. Therefore, locoregional control (disease recurrence at the primary site or the neck), quality of life and organ function are critical outcome considerations in describing and evaluating treatment (List & Bilir, 2004; BAO-HNS, 2011).

Nutrition is a fundamental long term prognostic factor (Brooks, 1985) and has become an increasingly important quality of life issue surrounding the psychosocial and rehabilitation needs of head and neck cancer patients (BAO-HNS, 2011).

Nutritional implications

Head and neck cancer patients present a significant nutritional challenge due to their risk of malnutrition associated with lifestyle choices, site of their cancer, the disease process and treatment. It is estimated that approximately 50–75% of diagnosed patients experience moderate to severe malnutrition (van Bokhorst-de van der Scheuren

Table 7.15.3 Factors contributing to malnutrition in head and neck cancer (source: Talwar 2010. Reproduced with permission of Wiley-Blackwell Publishing)

Contributory factors	Cause
Poor dietary habits	Consumption of unbalanced meals can lead to energy, protein and micronutrient deficiency
Excessive alcohol intake	Associated with appetite suppression, inadequate nutrient intake and micronutrient deficiency
Depression and anxiety	These can result in aversion to food and/or loss of appetite with reduced quality of life
Difficulty with chewing	Lack of teeth, ill fitting dentures and physical problems with jaw movement can markedly affect food choice in favour of a limited range of soft or liquid foods
Difficulty with swallowing	Presence of the tumour mass, pain on eating, ulcerated mouth and fear of choking can compromise the safety of swallowing and result in the consumption of a diet restricted in variety, texture and nutritional content
Cachexia	Altered nutritional and metabolic response due to the presence of the tumour can result in symptoms such as anorexia, loss of appetite, early satiety and marked weight loss associated with muscle wasting and increased production of acute phase protein
Changes in body composition	Disturbance in energy balance with changes in resting energy expenditure, glucose uptake, mobilisation of fat and protein stores, and muscle protein release
Halitosis	Anaerobic respiration with the production of lactic acid and subsequent build-up of ammonia released via the mouth
High risk of refeeding syndrome	Combined effect of the causes and consequences of malnutrition in this patient group, leading to risk of starvation for longer than 7–10 days and unintentional significant weight loss
Limited support network	Patients who live alone or have no family can be less motivated and often find it more challenging to maintain adequate nutrition
Impaired wound healing	Increased risk of infection due to decreased muscle, respiratory, gut and immune functions
Higher risk of hospital admission	Nutritional deterioration requiring feeding management with greater length and cost of hospital stay
Poor functional status and quality of life	Increased lethargy and decreased ability to mobilise, work and socialise
Increased morbidity and mortality	Poor nutritional status at presentation combined with malnutrition and its associated consequences, limiting the options and choice of cancer therapy due to tolerance and therefore contributing towards poorer tumour control and survival

et al., 1997; Hammerlid *et al.*, 1998), and 80% will lose weight during multimodality treatment (BAO-HNS, 2011). Malnutrition is discussed in more detail in Chapter 6.2. However, the causes and consequences of malnutrition in head and neck cancer patients at presentation are multifactorial (Table 7.15.3). It is evident from the above that nutrition influences patients' functional, oncological and quality of life outcomes, which have an impact on health economics.

Nutritional effects of treatment

Treatment options for head and neck cancers involve single- or multi-modality regimens with surgery, radiotherapy and, more recently, the advances that have been made with the use of chemotherapy and biological targeted treatment (BAO-HNS, 2011). The International Union Against Cancer (2007) TNM classification of head and neck tumours describes the anatomical extent of disease based on the size of the primary tumour (T1 4), the absence or presence and extent of regional lymph node metastasis (N1 3), and the absence or presence of distant metastasis (M site). The main anatomical sites in the head and neck region are shown in Figure 7.15.1.

Curative treatment options differ according to the staging and primary tumour site with stage I or II disease managed with single modality treatment using surgery or radiotherapy, and stage III and IV disease requiring multimodality therapy with surgery, radiotherapy and chemotherapy (Argiris *et al.*, 2008). The different combination treatments have led to several competing management strategies, each with different advantages and disadvantages, and initial treatment can vary significantly between institutions (BAO-HNS, 2011).

Over the past decade there have been significant advances in treatments. Surgical resection and reconstruction techniques have evolved and now include minimally invasive approaches such as trans oral laser. Radiotherapy fractionation schedules have been modified to promote organ preservation with induction and/or concurrent chemotherapy sparing healthy tissue by targeted coverage (BAO-HNS, 2011). Chemoradiotherapy results in an absolute survival improvement of 8% at 5 years and is currently recognised as the gold standard treatment for advanced cancers requiring combined modality treatment. These chemotherapeutic agents are platinum based, with the dose, delivery method and timing varying between institutions (Pignon *et al.*, 2009). Cancer treatments delivered as single or multimodality therapy to the head and neck region have a permanent effect on organs essential for normal human activities like breathing, speaking, eating and drinking (NICE, 2004). This creates further nutritional problems and increases

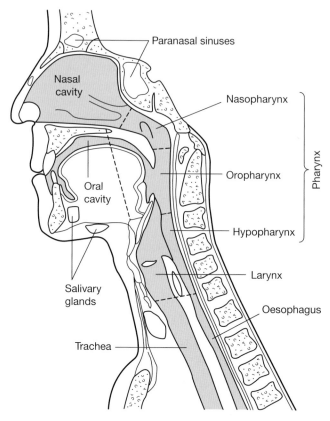

Figure 7.15.1 Main sites of head and neck cancers (adapted from Talwar 2010. Reproduced with permission of Wiley-Blackwell Publishing)

the risk of nutritional depletion requiring appropriate and timely intervention (Talwar, 2010).

Surgery

Surgical resection can severely restrict or even eliminate the patient's ability to consume oral nutrition. Van Bokhorst-de van der Schueren *et al.* (1997) assessed a variety of malnutrition parameters in patients undergoing major surgery for advanced cancer and identified weight loss as the most significant. Patients with a weight loss of >10% during the 6 months presurgery had a greater risk of postoperative complications, with an incidence of between 20% and 50% (Bertrand *et al.*, 2002). A follow-on study to evaluate nutritional status as a prognostic value found no influence of any of the investigated nutritional parameters for the whole group. However, preoperative weight loss and occurrence of major postoperative complications showed a marked negative influence on the survival of male patients with head and neck cancers (van-Bokhurst-de van der Schueren *et al.*, 1999).

Based on the above findings, the same researchers conducted a randomised controlled trial to study the effect of perioperative nutritional support on nutritional status, immune status, postoperative outcome and survival in severely malnourished patients undergoing major surgery. Although the trial concluded that 7–10 days preoperative feeding did not improve nutritional status, it did find that preoperative enteral nutrition in patients with head and

> **Box 7.15.1** High risk selection criteria for preoperative feeding of head and neck cancer patients (Weimann *et al.*, 2006)
>
> - Weight loss >10–15% in 6 months
> - Body mass index <18.5 kg/m^2
> - Subjective Global Assessment Grade C
> - Serum albumin <30 g/L
> - Unable to maintain intake above 60% of recommended intake for >10 days

neck cancer improved their functional and emotional status in the preoperative period, although this was not evident at 6 months (Van Bokhorst-de van der Schueren *et al.*, 2000). This raised the question of whether preoperative enteral feeding should commence at clinical presentation when there is a strong suspicion that the diagnosis is likely to be a malignancy, to evaluate if there is a beneficial effect on nutritional status (Bradley & Donaldson, 2000).

Immunonutrition is supported by limited evidence in the literature and therefore is recommended in this patient group, with some benefit observed if administered in the pre- or post-operative period to reduce fistulae rates and length of stay, and improve 10-year survival (Findlay *et al.*, 2011). Further research is required. However, there is consensus guidance at an international level for best practice, recommending preoperative nutrition in patients at severe nutritional risk (BAO-HNS, 2011; Findlay *et al.*, 2011) as identified in Box 7.15.1. Consequences of surgery are outlined in Table 7.15.4.

Radiotherapy

Side effects of radiotherapy are due to the direct effect of radiation upon the tumour, or because of involvement of healthy tissue within the field of treatment in the head and neck region (Figure 7.15.1). The severity of the reaction depends on the radiation schedule, volume and cumulative dose given to the anatomical structures in the treatment field. This treatment can be given as a single or cumulative dose, and a radical course involves the patient attending daily treatments for up to 6–7 weeks and receiving a total dose of 60–70 Gray (Kelly, 2007). Radiotherapy side effects impact on the patient from the second week of treatment, peaking during the fourth to fifth week and continuing for on average 3 weeks after completing the course (Polisena, 2010). Radiotherapy can further compromise the patient's nutritional status and make the management particularly challenging. The treatment side effects can occur in the acute stage with permanent changes, or as a late reaction during the patient's follow-up and rehabilitation (Talwar, 2010). These side effects are summarised in Table 7.15.5. Prior to starting radiotherapy, it is estimated that 44% of patients present with common symptoms associated with eating, including difficulty with mastication, swallowing and odynophagia, loss of appetite and nausea, and by the third week of

Table 7.15.4 Effects of surgery and nutritional consequences (source: Talwar 2010. Reproduced with permission of Wiley-Blackwell Publishing)

Effects of surgery	Nutritional consequences
Loss of taste	Surgery to the tongue, salivary glands or olfactory nerve negatively influence taste acuity, leading to reduced appetite and gustation
Loss of smell	Loss of nasal airflow via the olfactory receptors in the nasal cavity leading to reduced enjoyment of meal times and social interaction
Difficulty chewing	Partial or total inability to masticate due to loss of bony supporting structure (mandible), exacerbated by dental extraction, misalignment of the jaw and trismus, leading to the requirement for texture modification, increased effort and reduced enjoyment of food, and social isolation
Drooling and pocketing of food and fluid	Reduced pressure to move the bolus into the pharynx occurs due to surgery or nerve damage, and can be embarrassing and isolating, causing anxiety and depression
Reduced peristalsis	Prolonged meal times with risk of avoiding food and fluid, leading to inadequate diet, dehydration, constipation and weight loss
Oral regurgitation	Due to reconstruction or gastric transposition (pharyngolaryngo-oesophagectomy) requiring small frequent meals, remaining upright for 1 hour post meal, and lying down with the head elevated
Nasal regurgitation	Functional impairment of the soft palate or motor activity of the graft can be embarrassing and distressing, and require to be maintained whilst eating and drinking
Dumping syndrome (pharyngolaryngo-oesophagectomy)	Causes nausea, bloating, abdominal cramps and explosive diarrhoea; fear of food and eating is common and changes in eating habits are required due to prolonged meal times and early satiety
Poor wound healing	Examples include flap failure, dehiscence at anastomosis, necrosis and infection. Contributing factors include previous radiotherapy, malnutrition and increased nutritional requirements, necessitating assessment for vitamin and mineral supplementation
Fistulae	Occur in the oral cavity, pharynx or larynx, caused by previous radiotherapy and affect tissue healing and swallowing, requiring alternative feeding
Risk of wound infection	At wound site or chest with extensive or revision surgery and lengthy operations when entering into or resecting part of the upper aerodigestive tract, increasing nutritional requirements
Nerve injury	Damage to the trigeminal, facial, glossopharyngeal, vagus, accessory, hyoglossal and recurrent laryngeal nerves affect swallowing coordination, chewing and taste, increasing the risk of aspiration and fatigue during meals, as well as facial disfigurement
Aspiration	Can be a silent or reactive cough with food or fluid entering the lungs, requiring the patient to be nil by mouth and needing alternative feeding
Chylous fistulae	Tumour invasion or surgical trauma of the thoracic duct with <500 mL/day lymphatic drainage, requiring conservative management or >600 mL/day over a prolonged period and suggesting surgical repair
Strictures and stenosis	Complete or partial obstruction of the food bolus, requiring dilatation with texture modification, and smaller size food bolus with plenty of fluid and multiple swallows
Patient comorbidity factors	Diabetes, renal impairment, malnutrition, previous surgery or radiotherapy, anaesthetics for procedure and duration of the surgery

treatment patients report three or more eating problems (Larsson *et al.*, 2005).

In a small study (Larsson *et al.*, 2003) using qualitative measures to examine patient experiences during radiotherapy, the following symptoms were reported to affect quality of life:

- Ability to chew and swallow.
- Will and desire to eat.
- Changes in saliva quantity and consistency.
- Narrowing in the throat and pain.
- Nausea.
- Taste changes.

Patients felt their way of life was disturbed as a result of having to cope with the effects of their symptoms at meal times, leading to loss of togetherness with family and friends. Additionally, they experienced extreme fatigue and loss of self confidence (Larsson *et al.*, 2003).

Up to 57% of head and neck cancer patients experience weight loss before starting radiotherapy, 95% of whom report this as being unintentional weight loss. Radiotherapy treatment may result in a further loss of approximately 10% of body weight (Lees, 1999).

Chemoradiation

Chemotherapy is particularly likely to affect the rapidly dividing cells of the buccal and gastrointestinal mucosa, causing damage to the mucosal lining of the mouth (Van Cutsen & Arends, 2005). Chemotherapy alone is not used widely, but is administered as a neoadjuvant (before radiotherapy) and/or concurrently with radiotherapy; although it has been shown to improve survival, this is at the cost of increased toxicity (Pignon *et al.*, 2009). Chemoradiation results in more severe acute adverse effects than radiotherapy alone, and the long term effects of

Table 7.15.5 Side effects of radiotherapy and nutritional consequences (source: Talwar 2010. Reproduced with permission of Wiley-Blackwell Publishing)

Side effect	Nutritional consequences
Taste changes	Diminished, distorted, abnormal and/or loss of taste (described as cardboard, metallic or sandpaper) leading to food aversion and reduced intake
Mucositis	Oral mucosal reaction that can result in pain, infection or retching
Xerostomia	Requires good oral hygiene, artificial saliva and food texture modification
Dysphagia	Pre-existing or post treatment with tissue damage impairing wound healing
Swallowing impairment of oral phase	Reduced range of lingual motion and strength, impaired bolus formation and transport through the oral cavity, prolonged transit time and increased residue occur in floor of mouth resections, causing difficulty with chewing, taste changes and fatigue during meals
Swallowing impairment of pharyngeal phase	Impaired tongue base movement, delayed trigger of the swallow, reduced pharyngeal contraction, reduced laryngeal function, reduced opening of the oesophageal sphincter, resulting in impaired bolus clearance and aspiration
Aspiration	Silent or reactive coughing on food and fluid associated with fear of eating; can be due to lethargy, weakness and reduced alertness secondary to malnutrition
Trismus	Restricted ability to open the mouth, which can be due to pre-existing tumour obstruction, radiation induced or reduced mastication over a prolonged period
Osteoradionecrosis	Mandible incapable of healing itself or fighting infection due to poor blood supply, resulting in reduced ability to masticate and limited mouth opening
Impaired wound healing	Permanent tissue damage increasing risk of poor wound healing
Fatigue	Apathy and severe tiredness limiting physical function, as well as motivation with swallowing increasing time and effort at meals with an overall reduced nutrient intake
Dental caries	Due to poor oral hygiene or exacerbated in the presence of xerostomia as food and fluid stick to the teeth, there is no flushing effect from saliva and the teeth rapidly decay
Dehydration	Decreased salivary flow resulting in altered colonisation of the oropharynx, impaired bolus preparation due to lack of saliva and increased thickness of sputum

radiation are also increased and can profoundly affect nutritional intake and swallowing physiology, causing significant morbidity and diminished quality of life (Shiley et al., 2006). In head and neck cancer the chemotherapeutic agents most commonly used are platinum based and where patient comorbidities present a risk for administering systemic agents, an alternative monoclonal epidermal growth factor receptor (EGFR) inhibitor is used (cetuxmab) (BAO-HNS, 2011).

Chemoradiation is known to exacerbate weight loss during treatment by>5% of pretreatment weight (Nugent et al., 2010b). Odynophagia (pain on swallowing food and fluids) caused by severe mucositis and nausea can markedly impair the intake and enjoyment of food, and are thought to be significant factors associated with the weight loss and difficulties experienced with eating (Kelly, 2007).

Poor symptom control during radiotherapy and/or chemotherapy will result in dehydration, lethargy and severe weight loss if nutrition support is inadequate, and contribute to inadequate treatment delivery and efficacy for local regional control and survival (BAO-HNS, 2011; Findlay et al., 2011). The side effects of chemotherapy on nutritional consequences are listed in Table 7.15.6.

Current treatments for head and neck cancer have an adverse effect on many nutritional aspects. A prospective cross sectional study, taking account of the stage of disease and therapeutic intervention, evaluated quality of life, nutritional status and dietary intake, and found that reduced energy and protein intakes, together with weight loss, were independent determinants of quality of life (Ravasco et al., 2004). Patients at risk of severe weight loss at diagnosis and during treatment can be identified with health related quality of life questionnaires (Karin et al., 2005), although there is no nutrition specific module to assess the relationship between malnutrition, nutritional status, dietary counselling and nutrition support in this patient group (Talwar, 2010).

New treatments for head and neck cancer currently being examined include robotic surgery, photodynamic therapy and biological targeted therapy focussing on tumour suppression genes and EGFRs using cetuximab (Argiris et al., 2008). The nutritional consequences have yet to be evaluated.

Principles of nutritional management

The organisation and structure of nutrition and dietetic services should aim to provide a quality centred, seamless service at all stages of the patient pathway, with access to site specific dietitians throughout the patient journey and recognising that they are core members of the multidisciplinary head and neck cancer team (BAO-HNS, 2011). The publication of evidence based practice guidelines based on a systematic review of literature across the entire nutritional care pathway sets the benchmark for quality rated nutritional interventions and outcomes (Findlay et al., 2011). Best practice nutritional care should

Table 7.15.6 Side effects of chemotherapy and nutritional consequences (source: Talwar 2010. Reproduced with permission of Wiley-Blackwell Publishing)

Side effect	Nutritional consequences
Severe mucositis	Although radiation induced, this can be exacerbated by the systemic effects of the drug and can impair wound healing
Nausea and vomiting	Systemic or anticipatory; triggered by taste, smell and anxiety
Anorexia	Reduced appetite accompanied by reduced intake
Taste and smell alterations	Diminished, distorted, abnormal and/or loss of taste (described as cardboard, metallic or sandpaper), leading to food aversion and reduced intake
Diarrhoea	Risk of dehydration and distressing to the patient
Stomatitis	Sore mouth significantly affecting food intake
Nephrotoxicity/ ototoxicity	Renal impairment can lead to nausea and loss of appetite
Metabolic abnormalities	Can lead to increased energy expenditure and micronutrient deficiency

incorporate implementation of appropriate validated tools for routine malnutrition screening, early referral to the dietitian, and regular comprehensive nutritional assessment and monitoring to optimise nutritional status (Talwar & Findlay, 2012). The patient pathway and dietetic clinical model of care is shown in in Box 7.15.2.

Nutritional screening

It is crucial that all head and neck cancer patients undergo nutritional screening to identify those who have, or are at risk of developing,, malnutrition at any stage of the patient pathway, and it should be an integral part of multidisciplinary clinical practice (NICE, 2004; BAO-HNS, 2011; Findlay *et al.*, 2011). Nutritional screening tools should be validated in oncology patients and where used for head and neck cancer patients should be able to identify the following groups who may benefit from full nutritional assessment (BAO-HNS, 2011; Findlay *et al.*, 2011):

- Patients who are not nutritionally compromised at diagnosis, but who are at risk of malnutrition during treatment. These patients would benefit from a dietetic assessment during the planning of their cancer treatment in order to recommend an appropriate nutritional management plan.
- Patients who are disease free post treatment, but who present with late side effects from both surgery and radiotherapy that may impact on their oral intake and increase the patients' risk of developing malnutrition.

Nutritional assessment

Effective nutritional management is dependent upon appropriate nutritional assessment. Useful factors to con-

sider include clinical observation, dietary history, and calculation of requirements, proposed treatment, anthropometry, biochemistry and social information. The specific parameters for this patient group are summarised in national clinical guidance (BAO-HNS, 2011) with key reflective questions that should be considered as part of the assessment. These should include the following.

Nutritional aspects

- What is the nutritional status of the patient? Consider the percentage energy intake from alcohol, percentage body weight loss in the previous 6 months, and body mass index (BMI).
- Is the patient at risk of refeeding syndrome?
- How many cups of fluid is the patient drinking during the day?
- How long is it taking the patient to consume a meal?
- Is the patient feeling hungry or thirsty after a meal?
- Which types of food is the patient finding easy/difficult to manage?
- Is the patient chewing food for longer before swallowing?
- Consider the effort and time taken to eat or drink and how this is impacting on the patients quality of life.
- Does drinking sips of liquids between bites of food make it easier to swallow?
- Has the patient adapted their eating habits to make it easier to swallow? If so, how?
- Is it taking more time and effort to eat and drink throughout the day?
- Are there any problems with the patient's dentition?

Clinical aspects

- What is the size of the tumour?
- What part(s) of the anatomy does the tumour involve?
- What are the aims of treatment – cure, symptom control, palliation?
- Does the treatment plan involve combined modality treatment?
- Has the patient had previous oncological treatment?
- What is the extent of any surgical resection and is reconstruction planned?
- What are the risk factors for postoperative complications?
- What is the radiotherapy dose and treatment field?
- What is the patient's performance status?
- Does the patient have comorbidities or contraindications if considering alternative feeding?
- What is the patient's social support network?
- What are the patient's lifestyle choices for smoking, drinking and recreational drugs?

Dietetic management

Dietetic input throughout the patient pathway is needed to assess and correct nutritional deficiencies, evaluate how different treatment modalities will impact on a patient's nutritional status, and recommend the most appropriate short and long term nutritional interventions to meet the nutritional needs of the patient and/or achieve

Box 7.15.2 Patient pathway and dietetic clinical model of care (Talwar, 2010)

Diagnosis

Intervention

Assess risk factors for patient compliance

Negotiate feeding options with team and patient

Assess need for artificial feeding to include screening for suitability and method of insertion

Screening of nutritional status

Outcome

Improve or maintain nutritional status

Identify need and determine timing and type of prophylactic tube placement

Pretreatment

Intervention

Discuss outcomes of intensive nutritional counselling with dietary intake, oral and enteral nutrition support

Assess presenting symptoms from previous treatment

Discuss effects of treatment and possible impact on ability to eat and drink in the short and long term

Discuss method of feeding options and types of feeding tubes using visual aids, psychosocial aspects relating to body image, feeding in public, physical activity

Outcome

Assess need for pretreatment reconditioning

Provide realistic expectations of eating and feeding issues

Establish rapport to promote patient motivation and compliance

Support consent process for placement and use of feeding tubes, timelines for oral and enteral nutrition and rehabilitation programme to ensure timely and appropriate tube removal

Treatment: Surgery

Intervention

Discuss effects of surgery on ability to eat and drink

Advise patient on how to overcome dietary problems and use the feeding tube

Tailor feeding regimen to meet patient's individual requirements

Adjust feeding regimen accordingly following introduction of oral diet so that optimum intake is maintained

Prepare patient for discharge on enteral feeding, including necessary training of patient and carers, practical feeding tube management

Liaise with all relevant community staff and feed company to ensure that discharge home on enteral feed is safe and efficient

Outcome

Improve or maintain nutritional status to reduce risk of developing postoperative complications

Prepare patient for safe and effective discharge, allaying any anxieties

Adequate preparation for discharge reduces likelihood of readmission for feeding tube related problems

Treatment: Radiotherapy and/or chemoradiation

Intervention

Discuss any presenting or ongoing problems with eating and drinking, and potential impact of further treatment

Advise patient on overcoming problems associated with chemoradiation

Monitor dietary adequacy and tolerance to treatment

Outcome

Optimise nutritional status to minimise risk of treatment interruptions (and subsequent admission)

Provide support and advice to enhance motivation and compliance with oral nutrition support and appropriate use of enteral feeding to prevent tube reliance

Post treatment

Intervention

Assess/monitor post treatment effect on ability to eat and drink

Adjust dietary feeding regimen accordingly with oral diet to maintain adequate nutritional intake

Provide advice on modifying texture of diet and symptom control for side effects

Negotiate feeding tube removal as appropriate

Outcome

Maintain adequate nutritional status

Maximise patient motivation and compliance

Assist patient to re-establish eating and drinking, thus improving quality of life

Long term care/survivorship

Intervention

Provide ongoing nutritional care with dietary advice for oral nutrition support and enteral nutrition

Provide psychosocial support for enteral feeding

Outcome

Establish goals for weight management and maintaining adequate nutrition support

Support the patient and carers living with the effects of treatment outcomes (BAO-HNS, 2011; Findlay *et al.*, 2011). Key questions that need to be asked in order to determine the nutritional management:

- Is it safe for the patient to consume oral nutrition and/or does the patient need to be referred to a speech and language therapist?
- Is the patient maintaining their nutritional status with oral intake alone or is an alternative system of feeding required?
- Do the patient's symptoms and/or treatment plan indicate the need for alternative feeding in the short or long term?
- If the patient requires enteral feeding, what is the type of tube and safest technique for placement to meet the patient nutritional needs?
- If the patient requires tube feeding, is there continuity with dietetic support and management until it is appropriate to remove the feeding?

Dysphagia can lead to an inadequate energy, nutrient and fluid intake, and can have a severe adverse effect on the patient's health, nutritional status and quality of life unless the cause is identified and appropriately managed. If unrecognised over a prolonged period of time, dysphagia can place the patient at risk of malnutrition or dehydration and their associated complications (Table 7.15.7).

The speech and language therapist will assess the degree of dysphagia, including the risk of aspiration, and recommend management that may include alternative texture modification and the use of swallowing techniques or postures where appropriate (RCSLT, 2002) (see Chapter 7.3). The dietitian should be part of the dysphagia team, providing nutrition information to support the diagnosis of swallowing problems and subsequent management (Lundy *et al.*, 2009).

Nutritional support

Choice of cancer treatment will influence the need for preoperative nutrition, and may also increase the nutritional requirements for postoperative recovery and hence the need for nutritional support during radiotherapy or chemoradiation. Recently there have been a number of systematic reviews to evaluate the outcomes of dietary counselling and methods of nutritional support in patients receiving treatment for head and neck cancer (Garg, 2010; Nugent *et al.*, 2010a; Findlay *et al.*, 2011).

First line nutritional support intervention is often food fortification, but it is imperative to evaluate the appropriateness of this given the intensity of treatment regimens and the consequences on the patient's ability to consume and sustain adequate oral nutrition. Each patient should be individualised to receive nutritional support that is tailored to their diagnosis and treatment plan, including early oral nutritional support and enteral nutrition (BAO-HNS, 2011).

Oral nutritional support

It is challenging for patients to remain motivated and committed to sustaining adequate nutrition whilst experiencing side effects of treatment (Cady, 2007; Mayre-Chilton *et al.*, 2011). It is important that patients maintain an intake as close as possible to a normal diet in order to maintain muscle function for swallowing and minimise feelings of loss of control with oral nutrition during their cancer care (BAO-HNS, 2011). However, a patient's ability to sustain an adequate oral intake over an extended period of time is underestimated (Talwar, 2010). Randomised controlled trials evaluating the impact of dietary counselling demonstrated improvements in patients' nutritional status, dietary compliance and quality of life (Isenring *et al.*, 2004; Ravasco *et al.*, 2005). (see Chapter 6.3).

Enteral nutritional support

If oral nutrition is inadequate or not possible, enteral feeding should be considered without delay as otherwise the patient's nutritional status will be compromised, leading to poor patient centred, clinical and financial outcomes (Findlay *et al.*, 2011). Assessing the need for early instigation of partial or total artificial support should be included when treatment options are being considered for head and neck cancer patient (Grobbelaar *et al.*, 2004; BAO-HNS, 2011). Details of the principles and practice of artificial nutritional support are given in Chapter 6.4.

The benefits of increased energy and protein intake, and reduced weight loss in patients receiving enteral nutrition compared with oral nutrition has been known for decades from randomised controlled trials (Daly *et al.*, 1984; Hearne *et al.*, 1985). Early referral to the

Table 7.15.7 Consequences of malnutrition and dehydration in head and neck cancer patients

Consequences of malnutrition	Swallowing impairment and increased risk of aspiration due to lethargy, weakness and reduced alertness Reduced strength of the cough and mechanical clearance in the lungs Impaired wound healing and increased risk of infection due to decreased muscle, respiratory, gut and immune functions Higher risk of admission to hospital and greater length and cost of hospital stay Poor functional status and quality of life due to lethargy and decreased ability to mobilise, work and socialise Increased morbidity and mortality
Consequences of dehydration	Decreased salivary flow resulting in altered colonisation of the oropharynx Impaired bolus preparation due to lack of saliva and increased thickness of sputum Increased risk of aspiration due to lethargy and mental confusion

dietitian within a nutritional support programme and dietary counselling have also been shown to improve outcomes for enteral nutrition, with less weight loss, and fewer treatment interruptions and unplanned hospital admissions (Wood, 2005; Mangar *et al.*, 2006; Paccagnella *et al.*, 2010).

Early studies showed gastrostomy feeding to be more advantageous than nasogastric tube feeding, with patients experiencing increased mobility, reduced anxiety with altered body image, higher energy intakes and improved quality of life scores with the former (Lees, 1997; Mekhail *et al.*, 2001; Piquet *et al.*, 2002). Patients and their carers need to be supported to establish a feeding pattern and to improve their confidence with tube care before having to cope with the debilitating effects of the treatment (Scolapio *et al.*, 2001).

The relative advantages of gastrostomy placement have been challenged over the past 5 years, with much debate regarding the optimal timing and route of enteral tube feeding (Talwar & Findlay, 2012). Prophylactic placement is gastrostomy insertion before treatment and differs from interventional gastrostomy, which refers to placement as required during treatment. In a non-prospective randomised controlled trial, nasogastric tubes were compared with non-prophylactic gastrostomy placement (Corry *et al.*, 2009). The gastrostomy group used tubes for longer and had better weight outcomes compared with the nasogastric group who experienced greater tube dislodgement and increasing patient and carer dissatisfaction as the study progressed. These findings have been supported in a large retrospective review that showed weight loss was less with prophylactic gastrostomy placement compared with placement as an intervention during treatment (Nugent *et al.*, 2010a). In a randomised controlled trial, improved quality of life scores at 6 months have also been reported with prophylactic gastrostomy placement compared with interventional gastrostomy placement (Salas *et al.*, 2008). A Cochrane review concluded that the method of enteral feeding remains unclear in patients receiving radiotherapy or chemoradiotherapy, but this review only included one study and this study had a high degree of bias (Nugent *et al.*, 2010b). However, another systematic review that included 10 randomised controlled trials concluded that both dietary counselling and prophylactic gastrostomy maintained or improved nutritional status (Garg, 2010). All of these studies used weight as a nutrition outcome, but more recently a prospective longitudinal case series evaluated other anthropometrical measures and found improvements with prophylactic tube placement before, during and after treatment (Silander *et al.*, 2010).

Despite the evidence supporting the benefits of prophylactic tube feeding, mainly with gastrostomy placement, there are no consensus guidelines and decision making is based on the clinical expertise and experience of the institution (Talwar, 2010). The optimal timing for decision making is at diagnosis and all factors impacting on nutrition should be considered, including patient demographics, tumour site and staging, treatment modalities, nutritional status, type and placement technique of feeding tube, and associated morbidity (Talwar & Findlay, 2012).

Careful consideration needs to be given to the timing and method of gastrostomy placement, with appropriate screening and selection for endoscopic, radiological or surgical placement based on comorbidities and contraindications. Organisational needs include a coordinated approach across the head and neck, gastroenterology and radiology services for appropriate screening and selection of placement method. Close monitoring to minimise the risk of morbidity or mortality from postoperative complications and accountable services for insertion and removal of the feeding tube are essential (Talwar, 2010; BAO-HNS, 2011; Findlay *et al.*, 2011; Talwar & Findlay, 2012).

Practical and psychosocial aspects of gastrostomy feeding

The emotional, psychological and physical stresses associated with the diagnosis and treatment of head and neck cancer can be substantial for patients and their partners (Vickery *et al.*, 2003). Patients and carers reported that the gastrostomy improved nutritional status, provided relief from the pressure of coping with the side effects of treatment during periods of extreme fatigue, and was a lifesaver; they would confidently make the same decision regarding gastrostomy placement (Mayre-Chilton *et al.*, 2011). However, a gastrostomy is not without a burden in day to day living and negative experiences have also been reported (Silver *et al.*, 2004; Jordan *et al.*, 2006; Brotherton & Judd, 2007; Mayre-Chilton *et al.*, 2011). These studies found the following key elements to influence the patient and/or carers' daily activities, lifestyle choices, relationship dynamics and quality of life (Talwar, 2010):

- *Practical limitations* – imposed physical restrictions on going out or staying at home during the day, as well as disturbed sleep at night.
- *Lifestyle restrictions* – restricted choice of clothing and going on holiday.
- *Social adjustments* – difficulties finding a place to feed, effect on eating patterns and interference with family life.
- *Psychological issues* – avoiding or missing meal times with others; dealing with the negative attitudes of others towards feeding; changes in body image; effect of setting up the feeds; confidence with feeding in front of others; inability to act affectionately; understanding of why the tube is necessary.
- *Impact on carers* – interaction at meal times; burden of care, with an estimated 15–30 hours/week dedicated to feeding issues.
- *Feeding tube management* – limited knowledge of and support for technical difficulties, leading to complications and hospital readmission.

The above findings have been confirmed in a quality of life study that also identified the importance of effective gastrostomy counselling in the pretreatment phase, with the use of appropriate literature and visual aids, and ongoing support until the tube is removed (Rogers *et al.*, 2007). A specialist dietitian should undertake this role

SECTION 7

from the point of deciding on tube placement until tube removal (Talwar, 2010).

Nutritional monitoring

Continuous feeding can markedly restrict a patient's independence but may be necessary to meet nutritional requirements when experiencing treatment related side effects. Patients established on a feeding regimen should be encouraged to bolus feed during the day with or without overnight pump feeding. This will prevent nutritional inadequacy, e.g. when attending radiotherapy on a daily basis, encourage a normal eating pattern, help the transition to oral feeding and, most importantly, release the patient from being attached to a pump and thus improve their sense of being in control over feeding issues (Talwar, 2010).

Nutritional intervention post treatment improves and maintains nutritional status and quality of life (Findlay *et al.*, 2011). The majority of patients continue to experience eating difficulties after treatment (Pauloski *et al.*, 2006) and places them at risk of ongoing weight loss; therefore, dietary manipulation and optimisation of nutritional support should continue as a priority (Schattner *et al.*, 2005). Weight loss and functional status are important predictors of quality of life in head and neck cancer patients (Karin *et al.*, 2005). Patient weight should be monitored weekly during treatment, or on admission and at each outpatient appointment (BAO-HNS, 2011). It should be routine practice to use anthropometric tools that measure functional muscle status in this patient group, especially in those on long term nutritional support (see Chapter 2.2). The specialist dietitian and speech and language therapist should set collaborative goals to optimise nutrition and swallowing outcomes, dispelling the misinterpreted concept of gastrostomy dependency and optimising safe transition with swallowing from enteral to oral nutrition without compromising the patient's quality of life in the presence of side effects from treatment (Talwar & Findlay, 2012).

Palliative care issues

The incidence of distant metastasis at initial diagnosis is 10%, with the lung, mediastinal lymph nodes, liver and bone being the most common sites of presentation (Argiris *et al.*, 2008). The incidence of developing a second primary is 3–5% on a yearly basis (Khuri *et al.*, 2006) and the 5-year survival for all stages combined is 60% (Ries *et al.*, 2006). Mortality is usually associated with recurrent disease from the primary site. The patient's ability to consume oral intake can be severely restricted or eliminated due to the progressive nature of the disease causing swallowing difficulties. This can lead to malnutrition and its associated consequences, and is further exacerbated by tumour induced metabolic changes (cancer cachexia) for which the incidence in this patient group is not known (Talwar, 2010). The treatment options at this stage are the same as for curative intent, with the aim of symptom control and the goal of improving quality and quantity of life (BAO-HNS, 2011).

Oral and/or artificial supportive nutrition should be offered as part of palliative care for symptom control. The specialist dietitian should discuss nutritional support and facilitate the decision making process for appropriate nutritional management with other members of the head and neck cancer care team (NICE, 2004; Findlay *et al.*, 2011; BAO-HNS, 2011) (see Chapter 7.16).

Further reading

British Association of Otorhinolaryngologists – Head and Neck Surgeons (BAO-HNS). (2011) *Effective Head and Neck Cancer Multidisciplinary Management 4th consensus document*. London: BAO-HNS.

Findlay M, Bauer J, Brown T, *et al.* (2011) Evidence based practice guidelines for the nutritional management of adult patients with head and neck cancer. Sydney, Australia: Clinical Oncological Society of Australia. Available at http://wiki.cancer.org.au/australia/COSA:Head_and_neck_cancer_nutrition_guidelines.

National Institute for Health and Care Excellence (NICE). (2004) *Improving Outcomes in Head and Neck Cancers – The Manual*. London: NICE.

Talwar B. (2010) Head & neck cancer. In: Shaw C (ed) *Nutrition and Cancer*. Vol 1. Oxford: Blackwell Wiley, pp. 188–220.

Internet resources

Head & Neck Sub Group, Oncology Group of the British Dietetic Association www.bda.uk.com

British Association of Head & Neck Oncology Nurses (BAHNON) www.bahnon.org.uk

National Association of Laryngectomee Clubs   www.laryngectomy.org.uk

References

Argiris A, Karamouzis M, Raben D, *et al.* (2008) Head and neck cancer. *Lancet* 371: 1695–1709.

Bertrand P, Piquet M, Bordier I, Monnier P, Roulet M. (2002) Preoperative nutritional support at home in head and neck cancer patients: from nutritional benefits to the prevention of the alcohol withdrawal syndrome. *Clinical Nutrition and Metabolic Care* 5(4): 435–440.

Bradley P, Donaldson M. (2000) Current management of the nutritional needs of the head and neck cancer patient. *Current Opinion in Otolaryngology Head & Neck Surgery* 8(2): 107–112.

British Association of Otorhinolaryngologists – Head and Neck Surgeons (BAO-HNS). (2011) *Effective Head and Neck Cancer Multidisciplinary Management 4th consensus document*. London: BAO-HNS.

Brookes G. (1985) Nutritional status- a prognostic indicator in head and neck cancer. *Otolaryngology Head and Neck Surgery* 93: 69–74.

Brotherton AM, Judd PA. (2007) Quality of life in adult enteral tube feeding patients. *Journal of Human Nutrition and Dietetic* 20(6): 513–522.

Cady J. (2007) Nutritional support during radiotherapy for head and neck cancer: The role of prophylactic feeding tube placement. *Clinical Journal of Oncology Nursing* 11(6): 875–880.

Corry J, Poon, W, McPhee N, *et al.* (2009) Prospective study of percutaneous endoscopic gastrostomy tubes versus nasogastric tubes for enteral feeding in patients with head and neck cancer undergoing (chemo)radiation. *Head & Neck* 31(7): 944–948.

SECTION 7

Daly JM, Hearne B, Dunaj J, et al. (1984) Nutritional rehabilitation in patients with advanced head and neck cancer receiving radiation therapy. *American Journal of Surgery* 148: 514–520.

Findlay M, Bauer J, Brown T, et al. (2011) Evidence based practice guidelines for the nutritional management of adult patients with head and neck cancer. Sydney, Australia: Clinical Oncological Society of Australia. Available at http://wiki.cancer.org.au/australia/COSA:Head_and_neck_cancer_nutrition_guidelines. Accessed 27 October 2012.

Garg S. (2010) Nutritional support for head and neck cancer patients receiving radiotherapy: a systematic review. *Support Care in Cancer* 18(6): 667–677.

Grobbelaar E, Owen S, Torrance A, Wilson J. (2004) Nutritional challenges in head and neck cancer. *Clinical Otolaryngology* 29: 307–313.

Hammerlid E, Wirblad B, Sandin C, et al. (1998). Malnutrition and food intake in relation to quality of life in head and neck cancer patients. *Head & Neck* 20(6): 540–548.

Hearne BE, Dunaj JM, Daly JM, et al. (1985) Enteral nutrition support in head and neck cancer: tube vs. oral feeding during radiation therapy. *Journal of the American Dietetic Association* 85: 669–674.

International Union Against Cancer. (2007) TNM classification. Available at www.uicc.org/resources/tnm. Accessed 6 September 2013.

Isenring I, Capra S, Bauer J. (2004) Nutrition intervention is beneficial in oncology outpatients receiving radiotherapy to the gastrointestinal or head and neck area. *British Journal of Cancer* 91(3): 447–452.

Jordan S, Philpin S, Warring J, et al. (2006) Percutaneous endoscopic gastrostomies: the burden of treatment from a patient perspective. *Journal of Advanced Nursing* 56(3): 270–281.

Karin P, Ewa S, Hammerlid E. (2005) Quality of life as predictor of weight loss in patients with head and neck cancer. *Head & Neck* 27(4): 302–310.

Kelly LE. (2007) Radiation and chemotherapy. In: Ward E, van As-Brooks CJ (eds) *Head & Neck Cancer: Treatment, Rehabilitation and Outcomes*. San Diego: Plural Publishing Inc, pp. 57–86.

Khuri FR, Lee JJ, Lippman SM, et al. (2006) Randomised phase III trial of low-dose isotretinoin for prevention of second primary tumours in stage I and II head and neck cancer patients. *Journal of National Cancer Institute* 98(7): 441–450.

Larsson M, Hedelin B, Athlin E. (2003) Lived experiences of eating problems for patients with head and neck cancer during radiotherapy. *Journal of Clinical Nutrition* (4): 562–570.

Larsson M, Hedelin B, Johansson I, et al. (2005) Eating problems and weight loss for patients with head and neck cancer. *Cancer Nursing* 28(6): 425–435.

Lees J. (1997) Nasogastric and percutaneous endoscopic gastrostomy feeding in head and neck cancer patients receiving radiotherapy treatment at a regional oncology unit: a two year study. *European Journal of Cancer Care* 6(1): 45–49.

Lees J. (1999) Incidence of weight loss in head and neck cancer patients on commencing radiotherapy treatment at a regional oncology centre. *European Journal of Cancer Care* 8(3): 133–136.

List M, Bilir P. (2004) Evaluations of quality of life and organ function. *Seminars in Oncology* 31: 827–835.

Lundy D, Sullivan P, Bernstein MG. (2009). Rehabilitation of Swallowing and Speech Following Treatment of Head & Neck Malignancies. In: Petruzzelli GP (ed) *Practical Head and Neck Oncology*. San Diego: Plural Publishing Inc, pp. 591–611.

Mangar S, Slevin N, Mais K, Sykes A. (2006) Evaluating predictive factors for determining enteral nutrition in patients receiving radical radiotherapy for head and neck cancer: a retrospective review. *Radiotherapy & Oncology* 78: 152–158.

Marron M, Boffetta P, Zhang Z, et al. (2010) Cessation of alcohol drinking, tobacco smoking and the reversal of head and neck cancer risk. *International Journal of Epidemiology* 39(1): 182–196.

Mayre-Chilton K, Talwar B, Goff L. (2011) Different experiences and perspectives between head and neck cancer patients and their care-givers on their daily impact of a gastrostomy tube. *Journal of Human Nutrition and Dietetics* 24: 449–459.

Mekhail TM, Adelstein D, Rybicki L, Laroto M, Saxton J, Lavertu P. (2001) Enteral nutrition during the treatment of head and neck carcinoma. *Cancer* 91: 1785–1790.

National Institute for Health and Care Excellence (NICE). (2004) *Improving outcomes in head and neck cancers – The Manual.* London: NICE.

Nugent B, Parker MJ, McIntyre IA. (2010a) Nasogastric tube feeding and percutaneous endoscopic gastrostomy tube feeding in patients with head and neck cancer. *Journal of Human Nutrition and Dietetics* 23: 277–284.

Nugent B, Lewis S, O'Sullivan JM. (2010b) Enteral feeding methods for nutritional management in patients with head and neck cancers being treated with radiotherapy and/or chemotherapy. *Cochrane Database of Systematic Reviews* 3: CD007904.

Paccagnella A, Morello M, Da Mosto MC, et al. (2010) Early nutritional intervention improves treatment tolerance and outcomes in head and neck cancer patients undergoing concurrent chemoradiotherapy. *Support Care in Cancer* 18: 837–845.

Pauloski BR, Rademaker AW, Logemann JA, et al. (2006) Relationship between swallow motility disorders on videofluorography and oral intake in patients treated for head and neck cancer with radiotherapy with or without chemotherapy. *Head & Neck* 28(12): 1069–1076.

Piquet M-A, Ozsahin M, Larpin I, et al. (2002) Early nutritional intervention in oropharyngeal cancer patients undergoing radiotherapy. *Support Care in Cancer* 10: 502–504.

Pignon J, le Maître A, Maillard E, Bourhis J; MACH-NC Collaborative Group. (2009) Meta-analysis of chemotherapy in head and neck cancer (MACH-NC): an update on 93 randomised trials and 17,346 patients. *Radiotherapy & Oncology* 92(1): 4–14.

Polisena CG. (2010) Nutrition concerns with the radiation therapy patient. In: McCallum PD, Polisena CG (eds). *The Clinical Guide to Oncology Nutrition*. Chicago: The American Dietetic Association.

Proia N, Paszkiewicz G, Nasca M, Franke G, Pauly J. (2006) Smoking and smokeless tobacco-associated human buccal cell mutations and their association with oral cancer – a review. *Cancer Epidemiology, Biomarkers & Prevention* 15: 1061–1077.

Quinn M, Babb P, Brock A, Kirby L, Jones J. (2001) *Cancer Trends in England and Wales 1950–1999. Studies on Medical and Population Subjects no.66.* London: The Stationery Office.

Ravasco P, Monterio-Grillo I, Marques P, Camilo E. (2004) Cancer: Disease and nutrition are key determinants of patients' quality of life. *Supportive Care in Cancer* 12(4): 246–252.

Ravasco P, Monterio-Grillo I, Marques P, et al., (2005) Impact of nutrition on outcome: A prospective randomised controlled trial in patients with head and neck cancer undergoing radiotherapy. *Head & Neck* 27(8): 659–668.

Ries LG, Melbert D, Krapcho M, et al. (2006) SEER Cancer Statistics Review, 1975–2004. Bethesda, MD: National Cancer Institute.

Rogers SN, Thomson R, O'Toole P, et al. (2007) Patients experience with long-term percutaneous endoscopic gastrostomy feeding following primary surgery for oral and oropharyngeal cancer. *Oral Oncology* 43(5): 499–507.

Royal College of Speech and Language Therapists (RCSLT). (2002) *Communicating quality 2 professional standards for Speech and Language Therapists*. London: RCSLT.

Salas S, Deville J-L, Giorgi R, et al. (2008) Nutritional factors as predictors of response to radio-chemotherapy and survival in unresectable squamous head and neck carcinoma. *Radiotherapy & Oncology* 87: 195–200.

Schattner M, Willis H, Raykher A, et al. (2005) Long-term enteral nutrition facilitates optimization of body weight. *Journal of Parenteral and Enteral Nutrition* 29(3): 198–203.

SECTION 7

Scolapio J, Spangler P, Romano M, Mclaughlin M, Salassa J. (2001) Prophylactic placement of gastrostomy feeding tubes before radiotherapy in patients with head and neck cancer: Is it worthwhile? *Journal of Clinical Gastroenterology* 31(3): 215–217.

Shiley SG, HargunaniC, Skoner JM, *et al.* (2006) Swallowing function after chemoradiation for advanced stage oropharyngeal cancer. *American Academy of Otolaryngology-Head & Neck Surgery* 134(3): 455–459.

Silander E, Nyman J, Bove M, *et al.* (2010) The use of prophylactic percutaneous endoscopic gastrostomy and early enteral feeding in patients with advanced head and neck cancer – a prospective longitudinal study. *The European e-Journal of Clinical Nutrition and Metabolism* doi:10.1016.

Silver HJ, Wellman NS, Arnold DJ, *et al.* (2004) Older adults receiving home enteral nutrition: enteral regimen, provider involvement, and health care outcomes. *Journal of Parenteral and Enteral Nutrition* 28(2): 92–98.

Talwar B. (2010) Head & neck cancer. In: Shaw C (ed) *Nutrition and Cancer*. Vol 1, Oxford: Blackwell Wiley, pp. 188–220.

Talwar B, Findlay M. (2012) When is the optimal time for placing a gastrostomy in patients undergoing treatment for head and neck cancer? *Current Opinion in Supportive and Palliative Care* 6: 41–53.

Van Bokhorst-de van der Scheuren M, Van Leeuwen P, Sauerwein HP, *et al.* (1997) Assessment of malnutrition parameters in head and

neck cancer and their relation to postoperative complications. *Head & Neck* 19(5): 419–425.

Van Bokhorst-de van der Scheuren M, Van Leeuwen P, Kuik D, Klop M, Sauerwein H, Snow G, Quak J. (1999) The impact of nutritional status on the prognosis of patients with advanced head and neck cancer. *Cancer* 86(3): 519–527.

Van Bokhorst-de van der Scheuren M, Langendoen S, Vondeling H, Kuik D, Quak J, Van Leeuwen P. (2000) Perioperative enteral nutrition and quality of life of severely malnourished head and neck cancer patients: a randomised clinical trial. *Clinical Nutrition* 19(6): 437–444.

Van Cutsem E, Arends J. (2005). The causes and consequences of cancer-associated malnutrition. *European Journal of Oncology Nursing* 9 (Suppl 2): S51–63.

Vickery L, Psychol D, Latchford G, Hewison J, Bellew M, Feber T. (2003) The impact of head and neck cancer and facial disfigurement on the quality of life of patients and their partners. *Head & Neck* 25(4): 289–296.

Weimann A, Braga M, Harsanyi L, *et al.* (2006) ESPEN guidelines on Enteral Nutrition: Surgery including Organ Transplantation. *Clinical Nutrition* 25(2): 224–244.

Wood K. (2005) Audit of nutritional guidelines for head and neck cancer patients undergoing radiotherapy. *Journal of Human Nutrition and Dietetics* 18 (5): 148–155.

7.15.3   Cancer of the gastrointestinal tract

Eva Glass, Linda Murray, Lindsey Bottle

Key points

■ Cancers of the gastrointestinal tract (GIT) are associated with nutritional risk factors, including obesity.

■ A range of symptoms, which greatly affect food intake and utilisation, accompany GIT cancer.

■ Nutritional problems can be further exacerbated by treatment interventions such as major surgery, radiotherapy or chemotherapy.

■ Nutritional intervention may involve dietary counselling and nutritional support at all stages of cancer treatment, including palliation.

This chapter discusses cancer of the gastrointestinal tract (GIT) apart from hepatocellular carcinoma (liver cancer), which is discussed in Chapter 7.4.12.

Carcinoma of the oesophagus

Eva Glass

Oesophageal cancer is the ninth most common cancer in the UK, accounting for nearly 8000 new diagnoses/year (CSR, 2011; NHS Scotland, 2011; NISRA, 2008; 2010; Welsh CISU, 2010). The incidence is much higher in males, with a 2:1 male to female ratio. The World Health Organization (WHO) describes more than 20 histological subtypes of oesophageal carcinoma, although adenocarcinoma, arising from the glandular epithelium, and squamous cell carcinoma, arising from the epithelial cells, represent the majority of the diagnoses. In the western world, adenocarcinoma is on the rise, whereas the inci-

dence of squamous cell carcinoma is stable or even decreasing. However, adenocarcinoma remains the most dominant subtype in the developing world (Vizcaino *et al.*, 2002). Environmental factors for which there is convincing evidence of an increase in the risk of oesophageal cancer include reflux disease, consumption of tobacco and alcohol, and greater body fatness. There is probable evidence that non-starchy vegetables, fruit, foods containing beta-carotene and vitamin C decrease the risk of developing oesophageal cancer (WCRF, 2007).

Patients may present with loss of body weight, dysphagia and retrosternal pain on eating. The extent of weight loss tends to be related to the degree and duration of the dysphagia.

Cancer of the oesophagus is diagnosed by endoscopy, endoscopic ultrasound, computed tomography (CT) and positron emission tomography CT. Biopsy is required to confirm the histological diagnosis. By the time patients present with symptoms, the disease may be advanced and deterioration may occur rapidly. Treatment may involve chemotherapy, radiotherapy and surgery, depending on patient choice, fitness, location and stage of disease, and whether there is spread to adjacent lymph nodes or distant sites in the body. Endoscopic techniques such as dilatation or the insertion of a stent may also be required depending on the progression of disease or symptoms following treatment. If the cancer is advanced, palliative chemotherapy and/or supportive care may be appropriate.

Upper gastrointestinal (UGI) cancer patients present many dietetic challenges, as discussed in Chapter 7.15.2 and later in this chapter. The reported incidence of malnutrition in UGI patients ranges from 35% to 100% (Isenring *et al.*, 2003; Ravasco *et al.*, 2003). This reported variance is due to differences in the definition of malnutrition and in subjects included in studies. The highest incidences of malnutrition are normally found in those with advanced disease, with the majority of studies reporting an incidence of approximately 30–50% (Bozzetti & SCRINIO Working Group, 2009; Deans *et al.*, 2009; Khalid *et al.*, 2007).

Management

Oesophageal resection

Endoscopic mucosal resection is mainly used in severe dysplasia, but its use in treating very early carcinomas is increasing. Surgical treatment of carcinoma of the oesophagus may be by partial or total oesophagectomy or oesophagogastrectomy, depending on the site and extent of the cancer. Patients who are severely nutritionally depleted will require nutritional support prior to surgery. Patients who are able to swallow will require dietary advice, often with nutritional supplements. Those undergoing preoperative chemotherapy may experience an improvement in dysphagia during this time, which enables an improved dietary intake prior to surgery.

The Enhanced Recovery Programme is mainly used in other surgical areas, e.g. orthopaedics, but there is increasing usage in the UK with oesophagectomies and gastrectomies; this area is being developed. The main nutritional areas of this programme are:

- Preoperative assessment and education.
- Carbohydrate loading.
- Late nil by mouth status preoperatively.
- Early oral or enteral feeding postoperatively.

The programme has been shown to have positive benefits, including a lower lean body mass loss, decreased complications and decreased length of hospital stay (Varadhan *et al.*, 2010) (see Chapter 7.17.5).

Early postoperative nutritional support is essential. Enteral feeding by a route that bypasses the oesophagus and stomach is usually appropriate, e.g. jejunostomy feeding. Once the integrity of the anastomosis has been confirmed, oral feeding can resume, starting with oral fluids followed by gradual phasing in in of solid foods (see Chapter 7.3) as enteral nutrition is phased out.

Ongoing dietetic supervision is essential, both during hospitalisation and following discharge. Persistent postoperative nutritional problems can include:

- Poor appetite.
- Early satiety.
- Fear of eating, particularly foods that were difficult to eat preoperatively.
- Difficulty in regaining or maintaining body weight.
- Nausea.
- Reflux.
- Dysphagia (due to anastomotic stricture or recurrence of disease).

Dietary management should aim to prevent further nutritional deterioration and weight loss, and attempt to restore good nutritional status, which may have been severely compromised prior to surgery.

Practical guidance should focus on:

- Eating small, frequent meals.
- Taking time at meal times and chewing foods well.
- Drinking fluids separately from meals.
- Good choices of nutrient and energy dense foods, and useful food enrichment strategies (see Chapter 6.3).
- Good choices of nutrient rich beverages.
- Avoiding foods that cause discomfort or gastrointestinal symptoms.
- Adopting strategies that reduce the likelihood of reflux, e.g. not eating late at night, not lying down soon after eating and avoiding strong tea, coffee and alcohol.

Additional support measures, such as oral sip feed supplementation, may be indicated if nutritional needs cannot be met by these measures alone.

Radiotherapy

Radiation therapy, external beam radiation therapy (EBRT) or, occasionally, intraluminal radiation (brachytherapy) may be used to treat oesophageal carcinoma. One of these may be the sole treatment or used in combination with chemotherapy or surgery. During a course of radiotherapy, the tissues will become oedematous, inflamed and swollen, and it is therefore likely that dysphagia will worsen before it improves. These effects are usually temporary but, as these patients are often already severely malnourished and have suffered marked weight loss, it may be important for the dietitian to raise with the medical team whether enteral feeding is indicated prior to or during treatment. The need for enteral feeding is even more imperative in those patients presenting with an already high degree of dysphagia due to the anticipated side effects experienced with radiotherapy. Nutritional support at this stage via nasogastric tube, gastrostomy or jejunostomy may prevent further deterioration of an already poor nutritional status. If such support is implemented, it is important to explain to the patient why such intervention is advisable at this stage, i.e. to avert possible problems and not a sign that their condition has worsened.

During radiotherapy treatment, patients may experience a sore throat and/or an increase in dysphagia. Therefore, they may find that bland foods (avoiding strong flavours, artificial or natural acidity, and spices) are best tolerated. Foods may need to have a smooth consistency, e.g. liquidised meals, strained thickened soups, custard and milk pudding, or of a crumbly texture, e.g. crackers, crisp bread or savoury cheese snacks.

Reintroduction of a normal diet should be gradual. Meals will need to be well moistened and accompanied by frequent sips of drinks to assist the passage of food past the inflamed area. Sip feed supplements may be necessary to maintain adequate energy and nutrient intake. Most patients will continue with a soft diet for some time as some difficulties with swallowing often persist. Some will also be afraid to try foods they associate problems, particularly meat and bread. Patients may find that such foods can be well tolerated if consumed with plenty of sauce or gravy.

Chemotherapy

Side effects, such as nausea, vomiting and taste changes, commonly associated with this form of therapy, may have an additional impact on oral intake. General remedial measures to help alleviate these effects are discussed in Chapter 6.3 and Chapter 7.15.1.

Other treatment strategies

When radical surgery is contraindicated because of surgical risk due to medical history, metastatic spread or the patient being considered unfit or too weak to withstand its effects, endoscopic techniques such as dilatation, laser therapy or the insertion of a stent can be used as palliative procedures to relieve dysphagia. Intubation with an oesophageal stent is carried out under general anaesthesia or sedation. Often this will be a permanent self expanding metal stent, although it may be removed if the patient proceeds to surgery. These procedures have a high rate of complications, such as perforation or haemorrhage, and there is an increased risk of mortality. However, insertion of the device does usually bring about an immediate improvement in dysphagia and, with appropriate guidance, many patients are able to resume a fairly normal diet comprised of soft normal foods. The main complication is that of stent migration or overgrowth of tumour, which leads to a recurrence of dysphagia. If this occurs, laser therapy or placement of a further stent is required. A temporary (around 3 months) biodegradable stent is sometimes the preferred to a permanent stent or enteral feeding. This is a measure for those who are dysphagic, but who will be receiving treatment that may ultimately improve their swallow without the need for a permanent stent.

Guidelines for the dietary management of patients who have an oesophageal stent in place vary according to the type of device inserted and local policy. There is little evidence in the literature of the best advice for such patients. The British Dietetic Association's Oncology Group (2008) has constructed a consensus statement based on the available literature and current practice (Table 7.15.8).

Table 7.15.8 Professional consensus statement of dietetic advice post oesophageal stent placement (British Dietetic Association's Oncology Group, 2008)

Fluids	Fluids only for 24 hours post insertion of stent. Local policy needs to be agreed, as many areas extend this to 48 hours. Role of fluid thereafter is to wash away debris. There is no evidence base to support the advice to use fizzy fluids. Fizzy fluids may cause problems if acid reflux is experienced. A stent positioned at the distal end of the oesophagus may result in reflux. Advise frequent consumption of any type of fluid after consuming food
Food	Education will depend on extent of tumour, ability to chew, continuing dysphagia and position/posture of patient. Gradual introduction of small amounts of liquid/soft foods may be required. Importance of chewing well needs to be emphasised
Caution with certain foods	Dietitians should be aware of any limitations on food intake. Literature provided should reflect individual need for texture modification. Patients should be advised to chew all food well, to sit upright, not to rush eating and to drink plenty of fluids. They should also be aware of foods that are most likely to cause a problem. Controversy remains about the use of a standard list of foods to avoid, but observational reports point to risk from: • Bread and toast • Egg • Fish with bones • Stringy, pithy fruit • Stringy/hard raw vegetables • Chips
Nutrition support	Required by the majority of patients to some extent

Guidance on texture modification may be helpful in some cases (see Chapter 7.3). However, tolerance of different foods does vary between patients, and may even vary on a day to day basis in the same patient. It is therefore difficult to give precise guidance as to which foods will or will not cause problems, but the dietitian should give advice on ensuring small mouthfuls, positioning and chewing food well. Many patients establish a diet of suitable texture by a process of trial and error.

Nutritional support

Whether the treatment plan is for surgery, chemotherapy with or without radiotherapy or supportive care, many patients will be nutritionally compromised. A common complaint is reduced appetite, often accompanied by dysphagia and other issues already outlined (Khalid *et al.*, 2007). Consumption of a nutrient dense diet via appropriate food choice, food enrichment strategies and, if necessary, use of proprietary supplements should be encouraged (see Chapter 6.3). However, patients may present with cancer cachexia that cannot be fully reversed with an improvement in energy intake alone (Fearon *et al.*, 2011) (see Chapter 7.15.9).

The use of enteral nutrition in oesophageal cancer varies depending on the treatment planned and its expected outcome, i.e. radical or palliative treatment. As already discussed, patients with total dysphagia will often receive enteral nutrition (normally via a jejunostomy or radiologically placed gastrostomy), particularly if they are to undergo radical treatment with chemotherapy and surgery, or chemotherapy and radiotherapy. Those who undergo palliative chemotherapy may also receive enteral nutrition if a stent is not in place. There is much debate on the ethics of enteral nutrition in the palliative care setting for oesophageal cancer patients who are unable to meet their nutritional requirements for reasons other than dysphagia. The multidisciplinary team may decide it is in the patient's best interest to have stent placement in order to improve their swallow, allow them to eat and improve their quality of life.

Gastric carcinoma

Eva Glass

The incidence of gastric cancer is on the decline, mainly due to the decrease in *Helicobacter pylori*; however, it is the seventh most common cause of cancer death in the UK (ISD, 2011; NISRA, 2008; 2010; ONS, 2010a; Welsh CISU, 2010). There is evidence to suggest the probability of salt and foods with a high salt content being implicated in gastric cancer. In contrast, it is probable that non-starchy vegetables, allium vegetables, e.g. garlic, and fruit protect against gastric cancer, although the exact way in which they do this has not been confirmed (World Cancer Research Fund, 2007). Gastric carcinoma is closely associated with *Helicobacter pylori* infection, which leads to chronic atrophic gastritis and eventual gastric neoplasia (Bonenkamp *et al.*, 2002). In populations where infection occurs at an early age the prevalence of gastric carcinoma is 100% in early adulthood. This is probably related to poor socioeconomic conditions.

Gastric carcinoma is often diagnosed late because its early symptoms may be dismissed as indigestion or heartburn. By the time patients present with anorexia, nausea, vomiting, pain on eating and severe weight loss, the disease may be well advanced, possibly with metastatic spread. If the condition is operable (usually assessed by CT scanning and endoscopic laparoscopy), the preferred treatment is perioperative chemotherapy followed by partial or total gastrectomy as appropriate (Cunningham *et al.*, 2006) (*see* later). If a gastrectomy is contraindicated in patients with pyloric obstruction, then a gastroenterostomy may be performed or the pylorus stented, to allow the patient to eat foods that can be tolerated. If a stent is used, then patients will require dietary advice on a suitable soft diet with sufficient fluids. The additional use of supplements or other support measures is usually necessary to make up the shortfall in energy and

nutrient intake. However, if pyloric obstruction occurs in patients with a poor prognosis, medical management is normally conservative, involving medications such as prokinetics and end of life care. Jejunal feeding may be used for a small number of patients receiving palliative treatment for gastric outlet obstruction if their prognosis is not as poor as the aforementioned and a stent is not placed.

Gastric resection and reconstruction

Gastric surgery can have a considerable negative impact on subsequent food intake, weight recovery and quality of life. Gastric replacement with various enteric reservoirs has been used to improve the postprandial symptoms and nutrition of patients after total gastrectomy. To improve quality of life postoperatively, pouch and Roux en Y reconstructions have been shown to be the most useful of the commonly performed procedures (Gertler *et al.*, 2009). Increasingly, laparoscopic techniques are being used for the removal of early gastric cancers.

As a result of the combination of cancer related cachexia and chronic symptoms such as nausea, vomiting or discomfort on eating, patients with gastric carcinoma often present in a significantly malnourished state and therefore nutritional support measures should be instigated as early after diagnosis as possible, preferably before surgery or as soon as possible afterwards and preferably using the enteral rather than parenteral route.

Early postoperative enteral nutritional support (within 24 hours of surgery) can be safely established via a jejunostomy catheter or nasojejunal tube placed intraoperatively. However, some hospitals do not provide this routinely, keeping patients nil by mouth postoperatively with or without the provision of parenteral nutrition until oral diet can be commenced (Baker *et al.*, 2011). Standard feeds are commonly given, although the use of immunonutrition is on the rise; there is increasing evidence for the benefit of this following gastric resection, some debate on its use remains (Shrikhande *et al.*, 2009).

Disturbances in gastrointestinal function following gastric resection and reconstruction are common, and may affect nutritional intake and subsequently nutritional status. Gastrointestinal consequences of gastric resection and reconstruction include:

- Rapid emptying of the stomach remnant.
- Reduced secretion of intrinsic factor.
- Reduced secretion of pancreatic enzymes.
- Inadequate mixing of food with enzymes and bile.
- Reduced absorption of certain food substances, especially protein and fat.
- Rapid absorption of glucose.
- Abolition of the normal pH gradient in the small intestine.
- Increased intestinal motility.

Some of these problems occur soon after eating; others result from the long term consequences of disturbed gastric function. Early symptoms may include the following.

Small stomach syndrome

The majority of patients experience early satiety and may feel distended and uncomfortable during or after eating. This is particularly common after total or partial gastrectomy, but may also occur after vagotomy and pyloroplasty. Small, frequent meals should be eaten and fluids should be consumed separately from solid food (see Chapter 6.3).

Dumping syndrome

Early dumping

This occurs soon after eating and causes symptoms such as sweating, dizziness, faintness, rapid weak pulse and hypotension as a response to the rapid and early delivery of a hyperosmolar meal into the jejunum. The symptoms usually recede by 2–3 months after surgery, but in the meantime may be relieved by consuming small meals, limiting the consumption of refined carbohydrates and avoiding the consumption of liquids with meals.

Late dumping

Some patients may also experience symptoms similar to hypoglycaemia around 2 hours after a meal as a result of overproduction of insulin in response to the rapid absorption of glucose. Patients typically experience weakness, light headiness, and feelings of cold and sweating, and these symptoms can be minimised by following the advice for early dumping, with emphasis on the regular consumption of starchy carbohydrate foods.

Diarrhoea

Diarrhoea frequently occurs following vagotomy or total gastrectomy, but may reduce with increasing time after surgery. Antidiarrhoeal agents such as codeine phosphate or loperamide may alleviate the problem.

Vomiting bile

Pancreatic and biliary secretions may accumulate in the afferent loop and, after food has left the stomach, can enter the gastric remnant, causing nausea and vomiting. Prokinetics, e.g. metoclopramide, domperidone or erythromycin, may be useful, although surgical correction may be needed if vomiting bile is refractory to medical management.

Long term consequences

Weight loss and malnutrition

Weight loss and nutritional inadequacy are common occurrences after gastric surgery, and nearly always reflect poor food intake. Problems such as early satiety or dumping syndrome tend to make people reluctant to eat, and side effects of treatments such as radiotherapy or chemotherapy may further affect appetite and food consumption. Dietary guidance should focus on the improvement of meal frequency and nutrient density via appropriate food choice and enrichment measures (see Chapter 6.3). Additional oral nutritional supplementation may also be indicated. Patients should be monitored regularly so that progress can be assessed and nutritional support measures adjusted as necessary.

Malabsorption

Malabsorption, particularly of fat, may result from a number of alterations in gastrointestinal function following gastrectomy as listed earlier. If this occurs, it is important to ensure that energy intake is increased to compensate for faecal energy losses and that micronutrient intake does not become compromised, particularly that of calcium, iron and fat soluble vitamins. Treatment of steatorrhoea by dietary fat restriction alone is not recommended as the resultant dietary energy content will be too low to meet energy needs. If symptoms of steatorrhoea are particularly troublesome, a proportion of dietary fat can be isocalorically substituted by either glucose polymers or medium chain triglycerides (MCTs). Medical management involves the use of antidiarrhoeal medication, bile acid binders and possibly pancreatic enzyme replacements.

Anaemias

Iron deficiency anaemia is a common and particular risk following gastrectomy as a result of the combination of poor iron intake and poor absorption. Haematological status should be regularly assessed and treated if necessary. Pernicious anaemia can be a secondary consequence of gastrectomy as a result of the loss of intrinsic factor (produced by gastric parietal cells) and other local conditions necessary for the absorption of vitamin B_{12}. Vitamin B_{12} should be given by injection at intervals to those considered to be at risk. Megaloblastic anaemia may also result from folate deficiency, particularly if dietary intake is poor and malabsorption is present. Oral folate supplementation may be necessary.

Dietetic management

Dietary guidance following gastric reconstruction should focus on the need for:

- Small, frequent, regular meals.
- Avoiding large quantities of fluid.
- Consuming fluids between meals rather than with them.
- Eating a variety of nutrient dense foods, e.g. milk, dairy products, lean meat and eggs. Non-bulky, i.e. not high fibre, cereal foods and small amounts of fruit and vegetables should also be included in the daily diet.
- Boosting nutrient intake via food enrichment strategies if food intake is, or has been, particularly poor.
- Taking recommended nutritional supplements (either energy/nutrient supplements or vitamin /mineral preparations) if indicated.
- Advising remedial dietary measures for dumping syndrome or malabsorption if present.

Cancer of the pancreas

Linda Murray

Pancreatic cancer is the tenth most common cancer in the UK, but the fifth most common cause of cancer death. The prognosis is very poor; >80% of pancreatic cancers are unresectable at diagnosis, with only 3% of patients surviving 5 years (ISD, 2010; NISRA, 2008; 2010; ONS, 2010b; Welsh CISU, 2010). The disease is often diagnosed at a stage when neither surgery, chemotherapy nor radiotherapy will prolong survival time for more than a few weeks.

Pancreatic cancer is accompanied by a range of symptoms that can affect food intake or utilisation, including pain, nausea, anorexia, early satiety and pancreatic insufficiency (Davidson *et al.*, 2004). Due to the retroperitoneal site of the pancreas and symptoms that are usually vague, delay in presentation and diagnosis is common. All too often the patient presents with features of advanced disease. Common modes of presentation include weight loss (70–90% of cases), pain (often relieved by sitting forward), jaundice (presenting feature in 75% of pancreatic head tumours) and diabetes mellitus (sudden onset in middle age with no family history). Only around 16% of patients survive for 1 year from diagnosis, which reflects the fact that most cases of pancreatic cancer are not suitable for potentially curative treatment (ONS, 2010b).

Curative resection

Curative resection, when possible, usually takes the form of a pancreaticoduodenectomy (Whipple's procedure). The extent of this resection ranges from preservation of the pylorus to radical surgery, combining Whipple's procedure with extensive lymph node dissection. Extensive surgery of this nature may be undertaken in patients who are already nutritionally compromised, and early nutritional assessment and intervention both pre- and post-operatively are essential. Postoperative nutritional problems vary and can include pancreatic fistulae, abdominal chyle leaks, delayed gastric emptying, diabetes mellitus and steatorrhoea. Early dietetic intervention from diagnosis and staging, through surgery and possible chemotherapy, is essential to maintain good nutritional intake, promote recovery and help improve quality of life. It is increasingly recognised that pre- and post-operative nutritional support via the enteral or parenteral route may make a considerable difference to recovery time and outcome (see Chapter 7.15.5). This aspect of care has often been overlooked in the past (Ulander *et al.*, 1991). Postoperatively, nutritional monitoring on a frequent basis remains important. Since enzyme supplementation and insulin are commonly required following pancreatic resection, dietary guidance on these aspects is also likely to be needed. Dietary fat should be included to tolerance as some patients, despite commencing pancreatic enzyme supplementation after surgery, often report symptoms of steatorrhoea. Recovery after major resective surgery of this type may take up to a year.

Palliative treatment

The aim of management in palliative care is to improve quality of life via pain and symptom control, such as malabsorption. Surgical treatments include biliary stenting to relieve jaundice and accompanying symptoms of anorexia and poor intake. Gastric or duodenal obstruction, evident by intractable vomiting, is common in pancreatic cancer and is relieved by palliative bypass procedures such as gastrojejunostomy, or a stent. However, as in gastric cancer, if the patient has a very poor prognosis and neither of these procedures is appropriate, then management is conservative. Where there is hepatic or biliary obstruction, biliary bypass procedures may be possible, but as with above, the surgical risk needs to be measured against the benefit. Ascites can often be a problem in this group of patients and they may require regular paracentesis.

Nutritional support should be sufficient to prevent unnecessary nutritional debilitation while not being over-invasive. Proprietary supplements may be useful to help maintain adequate energy and nutrient intake. Davidson *et al.* (2004) have shown that weight stabilisation with intensive nutritional intervention is associated with improved survival duration and quality of life in unresectable cancer patients. There has been evidence demonstrating the benefits of fish oil supplements in this group of patients to reverse the effects of cancer cachexia (Barber, 2001). Yet, a recent Cochrane review showed that there is currently insufficient evidence to support the use of supplement drinks containing eicosapentaenoic acid (EPA) (Dewey *et al.*, 2007) (see Chapter 7.15.9). Multidisciplinary team input is essential to improve symptoms of pain, nausea, steatorrhoea and early satiety. Good compliance with enzyme replacement therapy and pain control is required. The overall nutritional objective is to ensure that eating remains a pleasurable aspect of life for as long as possible, while preserving as much of the patient's strength and wellbeing as is practicable.

As well as these consequences, patients with pancreatic cancer also have to cope with the psychological effects of the diagnosis itself and its poor prognosis. The resulting depression and anxiety can profoundly impair the desire to eat. Since the rapid advancement of the disease can also result in high nutrient losses and poor nutrient intake if symptoms are not adequately controlled, the risk of debilitating malnutrition is high.

Colorectal cancer

Lindsey Bottle

Colorectal cancers include those that affect the colon, rectum (including the anus) and appendix. These are the third most common cancers in the UK, after breast and lung cancer, with approximately 40 000 new diagnoses/year (ISD, 2010; NISRA, 2008; 2010; ONS, 2010a; Welsh CISU, 2010). Incidence increased by 33% in men and 14% in women between 1971 and 2009 (ONS, 2011). Diagnosis is strongly related to age, and although three-quarters of all new cases are found in these aged over 65 years (NICE, 2011), it is not uncommon to encounter much younger patients. The introduction of the NHS Bowel Screening Programme in 2006 has led to earlier diagnosis, and is predicted to reduce mortality rates by 16% (NHS Bowel Screening Programme, 2011).

SECTION 7

Aetiology

A number of risk factors have been implicated in the development and progression of colorectal cancer. These include genetic predisposition, inflammatory bowel disease, smoking, excess alcohol, lack of physical activity, obesity and diet (WCRF/AICR, 2011). Most (95%) cases are adenocarcinomas that develop from adenomatous polyps; many of these can be detected early prior to molecular changes that can result in malignancies (Manne et al., 2010). Obesity has been associated with increased risk (Harriss et al., 2009) and there is conclusive evidence to show that increased levels of physical activity lower risk (Boyle et al., 2012). A positive association between intake of red and processed meat and colorectal cancer has been established (Xu et al., 2013) and there is evidence to show that dietary fibre can have a protective effect (Murphy et al., 2012), in particular wholegrain intake (Larsson et al., 2005). The effect of lifestyle factors has become more convincing over the past few years and in theory some cancers could be theoretically avoidable if these factors are addressed (WCRF, 2007).

Diagnosis

Colorectal cancer usually presents with symptoms of a persistent change in bowel habit (including unresolved diarrhoea for several weeks), rectal bleeding, abdominal pain, a lump in the abdomen, unexplained tiredness, anorexia and loss of weight. If the disease is detected at an early stage, it can be completely cured by surgery. One-year survival rates have significantly improved over the past 40 years from 39% to 73% in men and 40% to 72.2% in women (Coleman et al., 1999; ONS, 2011).

Management

The prognosis and treatment modality depend on the type and grade of tumour and its degree of spread. This is determined by the Duke's clinicopathological classification as well as the Royal College of Pathologists TNM5 staging (see Chapter 7.15.1).

Surgical resection is the principal first line treatment for the majority of patients. It is undertaken either as a curative treatment or as a palliative measure to improve quality of life in those with bowel obstruction. Carbohydrate loading as part of Enhanced Recovery Programmes is now common practice (see Chapter 7.17.5) will involve end to end anastamoses or stoma formation (ileostomy or colostomy), depending on the degree of tumour infiltration.

Chemotherapy and/or radiotherapy can be used neodjuvantly to reduce the tumour burden prior to surgery, and chemotherapy is used adjuvantly postoperatively to prevent the risk of recurrence. In the case of advanced metastatic disease, palliative chemotherapy is routinely offered. New surgical techniques and treatment modalities, including targeted therapies, e.g. cetuximab and bevacizumab, are being developed and it is now recognised that optimum outcomes for patients with colorectal cancer require specialised multidisciplinary care (NICE, 2011).

Dietary management

People with colorectal cancer may present in a nutritionally depleted state as a result of chronic symptoms, side effects from treatment and the cancer process itself. In such patients, appropriate nutritional support should be instituted as soon as possible to help manage the effects of treatment. An appropriate nutritional screening tool and dietetic referral system should be in place to identify at an early stage those who are malnourished (NICE, 2006).

Nutritional support should aim to prevent weight loss during treatment as undernutrition and cachexia are indicators of poor prognosis (Dewys et al., 1980) and can increase the risk of treatment related toxicity (Andreyev et al., 1998). Side effects experienced by colorectal cancer patients undergoing chemotherapy can include diarrhoea, nausea, taste changes and anorexia. In the first instance, it is essential to ensure that such symptoms are controlled with medication. Diet should then be manipulated accordingly to ensure that patients maximise their intake (see Chapter 7.15.1). Dietary counselling during chemotherapy has been shown to improve nutritional status (Dobrila-Dintinjana et al., 2012), and the use of oral nutritional supplements may be necessary if intake remains suboptimal and weight loss is ongoing. Supplements can result in increased energy intake and improved quality of life (Ravasco et al., 2005).

Pelvic radiotherapy related symptoms can include diarrhoea, faecal incontinence, increased urgency and pain. Approximately 70% of patients experience acute small intestinal changes that can lead to gastrointestinal symptoms both during and after treatment (Andreyev et al., 1998). Nutritional support is essential to prevent weight loss and manage these effects. Various approaches have been investigated, including elemental diets, probiotic supplementation, low fat diets and reducing insoluble fibre in the form of raw vegetables, but more research is recommended (McGough et al., 2004). Late onset of symptoms is not always initially linked to previous cancer treatment, and dietetic input may be required for up to 6 months after radiotherapy finishes. If a definitive cause cannot be established and symptoms persist, referral to a gastroenterologist for further investigation is advisable.

If the tumour or peritoneal metastases are causing a partial obstruction, a trial of a low fibre diet may be effective in reducing symptoms in the short term, but no research is available to support this approach. Patients undertaking such dietary restrictions should be advised, monitored and reviewed regularly by a dietitian. The aim is to maintain nutritional status whilst the obstruction is treated or palliated. This may involve placement of a colonic stent or insertion of a stoma if the patient is well enough to undergo surgery.

Patients who are undergoing colorectal surgery do not routinely require artificial nutritional support postoperatively. Oral fluids and diet should be initiated at an early stage (see Chapter 7.17.5). Nevertheless, as with all patients, nutritional status during the recovery period should be monitored, particularly if patients were malnourished preoperatively or experience postsurgical complications, or if resumption of oral food intake is slow. In such cases, appropriate nutritional support should be instigated (see Chapter 6.3, Chapter 6.4 and Chapter 6.5). Symptom control, including adequate pain relief, is important as part of the overall management plan because continuous pain, discomfort or nausea can markedly suppress appetite.

Specific dietary measures may be required during the initial phase of adjustment to the effects of intestinal resection and possible creation or reversal of a stoma (see Chapter 7.4.9).

In the palliative care setting, if nutrition is highlighted as an issue for either the patient or family and carers, this should be addressed as for advanced cancer of any site (see Chapter 7.16). Dietary advice for colorectal cancer survivors should be to increase dietary fibre, limit red and processed meat, maintain a healthy body weight and be regularly physical active (WCRF/AICR, 2011).

Further reading

National Institute for Health and Care Excellence (NICE). (2004) *Management of Dyspepsia in Adults in Primary Care*. London: NICE.

National Institute for Health and Care Excellence (NICE). (2004) *Photodynamic Therapy for Barrett's Oesophagus*. London: NICE.

Shaw C. (2000) *Current Thinking: Nutrition and Cancer*. Novartis Consumer Health, Medical Nutrition Division.

Shaw C (ed). (2011) *Nutrition and Cancer*. Oxford: Wiley Blackwell.

Internet resources

Macmillam Cancer Support   www.macmillan.org.uk
Oesophageal Patients Association   www.opa.org.uk
Pancreatic Cancer UK   www.pancreaticcancer.org.uk

References

Andreyev HJN, Norman AR, Oates J, Cunningham D. (1998) Why do patients with weight loss have a worse outcome when undergoing chemotherapy for gastrointestinal malignancies? *European Journal of Cancer* 34(4): 503–509.

Baker A, Wooten L-A, Malloy M. (2011) Nutritional considerations after gastrectomy and esophagectomy for malignancy. *Current Treatment Options in Oncology* 12(1): 85–95.

Barber MD. (2001) Cancer cachexia and its treatment with fish-oil-enriched nutritional supplementation. *Nutrition* 17(9): 751–755.

Bonenkamp JJ, van Krieken H, Kuipers EJ, *et al.* (2002) Gastric cancer. In: Souhami RL, Tannock I, Hohenberger P, Horiot JC. (eds) *Oxford Textbook of Oncology*, vol 2, 2nd edn. Oxford: Oxford University Press, pp. 1517– 1536.

Boyle T, Keegel T, Bull F, Heyworth J, Fritschi L. (2012) Physical activity and risks of proximal and distal colon cancers: a systematic review and meta-analysis. *Journal of the National Cancer Institute* 104(20): 1548–1561.

Bozzetti F; SCRINIO Working Group. (2009) Screening the nutritional status in oncology: a preliminary report on 1,000 out patients. *Supportive Care in Cancer* 17: 279–284.

British Dietetic Association's Oncology Group. (2008) Professional consensus statement of dietetic advice post oesophageal stent placement. Available at www.mccn.nhs.uk/userfiles/documents/Dietetic%20Advice%20Stent%20Replacement.pdf.

Cancer Statistics Registrations (CSR). (2011) *Registrations of Cancer Diagnosed in 2008, England*. London: MB1, no 38.

Coleman MP, Babb P, Damiecki P, *et al.* (1999) *Cancer Survival Trends in England and Wales, 1971–1995: Deprivation and NHS Region*. Series SMPS No 61. London: Stationery Office.

Cunningham D, Allum WH, Stenning SP, *et al.* (2006) Perioperative chemotherapy versus surgery alone for resectable gastroesophageal cancer. *New England Journal of Medicine* 355: 11–20.

Davidson W, Ash S, Capra S, Bauer J; Cancer Cachexia Study Group. (2004) Weight stabilisation is associated with improved survival duration and quality of life in unresectable pancreatic cancer. *Clinical Nutrition* 23(2): 239–247.

Deans DA, Tan BH, Wigmore SJ, *et al.* (2009) The influence of systemic inflammation, dietary intake and stage of disease on rate of weight loss in patients with gastro-oesophageal cancer. *British Journal of Cancer* 100: 63–69.

Dewey A, Baughan C, Dean T, Higgins B, Johnson I. (2007) Eicosapentaenoic acid (EPA, an omega-3 fatty acid from fish oils) for the treatment of cancer cachexia. *Cochrane Database of Systematic Reviews* 1: CD004597.

Dewys WD, Begg C, Lavin PT, *et al.* (1980) Prognostic effect of weight loss prior to chemotherapy in cancer patients. *American Journal of Medicine* 69: 491–497.

Dobrila-Dintinjana R, Trivanovic D, Zelic M, *et al.* (2012) Nutritional support in patients with colorectal cancer during chemotherapy: Does it work? *Hepatogastroenterology* 60(123) [Epub ahead of print].

Fearon K, Strasser F, Anker SD, *et al.* (2011) Definition and classification of cancer cachexia: an international consensus. *Lancet Oncology* 12(5): 489–495.

Gertler R, Rosenberg R, Feith M, Schuster T, Friess H. (2009) Pouch vs. no pouch following total gastrectomy: meta-analysis and systematic review. *American Journal of Gastroenterology* 104(11): 2838–2851.

Harriss DJ, Atkinson G, George K, *et al.*; C-CLEAR Group. (2009) Lifestyle factors and colorectal cancer risk(1): systematic review and meta-analysis of associations with body mass index. *Colorectal Disease* 11: 547–563.

Information Services Division (ISD). (2010) *Cancer in Scotland*. Available at www.isdscotland.org/Health-Topics/Cancer/Cancer-Statistics/Cancer_in_Scotland_summary_m.pdf. Accessed 2 December 2013.

Information Services Division (ISD). (2011) *Cancer in Scotland*. Available at www.isdscotland.org/Health-Topics/Cancer/Cancer-Statistics/Cancer_in_Scotland_summary_m.pdf. Accessed 2 December 2013.

Isenring E, Bauer J, Capra S. (2003) The scored Patient-Generated-Subjective Global Assessment (PG-SGA) and its association with quality of life in ambulatory patients receiving radiotherapy. *European Journal of Clinical Nutrition* 57: 305–309.

Khalid U, Spiro A, Baldwin C, *et al.* (2007) Symptoms and weight loss in patients with gastrointestinal and lung cancer at presentation. *Supportive Care in Cancer* 15(1): 39–46.

Larsson SC, Giovannucci E, Bergkvist L, Wolk A. (2005) Whole grain consumption and risk of colorectal cancer: a population-based cohort of 60 000 women. *British Journal of Cancer* 92: 1803–1807.

Manne U, Shanmugam C, Katkoori VR, Bumpers HL, Grizzle WE. (2010) Development and progression of colorectal neoplasia. *Cancer Biomarkers* 9(1–6): 235–265.

McGough C, Baldwin C, Frost G, Andreyev HJN. (2004) Role of nutritional intervention in patients treated with radiotherapy for pelvic malignancy. *British Journal of Cancer* 90(12): 2278–2287.

Murphy N, Norat T, Ferrari P, *et al.* (2012) Dietary Fibre intake and risks of cancers of the colon and rectum in the European prospective investigation into cancer and nutrition (EPIC). *Public Library of Science* 7(6): e39361.

National Institute for Health and Care Excellence (NICE). (2006) *Nutrition Support in Adults*. Clinical Guideline 32. London: NICE. Available at www.nice.org.uk. Accessed 21 December 2012.

National Institute for Health and Clinical Excellence (NICE). (2011) *The Diagnosis and Management of Colorectal Cancer*. London: NICE. Available at www.nice.org.uk. Accessed 21 December 2012.

NHS Bowel Screening Programme. (2011) Press release issued on 8.12.2011. Available at www.cancerscreening.nhs.uk/bowel/news/010.html. Accessed 21 December 2012.

NHS Scotland. (2011) Information and Statistics Division (ISD) (2011) Cancer incidence data. Available at www.isdscotland.org/Health-Topics/Cancer/Cancer-Statistics/Cancer_in_Scotland_summary_m.pdf. Accessed 9 September.

Northern Ireland Statistics and Research Agency (NISRA). (2008) Northern Ireland incidence data. *Northern Ireland Statistics and Research* ICD-9 151.

Northern Ireland Statistics and Research Agency (NISRA). (2010) Northern Ireland Mortality data, 2008. *Northern Ireland Statistics and Research* C16.

Office for National Statistics (ONS). (2010a) *Mortality Statistics: Cause. England and Wales 2008*. UK National Statistics. London: ONS.

Office for National Statistics (ONS). (2010b) *Cancer Statistics Registrations: Registrations of Cancer Diagnosed in 2008, England*. Office for National Statistics: MB1 Series No. 39. London: ONS.

Office for National Statistics (ONS). (2011) *Statistical Bulletin: Cancer survival in England: Patients Diagnosed 2005–2009 and Followed up to 2010*. Released 15 November 2011. Available at www.ons.gov.uk/ons/publications/re-reference-tables.html?edition=tcm%3A77-239726. Accessed 21 December 2012.

Ravasco P, Monteiro-Grillo I, Vidal PM, Camilo ME. (2003) Nutritional deterioration in cancer: The role of disease and diet. *Clinical Oncology (Royal College of Radiologists)* 15(8): 443–450.

Ravasco P, Monteiro-Grillo I, Vidal PM, Camilo ME. (2005) Dietary counseling improves patient outcomes: a prospective, randomized, controlled trial in colorectal cancer patients undergoing radiotherapy. *Journal of Clinical Oncology* 23(7): 1431–1438.

Shrikhande SV, Shetty GS, Singh K, Ingle S. (2009) Is early feeding after major gastrointestinal surgery a fashion or an advance evidence-based review of literature. *Journal of Cancer Research and Therapeutics* 5(4): 232–239.

Ulander K, Grahn G, Sundahl G, Jeppsson B. (1991) Needs and care of patients undergoing subtotal pancreatectomy for cancer. *Cancer Nursing* 14(1): 27–34.

Varadhan KK, Neal KR, Dejong CH, Fearon KC, Ljungqvist O, Lobo DN. (2010) The enhanced recovery after surgery (ERAS) pathway for patients undergoing major elective open colorectal surgery: a meta-analysis of randomized controlled trials. *Clinical Nutrition* 29(4): 434–440.

Vizcaino AP, Moreno V, Lambert R, Parkin DM. (2002) Time trends incidence of both major histologic types of esophageal carcinomas in selected countries, 1973–1995. *International Journal of Cancer* 99(6): 860–868.

Welsh Cancer Intelligence and Surveillance Unit (CISU). (2010) *Cancer Registrations in Wales 2008*. Welsh Cancer Intelligence and Surveillance Unit.

World Cancer Research Fund (WHO)/American Institute For Cancer Research (2007). *Food, Nutrition, Physical Activity, and the Prevention of Cancer: a Global Perspective*. Washington DC: AICR. Available at www.wcrf.org. Accessed 21 December 2012.

World Cancer Research Fund/American Institute for Cancer Research (WCRF/AICR). (2011) Continuous update project report summary. *Food, Nutrition, Physical Activity, and the Prevention of Colorectal Cancer*. Available at www.wcrf.org. Accessed 21 December 2012.

Xu X, Yu E, Gao X, *et al*. (2013) Red and processed meat intake and risk of colorectal adenomas: A meta-analysis of observational studies. *International Journal of Cancer* 132(2): 437–448.

7.15.4   Breast cancer

Michelle Harvie

Key points

■ Breast cancer is the most common malignancy amongst women.

■ Increasing rates of breast cancer are linked to trends in overweight and obesity, sedentary lifestyle and increased alcohol intakes.

■ Weight control and exercise are recommended to improve survival after a diagnosis of breast cancer.

Breast cancer accounts for a third of cancer cases in women in the UK. In 2008, 47 693 women and 341 men were diagnosed in the UK, and 12 047 died from the disease. Earlier detection and improved adjuvant treatment has reduced breast cancer mortality by 37% in the past 20 years. The most recent, and undoubtedly conservative, estimates indicate there are approximately 550 000 women living with a history of breast cancer in the UK. This equates to almost 2% of the total female population and nearly 10% of the population aged 65 years and older. The long term health and wellbeing of breast cancer patients is therefore an increasingly important consideration for researchers and healthcare professionals [Cancer Research UK (CRUK), 2011b].

Risk factors and prevention

Estimated lifetime risk of breast cancer in the UK is 1 in 8 for women and 1 in 1014 for men. Female UK breast cancer rates doubled between 1979 and 2008, with similar increases globally, particularly within Asian and developing countries that traditionally have had low rates (Bray *et al.*, 2004). These increases have been linked to adverse trends in a number of lifestyle, hormonal and reproductive risk factors.

Hormonal and reproductive risk factors

The majority of breast cancers (81%) occur in postmenopausal women. Both earlier age of menarche (20% risk reduction for 5-year delay) and later age of menopause (3% for each year older at menopause) increase risk. The average age of menarche in developed countries has fallen from 16–17 years in the mid 19th century to 12–13 years today. Risk of breast cancer reduces by 7% with each full term pregnancy and by 4% for every 12 months of breastfeeding. Women currently taking hormone replacement therapy (HRT), particularly combined oestrogen–progestogen therapy, have a two-fold increased risk of breast cancer compared with non-users. Once HRT use ceases, a woman's risk returns to that of a never user within 5 years.

Lifestyle risk factors

Observational data consistently link overweight and obesity, adult weight gain, sedentary lifestyle and alcohol intake to increased risk amongst women; excess weight is linked to post-, but not pre-menopausal, breast cancer. A weight gain of 20 kg during adulthood doubles the risk of postmenopausal breast cancer (Vrieling et al., 2010). Alcohol and sedentary behaviour increase the risk of both pre- and post-menopausal breast cancer. An additional 10 g of alcohol (1 unit) on a daily basis increases risk by 10% (Key et al., 2006), whilst each additional hour of moderate exercise (65–80% maximum heart rate) per week can reduce risk by 6% (Monninkhof et al., 2007). Observational studies and recent bariatric data suggest cancer risk reduction with weight loss and energy restriction, even with modest weight loss (5–10%) (Christou et al., 2008; Eliassen et al., 2006; Harvie et al., 2005a). Energy restriction appears to be more important for prevention of breast cancer compared with modification of dietary composition (Brennan et al., 2010). Weight is the only identified lifestyle risk factor amongst men, where a body mass index (BMI) of >30 kg/m^2 doubles risk (Johansen Taber et al., 2010).

The proportion of breast cancer cases estimated to be preventable with weight control, exercise and limiting alcohol is contentious, but has recently been cited to be between 18% and 40% in the UK (Department of Health, 2007; WCRF, 2007).

Genetic factors

Fifteen per cent of breast cancer cases occur in women with a family history of the disease, and 2% occur in women with mutations in the breast cancer susceptibility genes BRCA1 and BRCA2. These mutation carriers have a 45–65% chance of developing breast cancer in their lifetime. As with the general population, excess weight and lack of exercise increase the risk of developing postmenopausal breast cancer amongst women with a family history and known BRCA mutation carriers (Begum et al., 2009; Manders et al., 2011).

Treatment

In countries with breast screening, approximately 60% of cancers are localised to the breast at the time of diagnosis (stages 1 and 2), 30% have local lymph involvement (stage 3) and 10% are metastatic (stage 4) (CRUK, 2011a). Patients with early breast cancer (stage 1–3) generally have some form of breast and axillary lymph node surgery, followed by 15 or 19 daily sessions of radiotherapy for women who have had conservation surgery, i.e. not a mastectomy. Three-quarters of breast cancers in the UK are oestrogen receptor positive (ER positive) and these patients receive adjuvant endocrine (hormone) therapy. Standard treatment is a 5-year course of the selective ER receptor modulator tamoxifen. Aromatase inhibitors (anastrozole, exemestane and letrozole) are increasingly prescribed after surgery instead of tamoxifen for women at high risk of recurrence, or after 2–5 years on tamoxifen.

Approximately 25% of breast cancer patients receive adjuvant chemotherapy (after breast surgery) and 3% receive neoadjuvant chemotherapy (before breast surgery). The 20% of patients with cancers that express the human epidermal growth factor receptor 2 (HER 2) receive a targeted monoclonal antibody therapy, e.g. trastuzumab or lapatinib. Women diagnosed with advanced metastatic disease receive either endocrine therapy or chemotherapy.

Most men diagnosed with breast cancer undergo mastectomy with axillary lymph node clearance or sentinel node biopsy, where fewer than five lymph nodes are generally removed. Indications for radiotherapy are similar to those for female breast cancer. The majority of male breast tumours are ER positive and are treated with either tamoxifen or aromatase inhibitors, whilst some individuals receive chemotherapy. Men with metastatic disease typically receive endocrine treatment.

Body weight

An estimated 50–65% of breast cancer patients are overweight or obese at the time of diagnosis, whilst 60–75%, including those with previous healthy weight, gain weight during adjuvant treatment. Gains in fat mass are usually accompanied by a loss of fat free mass (sarcopenic obesity) (Irwin et al., 2005). Excess weight at diagnosis has been consistently linked to poorer outcome (Vance et al., 2010), whilst weight gain has been linked to increased risk of recurrence and poorer overall survival in many (Chen et al., 2010; Nichols et al., 2009); however, not all studies are consistent (Caan et al., 2006; 2008). Gains in body fat are greater during adjuvant chemotherapy compared with endocrine therapy (3–7 kg versus 1–4 kg, respectively) (Harvie et al., 2004; Irwin et al., 2005). Gains occur both during and after chemotherapy due to increased energy intake and decreased energy expenditure linked to treatment (chemotherapy and steroids), hormonal (chemotherapy induced menopause), psychosocial and anxiety related factors. Part of the adverse effects of adiposity is linked to increased levels of insulin; therefore, the insulin sensitising drug metformin is currently being tested as a potential treatment for breast cancer (Goodwin, 2008).

Unlike other cancer patients, women with advanced breast cancer do not generally develop weight loss and cachexia, i.e. hypermetabolism and anorexia. These metastatic patients often maintain good energy intakes, which lead to gains in body fat of 2%, but do not prevent declines in lean body mass (Harvie *et al.*, 2005b).

Evidence based diet and exercise recommendations after diagnosis

As for breast cancer prevention, weight control, energy restriction and exercise rather than specific dietary constituents influence outcome after diagnosis. The randomised Women's Intervention Nutrition Study (WINS) reported a 23% reduction in breast cancer relapse in women losing modest amounts of weight compared with a control group who had gained weight (3% difference in weight between the groups) (Chlebowski *et al.*, 2006). The weight losing women had consumed a low fat diet (30 g of fat/day; 20% of energy as fat) compared with control women consuming on average 50 g of fat/day (30% of energy as fat). The lack of effect on outcome of a comparable low fat intervention in the Women's Healthy Eating and Living study (WHELS), in which women did not lose weight (Pierce *et al.*, 2007), suggests energy restriction and weight loss are more important than fat restriction for outcome. Moderate fat diets (30–35% of energy from fat) are likely to be superior to low fat eating plans (20% of energy from fat) for breast cancer patients, as in other settings they are better for limiting calorie intake and weight, improving insulin sensitivity and reducing risk of cardiovascular disease (Shai *et al.*, 2008) (see Chapter 7.14.1).

There is much interest in the potential anticancer effects of fruit and vegetables, specifically carotenoids and brassicas. However, a recent large randomised trial of a high fruit and vegetable diet (13 servings/day) and low fat diet plan (20% of energy from fat) amongst 3088 early breast cancer patients did not find beneficial effects in terms of breast cancer recurrence or mortality (Pierce *et al.*, 2007). Alcohol is consistently linked to risk, but not with survival after diagnosis (McTiernan *et al.*, 2010). Exercise alone does not control weight amongst breast cancer survivors (Markes *et al.*, 2006). However, exercise is a vital part of energy restricted weight control programmes. Exercise has been associated with greater disease free survival, quality of life, cardiovascular fitness and bone density (McTiernan *et al.*, 2010).

Popular dietary practices

Soya and phytoestrogens

Many breast cancer patients deliberately increase their intake of soya foods or phytoestrogen supplements, i.e. black cohosh, agnus castus and red clover, in the belief that this will either reduce their risk of breast cancer recurrence or reduce hot flushes. However, soya has no proven benefits for hot flushes (Lethaby *et al.*, 2007). There have been concerns that soya may limit the efficacy of antioestrogen therapies such as tamoxifen (van Duursen *et al.*, 2011). Recent Asian population studies report 10–15 g of soya protein/day to be safe as part of a healthy lifestyle amongst patients taking tamoxifen (250 mL of soya milk = 7.5 g of soya protein) (Guha *et al.*, 2009; Shu *et al.*, 2009) and aromatase inhibitors. These

studies do not however conclusively suggest soya has benefits for patients (Kang *et al.*, 2010).

Dairy free diets

An estimated 20% of UK breast cancer patients avoid or limit dairy foods after diagnosis (Breast Cancer Care, 2005). This populist approach is not supported by evidence. A recent meta analyses including 24 187 cases and 1 063 471 participants found 15% fewer breast cancers amongst high (>3 servings/day) versus low dairy consumers (<1 serving/day). Likewise, a prudent diet that includes low fat dairy foods has been linked to reduced recurrence and all cause mortality amongst breast cancer patients (Kroenke *et al.*, 2005; Kwan *et al.*, 2009).

High dose vitamin supplements

An estimated 10% of breast cancer patients self prescribe high dose antioxidant supplements (beta-carotene, vitamins C and E, and selenium). There are concerns that antioxidants may protect tumour cells from the targeted oxidative damage during radiotherapy and chemotherapy, and potentially reduce the effectiveness of these treatments. Studies to date have not resolved this issue and further research is required (Greenlee *et al.*, 2009; Nechuta *et al.*, 2011).

Late treatment effects

Lymphoedema (arm swelling) is an undesirable complication following axillary clearance or radiotherapy to the axilla, which can have negative physical and psychological effects on women. Obesity is a risk factor for the development of lymphoedema and recent data suggest weight loss may reduce arm swelling and is likely to increase overall wellbeing and quality of life (Shaw *et al.*, 2007).

Bone health

Bone density is an important consideration amongst patients with chemotherapy induced menopause or for those prescribed aromatase inhibitors. Lifestyle recommendations to limit reduction in bone density include increasing weight bearing exercise, reducing alcohol intake, smoking cessation and supplementation with vitamin D (400–800 IU/day). Calcium supplementation is only advised if dietary intake is less than the requirement of 1 g/day (Reid *et al.*, 2008).

Associated conditions and diseases

Both postmenopausal and menopausal breast cancer patients have obesity related comorbidities such as hypertension (18–50%), hyperlipidaemia (25%) (Manjer *et al.*, 2000), coronary heart disease (15–27%), vascular disease (3–5%) and type 2 diabetes mellitus (5–10%) (Yancik *et al.*, 2001). Comorbidities are a major cause of mortality amongst women diagnosed with localised breast cancer, particularly amongst older women in whom cardiovascular disease can account for over half of deaths (Schairer *et al.*, 2004). The consistent adverse effect of comorbidities on overall survival highlights the importance of managing comorbid conditions alongside breast cancer treatments (Barone *et al.*, 2008).

Further reading

Harvie M, Ackerman R. (2006) *The Genesis Breast Cancer Prevention Diet*. London: Rodale International Ltd.

Internet resources

Breast Cancer Care   www.breastcancercare.org.uk
Cancer Research UK   www.cancerresearch.uk.org
Genesis Breast Cancer Prevention Appeal   www.genesisuk.org
Natural Methods Quality Standard (The Authority on Integrative Medicine   http://naturalstandard.com
Memorial Sloan-Kettering Cancer Center   www.mskcc.org
National Cancer Survivorship Initiative   www.ncsi.org.uk
National Institute for Health and Care Excellence   www.nice.org.uk
    Breast cancer (early & locally advanced): Diagnosis and Treatment (CG80)
    Advanced Breast Cancer: Diagnosis and Treatment (CG81)
    Familial Breast Cancer: The classification and care of women at risk of familial breast cancer in primary, secondary and tertiary care (CG41)

References

Barone BB, Yeh HC, Snyder CF, *et al*. (2008) Long-term all-cause mortality in cancer patients with pre existing diabetes mellitus: a systematic review and meta-analysis. *JAMA* 300(23): 2754–2764.

Begum P, Richardson CE, Carmichael AR. (2009) Obesity in post menopausal women with a family history of breast cancer: prevalence and risk awareness. *International Seminars on Surgical Oncology* 6: 1.

Bray F, McCarron P, Parkin DM. (2004) The changing global patterns of female breast cancer incidence and mortality. *Breast Cancer Research* 6(6): 229–239.

Breast Cancer Care. (2005) Dietary practices of breast cancer patients. Available at www.breastcancercare.org.uk. Accessed 2 April 2005.

Brennan SF, Cantwell MM, Cardwell CR, Velentzis LS, Woodside JV. (2010) Dietary patterns and breast cancer risk: a systematic review and meta-analysis. *American Journal of Clinical Nutrition* 91(5): 1294–1302.

Caan BJ, Emond JA, Natarajan L, *et al*. (2006) Post-diagnosis weight gain and breast cancer recurrence in women with early stage breast cancer. *Breast Cancer Research and Treatment* 99(1): 47–57.

Caan BJ, Kwan ML, Hartzell G, *et al*. (2008) Pre-diagnosis body mass index, post-diagnosis weight change, and prognosis among women with early stage breast cancer", *Cancer Causes Control* 19(10): 1319–1328.

Cancer Research UK (CRUK). (2011a) Breast cancer – risk factors. Available at www.cancerresearch.org.uk. Accessed 6 September 2011.

Cancer Research UK. (2011b) Breast cancer – UK incidence statistics. Available at www.cancerresearch.org.uk. Accessed 15 April 2011.

Chen X, Lu W, Zheng W, *et al*. (2010) Obesity and weight change in relation to breast cancer survival. *Breast Cancer Research and Treatment* 122(3): 823–833.

Chlebowski, RT, Blackburn GL, Thomson CA, *et al*. (2006) Dietary fat reduction and breast cancer outcome: interim efficacy results from the Women's Intervention Nutrition Study. *Journal of the National Cancer Institute* 98(24): 1767–1776.

Christou NV, Lieberman M, Sampalis F, Sampalis JS. (2008) Bariatric surgery reduces cancer risk in morbidly obese patients. *Surgery for Obesity and Related Diseases* 4(6): 691–695.

Department of Health. (2007) *The Cancer Reform Strategy*. London: Department of Health.

Eliassen AH, Colditz GA, Rosner B, Willett WC, Hankinson SE. (2006) Adult weight change and risk of postmenopausal breast cancer. *JAMA* 296(2): 193–201.

Goodwin PJ. (2008) Insulin in the adjuvant breast cancer setting: a novel therapeutic target for lifestyle and pharmacologic interventions? *Journal of Clinical Oncology* 26(6): 833–834.

Greenlee H, Hershman DL, Jacobson JS. (2009) Use of antioxidant supplements during breast cancer treatment: a comprehensive review", *Breast Cancer Research and Treatment* 115(3): 437–452.

Guha N, Kwan ML, Quesenberry CP Jr, Weltzien EK, Castillo AL, Caan BJ. (2009) Soy isoflavones and risk of cancer recurrence in a cohort of breast cancer survivors: the Life After Cancer Epidemiology study. *Breast Cancer Research and Treatment* 118(2): 395–405.

Harvie MN, Campbell IT, Baildam A, Howell A. (2004) Energy balance in early breast cancer patients receiving adjuvant chemotherapy. *Breast Cancer in Research and Treatment* 83(3): 201–210.

Harvie M, Howell A, Vierkant RA, *et al*. (2005a) Association of gain and loss of weight before and after menopause with risk of postmenopausal breast cancer in the Iowa women's health study. *Cancer Epidemiology, Biomarkers and Prevention* 14(3): 656–661.

Harvie MN, Howell A, Thatcher N, Baildam A, Campbell I. (2005b) Energy balance in patients with advanced NSCLC, metastatic melanoma and metastatic breast cancer receiving chemotherapy–a longitudinal study. *British Journal of Cancer* 92(4): 673–680.

Irwin ML, McTiernan A, Baumgartner RN, *et al*. (2005) Changes in body fat and weight after a breast cancer diagnosis: influence of demographic, prognostic, and lifestyle factors. *Journal of Clinical Oncology* 23(4): 774–782.

Johansen Taber KA, Morisy LR, Osbahr AJ III, Dickinson BD. (2010) Male breast cancer: risk factors, diagnosis, and management (Review). *Oncology Reports* 24(5): 1115–1120.

Kang X, Zhang Q, Wang S, Huang X, Jin S. (2010) Effect of soy isoflavones on breast cancer recurrence and death for patients receiving adjuvant endocrine therapy. *CMAJ* 182(17): 1857–1862.

Key J, Hodgson S, Omar RZ, *et al*. (2006) Meta-analysis of studies of alcohol and breast cancer with consideration of the methodological issues. *Cancer Causes and Control* 17(6): 759–770.

Kroenke CH, Fung TT, Hu FB, Holmes MD. (2005) Dietary patterns and survival after breast cancer diagnosis. *Journal of Clinical Oncology* 23(36): 9295–9303.

Kwan ML, Weltzien E, Kushi LH, Castillo A, Slattery ML, Caan BJ. (2009) Dietary patterns and breast cancer recurrence and survival among women with early-stage breast cancer. *Journal of Clinical Oncology* 27(6): 919–926.

Lethaby AE, Brown J, Marjoribanks J, Kronenberg F, Roberts H, Eden J. (2007) Phytoestrogens for vasomotor menopausal symptoms", *Cochrane Database of Systematic Reviews* 4: CD001395.

Manders P, Pijpe A, Hooning MJ, *et al*. (2011) Body weight and risk of breast cancer in BRCA1/2 mutation carriers. *Breast Cancer Research and Treatment* 126(1): 193–202.

Manjer J, Andersson I, Berglund G, *et al*. (2000) Survival of women with breast cancer in relation to smoking. *European Journal of Surgery* 166(11): 852–858.

Markes M, Brockow T, Resch KL. (2006) Exercise for women receiving adjuvant therapy for breast cancer. *Cochrane Database of Systematic Reviews* 4: CD005001.

McTiernan A, Irwin M, Vongruenigen V. (2010) Weight, physical activity, diet, and prognosis in breast and gynecologic cancers. *Journal of Clinical Oncology* 28(26)L: 4074–4080.

Monninkhof EM, Elias SG, Vlems FA, *et al.* (2007) Physical activity and breast cancer: a systematic review. *Epidemiology* 18(1): 137–157.

Nechuta S, Lu W, Chen Z, *et al.* (2011) Vitamin supplement use during breast cancer treatment and survival: a prospective cohort study. *Cancer Epidemiology, Biomarkers and Prevention* 20(2): 262–271.

Nichols HB, Trentham-Dietz A, Egan KM, *et al.* (2009) Body mass index before and after breast cancer diagnosis: associations with all-cause, breast cancer, and cardiovascular disease mortality. *Cancer Epidemiology, Biomarkers and Prevention* 18(5): 1403–1409.

Pierce JP, Natarajan L, Caan B, *et al.* (2007) Influence of a diet very high in vegetables , fruit and fiber and low in fat on prognosis following treatment for breast cancer. *JAMA* 298(3): 289–298.

Reid DM, Doughty J, Eastell R, *et al.* (2008) Guidance for the management of breast cancer treatment-induced bone loss: A consensus position statement from a UK Expert Group. *Cancer Treatment Reviews* 34 (Suppl 1): S3–18.

Schairer C, Mink PJ, Carroll L, Devesa SS. (2004) Probabilities of death from breast cancer and other causes among female breast cancer patients. *Journal of the National Cancer Institute* 96(17): 1311–1321.

Shai I, Schwarzfuchs D, Henkin Y, *et al.* (2008) Weight loss with a low-carbohydrate, Mediterranean, or low-fat diet. *New England Journal of Medicine* 359(3): 229–241.

Shaw C, Mortimer P, Judd PA. (2007) A randomized controlled trial of weight reduction as a treatment for breast cancer-related lymphedema. *Cancer* vol. 110(8): 1868–1874.

Shu XO, Zheng Y, Cai H, *et al.* (2009) Soy food intake and breast cancer survival. *JAMA* 302(22): 2437–2443.

van Duursen MB, Nijmeijer SM, de Morree ES, de Jong PC, van den BM. (2011) Genistein induces breast cancer-associated aromatase and stimulates estrogen-dependent tumor cell growth in in vitro breast cancer model. *Toxicology* 289(2–3): 67–73.

Vance V, Mourtzakis M, McCargar L, Hanning R. (2010) Weight gain in breast cancer survivors: prevalence, pattern and health consequences. *Obesity Reviews* 12(4): 282–294.

Vrieling A, Buck K, Kaaks R, Chang-Claude J. (2010) Adult weight gain in relation to breast cancer risk by estrogen and progesterone receptor status: a meta-analysis. *Breast Cancer Research and Treatment* 123(3): 641–649.

World Cancer Research Fund (WCRF). (2007) *Food, Nutrition, Physical Activity and the Prevention of Cancer: a Global Perspective.* Available at www.wcrf-uk.org/research/cp_report.php. Accessed 15 April 2011.

Yancik R, Wesley MN, Ries LA, Havlik RJ, Edwards BK, Yates JW. (2001) Effect of age and comorbidity in postmenopausal breast cancer patients aged 55 years and older. *JAMA* 285(7): 885–892.

7.15.5 Lung cancer

Mhairi Donald

Key points

■ People with lung cancer should always be managed as part of a multidisciplinary team.

■ Patents experience a wide range of nutritional problems and require a full nutritional assessment at diagnosis.

■ Dietary adaptations should be implemented to help minimise specific nutritional symptoms and support quality of life.

Lung cancer is the most common type of cancer worldwide and in the UK it is the most frequent cause of cancer mortality death and the second most common cancer. Currently, it is more common in men than in women, although the incidence in men is falling as fewer men are smoking, while the incidence in women is rising as the number of women smoking has increased. The incidences are 58.8 and 39.3 per 100 000 population in men and women, respectively [Cancer Research UK (CRUK), 2011]. Cigarette smoking causes approximately 90% of lung cancers. Other factors thought to contribute are poor diet (lack of fruit and vegetables in particular), industrial carcinogens and air pollutants.

The symptoms of lung cancer may include:

• Continuing cough or change in a long standing cough.
• Chest infection that does not improve.
• Increasing breathlessness and wheezing.
• Coughing up blood stained phlegm.
• Hoarse voice.

• Dull ache or sharp pain on coughing or taking in a deep breath.
• Loss of appetite and weight loss.
• Difficulty swallowing.
• Excessive tiredness (fatigue) and lethargy.

There are two main types of primary lung cancer:

• Non small cell lung cancer (NSCLC), which accounts for 80% of cases.
• Small cell lung cancer (SCLC), which accounts for 20% of cases; this is more aggressive than NSCLC and can spread widely to other organs, including the brain.

The early stages of lung cancer do not usually produce symptoms, so the disease is generally at an advanced stage by the time it is diagnosed. It has one of the lowest survival outcomes of any cancer. Many patients are older, with 87% of those diagnosed being over 60 years old, and because of the association with smoking they may also have coexisting, comorbid problems such as chronic obstructive pulmonary disease (COPD). In England and Wales, only 27 of male and 30% of female lung cancer patients are alive after 1 year; this drops to 7% and 9%, respectively, at 5 years (CRUK, 2011).

Every patient with a diagnosis of lung cancer should have a management plan developed by a lung cancer multidisciplinary team (NICE, 2011). Treatment options are determined by the type and stage of cancer and medical fitness, but may include surgery, chemotherapy, radiation, biological therapies or a combination of these. There are many side effects associated with these treatments and nutritional compromises are pronounced in lung cancer.

Nutritional screening

Most patients with lung cancer will have multiple disease related symptoms, such as breathing difficulties, cough, pain, anorexia, fatigue and weight loss, that are likely to have an effect on nutritional status and overall quality of life. Knowledge of symptom prevalence and distress can be used to develop specific interventions that can reduce distressing symptoms and improve quality of life.

Unintentional weight loss is common in cancer patients. Weight loss is often the first sign of disease in patients with lung cancer and most patients will experience it as their disease progresses. To combat weight loss and malnutrition, best practice suggests that nutritional screening using a validated tool should form part of the initial assessment at the time of diagnosis. In a small study of lung cancer patients at the start of treatment (Khalid et al., 2007), 66% of patients were already reporting symptoms; loss of appetite was the most common, followed by nausea and early satiety. Unintentional weight loss was identified in 28%, with patients who experienced weight loss of 5% or more having significantly more symptoms than patients with no weight loss. Isenring et al. (2010) reported a similar association in a mixed group of cancer patients on treatment: those who experienced a greater number of symptoms affecting nutritional intake or status (otherwise referred to as nutrition impact symptoms) were more likely to be malnourished.

Weight loss in lung cancer patients has been reported as anything from 0% to 68% (Beckles et al., 2003). To adequately support a patient's nutritional status it is important to identify the nutrition impact symptoms and set up individual nutritional management plans. These plans must be monitored and adjusted throughout the patient pathway (National Cancer Action Team, 2009).

Treatment options and nutritional implications

Surgery

The type of operation required for lung cancer will depend on the size and position of the tumour. Procedures include a lobectomy (removal of a lobe of the lung), a pneumonectomy (removal of the whole lung or a wedge) and resection/segmentectomy (removal of a small wedge shaped section of cancerous lung and a margin of healthy tissue around the cancer). The outcome of surgery is closely related to the extent of the operation and preoperative lung function. The role of nutrition in predicting the outcome of lung cancer surgery has not been studied extensively. However, one study found that impaired nutritional status was an important predictor of death and need for postoperative ventilation. Impaired nutritional status was more common in patients with lower body mass index (BMI) and lower fat free mass (Jagoe et al., 2001).

Any surgical intervention is likely to affect nutritional status. Respiration requires energy and the work of breathing after surgery may increase expenditure in patients who may also be experiencing anorexia, early satiety and fatigue, which in combination contribute to an inadequate energy intake. Patients having surgery require ongoing monitoring and nutritional support (see Chapter 6.3).

Radiotherapy

Radiotherapy for lung cancer targets the mediastinal area, which includes the pharynx and the oesophagus, both of which are lined by highly radiosensitive epithelial cells that will be damaged by the treatment. This can lead to a range of radiation related side effects, including oesophagitis and resulting in dysphagia, epigastric pain, indigestion, heartburn and taste changes (Cranganu & Camporeale, 2009). It is important to relieve pain and discomfort caused by oesophagitis, both to support the patient and to maintain adequate nutrition and hydration. For pain control, topical medications, such as sucralfate and antacids may all need to be considered. Avoiding acidic or spicy ingredients and changing the texture of the diet to soft, semi solid or nutritious liquids, including oral nutritional supplements, may be recommended. A change in food temperature such as keeping foods cool or at body temperature can also help.

Administration of chemotherapy alongside radiotherapy improves local control by sensitising the tumour to radiation while treating the disease systemically. This treatment can accentuate the significant nutritional issues caused by the radiotherapy as well as adding chemotherapy specific symptoms such as taste changes and increased nausea.

Prophylactic cranial radiotherapy may be given to SCLC patients who have limited stage disease that has not progressed on first line treatment (NICE, 2011). It is given to the brain to reduce the risk of the lung cancer spreading to that area. Side effects of this therapy can include tiredness, headaches, nausea and vomiting.

Chemotherapy

When the tumour is not considered to be resectable, and in advanced SCLC, chemotherapy is considered the mainstay of treatment. The response is poor and the survival benefit marginal, although there may be a benefit in symptom management. The chemotherapy regimens are generally platinum based, with the most common

SECTION 7

nutrition related side effects being nausea and vomiting, early satiety, taste changes and dry mouth.

Biological therapies

Biological therapies are treatments that change the way cells signal each other, either by controlling the growth or switching growth off. Most of the potential side effects of biological therapies are likely to adversely affect nutritional intake, including:

- Tiredness and/or weakness.
- Diarrhoea.
- Sore mouth.
- Lack of appetite.
- Skin rashes.

Supplementation with fish oils

The addition of fish oil [2.5 g/day eicosapentaenoic acid (EPA) and docosahexaenoic acid (DHA)] to standard first line platinum based chemotherapy has been shown to increase response rates and offers clinical benefit in patients with advanced NSCLC without affecting treatment toxicity (Murphy et al., 2011a). The plasma phospholipid EPA concentration after supplementation was a significant predictor of response to chemotherapy, independent of age, sex, BMI, presence of sarcopenia (loss of muscle mass and strength associated with ageing), performance score and weight loss history. This is an important finding given the poor patient compliance often associated with these products. Nutritional intervention with 2.2 g of fish oil/day also resulted in weight and muscle mass maintenance during chemotherapy for NSCLC (Murphy et al., 2011b). However, these findings were from small trials; therefore, further investigation of fish oil supplementation is needed.

Fatigue

Fatigue, pain and dyspnoea (difficult or laboured respiration) have been identified as common symptoms associated with particular distress in lung cancer sufferers. Okuyama et al. (2001) found that 59% of patients with advanced lung cancer had experienced clinical fatigue (defined as fatigue that interferes with any daily activities). Clinical fatigue is not generally relieved with rest; it can turn everyday life and basic tasks such as cooking, cleaning and shopping into hard work.

Several factors may contribute to fatigue, including the disease itself. In inoperable NSCLC patients, the presence of a systemic inflammation (identified by elevated C-reactive protein) was associated with increased weight loss, a reduction in performance status, increased fatigue and reduced survival; the greater the inflammatory response, the worse those parameters were affected (Scott et al., 2002). Anaemia and problems maintaining an adequate oral intake may also contribute to fatigue. Patients may be unable to stand for long enough to prepare or cook food. Some lung cancer patients will need ambulatory oxygen, which must be disconnected whilst using a gas cooker. Supporting an adequate oral intake needs to be carefully considered; food and drinks must be nutritious and require minimal preparation effort from the patient. The patient's ability to manage provisions and cooking is crucial. Social support may be recommended, such as the use of Meals on Wheels, ready or prepared meals, and help with shopping and cooking through social services or Age UK. Menu planning with an understanding of the patient's social support, and including nutritious snacks, drinks and oral nutritional supplements, should help with physical symptoms and quality of life (see Chapter 6.3). When using oral nutritional supplements, the volume must be considered. In a study of patients with COPD (which has symptoms similar to those of lung cancer), voluntary intake was limited by the volume, frequency and energy density of food portions because those factors influenced symptoms such as early satiety and bloating. Weight gain was higher in patients who received 125 mL supplements compared with 200 mL cartons despite their lower total energy contribution (Broekhuizen et al., 2005). The optimum volume of supplements should be considered in the dietary management strategy. Gentle exercise, pulmonary rehabilitation and energy conservation techniques can also help; a specialist or palliative physiotherapist can plan a programme.

Recurrent laryngeal nerve palsy

Recurrent laryngeal nerve palsy has been reported in 2–15% of lung cancer patients and is more common in left sided tumours. It is associated with poor expectoration with coughing and an increased risk of aspiration (Beckles et al., 2003). A modified consistency diet may need to be implemented to help manage it.

Supportive and palliative care

Lung cancer is often diagnosed at an advanced stage and can progress rapidly; median survival from diagnosis is <4 months (NHS Executive, 1998). Palliative or best supportive care may need to be implemented from the outset. Patients with NSCL assigned to early palliative care reported better quality of life and fewer depressive symptoms, and their median survival time post diagnosis increased by 2.7 months (Temel et al., 2010). The early identification and proactive management of symptoms clearly offered a benefit. Identifying nutrition impact symptoms and offering supportive management strategies are an important focus for dietitians to help support quality of life in this setting (see Chapter 7.16).

Internet resources

British Lung Foundation   www.lunguk.org
The Roy Castle Lung Cancer Foundation   www.roycastle.org

References

Beckles MA, Spiro SG, Colice GL, Rudd RM. (2003) Initial evaluation of the patient with lung cancer: symptoms, signs, laboratory tests and paraneoplastic syndromes. *Chest* 123(1 Suppl): 97S–104S.

Broekhuizen B, Creutzberg EC, Weling-Scheepers CA, Wouters EF, Schols AM. (2005) Optimizing oral nutritional drink supplementation in patients with chronic obstructive pulmonary disease. *British Journal of Nutrition* 93: 965–971.

Cancer Research UK (CRUK). (2011) UK Summary table: Incidence and mortality rates for 40 types of cancer. Available at www.cancerresearchuk.org/cancer-info/cancerstats/incidence/. Accessed 2 September 2011.

Cranganu A, Camporeale J. (2009) Nutrition aspects of lung cancer. *Nutrition in Clinical Practice* 24(6): 688–700.

Isenring E, Cross G, Kellet E, Koczwara B, Daniels L. (2010) Nutritional status and information needs of medical oncology patients receiving treatment at an Australian public hospital. *Nutrition and Cancer* 62(2): 220–228.

Jagoe RT, Goodship TH, Gibson GJ. (2001) The influence of nutritional status on complications after operations for lung cancer. *Annals of Thoracic Surgery* 71(3): 936–943.

Khalid U, Spiro A, Baldwin C, et al. (2007) Symptoms and weight loss in patients with gastrointestinal and lung cancer at presentation. *Supportive Care in Cancer* 15(1): 39–46.

Murphy RA, Mourtzakis M, Chu QS, Baracos VE, Reiman T, Mazurak VC. (2011a) Nutritional intervention with fish oil provides a benefit over standard of care for weight and skeletal muscle mass in patients with nonsmall cell lung cancer receiving chemotherapy. *Cancer* 117(8): 1775–1782.

Murphy RA, Mourtzakis M, Chu QS, Baracos VE, Reiman T, Mazurak VC. (2011b) Supplementation with fish oil increases first-line chemotherapy efficacy in patients with advanced nonsmall cell lung cancer. *Cancer* 117(16): 3774–3780.

NHS Executive. (1998) Guidance on commissioning cancer services: improving outcomes in lung cancer. Available at www.dh.gov.uk. Accessed 23 May 2012.

National Institute for Health and Care Excellence (NICE). (2011) The diagnosis and treatment of lung cancer. Clinical Guideline 121. Available at www.nice.org.uk/guidance/CG121. Accessed 23 May 2012.

National Cancer Action Team (NCAT). (2009) Rehabilitation care pathway – lung. Available at www.ncat.nhs.uk. Accessed 2 September 2011.

Okuyama T, Tanaka K, Akechi T, et al. (2001) Fatigue in ambulatory patients with advanced lung cancer: prevalence, correlated factors, and screening. *Journal of Pain and Symptom Management* 22(1): 554–564.

Scott HR, McMillan DC, Forrest LM, Brown DJ, McArdle CS, Milroy R. (2002) The systemic inflammatory response, weight loss, performance status and survival in patients with inoperable non-small cell lung cancer. *British Journal of Cancer* 87(3): 264–267.

Temel JS, Greer JA, Muzikansky A, et al. (2010) Early palliative care for patients with metastatic non-small cell lung cancer. *New England Journal of Medicine* 36: 733–742.

7.15.6 Gynaecological cancers

Mhairi Donald

Key points

■ Gynaecological cancer includes a range of cancers originating from the female reproductive tract; these cancers have differing incidences, treatments and survivorship outcomes.

■ Women with gynaecological cancer experience many nutritional problems and require a full nutritional assessment at diagnosis.

■ Ongoing monitoring and responsive dietary management by a dietitian working within a multidisciplinary team is necessary throughout the treatment pathway, from diagnosis to survival or palliation.

Gynaecological cancer refers to cancers originating in the female reproductive organs, including the ovaries, cervix, endometrium, vagina and vulva. Different forms of gynaecological cancer have differing incidences, treatments and survival outcomes. Gynaecological cancers and their treatments usually have profound and often permanent effects on women, including:

• Rectal, bladder and sexual dysfunction.
• Infertility/onset of early menopause and associated symptoms.
• Changes in body image.

Ovarian cancer

Menstruating women ovulate monthly and it is thought that ovarian cancer may start when the cells on the surface of the ovary do not repair themselves after ovulation.

Ovarian cancer is the leading cause of death in women with gynaecological cancer, with an incidence of 16.2 per 100 000 population [Cancer Research UK (CRUK), 2009]. The incidence rates are higher in postmenopausal women, with the highest rate in the 60–64 year age group. The 5-year survival rate is 34% (CRUK, 2001).

Many women present with advanced disease because the symptoms are often attributed to other conditions, e.g. irritable bowel syndrome. Women (especially those aged 50 years or over) should undergo diagnostic tests if they report the following symptoms on a persistent or frequent basis (NICE, 2011):

• Persistent abdominal distension (referred to as bloating).
• Feeling full (early satiety) and or loss of appetite.
• Pelvic or abdominal pain.
• Increased urinary urgency and/or frequency.

SECTION 7

Endometrial cancer

Endometrial cancer involves the lining of the uterus and is the most common type of cancer of the uterus. The incidence rate is 19.4 per 100000 population (CRUK, 2009), with a 5-year survival rate of 76% (CRUK, 2001).

Risk factors for endometrial cancer include:

- Overweight or obesity (WCRF/AICR, 2007).
- Heightened exposure to oestrogen associated, with early menarche and/or late menopause.
- Pregnancy lowers the risk of endometrial cancer and more than one pregnancy will lower the risk further.

Cervical cancer

Cancer can occur in the cells or glands lining the cervix. The incidence rate is 8.5 per 100000 population (CRUK, 2009), with a 5-year survival rate of 68% (CRUK, 2001). Risk factors for cervical cancer include:

- Infection with human papilloma virus (HPV), particularly types 16 and 18.
- Unprotected sexual intercourse before the age of 17 years with multiple partners.
- Smoking.
- A weakened immune system, e.g. HIV/AIDS.

Vaccines to protect against the strains of HPV most likely to cause cervical cancer are routinely offered to schoolgirls aged 12–13 years in the UK.

Vulval and vaginal cancers

These are rarer cancers with a combined incidence rate of 3.1 per 100000 population (CRUK, 2013).

Nutrition

Malnutrition in cancer patients is associated with a variety of clinical consequences, including reduced quality of life, decreased response to treatment, increased risk of treatment induced toxicity and a reduction in overall survival. However, rates of malnutrition are lower with gynaecological cancers than with other cancers. Laky et al. (2007) identified malnutrition in 20% of gynaecological cancer patients at diagnosis; the prevalence varied between specific cancer sites, with the highest rate (67%) in ovarian cancer and the lowest rate (6%) in endometrial cancer.

Treatment

The management of gynaecological cancers includes surgery, radiotherapy, brachytherapy, chemotherapy, intraperitoneal (intra-abdominal) chemotherapy, hormone therapy or a combination of any of these. The nutritional needs of the patients are likely to vary through the course of treatment. It is important to nutritionally assess and manage the patient at all stages of the rehabilitation care pathway (National Cancer Action Team, 2009).

Surgery

Surgery is the definitive treatment for endometrial, cervical, ovarian and vulval cancers. The extent of the surgery, or choice of alternative treatment, depends on the stage, size and histology of the tumour and fitness of the patient. Gynaecological cancer surgery can be a major procedure that may also involve the gastrointestinal or urinary tracts. Surgery is undertaken as part of the Enhanced Recovery Programme (ERP) (Enhanced Recovery Partnership Programme, 2010), the underlying principle of which is to minimise the stress responses in the body during surgery, enabling quicker recovery and hospital discharge. The ERP involves preoperative assessment and management to ensure comorbidities such as anaemia, hypertension or diabetes are managed optimally. It also involves admission on the day of surgery, with minimal periods of preoperative starvation and carbohydrate loading. Postoperative management includes the early removal of nasogastric (NG) tubes and a rapid return to normal nutrition and hydration.

Women with gynaecological cancer will sometimes require formation of stomas (colostomy, ileostomy and/or urostomy) as a result of surgery for tumour removal, or debulking to deal with progression or complications of treatment such as obstruction. If the underlying problem cannot be cured, a palliative stoma may be required to make the woman more comfortable. Individual dietary advice should be offered to patients with new stomas to support an adequate fluid intake and a return to a normal mixed diet.

Chemotherapy

Chemotherapy may be used alone, particularly in the management of ovarian cancer, or in combination with radiotherapy for cervical and endometrial cancer. The nutritional impact symptoms associated with this therapy are oral mucositis, nausea, vomiting, loss of appetite, taste changes and early satiety. Several studies have examined nutritional status and weight changes as prognostic factors for ovarian cancer patients undergoing chemotherapy. Well nourished patients survived 12.6 months longer than severely malnourished women (Gupta et al., 2008); the risk of death increased by 7% for every 5% loss of body weight (Hess et al., 2007). Improving nutritional status from the start of chemotherapy is also associated with better survival (Gupta et al., 2010). Evidence supports the early implementation of strategies to minimise weight loss in women with ovarian cancer and shows that ongoing individualised nutritional input is vital. Further research is required to determine whether these findings apply to other gynaecological cancers.

Radiotherapy

Radiotherapy is predominantly used to treat cervical and endometrial cancer; it can be given externally or internally (brachytherapy) or as a combination of the two. It may be delivered alone or concurrently with chemotherapy, which can increase early toxicity and add to nutritional problems. The radiation treatment can encompass the entire pelvis, which means there may also be damage to the rapidly dividing cells lining the small and large bowel. It can cause side effects, including diarrhoea, irritable bladder, nausea and tiredness. Malnutrition occurs in approximately 33% of radiotherapy recipients and up to 83% of patients lose weight during treatment (McGough *et al.*, 2004). There is little convincing evidence to support dietary modifications to manage the gastrointestinal side effects of radiotherapy (particularly diarrhoea) (McGough *et al.*, 2004). More randomised controlled trials to establish the efficacy of low fat diets, the elemental diet and the use of probiotic supplementation are required. A current UK trial (CRUK) is investigating whether diets high or low in fibre have a beneficial effect on diarrhoea during pelvic radiotherapy. It is important to identify patients at risk of weight loss or specific nutrition related symptoms and implement individual nutrition support plans; it is likely this will require support from a specialist oncology dietitian.

Medical problems

Bowel obstruction

Bowel obstruction occurs most commonly as a complication of advanced or recurrent ovarian cancer; the bowel may be completely or partially blocked. Blockages can result from the tumour growing into the abdominal area or mesentery of bowel muscle or nerves and compromising bowel motility. The optimal management of bowel obstruction remains controversial and is dependent on the individual clinical picture. Much will depend on the patient's age, nutritional and tumour status, the presence and/or quantity of ascites, and history of chemotherapy or radiotherapy. The goals of treatment for bowel obstruction are to control or relieve symptoms and to optimise quality of life. Treatment may include:

- *Laparotomy with surgical bypass* (Feuer & Broadley, 2000; Pothuri *et al.*, 2003).
- *Pharmacological management* with drugs such as steroids, prokinetics or the antisecretory agent octreotide with NG drainage (Feuer & Broadley, 1999).
- *A venting percutaneous endoscopic gastrostomy* – offers gastric decompression and drainage, often with the resumption of a modified oral intake (Meyer & Pothuri, 2006).
- *Total parenteral nutrition (TPN)* – the risks, burdens and benefits of TPN must be discussed when considering its use. It seems to be of most benefit to women who have good performance status, i.e. the patient is capable of self care (Madhok *et al.*, 2011).
- *Low fibre diet* – the efficacy is not well studied, but patients anecdotally report benefits. In theory, less fibre reduces the amount of faeces and wind produced, resulting in a reduction in symptoms such as bloating and stomach cramps. Dietary information is available via the Ovacome website (Power, 2009).

Ascites

The peritoneum is a fine membrane lining the abdomen. It is made up of two layers: one encloses the organs such as the small bowel, and the other lines the muscle wall of the abdomen. Ascites is the build-up of excessive fluid in the abdominal cavity between these layers. It is commonly associated with ovarian cancer as a result of malignant cells shedding into the abdominal cavity and impairing normal drainage. The fluid can also accumulate around the lungs, causing a pleural effusion. The symptoms associated with ascites can significantly reduce quality of life. They are:

- Shortness of breath.
- Anorexia.
- Nausea, indigestion and heartburn.
- Discomfort and immobility.

The aim of nutritional management of ascites is to maximise oral intake and quality of life, whilst minimising any detrimental gastrointestinal effects. This largely involves encouraging frequent small meals and snacks, fortifying foods and using low volume oral nutritional supplements.

Survivorship

Although excess body weight does not appear to affect recurrence in endometrial cancer, 72% of endometrial survivors are overweight or obese (von Gruenigen *et al.*, 2008) and their mortality is affected by other comorbidities, e.g. hypertension, cardiac disease and diabetes. A healthy lifestyle after cancer is associated with improved physical and psychological wellbeing and improved survival. Positive lifestyle changes, including increased exercise and avoiding excess weight, should be encouraged.

Some women will develop late effects of pelvic radiotherapy that affect the bladder and/or bowel. In one study 47% of women reported post treatment symptoms, which they had tried to manage with dietary changes (Abayomi *et al.*, 2009). Women should be dissuaded from unnecessarily restricting nutritional intake as this could result in unbalanced diets in the long term. These late gastrointestinal effects and their causes require more detailed investigation and specialist management; women with these effects should be referred to a specialist centre.

Internet resources

Gynae C (Supporting Women with Gynaecological Cancer) www.gynaec.co.uk
Jo's Cervical Cancer Trust www.jostrust.org.uk
Ovacome (The Ovarian Cancer Support Network) www.ovacome.org.uk

References

Abayomi JC, Kirwan J, Hackett AF. (2009) Coping mechanisms used by women in an attempt to avoid symptoms of chronic radiation enteritis. *Journal of Human Nutrition and Dietetics* 22(4): 310–316.

Cancer Research UK (CRUK). (2001) *Relative Five Year Survival Estimates Based on Survival Probabilities Observed During 2000–2001, by Sex and Site, England and Wales*. London: CRUK.

Cancer Research UK (CRUK). (2009) Ovarian cancer incidence statistics. Available at www.cancerresearchuk.org/cancer-info/cancerstats/types/ovary/incidence/uk-ovarian-cancer-incidence-statistics. Accessed 9 September 2013.

Cancer Research UK (CRUK). (2013) UK Cancer incidence (2010) and mortality (2010) summary. Available at http://publications.cancerresearchuk.org/downloads/Product/CS_DT_INCMORTRATES.pdf. Accessed 9 September 2013.

Enhanced Recovery Partnership Programme. (2010). Delivery Enhanced Recovery – Helping patients to get better sooner after surgery. Available at www.improvement.nhs.uk/cancer/LinkClick.aspx?fileticket=PZtQT%2F8LAdw%3D&tabid=105. Accessed 3 September 2011.

Feuer DDJ, Broadley KE. (1999) Corticosteroids for the resolution of malignant bowel obstruction in advanced gynaecological and gastrointestinal cancer. *Cochrane Database of Systematic Reviews* 3: CD001219.

Feuer DDJ, Broadley KE. (2000) Surgery for the resolution of malignant bowel obstruction in advanced gynaecological and gastrointestinal cancer. *Cochrane Database of Systematic Reviews* 3: CD002764.

Gupta D, Lammersfeld CA, Vashi PG, Dahlk SL, Lis CG. (2008) Can subjective global assessment of nutritional status predict survival in ovarian cancer *Journal of Ovarian Research* 15(1): 5.

Gupta D, Lis CG, Vashi PG, Lammersfeld CA. (2010) Impact of improved nutritional status on survival in ovarian cancer. *Supportive Care in Cancer* 18(3): 373–381.

Hess LM, Barakat R, Tian C. (2007) Weight change during chemotherapy as a potential prognostic factor for stage III epithelial ovarian carcinoma: A Gynaecological Oncology Group Study. *Gynecologic Oncology* 107(2): 260–265.

Laky B, Janda M, Bauer J, Vavra C, Cleghorn G, Obermair A. (2007) Malnutrition among gynaecological cancer patients. *European Journal of Clinical Nutrition* 61(5): 642–646.

Madhok BM, Yeluri S, Haigh K, Burton A, Broadhead T, Jayne DG. (2011) Parenteral nutrition for patients with advanced ovarian malignancy. *Journal of Human Nutrition and Dietetics* 24(2): 187–191.

McGough C, Baldwin C, Frost G, Andreyev HJ. (2004) Role of nutritional intervention in patients treated with radiotherapy for pelvic malignancy. *British Journal of Cancer* 90(12): 2278–2287.

Meyer L, Pothuri B. (2006) Decompressive percutaneous gastrostomy tube use in gynaecologic malignancies. *Current Treatment Options in Oncology* 7(2): 111–120.

National Cancer Action Team (NCAT). (2009) *Rehabilitation Care Pathway-Gynae General*. London: NCAT.

National Institute for Health and Care Excellence (NICE). (2011) *Ovarian Cancer: The Recognition and Initial Management of Ovarian Cancer*. CG 122. London: NICE.

Pothuri B, Vaidya A, Aghajanian C, Venkatraman R, Barakat R, Chi D. (2003) Palliative surgery for bowel obstruction in recurrent ovarian cancer:-an updated series. *Gynecologic Oncology* 89(2): 306–313.

Power J. (2009) *Fact sheet 14: If your bowel is blocked*. London: Ovacome.

World Cancer Research Fund/American Institute for Cancer Research (WCRF/AICR). (2007) *Food, Nutrition, Physical Activity, and the Prevention of Cancer: A Global Perspective*. Washington DC: AICR.

Von Gruenigen VE, Courneya KS, Gibbons HE, *et al*. (2008) Feasibility and effectiveness of a lifestyle intervention program in obese endometrial cancer patients: a randomized trial. *Gynecologic Oncology* 109(1): 19–26.

7.15.7 Prostate cancer

Saira Chowdhury

Key points

- Prostate cancer is one of the most common malignancies amongst men, with the majority of new diagnoses undergoing curative treatment.

- Diet may play a role in the aetiology of prostate cancer.

- Hormone therapy can cause symptoms of metabolic syndrome and bone thinning; both warrant changes in diet and lifestyle.

- Dietary modifications may be beneficial in managing symptoms of radiation enteritis.

The prostate gland is part of the male reproductive system and makes some of the alkaline fluid that constitutes 20–30% of semen. It is the size of a walnut, located below the bladder and in front of the rectum, with the urethra running through its centre. Prostate cancer is the most common malignancy amongst men in England, with 34 892 new diagnoses made in 2010. This accounted for 26% of all cancer diagnoses in men [Office for National Statistics (ONS), 2012a]. Survival has increased in the past 30 years with 93% and 81% of men now surviving 1 and 5 years after diagnosis, respectively (ONS, 2012b). Incidence is greater in western countries, with the highest rate observed in the USA (124.8 per 100 000 population) and the lowest in Bangladesh (0.3 per 100 000 population) (Hsing *et al.*, 2000; Quinn & Babb, 2002; Baade *et al.*, 2009). Prostate cancer risk increases in migrants to western countries when compared with those in their native countries. This could be the result of migrants adopting western dietary practices (Giovanucci *et al.*, 2007). Ninety per cent of new diagnoses undergo treatment with curative intent (Greene *et al.*, 2005). Treatment may be a combination of surgery, radiotherapy, chemotherapy and hormones. Some adjunct treatments include the use of bisphosphonates and steroids.

Nutrition

Diet plays a role in disease aetiology, supporting nutritional difficulties during treatment and managing long term side effects resulting from treatment. The incidence of undernutrition in prostate cancer is relatively low compared with other cancers and occurs more commonly in advanced disease (Segura *et al.*, 2005). Weight gain and features of metabolic syndrome are important side effects of hormone treatment and lend a role for dietetics in survivorship.

Nutrition and aetiology

Age, race, family history and diet may influence prostate cancer development. The effect of various nutrients in prostate cancer incidence has been investigated and currently, results mainly suggest a causal relationship. Whilst there is insufficient evidence to translate these findings into public health recommendations, the studies conducted up to now provide a platform for further research. Two reviews explain the role of dietary constituents in prostate cancer prevention (WCRF/AICR, 2007; Ma & Chapman, 2009); the findings are summarised in Table 7.15.9.

The World Cancer Research Fund (WCRF) expert panel concluded that the antioxidants, lycopene and selenium, have the strongest dietary influences in prostate cancer prevention (WCRF/AICR, 2007). Lycopene is found in tomatoes, watermelon, grapefruit, guava and apricot. Cooked tomato products, e.g. tomato ketchup and tomato sauces, have a greater bioavailability of lycopene compared with raw tomato. In 2004, a meta analysis of observational studies suggested a beneficial role for lycopene. It identified a 6% prostate cancer risk reduction in men consuming raw tomatoes and 1% reduction in men consuming lycopene (Etminan *et al.*, 2004). Since this, a Cochrane meta analysis of three randomised controlled trials of lycopene supplements concluded there was insufficient evidence to support or refute the use of lycopene in prostate cancer prevention and that better quality randomised, controlled studies are needed (Ilic *et al.*, 2011). There were several limitations to the studies included in this review, including poorly powered studies and a high risk of bias. More studies into whether dietary lycopene is better than lycopene supplementation and whether any observed benefits of dietary lycopene are due to lycopene alone or the effect of lycopene combined with another nutrient are needed.

A protective role of selenium was suggested by the results of the Nutritional Prevention of Cancer (NPC) study. Between 50% and 60% fewer prostate cancer cases were observed in selenium deficient men taking selenium supplements, compared with those taking a placebo (Clark *et al.*, 1996; Duffield-Lillico *et al.*, 2003). Two studies report a 50–65% increased prostate cancer incidence in men with low selenium levels (Chan *et al.*, 2005; Brinkman *et al.*, 2006). The effect of vitamin E was observed in the Alpha-T, Beta-Carotene (ATBC) Cancer Prevention Study; a randomised, double blind placebo controlled trial where alpha-tocopherol supplementation in smokers showed a reduced prostate cancer incidence (ATBC Study Group, 2003). The Selenium and Vitamin E Cancer Prevention Trial (SELECT), a double blind, randomised controlled trial, examined the role of dietary supplementation of these two nutrients in prostate cancer prevention. Initial results showed that selenium and vitamin E taken alone or together did not prevent prostate cancer and subjects were advised to stop taking supplements. These was a non-statistically significant increase in prostate cancer incidence with vitamin E supplementation (Lippman *et al.*, 2009). The results of additional follow-up 3 years after the participants had stopped supplementation showed that men who had been taking selenium or vitamin E alone or in combination had increased prostate cancer incidence compared with the placebo group. However, this finding only reached statistical significance in the vitamin E group, with a 17% increased incidence of prostate cancer (Klein *et al.*, 2011). The reasons for the contrasting results for vitamin E in SELECT compared with the ATBC study are not fully understood. The reduced prostate cancer incidence with vitamin E supplementation in the ATBC study could be due to chance as it was a secondary finding in a trial not designed to investigate supplementation on prostate cancer. The dose of vitamin E used in SELECT was much higher than in the ATBC study and could be too high to provide benefit.

A recent Cochrane review has concluded that while an inverse relationship between selenium levels and prostate cancer incidence exists, further research is needed to provide more convincing evidence of a role (Dennert

Table 7.15.9 Influence of dietary components on prostate cancer risk [source: WCRF/AICR Report 2007. Reproduced with permission of the World Cancer Research Fund International (www.dietandcancerreport.org)]

Strength of evidence	Decreases risk	Increases risk
Convincing	Nil	Nil
Probable	Foods containing lycopene Foods containing selenium Selenium supplements	Calcium
Limited (suggestive)	Pulses (legumes) Foods containing vitamin E Alpha-tocopherol	Milk and dairy products

Limited – no conclusion
Alpha-tocopherol, cereals (grains) and their products; dietary fibre; potatoes; non-starchy vegetables; fruit; meats; poultry; eggs; total fat; plant oils; sugar (sucrose); sugary foods and drinks; coffee; tea; alcohol; carbohydrate; protein; vitamin A; retinol; thiamine; riboflavin; niacin; vitamin C; vitamin D; delta-tocopherol; vitamin supplements; multivitamins; iron; phosphorus; zinc; other carotenoids; physical activity; energy expenditure; vegetarian diets; Seventh Day Adventist diets; body fatness; abdominal fatness; birth weight; energy intake

et al., 2011). A recent meta analysis has examined selenium status in relation to prostate cancer incidence (Hurst *et al.*, 2012). It showed decreasing prostate cancer incidence with selenium serum or plasma levels up to 170 ng/mL and selenium toenail concentrations of 0.85–0.94 µg/g. However, as the observed relation was over a relatively narrow range of selenium status, further studies in low selenium populations are recommended. In contrast to the NPC study and the studies in the Hurst *et al.* (2012) meta analysis, the participants in the SELECT trial were not selenium deficient. Whilst SELECT did not demonstrate a preventative role for selenium in a non-selenium deficient population of men, there may be a beneficial role for supplementation in selenium deficient men. At present, selenium supplementation for prostate cancer prevention has not been proven, and therefore its use cannot be recommended based on current evidence.

The WCRF/AICR (2007) reported limited evidence to suggest that pulses (including soya and soya products) reduce prostate cancer risk. Part of the protective role from soya is related to the oestrogen-like effects of its isoflavone component. Two meta analyses published since 2007 concluded there was evidence of a protective role from soya, related to the quantity and type of soya consumed. Non-fermented soya (e.g. soyabeans, tofu and soya milk) appears to offer a protective role, whilst the role of fermented soya, e.g. miso, is less clear. The protective effect of soya is seen in groups with the highest intake when compared with groups with the lowest intake. However, the level of soya intake required to acquire benefit has not been established. It is important to highlight that soya encompasses a number of foods and the magnitude of the effect of soya on prostate cancer incidence may be variable with soya type. This can influence the results of research where a variety of soya products are investigated (Hwang *et al.*, 2009; Yan Spitznagal, 2009).

Other foods demonstrating protective properties are shown in Table 7.15.9; however, evidence for these are weak and variable. There is a positive correlation for calcium, grilled and processed meats, milk and dairy products, and fat intake with increased prostate cancer risk. The strongest and most convincing correlation is with calcium, where intakes above 1.5 g/day were associated with increased risk, but no increase in risk was observed with intakes up to 1.2 g/day (Baron *et al.*, 2005; WCRF/AICR, 2007). Limited evidence suggests an increased prostate cancer risk with grilled and processed meats (particularly at over five servings a week), milk and dairy products (irrespective of fat content) and increased fat intake. This is particularly the case with animal and saturated fats (WCRF/AICR, 2007; Ma & Chapman, 2009). These findings reinforce the importance of following guidelines for healthy eating for the general population as part of prostate cancer prevention.

Treatment

Surgery

A prostatectomy may be undertaken in the curative setting. Nutritional difficulties preoperatively are gener-ally uncommon. In the postoperative setting, ileus is an important although infrequent complication, occurring in <5% of all patients, but more commonly following an anastomotic leak with an incidence of 55% (Sukkarie *et al.*, 2007). Where a prolonged ileus occurs, the timely instigation of parenteral nutrition should be considered to support postoperative recovery.

Radiotherapy

Radiotherapy is often used in a curative setting. While treatment is directed at the prostate gland, the bowel and rectum sometimes receive radiotherapy. As a consequence of this, diarrhoea due to mucosal damage may occur. This is known as acute radiation enteritis. Temporary changes in bowel motility, lactose intolerance, bile acid malabsorption, bile acid and pancreatic enzyme damage to bowel mucosa, and bacterial overgrowth may also be observed. There is some research showing dietary modifications may improve symptoms of acute radiation enteritis, e.g. a low fat or elemental diet, probiotic supplementation and reducing fibre intake. Whilst the evidence supporting these therapeutic diets is weak due to inadequacies in research methodology with results confounded by poor compliance in treatment groups, a trial may nonetheless be beneficial in symptomatic patients (McGough *et al.*, 2004; Wedlake *et al.*, 2012). A limited number of patients may experience longer term gastrointestinal disturbances due to chronic radiation enteritis, causing impaired quality of life. Andreyev *et al.* (2012) provide guidance on managing the acute and chronic gastrointestinal problems arising from cancer treatment. In planning radiotherapy, and throughout treatment, patients may be required to make dietary changes, e.g. a low fibre diet, avoidance of carbonated drinks and reduced consumption of foods known to cause wind. Bowel gas can influence the position of the prostate gland and therefore affect treatment. More research is needed to assess the effectiveness of this intervention, although some centres may already recommend patients follow advice (McNair *et al.*, 2011).

Hormone treatment

Hormone treatment may use antiandrogen therapy, lutein hormone releasing hormone analogues and oestrogen. Hormones treat prostate cancer by reducing the effects of testosterone in the body to shrink or delay tumour growth and reduce symptoms; hormone treatment may continue for a number of years. Nutritional consequences include weight gain and features of metabolic syndrome, e.g. abdominal obesity, increased total body fat mass, dyslipidaemia, increased diabetes risk and hyperinsulinaemia (Tayek *et al.*, 1990; Smith *et al.*, 2002). The effect of hormone treatment on lipid profile is summarised in Table 7.15.10. Tailored interventions for weight management and advice on principles of healthy eating to manage these side effects can be effective (Jones & Demark-Wahnefried, 2006; Demark-Wahnefried *et al.*, 2012) (see Chapter 7.12 and 7.14.3).

Reduced bone density is another important implication of antiandrogen therapy. Consideration should be given

Table 7.15.10 Effect of hormone therapy on lipid profile (Fillippatos *et al.*, 2008)

Hormone therapy type	Total cholesterol	Low density lipoprotein	High density lipoprotein	Triglyceride
Oestrogen	↓	↓	↑	↑
Anti-androgen	↓	↓	↑	↑
Lutein hormone releasing hormone analogues	↑	Unchanged	↑	Not available

to vitamin D and calcium supplementation. Bisphosphonates may be prescribed to preserve bone density by reducing osteoclast activity and increasing osteoblast activity in bone (see Chapter 7.9.1).

Chemotherapy

Chemotherapy is given where cure is no longer possible, and aims to shrink and slow the growth of the cancer, control symptoms such as pain and improve quality of life. Side effects with potential nutritional implications include stomatitis, taste changes, anorexia, nausea, vomiting, changes in bowel habit and fatigue. These side effects are temporary and resolve shortly after completing treatment. Short term dietary changes and oral supplementation may be necessary to help manage eating more easily. Advanced cancer can influence appetite and cause difficulties with eating. Dietary advice and supplementation should be considered with the aim of preserving quality of life. Steroids may sometimes be given with chemotherapy to make treatment more effective and this can also help improve appetite.

Disease progression and survivorship

Men with prostate cancer can live for many years with the disease. Foods and dietary supplements for this patient group that have been investigated include: processed meats, eggs, plant based diets, lycopene and/or tomato, vitamin E, alpha-tocopherol, beta-carotene, soya/isoflavones, soya (in conjunction with other supplements), low fat diets, pomegranate juice and green tea. A number of review articles all provide similar conclusions in that further research is needed to prove a definitive role for diet in this patient population (Chan *et al.*, 2005; Bekkering *et al.*, 2006; Van Patten *et al.*, 2008; Ma & Chapman, 2009; Davies *et al.*, 2011).

Dietary changes can help manage the long term health implications of hormone treatment and radiotherapy. To reduce the risk of developing comorbidities associated with weight gain and dyslipidaemia, advice on healthy eating and lifestyle measures, including exercise, should be integrated into the patient's care. It is possible that the benefits of this may also extend to a positive impact on disease progression and survival (Davies *et al.*, 2011).

Conclusion

There is great consumer interest in the role of diet in disease prevention and management. When a cancer diagnosis is received, diet provides individuals with a readily available method to actively control their own health. Whilst evidence points towards certain correlations with prostate cancer, diet and use of dietary supplements, the lack of high quality studies and publication of consistent results has not provided sufficient evidence to translate these into public health or clinical practice recommendations. Individuals may seek advice on diet and prostate cancer and it is important for dietetic professionals to understand the evidence available. Further research is needed to substantiate current findings. However, the existing knowledge from studies provides a basis for dietitians in giving patients and the general public guidance on diet and prostate cancer.

Internet resources

Prostate Cancer Charity   www.prostate-cancer.org.uk

References

Andreyev HN, Davidson SE, Gillespie C, *et al.* (2012) Practice guidance on the management of acute and chronic gastrointestinal problems arising as a result of treatment for cancer. *Gut* 61(2): 179–192.

ATBC Study Group. (2003) Incidence of cancer and mortality following α-tocopherol and β-carotene supplementation: A post intervention follow-up. *JAMA* 290(4): 476–485.

Baade PD, Yulden DR, Krnjacki LJ. (2009) International epidemiology of prostate cancer: Geographical distribution and secular trends. *Molecular Nutrition & Food Research* 53(2): 171–184.

Baron JA, Beach M, Wallace K, *et al.* (2005) Risk of prostate cancer in a randomised clinical trial of calcium supplementation. *Cancer Epidemiology, Biomarkers & Prevention* 14: 586–589.

Bekkering T, Beynon R, Davey Smith G, *et al.* (2006) *A Systematic Review of RCTs Investigating the Effect of Dietal and Physical Activity Interventions on Cancer Survival, Updated Report.* World Cancer Research Fund. Available at www.dietandcancerreport.org/cancer_resource_center/downloads/SLR/Cancer_survivors_SLR.pdf. Accessed 3 March 2013.

Brinkman M, Reulen RC, Kellen E, *et al.* (2006) Are men with low selenium levels at increased risk of prostate cancer? *European Journal of Cancer* 42: 2463–2471.

Chan JM, Gann PH, Giovannucci EL. (2005) Role of diet in prostate cancer and progression. *Journal of Clinical Oncology* 23: 8152–8160.

Clark LC, Combs GF Jr, Turnbull BW, *et al.* (1996) Effects of selenium supplementation for cancer prevention in carcinoma of the skin. A randomized controlled trial: Nutritional Prevention of Cancer Study Group. *JAMA* 276(24): 1957–1963.

Davies NJ, Batehup L, Thomas R. (2011) The role of diet and physical activity in breast, colorectal, and prostate cancer survivorship: a review of the literature. *British Journal of Cancer* 105(S1): S52–S73.

Demark-Wahnefried W, More MC, Sloane R, *et al.* (2012) Reach Out to Enhance Wellness Home-Based Diet-Exercise Intervention promotes reproducible and sustainable long-term Improvements in health behaviors, body weight, and physical functioning in older, overweight/obese cancer survivors. *Journal of Clinical Oncology* 30(19): 2354–2361.

Dennert G, Zwahlen M, Brinkman M, *et al.* (2011) Selenium for preventing cancer. *Cochrane Database of Systematic Reviews* 5: CD005195.

Duffield-Lillico AJ, Dalkin BL, Reid ME, *et al.* (2003) Selenium supplementation, baseline plasma selenium status and incidence of prostate cancer: an analysis of the complete treatment period of the Nutritional Prevention of Cancer Trial. *BJU International* 91: 608–612.

Etminan M, Takkouche B, Caamaño-Isorna F. (2004) The role of tomato products and lycopene in the prevention of prostate cancer: a meta-analysis of observational studies. *Cancer Epidemiology, Biomarkers and Prevention* 13(3): 340–345.

Filippatos TD, Liberopoulos EN, Pavlidis N, *et al.* (2008) Effects of hormonal treatment on lipids in patients with cancer. *Cancer Treatment Reviews* 35(2): 175–184.

Giovannucci E, Liu Y, Platz EA, *et al.* (2007) Risk factors for prostate cancer incidence and progression in the health professionals follow-up study. *International Journal of Cancer* 121: 1571–1578.

Greene K, Cowan JE, Cooperberg MR. (2005) Who is the average patient presenting with prostate cancer? *Urology* 6(5): 76–82.

Hsing AW, Tsao L, Devesa SS. (2000) International trends and patterns of prostate cancer incidence and mortality. *International Journal of Cancer* 85(1): 60–67.

Hurst R, Hooper L, Norat T, *et al.* (2012) Selenium and prostate cancer: systematic review and meta-analysis. *American Journal of Clinical Nutrition* 96(1): 111–122.

Hwang YW, Kim SY, Jee SH, *et al.* (2009) Soy food consumption and risk of prostate cancer: A meta-analysis of observational studies. *Nutrition and Cancer* 61(5): 598–606.

Ilic D, Forbes KM, Hassed C. (2011) Lycopene for the prevention of prostate cancer. *Cochrane Database of Systematic Reviews* 11: CD008007.

Jones JW, Demark-Wahnefried W. (2006) Diet, exercise, and complementary therapies after primary treatment for cancer. *Lancet Oncology* 7(12): 1017–1026.

Klein EA, Thompson IM, Tangen CM, *et al.* (2011) Vitamin E and the risk of prostate cancer. The Selenium and Vitamin E Cancer Prevention Trial (SELECT). *JAMA* 306(14): 1549–1556.

Lippman SM, Klein EA, Goodman PJ, *et al.* (2009) Effect of selenium and vitamin E on risk of prostate cancer and other cancers. The Selenium and Vitamin E Cancer Prevention Trial (SELECT). *JAMA* 301(1): 39–51.

Ma RWL, Chapman K. (2009) A systematic review of the effect of diet in prostate cancer prevention and treatment. *Journal of Human Nutrition and Dietetics* 22(3): 187–199.

McGough C, Baldwin C, Frost G, *et al.* (2004) Role of nutritional intervention in patients treated with radiotherapy for pelvic malignancy. *British Journal of Cancer* 90(12): 2278–2287.

McNair HA, Wedlake L, McVey GP, *et al.* (2011) Can diet combined with treatment scheduling achieve consistency of rectal filling in patients receiving radiotherapy to the prostate. *Radiotherapy & Oncology* 101(3): 471–478 (Abstract).

Office for National Statistics (ONS). (2012a) *Cancer Statistics Registrations. Registrations of cancer diagnosed in 2010, England.* Edition No MB1 41. London. The Stationery Office. Available at www.ons.gov.uk/ons/dcp171778_267154.pdf. Accessed 3 March 2013.

Office for National Statistics (ONS). (2012b) *Summary: Cancer survival in England: Patients Diagnosed 2006–2010, Followed up to 2011. Statistical Bulletin.* London. The Stationery Office. Available at www.ons.gov.uk/ons/dcp171780_283943.pdf. Accessed 3 March 2013.

Quinn M, Babb P. (2002) Patterns and trends in prostate cancer incidence, survival, prevalence and mortality. Part I: international comparisons. *BJU International* 90: 162–173.

Segura A, Pardo J, Jara C, *et al.* (2005) An epidemiological evaluation of the prevalence of malnutrition in Spanish patients with locally advanced or metastatic cancer. *Clinical Nutrition* 24: 801–814.

Smith MR, Finkelstein JS, McGovern FJ, *et al.* (2002) Changes in Body Composition during Androgen Deprivation Therapy for Prostate Cancer. *Journal of Clinical Endocrinology and Metabolism* 87: 599–603.

Sukkarie T, Harmon J, Penna F, *et al.* (2007) Incidence and management of anastomotic leakage following laparoscopic prostatectomy with implementation of a new anastomotic technique incorporating posterior bladder neck tailoring. *Journal of Robotic Surgery* 1: 213–215.

Tayek JA, Heber D, Byerley LO, *et al.* (1990) Nutritional and metabolic effects of gonadotropin-releasing hormone agonist treatment for prostate cancer. *Metabolism* 39(12): 1314–1319.

Van Patten CL, de Boer JG, Tomlinson Guns ES. (2008) Diet and Dietary Supplement Intervention Trials for the Prevention of Prostate Cancer Recurrence: A Review of the Randomized Controlled Trial Evidence. *Journal of Urology* 180(6): 2314–2321.

Wedlake LJ, McGough C, Shaw C, *et al.* (2012) Clinical trial: efficacy of a low or modified fat diet for the prevention of gastrointestinal toxicity in patients receiving radiotherapy treatment for pelvic malignancies. *Journal of Human Nutrition and Dietetics* 25: 247–259.

World Cancer Research Fund/American Institute for Cancer Research & (WCRF/AICR). (2007) *Food, Nutrition, Physical Activity and the Prevention of Cancer: A Global Perspective: A Project of World Cancer Research Fund International.* Washington, DC: AICR, pp. 305–306.

Yan L, Spitznagal EL. (2009) Soy consumption and prostate cancer risk in men: a revisit of a meta-analysis. *American Journal of Clinical Nutrition* 89: 1155–1163.

7.15.8 Haematological cancers and high dose therapy
Julie Beckerson

Key points

- High dose chemotherapy, radiotherapy and stem cell transplant provide potential cure or remission for many haematological cancers.

- Treatment associated side effects such as severe mucositis, nausea and vomiting can lead to rapid deterioration of nutritional status. Nutrition support is therefore recognised as an important adjunct to high dose therapy.

- The benefit of dietary restrictions during neutropenia is not clear, and advice should focus on minimising food poisoning risk whilst optimising choice at a time when nutritional intake may already be compromised.

Haematological cancers involve the blood or lymphatic system and include leukaemia, lymphoma, myeloma, myelodysplastic syndromes and lymphoproliferative disorders. These are rare in children and young adults, but become more common with increasing age and account for approximately 35 000 UK cases per year (www.hmrn .org/Statistics/Incidence.aspx). Non-Hodgkin's lymphoma, leukaemia and myeloma are the fifth, 12th and 17th most common cancer diagnoses, respectively (www .cancerresearchuk.org/cancer-info/cancerstats).

Leukaemia refers to a proliferation and accumulation of abnormal white blood cells in the bone marrow (abnormal blasts). As the disease progresses, abnormal cells spill out of the bone marrow and infiltrate and damage other tissues. Leukaemia is described as either myeloid or lymphoid according to the origin of the abnormal cells. Acute and chronic leukaemia are differentiated by the maturity of the cells affected. Acute leukaemia affects immature white blood cells that continue to divide after normal cells have stopped. In chronic leukaemia, mature cells are affected, increasing their lifespan and number in the marrow and circulation.

Lymphoma results from abnormal replication of cells within lymph nodes or other lymphoid tissues, such as the spleen, bone marrow and thymus. It is broadly classified into Hodgkin's or non-Hodgkin's lymphoma, but within these categories there are numerous disease subtypes according to the cell line that multiplies. High grade lymphomas replicate the quickest, whereas low grade or indolent lymphomas develop slowly and may be asymptomatic for many years.

Myeloma is a malignant proliferation of monoclonal plasma cells that often secrete large amounts of ineffective antibodies known as paraproteins. In addition to bone marrow involvement there maybe infiltration of bone, causing osteolytic lesions, kidney damage from elevated plasma paraprotein and/or hypercalcaemia, and isolated lesions known as plasmacytomas.

Diagnosis

The clinical presentation of haematological malignancies frequently reflects the underlying altered haematopoiesis (formation and development of blood cells). In leukaemia, suppressed or ineffective white blood cells increase susceptibility to infection. Patients may complain of fatigue due to anaemia caused by reduced red blood cells or increased bruising and bleeding resulting from thrombocytopenia (low platelets). Presenting symptoms such as fever, night sweats and weight loss occur in lymphoma and may suggest advanced disease.

Blood tests and bone marrow aspirate are used to determine the type and extent of blood cell abnormalities. Cytogenetic testing of chromosomal changes and immunophenotyping to detect specific molecules on the surface of malignant cells are also used to guide treatment decisions. Other tests include urinary paraprotein, lymph node biopsy and imaging. Subsequent staging and prognosis of haematological cancers will vary significantly according to the disease subtype.

Treatment

Protocols used in haemato-oncology frequently involve the most intensive and high dose regimens. In acute leukaemia, disease onset is rapid and induction chemotherapy must be initiated immediately. However, for some chronic leukaemias, low grade lymphomas and myeloma, treatment may be delayed until symptoms present. The treatment goal is to control disease and maximise quality of life, whilst minimising treatment side effects. Bone marrow, or increasingly stem cell transplants (SCT), can be used to enable higher doses of chemotherapy and radiotherapy with the aim of achieving long term remission or cure. These are usually performed after several courses of induction chemotherapy to control disease or achieve remission.

There are two main types of SCT; autologous (the patient is given back their own cells) and allogeneic (using donor cells). Donor transplants provide the greatest likelihood of long term remission or cure due to the immunological effects of the donor cells against the host's disease. However, autologous SCTs are considered standard care for some conditions, such as myeloma, due to the high morbidity associated with allogeneic transplantation (Bensinger, 2009).

Prior to an infusion of stem cells, a conditioning regimen that may include chemotherapy, radiation and immunosuppressive therapy is given. Cytotoxic agents are given to eradicate tumour cells and destroy host haematopoiesis in preparation for the donor stem cells. Reduced intensity conditioned (RIC) transplants have been developed for older patients less able to withstand high dose myeloablative chemotherapy. Early toxicities are reduced but there is an increased risk of subsequent relapse (Gratwohl, 2005). The choice of SCT depends on the disease, stage, fitness of the recipient and donor availability.

Consequences of high dose therapies and stem cell transplant

Neutropenia and infectious complications

Myeloablative therapy causes neutrophil levels to fall, increasing the risk of bacterial sepsis, pneumonia and fungal infections. This is a major cause of morbidity and mortality; therefore, antimicrobial, antifungal and antiviral medications are routine (Gratwohl et al., 2005). Other preventative measures include contact precautions, hand washing, air filtration and positive pressure isolation rooms.

Infection risk is highest in allogeneic SCT where the period of neutropenia is longer than in autologous SCT. Immunosuppressive therapy and immune reconstitution continue for several months after neutrophil recovery following allogeneic SCT. Viral infections are common during this phase and can be fatal (Cordonnier, 2008).

Mucositis

Mucositis after SCT typically lasts for 1–3 weeks, dependent on the conditioning regimen. It can affect any part of the gastrointestinal tract, resulting in mouth or throat pain, ulceration, abdominal pain, nausea, vomiting and diarrhoea. Up to 80% of SCT recipients will experience severe mucositis, frequently requiring intravenous opioid analgesia (Rubenstein et al., 2004; Keefe et al., 2007). The breakdown of mucosal barriers during mucositis significantly increases infection risk and is associated with worse clinical and economic outcomes (Keefe, 2006; Sonis et al., 2001; Fanning et al, 2006).

Organ toxicity

The high dose chemotherapy and/or radiotherapy used in SCT can cause gastrointestinal, renal, bladder, pulmonary, cardiac, neurological and hepatic complications, resulting in significant morbidity and mortality (Gratwohl, 2008). Around 14% of SCT recipients will develop hepatic veno-occlusive disease (also known as sinusoidal obstructive syndrome), which is characterised by occlusion and injury to hepatic venules and hepatocytes induced by chemotherapy. It often leads to multiorgan failure and is associated with high mortality rates (Coppell et al., 2010).

Graft versus host disease

Immunosuppression is given to allogeneic SCT patients to avoid the potentially fatal complication of graft versus host disease (GvHD). This occurs as a consequence of interactions between mature donor immune cells (T cells) and antigen presenting cells of the recipient. There are two types. Acute GvHD usually occurs within 100 days of SCT and may affect the skin, gut or liver, manifesting as rash, nausea, vomiting, diarrhoea, ileus and deranged liver function or liver failure. Chronic GvHD is a major long term complication of allogeneic SCT and occurs in 30–70% of transplant recipients. It occurs more than 100 days after transplant and can affect numerous organs and tissues. About 50% of patients will have three or more involved organs (Lee 2010).

Psychological effects

Extended periods in isolation, separation from family and the experience of transplant have major psychological effects (Wagner & Cella, 2004). Reduced attention span and slower cognitive processing can occur as a result of fatigue following high dose therapy, further impacting on mood.

Survivorship

Continued hospital appointments, fatigue and susceptibility to infection significantly impact rehabilitation after high dose therapy. Full return to normal functioning and nutritional status can take >1 year after transplantation (Iestra et al., 2002).

Nutritional assessment

Nutritional screening is recommended to identify subjects for whom nutritional assessment and care planning is necessary (August et al., 2009). Assessment prior to high dose treatment is useful to establish pre-existing malnutrition, discuss potential side effects of treatment, develop rapport and improve compliance with recommended interventions (Iestra et al., 2002). High dose therapies, particularly SCT, have marked effects on metabolic demands and significantly impair nutritional intake. Furthermore, reduced physical activity and loss of mobility due to hospitalisation and prolonged isolation result in reduced muscle mass, particularly in a previously active patient (Coleman et al., 2003).

Optimum nutrition improves tolerance to treatment and outcome in malnourished patients, and well nourished individuals experience shorter treatment delays, less myelosuppression and fewer infections (Aviles et al., 1995). Studies in SCT indicate that poor nutritional status and low body mass index (BMI) are negative prognostic factors in terms of time to engraftment and survival (Hadjibabaie et al., 2008; Schulte et al., 1998). Conversely, high BMI prior to SCT is linked with acute GvHD, infections and poorer 5-year survival rates (Bulley et al., 2008; Fuji et al., 2009).

Anthropometry

Weighing may be inaccurate due to large intravenous infusions given during treatment and changes in organ function. Pathological fractures or vertebral collapse in

Table 7.15.11 Mineral and electrolyte changes with drugs commonly used in stem cell transplantation

Drug	Therapeutic use	Biochemical side effect
Ciclosporin	Immunosuppression	Hyperkalaemia, hypomagnesaemia
Tacrolimus		Hyperkalaemia, hypokalaemia
Amphotericin Ambisome	Antifungal	Hypokalaemia, hypomagnesaemia
Foscarnet	Antiviral	Hypocalcaemia, other electrolyte disturbances

myeloma patients may introduce errors in measuring height. Other anthropometry may provide a better indication of nutritional status, but the use of skinfold callipers is limited during thrombocytopenia due to bleeding risk.

Biochemistry

Regular laboratory monitoring is essential to detect changes in organ function, mineral and electrolyte imbalances, hyperglycaemia or hyperlipidaemia (Lipkin *et al.*, 2005). Biochemistry alone cannot accurately reflect nutritional status. The underlying disease and complications, such as sepsis and GvHD, will confound the interpretation of albumin. In advanced myeloma, this is also lowered at the expense of raised paraprotein.

Mineral and electrolyte losses are common and often exacerbated by antimicrobial and immunosuppressive drugs, examples of which are shown in Table 7.15.11. Multiple blood transfusions may elevate ferritin levels, indicating iron overload. Repeated hospital stays for treatment can result in suboptimal vitamin D status and low calcium levels, which are of particular relevance for those receiving corticosteroid therapy (Lipkin *et al.*, 2005).

Nutritional requirements

Energy expenditure differs between transplant type and the presence of complications, although evidence is limited. Metabolic rate will vary with the phase of illness or stage of treatment, and older studies may not be relevant to current treatment modalities. Current recommendations for energy suggest disease specific elevations in basal metabolic rate of 25–34% in leukaemia and of 0–25% in lymphoma (Weekes, 2011). However, these studies include few haematology subjects and measurements were taken whilst a proportion of subjects were receiving artificial nutrition (Barak *et al.*, 2002).

Nutritional requirements are raised in acute GvHD and there may be significant gastrointestinal losses, resulting in a negative balance for many nutrients, including nitrogen. Chronic GvHD patients have an elevated tumour necrosis factor alpha and elevated resting energy expenditure, which may contribute to chronic weight loss (Zauner *et al.*, 2001).

Evidence is lacking to support specific recommendations for nitrogen intake at different stages of treatment. Negative nitrogen balance is likely during high dose therapy and the catabolic effects of disease, treatment and complications should be considered when estimating protein requirements (Muscaritoli *et al.*, 2002).

Micronutrient requirements may be raised during high dose therapy due to increased oxidation and tissue damage; however, there is no evidence to support routine antioxidant or trace element supplementation (Lipkin *et al.*, 2005). Losses of fluid, electrolytes and other nutrients frequently occur; however, intravenous input from medications, blood products and electrolyte replacement can predispose to fluid overload.

Nutritional intervention in stem cell transplant

The dietitian and appropriate nutritional support are recognised as vital components of the transplant process (August *et al.*, 2009; NICE, 2003). Appropriate nutritional interventions for symptom management during chemotherapy and radiotherapy are discussed in Chapter 7.15.1. The side effects from SCT that impair nutritional intake are frequently severe and may occur concurrently (Figure 7.15.2), and despite aggressive medical management, the SCT patient is often unable to maintain adequate oral nutritional intake.

Artificial nutrition support

The type of transplant, intensity of conditioning and mucositis are the biggest determinants for artificial nutrition support (Iestra *et al.*, 1999). Transplant patients may experience nausea, anorexia and mucositis following chemotherapy, and these side effects are most severe during myeloablative allogeneic SCT. The use of reduced intensity conditioning causes fewer side effects, reducing the need for artificial nutrition (Parker *et al.*, 2002; Topcuoglu *et al.*, 2012; Johansson *et al.*, 2001).

Parenteral nutrition (PN) is recommended for those with severe mucositis, prolonged ileus, intractable vomiting or diarrhoea, those who are malnourished or those for whom it is anticipated that enteral nutrition (EN) will not be tolerated for 7–14 days (August *et al.*, 2009). Further studies in SCT recipients are required to confirm the optimum time without nutrition after which PN demonstrates a survival benefit.

Historically, PN was used extensively during SCT. This was partly due to the high gastrointestinal toxicities of older conditioning regimens and the availability of central access, already established for chemotherapy and stem cell infusion. Recently, better pharmacological management of treatment side effects has allowed safe and effective use of EN during SCT (August *et al.*, 2009; Thompson & Duffy, 2008). Although there is a lack of evaluable data to compare EN with PN (Thompson & Duffy, 2008), EN is recommended for situations where the GI tract remains accessible and functioning (August *et al.*, 2009).

The known infectious risks of PN are likely to be amplified in this immunocompromised group (Black, 2011).

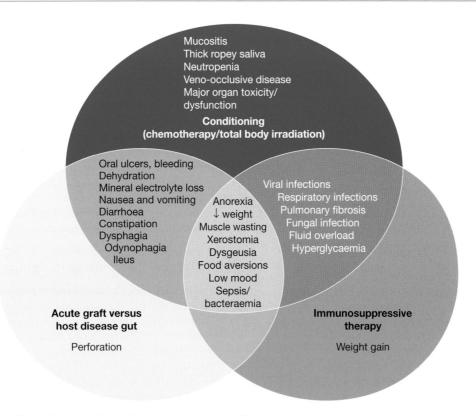

Figure 7.15.2   Side effects of stem cell transplant impacting on nutritional status

During SCT, EN may reduce infectious complications by promoting intestinal recovery since disruption of the mucosal barrier is thought to contribute to the development of 25–75% of bacteraemias during neutropenia (Stiff, 2001). There is also some evidence that the provision of nutrition via the enteral rather than the parenteral route during SCT may reduce acute GvHD incidence (Seguy *et al.*, 2006; Cheney *et al.*, 1991).

Enteral feeding tubes need to be placed prior to the development of mucositis to avoid pain and further mucosal damage. Thrombocytopenia is common and tube placement presents a risk of haemorrhage. Local guidelines will vary, but a platelet count of >20 × 10⁹/L may be adequate (Lipkin *et al.*, 2005). Since feeding tubes are sterile, neutropenia *per se* is not a contraindication to placement of a nasoenteric tube. Waiting until the acute emetic effects of conditioning have settled will reduce the risk of tube dislodgement.

Post pyloric feeding (nasojejunal) feeding may be useful if there is protracted vomiting or gastric stasis and this approach has been adopted by some UK transplant centres (Black, 2011). The prophylactic insertion of gastrostomy or jejunostomy tubes to overcome repeated nasoenteric tube displacements due to vomiting has been trialled. However, stoma site infections resulting in peritonitis and associated treatment delays have limited the use of these tubes (Black, 2011).

Evidence for the optimum enteral feed composition during SCT is lacking; hence, choice should be made according to clinical parameters such as renal function, fluid status and gastrointestinal side effects. Polymeric feeds may be suitable, but if malabsorption is suspected, then semi elemental or peptide feeds may be better tolerated (Lipkin *et al.*, 2005; Black, 2011).

During gut GvHD, destruction of intestinal crypts, profuse diarrhoea and ulceration can lead to perforation. Acute GvHD can occur in conjunction with mucositis, and in severe cases the most appropriate form of nutrition is PN (Muscaritoli *et al.*, 2002). However, EN was shown to be safe and beneficial in one small controlled cohort study (Imataki *et al.*, 2006) and the use of peptide based and low osmolality feed can be considered for low grade gut GvHD.

The neutropenic diet

The need for and efficacy of a neutropenic diet is controversial (August *et al.*, 2009; Jubelirer, 2011; Mank & Davies, 2008). Damage to the gut mucosal barrier by high dose therapy, bacterial overgrowth and opioid related impairment of peristalsis may increase the risk of translocation and bacteraemia (Black, 2011; Berg, 1999). Recommendations for a low bacterial diet arise from known sources of food borne microorganisms in the food chain (National Digestive Diseases Information Clearing House, 2011) and published case reports of infections, as well as outbreaks of food poisoning in the general population and immunocompromised individuals.

Early studies that placed leukaemia patients on a sterile diet suggested a reduction in infections; however, these results maybe confounded by the use of protective isolation, laminar airflow and antimicrobial gut decontamination. Subsequent small studies have not confirmed the

Table 7.15.12 Dietary restrictions according to neutrophil count (Leukaemia and Lymphoma Research, 2012)

Neutrophil count	Foods to restrict
$<2.0 \times 10^9$	Mould ripened or blue veined cheeses Unpasteurised dairy products Raw or lightly cooked shellfish Raw or undercooked meat, poultry or fish Raw or undercooked eggs Probiotic products Fresh pâté
$< 0.5 \times 10^9$	Raw or unpeeled fruit, dried fruit, vegetables and salad Unpasteurised fruit or vegetable juices or smoothies Water or ice from wells, coolers or bottled water Ice cream from ice cream vans Fresh nuts Uncooked herbs, spices and pepper Unpasteurised honey Unnecessarily large packets of food items

benefit of excluding uncooked fruit and vegetables (Gardner *et al.*, 2008; DeMille *et al.*, 2006) or following a low bacterial diet (van Tiel *et al.*, 2007), and some institutions have removed restrictions without any corresponding increase in infection rates (Tarr & Allen, 2009).

Many UK centres follow recommendations published by Lymphoma and Leukaemia Research (2012) on behalf of the Haematology subgroup of the British Dietetic Association (BDA) Oncology Group. This includes food safety advice on preparation and storage and foods to restrict according to neutrophil count, as shown in Table 7.15.12. Due to contamination of bottled mineral water by coliforms and listeria (Hunter, 1993), freshly run tap water is recommend during neutropenia. Commercial quality water filtration is recommended where institutional tap water is at risk of contamination from *Legionella spp* (Cordonnier 2008).

The American Society for Parenteral and Enteral Nutrition (ASPEN) guidelines for nutrition support during SCT recommend advice regarding safe food handling and avoidance of specific foods that may increase the risk of infection during neutropenia (August *et al.*, 2009). In practice, advice varies significantly between different transplant centres, with inconsistencies around the type of foods restricted, when and for how long to restrict these foods, and guidance for non-neutropenic patients on post transplant immunosuppression (Mank & Davies, 2008).

Glutamine

Radiation or chemotherapy induced tissue damage may be attenuated by adequate tissue glutamine, suggesting a potential role in the prevention of tissue toxicity during myeloblative treatments (Wischmeyer, 2003). A meta analysis of three studies suggests oral glutamine may reduce mucositis and GvHD, but robust evidence in this area is lacking (Crowther *et al.*, 2009).

Currently, ASPEN suggests pharmacological doses of parenteral glutamine may benefit patients undergoing SCT (August *et al.*, 2009) . A Cochrane review in 2002 indicated beneficial effects of glutamine supplemented PN versus standard PN on length of stay and incidence of positive blood cultures (Murray & Pindoria, 2002). However, subsequent studies and meta analyses suggest the benefits may be limited to the allogeneic SCT population in whom the need for artificial support is likely to be the greatest (Murray & Pindoria, 2008; Crowther *et al.*, 2009; Gama Torres *et al.*, 2008). Further studies of both oral and parenteral glutamine are required to confirm the dose, duration and patient group that will benefit.

Drug–nutrient interactions

The following drugs reduce bioavailability or absorption with oral and enteral nutrition (Wohlt *et al.*, 2009):

- Alendronic acid.
- Ciprofloxacin.
- Lansoprazole.
- Omeprazole.
- Pantoprazole.
- Penicillin V.
- Phenytoin.
- Sucralfate.
- Voriconazole.

Other drugs of note used in this patient group include:

- Ciclosporin – avoid all grapefruit containing foods.
- Posaconazole – requires concurrent oral or enteral nutrition.

Exact recommendations may vary according to formulation and local policy.

References

August DA, Huhmann MB. (2009) A.S.P.E.N. clinical guidelines: nutrition support therapy during adult anticancer treatment and in hematopoietic cell transplantation. *Journal of Parenteral and Enteral Nutrition* 33(5):472–500.

Aviles A, Yanez J, Lopez T, Garcia EL, Guzman R, Diaz-Maqueo JC. (1995) Malnutrition as an adverse prognostic factor in patients with diffuse large cell lymphoma. *Archives of Medical Research* 26(1): 31–34.

Barak N, Wall-Alonso E, Sitrin MD. (2002) Evaluation of stress factors and body weight adjustments currently used to estimate energy expenditure in hospitalized patients. *Journal of Parenteral and Enteral Nutrition* 26(4): 231–238.

Bensinger WI. (2009) Role of autologous and allogeneic stem cell transplantation in myeloma. *Leukemia* 23(3): 442–448.

Berg RD. (1999) Bacterial translocation from the gastrointestinal tract. *Advances in Experimental Medical Biology* 473: 11–30.

Black G. (2011) Haemato-Oncology. In: Shaw C (ed) *Nutrition and Cancer*. Chichester: Wiley Blackwell, pp. 287–310.

Bulley S, Gassas A, Dupuis LL, *et al.* (2008) Inferior outcomes for overweight children undergoing allogeneic stem cell transplantation. *British Journal of Haematology* 140(2): 214–217.

Cheney CL, Weiss NS, Fisher LD, Sanders JE, Davis S, Worthington-Roberts B. (1991) Oral protein intake and the risk of acute graft-versus-host disease after allogeneic marrow transplantation. *Bone Marrow Transplantation* 8(3): 203–210.

Coleman EA, Coon S, Hall-Barrow J, Richards K, Gaylor D, Stewart B. (2003) Feasibility of exercise during treatment for multiple myeloma. *Cancer Nursing* 26(5): 410–419.

Coppell JA, Richardson PG, Soiffer R, *et al.* (2010) Hepatic veno-occlusive disease following stem cell transplantation: incidence, clinical course, and outcome. *Biology of Blood and Marrow Transplantation* 16(2): 157–168.

Cordonnier C. (2008) Infections after HSCT. In: Apperley J, Carreras E, Gluckman E, Gratwohl A, Masszi T (eds) *Haematopoietic Stem Cell Transplantation*. France: European School of Haematology, pp. 198–217.

Crowther M, Avenell A, Culligan DJ. (2009) Systematic review and meta-analyses of studies of glutamine supplementation in haematopoietic stem cell transplantation. *Bone Marrow Transplantation* 44(7): 413–425.

DeMille D, Deming P, Lupinacci P, Jacobs LA. (2006) The effect of the neutropenic diet in the outpatient setting: a pilot study. *Oncology Nursing Forum* 33(2): 337–343.

Fanning SR, Rybicki L, Kalaycio M, *et al.* (2006) Severe mucositis is associated with reduced survival after autologous stem cell transplantation for lymphoid malignancies. *British Journal of Haematology* 135(3): 374–381.

Fuji S, Kim SW, Yoshimura K, *et al.* (2009) Possible association between obesity and posttransplantation complications including infectious diseases and acute graft-versus-host disease. *Biology of Blood and Marrow Transplantation* 15(1): 73–82.

Gama Torres HO, Vilela EG, da Cunha AS, *et al.* (2008) Efficacy of glutamine-supplemented parenteral nutrition on short-term survival following allo-SCT: a randomized study. *Bone Marrow Transplantation* 41(12): 1021–1027.

Gardner A, Mattiuzzi G, Faderl S, *et al.* (2008) Randomized comparison of cooked and noncooked diets in patients undergoing remission induction therapy for acute myeloid leukemia. *Journal of Clinical Oncology* 26(35): 5684–5688.

Gratwohl A, Brand R, Frassoni F, *et al.* (2005) Cause of death after allogeneic haematopoietic stem cell transplantation (HSCT) in early leukaemias: an EBMT analysis of lethal infectious complications and changes over calendar time. *Bone Marrow Transplantation* 36(9): 757–769.

Gratwohl A. Principles of conditioning. In: Apperley J, Carreras E, Gluckman E, Gratwohl A, Masszi T (eds) *Haematopoietic Stem Cell Transplantation*. France: European School of Haematology, pp. 128–145.

Hadjibabaie M, Iravani M, Taghizadeh M, *et al.* (2008) Evaluation of nutritional status in patients undergoing hematopoietic SCT. *Bone Marrow Transplantation* 42(7): 469–473.

Hunter PR. (1993) The microbiology of bottled natural mineral waters. *Journal of Applied Bacteriology* 74(4): 345–352.

Iestra JA, Fibbe WE, Zwinderman AH, Romijn JA, Kromhout D. (1999) Parenteral nutrition following intensive cytotoxic therapy: an exploratory study on the need for parenteral nutrition after various treatment approaches for haematological malignancies. *Bone Marrow Transplantation* 23(9): 933–939.

Iestra JA, Fibbe WE, Zwinderman AH, van Staveren WA, Kromhout D. (2002) Body weight recovery, eating difficulties and compliance with dietary advice in the first year after stem cell transplantation: a prospective study. *Bone Marrow Transplantation* 29(5): 417–424.

Imataki O, Nakatani S, Hasegawa T, *et al.* (2006) Nutritional support for patients suffering from intestinal graft-versus-host disease after

allogeneic hematopoietic stem cell transplantation. *American Journal of Hematology* 81(10): 747–752.

Jubelirer SJ. (2011) The benefit of the neutropenic diet: fact or fiction? *Oncologist* 16(5): 704–707.

Johansson JE, Brune M, Ekman T. (2001) The gut mucosa barrier is preserved during allogeneic, haemopoietic stem cell transplantation with reduced intensity conditioning. *Bone Marrow Transplantation* 28(8): 737–742.

Keefe DM. (2006) Mucositis management in patients with cancer. *Support in Cancer Therapy* 3(3): 154–157.

Keefe DM, Rassias G, O'Neil L, Gibson RJ. (2007) Severe mucositis: how can nutrition help? *Current Opinion in Clinical Nutrition and Metabolic Care* 10(5): 627–631.

Lee SJ. (2010) Have we made progress in the management of chronic graft-vs-host disease? *Best Practice and Research in Clinical Haematology* 23(4): 529–535.

Leukaemia and Lymphoma Research. (2012) Dietary advice for patients with neutropenia. Available at http://leukaemialympho maresearch.org.uk/sites/default/files/dapn_jan_2012.pdf. Accessed 25 February 2013.

Lipkin AC, Lenssen P, Dickson BJ. (2005) Nutrition issues in hematopoietic stem cell transplantation: state of the art. *Nutrition in Clinical Practice* 20(4): 423–439.

Mank AP, Davies M. (2008) Examining low bacterial dietary practice: a survey on low bacterial food. *European Journal of Oncology Nursing* 12(4): 342–348.

Murray SM, Pindoria S. (2002) Nutrition support for bone marrow transplant patients. *Cochrane Database of Systematic Reviews* 2: CD002920.

Murray SM, Pindoria S. (2008) Nutrition support for bone marrow transplant patients. *Cochrane Database of Systematic Reviews* 4: CD002920.

Muscaritoli M, Grieco G, Capria S, Iori AP, Rossi FF. (2002) Nutritional and metabolic support in patients undergoing bone marrow transplantation. *American Journal of Clinical Nutrition* 75(2): 183–190.

National Digestive Diseases Information Clearing House. (2011) Bacteria and foodborne illness. Available at http://digestive.niddk .nih.gov/ddiseases/pubs/bacteria/. Accessed October 2011.

National Institute for Health and Care Excellence (NICE). (2003) Improving outcomes in haematological cancers. Available at www.nice.org.

Parker JE, Shafi T, Pagliuca A, *et al.* (2002) Allogeneic stem cell transplantation in the myelodysplastic syndromes: interim results of outcome following reduced-intensity conditioning compared with standard preparative regimens. *British Journal of Haematology* 119(1): 144–154.

Rubenstein EB, Peterson DE, Schubert M, *et al.* (2004) Clinical practice guidelines for the prevention and treatment of cancer therapy-induced oral and gastrointestinal mucositis. *Cancer* 100 (9 Suppl): 2026–2046.

Schulte C, Reinhardt W, Beelen D, Mann K, Schaefer U. (1998) Low T3-syndrome and nutritional status as prognostic factors in patients undergoing bone marrow transplantation. *Bone Marrow Transplantation* 22(12): 1171–1178.

Seguy D, Berthon C, Micol JB, *et al.* (2006) Enteral feeding and early outcomes of patients undergoing allogeneic stem cell transplantation following myeloablative conditioning. *Transplantation* 82(6): 835–839.

Stiff P. (2001) Mucositis associated with stem cell transplantation: current status and innovative approaches to management. *Bone Marrow Transplantation* 27 (Suppl 2): S3–S11.

Sonis ST, Oster G, Fuchs H, *et al.* (2001) Oral mucositis and the clinical and economic outcomes of hematopoietic stem-cell transplantation. *Journal of Clinical Oncology* 19(8): 2201–2205.

Tarr S, Allen DH. (2009) Evidence does not support the use of a neutropenic diet. *Clinical Journal of Oncology Nursing* 13(6): 617–618.

Thompson JL, Duffy J. (2008) Nutrition support challenges in hematopoietic stem cell transplant patients. *Nutrition in Clinical Practice* 23(5): 533–546.

Topcuoglu P, Arat M, Ozcan M, *et al.* (2012) Case-matched comparison with standard versus reduced intensity conditioning regimen in chronic myeloid leukemia patients. *Annals of Hematology* 91(4): 577–586.

van Tiel F, Harbers MM, Terporten PH, *et al.* (2007) Normal hospital and low-bacterial diet in patients with cytopenia after intensive chemotherapy for hematological malignancy: a study of safety. *Annals of Oncology* 18(6): 1080–1084.

Wagner LI, Cella D.(2004) Fatigue and cancer: causes, prevalence and treatment approaches. *British Journal of Cancer* 91(5): 822–828.

Weekes CE. (2011) Adult macro and micro nutrient requirements. In: Todorovic VE, Micklewright A (eds). *A Pocket Guide to Clinical Nutrition*. Birmingham: British Dietetic Association, pp. 3.1–3.20.

Wischmeyer PE. (2003) Clinical applications of L-glutamine: past, present, and future. *Nutrition in Clinical Practice* 18(5): 377–385.

Wohlt PD, Zheng L, Gunderson S, Balzar SA, Johnson BD, Fish JT. (2009) Recommendations for the use of medications with continuous enteral nutrition. *American Journal of Health Systems Pharmacy* 66(16): 1458–1467.

Zauner C, Rabitsch W, Schneeweiss B, *et al.* (2001) Energy and substrate metabolism in patients with chronic extensive graft-versus-host disease. *Transplantation* 71(4): 524–528.

7.15.9 Cancer cachexia

Deborah Howland

Key points

- Cachexia is a complex syndrome associated with muscle loss, which is frequently accompanied by increased muscle catabolism, inflammation and anorexia.

- All cachetic patients are malnourished.

- Nutrition support can increase body weight; however, it does not have a demonstrable effect on lean body mass and therefore does not improve functional status or quality of life.

- Nutrition support may reduce carer anxiety and improve a patient's psychological condition.

Cachexia has been described throughout history as a condition associated with illness (Katz & Katz, 1962). The term cachexia is Greek in origin and is a combination of *kakós* (bad) and *hexis* (condition or appearance) (Doehner & Anker, 2002). More than 30% of cancer patients die due to cachexia and >50% die with cachexia (von Haehling & Anker, 2010).

Diagnostic criteria and classification

The causes of cachexia are complex and not fully elucidated. Therefore, there is no agreed definition, criteria or treatment despite several suggestions. A group of experts (Evans *et al.*, 2008) defined cachexia as '*a complex multifactorial syndrome associated with underlying illness and characterised by muscle loss with or without loss of fat mass, frequently accompanied by increased muscle catabolism, anorexia and inflammation*'. They suggested the following diagnostic criteria:

- Presence of a chronic disease with weight loss of at least 5% within a 12-month period.
- And three of the following:
  ○ Decreased muscle strength.
  ○ Reduced muscle mass.
  ○ Fatigue.
  ○ Anorexia.

  ○ Biochemical alterations (anaemia, markers of inflammation, low albumin).

The Cancer Cachexia Study Group (Fearon *et al.*, 2006) proposed a definition of cachexia based on the simultaneous presence of weight loss (>10%), low food intake (<1500 kcal/day) and an increased C-reactive protein (CRP) level (>10 mg/L) indicative of systemic inflammation. The Screening the Nutritional Status In Oncology (SCRINIO) Working Group (Bozzetti & Mariani, 2009) has proposed a classification system and defined four stages of severity (at risk of cachexia to symptomatic cachetic) based on weight loss of >10% or <10% with anorexia, early satiety or fatigue.

Disease process

Cancer cachexia is caused by complex interactions between inflammatory processes, neurohormonal alterations and lipolytic responses (Baracos, 2006; Tisdale, 2008). Inflammation has an important role in cachexia, with increased circulating proinflammatory cytokines, e.g. tumour necrosis factor alpha, and reduced anti-inflammatory cytokines, e.g. interleukin 4, contributing to inappropriate appetite suppression, increased resting energy expenditure and catabolism of skeletal muscle

SECTION 7

mass. Chemotherapy increases oxidative stress, thereby exacerbating the inflammatory process.

Muscle proteins are normally in constant flux with a balance between their anabolism and catabolism such that there is no change in muscle mass. However, in cancer cachexia protein synthesis is decreased, protein catabolism is increased and muscle wasting occurs (Baracos, 2001). Muscle wasting is perhaps the most devastating component of cancer cachexia because it results in functional decline, reduced ambulation and reduced quality of life (Dodson et al., 2011).

The incidence of cachexia is highly dependent on the underlying tumour type, with weight loss accompanying the majority of lung, colorectal and pancreatic cancers. It is less common in haematological malignancies, breast cancer and sarcomas (Tisdale, 2009).

Nutritional assessment

Malnutrition is frequently seen in cancer patients and may be the first indication of the presence of the disease. In addition, macro- and micro-nutrient requirements may be increased in cancer (Fearon et al., 2006). Side effects of cancer treatments can cause weight loss and lead to malnutrition; however, the mechanism is distinct from that of cachexia (Coss et al., 2011). Response to chemotherapy can reduce the catabolic stimulus of the tumour and ameliorate cachexia (Giordano & Jatoi, 2005). Not all malnourished patients are cachetic, but all cachetic patients are malnourished (Muscaritoli et al., 2010). Malnutrition is reversible when adequate nutrition is provided; however, cachexia is not treatable by this approach.

The patient generated subjective global assessment (PGSGA) is widely used as an assessment of nutritional risk in cancer patients (Bauer et al., 2002; Thoresen et al., 2002) and includes cachexia related variables. The PGSGA scores several aspects including:

- Weight loss – generated from weight history.
- Amount and type of food intake, including a list of 13 symptoms related to food intake.
- Functional status score.
- Body composition – fat and muscle mass measurement.
- Comorbid conditions.
- Age.
- Cancer stage.
- Presence of fever.
- Corticosteroid use.

The European Palliative Care Research Collaboration (EPCRC) is reviewing cachexia definition and classification, nutritional impact of symptoms and the psychosocial consequences of involuntary loss of appetite or weight in patients with advanced cancer in order to produce a new cachexia assessment instrument (Radbruch et al., 2010). A clear definition of cancer cachexia may inform clinical decision making, so improving treatment plans and assisting further research (Blum et al., 2010). It is essential to adopt a multidisciplinary approach in the management of cachexia (Santarpia et al., 2011).

Nutritional management

Nutrition support (oral nutrition supplements, enteral and parenteral feeding) can increase body weight; however, it does not have a demonstrable effect on lean body mass and therefore does not improve functional status or quality of life (Dodson et al., 2011; Kotler, 2000). However, artificial nutrition support may reduce carer anxiety and improve a patient's psychological condition (Bruera & Sweeney, 2000). Cachexia can be distressing to both the patient and carers. In the absence of starvation and given normal gastrointestinal function and integrity, parenteral nutrition should not be used in patients who are catabolic (Blum et al., 2010). However, patients with active tumours and significant starvation from bowel obstruction or short bowel syndrome benefit from total parenteral nutrition (Hoda et al., 2005). Parenteral nutrition may prevent further deterioration in nutritional status, but will not treat cachexia (Bozzetti et al., 1999) and its use should be considered carefully (see Chapter 6.5).

Nutritional supplements enriched with n-3 polyunsaturated fatty acids and antioxidants are available. Eicosapentaenoic acid (EPA), an n-3 polyunsaturated fatty acid, is found in oily fish. It appears to attenuate weight loss, particularly loss of skeletal muscle mass, by reducing inflammatory processes (Fearon et al., 2003; Cerchietti et al., 2007; Dewey et al., 2007). However, it does not affect muscle protein synthesis, although combined with protein and energy rich supplements to optimise intake it may regulate inflammatory activity (Siddiqui et al., 2006). The use of fish oil rich in EPA and docosahexaenoic acid (DHA) in pancreatic and lung cancer has been shown to reduce the rate of weight loss (Barber et al., 1999; Bauer et al., 2005; Fearon et al., 2003; Moses et al., 2004). Compliance is often limited by anorexia and an unpleasant aftertaste. Improved palatability may help to improve patient compliance and therefore effectiveness (Arends et al., 2006).

Clinical management

Cancer cachexia treatment may include appetite stimulation, energy intake supplementation, control of catabolism and stimulation of protein anabolism (MacDonald et al., 2003), which are often be used in combination. Many approaches in the treatment of patients with cancer cachexia are required.

Several types of drug have been used in patients with poor appetite, including progestins, glucocorticoids and cannabinoids, (Mantovani & Madeddu, 2009; Muscaritoli et al., 2006), which may successfully stimulate appetite and increase food intake, but any weight gain is usually short lived, consists primarily of fat or water and offers limited benefit for quality of life (Maltoni et al., 2001; Behl & Jatoi, 2007). Table 7.15.13 summarises examples of drugs used in the management of cachexia.

Research is continuing into other agents, including ghrelin (DeBoer, 2008; Kamiji & Inui, 2008). Administration of synthetic ghrelin to cachetic cancer patients

Table 7.15.13 Examples of drugs used in the management of cancer cachexia

Drug	Actions	Disadvantages	Further reading
Megestrol acetate	A synthetic progestogen, which stimulates appetite; mechanisms not fully known but may induce neuropeptide Y and suppress proinflammatory cytokines	Increases resting energy expenditure Increases risk of thromboembolic events Suppresses testosterone production in men No improvements have been shown in physical function, fatigue or lean body mass	Berenstein & Ortiz (2005) Loprinzi et al. (1999) Mantovanu et al. (2009)
Corticosteroids (glucocorticoids)	Improve appetite/ oral intake	Can exacerbate cachexia due to myopathy, insulin resistance and infections	
Cannabinoids	Stimulate appetite	Lower gastrointestinal motility, which undermines the effect on appetite stimulation No quality of life improvement	Jatoi et al. (2002) Sarhill et al. (2003) Strasser et al. (2006)
Thalidomide	Maintains lean body mass through affecting proinflammatory cytokines	No quality of life or survival benefit	Khan et al. (2003) Gordon et al. (2005)

elicited a small non-significant increase in food intake (Strasser *et al.*, 2008). Animal models have shown some success with melanocortin antagonists in disease associated cachexia, but this has not been tested in humans (DeBoer, 2010). Despite ongoing research, drug therapies have not shown significant clinical benefits.

Cachexia management must be considered as part of the overall management plan of patients with cachetic cancer. The aim of nutritional intervention at this stage should be to optimise quality of life rather than nutritional status. Palliation of symptoms is vital and a multidisciplinary approach, involving hospital and community professionals, including dietitians, other therapists and palliative care specialists, is essential. Treatment plans should consider both physiological and psychosocial factors and their impact on the patient and their carers in the widest sense (see Chapter 7.16). Cachexia is particularly distressing and will require sensitive management due to the often conflicting needs and desires of patients and carers.

Further reading

Shaw C (ed). (2010) *Nutrition and cancer*. Oxford: Wiley Blackwell.

Internet resources

European Palliative Care Research Collaborative www.epcrc.org/guidelines.php?p=cachexia
(Radbruch L, Elsner F, Trottenberg P, Strasser F, Fearon K. Clinical practice guidelines on cancer cachexia in advanced cancer patients. Aachen, Department of Palliative Medicine. European Palliative Care Research Collaborative; 2010.)

References

Arends J, Bodoky G, Bozzetti F, *et al.*; DGEM (German Society for Nutritional Medicine) (2006) ESPEN Guidelines on Enteral Nutrition: Non-surgical oncology. *Clinical Nutrition* 25: 245–259.

Baracos V. (2001) Management of muscle wasting in cancer associated cachexia: understanding gained from experimental studies. *Cancer* 92: 1669–1677.

Baracos V. (2006) Cancer-associated cachexia and underlying biological mechanisms. *Annual Reviews of Nutrition* 26: 435–461.

Barber M, Ross J, Preston T, Shenkin A, Fearon K. (1999) Fish oil-enriched nutritional supplements attenuates progression of the acute phase response in weight-losing patients with advanced pancreatic cancer. *Journal of Nutrition* 129: 1120–1125.

Bauer J, Capra S, Ferguson M. (2002) Use of the scored Patient-Generated Subjective Global Assessment (PG-SGA) as a nutrition assessment tool in patients with cancer. *European Journal of Clinical Nutrition* 56: 779–785.

Bauer J, Capra S, Battistutta D, Davidson W, Ash S, on behalf of the Cancer Cachexia Study Group. (2005) Compliance with nutrition prescription improves outcomes in patients with unresectable pancreatic cancer. *Clinical Nutrition* 24: 998–1004.

Behl D, Jatoi A. (2007) Pharmacological options for advanced cancer patients with loss of appetite and weight. *Expert Opinion in Pharmacotherapy* 8: 1085–1090.

Berenstein E, Ortiz Z. (2005) Megestrol acetate for the treatment of anorexia-cachexia syndrome. *The Cochrane Database of Systematic Reviews* 2: CD004310.

Blum D, Omlin A, Fearson K, *et al.* (2010) Evolving classification systems for cancer cachexia: ready for clinical practice? *Support in Cancer Care* 18: 273–279.

Bozzetti F, Mariani L. (2009) Defining and classifying cancer cachexia: a proposal by the SCRINIO working group. *Journal of Parenteral and Enteral Nutrition* 33(4): 361–367.

Bozzetti F, Gavazzi C, Mariani L, Crippa F. (1999) Artificial nutrition in cancer patients: which route, what composition? *World Journal of Surgery* 23: 577–583.

Bruera E, Sweeney C. (2000) Cachexia and asthenia in cancer patients. *Lancet Oncology* 1: 138–147.

Cerchietti L, Navigante A, Castro M. (2007) Effects of eicosapentaenoic and docosahexaenoic n-3 fatty acids from fish oil and preferential Cox-2 inhibitor on systemic syndromes in patients with advanced lung cancer. *Nutrition in Cancer* 59: 14–20.

Coss C, Bohl C, Dalton J. (2011) Cancer cachexia therapy: a key weapon in the fight against cancer. *Current Opinion in Clinical Nutrition and Metabolic Care* 14: 268–273.

DeBoer M. (2008) Emergence of ghrelin as a treatment for cachexia syndromes. *Nutrition* 24: 806–814.

DeBoer M. (2010) Update on melanocortin interventions for cachexia: Progress toward clinical application. *Nutrition* 26: 146–151.

Dewey A, Baughan C, Dean T, Higgins B, Johnson I. (2007) Eicosapentaenoic acid (EPA, an omega-3 fatty acid from fish oils) for the treatment of cancer cachexia. *Cochrane Database Systematic Reviews* 4: CD004597.

Dodson S, Baracos VE, Jatoi A, *et al.* (2011) Muscle wasting in cancer cachexia: clinical implications, diagnosis, and emerging treatment strategies. *Annual Review of Medicine* 62: 265–279.

Doehner W, Anker S. (2002) Cardiac cachexia in early literature: a review of research prior to Medline. *International Journal of Cardiology* 85: 7–14.

Evans WJ, Morley JE, Argilés J, *et al.* (2008) Cachexia: a new definition. *Clinical Nutrition* 27: 793–799.

Fearon KC, Von Meyenfeldt MF, Moses AG, *et al.* (2003) Effect of a protein and energy dense N-3 fatty acid enriched oral supplement on loss of weight and lean tissue in cancer cachexia: a randomised double blind trial. *Gut* 52: 1479–1486.

Fearon K, Voss A, Hustead D. (2006) Cancer Cachexia Study Group. Definition of cancer cachexia: effect of weight loss, reduced food intake, and systemic inflammation on functional status and prognosis. *American Journal of Clinical Nutrition* 83(6): 1345–1350.

Giordano K, Jatoi A. (2005) The cancer anorexia/weight loss syndrome: therapeutic challenges. *Current Oncology Reports* 7(4): 271–276.

Gordon J, Trebble T, Ellis R, Duncan HD, Johns T, Goggin PM. (2005) Thalidomide in the treatment of cancer cachexia: a randomised placebo controlled trial. *Gut* 54: 540–545.

Hoda D, Jatoi A, Burnes J, Loprinzi C, Kelly D. (2005) Should patients with advanced, incurable cancers ever be sent home with total parenteral nutrition? A single institution's 20 year experience. *Cancer* 103(4): 863–868.

Jatoi A, Windschitl HE, Loprinzi CL, *et al.* (2002) Dronabinol versus megestrol acetate versus combination therapy for cancer-associated anorexia: a North Central Cancer Treatment Group study. *Journal of Clinical Oncology* 20(2): 567–573.

Kamiji M, Inui A. (2008) The role of ghrelin and ghrelin analogues in wasting disease. *Current Opinion in Clinical Nutrition and Metabolic Care* 11: 443–451.

Katz A, Katz P. (1962) Diseases of the heart in the works of Hippocrates. *British Heart Journal* 24: 257–264.

Khan ZH, Simpson EJ, Cole AT, *et al.* (2003) Oesophageal cancer and cachexia: the effect of short-term treatment with thalidomide on weight loss and lean body mass. *Alimentary Pharmacology and Therapy* 17: 677–682.

Kotler D. (2000) Cachexia. *Annals of Internal Medicine* 133: 622–634.

Loprinzi CL, Kugler JW, Sloan JA, *et al.* (1999) Randomised comparison of megestrol acetate versus dexamethasone versus fluoxymesterone for the treatment of cancer anorexia/cachexia. *Journal of Clinical Oncology* 17: 3299–3306.

MacDonald N, Easson A, Mazurak V *et al.* (2003) Understanding and managing cancer cachexia. *Journal of the American College of Surgery* 197: 143–161.

Maltoni M, Nanni O, Scarpi E, Rossi D, Serra P, Amadori D. (2001) High-dose progestins for the treatment of anorexia-cachexia syndrome: a systematic review of randomised clinical trials. *Annals of Oncology* 12: 289–300.

Mantovani G, Madeddu C. (2009) Cancer cachexia: medical management. *Support in Cancer Care* 2009; 18: 1–9.

Moses A, Slater C, Preston T, Barber M, Fearon K. (2004) Reduced total energy expenditure and physical activity in cachetic patients with pancreatic cancer can be modulated by an energy and protein dense oral supplement enriched with n-3 fatty acids. *British Journal of Cancer* 90(5): 996–1002.

Muscaritoli M, Bossola M, Aversa Z, Bellantone R, Rossi Fanelli F. (2006) Prevention and treatment of cancer cachexia: new insights into an old problem. *European Journal of Cancer* 42: 31–41.

Muscaritoli M, Anker SD, Argilés J, *et al.* (2010) Consensus definition of sarcopenia, cachexia and pre-cachexia: joint document elaborated by Special Interest Groups (SIG) 'cachexia-anorexia in chronic wasting diseases' and 'nutrition in geriatrics'. *Clinical Nutrition* 29: 154–159.

Radbruch L, Elsner F, Trottenberg P, Strasser F, Fearon K. (2010) *Clinical Practice Guidelines on Cancer Cachexia in Advanced Cancer Patients*. Aachen, Department of Palliative Medicinen/ European Palliative Care Research Collaborative.

Santarpia L, Contaldo F, Pasanisi F. (2011) Nutritional screening and early treatment of malnutrition in cancer patients. *Journal of Cachexia, Sarcopenia and Muscle* 2: 27–35.

Sarhill N, Mahmoud F, Walsh D, *et al.* (2003) Evaluation of nutritional status in advanced metastatic cancer. *Support in Cancer Care* 11(10): 652–659.

Siddiqui R, Pandya D, Harey K, Zaloga GP. (2006) Nutrition modulation of cachexia/proteolysis. *Nutrition in Clinical Practice* 21: 155–167.

Strasser F, Luftner D, Possinger K, *et al.* (2006) Comparison of orally administered cannabis extract and delta-9-tetrahydrocannabinol in treating patients with cancer related anorexia-cachexia syndrome: a multicentre, phase III, randomised, double-blind, placebo-controlled clinical trial from the Cannabis-In-Cachexia-Study-Group. *Journal of Clinical Oncology* 24: 3394–3400.

Strasser F, Lutz TA, Maeder MT, *et al.* (2008) Safety, tolerability and pharmacokinetics of intravenous ghrelin for cancer-related anorexia/cachexia: a randomised, placebo controlled, double-blind, double crossover study. *British Journal of Cancer* 98: 300–308.

Thoresen L, Fjeldstad I, Krogstad K, Kaasa S, Falkmer UG. (2002) Nutritional status of patients with advanced cancer: the value of using the Subjective Global Assessment of nutritional status as a screening tool. *Palliative Medicine* 16: 33–42.

Tisdale M. (2008) Catabolic mediators of cancer cachexia. *Current Opinion in Supportive Palliative Care* 2(4): 256–261.

Tisdale M. (2009) Mechanisms of cancer cachexia. *Physiology Review* 89: 381–410.

von Haehling S, Anker D. (2010) Cachexia as a major underestimated and unmet medical need: facts and numbers. *Journal of Cachexia, Sarcopenia and Muscle* 1: 1–5.

7.16

Palliative care and terminal illness

Lucy Eldridge and Jane Power

Key points

■ Palliative care is the active holistic care of patients with advanced progressive illness, providing management of pain and other symptoms as well as psychological, social and spiritual support.

■ The primary nutritional objective is to maintain or improve the quality of life.

■ Decisions concerning nutrition should always be patient centred, individualised and open to change in line with the patient's condition.

■ Artificial nutritional support is a medical intervention and therefore decision making should consider benefits, burdens, harms and risks.

Palliative care is the active holistic care of patients with advanced progressive illness. There are various definitions of palliative care (Walshe, 2011). The World Health Organization (WHO, 2011) currently describes it as *an 'approach that aims to improve the quality of life of patients and their families facing the problems associated with life-threatening illness, through the prevention and relief of suffering by means of early identification and impeccable assessment and treatment of pain and other problems whether physical, psychosocial or spiritual'.*

Palliative care is based on a number of principles (WHO, 2011), which aim to:

- Provide relief from pain and other distressing symptoms.
- Affirm life and regard dying as a normal process.
- Neither hasten nor postpone death.
- Integrate the psychological and spiritual aspects of patient care.
- Offer a support system to help patients to live as actively as possible until death.
- Offer a support system to help the family cope during the patient's illness and in their bereavement.
- Use a team approach to address the needs of patients and their families, including bereavement counselling if indicated.
- Enhance quality of life, and may also positively influence the course of illness.

Palliative care is applicable early in the course of illness; in conjunction with other therapies that are intended to prolong life or symptom control, e.g. chemotherapy or radiation therapy. Patients may be in the palliative stage of their disease for months or years. It may be difficult to define what stage a patient has reached and, although clear that life expectancy is limited, identifying the length of time remaining may be impossible. Terminal care is a part of palliative care and usually refers to the last few days of life. Patients, carers and some health and social care professionals may associate palliative care specifically with care for dying people, which consequently may have significant implications for acceptability and access (NICE, 2004).

During the past four decades, the emergence of the modern hospice movement has led to the development of a model of care that is now used throughout the health service in the UK and has been adopted worldwide (Help the Hospices, 2011). Palliative and terminal care can be provided at home, in day care centres, nursing homes and hospitals, as well as within a hospice or palliative care unit. It involves a multiprofessional approach that may include healthcare and social professionals, as well as members of charitable, voluntary and independent organisations (NICE, 2004). The aim is to provide care based on individual needs and personal choice. Although palliative care is focused on the patient, providing support to the patient's relatives and carers is recognised as being an integral part of care.

Professionals involved in providing palliative care are either specialist or non-specialist. Specialist providers of palliative care have the expertise to address patient's complex needs. However, it is the responsibility of all health and social care professionals who provide day to day care to assess and meet the needs of each patient and

Manual of Dietetic Practice, Fifth Edition. Edited by Joan Gandy.
© 2014 The British Dietetic Association. Published 2014 by John Wiley & Sons, Ltd.
Companion Website: www.manualofdieteticpractice.com

their families within their limits, and know when to seek advice from or refer to a specialist palliative care service (NICE, 2004). The role of the dietitian within the palliative care setting is to help identify and address nutritional factors that impair a patient's physical and psychological wellbeing, with the primary nutritional objective of maintaining or improving the quality of life for that individual. The dietitian in this setting should:

- Assess the nutritional needs and problems of the patient.
- Establish when nutritional support measures may be appropriate.
- Advise on how the nutritional requirements of the patient may be met.
- Suggest ways in which nutrition related problems caused by the physical or psychological effects of the disease or its treatment may be alleviated.
- Provide advice and guidance for carers.
- Liaise with catering services to provide a flexible approach to food provision.
- Identify need for eating aids to assist independent eating.
- Provide training and support for professional colleagues.

Dietitians working in the field of palliative care require good communication skills in order to create an empathic relationship with patients and carers. Whilst dietitians can play a vital role in the palliative care setting, most palliative care teams or hospices do not currently have an identified specialist dietitian as a core member (Help the Hospices, 2009). However, it is the responsibility of all dietitians involved in the care of those with life limiting illnesses to facilitate the provision of appropriate nutritional care. They should have access to support and advice within the dietetic and multidisciplinary team for more complex cases.

Diagnostic criteria and classification

The target population for palliative care is wide and should not be constrained by diagnosis. Although historically associated with cancer, it is now recognised that palliative care equally applies to those with other nonmalignant life limiting conditions, e.g. motor neurone disease, dementia, heart failure, end stage diabetes and renal disease.

In order to provide high quality palliative care regardless of diagnosis, a whole system, involving all providers of palliative care in all locations, coordinated care pathway approach has been strongly recommended (Department of Health, 2008). This requires identification of people approaching the end of life, assessing their needs, initiating discussions surrounding preferences and wishes for end of life care, agreeing a care plan to reflect these and supporting carers both during a person's illness and after their death. Three care models have been recommended by the National Institute for Health and Care Excellence (NICE, 2004) and as part of the national End of Life Programme (Department of Health, 2008); Gold Standards

Framework, Liverpool Care Pathway for the Dying Patient and Preferred Priorities for Care.

Nutritional aspects

In addition to providing nutrients, nutrition has an important psychological, social, spiritual and cultural role in the palliative stages of illness. Eating can help maintain a sense of normality within a patient's life. As food intake is also associated with health and wellbeing, it may evoke feelings of fear and despair in those who are struggling to eat. This can have a major effect on an individual's self esteem and confidence, leading to social isolation and depression. Progressive illness may also affect nutritional status in a number of ways:

- The psychological effect of being diagnosed with an incurable and progressive illness is profound, especially if the diagnosis is unexpected. The consequent anxiety, depression and perhaps sense of hopelessness can markedly impair food intake.
- Worsening symptoms of the disease, particularly those of a fatigue, dysphagic or gastrointestinal nature, may make eating physically difficult and lead to associations with discomfort.
- Medication may cause side effects, e.g. nausea, vomiting or diarrhoea, that reduce food intake. Drowsiness induced by sedatives or pain relievers, such as opioids or narcotics, may make patients disinclined to eat.
- Treatments such as chemotherapy or radiotherapy and associated side effects can markedly affect food intake and increase the likelihood of nutritional deficiencies.
- Nutritional requirements may be increased by the physiological effects of the illness, e.g. pyrexia, secondary infection, increasing tumour mass, or by nutrient losses, e.g. malabsorption.
- As the final phase of the illness develops, physiological functions such as gastric emptying, digestion, absorption and peristalsis may decline. Both appetite and the ability to tolerate food will decrease.

Nutritional assessment

It is important that patients are assessed throughout their illness trajectory to ensure that nutritional support is proactive instead of reactive, thus ensuring that patients do not enter the terminal phases of their illness seriously nutritionally depleted. The assessment of palliative patients will vary according to individual needs, problems and clinical circumstances, but will primarily follow a stepwise process of:

- Defining the clinical condition, prognosis and aim of any medical intervention.
- Assessing eating habits.
- Establishing current nutritional status; it may not always be appropriate to regularly weigh a patient as this can cause anxiety.
- Identifying nutrition related problems or barriers to food and fluid intake, and evaluating their physical and psychological impact.

- Exploring the nutritional concerns of the patient and their family and/or carers.
- Discussing with patients and carers dietary goals that are appropriate and achievable.
- Integrating these goals into the care plan in a way that is compatible with medical and nursing objectives.
- Regularly reviewing progress, evaluating the effectiveness of any measures implemented and modifying them as necessary.

Screening tools and the weighing of patients will vary depending on where the patient is based and local policy and practice; there are no specific palliative care nutrition screening tools. Within a palliative care setting, it is important to assess both quantitative and qualitative issues, including what food means to the individual at any particular stage. Food issues, especially weight loss, can be more distressing to carers than patients (Poole & Froggatt, 2002). The relevance of biochemistry and weighing patients will depend on the prognosis, the medical intent at that stage of palliative care and the patient's preference.

Nutritional management

The principal objectives are to maximise food enjoyment and minimise food related discomfort. It is also important to prevent or treat avoidable and unnecessary malnutrition since this can affect both physical and psychological wellbeing. However, it is equally important that nutritional support measures are not so invasive or unacceptable to the patient that they impair quality of life. The objectives should always be one or more of the following:

- Retain the ability to derive pleasure from food and the social aspects of eating.
- Retain physical strength long enough to fulfil final wishes and ambitions.
- Have sufficient physical strength to obtain benefit from rehabilitation.
- Retain some control over the disease process through attention to nutrition.
- Die with dignity and not as a result of starvation.

Patients should be encouraged to retain an interest in food, and to regard good nutrition as a positive aid to help maintain strength and improve wellbeing. Nutritional counselling on both the use of nutrient dense foods and finding foods the patient enjoys is important, and should consider symptoms, emotional adaptation to illness and social circumstances (Hopkinson *et al.*, 2011). If nutritional needs are not being met, suggestions to improve nutrient intake by increasing frequency of food consumption and choosing foods of greater nutrient density are a useful first step. Fortification strategies to boost energy intake can be effective, but if these prove inadequate or food intake is particularly poor, oral supplements may be helpful. However, it is important to be aware that although nutritional supplements can be useful, they can divert patients from the foods they want to eat. In addition, patients do not always like supple-

ments and may feel guilty if they are unable to take them (Hill & Hart, 2001). Forcing food on those who have no desire to eat and drink can cause distress (McClement *et al.*, 2003; Strasser *et al.*, 2007).

Patients may have reduced their dietary intake for a variety of reasons; however, simple measures can often make an enormous difference to nutrient intake. Ideally, food should be offered that is of high quality and attractively presented. Menus should be tempting and varied, with snacks that can be provided at any time. The giving and receiving of nourishment is a means of showing love and affection, and consequently food refusal can cause offence and create barriers within the family unit. Involving carers in discussions about the nutritional needs and difficulties of the patient and establishing realistic expectations can help defuse problems. Table 7.16.1 gives suggestions that may be particularly helpful for people with palliative care (see Chapter 6.3).

Maintaining good hydration

Good hydration is essential, but it is important that adequate fluid provision is not achieved in such a way that it impairs appetite and compromises nutrient intake from food. If food intake is generally poor, nutrient rich sources of fluids should be encouraged.

Dysphagia

Dysphagia requires expert assessment and management in order to provide food of an appropriate consistency, while also maintaining nutrient intake (see Chapter 7.3). It is important to ensure these are nutrient dense as appropriate. At the end of life, a risk management approach allowing patients to eat and drink even with an unsafe swallow is deemed the most appropriate route, and may offer quality of life [Royal College of Physicians (RCP), 2010].

Therapeutic diets

For patients who have pre-existing conditions that require special diets, e.g. diabetes mellitus and hyperlipidaemia, consideration should be given to the appropriateness of the dietary restriction. For individuals in the advanced stages of disease, the restrictions can be relaxed or stopped; however, this needs to be done with reassurance and encouragement (Diabetes UK Nutrition Working Group, 2011). The priority is symptom management and therefore alteration of drug regimens may be required (Rowles *et al.*, 2010).

Artificial nutritional support

As a result of increasing debility, dysphagia or intestinal failure, a point may be reached when adequate nutrition can only be maintained by enteral or parenteral feeding. However, it is important to remember that for some, artificial nutrition support (ANS) may cause more harm than good and have potentially limited success; therefore,

Table 7.16.1 Dietary guidance for people with palliative care needs

Symptom	Dietary guidance
Poor appetite	Eat small, frequent, attractively presented foods Eat favourite foods or those found to be most enjoyable Consume fluids after, rather than with, meals to maximise food intake Ensure posture helps rather than hinders eating Eat in surroundings that are as pleasant as possible Eat in the company of others unless a preference is expressed to eat alone Consider appetite stimulants, e.g. alcohol, megestrol acetate or low dose steroids
Sore mouth	Replace salty, spicy or acidic foods with blander, less astringent alternatives Eat soft moist foods Cold foods are more soothing
Dry mouth (xerostomia)	Take frequent small sips of water Suck ice cubes, ice lollies or citrus flavoured boiled sweets Chew fruit flavoured sweets Meals should be moist in texture Consider artificial saliva
Taste changes	Problematic foods should be substituted with nutritionally similar alternatives: • Poultry or fish instead of red meat • Soft drinks or milk instead of tea or coffee • Boiled sweets or pastilles instead of chocolate Experiment with herbs and spices in cooking
Early satiety	Consume small, frequent amounts of nutrient dense foods
Belching and/or flatulence	Avoid foods and drinks that exacerbate gas production such as: • Carbonated beverages, beer, brassicas (broccoli, spinach, cauliflower, Brussels sprouts), peas, beans, sweetcorn, onion and radish Reduce the amount of ingested air by: • Eating slowly • Keeping the mouth shut when chewing and swallowing • Avoiding sucking drinks through a straw
Constipation	Ensure adequate medical intervention Increase fluid intake without compromising nutritional intake Clarify the patient does not have an intestinal obstruction or is dehydrated If appropriate, increase fibre rich foods, but care should be taken with patients whose appetite is decreased
Diarrhoea	Establish cause Avoid foods that appear to exacerbate symptoms If appropriate, ensure that antidiarrhoeal drugs have been prescribed Encourage a wide variety of foods
Hypercalcaemia	Do not reduce or restrict dietary sources of calcium Encourage carbonated drinks containing phosphoric acid

quality of life always needs to be considered (Raijmakers *et al.*, 2011). Cochrane reviews assessing the effects of ANS (Good *et al.*, 2010) and hydration (Good *et al.*, 2011) in palliative patients concluded that there was a lack of randomised controlled studies and therefore n recommendations for practices could be made. Clinicians need to make a decision based on the perceived benefits, harms, risks and burdens of ANS in individual patient circumstances (Table 7.16.2).

Ethical and legal considerations

The RCP (2010) and the General Medical Council (GMC, 2010) provide guidance on end of life care, which includes nutritional advice.

Oral nutrition

Oral nutrition and hydration are considered basic care, both ethically and legally, and should always be provided

unless actively resisted by the patient. It is important that patients are monitored and if a patient refuses food, this issue should be explored with the patient and documented (GMC, 2010). Food should not be forced upon a patient where this causes unavoidable choking or aspiration (Lennard-Jones, 1998).

Artificial nutritional support

All forms of ANS and hydration are deemed medical treatment and as such can be treated as any other form of medical intervention. It is vital that each patient is considered individually, the goals of care are clear and the resulting decision is a joint one involving both the care team and the patient. A patient cannot insist on artificial nutrition if the doctor feels it is not in their best interests (GMC, 2010). However, a patient's wishes are paramount and a competent patient has the absolute right to decide what nutritional support they will or will not accept, even if it may be considered to be of clinical benefit and refusal

Table 7.16.2 Potential benefits, harms, risks and burdens of artificial nutrition support in palliative care (Brotherton & Judd, 2007; Dy, 2006; Raijmakers *et al.*, 2011; Shaw, 2011)

Benefits	Assess for nutrition, fluid and medication May improve quality of life, functional status and a sense of wellbeing May prevent deterioration and reduce fatigue and chronic nausea Support religious beliefs Decrease the pressure to eat
Harms	False hope Exacerbation or cause of symptoms, e.g. gastrointestinal, fluid overload or ascities Altered body image
Risks	Complications of placement, metabolic disturbances, wound infection, abdominal pain, leakage Sepsis
Burdens	Possibly delays discharge or requires hospital admission Period of time required for training and/or to arrange home package of care Carers have greater responsibility Limitations of activities of daily living and of social life Additional monitoring

could lead to starvation or exacerbation of their symptoms. Incompetent patients retain this right through a valid advance refusal (Mental Capacity Act, 2005). In patients for whom death is believed to be inevitable and nutrition intervention is not considered to be of benefit, it can be withheld or withdrawn (GMC, 2010). However, if ANS is withheld or withdrawn, it is important that the anxieties of patients, relatives and carers are addressed. The primary goal of treatment in terminal care is the comfort of the patient; therefore, the decision concerning whether or not to feed must be made on this basis (GMC, 2010; RCP, 2010).

Artificial hydration

In the last few days of life, patients may be too weak to take oral foods and fluids. This may be due in part to declining physical function, but is often attributable to a reduced level of consciousness resulting from the use of sedatives and pain relieving drugs. The use of intravenous hydration at this stage has been a matter of debate and raises a number of ethical issues (Thorns & Garrard, 2003). The extent to which intravenous fluids offer symptomatic relief is unknown as comparative studies are not possible to conduct for ethical reasons. It has been argued that artificial rehydration is necessary to satisfy thirst and other symptoms, such as confusion and headaches (Dalal & Bruera, 2004). Others consider that simpler measures such as attention to oral hygiene are sufficient to prevent discomfort. It is also argued that intravenous hydration at this stage is unnecessarily invasive and can cause a physical barrier between the patient and their family at an important time (Thorns & Garrard, 2003).

Conclusion

The principal conclusion is that a blanket policy of artificial nutrition and hydration or no artificial nutrition and hydration is ethically indefensible. Deciding what is appropriate for each case must be based on an individual basis according to the likely benefits and burdens of such intervention. Good practice decisions concerning artificial nutrition and hydration should involve a multidisciplinary team, the patient and relatives and carers.

Further reading

Ellershaw J, Wilkinson S (eds). (2003) *Care of the Dying. A Pathway to Excellence*. Oxford: Oxford University Press.

Help the Hospices. (2007) Food and Nutrition Group Survey. Available at www.helpthehospices.org.uk.

Holmes S. (1998) The challenge of providing nutrition support to the dying. *International Journal of Palliative Medicine* 4(1): 26–31.

Meares CJ. (2000) Nutritional issues in palliative care. *Seminars in Oncology Nursing* 16(2): 135–145.

Planas M, Camilo M. (2002) Artificial nutrition: dilemmas in decision-making. *Clinical Nutrition* 21(4): 355–361.

Preedy V. (2011) *Diet and Nutrition in Palliative Care*. New York: CRC Press.

Randall F, Downie R. (1999) *Palliative Care Ethics. A Companion for all Specialities*, 2nd edn. Oxford: Oxford University Press.

Watson M, Lucas C, Hoy A, Back I, Armstrong P. (2011) Palliative adult network guidelines, 3rd edn. Available at www.book .pallcare.info.

Woodruff R. (1999) *Palliative Medicine. Symptomatic and Supportive Care for Patients with Advanced Cancer and AIDS*, 3rd edn. Oxford: Oxford University Press.

Internet resources

British Dietetic Association   www.bda.uk.com
    Palliative Care Sub Group of the Oncology Group
Cruse Bereavement Care   www.crusebereavementcare.org.uk
European Association for Palliative Care   www.eapcnet.eu
Gold Standards Framework   www.goldstandardsframework.org.uk
Help the Hospices   www.helpthehospices.org.uk
Liverpool Care Pathway for the Dying   www.liv.ac.uk/mcpcil/liverpool-care-pathway/
Macmillan Cancer Support   www.macmillan.org.uk
Marie Curie Cancer Care   www.mariecurie.org.uk
The National Council for Palliative Care   www.ncpc.org.uk
NHS National End of Life Care Programme   www .endoflifecareforadults.nhs.uk
The Scottish Partnership for Palliative Care   www .palliativecarescotland.org.uk

References

Brotherton AM, Judd PA. (2007) Quality of life in adult enteral tube feeding patients. *Journal of Human Nutrition and Dietetics* 20: 513–522.

Dalal S, Bruera E. (2004) Dehydration in cancer patients: to treat or not to treat. *Supportive Oncology* 2(6): 467–479.

Department of Health. (2008) End of life care strategy: promoting high quality care for all adults at the end of life, July 2008. Available at www.dh.gov.uk. Accessed 27 November 2011.

Diabetes UK Nutrition Working Group. (2011) Evidence-based nutrition guidelines for the prevention and management of diabetes. Available at www.diabetes.org.uk/nutrition-guidelines. Accessed 20 May 2012.

SECTION 7

Dy S. (2006) Enteral and parenteral nutrition in terminally ill cancer patients: A review of the literature. *American Journal of Hospice and Palliative Medicine* 23: 369–377.

General Medical Council. (2010) Treatment and care towards the end of life: Good practise in decision making. Available at www.gmc-uk.org/End_of_life.pdf_32486688.pdf. Accessed 20 May 2012.

Good P, Cavenagh J, Mather M, Ravencroft P (2010) Medically assisted nutrition for palliative care in adult patients (review). *The Cochrane Collaboration* 8(4): CD006274.

Good P, Cavenagh J, Mather M, Ravencroft P. (2011) Medically assisted hydration for palliative care in adult patients (review). *The Cochrane Collaboration* 2: CD006273.

Help the Hospices. (2009) Professional consensus statement of nutritional care in palliative care patients. Available at www.helpthehospices.org.uk. Accessed 6 September 2013

Help the Hospices. (2011) *The History of the Hospice Movement.* Available at www.helpthehospices.org.uk. Accessed 27 November 2011.

Hill D, Hart K. (2001) A practical approach to nutritional support for patients with advanced cancer. *International Journal of Palliative Nursing* 7(7): 317–321.

Hopkinson JB, Okamoto I, Addington-Hall JM. (2011) What to eat when off treatment and living with involuntary weight loss and cancer: a systematic search and narrative review. *Support in Care Cancer* 19(1): 1–17.

Lennard-Jones J. (1998) *Ethical and Legal Aspects of Clinical Hydration and Nutrition Support.* Maidenhead: BAPEN.

McClement SE, Degner LF, Harlos MS. (2003) Family beliefs regarding the nutritional care of a terminally ill relative: a qualitative study. *Journal of Palliative Medicine* 6(5): 737–748.

National Institute for Health and Care Excellence (NICE). (2004) *Guidance on Cancer Services: Improving Supportive and Palliative Care for Adults with Cancer.* London: NICE. Available at www.nice.org.uk. Accessed 20 May 2012.

Poole K, Froggatt K. (2002) Loss of weight and loss of appetite in advanced cancer: a problem for the patient, the carer, or the health professional? *Palliative Medicine* 16: 499–506.

Raijmakers N, Zuylen L, Costantini M, *et al.* (2011) Artificial nutrition and hydration in the last week of life in cancer patients. A systematic literature review of practices and effects. *Annals of Oncology* 22(7): 1478–1486.

Rowles S, Kilvert A, Sinclair A, *et al.* (2010) ABCD positions statement on diabetes and end of life care. *Practical Diabetes International* 28: 26–27.

Royal College of Physicians (RCP). (2010) *Oral Feeding Difficulties and Dilemmas. A Guide to Practical Care Particularly Towards the End of Life.* London: RCP.

Shaw C. (2011) Nutrition in palliative care. In: Shaw C (ed) *Nutrition and Cancer.* Oxford: Wiley Blackwell, pp. 173–187.

Strasser F, Binswanger J, Cerny T, Kesselring A. (2007) Fighting a losing battle: eating-related distress of men with advanced cancer and their female partners. A mixed-methods study. *Palliative Medicine* 21: 129–137.

Thorns A, Garrard E. (2003) Ethical issues in care of the dying. In: Ellershaw J, Wilkinson S (eds). *Care of the Dying. A Pathway to Excellence.* Oxford: Oxford University Press.

Walshe C. (2011) What do we mean by palliative care? In: Preedy V (ed) *Diet and Nutrition in Palliative Care.* New York: CRC Press, pp. 17–30.

World Health Organization. (2011) WHO definition of palliative care. Available at www.who.int/cancer/palliative/definition/en/. Accessed 26 November 2011.

7.17.1 Critical care

Ella Segaran

Key points

■ Up to 75% of patients survive an intensive care unit (ICU) admission; however many are left with severe weakness and delayed recovery.

■ The critical illness, ICU procedures, equipment and medications all influence nutritional provision and need to be accounted for in nutritional assessments.

■ Enteral feeding is the route of choice and feeding should commence within 48 hours of admission to positively influence outcome.

■ Controversy exists regarding the optimal timing for supplementing poor enteral feeding with parenteral nutrition.

■ One of the biggest dilemmas facing ICU dietitians is the accurate assessment of energy and protein requirements.

■ Approximately half of prescribed feed is delivered to patients whilst on an ICU. Strategies need to be employed, e.g. algorithms and prokinetic agents, to reduce interruptions and overcome delayed gastric emptying.

Critical care medicine is primarily concerned with the management of patients with acute life threatening disorders. Compared with other medical specialities it is a relatively new and developing area. The term critical care medicine was first introduced in the late 1950s. During the poliomyelitis epidemic in 1947–1948, manual ventilation evolved and prevented patients dying from respiratory paralysis. By the mid 1950s primitive ventilators were developed, thus allowing the establishment of intensive care units (ICU) and the birth of critical care medicine. Between the 1980s and 1990s huge advancements took place in computer technology and ventilator development. Multidisciplinary critical care teams were formed as well as national and international societies for critical care. Today, ICUs are modern high tech units with a vast array of equipment designed to support each of the body systems. The immediate objective of care is to preserve life and to prevent, minimise or reverse damage to vital organs. The ICU multidisciplinary team usually includes consultant intensivists, medical and nursing staff, pharmacists, dietitians and physiotherapists. To ensure nutritional support is appropriate, the dietitian needs to appreciate all aspects of patient care. The dietitian provides input into:

• The route and timing of nutritional support.
• The most appropriate access route.
• An assessment of the patient's nutritional requirements.
• The use of specialised enteral and parenteral products.
• Adjustments to the nutritional care plan, secondary to the disease state and changes in the patient's condition (Taylor *et al.*, 2005).

Diagnostic criteria and classification

Approximately 160000 patients a year require admission to English ICUs (NHS, 2011). The Department of Health guidelines (2000) suggest that 1–2% of acute beds in a general hospital should be designated ICU beds, and that this number should be greater where there are specialist units, e.g. cardiac or major vascular surgery, or neurosurgery. Patients are classified according to the severity of the illness and the level of support that is needed rather than their hospital location, e.g. ICU or high dependency unit (HDU) (Table 7.17.1). Typically, there are three groups of patients in the ICU:

• Postoperative, e.g. major elective and emergency surgery.
• Major trauma, e.g. head injuries, road traffic accidents, burns, penetrating injuries.
• Serious sepsis, e.g. respiratory failures, HIV infection.

SECTION 7

Table 7.17.1 Classification of patients in the acute hospital setting

Classification	Level of support required
Level 0	Patients whose needs can be met through normal ward care in an acute hospital
Level 1	Patients at risk of their condition deteriorating, or those recently relocated from higher levels of care, whose needs can be met on an acute ward with additional advice and support from the critical care team
Level 2	Patients requiring more detailed observation or intervention, including support for a single failed organ system or postoperative care and those stepping down from higher levels of care
Level 3	Patients requiring advanced respiratory support alone or basic respiratory support together with support of at least two organ systems

Metabolic response to injury, trauma and sepsis

The changes that occur following stress (injury, trauma or sepsis) are different from those to starvation, being designed to mobilise tissues for defence and repair in an attempt to survive. This mechanism takes priority even in the presence of starvation. Cuthbertson's (Cuthbertson *et al*., 2001) pioneering work introduced the terms *ebb* and *flow* to describe the metabolic response. The response is complex and involves interactions and physiological responses, including counter regulatory hormones and cytokines.

Ebb phase

This occurs immediately after the injury and lasts approximately 24–48 hours. There is a reduction in metabolic activity and oxygen consumption, and a fall in body temperature. Energy reserves, e.g. glucose from liver glycogen and free fatty acids from adipose tissue, are mobilised, but there is impairment in the ability to use them.

Flow phase

Following the ebb phase, there is a second phase called the flow or acute phase. This is characterised by hypermetabolism, catabolism and increased oxygen consumption. These mechanisms are mediated by cytokines, hormones and changes in nutrient metabolism. The length of the flow phase depends on the severity of the injury and the resolution (treatment) of the traumatic or septic insult. After uncomplicated major surgery, the patient can be expected to enter the anabolic phase within 2–3 weeks, but with major burns or unresolved sepsis the breakdown of lean tissue continues for as long as the pathological stimulus is present.

Counter regulatory hormones

The levels of these hormones, catecholamines, glucagon and cortisol, increase, resulting in increased protein mobilisation and the ensuing catabolism. They are responsible for the hyperglycaemia and insulin resistance commonly seen in critically ill patients. Glucagon stimulates gluconeogenesis, cortisol increases net protein catabolism and the catecholamines lead to glucose intolerance.

Cytokines

Circulating levels of pro- and anti-inflammatory cytokines also increase. Interleukin (IL)-1, IL-6 and tumour necrosis factor alpha (TNFα) are the major proinflammatory mediators. They act in conjunction with the various hormones on hepatic and peripheral tissue to increase lean tissue breakdown and loss.

Gluconeogenesis and protein metabolism

Following injury, glucose is an important fuel for the central nervous system, wounds and the immune system, all of which are metabolically active during stress. Glycogen stores are quickly depleted so the need for available glucose is met from muscle protein breakdown for hepatic gluconeogenesis. Amino acids derived from muscle breakdown are also required for the synthesis of the acute phase proteins, e.g. C-reactive protein (CRP).

During the flow phase, achievement of energy balance (non-protein or total energy) fails to alleviate catabolism in critically ill patients (Frankenfield *et al*., 1997). In sepsis and trauma, provision of glucose only partially reduces gluconeogenesis, even at maximum rates of glucose provision of 5 mg/kg/min. Therefore, supplying energy to the severely septic or injured patient will never preserve lean tissue and the most that can be hoped for is to attenuate the rate at which it is lost.

Anabolic phase

Eventually catabolism declines and the flow phase passes into the anabolic or recovery phase. Metabolic rate decreases, and fluid status and insulin sensitivity return to preinjury levels, which are usually coupled with an increase in appetite and ambulation. Nutritional therapy should now aim to increase protein synthesis and restore muscle mass.

Disease consequences

Although 75% of patients return home after an ICU stay (NICE, 2009), many are left with multiple health problems and delayed recovery, e.g. severe weakness and fatigue (commonly termed ICU acquired weakness), which typically occurs in a third of patients who have a prolonged stay (Hermans *et al*., 2008); a third of patients never work again (Hayes *et al*., 2000; Herridge *et al*., 2003). Patients in an ICU can lose up to 2% of their muscle mass a day (Griffiths & Jones, 1999). The related respiratory muscle weakness is associated with prolonged ventilation (De Jonghe *et al*., 2004). Patients can be so weak on discharge to a ward that they are unable to feed themselves. Impaired coughing and swallowing can place them at risk of aspiration and taste changes can further compromise nutritional status. Poor recovery post ICU is a major public health issue and the subject of guidelines (NICE, 2009). The cause of the ICU acquired muscle weakness is multifactorial (Griffiths & Hall, 2010) and the risk factors include:

- Prolonged controlled mechanical ventilation.
- Inflammation, systemic inflammatory response syndrome.
- Sepsis or septic shock.
- Illness severity.
- Bed rest, immobilisation.
- Neuromuscular blockage, paralysing agents.
- Corticosteroid medication.

Nutritional consequences

At first the ICU environment can be appear very daunting; patients are extremely ill and surrounded with multiple pieces of equipment. Dietitians working in critical care need to take time to familiarise themselves with the equipment, procedures and medications used, to ensure their nutritional assessments and therapy recommendations are safe and appropriate. Table 7.17.2 and Table 7.17.3 give details of equipment and medications commonly used in the ICU and their nutritional implications.

Nutritional assessment

Anthropometry

Many patients are admitted to the ICU as emergencies and therefore cannot give their weight or height. Also, patients are often bedbound and immobile, so obtaining an accurate weight and height is challenging. Some ICU beds have an facility to weigh patients but weights so obtained need to be interpreted with caution. Oedema and fluid retention can cause weight to increase by 10–20% in a single day (Lowell et al., 1990), thus making anthropometric measures commonly used elsewhere inaccurate. Surrogate measures for height can be used, e.g. ulna length or knee height, although it should be noted that these have not been validated for use with critically ill patients and therefore should be used as a guide only.

Biochemistry

Assessment of biochemistry is carried out frequently in the ICU, often twice a day. Many factors during critical illness, e.g. losses from the gut, excess diuresis, volume expansion and internal redistribution, and renal replacement therapy, alter biochemical values such as potassium, magnesium and phosphate. Low levels of these are not always related to nutritional status or refeeding syndrome. Twenty four hours is a long time in the ICU, thus blood results from 3 days previously may be of little help in assessing the current picture (Runcie & Dougall, 1990).

Table 7.17.2 Commonly used equipment in the intensive care unit (ICU) and their nutritional implications

Equipment	Purpose	Nutritional considerations
Mechanical ventilator	Controls the breathing pattern Different settings to suit patient's needs, e.g. mandatory ventilation (machine doing all the breathing) and spontaneous ventilation (the patient initiates the breaths)	The different ventilator settings can either reduce (mandatory ventilation) or increase (spontaneous ventilation) the work of breathing, which influences energy expenditure and energy requirements (Hoher et al., 2008)
Endotracheal tubes (ETT)	Tubes used to provide mechanical ventilation The ETT is passed through the mouth or nose into the trachea. Used for short term ventilation	The tube makes it difficult to coordinate swallowing Oral intake is usually avoided Can cause temporary dysphagia when removed
Tracheostomy	Tracheostomy is inserted (endoscopically or surgically) into the trachea via the neck Used for mid to long term ventilation	Swallowing difficulties as above In special circumstances oral trials can be facilitated, usually with the help of an experienced speech and language therapist
Airflow cooling blanket	Used to decrease body temperature Aims to achieve body temperature of 35°C Used as a treatment for traumatic brain injury, following cardiac surgery and after cardiac arrest	Significantly lowers energy expenditure and energy requirements. Use a predictive equation that takes temperature into consideration (Faisy et al., 2003; Frankenfield et al., 2004)
Continuous renal replacement therapy	Used to treat acute kidney injury in ICU patients Clears unwanted solutes and large volumes of fluid	Loss of electrolytes, e.g. phosphate and magnesium Loss of 5–10 g of protein/day dependent on modality type Loss of water soluble vitamins Loss of trace elements, e.g. selenium (Cano et al., 2009)

Table 7.17.3 Drug–nutrient interactions

Drug	Nutritional consideration
Opioid analgesia/sedation agents, e.g. fentanyl and morphine	Can cause constipation and decrease gut motility, resulting in reduced gastric emptying
Propofol	1.1 kcal/mL – contributes additional energy Only take into consideration if taken over a prolonged period Risk of fat overload
Paralysing agents, e.g. atracurium and pancuronium	Decrease energy expenditure and gut motility
Phenytoin/rifampicin/ ciprofloxin	If given via the enteral route, require a break from feed to allow drug absorption
Intravenous fluids, e.g. crystalloids and colloids	Can contribute to sodium overload
Inotropes and vasopressors, e.g. noradrenaline (norepinephrine), adrenaline (epinephrine), dobutamine and vasopressin	High doses cause a reduction of hepatic, renal and splanchnic blood flow Can lead to risk of gut ischaemia
Prokinetics, e.g. metoclopramide and erythromycin	Enhance gut motility and help overcome delayed gastric emptying
Sliding scale insulin therapy	Hypoglycaemia risk with interruptions to feeding
Stress ulcer prophylaxis, e.g. lansoprazole, esomeprazole, omeprazole and ranitidine	Alters pH and can make nasogastric tube placement confirmation by pH paper unreliable

Table 7.17.4 Factors commonly associated with either an increase or decrease in energy expenditure in hospitalised patients

Factors increasing energy expenditure	Factors reducing energy expenditure
Pyrexia Disease state Surgery Abnormal losses, e.g. wound exudate, diarrhoea and vomiting Infection Pain Extraneous movements, e.g. following head injury Spontaneous ventilation and weaning from ventilator	Sedation Anaesthesia Neuromuscular blocking agents, barbiturates, coma Mandatory ventilation Hypothermia, active cooling Starvation Reduced mobility

All values need to be interpreted with care, taking the clinical situation into consideration.

Clinical assessment

Clinical condition and treatments will influence the assessment of nutritional status, nutritional requirements, and route and tolerance of the nutritional support provided (Table 7.17.4). The reason for the patient's admission often relates to preadmission nutritional status:

- *Following major elective surgery*, e.g. surgery to the gastrointestinal tract – the patients tend to be moderately depleted of body protein preoperatively and, without nutritional support, lose approximately another 5% (approximately ~43 g/day) body protein in the first 2 weeks postoperatively (Hill, 1992).
- *Trauma or brain injury* – most of these patients are young and in good health prior to injury. Initially they are not protein depleted but do lose a large amount of body protein (approximately 110 g/day) in the first 10 days after trauma, despite provision of nutritional support (Monk *et al.*, 1996).
- *Serious sepsis* – these patients may be older and have pre-existing nutritional depletion and chronic medical

conditions. Large protein losses occur (approximately 150 g/day) despite aggressive nutritional support (Streat *et al.*, 1987).

Dietary assessment

Up to 61% of ICU patients have been shown to be moderately malnourished, with 23% severely malnourished on admission (Barr *et al.*, 2004). Patients with malnutrition develop poor muscle function and their immunological function becomes depressed, placing them at increased mortality risk and worsened hospital discharge functional status (Tremblay & Bandi, 2003). Patients with a body mass index (BMI) of <18.5 kg/m^2 have an significantly increased 60-day mortality after developing acute respiratory distress syndrome (ARDS) compared with normal and obese patients (Gong *et al.*, 2010).

Nutritional assessment informs the selection of the most appropriate route for nutritional supportand the dietitian can further advise on the best route of delivery. Most ICUs will have an enteral feeding starter regimen, where feed is started and a goal target reached. The dietitian is usually responsible for assessing if this meets the patient's requirements or if modifications are necessary.

Nutritional management

Route of nutrient delivery

International guidelines consider enteral feeding to be the best way to feed critically ill patients (Kreymann *et al.*, 2006; McClave *et al.*, 2009). However, the evidence is conflicting regarding the optimum route (enteral or parenteral) of delivery. Three meta analyses of trials comparing enteral nutrition (EN) with parenteral nutrition (PN) in critically ill patients have been published (Gramlich *et al.*, 2004; Heyland *et al.*, 2003; Simpson & Doig, 2005). Heyland *et al.* (2003) reported no difference in mortality between EN and PN, but EN was associated with a significant reduction in infections. Gramlich *et al.*

(2004) also found no difference in mortality and a significant reduction in infections with EN. Simpson & Doig (2005) found a significant reduction in mortality with PN, but this appears to exist when the provision of EN was delayed, i.e. started after 48 hours. They also found a significant increase in infections in the PN group. Simpson & Doig concluded that EN remains the feeding route of choice until more evidence is available. Critically ill patients relying solely on EN do not often achieve energy intake targets (Reid, 2006), leading to significant underfeeding. Underfeeding is associated with increased infections (Rubinson et al., 2004) and other complications such as prolonged ventilation, prolonged length of stay and pressure ulcers (Dvir et al., 2006; Villet et al., 2005).

In European ICUs the consensus is for the combined use of EN with PN to optimise nutritional support early in a patient's admission (Kreymann et al., 2006). However, there are important differences between the American and European societies' recommendations for the use of PN in critically ill patients. The joint American Society for Parenteral and Enteral Nutrition (ASPEN) and Society of Critical Care Medicine (SCCM) (McClave et al., 2009) guidelines recommend PN is given to non-malnourished ICU patients during the first 7 days, to reduce the risk of infectious morbidity and mortality. In contrast, the European Society for Parenteral and Enteral Nutrition (ESPEN) guidelines (Kreymann et al., 2006) focus on preventing an early energy deficit by preferentially using EN and supplementing with PN if needs are not met by the fourth day.

The two different approaches have been compared in the recent EPaNIC trial (Casaer et al., 2011), which aimed to study the impact of early initiation of PN (European guidelines) with late initiation (American guidelines) to supplement inadequate EN. The findings suggest that early supplementation of PN is associated with worse outcomes than those where PN initiation is delayed for 7 days. The late initiation group had a significantly shorter ICU stay and fewer infectious complications, and shorter duration of mechanical ventilation and renal replacement therapy; no differences in mortality were observed. The results need to be interpreted with caution as there were study design limitations. The eight centres were all from one European country and the majority of patients were admitted following cardiac surgery, which make the generalisability of the results questionable. Also, the energy targets appear higher than used elsewhere and these were not individualised. Tight glycaemic control was employed in both groups, which is no longer standard practice. Finally, it was unclear how many patients were still on the ICU at day 8 to receive late PN, or how many actually needed either early or late PN.

Timing of initiation of nutritional support

Early nutritional support is commonly defined as commencing 24–48 hours after admission and assumes that the patient has been adequately resuscitated and is haemodynamically stable. It is associated with signifi-

cantly shorter hospital stays and a trend towards reduced mortality (Martin et al., 2004). It is now standard care to implement EN within 24–48 hours following ICU admission (Singer et al., 2009).

Estimated energy requirements

One of the biggest dilemmas facing ICU dietitians is the accurate assessment of metabolic rate for critically ill patients. The most accurate method for this is indirect calorimetry, although very few dietitians have access to this equipment in the clinical setting. Therefore, standardised equations are used to estimate the metabolic rate. Many equations are available, but data are sparse on how they compare against measured energy expenditure (MEE) in a range of critically ill patients, e.g. sepsis, trauma and obesity. The energy expenditure (EE) of critically ill patients is variable, influenced by the impact of the illness and its treatment. Several factors other than the severity of illness modify EE (Table 7.17.4) (see Chapter 6.1).

There are published predictive equations for use in critically ill patients, including Swinamer (Swinamer, et al., 1990), Ireton-Jones (Ireton-Jones et al., 1992), Penn State (Frankenfield et al., 2004), Brandi (Brandi et al., 1999) and Faisy (Faisy et al., 2003). With the exception of the Ireton-Jones equation, the others incorporate physiological factors such as temperature and ventilation settings, making them more applicable to this group of patients. Frankenfield et al. (2009) carried out the largest and most complete validation study of metabolic rate equations for critical care use. Nine different equations were compared with MEE via indirect calorimetry in 202 critically ill patients. The Penn State equation was the most consistent, being able to predict EE within a 10% range on 67% of occasions. When using a predictive equation it is preferable to use one that is designed for critical care use, taking clinical parameters into consideration (Table 7.17.5).

Estimated protein requirements

Optimal protein requirements are a challenge to determine during critical illness. The nitrogen balance obtained from 24-hour urine collections does not reflect whole body protein balance. Protein is synthesised and lost via the liver, gut and immune system, and estimations of these losses are needed. As discussed above, in healthy individuals muscle mass is controlled by a balance between muscle protein synthesis (MPS) and muscle protein catabolism (MPB), so that it remains constant. However, in critical illness this balance is altered (Rennie, 1985); there is a decrease in MPS and increase in MPB (Puthucheary et al., 2010). The ability of protein or amino acids to stimulate MPS is positively correlated with physical exercise, which is not possible in bed bound critically ill patients (Barazzoni et al., 2004; Biolo & De Cicco, 2004; Biolo et al., 1997). Patients are unlikely to achieve a positive nitrogen balance whilst critically ill (Wolfe & Miller, 1999). Protein dynamics are

SECTION 7

Table 7.17.5 Predictive equations for use in critical care

Equation	Reference:	Advantages	Disadvantages
20–25 kcal/kg (84–105 kJ/kg) 25–30 kcal/kg (105–126 kJ/kg)	ACCP (Cerra et al., 1997), ESPEN (Singer et al., 2009)	Quick and easy Designed to avoid harmful overfeeding	Consensus decision Not age, gender, condition specific Ambiguity over which weight to use Individual interpretation as to when patient is in the recovery phase Very low accuracy compared with MEE (Reid, 2007)
Schofield and stress factors (SFs)	Schofield (1985)	Gender, age, disease and activity specific	Based on data from healthy individuals Use of SFs introduces substantial error SFs based on outdated references – ICU practices have improved considerably since, thus impacting on energy expenditure Does not reflect clinical parameters Associated with under- and over-feeding when compared with MEE (Reid, 2007)
Penn State University	Frankenfield (2011), Frankenfield et al. (2009)	Gender, age, height specific Includes clinical parameters specific to ICU, i.e. temperature and ventilation settings 67% accuracy within 10% of MEE in 202 patients (Frankenfield et al., 2009) Useful for obese patients	Day to day variability due to clinical parameters Time required Needs familiarity with ventilation settings Does not capture activity – need to add a factor for physical activity
Ireton-Jones	Ireton-Jones et al. (1992)	Best known ICU specific equation Gender and age specific Includes factors for trauma and burns	Developed on burns and trauma patients Overestimates in non-obese and underestimates in obese patients 46% accuracy compared with MEE (Frankenfield, et al., 2009)
Faisy	Faisy et al. (2003)	Age, height specific Includes clinical parameters specific to ICU, i.e. temperature and ventilation settings	Developed on medical critical care patients only Mean age 61 years Not gender specific 53% accuracy compared with MEE (Frankenfield, et al., 2009)

MEE, measured energy expenditure; ICU, intensive care unit; ACCP, American College of Chest Physicians; ESPEN, European Society for Parenteral and Enteral Nutrition.

influenced by both severity of injury and underlying nutritional status.

Several studies have investigated the influence of differing levels of protein intakes on protein metabolism (Larsson et al., 1990; Shaw et al., 1987; Ishibashi et al., 1998). Larsson et al. (1990) found that nitrogen balance was improved in patients who received 1.3 g/kg of protein for the first week following injury. Ishibashi et al. conducted a similar study in general ICU patients (including trauma, head injury and sepsis patients) using enteral feeds and found that protein losses were minimised at intakes of 1.2 g/kg, with intakes in excess of 1.5 g/kg conferring no further benefit.

In septic patients, Streat et al. (1987) demonstrated a 12.5% loss of total body protein (TBP) during the first 10 days of the illness, despite apparently adequate nutritional support. Trauma patients appear to show even greater protein losses, with TBP losses of 16% seen over a 21-day study period (Monk et al., 1996). In these studies, approximately 70% of protein losses came from skeletal muscle, which has serious implications for patient recovery and rehabilitation.

The recommendations for protein requirements are summarised in Table 7.17.6.

Obese patients

Obesity impacts on acute illnesses, with increased numbers of obese patients requiring intensive care. Internationally approximately 20% of mechanically ventilated ICU patients are obese (BMI 30–40 kg/m²) and 4–7% morbidly obese (BMI >40 kg/m²) (Akinnusi et al., 2008; Anzueto et al., 2011; Oliveros & Villamor, 2008). As BMI increases, patients are more likely to experience complications than non-obese patients, e.g. increased ventilator days, higher incidence of ARDS, increased infections, acute kidney injury and longer ICU and hospital stays (Akinnusi et al., 2008; Dossett et al., 2008; Hogue et al., 2009; Morris et al., 2007; Oliveros & Villamor, 2008). On discharge obese patients are more likely to require rehabilitation facilities or enter a nursing home (Morris et al., 2007). However, obesity is not associated with increased ICU mortality (Akinnusi et al., 2008; Anzueto et al., 2011; Frat et al., 2008; Gong et al., 2010; Hogue et al., 2009;

Table 7.17.6 Protein requirements in critical care patients

Patient group	Protein recommendation (g/kg/day)	Reference	Comments
Trauma and burns	1.3	Larsson et al. (1990)	Used parenteral nutrition
General intensive care unit (ICU)	1.2	Ishibashi et al. (1998)	Used enteral nutrition
Severe sepsis	1.5	Shaw et al. (1987)	Used parenteral nutrition
ICU on continuous renal replacement therapy (CRRT)	1.5 up to 2.5	Cano et al. (2009), Bellomo et al. (2002), Scheinkestel et al. (2003)	Increased requirements to compensate for losses via the filtering process

Morris et al., 2007; Oliveros & Villamor, 2008; Sakr et al., 2008).

The increasing numbers of obese patients in ICUs has not led to an increase in studies regarding their nutritional needs; therefore, the best way to nourish these patients is under debate. However, it is agreed that the preservation of muscle mass is vitally importance. Due to the multiple comorbidities associated with obesity, the avoidance of overfeeding has been proposed (McClave et al., 2009).

Estimated energy requirements

Controversy remains surrounding the most appropriate weight to use in predictive equations for obese patients. Determining body composition in obese patients is difficult, as actual weight does not reflect the amount of metabolically inactive body fat. Resting metabolic rate is mainly dependent upon fat free mass (Miller & Blyth, 1953; Webb, 1981). However, while weight is gained from both fat and lean body mass (Horgan & Stubbs, 2003), in severe obesity there is a greater proportion of fat tissue deposited (Forbes, 1982; 1987). These differences in body composition make it challenging to determine which weight to use in predictive equations. As a result of the larger fat free mass, using ideal body mass (IBW) in obese patients is likely to underestimate energy needs, and the use of actual body weight (ABW) will overestimate this as a consequence of the metabolically inactive fat mass. Adjusted body weight (AdjBW) has been proposed (Amato et al., 1995) on the assumption that the obese have a lean body mass that equates to 25% more than that of the non-obese. This approach has not been validated and is not recommended as the original predictive equations were developed using ABW and the use of an AdjBW for predicting EE in obese patients will result in an underestimation (Frankenfield et al., 2003).

Anderegg et al. (2009) compared 13 different prediction methods against MEE in obese hospitalised adults and found that the Harris–Benedict equation (HBE) (Harris & Benedict, 1919) with AdjBW plus a stress factors and 21 kcal/kg of ABW most frequently predicted the EE within ±10% of the MEE, albeit only in 50% of participants. This was a single centred small trial of only 36 patients and not all patients were mechanically ventilated. Measured energy expenditure was assessed once per individual and it is unclear on what day from admission the

readings were undertaken. The authors concluded that the agreement between all predictive equations and MEE was poor and no equation could be recommended over the others.

In a study by Frankenfield et al. (2009) half of the 100 participants were obese (BMI 30–112 kg/m^2); the Penn State equation had an accuracy rate of 70% in the young obese but only 53% in the elderly obese. The MEE readings were only undertaken once per patient and the mean day of measurement was day 6 of the ICU stay (range day 2–27). In a follow-up study, a revised Penn State equation devised for use in those aged over 60 years with a BMI of >30 kg/m^2 achieved an accuracy rate of 74% when compared with MEE (Frankenfield, 2011).

The ASPEN/SCCM guidelines (McClave et al., 2009), recommend that energy requirements for those with a BMI of >30 kg/m^2 are calculated as 11–14 kcal/kg of ABW or 22–25 kcal/kg of IBW. This recommendation is based on pooled findings of six studies undertaken in obese patients (Dickerson, 2004). Patients experienced shorter ICU lengths of stays, and fewer antibiotic days when fed 11–14 kcal/kg of ABW compared with those who received 19–25 kcal/kg of ABW. This recommendation needs to be interpreted with caution as the studies used very different protocols; only one was conducted in ICU patients. All of the studies were inadequately powered to evaluate major end points such as morbidity and mortality; nitrogen balance was the primary outcome assessed. Only two studies were randomised and used PN, and one that collected data retrospectively investigated the use of EN. None of the studies looked at body composition, protein turnover or muscle function. Due to these severe limitations, it can be concluded that there is inadequate evidence to make any recommendation.

To conclude, predictive equations in obese critically ill patients are inaccurate and can result in significant under- and over-feeding. Indirect calorimetry (IC) remains the best way of ascertaining EE, but without this the Penn State predictive equations, which include a specific equation for obese elderly patients, may be the best option.

Estimated protein requirements

No trials have evaluated a range of protein intakes, so the optimal protein requirements for obese patients remain unknown. The ASPEN/SCCM guidance (McClave et al., 2009) of 2 g/kg of IBW for those with a BMI of

SECTION 7

30–40 kg/m² and 2.5 g/kg of IBW for those with a BMI of >40 kg/m² is based on the six trials of nutritional support in hospitalised patients (Dickerson, 2004). The severe limitations of these studies have been discussed above. In addition, it should be noted that five of the trials used PN and only the retrospective EN study was in critically ill patients. Only the PN trials achieved a positive nitrogen balance, but these patients were not critically ill. The Parenteral and Enteral Nutrition Group of the British Dietetic Association (Todorovic & Micklewright, 2007) recommends that for patents with a BMI of >30 kg/m², approximately 75% of the value should be estimated from weight and for those with a BMI of 50 kg/m² this should be approximately 65%. It is unclear how this recommendation was derived as no studies are referenced. Further studies investigating the optimum protein intake for obese patients need to be undertaken. Until such time, expert guidelines should be consulted and clinical judgement used.

Overfeeding

Overfeeding macronutrients to critically ill patients can negatively affect organ function, particularly that of the lungs, liver and kidneys. Any excessive intake, but particularly excessive carbohydrate, can result in hypercapnia (carbon dioxide retention), which increases the work of the lungs and potentially prolongs the need for mechanical ventilation (Liposky & Nelson, 1994). Additionally, overfeeding carbohydrate can lead to hyperglycaemia, hypertriglyceridaemia and an accumulation of fat in the liver. Overfeeding protein can lead to azotaemia, uraemia, hypertonic dehydration and metabolic acidosis if the kidneys are unable to sufficiently adjust urea excretion or acid–base balance. Excessive fat infusions can result in hypertriglyceridaemia and fat overload (Klein et al., 1998).

Non-feed energy sources need to be considered when they make a significant energy contribution. The anaesthetic propofol is administered in a lipid base (Intralipid) and contributes 1.1 kcal/mL of additional energy. In addition, this high fat infusion can cause hypertriglyceridaemia and fat overload syndrome when used in excessive doses. Intravenous 5% dextrose is also frequently used in the ICU and contributes 200 kcal/L.

In underweight patients, rapid attempts to restore body mass and nutritional status may have adverse metabolic consequences (Klein et al., 1998). The underweight, overweight and elderly are particularly vulnerable to overfeeding, because of the difficulties in assessing their true requirements.

Feeding protocols

The use of ICU feeding protocols to promote early and safe enteral feeding is encouraged. Units that follow simple algorithms are able to feed patients earlier and achieve calorie goals sooner (Doig et al., 2008; Heyland et al., 2004). Their use has been shown to increase the number of patients receiving EN, and reduce the number

receiving PN or not being fed at all (Heyland et al., 2004). Feeding protocols positively influenced outcomes, including a reduction in hospital stay and in hospital mortality rate (Martin et al., 2004). The combination of a feeding protocol and dietetic input on ward rounds was an effective method of increasing enteral feed delivery in intensive care (Adam & Batson, 1997). The key to successful protocol/algorithm implementation is simplicity, as cumbersome protocols are more likely to be ignored or incorrectly applied (Doig et al., 2008). Although feeding protocols may vary between institutions, they have the following features in common:

- Aim to promote early, safe EN.
- Advocate use of prokinetics to improve tolerance.
- Recommend alternative routes of feeding if any intolerance persists, e.g. post pyloric feeding or PN.

Interruptions to feed

The unpredictable nature of critical illness and the medical management of these patients frequently lead to disruption in the delivery of nutritional support, especially EN. In practice, it is rare for all the prescribed daily feed to be delivered. On average, between 43% and 58% of prescribed feed is delivered (Heyland et al., 2004; Reid, 2006). A large multicentre study found that ICU patients were uniformly underfed, with an average of 59% of energy and 56% of protein prescriptions being received (Alberda et al., 2009). Two thirds of feed cessations are attributable to avoidable causes (McClave et al., 1999). Reasons for the discontinuation of feeds on the ICU are listed in Table 7.17.7.

Gastric residual volumes

Feeding intolerance is frequently responsible for poor enteral feed delivery. Large gastric residual volumes (GRVs) are used as a marker of gastric emptying and assumed to reflect enteral feed intolerance. Other symptoms of delayed gastric emptying are nausea, vomiting, abdominal distension and discomfort. The incidence of patients experiencing large GRVs varies between 22% and 56% (Adam & Batson, 1997; Heyland et al., 1995; Reintam et al., 2009). There is no agreement in the literature for the definition of a large GRV or their management, such as whether feed should be withheld after a single high GRV or how long feeds should be withheld for before checking GRVs. The reported values for the designated cut-off for withholding feed vary from 150 mL up to 500 mL. The main concern with GRVs of >200 mL is the associated risk of pulmonary aspiration of gastric contents, resulting in the development of pneumonia. However, it has been suggested that GRVs may have very little clinical meaning and do not consistently correlate with aspiration risk (McClave et al., 2005). However, the perceived risk often causes unnecessary delays and frequent interruptions of EN.

McClave et al. (2005) reported that increasing the designated GRV cut-off for cessation of enteral feeding from 200 mL to 400 mL did not increase the risk of aspiration.

Table 7.17.7 Reasons for discontinuation of enteral feed on the intensive care unit

Category	Example	Frequency of occurrence (%)	Considered potentially avoidable (%)
High gastric residual volumes (GRVs)	Volumes >200 mL – even though commonly isolated events	45	70
Tube displacement	Patient or staff removal	41	66
Procedures	Bronchoscopy, tracheostomy, transoesophageal echo, endoscopy, surgical intervention	39	80
Diagnostic tests	Chest X ray, CT or MRI scan, ultrasound	27	52
Nursing care	Patient baths, changing bedding, tracheostomy care	30	99
Other	Haemodynamic instability, nausea, vomiting and ileus	32	52

CT, computed tomography; MRI, magnetic resonance imaging.

Conversely, dropping the designated GRV cut-off from 400 mL to 200 mL failed to reduce the risk and protect patients from aspiration. Recommendations were that feeds should not be stopped for GRVs below 400–500 mL in the absence of other signs of intolerance. The recent REGANE study (Montejo *et al.*, 2010) compared GRV cut-offs of 200 mL and 500 mL. High GRVs were experienced in 42% of control (200-mL GRV) and 26% of intervention (500-mL GRV) patients. The mean enteral feed delivery was significantly higher in the intervention group, although the incidence of pneumonia, duration of mechanical ventilation and ICU length of stay were similar in both groups. It appears that increasing the volume of the GRV cut-off to 500 mL is not associated with worse complications or outcomes and can be recommended as a normal limit for GRV.

As 80% of high GRVs are isolated events (McClave *et al.*, 1999), clinicians should be encouraged to look for a trend of gradually increasing GRVs, with abrupt cessation of feeds being reserved for those patients with overt regurgitation and aspiration. Causes of large GRVs are:

* Mechanical ventilation.
* Sedation.
* Use of paralysing agents.
* Use of vasopressors.
* Sepsis.
* Traumatic brain injury.

Prokinetic agent treatment

Delayed gastric emptying may be overcome by the regular administration of prokinetic agents, which increase gastrointestinal motility. It is hypothesised that their use leads to improved tolerance to feeds and nutritional indices, and reduced infectious morbidity. However, studies of their use have often been small and have methodological weaknesses, such as varying doses of drugs and a range of GRV cut-off values (Booth *et al.*, 2002) Metoclopramide and erythromycin are used most frequently. Their intravenous use has been found to promote gastric emptying, but erythromycin appears to be the more effective (MacLaren *et al.*, 2008; Nguyen *et al.*,

2007b). However, the effect on gut motility is short lived, with the effect wearing off after 24–72 hours (Chapman *et al.*, 2000; Nguyen *et al.*, 2007b). When the two drugs are combined, the effect is superior to erythromycin alone (Nguyen *et al.*, 2007a).

It should be noted that there are safety concerns regarding the use of erythromycin, an antibiotic, as its routine use may result in antibiotic resistance. However, for a prokinetic effect erythromycin is administered at a subantibiotic dose and there is no evidence that short term use results in adverse effects.

Reducing the risk of aspiration

Preventative measures include (McClave *et al.*, 2009; Metheny *et al.*, 2004):

* Elevate the head of the bed to ≥45° and if this is not possible, position the patient in reverse Trendelenburg.
* Consider the use of prokinetic agents, e.g. metoclopramide and erythromycin.
* Change formula delivery method from bolus or intermittent to continuous.
* Consider the placement of a post pyloric tube; regularly assess feeding tube placement to ensure that it has remained in the correct position.
* Consider the use of chlorhexidine mouthwash.
* Reduce the level of sedation when possible.
* Minimise the transport out of the ICU for diagnostic tests and procedures.

Post pyloric enteral nutrition

Post pyloric enteral feeding is often considered an effective way of overcoming large GRVs and therefore reducing the risk of aspiration; however, studies to support this assumption are limited. Nasoduodenal or nasojejunal tubes are difficult to place and to keep in the correct position; endoscopic placement can be time consuming and labour intensive. Self propelling tubes are available, but in one study only 26–38% of tubes placed in to the stomach moved spontaneously into the duodenum and the majority retroperistalsed back into the stomach (Rees *et al.*, 1988). The use of a fluoroscopic technique to place tubes has been shown to be successful in critically ill patients (Welpe *et al.*, 2010). Others have also achieved successful tube placement with an electromagnetic tracking system (Taylor *et al.*, 2010).

There is conflicting advice regarding the use of jejunal feeding. The ASPEN/SCCM guidelines (McClave *et al.*, 2009) support their use, whilst the European guidelines (Kreymann *et al.*, 2006) concluded that the results of 11 randomised controlled trials do not justify general recommendations. The studies described in both guidelines comparing gastric with jejunal feeding are small and report on differing outcomes. The adequacy of nutritional support provided was only discussed in six of the trials; these demonstrated superior nutrient delivery with jejunal feeding. There was no difference observed between jejunal and gastric routes with regards to the time to achieve nutritional goals. The ICU length of stay was significantly reduced in two of the six studies, but there was no difference in mortality or pneumonia incidence between the two groups. Despite this, both guidelines recommend the use of post pyloric feeding in those who are intolerant to gastric feeding, providing access can be easily gained.

Glycaemic control

An acute state of insulin resistance and hyperglycaemia is characteristically seen following the metabolic effects of sepsis and injury, although the exact mechanisms precipitating this response remain unclear (Carlson, 2001). It is considered to occur secondary to raised endogenous production or exogenous provision of insulin antagonists, e.g. noradrenaline (norepinephrine), adrenaline (epinephrine), cortisol and glucagon (Bessey *et al.*, 1984). Proinflammatory cytokines are also thought to play a key role in the development of insulin resistance (Carlson, 2004). Insulin resistance can be correlated directly with the severity of illness and determines the speed of recovery (Carlson, 2001). Hyperglycaemia is not exclusive to patients with pre-existing diabetes, but appears to be related to the extent of critical illness. In most cases, it will resolve as the clinical condition improves. Excessive carbohydrate intake (particularly from PN) will result in hyperglycaemia, but this is rarely the primary cause.

Following the study by van den Berghe *et al.* (2001), close attention has been paid to glycaemic control in the critically ill. A significant reduction in the morbidity and mortality of surgical ICU patients was achieved with the aggressive use of insulin to maintain normoglycaemia. Favourable outcomes were attributed to the tight control of blood glucose levels between 4.4 and 6.1 mmol/L compared with a control group where the target blood glucose was 10.0–11.1 mmol/L. It was concluded that this tight glycaemic control and early aggressive feeding resulted in a reduction in mortality by 33% in surgical ICU patients.

Since the publication of this trial, six independent prospective randomised controlled trials involving nearly 10 000 patients have been unable to reproduce the same mortality benefits, leading to international controversy surrounding the benefits of tight glycaemic control. The Normoglycaemia in Intensive Care Evaluation-Survival Using Glucose Algorithm Regulation trial (NICE SUGAR) (Finfer *et al.*, 2009), compared intensive glucose control (4.5–6 mmol/L) with a conventional glucose control target of 10 mmol/L; the end point was death from any cause within 90 days of randomisation. Mortality was 27.5% in the intensive glucose group and 24.9% in the conventional group, which was a statistically significant difference. The study concluded that intensively treated patients experienced more periods of hypoglycaemia and these contributed to the increased mortality.

The original Van den Berge *et al.* study has limitations; it was conducted in a single centre, in cardiac surgery patients and was not blinded. Participants were given large doses of intravenous glucose on day 1 and nutrition was commenced within 24 hours of admission to the ICU, predominantly as PN. All of these factors result in a lack of applicability to other critical care populations. The NICE SUGAR trial on the other hand was a multicentre trial involving 42 hospitals, had a robust study design and was conducted in a mixed ICU population. In light of the conflicting findings, there is still a lack of international recommendations of the optimal glucose range for critically ill patients. Until further guidance is provided, many have opted for a moderate range of blood glucose management of 6–10 mmol/L (Bellomo & Egi, 2005).

Immune modulating nutritional support

Enteral formulations

Immune modulating enteral feeds are characterised by increased quantities of specific nutrients that may have the potential to improve immune function and modulate the inflammatory response. Such nutrients include arginine, n-3 polyunsaturated fatty acids, glutamine, ribonucleic acid (RNA) and antioxidants, including vitamin C and selenium. Although the use of immune modulating enteral feeds is recommended in international guidelines (ASPEN, Canadian), their routine use in UK clinical practice is still controversial. Factors influencing uptake include the lack of a definitive optimum time for starting these products, and evidence for the most advantageous combination of nutrients and which patients are likely to gain benefit.

Meta analyses (Heyland *et al.*, 2001; Montejo *et al.*, 2003; Waitzberg *et al.*, 2006) and systematic reviews (Marik & Zaloga, 2008; 2010) suggest that immune modulating enteral feeds are of benefit in reducing duration of mechanical ventilation, infections, wound complications and length of stay compared with standard enteral feeds. There is no overall impact on mortality. It appears that the benefits are seen in those undergoing major surgery rather than trauma and septic ICU patients.

Specific nutrients

Fish oils

Three studies have investigated enteral feed enhanced with eicosapentaenoic acid (EPA), δ-linolenic acid (GLA) and antioxidants in septic ICU patients with ARDS (Gadek *et al.*, 1999; Pontes-Arruda *et al.*, 2006; Singer *et al.*, 2006) The findings were combined in a meta analysis that showed a reduction in mechanical ventilation and intensive care days, as well as a decreased risk of developing new organ failures and mortality in those who received the EPA/GLA enteral feed (Pontes-Arruda *et al.*, 2008). The original studies have a number of limitations; no power calculations were undertaken to determine appropriate study size, there was a lack of blinding and the studies were conducted over a short time period (4–7 days). In addition, the sickest patients were excluded, bronchoscopy was used to diagnose ARDS, differing levels of EPA and GLA were used, and a high fat, low carbohydrate control feed was used, which is not representative of a standard ICU enteral feed. The source of fat was rich in n-6 fatty acids, i.e. linoleic acid, which could potentially produce an upregulation of the inflammatory response. All of these limitations inhibit the applicability of the studies.

In 2011, Pontes-Arruda *et al.* used a high carbohydrate, high protein feed as the control, aiming to better represent a standard ICU enteral feed and overcome the criticisms of the earlier studies. However, the study's aim was different from the original studies as it investigated if EPA/GLA supplemented enteral feed could prevent early sepsis progressing to severe sepsis. The results suggested that the intervention group (EPA/GLA) developed significantly less sepsis, and cardiac and respiratory failures, and experienced 6.5 fewer ICU days and 8.9 fewer hospital days. The results seem remarkable, but there are also limitations to this study. It was single centred and despite being conducted in ICU patients, the majority of these were not intubated and had no organ failure. They received in excess of 95% of prescribed volume of feed and had a mean age of 70 years, which are not representative of most ICU patients. Another trial, the EDEN-Omega study, investigated whether administering n-3 fatty acids and antioxidants as a bolus was more beneficial than within an enteral feed in patients with acute lung injury/ARDS (Clinicaltrials.gov 2011). However, this study was stopped early for futility in the treatment effect.

Arginine

Arginine is one of the most controversial immunomodulatory nutrients. Studies show improvements in clinical outcomes and reduced mortality with arginine supplementation of enteral feeds (Atkinson *et al.*, 1998; Caparros *et al.*, 2001; Galban *et al.*, 2000), although some investigators have suggested that it can be detrimental. An increase in the inflammatory response and greater mortality have been observed in severely septic patients (Bertolini *et al.*, 2003; Heyland & Samis, 2003). The proposed mechanism is that in severe sepsis, arginine may be converted to nitric oxide, which contributes to haemodynamic instability. For this reason, recent international guidelines suggest caution or avoidance of arginine in severe sepsis (Critical Care Nutrition, 2009; McClave *et al.*, 2009).

Glutamine and selenium

Parenteral route

The systematic review conducted as part of the Canadian guidelines suggests that parenteral administration of glutamine to critically ill patients reduces mortality and new infections, whilst selenium supplementation can reduce mortality but has little effect on infections (Critical Care Nutrition, 2009). However, the trials included in the systematic review were small and many were of poor quality.

The results of the recent SIGNET trial (Andrews *et al.*, 2011), a large multicentre randomised double blind trial, examined the influence of glutamine, selenium or both added to PN on new infections and mortality in critically ill patients. The trial intervention was for a maximum of 7 days. The findings suggested that addition of glutamine (0.2–0.3 g/kg) and/or selenium (500 µg) to PN did not decrease new infections or mortality. In the subgroup analysis of those who received the intervention for 5 or more days (46% of the original population), selenium supplementation significantly reduced new infections. There was no effect of glutamine on new infections. The median duration of PN in the trial was 5 days and it is possible that timing of administration (especially for glutamine) was not optimal and it needed to be continued for longer. The PN was commenced at the ICU team's discretion and it could be argued that the treatment might have offered more benefit if it had been commenced earlier. The dose was also low and probably subtherapeutic compared with the recommendation of 0.5 g/kg/day in the ESPEN/SCCM guidelines (McClave *et al.*, 2009).

Enteral route

Enteral nutrition supplemented with glutamine is recommended by the ESPEN and ASPEN/SCCM guidelines in trauma and burns patients only. Its use in general ICU patients or surgical patients is not recommended as no benefits have been found over standard EN (Schulman *et al.*, 2005). Enteral glutamine may be associated with a decrease in mortality in burns patients, and reduced infections and length of stay in both burns and trauma patients. However, these findings are based on a meta analysis of six studies that were all carried out in single centres, and the likelihood of the results being replicated in other settings is low. It is not possible to confirm the optimal dose of enteral glutamine (Critical Care Nutrition, 2009).

Vitamin and mineral requirements

In critically ill adults who do not otherwise have extraordinary needs for particular micronutrients, the majority of standard enteral and parenteral formulae contain suitable quantities of vitamins and minerals. The micronutrient needs of most patients can be met if target energy intakes are achieved. The reference nutrient intake (RNI) should be the minimum aim, bearing in mind that excessive amounts of trace elements may compromise the response to infection. Thiamine and vitamin C deficits seen in patients who abuse alcohol can pose risks on admission to the ICU. Thiamine supplementation should be provided during the first 3 days (Singer *et al.*, 2009). Patients with major burns and those on continuous renal replacement therapy will have additional vitamin and mineral needs (Berger *et al.*, 2004).

Fluid management

Fluid management in ICU patients is complex as it encompasses many factors. The medical team sets daily fluid balance targets. The simplistic tool of 30–35 mL/kg is not appropriate for use in this setting. Injured and postoperative patients find it more difficult to excrete sodium and water as there is an increase in capillary permeability to water and to the smaller plasma proteins, e.g. albumin, and a resulting loss of intravascular fluid into the extravascular space. Intravenous fluids given for resuscitation also pass into the interstitial space and are retained for the duration of the acute phase of the illness, causing interstitial oedema. Even in the absence of exogenous fluid administration, these compartmental shifts in fluid distribution occur. Fluid retention following surgery can amount up to 7 L (BAPEN, 2011). In severe sepsis and organ dysfunction, around 5–15 L are retained, although fluid retention of up to 35 L has been recorded (Foley *et al.*, 1999).

Fluid requirements are based on the following parameters:

- Clinical history.
- Changes in weight.
- Fluid balance charts.
- Urine output.
- Blood pressure.
- Capillary refill.
- Autonomic responses.
- Skin turgor and dry mouth.
- Serum and urine biochemistry.

Types of intravenous fluids

There are two different categories of intravenous fluids routinely used in the ICU:

- *Crystalloids* – small molecular weight salts or sugars dissolved in water.
- *Colloids* – larger molecular weight molecules, insoluble in water.

Crystalloids

The most commonly used crystalloids are normal saline (0.9% NaCl), dextrose (5–50% glucose), dextrose saline (4% glucose:0.18% NaCl) and Hartmann's solution (Ringer's lactate). All are approximately isotonic, but once infused distribute differently between the different fluid compartments that they are used to maintain.

Colloids

The most frequently used colloids contain gelatine (large molecular weight, approximately 35 000) dissolved in an isotonic crystalloid, e.g. Gelofusine. The large molecules do not dissolve completely and therefore can remain in the blood for longer, expanding the plasma volume. They are commonly used to resuscitate intravascular volume.

Electrolytes

For optimal physiological function, humans must maintain fluid and electrolytes within narrow limits. Homeostasis mechanisms function to maintain these balances; however, critically ill patients frequently have fluid and electrolyte abnormalities that overcome homeostatic mechanisms and may contribute to morbidity and mortality (Lobo, 2004). Sodium and chloride are the most common extracellular cation and anion, respectively, and potassium and inorganic phosphate the intracellular equivalents. No international guidance is available for electrolyte requirements or supplementation during artificial nutrition. The ESPEN guidelines for PN (Singer *et al.*, 2009) state that as requirements are highly variable, they should instead be determined by plasma electrolyte monitoring.

Sodium

The normal requirement for sodium is approximately 70–120 mmol/day. The BAPEN (2011) recommendation is 50–100 mmol/day in 1.5–2.5 L of water. However, additional amounts should only be given to correct deficit or continuing losses.

Hypernatraemia

Hypernatraemia is common in the critically ill patient and is usually caused by a combination of excessive sodium administration, inadequate fluid intake or excessive fluid losses. It is not uncommon for postoperative patients to have 700 mmol of sodium overloaded (BAPEN, 2011). Retention may occur in acute renal failure or as a stress induced syndrome of inappropriate antidiuretic hormone (SIADH). A 24-hour urine collection for measurement of urinary urea, electrolytes and osmolality can identify the cause of hypernatraemia.

The use of low sodium feeds to treat hypernatraemia is not recommended. Instead it is important to determine the cause of the high sodium level and to treat this. In many cases the use of additional enteral water can be effective at achieving a gradual improvement in biochemistry. However, treatment decisions should be made in consultation with the medical team, with overall fluid balance targets in mind.

Hyponatraemia

Hyponatraemia is commonly due to fluid overload, with or without inadequate sodium intake, or associated with hepatic failure (Arieff & Ayus, 1991). Fluid restriction to raise serum sodium levels is the first line treatment, but sodium supplementation may be necessary (Ayus & Arieff, 1999). Desired changes in serum sodium should not exceed 6–8 mmol/24 hours, as more rapid repletion and dehydration is associated with neurological damage.

Potassium

Dietary requirements are in the region of 80–120 mmol/day and the BAPEN (2011) recommendation is 40–80 mmol/day in 1.5–2.5 L of water.

Hyperkalaemia

Hyperkalaemia may be iatrogenic, or associated with excessive use of potassium sparing diuretics, potassium supplements (often administered intravenously), catabolic states such as rhabdomyolysis (where muscle tissue destruction releases intracellular potassium), or the metabolic acidosis of progressive renal failure.

Hypokalaemia

Hypokalaemia is associated with the use of steroids, diuretics, continuous renal replacement therapy or SIADH resulting in increased urinary losses of potassium. Hypokalaemia secondary to cellular uptake of glucose is more pronounced with insulin therapy. The body has no known potassium retaining hormone, so increased urinary or gastrointestinal losses may also induce hypokalaemia. A low potassium feed may be indicated if a patient has deteriorating renal function but is not to receive continuous renal replacement therapy. However, it is not indicated for patients on continuous renal replacement therapy; in addition to being low in potassium, the feed is also low in protein. Additional protein supply is required to counteract the protein losses from the haemofiltration process.

Internet resources

American Society for Parenteral & Enteral Nutrition www
.nutritioncare.org
British Dietetic Association   www.bda.co.uk
  Dietitians in Critical Care
British Society for Parenteral & Enteral Nutrition   www.bapen
.org.uk
  Critical Care Nutrition, at the Clinical Evaluation Research Unit
  (CERU)   www.criticalcarenutrition.com
European Society for Clinical Nutrition & Metabolism   www
.espen.org
Intensive Care Society   www.ics.ac.uk
Scottish Intensive Care Society   www.scottishintensivecare.org.uk
Society of Critical Care Medicine   www.sccm.org

References

Adam S, Batson S. (1997) A study of problems associated with the delivery of enteral feed in critically ill patients in five ICUs in the UK. *Intensive Care Medicine* 23(3): 261–266.

Akinnusi ME, Pineda LA, El Solh AA. (2008) Effect of obesity on intensive care morbidity and mortality: a meta-analysis. *Critical Care Medicine* 36(1): 151–158.

Alberda C, Gramlich L, Jones N, *et al.* (2009) The relationship between nutritional intake and clinical outcomes in critically ill patients: results of an international multicenter observational study. *Intensive Care Medicine* 35(10): 1728–1737.

Amato P, Keating KP, Quercia RA, Karbonic J. (1995) Formulaic methods of estimating calorie requirements in mechanically ventilated obese patients: a reappraisal. *Nutrition in Clinical Practice* 10(6): 229–232.

Anderegg BA, Worrall C, Barbour E, Simpson KN, Delegge M. (2009) Comparison of resting energy expenditure prediction methods with measured resting energy expenditure in obese, hospitalized adults. *Journal of Parenteral and Enteral Nutrition* 33(2): 168–175.

Andrews PJ, Avenell A, Noble DW, *et al.* (2011) Randomised trial of glutamine, selenium, or both, to supplement parenteral nutrition for critically ill patients. *BMJ* 342: d1542.

Anzueto A, Frutos-Vivar F, Esteban A, *et al.* (2011) Influence of body mass index on outcome of the mechanically ventilated patients. *Thorax* 66(1): 66–73.

Arieff AI, Ayus JC. (1991) Treatment of symptomatic hyponatremia: neither haste nor waste. *Critical Care Medicine* 19(6): 748–751.

Atkinson S, Sieffert E, Bihari, D. (1998) A prospective, randomized, double-blind, controlled clinical trial of enteral immunonutrition in the critically ill. Guy's Hospital Intensive Care Group. *Critical Care Medicine* 26(7): 1164–1172.

Ayus JC, Arieff AI. (1999) Chronic hyponatremic encephalopathy in postmenopausal women: association of therapies with morbidity and mortality. *JAMA* 281(24): 2299–2304.

Barazzoni R, Zanetti M, Bosutti A, *et al.* (2004) Myostatin expression is not altered by insulin deficiency and replacement in streptozotocin-diabetic rat skeletal muscles. *Clinical Nutrition* 23(6): 1413–1417.

Barr J, Hecht M, Flavin KE, Khorana A, Gould MK. (2004) Outcomes in critically ill patients before and after the implementation of an evidence-based nutritional management protocol. *Chest* 125(4): 1446–1457.

Bellomo R, Egi M. (2005) Glycemic control in the intensive care unit: why we should wait for NICE-SUGAR. *Mayo Clinic Proceedings* 80(12): 1546–1548.

Bellomo R, Tan HK, Bhonagiri S, *et al.* (2002) High protein intake during continuous hemodiafiltration: impact on amino acids and nitrogen balance. *International Journal of Artificial Organs* 25(4): 261–268.

Berger MM, Shenkin A, Revelly JP, *et al.* (2004) Copper, selenium, zinc, and thiamine balances during continuous venovenous hemodiafiltration in critically ill patients. *American Journal Clinical Nutrition* 80(2): 410–416.

Bertolini G, Iapichino G, Radrizzani D, *et al.* (2003) Early enteral immunonutrition in patients with severe sepsis: results of an interim analysis of a randomized multicentre clinical trial. *Intensive Care Medicine* 29(5): 834–840.

Bessey PQ, Watters JM, Aoki TT, Wilmore DW. (1984) Combined hormonal infusion simulates the metabolic response to injury. *Annals of Surgery* 200(3): 264–281.

Biolo G, De Cicco M. (2004) Muscle mass and protein metabolism. *Nestle Nutrition Workshop Series Clinical Performance Programme* 9: 111–120.

Biolo G, Tipton KD, Klein S, Wolfe RR. (1997) An abundant supply of amino acids enhances the metabolic effect of exercise on muscle protein. *American Journal of Physiology* 273(1 Pt 1): E122–E129.

Booth CM, Heyland DK, Paterson WG. (2002) Gastrointestinal promotility drugs in the critical care setting: a systematic review of the evidence. *Critical Care Medicine* 30(7): 1429–1435.

Brandi, LS, Bertolini R, Santini L, Cavani S. (1999) Effects of ventilator resetting on indirect calorimetry measurement in the critically ill surgical patient. *Crit Care Medicine* 27(3): 531–539.

British Society for Parenteral & Enteral Nutrition (BAPEN). (2011) *British Consensus Guidelines on IV Fluid Treatment for Adult Surgical Patients*. Redditch: BAPEN.

Cano NJ, Aparicio M, Brunori G, *et al.* (2009) ESPEN Guidelines on Parenteral Nutrition: adult renal failure. *Clinical Nutrition* 28(4): 401–414.

Caparros T, Lopez J, Grau T. (2001) Early enteral nutrition in critically ill patients with a high-protein diet enriched with arginine, fiber, and antioxidants compared with a standard high-protein diet. The effect on nosocomial infections and outcome. *Journal of Parenteral and Enteral Nutrition* 25(6): 299–308.

Carlson GL. (2001) Insulin resistance and glucose-induced thermogenesis in critical illness. *Proceedings of the Nutrition Society* 60(3): 381–388.

Carlson GL. (2004) Hunterian Lecture: Insulin resistance in human sepsis: implications for the nutritional and metabolic care of the critically ill surgical patient. *Annals of the Royal College of Surgery of England* 86(2): 75–81.

Casaer MP, Mesotten D, Hermans G, *et al.* (2011) Early versus late parenteral nutrition in critically ill adults. *New England Journal of Medicine* 365(6): 506–517.

Cerra FB, Benitez MR, Blackburn GL, *et al.* (1997) Applied nutrition in ICU patients. A consensus statement of the American College of Chest Physicians. *Chest* 111(3): 769–778.

Chapman MJ, Fraser RJ, Kluger MT, Buist MD, De Nichilo DJ. (2000) Erythromycin improves gastric emptying in critically ill patients intolerant of nasogastric feeding. *Critical Care Medicine* 28(7): 2334–2337.

Critical Care Nutrition. (2009) Canadian Critical Care Nutrition Practice Guidelines. Avaialble at www.criticalcarenutrition.com. Accessed 26 June 2012.

Cuthbertson DP, Valero A, Zanuy MA, Leon Sanz ML. (2001) Post-shock metabolic response, 1942. *Nutricion Hospitalaria* 16(5): 176–182.

De Jonghe B, Bastuji-Garin S, Sharshar T, Outin H, Brochard L. (2004) Does ICU-acquired paresis lengthen weaning from mechanical ventilation? *Intensive Care Medicine* 30(6): 1117–1121.

Department of Health. (2000) *Comprehensive Critical Care: A Review of Adult Critical Care Services*, London: Department of Health.

Dickerson RN. (2004) Specialized nutrition support in the hospitalized obese patient. *Nutrition in Clinical Practice* 19(3): 245–254.

Doig GS, Simpson F, Finfer S, *et al.* (2008) Effect of evidence-based feeding guidelines on mortality of critically ill adults: a cluster randomized controlled trial. *JAMA* 300(23): 2731–2741.

Dossett LA, Heffernan D, Lightfoot M, *et al.* (2008) Obesity and pulmonary complications in critically injured adults. *Chest* 134(5): 974–980.

Dvir D, Cohen J, Singer P. (2006) Computerized energy balance and complications in critically ill patients: an observational study. *Clinical Nutrition* 25(1): 37–44.

Faisy C, Guerot E, Diehl JL, Labrousse J, Fagon JY. (2003) Assessment of resting energy expenditure in mechanically ventilated patients. *American Journal of Clinical Nutrition* 78(2): 241–249.

Finfer S, Chittock DR, Su SY, *et al.* (2009) Intensive versus conventional glucose control in critically ill patients. *New England Journal of Medicine* 360(13): 1283–1297.

Foley K, Keegan M, Campbell I, Murby B, Hancox D, Pollard B. (1999) Use of single-frequency bioimpedance at 50 kHz to estimate total body water in patients with multiple organ failure and fluid overload. *Critical Care Medicine* 27(8): 1472–1477.

Forbes GB. (1982) Is obesity a genetic disease? *Journal of the Medical Society of New Jersey* 79(1): 47–48.

Forbes GB. (1987) Lean body mass-body fat interrelationships in humans. *Nutrition Reviews* 45(8): 225–231.

Frankenfield D. (2011) Validation of an equation for resting metabolic rate in older obese, critically ill patients. *Journal of Parenteral and Enteral Nutrition* 35(2): 264–269.

Frankenfield DC, Smith JS, Cooney RN. (1997) Accelerated nitrogen loss after traumatic injury is not attenuated by achievement of energy balance. *Journal of Parenteral and Enteral Nutrition* 21(6): 324–329.

Frankenfield DC, Rowe WA, Smith JS, Cooney RN. (2003) Validation of several established equations for resting metabolic rate in obese and nonobese people. *Journal of the American Dietetic Association* 103(9): 1152–1159.

Frankenfield D, Smith JS, Cooney RN. (2004) Validation of 2 approaches to predicting resting metabolic rate in critically ill patients. *Journal of Parenteral and Enteral Nutrition* 28(4): 259–264.

Frankenfield DC, Coleman A, Alam S, Cooney RN. (2009) Analysis of estimation methods for resting metabolic rate in critically ill adults. *Journal of Parenteral and Enteral Nutrition* 33(1): 27–36.

Frat JP, Gissot V, Ragot S, *et al.* (2008) Impact of obesity in mechanically ventilated patients: a prospective study. *Intensive Care Medicine* 34(11): 1991–1998.

Gadek JE, DeMichele SJ, Karlstad MD, *et al.* (1999) Effect of enteral feeding with eicosapentaenoic acid, gamma-linolenic acid, and antioxidants in patients with acute respiratory distress syndrome. Enteral Nutrition in ARDS Study Group. *Critical Care Medicine* 27(8): 1409–1420.

Galban C, Montejo JC, Mesejo A, *et al.* (2000) An immune-enhancing enteral diet reduces mortality rate and episodes of bacteremia in septic intensive care unit patients. *Critical Care Medicine* 28(3): 643–648.

Gong MN, Bajwa EK, Thompson BT, Christiani DC. (2010) Body mass index is associated with the development of acute respiratory distress syndrome. *Thorax* 65(1): 44–50.

Gramlich L, Kichian K, Pinilla J, Rodych NJ, Dhaliwal R, Heyland DK. (2004) Does enteral nutrition compared with parenteral nutrition result in better outcomes in critically ill adult patients? A systematic review of the literature. *Nutrition* 20(10): 843–848.

Griffiths RD, Hall JB. (2010) Intensive care unit-acquired weakness. *Critical Care Medicine* 38(3): 779–787.

Griffiths RD, Jones C. (1999) Recovery from intensive care. *BMJ* 319: 427–429.

Harris, JA, Benedict FG. (1919) *A Biometric Study of Basal Metabolism in Man*. No 279. Washington, DC: Carnegie Insitute of Washington.

Hayes JA, Black NA, Jenkinson C, *et al.* (2000) Outcome measures for adult critical care: a systematic review. *Health Technology Assessment* 4(24): 1–111.

Hermans G, De Jonghe B, Bruyninckx F, Van den Berghe G. (2008) Clinical review: Critical illness polyneuropathy and myopathy. *Critical Care* 12(6): 238.

Herridge MS, Cheung AM, Tansey CM, *et al.* (2003) One-year outcomes in survivors of the acute respiratory distress syndrome. *New England Journal of Medicine* 348(8): 683–693.

Heyland DK, Samis A. (2003) Does immunonutrition in patients with sepsis do more harm than good? *Intensive Care Medicine* 29(5): 669–671.

Heyland D, Cook DJ, Winder B, Brylowski L, Van DH, Guyatt G. (1995) Enteral nutrition in the critically ill patient: a prospective survey. *Critical Care Medicine* 23(6): 1055–1060.

Heyland DK, Novak F, Drover JW, Jain M, Su X, Suchner U. (2001) Should immunonutrition become routine in critically ill patients? A systematic review of the evidence. *JAMA* 286(8): 944–953.

Heyland DK, Dhaliwal R, Drover JW, Gramlich L, Dodek P. (2003) Canadian clinical practice guidelines for nutrition support in mechanically ventilated, critically ill adult patients. *Journal of Parenteral and Enteral Nutrition* 27(5): 355–373.

Heyland DK, Dhaliwal R, Day A, Jain M, Drover J. (2004) Validation of the Canadian clinical practice guidelines for nutrition support in mechanically ventilated, critically ill adult patients: results of a prospective observational study. *Critical Care Medicine* 32(11): 2260–2266.

Hill GL. (1992) Jonathan E. Rhoads Lecture. Body composition research: implications for the practice of clinical nutrition. *Journal of Parenteral and Enteral Nutrition* 16(3): 197–218.

Hogue CW Jr, Stearns JD, Colantuoni E, *et al.* (2009) The impact of obesity on outcomes after critical illness: a meta-analysis. *Intensive Care Medicine* 35(7): 1152–1170.

Hoher JA, Zimermann Teixeira PJ, Hertz F, da S Moreira A. (2008) A comparison between ventilation modes: how does activity level affect energy expenditure estimates? *Journal of Parenteral and Enteral Nutrition* 32(2): 176–183.

Horgan GW, Stubbs J. (2003) Predicting basal metabolic rate in the obese is difficult. *European Journal of Clinical Nutrition* 57(2): 335–340.

Ireton-Jones CS, Turner WW Jr, Liepa GU, Baxter CR. (1992) Equations for the estimation of energy expenditures in patients with burns with special reference to ventilatory status. *Journal of Burn Care and Rehabilitation* 13(3): 330–333.

Ishibashi N, Plank LD, Sando K, Hill GL. (1998) Optimal protein requirements during the first 2 weeks after the onset of critical illness. *Critical Care Medicine* 26(9): 1529–1535.

Klein CJ, Stanek GS, Wiles CE III. (1998) Overfeeding macronutrients to critically ill adults: metabolic complications. *Journal of the American Dietetic Association* 98(7): 795–806.

Kreymann KG, Berger MM, Deutz NE, *et al.* (2006) ESPEN Guidelines on Enteral Nutrition: Intensive care. *Clinical Nutrition* 25(2): 210–223.

Larsson J, Lennmarken C, Martensson J, Sandstedt S, Vinnars E. (1990) Nitrogen requirements in severely injured patients. *British Journal of Surgery* 77(4): 413–416.

Liposky JM, Nelson LD. (1994) Ventilatory response to high caloric loads in critically ill patients. *Critical Care Medicine* 22(5): 796–802.

Lobo DN. (2004) Fluid, electrolytes and nutrition: physiological and clinical aspects. *Proceedings of the Nutrition Society* 63(3): 453–466.

Lowell JA, Schifferdecker C, Driscoll DF, Benotti PN, Bistrian BR. (1990) Postoperative fluid overload: not a benign problem. *Critical Care Medicine* 18(7): 728–733.

MacLaren R, Kiser TH, Fish DN, Wischmeyer PE. (2008) Erythromycin vs metoclopramide for facilitating gastric emptying and tolerance to intragastric nutrition in critically ill patients. *Journal of Parenteral and Enteral Nutrition* 32(4): 412–419.

Marik PE, Zaloga GP. (2008) Immunonutrition in critically ill patients: a systematic review and analysis of the literature. *Intensive Care Medicine* 34(11): 1980–1990.

Marik PE, Zaloga GP. (2010) Immunonutrition in high-risk surgical patients: a systematic review and analysis of the literature. *Journal of Parenteral and Enteral Nutrition* 34(4): 378–386.

Martin CM, Doig GS, Heyland DK, Morrison T, Sibbald WJ. (2004) Multicentre, cluster-randomized clinical trial of algorithms for critical-care enteral and parenteral therapy (ACCEPT). *CMAJ* 170(2): 197–204.

McClave SA, Sexton LK, Spain DA, *et al.* (1999) Enteral tube feeding in the intensive care unit: factors impeding adequate delivery. *Critical Care Medicine* 27(7): 1252–1256.

McClave SA, Lukan JK, Stefater JA, *et al.* (2005) Poor validity of residual volumes as a marker for risk of aspiration in critically ill patients. *Critical Care Medicine* 33(2): 324–330.

McClave SA, Martindale RG, Vanek VW, *et al.* (2009) Guidelines for the Provision and Assessment of Nutrition Support Therapy in the Adult Critically Ill Patient: Society of Critical Care Medicine (SCCM) and American Society for Parenteral and Enteral Nutrition (A.S.P.E.N.). *Journal of Parenteral and Enteral Nutrition* 33(3): 277–316.

Metheny NA, Schallom ME, Edwards SJ. (2004) Effect of gastrointestinal motility and feeding tube site on aspiration risk in critically ill patients: a review. *Heart and Lung* 33(3): 131–145.

Miller AT Jr, Blyth CS. (1953) Lean body mass as a metabolic reference standard. *Journal of Applied Physiology* 5(7): 311–316.

Monk DN, Plank LD, Franch-Arcas G, Finn PJ, Streat SJ, Hill GL. (1996) Sequential changes in the metabolic response in critically injured patients during the first 25 days after blunt trauma. *Annals of Surgery* 223(4): 395–405.

Montejo JC, Zarazaga A, Lopez-Martinez J, *et al.* (2003) Immunonutrition in the intensive care unit. A systematic review and consensus statement. *Clinical Nutrition* 22(3): 221–233.

Montejo JC, Minambres E, Bordeje L, *et al.* (2010) Gastric residual volume during enteral nutrition in ICU patients: the REGANE study. *Intensive Care Medicine* 36(8): 1386–1393.

Morris AE, Stapleton RD, Rubenfeld GD, Hudson LD, Caldwell E, Steinberg KP. (2007) The association between body mass index and clinical outcomes in acute lung injury. *Chest* 131(2): 342–348.

National Institute for Health and Care Excellence (2009). *Rehabilitation after clinical illness.* CG83 Avaialble at www.nice.org.uk/cg83. Accessed 26 June 2012.

Nguyen NQ, Chapman M, Fraser RJ, Bryant LK, Burgstad C, Holloway RH. (2007a) Prokinetic therapy for feed intolerance in critical illness: one drug or two? *Critical Care Medicine* 35(11): 2561–2567.

Nguyen NQ, Chapman MJ, Fraser RJ, Bryant LK, Holloway RH. (2007b) Erythromycin is more effective than metoclopramide in the treatment of feed intolerance in critical illness. *Critical Care Medicine* 35(2): 483–489.

NHS. (2011) NHS Health Episode Statistics Online. Adult critical care in HES: England, 2009–10. Available at www.hscic.gov.uk/pubs/acc1011. Accessed 9 September 2013.

Oliveros H, Villamor E. (2008) Obesity and mortality in critically ill adults: a systematic review and meta-analysis. *Obesity(Silver Spring)* 16(3): 515–521.

Pontes-Arruda A, Aragao AM, Albuquerque JD. (2006) Effects of enteral feeding with eicosapentaenoic acid, gamma-linolenic acid, and antioxidants in mechanically ventilated patients with severe sepsis and septic shock. *Critical Care Medicine* 34(9): 2325–2333.

Pontes-Arruda A, Demichele S, Seth A, Singer P. (2008) The use of an inflammation-modulating diet in patients with acute lung injury or acute respiratory distress syndrome: a meta-analysis of outcome data. *Journal of Parenteral and Enteral Nutrition* 32(6): 596–605.

Pontes-Arruda A, Martins LF, de Lima SM, *et al.;* Investigating Nutritional Therapy with EPA, Gla and Antioxidants Role In Sepsis Treatment Study Group II. (2011) Enteral nutrition with eicosapentaenoic acid, gamma-linolenic acid and antioxidants in the early treatment of sepsis: results from a multicenter, prospective, randomized, double blinded and controlled Study – INTERSEPT study. *Critical Care* 15(3): R144.

Puthucheary Z, Montgomery H, Moxham J, Harridge S, Hart N. (2010) Structure to function: muscle failure in critically ill patients. *Journal of Physiology* 588, (Pt 23): 4641–4648.

Rees RG, Payne-James JJ, King C, Silk DB. (1988) Spontaneous transpyloric passage and performance of 'fine bore' polyurethane feeding tubes: a controlled clinical trial. *Journal of Parenteral and Enteral Nutrition* 12(5): 469–472.

Reid C. (2006) Frequency of under- and overfeeding in mechanically ventilated ICU patients: causes and possible consequences. *Journal of Human Nutrition and Dietetics* 19(1): 13–22.

Reid CL. (2007) Poor agreement between continuous measurements of energy expenditure and routinely used prediction equations in intensive care unit patients. *Clinical Nutrition* 26(5): 649–657.

Reintam A, Parm P, Kitus R, Kern H, Starkopf J. (2009) Gastrointestinal symptoms in intensive care patients. *Acta Anaesthesiologica Scandinavica* 53(3): 318–324.

Rennie MJ. (1985) Muscle protein turnover and the wasting due to injury and disease. *British Medical Bulletin* 41(3): 257–264.

Rubinson L, Diette GB, Song X, Brower RG, Krishnan JA. (2004) Low caloric intake is associated with nosocomial bloodstream infections in patients in the medical intensive care unit. *Critical Care Medicine* 32(2): 350–357.

Runcie CJ, Dougall JR. (1990) Assessment of the critically ill patient. *British Journal of Hospital Medicine* 43(1): 74–76.

Sakr Y, Madl C, Filipescu D, *et al.* (2008) Obesity is associated with increased morbidity but not mortality in critically ill patients. *Intensive Care Medicine* 34(11): 1999–2009.

Scheinkestel CD, Kar L, Marshall K, *et al.* (2003) Prospective randomized trial to assess caloric and protein needs of critically Ill, anuric, ventilated patients requiring continuous renal replacement therapy. *Nutrition* 19(11–12): 909–916.

Schofield WN. (1985) Predicting basal metabolic rate, new standards and review of previous work. *Human Nutrition and Clinical Nutrition* 39(Suppl 1): 5–41.

SECTION 7

Schulman AS, Willcutts KF, Claridge JA, *et al.* (2005) Does the addition of glutamine to enteral feeds affect patient mortality? *Critical Care Medicine* 33(11): 2501–2506.

Shaw JH, Wildbore M, Wolfe RR. (1987) Whole body protein kinetics in severely septic patients. The response to glucose infusion and total parenteral nutrition. *Annals of Surgery* 205(3): 288–294.

Simpson F, Doig GS. (2005) Parenteral vs. enteral nutrition in the critically ill patient: a meta-analysis of trials using the intention to treat principle. *Intensive Care Medicine* 31(1): 12–23.

Singer P, Theilla M, Fisher H, Gibstein L, Grozovski E, Cohen J. (2006) Benefit of an enteral diet enriched with eicosapentaenoic acid and gamma-linolenic acid in ventilated patients with acute lung injury. *Critical Care Medicine* 34(4): 1033–1038.

Singer P, Berger MM, van den BG, *et al.*; ESPEN. (2009) ESPEN Guidelines on Parenteral Nutrition: intensive care. *Clinical Nutrition* 28(4): 387–400.

Streat SJ, Beddoe AH, Hill GL. (1987) Aggressive nutritional support does not prevent protein loss despite fat gain in septic intensive care patients. *Journal of Trauma* 27(3): 262–266.

Swinamer DL, Grace MG, Hamilton SM, Jones RL, Roberts P, King EG. (1990) Predictive equation for assessing energy expenditure in mechanically ventilated critically ill patients. *Critical Care Medicine* 18(6): 657–661.

Taylor B, Renfro A, Mehringer L. (2005) The role of the dietitian in the intensive care unit. *Current Opinion in Clinical Nutrition and Metabolic Care* 8(2): 211–216.

Taylor SJ, Manara AR, Brown J. (2010) Treating delayed gastric emptying in critical illness: metoclopramide, erythromycin, and bedside (cortrak) nasointestinal tube placement. *Journal of Parenteral and Enteral Nutrition* 34(3): 289–294.

Todorovic V, Micklewright A. (2007) *A Pocket Guide to Clinical Nutrition.* Birmingham: British Dietetic Association.

Tremblay A, Bandi V. (2003) Impact of body mass index on outcomes following critical care. *Chest* 123(4): 1202–1207.

van den Berghe G, Wouters P, Weekers F, *et al.* (2001) Intensive insulin therapy in the critically ill patients. *New England Journal of Medicine* 345(19): 1359–1367.

Villet S, Chiolero RL, Bollmann MD, *et al.* (2005) Negative impact of hypocaloric feeding and energy balance on clinical outcome in ICU patients. *Clinical Nutrition* 24(4): 502–509.

Waitzberg DL, Saito H, Plank LD, *et al.* (2006) Postsurgical infections are reduced with specialized nutrition support. *World Journal of Surgery* 30(8): 1592–1604.

Webb P. (1981) Energy expenditure and fat-free mass in men and women. *American Journal of Clinical Nutrition* 34(9): 1816–1826.

Welpe P, Frutiger A, Vanek P, Kleger GR. (2010) Jejunal feeding tubes can be efficiently and independently placed by intensive care unit teams. *Journal of Parenteral and Enteral Nutrition* 34(2): 121–124.

Wolfe RR, Miller SL. (1999) Amino acid availability controls muscle protein metabolism. *Diabetes Nutrition and Metabolism* 12(5): 322–328.

7.17.2 Traumatic brain injury

Kirsty-Anna Mclaughlin and Gemma Moore

Key points

■ Early nutritional support is associated with better outcomes and full nutritional requirements should be safely met as soon as possible post injury.

■ Hypermetabolism and catabolism cause higher energy and protein requirements in the acute phase of traumatic brain injury over and above those seen in many other hypermetabolic conditions.

■ Regular monitoring of anthropometry, biochemistry, feed tolerance and nutritional intake will help to ensure appropriate nutritional management.

■ The multidisciplinary team is key throughout the acute and rehabilitation phases in ensuring optimal outcomes.

There are three stages of traumatic brain injury (TBI):

- *Acute* – intensive care aiming for medical stabilisation and prevention of secondary brain damage.
- *Post acute* – ward based care to provide transition from intensive care to rehabilitation.
- *Rehabilitation* – multidisciplinary therapy to maximise physical and cognitive functioning and to minimise chronic disability.

The duration of these stages will differ considerably between patients. Krakau *et al.* (2010) found that on average 73% of TBI patients remain in an intensive care unit (ICU) for 2–33 days, a mixed ward for 5–115 days and a rehabilitation unit for 7–299 days.

Traumatic brain injury is thought to be the leading cause of disability and mortality in young people and 30% of head injured patients are children under the age of 15 years (Maas *et al.*, 2008; NICE, 2007). Each year 600 000 people attend emergency departments with a head injury in England and Wales, with the majority of cases considered to be mild (NICE, 2007). Moderate and severe cases account for 15% of head injuries, with 113 000 people admitted to hospital annually in England (NICE, 2007; Krakau, 2010). The primary causes of head injury include falls (22–43%), assaults (30–50%) and road traffic accidents (approximately 25%). The incidence of head injury is greater in males (approximately 72% of cases). Alcohol consumption is thought to be involved in up to 65% of adult head injuries (NICE, 2007).

SECTION 7

Table 7.17.8 Commonly used terms in traumatic brain injury

Commonly used terms	Definition
Traumatic brain injury (TBI)	Specifically defined by the presence of symptoms ranging from behavioural and neuropsychological alterations in mild cases to altered consciousness, coma, seizure, focal sensory or motor neurological deficit or confusion in more severe cases (Bruns & Hauser, 2003)
Head injury	Less specifically defined by the presence of external injuries to the face, scalp and calvarium. TBI may not be present (Bruns & Hauser, 2003)
Coma	Unarousable with lack of spontaneous eye opening, and an inability to wake the patient even with vigorous sensory stimulation (Giacino et al., 2002)
Vegetative state	'A complete absence of behavioural evidence for self or environmental awareness. However, the presence of sleep wake cycles indicates that the capacity for spontaneous or stimulus induced arousal remains' (Giacino et al., 2002)
Minimally conscious state	Similar to vegetative state but with some consciousness preserved (Giacino et al., 2002)
Brain stem death	Irreversible coma: 'unresponsiveness and lack of receptivity, the absence of movement and breathing, the absence of brain stem reflexes, and coma whose cause has been identified' (Wijdicks, 2001)

Definition

There are many terms commonly used to classify TBI and head injury (HI) (Table 7.17.8). Head injury is classified as either closed or penetrative, and the damage from TBI either primary brain damage or secondary brain damage.

- *Closed head injury – 'A blow to the head or a severe shaking. The skull may be fractured but there is no penetration of the skull or brain tissue'* (NICE, 2007).
- *Penetrating head injury – 'Head injury where an object penetrates the scalp and skull and enters the brain or its lining'* (NICE, 2007).
- *Primary brain damage* – occurs immediately as a result of trauma. Factors that may cause brain damage include shearing of white matter tracts, focal contusions, haematomas and diffuse swelling (Maas *et al.*, 2008).
- *Secondary brain damage* – occurs hours or days after the initial trauma and is caused by inflammatory and stress responses (Maas *et al.*, 2008). It is possible to prevent secondary brain damage by controlling clinical parameters.

Diagnostic criteria and classification

Assessment and classification of TBI is primarily guided by the Glasgow Coma Score (GCS) (Teasdale & Jennett, 1974). The minimum possible GCS is 3 and the maximum is 15; severity of TBI is classified as severe (GCS 3–8), moderate (GCS 9–12) or mild (GCS 13–15).

Morbidity and mortality

Mortality rates from TBI have not been thoroughly researched in the UK. A systematic review by Tagliaferri *et al.* (2005) proposed an average mortality rate of 15 per 100 000 per year from TBI across Europe. Thornhill *et al.* (2000) reported that 38% of patients with severe head injury were deceased or vegetative at 1 year post injury. Morbidity varies considerably between patients, although long term effects are extensive and persistent (Tagliaferri *et al.*, 2005). Thornhill *et al.* (2000) found that 29% of patients with severe head injury had a severe disability and 19% had a moderate disability at 1 year post injury. One study found that 34% of patients reported difficulties subsequent to their injury and 11% were medically unfit for employment (McCartan *et al.*, 2008). Consequences may include memory problems, physical disability and neuropsychological difficulties.

Clinical investigation and management

Initial priorities include resuscitation and pain management, as pain can lead to a rise in intracranial pressure. Early imaging is also a priority, as this will ensure detection of complications, leading to better outcomes. Computed tomography imaging of the head forms the primary investigation to detect brain injuries. Neurosurgery may also be required depending on the nature of the injury. The medications frequently used in TBI and relevant nutritional considerations are collated in Table 7.17.9.

Multidisciplinary approach

It is essential that patients with TBI are treated by a multidisciplinary team (MDT). Table 7.17.10 describes the dietetic role within the MDT. Some rehabilitation units may include art and music therapists. The specialist MDT facilitates improvements in patient outcomes (Turner-Stokes *et al.*, 2011).

Nutritional consequences

Metabolic response to traumatic brain injury

Traumatic brain injury may cause an abnormal regulation of nervous, endocrine and inflammatory systems in order to enable a continuous supply of substrates for cell growth and repair (Agha *et al.*, 2004a; Ghirnikar *et al.*, 1997). These changes may be caused by a metabolic response to stress and by direct injury to the brain, the major organ responsible for regulation and homeostasis. Possible alterations in regulatory systems include:

Table 7.17.9 Medications used in traumatic brain injury that affect nutritional status

Use	Examples	Effect on nutritional status/treatment
Sedative – to manage raised ICP	Propofol	Causes reduced activity levels and suppression of cerebral metabolism, leading to reduced energy expenditure
		Propofol is formulated in 10% lipid emulsion, which provides 4.6 kJ/mL (1.1 kcal/mL). NB: Consider when calculating energy intake
		High dose and use for >48 hours may cause metabolic acidosis, hyperlipidaemia and hyperkalaemia
	Midazolam	Reduced activity levels leading to reduced energy expenditure
Barbiturate – to manage raised ICP	Pentobarbitual Thoipental sodium	May reduce metabolic rate to 80% of BMR (Gross et al., 2010)
Analgesia – to manage pain and potentiate effects of sedatives	Morphine Fentanyl Alfentanil Remifentanil	Long term analgesia may lead to constipation. Review fluid and fibre intake and consider laxatives
Intracranial hypertension treatment – reduces cerebral oedema and ICP	Mannitol	Osmotic effect can cause polyuria, leading to fluid and electrolyte loss. Monitor fluid balance to assess hydration and electrolyte levels. Liaise with the medical team to assess fluid requirement in line with medical treatment and correct electrolyte imbalance if necessary
	Hypertonic saline Solution	May increase serum osmolality and lead to acid–base abnormalities (Gross et al., 2010). Hypernatraemia may occur
Anticonvulsants	Sodium valproate	Consider vitamin D supplementation as long term use of antiepileptic drugs is associated with reduced bone mineral density
	Carbamazepine	Consider vitamin D supplementation in patients who are immobilised for long periods or who have inadequate sun exposure or dietary intake of calcium. May precipitate when administered with enteral nutrition and withholding EN pre and post administration will reduce this (Gross et al., 2010)
	Phenobarbital	Consider vitamin D supplementation
	Topiramate	Ensure adequate hydration to reduce the risk of nephrolithiasis
	Phenytoin	Consider vitamin D supplementation. Absorption is reduced when administered with enteral nutrition and therefore withholding enteral nutrition for 2 hours post and pre phenytoin administration is advised (Gross et al., 2010)
Musculoskeletal and skeletal muscle relaxants	Baclofen	Gastrointestinal disturbances
Thyroid hormones	Levothyroxine	Give at least 2 hours apart from iron supplementation as levothyroxine sodium reduces absorption of oral iron
Prokinetics	Erythromycin	May be more effective than metoclopramide at improving feed tolerance (AANN, 2009)
	Metoclopramide	May help to improve feed tolerance but evidence is not convincing (AANN, 2009)

ICP, intracranial pressure, BMR, basal metabolic rate.

- Increased production of proinflammatory cytokines tumour necrosis factor alpha (TNFα), interleukin 1 (IL-1) and IL-6 (Charrueau et al., 2009).
- Increased circulation of the counter regulatory hormones cortisol, glucagon and catecholamines (Vizzinni & Aranda-Michel, 2011).
- Production of acute phase proteins from the liver (Charrueau et al., 2009).
- Increased cardiac output and hypertension, leading to elevated CO_2 production and O_2 consumption (Vizzinni & Aranda-Michel, 2011).

The subsequent effects on metabolic processes are shown in Figure 7.17.1.

Energy expenditure 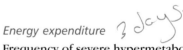 3 days.

Frequency of severe hypermetabolism in TBI ranges from 31% to 57% within 72 hours post injury (Ott et al., 1994; Raurich & Ibanez, 1994). Foley et al. (2008) reported that hypermetabolism continues for 30 days post injury; however, there is a lack of evidence examining measured energy expenditure (MEE) for longer than this period. Hypermetabolism is defined as the ratio of MEE to predicted energy expenditure (PEE), and can be expressed as a percentage of the PEE (Krakau et al., 2007):

- Hypometabolism <0.9 (90%).
- Hypermetabolism 1.1 (110%).
- Severe hypermetabolism 1.3 (130%).

Table 7.17.10 Link between the dietitian and other members of the multidisciplinary team (MDT)

MDT member	Liaise with dietitian regarding
Speech and language therapist	Method of communication Texture modification in dysphagia Joint sessions with patient to aid communication and understanding
Physiotherapist	Weaning and decannulation of tracheostomy tube and progression to oral feeding. Activity/mobility to assess energy requirements Positioning regarding potential impact on feeding and safety of delivery Possible member of the team who can weigh when hoisting patient
Occupational therapist	Functional ability to self feed Identification of issues such as hemineglect Practicalities of shopping, preparing and making meals Encouraging appropriate food shopping and cooking specific to the patient's nutritional needs
Nursing staff	Nutritional screening and regular monitoring Issues with feeding regimen practicalities Issues with gastrointestinal intolerances Dietary intake issues/progress Family concerns and comments Special diet awareness training
Psychologist	Regarding mood and behaviour and effect on nutritional intake
Doctor	Diagnosis, treatment and prognosis Discharge planning Safe enteral feeding tube removal date
Pharmacist	Medication and relevant drug–nutrient interactions Medications given via enteral feeding tubes Medications with gastrointestinal side effects Medications that affect appetite and weight
Coordinator/keyworker	Discharge planning – can provide information on transfer/discharge destination May need to transfer to another acute, community or home enteral feeding dietitian Carer training regarding special diets and/or enteral tube feeding Recommendations for monitoring of nutritional status and feeding Liaison with GP of dietary needs and any supplement prescriptions

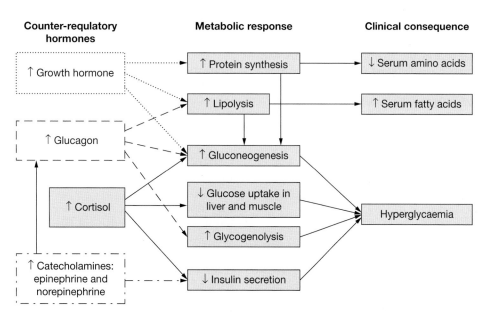

Figure 7.17.1 Metabolic response to traumatic brain injury

SECTION 7

The degree of hypermetabolism is believed to be proportional to the severity of head injury (Fruin *et al.*, 1986). A systematic review (Foley *et al.*, 2008) found that mean percentage of PEE ranged from 116% to 200% up to 7 days post injury in patients without sedation, paralysis or barbiturate induced coma (Raurich & Ibanez, 1994; Haider *et al.*, 1975), whereas patients with barbiturate induced coma, sedation or induced paralysis had a mean percentage of PEE of 80–123%. Coma reduces metabolism, whereas paralysis reduces motor activity, leading to a reduced energy requirement (Clifton *et al.*,1984; Dempsey *et al.*,1985; Bruder *et al.*, 1998). Other factors that may affect energy expenditure include:

* Morphine – may reduce energy expenditure by 8% (Raurich & Ibanez, 1994).
* Controlled mechanical ventilation – may reduce energy expenditure by 4–25% due to a reduction in motor activity (Lewis *et al.*, 1988; Bursztein *et al.*, 1978).
* Weaning from mechanical ventilation – may cause an increase in energy expenditure for a limited period (Bruder *et al.*, 1991).

In addition, some symptoms may affect energy expenditure, including pyrexia, which can increase energy expenditure by 13%/°C (Bruder *et al.*, 1998), muscle contractions and autonomic storming, a dramatic increase in activity of the sympathetic nervous system. Autonomic storming describes the consequences TBI can have on the sympathetic and parasympathetic (autonomic) nervous system. It results in a hyper stress response that can affect a number of processes, including regulation of digestion, perspiration, breathing, temperature and heart rate. Dietary induced thermogenesis and the use of steroids are unlikely to directly affect energy expenditure (Foley *et al.*, 2008).

Catabolism

Catabolism is observed in the majority of patients with TBI during the first 2 weeks post injury and nitrogen excretion is elevated (Krakau *et al.*, 2007; Young *et al.*, 1988; Clifton *et al.*, 1984). The severity of catabolism is reported as varying from a negative nitrogen balance of −3 to −16 g/day (Krakau *et al.*, 2007), although nitrogen losses have been reported to be as high as 30 g/day. This level of protein breakdown can cause a 10% loss of lean body mass within 7 days post injury, increasing to a 10–29% loss of total body mass within 2 months (Rajpal & Johnston, 2009; Krakau *et al.*, 2007).

Hyperglycaemia

Hyperglycaemia is frequently observed in the head injured patient as cells become insulin resistant to ensure glucose provision for brain functioning and to mobilise substrates for defence and repair. Hyperglycaemia occurs as a result of circulating counter regulatory hormones, which are released in response to trauma and cause an increase in gluconeogenesis despite persistent hyperglycaemia (Figure 7.17.1). Blood glucose levels above 11 mmol/L in the first 24 hours post TBI have been associated with poorer outcomes, including increased mortality, lower

GCS at day 5 post injury and increased length of hospital stay (Jeremitsky *et al.*, 2005; Vizzinni & Aranda-Michel, 2011). Intensive insulin therapy is an integral part of acute traumatic brain injury management. The dietitian plays a key role in monitoring and assessing the potential impact of feeding on glycaemic control and aims to avoid overfeeding that may exacerbate hyperglycaemia.

Gastroparesis and gut dysfunction

Gastroparesis is frequently reported in patients with head injury; with one study reporting delayed gastric emptying in 80% of patients (Kao *et al.*, 1998). The cause of gut dysfunction remains unclear, but theories include a possible suppression of vagal nerve activity caused by an increased intracranial pressure, which leads to delayed gastric emptying; and alteration in brain gut peptides, including vasoactive intestinal peptide and cholecystokinin, which is associated with enterogastric reflex (Tan *et al.*, 2011). In addition, hyperglycaemia, disordered intestinal flora, inflammation, electrolyte disturbances and medication are associated with gut dysfunction (Tan *et al.*, 2011) (see Chapter 7.4.4).

Nutritional assessment

Nutritional assessment of the head injured patient can be complex, as nutritional status is affected by many factors (Table 7.17.11). Thorough and frequent monitoring is essential due to the potential for rapid changes in clinical condition. Monitoring is also important to assess feed tolerance, which can be an ongoing issue for this patient group.

Nutritional management

Nutritional requirements

Estimating nutritional requirements in this patient group is extremely difficult due to rapid changes in clinical condition and a wide range of complex symptoms that can dramatically affect energy requirements (see Chapter 6.1 and Chapter 7.17.1).

Energy

Indirect calorimetry is considered the gold standard method of measuring energy requirement. However, this may not be realistic in practice due to cost and time implications. In practice, all factors contributing to fluctuations in energy requirement should be considered to estimate energy requirements for individual patients. Schofield or Harris–Benedict equations are frequently used to predict energy requirements, with an addition of 0–30% in the acute phase (Bruder *et al.*, 1991; Weekes & Elia, 1996). More recently, the Scientific Advisory Committee on Nutrition recommended the use of the Henry equations (2005). The key to establishing whether estimated requirements are accurate is to monitor weight changes or changes in body composition, amending the feeding regimen as appropriate. Overfeeding is associated

Table 7.17.11 Assessment and monitoring of nutritional status in the brain injured patient

Parameter		Relevance to dietetic practice
Biochemistry	Urea and electrolytes	Assess hydration status and potential effects of refeeding
		May indicate the need for a low sodium feed or fluid restriction
	White blood cells and C-reactive protein	Raised levels can indicate infection ± inflammation
		A stress factor should be added to BMR; energy and protein requirements will be increased
	Glucose	Hyperglycaemia may occur as a result of metabolic stress or overfeeding, and may be a side effect of chronic steroid use
		Hypoglycaemia may occur with suboptimal feeding/nutritional intake alongside intensive insulin therapy
Anthropometry		Anthropometry is useful to measure outcomes in nutritional goals
		Obtain a baseline measurement on admission, monitor regularly and on transfer/discharge
	Weight	Influences nutritional requirements
		If applicable, calculate weight loss percentage and highlight any significant risks
		Rapid weight gain/loss over 1–2 days can indicate oedema or fluid losses
	Body mass index	To assess and monitor nutritional status
		To formulate nutritional goals, e.g. weight gain, stability or reduction
	Triceps skin fold	Use with caution in hemineglect patients as muscle loss may not be directly attributable to nutrition
	Waist circumference	Used in rehabilitation to assess central adiposity and monitor changes
Gastrointestinal tolerance	Constipation	Sedation, paralysis and analgesia may result in reduction in bowel activity. A proactive approach to aperients therapy is required
		Review the fibre and fluid content of the feeding regimen
	Diarrhoea	Inappropriate continuation/overuse of laxatives and/or other medications, e.g. antibiotic therapy, may result in frequent and/or loose stools.
		A side effect of traumatic brain injury on the parasympathetic nervous system
		Consider increasing fibre in the feeding regimen
		Increased risk of dehydration
	Vomiting/reflux	Reducing the rate of feeding or bolus sizes and choosing a lower fibre feed may improve symptoms
		Review medications and the use of antiemetics
	Bloating	Review the fibre content, total volume of feed and fluid
		Consider bolus feeding versus continuous feeding
	Suspected infection	Stool samples should be analysed alongside a medicine review
	Gastric aspirates	Large residual volumes can be observed in the acute stage due to reduced gastric emptying. Prokinetics and/or proton pump inhibitors may be beneficial
Fluid balance	Hyperhydration Dehydration	Consider fluid used with drug administration when calculating fluid balance
		Consider diuretics and other drugs that may cause polyuria
		Tracheostomy patients may have a higher fluid requirement due to tracheostomy secretions. Consider volume, frequency and viscosity of secretions in order to replace fluid losses
		Monitor for perspiration (duration and frequency) in order to replace fluid losses
	Regulatory hormone disturbances	Diabetes insipidus, cerebral salt wasting (CSW) and syndrome of inappropriate antidiuretic hormone secretion (SIADH)
		Liaise with medical colleagues with regards to therapeutic fluid management plans. (see Table 7.17.12)
Medication		Drug–nutrient interactions, nausea, vomiting, diarrhoea, weight gain and loss can be common side effects (see Table 7.17.9)
Body temperature		Can fluctuate due to potential hypothalamus dysfunction
		Pyrexia may indicate the presence of infection or sepsis, which can affect energy expenditure and fluid requirements
Dietary intake	Increased requirements	Oral intake is likely to be insufficient without significant nutrition support. Thorough assessment of oral intake is paramount
	Respiratory infections	Recurrent infections may indicate aspiration of oral intake
	Sunlight exposure	In rehabilitation units, the patient may be at risk of reduced sunlight exposure
		Advise a diet high in vitamin D ± supplementation
Nutritional status prior to injury		Individuals, who overuse alcohol, are elderly or have coexisting medical conditions may be at increased risk of malnutrition
		Previous weight can help in formulating a patient specific weight goal in rehabilitation
Skin integrity		Long periods of immobility can increase the risk of pressure sores
		Regular positional changes, hygiene care and nutrition can help to minimise this risk

SECTION 7

with poorer outcomes, including prolonged ventilator dependency as a result of excessive carbon dioxide production; hyperglycaemia; metabolic acidosis; and impaired liver function (Griffiths, 2007).

Protein

Protein requirements for patients with TBI are controversial. Twyman *et al.* (1985) found that providing 2.2 g of protein/kg/day resulted in a positive nitrogen balance (9.9 g of nitrogen retained over 10 days), even though nitrogen losses were high compared with the control group who received 1.5 g of protein/kg/day and had a negative nitrogen balance (−31.2 g of nitrogen retained over the same period). However, this level of protein provision is not realistic in practice and lean tissue loss may be unavoidable in patients with TBI regardless of nutritional intervention (Hoffer, 2003). In addition, sufficient energy is required to maximise nitrogen retention and utilisation. Provision of high protein levels to meet requirements without adequate energy leads to an increased nitrogen loss (Hoffer, 2003). Caution is necessary to avoid excessive energy intake when aiming to meet elevated protein requirements as this may lead to the potentially detrimental effects of overfeeding. Minimising obligatory losses in lean body mass is a primary aim. The Brain Trauma Foundation (2007) recommends that protein should provide 15–20% of calories and evidence suggests that there may be little benefit in providing protein in excess of 1.5 g/kg/day for trauma patients (Hoffer, 2003).

Micronutrients

Dietary reference values (Department of Health, 1991) should be met; however, there are some amendments for specific nutrients in TBI in the critically ill (Vizzinni & Aranda-Michel, 2011) (see Chapter 17.7.1). Patients with TBI have increased urinary zinc excretion as well as a reduced serum zinc concentration (McClain *et al.*, 1986). Young *et al.* (1996) reported an improved GCS and visceral protein level in a zinc supplemented group of TBI patients. A recent study found that supplementation of zinc sulphate for 2 weeks led to a reduction in C-reactive protein (a marker of inflammation); however, there was no significant effect on GCS score (Meshkini *et al.*, 2009).

Fluid and electrolytes

Fluid and electrolyte levels may be depleted in acute TBI patients. In addition, nutritional intervention may be delayed post injury and therefore electrolytes should be monitored closely and promptly corrected if there is risk of refeeding syndrome. Drugs such as mannitol can cause fluid loss through polyuria and subsequent hypomagnesaemia, hypokalaemia and hypophosphataemia (Polderman *et al.*, 2001). Polderman *et al.* (2001) found that induced hypothermia via use of water circulating blankets was associated with severe electrolyte depletion as a result of increased urinary excretion during the cooling phase. In addition, damage to the brain can cause changes in regulatory systems, resulting in neurohypophyseal dysfunction in some patients. The resulting conditions are:

Table 7.17.12 Diagnostic criteria of cerebral salt wasting syndrome (CSWS) and syndrome of inappropriate antidiuretic hormone secretion (SIADH) (Cerda-Esteve *et al.*, 2008; Zafonte & Mann, 1997)

Parameter	CSWS	SIADH
Plasma volume	↓	↑ or normal
Salt balance	Negative	Variable
Water balance	Negative	↑ or normal
Signs and symptoms of dehydration	Present	Absent
Serum osmolality	↓	↓
Urine sodium	↑↑	↑
Urine volume	↑↑	↓ or normal
Serum potassium	↑ or normal	↓ or normal
Blood urea nitrogen	↑	Normal
Uric acid	Normal	↓
Weight	↑	↓
Treatment	Normal saline, hypertonic saline, fludrocortisone	Fluid restriction, hypertonic saline, democycline, furosemide

- *Diabetes insipidus (DI)* – can be caused by an insufficient secretion of vasopressin. Symptoms are polyuria and polydipsia; polyuria can lead to hypernatraemia (Tisdall *et al.*, 2006). A low sodium feed may be required.
- *Syndrome of inappropriate antidiuretic hormone secretion (SIADH)* – can be caused by an excessive secretion of the antidiuretic hormone vasopressin. Symptoms are reduced urine output, hyponatraemia presenting within 2–18 days post injury (Behan *et al.*, 2007) and, possibly, fluid overload. Fluid restriction and additional sodium may be necessary (Table 7.17.12).

Cerebral salt wasting syndrome (CSWS) is a rare endocrine condition secondary to TBI. Symptoms are polyuria, polydipsia and a strong desire for salt. This is in response to hyponatraemia due to renal loss of sodium (Cerda-Esteve *et al.*, 2008). The aetiology is not certain; however, reports suggest that neural activity on renal tubular function may be responsible (Zafonte & Mann, 1997). Treatment tends to be increased fluids and salt replacement using intravenous infusion or sodium chloride tablets (Table 7.17.12).

Nutritional support

There is a paucity of research examining the effects of nutritional support in TBI patients and the limited research that is available has not provided conclusive evidence.

Enteral feeding

Enteral feeding is the preferred route in head injured patients as it maintains the integrity of the intestinal mucosa and is also cheaper (see Chapter 6.4). Feeding into the stomach is the first line approach; this is generally via a nasogastric tube. Orogastric tubes are often placed when there is a (suspected) base of skull fracture.

Post pyloric feeding

Jejunal feeding may provide better outcomes in patients who cannot tolerate gastric feeding (Kreymann et al., 2006). The Sussex Critical Care Network (2009) recommends nasojejunal feeding if feed is not absorbed by day 4 of nasogastric feeding and after the use of prokinetic therapy. However, local policies regarding post pyloric feeding and prokinetic therapy may vary. Jejunal feeding has been associated with lower rates of pneumonia (Kreymann et al., 2006; Acosta-Escribano et al., 2010). A nutrition support team with input from a doctor, nutrition nurse, biochemist, pharmacist and dietitian is essential to ensure that an appropriate decision is made to feed post pylorically as this may further delay feeding if unsuccessful.

Parenteral feeding

Parenteral feeding is indicated if the gastrointestinal tract is not functioning and the patient cannot be fed sufficiently by enteral feeding (Kreymann et al., 2006) (see Chapter 6.5).

A Cochrane review (Perel et al., 2006) found that parenteral nutrition (PN) was associated with better outcomes; however, this may have been as a result of earlier initiation of feeding rather than PN itself. This review also reported a trend towards increased incidence of infection in parenteral feeding when compared with enteral feeding, and also an association with hyperglycaemia (Kreymann et al., 2006). Conversely, PN was associated with lower rates of pneumonia.

Initiation of feeding

A number of guidelines recommend initiation of feeding within 24–48 hours of TBI as the evidence suggests that early nutritional intervention is associated with better outcomes (Kreymann et al., 2006; Doig et al., 2009). However, feeding is often not initiated for >48 hours in 60% of patients on the ICU despite the well documented benefit of early intervention (Doig et al., 2008). A Cochrane review (Perel et al., 2006) found that earlier initiation of nutritional support resulted in improved survival and reduced disability. Furthermore, a meta analysis examining initiation of enteral nutrition (EN) within 24 hours found that earlier feeding resulted in a significant reduction in mortality and pneumonia (Doig et al., 2009). The American Brain Trauma Foundation (2007) suggests that brain injured patients should meet full nutritional requirements by day 7 post injury.

Rehabilitation

In rehabilitation, the overarching aim is to help patients regain their functional independence, which may take from many months to several years. Specialist head injury rehabilitation units offer high intensity rehabilitation that provides earlier physical and cognitive functional gains (Turner-Stokes et al., 2011). This is often accompanied by slow stream rehabilitation in the community that is thought to maintain the progress made in post acute rehabilitation. Multidisciplinary treatment focuses on physical, cognitive and behavioural rehabilitation, and psychosocial, vocational and recreational therapy and counselling.

Nutritional considerations

As in the acute phase of TBI, the brain injury will dominate the body's central and autonomic nervous system. The clinical parameters to consider for patients at nutritional risk are listed in Table 7.17.7. Where a nutrient requirement has not been identified as been altered, the dietary reference values are accepted (Department of Health, 1991).

There can be a marked increase in weight in TBI rehabilitation, possibly due to changes in energy requirements and altered eating behaviours. McEvoy et al. (2009) described 25% of rehabilitation patients as being hypermetabolic and 25% being hypometabolic. The mechanisms for hypermetabolism and weight loss are as discussed in the acute phase. Weight gain secondary to a reduction in metabolic rate is likely to be multifactorial including:

- Loss of lean body mass in the acute stage leads to decreased basal metabolic rate (McEvoy et al., 2009).
- Less physically activity than normal population (Patradoon-Ho et al., 2005).
- Hypothalamopituitary dysfunction (Medic-Stojanoska et al., 2007; Popovic, 2005) is found in 27.5–50.9% of TBI rehabilitation patients (Schneider et al., 2007; Tanriverdi et al., 2006; Agha et al., 2004b).
- Loss of neuronal integrity (Shiga et al., 2006).

Overweight and obesity have been observed by a number of researchers and experts (Greenwood, 2002; Voevodin & Haala, 2007). However, a pilot study by French & Merriman (1999) showed that obesity rates were similar to those for the normal population. In the TBI rehabilitation population, appropriate energy restriction is essential to minimise unnecessary weight gain. However, there is limited strong evidence for energy requirements in TBI rehabilitation (McEvoy et al., 2009), which suggests that regular holistic assessment by a dietitian to formulate the appropriate care plan is essential.

Dysphagia and enteral nutrition

Gastrostomy tube feeding is recommended as the optimal form of feeding in rehabilitation if tolerated (Cook et al., 2008–2009). In addition to the recommendations in Chapter 7.6.6 regarding enteral tube feeding, Table 7.17.7 shows the nutrition related issues within TBI rehabilitation to consider when assessing nutritional status. Designing a feeding regimen around therapy input, meeting nutritional requirements and managing any gastrointestinal intolerance issues can be complex. A good knowledge

SECTION 7

of commercially available feeds and the patient's therapy timetable combined with effective communication skills to involve the patient in decision making where possible are paramount in creating an optimum feeding regimen.

Dysphagia and oral nutrition

Approximately 40% of patients on admission are dysphagic, decreasing to 0.4% after 1 year in rehabilitation (Brown *et al.*, 2007). The complexity of regaining a safe swallow in head injury patients is affected by their cognitive, behavioural and communication related impairments (Cherney & Halper, 1996). A multidisciplinary approach facilitates the rehabilitation of dysphagia. The transition from enteral to oral diet has three defined stages:

- Enteral feeding only with regular swallow assessment by a specialist speech and language therapist (SLT).
- Enteral tube feeding and oral texture modified diet (TMD) as recommended by the SLT.
- TMD with nutritional supplementation or food fortification.

Regular formal assessment of oral intake to assess adequacy of energy and protein intakes is necessary (Rajpal & Johnston, 2009) (see Chapter 7.3). The enteral tube feed should then be reduced accordingly to ensure that enteral feeding plus oral intake meets the total estimated nutritional requirements. Oral intake tends to increase as swallow function improves and strengthens. More information on the enteral to oral transition period is given in Chapter 7.6.6. Dietetic intervention should maximise oral intake safely and minimise unnecessary weight gain.

Patients can accidentally remove or dislodge feeding tubes if agitated or confused. Also the feeding tube may be removed prematurely if dysphagia is seen to have improved, causing problems with receiving vital medication, adequate nutrition and hydration. It may be necessary to intervene if requirements cannot be met orally and with supplementation.

Eating behaviour

The senses of taste and smell can be distorted in occipital or frontal injuries (Greenwood, 2002). Advice on choosing foods to compensate for anosmia (loss of smell) and ageusia (loss of taste) should be provided (see Chapter 7.15.1). Visual problems can also result in changes in eating behaviour. Ensuring meals, snacks and drinks are presented in an appropriate manner, and prompting when necessary, can improve nutritional intake.

Disinhibition is another common consequence of frontal lobe damage in TBI (Oder *et al.*, 1992). This has a marked effect on a patient's behaviour and this can be very different from their preinjury persona. The following are common signs of disinhibition (Walker & Wickes 2005):

- Short attention span.
- Fatigue.
- Frustration and irritability.
- Inflexibility and argumentativeness.

- Reduced initiative.
- Impulsiveness.
- Socially and sexually inappropriate behaviour.
- Difficulty forming relationships.

Disinhibition can have nutritional consequences such as weight gain or loss and difficulties with compliance to dietetic advice. Kluver–Bucy syndrome is a rare neurobehaviour syndrome associated with TBI and exists when there is damage to both anterior temporal lobes of the brain (National Institutes of Health, 2008). A nutritional consequence is hyperphagia, which can potentially increase body weight. For both disinhibition and Kluver–Bucy syndrome, dietetic input should focus on managing portion size, choosing a balanced diet, and patient and carer education on the health benefits of a balanced diet.

Conclusion

Traumatic brain injury can have lasting and profound effects on the patient's physical and cognitive functioning. Providing adequate and safe nutritional support early post injury has been shown to promote better outcomes in recovery. Close monitoring of anthropometry, biochemistry, clinical and dietary aspects throughout the acute and rehabilitation stage will help to ensure the patient receives timely and apt adjustments in nutritional care.

Further reading

MRC CRASH Trial Collaborators. (2008) Predicting outcome after traumatic brain injury: practical prognostic models based on large cohort of international patients. *BMJ* 336: 1–10.

Internet resources

Brain Injury Rehabilitation Trust   www.birt.co.uk
Brainwave   www.brainwave.org.uk
Child Brain Injury Trust   www.childbraininjurytrust.org.uk
Headway   www.headway.org.uk
UK Acquired Brain Injury Forum   www.ukabif.org.uk

References

Acosta-Escribano J, Fernandez-Vivas M, Carmona T, *et al.* (2010) Gastric versus transpyloric feeding in severe traumatic brain injury: a prospective randomized trial. *Intensive Care Medicine* 36(9): 1532–1539.

Agha A, Rogers B, Mylotte D, *et al.* (2004a) Neuroendocrine dysfunction in the acute phase of traumatic brain injury. *Clinical Endocrinology* 60(5): 584–591.

Agha A, Rogers B, Sherlock M, *et al.* (2004b) Anterior pituitary dysfunction in survivors of traumatic brain injury. *Journal of Clinical Endocrinology and Metabolism* 89(10): 4929–2936.

American Association of Neuroscience Nurses (AANN). (2009) Nursing management of adults with severe traumatic brain injury: AANN Clinical Practice Guideline Series. Available at www.aann.org/pdf/cpg/aanntraumaticbraininjury.pdf. Accessed 26 April 2011.

Behan L, Phillips J, Thompson C, Agha A. (2007) Neuroendocrine disorders after traumatic brain injury. *Journal of Neurology, Neurosurgery and Psychiatry* 79(7): 753–759.

Brain Trauma Foundation. (2007) Guidelines for the management of severe traumatic brain injury, 3rd edn. Available at www.braintrauma.org/coma-guidelines/. Accessed 18 April 2011.

Brown A, Malec J, Diehl N, Englander J, Cifu D. (2007) Impairment at rehabilitation admission and 1 year after moderate-to-severe traumatic brain injury: a prospective multi-centre analysis. *Brain Injury* 27(7): 673–680.

Bruder N, Dumont JC, François G. (1991) Evolution of energy expenditure and nitrogen excretion in severe head-injured patients. *Critical Care Medicine* 19: 43–48.

Bruder N, Raynal M, Pellissier D, Courtinat C, Francois G. (1998) Influence of body temperature, with or without sedation, on energy expenditure in severe head injured patients. *Critical Care Medicine* 26(3): 568–572.

Bruns J, Hauser A. (2003) The epidemiology of traumatic brain injury: A review. *Epilepsia* 44(10): 2–10.

Bursztein S, Taitelman U, Myttenaere S, *et al.* (1978) Reduced oxygen consumption in catabolic states with mechanical ventilation. *Critical Care Medicine* 6(3): 162–164.

Cerda-Esteve M, Cuadrado-Godia E, Chillaron J, *et al.* (2008) Cerebral salt wasting syndrome: Review. *European Journal of Internal Medicine* 19(4): 249–254.

Charrueau C, Belabed L, Besson V, *et al.* (2009) Metabolic response and nutritional support in traumatic brain injury: evidence for resistance to renutrition. *Journal of Neurological Trauma* 26(11): 1911–1920.

Cherney L, Halper A. (1996) Swallowing problems in adults with traumatic brain injury. *Seminar in Neurology* 16(4): 349–353.

Clifton G, Robertson C, Grossman R, Hodge S, Foltz R, Garza C. (1984) The metabolic response to severe head injury. *Journal of Neurosurgery* 60(4): 687–696.

Cook A, Peppard A, Magnuson B. (2008–2009) Nutrition considerations in traumatic brain injury. *Nutrition in Clinical Practice* 23(6): 608–620.

Dempsey D, Guenter P, Mullen J, *et al.* (1985) Energy expenditure in acute trauma to the head with and without barbiturate therapy. *Surgery Gynaecology and Obstetrics* 160(2): 128–134.

Department of Health. (1991) *Dietary Reference Values for Food Energy and Nutrients for the United Kingdom.* (41) London: HSMO.

Doig G, Simpson F, Finfer S, *et al.*; Nutrition Guidelines Investigators of the ANZICS Clinical Trials Group. (2008) Effect of evidence based feeding guidelines on mortality of critically ill adults: a cluster randomised control trial. *JAMA* 300(23): 2731–2741.

Doig G, Heighes P, Simpson F, Sweetman E, Davies A. (2009) Early enteral nutrition, provided within 24 h of injury or intensive care unit admission, significantly reduces mortality in critically ill patients: a meta-analysis of randomised controlled trials. *Intensive Care Medicine* 35(12): 2018–2027.

Foley N, Marshall S, Pikul J, Salter K, Teasell R. (2008) Hypermetabolism following moderate to severe traumatic acute brain injury: A systematic review. *Journal of Neurotrauma* 25(12): 1415–1431.

French A, Merriman S. (1999) Nutritional status of a brain-injured population in a long-stay rehabilitation unit: a pilot study. *Journal of Human Nutrition and Dietetics* 12(1): 35–42.

Fruin A, Taylon C, Pettis M. (1986) Caloric requirements in patients with severe head injuries. *Surgical Neurology* 25(1): 25–28.

Ghirnikar R, Ling Lee Y, Eng L. (1997) Inflammation in traumatic brain injury: Role of cytokines and chemokines. *Neurochemical Research* 23(3): 329–330.

Giacino J, Ashwal S, Childs N, *et al.* (2002) The minimally conscious state: Definition and diagnostic criteria. *Neurology* 58(3): 349–353.

Greenwood R. (2002) Head injury For neurologists. *Journal of Neurology, Neurosurgery and Psychiatry with Practical Neurology* 73(1): 8–16.

Griffiths R. (2007) Too much of a good thing: the curse of overfeeding. *Critical Care* 11(6): 176.

Gross K, Norman J, Cook A. (2010) Contemporary pharmacologic issues in the management of traumatic brain injury. *Journal of Pharmacy Practice* 23(5): 425–440.

Haider W, Lackner F, Schlick W *et al.* (1975) Metabolic changes in the course of severe acute brain damage. *European Journal of Intensive Care Medicine* 1(1): 19–26.

Henry CJK. (2005) Basal metabolic rate studies in humans: measurement and development of new equations. *Public Health Nutrition* 8(7A): 1133–1152.

Hoffer L. (2003) Protein and energy provision in critical illness. *American Journal of Clinical Nutrition* 78(5): 906–911.

Jeremitsky E, Omert LA, Dunham MC, Wilberger J, Rodriguez A. (2005) The impact of hyperglycemia on patients with severe brain injury. *Journal of Trauma-Injury Infection & Critical Care* 58(1): 47–50.

Kao C, ChangLai S, Chieng P, Yen T. (1998) Gastric emptying in head-injured patients. *American Journal of Gastroenterology* 93(7): 1108–1112.

Krakau K. (2010) *Energy Balance Out of Balance After Severe Traumatic Brain Injury.* Digital Comprehensive Summaries of Uppsala Dissertations from the Faculty of Medicine 523. Uppsala Universitet.

Krakau K, Omne-Ponten M, Karlsson T, Borg J. (2007) Metabolism and nutrition in patients with moderate and severe traumatic brain injury: A systematic review. *Brain Injury* 20(4): 345–367.

Krakau K, Hansson A, Odlund Olin A, Karlsson T, De Boussard C, Borg J. (2010) Resources and routines for nutritional assessment of patients with severe traumatic brain injury. *Scandinavian Journal of Caring Sciences* 24(1): 3–13.

Kreymann K, Berger M, Deutz N, *et al.* (2006) ESPEN guidelines on Enteral Nutrition: Intensive Care. *Clinical Nutrition* 25(2): 210–223.

Lewis W, Chwals W, Benotti P, *et al.* (1988) Bedside assessment of the work of breathing. *Critical Care Medicine* 16(2): 117–122.

Maas A, Stocchetti N, Bullock R. (2008) Moderate and severe traumatic brain injury in adults. *Lancet Neurology* 7(8): 725–741.

McCartan D, Fleming F, Motherway C, Grace P (2008) Management and outcome in patients following head injury admitted to an Irish Regional Hospital. *Brain Injury* 22(4): 305–312.

McClain C, Twyman D, Ott L, *et al.* (1986) Serum and urine zinc response in head-injured patients. *Journal of Neurosurgery* 64(2): 224–230.

McEvoy C, Cran G, Cooke S, Young I. (2009) Resting energy expenditure in non-ventilated, non-sedated patients recovering from serious traumatic brain injury; Comparison of predicted equations with indirect calorimetry values. *Clinical Nutrition* 28(5): 526–532.

Medic-Stojanoska M, Pekic S, Curic N, Djilas-Ivanovic D, Popovic V. (2007) Evolving hypopituitarism as a consequence of traumatic brain injury (TBI) in childhood – call for attention. *Endocrine* 31(3): 268–271.

Meshkini A, Mahboubi B, Ostad R, Lotfinia E. (2009) Effect of zinc supplementation on recovery trend of head injury. *Medical Journal of Tabriz University Medical Sciences* 31(1): 61–65.

National Institutes of Health. (2008) National Institute of Neurological Disorders and Stroke. Available at www.ninds.nih.gov/disorders/kluver_bucy/kluver_bucy.htm. Accessed 12 April 2011.

National Institute for Health and Care Excellence (NICE). (2007) Triage, assessment, investigation and early management of head injury in infants, children and adults. Available at www.nice.org.uk. Accessed 25 April 2011.

Oder W, Goldenberg G, Spatt J, Podreka I, Binder H, Deecke L. (1992) behavioural and psychosocial sequelae of severe closed head injury and regional cerebral blood flow: a SPECT study. *Journal of Neurology, Neurosurgery and Psychiatry with Practical Neurology* 55(6): 475–480.

Ott L, McClain C, Gillespie M, Young B. (1994) Nutritional and metabolic variables correlate with amino acid forearm flux in

SECTION 7

patients with severe head injury. *Critical Care Medicine* 22(3): 393–398.

Patradoon-Ho P, Scheinberg A, Baur L. (2005) Obesity in Children and adolescents with acquired brain injury. *Paediatric Rehabilitation* 8(4): 303–308.

Perel P, Yanagawa T, Bunn F, Roberts IG, Wentz R. (2006) Nutritional support for head-injured patients. *Cochrane Database of Systematic Reviews* 4: CD001530.

Polderman K, Peerdeman S, Girbes A. (2001) Hypophosphatemia and hypomagnesemia induced by cooling in patients with severe head injury. *Journal of Neurosurgery* 94(5): 697–705.

Popovic V. (2005) GH Deficiency as The Most Common Pituitary Defect After TBI: Clinical Implications. *Pituitary* 3–4(8): 239–243.

Rajpal V, Johnston J. (2009) Nutrition management of traumatic brain injury patients. *Support Line* 31(1): 10–19.

Raurich J, Ibanez J. (1994) Metabolic rate in severe head trauma. *Journal of Parenteral and Enteral Nutrition* 18(6): 521–524.

Schneider H, Kreitschmann-Andermahr I, Ghigo E, Stalla G, Agha A. (2007) Hypothalamopituitary dysfunction following traumatic brain injury and aneurismal subarachnoid hemorrhage: a systematic review. *JAMA* 298(12): 1429–1438.

Shiga T, Ikoma K, Katoh C, *et al.* (2006) Loss of neuronal integrity: a cause of hypometabolism in patients with traumatic brain injury without MRI abnormality in the chronic stage. *European Journal of Nuclear Medicine and Molecular Imaging* 33(7): 817–822.

Sussex Critical Care Network. (2009) Guidelines for the management of the patient with severe traumatic head injury in ICU. Available at www.sussexcritcare.nhs.uk. Accessed 2 April 2011.

Tagliaferri F, Compagnone C, Korsic M, Servadei F, Kraus J. (2005) A systematic review of brain injury epidemiology in Europe. *European Journal of Neurosurgery* 148(3): 255–268.

Tan M, Zhu J, Yin H. (2011) Enteral nutrition in patients with severe traumatic brain injury: reasons for intolerance and medical management. *British Journal of Neurosurgery* 25(1): 2–8.

Tanriverdi F, Senyurek H, Unluhizarci K, Selcuklu A, Cassenueva F, Kelestimur F. (2006) High risk of hypopituitarism after traumatic brain injury: A prospective investigation of anterior pituitary function in the acute phase and 12 months after trauma. *Journal of Clinical Endocrinology & Metabolism* 91(6): 2105–2111.

Teasdale G, Jennett B. (1974). Assessment of coma and impaired consciousness. A practical scale. *Lancet* 2: 81–84.

Thornhill S, Teasdale G, Murray G, McEwan J, Roy C, Penny K. (2000) Disability in young people and adults one year after head injury: prospective cohort study. *BMJ* 320: 1631–1635.

Tisdall M, Crocker M, Watkiss J, Smith M. (2006) Disturbances of sodium in critically ill adult neurologic patients: a clinical review. *Journal of Neurosurgical Anesthesiology* 18(1): 57–63.

Turner-Stokes L, Nair A, Sedki I, Disler PB, Wade DT. (2011) Multidisciplinary rehabilitation for acquired brain injury in adults of working age. *Cochrane Collaboration*. Available at http://onlinelibrary.wiley.com/o/cochrane/clsysrev/articles/CD004170/pdf_fs.html. Accessed 12 April 2011.

Twyman D, Young B, Ott L, Norton J, Bivins B. (1985) High protein enteral feedings: A means of achieving positive nitrogen balance in head injured patients. *Journal of Parenteral and Enteral Nutrition* 9(6): 679–684.

Vizzinni A, Aranda-Michel J. (2011) Nutritional support in head injury. *Nutrition* 27(2): 129–132.

Voevodin M, Haala R. (2007) Eight years of nutrition intervention for a young person with an acquired brain injury. *Nutrition and Dietetics* 64(3): 207–211.

Walker S, Wickes B. (2005) *Educating children with Acquired Brain Injury*. The Brain and Spine Foundation. London. David Fulton Publishers.

Weekes E, Elia M. (1996) Observations on the patterns of 24-hour energy expenditure changes in body composition and gastric emptying in head-injured patients receiving nasogastric tube feeding. *Journal of Parenteral and Enteral Nutrition* 20(1): 31–37.

Wijdicks EFM. (2001) The diagnosis of brain death. *New England Journal of Medicine* 344(16): 1215–1216.

Young B, Ott L, Kasarskis E, *et al.* (1996) Zinc supplementation is associated with improved neurologic recovery rate and visceral protein levels of patients with severe closed head injury. *Journal of Neurotrauma* 13(1): 25–34.

Young A, Ott L, Beard D, Dempsey R, Tibbs P, McClain C. (1988) The acute-phase response of the brain injured patient. *Journal of Neurosurgery* 69(3): 375–380.

Zafonte R, Mann N. (1997) Cerebral salt wasting syndrome in brain injury patients: A potential cause of hyponatremia. *Archives of Physical Medicine and Rehabilitation* 78(5): 540–542.

7.17.3   Spinal cord injury

Anthony Twist and Samford Wong

Key points

- Energy expenditure in the acute post injury period is reduced; care is needed to avoid overfeeding.

- Protein requirements may be high.

- A reduction in energy expenditure during rehabilitation increases the risk of excessive weight gain.

- Neurogenic bowel dysfunction may require dietary fibre intake adjustment.

- There is a high risk of pressure ulcers; therefore, nutritionally balanced diets are essential.

There are approximately 40 000 people living in the UK with spinal cord injuries (SCIs) (Spinal Injuries Association, 2009), with an incidence of approximately 8–12 cases per million population. In 2001 (the most recent year for which figures are available), 744 people experienced spinal pathology sufficiently serious to require admission to a spinal unit in the UK or Ireland. The most common causes of SCI were falls and road traffic accidents (Table 7.17.13). Other injuries such as head and chest injury often coexist and may complicate management and

Table 7.17.13 Causes of spinal pathology in the UK and Ireland in people admitted to spinal cord injury centres in 2001 [from Inman, the British Association of Spinal Cord Injury Specialists (BASCIS)]

Cause of injury	Number	%
Trauma		
Road traffic accidents	230	39.0
Falls	269	45.5
Sharp trauma/assaults	14	2.4
Sports	46	7.8
Knocked over/object falling	13	2.2
Collision/lifting	2	0.3
Trauma (not specified)	15	2.5
Total trauma	*589*	*100*
Non-trauma		
Epidural injections	3	1.9
Transverse myelitis	12	7.7
Vascular causes	30	19.3
Tumour	23	14.8
Infection	19	12.3
Disc (thoracic and lumbar)	10	6.5
Cervical myelopathy	15	9.7
Guillain–Barré	8	5.2
Stenosis (lumbar and thoracic)	7	4.5
Spondylolisthesis	1	0.6
Haematoma	9	5.8
Unnecessary	2	1.3
Congenital	1	0.6
Radiation myelitis	2	1.3
Rheumatoid arthritis/systemic lupus erythematosus	3	1.9
Syringomyelia/arachnoid cysts	7	4.5
Scoliosis/spinal cysts	2	1.3
Intubation	1	0.6
Total non-trauma	*155*	*100*

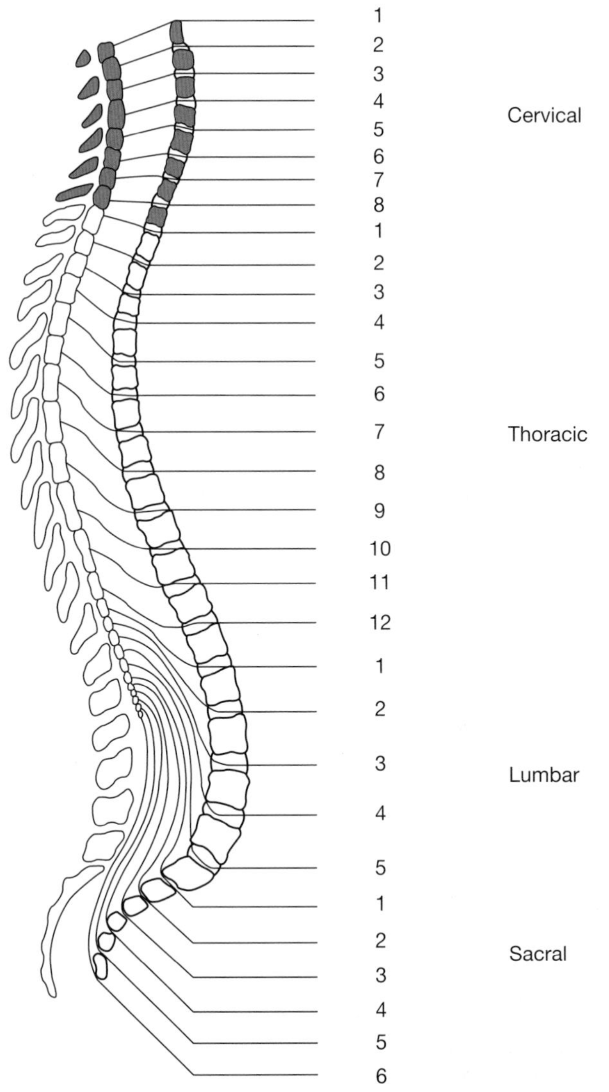

Figure 7.17.2   The spinal cord

rehabilitation. The UK has eleven SCI centres, which have a total of 458 beds for the rehabilitation of people with a SCI. The first UK SCI centre was opened in Stoke Mandeville in 1944.

The metabolic response to injury is well documented (see Chapter 7.17.1) and the prevalence of malnutrition and its effects on the person with SCI have been recognised since the time of Hippocrates (Guttmann, 1973). Prior to World War II, few people with SCI survived more than 2 years. Today long term survival is normal and the mean age for sustaining a SCI appears to be increasing. For example, the Northern General Hospital, Sheffield's SCI centre showed a rise in mean age for new admissions from 32 years in 2007/8 to 48 years in 2009/10 (personal communication).

As with anyone suffering acute injury necessitating subsequent rehabilitation, dietetic care should be an integral part of management. Dietetic provision in UK spinal injury centres is very variable, ranging from 7.5 to 31 hours/week (Wong *et al.*, 2012a). The level of experience of the dietitians is also variable, with some units employing specialist dietitians (NHS band 8a) and others using relatively less experienced staff (NHS band 5).

Definitions

The effects of a SCI depends on which segments of the spinal cord are damaged (Figure 7.17.2). The American Spinal Injury Association Impairment Scale (ASIA, 2002) focuses on 10 key muscles and 10 key sensory points to be tested during neurological assessment. Figure 7.17.3 shows the likely consequences of SCI on both motor and sensory dermatomes (areas of skin supplied with afferent nerve fibres by a single posterior spinal root) as define by the International Spinal Cord Society (ISCOS, 2006). These consequences may include:

SECTION 7

Patient Name _____

Examiner Name _____ Date/Time of Exam_____

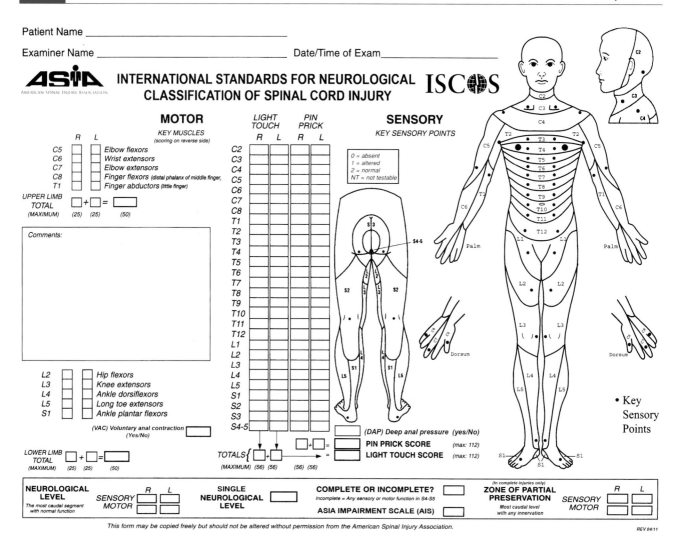

Figure 7.17.3 International standards for neurological classification of spinal cord injury (source: International Standards for Neurological Classification of Spinal Cord Injury 2013. Reproduced with permission of the American Spinal Injury Association)

- *Complete and incomplete lesions:*
  - In a complete lesion, all neurological function is lost below the level of the lesion.
  - In an incomplete lesion, there is partial preservation of neurological function and any combination of motor (muscle), sensory (feeling) or autonomic function may be spared (nerves of the autonomic system control those body functions, which are not under conscious control).
  - Brown–Séquard syndrome or central cord syndrome describes different patterns of incomplete lesion, usually occurring as a result of neck injuries. These and other syndromes are described in the ABC of Spinal Cord Injury (*see* Further reading).
- *Paraplegia* – function of the lower limbs is lost as a result of damage to the thoracic, lumbar or, to a lesser extent, sacral cord segments.
- *Tetraplegia (quadriplegia)* – this results from damage to cervical cord segments causing loss of function in all four limbs.

- In both paraplegia and tetraplegia there is impairment of autonomic function, including bladder and bowel control.
- *Muscle wasting* – post injury this results in a reduction of lean body mass and, in the longer term, immobility encourages an increase in total body fat (Shizgal *et al.*, 1986; Rasmann Nuhlicek *et al.*, 1988; Spungen *et al.*, 2003).
- *Autonomic dysreflexia (AD)* – people with SCI above the T6 level (thoracic vertebra) can experience AD. It is a group of abnormal signs and symptoms triggered by a noxious stimulus below the level of the lesion that causes an increase in autonomic activity (Consortium for Spinal Cord Medicine, 2008). It is characterised by a sudden, severe headache secondary to an uncontrolled elevation of blood pressure, flushing and profuse sweating. If untreated, the hypertension may progress to fatal complications, such as cerebral haemorrhage or acute myocardial infarction. The most common nutrition related stimuli are an over

Muscle Function Grading

0 = total paralysis

1 = palpable or visible contraction

2 = active movement, full range of motion (ROM) with gravity eliminated

3 = active movement, full ROM against gravity

4 = active movement, full ROM against gravity and moderate resistance in a muscle specific position.

5 = (normal) active movement, full ROM against gravity and full resistance in a muscle specific position expected from an otherwise unimpaired peson.

5* = (normal) active movement, full ROM against gravity and sufficient resistance to be considered normal if identified inhibiting factors (i.e. pain, disuse) were not present.

NT = not testable (i.e. due to immobilization, severe pain such that the patient cannot be graded, amputation of limb, or contracture of >50% of the range of motion).

ASIA Impairment (AIS) Scale

☐ **A = Complete.** No sensory or motor function is preserved in the sacral segments S4-S5.

☐ **B = Sensory Incomplete.** Sensory but not motor function is preserved below the neurological level and includes the sacral segments S4-S5 (light touch, pin prick at S4-S5: or deep anal pressure (DAP)), AND no motor function is preserved more than three levels below the motor level on either side of the body.

☐ **C = Motor Incomplete.** Motor function is preserved below the neurological level**, and more than half of key muscle functions below the single neurological level of injury (NLI) have a muscle grade less than 3 (Grades 0-2).

☐ **D = Motor Incomplete.** Motor function is preserved below the neurological level**, and at least half (half or more) of key muscle functions below the NLI have a muscle grade ≥ 3.

☐ **E = Normal.** If sensation and motor function as tested with the ISNCSCI are graded as normal in all segments, and the patient had prior deficits, then the AIS grade is E. Someone without an initial SCI does not receive an AIS grade.

**For an individual to receive a grade of C or D, i.e. motor incomplete status, they must have either (1) voluntary anal sphincter contraction or (2) sacral sensory sparing <u>with</u> sparing of motor function more than three levels below the motor level for that side of the body. The Standards at this time allows even non-key muscle function more than 3 levels below the motor level to be used in determining motor incomplete status (AIS B versus C).

NOTE: When assessing the extent of motor sparing below the level for distinguishing between AIS B and C, the **motor level** on each side is used; whereas to differentiate between AIS C and D (based on proportion of key muscle functions with strength grade 3 or greater) the **single neurological level** is used.

Steps in Classification

The following order is recommended in determining the classification of individuals with SCI.

1. Determine sensory levels for right and left sides.
2. Determine motor levels for right and left sides.
   Note: in regions where there is no myotome to test, the motor level is presumed to be the same as the sensory level, if testable motor function above that level is also normal.
3. Determine the single neurological level.
   This is the lowest segment where motor and sensory function is normal on both sides, and is the most cephalad of the sensory and motor levels determined in steps 1 and 2.
4. Determine whether the injury is Complete or Incomplete. (i.e. absence or presence of sacral sparing)
   *If voluntary anal contraction = **No** AND all S4-5 sensory scores = **0** AND deep anal pressure = **No**, then injury is COMPLETE. Otherwise, injury is incomplete.*
5. Determine ASIA Impairment Scale (AIS) Grade:

Is injury **Complete**?   If **YES**, AIS=A and can record ZPP
NO ↓   (lowest dermatome or myotome on each side with some preservation)

Is injury
motor **Incomplete**?   If **NO**, AIS=B
YES ↓   (Yes=voluntary anal contraction OR motor function more than three levels below the motor level on a given side, if the patient has sensory incomplete classification)

Are <u>at least</u> half of the key muscles below the single <u>neurological</u> level graded 3 or better?

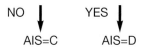

If sensation and motor function is normal in all segments, **AIS=E**
Note: AIS E is used in follow-up testing when an individual with a documented SCI has recovered normal function. If at initial testing no deficits are found, the individual is neurologically intact; the ASIA Impairment Scale does not apply.

Figure 7.17.3 *(Continued)*

---

distended bladder, bowel impaction, urinary infection and pressure ulcers.

Management

Initial post injury period (within the first week of injury)

Complex physiological changes occur following SCI and these vary with:

- Level of the lesion.
- ASIA scale or Frankel classification (extent of damage to the spinal cord).
- Presence of concomitant injury or illness.
- Time elapsed since injury.

These physiological changes result in a dynamic metabolic state that may adversely affect the nutritional status at any time (Worthington *et al.*, 1993). If left untreated, this catabolic state can lead to loss of lean muscle mass and poorer clinical outcomes, including impaired wound healing, and increased risk of infection, premature mortality and healthcare costs. The association between acute SCI and deterioration in nutritional status can persist for several months post injury (Marian, 2004).

The presence of delayed gastric emptying and paralytic ileus during this initial post injury period often preclude or complicate enteral feeding (see Chapter 7.17.1). Unfortunately, other priorities in clinical care may result in neglect of nutritional needs. Additionally, weighing the SCI individual is often difficult, as is interpretation of anthropometry. However, most people with SCI transferred from a general hospital to a spinal injury centre should have had at least a nutritional risk assessment by a validated nutrition screening tool, such as the Spinal Nutrition Screening Tool (SNST) (Wong *et al.*, 2012b) (see Appendix A11), in order to identify the need for further nutritional interventions; this assessment should have been repeated periodically unless transfer occurred very quickly.

Nutritional requirements

Energy requirements

The energy needs of SCI individuals are far from clear (Cox *et al.*, 1985; Kearns *et al.*, 1992; Peruzzi *et al.*, 1994; Rodriguez *et al.*, 1997; Barco *et al.*, 2002). However, in contrast to people with trauma or head injury, it appears that energy expenditure is reduced after SCI (Shedlock & Laventures, 1990; Buchholz & Pencharz, 2004). Patients with SCI have reduced metabolic activity due to denervated muscle and actual energy needs are at least 10% below predicted needs [American Dietetic Association (ADA), 2009]. Indirect calorimetry (IC) is more accurate than estimation of energy needs, but in the absence of IC, interpreting predicted energy requirements with caution is recommended. This should avoid overfeeding, which can have adverse effects on glucose tolerance and lead to respiratory dysfunction due to excessive carbon dioxide production (EAST, 2003). Dietitians must exercise judgement and be alert to emerging research on energy requirements in SCI.

Iron

Anaemia is common in acute SCI even without visible blood losses (Huang *et al.*, 1990). Providing an adequate nutritional intake of iron is essential. Adequate vitamin C intakes help improve iron absorption from non-haem sources.

Vitamins

Laven *et al.* (1989) demonstrated deficiencies in a variety of vitamins, including vitamin C, folate and thiamine, which drop to their lowest level 2 weeks following injury and remain low for some weeks. They suggested full vitamin screens to ensure these deficiencies are recognised and rectified. Rice *et al.* (1995) recommended that a daily multivitamin should be given to all acute SCI individuals.

Subsequent post injury period (within the first 12 weeks following injury)

An SCI individual should be transferred as soon as possible to an SCI centre, where the importance of nutritional assessment, early identification of those at nutritional risk and appropriate nutritional support is being increasingly recognised (RCP, 2008; MASCIP, 2010). Dietitians who manage people with SCI need to understand the extent of their injuries (Figure 7.17.2) and acknowledge the profound psychological effects of these injuries. Whenever clinically possible, SCI individuals should be fed in a semi recumbent position; this may not be possible if they have not undergone spinal fixation. Consideration then needs to be given to options for safely feeding SCI individuals in a fully recumbent position.

Nutritional status is adversely affected by SCI, particularly during the first 2–4 weeks (Cheshire & Coats, 1969; Laven *et al.*, 1989), and nutritional depletion resulting from the initial metabolic response to trauma may be severe. Negative nitrogen balance after SCI is inevitable, correlating with the level and extent of injury, and may persist for as long as 7 weeks (Hadley, 2002). Protein needs are unclear but 2 g of protein /kg/day is suggested (Kearns *et al.*, 1992; Peruzzi *et al.*, 1994; Marian 2004; ADA, 2009).

Gastrointestinal problems arise in both the acute and long term setting, with paralytic ileus and gastric ulcers commonly occurring during the first 4 weeks post injury, and lower tract dysfunction thereafter (Frost, 1998).

Table 7.17.14 Factors that may reduce dietary intake in spinal cord injury (SCI)

Category	Factors
Neurological	Extent of SCI Pain associated with SCI Surgical intervention of spinal cord
Psychological	Depression due to SCI Social isolation Confusion
Infections	Urinary tract Bladder Chest Catheter related Infected pressure ulcers
Drugs	Polypharmacy Nausea and vomiting Diarrhoea
Physical difficulties	Bed rest post SCI Refusal or reluctance to eat and drink Mechanical dysphagia due to ventilator
Respiratory	Chest infections Ventilating support Tracheostomy tube
Gastrointestinal	Neurological or mechanical dysphagia Paralytic ileus Nausea and vomiting Gastrointestinal bleeding; Diarrhoea or constipation Early satiety Abdominal injuries
Social	Recreational drug use Alcohol abuse Stress Lack of social support

Nutritional assessment

The prevalence of malnutrition is common amongst SCI individuals. A recent study of people admitted to UK SCI centres found that approximately 40% were at risk of undernutrition and 45% were overweight (Wong *et al.*, 2011a). Factors that are likely to reduce dietary intake are summarised in Table 7.17.14. Factors likely to increase nutritional requirements include:

- Associated injuries, e.g. long bone fractures and head injuries.
- Pressure ulcers.
- Fever, infection and sepsis.

Use of the disease specific nutrition screening tool

National and international reports (NICE, 2006; RCP, 2008; Council of Europe, 2003) have highlighted the importance of nutritional screening as an important step to address malnutrition. The SNS tool (see Appendix A11) has been developed for use in people with SCI and externally validated in this population (Wong *et al.*, 2012b). It is based on eight parameters:

- Body mass index (BMI).
- Age.

- Level of SCI.
- Presence of comorbidities.
- Skin conditions.
- Diet.
- Appetite.
- Ability to eat.

Assessing weight loss since injury

The degree of weight loss since SCI is an important indicator of nutritional depletion; most individuals will be able to recall their preinjury weight. Obtaining current weight can be difficult even if bed weighing scales are available. It is recommended that weight be taken on admission, and this repeated periodically for those identified to be at nutritional risk (NICE, 2006). In some cases, estimation of weight loss has to be done visually; however, it should be borne in mind that muscle wasting may have resulted from denervation following the SCI and bed rest rather than nutritional depletion.

Other assessments

Estimates of muscle mass from measurements such as mid arm muscle circumference are likely to be distorted by the effects of the SCI and any consequent paraplegia. Estimates of adiposity from BMI will be dependent on the ability to obtain a meaningful estimate of current body weight. While direct measurement of height is likely to be impossible, a reliable estimate of height can be estimated from ulna length measurements (see Appendix A7); knee height or ulna length should be acceptable. A 24-hour urine collection to measure urea nitrogen can be useful in determining protein status (Agarwal *et al.*, 1987). Bioelectrical impedance measurement is potentially useful, although hydration states can fluctuate in the acute period.

Current dietary intake

Although it is often possible to obtain estimates of previous and current dietary intake from the SCI individual, records of food and fluid intake and changes in appetite noted by care staff should also be taken into account. People with SCI appear to have a reduced dietary intake in SCI centres, but due to the enforced immobility, they may be meeting their energy requirement (personal communication).

Continuing rehabilitation phase (after 12 weeks post injury)

The aim of rehabilitation is to enable the individual to develop the maximum potential possible for their disability (Chapter 7.6.6). For the person who has lost weight during the immediate post injury period, weight regain and restoration of muscle mass are a priority so that the person is are able to derive maximum benefit from physiotherapy and occupational therapy sessions. Where normal food intake is insufficient, additional nutritious snacks and prescribed oral nutritional supplements may be required. Reduction in energy needs is proportional to the amount of denervated muscle a SCI individual has.

Table 7.17.15 Guide to weighing individuals with spinal cord injuries

Degree of mobility	Suitable weighing method
Fully mobile SCI individuals	
Good balance	Standing scales
Poor balance	Sit down scales
Wheelchair dependent	
Able to transfer and can hold legs free from the floor	Sit down scales
Unable/inconvenient to transfer from wheelchair	Wheelchair weighing scales
Able to transfer but cannot hold legs free from the chair	Weighbridge Wheelchair weighing scales Weighbridge
On bed or trolley and can be lifted by hoist	Hoist scale with sling or stretcher attachment
Bed bound and bed not easily moved	Weighbridge
Bed bound, bed cannot be moved	Bed with weighing device Portable bed weighing scales

Manufacturers of this equipment are given at the end of this chapter.

The ADA (2009) suggested using 22 kcal/kg of body weight for those with quadriplegia and 28 kcal/kg for those with paraplegia to estimate (with caution) energy needs. If individuals are unable to meet their nutritional needs by oral intake alone, overnight enteral feeding may be a useful method of nutritional support, as this strategy does not interfere with daytime therapy sessions (see Chapter 6.4).

At this rehabilitation stage it is usually easier to measure and monitor SCI individuals than in earlier stages; Table 7.17.15 lists methods of weighing. However, due to the associated muscle wasting, the ideal BMI range is suggested to be 18.5–22 kg/m^2 (Laughton *et al.*, 2009).

Obesity

As rehabilitation progresses, becoming overweight is an increasing risk as appetite and food intake return to, or even exceed, preinjury levels. Body composition changes occur after SCI in response to reduced physical activity, immobilisation and muscle atrophy, resulting in basal metabolic rate (BMR) reduction by 7–48% (Mollinger *et al.*, 1985), depending on the level of injury. Predicting energy expenditure with the use of standard equations can therefore lead to overestimation of energy requirements (Cox *et al.*, 1985; Monroe *et al.*, 1998). In a cross sectional study of 133 men with SCI, Spungen *et al.* (2003) found that body composition changes were exaggerated with advancing age and resulted in adiposity levels and loss of muscle mass significantly greater than those of an ethnicity matched able bodied cohort.

The management of obesity in individuals with SCI is very important due its high prevalence (Groah *et al.*, 2009). There is limited data on the rate of weight gain after SCI in the UK, but in comparison with the UK

SECTION 7

national survey data (Henderson *et al.*, 2003), SCI individuals (Groah *et al.*, 2009) seem more likely to become overweight and obese than the able bodied population (74% and 40%, respectively).

The detrimental health consequences of obesity are well documented (see Chapter 7.13.1). The risk of mortality associated with cardiovascular disease (CVD) is twice as high in SCI individuals compared with able bodied individuals (Myers *et al.*, 2007). In long term SCI individuals, CVD morbidity and mortality now exceeds that caused by renal and pulmonary conditions, with CVD becoming the primary cause of death (Myers *et al.*, 2007). In addition, overweight SCI individuals are higher risk of developing pressure ulcers (Elsner & Gefen, 2008), and have increased difficulties in managing daily life compared with overweight individuals without SCI (Abresch *et al.*, 2007).

Evidence suggests a simple dietetic intervention (Chen *et al.*, 2006; Wong *et al.*, 2011b) can help individuals with SCI to lose weight without compromising lean body mass. Although the intervention incurs additional cost, it has the potential to significantly decrease long term healthcare expenditure if health outcome and quality of life are improved. Dietetic intervention, including comprehensive nutrition education and counselling on a cardioprotective diet, should be offered to at risk individuals. This is particularly important for those who may previously have had little interest or knowledge of nutritional issues.

Other nutrition related problems

Neurogenic bowel dysfunction

Neurogenic bowel dysfunction (NBD) is one of many impairments that result from SCI and is often quoted as being one of the most distressing problems (Lynch *et al.*, 2000). According to Stiens *et al.*, (1997) two patterns of NBD occur post SCI:

- *Upper motor neurone (UMN) or reflexic bowel syndrome* – generally occurs in cervical and thoracic injury. It results in constipation with faecal retention behind a spastic anal sphincter.
- *Lower motor neurone (LMN) or areflexic bowel syndrome* – generally occurs in lumbar or sacral injury where the conus (the conical end of the spinal cord) or nerve roots are damaged. It produces constipation with a high risk of frequent incontinence through a lax external sphincter mechanism.

Each type of NBD requires different bowel management and adjustments to dietary intake (particularly dietary fibre) may be required to produce an ideal stool consistency. Chemical stimulants are commonly used in UMN where a softer stool is required. A high fibre intake with adequate fluids may be helpful. Manual evacuation is commonly used if a harder or drier stool is required and a reduced fibre intake may be more appropriate.

The SCI centres have produced guidelines on bowel management (SCIC-UK&I, 2009), which emphasise that, whilst it is important to maintain a balanced diet, either an increase or decrease in dietary fibre intake (particularly insoluble fibre intake) may be helpful and that each

person with SCI should be individually assessed. Further research is needed to determine the exact optimal dietary fibre intake for individuals with SCI.

If enteral feeding is required, it has been found anecdotally to be best tolerated if started with a non-fibre feed and then introducing fibre containing feed gradually to toleration, perhaps ending with a feed that is a mixture of fibre and non-fibre. Additional fluids may be necessary due to the slower colonic transit time that results in increased resorption of fluid. In practice, at least 2 L or more of fluid is usually recommended.

Pressure ulcers

Individuals with SCI are at high risk of pressure ulcers due to the loss of sensation of pressure, skin ischaemia, incontinence, poor nutritional intake and inability or reluctance to change position. Both underweight and overweight increase the likelihood of pressure sore development. Pressure ulcers can significantly increase nutritional requirements due to protein rich exudate and also expose tissue to infection. Antibiotic treatment of pressure sores may also reduce food intake as a result of associated side effects (see Chapter 7.17.6).

Metabolic syndrome

The SCI population is at higher risk of diabetes mellitus, metabolic syndrome and coronary heart disease due to decreased mobility, increased obesity and, in particular, central obesity. Early lifestyle modification and dietetic intervention targeted for at risk individuals to prevent the development of nutrition related complications should be part of the rehabilitation programme.

Renal calculi

The SCI population has a greater risk of renal calculi, primarily as a result of recurrent bladder infections, increased retention of calcium by the bladder and kidneys, and immobility. To help prevent bladder infections, SCI individuals are normally recommended to drink at least 2 L/day of water based fluids; restriction of calcium is not indicated (Rice *et al.*, 1995).

Some people take cranberry juice in the belief that it might help in preventing bladder infections; however, there little research on this topic. A Cochrane review (Jepson *et al.*, 2004) in otherwise healthy adults indicated that, while there is some evidence of beneficial effects from regular cranberry consumption in women, the optimum dosage or method of administration, e.g. juice or tablets, remains unknown and that further better designed trials are needed. Since cranberry juice may enhance the anticoagulant effect of warfarin, those on warfarin should avoid it. In addition, it may provide a significant amount of energy and contribute to weight gain.

Osteoporosis

Individuals are at increased risk of osteoporosis due to lack of weight bearing exercise; therefore, osteoporotic fractures occur mostly in the lower limbs and pelvis. Risk is greatest within the first post injury year (Harrison,

2006). A well balanced diet incorporating sufficient calcium is recommended (see Chapter 7.9.1).

Nutritional support may be required at any stage following a SCI to offset catabolic losses and commence the process of nutritional repletion (see Chapters 6.3).

Further reading

Campagnolo DI, Kirshbaum S. (2011) *Spinal Cord Medicine*, 2nd edn. Philadelphia: Lippincott, Williams and Wilkins.

Grundy D, Swain A. (2002) *The ABC of Spinal Cord Injury*, 4th edn. London: BMJ Publications.

Harrison P (ed). (2006) *Managing Spinal Cord Injuries: Continuing Care*. Milton Keynes: SIA.

Harrison P (ed). (2007) *Managing Spinal Cord Injuries: The First 48 Hours*, 2nd edn. Milton Keynes: SIA.

Lin WV (ed in chief). (2010) *Spinal Cord Medicine Principles and Practice*, 2nd edn. New York: Demos.

Multidisciplinary Association of Spinal Cord Injury Professionals (MASCIP). (2010) *Management of the Older Person with a New Spinal Cord Injury*. Stanmore: MASCIP.

Internet resources

British Association of Spinal Cord Injury Specialist (BASCIS) www.bascis.pwp.blueyonder.co.uk

International Spinal Cord Society (ISCOS) www.iscos.org.uk

Locations of the SCI Centres in the UK and Ireland www.bascis.org.uk/?page_id=171

Multidisciplinary Association of Spinal Cord Injury Professionals (MASCIP) www.mascip.co.uk

Spinal Injuries Association www.spinal.co.uk

Spinal Injuries Scotland www.sisonline.org

Weighing equipment manufacturers

Arjohuntleigh UK and Ireland www.arjo.com.uk

Avery Weigh-Tronix www.averyweigh-tronix.com

Marsden Weighing Machine Group Ltd www.marsden-weighing.co.uk

Seca www.seca.com

References

Abresch RT, McDonald DA, Widman LM, McGinnis K, Hickey KJ. (2007) Impact of spinal cord dysfunction and obesity on the health-related quality of life of children and adolescents. *Journal of Spinal Cord Medicine* 30(Suppl 1): S112–S118.

Agarwal N, Lee BY, Del Guercio LRM. (1987) Urinary creatinine excretion in spinal cord injury patients. *Nutrition* 3: 192.

American Spinal Injury Association (ASIA). (2002) *International Standards for Neurological Classification of Spinal Cord Injury* (revised 2000). Chicago: ASIA.

American Dietetic Association. (2009) Spinal cord injury (SCI). Evidence-based nutrition practice guideline. Available at www.adaevidencelibrary.com.

Barco KT, Smith RA, Peerless JR, Plaisier BR, Chima CS. (2002) Energy expenditure assessment and validation after acute spinal injury. *Nutrition in Clinical Practice* 17: 309–313.

Buchholz AC, Pencharz PB. (2004) Energy expenditure in chronic spinal cord injury. *Current Opinion in Clinical Nutrition and Metabolism Care* 7: 635–639.

Chen Y, Henson S, Jackson AB, Richards JS. (2006) Obesity Intervention in persons with spinal cord injury. *Spinal Cord* 44: 82–91.

Cheshire DJE, Coats DA. (1969) Respiratory and metabolic management in acute tetraplegia. *Paraplegia* 4: 1–23.

Consortium for Spinal Cord Medicine. (2008) *Early Acute Management in Adults with Spinal Cord Injury: A Clinical Practice Guideline for Health-Care Providers*. Washington, DC: Paralyzed Veterans of America.

Cox SAR, Weiss SM, Posuniak EA, Worthington P, Prioleau M, Heffley G. (1985) Energy expenditure after spinal cord injury: an evaluation of stable rehabilitating patients. *Journal of Trauma* 25: 419–423.

Council of Europe Committee of Ministers (2003) Resolution RESAP on food and nutritional care in hospitals. Available at https://wcd.coe.int/ViewDoc.jsp?id=85747. Accessed 26 July 2012.

Eastern Association for the Surgery of Trauma (EAST). (2003) *Practice Management Guidelines Work Group. Practice Management Guidelines for Nutritional Support of the Trauma Patient*. Allentown, PA: EAST.

Elsner JJ, Gefen A. (2008) Is obesity a risk factor for deep tissue injury in patients with spinal cord injury? *Journal of Biomechanics* 41: 3322–3331.

Frost FS. (1998) Spinal cord injury: Gastrointestinal implications and management. *Topics in Spinal Cord Injury Rehabilitation* 4(2): 56–80.

Groah SL, Nash MS, Ljungberg IH, *et al*. (2009) Nutrient intake and body habits after spinal cord injury: an analysis by sex and level of injury. *Journal of Spinal Cord Medicine* 32: 25–33.

Guttmann L. (1973) *Spinal Cord Injuries: Comprehensive Management and Research*. Oxford: Blackwell Scientific Publications.

Hadley MN. (2002) Nutrition support after spinal cord injury. *Neurosurgery* 50: S81–S84.

Harrison P. (ed). (2006) *Managing Spinal Cord Injuries: Continuing Care*. Milton Keynes: SIA.

Henderson L, Gregory J, Irving K, Swan G. (2003) *The National Diet and Nutritional Survey: Adults Aged 19–64 years. Volume 2: Energy, Protein, Carbohydrates, Fat and Alcohol Intake*. London: HMSO.

Huang CT, DeVivo, Stover SL. (1990) Anemia in acute phase of spinal cord injury. *Archives of Physical and Medical Rehabilitation* 71(1): 3–7.

International Spinal Cord Society (ISCOS). (2006) International standards for neurological classification of spinal cord injury. Available at www.iscos.org.uk. Accessed 10 September 2013.

Jepson RG, Mihaljevic L, Craig J. (2004) Cranberries for preventing urinary tract infection. *Cochrane Database of Systematic Reviews* 2: CD001321.

Kearns PJ, Thompson JD, Werner PC, Pipp TL, Wilmot CB. (1992) Nutritional and metabolic response to acute spinal cord injury. *Journal of Parenteral and Enteral Nutrition* 16(1): 11–15.

Laughton GE, Buchholz AC, Martin Ginis KA, Goy RE. (2009) Lowering body mass index cutoffs better identifies obese persons with spinal cord injury. *Spinal Cord* 47: 757–762.

Laven GT, Huang CT, DeVivo MJ, Stover SL, Kuhlemeier KV, Fine PR. (1989) Nutritional status during the acute stage of spinal cord injury. *Archives of Physical Medicine and Rehabilitation* 70: 277–282.

Lynch AC, Wong C, Anthony A, Dobbs BR, Frizelle FA. (2000) Bowel dysfunction following spinal cord injury: a description of bowel function in a spinal cord injured population and comparison with age and gender matched controls. *Spinal Cord* 38(12): 717–723.

Marian M. (2004) Acute spinal cord injuries: nutrition management. *Support Line* 26(2): 3–8.

Mollinger LA, Spurr GB, Elghatit AZ, Barboriak JJ, Rooney CB. (1985) Daily energy expenditure and basal metabolic rates of patients with spinal cord injury. *Archives of Physical Medicine and Rehabilitation* 66(7): 420–426.

Monroe MB, Tataranni PA, Pratley R, Manore MM, Skinner JS, Ravussin E. (1998) Lower daily expenditure as measured by a respiratory chamber in subjects with spinal cord injury compared with control subjects. *American Journal of Clinical Nutrition* 68(Dec): 1223–1227.

SECTION 7

Multidisciplinary Association of Spinal Cord Injury Professionals (MASCIP). (2010) *Management of the Older Person with a New Spinal Cord Injury*. Stanmore: MASCIP.

Myers J, Lee M, Kiratli J. (2007) Cardiovascular Disease in Spinal Cord Injury: An overview of prevalence, risk, evaluation and management. *American Journal of Physical and Medical Rehabilitation* 86: 142–152.

National Institute for Health and Care Excellence (NICE). (2006) *Nutrition Support in Adults: Oral Nutrition Support, Enteral Tube Feeding and Parenteral Nutrition*. London: NICE.

Peruzzi W, Shapiro B, Cane R, Meyer P. (1994) Resting energy expenditure in the acute phase of spinal cord injury (oral presentation). *Critical Care Medicine* 22(1): A208.

Rasmann Nuhlicek DN, Spurr GB, Barboriak JJ, Rooney CB, Elghatit AZ, Bangard RD. (1988) Body composition of patients with spinal cord injury. *European Journal of Clinical Nutrition* 42: 765–773.

Royal College of Physicians (RCP). (2008) *Chronic Spinal Cord Injury: Management of Patients in Acute Hospital Setting: National Guidelines*. London: RCP.

Rice HB, Ponichtera-Mulcare JA, Glaser RM. (1995) Nutrition and the spinal cord injured individual. *Clinical Kinesiology* 49: 21–27.

Rodriguez DJ, Benzel EC, Clevenger FW. (1997) The metabolic response to spinal cord injury. *Spinal Cord* 35(9): 599–604.

Shedlock DA, Laventures SJ. (1990) Body composition and resting energy expenditure in long term spinal cord injury. *Paraplegia* 28: 448–454.

Shizgal HM, Roza A, Leduc B, Drouien G, Villemure JG, Yaffe C. (1986) Body composition in quadriplegic patients. *Journal of Parenteral and Enteral Nutrition* 10(4): 364–368.

Spinal Injuries Association. (2009) Some basic facts about SCI. Available at www.spinal.co.uk/page/Some-basic-facts-about-SCI. Accessed 8 February 2012.

The Spinal Cord Injury Centres of United Kingdom and Ireland (SCIC-UK&I). (2009) Guidelines for the management of neurogenic bowel dysfunction after SCI. Available at www.rcn.org.uk.

Spungen A, Adkins RH, Stewart CA, *et al.* (2003) Factors influencing body composition in persons with spinal cord injury: a cross-sectional study. *Journal of Applied Physiology* 95: 2398–2407.

Stiens SA, Bergman SB, Goetz LL. (1997) Neurogenic bowel dysfunction after spinal cord injury: clinical evaluation and rehabilitative management. *Archives of Physical Medicine and Rehabilitation* 78(3 Suppl): S86–101.

Wong S, Derry F, Jamous A, Hirani SP, Grimble G, Forbes A. (2011a) The prevalence of malnutrition in spinal cord injured patients – a UK multicentre study. *British Journal of Nutrition* 108(5): 918–923.

Wong S, Graham A, Grimble G, Forbes A. (2011b) Spinal Clinic for Obese Out-patient Project (SCOOP) – a 1 year report. *Food Nutrition and Science* 2: 901–907.

Wong S, Derry F, Grimble G, Forbes A. (2012a) How do spinal cord injury centres manage malnutrition? A cross-sectional survey of 12 SCIC in the UK and Ireland. *Spinal Cord* 50: 132–135.

Wong S, Derry F, Jamous A, Hirani SP, Grimble G, Forbes A. (2012b) Validation of the Spinal Nutrition Screening Tool (SNST) in patients with spinal cord injuries (SCI) – result from a multicentre study. *European Journal of Clinical Nutrition* 66: 382–387.

Worthington P, Crowe MA, Armenti V. (1993) Nutritional support for patients with spinal cord injury. *Trauma Quarterly* 9(2): 82–92.

7.17.4   Burn injury

Mark Windle

Key points

- Severe burn injury elicits one of the most pronounced inflammatory responses likely to be encountered in a clinical setting.

- Goals are to minimise loss of lean body mass and to optimise immune function, skin graft take and wound healing.

- Early nutritional support may reduce wound infection rates, catabolism and incidence of stress ulceration.

- Glutamine supplementation is now recommended for critically ill burns patients.

Burn injury accounts for approximately 16 000 admissions to hospital per year in the UK (National Burn Care Committee, 2001). Care may be provided in a range of clinical settings, including general surgery wards, plastic surgery wards and intensive care units, depending on the severity of illness and availability of services. Those with severe burn injuries may be managed in a specialist burns centre. Burns patients typically spend longer, often up to 3 weeks or more, in a critical care environment than the general intensive care population (Windle, 2006).

Young children present with a range of burn injuries, although scalds are the most frequently encountered (Hettiaratchy & Dziewulski, 2004). Whilst this chapter focuses on the management of adults with severe burns, metabolic and physiological consequences and interventional approaches in paediatric burns are similar in many respects. Dietetic management of children with severe burns is discussed comprehensively elsewhere (McCarthy & Gurry, 2007).

Adult admissions may be more mixed. Types of burn injury are diverse and include flame, fat and water scalds; chemical, friction and contact burns; and electrical injury.

Diagnostic criteria and classification

A major burn injury in adults is defined as one affecting around 20% total body surface area (TBSA) or greater (Saffle & Graves, 2007). Regular assessment of size, distribution and depth of burn is essential for surgical planning; TBSA is assessed with the aid of pictorial charts

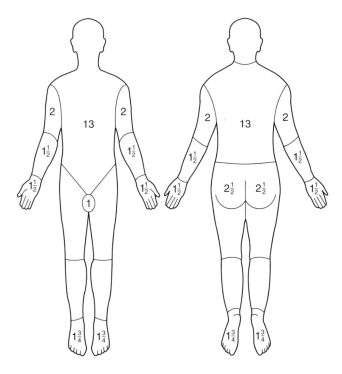

Age	Age (years)					
	0	1	5	10	15	Adult
Head and neck	21	19	15	13	11	9
Thigh	$5\frac{1}{2}$	$6\frac{1}{2}$	8	9	9	$9\frac{1}{2}$
Calf	5	5	$5\frac{1}{2}$	6	$6\frac{1}{2}$	7

Figure 7.17.4   *Percentage of different parts of the body at different ages (source: Kemble & Lamb, 1984. Reproduced with permission of Elsevier)*

(Figure 7.17.4). Wound depth is described as partial thickness (affecting superficial dermal or deeper dermal areas) or full thickness, which may extend to muscle and bone.

Metabolism and physiology

Major burn injury is characterised by an extreme systemic inflammatory response syndrome (SIRS). Tissue damage releases proinflammatory cytokines that initiate several metabolic, haemodynamic and systemic effects, including activation of the clotting cascade. Systemic inflammatory response syndrome is characterised by increases in temperature, heart rate and respiratory rate (Bone *et al.*, 1992). Increased vascular permeability, transcapillary escape and exudate loss leads to rapid hypovolaemia, hypoperfusion and organ failure if uncorrected. Adrenaline (epinephrine) increases amino acid utilisation from skeletal muscle for gluconeogenesis, cellular immunity, tissue repair and positive acute phase protein synthesis. Secondary inflammatory hits may also occur from local infection, sepsis and repeated surgical insults.

Public health aspects of burns

Any individual in society may sustain a burn injury. However, the profile of major burns admissions often includes patients with complex social needs, physical disability, mental health issues (self immolation), the very young, elderly, those with chronic disease and those who abuse alcohol. Some of these patients may also be nutritionally at risk. Fifteen per cent of patients in a UK burn centre were found to have a body mass index (BMI) on admission of $<20\,\mathrm{kg/m^2}$ (Windle, 2004).

Consequences of injury

Risk of death increases with injury severity, age and chronic disease. Burns survivors are often left with long term physical disfigurement, disability and psychological disorders. Large burns are now more survivable with refinements in a range of surgical, medical, nursing and nutritional interventions. This increases the need for intense multidisciplinary rehabilitation input and long term follow-up.

Hydration and nutritional consequences

Fluid losses via exudate can be massive; immediate and aggressive intravenous fluid resuscitation is required to minimise potentially fatal hypovolaemia. Exudate is albumin and micronutrient rich, and contributes to rapid zinc and copper loss (Berger *et al.*, 1992). Even with aggressive nutritional support, weight loss can be considerable. Around a third of adults admitted to a UK burn unit were unable to maintain weight within an acceptable limit, losing up to 22% of their admission or reported preinjury weight (Windle, 2004). Catch-up growth may be delayed in children with significant burn injuries (Rutan & Herndon, 1990). Metabolic rate may be raised above baseline for up to a year post burn injury (Hart *et al.*, 2000). Factors contributing to malnutrition are listed in Table 7.17.16.

Nutritional assessment and monitoring

Due to the often prolonged nature of critical illness and the often constantly changing clinical picture, dietetic assessment, monitoring and intervention can be time consuming in major burns (Windle, 2008). No evidence is available in burns regarding the benefits of monitoring frequency for the prevention of related complications. However, guidelines set by the NICE (2006) and the Parenteral and Enteral Nutrition Group (2007) of the British Dietetic Association for frequency of nutritional, biochemical and clinical monitoring may be suitable for most burn patients.

Weight

Some units have a weighbridge or weighing beds for assessing patients on admission for fluid resuscitation, drug dosage calculation and nutritional assessment

SECTION 7

Table 7.17.16 Potential factors contributing to malnutrition and loss of lean body mass after burn injury

Metabolic	Catecholamine and inflammatory cytokine mediated effects: hypermetabolism, muscle proteolysis (mobilisation of amino acid from skeletal muscle for gluconeogenesis, cellular immunity, tissue repair and acute phase protein synthesis) Reduced growth hormone Secondary inflammatory hits from local infection and sepsis
Physiological/ functional	Loss of micronutrients via burn wound exudate Increased urinary loss of copper and zinc Gastroparesis in critical illness phase reducing feed delivery Burn injury affecting oral cavity/oesophagus Severe inhalation injury – shortness of breath limiting intake Loss of lean body mass as a result of muscle necrosis from electrical injury
Interventions	Fasting for sedation related procedures for wound debridement and skin grafting Fasting for dressing change sessions which may require sedation (frequently on alternative days) Analgesia (constipation) Antibiotics (diarrhoea, nausea)
Psychological	Psychological effects on appetite (hospital environment, low mood, anxiety, post traumatic stress disorder, pain)

purposes. However, patients are usually transferred from an accident and emergency department in a referring hospital and considerable time may have lapsed between injury and admission to the burn care setting. Initial weight may therefore reflect under or over fluid resuscitation, wound exudate loss and (later) oedema. Nevertheless, an admission weight is useful as a starting point for calculation of nutritional needs if no history can be obtained. In the post extubation rehabilitation phase, regular weighing remains an important part of ongoing monitoring and screening until and beyond discharge from hospital.

Nitrogen economy and catabolism

Urinary nitrogen output is the result of internal nitrogen processing and so may assist in determining changes in protein economy and metabolism. Urinary urea nitrogen (UUN) is used to assess nitrogen balance (see Chapter 6.1) and severity of catabolism. In turn, these may help direct nutritional therapy. Eighty per cent of surveyed Australian and US burn centres regularly utilise nitrogen balance studies (Masters & Wood, 2008). Limitations exist in that protein intake must be accurately assessed and an accurate urine collection is required for use in the assessment of urinary urea excretion to facilitate calculation of nitrogen output. In the sedated critically ill burns patient, some potential barriers may be overcome. Nitrogen

intake can be calculated from observation charts documenting the administration of nutritional support, and urinary catheterisation facilitates an accurate urine collection. However, nitrogen loss from burn wound exudate may be significant and difficult to quantify. The usefulness of accounting for loss from exudate, i.e. loss other than from metabolism, in nitrogen balance calculations is unclear. In addition, ureagenesis is itself influenced in part by nitrogen intake. The catabolic index (CI) takes this into account when categorising the severity of metabolic stress (Bristan, 1979):

$$CI = [UUN, \text{ i.e. urea} (mmol/L) \times 0.028] \\ - (0.5 \times \text{nitrogen input} + 3\,g)$$

where <0 = no stress, 0–5 = moderate stress and >5 = severe stress.

Overestimation of CI may occur at high levels of nitrogen intake or where protein utilisation is lower than the assumed rate of 50% of intake. A further limit is the factors used to convert UUN to total urea nitrogen. Current factors used may not account for increased non-urea components in metabolically stressed patients, and higher conversion factors may be required for burns (Konstantinides *et al.*, 1992).

Biochemistry

Serum albumin concentration is a poor marker of nutritional status. Levels may reflect the extent of the inflammatory response and physiological insult in burns. Hypoalbuminaemia is the consequence of transcapillary escape, wound exudate loss and reduced albumin synthesis in preference for positive acute phase protein production. Serum concentration trends should be interpreted alongside inflammatory markers such as C-reactive protein. Anaemia may be related to acute blood loss from injury and surgery, and to cytokine effects on bone marrow suppression (Posluszny & Gamelli, 2011). However, in view of the potential for preburn suboptimal nutritional status in some patients, a nutritional cause should be excluded if possible. Again, interpretation of test results for specific nutrient or biomarker assays (such as ferritin for suspected iron deficiency, or zinc, copper and selenium status) is unfortunately difficult in a setting of inflammation. These limitations place emphasis on full consideration of clinical and diet history, lifestyle factors, nutritional intake since admission, and inflammatory markers.

Clinical management

Clinical goals concern survival from acute injury, recovery to the preinjured state and return to society with unaltered potential as far as possible. The 7 'Rs' to clinical management are as follows (National Burn Care Committee, 2001):

- *Rescue, resuscitation and retrieval* – the injured individual is removed from the location of injury, formal intravenous fluid resuscitation is initiated where necessary to minimise hypovolaemia, and the patient is transferred to the specialist area of care.

- *Resurfacing of skin* – debridement and dressing application, temporary or permanent skin coverage or grafting as soon as possible after injury, in order to reduce the inflammatory stimulus. Repeated theatre visits may be required for weeks or months. Full thickness areas will require skin grafting. Some partial thickness injuries may heal with conservative management or without surgery beyond initial removal of burned tissue. However, depth is often mixed and the surgical approach is often influenced by wound distribution and clinical stability. Other skin treatments may include application of cultured skin cells and synthetic skin replacement.
- *Rehabilitation* – this includes nutritional support, physical therapy, scar modulation, psychological management and discharge planning back into society. A multidisciplinary approach is required, including the involvement of dietitians, physiotherapists, occupational therapists and clinical psychologists.
- *Reconstruction and review* – surgical reconstruction may be required for years post injury for contracture release and cosmetic purposes. Outpatient monitoring is likely to be required for a number of years following major burn injury.

Nutritional management

Routes of feeding and timing of nutritional support

Parenteral nutrition may be associated with increased morbidity and mortality in critically ill patients, including those with burns (Gramlich *et al.*, 2004). This may be related to metabolic characteristics specific to burns; bacterial translocation and exacerbation of hepatobiliary complications have been observed in major burn injury (Herndon, 2007). Enteral feeding remains the route of choice, and all steps to utilise the gastrointestinal tract should be pursued. Gastroparesis may be managed by prokinetic therapy, or post pyloric tube placement where this fails (see Chapter 7.4.4).

Early initiation of nutritional support in burns patients appears safe, and may confer advantages in terms of avoiding stress ulceration, reducing incidence of wound infections, and when in combination with early surgical excision of wounds, reduction in skeletal muscle catabolism (Hart *et al.*, 2003, Mosier *et al.*, 2011). However, it is unclear how early this should commence and what the extent of clinical benefit is (Wasiak *et al.*, 2007). There has been concern regarding the risk of ischaemic injury in initiating enteral nutrition (EN) support in underperfused patients (Andel *et al.*, 2002). In practice however, by the time the patient is admitted, fluid resuscitation is usually well underway. Most units commence EN support within 24–48 hours of injury and benefit continues to be demonstrated in terms of reduced wound infection rates and intensive care unit length of stay (Mosier *et al.*, 2011).

Nutritional requirements

Energy

Energy requirements are largely influenced by the extent of inflammation. After an initial hypometabolic phase (ebb), an extended period of hypermetabolism (flow) occurs (see Chapter 7.17.1). The extent of the rise may vary depending on additional events such as dressing changes, septic episodes, surgical interventions, infectious complications and time post injury, and is not always related to injury severity. At one time energy prescriptions of up to 33.4 MJ (8000 kcal)/day were advocated for burns patients (Wilmore *et al.*, 1971). Since then, more conservative prediction formulae have been developed. These are particularly important in light of more recent knowledge gained of energy expenditure, complications of overzealous energy provision such as prolonged ventilator dependency, and higher septic mortality rates in hyperglycaemic critically ill patients. Interventions such as early surgery and initiation of nutritional support have contributed to a reduction in the hypermetabolic response (Hart *et al.*, 2003). Nevertheless, no consensus on the predictive equation to use for energy requirements exists.

A range of formulae have been proposed to estimate requirements. Some well known and traditionally used burns formulae were proposed before a range of treatment approaches were developed that blunt the hypermetabolic response, and so are likely to overestimate energy requirements. The Schofield formula (Schofield, 1985) with stress factors related to burn size was previously recommended, but this approach is not specifically validated in burns. Examples of prediction formulae used for burns patients today are shown in Table 7.17.17. Some authors have commented that many equations do not accurately predict measured energy expenditure for the reasons described above, and recommend equations that consider a range of parameters to reflect changing physiology, or the use of indirect calorimetry where facilities are available (Taylor, 2007; Herndon, 2007; Prelack *et al.*, 2007). Whilst the use of indirect calorimetry in US burn units has increased four fold over the last 20 years (Graves *et al.*, 2009), use is less common in the UK and ultimately the technique has its own limitations (Simonson & DeFronzo, 1990).

Protein

Intake of at least 1.5 g/kg protein/day has been suggested to ensure adequate provision in adults, following the observations that amino acid oxidation rates can be increased by 50% in burns patients compared with healthy individuals (Herndon, 2007). Intakes of 0.24 g nitrogen/kg (or 1.5 g/kg) of protein/day is likely to improve nitrogen balance in adults with burns covering >20% of TBSA, and further benefit may be achieved at higher intakes, although optimum levels are unknown due to study limitations (Taylor, 2007). The actual protein level used in surveyed US and Australian burn centres was 2 g/kg of body weight/day (Masters & Wood, 2008). The anabolic steroid oxandrolone is increasingly being used in severe burns. Benefits include improvements in preservation of

Table 7.17.17 Equations for estimating energy requirements in burns patients (kcal/day)

Author	Formula	Comments

Ireton-Jones & Jones (2002)	Spontaneous, breathing
	  $629 - 11(A) + 25(W) + 609(O)$
	Ventilator dependency
	  $1784 - 11(A) + 5(W) + 244(G) +$
	  $239(T) + 840(B)$
		Does not account for changes in physiology over time affected by, for example, interventions, pharmacology, reducing burn wound size, presence or absence of sepsis
		May overestimate in the obese and underestimate in the non-obese

Allard et al. (1990) Toronto formula	REE = $-4343 + (10.5 \times \%$ TBSA burn) $+ (0.23 \times$ kcal intake) $+ (0.84 \times$ HB) $+ (114 \times t) - (4.5 \times$ post burn days)	Complex, requires calculation of HB formula, which itself is an estimate of basal energy expenditure and requires multiplication by a 'static' factor, but for spontaneous breathing patients at least takes account of healing over time
Kreymann et al. (2006)	Maximum 20–25 kcal/kg of body weight in acute phase of critical illness 25–30 kcal/kg of body weight in flow phase	ESPEN generic guidelines for critically ill patients Does not track physiological changes Acute and recovery phases not clearly defined

Frankenfield et al. (2009), Frankenfield; (2011)
Modified Penn State formula
	Ventilator dependency
	RMR = Male: $10(W) + 6.25(ht) - 5(A) + 5$ or
	    Female: $10(W) + 6.25(ht) - 5(A) - 161$
	then
	BMI <30 kg/m^2
	  $\times 0.96 + T_{max}(167) + Ve(31) - 6212$
	or
	BMI ≥30 kg/m^2
	  $\times 0.71 + T_{max}(85) + Ve(64) - 3085$
		Considers physiological parameters associated with changes in metabolic rate
		Not validated specifically in burns patients but predictive ability higher than current validated equations for ventilated patients

A, age (years); B, burn (absent 0; present1); G, gender (female 0; male 1); O, obesity (absent 0; present 1); W, weight (kg); REE, resting energy expenditure; HB, Harris–Benedict equation; TBSA, total body surface area; t, temperature (°C); ESPEN, European Society for Parenteral and Enteral Nutrition; RMR, resting metabolic rate; T_{max}, maximum body temperature in past 24 hours (°C); Ve, expired minute volume (L/m) at time of reading from ventilator.

lean body mass and muscle function, and shorter hospital length of stay (Demling & DeSanti, 1998; Wolf et al., 2006). Maintenance of nutritional intake whilst on treatment may be essential as restoration of body weight and muscle function has been demonstrated at protein intakes of 2 g/kg/day compared with lower levels (Demling & DeSanti, 1998).

Micronutrient supplementation

Almost all vitamins, minerals and trace elements play a direct or indirect role in wound healing. Important nutrients are listed in Table 7.17.18 (see Chapter 7.17.6). Research interest in trace element supplementation in burns is not surprising when it is considered that 10% of total body zinc and 40% of total body copper may be lost in exudate (Berger et al., 1992), and the role that they play as cofactors for enzyme systems involved in immunity and wound healing. European practice guidelines for adults (Kreymann et al., 2006) support the use of copper, selenium and zinc supplementation at a dose higher than standard, following a randomised controlled trial that demonstrated that administration of 40.4 µmol of copper, 2.9 µmol selenium and 406 µmol of zinc for 30 days after burn injury reduced chest infection rates and length of hospital stay. Other guidelines suggest reserving specific micronutrient supplementation for correcting deficiency states, and note that regular nutritional therapy often provides well in excess of baseline amounts (Prelack et al., 2007). Nevertheless, most US centres routinely

administer additional micronutrient supplements (Graves et al., 2009). This practice is also increasing in the UK with some burn units agreeing a policy of routinely giving intravenous trace elements to all burns patients from admission up to at least day 7. It may be prudent to avoid routine iron supplementation for correction of anaemia in the critically ill as free iron can encourage bacteria growth and may be associated with an increased risk of sepsis and mortality (Lapointe, 2004). In burns patients, high dose ascorbic acid has been used for its antioxidant properties as an additive to intravenous resuscitation fluid. Reduced free radical production leads to less vascular permeability and oedema, although outcomes are inconsistent between studies (Kahn et al., 2011). Enteral supplementation with up to 800–1000 mg/day of vitamin C is likely to be safe (Department of Health, 1991) and vitamin C toxicity issues are generally minor. Perhaps for these reasons, a number of centres include specific supplementation as part of their protocol (Masters & Wood, 2008; Graves et al., 2009). Evidence in burns patients to support routine supplementation is however limited at present.

Immune modulating nutrition

Glutamine

Glutamine, a conditionally essential amino acid in metabolic stress, has a number of roles, including providing an oxidative fuel for lymphocytes and gastrointestinal

Table 7.17.18 Role of micronutrients in burn wound healing

Micronutrient	Role	Notes
Vitamin A	Needed for epithelialisation and stimulation of fibroblasts Antioxidant effect of beta-carotene prevents damage by free radicals in SIRS	
B vitamin	Role in oxidative pathways Cofactor for collagen deposition	
Vitamin C	Cofactor in hydroxylation of proline and lysine Collagen synthesis Antioxidant properties protect metalloenzymes from oxidation	As a free radical scavenger, may reduce vascular permeability and therefore reduce fluid resuscitation requirements
Iron	Promotes collagen synthesis Optimises tissue perfusion	Avoid iron supplements in acute illness – possible increased risk of infection and mortality
Zinc	Role in RNA/DNA replication, lymphocyte function and collagenase enzyme systems	Up to 10% total body zinc lost via wound exudate
Copper	Cofactor in the lysyl oxidase enzyme system, essential for collagen synthesis and maturation	Up to 40% of total body copper lost via wound exudate
Selenium	Component of glutathione peroxidase (antioxidant)	Lost through skin following burn injury

mucosa. Severe glutamine depletion through reduced endogenous production and increased central consumption persists for at least 11 days after burn injury (Gore & Jahoor, 2000). A review of randomised controlled trials and practice guidelines in burns highlighted improvements in biomarkers of intestinal permeability, improved wound healing rates, length of stay, reduction in *Pseudomonas aeruginosa* infection and cost savings following glutamine supplementation (Windle, 2006). Most studies have investigated enteral supplementation, reflecting the primary nutritional approach in burns, although intravenous glutamine has been associated with a decrease in Gram negative bacteraemia and quicker resolution of inflammatory markers (Wischmeyer *et al.*, 2001). Use of glutamine in burn units is increasing and critical care practice guidelines now endorse enteral glutamine for mechanically ventilated burns patients (Heyland *et al.*, 2003; Kreymann *et al.*, 2006; McClave *et al.*, 2009). The optimum dose and duration of supplementation in burns patients is still unknown, although a dose of 0.3–0.57 g/kg of body weight/day for up to 3 weeks post burn injury may be appropriate (Windle, 2006; Kurmis *et al.*, 2010).

Arginine

Arginine has a role in T lymphocyte synthesis and promotes wound healing. However, arginine rich feeds have been associated with increased mortality in patients with sepsis (Heyland *et al.*, 2003). This may be related to an exacerbation of nitric oxide production, which can cause profound hypotension, hypoperfusion and ultimately multiorgan failure. However, others have noted that this mortality effect has not been observed in burns patients (Kurmis *et al.*, 2010).

Omega 3 fatty acids

n-3 Fatty acids compete with n-6 fatty acids for incorporation into cell membranes. A high ratio of n-3 to n-6 fatty acids gives rise to fewer proinflammatory mediators. It is plausible that burns patients may be among the group most likely to benefit from n-3 fatty acid supplementation, although research in this group is surprisingly sparse. Existing studies in burns patients suffer from design limitations, such as small sample size or use of n-3 fatty acids in combination with other nutrients (Kurmis *et al.*, 2010).

Some commercially available enteral feeds provide immune modulating nutrients in combination. A major disadvantage is that the relative effects of constituents are unknown. A review of burns studies has noted mixed results and suggests that the priority should be for defining optimal doses and safety before developing such products (Kurmis *et al.*, 2010).

Follow up post discharge

Dietetic follow-up may be required beyond inpatient discharge to monitor weight maintenance and to support any functional difficulties with eating as a result of injury. Physiotherapy and occupational therapists are inevitably engaged in long term follow-up and may assist in flagging up developing nutritional problems. As regional burn centres tend to serve wide populations geographically, sometimes transfer of or shared dietetic care with a local department is required for logistical reasons. When wounds fully heal, transfer from a high protein high energy diet to a longer term healthy eating approach may require further ongoing support.

Drug–nutrient interactions

The following drugs affect nutritional status:

- Oxandrolone (testosterone analogue steroid) – hyperglycaemia, nausea, vomiting and diarrhoea.
- Morphine salts (opioid analgesic) – paralytic ileus, abdominal pain, anorexia and taste disturbance.
- Meropenem (antibiotic) – nausea, vomiting, diarrhoea and abdominal pain.
- Piperacillin with tazobactam (Tazocin; antibiotic) – nausea, vomiting and diarrhoea; less commonly – stomatitis and dyspepsia; rarely – abdominal pain; and very rarely – hypoglycaemia and hypokalaemia.

SECTION 7

Internet resources

British Burns Association   www.britishburnsassociation.org

References

Allard JP, Pichard C, Hoshino E, *et al.* (1990) Validation of a new formula for calculating the energy requirements of burn patients. *Journal of Parenteral and Enteral Nutrition* 14: 115–118.

Andel H, Rab M, Andel D, *et al.* (2002) Impact of duodenal feeding on the oxygen balance of the splanchnic region during different phases of severe burn injury. *Burns* 28: 60–64.

Berger M, Cavadini C, Bart A, *et al.* (1992) Cutaneous copper and zinc losses in burns. *Burns* 18: 373–380.

Bone RC, Balk RA, Cerra FB, *et al.* (1992) Definitions for sepsis and organ failure and guidelines for the use of innovative therapies in sepsis. *Chest* 101: 1644–1655.

Bristan B. (1979) A simple estimate technique to estimate severity of stress. *Surgery, Gynecology & Obstetrics* 148: 675–678.

Department of Health. (1991) *Dietary Reference Values: A guide.* London: HMSO.

Demling RH, DeSanti L. (1998) Increased protein intake during the recovery phase after severe burns increases body weight gain and muscle function. *Journal of Burn Care and Rehabilitation* 19: 161–168.

Frankenfield D. (2011) Validation of an equation for resting metabolic rate in older obese, critically ill patients. *Journal of Parenteral and Enteral Nutrition* 35: 264–269.

Frankenfield DC, Coleman A, Alam S, Cooney RN. (2009) Analysis of estimation methods for resting metabolic rate in critically ill adults. *Journal of Parenteral and Enteral Nutrition* 33: 27–36.

Gore DC, Jahoor F. (2000) Deficiency in peripheral glutamine production in paediatric patients with burns. *Journal of Burn Care and Rehabilitation* 21: 172–177.

Gramlich LK, Kichian J, Pinilla J, Rodych NJ, Dhaliwal R, Heyland DK. (2004) Does enteral nutrition compared to parenteral nutrition result in better outcomes in critically ill adult patients? A systematic review of the literature. *Nutrition* 20: 843–848.

Graves C, Saffle J, Cochran A. (2009) Actual burn nutrition care practices: an update. *Journal of Burn Care and Research* 30: 77–82.

Hart DW, Wolf SE, Mlack R, *et al.* (2000) Persistence of muscle catabolism after severe burn. *Surgery* 128: 312–319.

Hart DW, Wolf SE, Chinkes DL, *et al.* (2003) Effects of early excision and aggressive enteral feeding on hypermetabolism, catabolism and sepsis after severe burn. *Journal of Trauma* 54: 755–761.

Herndon DN. (2007) *Total Burn Care*, 3rd edn. Philadelphia: Saunders Elsevier.

Hettiaratchy S, Dziewulski P. (2004) ABC of burns. Pathophysiology and types of burns. *BMJ* 328: 1427–1429.

Heyland DK, Dhaliwal R, Drover JW, Gramlich L, Dodek P; Canadian Critical Care Clinical Practice Guidelines Committee. (2003) Canadian clinical practice guidelines for nutrition support in mechanically ventilated, critically ill patients. *Journal of Parenteral and Enteral Nutrition* 27: 355–373.

Ireton-Jones C, Jones JD. (2002) Improved equations for predicting energy expenditure in patients: the Ireton-Jones Equations. *Nutrition in Clinical Practice* 17: 29–31.

Kahn SA, Beers RJ, Lentz CW. (2011) Resuscitation after severe burn injury using high dose ascorbic acid: a retrospective review. *Journal of Burn Care and Research* 32: 100–117.

Konstantinides FN, Radmer WJ, Becker WK, *et al.* (1992) Inaccuracy of nitrogen balance determinations in thermal injury with calculated total urinary nitrogen. *Journal of Burn Care and Rehabilitation* 13: 254–260.

Kreymann KG, Berger MM, Deutz C, *et al.* (2006) ESPEN guidelines on enteral nutrition: intensive care. *Clinical Nutrition* 25: 210–223.

Kurmis R, Parker A, Greenwood J. (2010) The use of immunonutrition in burn injury care: where are we? *Journal of Burn Care and Research* 31: 677–691.

Lapointe M. (2004) Iron supplementation in the intensive care unit: when, how much and by what route? *Critical Care* 8: S37–S41.

Masters B, Wood F. (2008) Nutrition support in burns – is there consistency in practice? *Journal of Burn Care and Research* 29: 561–571.

McCarthy H, Guury C. (2007) Burns. In: Shaw V, Lawson M (eds) *Clinical Paediatric Dietetics*, 3rd edn. Oxford: Blackwell Publishing.

McClave SA, Martindale RG, Vanek VW, *et al.*; ASPEN Board of Directors, American College of Critical Care Medicine. (2009) Guidelines for the provision and assessment of nutrition support therapy in the adult critically ill patient. *Journal of Parenteral and Enteral Nutrition* 33: 277–316.

Mosier MJ, Pham TN, Klein MB, *et al.* (2011) Early enteral nutrition in burns: compliance with guidelines and associated outcomes in a multicenter study. *Journal of Burn Care and Research* 32: 104–109.

National Burn Care Committee. (2001) *National Burn Care Review: Standards and Strategy for Burn Care. A Review of Burn Care in the British Isles.* UK: Committee Report.

National Institute for Health and Care Excellence (NICE). (2006) *Nutrition Support in Adults. Oral Nutrition Support, Enteral Tube Feeding and Parenteral Nutrition.* London: NICE.

Parenteral and Enteral Nutrition Group. (2007) *A Pocket Guide to Clinical Nutrition*, 3rd edn. British Dietetic Association.

Posluszny JA, Gamelli RL. (2011) Anaemia of thermal injury: combined acute blood loss anaemia and anaemia of chronic illness. *Journal of Burn Care Research* 31: 229–242.

Prelack K, Dylewski M, Sheridan RL. (2007) Practical guidelines for the nutritional management of burn injury and recovery. *Burns* 33: 14–24.

Rutan RL, Herndon DN. (1990) Growth delay in postburn paediatric patients. *Archives of Surgery* 125: 392–395.

Saffle JR, Graves C. (2007) Nutritional support of the burned patient. In: Herndon DN (ed) *Total Burn Care*. Philadelphia: Saunders Elsevier, pp. 398–419.

Schofield WN. (1985) Predicting basal metabolic rate, new standards and review of previous work. *Human Nutrition and Clinical Nutrition* 39C(Suppl 1): 5–41.

Simonson DC, DeFronzo RA. (1990) Indirect calorimetry: methodological and interpretative problems. *American Journal of Physiology* 258: E399–E412.

Taylor SJ. (2007) *Energy and Nitrogen Requirements in Disease States.* West Sussex: Smith-Gordon & Company Ltd.

Wasiak J, Cleland H, Jeffrey R. (2007) Early versus late enteral nutritional support in adults with burn injury: a systematic review. *Journal of Human Nutrition and Dietetics* 20: 75–83.

Wilmore DW, Currerri PW, Spitzer KW, Pruit BA Jr. (1971) Supranormal dietary intake in thermally injured hypermetabolic patients. *Surgery, Gynecology & Obstetrics* 132: 881–886.

Windle EM. (2004) Audit of successful weight maintenance in adult and paediatric survivors of thermal injury at a UK regional burn centre. *Journal of Human Nutrition and Dietetics* 17: 435–441.

Windle EM. (2006) Glutamine supplementation in critical illness: evidence, recommendations and implications for clinical practice in burn care. *Journal of Burn Care and Research* 27: 764–772.

Windle EM. (2008) Nutrition support in major burn injury: case analysis of dietetic activity, resource use and cost implications. *Journal of Human Nutrition and Dietetics* 21: 165–173.

Wischmeyer PE, Lynch J, Liedel J, *et al.* (2001) Glutamine administration reduces Gram-negative bacteraemia in severely burned patients: a prospective, controlled, randomised, double-blind trial versus isonitrogenous control. *Critical Care Medicine* 29: 2075–2080.

Wolf SE, Edelman LS, Kemalyan N, *et al.* (2006) Effects of oxandrolone on outcome measures in the severely burned: a multicenter prospective randomised double-blind trial. *Journal of Burn Care and Research* 27: 131–139.

7.17.5 Surgery

Rachael Barlow

Key points

■ Surgical trauma causes physiological stress, which is related to the severity of the procedure and results in an increase in energy expenditure and protein mobilisation.

■ Preoperative weight loss is a recognised cause of postoperative morbidity and mortality.

■ Malnutrition is associated with a significantly higher risk of postoperative complications.

■ Nutritional screening, assessment and early enteral nutrition are key components of the Enhanced Recovery After Surgery (ERAS) programme; a patient centred pathway that optimises surgical outcome by improving clinical outcomes and patient experience.

Approximately 3 million surgical operations are performed in the UK each year, with an average hospital mortality of 0.8–1%. This equates to over 20000 deaths following surgery a year (NECPOD, 2011). The range of surgical procedures now practised, along with the diversity of patients undergoing surgery, make it difficult to generalise the metabolic and nutritional responses following surgery. Procedures vary from elective (planned) to emergency surgery, and from laparoscopic (keyhole) to prolonged procedures taking many hours. The type and duration of surgery influence the speed of postoperative recovery. The health status of the patient and the reason for surgery also require much consideration. An emergency appendicectomy in an otherwise fit, healthy adult carries little implication for nutritional intervention, whereas a malnourished, cachectic patient requires nutritional support pre and post surgery if compromised nutritional status is not to adversely affect clinical progress. The majority of this chapter focuses on major surgery patients.

The clinical management of surgical patients has progressed radically over the last 100 years with the availability of prophylactic antibiotics, intravenous fluids and colloids, increased understanding of anaesthetic agents and analgesics, specialist critical care units and an increased understanding of organ function perioperatively. Nutrition is now an integrated component of surgical care.

Effects of surgery

Any surgical trauma causes physiological stress, which is related to the severity of the procedure. An initial surge in sympathetic activity generates a transient rise in catecholamine secretion post trauma. The resultant increase in energy expenditure and protein mobilisation is moderated through cytokine release, especially tumour necrosis factor (TNF) and proinflammatory interleukins (particularly IL-1 and IL-6) (Inui, 1999). A delay in postoperative feeding, coupled with preoperative starvation, often results in significant negative nitrogen balance. Protein depletion postoperatively results in loss of lean body mass

and reduced muscle strength, and thus increased risk of cardiorespiratory impairment; in addition, impaired immunity increases the likelihood of infectious complications (Inui, 1999). Impaired immunity and associated sepsis may also be linked to the altered intestinal permeability seen in the postoperative period (Beattie *et al.*, 2000). A compromised supply of oxygen to the gut during surgery (splanchnic hypoperfusion) has been shown to downregulate local and systemic immune function, increase intestinal permeability and exaggerate the acute phase response. Thus, wherever the site of surgery, the gut has a central modulatory role in the inflammatory and immune responses to major surgery (Holland *et al.*, 2005).

Traditionally, malnourished surgical patients were classified into four groups; depleted, hypercatabolic, hypercatabolic and depleted, or chronic malabsorption (Elwyn, 1980). This is of limited use today, as routine use of a nutritional support and associated pain management strategy has been shown to attenuate the catabolic response to surgical injury (Kehlet, 1999).

Pre-existing malnutrition

Several prospective studies have concluded that patients undergoing surgery are at increased risk and this can have a negative impact on clinical outcome. Malnutrition is of widespread concern in hospitalised patients (see Chapter 6.1). Evidence suggests that the preoperative nutritional status of many surgical patients is poorly documented (Kudsk *et al.*, 2003), despite preoperative weight loss being a recognised cause of postoperative morbidity and mortality. However, poor documentation should be addressed via the Enhanced Recovery After Surgery (ERAS) programme (see later).

Although it is difficult to establish a causal relationship, malnutrition is associated with a significantly higher risk of postoperative complications (Allison, 2000; Salvino *et al.*, 2004) and impaired quality of life (Ferguson & Capra, 1998). Therefore, it is thought that the correction or prevention of malnutrition with the use of nutritional support may impact on health related quality of life (McKenna & Thorig, 1995).

SECTION 7

Stages of nutritional support delivery

The delivery of nutritional support in the surgical patient can be divided into preoperative and postoperative stages.

Preoperative nutritional intervention

Evidence suggests that 25–40% of all patients are malnourished on hospital admission (Kruizenga et al., 2005). A low admission body mass index (BMI) increases the relative risk of death from cardiac procedures in the older age group (Rapp-Kesek et al., 2004). The nutritional risk increases in many patients during their hospital stay (Kyle et al., 2005) and up to a third of postsurgical patients experience clinically significant weight loss (Fettes et al., 2002). Many patients presenting for surgery may be malnourished as a consequence of underlying pathology, e.g. cancer related cachexia or Crohn's disease, or of associated symptoms such as diarrhoea, nausea or vomiting. All causes of excessive nutrient loss and/or increased metabolic needs will influence nutritional status. Nutritionally at risk patients include those who:

- Are of advanced age.
- Are currently or predicted to eat little or nothing for >5 days.
- Have taken <60% of nutritional requirements over the previous 10 days.
- Are unable to eat the normal hospital diet.
- Have increased but unmet nutritional needs.

These groups of patients are deemed at risk of malnutrition and should be the focus of early nutritional support (Weimann et al., 2006), as optimisation of nutritional status preoperatively reduces postoperative infectious complications (Windsor et al., 2004) and enhances wound healing rates (see Chapter 7.17.6).

Nutritional screening

A variety of tools have been developed to assess the nutritional status of patients awaiting surgery, such as the Mini Nutritional Assessment (MNA), Subjective Global Index (SGI), Nutritional Risk Index (NRI), and Malnutrition Universal Screening Tool ('MUST') (see Chapter 7.17.2). Whilst the sensitivity and specificity of the tools vary, the consistency of the predictive value for each tool means that any one can be used for nutritional risk assessment (Kuzu et al., 2006). It is recommended that all surgical inpatients should be screened for nutritional and physical status on admission, and reviewed weekly thereafter (NICE, 2006).

Preoperative nutritional support

Active nutritional support by provision of oral nutritional supplements or enteral feeding should be routinely considered in patients with a BMI of <18.5 kg/m² or those who present with unintentional weight loss within the last 3 months of >10% of body weight. A BMI below 20 kg/m² with unintentional weight loss of >5% of body weight within the previous 3–6 months is also predictive of malnutrition (NICE, 2006).

Fasting guidelines

Prolonged preoperative fasting has until recently been a time honoured tradition, although over 100 years ago the British surgeon Joseph Lister (1827–1912) stated, *'While it's desirable that there should be no solid matter in the stomach when chloroform is administered, it will be found very salutary to give a cup of tea or beef-tea about two hours previously'*. The need for a short period of starvation has recently come to the forefront, with work suggesting better postoperative recovery with oral fluid intake up to 2 hours before surgery.

The rationale for preoperative fasting is to reduce the volume and acidity of gastric contents, thus reducing the risks of intraoperative regurgitation and aspiration of gastric contents into the lungs, yet evidence supporting this rationale is lacking. *'Nil by mouth from midnight'* is a slowly changing practice as evidence increases that patients fasted from liquids and solids for an average of 12–14 hours have a compromised fluid and nutritional intake (Crenshaw & Winslow, 2002). Patients remain exposed to unnecessary starvation, suboptimal stress reduction and intravenous fluid overload preoperatively (Lassen et al., 2005).

Guidelines from the American Society of Anesthesiologists (ASA, 1999) have revised these recommendations, allowing consumption of clear liquids (including fruit juices without pulp) up to 2 hours before elective surgery, a light breakfast, e.g. tea and toast, 6 hours before the procedure and a heavier meal 8 hours beforehand. These newer practices improve patient comfort and reduce adverse outcomes (Saqr & Chambers, 2006).

The recent Royal College of Nursing guidelines (RCN, 2005) for preoperative fasting in the UK permit low risk patients to take water, clear tea and black coffee up to 2 hours before anaesthetic induction, and milky drinks and food up to 6 hours before induction. Patients considered at high risk of aspiration (those who are obese, diabetic or with gastrointestinal reflux) can follow a similar fasting regimen, but this should be at the anaesthetist's discretion (Maltby et al., 2004; Jellish et al., 2005).

Carbohydrate loading

Carbohydrate loading has gained widespread popularity in the preoperative management of major surgical patients over the past decade. The surge in popularity is due to its integral role in the ERAS Programme. The use of carbohydrate rich drinks prior to surgery has been shown to alter the metabolic state from fasted to fed. This modulates the postoperative insulin response by improving the insulin sensitivity, leading to improved muscle strength and mass in particularly lean body tissue (Ljungqvist & Søreide, 2003), which is thought to help with early mobilisation and rehabilitation (Yuill et al., 2005; Melis et al., 2006a). A detailed review of the physiological action of the mechanism of carbohydrate and insulin resistance is given by Ljungqvist & Søreide (2003). However, carbohydrate rich drinks given prior to laparoscopic procedures such as cholecystectomy produce conflicting outcomes (Bisgaard et al., 2004; Hausel et al., 2005).

The use of preoperative carbohydrates has a positive effect on patient experience, reducing anxiety, thirst and hunger. Practically, carbohydrate solutions should be administered 4–12 hours preoperatively. Caution is required for diabetics due to possible impaired glycaemic control and impaired gastric emptying.

Postoperative nutritional support

The routine use of early nutritional support remains a controversial postoperative, therapeutic intervention in surgical patients; however, the advent of the ERAS programme seems to be resolving this controversy. Commencement of enteral or oral feeding within 24 hours of surgery is associated with optimal clinical outcome (Allison, 2005). Immediate postoperative enteral feeding, commenced within 6–12 hours post procedure, is associated with a significant reduction in postoperative complications, reducing both intensive care unit (ICU) and total hospital length of stay (Gabor et al., 2005; Kreymann et al., 2006). The recommendation to commence early enteral feeding is often tempered by the possibility of postoperative complications.

Several meta analyses have suggested that normal food intake or enteral nutrition (EN) may be beneficial in reducing infective complications and hospital stay in general surgical patients (Møiniche et al., 1995; Schilder et al., 1997; Marik & Zaloga, 2001). However, the issue of the early introduction of oral food intake in patients with an upper gastrointestinal tract anastomosis is not straightforward. Lassen et al. (2005) advocated the use of early oral food after upper gastrointestinal tract resection at will; however, for many patients this may not be the preferred method. This may not be a viable option for patients with anorexia or who lack confidence with eating in the first few days postoperatively. The use of jejunostomy feeding for immediate early EN has been reported to be safe, well tolerated and to have advantages over traditional management with intravenous fluids or parenteral nutrition (PN) (Aiko et al., 2001; Sand et al., 1997). For a detailed review of the proposed mechanism of action of early EN, see Kudsk (2002) and Genton & Kudsk (2003).

Early enteral feeding post surgery reduces the risk of anastomotic dehiscence, pneumonia, wound infection and intra-abdominal abscess (Lewis et al., 2001). This has been reiterated in a recent study (Barlow et al., 2011). The recommendation for clinical practice should be to use EN (either oral or enteral tube feeding) where the gastrointestinal tract is accessible and functioning. Nutritional support intervention in the perioperative period has been evaluated using standard oral nutritional supplements in mixed patient populations (Beattie et al., 2000; Macfie et al., 2000; Smedley et al., 2004). In these trials, oral nutritional intervention positively influenced the clinical course by reducing postoperative complications. There is evidence to support the integration of nutrition into the care pathway for colorectal cancer (CRC) patients (see Chapter 7.15.3).

Immunonutrition

Immune enhancing supplementation is an expensive alternative to standard formula products. Although benefit from these has been demonstrated, their cost currently prohibits large scale implementation into routine practice in the preoperative period for elective surgical patients. Several studies on the use of immune nutrition perioperatively have indicated that immune enhanced EN is superior to EN in lowering incidence of infections and complications (Daly et al., 1995; Braga et al., 1999; 2002; Gianotti et al., 2002).

The use of preoperative immune enhancing oral supplementation has been shown to reduce complication rates in CRC patients (Waitzberg et al., 2006). A recent study (Burden et al., 2011) concluded that there is no advantage in providing routine immune nutritional supplements to all patients, but did suggest these may be beneficial in patients who are weight losing preoperatively (see Chapter 7.11.1).

Route of feeding

Jejunostomy

Jejunostomy is a surgical procedure by which a tube is situated in the lumen of the proximal jejunum, primarily to administer nutrition, fluid and medication (Sarr, 1988), reducing the need for central venous access for administration of nutrition and drugs (see Chapter 6.4). Delany et al. (1973) inserted the first needle catheter jejunostomy (NCJ) in 1973. They described the delivery of feeding and fluids via a NCJ in patients undergoing upper gastrointestinal tract surgery. Since this, many cohort and feasibility studies have reviewed jejunostomy feeding, with many reporting serious and occasionally life threatening complications (Biffi et al., 2000; Eddy et al., 1996; Ryan et al., 2006). The complications seen with jejunostomy can be classified into:

- *Mechanical* – such as tube dislocation, occlusion or migration.
- *Surgical* – such as cutaneous or intrabdominal abscesses, enterocutaneous fistulae, pneumatosis, small bowel obstruction and intestinal ischaemia.
- *Infectious* – can occur such as aspiration pneumonia or contamination of the enteral feed.
- *Gastrointestinal intolerance* to jejunal feeding is reported to be between 2.3% and 6.8% and includes abdominal distension, colic, constipation, nausea and vomiting.
- *Metabolic* – including hyperglycaemia, hypokalaemia, water and electrolyte imbalance, hypophosphataemia and hypomagnesaemia.

The largest prospective study over 9 years was reported by Braga et al. (2002) who studied 650 patients undergoing gastrointestinal tract surgery. All patients had either a NCJ (61.8%) or nasojejunal feeding tube (NJT) (38.2%). Severe jejunostomy related complications were noted in 1.7% of patients and EN related mortality was 0.1%. Refractory intolerance of the enteral feed was reported in

48% of patients. The authors recommended that intolerance could be minimised with a slow increase in feed rate in the first postoperative week and close monitoring. They concluded that EN was safe, well tolerated and not detrimental to anastomotic healing. The authors suggested that intolerance of EN was an early predictor of impending surgical complications.

In a recent study Ryan *et al.* (2006) prospectively studied 205 patients post oesophagectomy. They concluded that early EN via a NCJ was tolerated in 92% of patients. Patients were fed on average for 15 days, with 26% requiring long term nutritional support, i.e. for longer than 20 days. Serious complications were reported in 1.4% of patients, all of whom required repeat laparotomy. There was one death directly attributed to jejunostomy feeding.

Clearly, the choice of feeding jejunostomy is crucial and it may be a major factor in the development of complications, alongside the insertion technique used by the surgeon. The use of aggressive feeding, such as using high rates to initiate the enteral feed, coupled with the rapid increase in rate of the feed and the osmolarity of the feed, are all important (Melis *et al.*, 2006b). The too rapid delivery of EN coupled with the overzealous use of opioids, which slow gastrointestinal peristalsis, could lead to increased intra-abdominal pressure and exacerbate gastrointestinal oedema, reducing splanchnic blood flow and increasing the likelihood of gastrointestinal ischaemia (Melis *et al.*, 2006b). The volume of EN delivered is vital. A study by Watters *et al.* (1997) reported that EN delivered to nutritional requirements within 3 days in major surgical patients lead to respiratory problems secondary to increased abdominal distension.

Parenteral nutrition

Parenteral nutrition is discussed in Chapter 6.5.

Postoperative gastrointestinal motility

The three most common reasons for the delay of feed commencement are the absence of bowel sounds (with presumed ileus), risk of gastrointestinal anastamoses dehiscence and haemodynamic instability, especially in the ICU patient, but evidence does not support the necessity for delay.

After surgery, postoperative gastrointestinal dysfunction or ileus is commonly reported to occur. It is thought to occur in 90% of patients undergoing intra-abdominal surgery. Livingston & Passaro (1990) defined ileus as '*The inhibition of propulsive bowel motility, irrespective of pathological mechanisms*'.

Ileus is characterised by the development of nausea, vomiting, delayed gastric emptying, bowel distension, decreased bowel sounds, delay in passage of stools and pain after a surgical procedure. The pathogenesis of ileus is multifactorial; however, it is thought to stem from the high concentration of inflammatory mediators following any injury to the intestinal muscularis of the gastrointestinal tract. These act locally to initiate morphological

changes in the bowel wall. In addition, these immunological cells cause an increase in free radical production, which disrupts the membrane ion channels (potassium and calcium) that regulate smooth muscle contraction and rhythm. The result is a decrease in circular muscle contraction and thus a reduced intestinal transit time (Livingston & Passaro, 1990). Subsequently, systemic cytokines, prostaglandins and catecholamines are released that activate the autonomic nervous system. This produces inhibitory effects that alter motility and reduce mesenteric blood flow.

There are many other factors that have been linked to ileus, such as nitric oxide, nasogastric intubation, gum chewing, use of laparoscopic procedures, and pharmacological agents such as non-steroidal anti-inflammatory drugs, prokinetics such as metaclopramide hydrochloride, erythromycin, ceruletide and octreotide, a somatostatin analogue that inhibits the secretion of gastrointestinal hormones. These factors were reviewed extensively by Mythen (2005).

Traditionally, it has been considered that ileus prevents the safe delivery of EN. Barium studies have demonstrated that small bowel motility continues in the postoperative phase, despite delayed gastric emptying taking 24–48 hours to recover and colonic motility taking 3–5 days to return (Livingston & Passaro, 1990). Clinicians often use the traditional practice of auscultation of bowel sounds to gain information on intestinal function and motility. However, bowels sounds have not been shown to correlate with motor patterns of function or dysfunction (Madsen *et al.*, 2005). The administration of EN has been shown to promote gastrointestinal motility in several studies (Stewart *et al.*, 1998; Beier-Holgersen & Boesby, 1996). Delivery of EN in clinical practice is not simple. Attention to the feed rate of EN delivery is important, as failure to increase this may not produce a postprandial motility response and without this there will be no normal small bowel contraction and peristalses, resulting in undigested EN passing into the colon.

Nutrition requirements

It is important to remember that the aim of nutritional support in the surgical patient is to reduce postoperative complications, whilst optimising recovery and quality of life. Postsurgical energy requirements vary according to the degree of trauma and concurrent clinical factors. After minor surgical procedures, normal energy expenditure will hardly be affected, whereas major procedures with resultant sepsis and high output stoma or drain losses potentially increase energy and protein requirements. Postoperative management of head and neck cancer patients has been shown to be improved if a dietitian is part of the multidisciplinary team (Wood, 2005).

The quality of nutritional support rather than the quantity is now considered the more relevant for postsurgical patients. An intake of 25–35 kcal/kg/day of total energy with 0.8–1.5 g of protein (0.13–0.24 g of nitrogen)/kg/day is a starting point. However, overzealous, aggressive nutritional support is not helpful if it leads to complications.

Fluid requirements can be met by 30–35 mL/kg/day, with additional fluid provided to compensate for pyrexia and increased drain, fistulae or stoma losses. Serum biochemistry and anthropometry are usually the only tools available to estimate the nutritional adequacy of a prescribed regimen, but it should be noted that these may not be representative of nutritional status in the postsurgical patient (Bachrach-Lindstrom et al., 2001).

It is widely known that postoperative fluid and electrolyte balance has been traditionally suboptimal (Lobo et al., 2001). Optimal fluid balance is central to the return of normal physiological function postoperatively. Suboptimal fluid balance can impair respiratory function and wound healing by affecting tissue oxygenation due to interstitial oedema. A positive fluid balance causes gut oedema. Lobo et al. (2001) concluded that fluid and sodium restriction in patients undergoing major colonic resection significantly reduced the duration of ileus and improved gut perfusion. Additionally, disturbances in acid–base balance, glucose or electrolytes affect gut function and motility, presumably due to altered cellular mechanics (Wilkes et al., 2001). The British Consensus Guidelines on Intravenous Fluid Therapy for Adult Surgical Patients (GIFTASUP) (Powell-Tuck et al., 2011) provide a useful consensus for the recommendations for perioperative fluid management, and these are now being incorporated into many hospital surgical and critical care units.

Glycaemic control

Postoperative insulin resistance and hyperglycaemia aggravate the inflammatory response, enhancing cytokine production and contributing to the surgical stress that negatively impacts on morbidity and mortality (Ljungqvist et al., 2005). Tight glycaemic control using sliding scale insulin therapy improves outcome (see Chapter 7.17.1). This appears to be due to a direct effect of insulin on blood glucose and an indirect effect of insulin in correcting abnormal serum lipid profile and downregulation of the catabolic state evoked in the surgically stressed patient (Vanhorebeek et al., 2005). Many ICUs adopting tight glycaemic control protocols require a 24-hour feed schedule to minimise the risk of catastrophic hypoglycaemia.

Nutritional management of surgical complications

Complications of feeding the surgical patient may relate to the presence of the underlying pathology (such as Crohn's disease, cachexia, pancreatitis or diabetes), the planned surgical outcome (such as ileostomy formation) or an adverse effect as a result of surgery (wound dehiscence, fistula formation, infection and pyrexia). The use of bariatric surgery as a method of weight management has increased dramatically in recent years and brings its own nutritional problems (Edwards et al., 2006), including late developing deficiencies of iron, vitamin B_{12}, calcium and vitamin D, in addition to protein energy malnutrition and fat malabsorption (Malinowski, 2006).

The immediate perioperative nutritional input for common complications of surgery is described below. Long term management of each condition may require a different approach.

Wound healing

Nutritional aspects of wound healing are discussed in Chapter 7.17.6. Malnutrition and recent nutritional intake are key factors in the complex mechanism of wound healing (Clark et al., 2000). However, up to date literature is scarce. Malnutrition has been linked to impaired wound healing in surgical patients. Even acute starvation for a few days is detrimental to wound healing (Hunt & Williams-Hopf, 1996). Goodson et al. (1987) showed that even 1–2 days of inadequate nutrient intake decreased hydroxyproline synthesis, one of the main components of collagen. Preoperative oral food intake is also important in wound healing (Windsor et al., 1988). The authors found a positive correlation between preoperative nutritional intake and improved postoperative wound healing. This is important as in clinical practice it is not uncommon for patients to have numerous radiological interventions and hence prolonged periods of nil by mouth in the week prior to surgical intervention.

Recent studies of the role of nutritional support in wound healing in surgical patients are limited; the majority are over 20 years old. Schroeder et al. (1991) concluded that EN in patients after gastrointestinal resection, compared with to nil by mouth and intravenous fluids, improved collagen synthesis and promoted wound strength. More recently, a meta analysis (Lewis et al., 2001) demonstrated that anastomotic dehiscence rates were reduced in patients receiving EN. A study by Braga et al. (2002) also suggested that EN is not detrimental to anastomotic healing even when early direct passage of nutrients over a fresh intestinal suture has occurred.

Enterocutaneous fistulae

These fistulae are tracts leading from the bowel to the skin surface. Low residue enteral feeds are well tolerated and do not contribute to losses from distal bowel fistula. Sodium and magnesium replacement may be necessary if the fistula drains small bowel contents. The use of antidiarrhoeal or antisecretory drugs may reduce fistula losses sufficient to allow healing. Enteral feeding with predigested formula may also be successful if a somatostatin analogue (octreotide) is given to reduce gastrointestinal secretions. Nutritional support decreases or modifies the composition of the gastrointestinal secretions and is considered to have a primary therapeutic role in the management of patients with a fistula (Dudrick et al., 1999).

Chylothorax

Chylothorax is the outcome of a rare but serious complication of thoracic surgery or major neck dissection, resulting in damage to the thoracic duct. Drainage of chyle from the thoracic duct injury into the pleural cavity results in chylothorax, which is relieved by chest drain insertion.

Most nutrients, including medium chain triglycerides (MCTs), are absorbed across the gastrointestinal tract into the portal circulation for transport to the liver. Dietary fats are insoluble in aqueous solutions such as blood, so are packaged into chylomicrons within the intestinal cells and then travel as chyle (fat rich lymph fluid) in the interstitial fluid within the lymphatic system. Chyle also contains quantities of protein, e.g. albumin, lymphocytes and antibodies and has an electrolyte composition similar to that of plasma. Chyle flow is reduced by fasting and increased by oral fluids, especially those high in long chain fatty acids. Intravenous fluids have no effect on chyle flow.

Chylothorax can be managed conservatively by following a very low fat diet (ideally providing <15 g of fat/day) and substituting MCTs for longer chain fatty acids in enteral or oral diets, or by bypassing the thoracic duct completely and using PN (which can contain long chain fatty acids). A chest drain relieves the chyle collection. If conservative management fails, ligation of the thoracic duct, traditionally carried out by thoracotomy is required. The advent of video assisted thoracoscopic surgery (VATS) permits a laparoscopic approach to ligation of the thoracic duct (Kumar *et al.*, 2004).

Acute pancreatitis

Early EN modulates the stress response, promotes more rapid resolution of pancreatitis and results in a better outcome compared to PN (McClave *et al.*, 2006). Enteral nutrition attenuates inflammation, reduces the incidence of septic complications and provides a more cost effective approach to postsurgical feeding than PN (Louie *et al.*, 2005) (see Chapter 7.4.5). The use of antioxidants has been shown to improve outcome (Braganza *et al.*, 2011), but this remains an area of controversy,

Open abdomen

Occasionally, patients undergoing abdominal surgery develop abdominal compartment syndrome (ACS); a massive intestinal oedema following abdominal laparotomy that renders the abdomen difficult to close surgically. Closure of the abdomen increases intra-abdominal pressure to such an extent that cardiovascular, respiratory and renal function is compromised. The abdomen is therefore left open but covered until swelling subsides and surgical closure can be achieved. It is possible to enterally feed a patient with an open abdomen without complication (Cothren *et al.*, 2004).

High output stomas and intestinal failure

The small intestine is initially maladapted to the uptake of sodium and water; a process usually confined to the large bowel. Net secretion occurs in the upper small intestine to increase the sodium content of luminal fluid and will have the effect of increasing stoma losses. Restricting the intake of salt poor fluids to <500 mL/day and sipping sodium rich oral rehydration solution, e.g. WHO rehydration solution or double strength Dioralyte or Rehydrat, can reduce small intestine secretions, minimise the fluid load through the small intestine and increase the chance of absorption. Alternatively, patients can take oral salt tablets *pro rata* with salt poor fluids for a similar effect (see Chapter 7.4.9).

The enhanced recovery after surgery programme

Traditionally, the use of nutritional support was a controversial postoperative therapeutic intervention. Perioperative use of nutritional support was reported to be *ad hoc* in many UK hospitals (Murphy *et al.*, 2006), with many patients remaining nil by mouth for the first week postoperatively. Parenteral nutrition was frequently used to provide nutritional support postoperatively. However, its use tended to be delayed and initiated only after the development of major surgical complications.

Over the past decade, the development of the ERAS programme has revolutionised the care of major elective surgical patients across Europe and the UK. This patient centred method optimises surgical outcome by improving clinical outcomes and patient experience. The ERAS programme was first described by Kehlet & Mogensen (1999) and it aims to improve the quality of care provided to patients who undergo major surgery. With improved care quality and reduced harm, it is assumed that the hospital stay will become more efficient and hospitals should benefit from the programme by savings in bed days (NHS Wales, 2010).

Enhanced recovery is sometimes referred to as fast track or accelerated surgery, and is supported by a growing base of clinical and research evidence (see the ESRA Society UK web site, www.erasuk.org). Enhanced recovery principles include:

- Optimising the patient's health/medical condition preoperatively.
- Assessing risk and fitness for surgery at preoperative assessment.
- Reducing starvation by using carbohydrate loading drinks up to 2 hours before surgery.
- Using minimally invasive surgery where possible.
- Using a clear and structured approach to postoperative management, including pain relief.
- Early mobilisation and early nutrition.

Enhanced recovery is dependent on the engagement, commitment and involvement of all members of the multidisciplinary team at all stages of the patient's care, starting at general practice surgery and continuing through the hospital stay and during recuperation in the patient's own home. Nutritional screening, assessment and early EN are key components of the ERAS pathway. The NHS enhanced recovery surgical pathway is shown in Figure 7.17.5; this is now embedded within the NHS.

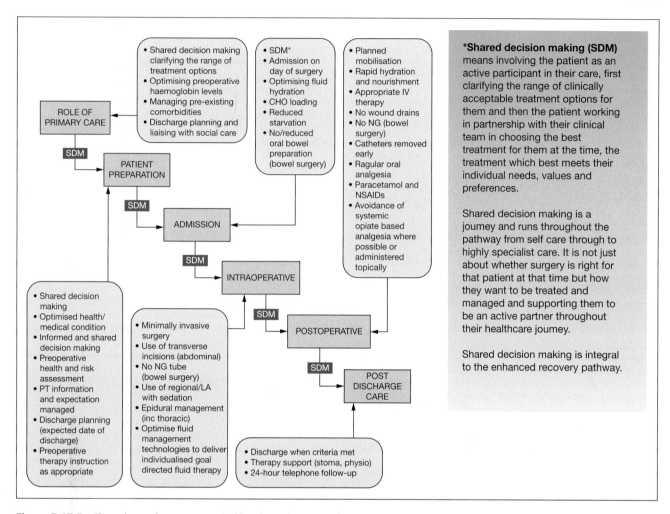

Figure 7.17.5 The enhanced recovery surgical l pathway (source: Enhanced Recovery Partnership. Reproduced with permission of the NHS) CHO, carbohydrate; IV, intravenous; NG, nasogastric; NSAIDs, non-steroidal anti-inflammatory drugs; PT, physiotherapy; LA, local anaesthetic

Internet resources

American Society of Anesthesiologists   www.asahq.org

Enhanced Recovery After Surgery in the NHS

   NHS Improvement   www.improvement.nhs.uk/
      enhancedrecovery2

   NHS Scotland   www.18weeks.scot.nhs.uk/service-redesign-and
     -transformation/enhanced-recovery/

   NHS Wales   www.1000livesplus.wales.nhs.uk

ESRA Society UK   www.erasuk.org

Royal College of Surgeons   www.rcsenf.ac.uk

References

Aiko S, Yoshizumi Y, Sugiura Y, *et al*. (2001) Beneficial effects of immediate enteral nutrition after esophageal cancer surgery. *Surgery Today* 31(11): 971–978.

Allison SP. (2000) Malnutrition, disease, and outcome. *Nutrition* 16: 590–593.

Allison SP. (2005) Integrated nutrition. *Proceedings of the Nutrition Society* 64(3): 319–323.

American Society of Anesthesiologists (ASA). (1999) Practice guidelines for preoperative fasting and the use of pharmacologic agents to reduce the risk of pulmonary aspiration. Application to healthy patients undergoing elective procedures. Anesthesiology 114:495*511.

Bachrach-Lindstrom M, Unosson M, Ek AC, Arnqvist HJ. (2001) Assessment of nutritional status using biochemical and anthropometric variables in a nutritional intervention study of women with hip fracture. *Clinical Nutrition* 20: 217–223.

Barlow R, Price P, Reid TD, *et al*. (2011) Prospective multicentre randomised controlled trial of early enteral nutrition for patients undergoing major upper GI resection. *Clinical Nutrition* 30(5): 560–566.

Beattie AH, Prach AT, Baxter JP, Pennington CR. (2000) A randomised controlled trial evaluating the use of enteral nutritional supplements postoperatively in malnourished surgical patients. *Gut* 46: 813–818.

Beier-Holgersen R, Boesby S. (1996) Influence of postoperative enteral nutrition on postsurgical infections. *Gut* 39(96): 833–835.

Biffi R, Lotti M, Cenciarelli S, *et al*. (2000) Complications and long-term outcome of 80 oncology patients undergoing needle catheter jejunostomy placement for early postoperative enteral feeding. *Clinical Nutrition* 19(4): 277–279.

Bisgaard T, Kristiansen VB, Hjortso NC, Jacobsen LS, Rosenberg J, Kehlet H. (2004) Randomized clinical trial comparing an oral carbohydrate beverage with placebo before laparoscopic cholecystectomy. *British Journal of Surgery* 91: 151–158.

Braga M, Gianotti L, Nespoli L, Radaelli G, Di Carlo V. (1999) Perioperative immunonutrition in patients undergoing cancer surgery: results of a randomized double-blind phase 3 trial. *Archives of Surgery* 134(4): 428–433.

Braga M, Gianotti L, Nespoli L, Radaelli G, Di Carlo V. (2002) Nutritional approach in malnourished surgical patients: a prospective randomized study. *Archives of Surgery* 137(2): 174–180.

Braganza J, Lee SH, McCloy RF, McMahon MJ. (2011) Chronic pancreatitis. *Lancet* 377: 1184–1197.

Burden ST, Hill J, Shaffer JL, Campbell M, Todd C. (2011) An unblended randomised controlled trial of preoperative oral supplements in colorectal cancer patients. *Journal of Human Nutrition and Dietetics* 24(5): 441–448.

Clark MA, Plank LD, Hill GL. (2000) *Wound healing associated with severe surgical illness. World Journal of Surgery* 24(6): 648–654.

Cothren CC, Moore EE, Ciesla DJ, et al. (2004) Postinjury abdominal compartment syndrome does not preclude early enteral feeding after definitive closure. *American Journal of Surgery* 188(6): 653–658.

Crenshaw JT, Winslow EH. (2002) Preoperative fasting: old habits die hard. *American Journal of Nursing* 102: 36–44.

Daly JM, Weintraub FN, Shou J, Rosato EF, Lucia M. (1995) Enteral nutrition during multimodality therapy in upper gastrointestinal cancer patients. *Annals of Surgery* 221(4): 327–338.

Delany HM, Carnevale NJ, Garvey JW. (1973) Jejunostomy by a needle catheter technique. *Surgery* 73(5): 786–790.

Dudrick SJ, Maharaj AR, McKelvey AA. (1999) Artificial nutritional support in patients with gastrointestinal fistulas. *World Journal of Surgery* 23: 570–576.

Eddy VA, Snell JE, Morris JA Jr. (1996) Analysis of complications and long-term outcome of trauma patients with needle catheter jejunostomy. *American Surgeon* 62(1): 40–44.

Edwards ED, Jacob BP, Gagner M, Pomp A. (2006) Presentation and management of common post-weight loss surgery problems in the emergency department. *Annals of Emergency Medicine* 47: 160–166.

Elwyn DH. (1980) Nutritional requirements of adult surgical patients. *Critical Care Medicine* 8: 9–20.

Ferguson M, Capra S. (1998) Quality of life in patients with malnutrition. *JAMA* 98: A–22.

Fettes SB, Davidson HI, Richardson RA, Pennington CR. (2002) Nutritional status of elective gastrointestinal surgery patients pre- and post-operatively. *Clinical Nutrition* 3: 249–254.

Gabor S, Renner H, Matzi V, Ratzenhofer B, et al. (2005) Early enteral feeding compared with parenteral nutrition after oesophageal or oesophago-gastric resection and reconstruction. *British Journal of Nutrition* 93: 509–513.

Genton L, Kudsk KA. (2003) Interactions between the enteric nervous system and the immune system: role of neuropeptides and nutrition. *American Journal of Surgery* 186(3): 253–258.

Gianotti L, Braga M, Nespoli L, Radaelli G, Beneduce A, Di Carlo V. (2002) A randomized controlled trial of preoperative oral supplementation with a specialized diet in patients with gastrointestinal cancer. *Gastroenterology* 122(7): 1763–1770.

Goodson WH, Lopez-Sarmiento A, Jensen JA, West J, Granja-Mena L, Chavez-Estrella J. (1987) The influence of a brief pre-operative illness on post-operative healing. *Annals of Surgery* 205: 250–255.

Hausel J, Nygren J, Thorell A, Lagerkranser M, Ljungqvist O. (2005) Randomized clinical trial of the effects of oral preoperative carbohydrates on postoperative nausea and vomiting after laparoscopic cholecystectomy. *British Journal of Surgery* 92: 415–421.

Holland J, Carey M, Hughes N, et al. (2005) Intraoperative splanchnic hypoperfusion, increased intestinal permeability, down-regulation of monocyte class II major histocompatibility complex expression, exaggerated acute phase response, and sepsis. *American Journal of Surgery* 190: 393–400.

Hunt K, Williams-Hopf I. (1996) Nutrition in wound healing. In: Fischer J (ed) *Nutrition and Metabolism in the Surgical Patient*. New York: Little, Brown and Company, p. 438.

Inui A. (1999) Cancer anorexia-cachexia syndrome: are neuropeptides the key? *Cancer Research* 59(18): 4493–4501.

Jellish WS, Kartha V, Fluder E, Slogoff S. (2005) Effect of metoclopramide on gastric fluid volumes in diabetic patients who have fasted before elective surgery. *Anesthesiology* 102(5): 904–909.

Kehlet H. (1999) Acute pain control and accelerated postoperative surgical recovery. *Surgical Clinics of North America* 79(2): 431–443.

Kehlet H, Mogensen T. (1999) Hospital stay of 2 days after open sigmoidectomy with a multimodal rehabilitation programme. *British Journal of Surgery* 86(2): 227–230.

Kreymann KG, Berger MM, Deutz NE, et al. (2006) ESPEN Guidelines on enteral nutrition: Intensive care. *Clinical Nutrition* 25(2): 210–223.

Kruizenga HM, Van Tulder MW, Seidell JC, Thijs A, Ader HJ, Van Bokhorst-de van der Schueren MA. (2005) Effectiveness and cost-effectiveness of early screening and treatment of malnourished patients. *American Journal of Clinical Nutrition* 82: 1082–1089.

Kudsk K. (2002) *Current aspects of mucosal immunology and its influence by nutrition. American Journal of Surgery* 183: 390–398.

Kudsk KA, Reddy SK, Sacks GS, Lai HC. (2003) Joint Commission for Accreditation of Health Care Organizations guidelines: too late to intervene for nutritionally at-risk surgical patients. *Journal of Parenteral and Enteral Nutrition* 27: 288–290.

Kumar S, Kumar A, Pawar DK. (2004) Thoracoscopic management of thoracic duct injury: Is there a place for conservatism? *Journal of Postgraduate Medicine* 50: 57–59.

Kuzu MA, Terzioglu H, Genc V, et al. (2006) Preoperative nutritional risk assessment in predicting postoperative outcome in patients undergoing major surgery. *World Journal of Surgery* 30: 378–390.

Kyle UG, Kossovsky MP, Karsegard VL, Pichard C. (2005) Comparison of tools for nutritional assessment and screening at hospital admission: A population study. *Clinical Nutrition* 2005 25(3): 409–417.

Lassen K, Hannemann P, Ljungqvist O, et al. Enhanced Recovery After Surgery Group. (2005) Patterns in current perioperative practice: survey of colorectal surgeons in five northern European countries. *BMJ* 330: 1420–1421.

Lewis SJ, Egger M, Sylvester PA, Thomas S. (2001) Early enteral feeding versus 'nil by mouth' after gastrointestinal surgery: systematic review and meta-analysis of controlled trials. *BMJ* 323: 773–776.

Livingston EH, Passaro EP Jr. (1990) Postoperative ileus. *Digestive Diseases & Sciences* 35(1): 121–132.

Ljungqvist O, Søreide E. (2003) Preoperative fasting. *British Journal of Surgery* 90: 400–406.

Ljungqvist O, Nygren J, Soop M, Thorell A. (2005) Metabolic perioperative management: novel concepts. *Current Opinion in Critical Care* 11: 295–299.

Lobo DN, Dube MG, Neal KR, Simpson J, Rowlands BJ, Allison SP. (2001) Problems with solutions: drowning in the brine of an inadequate knowledge base. *Clinical Nutrition* 20(2): 125–130.

Louie BE, Noseworthy T, Hailey D, Gramlich LM, Jacobs P, Warnock GL. (2005) 2004 MacLean-Mueller prize. Enteral or parenteral nutrition for severe pancreatitis: a randomized controlled trial and health technology assessment. *Canadian Journal of Surgery* 48: 298–306.

Macfie J, Woodcock NP, Palmer MD, Walker A, Townsend S, Mitchell CJ. (2000) Oral dietary supplements in pre- and postoperative surgical patients: a prospective and randomised control trial. *Nutrition* 16: 723–728.

McClave SA, Chang WK, Dhaliwal R, Heyland DK. (2006) Nutrition support in acute pancreatitis: a systematic review of the literature. *Journal of Parenteral and Enteral Nutrition* 30(2): 143–156.

Madsen D, Sebolt T, Cullen L, et al. (2005) Listening to bowel sounds: an evidence-based practice project: nurses find that a traditional practice isn't the best indicator of returning gastrointestinal motility in patients who've undergone abdominal surgery. *American Journal of Nursing* 105(12): 40–49.

Malinowski SS. (2006) Nutritional and metabolic complications of bariatric surgery. *American Journal of Medical Science* 331: 219–225.

Maltby JR, Pytka S, Watson NC, Cowan RA, Fick GH. (2004) Drinking 300 mL of clear fluid two hours before surgery has no effect on gastric fluid volume and pH in fasting and non-fasting obese patients. *Canadian Journal of Anaesthesia* 51: 111–115.

Marik PE, Zaloga GP. (2001) Early enteral nutrition in acutely ill patients: a systematic review. *Critical Care Medicine* 29(12): 2264–2270.

McKenna SP, Thorig L. (1995) Nutrition and quality of life. *Nutrition* 11(3): 308–309.

Melis GC, van Leeuwen PA, von Blomberg-van der Flier BM, *et al.* (2006a) A carbohydrate-rich beverage prior to surgery prevents surgery-induced immunodepression: a randomized, controlled, clinical trial. *Journal of Parenteral and Enteral Nutrition* 30: 21–26.

Melis M, Fichera, A, Ferguson, MK. (2006b) Bowel Necrosis associated with early jejunal tube feeding: A complication of postoperative enteral nutrition. *Archives of Surgery* 141(7): 701–704.

Møiniche S, Bülow S, Hesselfeldt P, Hestbaek A, Kehlet H. (1995) Convalescence and hospital stay after colonic surgery with balanced analgesia, early oral feeding, and enforced mobilisation. *European Journal of Surgery* 161(4): 283–288.

Murphy PM, Modi P, Rahamim J, Wheatley T, Lewis SJ. (2006) An Investigation into the Current Peri-Operative Nutritional Management of Oesophageal Carcinoma Patients in Major Carcinoma Centres in England. *Annals of the Royal College of Surgeons of England* 88(4): 358–362.

Mythen MG. (2005) Postoperative gastrointestinal tract dysfunction. *Anesthesia & Analgesia* 100(1): 196–204.

National Confidential Enquiry into Patient Outcome and Death (NECPOD). (2011) Knowing the risk; A review of the peri-operative care of surgical patients. Available at www.ncepod.org.uk/2011report2/downloads/POC_fullreport.pdf. Accessed 1 December 2012.

National Institute for Health and Care Excellence (NICE). (2006) *Nutrition support in adults*. Clinical Guideline 32. London: NICE. Available at www.nice.org.uk/CG032.

NHS Wales. (2011) How to guide (16). Enhances recovery after surgery. Available at www.wales.nhs.uk. Accessed 2 February 2012.

Powell-Tuck J, Gosling P, Lobo DN, *et al.* (2011) British Consensus Guidelines on intravenous fluid therapy for adult surgical patients GIFTASUP. Available at www.bapen.org.uk/pdfs/bapen_pubs/giftasup.pdf. Accessed 2 February 2012.

Rapp-Kesek D, Stahle E, Karlsson TT. (2004) Body mass index and albumin in the preoperative evaluation of cardiac surgery patients. *Clinical Nutrition* 23: 1398–1404.

Royal College of Nursing (RCN). (2005) *Perioperative fasting in adults and children*. A national guideline. London: RCN. Available at www.rcn.org.uk.

Ryan AM, Rowley SP, Healy LA, Flood PM, Ravi N, Reynolds JV. (2006) Post-oesophagectomy early enteral nutrition via a needle catheter jejunostomy: 8-year experience at a specialist unit. *Clinical Nutrition* 25(3): 386.

Salvino RM, Dechicco RS, Seidner DL. (2004) Perioperative nutrition support: who and how. *Cleveland Clinical Journal of Medicine* 71: 345–351.

Sand J, Luostarinen M, Matikainen M. (1997) Enteral or parenteral feeding after total gastrectomy: prospective randomised pilot study. *European Journal of Surgery* 163(10): 761–766.

Sarr MG. (1988) Needle catheter jejunostomy: an aid to postoperative care of the morbidly obese patient. *American Surgeon* 54(8): 510–512.

Saqr L, Chambers WA. (2006) Preventing excessive pre-operative fasting: national guideline or local protocol? *Anaesthesia* 61: 1–3.

Schilder JM, Hurteau JA, Look KY, *et al.* (1997) A prospective controlled trial of early postoperative oral intake following major abdominal gynecologic surgery. *Gynecologic Oncology* 67(3): 235–240.

Schroeder D, Gillanders L, Mahr K, Hill GL. (1991) Effects of immediate postoperative enteral nutrition on body composition, muscle function, and wound healing. *Journal of Parenteral and Enteral Nutrition* 15(4): 376–383.

Smedley F, Bowling T, James M, *et al.* (2004) Randomised clinical trial of the effects of preoperative and postoperative oral nutritional supplements on clinical course and cost of care. *British Journal of Surgery* 91: 983–990.

Stewart BT, Woods RJ, Collopy BT, Fink RJ, Mackay JR, Keck JO. (1998) Early feeding after elective open colorectal resections: a prospective randomized trial. *Australian & New Zealand Journal of Surgery* 68(2): 125–128.

Vanhorebeek I, Langouche L, Van den Berghe G. (2005) Glycemic and nonglycemic effects of insulin: how do they contribute to a better outcome of critical illness? *Current Opinion in Critical Care* 11: 304–311.

Waitzberg DL, Saito H, Plank LD, *et al.* (2006) Post surgical infections are reduced with specialised nutritional support. *World Journal of Surgery* 30: 1592–1604.

Watters JM, Kirkpatrick SM, Norris SB, Shamji FM, Wells GA. (1997) Immediate postoperative enteral feeding results in impaired respiratory mechanics and decreased mobility. *Annals of Surgery* 226(3): 369–377; discussion 377–380.

Weimann A, Braga M, Harsanyi L, *et al.* (2006) ESPEN Guidelines on enteral nutrition: Surgery including organ transplantation. *Clinical Nutrition* 25(2): 224–244.

Wilkes NJ, Woolf R, Mutch M, *et al.* (2001) The effects of balanced versus saline-based hetastarch and crystalloid solutions on acid-base and electrolyte status and gastric mucosal perfusion in elderly surgical patients. *Anesthesia and Analgesia* 93(4): 811–816.

Windsor J, Knight G, Hill GL. (1988) Wound healing responses in surgical patients: recent food intake is more important than nutritional status. *British Journal of Surgery* 75: 135.

Windsor A, Braga M, Martindale R, *et al.* (2004) Fit for surgery: an expert panel review on optimising patients prior to surgery, with a particular focus on nutrition. *Surgeon* 2: 315–319.

Wood K. (2005) Audit of nutritional guidelines for head and neck cancer patients undergoing radiotherapy. *Journal of Human Nutrition and Dietetics* 18: 343–351.

Yuill KA, Richardson RA, Davidson HI, Garden OJ, Parks RW. (2005) The administration of an oral carbohydrate-containing fluid prior to major elective upper-gastrointestinal surgery preserves skeletal muscle mass postoperatively – a randomised clinical trial. *Clinical Nutrition* 24: 32–37.

7.17.6 Wound healing, tissue viability and pressure sores
Christina Merryfield

Key points

■ Malnutrition impairs wound healing.

■ Micronutrient status should be checked and deficiencies corrected.

■ There is no additional benefit for supplemental intakes of micronutrients in the absence of deficiency.

■ It is important to identify other local and systemic factors that may delay or impede healing, e.g. medication, anaemia, smoking and age.

In the early 1990s wound care gained importance with a rapid expansion of outpatient clinics and the emergence of multidisciplinary team experts in wound care (Peirce, 2007). Today's clinical setting has a critical dependence on technology and rapid advancement of healthcare practice. Nutrition continues to be essential in dealing with wound care management; it was Florence Nightingale who defined the nursing role *as 'preparing the patient for the most favourable condition for healing'* (Hurd, 2003).

A wound may be described in many ways; by its aetiology, anatomical location and whether it is acute or chronic (Enoch & Price, 2004). A wound is a breakdown in the protective function of the skin, with the loss of continuity of epithelium with or without loss of underlying connective tissue (muscle, bone, nerves) (Leaper & Harding, 1998). Wounds occur following injury to the skin, underlying tissues or organs caused by surgery, trauma, cuts, chemicals, heat or cold, friction, shear force, pressure or disease, such as leg ulcers or carcinomas (Hutchinson, 1992). A pressure ulcer is defined as a localised injury to the skin and/or underlying tissue, usually over a bony prominence as a result of pressure, or pressure in combination with shear and/or fraction. A number of contributing or confounding factors are also associated with pressure ulcers; the significance of these factors has yet to be elucidated. Wound healing can be defined as the physiology by which the body replaces and restores function to damaged tissues (Shipperley & Martin, 2002).

Diagnostic criteria and classification

Skin wounds will commonly result in the exposure of dermal tissues to the environment, haemorrhage, and loss of body fluids (water and plasma), micronutrients and metabolites, thus disturbing intercellular relationships (Lansdown, 2001). Wounds are often divided into acute or chronic and heal by primary or secondary intention. Acute wounds result from surgery or trauma and usually have a relatively short, uneventful healing time. Chronic wounds such as leg ulcers, pressure ulcers, diabetic foot ulcers and malignant wounds have prolonged healing times, are prone to episodes of infection and may

have increased levels of exudate due to prolonged inflammation (Gray *et al.*, 2006). Common types of chronic wounds are venous, arterial, neuropathic and pressure. Other important causes include malignancy, drug induced ulcers and vasculitis (Fan Wai-Ping *et al.*, 2010).

A pressure ulcer is an area of damage that is caused by unrelieved pressure, friction and/or shear forces. Currently there are four stages of pressure ulcers, plus two additional stages for deep tissue injury and unstageable pressure ulcers (Black *et al.*, 2007]. Stage I and II ulcers generally are considered the least severe and stage IV ulcers are considered the most severe, but a broad range of skin damage or necrosis may be represented within the stage III classification. A stage III wound may appear shallow and superficial or as a full thickness wound (Tempest *et al.*, 2010).

Process of wound healing

The process of wound healing can be divided into three overlapping phases:

- Inflammatory.
- Proliferation.
- Maturation and remodelling.

Some wounds heal with routine wound care; however, those with rough edges and tissue deficit are likely to take longer to heal. The inflammatory stage occurs during the first few days and the wound area attempts to restore homeostasis by constricting blood vessels to control bleeding. Platelet aggregation and thromboplastin make a clot and inflammation occurs. The proliferative stage lasts 3 or more weeks. Granulation occurs and collagen is formed to fill the wound and new blood vessels are formed. The maturation and remodelling stage may last up to 2 years during which time new collagen is synthesised and eventually scar tissue is formed (RCN, 2005) (Figure 7.17.6).

Healing of wounds, whether from accidental injury or surgical intervention, involves the activity of an intricate network of blood cells, tissue types, cytokines and growth factors. This results in increased cellular activity, which intensifies the metabolic demand for nutrients (MacKay

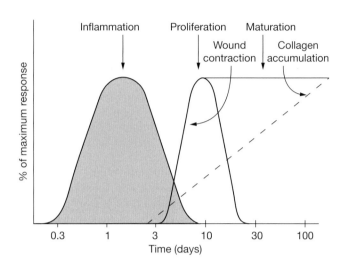

Figure 7.17.6 Stages of wound healing (source: Royal College of Nursing, 2005, figure 1, p. 30. Reproduced with permission of the Royal College of Nursing)

& Miller, 2003). The aim of wound healing management is to achieve a stable wound that has healthy granulation tissue tone characterised by a well vascularised wound bed. Good management should remove, or at least minimise, factors that delay healing (Enoch & Harding, 2003).

Disease consequence and public health

In the UK, chronic wounds represent a significant burden to patients and the NHS; approximately 200 000 patients have a chronic wound. Common symptoms of ulceration include pain, exudate and odour, and these symptoms are frequently associated with poor sleep, loss of mobility and social isolation. The cost of chronic wound care in an average general district hospital has been estimated to be £600 000 to £3 million per year (NHS Institute for Innovation and Improvement, 2009). It is estimated that one in five hospitalised patients have a pressure ulcer; this represent at least 20 000 hospital patients in the UK at any time (Posnett & Franks, 2008). Trends in patients with chronic wounds in the UK are likely to increase due to an ageing population. Care of pressure ulcers in nursing homes has been estimated to account for 4% of the NHS annual spending on budget (Bennett *et al.*, 2004). The scale of wound care in terms of the personnel and beds required per health district has been reported to be equivalent to 88.5 whole time equivalent nurses and up to 87 hospital beds (Drew *et al.*, 2007).

Good nutritional status is essential for wound healing to take place. Ignoring nutritional status may compromise the patient's ability to heal and subsequently prolong the stages of wound healing (Russell, 2001). Malnutrition is frequently undetected and untreated, causing a wide range of adverse consequences such as impaired wound healing and subsequently increased length of hospital stay. In 2010 34% of patients were found to be at risk of malnutrition (BAPEN, 2010), which is higher than the overall prevalence found in the 2008 and 2007 surveys. This represents a considerable number of people at risk of poor wound healing (see Chapter 6.2). The use of nutritional screening or assessment tools appears to be more prevalent in managing patients at risk of pressure ulcers. However, they should not replace clinical judgement (EPUAP, 2003).

Assessment

Assessment should include the following (see Chapter 2.2 and Chapter 2.3).

Anthropometry

This should include weight, height and calculated body mass index (BMI). Mid upper arm circumference (MUAC) is a useful alternative indicator of nutritional status if it is not possible to measure height or weight. Impaired hand grip strength has been shown to be a popular marker of nutritional status and is an indicator of increased postoperative complications, increased length of hospitalisation, higher rehospitalisation and decreased physical status (Norman *et al.*, 2011). It is essential that patients and care home residents be screened for the risk of malnutrition as recommended by the National Institute for Health and Care Excellence (NICE, 2006).

Biochemical assessment

In general, it is unlikely that biochemical measurements will provide more information than other indicators such as undesired weight loss, although there may be an association between albumin level and pressure ulcers.

Clinical assessment

Assessment tools such as the Waterlow pressure ulcer risk assessment tool is frequently used in the UK; it incorporates a scoring system and provides guidance associated with levels of risk status (Waterlow, 2005). The assessment incorporates BMI and a malnutrition screening tool such as the Malnutrition Universal Screening Tool ('MUST') (see Chapter 6.2).

Dietary assessment

It is fundamental to assess whether the patient has an optimum nutritional status to allow wounds to heal. A diet history and/or food chart at ward level will help to assess the patient's intake.

Clinical investigation and management

Factors that may delay or prevent wound healing can be localised or systemic throughout the body, as shown in Table 7.17.19.

An individual's potential to develop pressure ulcers may be influenced by various factors (NICE, 2005), including:

- Reduced mobility or immobility.
- Sensory impairment.
- Acute illness.
- Level of consciousness.

Table 7.17.19 Factors that may delay or impede wound healing (Gottrup *et al.*, 2007)

Local factors	Systemic factors
Primary	**Pivotal**
Blood supply (tissue perfusion)	Haemodynamic conditions
Tissue oxygen tension	(perfusion, hypovolaemia, hypoxia, pain, etc.)
Secondary	**Important**
Tissue damage	Age
Mechanical stress of the tissue	Smoking
Hypothermia	Medication
Pain	Diseases
Radiation	Nutritional status
Infection	Anaemia
Surgical technique	Alcoholism
Suture technique and materials	Radiation
Others (vasculitis, immunological, etc.)	Others (immunological, etc.)

- Extremes of age.
- Vascular disease.
- Severe chronic or terminal illness.
- Previous history of pressure damage.
- Malnutrition and dehydration.

Wound healing assessment is critical for the planning and evaluation of care, and should include (Gottrup *et al.*, 2007):

- Medical history.
- Cause of tissue damage.
- Medication and allergies.
- Other diseases, e.g. diabetes, vascular disease and immune compromise.
- Lifestyle and environment – obesity, tobacco and/or alcohol use.
- Impaired mobility.
- Inadequate social network, carer support.
- Psychological problems.

An infected pressure ulcer will also increase tissue damage, causing further strain, a deeper ulcer and an increase in nutritional demands (Hurd, 2003). The infection requires treatment in order for the wound to heal.

Nutritional management

Nutritional requirements increase in the presence of a chronic wound and if the demand is not met, this can have a significant impact on wound healing. Metabolic demand rises in the presence of a wound due to greatly increased cell activity in the region (Casey, 1998). Optimum nutrition is a key factor in maintaining all phases of wound healing. Protein energy malnutrition (PEM) in the presence of a wound will lead to the loss of lean body tissue or protein stores, which will impede the healing process (Demling, 2009). A balance of all food groups is required to meet the essential nutrient needs for wound healing. The role of specific nutrients in wound healing is shown in Table 7.17.20.

Macronutrients

Metabolic or energy demands rise significantly in the presence of a wound. It has been estimated that the basal metabolic rate rises by up to 10% following even minor surgery and can rise by 100% or more in the presence of severe burns (White & Baxter, 1998). It is estimated that an individual may require a minimum of 30–35 kcal/kg of body weight/day (EPUAP, 2003). Activation of the immune system and the action of white blood cells demand higher levels of energy. Intake of insufficient energy will lead to a decrease in fat stores and the loss of protective cushioning, thus increasing the likelihood of pressure injuries (Todorovic, 2003). Also, low energy intake is usually associated with a lower intake of micronutrients and resultant deficiencies may impact wound healing (Thomas, 2001).

Carbohydrates together with fats are the primary source of energy in the wound healing process. Glucose is the major source of fuel used to provide energy for new tissues and prevent depletion of protein (Guo & DiPietro, 2010). Fat has a role in cell membrane structure and function. n-3 Fatty acids may have a role in increasing proinflammatory cytokine production at wound sites and therefore have the potential to affect wound healing during the inflammatory stage (McDaniel *et al.*, 2010). There is also some evidence that n-3 fatty acids may have a benefit when administered pre- and post-operatively as immune feeds (Moskovitz & Kim, 2002).

There is a direct correlation between wounds that are non-healing and the indication of PEM. Therefore, wound healing depends on good wound management along with the reversal of PEM (Hurd, 2003). Protein malnutrition delays wound healing by impairing collagen synthesis and deposition, and decreasing scar strength (Arnold & Barbul, 2006). Prolonged inadequate protein intake may promote tissue oedema, which delays healing by slowing oxygen diffusion from capillaries to cell membranes. Available nutrients will be drawn to the wound site initially, with lean muscle mass used to provide the amino acids necessary for wound healing. A 15% or greater loss of lean body mass is associated with impaired wound healing; a 30% or greater loss is associated with development of new wounds (Demling, 2009). Minor surgery may not significantly increase protein requirement; however, if the patient is already malnourished, wound healing will be adversely affected unless dietary protein intake is increased (MacKay & Miller, 2003). Studies have shown that increasing the protein in the diet of patients with chronic ulcers leads to faster healing times when compared with low protein diets (Hurd, 2003).

There have been mixed results on the impact of using glutamine in burns patients. However, in some experimental studies there seems to be some positive impact on wound healing (Robert & Demling, 2009).

Micronutrients

Micronutrients serve a vital role in wound healing and metabolic functions. Vitamins A, B_1, B_2 and B_6 are vital to energy production and collagen deposition (Woodward

Table 7.17.20   Role of key nutrients in tissue viability and wound healing (Johnston, 2007)

Nutrient	Function	Comments
Fat	Energy Cell membrane component Involved in formation of inflammatory mediators and clotting components	
Carbohydrate	Energy	
Protein	Tissue synthesis and repair	Excess protein can stress the liver and kidney
Vitamin A	Enhances immune response Antioxidant Promotes collagen synthesis and epithelialisation	Excess toxic
Vitamin C	Antioxidant Promotes collagen synthesis and angiogenesis Enhances iron absorption Promotes immune function	Additional vitamin C not beneficial unless deficient
Selenium	Antioxidant	Deficiency relatively common
Copper	Collagen cross linkage	Deficiency rare
Manganese	Component of enzymes needed for tissue Regeneration	Deficiency rare Magnesium can substitute for manganese when manganese status is poor
Zinc	Fibroblast proliferation Component of enzyme systems Collagen synthesis Immune function	Zinc supplement will not accelerate healing if not deficient in patients Can cause toxicity
Iron	Promotes collagen synthesis Improves O_2, nutrient and components of healing delivery to tissue Component of many enzyme systems	Blood loss can lead to anaemia
B vitamins	Efficient energy usage Collagen formation Component of enzyme systems	
Vitamin E	Antioxidant Enhances immune response	Excess can impair wound healing
Vitamin K	Blood clotting	Deficiency very rare

et al., 2009). Copper, zinc and selenium have a role in immune function and can be lost in significant amounts in patients with wounds, particularly in the burn exudate and urine of patients with severe burns. Patients with total body surface area burns of 30% or greater should be given intravenous supplementation for the first 8 days from admission and serum levels monitored on a weekly basis (Berger et al., 1998).

Vitamin C is essential for collagen formation and critical for wound healing. An eight-fold increase in wound dehiscence has been reported in patients who had depleted concentrations of vitamin C compared with those who had adequate concentrations (Zaloga, 1994). It has been suggested that patients with stage III or IV pressure ulcers may benefit from supplementation with 500 mg twice daily for 14 days (Castellanos et al., 2003). However, discretion must be used when recommending vitamin C supplementation as toxicity may occur in patients who are at risk for oxalate stone formation, although the risk is low (Posthauer, 2006; Flanigan, 1997). To maximise wound healing but minimise soft tissue damage in patients with renal failure, a suggested maximum recommended intake is 100 mg/day (Winkler,

2000; Clark, 2002). Doses over 200 mg/day are not usually required as tissue saturation occurs at this level (Woodward et al., 2009). Some studies have shown that vitamin C supplementation at 60–200 mg/day only helps a pressure ulcer to heal if the patient is deficient in vitamin C. Vitamin C supplementation in non-deficient patients has not been shown to accelerate wound healing (Ringsdorf & Cheraskin, 1982).

Adequate concentrations of vitamin A appear to influence the body's therapeutic inflammatory response to wounds (Arnold & Barbul, 2006). Vitamin A plays a role in cell division, cell differentiation and immune system function (National Institutes of Health, 2009). Depletion of vitamin A, although rare, can result in impaired wound healing and susceptibility to infection (Ross, 2002).

Zinc has an identifiable role in all stages of wound healing (Bradbury, 2006). Deficiency has been associated with delayed wound healing by reducing the rate of epithelialisation, and decreasing scar strength and collagen synthesis (Andrews et al., 1999). Although zinc supplementation is often recommended, it does not appear to aid the healing of leg ulcers, although it may be beneficial in those with venous legs ulcers and low serum zinc

(Wilkinson, 2012). A suggested supplementation for non-healing pressure ulcers is 15 mg/day and 20–25 mg/day for larger non-healing wounds, but this should be limited to 14 days (Woodward *et al.*, 2009). It has been acknowledged that excess zinc in animals can have a detrimental effect on wound healing (Lim *et al.*, 2004). In humans, excess zinc has been shown to induce both copper and iron deficient anaemia, which could result in decreased oxygen delivery to the wound (Gray, 2003). There appears to be more support for supplementing zinc deficient patients in order to improve wound healing rather than routine zinc supplementation (Bradbury, 2006).

Iron

Iron is necessary for the formation of collagen and to support tissue oxygenation at the wound site. Low haemoglobin levels need to be corrected before healing can continue effectively (McClemont, 1984). Iron also provides oxygen to the site of the wound (Woodward *et al.* 2009).

Fluid

Adequate fluid is required to maintain good skin tone and blood flow to wounded tissues, which is critical for the prevention of skin breakdown. A general guide of 30–35 mL/kg of body weight/day (minimum of 1500 mL/day) is recommended, but should be adjusted depending on the patient's clinical condition, such as cardiac and renal problems for which fluid may be restricted (Todorovic, 2003). Dehydration is also a major risk factor for the development of pressure sores as the skin becomes inelastic, fragile and more susceptible to breakdown (Horns *et al.*, 2004).

Drug–nutrient interactions

Medications may have a positive or negative effect on wound healing. Drugs that impair wound healing include those that are frequently used in the clinical setting. Corticosteroids inhibit fibroplasia and the formation of granulation tissue. High doses have a major effect on wound healing because of their interference with vascular proliferation and their effect of delaying epithelialisation. Antiplatelet drugs, including aspirin and other non-steroidal anti-inflammatory drugs, have a dose dependant effect as they act as inflammatory mediators. Anticoagulants such as warfarin and heparin inhibit proper coagulation and adversely affect wounds. Conversely, drugs such as prostacyclin can be used to promote healing in arterial and vasculitic ulcers. Calcium antagonists can help improve blood flow (Sussman, 2007).

Internet resources

Coloplast Wound Care   www.coloplast.co.uk
European Pressure Ulcer Advisory Panel   www.epuap.org
National Institute for Health and Care Excellence
   Clinical Guideline (CG29) Pressure Ulcers – Prevention and Treatment   www.nice.org.uk/nicemedia/pdf/CG029publicinfo.pdf
The Waterlow Score card   www.judy-waterlow.co.uk
World Wide Wounds   www.worldwidewounds.com

References

Andrews M, Gallager-Allred C. (1999) The role of zinc in wound healing. *Advances in Wound Care* 12: 137–138.

Arnold M, Barbul A. (2006) Nutrition and wound healing. *Journal of Plastic and Reconstructive Surgery* 117 42–48.

Berger MM, Spertini F, Shenkin A, *et al.* (1998). Trace element supplementation modulates infection rates in major burns: A double blind placebo clinical trial. *American Journal of Clinical Nutrition* 68: 365–371.

Bennett G, Dealey C, Posnett J. (2004). The cost of pressure ulcers in the UK. *Age and Ageing* 33: 230–235.

Black J, Baharestani M, Cuddigan J, *et al.*, National Pressure Ulcer Advisory Panel (NPUAP). (2007) National Pressure Ulcer Advisory Panel's updated pressure ulcer staging system. *Dermatology Nursing* 19(4): 343–349.

Bradbury S. (2006) Wound healing: is oral zinc supplementation beneficial? *Wounds UK* 2(1): 54–61.

British Association of Parenteral and Enteral Nutrition (BAPEN). (2010). Nutrition Screening Survey in the UK and Republic of Ireland in 2010. Available at www.bapen.org.uk. Accessed 18 July 2012.

Casey G. (1998) The importance of nutrition in wound healing. *Nursing Standard* 13(3): 51–56.

Castellanos WH, Silver HJ, Gallagher-Allred C, Smith TR. (2003) Nutrition Issues in the Home, Community and Long-term Care Setting. *Nutrition in Clinical Practice* 18: 21–36.

Clark S. (2002) The biochemistry of antioxidants revisited. *Nutrition in Clinical Practice* 17: 5–17.

Demling RH. (2009) Nutrition, anabolism, and the wound healing process: an overview. *ePlasty* 9: 65–94.

Drew P, Posnett J, Rusling L. (2007). The cost of wound care for a local population in England. *International Wound Journal* 4(2): 149–155.

Enoch S, Harding K. (2003) Wound bed preparation: The science behind the removal of barriers to healing. *Wounds; A Compendium of Clinical Research and Practice* 15(7): 213–229.

Enoch S, Price P. (2004) Cellular, molecular and biochemical differences in the pathophysiology of healing between acute wounds, chronic wounds and wounds in the aged. Available at www.worldwidewounds.com.

European Pressure Ulcer Advisory Panel (EPUAP). (2003) Nutritional guidelines for pressure ulcer prevention and treatment. Available at www.epuap.org.

Fan Wai-Ping L, Rashid M, Enoch S. (2010) Current advances in modern wound healing. *Wounds UK* 6(93): 22–36.

Flanigan KH. (1997) Nutritional aspects of wound healing. *Advances in Wound Care* 10: 48–52.

Gottrup F, Kirsner R, Meaumes S, Münter C, Sibbald G. (2007) *Clinical Wound Assessment – A Pocket Guide*. Coloplast A/S, p. 6.

Gray M. (2003) Does oral zinc supplementation promote healing of chronic wounds. *Journal of Wound Ostomy and Continence Nursing* 30(6): 295–299.

Gray D, Cooper P, Timmons J (eds). (2006) *Essential Wound Management. An Introduction for Undergraduates*. Wounds UK Limited, p. 6.

Guo S, DiPietro L. (2010) Factors affecting wound healing. *Journal of Dental Research* 89(3): 219–229.

Horns D, Bender SA, Ferguson ML, *et al.* (2004) The National Pressure Ulcer Long-term Care Study: Pressure ulcer development in long-term care residents. *Journal of the American Geriatrics Society* 52: 359–367.

Hurd TA. (2003). Nutrition and wound-care management/prevention. *Wound Care Canada* 2(2): 20–24.

Hutchinson J. (1992) *The Wound Programme*. Dundee: Centre for Medical Education.

Johnston E. (2007) The role of nutrition in tissue viability. *Wound Essentials* 2: 10–21.

Lansdown ABG. (2001) Nutrition and the healing of skin wounds. *Wound Care Society Educational Booklets*, Oct, 8(2).

Leaper DJ, Harding KG. (1998) *Wounds: Biology and Management*. Oxford: Oxford University Press, pp. 23–40.

Lim Y, Levy M, Bray TM. (2004) Dietary zinc alters early inflammatory responses during cutaneous wound healing in weaning CD-1 mice. *Journal of Nutrition* 134(94): 811–816.

MacKay D, Miller AL. (2003) Nutritional support for wound healing. *Alternative Medicine Reviews* 8(4): 359–377.

McClemont E. (1984) Pressure sores. No pressure-no sore. *Nursing (London)* 2(21), Suppl 3.

McDaniel JC, Belury M, Ahijevych K, Blakely W. (2010) Omega-3 fatty acids effect on wound healing. *Journal of Dental Research* 89(3): 219–229.

Moskovitz AN, Kim YI. (2002) Does perioperative immunonutrition reduce postoperative complications in patients with gastrointestinal cancer undergoing operations? *Nutrition Reviews* 62: 443–447.

National Institute for Health and Care Excellence (NICE). (2005) *Pressure Ulcer Risk Assessment and Prevention*. CG 29. Available at www.nice.org.uk/nicemedia/pdf/CG029publicinfo.pdf. Accessed 18 July 2012.

National Institute for Health and Care Excellence (NICE). (2006) *Nutrition Support in Adults. Oral nutrition support, enteral tube feeding and parenteral nutrition*. Clinical Guideline 32. London: NICE. Accessed 1 March 2013.

National Institutes of Health (NIH). (2009) *Office of Dietary Supplements Vitamin A and Caroteniods*. Bethesda: NIH.

NHS Institute for Innovation and Improvement. (2009) High impact actions for nursing and midwifery, Coventry. Available at www.institute.nhs.uk. Accessed 18 July 2012.

Norman K, Stobäus N, Gonzalez MC, Schulzke JD, Pirlich M. (2011) Hand grip strength: Outcome predictor and marker of nutritional status. *Clinical Nutrition* 30(2): 135–142.

Peirce B. (2007) Wound care and the WOC nurse. How did we get here? *Journal of Wound Ostomy and Continence Nursing* 34(6): 602–604.

Posnett J, Franks PJ. (2008) The burden of chronic wounds in the UK. *Nursing Times* 104(3): 44–45.

Posthauer ME. (2006) The role of nutrition in wound care. Clinical management extra. *Advances in Skin Wound Care* 19: 43–52.

Ringsdorf WM Jr, Cheraskin E. (1982) Vitamin C and human wound healing. *Oral Surgery Oral Medicine Oral Pathology* 53: 231–236.

Ross V. (2002) Micronutrient recommendations for wound healing. *Support Line* 24(4): 3–9.

Robert H, Demling RH. (2009) Nutrition, anabolism and the wound healing process: An overview. *ePlasty* 9: 65–94.

Royal College of Nursing (RCN). (2005) *The Management of Pressure Ulcer's in Primary and Secondary Care. A Clinical Practice Guideline*. London: RCN.

Russell L. (2001) The importance of patients' nutritional status in wound healing. *British Journal of Nursing* 10(6 Suppl): S42, S44–49.

Shipperley T, Martin C. (2002) The physiology of wound healing: an Emergency Response. *Nursing Times.net* 98(8).

Sussman G. (2007) The impact of medicines on wound healing. *Pharmacist* 26(11): 874–878.

Tempest M, Siesennop E, Hartoin K. (2010) Nutrition, physical assessment, and wound healing. *Support Line* 22–28.

Thomas D. (2001) Issues and dilemmas in the prevention and treatment of pressure ulcers: A review. *Journal of Gerontology: A Biological Science and Medical Science* 56(6): M328–340.

Todorovic V. (2003) Food and wounds: nutritional factors in wound formation and healing. *Clinical Nutrition Update* 8(2): 6–8.

Waterlow J. (2005). *Pressure Ulcer Prevention Manual*. Available at www.judy-waterlow.co.uk. Accessed 18 July 2012.

White B, Baxter M. (1998) *Hormones and Metabolic Control*, 2nd edn. London: Edward Arnold

Wilkinson E. (2012) Oral zinc for arterial and venous leg ulcers. *Cochrane Database of Systematic Reviews* 8: CD001273.

Winkler MR. (2000) Inquire here: should vitamin C and zinc be administered as supplements for wound healing? *Support Line* 22: 20.

Woodward M, Sussman G, Rice J, Ellis T, Fazio V. (2009) *Nutrition and Wound Healing: Expert Guide for Healthcare Professionals*. Nestle Nutrition Healthcare.

Zaloga GP. (1994) *Nutrition in Critical Care*. St Louis: Mosby.

Appendix A1 Generic framework for critical appraisal

Table A1.1 Generic framework for critical appraisal

Article section	Example questions that should be answered
Title	Is it accurate?
Introduction	Does it put the study entirely into context? Is the literature used to support statements? Is it contemporary? Do the authors use the literature to justify why they did the study and how it was done? Does the topic relate to your area of practice? Is the research question or aim of the study clearly stated?
Methods	Is the design logical and clearly described? Has the correct methodology been used? Is the study design able to answer the research question or achieve the aim? Is the study population and recruitment clearly described? What was the sampling strategy? Is there a sample size calculation? Was ethical approval given for the study if appropriate? If not, why not? Is there a clear, logical description of the study? Has the correct data been collected to answer the research question or achieve the aim? How were the data collated and analysed? Did the authors test to see if the data were normally distributed or not? What statistical tests were used? Are they appropriate? Was a statistician involved in the analysis? If the study is qualitative, how have the data been collated and analysed? Did the authors validate their interpretations? Is there a clear audit trail? Was an analysis package used?
Results	Are the results reported clearly and concisely? Do the results relate to the research question or aim and literature review? Are there results for all the data described in the methods? Are results given for data collection that was not described in the methods? Are the tables and figures used appropriately? Is the statistical analysis interpreted correctly? For qualitative research are the themes appropriate and clearly described with examples? Was the method of analysis appropriate?
Discussion	Does the discussion discuss the actual results or what the authors would like to have found? Are the results discussed in the context of the literature? Was the research question answered or aim achieved? How well? Are the weaknesses in design acknowledged?
Conclusion	Do they relate directly to the study? What are the implications for practice and further research?

APPENDIX

Appendix A2 Micronutrients

Table A2.1 Vitamins

Vitamin	Function	Food sources	Recommended nutrient intake (RNI)	Deficiency	Toxicity
Fat soluble vitamins					
A (retinol, beta-carotene)	Rhodopsin production in retinal rods, which are involved in adaptation of vision in the dark Growth Cell differentiation Embryogenesis Immune response	Retinol – liver and liver products, kidney and offal, oily fish and fish liver oils, eggs Beta-carotene – carrots, red peppers, spinach, broccoli, tomatoes	0–1 – years 350 µg of retinol/day 1–3 years – 400 µg of retinol/day 4–10 years – 500 µg of retinol/day 11–14 years – 600 µg of retinol/day Males 15+ years – 700 µg of retinol equivalent/day Females 15+ years – 600 µg of retinol equivalent/day Pregnancy – +100 µg of retinol equivalent/day Lactation – +350 µg of retinol equivalent/day	Eye changes – night blindness xerophthalmia (conjunctival xerosis, Bitot's spots, corneal xerosis, corneal ulceration, corneal necrosis and scars) Epithelial tissues – skin keratinisation (horny plugs block the sebaceous glands, follicular hyperkeratosis Immunity – susceptibility to infectious diseases Can contribute to nutritional deficiency anaemia	Retinol Acute toxicity – >200 mg (0.7 mmol) adults; >100 mg children Vomiting, abdominal pain, anorexia, blurred vision, headache and irritability Chronic toxicity – >10 mg for >1 month Headache, muscle and bone pain, ataxia, skin disorders, alopecia, liver toxicity and hyperlipidaemia. Not all the chronic symptoms are reversible Pregnancy – teratogenic intakes >3 mg/day
D (calciferols)	Precursor of 1, 25-dihydroxyvitamin D controls calcium absorption and excretion; involved in bone mineralisation May inhibit cell proliferation in some forms of cancer	Cod liver oil Oily fish (salmon, mackerel, etc.) Milk Margarine Breakfast cereals Eggs Liver	0–6 months – 8.5 µg/day 7–12 months – 7.0 µg/day 1–3 years – 7.0 µg/day 4–65 years – 0* 65+ years – 10 µg/day Pregnancy – +10 µg/day Lactation – +10 µg/day *Certain at risk groups or individuals may require dietary vitamin D	Rickets (children) Osteomalacia (adults) Impaired immune function (corrected by the administration of vitamin D)	Excess D₃ from sunlight is converted to inert products Excess from supplements leads to hypercalcaemia, thirst, anorexia, soft tissue calcification, urinary calcium stones

APPENDIX

Table A2.1 (*Continued*)

Vitamin	Function	Food sources	Recommended nutrient intake (RNI)	Deficiency	Toxicity
E (tocopherols)	Protects cell membrane and lipoprotein from damages by free radicals Maintains cell membrane integrity Regulates prostaglandin synthesis DNA synthesis	Wheatgerm oil Almonds Sunflower seeds and oil Safflower oil Hazelnuts Peanuts and peanut butter Corn oil	Requirements are influenced by PUFA; 0.4 mg of α-tocopherol/g of dietary PUFAs intake is required Average UK adult diet has 7% energy from PUFAs; therefore, vitamin E requirement is 6 mg for women and 8 mg for men Milk formulae should not be <0.3 mg of α-tocopherol equivalents/100 mL of reconstituted feed and not <0.4 mg of α-tocopherol equivalents/g of PUFA	Reduced tendon reflexes by age 3–4 years In adolescence – loss of touch and pain sensations, unsteady gait, impaired coordination and eye movement Supplementation can reduce similar symptom experiences by those with chronic/severe fat malabsorption, cystic fibrosis, cholestatic liver disease and abetalipoproteinaemia (particularly in children)	At high doses vitamin E acts as an antagonist to vitamins A, D and K >900 mg/kg of diet leads to headaches, nausea, muscle weakness, double vision, creatinuria, gastrointestinal disturbances
K	Synthesis of gamma-carboxyglutamic acid in the liver Essential for blood coagulation and other proteins, including osteocalcin	Green leafy vegetables (spinach, broccoli, cabbage and kale) Vegetable oils especially soyabean oil Eggs Meat Dairy products	No RNI as it is difficulty to induce deficiency by dietary manipulation Suggested requirements are 0.5–1.0 µg/kg/day	Poor blood clotting – low prothrombin activity Newborns are given vitamin K injection at birth (infants do not have bacteria producing vitamin K) Obstructive jaundice (lack of bile leading to poor absorption) Warfarin and dicoumarol (anticoagulants) – block enzymes that recycle vitamin K in the liver	Synthetic preparation of vitamin K_3 (menadione) – used to treat intracranial and pulmonary haemorrhage in premature infants Overdosage – liver overload and brain toxicity Supplements containing vitamin K should not be taken with anticoagulant drugs

Water soluble vitamins

Vitamin	Function	Food sources	Recommended nutrient intake (RNI)	Deficiency	Toxicity
C (ascorbic acid)	Powerful reducing agent (antioxidant) Synthesis of collagen Hydroxylation of dopamine to noradrenaline (norepinephrine) Production of carnitine Activation of peptide hormones and releasing factors Synthesis of bile Metabolism of drugs and carcinogens Enhances absorption of iron when consumed in the same meal	Kiwi fruit Citrus fruit (oranges, lemons, satsumas, etc.) Blackcurrants Guava Mango Papaya Pepper Brussels sprouts Broccoli Sweet potato	0–1 years – 25 mg/day 1–10 years – 30 mg/day 11–14 years – 35 mg/day Adults (15+ years) – 40 mg/day Pregnancy – +10 mg/day (last trimester only) Lactation – +30 mg/day Regular smokers – 80 mg/day	Scurvy Connective tissue abnormalities, poor wound healing, weakness, fatigue, bleeding gums (gingival), hyperkeratosis and skin haemorrhages	No evidence to support high doses (1–10 g/day) to prevent the common cold (although they may reduce symptom severity) Sudden cessation of high dose supplements may precipitate rebound scurvy High doses associated with diarrhoea and risk of kidney oxalate stone formation

Table A2.1   (*Continued*)

Vitamin	Function	Food sources	Recommended nutrient intake (RNI)	Deficiency	Toxicity
Thiamine (B$_1$)	Thiamine forms part of the coenzyme thiamine pyrophosphate (TPP) involved in decarboxylation steps ∴ Metabolism of fat, carbohydrate and alcohol	Cereal products Yeast and yeast products Pulses Nuts Pork and other meats Vegetables Milk	0–12 months – 0.3 mg/1000 kcal 1–50 years – 0.4 mg/1000 kcal No increment for pregnancy or lactation	Beriberi Wet – cardiac: high output cardiac failure, bounding pulse, warm extremities, peripheral oedema and cardiac dilatation Dry – neurological: peripheral neuropathy, foot drop, absent knee jerk reflexes Wernicke–Korsakoff syndrome – Wernicke's encephalopathy and Korsakoff's psychosis	>3 g/day – headache, irritability, insomnia, weakness, tachycardia, pruritus Regular large intakes can cause an allergic reaction
Riboflavin (B$_2$)	Oxidation–reduction reactions in metabolic pathways Promotion of normal growth Assists the synthesis of steroids, red blood cells and glycogen Maintenance of mucous membrane, skin, eyes and nervous system Aids iron absorption	Eggs Milk and milk products Liver and kidney Yeast extract Fortified breakfast cereal	0–1 years – 0.4 mg/day 1–3 years – 0.6–1.0 mg/day 4–6 years – 0.8 mg/day 7–10 years –1.0 mg/day Males 11–14 years – 1.4 mg/day Males 15+ years – 1.3 mg/day Females 11+ years – 1 mg/day Pregnancy – +0.3 mg/day Lactation – +0.5 mg/day	Mucosal lesions of the mouth, angular stomatitis, cheilosis, glossitis and magenta tongue Lesions of the genitalia, seborrhoeic skin lesions and vascularisation of the cornea Poor growth in the young/neonates	Low risk as only small amounts absorbed through the gastrointestinal tract in a single dose
Niacin (nicotinamide, nicotinic acid) (B$_3$)	Incorporated into pyridine nucleotide coenzymes Nicotinamide adenine dinucleotide (NAD) Nicotinamide adenine dinucleotide phosphate (NADP) Glycolysis Fatty acid metabolism Tissue respiration Detoxification	Beef Pork Chicken Wheat flour Maize flour Eggs Milk	All ages – 6.6 mg/1000 kcal Pregnancy – no increment Lactation – +2.3 mg/day	Pellagra (the three Ds): Dermatitis – skin exposed to the sun becomes inflamed and pigmented, cracks and peels. Casal's collar Diarrhoea – often accompanied by an inflamed tongue Dementia – ranging from mild confusion and disorientation to mania, occasionally psychoses	Nicotinic acid ≥200 mg/day leads to vasodilatation and hypotension (1–2 g/day are used in the treatment of hypertriglyceridaemia and hypercholesterolaemia) 3–6 g/day leads to reversible liver toxicity, changes in liver function, carbohydrate tolerance and uric acid metabolism

Table A2.1 (*Continued*)

Vitamin	Function	Food sources	Recommended nutrient intake (RNI)	Deficiency	Toxicity
Folate (folic acid)	Involved in single carbon transfer reactions – synthesis of purines, pyrimidines, glycine and methionine Essential for the synthesis of DNA and RNA 5-methyl tetrahydrofolate (folate derivative) requires vitamin B_{12} to enable the use of methionine synthase in the synthesis of methionine and tetrahydrofolate	Rich sources (>100 μg/ serving) – Brussels sprouts, kale, spinach. Good sources (50–100 μg/ serving) – fortified bread and breakfast cereals, broccoli, cabbage, cauliflower, chickpeas, green beans, kidney, beans, peas, spring greens Moderate sources (15–15 μg/ serving) – potatoes, most other vegetables, most fruit, most nuts, brown rice, wholegrain pasta, oats, bran, some breakfast cereals, cheese, yoghurt, milk, eggs, salmon, beef, game	0–1 years – 50 μg/day 1–3 years – 70 μg/day 4–6 years – 100 μg/ day 7–10 years – 150 μg/ day Adults (11+ years) – 200 μg/day Pregnancy – +100 μg/ day Preconception and until 12th week of pregnancy – 400 μg/ day (to prevent first occurrence of neural tube defects); 5000 μg/day (to prevent recurrence of neural tube defects)	Secondary deficiency (from malabsorption, certain drugs, late pregnancy and some disease states) Megaloblastic anaemia Infertility Diarrhoea	Low toxicity Folate supplements given to patients with developing vitamin B_{12} deficiency may obscure diagnosis Folate supplements in early pregnancy reduce neural tube defects Large doses (200 μg/ day) reduce plasma homocysteine levels (raised plasma homocysteine – risk factor for cardiovascular disease)
Vitamin B_6 (pyridoxine)	The three naturally occurring forms of vitamin B_6 – pyridoxine, pyridoxal, and pyridoxamine – can be converted to the coenzyme pyridoxal-5-phosphate, which is involved in amino acid metabolism Also involved in the conversion of glycogen to glucose in muscles, the conversion of tryptophan to niacin, and in hormone metabolism	Meat Wholegrain cereals Fortified cereals Bananas Nuts Pulses	0–6 months – 8 μg/ day 7–9 months – 10 μg/ day 10–12 months – 13 μg/day 1–50+ years – 15 μg/ day	Severe deficiency of vitamin B_6 is rare. Patients suffering malabsorption, receiving dialysis or alcoholics are at risk of deficiency Deficiency symptoms – lesions of the lips and corners of the mouth, and inflammation of the tongue	Intakes of 500 mg/day and above have been associated with peripheral neuropathy The Department of Health recommends not to exceed a daily dose of 10 mg/day

Table A2.1 (*Continued*)

Vitamin	Function	Food sources	Recommended nutrient intake (RNI)	Deficiency	Toxicity
Cobalamin (B$_{12}$)	Recycles folate coenzymes. Normal myelination of nerves. Synthesis of methionine from homocysteine.	Meat and meat products Eggs Milk and dairy products Fish and fish products Yeast products and fortified vegetable extracts Fortified breakfast cereal	0–6 months – 0.3 μg/day 7–12 months – 0.4 μg/day 1–3 years – 0.5 μg/day 4–6 years – 0.8 μg/day 7–10 years – 1.0 μg/day 11–14 years – 1.2 μg/day 15+ years –1.5 μg/day 19–50+ years – 1.5 μg/day Lactation – +0.5 μg/day	Malabsorption secondary to atrophy of the gastric mucosa leads to reduced intrinsic factor/ileum disease Pernicious (megaloblastic) anaemia and/or neurological problems such as loss of sensation	No reports in humans
Biotin (B$_7$)	Coenzyme for several carboxylases including fatty acid synthesis and metabolism, gluconeogenesis, metabolism of branched chain amino acids	Liver Kidney Milk Eggs Dairy products	It is believed that intakes of between 10 and 200 μg/day are safe and adequate	Deficiency is rare. Reported in patients receiving total parenteral nutrition, when it should be added to the infusion solution Scaly dermatitis Glossitis Hair loss Anorexia Depression Hypercholesterolaemia Egg whites contain the protein avidin; eaten in great amounts this can bind with biotin and prevent absorption. Prevented by heating the egg whites	There have been no reports of biotin toxicity
Pantothenic acid (B$_5$)	Part of coenzyme A (CoA) and is involved in the tricarboxylic acid cycle Essential for carbohydrate and lipid metabolism	Yeast Offal Peanuts Meat Eggs Green vegetables	Information is not available to derive recommended intakes, but intake of 3–7 mg/day is considered adequate	Spontaneous deficiency has not been described Deficiency symptoms – burning sensation in the feet, depression, fatigue, vomiting and muscle weakness	No specific toxic effects, although large doses may cause gastrointestinal symptoms, such as diarrhoea

PUFA, polyunsaturated fatty acid.

Table A2.2 Minerals

Vitamin	Function	Food sources	Recommended nutrient intake (RNI)	Deficiency	Toxicity
Calcium (Ca)	Structural rigidity of bones and teeth, as hydroxyapatite Intracellular signalling control of muscles and nerves Blood clotting Cofactor for enzymes, e.g. lipase	Dairy sources – milk, cheese, yoghurt Cereals and cereal products, e.g. breakfast cereals, white bread Pulses e.g. baked beans, lentils, chickpeas	0–12 months – 525 mg/day 1–3 years – 350 mg/day 4–6 years – 450 mg/day 7–10 years – 550 mg/day Boys 11–18 years – 1000 mg/day Girls 11–18 years – 800 mg/day Men 19+ years – 700 mg/day Women 19+ years – 700 mg/day Lactation – +550 mg/day	Deficiency symptoms – Stunted growth in childhood, not reaching peak bone mass in early adulthood, higher risk of developing osteoporosis in later life	Tight homeostatic control of Ca generally prevents Ca accumulation in blood and tissues (hypercalcaemia) Intakes of up to 2 g of Ca/day have been shown to be safe Milk alkali syndrome (MAS) results from excessive intake of Ca and alkali as antacid tablets, Ca supplements and milk MAS has been reported at Ca carbonate intakes of ≥4 g/day or more. A rare cause of MAS is excessive intake of Ca by the ingestion of betel nut paste containing oyster shells
Phosphorus (P)	Skeletal rigidity – Ca compound hydroxyapatite Energy for metabolism – phosphate bonds in adenosine triphosphate (ADP) Constituent of phospholipids and membranes Constituent of nucleic acids	Milk and dairy products (except butter) Cereals and cereal products Meat and meat products Fish Nuts Fruit and vegetables	0–12 months – 525 mg/day 1–3 years – 350 mg/day 4–6 years – 450 mg/day 7–10 years – 550 mg/day Males 11–18 years – 1000 mg/day Females 11–18 years – 800 mg/day Adults 19+ years – 700 mg/day Lactation – +550 mg/day	Hypophosphataemia occurs in poorly managed parenteral nutrition and refeeding syndrome, sepsis, liver disease, alcoholism, diabetic ketoacidosis and excessive use of aluminium containing antacids Deficiency at birth possibly linked to rickets at a later age	>70 mg/kg leads to high serum levels that are above any likely to be taken in foods High intakes balanced by excretion in urine; disrupted in renal patients P:Ca ratio should not be above 2.2 mg of P to 1 mg of Ca
Iron (Fe)	As haemoglobin – transport of oxygen, cell respiration As myoglobin – oxygen storage in muscles Other functions – component of enzymes, including those involved in immune functions, and cytochromes, which are essential for energy production	Very good sources – meat, especially offal (but not during pregnancy due to high vitamin A level), fish, eggs, meat extracts Good sources – bread and flour, breakfast cereals, vegetables (dark green) and pulses, nuts and dried fruit (prunes, figs, apricots), yeast extract	0–3 months – 1.7 mg/day 4–6 months – 4.3 mg/day 7–12 months – 7.8 mg/day 1–3 years – 6.9 mg/day 4–6 years – 6.1 mg/day 7–10 years – 8.7 mg/day Boys 11–18 years – 11.3 mg/day Girls 11–18 years – 14.8 mg/day Men 19–50+ years – 8.7 mg/day Women: 19–50 years – 14.8 mg/day 50+ years – 8.7 mg/day	Deficiency symptoms Pallor of finger nails and mucous membranes in the mouth and under eyelids Koilonychia (spoon shaped nails) Tachycardia and in severe cases, oedema Fatigue, breathlessness on exertion, insomnia, giddiness, anorexia Paraesthesia of fingers and toes	Tight metabolic control prevents dietary excess. Toxicity due to Fe supplement overdose causing gastrointestinal symptoms, especially constipation. Absorption of other micronutrients, e.g. Zinc are reduced by high dose Fe supplements. The hereditary disease primary idiopathic haemochromatosis is characterised by high levels of Fe absorption and tissue deposition

Table A2.2   (*Continued*)

Vitamin	Function	Food sources	Recommended nutrient intake (RNI)	Deficiency	Toxicity
Zinc (Zn)	Enzymes – alcohol dehydrogenase, alkaline phosphate, aldolase and RNA polymerase Involved in digestion, carbohydrate and bone metabolism, oxygen transportation Immune response Stabilising the structure of DNA, RNA and ribosomes	Rich sources – whole grains, pork, poultry, milk and milk products, eggs and nuts Very rich sources – lamb, leafy/ root vegetables, crab and shellfish, beef and offal	0–6 months – 4.0 mg/day 7–months–3 years – 5.0 mg/day 4–6 years – 6.5 mg/ day 11–14 years – 9.0 mg/day Males 15+ years – 9.5 mg/day Females 15+ years – 7.0 mg/day Lactation: 0–4 months – +6 mg/day 4+ months – +2.5 mg/day	Deficiency symptoms Growth retardation Failure to thrive Delayed sexual maturation Sore throat and immune defects Circumoral and acral dermatitis Diarrhoea Alopecia and neuropsychiatric symptoms	Acute toxicity (>200 mg) – nausea, vomiting and fever 50 mg interferes with copper and iron metabolism 75–300 mg/day – symptoms of copper deficiency, e.g. microcytic anaemia and neutropenia
Copper (Cu)	Incorporated in many metalloenzymes	Offal Nuts Cereals and cereal products Meat and meat products	0–12 months – 0.3 mg/day 1–3 years – 0.4 mg/ day 4–6 years – 0.6 mg/ day 7–10 years – 0.7 mg/day 11–14 years – 0.8 mg/day 15–16 years – 1.0 mg/day 18+ years – 1.2 mg/ day Pregnancy – +0.3 mg/day	Deficiency is rare; can occur in premature infants and in patients receiving total parenteral nutrition Associated with cystic fibrosis, coeliac disease and chronic diarrhoea in children Occurs in the hereditary condition Menkes disease where Cu transport is impaired Deficiency symptoms Failure to thrive in babies Oedema with low serum albumin Fe resistant anaemia Impaired immunity with low neutrophil count Fractures and osteoporosis Abnormal blood vessels due to defects in collagen and elastin Hair and skin hypopigmentation with steely, uncrimped (kinky) hair Neurological abnormalities May be a risk factor for coronary heart disease Associated with raised plasma cholesterol levels and heart related abnormalities	Contamination by Cu water pipes or cooking utensils. Deliberate ingestion of Cu salts Nausea, vomiting, and diarrhoea May be fatal in extreme cases Liver cirrhosis; infants and young children are particularly vulnerable Wilson's disease

Table A2.2 (Continued)

Vitamin	Function	Food sources	Recommended nutrient intake (RNI)	Deficiency	Toxicity
Iodine	Maintain metabolic rate controlling energy production and oxygen consumption in cells Normal growth and development In foetus and neonate – normal protein metabolism in brain and central nervous system	Milk and dairy products Sea fish, e.g. haddock and cod Seaweed Iodised salt	0–3 months – 50 μg/day 4–12 months – 60 μg/day 1–3 years – 70 μg/day 4–6 years – 100 μg/day 7–10 years – 110 μg/day 11–14 years – 130 μg/day 15+ years – 140 μg/day	Goitre hypothyroidism symptoms include: lethargy, poor cold tolerance, bradycardia and myxoedema In foetus, causes cretinism. Symptoms include mental retardation, hearing and speech defect, squint, disordered stance and gait, growth retardation In infants and children, varying degrees of growth and mental retardation Associated with stillbirth, miscarriage and infertility	High doses lead to hyperthyroidism, toxic modular goitre and weak association with thyroid cancer if taken at persistently high intakes
Selenium (Se)	Integral part of >30 selenoproteins Glutathione peroxidases – protect against oxidative damage Iodothyronine deiodinases – production of triiodothyronine from thyroxine Selenoprotein P – antioxidant and transport functions	Offal Fish Brazil nuts Eggs Poultry Meat and meat products	0–3 months – 10 μg/day 4–6 months – 13 μg/day 7–12 months – 10 μg/day 1–3 years – 15 μg/day 4–6 years – 20 μg/day 7–10 years – 30 μg/day 11–14 years – 45 μg/day Men: 15–18 years – 70 μg/day 19+ years – 75 μg/day Women 15+ years – 60 μg/day Lactation – +15 μg/day	Endemic causes – Keshan disease (cardiomyopathy), Kashin–Beck disease (musculoskeletal disorder) Iatrogenic causes – TPN, phenylketonuric patients receiving a semi synthetic diet Deficiency symptoms Cardiomyopathy Musculoskeletal disorders	Acute – hypersalivation, nausea, vomiting, garlic smelling breath, diarrhoea, hair loss, restlessness, tachycardia and fatigue Chronic (selenosis) – nail and hair changes, skin lesions and neurological effects; numbness, pain and paralysis Recommended maximum safe intake – 6 μg/kg/day
Magnesium (Mg)	Integral part of bones and teeth; 60% is found in the skeleton Intracellular energy metabolism; a cofactor for enzymes requiring ATP in the replication of DNA, and synthesis of protein and RNA Essential for phosphate transferring systems Muscle and nerve cell function	Green vegetables Pulses and wholegrain cereals Meat Hard drinking water	0–3 months – 55 mg/day 4–6 months – 60 mg/day 7–9 months – 75 mg/day 10–12 months – 80 mg/day 1–3 years – 85 mg/day 4–6 years – 120 mg/day 7–10 years – 200 mg/day 11–14 years – 280 mg/day 15–18 years – 300 mg/day Men 19+ years – 300 mg/day Women 19+ years – 270 mg/day Lactation +50 mg/d	In healthy adults, dietary deficiency is unlikely to occur Low serum Mg levels occur when there are renal losses, malabsorption or changes in tissue distribution due to disease or use of some drugs, e.g. diuretics, refeeding syndrome Deficiency symptoms Cardiac arrhythmias and cardiac arrest Very low levels of Mg are associated with hypocalcaemia	Hypermagnesaemia can occur in renal or adrenal disease

Table A2.2 *(Continued)*

Vitamin	Function	Food sources	Recommended nutrient intake (RNI)	Deficiency	Toxicity
Manganese (Mn)	Component of several metalloenzymes (e.g. arginase and pyruvate), Needed for enzyme activity such as glutamine synthetase, various hydrolases, kinases, decarboxylases and phosphotransferases	Cereals and cereal products Tea Vegetables	Infants and children −16 µg/kg/day Men − 3.32 µg/day Women − 2.69 µg/day	In experimental studies, deficiency is linked to delayed growth of fingernails, reddened black hair and scaly dermatitis	Risk is low as high intakes are resolved by the excretion of manganese in bile and urine
Molybdenum (Mo)	Cofactor in xanthine oxidase, sulphite oxidase and aldehyde oxidase metabolism of purines, pyrimidines, quinolines and sulphites	Offal Nuts Cereals Bread	No RNIs Safe intakes believed to be 50–400 µg/day	Not observed in humans, single case reported following prolonged TPN which lead to mental disturbance and coma Inborn error of metabolism results in abnormal production of the coenzyme leading to abnormal urinary metabolites, neurological and ocular problems Failure to thrive Most severe cases can be fatal at 2–3 years	Little data are available for dietary excess Intakes >100 mg/kg/day have been reported to cause diarrhoea, anaemia and high blood uric acid levels associated with gout
Chromium (Cr)	Believed to be part of the 'glucose tolerance factor' (GTF) − potentiates the action of insulin May participate in lipoprotein metabolism	Meat Wholegrains Legumes Nuts	There are no RNIs for Cr Theoretical requirements: Children − 0.1–1.0 µg/kg/day Adults − 25–30 µg/day	Only observed with long term TPN: impaired glucose tolerance, weight loss, neuropathy, elevated plasma fatty acids, depressed respiratory quotient and abnormal nitrogen metabolism	Hexavalent form is very toxic Two fatalities reported following acute ingestion of large doses as dichromate (75 mg/kg) and chromic acid (4.1 mg/kg). Acute − gastrointestinal haemorrhages, renal and liver abnormalities Chronic − renal failure, liver failure, haemolysis and anaemia

TPN, total parenteral nutrition.

Appendix A3 Dietary reference values

Energy

Table A3.1 Estimated average requirements (EARs) for energy of children 0–18 years (SACN, 2011)

Age	EAR [MJ/day (kcal/day)]	
	Boys	Girls
0–3 months	2.6	2.4
4–6 months	2.7	2.5
7–9 months	2.9	2.7
10–12 months	3.2	3.0
1–3 years	4.1	3.8
4–6 years	6.2	5.8
7–10 years	7.6	7.2
11–14 years	9.8	9.1
15–18 years	12.6	10.2

Table A3.2 Estimated average requirements (EARs) according to height and weight at body mass index (BMI) of 22.5 kg/m² and assuming a physical activity level (PAL) of 1.63 (SACN, 2011)

Age (years)	Height (cm)	Weight (kg) BMI = 22.5 kg/m²	EAR (MJ/day)
Males			
19–24	178	71.5	11.6
25–34	178	71.0	11.5
35–44	176	69.7	11.0
45–54	175	68.8	10.8
55–64	174	68.3	10.8
65–74	173	67.0	9.8
75+	170	65.1	9.6
Females			
19–24	163	29.9	9.1
25–34	163	59.7	9.1
35–44	163	59.9	8.8
45–54	162	59.0	8.8
55–64	161	58.0	8.7
65–74	159	57.2	8.0
75+	155	54.3	7.7

Protein

Table A3.3 Reference nutrient intakes (RNIs) for protein (Department of Health, 1991)

Age	Weight (kg)	RNI (g/day)
0–3 months	5.9	12.5
4–6 months	7.7	12.7
7–9 months	8.8	13.7
10–12 months	9.7	14.9
1–3 years	12.5	14.5
4–6 years	17.8	19.7
7–10 years	28.3	28.3
Males		
11–14 years	43.0	42.1
15–18 years	64.5	55.2
19–50 years	74.0	55.5
50+ years	71.0	53.3
Females		
11–14 years	43.8	41.2
15–18 years	55.5	45.4
19–50 years	60.0	45.0
50+ years	62.0	46.5
Pregnancy		+6.0
Lactation		
0–4 months		+11.0
4+ months		+8.0

Manual of Dietetic Practice, Fifth Edition. Edited by Joan Gandy.
© 2014 The British Dietetic Association. Published 2014 by John Wiley & Sons, Ltd.
Companion Website: www.manualofdieteticpractice.com

Vitamins

Table A3.4   Reference nutrient intakes (RNIs) for vitamins

Age	Thiamin (mg/day)	Riboflavin (mg/day)	Niacin[1] (mg/day)	Vitamin B_6[2] (mg/day)	Vitamin B_{12} (μg/day)	Folate (μg/day)	Vitamin C (mg/day)	Vitamin A (μg/day)	Vitamin D (μg/day)
0–3 months	0.2	0.4	3	0.2	0.3	50	25	350	8.5
4–6 months	0.2	0.4	3	0.2	0.3	50	25	350	8.5
7–9 months	0.2	0.4	4	0.3	0.4	50	25	350	7
10–12 months	0.3	0.4	5	0.4	0.4	50	25	350	7
1–3 years	0.5	0.6	8	0.7	0.5	70	30	400	7
4–6 years	0.7	0.8	11	0.9	0.8	100	30	500	–
7–10 years	0.7	1.0	12	1.0	1.0	150	30	500	–
Males									
11–14 years	0.9	1.2	15	1.2	1.2	200	35	600	–
15–18 years	1.1	1.3	18	1.5	1.5	200	40	700	–
19–50 years	1.0	1.3	17	1.4	1.5	200	40	700	–
50+ years	0.9	1.3	16	1.4	1.5	200	40	700	[3]
Females									
11–14 years	0.7	1.1	12	1.0	1.2	200	35	600	–
15–18 years	0.8	1.1	14	1.2	1.5	200	40	600	–
19–50 years	0.8	1.1	13	1.2	1.5	200	40	600	–
50+ years	0.8	1.1	12	1.2	1.5	200	40	600	[3]
Pregnancy	+0.1[4]	+0.3	[5]	[5]	[5]	+100	+10	+100	10
Lactation									
0–4 months	+0.2	+0.5	+2	[5]	+0.5	+60	+30	+350	10
4+ months	+0.2	+0.5	+2	[5]	+0.5	+60	+30	+350	10

[1]Nicotinic acid equivalent.
[2]Based on protein providing 14.7% of the estimated average requirement (EAR) for energy.
[3]After the age of 65 years the RNI is 10 μg/day for men and women.
[4]For the last trimester only.
[5]No increment.
London: HMSO, 1991. Crown copyright material is reproduced with the permission of the Controller of Her Majesty's Stationery Office.
Source: Department of Health. *Dietary Reference Values for Food Energy and Nutrients for the United Kingdom*. Report on Health and Social Subjects 41.

Minerals and trace elements

Table A3.5 Reference nutrient intakes (RNIs) for minerals and trace elements

Age	Calcium (mg/day)	Phosphorus[1] (mg/day)	Magnesium (mg/day)	Sodium[2] (mg/day)	Potassium[3] (mg/day)	Chloride[4] (mg/day)	Iron (mg/day)	Zinc (mg/day)	Copper (mg/day)	Selenium (μg/day)	Iodine (μg/day)
0–3 months	525	400	55	210	800	320	1.7	4.0	0.2	10	50
4–6 months	525	400	60	280	850	400	4.3	4.0	0.3	13	60
7–9 months	525	400	75	320	700	500	7.8	5.0	0.3	10	60
10–12 months	525	400	80	350	700	500	7.8	5.0	0.3	10	60
1–3 years	350	270	85	500	800	800	6.9	5.0	0.4	15	70
4–6 years	450	350	120	700	1100	1100	6.1	6.5	0.6	20	100
7–10 years	550	450	200	1200	2000	1800	8.7	7.0	0.7	30	110
Males											
11–14 years	1000	775	280	1600	3100	2500	11.3	9.0	0.8	45	130
15–18 years	1000	775	300	1600	3500	2500	11.3	9.5	1.0	70	140
19–50 years	700	550	300	1600	3500	2500	8.7	9.5	1.2	75	140
50+ years	700	550	300	1600	3500	2500	8.7	9.5	1.2	75	140
Females											
11–14 years	800	625	280	1600	3100	2500	14.8[5]	9.0	0.8	45	130
15–18 years	800	625	300	1600	3500	2500	14.8[5]	7.0	1.0	60	140
19–50 years	700	550	270	1600	3500	2500	14.8[5]	7.0	1.2	60	140
50+ years	700	550	270	1600	3500	2500	8.7	7.0	1.2	60	140
Pregnancy	–*	–*	–*	–*	–*	–*	–*	–*	–*	–*	–*
Lactation											
0–4 months	+550	+440	+50	–*	–*	–*	–*	+6.0	+0.3	+15	–*
4+ months	+550	+440	+50								

[1] Phosphorus (P) RNI is set to equal to calcium (Ca) in mmol values; 1 mmol Ca = 40 mg, 1 mmol P = 30.9.
[2] 1 mmol = 23 mg sodium (Na): 1 g salt (NaCl) contains 17.1 mmol, Na.
[3] 1 mmol = 39.1 mg.
[4] Intakes of dietary chloride should equal sodium intakes in molar terms. 1 mmol chloride = 35.5 mg.
[5] Supplements may be required if menstrual losses are high.
*No increment.

References

Department of Health. (1991). *Dietary Reference Values for Food and Nutrients for the United Kingdom*. London: HMSO.

Scientific Advisory Committee on Nutrition (SACN). (2011) *Dietary Reference Values for Energy*. London: The Stationery Office.

Appendix A4 Weights and measures

Height/length

1 inch = 2.54 cm
1 foot (12 inches) = 30.48 cm (0.305 m)
1 yard (36 inches) = 91.44 cm
1 centimetre = 0.394 inch
1 metre = 39.37 inches

Table A4.1   Inches and centimetres conversion table

Inches to centimetres		Centimetres to inches	
Inches	Centimetres	Centimetres	Inches
1	2.54	1	0.39
2	5.08	2	0.79
3	7.62	3	1.18
4	10.16	4	1.57
5	12.70	5	1.97
6	15.25	6	2.36
7	17.78	7	2.76
8	20.32	8	3.15
9	22.86	9	3.54
10	25.40	10	3.94
20	50.8	20	7.87
30	76.2	30	11.81
40	101.6	40	15.75
50	127.0	50	19.69
60	152.4	60	23.62
70	177.8	70	27.56
80	203.2	80	31.50
90	228.6	90	35.43
100	254.0	100	39.37

Table A4.2   Height conversion table

Feet	Inches	Metres	Feet	Inches	Metres
4	0	1.22	5	3½	1.61
4	0½	1.23	5	4	1.63
4	1	1.24	5	4½	1.64
4	1½	1.26	5	5	1.65
4	2	1.27	5	5½	1.66
4	2½	1.28	5	6	1.68
4	3	1.29	5	6½	1.69
4	3½	1.31	5	7	1.70
4	4	1.32	5	7½	1.71
4	4½	1.33	5	8	1.73
4	5	1.35	5	8½	1.74
4	5½	1.36	5	9	1.75
4	6	1.37	5	9½	1.76
4	6½	1.38	5	10	1.78
4	7	1.40	5	10½	1.79
4	7½	1.41	5	11	1.80
4	8	1.42	5	11½	1.82
4	8½	1.43	6	0	1.83
4	9	1.45	6	½	1.84
4	9½	1.46	6	1	1.85
4	10	1.47	6	1½	1.87
4	10½	1.49	6	2	1.88
4	11	1.50	6	2½	1.89
4	11½	1.51	6	3	1.90
5	0	1.52	6	3½	1.92
5	0½	1.54	6	4	1.93
5	1	1.55	6	4½	1.94
5	1½	1.56	6	5	1.96
5	2	1.57	6	5½	1.97
5	2½	1.59	6	6	1.98
5	3	1.60			

Manual of Dietetic Practice, Fifth Edition. Edited by Joan Gandy.
© 2014 The British Dietetic Association. Published 2014 by John Wiley & Sons, Ltd.
Companion Website: www.manualofdieteticpractice.com

Weight

1 ounce = 28.35 g

1 pound (16 oz) = 454 g (0.45 kg)

1 stone (14 lb) = 6.35 kg

1 kilogram (1000 g) = 2.2 lb

Table A4.3 Ounces and grams conversion table (approximate rounded figures)

Ounces to grams			Grams to ounces	
Oz	g	(approximate conversion)	g	oz (approximate conversion)
1	28	(25–30)	10	0.35 (⅓ oz)
2	57	(50–60)	15	0.53 (½ oz)
3	85	(75–90)	20	0.71 (¾ oz)
4 (¼ lb)	113	(100–120)	30	1.06 (1 oz)
5	142	(150)	40	1.41
6	170	(175)	50	1.76 (1¾ oz)
7	198	(200)	60	2.12 (2 oz)
8 (½ lb)	227	(225)	70	2.47
9	255	(250)	80	2.82
10	284	(300)	90	3.17
11	312	(325)	100	3.53 (3½ oz)
12 (¾ lb)	340	(350)	110	3.88
13	368	(375)	120	4.23
14	397	(400)	130	4.58
15	425	(425)	140	4.94
16 (1 lb)	454	(450)	150	5.29
			175	6.31
			200	7.05
			225	7.94 (8 oz/½ lb)
			250	8.82
			300	10.58
			350	12.34 (12 oz/¾ lb)
			400	14.1
			450	15.9 (16 oz/1 lb)
			500	17.6
			1000	35.27 (2.2 lb)

APPENDIX

Table A4.4 Body weight conversion table (stones and pounds to kilograms)

St	lb	kg	St	lb	kg	St	lb	kg	St	lb	kg	St	lb	kg
0	1	0.45		5	40.37	9	13	63.05		7	85.73	17	1	108.41
	2	0.90		6	40.82	10	0	63.50		8	86.18		2	108.86
	3	1.36		7	41.28		1	63.96		9	86.64		3	109.32
	4	1.81		8	41.73		2	64.41		10	87.09		4	109.77
	5	2.27		9	42.18		3	64.86		11	87.54		5	110.22
	6	2.72		10	42.64		4	65.32		12	88.00		6	110.68
	7	3.17		11	43.09		5	65.77		13	88.45		7	111.13
	8	3.63		12	43.55		6	66.23	14	0	88.91		8	111.59
	9	4.08		13	44.00		7	66.68		1	89.36		9	112.04
	10	4.54	7	0	44.45		8	67.13		2	89.81		10	112.49
	11	4.99		1	44.91		9	67.59		3	90.27		11	112.95
	12	5.44		2	45.36		10	68.04		4	90.72		12	113.40
	13	5.90		3	45.81		11	68.49		5	91.17		13	113.85
				4	46.27		12	68.95		6	91.63	18	0	114.31
1	0	6.35		5	46.72		13	69.40		7	92.08		1	114.76
2	0	12.70		6	47.17	11	0	69.85		8	92.53		2	115.21
3	0	19.05		7	47.63		1	70.31		9	92.98		3	115.67
4	0	25.40		8	48.08		2	70.76		10	93.44		4	116.12
	1	25.86		9	48.54		3	71.22		11	93.90		5	116.58
	2	26.31		10	48.99		4	71.67		12	94.35		6	117.03
	3	26.76		11	49.44		5	72.12		13	94.80		7	117.48
	4	27.22		12	49.90		6	72.58	15	0	95.26		8	117.94
	5	27.67		13	50.35		7	73.03		1	95.71		9	118.39
	6	28.12	8	0	50.80		8	73.48		2	96.16		10	118.84
	7	28.57		1	51.26		9	73.94		3	96.62		11	119.30
	8	29.03		2	51.71		10	74.39		4	97.07		12	119.75
	9	29.48		3	52.16		11	74.84		5	97.52		13	120.20
	10	29.93		4	52.62		12	75.30		6	97.98	19	0	120.66
	11	30.39		5	53.07		13	75.75		7	98.43		1	121.11
	12	30.84		6	53.52	12	0	76.20		8	98.88		2	121.56
	13	31.30		7	53.98		1	76.66		9	99.34		3	122.02
5	0	31.75		8	54.43		2	77.11		10	99.79		4	122.47
	1	32.21		9	54.89		3	77.57		11	100.24		5	122.93
	2	32.66		10	55.34		4	78.02		12	100.70		6	123.38
	3	33.11		11	55.79		5	78.47		13	101.15		7	123.83
	4	33.57		12	56.25		6	78.93	16	0	101.61		8	124.29
	5	34.02		13	56.70		7	79.38		1	102.06		9	124.74
	6	34.47	9	0	57.15		8	79.83		2	102.51		10	125.19
	7	34.93		1	57.61		9	80.29		3	102.97		11	125.65
	8	35.38		2	58.06		10	80.74		4	103.42		12	126.10
	9	35.83		3	58.51		11	81.19		5	103.87		13	126.55
	10	36.29		4	58.97		12	81.65		6	104.33	20	0	127.27
	11	36.74		5	59.42		13	82.10		7	104.79		7	130.45
	12	37.19		6	59.88	13	0	82.55		8	105.24	21	0	133.64
	13	37.65		7	60.33		1	83.01		9	105.69		7	136.82
6	0	38.10		8	60.78		2	83.46		10	106.14	22	0	140.00
	1	38.56		9	61.24		3	83.92		11	106.60		7	143.18
	2	39.01		10	61.69		4	84.37		12	107.04	23	0	146.36
	3	39.46		11	62.14		5	84.82		13	107.50	24	0	152.73
	4	39.92		12	62.60		6	85.28	17	0	107.96	25	0	159.09

Volume

1 fluid oz = 28.41 mL

1 pint (20 fluid oz) = 568.3 mL (or 0.568 L)

1 litre (1000 mL) = 1.76 pints

Table A4.5 Pints and litres conversion table

fl oz/ pints	mL/L	mL/L	fl oz/pint
1 fl oz	28 mL	50 mL	1.75 fl oz
¼ pint (5 fl oz)	142 mL	100 mL	3.5 fl oz
½ pint (10 fl oz)	284 mL	200 mL	7 fl oz
¾ pint (15 fl oz)	426 mL	250 mL	8.8 fl oz
1 pint	568 mL	500 mL	17.6 fl oz
2 pints	1.1 L	750 mL	26.4 fl oz
3 pints	1.7 L	1000 mL	1.76 pints (1¾ pints)
4 pints	2.3 L		
5 pints	2.8 L		

Appendix A5 Dietary data

Conversion factors

Energy

1000 joules = 1 kJ

1000 kJ = 1 MJ

1 kcal = 4.184 kJ [The Royal Society (London) recommended conversion factor]

1 kJ = 0.239 kcal

1 W = 1 joule/second

0.06 W = 1 kJ/min

86.4 W = 1 kJ/24 h

Table A5.1   Nutrient energy yields

Nutrient	kcal/g	kJ/g
Protein	4	17
Fat	9	37
Carbohydrate	3.75	16
Su gar alcohols	2.4	10
Ethyl alcohol	7	29
Glycerol	4.31	18
Medium chain triglyceride (MCT)	8.4	35

Protein and nitrogen

Dietary protein (g) = dietary nitrogen (g) × 6.25

Dietary nitrogen (g) = dietary protein (g) ÷ 6.25

This conversion factor is only appropriate for a mixture of foods. For milk or cereals alone, the factors 6.4 or 5.7 should be used.

Vitamins

Vitamin A

The active vitamin A content of a diet is usually expressed in retinol equivalents.

1 µg of retinol equivalent
= 1 µg of retinol or 6 µg of beta-carotene

1 IU of vitamin A
= 0.3 µg of retinol or 0.6 µg of beta-carotene

Vitamin D

1 µg of vitamin D = 40 IU

1 IU = 0.025 µg of vitamin D

Nicotinic acid/tryptophan

1 mg of nicotinic acid = 60 mg of tryptophan

Nicotinic acid content mg equivalents
= nicotinic acid (mg) + [tryptophan (mg)/60]

Vitamin E

Vitamin E activity is expressed as D-alpha-tocopherol equivalents. Activity is expressed as international units (IU): 1 IU is equivalent to 0.67 mg D-alpha-tocopherol.

Table A5.2   Mineral content of compounds and solutions

Solution/compound	Mineral content	
1 g of sodium chloride	393 mg of Na	17 mmol of Na
1 g of sodium bicarbonate	273 mg of Na	12 mmol of Na
1 g of potassium bicarbonate	524 mg of K	13.4 mmol of K
1 g of calcium chloride (hydrated)	273 mg of Ca	7 mmol of Ca
1 g of calcium carbonate	400 mg of Ca	10 mmol of Ca
1 g of calcium gluconate	93 mg of Ca	2.3 mmol of Ca
1 L of normal saline	3450 mg of Na	150 mmol of Na

Manual of Dietetic Practice, Fifth Edition. Edited by Joan Gandy.
© 2014 The British Dietetic Association. Published 2014 by John Wiley & Sons, Ltd.
Companion Website: www.manualofdieteticpractice.com

Food exchange lists

Carbohydrate

Table A5.3 Food portions containing approximately 10 g of carbohydrate (CHO)

Food	Weight (g)	Description
Wholemeal bread	25	1 thin slice/large loaf
White bread	20	1 thin slice/small loaf
Potatoes – boiled	60	1 size of hen's egg
Potatoes – mashed	60	1 scoop
Potatoes – roast	40	1 very small
Sweet potatoes – boiled	50	1 size of hen's egg
Rice – boiled, brown, white	30	¾ tablespoon
Pasta – boiled, e.g. spaghetti, macaroni	50	1 tablespoon
Pulses, e.g. lentils	60	2 tablespoons
Peas – frozen	100	3 tablespoons
Parsnip – boiled	80	1 medium
Sweetcorn – boiled	50	2 tablespoons
Thick soup, e.g. tinned vegetable	100	1 small tin
Thin soup, e.g. minestrone	250	1 standard mug
Sausages	100	2 large sausages
Beefburger, economy	100	1 economy burger
Beefburger, 100% meat = no CHO	–	–
Fish fingers	60	2 fish fingers
Breakfast cereals, e.g. branflakes	15	2 tablespoons
Breakfast cereals, e.g. wheat bisk type	20	1 bisk
Muesli, no added sugar	15	¾ tablespoon
Porridge – made with water	125	Small average portion
Biscuits – plain digestive	15	1 digestive
Apple, pear	100	1 medium
Orange	120	1 small
Banana	45	½ small banana
Melon – galia, honeydew	200	1 medium slice
Pineapple, fresh	100	1 large slice
Grapes	70	15 large grapes
Orange juice – no added sugar	110	½ average glass
Apple juice – no added sugar	100	½ average glass
Cranberry juice	70	⅓ average glass
Milk – full fat, semi or skimmed	200	1 average glass
Yogurt – low fat, fruit	70	½ small pot
Yogurt – low fat, plain	135	1 small pot
Ice cream – plain dairy, vanilla	50	1 small scoop
Lemonade	170	1 small glass
Lucozade®	60	⅓ average glass
Cola	90	½ average glass
Beer – best bitter	450	¾ pint glass
Lager – premium	400	¾ pint glass
Wine – medium white	330	2½ small wine glasses
Wine – red contains 0.2 g CHO/100 mL	–	–
Crisps	20	¾ small packet
Peanuts – dry roasted	100	1 large packet

Protein

Table A5.4 Food portions containing approximately 6 g or 2 g of protein

Food	Portion size	Protein per portion (g)	Approximate energy per portion (kcal)
Milk	180 mL	6	115 (full-fat) 85 (semi skimmed) 60 (skimmed)
Cheddar cheese	25 g	6	100
Yoghurt	125 g	6	125
Egg	50 g (one average hen's egg)	6	70
Meat/poultry lean cooked	25 g	6	40
White fish	35 g	6	30
Baked beans	120 g	6	100
Peas	100 g	6	70
Bread (1 large thin slice)	25 g	2	50
Pasta (boiled)	50 g	2	50
Rice (boiled)	100 g	2	140
Most breakfast cereals	25 g	2	90
Digestive biscuits	15 g (one biscuit)	2	70
Potatoes	140 g	2	100
Crisps	30 g	2	160

Potassium

Table A5.5 Food portions containing approximately 4 mmol of potassium

Food	Portion size providing approximately 4 mmol potassium
Milk	100 mL
Yoghurt	60 g
Cheddar cheese	130 g
Egg	100 g (2 small eggs)
Meat/fish	50 g
White flour	120 g
Wholemeal flour	45 g
White bread	160 g
Wholemeal bread	70 g
Apple	125 g
Orange with skin	100 g
Grapes / Orange without skin	50 g
Potato boiled	50 g
Orange juice	100 mL
Tomato juice	60 mL

Sodium

Table A5.6 No added salt and 40 mmol of sodium diets

No added salt	40 mmol of sodium diet
This restricts sodium intake to <100 mmol of Na⁺/day A pinch of salt may be used in cooking, but none should be added to food at the table The following foods must be avoided: • Bacon, ham, sausages, pâté • Tinned fish and meat • Smoked fish and meat • Fish and meat pastes • Tinned and packet soups • Sauce mixes • Tinned vegetables • Bottled sauces and chutneys • Meat and vegetable extracts, stock cubes • Salted nuts and crisps • Soya sauce • Monosodium glutamate • Cheese – up to 100 g/week • Bread – up to 4 slices/day	In addition to the foods listed opposite, the following restrictions apply: • No salt to be used in cooking or at table • Salt free butter or margarine must be used • Milk should be restricted to 300 mL/day • Breakfast cereals must be salt free

E number classification system (see Chapter 4.5)

El00–180	Colours
E200–283	Preservatives
E300–321	Antioxidants
E322–495	Emulsifiers, stabilisers, acidity regulators, thickeners
E950–969	Artificial sweeteners

Table A5.7 Commonly used additives

Type of additive	E number	Chemical name
Colours		
Natural and nature identical colours	E101	Riboflavin (yellow)
	E100	Curcumin (yellow)
	E120	Cochineal (red)
	E140	Chlorophyll (green)
	E150a	Plain caramel (brown/black)
	E153	Carbon (black)
	E160a	Alpha-, beta- and gamma-carotene (yellow/orange)
	E160b	Annatto (yellow/red)
	E160c	Capsanthin (paprika extract) (red/orange)
	E160d	Lycopene (red extract from tomatoes)
	E162	Beetroot red (betanin) (purple/red)
	E163	Anthocyanins (red/blue/violet)
Synthetic colours	E102	Tartrazine* (yellow)
	E104	Quinoline Yellow*
	E110	Sunset Yellow FCF*
	E122	Carmoisine (Azorubine)* (red)
	E123	Amaranth* (purple red)
	E124	Ponceau 4R* (red)
	E127	Erythrosine* (pink/red)
	E128	Red 2 G*
	E129	Allura Red AC*
	E132	Indi go carmine (Indigotine) * (blue)
	E142	Green S*
	E150 b–d	Caustic sulphite caramel; ammonia caramel; sulphite ammonia caramel (brown/black)
	E151	Black PN*
	E154	Brown FK*
	E155	Brown HT*
	E180	Litholrubine BK (Pigment Rubine; Rubine)*
Preservatives		
Sorbic acid and its derivatives	E200	Sorbic acid
	E201–203	Sodium, potassium and calcium sorbates
Benzoic acid and derivatives	E210	Benzoic acid
	E211–213	Sodium, potassium and calcium benzoates
	E214 – E219	Ethyl, methyl or propyl hydroxybenzoates
Sulphur dioxide and derivatives	E220	Sulphur dioxide
	E221	Sodium sulphite
	E222	Sodium hydrogen sulphite (sodium bisulphite)
	E223	Sodium metabisulfite
	E224	Potassium metabisulphite
	E226	Calcium sulphite
	E227	Calcium hydrogen sulphite (calcium bisulphite)
Nitrites and nitrates	E249	Potassium nitrite
	E250	Sodium nitrite
	E251	Sodium nitrate
	E252	Potassium nitrate
Acetic, lactic and propionic acid derivatives	E260–E263	Acetic acid and acetates
	E270	Lactic acid
	E280–E283	Propionic acid and propionates

(Continued)

Table A5.7 (*Continued*)

Type of additive	E number	Chemical name
Antioxidants		
Ascorbic acid and derivatives	E300 E301–304	Ascorbic acid (vitamin C) Ascorbates and ascorbyl palmitate
Tocopherols	E306 E307–309	Vitamin E Synthetic tocopherols
Gallates	E310–312	Propyl, octyl and dodecyl gallates
BHA/BHT	E320 E321	Butylated hydroxyanisole (BHA) Butylated hydroxytoluence (BHT)
Emulsifiers and stabilisers		
Emulsifier	E322	Lecithins
Acidity regulators, buffers, stabilisers	E325–327 E330–333 E334–337 E338–341 E350–352	Sodium, potassium and calcium lactate Citric acid; sodium, potassium and calcium citrates Tartaric acid; sodium and potassium tartrates Phosphoric acid; sodium, potassium and calcium phosphates and orthophosphates Sodium, potassium and calcium malates
Gelling agents	E401–405 E406 E407	Sodium, ammonium, potassium and calcium alginates Agar Carrageenan
Gums	E410 E412 E413 E414 E415	Locust bean gum Guar gum Tragacanth Gum arabic Xanthan gum
Emulsifiers/stabilisers	E471–E477	Esters and glycerides of fatty acids, e.g. mono- and di-glycerides of fatty acids or glyceryl monostearate and distearate

*Azo dye.

Appendix A6 Body mass index (BMI)

APPENDIX

Manual of Dietetic Practice, Fifth Edition. Edited by Joan Gandy.
© 2014 The British Dietetic Association. Published 2014 by John Wiley & Sons, Ltd.
Companion Website: www.manualofdieteticpractice.com

Table A6.1 BMI ready reference table

Weight (kg)

BMI	BMI value	1.5	1.52	1.54	1.56	1.58	1.6	1.62	1.64	1.66	1.68	1.7	1.72	1.74	1.76	1.78	1.8	1.82	1.84	1.86	1.88	1.9	1.94	1.96
Morbidly obese (BMI > 40)	45	102	104	107	110	113	116	119	121	124	127	131	134	137	140	143	146	150	153	156	159	163	170	173
	44	99	102	105	108	110	113	116	119	122	125	128	131	134	137	140	143	146	149	153	156	159	166	169
	43	97	100	102	105	108	111	113	116	119	122	125	128	131	134	137	140	143	146	149	152	156	162	166
	42	95	97	100	103	105	108	111	113	116	119	122	125	128	131	134	137	140	143	146	149	152	159	162
	41	93	95	98	100	103	105	108	111	113	116	119	122	125	127	130	133	136	139	142	145	148	155	158
Obese (BMI 31–40)	40	90	93	95	98	100	103	105	108	111	113	116	119	122	124	127	130	133	136	139	142	145	151	154
	39	88	91	93	95	98	100	103	105	108	111	113	116	119	121	124	127	130	132	135	138	141	147	150
	38	86	88	91	93	95	98	100	103	105	108	110	113	115	118	120	123	126	129	132	135	138	143	146
	37	84	86	88	91	93	95	97	100	102	105	107	110	112	115	117	120	123	126	128	131	134	140	143
	36	81	84	86	88	90	93	95	97	100	102	104	107	109	112	115	117	120	122	125	128	130	136	139
	35	79	81	83	86	88	90	92	95	97	99	102	104	106	109	111	114	116	119	122	124	127	132	135
	34	77	79	81	83	85	87	90	92	94	96	99	101	103	106	108	111	113	116	118	121	123	128	131
	33	75	77	79	81	83	85	87	89	91	94	96	98	100	103	105	107	110	112	115	117	120	125	127
	32	72	74	76	78	80	82	84	87	89	91	93	95	97	100	102	104	106	109	111	114	116	121	123
	31	70	72	74	76	78	80	82	84	86	88	90	92	94	96	99	101	103	105	108	110	112	117	120
Overweight (BMI 26–30)	30	68	70	72	73	75	77	79	81	83	85	87	89	91	93	96	98	100	102	104	106	109	113	116
	29	66	67	69	71	73	75	77	78	80	82	84	86	88	90	92	94	97	99	101	103	105	110	112
	28	63	65	67	69	70	72	74	76	78	79	81	83	85	87	89	91	93	95	97	99	102	106	108
	27	61	63	64	66	68	70	71	73	75	77	78	80	82	84	86	88	90	92	94	96	98	102	104
	26	59	61	62	64	65	67	69	70	72	74	76	77	79	81	83	85	87	88	90	92	94	98	100
Normal weight (BMI 20–25)	25	57	58	60	61	63	64	66	68	69	71	73	74	76	78	80	81	83	85	87	89	91	95	96
	24	54	56	57	59	60	62	63	65	67	68	70	71	73	75	76	78	80	82	83	85	87	91	93
	23	52	54	55	56	58	59	61	62	64	65	67	68	70	72	73	75	77	78	80	82	83	87	89
	22	50	51	53	54	55	57	58	60	61	63	64	66	67	69	70	72	73	75	77	78	80	83	85
	21	48	49	50	52	53	54	56	57	58	60	61	63	64	65	67	68	70	72	73	75	76	79	81
	20	45	47	48	49	50	52	53	54	56	57	58	60	61	62	64	65	67	68	70	71	73	76	77
Underweight (BMI 16–19)	19	43	44	46	47	48	49	50	52	53	54	55	57	58	59	61	62	63	65	66	68	69	72	73
	18	41	42	43	44	45	47	48	49	50	51	52	54	55	56	57	59	60	61	63	64	65	68	70
	17	39	40	41	42	43	44	45	46	47	48	50	51	52	53	54	56	57	58	59	61	62	64	66
	16	36	37	38	40	41	42	43	44	45	46	47	48	49	50	51	52	53	55	56	57	58	61	62
Severely underweight (BMI < 16)	15	34	35	36	37	38	39	40	41	42	43	44	45	46	47	48	49	50	51	52	54	55	57	58
	14	32	33	34	35	36	36	37	38	39	40	41	42	43	44	45	46	47	48	49	50	51	53	54
	13	30	31	31	32	33	34	35	35	36	37	38	39	40	41	42	43	44	45	45	46	47	49	50
	12	27	28	29	30	30	31	32	33	34	34	35	36	37	38	39	39	40	41	42	43	44	46	47
	11	25	26	27	27	28	29	29	30	31	32	32	33	34	35	35	36	37	38	39	39	40	42	43
	10	23	24	24	25	25	26	27	27	28	29	29	30	31	31	32	33	34	34	35	36	37	38	39
Height (m)		1.5	1.52	1.54	1.56	1.58	1.6	1.62	1.64	1.66	1.68	1.7	1.72	1.74	1.76	1.78	1.8	1.82	1.84	1.86	1.88	1.9	1.94	1.96
Height (feet inches)		4'11"	5'0"	5'1"	5'1½"	5'2¼"	5'3"	5'3¼"	5'4½"	5'5½"	5'6"	5'7"	5'7¼"	5'8½"	5'9¼"	5'10"	5'11"	5'11¾"	6'0½"	6'1¼"	6'2"	6'3"	6'4½"	6'5½"

Appendix A7 Anthropometric data

Demiquet and Mindex

These can be used as an index of adiposity in elderly people (see Chapter 2.2).

$$\text{Demiquet} = \frac{\text{Weight (kg)}}{\text{Demispan (m)}^2}$$

$$\text{Mindex} = \frac{\text{Weight (kg)}}{\text{Demispan (m)}}$$

Table A7.1   Distribution of Demiquet and Mindex in a normal population over the age 65 years [data derived from Lehmann et al. (1991)]

	Percentiles				
	10th	30th	50th	70th	90th
Men (Demiquet kg/m²)					
64–74 years	87.6	99.6	106.7	117.1	130.7
75+ years	84.5	98.9	106.3	113.4	125.0
Women (Mindex kg/m)					
64–74 years	68.3	77.8	84.8	92.3	110.6
75+ years	63.1	73.6	81.7	88.4	102.2

Upper arm anthropometry

For measurement techniques and discussion see Chapter 2.2.

Table A7.2   Triceps skinfold thickness (TSF) [data derived from Bishop et al. (1981)]

		Centiles						
	Mean (mm)	5th	10th	25th	50th	75th	90th	95th
Men								
18–74 years	12.0	4.5	6.0	8.0	11.0	15.0	20.0	23.0
18–24 years	11.2	4.0	5.0	7.0	9.5	14.0	20.0	23.0
25–34 years	12.6	4.5	5.5	8.0	12.0	16.0	21.5	24.0
35–44 years	12.4	5.0	6.0	8.5	12.0	15.5	20.0	23.0
45–54 years	12.4	5.0	6.0	8.0	11.0	15.0	20.0	25.5
55–64 years	11.6	5.0	6.0	8.0	11.0	14.0	18.0	21.5
65–74 years	11.8	4.5	5.5	8.0	11.0	15.0	19.0	22.0
Women								
18–74 years	23.0	11.0	13.0	17.0	22.0	28.0	34.0	37.5
18–24 years	19.4	9.4	11.0	14.0	18.0	24.0	30.0	34.0
25–34 years	21.9	10.5	12.0	16.0	21.0	26.5	33.5	37.0
35–44 years	24.0	12.0	14.0	18.0	23.0	29.5	35.5	39.0
45–54 years	25.4	13.0	15.0	20.0	25.0	30.0	36.0	40.0
55–64 years	24.9	11.0	14.0	19.0	25.0	30.5	35.0	39.0
65–74 years	23.3	11.5	14.0	18.0	23.0	28.0	33.0	36.0

Manual of Dietetic Practice, Fifth Edition. Edited by Joan Gandy.
© 2014 The British Dietetic Association. Published 2014 by John Wiley & Sons, Ltd.
Companion Website: www.manualofdieteticpractice.com

APPENDIX

Table A7.3   Mid arm circumference (MAC) [data derived from Bishop *et al.* (1981)]

	Centiles							
	Mean (cm)	5th	10th	25th	50th	75th	90th	95th
Men								
18–74 years	31.8	26.4	27.6	29.6	31.7	33.9	36.0	37.3
18–24 years	30.9	25.7	27.1	28.7	30.7	32.9	35.5	37.4
25–34 years	30.5	25.3	26.5	28.5	30.7	32.4	34.4	35.5
35–44 years	32.3	27.0	28.2	30.0	32.0	34.4	36.5	37.6
45–54 years	32.7	27.8	28.7	30.7	32.7	34.8	36.3	37.1
55–64 years	32.1	26.7	27.8	30.0	32.0	34.2	36.2	37.6
65–74 years	31.5	25.6	27.3	29.6	31.7	33.4	35.2	36.6
Women								
18–74 years	29.4	23.2	24.3	26.2	28.7	31.9	35.2	37.8
18–24 years	27.0	22.1	23.0	24.5	26.4	28.8	31.7	34.3
25–34 years	28.6	23.3	24.2	25.7	27.8	30.4	34.1	37.2
35–44 years	30.0	24.1	25.2	26.8	29.2	32.2	36.2	38.5
45–54 years	30.7	24.3	25.7	27.5	30.3	32.9	36.8	39.3
55–64 years	30.7	23.9	25.1	27.7	30.2	33.3	36.3	38.2
65–74 years	30.1	23.8	25.2	27.4	29.9	32.5	35.3	37.2

Table A7.4   Mid arm muscle circumference (MAMC) [data derived from Bishop *et al.* (1981)]

$$MAMC\ (cm) = MAC\ (cm) - [TSF\ (mm) \times 0.314]$$

	Centiles							
	Mean (cm)	5th	10th	25th	50th	75th	90th	95th
Men								
18–74 years	28.0	23.8	24.8	26.3	27.9	29.6	31.4	32.5
18–24 years	27.4	23.5	24.4	25.8	27.2	28.9	30.8	32.3
25–34 years	28.3	24.2	25.3	26.5	28.0	30.0	31.7	32.9
35–44 years	28.8	25.0	25.6	27.1	28.7	30.3	32.1	33.0
45–54 years	28.2	24.0	24.9	26.5	28.1	29.8	31.5	32.6
55–64 years	27.8	22.8	24.4	26.2	27.9	29.6	31.0	31.8
65–74 years	26.8	22.5	23.7	25.3	26.9	28.5	29.9	30.7
Women								
18–74 years	22.2	18.4	19.0	20.2	21.8	23.6	25.8	27.4
18–24 years	20.9	17.7	18.5	19.4	20.6	22.1	23.6	24.9
25–34 years	21.7	18.3	18.9	20.0	21.4	22.9	24.9	26.6
35–44 years	22.5	18.5	19.2	20.6	22.0	24.0	26.1	27.4
45–54 years	22.7	18.8	19.5	20.7	22.2	24.3	26.6	27.8
55–64 years	22.8	18.6	19.5	20.8	22.6	24.4	26.3	28.1
65–74 years	22.8	18.6	19.5	20,8	22.5	24.4	26.5	28.1

Estimating height from ulna length (see Figure A7.1)

Table A7.5 Estimates of height from ulna length (Elia, 2003)

Men Height (m)		Ulna length (cm)	Women Height (m)	
<65 years	>65 years		<65 years	>65 years
1.94	1.87	**32.0**	1.84	1.84
1.93	1.86	**31.5**	1.83	1.83
1.91	1.84	**31.0**	1.81	1.81
1.89	1.82	**30.5**	1.80	1.79
1.87	1.81	**30.0**	1.79	1.78
1.85	1.79	**29.5**	1.77	1.76
1.84	1.78	**29.0**	1.76	1.75
1.82	1.76	**28.5**	1.75	1.73
1.80	1.75	**28.0**	1.73	1.71
1.78	1.73	**27.5**	1.72	1.70
1.76	1.71	**27.0**	1.70	1.68
1.75	1.70	**26.5**	1.69	1.66
1.73	1.68	**26.0**	1.68	1.65
1.71	1.67	**25.5**	1.66	1.63
1.69	1.65	**25.0**	1.65	1.61
1.67	1.63	**24.5**	1.63	1.60
1.66	1.62	**24.0**	1.62	1.58
1.64	1.60	**23.5**	1.61	1.56
1.62	1.59	**23.0**	1.59	1.55
1.60	1.57	**22.5**	1.58	1.53
1.58	1.56	**22.0**	1.56	1.52
1.57	1.54	**21.5**	1.55	1.50
1.55	1.52	**21.0**	1.54	1.48
1.53	1.51	**20.5**	1.52	1.47
1.51	1.49	**20.0**	1.51	1.45
1.49	1.48	**19.5**	1.50	1.44
1.48	1.46	**19.0**	1.48	1.42
1.46	1.45	**18.5**	1.47	1.40

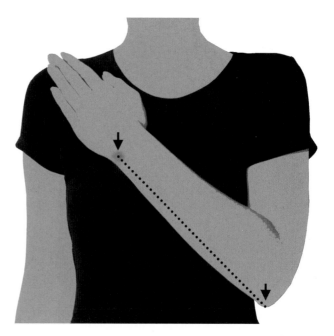

Figure A7.1 How to measure ulna length
Measure between the point of the elbow (olecranon process) and the mid point of the prominent bone of the wrist (styloid process) (left side if possible)

Table A7.7 Waist measurements in adults as a predictor of health risk (WHO, 2008)

	Men	Asian men	Women	Asian women
Waist circumference				
Increased risk	≥94 cm		≥80 cm	
Substantially increased risk	≥102 cm	≥90 cm	≥88 cm	≥80 cm
Waist to hip ratio				
Increased risk	≥0.9		≥0.0.85	

Table A7.6 Classification of body mass index (BMI) and risk of comorbidities in adults (WHO, 1998; 2004)

Classification	BMI (kg/m²)	BMI (kg/m²) Asian origin	Risk of comorbidities
Underweight	<18.5	<18.5	Low (but risk of other clinical problems increased)
Normal range	18.5–24.9	18.5–22.9	Average
Overweight	25.0–29.9	23–27.4	Increased risk
Obese class I	30.0–34.9	27.5–32.4	Moderate
Obese class II	35.0–39.9	32.5–37.4	Severe
Obese class III	>40.0	>37.5	Morbid obesity

References

Bishop CW, Bowen PE, Ritchey SJ. (1981) Norms for nutritional assessment of American adults by upper arm anthropometry. *American Journal of Clinical Nutrition* 34: 2530–2539.

Elia M. (2003) *Development and use of the Malnutrition Universal Screening Tool ('MUST') for adults*. Basingstoke: BAPEN.

Lehmann AB, Bassey EJ, Morgan K, Dallosso HM. (1991) Normal values for weight, skeletal size and body mass indices in 890 men and women aged over 65 years. *Clinical Nutrition* 10: 18–22.

World Health Organization (WHO). (1998) *Obesity: Preventing and Managing the Global Epidemic*. Report of a WHO consultation on obesity. Geneva: WHO.

World Health Organization Expert Consultation. (2004) Appropriate body mass index for Asian Populations and its implications for policy and intervention strategies. *Lancet* 363: 157–164.

World Health Organization. (2008) Waist circumference and waist-hip ratio. Report of a WHO expert consultation. Available at www .who.int. Accessed 16 February 2013.

Appendix A8 Predicting energy requirements

For a discussion on stress factors and physical activity levels (PALs) in clinical practice, see Chapter 6.1 and the specific clinical chapters in Section 7 for detailed discussion as appropriate.

In 2011, the Scientific Advisory Committee on Nutrition (SACN) published the report *Dietary Reference Values for Energy*. Energy requirements for the UK were last reviewed by the Committee on Medical Aspects of Food Policy (COMA) in their 1991 report *Dietary Reference Values for Food and Energy and Nutrients for the United Kingdom*. Following careful consideration of the evidence, SACN has recommended a revision to the estimated average requirements (EAR) for food energy for infants, children, adolescents and adults. However, these are intended only for use in healthy populations and not individuals or groups who require clinical management. Although exclusive breastfeeding is recommended for about the first 6 months of life, it is recognised that infants are fed in a variety of ways. Therefore, separate recommendations have been made for exclusively breast-fed infants, breast milk substitute fed infants and those for whom the method of feeding is mixed or unknown. For the full report, refer to SACN (2011), particularly Tables 14 and 15.

References

Henry CJ. (2005) Basal metabolic rate studies in humans: measurement and development of new equations. *Public Health Nutrition* 8: 1133–1152.

Scientific Advisory Committee on Nutrition (SACN). (2011) Dietary recommendations for energy. Working Group Report. Available at www.sacn.gov.uk/pdfs/sacn_energy_report_author_date_10th _oct_fin.pdf. Accessed 22 March 2012.

Table A8.1 Basal metabolic rate (BMR) [Henry, (2005); as recommended by SACN (2011)]

	Age (years)	BMR prediction equation (MJ/day)
Males	<3	$0.255 (w) - 0.141$
	3–10	$0.0937 (w) + 2.15$
	10–18	$0.0769 (w) + 2.43$
	18–30	$0.0669 (w) + 2.28$
	30–60	$0.0592 (w) + 2.48$
	>60	$0.0563 (w) + 2.15$
Females	<3	$0.246 (w) - 0.0965$
	3–10	$0.0842 (w) + 2.12$
	10–18	$0.0465 (w) + 3.18$
	18–30	$0.0546 (w) + 2.33$
	30–60	$0.0407 (w) + 2.90$
	>60	$0.0424 (w) + 2.38$

w, weight in kg.

Appendix A9 Clinical chemistry

Conversion calculations

mg to mmol

$$\frac{mg}{\text{atomic weight}}$$

mmol to mg $\quad$ mmol $\times$ atomic weight

Milliequivalents (mEq)

$$1\ mEq = \frac{\text{atomic weight (mg)}}{\text{valency}}$$

To convert

mg to mEq $\quad$ (mg $\times$ valency)/atomic weight
mEq to mg $\quad$ (mEq $\times$ atomic weight)/valency

For minerals with a valency of 1, mEq = mmol
For minerals with a valency of 2, mEq = mmol $\times$ 2

Table A9.1 Atomic weights and valencies

Mineral	Atomic weight	Valency
Sodium	23.0	1
Potassium	39.0	1
Phosphorus	31.0	2
Calcium	40.0	2
Magnesium	24.3	2
Chlorine	35.4	1
Sulphur	32.0	2
Zinc	65.4	2

Table A9.2 Mineral content of compounds and solutions

Solution/compound	Mineral content	
1 g sodium chloride	393 mg Na	(17.1 mmol Na$^+$)
1 g sodium bicarbonate	274 mg Na	(12 mmol Na$^+$)
1 g potassium bicarbonate	390 mg K	(10 mmol K$^+$)
1 g calcium chloride (dihydrate)	273 mg Ca	(6.8 mmol Ca^{2+})
1 g calcium carbonate	400 mg Ca	(10 mmol Ca^{2+})
1 g calcium gluconate	89 mg Ca	(2.2 mmol Ca^{2+})
1 litre normal saline	3450 mg Na	(150 mmol Na$^+$)

Table A9.3 Conversion factors for mmol/mg/mEq

Mineral	mg/mmol		mg/mEq		mmol/mEq	
	mg=	mmol=	mg=	mEq=	mmol=	mEq=
Sodium	mmol $\times$ 23	mg $\div$ 23	mEq $\times$ 23	mg $\div$ 23	mEq	mmol
Potassium	mmol $\times$ 39	mg $\div$ 39	mEq $\times$ 39	mg $\div$ 39	mEq	mmol
Phosphorus	mmol $\times$ 31	mg $\div$ 31	mEq $\times$ 15.5	mg $\div$ 15.5	mEq $\div$ 2	mmol $\times$ 2
Calcium	mmol $\times$ 40	mg $\div$ 40	mEq $\times$ 20	mg $\div$ 20	mEq $\div$ 2	mmol $\times$ 2
Magnesium	mmol $\times$ 24.3	mg $\div$ 24.3	mEq $\times$ 12.15	mg $\div$ 12.15	mEq $\div$ 2	mmol $\times$ 2
Chlorine	mmol $\times$ 35.4	mg $\div$ 35.4	mEq $\times$ 35.4	mg $\div$ 35.4	mEq	mmol
Sulphur	mmol $\times$ 32	mg $\div$ 32	mEq $\times$ 16	mg $\div$ 16	mEq $\div$ 2	mmol $\times$ 2
Zinc	mmol $\times$ 65.4	mg $\div$ 65.4	mEq $\times$ 32.7	mg $\div$ 32.7	mEq $\div$ 2	mmol $\times$ 2

Manual of Dietetic Practice, Fifth Edition. Edited by Joan Gandy.
© 2014 The British Dietetic Association. Published 2014 by John Wiley & Sons, Ltd.
Companion Website: www.manualofdieteticpractice.com

APPENDIX

Osmolarity and osmolality

Osmolality is the number of osmotically active particles (milliosmoles) in a *kilogram* of *solvent*. Osmolarity is the number of osmotically active particles in a *litre* of *solution* (i.e. solvent + solute).

In body fluids, there is only a small difference between the two. However, in commercially prepared feeds, osmolality is always much higher than osmolarity. Osmolality is therefore the preferred term for comparing the potential hypertonic effect of liquid diets (although, in practice, it is often osmolarity which is stated).

The osmolality of a liquid feed is considerably influenced by the content of amino acids and electrolytes such as sodium and potassium. Carbohydrates with a small particle size (e.g. simple sugars) increase osmolality more than complex carbohydrates with a higher molecular weight. Fats do not increase the osmolality of solutions because of their insolubility in water.

The osmolality of plasma is normally in the range 280–300 mosmol/kg and the body attempts to keep the osmolality of the contents of the stomach and intestine at an isotonic level. It does this by producing intestinal secretions which dilute a concentrated meal or drink. If enteral feeds with a high osmolality are administered, large quantities of intestinal secretions will be produced rapidly in order to reduce the osmolality. In order to avoid diarrhoea, it is therefore important to administer such feeds slowly; the number of mosmoles given per unit of time is more important than the number of mosmoles per unit of volume.

Biochemical and haematological reference ranges

The results of laboratory tests are interpreted by comparison with reference or normal ranges. These are usually defined as the mean ±2 SD (standard deviation), which assumes a Gaussian or normal (symmetrical) type distribution (Figure A9.1). Unfortunately, most biological data have a skewed rather than a symmetrical distribution and more complex statistical calculations are required to define the reference ranges.

The reference ranges as defined usually include approximately 95% of the normal 'healthy' population; consequently, 5% of this population will have values outside the reference range but cannot be said to be abnormal. The use of reference ranges may be illustrated by taking the reference range of blood urea as 3.3–6.7 mmol/L. Approximately 95% of the normal 'healthy' population would come within these limits. However, it would be wrong to interpret a value of 6.4 mmol/L as normal while assuming a value of 7.0 mmol/L to be abnormal. Nature 'abhors abrupt transitions', so there is no clear-cut division between 'normal' and 'abnormal'. This applies equally well to body weight and height and also to measurements undertaken in the laboratory.

The majority of the normal 'healthy' population will have results close to the mean value for the population as a whole and all values will be distributed around

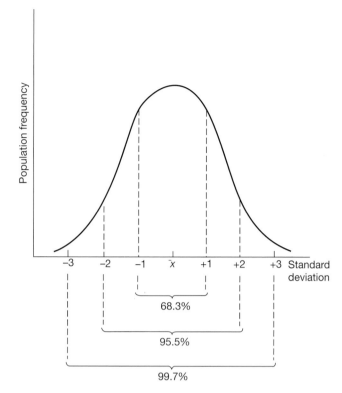

Figure A9.1 Normal distribution curve

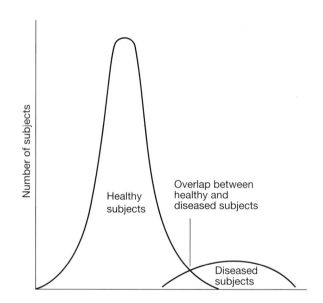

Figure A9.2 Theoretical distribution of values in health and disease

that mean. Therefore, the probability that a value is abnormal increases the further it is from the mean value (Figure A9.2).

A variety of factors can cause variation in the biochemical and haematological constituents present within the blood. These can be conveniently divided into factors causing variation within an individual and those causing variation between groups of individuals.

Variations within individuals

The following factors can cause significant variation in clinical biochemical and haematological data and should be considered when interpreting individual results.

Diet

Variation in diet can affect the levels of triglycerides, cholesterol, glucose, urea and other blood constituents.

Drugs

These can have significant effects on a number of biochemical determinations, often resulting from secondary effects on sensitive organs, e.g. liver, kidney and endocrine glands. Steroids, including oral contraceptives, can cause variations in a number of biochemical and haematological parameters, including a reduction in albumin, increases in several carrier proteins, e.g. transcortin, thyroxine-binding globulin, caeruloplasmin and transferrin, and also increases in coagulation factors, e.g. fibrinogen, factor VII and factor X.

Menstrual cycle

Several biochemical constituents show marked variations with the phase of the cycle; these include the pituitary gonadotrophins, ovarian steroids and their metabolites. There is also a marked fall in plasma iron just before and during menstruation. This is probably caused by hormonal changes rather than blood loss.

Muscular exercise

Moderate exercise can cause increases in levels of potassium, together with a number of enzymes including aspartate transferase, lactate dehydrogenase, creatine kinase and hydroxybutyrate dehydrogenase.

Posture

Significant differences in the concentration of many blood constituents may be obtained by collecting blood samples from ambulant compared with recumbent individuals. The red cell and white cell counts, together with the concentration of proteins (e.g. albumin, immunoglobulins) and protein-bound substances (e.g. calcium, cholesterol, T4, cortisol), may decrease by up to 15% following 30 minutes of recumbency. This is probably due to fluid redistribution within the body. Hospitalised patients usually have their blood samples collected early in the morning following overnight recumbency, and consequently have significantly lower values than the normal ambulant (outpatient) population.

Stress

Both emotional and physical stress can alter circulating biochemical constituents, causing increases in the levels of pituitary hormones [e.g. adrenocorticotropic hormone (ACTH), prolactin, growth hormone] and adrenal steroids (cortisol).

Time of day

Some substances exhibit a marked circadian (diurnal) variation which is independent of meals or other activities, e.g. serum cortisol, iron and the amino acids tyrosine, phenylalanine and tryptophan. Cortisol levels are at their highest in the morning (9 am) and at their lowest levels at midnight, while iron concentration may decrease by 50% between the morning and evening. Plasma phenylalanine levels are at their lowest after midnight and reach their highest concentrations between 8.30 and 10.30 am.

Variations between groups of individuals

Several factors influence the reference values quoted for individuals. These include age, sex and race.

Age

The blood levels of many biochemical and haematological constituents are age related; these include haemoglobin, total leucocyte count, creatinine, urea, inorganic phosphate and many enzymes, e.g. alkaline phosphatase, creatine kinase and γ-glutamyl transferase. Haemoglobin levels and total leucocyte counts are highest in the newborn and gradually decrease through childhood, reaching the adult reference range at puberty. As creatinine is related to muscle mass, paediatric reference ranges are lower than those of adults. Urea levels rise slightly with age but this may well indicate impaired renal function. Alkaline phosphatase activity and inorganic phosphate levels are at their highest during childhood, reaching peak levels at puberty.

Gender

Many biochemical and haematological parameters show concentration differences which are sex dependent, including creatinine, iron, urea, urea and the various sex hormones. Ferritin, haemoglobin and red cell counts are slightly higher in males than in females. Creatinine and urea levels are 15–20% lower in premenopausal females than in males. Premenopausal females also have lower serum iron levels than males, but after the menopause iron levels are similar in both sexes.

Race

Racial differences have been reported in some biochemical constituents, including cholesterol and protein. The reference ranges for cholesterol are higher in Europeans than in similar groups of Japanese. Similarly, the Bantu Africans have higher serum globulins than corresponding Europeans. African and Middle-Eastern individuals have lower total leucocyte and neutrophil counts than other races. Some of these racial differences are probably genetic in origin, although the environment and diet may also be contributory factors.

Laboratory variations

Methods of analysis and standardisations vary considerably from laboratory to laboratory. These differences will influence the quoted reference ranges, and therefore readers are advised to use only those quoted by their local laboratory. Local reference ranges may be at variance with the levels quoted in the following tables.

Correction of serum calcium for low albumin

Corrected serum calcium level (mmol/L)

$$= \frac{\text{measured serum}}{\text{calcium (mmol/L)}} + \left(\frac{40 - \text{measured albumin}}{40} \right)$$

An alternative (and possibly more accurate) equation is:

Corrected serum calcium level (mmol/L)

$$= \frac{\text{measured serum}}{\text{calcium (mmol/L)}} + \left[\left(40 - \frac{\text{measured}}{\text{albumin}} \right) \times 0.02 \right]$$

To be even more accurate, the serum protein level should also be considered:

Corrected serum calcium level (mmol/L)

$$= \frac{\text{measured serum}}{\text{calcium (mmol/L)}} + \left[\left(72 - \frac{\text{measured}}{\text{protein}} \right) \times 0.02 \right]$$

This corrected calcium value should be added to that obtained from the correction for low albumin, and a mean of the two levels obtained, calculated to two decimal places.

Table A9.4 Adult normal values [adapted from Provan (2005)] Oxford Handbook of Clinical and laboratory investigation, 2nd edn

Substance	Value	Substance	Value
Albumin	32–50 g/L	Red cell count	
Bicarbonate	20–29 mmol/L	Males	$4.5–6.5 \times 10^{12}$/L
Bilirubin	<17 µmol/L	Females	$3.8–5.8 \times 10^{12}$/L
Calcium	2.15–2.55 mmol/L	Mean cell haemoglobin (MCH)	27–32 pg
Chloride	97–107 mmol/L	Mean cell volume (MCV)	77–95 fl
Total cholesterol	<5 mmol/L	Mean cell haemoglobin concentration	32–36 g/dL
Creatinine	60–125 mmol/L	White blood count (WBC)	$4.0–11.0 \times 10^9$/L
Glucose (fasting)	<6.1 mmol/L	Neutrophils	$2.0–7.5 \times 10^9$/L
Phosphate	0.7–1.5 mmol/L	Eosinophils	$0.04–0.4 \times 10^9$/L
Magnesium	0.7–1.0 mmol/L	Monocytes	$0.2–0.8 \times 10^9$/L
Osmolality	278–305 mOsmol/kg	Basophils	$0.0–0.1 \times 10^9$/L
Potassium	3.5–5.0 mmol/L	Lymphocytes	$1.5–4.5 \times 10^9$/L
Sodium	135–150 mmol/L	Platelets	$150–400 \times 10^9$/L
Total protein	63–80 g/L	Erythrocyte sedimentation rate	2–12 mm/1st hour
Triglycerides	0.55–1.90 mmol/L	Ferritin (varies with age)	14–200 µg/L
Urate	0.14–0.46 mmol/L	Premenopausal women	14–148 µg/L
Urea	3.0–6.5 mmol/L	Serum B_{12}	150–700 ng/L
Haemoglobin		Serum folate	2.0–11.0 µg/L
Males	13.0–18.0 g/dL	Red cell folate	150–700 µg/L
Females	11.5–16.5 g/dL	Prothrombin time (PT)	12–14 s
Haematocrit (PCV)		Activated partial thromboplastin	26.0–33.5 s
Males	0.40–0.52	time (APTT)	
Females	0.36–0.47	Thrombin time (TT)	+3 s of control

Table A9.5 Normal adult urine values

Substance	Value
Albumin	<20 mg/24 hours
Calcium	<7.5 mmol/24 hours
Creatinine	9–15 mmol/24 hours
Phosphate	15–50 mmol/24 hours
Osmolality	50–1500 mOsmol/24 hours
Potassium	14–120 mmol/24 hours
Protein	<150 mg/24 hours
Sodium	100–250 mmol/24 hours
Urate	<3.0 mmol/24 hours
Urea	250–600 mmol/24 hours

Table A9.6 Normal adult faecal values

Substance	Value
Faecal fat	<18 mmol/24 hours
Nitrogen	70–140 mmol/24 hours

Table A9.7 Conversion chart for HbA1$_c$ from % to International Federation of Clinical Federation (IFCC) mmol/mol

%	mmol/mol	%	mmol/mol	%	mmol/mol	%	mmol/mol	%	mmol/mol	%	mmol/mol	%	mmol/mol	%	mmol/mol	%	mmol/mol	%	mmol/mol
4.0	20	5.0	31	6.0	42	7.0	53	8.0	64	9.0	75	10.0	86	11.0	97	12.0	108	13.0	119
4.1	21	5.1	32	6.1	43	7.1	54	8.1	65	9.1	76	10.1	87	11.1	98	12.1	109	13.1	120
4.2	22	5.2	33	6.2	44	7.2	55	8.2	66	9.2	77	10.2	88	11.2	99	12.2	110	13.2	121
4.3	23	5.3	34	6.3	45	7.3	56	8.3	67	9.3	78	10.3	89	11.3	100	12.3	111	13.3	122
4.4	25	5.4	36	6.4	46	7.4	57	8.4	68	9.4	79	10.4	90	11.4	101	12.4	112	13.4	123
4.5	26	5.5	37	6.5	48	7.5	58	8.5	69	9.5	80	10.5	91	11.5	102	12.5	113	13.5	124
4.6	27	5.6	38	6.6	49	7.6	60	8.6	70	9.6	81	10.6	92	11.6	103	12.6	114	13.6	125
4.7	28	5.7	39	6.7	50	7.7	61	8.7	72	9.7	83	10.7	93	11.7	104	12.7	115	13.7	126
4.8	29	5.8	40	6.8	51	7.8	62	8.8	73	9.8	84	10.8	95	11.8	105	12.8	116	13.8	127

References

Provan J. (2005) *Oxford Handbook of Clinical and Laboratory Investigation*, 2nd edn. Oxford: Oxford University Press.

Appendix A10 Nutritional supplements and enteral feeds

Patients at risk of malnutrition may be prescribed oral nutritional supplements (ONS) or enteral feeds as long as they have a functional gastrointestinal tract. Many of these products are prescribed only in specified clinical circumstances defined by the Advisory Committee on Borderline Substances (ACBS); they are termed ACBS prescribable. Standard ACBS indications are disease related malnutrition, intractable malabsorption, preoperative preparation of malnourished patients, dysphagia, proven inflammatory bowel disease, following total gastrectomy, short bowel syndrome and bowel fistula. The following tables provide a guide to the range of proprietary supplements, feeds and other nutritional support products currently available in the UK.

Product composition within a particular category will differ; some products may be more appropriate than others in particular clinical circumstances. Ongoing product development by the manufacturers inevitably means that over time the availability and composition of some products may change and new products will appear. The information given here is for guidance only and product details should be checked before clinical usage.

For current product availability, composition and prescribing indications, consult the *British National Formulary (BNF)*, the *Monthly Index of Medical Specialities (MIMS)* or the manufacturers (for web addresses, see Table A10.1.11 and Table A10.2.6). Information on which products are suitable for special diets, e.g. kosher, halal, gluten free, lactose free, vegetarian or vegan, can also be obtained directly from the manufacturers.

Appendix A10.1 Adult nutritional supplements and enteral feeds

Table A10.1.1 Prescribable liquid (sip feed) supplements

Note: Many sip feed supplements are available in a variety of flavours to offset taste fatigue. Some, but not all, are nutritionally complete; check compositional details before use. Some products can also be used for tube feeding.

Product type	Product name (manufacturer) Quantity	Per bottle/can			
		kJ	kcal	Protein (g)	Fibre (g)
Standard energy (1 kcal/mL)	Ensure (Abbott) 250 mL	1058	251	10.0	0.0
	Fresubin Original (Fresenius Kabi) 200 mL	840	200	7.6	0.0
Juice type (low fat) (1.25–1.5 kcal/mL)	Ensure Plus Juce (Abbott) 220 mL	1404	330	10.6	0.0
	Fortijuce (Nutricia Clinical) 200 mL	1280	300	8.0	0.0
	Provide Xtra Juice Drink (Fresenius Kabi) 200 mL	1260	250	7.5	0.0
	Resource Fruit (Nestlé) 200 mL	1040	250	8.0	0.0
High energy (1.5–2.4 kcal/mL)	Ensure Plus Milkshake style (Abbott) 220 mL	1390	330	13.8	0.0
	Ensure Plus Savoury (Abbott) 220 mL	1390	330	14.0	0.0
	Ensure Plus Yoghurt style (Abbott) 220 mL	1390	330	13.8	0.0
	Ensure Twocal (Abbott) 200 mL	1675	400	16.8	2.0
	Fortisip Bottle (Nutricia Clinical) 200 mL	1260	300	12.0	0.0

Manual of Dietetic Practice, Fifth Edition. Edited by Joan Gandy.
© 2014 The British Dietetic Association. Published 2014 by John Wiley & Sons, Ltd.
Companion Website: www.manualofdieteticpractice.com

Table A10.1.1 (*Continued*)

Product type	Product name (manufacturer) Quantity	Per bottle/can			
		kJ	kcal	Protein (g)	Fibre (g)
	Fortisip Compact (Nutricia Clinical) 125 mL	1250	300	12.0	0.0
	Fortisip Extra (Nutricia Clinical) 200 mL	1350	320	20.0	0.0
	Fortisip Yogurt Style (Nutricia Clinical) 200 mL	1260	300	12.0	0.4
	Fresubin 2 kcal Drink (Fresenius Kabi) 200 mL	1680	400	20.0	0.0
	Fresubin Energy (Fresenius Kabi) 200 mL	1260	300	11.2	0.0
	Renilon 7.5 (Nutricia Clinical) 125 mL	1050	250	9.4	0.0
High energy + fibre (1.5–2.0 kcal/mL)	Ensure Plus Fibre (Abbott) 200 mL	1284	300	13.0	5.0
	Fresubin 2 kcal Fibre Drink (Fresenius Kabi) 200 mL	1680	400	20	3.2
	Fresubin Energy Fibre (Fresenius Kabi) 200 mL	1260	300	11.2	4.0
	Fortisip Compact Fibre (Nutricia Clinical) 125 mL	1250	300	11.8	4.5
	Fortisip Multi Fibre (Nutricia Clinical) 200 mL	1260	300	12.0	4.6
	Resource 2.0 Fibre (Nestlé) 200 mL	1672	400	18.0	5.0
High protein (1.0–1.5 kcal/mL)	Fortimel Regular (Nutricia Clinical) 200 mL	840	200	20.0	0.0
	Fresubin Protein Energy Drink (Fresenius Kabi) 200 mL	1260	300	20.0	0.0
	Resource Protein (Nestlé) 200 mL	1060	250	18.8	0.0
Thickened (1.5–2.4 kcal/mL)	Fresubin Thickened (Fresenius Kabi) 200 mL Syrup (stage 1) and custard (stage 2)	1260	300	20.0	*
	Nutilis Complete Stage 1 (Nutricia) 125 mL	1263	300	12.0	4.0
	Resource Thickened Drink (Nestlé) 114 mL Syrup and custard consistencies	435	103	0.0	0.0
	SLO Drinks (SLO Drinks) Syrup, custard and pudding consistencies		*	*	*
	Thick & Easy Thickened Juices (Fresubin Kabi) 118-mL pot or 1.42-L bottle Custard consistency		*	*	*
Powdered	Complan Shake (Complan Foods) 57-g sachet In 250 mL of water	1057	251	8.8	0.0
	In 200 mL of whole milk	1621	387	15.6	0.0
	Foodlink Complete (Foodlink) 3 heaped tablespoonfuls in 250 mL of water	1048	249*	12.5*	0.0
	Foodlink Complete with Fibre (Foodlink) 4 heaped tablespoonfuls in 250 mL of water	1137	270	12.3	5.0
	Oral Impact (Nestlé) 74 g in 250 mL of water		*	*	*
	Vegenat-med Balanced Protein (Vegenat) 110-g sachet	1924	458	18.0	5.8
	Vegenat-med High Protein (Vegenat) 110-g sachet	1940	463	23.3	6.0

*Exact composition varies – see manufacturer's data.

Table A10.1.2 Non-prescribable liquid supplements

These products can be purchased by patients from supermarkets and chemists, and are useful at times when dietary intake is poor. None is nutritionally complete.

Product name (manufacturer) Quantity	Per sachet + 200 mL of whole milk			
	kJ	kcal	Protein (g)	Fibre (g)
Build-Up Nutrition Shake (Nestlé) 38-g sachet in 200 mL of whole milk	1105	263	14.9	3.0
Complan (Complan Foods) 57-g sachet in 200 mL of whole milk	1596	380	14.9	0.2

Table A10.1.3 Prescribable solid/semi solid supplements

Dessert style – also useful for dysphagic patients.

Product type	Product name (manufacturer) Quantity	Per bottle/can			
		kJ	kcal	Protein (g)	Fibre (g)
Solid/semi solid desserts	Clinutren Dessert (Nestlé) 125 g	650	156	11.9	0.0
	Ensure Plus Crème (Abbott) 125 g	718	171	7.1	0.0
	Forticreme Complete (Nutricia Clinical) 125 g	844	200	11.9	0.0
	Fortisip Fruit Dessert (Nutricia Clinical) 150 g	840	200	10.5	3.9
	Fresubin Crème (Fresenius Kabi) 125 g	945	225	12.5	2.5
	Resource Dessert Energy (Nestlé) 125 g	839	200	6.0	0.0
	Resource Dessert Fruit (Nestlé) 125 g	848	200	6.3	1.8

Table A10.1.4   Single nutrient component supplements

Component	Product name (manufacturer)	Notes, ACBS indications and nutritional values	
Carbohydrate	Caloreen (Nestlé) Powder	1640 kJ (390 kcal)/100 g	Disease related malnutrition or malabsorption states or other conditions requiring fortification with a high or readily available carbohydrate supplement
	Maxijul Liquid (SHS) Liquid	850 kJ (200 kcal)/100 mL	
	Maxijul Super Soluble (SHS) Powder	1615 kJ (380 kcal)/100 g	
	Polycal (Nutricia Clinical) Powder	1630 kJ (384 kcal)/100 g	
	Polycal Liquid (Nutricia Clinical) Liquid	1050 kJ (247 kcal)/100 mL	
	Resource Optifibre (Nestlé) Powder	323 kJ (76 kcal) and 78 g of fibre/100 g	
	S.O.S. 10, 15, 20, 25 (Vitaflo) Powder	1590 kJ (380 kcal)/100 g	
	Vitajoule (Vitaflo) Powder	1610 kJ (380 kcal)/100 g	
Fat	Calogen (Nutricia Clinical) Liquid (100% LCTs fat emulsion)	1850 kJ (450 kcal)/100 mL	Disease related malnutrition or malabsorption states or other conditions requiring fortification with a high fat supplement
	Fresubin 5kcal Shot (Fresenius Kabi) Liquid	2100 kJ (500 kcal)100 mL	Steatorrhoea associated with cystic fibrosis (pancreas), intestinal lymphangiectasia, intestinal surgery, chronic liver disease/cirrhosis and other proven malabsorption syndromes
	Liquigen (SHS) Liquid (97% MCTs)	1850 kJ (450 kcal)/100 mL	
	Medium-Chain Triglyceride (MCT) Oil (SHS) Liquid (100% MCTs)	3515 kJ (855 kcal)/100 mL	
Protein	Casilan 90 (Heinz) Powder (90% protein)	1572 kJ (370 kcal)/100 g	Disease related malnutrition or malabsorption states or other conditions requiring fortification with a high protein supplement
	Protifar (Nutricia Clinical) Powder (89% protein)	1580 kJ (373 kcal)/100 g	
	Vitapro (Vitaflo) Powder (75% protein)	1506 kJ (360 kcal)/100 g	Protein energy malnutrition or malabsorption states, hypoproteinaemia and as a protein source in modular feed

LCTs, long chain triglycerides; MCTs, medium chain triglycerides.

Table A10.1.5 Multiple nutrient component supplements

Components	Product name (manufacturer)	Notes, ACBS indications and nutritional values	
Fat/ carbohydrate	MCT Duocal (SHS) Powder	Conditions requiring extra calories, e.g. fat malabsorption or where assimilation of LCTs is impaired	50 g in 150 mL of water provides 1041 kJ (249 kcal), 36 g of CHO and 11.6 g of fat
	Duocal (SHS) Liquid	Conditions requiring extra calories	Per 100 mL: 695 kJ (166 kcal), 23.7 g of CHO and 7.9 g of fat (30% MCTs)
Protein/ carbohydrate	ProSource (Nutrinovo) Liquid	Protein energy malnutrition and patients on a fluid restricted diet	Per 30 mL: 420 kJ (100 kcal), 10 g of protein and 15 g of CHO
	Calogen Extra (Nutricia Clinical) Liquid	High energy fat emulsion with protein, carbohydrate, vitamins and minerals	Per 100 mL: 1650 kJ (400 kcal), 5.0 g of protein, 4.5 g of CHO and 40.3 g of fat
Protein/fat/ carbohydrate	Calshake (Fresenius Kabi) Powder	For increased energy requirements, e.g. patients with cystic fibrosis, cancer or HIV/AIDS	87-g sachet + 240 mL of whole milk provides approx. 2495 kJ (596 kcal), 11.6 g of protein, 68.4 g of CHO and 30.8 g of fat
	Enshake (Abbott) Powder	High energy, high protein drink for patients with involuntary weight loss	96.5-g sachet + 240 mL of whole milk provides approx. 2519 kJ (600 kcal), 16 g of protein, 78.4 g of CHO and 24.7 g of fat
	Pro-Cal (Vitaflo) Powder	Disease related malnutrition or malabsorption states and other conditions requiring fortification with energy and protein, e.g. burns	15-g sachet provides 418 kJ (/100 kcal), 2 g of protein, 4 g of CHO and 8.4 g of fat
	Pro-Cal Shot (Vitaflo) Liquid		Per 30 mL: 418 kJ (/100 kcal), 2 g of protein, 4 g of CHO and 8.5 g of fat
	QuickCal (Vitaflo) Powder		13-g sachet provides 418 kJ (100 kcal), 0.6 g of protein, 2.2 g of CHO and 10 g of fat
	Scandishake Mix (Nutricia Clinical) Powder	High energy supplement for disease related malnutrition based on skimmed milk powder, carbohydrate and fat	85-g sachet + 240 mL of whole milk provides 2457 kJ (588 kcal), 11.7 g of protein, 66.8 g of CHO and 30.4 g of fat
	Vitasavoury 200 (Vitaflo) Powder	Low volume, high energy supplements for disease related malnutrition or malabsorption states or other conditions requiring additional energy and protein	33-g sachet provides 855 kJ (200 kcal), 4 g of protein, 7.4 g of CHO and 17.2 g of fat
	Vitasavoury 300 (Vitaflo) Powder		50-g sachet provides 1295 kJ (300 kcal), 6 g of protein, 11.3 g of CHO and 26.0 g of fat

CHO, carbohydrate; MCTs, medium chain triglycerides; LCTs, long chain triglycerides.

Table A10.1.6 Food and fluid thickeners

For thickening of food and drinks of patients with dysphagia.

Type of product	Product name (manufacturer)
Modified maize starch powder*	Multi Thick (Abbott) Nutilis (Nutricia Clinical) Resource ThickenUp (Nestlé) Thick and Easy (Fresenius Kabi) Thixo-D (Sutherland) Vitaquick (Vitaflo)
Maltodextrin and xanthan gum	Resource ThickenUp Clear (Nestlé)

*See individual manufacturer's recommendations for the quantities required to achieve various textures.

Table A10.1.7 Enteral feeds – standard indications

Product type	Product name (manufacturer)	Per 100 mL			
		kJ	kcal	Protein (g)	Fibre (g)
Standard energy (1 kcal/mL)	Fresubin Original (Fresenius Kabi)	420	100	3.8	0.0
	Fresubin Original Fibre (Fresenius Kabi)	420	100	3.8	2.0
	Isosource Fibre (Nestlé)	422	100	3.8	1.4
	Isosource Standard (Nestlé)	420	100	4.0	0.0
	Jevity (Abbott)	441	106	4.0	1.8
	Jevity Promote (Abbott)	427	101	5.6	1.7
	Novasource GI Control (Nestlé) 40% MCTs	444	106	4.1	2.2
	Nutrison (Nutricia Clinical)	420	100	4.0	0.0
	Nutrison MCT (Nutricia Clinical) 61% MCTs	420	100	5.0	0.0
	Nutrison Multi Fibre (Nutricia Clinical)	420	100	4.0	1.5
	Osmolite (Abbott)	424	100	4.0	0.0
Nutritionally complete (1.0–1.2 kcal/mL)	Fresubin 1000 Complete (Fresenius Kabi) Complete in 1000 mL	420	100	5.5	2.0
	Fresubin 1200 Complete (Fresenius Kabi) Complete in 1000 mL	500	120	6.0	2.0
	Fresubin 1800 Complete (Fresenius Kabi) Complete in 1500 mL	500	120	6.0	2.0
	Fresubin 2250 Complete (Fresenius Kabi) Complete in 1500 mL	630	150	5.6	2.0
	Nutrison 1000 Complete Multi Fibre (Nutricia Clinical) Complete in 1000 mL	420	100	5.5	2.0
	Nutrison 1200 Complete Multi Fibre (Nutricia Clinical) Complete in 1000 mL	505	120	5.5	2.0
Medium energy (1.2–1.3 kcal/mL)	Jevity Plus (Abbott)	504	120	5.5	2.2
	Jevity Plus HP (Abbott)	547	130	8.1	1.5
	Nutrison Protein Plus (Nutricia Clinical)	525	125	6.3	0.0
	Nutrison Protein Plus Multi Fibre (Nutricia Clinical)	525	125	6.3	1.5
	Osmolite Plus (Abbott)	508	121	5.6	0.0
High energy (1.5–2.0 kcal/mL)	Ensure Twocal (Abbott)	838	200	8.4	1.0
	Fresubin Energy (Fresenius Kabi)	630	150	5.6	0.0
	Fresubin Energy Fibre (Fresenius Kabi)	630	150	5.6	2.0
	Fresubin HP Energy (Fresenius Kabi)	630	150	7.5	0.0
	Isosource Energy (Nestlé)	670	160	5.7	0.0
	Isosource Energy Fibre (Nestlé)	630	150	4.9	1.5
	Jevity 1.5 kcal (Abbott)	640	152	6.4	2.2
	Novasource GI Forte (Nestlé)	631	150	6.0	2.2
	Nutrison Energy (Nutricia Clinical)	630	150	6.0	0.0
	Nutrison Energy Multi Fibre (Nutricia Clinical)	630	150	6.0	1.5
	Osmolite 1.5 kcal (Abbott)	632	150	6.3	0.0
	Resource Energy (Nestlé)	630	150	5.6	<0.5

MCTs, medium chain triglycerides.

Table A10.1.8 Specialist indication enteral feeds and supplements

Product type	Product name (manufacturer)	Per 100 mL			
		kJ	kcal	Protein (g)	Fibre (g)
Amino acid liquid formula	Elemental 028 Extra (SHS) Sip feed	360	86	2.5	0.0
Low sodium liquid formula	Nutrison Low Sodium (Nutricia Clinical)	420	100	4.0	0.0
Peptide based liquid formula	Peptamen (Nestlé)	420	100	4.0	0.0
	Peptamen HN (Nestlé)	556	133	6.6	0.0
	Peptisorb (Nutricia Clinical)	425	100	4.0	0.0
	Perative (Abbott)	552	131	6.7	0.0
	Survimed OPD (Fresenius Kabi)	420	100	4.5	0.0
Soya protein liquid formula	Fresubin Soya Fibre (Fresenius Kabi)	420	100	3.8	2.0
	Nutrison Soya (Nutricia Clinical)	420	100	4.0	0.0
	Nutrison Soya Multi Fibre (Nutricia Clinical)	420	100	4.0	1.5

Table A10.1.9 Specialised formulae for specific clinical conditions

Condition	Product (manufacturer)	Notes and ACBS indications
Cancer	Forticare (Nutricia Clinical) Liquid	Pancreatic cancer Lung cancer undergoing chemotherapy
	Supportan (Fresenius Kabi) Liquid	
	ProSure (Abbott) Liquid	Pancreatic cancer Contains EPA
Crohn's disease	Alicalm (SHS) Powder	Crohn's disease
	Modulen IBD (Nestlé) Powder Can be flavoured with Flavour Mix (Nestlé) Powder	Active Crohn's disease/nutritional support during Crohn's remission
Epilepsy	KetoCal (SHS) Powder	Part of ketogenic diet in management of drug therapy resistant epilepsy
Liver disease	Generaid (SHS) Powder	Whey protein + BCAA Chronic liver disease and/or portohepatic encephalopathy
Pulmonary disease	Oxepa (Abbott) Liquid	Acute lung injury, ARDS and SIRS
	Pulmocare (Abbott) Liquid	COPD, cystic fibrosis or respiratory failure
	Respifor (Nutricia Clinical) Liquid	Disease related malnutrition in COPD + BMI <20 kg/m^2
Renal disease	Nepro (Abbott) Liquid	Chronic renal failure with haemodialysis or continuous ambulatory peritoneal dialysis Cirrhosis
	Renamil (KoRa) Powder	Chronic renal failure
	Renapro (KoRa) Powder	Biochemically proven hypoproteinaemia Patients on dialysis
Renal/liver disease	Duocal Super Soluble (SHS) Powder	For use where a high energy, low fluid and low electrolyte diet is required
	Suplena (Abbott) Liquid	Chronic/acute renal failure without dialysis Chronic/acute liver disease with fluid restriction
Short bowel syndrome	Elemental 028 Extra (SHS) Powder	Intractable malabsorption and proven irritable bowel disease
Synthetic diets	Metabolic Mineral Mixture (SHS) Powder	Mineral and trace element supplement for synthetic diets

ARDS, acute respiratory distress syndrome; BCAA, branched chain amino acids; COPD, chronic obstructive pulmonary disease; SIRS, systemic inflammatory response syndrome; BMI, body mass index; EPA, eicosapentaenoic acid.

Table A10.1.10 Nutritional supplements for metabolic diseases

Condition	Product (manufacturer)	Notes and ACBS indications
Glutaric aciduria	XLYS, TRY Glutaridon* (SHS) Powder	Type 1 glutaric aciduria
Glycogen storage diseases	Glycosade (Vitaflo) Powder	Plus other metabolic conditions where a constant glucose supply is essential
Homocystinuria	HCU cooler (Vitaflo) Liquid HCU Express (Vitaflo) Powder	Methionine free protein substitute
Hypermethioninaemia	HCU LV (SHS) Powder	And vitamin B_6 non-responsive homocystinuria
Hypermethioninaemia or homocystinuria	XMET Homidon* (SHS) Powder XMET Maxamum (SHS) Powder	Essential and non-essential amino acids except methionine
Isovaleric acidaemia	XLEU Faladon (SHS) Powder	Essential and non-essential amino acids except leucine
Maple syrup urine disease	Isoleucine Amino Acid Supplement (Vitaflo) Powder Valine Amino Acid Supplement (Vitaflo) Powder	Use in low protein diets by mixing with protein substitute, adding to modular feeds, or incorporating into other permitted food or drink
	MSUD Aid III (SHS) Powder MSUD cooler (Vitaflo) Liquid MSUD express (Vitaflo) Powder MSUD Maxamum (SHS) Powder	Essential and non-essential amino acids except isoleucine, leucine and valine
Methylmalonic acidaemia Propionic acidaemia	XMTVI Asadon (SHS) Powder XMTVI Maxamum (SHS) Powder	Essential and non-essential amino acids except methionine, threonine, valine and low isoleucine
Other errors of protein metabolism	Cystine Amino Acid Supplement (Vitaflo) Powder Leucine Amino Acid Supplement (Vitaflo) Powder Phenylalanine Amino Acid Supplement (Vitaflo) Powder	Use in low protein diets by mixing with protein substitute, adding to modular feeds, or incorporating into other permitted food or drink
Other inborn errors of metabolism	DocOmega (Vitaflo) Powder KeyOmega (Vitaflo) Powder	n-3 supplement containing DHA n-3 and supplement containing AA and DHA
Phenylketonuria (PKU)	Add-Ins (SHS) Powder Easiphen (SHS) Liquid Lophlex (SHS) Powder L-Tyrosine (SHS) Powder Milupa PKU 3-advanta (Milupa) Powder Phlexy-10 Exchange System (SHS) Capsule/tablet/drink PK Aid-4 (SHS) Powder	Phenylalanine free protein substitute Ready to drink phenylalanine free liquid product Phenylalanine free drink mix For use in maternal PKU where there are low plasma tyrosine concentrations Phenylalanine free protein supplement Each unit (1 sachet, 10 tablets or 20 capsules) provides 10 g of amino acids except phenylalanine Unflavoured blend of essential and non-essential amino acids

(Continued)

Table A10.1.10 (*Continued*)

Condition	Product (manufacturer)	Notes and ACBS indications
	PKU cooler10 (Vitaflo) Liquid Provides 10 g of protein equivalent PKU cooler15 (Vitaflo) Liquid Provides 15 g of protein equivalent PKU cooler20 (Vitaflo) Liquid Provides 20 g of protein equivalent	Ready to drink phenylalanine free protein substitutes, including n-3 LCPs, DHA and EPA
	PKU express (Vitaflo) *powder* 1 × 25 g sachet provides 15 g of protein equivalent	Phenylalanine free protein substitute
	PKU Lophlex LQ 10 (SHS) Liquid Provides 10 g of protein equivalent PKU Lophlex LQ 20 (SHS) Liquid Provides 20 g of protein equivalent	Phenylalanine free liquid containing a balanced mixture of essential and non-essential amino acids, carbohydrates, vitamins, trace elements and some minerals
	Tyrosine Amino Acid Supplement (Vitaflo) Powder	For use in low protein diets
	XP Maxamum (SHS) Powder	Phenylalanine free protein substitute drink mix
Tyrosinaemia	TYR cooler (Vitaflo) Liquid	Ready to drink tyrosine and phenylalanine free protein substitute
	TYR express (Vitaflo) *powder* 25-g sachet provides 15 g of protein equivalent	Unflavoured, powdered tyrosine and phenylalanine free protein substitute
	XPHEN TYR Tyrosidon (SHS) Powder	Normal plasma methionine concentrations
	XPTM Tyrosidon (SHS) Powder	Above normal plasma methionine concentrations
Urea cycle disorders	L-Arginine (SHS) Powder	Except arginase deficiency
	Dialamine (SHS) Powder	Essential amino acid supplement
	EAA Supplement (Vitaflo) Powder	
Low protein milk replacement drinks	Loprofin PKU Drink (SHS) Liquid	Low protein, low phenylalanine drink based on cow's milk
	Milupa lp-drink (Milupa) Powder	Suitable for dietary management of amino acid metabolism disorders
	ProZero (Vitaflo) Liquid	Liquid blend of carbohydrate and fat
	Sno-Pro (SHS) Liquid	Low protein, low phenylalanine drink based on milk extracts
Vitamin and mineral component	Phlexy-Vits (SHS) Powder/tablet	For use with restricted diets for PKU and similar amino acid abnormalities
Flavouring preparations	FlavourPac (Vitaflo) Powder Blackcurrant, lemon, orange, tropical, raspberry	For use with unflavoured protein substitutes
	Modjul Flavour System (SHS) Powder Blackcurrant, orange, pineapple	

*A source of vitamins, minerals and trace elements is also required, e.g. **Phlexy-Vits**.
AA, arachidonic acid; DHA, docosahexaenoic acid; EPA, eicosapentanoic acid; LCPs, long chain polyunsaturated fatty acids.

Table A10.1.11 Manufacturers' websites

Abbott, Abbott Laboratories Ltd	www.abbott.co.uk
Complan Foods, Complan Foods Ltd	www.complanfoods.com
Foodlink, Foodlink (UK) Ltd	www.foodlinkltd.co.uk
Fresenius Kabi, Fresenius Kabi Ltd	www.fresenius-kabi.co.uk/
Heinz, H. J. Heinz Company Ltd	www.heinz.co.uk
KoRa, KoRa Healthcare Ltd	www.kora-health.com/
Milupa, Milupa Aptamil	www.milupa-metabolics.com
Nestlé, Nestlé Nutrition	www.nestlenutrition.com
Nutricia Clinical, Nutricia Clinical Care	www.nutricia.co.uk
Nutrinovo, Nutrinovo Ltd	www.nutrinovo.com
SHS, SHS International Ltd	www.shs-nutrition.com
SLO Drinks, SLO Drinks Ltd	www.slodrinks.com
Sutherland, Sutherland Health Ltd	www.sutherlandhealth.com
Vegenat, Vegenat	www.vegenat.es/e_default.asp
Vitaflo, Vitaflo International Ltd	www.vitaflo.co.uk

Appendix A10.2 Paediatric nutritional supplements and enteral feeds

This appendix was compiled as a guide; it is not definitive. For further details, see Shaw & Lawson (2007).

Table A10.2.1 Paediatric sip feeds

Product type	Product name (manufacturer)	Per 100 mL of ready to drink product/standard dilution				Notes
		kJ	kcal	Protein (g)	Fibre (g)	
Low energy (<1 kcal/mL)	Nutriprem 1 (Cow & Gate) Liquid	201	48	1.5	0.5	60-mL bottle, formula for low birth weight babies <1.8 kg only available in hospital
	Nutriprem 2 (Cow & Gate) Liquid	310	75	2.0	0.6	Catch-up growth in preterm infants (<35 weeks' gestation at birth) and small for gestational age infants up to 6 months corrected age
	SMA Gold Prem 2 (SMA Nutrition) Powder	305	73	1.9	0.0	
	SMA High Energy (SMA Nutrition) Liquid	382	91	2.0	0.0	250-mL carton, disease related malnutrition, malabsorption, growth failure from birth to 18 months
Standard energy (1 kcal/mL)	Clinutren Junior (Nestlé) Powder	420	100	3.0	0.0	Growth failure*†
	Infatrini (Nutricia Clinical) Liquid	415	100	2.6	0.8	100-mL bottle, failure to thrive, disease related malnutrition and malabsorption, from birth up to body weight of 8 kg
	Paediasure (Abbott) Liquid	422	100	2.8	0.0	200-mL bottle*†
	Paediasure Fibre (Abbott) Liquid	420	100	2.8	0.8	
	Paediasure Peptide (Abbott) Liquid	420	100	3.0	0.0	
	Similac High Energy (Abbott) Liquid	419	100	2.6	0.4	120-mL bottle, increased energy requirements, faltering growth and/or need for fluid restriction, body weight up to 8 kg

(Continued)

Table A10.2.1 (*Continued*)

Product type	Product name (manufacturer)	Per 100 mL of ready to drink product/standard dilution				Notes
		kJ	kcal	Protein (g)	Fibre (g)	
High energy (1.5 kcal/mL)	Fortini (Nutricia Clinical) Liquid	630	150	3.4	0.0	Disease related malnutrition and growth failure in children aged 1–6 years,* body weight 8–20 kg
	Fortini Multifibre (Nutricia Clinical) Liquid	630	150	3.4	1.5	
	Fortini Smoothie Multifibre (Nutricia Clinical) Liquid	625	150	3.4	1.4	
	Frebini Energy Drink (Fresenius Kabi) Liquid	630	150	3.8	0.0	Disease related malnutrition and growth failure in children aged 1–10 years,* body weight 8–30 kg
	Frebini Energy Fibre Drink (Fresenius Kabi) Liquid	630	150	3.8	1.1	
	Paediasure Plus (Abbott) Liquid	632	151	4.2	0.0	*†
	Paediasure Plus Fibre (Abbott) Liquid	626	150	4.2	1.1	*†
	Paediasure Plus Juce (Abbott) Liquid	638	150	4.2	0.0	Low fat*†
	Resource Junior (Nestlé) Liquid	630	150	3.0	0.0	For children aged 1–10 years*

*Not suitable for use in children under 1 year of age.
†For children aged 1–10 years, body weight 8–30 kg.

Table A10.2.2   Feed thickener

Product name (manufacturer)	Notes
Carobel Instant (Cow & Gate)	Instant thickening agent, prepared from carob seed flour, suitable from birth. Prescribable for thickening feeds in the treatment of habitual and recurrent vomiting

Table A10.2.3 Paediatric enteral feeds – standard indications

Product type	Product name (manufacturer)	Per 100 mL				Notes
		kJ	kcal	Protein (g)	Fibre (g)	
Low energy (<1 kcal/mL)	Nutrini Low Energy Multi Fibre (Nutricia Clinical) Liquid	315	75	2.1	0.8	For children aged 1–6 years, except bowel fistula, body weight 8–20 kg
Standard energy (1 kcal/mL)	Clinutren Junior (Nestlé) Powder	420	100	3.0	0.0	For growth failure*†
	Frebini Original (Fresenius Kabi) Liquid	420	100	2.5	0.0	
	Frebini Original Fibre (Fresenius Kabi) Liquid	420	100	2.5	0.8	
	Infatrini (Nutricia Clinical) Liquid	415	100	2.6	0.8	Failure to thrive, disease related malnutrition and malabsorption, from birth up to body weight 8 kg
	Nutrini (Nutricia Clinical) Liquid	420	100	2.8	0.0	For growth failure in children aged 1–6 years, body weight 8–20 kg*
	Nutrini Multi Fibre (Nutricia Clinical) Liquid	420	100	2.8	0.8	
	Paediasure (Abbott) Liquid	422	100	2.8	0.0	*†
	Paediasure Fibre (Abbott) Liquid	420	100	2.8	0.8	
	Similac High Energy (Abbott) Liquid	419	100	2.6	0.4	Increased energy requirements, faltering growth and/or need for fluid restriction, body weight up to 8 kg
	Tentrini (Nutricia Clinical) Liquid	420	100	3.3	0.0	For growth failure in children aged 7–12 years, body weight 21–45 kg
	Tentrini Multi Fibre (Nutricia Clinical) Liquid	420	100	3.3	1.1	
Medium energy (1.2 kcal/mL)	Isosource Junior (Nestlé) Liquid	512	122	2.7	0.0	For growth failure in children aged 1–6 years, body weight 8–20 kg*
High energy (1.5 kcal/mL)	Frebini Energy (Fresenius Kabi) Liquid	630	150	3.8	0.0	For growth failure in children aged 1–10 years, body weight 8–30 kg*
	Frebini Energy Fibre (Fresenius Kabi) Liquid	630	150	3.8	1.1	
	Nutrini Energy (Nutricia Clinical) Liquid	630	150	4.1	0.0	For growth failure in children aged 1–6 years, body weight 8–20 kg*
	Nutrini Energy Multi Fibre (Nutricia Clinical) Liquid)	630	150	4.1	0.8	For children aged 1–6 years, body weight 8–20 kg* and total gastrectomy, not with bowel fistula
	Paediasure Plus (Abbott) Liquid	632	151	4.2	0.0	*†
	Paediasure Plus Fibre (Abbott) Liquid	626	150	4.2	1.1	
	Tentrini Energy (Nutricia Clinical) Liquid	630	150	4.9	0.0	For growth failure in children aged 7–12 years, body weight 21–45 kg
	Tentrini Energy Multi Fibre (Nutricia Clinical) Liquid	630	150	4.9	1.1	For children aged 7–12 years, body weight 21–45 kg and proven inflammatory bowel disease

*Not suitable for use in children under 1 year of age.
†For children aged 1–10 years, body weight 8–30 kg.

APPENDIX

Table A10.2.4 Specialist paediatric formulae

Formula type	Product name (manufacturer)	Per 100 mL of ready to drink product (standard dilution)				Notes
		kJ	kcal	Protein (g)	Fibre (g)	
Amino acid based	Emsogen (SHS) Powder	368	88	2.5	0.0	Short bowel syndrome, intractable malabsorption, proven inflammatory bowel disease, bowel fistula. Not suitable as sole source of nutrition for children aged 1–5 years*
	Neocate Active (SHS) Powder	418	100	2.8	0.0	For children aged 1–12 years*
	Neocate Advance (SHS) Powder	420	100	2.5	0.0	
	Neocate LCP (SHS) Powder	293	70	1.9	0.0	‡
	Nutramigen AA (Mead Johnson) Powder	286	68	4.9	0.0	
Fructose based	Galactomin 19 (SHS) Powder	288	69	1.9	0.0	Conditions of glucose plus galactose intolerance
Hydrolysate	Aptamil Pepti 1 (Allergy) (Milupa) Powder	280	67	1.6	0.6	Established cow's milk protein intolerance with or without secondary lactose intolerance‡
	Aptamil Pepti 2 (Allergy) (Milupa) Powder	285	68	1.6	0.6	Established cow's milk protein allergy or intolerance. Not suitable for children aged <6 months; suitable for children aged 6 months–12 years
	Cow & Gate Pepti-Junior (Cow & Gate) Powder	275	66	1.8	0.0	Disaccharide and/or whole protein intolerance, or where amino acids and peptides are indicated in conjunction with MCTs‡
	Nutramigen Lipil 1 (Mead Johnson) Powder	280	68	1.9	0.0	Disaccharide and/or whole protein intolerance where additional MCTs are not indicated‡
	Nutramigen Lipil 2 (Mead Johnson) Powder	285	68	1.7	0.0	Established disaccharide and/or whole protein intolerance where additional MCTs are not indicated. Not suitable for children aged <6 months; suitable for children aged 6 months–12 years
	Nutrini Peptisorb (Nutricia Clinical) Liquid	420	100	2.8	0.0	For growth failure in children aged 1–6 years,* body weight 8–20 kg
	Pepdite (SHS) Powder	297	71	2.1	0.0	Disaccharide and/or whole protein intolerance‡
	Pepdite 1+ (SHS) Powder	423	100	3.1	0.0	Disaccharide and/or whole protein intolerance, or where amino acids or peptides are indicated in conjunction with MCTs. For children aged 1–12 years*
	Peptamen Junior (Nestlé) Liquid	420	100	3.0	0.0	Short bowel syndrome, intractable malabsorption, proven inflammatory bowel disease, bowel fistula, in children aged 1–10 years*
	Pregestimil Lipil (Mead Johnson) Powder	280	68	1.9	0.0	Disaccharide and/or whole protein intolerance, or where amino acids or peptides are indicated in conjunction with MCTs and hydrolysed casein‡
Low calcium	Locasol (SHS) Powder	278	66	1.9	0.0	Conditions of calcium intolerance requiring restriction of calcium and vitamin D intake‡

Table A10.2.4 (*Continued*)

Formula type	Product name (manufacturer)	Per 100 mL of ready to drink product (standard dilution)				Notes
		kJ	kcal	Protein (g)	Fibre (g)	
MCT enhanced	Caprilon (SHS) Powder	277	66	1.5	0.0	Fat 3.6 g (MCTs 75%)[d‡]
	MCT Pepdite (SHS) Powder	286	68	2.0	0.0	Fat 2.7 g, (MCTs 75%)[d‡]
	MCT Pepdite +1 (SHS) Powder	381	91	2.8	0.0	Fat 3.6 g, (MCTs 75%)[d] for children aged 1–12 years*
	Monogen (SHS) Powder	313	74	2.0	0.0	LCAD , CPTD, and primary and secondary lipoprotein lipase deficiency. Fat 2.1 g (MCTs 90%)[‡]
Peptide-based	Paediasure Peptide (Abbott) Liquid	420	100	3.0	0.0	*[†]
	Peptamen Junior (Nestlé) Liquid	420	100	3.0	0.0	Short bowel syndrome, intractable malabsorption, proven inflammatory bowel disease, bowel fistula*[†]
Pre-thickened infant feeds	Enfamil AR (Mead Johnson) Powder	285	68	1.7	0.0	Significant gastro-oesophageal reflux[‡]
	SMA Staydown (SMA Nutrition) Powder	279	67	1.6	0.0	
Residual lactose	Enfamil O-Lac (Mead Johnson) Powder	280	68	1.4	0.0	Proven lactose intolerance[‡]
	Galactomin 17 (SHS) Powder	295	70	1.7	0.0	Proven lactose intolerance in preschool children, galactosaemia and galactokinase deficiency[‡]
	SMA LF (SMA Nutrition) Powder	281	67	1.5	0.0	Proven lactose intolerance[‡]
Soya based	InfaSoy (Cow & Gate) Powder	275	66	1.6	0.0	Proven lactose and associated sucrose intolerance in preschool children, galactokinase deficiency, galactosaemia and proven whole cow's milk sensitivity[‡]
	SMA Wysoy (SMA Nutrition) Powder	280	66	1.8	0.0	

*Not suitable for use in children under 1 year of age.
†For children aged 1–10 years, body weight 8–30 kg.
‡Suitable from birth to 12 years of age.
[d]Disorders in which a high intake of MCTs is beneficial (MCTs 75%).
MCT, medium chain triglycerides; LCAD, long chain acyl-CoA deficiency; CPTD, carnitine palmitoyl transferase deficiency.

Table A10.2.5 Nutritional supplements for metabolic diseases (products in italics are also listed in the adult Appendix A10.1)

Metabolic disease	Product name (manufacturer)	Age range	Notes
Glutaric aciduria (type 1)	GA1 Anamix Infant (SHS) Powder	Birth–3 years	Contains vitamins, minerals, trace elements, essential and non-essential amino acids except lysine and low tryptophan
	GA Gel (Vitaflo) Gel	1–10 years	
	XLYS, Low TRY, Maxamaid (SHS) Powder	1–8 years	
Glycogen storage disease	Glycosade (Vitaflo) Powder	>2 years	Also other metabolic conditions where a constant glucose supply is essential
Homocystinuria	Cystine Amino Acid Supplement (Vitaflo) Powder	>1 year	
	HCU cooler (Vitaflo) *Liquid*	>3 years	Methionine free protein substitutes for use as nutritional supplements
	HCU Express (Vitaflo) *Liquid*	>8 years	
	HCU gel (Vitaflo) Powder	1–10 years	
Hypermethioninaemia or homocystinuria	*XMET Homidon (SHS)* *Powder*		Methionine free, unflavoured, powdered drink mixes
	XMET Maxamaid (SHS) Powder	1–8 years	
	XMET Maxamum (SHS) *Powder*	>8 years	Methionine free, unflavoured, powdered drink mix with vitamins, minerals and trace elements
	HCU Anamix Infant (SHS) Powder	Birth–3 years	Essential and non-essential amino acids except methionine for proven vitamin B_6 non-responsive homocystinuria or hypermethioninaemia
	HCU LV (SHS) *Powder*	>8 years	For hypermethioninaemia or vitamin B_6 non-responsive homocystinuria
High energy fat/carbohydrate supplement	Energivit (SHS) Powder		For children requiring additional energy, vitamins, minerals and trace elements following a protein restricted diet
Hyperlysinaemia	HYPER LYS Anamix Infant (SHS) Powder	Birth–3 years	Essential and non-essential amino acids except lysine
	XLYS Maxamaid (SHS) Powder	1–8 years	
Isovaleric acidaemia	IVA Anamix Infant (SHS) Powder	Birth–3 years	Isovaleric acidaemia and other proven disorders of leucine metabolism
	XLEU Faladon (SHS) *Powder*		*XLEU Faladon can be used as part of a modular feed or added as an amino acid supplement to XLEU Analog in the latter stages of weaning*
	XLEU Maxamaid (SHS) Powder	1–8 years	
Low protein milk replacement drinks	Loprofin PKU Drink (SHS) Liquid	>1 year	Low protein, low phenylalanine drink based on cow's milk for use in PKU
	Low protein drink (Milupa) Powder	>1 year	For inborn errors of amino acid metabolism
	Milupa lp-drink (Milupa) Powder	>1 year	For dietary management of amino acid metabolism disorders
	ProZero (Vitaflo) Liquid	>6 months	Liquid blend of carbohydrate and fat
	Sno-Pro (SHS) Liquid		Low protein, low phenylalanine drink based on milk extracts for PKU, chronic renal failure and other inborn errors of amino acid metabolism

Table A10.2.5 (Continued)

Metabolic disease	Product name (manufacturer)	Age range	Notes
Maple syrup urine disease	MSUD Aid III (SHS) Powder		Also related conditions where intake of branched chain amino acids must be limited
	MSUD Anamix Infant (SHS) Powder	Birth–3 years	
	MSUD Anamix Junior (SHS) Powder	1–10 years	
	MSUD Anamix Junior LQ (SHS) Liquid	1–10 years	
	MSUD cooler (Vitaflo) Liquid	>3 years	
	MSUD express (Vitaflo) Powder	>8 years	
	MSUD Gel (Vitaflo) Powder	1–10 years	
	MSUD Maxamaid (SHS) Powder	1–8 years	
	MSUD Maxamum (SHS) Powder	>8 years	
Methylmalonic acidaemia and propionic acidaemia	MMA/PA Anamix Infant (SHS) Powder	Birth–3 years	Essential and non-essential amino acids except methionine, threonine, and valine, low isoleucine content
	XMTVI Asadon (SHS) Powder	Infants and children	
	XMTVI Maxamaid (SHS) Powder	1–8 years	
	XMTVI Maxamum (SHS) Powder	>8 years	
Phenylketonuria (PKU) PKU	Add-Ins (SHS) Powder	>4 years	Essential and non-essential amino acids except phenylalanine
	Easiphen (SHS) Liquid	>8 years	
	Lophlex (SHS) Powder	>8 years	
	Milupa PKU 2-prima (Milupa) Powder	1–8 years	
	Milupa PKU 2-secunda (Milupa) Powder	9–15 years	
	Milupa PKU 3-advanta (Milupa) Powder	>15 years	
	Phlexy-10 Exchange System (SHS) Capsule/tablet/drink	>8 years	Each unit (1 sachet, 10 tablets or 20 capsules) provides 10 g of amino acids except phenylalanine
	Phlexy-Vits (SHS) Powder/tablet	>11 years	Vitamin and mineral component of restricted therapeutic diets in PKU and similar amino acid abnormalities
	PKU Anamix First Spoon (SHS) Powder	6 months–5 years	Contains DHA, essential and non-essential amino acids except phenylalanine
	PKU Anamix Infant (SHS) Powder	Birth–3 years	Contains prebiotic oligosaccharides, AA and DHA
	PKU Anamix Junior (SHS) Powder	1–10 years	Contains AA, DHA, vitamins and minerals
	PKU Anamix Junior LQ (SHS) Liquid	1–10 years	
	PKU cooler 10, 15, 20 (Vitaflo) Liquid	>3 years	Ready to drink phenylalanine free protein substitute containing DHA and EPA, vitamins, minerals and trace elements.

(Continued)

Table A10.2.5   *(Continued)*

Metabolic disease	Product name (manufacturer)	Age range	Notes
	PKU express (Vitaflo) Powder	*>3 years*	Contains essential and non-essential amino acids except phenylalanine, carbohydrate, vitamins, minerals and trace elements
	PKU gel (Vitaflo) Powder	1–10 years	
Phenylketonuria	*PKU Lophlex LQ 10, 20 (SHS)* Liquid	*>4 years*	*Ready to drink, phenylalanine free protein substitute containing essential and non-essential amino acids, carbohydrates, vitamins, trace elements and some minerals*
	PKU Start (Vitaflo) Liquid	<12 months	Ready to feed phenylalanine free infant formula containing essential and non-essential amino acids, carbohydrate, fat, vitamins, minerals, trace elements, AA and DHA
	XP Maxamaid (SHS) Powder	1–8 years	Phenylalanine free drink mix containing essential and non-essential amino acids, carbohydrate, vitamins, minerals and trace elements
	XP Maxamum (SHS) Powder	*>8 years*	
Tyrosinaemia	Methionine-free TYR Anamix Infant (SHS) Powder	Birth–3 years	For proven tyrosinaemia type 1
	TYR Anamix Infant (SHS) Powder	Birth–3 years	Proven tyrosinaemia where plasma methionine concentrations are normal
	TYR Anamix Junior (SHS) Powder	1–10 years	Proven tyrosinaemia
	TYR Anamix Junior LQ (SHS) Liquid	>1 year	Tyrosinaemia type 1 (when NTBC is used), type 2 and type 3
	TYR cooler (Vitaflo) Liquid	*>3 years*	Contains carbohydrates, minerals, trace elements and vitamins, essential and non-essential amino acids except tyrosine and phenylalanine
	TYR express (Vitaflo) Powder	*>8 years*	
	TYR Gel (Vitaflo) Gel	1–10 years	
	XPHEN TYR Maxamaid (SHS) Powder	1–8 years	Tyrosinaemia type 1 (when NTBC is used), type 2 and type 3
Flavouring preparations	*FlavourPac (Vitaflo)* Powder *Modjul Flavour System (SHS)* Powder		*For use with unflavoured protein substitutes*

AA, arachidonic acid; DHA, docosahexaenoic acid; EPA, eicosapentaenoic acid; NTBC, nitisone.

Table A10.2.6   Manufacturers' websites

Abbott, Abbott Laboratories Ltd	www.abbott.co.uk
Cow & Gate, Nutricia Ltd	www.cowandgate.co.uk
Fresenius Kabi, Fresenius Kabi Ltd	www.fresenius-kabi.co.uk/
Mead Johnson, Mead Johnson Nutrition	www.meadjohnson.com
Milupa, Milupa Aptamil	www.milupa-metabolics.com
Nestlé, Nestlé Nutrition	www.nestlenutrition.com
Nutricia Clinical, Nutricia Clinical Care	www.nutricia.co.uk
SHS, SHS International Ltd	www.shs-nutrition.com
SMA Nutrition, Pfizer Ltd	www.smanutrition.co.uk
Vitaflo, Vitaflo International Ltd	www.vitaflo.co.uk

APPENDIX

References

Shaw V, Lawson M. (2007) *Clinical Paediatric Dietetics*, 3rd edn.
  Oxford: Blackwell Publishing.

Appendix A11 Nutrition screening tools

This appendix contains screening tools that are discussed in detail in the text; many other tools are available that are applicable to dietetic practice. For details on paediatric screening tools, refer to Shaw & Lawson (2007).

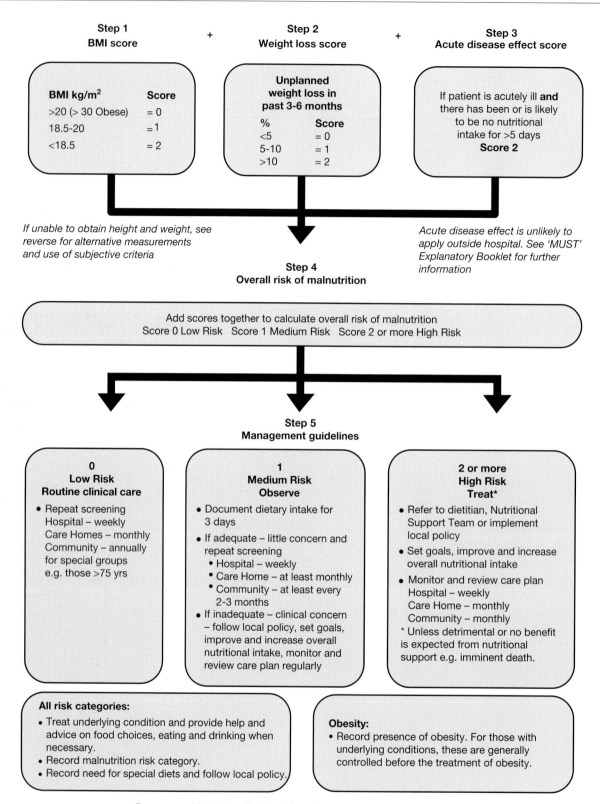

Step 1
BMI score

+

Step 2
Weight loss score

+

Step 3
Acute disease effect score

BMI kg/m²   Score
>20 (> 30 Obese)   = 0
18.5-20   =1
<18.5   =2

Unplanned weight loss in past 3-6 months

%   Score
<5   = 0
5-10   = 1
>10   = 2

If patient is acutely ill **and** there has been or is likely to be no nutritional intake for >5 days
Score 2

If unable to obtain height and weight, see reverse for alternative measurements and use of subjective criteria

Acute disease effect is unlikely to apply outside hospital. See 'MUST' Explanatory Booklet for further information

Step 4
Overall risk of malnutrition

Add scores together to calculate overall risk of malnutrition
Score 0 Low Risk   Score 1 Medium Risk   Score 2 or more High Risk

Step 5
Management guidelines

0
Low Risk
Routine clinical care

- Repeat screening
  Hospital – weekly
  Care Homes – monthly
  Community – annually
  for special groups
  e.g. those >75 yrs

1
Medium Risk
Observe

- Document dietary intake for 3 days
- If adequate – little concern and repeat screening
  - Hospital – weekly
  - Care Home – at least monthly
  - Community – at least every 2-3 months
- If inadequate – clinical concern – follow local policy, set goals, improve and increase overall nutritional intake, monitor and review care plan regularly

2 or more
High Risk
Treat*

- Refer to dietitian, Nutritional Support Team or implement local policy
- Set goals, improve and increase overall nutritional intake
- Monitor and review care plan
  Hospital – weekly
  Care Home – monthly
  Community – monthly
* Unless detrimental or no benefit is expected from nutritional support e.g. imminent death.

All risk categories:
- Treat underlying condition and provide help and advice on food choices, eating and drinking when necessary.
- Record malnutrition risk category.
- Record need for special diets and follow local policy.

Obesity:
- Record presence of obesity. For those with underlying conditions, these are generally controlled before the treatment of obesity.

Reassess subjects identified at risk as they move through care settings
See The 'MUST' Explanatory Booklet for further details and The 'MUST' Report for supporting evidence.

Figure A11.1   Malnutrition Universal Screening Tool 'MUST' (from www.bapen.org.uk/pdfs/must/must_page3.pdf)

Complete all boxes on admission and action as indicated by score

Estimated/reported Weight (kg)	Estimated/reported Height (m)	Body mass index (BMI) (use BMI chart to calculate)

Score each risk factor, using highest score if more than one is relevant.
Total up column scores to obtain final score and record below.

Weight loss in last 3 months and current BMI (choose highest score)	Age (years)	Level of SCI	Other medical conditions	Skin conditions	Diet	Intake	Ability to eat
0 'Minimal' (under 5%) MI ≥22.5 kg/m²	1 18–30	1 S1–S5	0 None	0 Intact	0 Normal diet and fluids or established NG/PEG feed	0 Eating all meals or tolerating full enteral feed	0 Not applicable as on NG/PEG feed
1 'Some' (5–10%) BMI 18.5–22.5 kg/m²	2 31–60	2 L1–L5	1 Chronic conditions, e.g. pain/substance abuse	1 Grade 1 ulcer	1 Introductory NG/PEG feed	1 Under half meal or NG/PEG feed tolerated	0 Able to eat independently
3 'Moderate' (11–15%) BMI 16.5–18.4 kg/m²	3 >60	3 T1–T12	2 Acute trauma, e.g. head injury/fractures	2 Grade 2 ulcer	2 Modified texture diet	2 Minimal diet or enteral feed	2 Requires some help
4 'Marked' (>15%) BMI <16.4 kg/m²	4 Under 18	5 C1–C8	3 Within 1 week of surgery/ongoing infection	3 Grade 3 ulcer	3 Nil by mouth for >5 days	3* Vomiting and diarrhoea or not tolerating NG/PEG feed	3 Needs to be fed
			4 Ventilated (non-invasive)	5 Grade 4 ulcer			
			5 Fully ventilated with tracheostomy			Investigate cause and treat	

Date	Column score	Column score	Column score	Column score	Column score	Column score	Column score	Column score	TOTAL SCORE

Figure A11.2 Spinal nutritional screening tool

Transfer total score overleaf and choose appropriate action plan according to identified risk category.

Complete table below to update nutritional risk scores and document weight changes.

Date	Total score	Risk (L/M/H)	Latest weight Actual/estimate	Weight Change (± kg)	Variance and comments	Referred to dietitian	Review date	Nurse's signature

Follow local action plan according to risk score. Document actions in nursing notes.

Score	Risk	Action plan	
10 and under	Low Rehab	Encourage healthy food and drink choices Assist with feeding if needed	**Monthly weight if possible Repeat score monthly**
	Low Acute	Encourage appropriate menu choices If eating less than half meals complete 3-day food chart and offer two nutritional supplements /sip feeds* a day **If no improvement in eating refer to dietitian**	**Weekly weight if possible Repeat score weekly**
11–15	**Moderate Rehab and Acute**	Encourage appropriate menu choices Assist with feeding if needed Complete 3-day food chart. Implement 'Red Tray' Replace missed meals with nutritional supplements /sip feeds* a day **If no improvement in eating refer to dietitian**	**Weekly weight if possible Repeat score weekly**
Above 15	**High Rehab and Acute**	Encourage high energy/protein menu choices Assist with feeding if needed Complete 3-day food chart. Implement 'Red Tray' Replace missed meals with nutritional supplements as prescribed by doctor or dietitian **Refer to dietitian**	**Weekly weight if possible Repeat score weekly**

Patients N.B.M. for over 5 days or requiring NG/PEG feeding need automatic referral to dietitian. If 'out of hours' feeding regimens for the prevention of refeeding syndrome guidance is available on ....

*Supplement drinks; if the patient has diabetes monitor blood glucose levels and refer to dietitian and diabetes advisor.
If the patient has renal problems, monitor bloods closely and refer to dietitian and medical team.
If too much weight is being gained or BMI above 30 kg/m^2: (1) give patient #Why Weight Matters' diet sheet, (2) Suggest patient attends 'drop-in' weight clinic to monitor weight trend and (3) offer referral to dietitian.

PLEASE RING EXT .... TO FORMALLY REFER PATIENTS TO DIETITIAN FROM NUTRITIONAL SCREENING

Figure A11.2   (Continued)

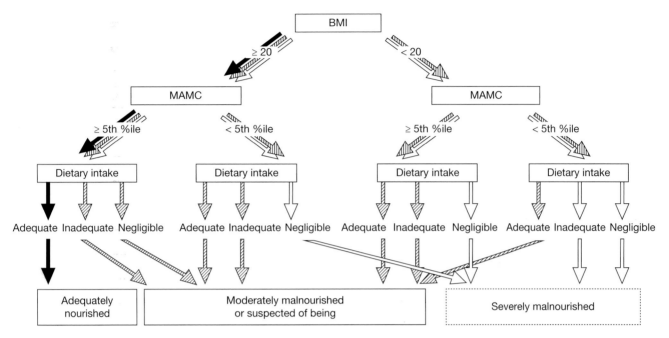

Figure A11.3 Royal Free Hospital Global Assessment (RFH-GA) scheme for determining nutritional status in patients with cirrhosis [from Morgan *et al.* (2006) Derivation and validation of a new global method for assessing nutritional status in patients with cirrhosis. *Hepatology* 44: 823–835]

N.B. This Figure shows an assessment tool rather than a screening tool but is added for completeness.

Index

Page numbers in *italic* denote figures, those in **bold** denote tables.

Note: As certain general terms such as dietary or nutritional management apply to every clinical condition, the reader should refer to specific conditions for more detailed information.